Mercer's Orthopaedic Surgery

Mercer's Orthopaedic Surgery

Ninth Edition

Edited by

ROBERT B. DUTHIE
CBE, MA, ChM, FRCS, FACS (Hon), DSc (Hon), CSOM

Professor Emeritus, Oxford University,
Nuffield Orthopaedic Centre, Headington,
Oxford, UK

and

GEORGE BENTLEY
MB ChM, FRCS

Director and Professor of Orthopaedics,
Institute of Orthopaedics, University College London,
Royal National Orthopaedic Hospital Trust, Stanmore,
Middlesex, UK

ARNOLD

A member of the Hodder Headline Group
LONDON • SYDNEY • AUCKLAND
Co-published in the USA by Oxford University Press, Inc., New York

First published in Great Britain in 1996 by Arnold,
a member of the Hodder Headline Group,
338 Euston Road, London NW1 3BH

Co-published in the United States of America by
Oxford University Press, Inc.,
198 Madison Avenue, New York, NY10016
Oxford is a registered trademark of Oxford University Press

British Library Cataloguing in Publication Data
A catalogue record for this book is available from the British Library

Library of Congress Cataloging-in-Publication Data
A catalog record for this book is available from the Library of Congress

ISBN 0 340 55163 1

Typeset in 10/11 Times by Keyboard Services, Luton, Bedfordshire
Printed and bound in Great Britain by The Bath Press, Avon

Contents

Preface to the Ninth Edition

It is over sixty years now since 'Mercer' first appeared. It has been a successful publication for undergraduates, but more particularly for postgraduates in training to become orthopaedic surgeons. Mercer described it in the first preface as 'a volume of modest size containing the essentials of the old and a summary of the new'. (Mercer had a unity of thought and expression, and knew exactly what should be emphasised and to be trained by him was a privilege.)

In 1964 the senior editor, Professor Robert B. Duthie (RBD), joined Sir Walter Mercer as an author and introduced the chapter on Basic Sciences of the Musculo-Skeletal System, probably the first chapter of its kind in any standard textbook of surgery.

Ten years later RBD became the senior author and had the pleasure of Professor Albert B. Ferguson, Jr of Pittsburgh, USA joining him as co-author. Because of tariff laws, this sadly lasted for only one edition, and in 1983 RBD was joined by Professor George Bentley (GB) then of Liverpool, now of London, having trained and worked in Oxford for 9 years.

The academic world is changing rapidly in orthopaedics and RBD and GB have been joined in this ninth edition by world authorities, teachers and friends, all of whom have been working colleagues of the Editors. It has been a particular pleasure to see them developing international authority in their various subjects.

Both teaching and learning are now international and therefore material based upon personal experience has to be of that nature also. At the same time, postgraduate education must be balanced and not based upon reading a single article or monograph but derived from a consensus of experts and teachers. Authors have a responsibility to synthesise and prioritise the importance of considered knowledge. The Editors have maintained this balance and included all aspects of elective orthopaedics in both children and adults within a single volume. The wizardry of modern technology can achieve its excellent results only when based upon good patient selection. This, in turn, requires an excellent knowledge of orthopaedic physiology and pathology with real understanding particularly of the onset, course and outcome of a disorder or disease. This understanding is essential for residents and registrars both for taking examinations and as a background to their future practice. They will find the ninth edition an invaluable guide to this, while it will also serve as a reference for practising orthopaedic surgeons who can consider a subject in totality rather than simply as a technique and thereby have a basis for future work and research.

All illustrations have been redrawn and developed, particularly the line artwork, which is of the highest standard. There has been great change in attitudes and in innovative technologies and the new edition reflects this. Once again the Editors have emphasised that knowledge of the diseases and disorders found in developing countries is essential not only for postgraduates working in those countries long term but equally for those in the so-called developed countries, allowing them to make a contribution in places that are less well off in technology. The privilege of teaching young surgeons from the developing world has shown the Editors the importance of imparting a process of reasoning, based upon accepted basic scientific information. Technological developments are of only superficial importance by comparison. In orthopaedics the surgeon is dealing with a changing individual who is either developing, as in childhood, or degenerating, as in adulthood. This lesson was accepted many years ago when orthopaedics developed as a separate specialty from so-called general surgery.

A textbook such as Mercer's is a mainstay of orthopaedic education, holding its own alongside other forms of learning via journals and monographs, courses, video tapes, and computer-based programmes. Changes in the format and authorship of this long standing, successful textbook will maintain this position. Its breadth has continued with the inclusion of subjects such as amputations, rehabilitation, physiotherapy, and neurocirculatory disturbances. All of these play an important part in the everyday activity of an orthopaedic surgeon. This scope should ensure the book will continue as an essential companion to orthopaedic training.

RBD GB

ACKNOWLEDGEMENTS

Among the many individuals who have helped us with this new edition we would particularly like to thank the following at the Institute of Orthopaedics: Peter Smith, the librarian; Rosemary Dutton, Helen Gale and Michelle Procter, secretaries; and Uta Boundy and the staff of the Photographic Department.

Contributors

Roger M. Atkins MA, DM, FRCS
Consultant Orthopaedic Surgeon, Department of Orthopaedic Surgery, Bristol Royal Infirmary, Bristol, UK

Thomas W. Bauer MD, PhD
Departments of Anatomic Pathology and Orthopaedic Surgery, The Cleveland Clinic Foundation, Cleveland, Ohio, USA

George H. Belhobek MD
Chairman, Department of Clinic Radiology, Section of Musculoskeletal Radiology, The Cleveland Clinic Foundation, Cleveland, Ohio, USA

George Bentley MB ChM, FRCS
Director and Professor of Orthopaedics, Institute of Orthopaedics, Royal National Orthopaedic Hospital Trust, Stanmore, Middlesex, UK; Member (and Past President) of British Orthopaedic Research Society; Fellow (and Past President) of the British Orthopaedic Association; Member of the Société Internationale de Chirugie Orthopèdique et de Traumatologie; Formerly Professor of Orthopaedic and Accident Surgery, University of Liverpool; Formerly Honorary Consultant Surgeon to the Royal Liverpool Hospital, the Royal Liverpool Children's Hospital and Broadgreen Hospital, Liverpool

Sáuria M. Burnett MD
Director of Pediatrics and Infantile Rehabilitation, SARAH Network of Hospitals for the Locomotor System, Brasilia, Brazil

R. I. Burton MD
Wehle Professor and Chairman, Department of Orthopedics, University of Rochester Medical Center, Rochester, New York, USA

A. Campos da Paz Jr MD
Surgeon-in-Chief, Medical Director, SARAH Network of Hospitals for the Locomotor System, Brasilia, Brazil

J. P. Cullen MD
Department of Orthopedic Surgery, University of Rochester Medical Center, Rochester, New York, USA

Robert A. Dickson MA, ChM, FRCS, DSc
Professor of Orthopaedics and Director, Department of Orthopaedic Surgery, University of Leeds, St James Hospital, Leeds, UK

S. H. Doerschuk MD
Department of Orthopedic Surgery, University of Rochester Medical Center, Rochester, New York, USA

Robert B. Duthie CBE, MA, ChM, FRCS, FACS (Hon), DSc (Hon), CSOM
Professor Emeritus, Nuffield Orthopaedic Centre, Headington, Oxford, UK; Late Nuffield Professor of Orthopaedic Surgery, Oxford University; Civil Consultant Adviser in Orthopaedic Surgery to the Royal Navy; Fellow and President of the British Orthopaedic Association; Fellow of the Royal Society of Medicine; Member and President of the Société Internationale Recherche d'Orthopédie et de Traumatologie; Member of the Société Internationale d'Orthopédie et de Traumatologie; Corresponding Member of the American Orthopaedic Association; Formerly Professor of Orthopaedic Surgery and Orthopaedic Surgeon-in-Chief, University of Rochester Medical Center, Rochester, New York, USA; Honorary Fellow of the Yugoslavian Orthopaedic Society, the Japanese Orthopaedic Association, the Portugese, the German, the Austrian Orthopaedic and Traumatology Societies

Aresh Hashemi-Nejad MB, FRCS (Orth)
Lecturer, Institute of Orthopaedics, Royal National Orthopaedic Hospital Trust, Stanmore, Middlesex, UK

I. M. R. Lowdon MB, FRCS
Consultant Orthopaedic Surgeon, Department of Orthopaedic Surgery, Princess Margaret Rose Hospital, Swindon, Wiltshire, UK

Kenneth E. Marks MD
Head of Musculoskeletal Oncology, The Cleveland Clinic Foundation, Cleveland, Ohio, USA

J. Dougall Morrison MA (Oxon), BM, FRCS (Edin & Eng)
Consultant in Rehabilitation, Prosthetic Service, Mary Marlborough Centre, Nuffield Orthopaedic Centre, Headington, Oxford, UK

Carl L. Nelson MD
Professor and Chairman, Department of Orthopedic Surgery, University of Arkansas for Medical Sciences, Little Rock, Arkansas, USA

Alvaro M. Nomura MD
SARAH Network of Hospitals for the Locomotor System, Brasilia, Brazil

David C. Reid MD, MCh (Orth), FRCSC
Professor and Chairman, The Glen Sather University of Alberta Sports Medicine Clinic and Faculty of Medicine, University of Alberta, Edmonton, Alberta, Canada

John R. Shearer PhD, FRCS
Professor of Orthopaedics and Head of Academic Orthopaedic Unit, Southampton General Hospital, Southampton, UK

Roger Smith PhD, MD, FRCP
Consultant Physician, Nuffield Orthopaedic Centre, Headington, Oxford, UK

David J. Wilson BSc, MB BS, FRCR, MRCP
Consultant Radiologist, Nuffield Orthopaedic Centre, Headington, Oxford, UK

CHAPTER 1

Introduction

ROBERT B. DUTHIE AND DAVID J. WILSON

The term 'orthopaedy', adapted from the Greek words, ὀρθός, meaning straight, upright or free from deformity, and παιδιον, a child, was originally used by Nicholas Andry, whose work, *L'Orthopédie ou l'art de prévenir et de corriger dans les enfants les déformatés du corps*, first appeared in 1741. The elder Sayre considered that the word Orthopaedics was derived from ὀρθός and παιδευω, meaning 'to educate', and as such emphasizes the preventive and advisory nature of the specialty.

Modern orthopaedics is concerned with the study of the form and function of the musculoskeletal system; its attack is directed against those affections that deform the architecture or arrest the balanced mechanisms of man's body, injuries and diseases of bones, muscles, nerves and soft structures which result in loss of form or function.

Andry originally taught orthopaedics as a branch of preventive medicine rather than as an offshoot of surgery, and the various methods he described of preventing and correcting bodily deformities in children were, in his own words, within the reach of 'fathers, mothers, nurses, and others entrusted with the bringing up of children'. Andry's words need not be passed over lightly: prevention is always better than cure, and if the principles and practice of preventive orthopaedics were more liberally applied today, many of the severer degrees of flat foot, scoliosis and similar deformities would disappear. But the timely institution of preventive measures demands the early recognition of loss of form or function.

The solution of the problems of an orthopaedic case depends on a clear understanding of the pathological nature of each lesion. Those who escape contact with the deformed do not appreciate the keen mental anguish which they suffer – a mental anguish that led Gloucester, when bewailing his fate in his sad monologue in *Richard III*, to exclaim:

> Cheated of feature by dissembling nature,
> Deformed, unfinished, sent before my time
> Into this breathing world, scarce half made up,
> And that so lamely and unfashionable,
> That dogs bark at me as I halt by them.

The scope of orthopaedic surgery

Orthopaedics as a specialized branch of surgery, though it has been growing progressively since the days of its great pioneers, achieved its present prominence largely as a result of the casualties of the two world wars and the accidents incidental to the present mechanical age, the management of acute infections of bones and joints, the result of poliomyelitis and other neurological disorders and the emergence of congenital and developmental disorders both of bone and of muscle.

Orthopaedic affections fall into one or other of six groups:

1. Congenital anomalies.
2. Affections of joints.
3. Affections of bones.
4. Affections of muscles, tendons and other soft tissues.
5. Affections of the nervous system.
6. Static deformities.

While many of the lesions have a definite pathological basis, it is being realized more and more that a large number of orthopaedic disorders are the end result of postural or static anomalies. These are anomalies which are produced by either *postural* forces which result from habit, occupational attitudes or body carriage or *static* forces which are concerned with bodies at rest, or in equilibrium, or acting as weights which are not moving.

Peabody (1938) differentiated between a *postural* deformity which is dynamic in origin occurring in young children with the possibility of continuing growth aggravating it and a *static* deformity in which, because of weakened musculature, structural abnormalities are aggravated by the forces or gravity in all ages. Dunn (1976) in defining congenital postural deformities (e.g. torticollis, scoliosis, club foot) has emphasized the importance of intrauterine moulding due to extrinsic forces arising in the later weeks of pregnancy when the amount of amniotic fluid is reducing and the enlarging fetus is being constrained. Intrinsic forces because of muscle imbalance secondary to neuromuscular disease (e.g. arthrogryposis multiplex congenita) are also usual causes of abnormal moulding.

Posture is dependent upon the tone of the skeletal muscles which is under the control of the sympathetic and somatic nervous systems necessary to maintain position against the forces of gravity. Posture abnormalities arise from abnormal forces, particularly during growth. This is particularly seen in adolescent kyphosis or round shoulders, and is correctable before any bony and disc deformities develop. It is also seen in the genu valgum deformity which usually is accompanied by laxity of ligaments and quadriceps muscle insufficiency. Forces of gravity during growth will produce deformity of bone and this is commonly seen in the overgrowth of medial condyles of the tibiae (Figure 1.1). Many cases of acquired flat foot deformity or pes planus are postural in nature.

Many of the following pages are occupied with this aspect of the orthopaedic problem; its intrinsic importance is great, and, further, it has

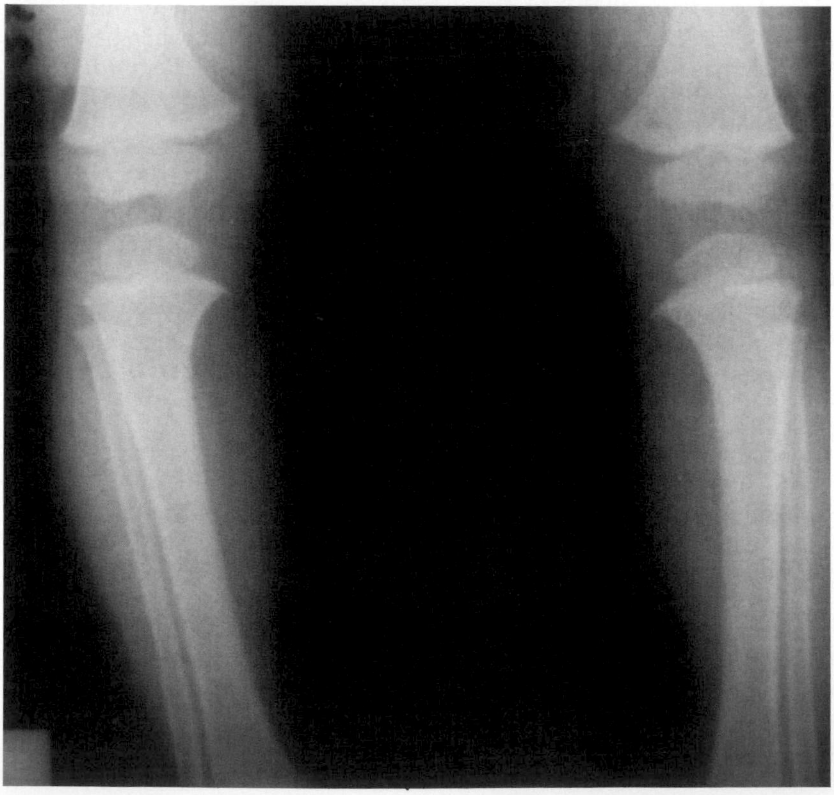

Figure 1.1 A standing radiograph of a young girl aged 6 years, showing genu varum and overgrowth of the medial condyles of both tibiae.

an important lesson to teach – that, from the orthopaedic standpoint, the body must be viewed as a whole, even though the actual complaint is a local one.

The clinical examination of an orthopaedic case

No part of orthopaedic training is more important than developing a systematized method of examination. It cannot be too strongly urged that a true knowledge of disease, which forms the basis of successful diagnosis and treatment, can be found only on the careful and accurate study of individual cases. Scientific and orderly investigation is essential in orthopaedic conditions.

THE HISTORY

At the first consultation it is necessary to elicit a complete and accurate history of the patient's complaint, the mode of its onset and the order in which the symptoms were first observed.

The complaint

The chief complaint may suggest to some extent the nature of the affection, while it always focuses attention on some definite part of the body.

Manner of onset

The illness may begin suddenly, or it may be gradual and insidious in its development. Apart from trauma, the most likely cause of sudden derangement is acute infection. When the onset is insidious, it may be due to a low-grade inflammation, granuloma or tumour, a slow degenerative process or a postural anomaly.

Typical symptoms

The typical symptoms to be inquired for in any injury, disease or deformity (congenital or acquired) of the musculoskeletal system and its associated structures are:

1. pain and its features;
2. disturbed sensation (e.g. paraesthesia);
3. deformity: its onset and progress;
4. weakness or paralysis of muscle power;
5. limitation of movement of a joint;
6. instability of a joint;
7. crepitus.

The question of preceding injury

There is a distinct tendency to ascribe all orthopaedic symptoms and errors to some injury, often sustained at a date considerably remote. An attempt should always be made to ascertain the exact details of any alleged trauma, and to establish its exact relation to the actual lesion as this may have important medicolegal aspects. Such an inquiry should be directed towards discovering whether the symptoms arose at the time of the injury, existed previously, or only appeared subsequently.

Pain and its features

Pain is one of the more common features of many orthopaedic conditions, and therefore some understanding of its nature and its properties is important for their management.

Aristotle described pain as 'an agony of the mind or a feeling state' excluding it from the five classical senses of vision, hearing, smell, taste and touch.

Pain was defined by Sherrington as 'the psychical adjunct of an imperative protective reflex' and is the sensation one feels when injured. However, any precise definition is very difficult because of the difficulty of describing where the afferent nociceptive impulses produced by injurious agents arise, before they pass up into the central nervous system to be given meaning by the emotional and psychological state of the individual based upon the past and present experience. Pain must be regarded as an *experience* rather than a sensory change in the strict neurological sense.

Pain is not a sensation with specific nerve endings, central nervous pathways and higher centres in the brain – the 'specific theory'. But there are nervous pathways largely (if not exclusively) devoted for neuroactive traffic of impulses associated with pain, with higher centres being located in the areas of the brain which subserve emotion. This is why chronic pain can lead to profound behavioural changes in emotion and personality.

THE ANATOMY OF PAIN

The painful stimulus

Pain was believed to have arisen by 'normal' stimuli exceeding the intensity threshold for sensory nerve endings. This is no longer accepted in the light of modern neurophysiological studies. Weddel suggested that stimulation of peripheral receptors by noxious agents produces a spatiotemporal pattern of nervous impulses, which is interpreted as pain within the higher cerebral centres, i.e. the 'pattern theory'. Such patterns of nervous activity may be produced by many physical phenomena such as pressure, puncturing, squeezing, tension and alteration in temperature or by chemical effects such as the alteration of pH or the concentration of histamine-like substances, serotonin, bradykinin and other polypeptide compounds. Bradykinin is formed in extracellular fluid whenever there is tissue damage and mainly accounts for the vascular and exudative changes of inflammation: it sensitizes and stimulates nerve endings and causes pain in minute concentration. Its actions are blocked by aspirin.

Chemical pain-producing substances, called allogens, have been investigated in human skin by Armstrong. Allogens may be intra- or extracellular; for example, the metabolites of anoxia such as lactic acid or a low pH. Kinogen can be acted upon by damaged cells, urate crystals and foreign materials to form kinin, of which bradykinin is one of the most potent allogens. Its effect is potentiated by 5-hydroxytryptamine and histamine. Prostaglandin E is synthesized locally by slight trauma and appears to lower the pain threshold for other physical and chemical stimuli, to create a hyperalgesic state.

Peripheral receptors

There is no doubt that specialized receptor organs for pressure and stress do occur in skin, tendons and ligaments. But the old concept of absolute *specificity* of end organs for pressure (Pacini), cold (Krause) and traction (Meissner and Ruffini), is no longer acceptable. Weddel and Winkelman demonstrated in the dermis that most cutaneous sensory nerve endings are made up of a dense network of unmyelinated fibres. Sensations of pressure, touch or pain, depending upon the impulse pattern invoked, may occur when these are stimulated. Similar networks of unmyelinated nerve fibres have been described in the walls of blood vessels, particularly arteries, in periosteum, bone, synovium and joint capsule. In muscles, a similar role is conducted by small myelinated fibres. Cartilage has no sensory end organs. Also, end organs of Golgi, Vater–Pacini corpuscles, etc., can be identified in ligaments and tendons where they act as stretch receptors, for muscle control and perhaps for pain. Bone and periosteum respond to pressure, percussion or tension. Identifiable nerve endings have been described in the annulus fibrosus of the intervertebral disc but not in the nucleus pulposus. When the annulus fibrosus is disrupted this is believed to result in the pain of 'lumbago' and paravertebral muscular spasm (Hirsch and Schajowicz, 1953). Capsule responds to both tension and traction, and is certainly the most sensitive of all joint structures. Although synovium contains scattered free new endings in two plexuses – deep and superficial – it is difficult to elicit their function experimentally because of the proximity to capsule. In muscle, pressure and pain receptors are related to the presence of small myelinated fibres. Wyke and his co-workers built up a very detailed picture of articular receptor systems (Table 1.1) as well as the articular nerves (Table 1.2) feeding back from the system. In this they identified 'pain' receptors of the high threshold, non-adapting type, and impulses from these nerves pass along both the small myelinated and unmyelinated articular nerves.

The complexity of pain receptor systems in the thoracic spinal tissues has been described and summarized by Wyke (1969) and are applicable to elsewhere in the vertebral column. Pain-sensitive nerve endings have been found in fibrous capsule of apophyseal joints, in the longitudinal (particularly the posterior) flaval and interspinal ligaments, in the periosteum of vertebral bony structures, in the dura mater and epidural adipose tissue, and in the walls of blood vessels – arteriolar as well as venous.

Nerve pathways

Peripheral nerves

The conduction velocity and frequency of pain impulses in afferent nerve fibres are dependent upon fibre diameter and have been described in at least two groups of sensory pathways (Table 1.3).

In the conditions of tabes dorsalis and of ischaemia, the A fibres are damaged and there is always a delay in painful stimuli. The C fibres are particularly sensitive to the application of local anaesthetic agents. The small myelinated and unmyelinated pain fibres end in synapses in the marginal zone and substantia gelatinosa at the apex of the posterior horn of the spinal grey matter. There is released from the C fibres a transmitter substance of a simple peptide known as substance P. Many years ago an 11 amino acid sequence was isolated from the gut and

Table 1.1 Articular receptor system

Type	Morphology	Location	Nerve fibres	Behaviour
I	Encapsulated globular corpuscles (100 × 40 μm)	Fibrous capsule (superficial layers)	Myelinated (6–9 μm)	Static and dynamic mechanoreceptors; low threshold, slowly adapting
II	Encapsulated conical corpuscles (280 × 120 μm)	Fibrous capsule, deeper layers, fat pads	Myelinated (9–12 μm)	Dynamic mechanoreceptors; low threshold, rapidly adapting
III	Encapsulated fusiform corpuscles (600 × 100 μm)	Joint ligaments	Myelinated (13–17 μm)	Dynamic mechanoreceptors, high threshold, very slowly adapting
IV	Plexuses and free nerve endings	Fibrous capsule, fat pads, ligaments, vessels	Myelinated (2–5 μm) Unmyelmated (<2 μm)	Pain receptors; high threshold, non-adapting

After B. Wyke, 1969.

called substance P because it was prepared as a powder. It might have been more appropriate if it had been P for pain because this substance has now been shown by immunofluorescence to be present in the central terminals of the C fibres and in other strategic sites in the pain pathway. It is absent from the dorsal column nuclei which carry the A beta (Aβ) fibres and it seems very likely that it is the primary transmitter in the pain pathway.

Spinal cord

The afferent impulses are carried within the peripheral nerves to spinal root ganglia and then to the cord where they synapse within one or two segments of the dorsal column before crossing the midline to form the contralateral, lateral spinothalamic tract. At the site of dorsal column synapse the pathway of pain fibres is regulated by fibres descending in the ipsilateral corticospinal tract. Melzack and Wall (1965) described a controlling mechanism acting at every junction in the substantia gelatinosa at which nerve impulses are relayed from one neuron to the next on their cerebral ascent utilizing psychological or emotional events in order to appreciate the quality and quantity of ultimate perception of pain.

The 'gate control' system as described by Melzack and by Wall has gradually replaced the classical description about the spinal cord dorsal column specificity for location, intensity and even shape of mechanical stimuli of the skin. 'Injury stimuli' are transmitted to the cord by the peripheral nerves carrying the A delta (Aδ) and C fibres. For example, light pressure on the skin selectively stimulates the Aβ fibres which have a lower threshold than the thin myelinated or unmyelinated nerve fibres. Activity predominantly in the Aδ fibres causes negative feedback from the neurons of the substantia gelatinosa, which all impulses entering the dorsal horn must pass through; thus the gate is *closed*. Heavier

Table 1.2 Articular nerves

Group number	Diameter range	Structure	Function
I	13–17	Large myelinated	Mechanoreceptor afferent (from ligaments)
II	6–12	Medium myelinated	Mechanoreceptor afferent (from capsule and fat pads)
III	2–5	Small myelinated	Pain afferent
	<2	Unmyelinated	Pain afferent Vasomotor efferent

After B. Wyke, 1969.

Table 1.3

Type of fibre for painful stimuli	Velocity (m/s)	Site	Stimuli
A Beta, thick myelinated	10–15	Skin and membranes	Light touch, pressure
B Delta, small myelinated	5–10		High intensity, mechanical (e.g. pinprick) Thermal 45°C+
C Unmyelinated	0.5–2	Skin and all deep tissues	High intensity, mechanical Chemical Thermal Pain

pressure progressively fires off Aδ and C fibres which have an intrinsically higher threshold. This results in proportionally greater activity in thin myelinated and unmyelinated fibres. This high proportion of activity in Aδ and C fibres causes a position feedback from the substantia gelatinosa, the gate is *opened* and a flood of neural traffic reaches the first transmission cell deeper in the dorsal horn (the T cell). The resulting high level of activity in the T cell may be interpreted as pain by the higher centres.

A feedback loop, and activity from these centres can override local neural input. This explains why attention and distraction, emotion and rational thought, etc., can determine whether or not pain is felt. Specific cells in the spinal cord are excited by injury signals, and are facilitated and inhibited by stimuli from other external events (e.g. touch, pressure, heat and cold). The excitability of these cells, transmitting information about the injury, is modified by descending stimuli from the brain. The 'gate-control' theory of Melzack and Wall (1965) has been criticized for being too specific about the function of the substantia gelatinosa, the presynaptic mechanisms and failing to account for the known stimulus specificity of nerve fibres, i.e. C fibres. However, the effect of descending inhibitory systems is now established as well as the modulation of the nociceptive inputs in the spinal cord at a lower level (Wall and Melzack, 1989). Such knowledge has substantiated the use of transcutaneous electrical nerve stimulation (TENS) for many painful conditions.

Noordenebos (1959) has emphasized the importance of short chain polysynaptic systems which would mean that there are 'gates' at all levels of the CNS.

In the spinothalamic tract, Willis and colleagues have shown that 59% of its fibres are carrying tactile information, 11% articular receptors and 30% high-intensity stimuli.

Obviously, with only 1500 fibres, this lateral tract cannot monitor pain for the entire periphery. The nociceptive input from the periphery is found within the grey matter of the spinal cord and still has not been completely charted. However, from an unknown number of interneuronal synapses, a number of axons arise from the intermediate grey matter and deeper layers of the dorsal horn, cross to the other side and ascend in the anterolateral columns of the spinal cord white matter alongside the spinothalamic tract. The spino-reticular fibres are more numerous than the spinothalamic and terminate in the reticular formation of the brain stem. Stimuli along this pathway reach the hypothalamus and the limbus – this, as well as the intralaminar thalamic nuclei, may account for the autonomic and positive effects which accompany the pain. From these diffuse structures, pain impulse reaches the whole cortex – more frontal than occipital – in which a complex inter-relationship exists.

The brain

In the cerebral cortex, pain is localized mainly in the posterior central gyrus of the parietal lobe. The frontal lobe is mainly concerned with emotion, attention and appreciation of pain. After a prefrontal leucotomy, pain is felt normally but the patient is no longer bothered by it. The temporal lobe is believed to act as a memory bank for pain and the hypothalmus for the autonomic effects of pain. Cerebral function in painful situations has been studied using electroencephalography; and there are three phases:

1. A positive complex associated with the arrival of impulses.
2. A negative complex during the period of excitation of the cortex.
3. A secondary positive complex as the stimuli disperses.

However, these studies are of little clinical value in studying pain *per se*.

Bowsher (1979) has described extensively with others how the spinoreticulothalamocortical system appears to be the 'morphological substrate' of chronic pain and is quite separate from the spinothalamic post-central system. Anterolateral cordotomy abolishes real pain as well as pinprick sensation from the opposite side of the body because both these systems pass together in the anterolateral segments of the cord. Ischaemia resulting from disease of the medullary branch of the posterior inferocerebellar artery may damage the spinothalamic tract while sparing the reticular portion, or by destroying the posterior thalamic nuclei but sparing the intralaminar nuclei; there is loss of pinprick and temperature sensations but not chronic pain. Tactile and joint sensation may be lost as well.

'Opiate receptors' have been found in the brain stem and thalamic relays of the spinoreticulothalamic system, particularly around the periaqueductal grey matter of the mid-brain where there is naturally occurring enkephalin – the opiate neurotransmitter substance of Hughes and Kosterlitz. From the periventricular and periaqueductal grey matter, serotoninergic fibres (using 5-hydroxytryptamine as a transmitter) descend through the posterolateral spinal cord, to end in the substantia gelatinosa. These 'raphe spinal' axons synapse with other neurons through the enkephalin neurotransmitter or modulator mechanism to inhibit the impulses of gelatinosa. It has now been shown that the hypothalamus, as well as the intermediate lobe of the pituitary, releases the neurohormone endorphin – which also contains an enkephalin complex and therefore has an opiate-like effect and acts as a hormone.

The enkephalin sequence of amino acids was detected in beta-lipotropin, a pituitary peptide hormone (and fragments of this substance were subsequently tested for analgesic activity). Thus, a 31 amino acid fragment – beta-endorphin – was discovered which is 48 times stronger than morphine in analgesic activity when injected into the brain. Intravenously it is three times stronger than morphine. Like morphine its effects are reversed by the specific antagonist naloxone.

Types of pain

Pain may be:

1. *Local:* when felt at the site of pathological processes in superficial structures. It is usually associated with local tenderness to palpation or percussion.
2. *Diffuse:* appears to be more characteristic of deeply lying tissues and has a more or less segmental distribution.
3. *Radicular:* commonly expressed as sciatica or brachialgia. This paroxysmal pain is characterized by its radiation from the centre to the periphery in a strict anatomical sense but not necessarily in continuity. It is often associated with paraesthesia and tenderness along the nerve root. Clinical examination will frequently show neurological disturbances of sensory loss, reflex depression or loss and muscle weakness. This will be described in greater detail under various clinical conditions. However, it does differ from the pain due to a neuritis (from an infective agent, e.g. herpes zoster; from a metabolic disturbance, e.g. lead or mercury poisoning) which is more continuous until relief of the disease process or total destruction of the neural tissues occurs.
4. *Referred:* or pain which is experienced in other areas, besides that felt in the area of initial stimulation. This is seen when there is injury or disease affecting either somatic or visceral structures, and results from 'misplaced pain projection because of cortical misrepresentation'. This occurs because of the convergence of sensory pathways onto a single cell within the cord or higher centres. Gaze and Gordon (1954) and McLeod (1958) demonstrated such confluence of visceral and cutaneous impulses in the thalamus of the cat. Whitty and Hockaday (1967) suggested that there is possible influence upon such convergence points of stored 'pain experience', from cells within the brain, rather than only at the spinal cord level.

The early experiments of Kellgren and Samuel (1950) and of Whitty and Willison (1958) have helped to define some characteristics of referred pain in different body tissues, particularly that arising from spinal disturbances. This will be described in Chapter 13.

Feinstein *et al.* (1954) described how the injection of muscle into intervertebral articulations produced gripping, boring and cramp-like pain in a segmental plane but often with overlapping accompanied by muscle spasm and autonomic effects such as hypotension, nausea and bradycardia. They found that in such cases there was less segmental distribution because of extensive arborization of nerve endings and the excitation within the internuncial pools which allowed extensive overflow into neighbouring segments. Whitty and Hockaday (1967), in repeating these experiments in 28 normal subjects, did manage to produce referred deep pain although not common and usually only specific to each of the individuals and not to the group as a whole.

Anaesthetizing the site of the stimulus by local analgesia did abolish the referred reflexes. Skin hyperalgesia was not a constant feature.

There still remains much uncertainty about the true nature of referred pain, especially if one believes that pain is part of a specialized system, or that the convergence is only at the cord level or only in the cortex or central area of the brain.

SPECIFIC TYPES OF PAIN

Bone pain

Bone pain has a deep boring quality usually attributable to the stimulus of internal tension as seen in osteomyelitis, expanding tumours and vascular lesions of bone such as Paget's disease. The deep boring night pain of osteoarthritis is thought to be of vascular origin – particularly an increase on the venous side. However, one must differentiate this type of pain in osteoarthritis from that due to soft tissue disturbances of capsular fibrosis and muscle spasm which can be often aggravated by unguarded movements. Pain of a similar 'boring' nature but perhaps more diffuse occurs in generalized osseous diseases such as osteomalacia, osteoporosis and hyperparathyroidism or metastatic lesions (myelomatosis, carcinomatosis) of the vertebral column, ribs, pelvic and shoulder girdles. Such pain may become more severe due to pathological fractures either macro or micro in severity.

Fracture pain has a different character and is often sharp or piercing and is characteristically relieved by rest. Pain which is unrelieved is ominous and suggests serious disease processes.

Muscle and tendon pain

Many unmyelinated nerve fibres are associated with the rich blood supply to muscle. In addition, there are many efferent motor fibres to the muscle end plate which can subserve a sensory function by virtue of their control over muscle contraction, which, when abnormal, is experienced as pain.

Muscle pain

In healthy individuals, local pain can be experienced during prolonged voluntary contraction and persist for hours or even days after the effort has ceased. Cramp also is a common experience on or after exercise. In 1927, Lewis described these as pains arising from the release of pain-stimulating substances which then accumulate. Although such substances as potassium ions, serotonin, histamine, bradykinin and other peptides have all been identified, there can be no direct implication of these substances as yet. A low pH or oxygen depletion also have been considered, specially in intermittent claudication with a reduced blood flow through muscle. Muscle oedema and swelling with muscle fibre damage may well result from metabolic failure; indeed, Brooke *et al.* (1979) have found elevated creatinine phosphokinase levels after forced exercise in healthy subjects. A severe example of this type of pain is seen in the anterior compartment syndrome of leg in which after moderately active exercise there is marked pain in the legs accompanied subsequently by necrosis of the compartment's musculature.

Direct tearing of muscle fibres within their epi- and perimysium which contain nerve fibres and blood vessels will also cause pain although the muscle fibres are believed to be insensitive. Morgan Hughes (1979) has described muscle pain in various diseases as arising at any level of the neuroaxis; for example, cramp or painful muscle stiffness in pyramidal or extrapyramidal lesions, in tetanus, in anterior horn cell diseases (e.g. poliomyelitis) and in peripheral neuritis. He emphasizes that pain is rare in muscular dystrophies and in myotonic disorders but common in the inflammatory myopathies (rheumatoid arthritis, polyarteritis nodosa, lupus, etc.) or in such conditions as polymyalgia rheumatica when there is rapid destruction of muscle cells, involvement of intramuscular blood vessels and/or defects in muscle energy metabolism. Rare conditions such as nodular myositis, viral polymyositis from influenza A and B, mumps and the Coxsackie group all present with very painful muscle swelling.

Morgan Hughes, in his excellent review, also emphasizes how in metabolic bone disease (e.g. dietary vitamin D deficiency rickets, primary hyperparathyroidism) the symptoms of painful weakness of certain muscle groups may well be overlooked until careful clinical, radiological and biochemical examinations are carried out.

The nocturnal cramps in the lower extremities of the elderly are quite characteristic in being relieved or prevented by the taking of quinine derivatives.

Joint pain

Joint pain is difficult because of the complexity and number of tissues involved in its structure.

In addition, the synovium is known to have two plexuses of nerve fibres – a superficial plexus lying in close proximity to the capsule and a deeper one running in the synovial villi, where it is intimately related to the blood vessels.

The capsule has a rich supply of somatic sensory

fibres and proprioceptive fibres in the form of specialized Golgi apparatus, Vater–Pacini corpuscles and Ruffini-like endings. Leriche clearly demonstrated that the capsule is obviously concerned in joint pain appreciation by showing that local anaesthetic injected into the capsule was more effective than an intra-articular injection.

Coomes (1963), by injecting hypertonic saline into joint capsule and the periosteum of the femoral neck, produced patterns of pain around the hip. Irritation of the anterior capsule produced pain in the groin, buttock, anterior thigh and knee, whereas irritation of the posterior capsule produced pain in the buttock, posterior aspect of the thigh and heel. Articular cartilage has been shown to be insensitive to stimuli. Bone contains many sensory endings in the periosteum and entering blood vessels.

Numerous pathological states can be a source of stimuli to the various receptor systems. For example:

1. Vascular – especially arteriolar hyperaemia or venous engorgements; the deep burning pain of a Sudeck's atrophy may be of this nature, especially in some disturbance of the local arterial nerve endings or a reflex central sympathetic system effect.
2. Mechanical, due to instability, asymmetry of surfaces, distension of the capsule by a sudden effusion (e.g. a septic arthritis) or distension within a bone by subchondral cyst formation.

Clinically pain can be described as either acute or chronic with an intermingling of these two states. However, in general terms of management, the *acute* state will respond to appropriate treatment and has a known and recognized cause. The *chronic* state is variable in its response to acceptable treatment and often the cause is difficult to determine, with differing physiological, pathological and psychological causes.

It is possible to divide all types of pains into a simple clinical classification with therapeutic implications:

1. Neuropathic – in which there is nerve or root or meningitic irritation or deformation with the interpretation of the abnormal signals as pain, e.g. disc protrusion, neuritis, etc.
2. Nociceptive – the stimulus arises from tissue damage or deformation, e.g. arthritis, trauma, postoperative orthopaedic pain, tumours.
3. Idiopathic – no local or distant pathology can be found, e.g. the low back pain syndrome.

Obviously the treatment of choice is to remove the local pathology by drugs or surgery and these will be discussed in the following chapters. In general drugs used to treat neuropathic pain are opioids, antiemetics, etc. and TENS is now an important adjunct. For nociceptive pain, non-steroidal anti-inflammatory drugs and opioids are used. For idiopathic pain, benzodiazepines, because of their addictive properties, must be avoided as indeed should opioids, except in the early acute phase. Other neurosurgical treatments have to be considered, e.g. ablative procedures on the peripheral nervous system (e.g. section: root blockade) or on the CNS, e.g. section, cordotomy, tractotomy, etc.

Postoperative orthopaedic pain requires special mention because it is a common problem requiring a team approach as well as an understanding of the unpredictable variation between patients. McQuay *et al.* (1988) have shown the advantages of opiate premedication, with or without the use of benzodiazepines, and with or without the use of regional and spinal, local anaesthesia as well as an intraoperative opiate.

CONGENITAL ABSENCE OF OR INDIFFERENCE TO PAIN

This was first described by Dearborn in 1932, and within 25 years there were over 50 such patients with a clear differentiation from those patients who have a peripheral sensory neuropathy (Chambers *et al.*, 1959).

All sensory modalities are usually intact except for loss of pain over the total skin surface, but as yet there has been no demonstrable abnormality of nerve elements in skin, fascia, bone or central nervous systems.

The orthopaedic problems arise early from injury to the tongue, chewing the ends of fingers, laceration of skin, burning and bony injuries with resultant skeletal deformities as described by Silverman and Gilden (1959) – valgus deformities of knees, exostosis formation, epiphyseal premature closures, abnormal body development in the metaphysis and painless fractures in various stages of repair.

Clinical features: symptoms and signs

The clinical features may be objective or subjective. The objective features, or signs, are those – such as deformity, errors in attitude or gait, and limitations of movement – which are obvious to the examiner.

The subjective symptoms are those of which the patient complains but of which the surgeon has no definite positive evidence. Considerable tact and discrimination are often required to disentangle the truth from the complaints of patients who are neurotic, hysterical or malingering.

The examination of the case

The examination of an orthopaedic case must include not only the physical condition of the patient but any laboratory tests and special investigations suggested by the clinical findings. Unless the complaint is a minor one, limited to one extremity, it is wise to make the examination with the patient wearing little clothing. The examination may be conveniently considered in two parts:

1. Examination of the body as a whole.
2. Examination of the affected member or part.

METHOD OF EXAMINATION

Inspection

The attitude in which the part is held, its general appearance and colour, and the presence of deformity are noted. In the case of a limb, a comparison should always be made between the affected and the presumably healthy side, especially for swelling or wastage.

Palpation

Handling of the affected part will elicit such objective phenomena as abnormal anatomical relationships, muscle tone, pulsations, tenderness, fluctuation, elevation of local temperature, induration or gross alteration in shape. Crepitus within a joint may be discovered by combining palpation with passive movement.

Passive motion

Valuable information may be obtained by carrying out the movements of which the part is normally capable, and by comparing this range with that on the normal side. The amount and quality of the movements are assessed in degrees, and the presence or absence of pain determined.

Limited joint movement may be due to some bony block, to adhesions between the joint surfaces or to reflex spasm of the related muscles, as in early cases of tuberculosis. During movement there may be a grating or crackling sensation, comparable to that produced between the ends of a broken bone. Such crepitation is characteristic of osteoarthritis.

Joint contracture

Joint contracture is defined as a chronic loss of the full passive range of movement of a joint (usually loss of full extension) due to structural changes in the non-bony tissues (Duthie and Young, 1987).

Structural changes may result from a failure of normal muscle growth, imbalance of antagonistic muscle groups acting across the joint (e.g. weakness of extensors and in poliomyelitis or dystrophies or hyperexcitability of flexors), immobilization, muscle degeneration and fibrosis, intra-articular haemorrhage in haemophilia and fibrosis, or skin scarring.

Perry (1987) has described physiological posturing of inflamed arthritic or swollen joints to minimize tissue strain, by the resting position of 15° plantar flexion at the ankle, and 30° flexion at the knee and hip. But these positions will be perpetuated by contractures if not counteracted by timely mobilizing procedures. Each of these joint positions is a serious deterrent to walking without stressful substitutive posturing, and the patient's ability to function is impaired.

Muscle strength rapidly declines during limb immobilization for pain because of a decrease in muscle size and a decrease in tension per unit of muscle cross-sectional area (Booth, 1987). Muscle fatiguability also increases rapidly after limb immobilization. Muscles within limbs fixed by plaster casts have:

1. lower levels of resting glycogen and adenosine triphosphate (ATP);
2. a more rapid depletion of muscle glycogen and ATP during work;
3. a greater increase in lactate during work; and
4. a decreased capacity to oxidize fatty acids during work.

The greatest loss of absolute muscle mass occurs at the beginning of muscle wasting with subsequent loss of muscle being exponential. A significant decrease in the rate of protein synthesis in muscles is observable at the sixth hour of limb immobilization, which most likely initiates the net loss of muscle protein.

The muscle wasting associated with joint damage may be highly selective; knee disorders produce quadriceps wasting but little change in the size of the hamstrings (Young, 1987). This causes isolated quadriceps weakness, so predisposing to a position of knee flexion. Nociceptors and other receptors in and around the joint can produce flexor excitatory and extensor inhibitory actions. At the knee these receptors are likely to excite hamstrings and inhibit quadriceps. Although other actions could occur, quadriceps inhibition may be favoured by a position of knee extension. Quadriceps inhibition will weaken voluntary contraction, reduce tone, and contribute to wasting of the muscle, further predisposing to a position of knee flexion. The potency of quadriceps inhibition may be considerable even in the absence of perceived pain. A small, apparently trivial, effusion (or even a clinically undetectable effusion) may cause important inhibition. In order to improve the orthopaedist's ability to prevent flexion contracture of the injured or operated joint, he/she must look not only for ways of reducing joint pain, but also for ways of preventing activity in other joint afferents. For example, he/she must consider the possible effects of joint position, intra-articular pressure, suture line tension after an operation, and afferent blockade.

Abnormal joint movement may take the form either of excessive mobility or of false mobility. In the former, the normal range of movement is exaggerated in every direction; in the latter, the joint moves in a new or abnormal direction.

Joint mobility, stability and laxity

Many factors contribute to the range of movement of a joint – e.g. the articular surfaces, cartilage, muscle and tendon stretch, the quality of skin, ligaments and joint capsule – these have been reviewed by Bird (1979). In the joint, an effusion or tendon rupture may affect movement.

Joint laxity varies considerably in normal healthy individuals. Some will be 'supple' or even 'double jointed' while others are 'stiff'. 'Supple' individuals are more likely to dislocate than are 'stiff' individuals with identical local factors, suggesting that generalized joint laxity also contributes to dislocation. In man, capsular laxity, ligamentous stretch and muscle tone are the main determinants of the range of movement in normal joints.

Laxity progressively decreases from the age of 5 years. The fall is rapid in late childhood, slow in a teenager and then gradual throughout adult life. Laxity is more marked in females than in males from the same ethnic group. It also varies with race; for example, the joints of individuals from the Indian subcontinent are more lax than those of Africans and Europeans.

Laxity may be altered with regular athletic training, when it can be increased by stretching ligaments and co-ordinating muscular relaxation or reduced by co-ordinating muscular contraction.

The following passive movements (after Bird, 1979) are made to determine abnormal degrees of laxity:

1. Bending the little finger back to 90°.
2. Extending the fingers parallel to the forearm.
3. Placing the thumb against the ulnar aspect of the wrist.
4. Hyperextending the elbow by more than 10°.
5. Hyperextending the knee by more than 10°.
6. Placing the hands flat on the floor while standing with the knees straight.
7. Dorsiflexion of the foot at the ankle to over 45°.

Clinical conditions of increased joint laxity include Marfan's and the Ehlers–Danlos syndromes. The former is easily recognized in its complete form by arachnodactyly, heart disorder and increased hydroxyproline in the urine, but the latter – particularly in the benign hypermobile variant – is often hard to distinguish from familial hypermobility. Patients with Ehlers–Danlos syndrome develop aneurysms and keloid formation not seen in familial hypermobility. Acromegaly may predispose to joint laxity. Mechanical causes include ligamentous damage after trauma (e.g. collateral ligamentous instability of the knee). Neurological disorder (e.g. dorsal column destruction in tabes dorsalis) leads to joint laxity, presumably through neurological loss of muscular tone rather than through damaged ligaments. The lax joints sometimes found in Down's syndrome may be caused by muscular hypotonia. Lax joints are seen after excessive corticosteroid therapy. Localized joint laxity results from tissue destruction subsequently seen in inflammatory conditions such as rheumatoid arthritis.

Active motion

This represents the degree to which the patient can, without assistance, move the affected part. It is usually considerably less than the amount of passive motion, the limitation being due to a similar cause, aggravated by a greater degree of spasm or weakness or paralysis of the associated muscle groups.

It is advisable to record accurate observations of the range of active mobility; this is usually done by employing an apparatus such as an arthrometer. It is often instructive to compare the readings on subsequent occasions, as in this way an index of improvement is provided. The instrument is a simple one, consisting essentially of two metal strips joined by a hinge. Opposite the joint there is a protractor, graduated in degrees. The joint is controlled by a thumb-screw, so that after the angle or arc of movement has been estimated, the arthrometer can be fixed until the reading is made. Other methods may be employed, but it is important always to adopt the same technique to eliminate possible sources of error.

Muscle power

Muscle power of individual muscles or groups of muscles must be carefully observed and recorded, and the following MRC grades are commonly used:

- 5 complete range of active motion against gravity and full resistance.
- 4 complete range of active motion against gravity and some resistance.
- 3 complete range of active motion against gravity.
- 2 complete range of active motion with gravity absent.
- 1 evidence of muscle contraction but no joint movement.
- 0 no muscle contraction seen or palpable.

Unfortunately, a wide range of degrees of weakness is covered by MRC grade 4, and manual muscle testing is insufficiently sensitive to identify minor to moderate changes. As a result, even patients with significant weakness as confirmed by dynamometry may be classified as MRC grade 5. This can be partially overcome by using the patient's own body weight to resist his muscle action. For example, unilateral foot plantar flexion should be strong enough to raise the patient's body weight, although no examiner is capable of exerting some 70 kg force when testing plantar flexion manually.

Dynamometry

The function of muscle is to produce forces, and therefore the objective evaluation of muscle function should include dynamometry. Force production can be recorded and measured under conditions where the muscle does not shorten (*isometric*), where the rate of shortening is controlled (*isokinetic*) or where the resistance to shortening is controlled (*isotonic*). The measurement of muscle power (as opposed to muscle strength) requires isokinetic or isotonic dynamometry, since isometric apparatus measures force, not work.

In the absence of pain, the skilled investigator can persuade most patients and normal subjects to produce maximal muscle activation in a voluntary isometric contraction. The simpler the action, the better is the reproducibility of the measurement.

Strength (especially in weight-bearing muscles) is usually closely related to body weight. Strength comparisons made between patients and normal subjects must take account of differences in body weight.

Weakness due to muscle disease or injury can be:

1. *Acute* – local – resulting from direct and obvious injury to a nerve or other causes of a lower motor neuron disease, e.g. compression or stretching. There is segmental demyelination which may or may not be reversible.

   Stimulation of the nerve distal to the lesion may produce contraction of the involved muscle or muscles. Pain may well be present, e.g. in diabetic radiculopathy.
2. *Acute* – general – sudden onset of weakness can result from nerve, motor end plate or muscle disease, e.g. anterior poliomyelitis (with spasm), Guillain–Barré syndrome (with marked paraesthesiae), acute polymyositis and myasthenia gravis.
3. *Chronic* – local – can be secondary to joint disease with associated muscle atrophy or nerve disruption.
4. *Chronic* – general – can be seen in anterior form cell disease of the cord or from primary muscle disease, e.g. spinal muscle atrophy or dystrophies or long standing collagen disease or malnutrition, or steroid-induced myopathy. Electrodiagnostic testing by EMG motor action potential studies and even muscle biopsy may be required.

Wasting commonly results from disuse or immobilization, or acute joint disease, or in the presence of pain. Akeson *et al.* (1987) have described the changes of proliferation of fibro-fatty connective tissue within the joint space, adhesions between synovial folds, adherence of fibro-fatty connective tissue to cartilage surfaces, atrophy of cartilage, 'ulceration' at points of cartilage–cartilage contact, disorganization of cellular and fibrillar ligament alignment, weakening of ligament insertion sites owing to osteoclastic resorption of bone and Sharpey's fibres, regional osteoporosis of the involved extremity, increased force requirement for joint cycling, and increased ligament compliance. Collagen mass in muscle declines by about 10% with collagen turnover increasing because of accelerated degradation and synthesis and formation of reducible collagen cross-links increases. Content of proteoglycan, notably hyaluronic acid, falls and water content is correspondingly reduced, all resulting in marked muscle wasting.

Innervation to muscle is important to maintain the spontaneous and active muscle contraction and when denervation occurs muscle atrophy can either be focal or general. Electrodiagnostic testing is of value.

Measurement

Careful comparison of the measurements of the affected part with those of the opposite healthy side will often demonstrate atrophy or hypertrophy.

The length of the limbs is measured in order to assess any inequality that may be present. In the leg, the measurement is taken from the anterior superior spine to the level of the knee joint, or to the medial malleolus. Certain lines may be drawn in the neighbourhood of the hip joint which are of value in discovering the site of any shortening in that region.

Nélaton's line extends from the anterior superior spine to the tuberosity of the ischium. Normally it passes through the tip of the greater trochanter, but in pathological conditions of the head or neck of the femur the trochanter is displaced upwards and lies above Nélaton's line.

Bryant's triangle is formed by the perpendicular dropped from the anterior superior spine when the patient is lying on his back. The base is the line extending from the tip of the trochanter to this perpendicular, while the hypotenuse is represented by the line joining the trochanter and the anterior superior spine. Here again, in pathological conditions of the femoral neck or head, the base of the triangle is shortened, whereas in fractures of the shaft or shortening situated in parts other than in the base and neck, the normal relations are maintained.

Schoemaker's line is valuable in that its demonstration requires no movement of the patient. It is drawn from the tip of the greater trochanter through the anterior superior spine and prolonged towards the midline. Where the trochanter is displaced upwards, the continuation of the line meets the middle line of the body below the umbilicus, whereas in the normal case the midline is reached above the umbilicus. Measurements should also be made of girths at fixed levels of the limbs.

Auscultation

This may be of value, particularly in the neighbourhood of joints, for locating crepitation, snaps and friction-rubs. As a rule, however, these can be detected without the aid of the stethoscope. McCoy *et al.* (1988) have reported on the use of vibration-sensitive sensors, attached to bony points around knee joints. They could diagnose and type meniscal tears 150/170 (proven by arthroscopic examination) as well as a physiological patellofemoral crepitus signal which would be of use in determining the integrity of articular cartilage. Mollan *et al.* (1982) have written extensively on modern amplifying methods of auscultating joints.

Neuromuscular examination

The examination of the central nervous system must be carried out when there are motor symptoms such as loss of power or paralysis involving voluntary movements, or sensory symptoms such as pain, numbness, tingling, altered sensation to touch or temperature, or loss of sense of position.

The motor components

For motor disturbance, one must examine for atrophy or hypertrophy of muscle mass, passive and active ranges of movements of joints, fibrillations or fasciculations as seen in progressive muscular atrophy, amyotrophic lateral sclerosis and, less frequently, in syringomyelia. There may be spasm of muscle or irritability of the muscle mass as well as soft tissue contractures to produce characteristic deformities of joints.

Involuntary movements
Involuntary movements may be present, either as irregular and spontaneous (e.g. in chorea and in athetosis of a cerebral palsy child) or they can be purposeful and regular such as spasms, tics and tremors arising from such conditions as multiple sclerosis and other diseases affecting particularly the *extrapyramidal system*. This consists of the vestibilar system and eyes, the spinocerebellar tracts and connections with the superior corpus quadrigeminum of the mid-brain and the cerebellum. It is concerned with the regulation of muscle tone and the co-ordination of muscle movements. Disease of the extrapyramidal tract is also seen as muscle rigidity, but with the presence of normal tendon and cutaneous reflexes and disturbed gait. One should examine for irregularity of gait (e.g. ataxia, the steppage gait). The examination of muscle mass, active movements, tone and reflexes should determine whether the lesion is in the *upper motor neuron*. This involves the pyramidal tract which is concerned with the execution of voluntary movements as well as the control of muscle groups. Disturbance is seen as paralysis, increase in muscle tone or spasticity, exaggeration of tendon reflexes, an extensor plantar reflex, but no atrophy of muscle. With a *lower motor neuron lesion* there is weakness or paralysis of individual muscles with tenderness and pain, decrease or absence of tendon and cutaneous reflexes.

Reflexes result from sudden stretching of tendons or associated structures, and require the presence of a sensory neuron, an internuncial connection in the spinal cord and finally an executing motor neuron. In the upper extremities, the biceps reflex results from integrity of C5 and 6, the triceps reflex from C6 and 7, and the supinator jerk from C7 and 8 segments. In the lower extremities, the knee reflex results from integrity of segments L2, 3 and 4, and the ankle reflex through S1 and 2 segments. Superficial or cutaneous reflexes are seen in the abdominal reflexes of T8 to 12, the plantar reflex from S1 and 2, cremasteric reflex from S1 and 2, bulbar cavernosus from S1 and 2, and anal reflex from S5. The jaw reflex depends upon the integrity of the fifth cranial nerve.

The sensory components

On examination of the sensory component of the central nervous system one examines for touch, pressure, pain, temperature, vibration and proprioceptive sensation. With involvement of the posterior nerve root and peripheral nerve, there is loss and impairment of all forms of superficial and deep sensation, with alteration in tendon reflexes and flaccidity of muscle. In disturbances in the posterior columns there is reduction or absence of the deep senses as well as proprioceptive and vibration sense, and tendon reflex changes. Alterations in touch, pain and temperature sensations are usually on the opposite side except for the areas of skin and present as the typical Brown-Séquard syndrome. With involvement of the sensory cortex one has a contralateral alteration in peripheral sensation and the decreased ability to recognize common objects by prehension, which is termed astereognosis. Examination of the cranial nerves is important and should be carried out.

Lumbar puncture

Lumbar puncture for examination of pressures (20–50 mmHg), Queckenstedt test for complete or partial blocks (particularly of the subarachnoid space) and examination of specimens of the cerebrospinal fluid should be carried out for colour, cell content (normal >5 lymphocytes/monocyte), protein (2.5–4.5 mmol/l), sugar (0.15–0.5 g/l), globulin fractions and bacteriological investigations. It is particularly indicated for bacterial as well as carcinogenic/leukaemic meningitis; for intracranial bleeding; for brain and spinal cord tumours; for unexplained fits and seizures, multiple sclerosis and other demyelinating diseases.

Contraindications are unrecognized brain herniation syndrome with intracranial hypertension and papilloedema and any overlying skin infection.

Complications are headaches (5–10%), backache, radicular pain, worsening of subarachnoid bleeding or brain herniation.

Serological testing of the cerebrospinal fluid for syphilis includes specific treponemal antibody tests and reagin antibody tests.

Electrodiagnostic methods

The electrical examination of a neuromuscular unit has its basis in the character and degree of the response of nervous and muscular tissue to electrical stimuli. An effective electrical stimulus is one which results in muscle contraction. Electrodiagnosis can, therefore, be helpful as follows:

1. To detect denervation and its degree.
2. To observe reinnervation before clinical signs are apparent.
3. To assess the progress of a lesion, whether or not recovery is occurring.
4. To localize the lesion in the spinal cord structures (myelopathic), in the motor root or peripheral nerve (neuropathic), and the neuromuscular junction or in muscle (myopathic) (Figure 1.2).

Peripheral nerve lesion

A muscle will contract in response to direct current of long duration (galvanic stimulus) or to a current in which duration is very brief (faradic stimulus) when applied to its motor point. With interruption of peripheral nerve supply, all response to faradic stimulation is lost within a few days. However, there remains a sluggish response to galvanic stimulation. Erb's reaction of degeneration (RD) is the loss of response to faradism with retention of the galvanic response. The value of this reaction is limited because of its lack of quantification, as well as its inability to define change in the state of denervation and, hence, prognosis.

Intensity/duration curves

These are obtained by stimulating the muscle mass with individual square waves or pulses, the duration and intensity of which can be varied, under control. The rheobase, which is defined as the minimal current required to give a slight muscle contraction or twitch (this requiring certain experience to detect), is determined; the current intensity is gradually reduced and characteristic curves can be obtained (Figure 1.3).

Very few workers in electrodiagnosis now use strength/duration curves; most prefer to use conventional electromyography to demonstrate denervation and/or reinnervation, nerve conduction velocity studies and somatosensory evoked responses.

Electromyography

Voluntary muscles, while at rest and during contraction, develop certain action-motor unit (consisting of a motor neuron, its nerve and the muscle fibres it supplies) potentials which can be picked up by surface electrodes or by a needle electrode inserted

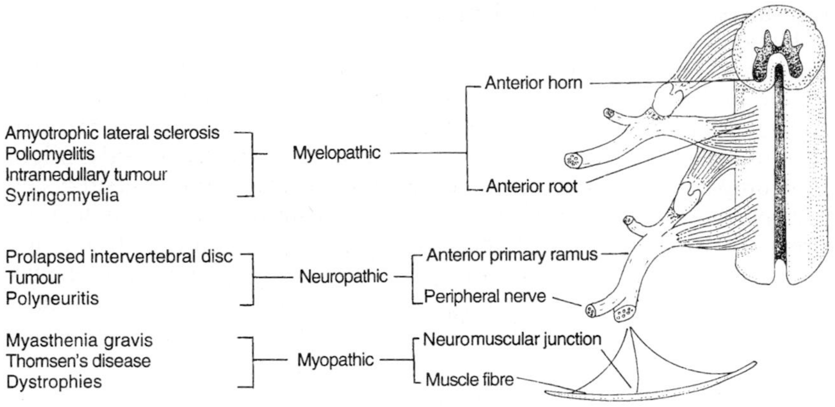

Figure 1.2 Lesions most commonly affecting the spinal cord structures, the motor root or peripheral nerve, the neuromuscular junction and muscle.

into muscle. Surface electrodes give much information about the activity of the muscle mass underlying the skin, but they produce many artefacts which may obscure the true patterns of activity. Therefore, needle electrodes inserted into the muscles are more accurate, but record the sum of the action potential from numerous motor muscle fibres lying near the tip of the needle electrode. The average area recorded is 0.07 mm^2. The 'single fibre' electrode has now been developed with only a very small recording surface of 0.0005 mm^2 (see Chapter 12). A characteristic normal muscle fibre potential can be obtained on the insertion or the removal of the electrode and readily identified (Figure 1.4). A fibrillation potential occurs after Wallerian degeneration

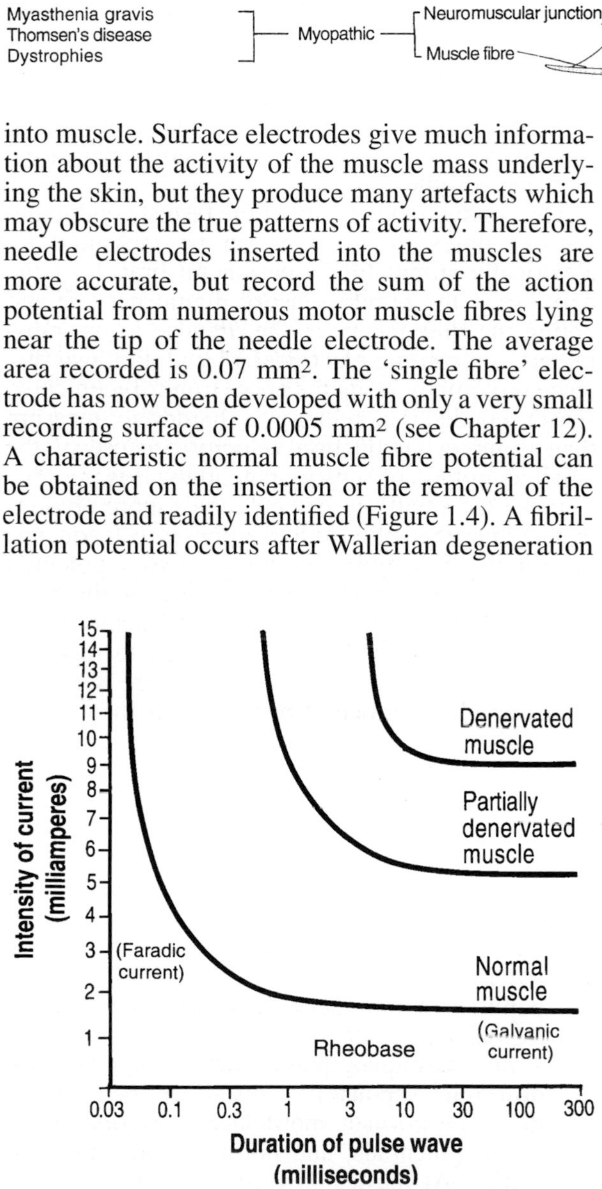

Figure 1.3 Contrasting the intensity/duration curves of denervated and of normal muscle. When the duration of the pulse rate is shortened, it becomes Faradic in type, whereas when prolonged sufficiently it becomes Galvanic.

of a nerve fibre and is seen as spontaneous contractions of the individual muscle fibres making up the motor unit. On denervation, small amounts of circulating acetyecholine cause spontaneous discharges in the hypersensitive fibres. It should be noted that fibrillation potentials are most common in trauma or compression of nerves and certain neuropathies associated with axonal loss. They may also be found in polymyositis and muscle dystrophies where there is focal necrosis separating the fibre segments from their nerve supply. With partial denervation, fibrillation will be present both at rest and on any attempt at movement (i.e. volitional activity). During regeneration, recovery potentials can also be identified and, therefore, this method is of great help in determining the degree and change in peripheral nerve injuries. Spontaneous activity with the muscles at rest is always abnormal.

In myelopathic diseases involving the anterior horn cells within the spinal cord, fibrillations can be seen clinically as well as by electromyography; these arise from fasciculation of muscle bundles rather than spontaneous contraction of the muscle

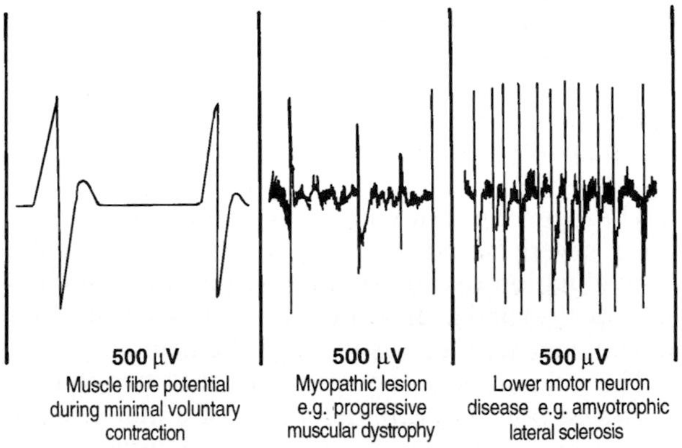

Figure 1.4 Typical electromyographic patterns of the muscle fibre potentials in normal muscle, in a myopathic and in a myelopathic lesion.

fibres. Fasciculation potentials are the result of spontaneous contractions of many muscle fibres, but their precise cause or pathology is uncertain. Their presence indicates denervation as seen in lower motor neuron damage, in amyotrophic lateral sclerosis, spinal muscle atrophy, syringomyelia, anterior horn cell disease (poliomyelitis) and neuropathies. Different patterns can be identified when there is involvement of a neuropathic nature or a lower motor neuron lesion and in primary muscle disease or myopathy.

More complex repetitive discharges, e.g. myotonic from myotonia congenita/dystrophy or polymyositis, result from several or more muscle fibres firing in sequence but rapidly and in quantity.

Surface EMG recordings can detect from a large area of muscle activity from several groups of muscle and are being used extensively in studying the kinetics of gait.

Electromyographic studies provide useful information alongside a careful clinical examination, nerve conduction studies and of course muscle biopsy. It should be noted that needle EMG studies will produce a rise in the serum creatine kinase and should not be carried out anywhere near the site of a muscle biopsy. Buchthal and Kamieniecka (1982) have found in myopathy patients the EMG agreed with the clinical classification in 81% of the patients (the muscle biopsy in 79%) and in neurogenic disease, the results agreed with 91% (biopsy 92%). The main differences were found in patients with neuromuscular transmission disorders.

Nerve conduction velocity

This combines stimulation of a peripheral nerve by an electrode with recording of the time of the muscle response. It is useful in differentiating between diseases of the axons and of the anterior horn cells, as well as abnormal fatiguability (Eaton and Lambert, 1957). It is also useful in determining the level of interruption of a peripheral nerve lesion (e.g. an ulnar nerve palsy occurring at the elbow or at the wrist), the site of the median nerve lesion producing a carpal tunnel syndrome or a lesion involving the lateral popliteal nerve in the leg.

The degree of slowing may also be important, since severe slowing is suggestive of segmental demyelination (as in a compression or entrapment neuropathy) and a lesser degree of slowing suggests axonal degeneration (as in alcoholic neuropathy).

The velocity of conduction between two widely separated points along the course of a motor nerve can be measured by recording the muscle action potential evoked by electrical stimulation at each of the two points. The time elapsing between stimulation and the onset of the muscle response, divided by the length of nerve between the two stimulation sites corresponds to the conduction velocity of the fastest conducting motor nerve fibres calculated in metres per second. Prominent slowing of conduction suggests a disorder of the peripheral nerve rather than of the muscle cell or the anterior horn cell body. Slight slowing may occur with lower motor neuron cell death (e.g. in motor neuron disease), indicating loss of the fastest conducting fibres. Stimulation proximal to an area of segmental demyelination may lower and broaden the muscle action potential recorded with surface electrodes. When interpreting nerve conduction velocities, it must be remembered that age and temperature can profoundly affect the values recorded for perfectly normal axons. Also, unrecognized anomalous innervation may be present, e.g. Martin–Gruber anastomosis and carpal tunnel syndrome.

The conduction velocity of the fastest conducting sensory fibres in a nerve can be measured by electrically stimulating a peripheral branch of the nerve (e.g. the purely sensory digital nerves) and noting the time taken for the impulse to be transmitted to recording electrodes placed a known distance proximally along the nerve trunk. Technically, sensor conduction velocity is harder to measure than is motor conduction velocity because of the small amplitude of sensory potentials. It is possible to make the small sensory potentials more obvious by the superimposition of the responses to a sequence of stimuli, thus giving prominence to a potential occurring at a constant point in the oscilloscope sweep. Much the same effect can be achieved by electronic averaging of the responses to repeated stimuli. Sensory conduction is a more sensitive indicator of a peripheral nerve lesion than motor conduction.

Nerve conduction velocities in:

1. *Acute compression neuropathy* – if prolonged there is displacement of myelin at the nodes of Ranvier, followed by demyelination at the margin of the compression site, e.g. radial nerve ‘Saturday night palsy’; lateral popliteal nerve ‘deck chair palsy’ or ‘cross-leg palsy’.

   In tourniquet palsy there may be two differing responses – distal to the damage there is normal motor and sensory nerve action potentials, and normal conduction velocities. At the lesion level there is a conduction block with slowed motor and sensory velocities.

   Slow recovery is evidence of Wallerian degeneration and there will be accompanying EMG signs of denervation.

2. *Chronic compression or entrapment neuropathy* – the mechanical constriction is sufficient to produce mechanical damage with paranodal to segmental demyelination and even Wallerian degeneration of the distal segment. There is slowing of the nerve conduction velocities and EMG changes of denervation in the involved muscle, e.g. median nerve at the wrist, the ulnar nerve in Guyon's canal of the palm or at the elbow, the radial nerve in the spiral groove, long thoracic nerve of Bell to the serratus anterior muscle; and the lateral popliteal nerve at the neck of the fibula. The lateral cutaneous nerve of the thigh, when compressed under the inguinal ligament anterior to the anterior superior iliac spine, although has no muscle weakness or wasting, characteristically gives rise of paraesthesiae and numbness over the anterolateral thigh with a local nerve conduction velocity decrease. Using these conduction techniques is often slow and indeterminate when used to measure recovery of success following surgical decompression.
3. *Peripheral neuropathies* – several nerves in both arms and legs require to be tested. In mixed motor and sensory neuropathy, e.g. diabetic neuropathy or Guillain–Barré syndrome, the motor nerve conduction velocity is very slowed proportional to the severity of the disease with abnormalities in the sensory nerve action potentials – particularly of the popliteal and the sural nerves.
4. *Traumatic nerve lesions* – there is a recognizable time sequence of conduction abnormalities described by Morgan (1989) as shown in Table 1.4. Such findings help to determine the severity of injury and the subsequent prognosis. It should be noted that Wallerian degeneration indicates much more severe damage, necessitating nerve regrowth and a much longer timetable for any recovery.

Somatosensory evoked potentials (SEPs)

Although surface recorded sensory evoked potentials resulting in the afferent pathways of the cord, brain stem or cortex are significantly smaller in amplitude and are easily obscured by larger ongoing potentials, the averaging computer technique of Dawson now makes these testings clinically significant (Halliday, 1989). It is now possible to detect and identify lesions of the sensory pathways in the CNS. Percutaneous electrical stimulation of a peripheral nerve:, e.g. median or ulnar nerves at the wrist or the posterior tibial at the ankle, is carried out and the potential waves picked up supraclavicularly for latency, upper end of cervical spine and then on the scalp overlying the frontal, the brain stem and the polandic cortex. Light touch, vibration, joint position modalities of sensation can be tested for but not as yet, except in research, testing for the pain and temperature potentials.

These tests do provide an objective test of sensory, function and can differentiate 'functional' and 'organic' sensory loss. They have been used in patients with peripheral neuropathy and trauma, in Friedreich's ataxia, Charcot–Marie–Tooth disease, in demyelinating diseases, e.g. multiple sclerosis (particularly 'silent' lesions) and in spinal cord monitoring during surgery.

Aspiration of joint fluid and cystic swellings

This procedure is often of great help in diagnosis of many effusions producing arthropathies and should be used routinely. The anatomy of aspiration in various joints is shown in Figure 1.5. A 20-gauge needle should be inserted after injecting the skin and soft tissues with a local anaesthetic agent such as 1% procaine, and all available fluid withdrawn from the joint. A larger-bore needle can be used if the fluid is too viscous.

Table 1.4 Time sequence of conduction abnormalities described by Morgan (1989)

Time after injury	Motor conduction	Site
Immediate	No response proximal, normal response distal	Absent nerve action potential across site
1–3 days	No change in conduction velocity	Decrease in nerve action
	Decrease in nerve excitability	Decrease in amplitude
	Decrease in motor action potential	No change in velocity
4–5 days	Absent motor action potential distally	Decrease in amplitude
10–21 days	Fibrillation potential on EMG	Decrease in amplitude

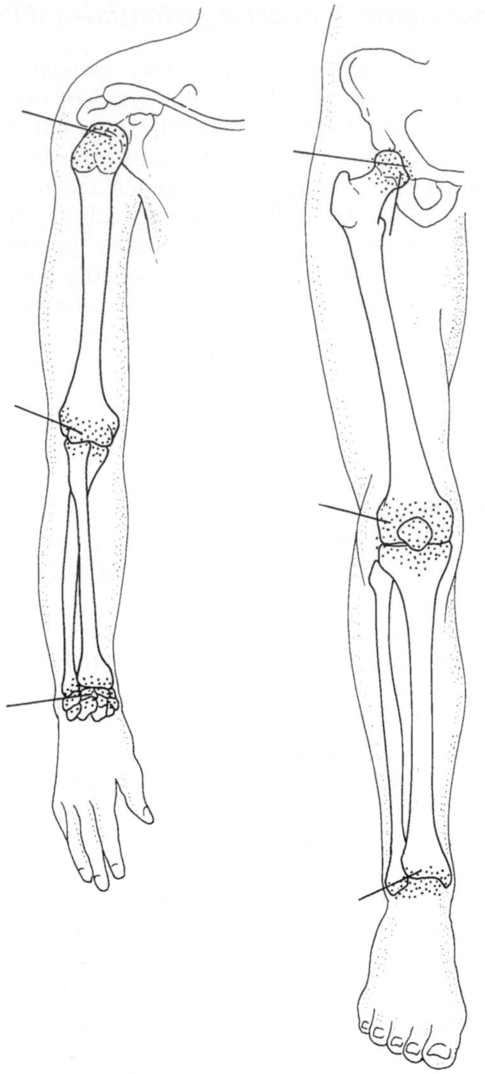

Figure 1.5 Sites of aspiration of joints of both upper and lower extremities.

The characteristics of synovial fluid are shown in Table 1.5. Its appearance should be noted. Then erythrocyte and white cell counts are carried out using a white cell counting pipette with physiological saline solution as the diluent in a standard counting chamber. Typical cell counts and the predominant cell type after Wright staining are shown. Uric acid crystals may be seen, particularly on using polarized light microscopy. The mucin clot test and the viscosity of the joint fluid are indicative of the degree of polymerization and the state of the hyaluronic acid content. Ropes and Bauer (1953) described a worthwhile test in which a few drops of joint fluid are shaken up with about 10 ml of 5% acetic acid and the clot formation noted. A poor or friable clot is usually seen in rheumatoid, gouty or septic arthritis, whereas rheumatic fever and osteoarthritis have good clot formation.

Sugar and total protein content should be measured and compared with the corresponding blood or serum levels. In septic arthritis there is a marked differential between joint and serum, sugar and protein levels – the former being markedly reduced and the latter increased.

The importance of aspirating joint fluids, both traumatic and inflammatory, is not sufficiently recognized. The accumulation of fluid expands the capsule, stretches the ligaments of the joint, interferes with the circulation, and irritates the nerve endings, which in turn causes muscular spasm. Following trauma, blood is absorbed slowly from the joint and produces inflammatory changes of the synovial membrane. Fibrin is precipitated and organized and may form a nucleus for the development of loose bodies. The cartilage undergoes degeneration. The immobilization of the joints may finally give rise to atrophy of muscles and bone.

In traumatic effusions, aspiration is carried out 24 hours after the injury. The severity and the type of injury are then determined by examination of the fluid and by clinical methods. In cases of simple traumatic synovitis, non-weight-bearing movement is allowed at once, and weight bearing after a few days if the effusion does not recur.

Aspiration is indicated in inflammatory effusions if treatment for I week does not produce a marked decrease in the swelling. Reaspiration should be done at weekly or biweekly intervals as long as necessary. As a precaution, a different point of entrance should be used at each aspiration.

Even less recognized than the therapeutic value is the diagnostic importance of the aspiration of joint fluids. In slight injuries with a tear in the capsule only blood is found in the effusion. In cases of rupture of the semilunar cartilages of the knee and intra-articular fractures the effusion may contain fat which has been torn from the fat deposits in the joint or from the bone marrow.

Examination of inflammatory effusions makes it possible to differentiate specific from non-specific forms of synovitis and arthritis. Luetic arthritis can be diagnosed most accurately from the Wassermann reaction of the joint fluids. Reschke and others have reported positive Wassermann reactions in joint fluid in cases in which the Wassermann test of the blood was negative. In a study of 121 synovial fluids in cases of gonococcal arthritis, Kling and Pinkus found the gonococcal complement-fixation test to be specific and to give stronger and more positive reactions than the blood serum. In tuberculous arthritis the effusion sometimes

Table 1.5

Synovial fluid changes in joint disease	Gross appearance	Total erythrocytes	Total leucocytes	Predominant WBC type test	Mucin clot	Sugar (mmol/l) (g/l)	Total protein	Urate crystals	Organisms
Normal	Clear	Some	100	Mononuclear	Good	5.0	17		
Traumatic arthritis	Slightly turbid	2000	1500	Mononuclear	Good	5.0	40		
Neuropathic or Charcot joints	Clear (red)	90 000	750	Mononuclear	Fair	4.5	34		
Osteoarthritis	Clear or slightly turbid	11 000	750	Mononuclear	Good	5.0	30		
Haemophilic arthritis	Turbid (red)	2 500 000	5000	Polymorphonuclear	Poor	3.4	59		
Gouty arthritis	Turbid	50 000	30 000	Polymorphonuclear	Poor	4.8	40	+	
Rheumatic fever	Turbid	60 000	50 000	Polymorphonuclear	Good	5.0	37		
Rheumatoid arthritis	Clear	2 000	15 000	Polymorphonuclear	Poor	4.4	47		
Tuberculous arthritis	Turbid	28 000	20 000	Polymorphonuclear	Poor	1.5	53		
Septic arthritis	Very turbid	30 000	80 000	Polymorphonuclear	Poor	1.2	48		+
Gonococcal arthritis	Turbid	1 000	100 000	Polymorphonuclear	Poor	1.6	56		+

+ = present.
Modified from Ropes and Bauer, 1953.

contains so many organisms that they can be demonstrated in the sediment, but for diagnostic purposes it is usually necessary to resort to animal inoculation of the fluid.

Arthrography examination

After aspiration, the injection of a water-soluble iodine-containing material with or without air is often carried out in order to visualize the non-osseous components of a joint: the articular surfaces, the menisci, capsular and ligaments, bursae communicating with the joint, loose bodies, any cartilaginous anlage and synovial folds and surfaces. It can be used to confirm the position of the needle before aspirating the contents or injecting any material. The knee and the hip are the most common joints to undergo arthrography.

Before undertaking the treatment of acute arthritis in any joint it is essential to know the method and the site of aspiration, the mode of approach for drainage, and the optimum position should ankylosis supervene.

Hip joint

The hip joint may be aspirated through either a lateral or an anterior route.

1. The needle is entered at a point 5 cm below the anterior inferior iliac spine and pushed upwards, backwards and medially.
2. The needle is inserted from the side just above the upper border of the greater trochanter, and thrust inwards and slightly upwards in a line almost parallel with the femoral neck.

Knee joint

A needle can be introduced into the knee joint at any point along the medial or lateral border of the patella. The patella should first be grasped, pulled to the opposite side, and the needle passed obliquely between the femur and the patella, while the quadriceps muscle is relaxed.

Ankle joint

The ankle joint is entered from the front, between the lateral border of the peroneus tertius and the lateral malleolus, or between the medial border of the tibialis anterior and the medial malleolus. The needle is thrust backwards and slightly downwards, and should gain the interval between the tibia and the talus, which has been previously identified by palpation. The joint may also be aspirated from the back, between the tendo calcaneus and the peroneal muscles.

Shoulder joint

Apiration of the shoulder joint is carried out by inserting the needle at some point in the delto-pectoral triangle, and thrusting it through the anterior part of the capsule. The joint may also be punctured between the acromion process and the head of the humerus, the needle being inserted below the anterior border of the acromion, and pushed downwards and backwards. On the lateral aspect, the subacromial bursa, when distended, offers a convenient route of aspiration, the needle being inserted just below the lateral edge of the acromion, either at its mid-point or towards the posterior end.

Elbow joint

The elbow joint may be approached from the back. The needle is introduced immediately above the olecranon and equidistant from the epicondyles, with the elbow flexed to about 135°.

An alternative and better route is to insert the needle at the lateral side of the olecranon, with the elbow at a right angle. This lateral approach is easier, since the head of the radius can be readily rotated and, in this way, the position of the joint defined.

Wrist joint

The needle is introduced posteriorly immediately below the lower end of the radius, between the extensor indicis proprius and the extensor pollicis longus. It passes directly into the radiocarpal joint.

Arthroscopic examination

Internal visual examination of joints by fibreoptic arthroscopes has been developed in the past 25 years, particularly for the knee, and first described by Watanabe *et al.*, 1969 and Jackson and Abe, 1972, but also for the shoulder and small joints such as the metacarpophalangeal. In small joints, the surface of the articular cartilage and defects or inflammation in the synovium and capsule caused by injury or rheumatoid arthritis can be recognized and tissue removed for biopsy.

In the knee the following structures can be recognized:

1. Loose bodies in the joint cavity.
2. Synovial membrane – tearing, inflammation, cartilage metaplasia.
3. Articular surfaces of patella – osteochondral fractures, chondromalacia, osteoarthrosis.
4. Articular surface of femur and tibia – osteochondral fractures, osteochondritis dissecans, osteoarthrosis.
5. Medial and lateral menisci – congenital abnormalities, tears, degenerative changes.
6. Anterior cruciate ligaments – tearing or stretching.
7. Infrapatellar fat pad – abnormal folds, entrapment.

In the shoulder adequate visualization of the articular cartilage, the biceps tendon, the underneath surface of the rotator cuff, the anterior half of the glenoid labrum and the capsular ligaments can be obtained. Diagnosis of anterior instability, frozen shoulder, impingement syndrome are now possible.

Arthroscopic examination of the elbow is rarely performed and is of greatest value for osteochondritis dissecans, loose bodies, synovial biopsy and assessment of osteochondral fractures.

Arthroscopic examination of the wrist is still being developed, particularly for wrist pain syndrome.

Examination of the hip is performed for unexplained pain, removal of loose bodies, synovial biopsy, torn acetabular labrum.

Because the structures are tight and small, arthroscopic examination of the ankle is usually a difficult procedure. It has proven to be of value for osteochondral disorder.

The examination of the newborn, the infant and the child

There are certain landmarks of growth and development during the first 2 years of life which are important to understand. With the child in the supine position, the tonic neck attitudes develop between 4 and 12 weeks, but it is not until 18 weeks that the child is able to raise the head. The head can be held erect and steady at 20 weeks. From the prone position the child can roll over by the age of approximately 5 months, but only begins to creep at the age of 40 weeks. By 28 weeks the child can usually sit alone, by leaning forward on his hands. By 40 weeks he is quite steady without any kyphosis of the back.

As regards the hand functions, the child will grasp from birth to age 8 weeks and will hold on tight until the age of 12 weeks. Up to 24 weeks he will reach out to grasp, using the palm, and will transfer to the other hand any object by 28 weeks. However, he does not use the pinch movement of the thumb and index fingers until 40 weeks, and this does not become efficient until the age of 1 year. On examining newborns and infants, certain techniques must be used in order to elicit such features as muscle weakness, soft tissue contractures, limitation of joint motion, ligamentous instability, etc. There are many childhood conditions which are important to diagnose early, such as lower motor neuron diseases, a brachial plexus injury, poliomyelitis and progressive muscular dystrophy. There are also upper motor neuron disturbances with spasticity and reflex changes, as seen in cerebral palsy (Johnson, 1958).

The first step is the inspection of the child for any spontaneous movements of the extremities as he lies on the examining couch. A specific reflex, the *Moro embrace* (Figure 1.6) is present at birth and usually disappears before the age of 4 months. It can be elicited by striking the examining couch on each side of the child or by active movement allowing the child's head to fall backwards for a few centimetres. This causes the child to reach around in an embrace attitude of abduction and extension, and often is accompanied by a tremor and closing of the fists.

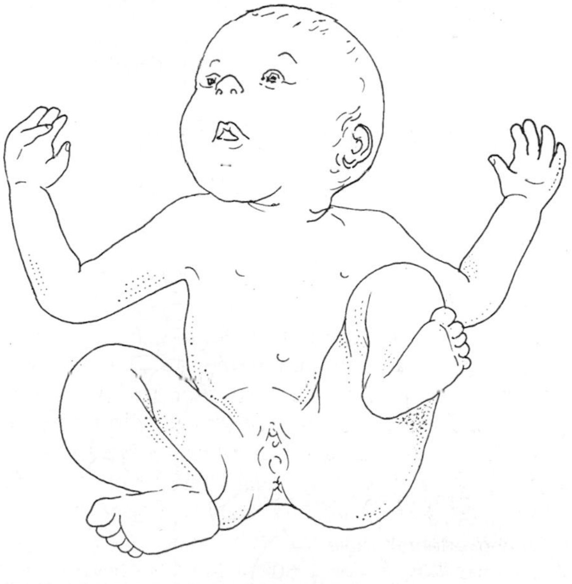

Figure 1.6 The Moro embrace reflex in which the upper extremities of the child move around in abduction and flexion accompanied by irregular movements of the lower extremities.

Movements will also take place in the lower extremities. Any asymmetrical movement or weakness of one extremity is recorded.

Palpation for tenderness, consistency and tone of muscle masses is next carried out to differentiate normal muscles from those of any flaccid hypotonic conditions or those which have failed to develop or have undergone fibrosis or contraction.

Gentle movements of the upper extremities and the lower extremities together will reveal asymmetrical tightness or weakness of the muscles, as well as any joint disturbance. The usual routine is to dorsiflex the foot until the shin is reached, then flex the knees and the hips, folding both thighs out into full abduction horizontal on the table top, then gradually extend the lower limbs. Limitation in any of these normal ranges must be recorded and fully examined for its cause. There are certain reflexes during infancy which should be looked for:

1. The tonic neck reflex, which is present at birth and disappears at about 4 months of age. If the head is turned sharply to one side the ipsilateral arm and leg flex, whereas the contralateral arm and leg extend (Figure 1.7).
2. The grasp reflex, which is present at birth and persists to about 4 months of age. The infant's fingers will grasp the examiner's fingers and should be strong enough to pull the child up into a sitting position. For the first 2 months the head will lag behind; then the head and trunk will come up together under control.
3. The Landau reflex is present from age 6 to 12 months and disappears before the age of 3 years, and is seen when the child is rolled over and held in the prone position: the head, trunk and legs extend (Figure 1.8); or, when the head is flexed, the legs flex.

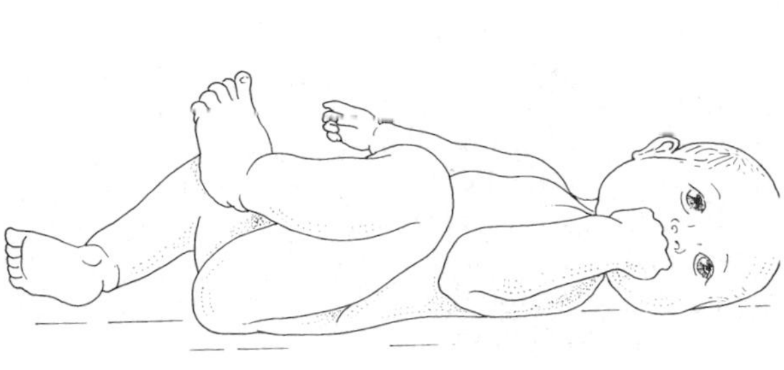

Figure 1.7 Tonic neck reflex of flexion of the ipsilateral arm and leg with extension of the opposite arm and leg produced by sharply turning the head to one side.

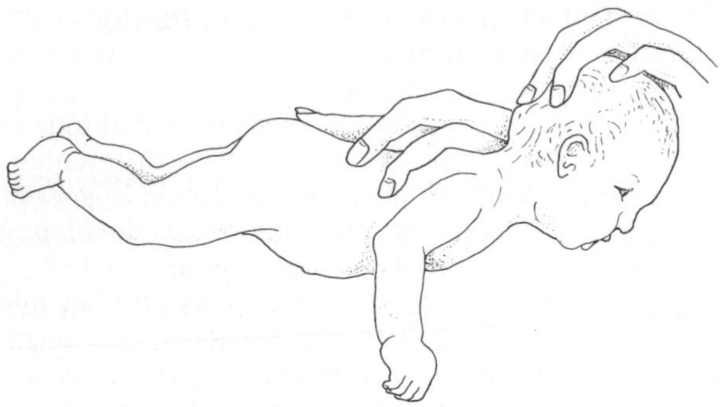

Figure 1.8 Landau reflex of extension of the trunk and legs on the child being placed into a prone position, or when the head is flexed, the legs flex.

4. Stroking the sole of the foot along the medial side will cause strong inversion, whereas stroking along the lateral side will cause eversion. Alteration in these as well as active movements may indicate neuromuscular disturbance and is useful in discovering such congenital static or postural lesions as metatarsus varus, various degrees of club foot, etc.

Examination of the gait is also very helpful, although the time of onset of walking has very little significance. By the age of 2 years the child can usually run, but is 3–4 before he can run well. The width between the walking base of the child has some significance and the toe push-off should present.

Posture – standing; walking

In regard to standing, the child will support the weight of the body and extend legs often by 20 weeks on being lifted up and will 'bounce' by 28 weeks. He will stand steady for a short while with supporting hands at the age of 36 weeks, but does not walk alone without support before the age of 12 months. During the following 3–6 months, the child will walk without support. It is not until the age of 18 months that the child can run, still stiffly, and 24 months before he runs without falling. At 18 months the child will start to climb stairs, particularly with one hand held. Going down stairs does not occur until the age of 21 months or older, particularly with support, and it is not until 36 months that the child is able to use alternate feet going upstairs and 48 months before coming downstairs without support.

Posture

Posture is the position of the body undergoing gravitational forces arising from its environment. In the standing position, the lines of forces making up the centre or gravity lie through the dens of the axis vertebra, the front of the body of the second thoracic vertebra and the back of the fifth lumbar vertebra. They then pass down behind the hip joint, in front of the ankle, and halfway between heel and the metatarsal heads.

The tilt of the pelvis contributes greatly to the postural position and is normally about 60°. This can be measured by meeting a horizontal line and a line through the sacral promontory, joining the upper border of the pubic symphysis (Figure 1.9).

In the coronal plane along the line adjoining the mastoid process, the greater trochanters and the tibial tubercles reach the ground at the base of the

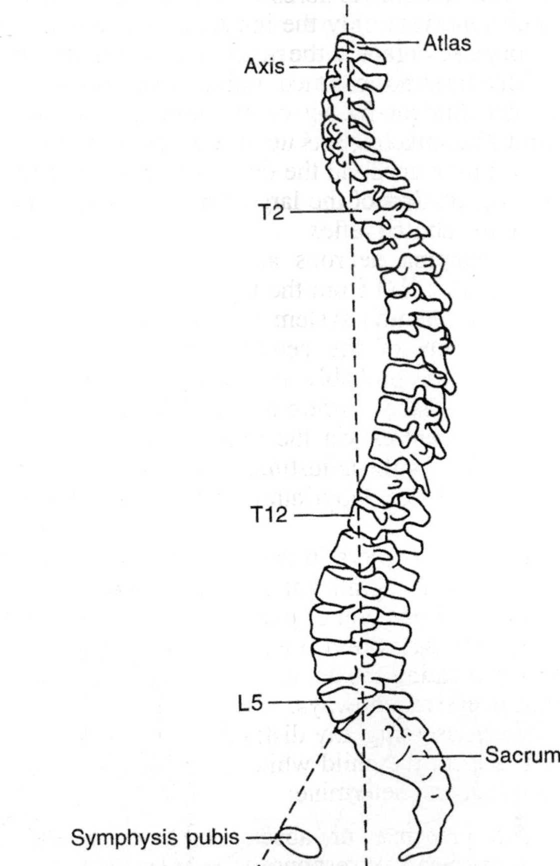

Figure 1.9 The line of gravity passing anterior to C1, posterior to L5 of the vertebral column, with the sacrovertebral angle of 60°.

fifth metatarsal bones. A state of equilibrium is achieved when a vertical line passes through the centre of gravity but falls within the boundary of a supporting base, and this occurs in the standing position. Regulation of normal posture depends upon the integrated activity of many reflex mechanisms. The anterior horn cell forms a convergent point for fibres from many dorsal nerve roots and for fibres from all levels of the brain and spinal cord. Activity of anterior horn cells, dorsal nerve roots, fibres at all levels without brain and spinal cord in a properly co-ordinated manner is required for normal posture.

In the spinal cord there are many reflex mechanisms for the variety of movements, but the maintenance of posture is a function of reflex arcs that have centres in the pons, medulla and mid-brain. The motor control of posture and movement requires common pathways from the anterior horn cells in the cord to the muscles which have been found to contain both large alpha neurons, which directly innervate the muscle fibres, and small gamma fibres, which innervate only the intrafusal muscles of the sensory end organs in the muscle spindle. Excitation of these does not produce ordinary muscle contraction but, by producing contraction of the muscle within the spindles, sets up afferent impulses which return to the cord via the dorsal roots to produce a tonic facilitation of the large alpha neurons, giving rise to the stretch reflex.

The gamma neurons are stimulated from the motor cortex and from the tegmentum of the brain stem. The gamma system of neurons passes from higher levels of the central nervous system by many routes, probably in the pyramidal or corticospinal system. Afferents which modify the discharge of centres via the reticulospinal tracts are responsible for the adjustments of posture produced by neck reflexes, labyrinthine reflexes and righting reflexes.

Mechanoreceptors in capsule, tendons and ligaments play a significant role in maintaining the stability and position of joints (Wyke, 1967). These act by limiting extreme ranges of movement as well as by indicating the actual position of the joint via proprioceptive pathways.

When assessing any disturbance of posture, one must inspect the child while he is standing, sitting and lying, and determine:

1. the presence or absence of any abnormal movements or response to movements;
2. any laxity of joints or hypertonia of muscles;
3. with the child standing erect, changes in the spinal column for cervical lordosis, a thoracic kyphosis and a lumbar lordosis.

DISTURBANCE IN GAIT OR LIMPING

In normal gait there are three major phases in which the lower limbs alternate:

1. Propulsion from the limb on the ground with plantar flexion of the foot and toes, and extension of the knee and hip joints. It has been estimated that in a human adult man the amount of work load through the hip joint on full weight bearing is about 350 lb per square inch (c. 25 kg/cm^2) (Denham, 1959). Therefore, there must be some locking mechanism to aid the joint stability as well as the strength of the soft tissues around the hip, knee and ankle joints. With full extension in the hip joint, there is a screwing home mechanism with internal rotation and some abduction so that the largest diameter of the head is accommodated within the acetabular margin. There has been described a gripping mechanism of the cotyloid ring cartilage or glenoid margin, the capsule and a 'fluid cushion' of synovial fluid. With full extension of knee, which is achieved by the vastus medialis component of the quadriceps musculature, there is internal rotation of the femoral condyles on the tibial plateau produced by the popliteus muscle, to complete the locking of the joint.
2. Pendulum swing-through of the opposite limb with dorsiflexion of the foot and toe, and flexion of the knee and hip joints.
3. Abduction and external rotation of the limbs – mainly at the hip joints with some abduction of the forefoot, with rotation of the pelvis and trunk in preparation for the next phase.

Normal gait in children requires:

1. Normal joints, stable and orientated congruently, with normal range of motion and muscle power.
2. Normal muscle tone with co-ordinated action cortical control of voluntary muscle action, as well as cerebellar control and intact ocular and auditory balance mechanisms.

Abnormal or disturbed gait must be clearly distinguished from an *ataxic gait*. The latter consists of an unco-ordinated, awkward, unbalanced, wide-based form of gait which has only fair symmetry or repetition of pattern. Ataxia usually results from a disturbance involving the central nervous system, particularly of the cerebellum or within the posterior cranial fossae (e.g. thrombosis of the cerebellar artery or tumour) or cerebrospinal cord disease (e.g.

multiple sclerosis, Guillain–Barré syndrome, poliomyelitis and Friedreich's ataxia).

Abnormal gait in children can arise from biomechanical or neurological disorders or from associated diseases as follows.

Biomechanical disorders

1. *Discrepancy of the lower limb caused by:*
   (a) shortness of either femur or tibia;
   (b) soft-tissue contractures involving either hip, knee or ankle joints, which may result from infection involving any of these joints or secondarily to synovitis of injury of Perthes' disease, etc.
2. *Joint disease involving the hip* such as congenital dysplasia or dislocation, slipping femoral epiphysis or Perthes' disease.
3. *Knee disorders* such as Osgood–Schlatter's disease, juvenile rheumatoid arthritis, osteochondritis dissecans, a discoid meniscus, congenital genu valgum or varus deformities.
4. *Foot conditions* such as congenital metatarsus peroneal spastic foot or club foot deformities.

Neurological disorders

1. Muscle imbalance due to paralysis of gluteus maximus or medius, or of gastrocnemius or tibialis anterior.
2. Muscle imbalance due to spasticity; e.g. cerebral palsy.
3. Muscle imbalance leading to ataxia due to cerebellar disease or tumour, posterior column disease; e.g. disseminated sclerosis, Friedreich's ataxia or the Guillain–Barré syndrome.
4. Muscle imbalance due to altered sensation and proprioceptive senses in tabes dorsalis neuritis, etc.

Associated diseases

These include associated conditions such as lymphadenitis, balanitis, inflammatory sacroiliac disease and osteomyelitis. The clinical condition of 'transient traumatic synovitis' of the hip joint can be excluded only by adequate clinical and radiographic investigation.

In acute infections or irritation around or within the hip joint, the hip is in a position of flexion, abduction or adduction and external rotation for maximum comfort and protection. This produces some degree of increased lumbar lordosis, and a lurching gait over the top of the involved hip in order to lessen the impact of the gait.

Any pain associated with limp and localized to a particular joint must be thoroughly investigated. Cameron and Isat (1960) described, from their series of Perthes' disease, the following features: a limp in 46% of the cases; a limp with pain in the hip, or a limp with pain in the knee in 31%; pain in the hip or pain in the knee alone in 10%; and miscellaneous in 12%. The referral of pain from hip joint disease to the knee is well recognized down along the descending genicular branch of the obturator nerve from lumbar segments 2, 3 and 4, and must be clearly differentiated from pain arising locally. Inspection for fixed flexion contractures of the hip should be carried out by the Thomas hip flexion test, for wasting of muscles and for the presence of a psoas abscess, etc. In examination of an unco-ordinated gait, one must try to determine the cause of the unsteadiness and whether it is related to weakness, pain or loss of proprioceptive sense. The reeling gaits of a cerebellar lesion, the dragging gait of a weakness or paralysis and the scissors gait of a cerebral spastic child require to be differentiated.

The hypermobility syndrome

Babies and infants normally have hypermobility of their limb joints, which gradually disappears by school age. However, in about 15% of 6–10-year-olds – particularly in girls – hypermobility persists (Gedalia and Press, 1991) It is diagnosed by having more than three of the following criteria:

1. Passive extension of the wrist and hyperextension at the metacarpophalangeal joints so that the fingers are parallel to the back of the forearm.
2. Passive flexion of the wrist and thumb so that the thumb can touch the front of the forearm.
3. Hyperextension of the elbows – greater than 10°.
4. Hyperextension of the knees – greater than 10°.
5. Ability to place palms of hands flat on the ground with knees extended.

Forty per cent of these children may have episodes of limb pain due to repetitive subclinical trauma, increased muscle tension, abnormal posture and weight at knee, ankle or feet. Reassurance is essential with explanation that this is self-limiting. Physiotherapy and orthotic support are rarely indicated.

'Growing pains' or nocturnal idiopathic musculoskeletal pain syndrome is a common complaint in 5–10-year-old children (Southwood and Sills, 1993). The child can be awakened from sleep because of pains around the knee joints and in the calf and ankle areas, which usually lasts for 15–30 minutes. Its frequency is very variable but usually subsides with the parent's reassurance, heat and massage, and children's aspirin. There is no clinical abnormality present and the next morning the child is normal without pain. The parents and child should be reassured that the condition will disappear in time, without developing any organic disease. It is an example of a chronic localized idiopathic musculoskeletal pain syndrome.

Radiological diagnosis – skeletal imaging (by David J. Wilson)

It is a century since Roentgen discovered 'x-rays' and there continues to be an explosion in new technology for imaging the human body. Despite these innovations, plain radiographs remain the mainstay of musculoskeletal imaging. The newer methods either enhance the value of standard radiographs or provide information not available from traditional methods. The uneven distribution of new equipment demands that clinicians learn the strengths of locally available methods whilst understanding when to look further afield for help.

PLAIN RADIOGRAPHS

Almost imperceptibly to the clinical user, film, intensifying screen and x-ray equipment have all improved in quality. This allows high definition radiographs using a considerably reduced radiation dose. Therefore the benefits accrued more often offset the risk. However, the public are increasingly aware of the hazards of ionizing radiation and they rightly demand vigilance from radiographic, clinical and medical staff to avoid unnecessary exposures. It is a prime role of radiologists to provide diagnostic information at minimum risk. Simple measures are most effective. For example, it is essential to trace old radiographs and it is not acceptable to examine the opposite side of the body when an atlas of normal Roentgen anatomy would suffice for comparison.

Experience has shown that interpretation of films depends on a systematic approach. Radiographs should be technically sound and the examination must include two projections of any part of the skeleton. Films are best studied on a light box with a bright light nearby to illuminate dark areas. The patient's name and the side examined should be marked on each film and the examiner should check these details first. It is strongly recommended that there is systematic study of soft tissues, air-filled spaces, bony outline and then bone texture.

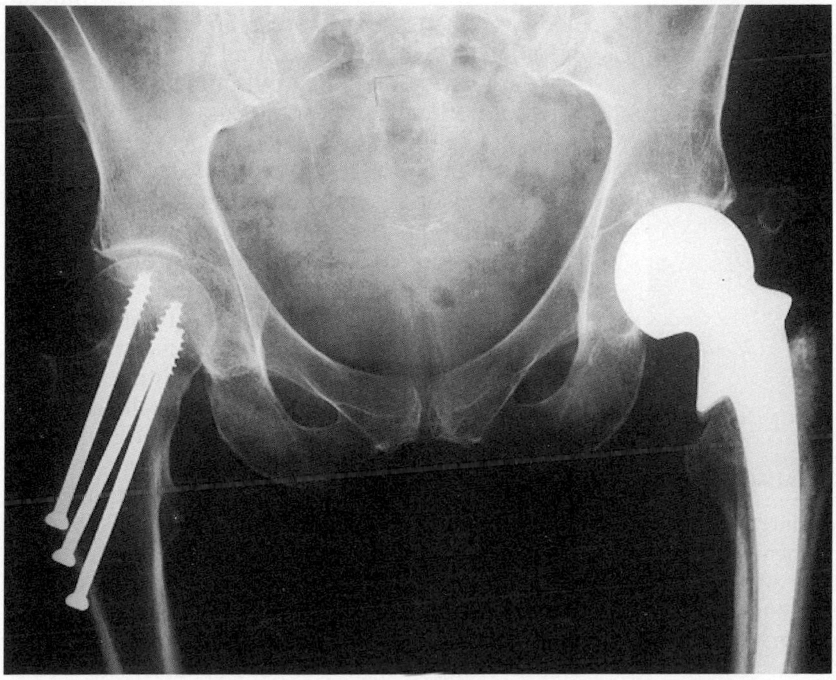

Figure 1.10 A plain radiograph of a left hemiarthroplasty and three screws within the femoral neck on the right. Note the intense white of metal, the white of bone, the grey of muscle, the dark grey of abdominal fat and the intense black of air in bowel and surrounding the patient.

There are four main densities seen on plain radiographs (Figure 1.10):

- Air (black)
- Soft tissue (grey)
- Bone (white)
- Metal (intense white).

Within these densities there are small variations. Fluid is identical to soft tissue but fat is darker. The thick areas of bone may mask trabecular destruction. Similarly, summation of shadows from normal overlying bone may cause substantial areas of destruction to disappear. Plain or computed tomography overcomes some of these deficiencies but at the expense of increased cost, time and radiation dose.

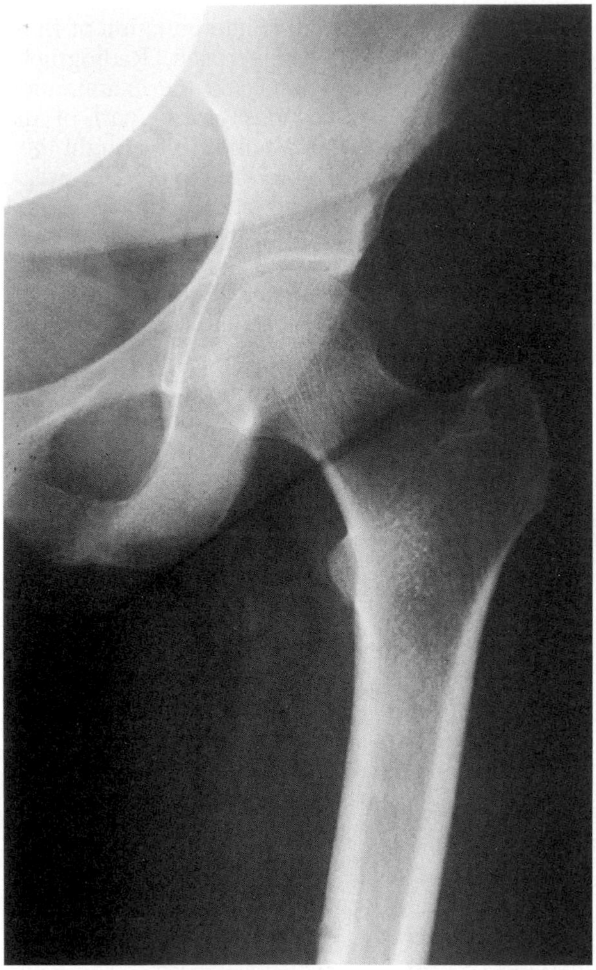

Figure 1.11 A 58-year-old woman complained of a swelling on the thigh. On this plain radiograph there is a subtle cortical spur just below the lesser trochanter and a second similar lesion on the medial aspect of the femur several centimetres away. These represent the bony reaction to the soft tissue mass seen in Figure 1.12.

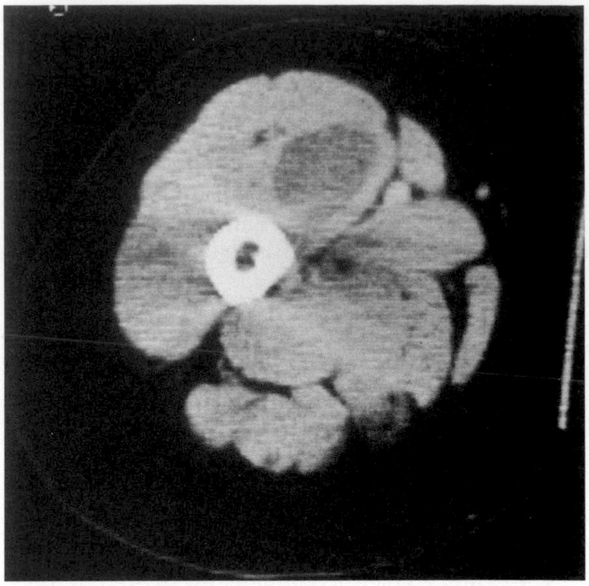

Figure 1.12 Axial computed tomography of the patient in Figure 1.11 shows a substantial soft tissue mass that was causing minor pressure effects on bone. Biopsy demonstrated a soft tissue sarcoma.

Soft tissues

In practice most mass lesions in the periphery are more readily palpable than they are visible on radiographs (Figures 1.11, 1.12). Plain films are most useful in the detection of bone destruction, soft tissue calcification or ossification. Peripheral calcification suggests an established haematoma whilst flecks of calcium centrally may indicate a cartilage tumour. Calcification in tendon sheaths is typical of pericapsulitis; some parasites give pathomnemonic features; myositis ossificans gives sheets of ossified material replacing muscle; and crystal deposition disorders associate with chondrocalcinosis. Ultrasound, computed tomography (CT) and magnetic resonance imaging (MRI) are all employed in the diagnosis of soft tissue mass lesions.

It is important to distinguish a soft tissue *swelling* from that of a soft tissue *mass*. A soft tissue *swelling* on radiography has a poorly defined limit which is caused by extracellular fluid infiltrating the area and obscuring the normal soft tissue outlines and perhaps enlarging the part. It may fade gradually into the normal more contrasted area at either end. Once a soft tissue swelling has been recognized the next important feature is 'where is it located?' Is it primarily in the deep tissues with the fat lines obscured by the muscle density? The importance of this is apparent when one realizes that a deep soft tissue swelling identified about a metaphyseal area is osteomyelitis until proved otherwise. A contusion may involve all soft tissue areas – superficial and deep.

A soft tissue *mass* is clearly delineated, obscuring by its own density the normal anatomy of vessel and fat lines. A cyst or a tumour will also produce such a finding. The shape of the mass may be significant; for example, when gravity enlarges its inferior portion because of its fluid or purulent content.

Calcification is characterized by its uniform amorphous appearance whereas *ossification* may be mature enough in formation to show cortex and trabecular pattern. Both may be seen in muscle (myositis ossificans), tendon (supraspinatus calcification), joint capsule or ligament, or joint menisci.

Bone

Focal lysis

Destruction of bone indicates trauma infection or neoplasm. Cancellous bone is more rapidly destroyed and large quantities may disappear with little radiographic evidence. Cortical destruction is more readily recognized. Lodwick (1965) described a method of analysing the type of destruction to predict the malignancy in bone lesions. In increasing order of aggressiveness he described:

1. Geographic defects – with well defined, sharp margins (Figure 1.13).
2. Moth eaten defects – multiple holes with blurred margins.
3. Permeative defects – multiple holes with cortical and destruction and ill-defined margins.

Expansion of bone implies slow growth but soft tissue invasion is a sinister sign. Using this method it is possible to divide lesions into definitely slow growing (probably benign), uncertain and definitely aggressive (probably malignant). Hence management is determined, the uncertain and aggressive lesions demanding biopsy.

In predicting the nature and types of lytic lesion the patient's age and the location within the bone are important. For example, giant cell tumours arise at the ends of bones and are most common between the ages of 20 and 40 years. Simple bone cysts involve the metaphyses and occur in younger patients.

Generalized lysis

Osteoporosis must be severe (over 1% bone volume loss) to be apparent by plain film signs of cortical thinning and osteopenia. Other methods are necessary to detect smaller changes. Quantitative CT and dual energy x-ray absorptimetry (DEXA) are the current preferred methods. In disuse and reflex algodystrophy the bone loss may be sufficient to be recognized as periarticular porosis, cortical tunnelling or loss of corticomedullary differentiation but the condition will have been present

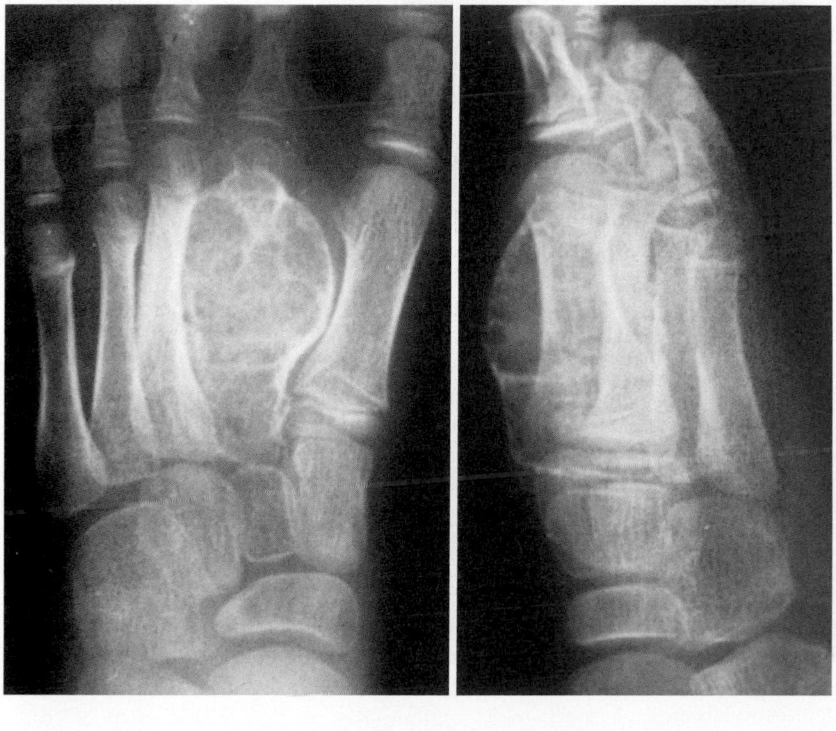

Figure 1.13 This aneurysmal bone cyst has destroyed the second metatarsal bone throughout the diaphysis. New bone has been laid down about the lesion. Increased bone deposition gives the appearance of sclerosis in the third metatarsal. Simple cysts are always metaphyseal and occupy the entire width of the bone.

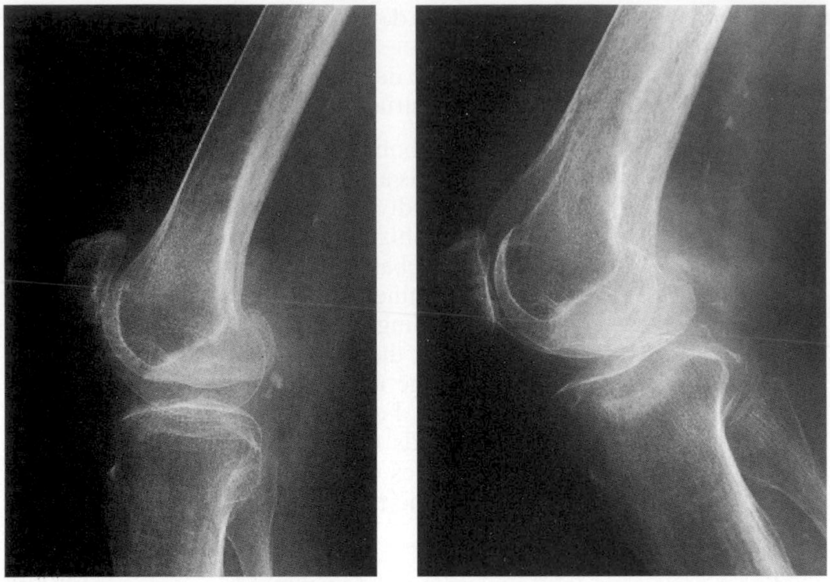

(a) (b)

Figure 1.14 (a) Thinning of the cortex and loss of differentiation between cortex and medulla are features of generalized bone loss in the elderly patient. (b) Radiograph taken a few weeks later shows that the tibial plateau has collapsed following minor trauma and a sclerotic line indicates repair.

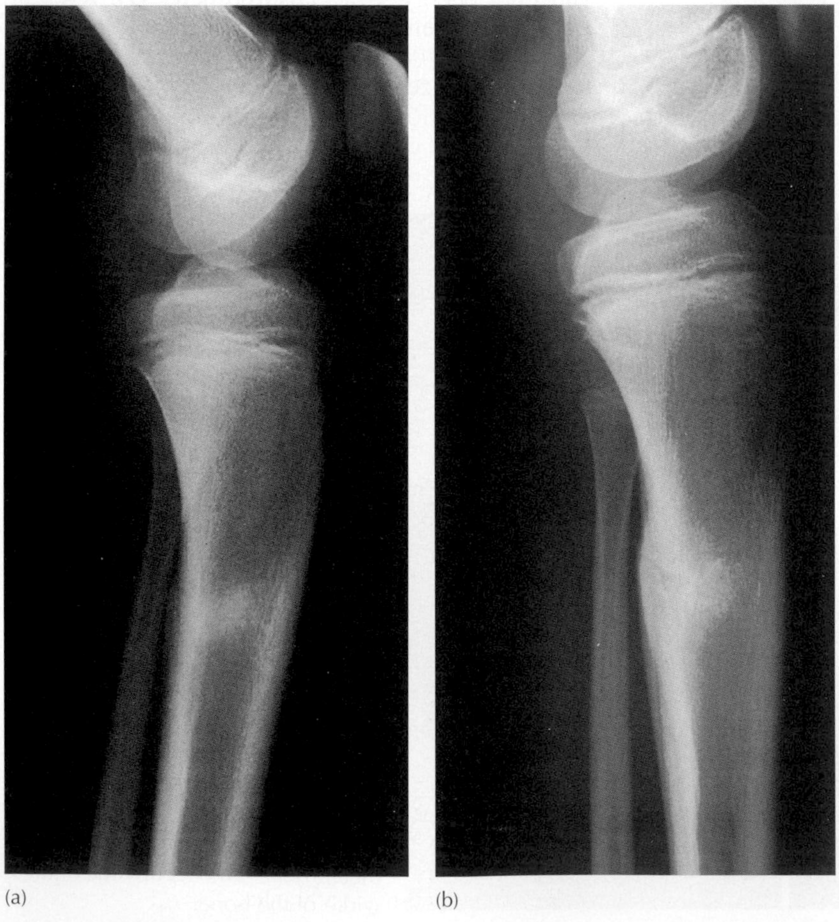

(a) (b)

Figure 1.15 (a) There is a sclerotic area in the proximal tibia with an adjacent periosteal reaction. (b) A few weeks later the lesion has considerably enlarged. This location and appearance is typical of a stress fracture. Unadvised biopsy may show frequent mitoses leading to the erroneous diagnosis of malignancy.

long before these radiographic signs occur (Figure 1.14).

Sclerosis

Focal
New bone may form in healing fractures, resolving infection, chronic osteomyelitis or bone-forming neoplasms. Rare conditions such as melorheostosis or osteopoikilosis are recognized by their typical patterns of increased density. Paget's disease of bone follows lytic then sclerotic phases and leads to expansion of the affected bone. Some secondary deposits are sclerotic, typically those from prostatic carcinoma. Renal, stomach, breast and bronchial deposits may be sclerotic especially after chemotherapy.

Periosteal reaction implies underlying bone disease but is a non-specific finding. It may occur in trauma (Figure 1.15), infection, metabolic disorders and benign or malignant neoplasia.

Generalized
Myelofibrosis, diffuse sclerotic deposits and fluorosis are recognized causes of a generalized increase in bone density.

Dysplasia

Disturbance of growth leading to abnormal bone shape is loosely termed dysplasia. These disorder are characterized by the area principally involved, i.e. epiphysis, metaphysis, diaphysis or the spine. Some are inherited and some arise *de novo*. The recognition and classification are important in genetic counselling as well as in advising on prognosis.

Local disturbance in growth occurs after damage to the epiphyseal plate from trauma, infection, radiation or neoplasm.

Arthropathy

Synovial disease affects both sides of a joint. Early radiographic signs include periarticular osteopenia, joint space narrowing and soft tissue swelling. Aggressive synovitis will lead to erosion of adjacent bone that the viewer sees as an open-ended cavity. Erosions are often seen earlier in the feet than in the hands despite greater symptoms in the upper limbs. Uncomplicated subchondral cysts do not open into the joint space. In its early stages osteoarthritis narrows the joint space and later produces both subchondral sclerosis and marginal osteophytes. The distribution and symmetry of an arthropathy are useful in diagnosis but note that the MRC criteria for the diagnosis of rheumatoid arthritis allow a firm decision that the disease is RA without recourse to radiographs. Erosions are a useful positive sign but their absence does not exclude synovial disease.

Osteonecrosis

Osteonecrosis affects areas of bone with fragile blood supply. The femoral head, talus and scaphoid are especially at risk. There are no plain film changes in the early stages and more sensitive methods are necessary to make this important diagnosis (scintigraphy or preferably MRI). The first plain film sign is lucency below the articular surface often in a crescent shape. Repair leads to sclerosis and weakening may allow collapse and fragmentation (Figure 1.16). MRI is normally positive within days of the insult, scintigraphy within weeks but plain films may take 4–12 months to show any abnormality (Figure 1.17). In ununited scaphoid fractures an entirely avascular proximal pole will not show any reparative sclerosis. However, it is more common to see increased density in a relatively ischaemic fragment indicating some attempt at repair.

TOMOGRAPHY

Simple or complex motion tomography allows improved clarity of bony structure by a technique that blurs out structures above and below the selected plane of focus. It cannot improve contrast and does not show the soft tissues. CT has largely replaced this technique although there is some residual use when metal implants are near to the area of interest and CT would be degraded by artefact.

NUCLEAR MEDICINE

Radiopharmaceuticals are introduced into the body and detected by a variety of scintillation detectors. The most commonly used instrument is a gamma camera that uses a sodium iodide crystal and photomultiplier tubes to enhance the fluorescence that γ-ray photons excite in the crystal. Collimation reduces the effect of scattered radiation that would otherwise degrade the image.

A variety of radioactive elements have been used for musculoskeletal imaging but by far the most useful is ^{99m}Tc linked to a diphosphonate. This isotope has a half-life of 6 hours and an energy of 140 kV_p ideally suited for camera imaging. It is readily produced in a molybdenum generator that lasts several days (half-life 67 hours). The ^{99m}Tc diphosphonate is injected intravenously and over 2–4 hours is allowed to equilibrate with the body's phosphate. Imaging shows the blood distribution

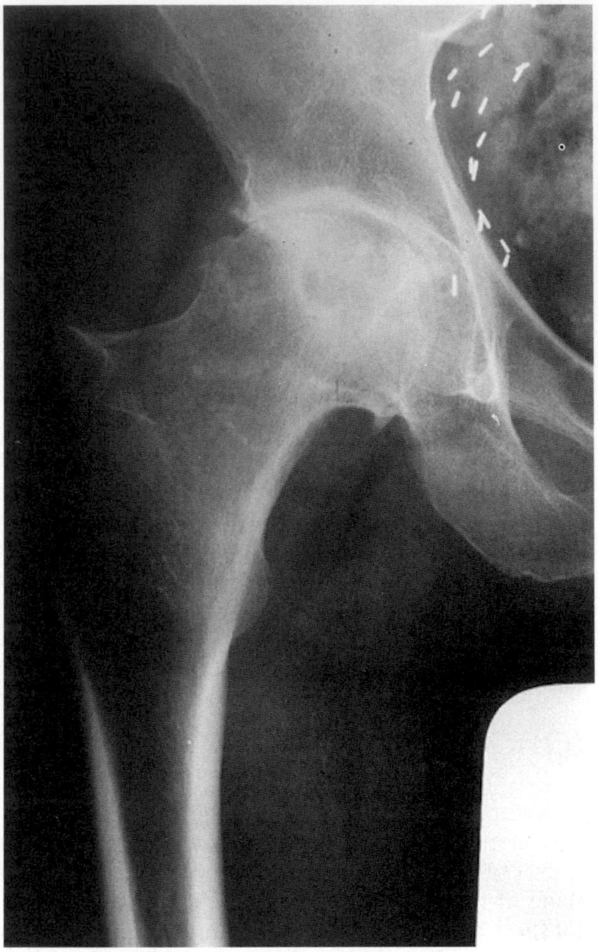

Figure 1.16 A plain radiograph of a patient who has undergone a renal transplant shows the surgical fragments from the graft and osteonecrosis of the femoral head in an advanced stage. There is fragmentation and collapse with some repair sclerosis and secondary osteoarthritis. No further imaging is needed to make this diagnosis.

over the first few minutes, concentrating in the bone within a few hours. Excess activity implies increased bone turnover or an area of necrotic soft tissue. The studies are usually non-specific and are of most value in guiding further more specific imaging (plain x-ray, CT, MRI) or biopsy. Lentle *et al.* (1975) have described an affinity of the ^{99m}Tc for immature collagen in areas of osteoblastic activity. Increased local blood flow is also an important factor in the deposition but its actual deposition, i.e. on the bone mineral surface, or being incorporated is not known.

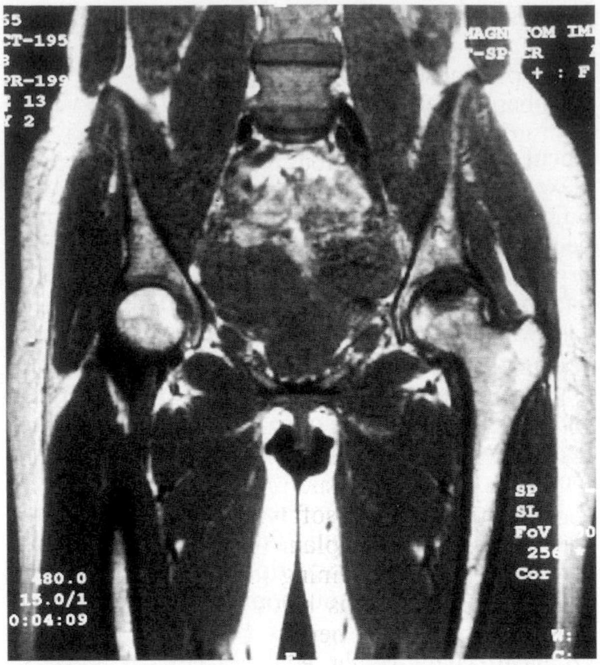

Figure 1.17 Magnetic resonance imaging of a different patient to Figure 1.16 shows a dark area within the normal bone marrow of the left femoral head. On this type of sequence (T1 weighted conventional spin echo) low signal indicates bone, fibrous tissue or necrotic material whilst normal fat and therefore bone marrow are white. These are early signs of osteonecrosis which are reliably present within a few days of the insult. This sensitivity allows early orthopaedic intervention.

Uses

The main role is the detection of metastases to the skeleton although some lesions are not active on scintigraphy, typically cases of multiple myeloma.

As stress fractures, neoplasms such as osteoid osteoma, and infection are active on scintigraphy, a ^{99m}Tc HMDP study is useful in cases of unexplained pain. Again the findings are non-specific.

Bone scintigraphy may be used to detect osteonecrosis but MRI is more sensitive and more specific. It is also useful in defining the extent of a tumour or osteomyelitis although MRI is also the preferred technique for these cases.

In osteomyelitis/infection scanning will be abnormal several days before radiology and has a sensitivity of 95% and specificity of 92% when compared with conventional radiology – 32% and 89%. The use of the early 'blood phase' and the delayed 'crystal' phase helps to distinguish other conditions, e.g. cellulitis, septic arthritis and the healing phase of sickle cell anaemia with salmonella infection.

Radioactive gallium can be combined with technetium scanning particularly to differentiate aseptic and septic loosening of hip arthroplasties.

Indium-labelled white cells and gallium citrate scintigraphy have been used in the detection of occult bone infection but with mixed reports on sensitivity. Many clinicians prefer to rely on ^{99m}Tc HMDP studies.

ULTRASOUND

Diagnostic ultrasound (US) equipment uses a piezoelectric crystal to convert electrical energy into mechanical movement generating focused sound waves. The same crystal is used to detect the reflected sound from soft tissue interfaces. Ultrasound is suitable for examining soft tissues and bone surfaces although for the latter plain x-rays are the preferred technique. Fluid-containing structures do not reflect sound and are seen as black areas on the image. Muscle is seen as a 'herring bone' pattern and fat produces many bright echoes. The technique is very dependent on the skill of the observer and it is unwise to attempt to interpret images away from the patient.

Uses

Mass lesions

US is a cheap, rapid and safe method for the diagnosis of lumps. It is highly sensitive to the presence of a mass and in experienced hands is probably as sensitive as MRI and better than CT. Fluid-filled cavities are detected more easily and with greater certainty than with CT or MRI. However, the anatomical definition is less clear and demonstration of a solid lesion should lead to CT or preferably MRI to follow. US is therefore a useful screening tool to exclude patients with no mass lesion and to show cysts that may require no further analysis. It is an easy and cheap way of following the resolution of haematoma, especially in coagulation disorders where the characteristics of the US image may be used to date the origin and to determine whether recent extension of the haemorrhage has occurred (Figure 1.18).

Tendon

US is the technique of choice in detecting tendon swelling or rupture. Tendonitis, paratendonitis and synovitis are readily apparent. Occasionally MRI will be useful in complex anatomical sites and for measuring the gap between the ends of a torn tendon.

Joints

US is very sensitive to joint effusion. In practice this is of most value in the hip when the exclusion of an effusion is of particular help in children with irritable hips (Figure 1.19). If fluid is found it is not possible to determine its nature by US but the method may be used to guide aspiration of the joint.

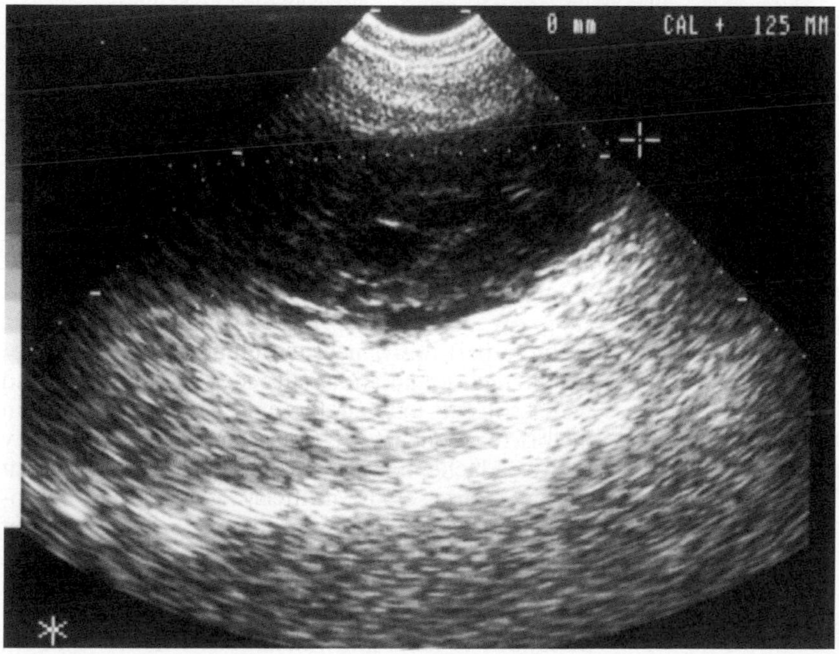

Figure 1.18 An ultrasound examination of a soft tissue haematoma in a patient with 0% factor VIII haemophilia. The small, dark cavities in the centre of the mass indicate liquefaction in a fairly solid bleed that is therefore around a week old. The dotted line is an electronic calliper used to measure the lesion.

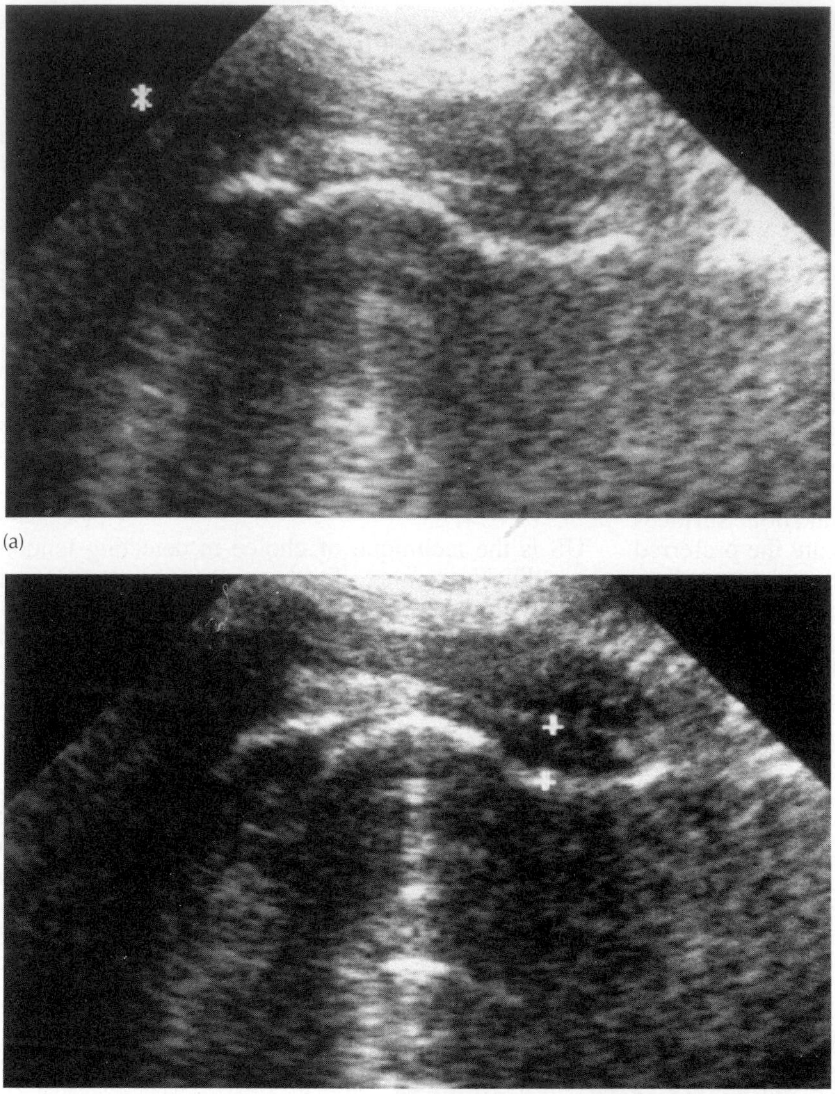

(a)

(b)

Figure 1.19 This ultrasound examination of the (a) normal and (b) abnormal hips of an 8-year-old child with pain and limitation show a dark area above the bright line that is the surface reflection of the femoral head and neck. This is a moderate sized joint effusion. Aspiration is essential to exclude infection and haemarthrosis as the ultrasound study cannot determine the nature of the fluid. This may easily be achieved using ultrasound guided needle placement after the application of local anaesthetic jelly. General anaesthesia is no longer required.

In neonates the unossified femoral head and acetabulum are easily seen by US. This allows detection of dislocation and dynamic instability. US has become an important dynamic technique in screening infants at risk of hip dysplasia and for follow-up of those undergoing treatment (Figure 1.20).

Deep venous thrombosis

US is an accurate method for the detection of femoral and popliteal vein thrombosis especially with the addition of Doppler flow studies. It is less accurate for calf vein thrombosis where venography remains the technique of choice.

MYELOGRAPHY

By introducing a contrast agent into the spinal canal by lumbar puncture, plain radiographs may be employed to show the cord and nerve roots. Impressions are caused by prolapsed intervertebral disc, bony hypertrophy, nerve tumours, metastatic deposits and granulation tissue. Air, oil-based and water-soluble iodinated agents have been used in historical sequence. There is moderate morbidity with headache, nausea and vomiting in a significant minority of cases. Death from infection and neurological complications is rare. More recently it has become apparent that some of the iodinated agents may excite an adhesive arachnoiditis with long-term sequelae. The incidence of this complication is not known although it is thought

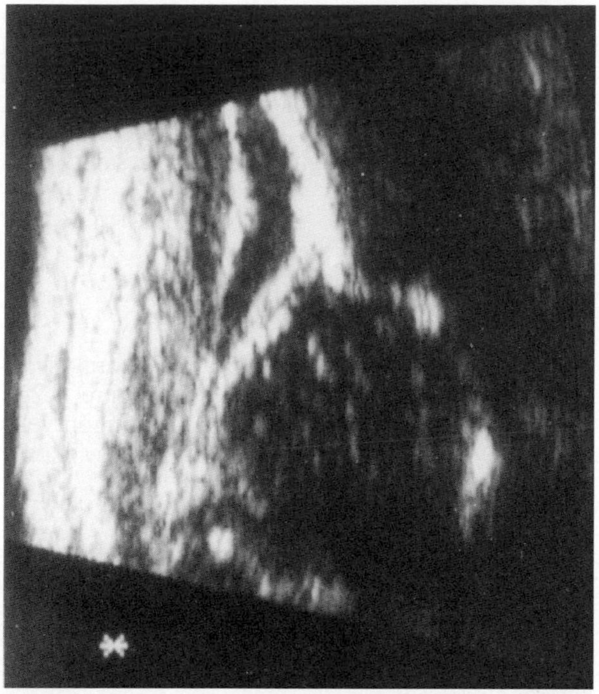

Figure 1.20 A coronal plane ultrasound examination of a new born infant's hip. Measuring shape and looking for dynamic instability considerably increases the sensitivity of clinical screening protocols for the detection of developmental dysplasia of the hip.

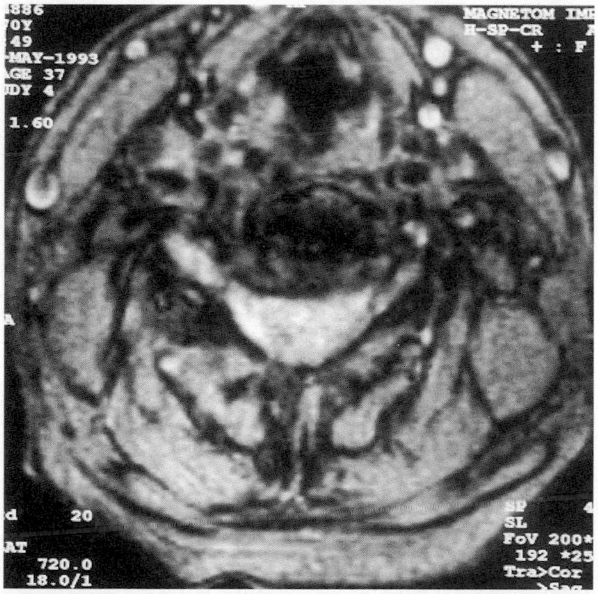

Figure 1.21 Axial MRI (T2* weighted gradient echo) shows the cord, canal and CSF but it is not precise in demonstrating bony anatomy especially in the root canals.

to be more common with the older oil-based agents.

Uses

MRI has replaced myelography in the majority of lumbar and thoracic investigations. MRI is cheaper than myelography. CT after myelography is currently more sensitive than MRI (Figure 1.21) in the detection of cervical root entrapment and there are occasional cases where spinal instrumentation prevents adequate MR images and myelography is of value.

COMPUTED TOMOGRAPHY

For their work in the development of CT, Dr Godfrey Hounsfield and Professor A. M. Cormick won the 1979 Nobel Prize for Medicine. Initially regarded as a prohibitively expensive method, CT has become widely available and is now a routine investigation in most institutions. Costs now are similar to plain radiographic studies.

A highly collimated x-ray beam traverses the patient and is detected by a photomultiplier tube or solid state detector on the opposite site. This beam is rotated around the patient resulting in multiple absorption values. A mathematical algorithm is applied to these data to calculate the density of tissue at the intersections. The unit of density is named after Hounsfield. A CT image is therefore a density map which, unlike plain x-ray techniques, is sensitive to variations in soft tissues. Unfortunately, although later machines are much faster (slice scanning time of 1 or 2 seconds), the radiation dose remains high and has increased since earlier generation equipment. CT is now the major source of medical radiation dose to patients.

Uses

Spine

In musculoskeletal practice CT is probably of greatest value in the spine. Although the cord cannot be distinguished from CSF the discs are identified as a separate density to the epidural fat and the technique is a very effective method for showing disc protrusion in the lumbar spine. In the thoracic and cervical cord there is less fat and CT is much less accurate. Bony hypertrophy, osteophytes and spondylosis are all seen and the spinal diameter may be assessed. Unlike myelography, CT is effective in detecting lateral disc protrusion. Radiation exposure limits the area that can be examined to three or sometimes four interspaces that may be a problem in cases where the neurological level is difficult to define.

Mass lesions

CT is an effective way of showing the extent of a mass lesion (see Figure 1.12). It may occasionally fail to show tumours that have the same attenuation as muscle although this risk is reduced by the routine use of intravenous contrast enhancement. Fat-containing lesions are especially well defined and difficult bony anatomy is usefully examined by CT. Bony fusion, either surgical or congenital (e.g. subtalar fusion) is well defined. Low-dose CT allows accurate measurement of the torsion or rotation of long bones although if MRI is available it gives equally precise measurement without ionizing radiation. CT shoulder arthrography shows the extent of capsule and bone damage in recurrent dislocation although MRI is a close rival as the technique of choice.

MRI

The first images using the nuclear magnetic resonance properties were published by Lauterbur (1973) and Hounsfield (1980). The principle behind this technique is that mobile protons of the hydrogen atom can be excited on an angled rotation motion by the interaction of a static and an oscillating magnetic field through a patient. When the oscillated field is stopped, the excited protons relax and induce a radiosequence signal which is reconstructed as a grey scale image on a computer. 'Magnetic resonance' occurs when the frequency of the spin and the frequency of the radio wave are matching or are proportional with the imparting of energy. Difference radio frequency pulses (T1, T2) are used to stimulate proton signals with selective measurement of proton density (Kent and Larson, 1988). Specific coils for anatomical areas are used: forehead, body, surface or limbs. Special angle slides can be taken and the use of contrast agents, e.g. gadolinium (DTPA dimeglumine) greatly increases the sensitivity and the specificity of the technique.

MRI uses the intrinsic paramagnetic property of hydrogen ion nuclei to produce cross-sectional images of the body in multiple planes. A strong magnetic field and radio signals are required but there is no ionizing radiation. Patients with pacemakers, neurostimulators and those with intracranial surgical clips must be excluded but there are no known deleterious biological effects from diagnostic MRI. Implanted metals, such as joint replacements, will lead to artefacts on the image but do not preclude imaging of nearby structures. Metal artefact is much less of a problem with MRI than it is in CT. High-field systems have a narrow bore and claustrophobic individuals may require sedation. There is a risk of loose metal objects becoming projectiles near the magnet but simple safety procedures avoid this risk.

Uses

Spine

MRI directly visualizes the cord and neural structures unlike myelography and CT (Figure 1.22). Intracord lesions such as tumour and syringomyelia are best seen on MRI. Disc disease is readily

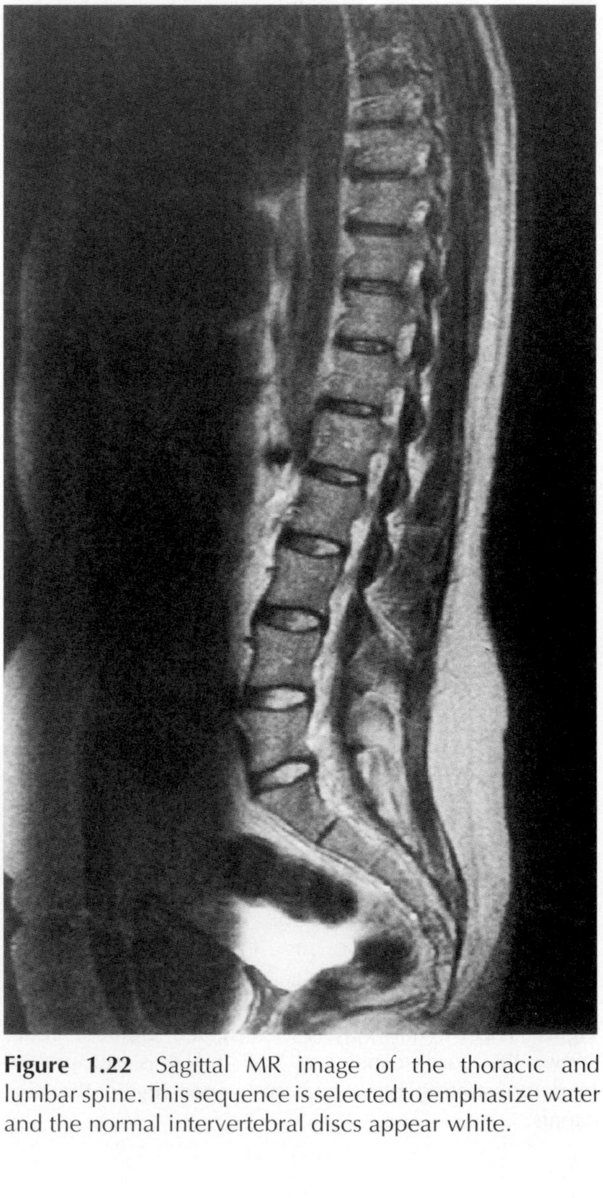

Figure 1.22 Sagittal MR image of the thoracic and lumbar spine. This sequence is selected to emphasize water and the normal intervertebral discs appear white.

Table 1.6

Tissue differentiation	Clinical indication
Recurrent disc herniation, from scar tissue	Persistent pain after lumbar discectomy
Intrathecal lesions, from cerebrospinal fluid	Intrathecal tumour and post-operative arachnoiditis
Bone tumour, from post-traumatic changes	Benign or malignant acute non-traumatic vertebral collapse
Tumour, from normal soft tissue	Spread of bone tumour into muscle
	Spread of soft tissue tumour
	Extension of vertebral lesions into the spinal canal
Recurrent tumour, from scar tissue	Post-treatment evaluation of bone and soft tissue tumours
Viable bone, from necrotic bone	Atypical avascular necrosis (AVN), from transient osteoporosis
	Post-traumatic fracture AVN of the scaphoid
	True AVN of the femoral condyle and tibial plateau, from subchondral insufficiency fractures
Necrotic tissues, from vascularized tissues in tumour or infection	Extent of tumour necrosis
	Need for drainage of musculoskeletal infection
Bone fissures, from surrounding bone oedema	Stress and insufficiency fractures

Reproduced from Laredo, J. D. (1993) *Journal of Bone and Joint Surgery* **75B**, 521–3 with the permission of the author and editor.

visualized and sagittal plane imaging allows many levels to be examined simultaneously. Arachnoid granulation tissue is well defined although intravenous enhancement with gadolinium DTPA may be necessary (Laredo, 1993; see Table 1.6).

Bone and facet joint changes are less clear and CT is preferred for these regions, although for most cases MRI gives an adequate image (Figure 1.23).

MRI, CT and myelography in the imaging of spinal diseases/disorders has become widespread in use. It is important for the clinician to understand their relative value and to appreciate their uncovering of non-symptomatic disorders. Boden *et al.* (1990) carried out MRI examination of the lumbar spine in 67 volunteers without evidence of any disease and found that in the 20–39-year-old age groups 35% had degeneration or bulging of a disc at at least one level and over the age of 60 years 57% of scans were diagnosed of either having a prolapsed disc or spinal stenosis. Similarly, when they studied the MRI scans of 63 volunteers without any history of cervical spinal diseases and mixed them at random with 37 scans of patients with a symptomatic lesion of the cervical spine, 19% of scans were positive of abnormality and in those patients over the age of 40 years 60% showed significant disc degeneration.

On examining the incidence of positive CT scans of the lumbar spine in asymptomatic groups of patients, 35.4% of the films were interpreted as being abnormal and for those over the age of 40 years 50% were abnormal with diagnosis of prolapsed disc, facet joint degeneration and spinal stenosis. Myelography gave a defect in 24% of people who had never complained of sciatica (Wiesel *et al.*, 1984). This means that these discovered pathologies are only significant when supported by appropriate and accurate clinical signs and symptoms and false positives have been excluded. The place of these techniques in some orthopaedic conditions is as follows:

1. *Disc herniation:* on comparing metrizamide myelography with CT, Bell *et al.* (1984) found that myelography was more accurate than CT, 83% vs. 72%, and suggested that an additional advantage was the ability to visualize up to the thoracolumbar junction to exclude occult spinal tumours. However, CT provided better visualization of any lateral pathology, had less adverse reactions and did not require in-patient care. In comparing MRI, myelography/CT, CT and myelography alone Jackson *et al.* (1989) found that the accuracy was quite similar, MRI 76.5%, myelography/CT 76%, CT 73.6% and myelography 71.4%. However, false positives were 13.5% for MRI, 21.1% for myelography/CT and the false negative rates were myelography/CT 27.2%, MRI 35.7%, CT 40.2% and myelography 41%. Therefore they recommended MRI as a procedure of choice in the diagnosis of disc disorder as it is non-invasive, without radiation and painless although more costly.

   For lateral disc herniation CT myelography is still the most valuable.
2. *Metastic disease:* obviously MRI has proven

to be very sensitive in picking up intraosseous lesions but Carmody *et al.* (1989) have shown that in spinal cord compression with extradural masses, the sensitivity and specificity of MRI was 92% and 90% vs. 95% and 88% for myelography. For extradural masses without spinal cord compression the sensitivity and specificity were better with MRI. MRI is of great value in delineating the site, the nature of spinal cord compression, any bone marrow involvement and any paravertebral soft tissue lesions.

3. *Infection:* the exact anatomical definition of infection such as tuberculosis in both osseous and paravertebral sites is now possible by MRI (Bell *et al.*, 1990). Indeed Sharif *et al.* (1990) found that MRI scanning predicted the presence of neurological complication in 93% of patients and the type of infection in 94% with gadolinium diethyl betriamine penta-acetic acid enhancement. The involvement of the meninges, spread under ligaments, into paraspinal locations, as well as intraosseous abscesses, are clearly seen and therefore are important, not only for initial diagnosis, but also for the effect of treatment by drugs and/or surgery.

Joints

In the knee MRI has made a major impact on medical practice. Meniscal, cartilage, ligament bone and soft tissue disorders may all be accurately assessed. MRI has replaced knee arthrography when it is available. A number of comparative studies have demonstrated that MRI rivals arthroscopy in precision and may be more accurate in the posterior portion of the medial meniscus. As experience widens it seems likely that MRI will be the initial method for examining patients with internal derangement of the knee, deciding who should undergo therapeutic arthroscopy and who should be treated conservatively. Currently meniscus tears, ligament rupture or partial tears and bone lesions are reliably detected by MRI. Articular cartilage is less well seen and only the larger lesions are reproducibly detected by MRI. However, if they are detected the finding is highly significant.

Most examinations of the hip are to detect occult osteonecrosis not seen on plain radiographs. This is particularly useful when one hip is affected, as MRI is the most reliable method of excluding asymptomatic disease in the opposite side. MRI changes include a crescent-shaped area of signal loss with signs of oedema, haemorrhage and bone repair. It is possible to stage the disease and monitor response to therapy. There is some overlap in the signs with those seen in Legg–Calvé–Perthes disease that is also detected earlier on MRI than by other techniques. Early work on the detection of acetabular labral tears is promising.

MRI has been used extensively in the detection of rotator cuff disease of the shoulder. It is arguably superior to ultrasound and although arthrography probably remains the gold standard it has the major advantage of being non-invasive. Signal changes in the rotator cuff may indicate tendonitis or myxomatous degeneration that is thought to be a precursor of tears. However, these changes are also seen in asymptomatic volunteers and there is debate regarding their significance. Labral and capsule damage after dislocation may be seen although CT is the method of choice.

In the wrist, applications include the staging of osteonecrosis in delayed union of scaphoid fractures, ligament injuries and triangular cartilage tears. MRI may be used to exclude mass lesions or anatomical anomalies as the cause of carpal tunnel syndrome. Similar indications apply to other joints including the ankle and elbow.

Temporomandibular joints are frequently studied to detect meniscal subluxation. Currently MRI does not provide images of a joint in motion. A series of sections in increasing degrees of opening may be linked to give a 'cine sequence'; unfortunately a number of cases of temporomandibular joint dysfunction involve transient subluxation that reduces with a click during opening. These may not be detected by MRI. Arthrography remains the most precise technique although MRI may be used as an initial test to detect the more striking cases of meniscal derangement avoiding a relatively complex and invasive test in many of patients. All those managing these cases should arrange access to MRI.

Tumours

MRI is the method of choice in staging the local extent of soft tissue or bone tumours (Figure 1.24). Signal characteristics are an adjunct to plain x-ray and ultrasound characterization of the tumour type, but they are not sufficiently reliable to avoid the necessity of biopsy. In particular it is hazardous to predict whether a lesion is malignant or benign using MRI appearances alone.

Osteomyelitis

MRI is valuable in showing the extent of bone infection and will show which areas of bone are involved in active suppuration. A normal MR study excludes established osteomyelitis.

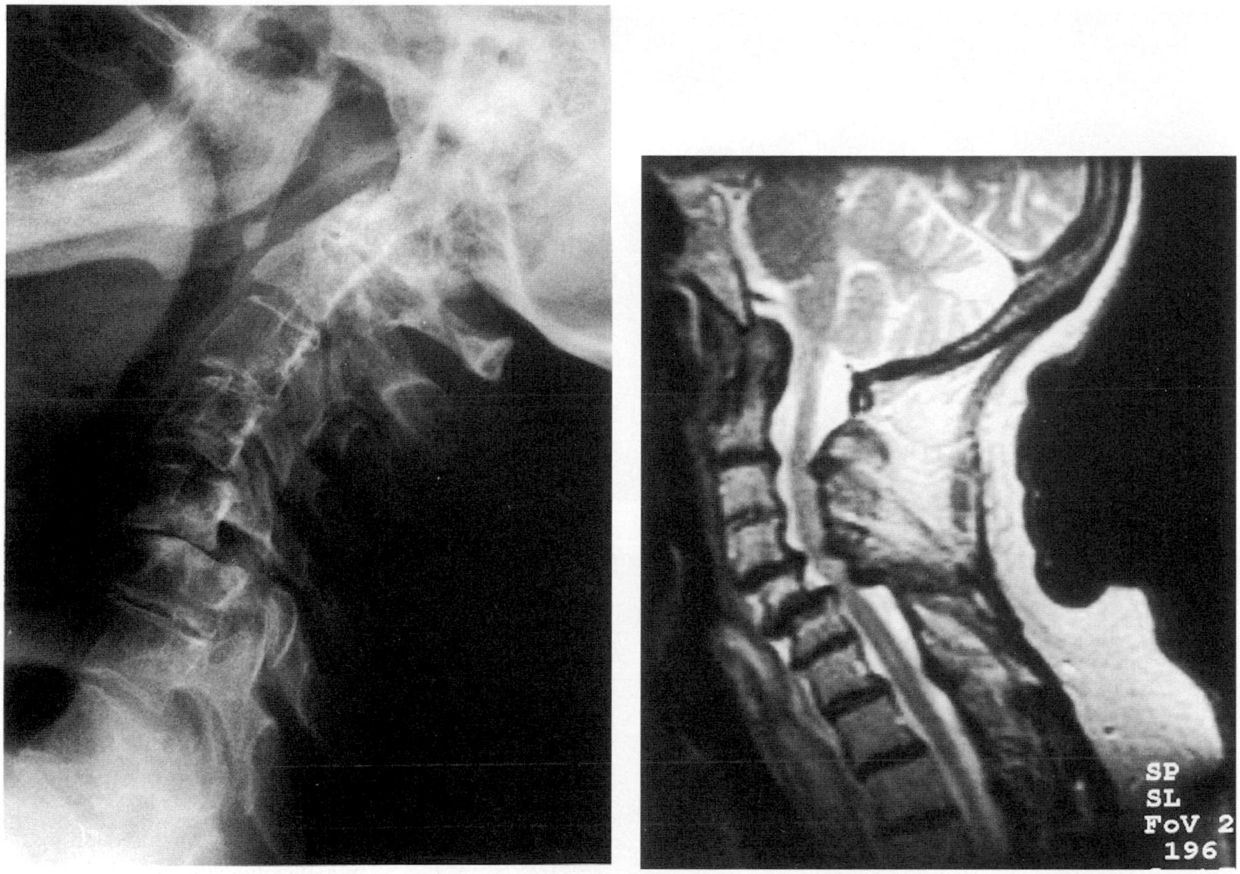

(a) (b)

Figure 1.23 (a) Plain radiograph of the cervical spine shows spondylolisthesis which was associated with amyloid deposition disease secondary to renal failure. (b) MRI (T2 weighted fast spine echo) shows that the cord compression is more extensive than suggested by the plain film.

Tendons

Ultrasound remains the easiest method of detecting tendon disease. However, MRI rivals this precision albeit at greater expense.

INTERVENTIONAL RADIOLOGY

Biopsy

Imaging techniques permit safe access to bone and soft tissue by percutaneous techniques. Fluoroscopy (Figure 1.25), CT (Figure 1.26), US and MRI may be used. There are a wide variety of needles available for biopsy of bone and soft tissue lesions. Many biopsies may be performed under mild sedation when previously a general anaesthetic for open biopsy would have been essential. Close collaboration between the surgeon, radiologist and pathologist is a prerequisite and it is wise to confine biopsy of tumours to the hospital where the definitive surgery will be performed. Otherwise the needle tract may contaminate areas that would not normally be excised or the sample may be inadequate for diagnosis.

Disc therapy

In the last few years a number of percutaneous methods have been developed for the treatment of disc prolapse. These include chymopapain nucleolysis and automated percutaneous discectomy. The indications for these procedures are similar to those for open disc surgery. They are not minor procedures but most series report lower complication rates than open surgery and an overall success of between 75% and 80%. These methods cannot treat bony compression and those patients technically suitable are a limited subgroup of those presenting with sciatica.

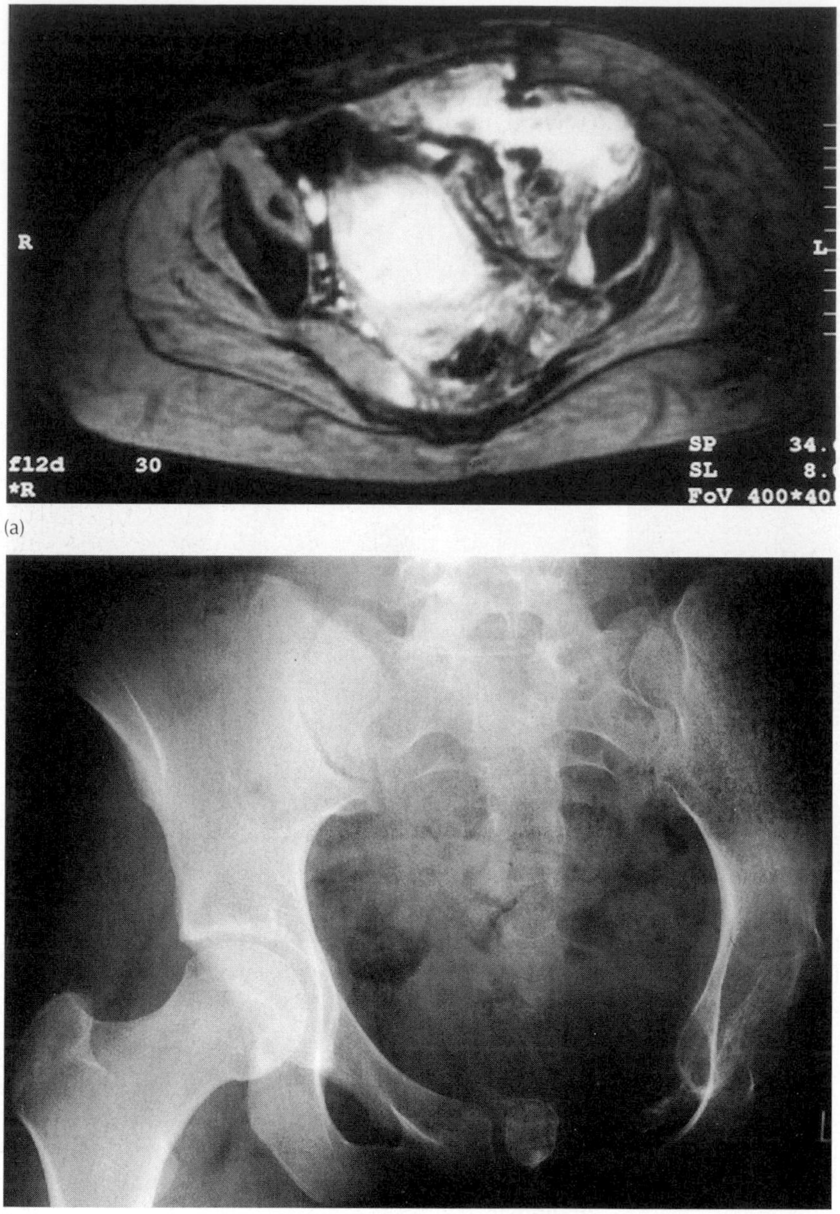

(a)

(b)

Figure 1.24 (a) Magnetic resonance imaging (axial T2* weighted gradient echo) shows a large aggressive neoplasm arising from the pubic ramus. Imaging is essential to define the local extent but the definitive diagnosis should be made by biopsy using the MRI to select the appropriate approach and area to sample. (b) This osteosarcoma was treated successfully by disarticulation and wide excision.

Pain diagnosis

Imaging is used to guide local anaesthetic injections that may determine whether a joint is the source of pain and to provoke disc pain by injection into the nucleus. Discography is now most often used to decide which level is painful and therefore whether fusion is likely to succeed.

Bone biopsy

Using trephine needle, under sedation and local anaesthesia, cortical and cancellous material can be readily obtained from the ilium for identifying and diagnosing demineralization disorders (e.g. osteoporosis, osteomalacia and Paget's disease). Elsewhere, needle biopsy can obtain bony abnormalities for histological and bacteriological diagnosis of tumours or infections. Biopsy to obtain sufficient material by operation is also indicated when larger amounts of material are required for greater accuracy in pathological interpretation.

Muscle biopsy

For needle biopsy a 4.5 mm needle should usually

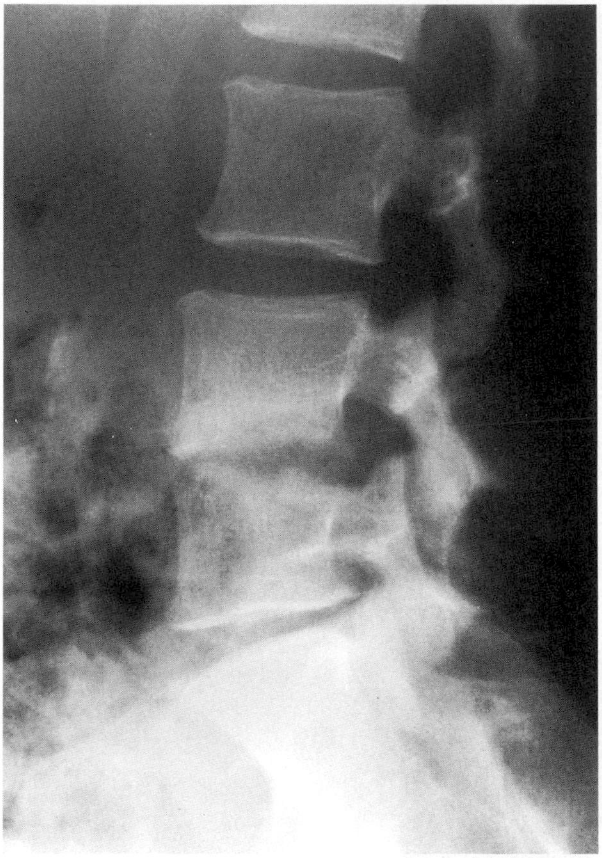

(a)

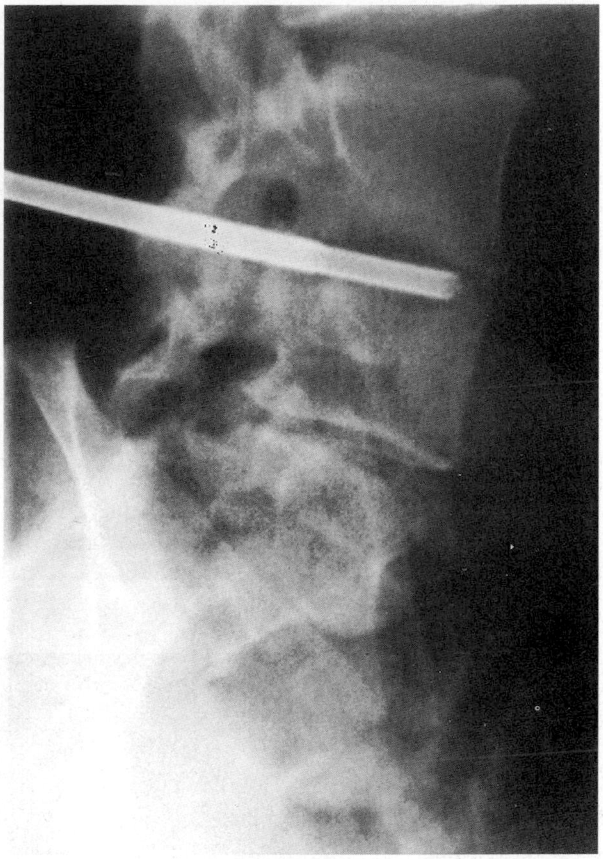

(b)

Figure 1.25 (a) An infected disc space is easily detected on plain radiographs but precise histological and microbiological diagnosis require biopsy. (b) This is best performed in the lumbar spine by fluoroscopic guided percutaneous needle trephine. The cultures are often disappointing and specimen should always be sent for histopathological studies as they are commonly more productive.

yield 35–50 mg of muscle, allowing at least 400 fibres to be examined in transverse section. If required, larger specimens can be obtained through an 8 mm skin incision with a conchotome technique, described by A. Young.

With certain specific exceptions, needle biopsy and open surgical biopsy of muscle are diagnostically equivalent. An open approach is necessary if it is important to obtain a motor point biopsy for examination of motor end plates or intramuscular nerves or if a large sample is required to allow examination of medium-sized intramuscular arterioles (e.g. in suspected polyarteritis nodosa).

The choice of muscle to be biopsied depends on the patient's symptoms and the clinical evidence of involvement by the pathological process. The muscle selected should be significantly affected but not so severely damaged that the biopsy merely shows the non-specific histopathology of end-stage muscle destruction. The muscle must not have been used for electromyography with a needle electrode. The lateral mass of the quadriceps femoris is a particularly suitable biopsy site since not only is it commonly involved in many neuromuscular disorders, but it is free of large blood vessels and nerves and may therefore be biopsied safely. Other muscles which may he studied include deltoid, supraspinatus, biceps and triceps brachii, pectoralis, gastrocnemius, soleus, tibialis anterior and erector spinae.

Adequate diagnostic microscopy requires the examination of frozen sections with the technique of enzyme histochemistry in addition to the more traditional strains as haemaloxylin and eosin, periodic acid–Schiff and Van Gieson. A piece from the biopsy should be fixed separately in glutaraldehyde for electron microscopy.

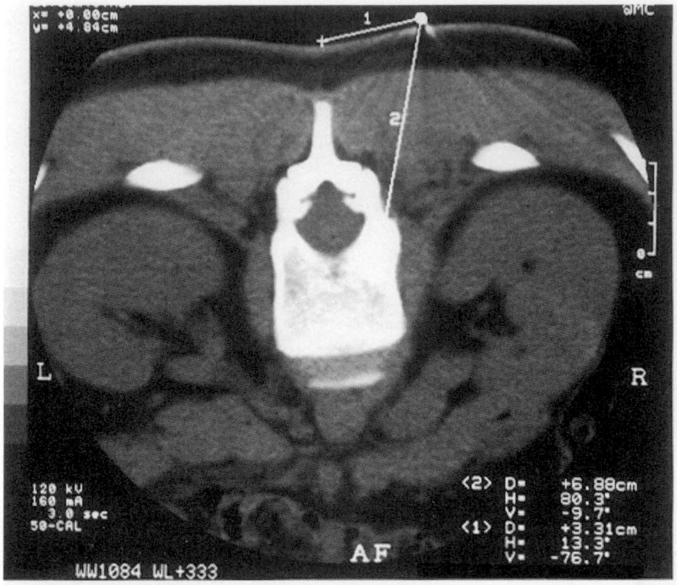

(a)

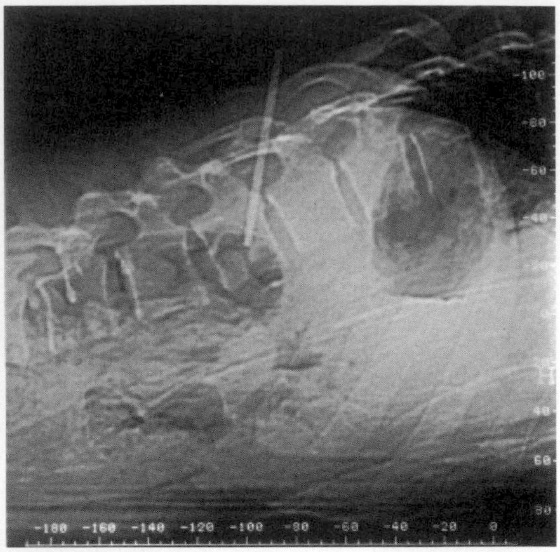

(b)

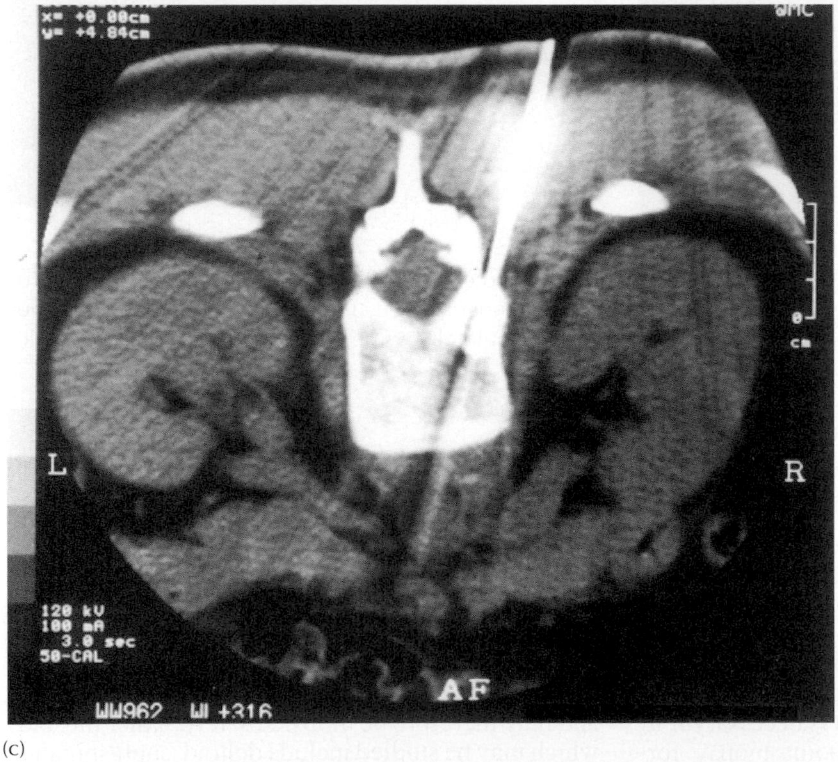

(c)

Figure 1.26 CT guidance is preferred for biopsies of the thoracic spine. Precise measurements may be made to plan the procedure (a). If the needle must run obliquely the pilot or scout digital radiograph (b) allows the gantry of the scanner to be orientated to give a slice along the needle track (c). In this case an osteoid osteoma was diagnosed and excised by multiple needle passes.

References

Akeson, W. H., Amiel, D., Ahel, M. F., Gartin, S. R. and Woo, L. Y. (1987) Effects of immobilisation of joints. *Clinical Orthopaedics and Related Research* **219**, 28–38

Bell, G. R., Rothman, R. H., Booth, R. E. *et al.* (1984) A study of computed axial tomography. II. Comparison of metrizamide myelography and computed tomography in the diagnosis of herniated lumbar disc and spinal stenosis. *Spine* **9**, 552–556

Bell, G. R., Stearns, K. L., Bonulti, P. M. and Boumphrey, F. R. (1990) MRI diagnosis of tuberculosis vertebral osteomyelitis. *Spine* **15**, 462–465

Bird, H. A. (1979) Joint laxity. *Reports on Rheumatic Diseases* **68**

Boden, S. D., Davies, D. O., Dina, T. S., Patronas, N. J. and Wiesel, S. W. (1990) Abnormal magnetic resonance scans of the lumbar spine in asymptomatic subjects. A prospective investigation. *Journal of Bone and Joint Surgery* **72A**, 403–408

Booth, F. W. (1987) Physiological and biochemical effects of immobilisation on muscle. *Clinical Orthopaedics and Related Research* **219**, 15–21

Bowsher, D. (1979) Spinal cord and brain. In: *Scientific Foundations of Surgery*, 4th edn, pp.177–190. Edited by J. Ryle and L. C. Carey. Heinemann: London

Brooke, M. H., Carroll, J. E., Davis, J. E. and Hagberg, J. M. (1979) The prolonged exercise test. *Neurology* **29**, 636–643

Buchthal, F. and Kamieniecka, Z. (1982) The diagnostic yield of quantified electromyography and quantified muscle biopsy in neuromuscular disorders. *Muscle and Nerve* **5**, 265–280

Cameron, J. M. and Isat, M. W. (1960) Legg–Calvé–Perthes' disease. *Scottish Medical Journal* **5**, 148–154

Carmody, R. F., Yang, P. J., Seeley, G. W., Seeger, J. F., Unger, E. C. and Johnson, J. E. (1989) Spinal cord compression due to metastatic disease: diagnosis with MR imaging versus myelography. *Radiology* **173**, 225–229

Chambers, N. G. E., Ogden, H. S., Coggs, G. C. and Crane, J. T. (1959) Osteomyelitis of the mandible following irradiation; an experimental study. *Radiology* **72**, 68–74

Coomes, E. N. (1963) Experimental pain from the hip. *Annals of Physical Medicine* **7**, 100

Denham, R. A. (1959) Hip mechanics. *Journal of Bone and Joint Surgery* **41B**, 550–557

Dunn, P. M. (1976) Congenital postural deformities. *British Medical Bulletin* **32**, 71–76

Duthie, R. B. and Young, A. (1987) Pathophysiology of joint contractures and their correction. *Clinical Orthopaedics and Related Research* **219**, 2–4

Eaton, L. M. and Lambert, E. H. (1957) *Journal of the American Medical Association* **163**, 117

Feinstein, B., Langston, J. W. K., Jamison, R. M. and Schiller, F. (1954) Experiments on pain (produced by intervertebral injections). *Journal of Bone and Joint Surgery* **36A**, 981

Gaze, R. M. and Gordon, G. (1954) *Quarterly Journal of Experimental Physiology* **39**, 279

Gedalia, A. and Press, J. (1991) Articular symptoms in hypermobile school children. *Journal of Pediatrics* **119**, 944–946

Halliday, A. M. (1989) Sensory evoked potentials. *British Journal of Hospital Medicine* **41**, 50–59

Hirsch, C. and Schajowicz, F. (1953) *Acta Orthopaedica Scandinavica* **22**, 184

Hounsfield, C. N. (1980) Computer medical imaging. Nobel lecture. *Journal of Computer Assisted Tomography* **5**, 665–674

Jackson, R. P., Becker, G. J., Jacobs, R. R., Montesano, P. X., Cooper, B. R. and McManus, G. E. (1989) The neuroradiographic diagnosis of lumbar herniated nucleus pulposus. I. A comparison of computed tomography (CT), myelography, CT-myelography, discography, and CT-discography. *Spine* **14**, 1356–1361

Jackson, R. W. and Abe, I. (1972) The role of arthroscopy in management of disorders of the knee. *Journal of Bone and Joint Surgery* **54B**, 310

Johnson, E. W. (1958) *Journal of the American Medical Association* **18**, 1306

Kellgren, J. H. and Samuel, E. P. (1950) The sensitivity and innervation of the articular capsule. *Journal of Bone and Joint Surgery* **32B**, 84

Kent, D. L. and Larson, E. B. (1988) Magnetic resonance imaging of the brain and spine. *Annals of Internal Medicine* **108**, 402–424

Laredo, J. D. (1993) Gadolinium-enhanced MRI in orthopaedic surgery. *Journal of Bone and Joint Surgery* **75B**, 521–523

Lauterbur, P. G. (1973) Image formation by induced local reactions: examples employing nuclear magnetic resonance. *Nature* **242**, 190–191

Lentle, B. C., Burns, P. E., Dierich, H. and Jackson, F. I. (1975) Bone scintiscanning in the initial assessment of carcinoma of the breast. *Surgery, Gynecology and Obstetrics* **141**, 43

Lodwick, G. S. (1965) A prognostic approach to the diagnosis of bone tumours. *Radiological Clinics of North America* **3**, 987–997

McCoy, F., Beverland, D. E., Kernohan, W. G., Agahi, A. and Mollan, R. A. B. (1988) Vibration arthrography in the diagnosis of knee joint disease. *Journal of Bone and Joint Surgery* **70B**, 332

McLeod, J. G. (1958) *Journal of Physiology* **140**, 642.

McQuay, H. J., Carroll, D. and Moore, P. A. (1988) Postoperative orthopaedic pain – the effect of opiate anaesthetic blocks. *Pain* **33**, 291–295

Melzack, R. and Wall, P. D. (1965) Pain mechanisms: a new theory. *Science* **150**, 971–979

Mollan, R. A. B., McCollagh, G. C. and Wilson, R. I. (1982) A critical appraisal of the auscultation of joints. *Clinical Orthopaedics and Related Research* **170**, 231–237

Morgan, M. H. (1989) Nerve conduction studies. *British Journal of Hospital Medicine* **41**, 22–36

Morgan Hughes, J. A. (1979) Painful disorders of muscle. *British Journal of Hospital Medicine* **22**, 360–365

Peabody, J. (1938) *Journal of Bone and Joint Surgery* **20**, 193.

Perry, J. (1987) Contractures. A historical perspective. *Clinical Orthopaedics and Related Research* **219**, 8–15

Ropes, H. M. and Bauer, W. (1953) *Synovial Fluid Changes in Joint Disease*. Harvard University Press: Cambridge, MA

Sharif, H. S., Clark, D. C., Aabed, M. Y. *et al.* (1990) Granulomatous spinal infections. MR imaging. *Radiology* **177**, 101–107

Silverman, F. N. and Gilden, J. J. (1959) Congenital insensitivity to pain: a neurological syndrome with bizarre skeletal lesions. *Radiology* **72**, 176–190

Southwood, T. R. and Sills, J. A. (1993) Non-arthritic locomotor disorders in childhood. *Report on Rheumatic Diseases, Series 2*, No. 24, 1

Wall, P. D. and Melzack, R. (1989) *Textbook of Pain*. Churchill Livingstone: Edinburgh

Watanabe, M., Takeda, S. and Ikeuchi, H. (1969) *Atlas of Arthroscopy*, 2nd edn. Igaku Shoin: Tokyo

Whitty, C. W. M. and Hockaday, J. M. (1967) Patterns of referred pain in the normal subject. *Brain* **90**, 481

Whitty, C. W. M. and Willison, R. G. (1958) Some aspects of referred pain. *Lancet* **1**, 226–231
Wiesel, S. W., Tsourmas, N., Feffer, M. L., Citrin, C. M. and Patronas, N. (1984) A study of computed axial tomography. I. The incidence of positive CAT scans in an asymptomatic group of patients. *Spine* **9**, 549–551
Wyke, B. (1967) *Annals of the Royal College of Surgeons of England* **41**, 25
Wyke, B. (1969) The neurological basis of thoracospinal pain. *Rheumatology and Physical Medicine* **10**, 356, 367
Young, A. (1987) Effects of joint pathology on muscle. *Clinical Orthopaedics and Related Research* **219**, 21–28

CHAPTER 2

The Musculoskeletal System

ROGER M. ATKINS

Orthopaedic surgery is concerned with manipulation of the musculoskeletal tissues which may become deranged by a variety of mechanisms including abnormalities of growth, inflammation, neoplasia and trauma. For a full understanding of the subject, therefore, it is essential to have a working knowledge of the anatomy, physiology, development and control of the mature musculoskeletal system.

BONE

Bone is a specialized connective tissue organized to form an endoskeleton, which arises by intramembranous or endochondral ossification. Its primary functions are structural support of the body, protection of vital organs, the formation of a series of mechanical levers through which attached muscles and ligaments can move the body and the provision of a store of calcium and phosphate.

To gross inspection, bone is made up of two components, the outer dense compact or cortical bone and the inner spongiosa or cancellous bone. The cortical bone forms the outer walls or supporting structures which, because of their tubular structure, provide maximum strength for a given weight. The cancellous bone is found within the cortex and consists of a network of bony trabeculae lying within the medullary cavity. The arrangement of these trabeculae follows closely the pressure and tension stress lines within the bone, adding to its mechanical strength (Figure 2.1).

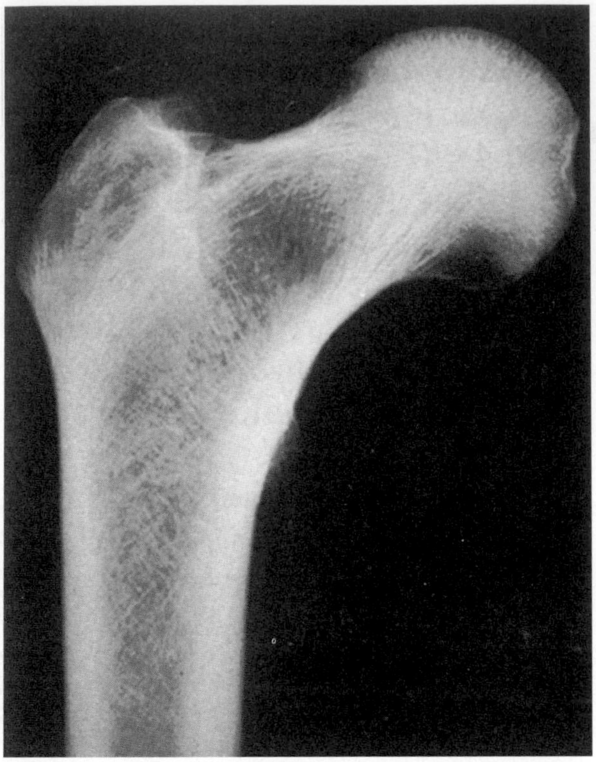

Figure 2.1 Frontal radiograph of the upper femur. The trabecular patterns which reflect the lines of stress within the bone are clearly shown.

Structure of bone

The basic structural unit of bone is the Haversian system or osteon, which consists of a series of concentric laminations or lamellae surrounding a central canal approximately 20 μm in diameter. Between these lamellae there are more irregularly arranged layers of bone called interstitial lamellae (Figures 2.2, 2.3). This lamellar appearance is produced by changing orientation of mineralized collagen fibres which is clearly seen under polarized light (Figures 2.4, 2.5). The arrangement of the bony tissue in lamellae is explained by the way in which bone is laid down by the addition of new layers onto the surface of that already formed. Between the lamellae, flattened bone cells (osteocytes) lie in spaces called lacunae from which arise innumerable fine passages, the canaliculae, which penetrate the interstitial matrix, branching and anastomosing and connecting all the lacunae into one continuous system. The canaliculae contain fine projections which arise from the osteocytes which are, therefore, in communication with each other (Cohen and Harris, 1958).

In the centre of each Haversian system is a central canal which is between 3 and 9 mm in length and contains interlacing reticular tissue, osteoblasts and osteoclasts in various stages of activity and a neurovascular bundle. The central canals run parallel to the long axis of the bone and are united by communication with the canaliculae and by Volkmann's canals which pierce the bone from the outer and inner surfaces.

The bone is surrounded by periosteum which is made up of an outer layer of white fibrous and elastic tissue and an inner cambium layer which has a looser composition, is more vascular and contains cells with osteogenic potency. The periosteum serves as a limiting membrane for bone and is responsible for periosteal osteogenesis, in which the bone substance is increased by a process of accretion. It also forms intimate contact for the attachment of muscles and other structures to establish continuity throughout the musculoskeletal system. Another limiting membrane, the endosteum, lines the surfaces of the cancellous bone.

Neurovascular structure of bone

Circulation through the vascular bed of bone is essential for maintaining its viability. Under normal physiological conditions, bone receives between 5 and 10% of the cardiac output (Shim, 1968), with the supply being relatively greater at the bone ends than in the diaphysis.

In the metaphyseal region near the capsular attachment and synovial reflections there are rich capillary plexuses from which vessels enter the bone, dividing to supply the epiphysis and metaphysis. The extent to which these vessels anastomose with the diaphyseal supply is unclear.

The arterial supply to the diaphyseal segment comes primarily via the nutrient artery (Figure 2.6), one or more of which enter the medulla through the nutrient foramen and divide into ascending and descending branches which ramify within the medullary cavity. The terminal branches consist only of an endothelium coated with a single layer of smooth muscle cells and diminish in size to a diameter of 5 μm. The capillaries of bone marrow are sinusoidal and consist of incomplete endothelial tubes without a basement membrane. At the junction of the terminal arteriole with the marrow sinusoid, the arteriolar pericytes are lost. Some of these junctions may represent arteriovenous anastomoses.

Valveless nutrient veins accompany the nutrient arteries outside the bone. Within the medullary

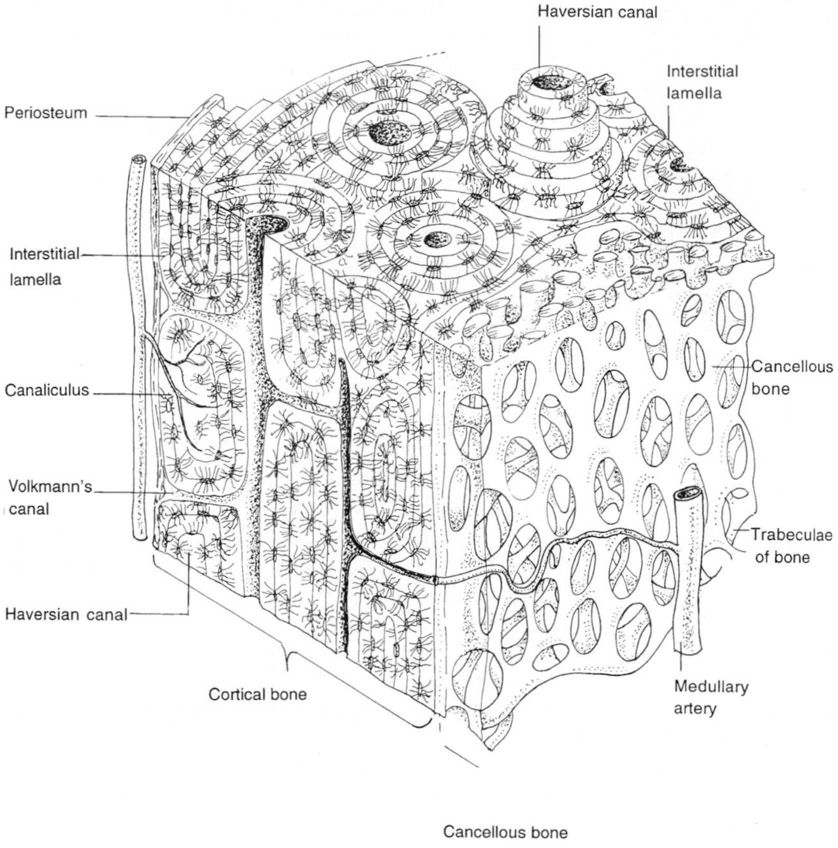

Figure 2.2 A diagrammatic view of part of the shaft of a long bone. Peripherally, immediately beneath the periosteal membrane are several circumferential lamellae. The majority of the cortex is made up of a series of osteons with a central Haversian canal and several lamellae. Interstitial lamellae fill in the space between the osteons while cross-connections are established by Volkmann's canals.

canal, the nutrient vein is continuous with a central longitudinal venous sinus which is served by radial connecting sinuses. These consist of endothelial tubes covered by thin supporting tissue without smooth muscle. The medullary sinusoids drain into the radial connecting sinuses. The general layout of the vascular supply of the cortex is fan shaped with cortical sinusoids radiating outwards towards the periosteal surface. The sinusoids are wider endosteally, becoming smaller towards the outer cortex of the bone and each Haversian canal is supplied with a solitary sinusoid (Figure 2.7).

Periosteal arteries penetrate bone at sites where

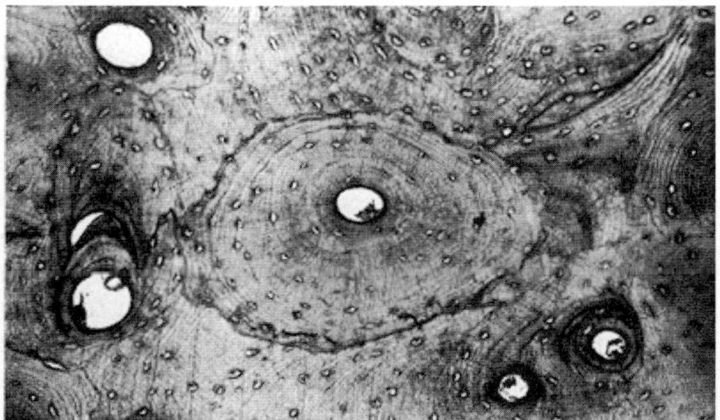

Figure 2.3 Photomicrograph showing the formation of a Haversian system with its central canal and surrounding concentric lamellae. The irregularly arranged layers or interstitial lamellae are seen between these systems.

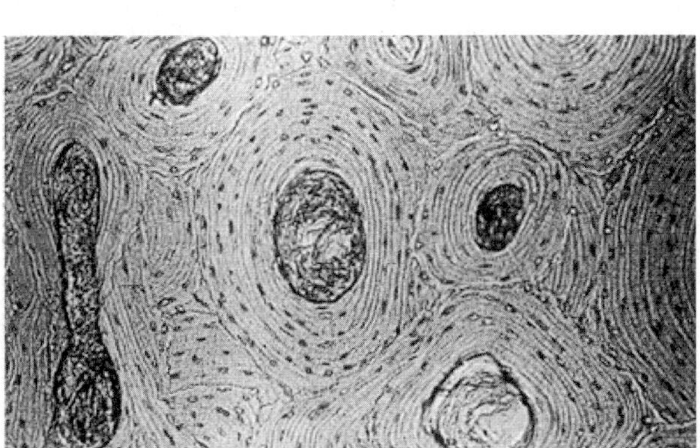

Figure 2.4 Photomicrograph of an area of bone produced by direct microscopy.

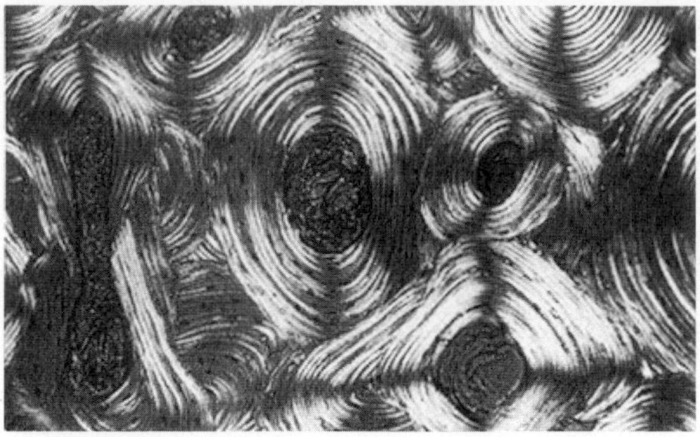

Figure 2.5 Photomicrograph of the area illustrated in Figure 2.4 but taken using polarized light. The characteristic biorefringements which appear as alternating bright and dark areas indicate the regular arrangement of collagen fibres in the lamellae.

fascial sheaths and aponeuroses gain attachment to the shaft (Rhinelander, 1980). However, the physiological function of these is unclear since terminal arterioles deriving from them have not been demonstrated in the outer layers of normal bone cortex. Brookes (1971) has suggested that the blood supply of bone is completely centrifugal, blood passing from the endosteal to the periosteal surface. This view has prevailed, although there is debate concerning the extent of the contribution of blood supply to the outer part of the cortex from the periosteum under normal conditions. It seems probable, however, that under conditions of pathological alteration of bone blood flow, such as a fracture treated by intramedullary nailing, the periosteal source is capable of increasing to supply the whole bone.

Arterial inflow into the medullary canal of the femur is taken up by central venous channels and then passes outwards through the diaphyseal bone into muscle and ligamentous venous outflow vessels (Dickerson and Duthie, 1963).

Other injection studies confirm that the venous drainage from bone is also centrifugal, passing into periosteal and muscular veins leaving the central venous sinus and nutrient vein unfilled (Cuthbertson *et al.*, 1965; Brookes, 1971; Oni and Gregg, 1990). This finding raises the possibility that the central venous sinus and nutrient veins may constitute a separate venous system. It has been suggested that circulating adrenaline may open arteriovenous shunts between the nutrient arterials and sinusoids draining into the central venous sinus which would provide a mechanism for increased transosseous venous return during exercise (Pooley *et al.*, 1990).

The primary resistance vessels of the osseous circulation are the medullary arteries and the diastolic marrow pressure is approximately 50 mmHg with a pulse pressure of approximately 8 mmHg in the dog (Brookes, 1986).

Accompanying the blood vessels there are usually fine medullated and non-medullated nerve fibres which extend into the Haversian systems and are present in the periosteum in even larger numbers. These nerve fibres are thought to be mainly concerned with the innervation of blood vessels, although periosteum and bone tissue have been described as being sensitive to painful stimuli and vibration. Following anterior motor-cell disease, such as poliomyelitis, or peripheral denervation, there is disturbance in both growth and bone density which appears to be due to altered vascularity. It is not clear whether there is a direct neural input into the cells of bone.

In the embryo, the medullary cavity is filled with red marrow and bony cancellous tissue. This gradually changes to fatty marrow during development and by the age of 12, red marrow is seen only in the metaphyseal regions of long bones. However, in the cancellous tissue of ribs, vertebrae, sternum, skull and innominate bones, the red marrow persists with active haemopoietic tissue present throughout life. Marrow is made up of a retinacular network of loose stroma filled with haemopoietic cells. In adults, the fatty marrow may revert back to its haemopoietic function in conditions where normal haemopoietic marrow is deficient, such as myelosclerosis.

Owen (1977, 1978), in her studies of the histogenesis of bone cells, has reviewed the description of these cellular systems and their interrelations.

Marrow stroma is made up of a network of reticular cells and their fibres with endothelial cells lining the sinusoidal blood vessel walls (Weiss, 1976). Haemopoietic cells are loosely held within the network, but the macrophages, although intertwining and enwrapping the stromal cells, are physically separate and are of a different histogenetic cell type (see Figure 2.7). The reticular or endothelial cells are members of the fibroblast family capable of forming extracellular connective tissue fibres, whereas the macrophages, monocytes and their precursors are part of the macrophage-monocyte system.

From ultrastructural studies, the stromal components of marrow are now believed to be continuous with the osteogenic connective-tissue cells (e.g. osteoblasts and pre-osteoblasts) of the periosteal and endosteal surfaces and Haversian canals of bone. It has been shown that the marrow stromal cells as well as osteogenic canal tissue can form bone. Evidence from cell marker experiments in osteopetrotic animals and parabiotic systems, indicates that the osteoclast is a member of the mononuclear-phagocyte cell system. However, it is still not yet known whether osteoclasts arise directly from tissue macrophagoes or blood monocytes, or both. What is less sure is whether

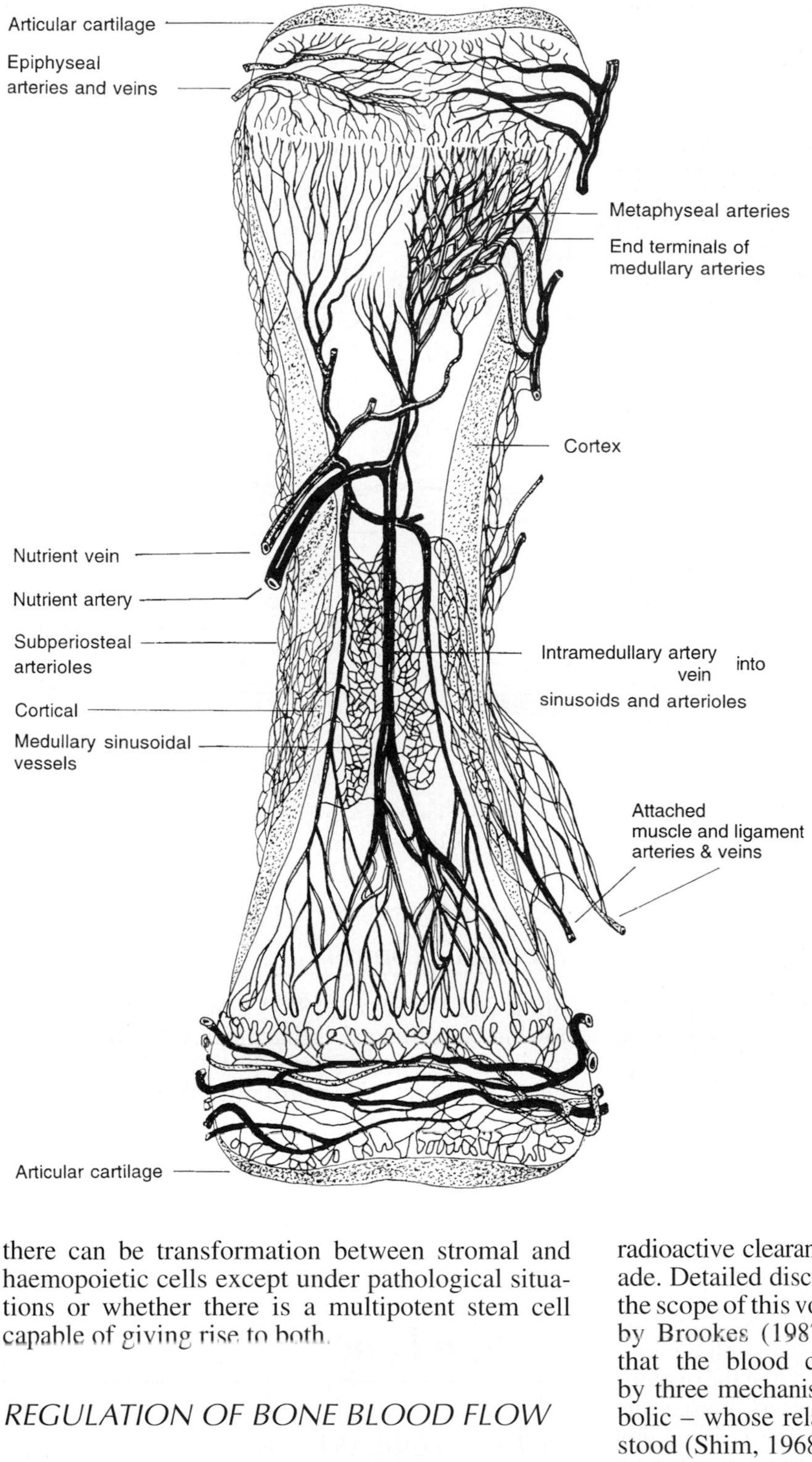

Figure 2.6 Longitudinal section of a long bone showing the vascular supply. (After Dr Murray Brookes)

there can be transformation between stromal and haemopoietic cells except under pathological situations or whether there is a multipotent stem cell capable of giving rise to both.

REGULATION OF BONE BLOOD FLOW

Although anatomical information can be obtained from radiopaque injection studies, investigation of the haemodynamics of bone blood flow requires more sophisticated techniques. These include venous effluent collection, red cell velocity measurement, radioactive clearance techniques and arteriolar blockade. Detailed discussion of these methods is beyond the scope of this volume but they have been reviewed by Brookes (1987a,b). Evidence has accumulated that the blood circulation of bone is regulated by three mechanisms – neural, hormonal and metabolic – whose relative importance is poorly understood (Shim, 1968).

Neural control

Drinker and Drinker (1916) were the first to demonstrate neural control of the circulation of bone. Using

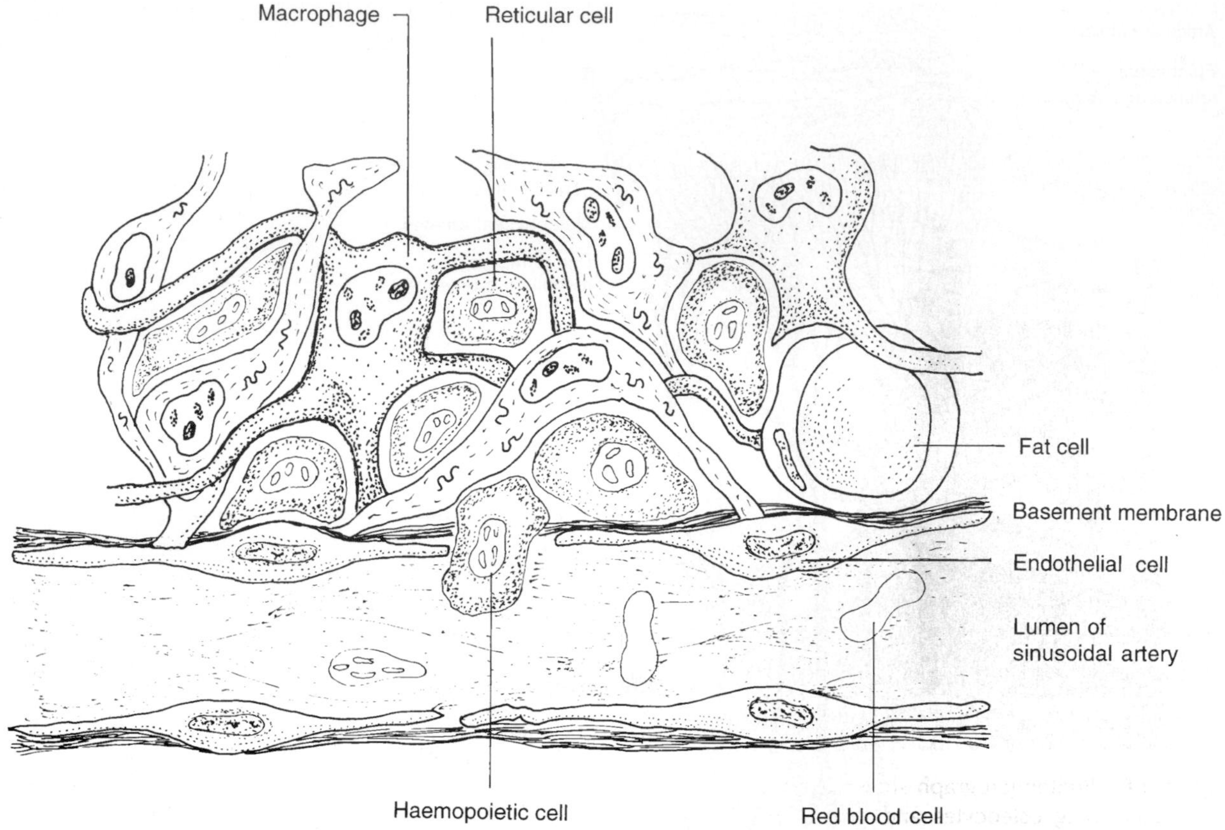

Figure 2.7 Diagrammatic representation of reticular and endothelial cells forming a stromal network. Macrophages are large bulky cells with long processes intertwining with the reticular and endothelial cells. Other haemopoietic cells are loosely held in the stroma.

an isolated dog tibia in which the nutrient artery was perfused, they showed that blood flow was decreased by electrical stimulation of nerve fibres to the bone. This observation has been repeated on a number of occasions. Stimulation of the sympathetic nerve trunk in a rabbit has also been shown to reduce bone blood flow (Shim and Patterson, 1967), while sympathectomy causes an increase (Trottman and Kelly, 1963).

Hormonal control

Since the original observation by Drinker and Drinker (1916), numerous authors have confirmed that administration of adrenaline reduces blood flow. Brinker *et al.* (1990) have suggested that the osseous circulation contains α_1-adrenoreceptors, muscarinic receptors and prostaglandin receptors. Using a dog tibia model in which the rate of perfusion was kept constant, they demonstrated that the predominant effect of pharmacological agents was vasoconstrictive.

Metabolic control

Shim and Patterson (1967) demonstrated that following a period of ischaemia, restoration of the circulation leads to a two- to threefold increase in blood flow over the control rate. This reactive bone hyperaemia was not abolished either by electrical stimulation or administration of vasopressor substances, suggesting that the metabolic control of bone blood flow is more important than the neural or hormonal control.

Cells of bone

THE OSTEOBLAST

Osteoblasts are cuboidal mononuclear cells 15–30 μm in length, which form a contiguous monolayer over the surface of bone. They are derived from marrow stromal cells by differentiation of pre-osteoblasts

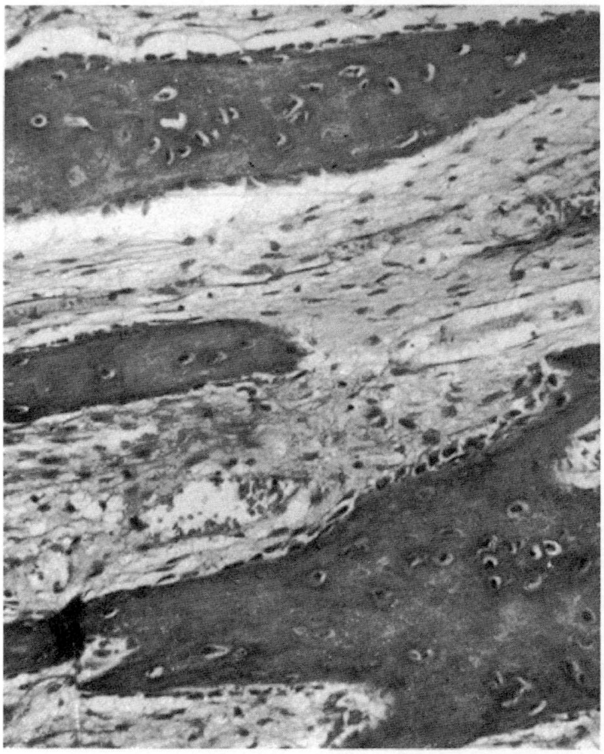

Figure 2.8 Photomicrograph showing the trabeculae of bone containing osteocytes and lined either by active osteoblasts or flattened cells (× 170).

and do not themselves undergo mitosis. The single nucleus is eccentrically placed and the abundant rough endoplasmic reticulum is characteristic of a cell engaged in protein synthesis (Figures 2.8, 2.9). There is also a high level of alkaline phosphatase. Vesicles containing amorphous calcium phosphate may also be present. The cells are connected together and to the processes of subjacent osteocytes by gap junctions. Inactive bone surfaces are lined by a monolayer of flattened cells which histological studies suggest are resting osteoblasts.

The osteoblast is responsible for the synthesis of the major proteins of bone including type I collagen and the non-collagenous proteins of bone such as osteocalcin (bone Gla protein) and osteonectin. The cell is also involved in the mineralization of bone and produces the enzyme alkaline phosphatase, which may be important for this.

Recent evidence suggests that the osteoblast plays a central role in controlling osteoclastic function. Thus osteoblasts and not osteoclasts have specific surface receptors for agents which stimulate bone resorption, such as 1,25-dihydroxyvitamin D_3 and parathyroid hormone. Furthermore, osteoclasts in culture, which are therefore not in contact with osteoblasts, do not respond to these agents.

The mechanism by which the osteoblast signals the osteoclast to resorb bone is unclear. There is evidence that the osteoblast secretes soluble substan-

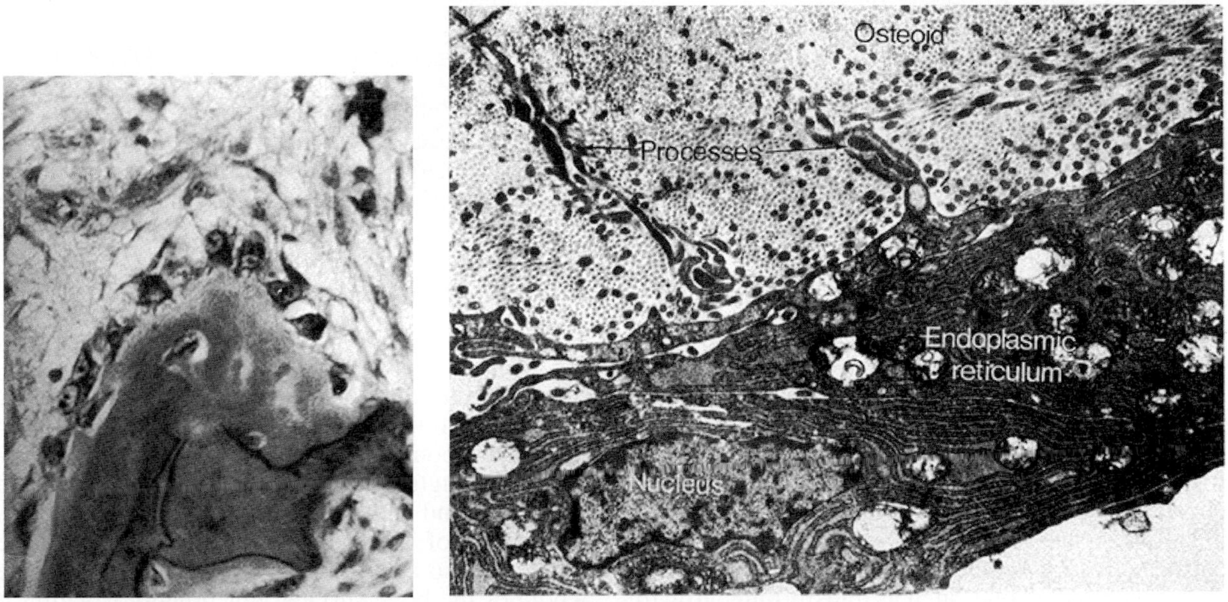

(a) (b)

Figure 2.9 (a) High power micrograph showing detail of active osteoblasts with large nucleus and centrosomes with reduced cytoplasmic content (× 365). (b) Electron micrograph of a wall of an osteoblast, showing the processes extending outwards into the osteoid tissue. Adjacent to the nucleus are masses of external reticulum (× 8750).

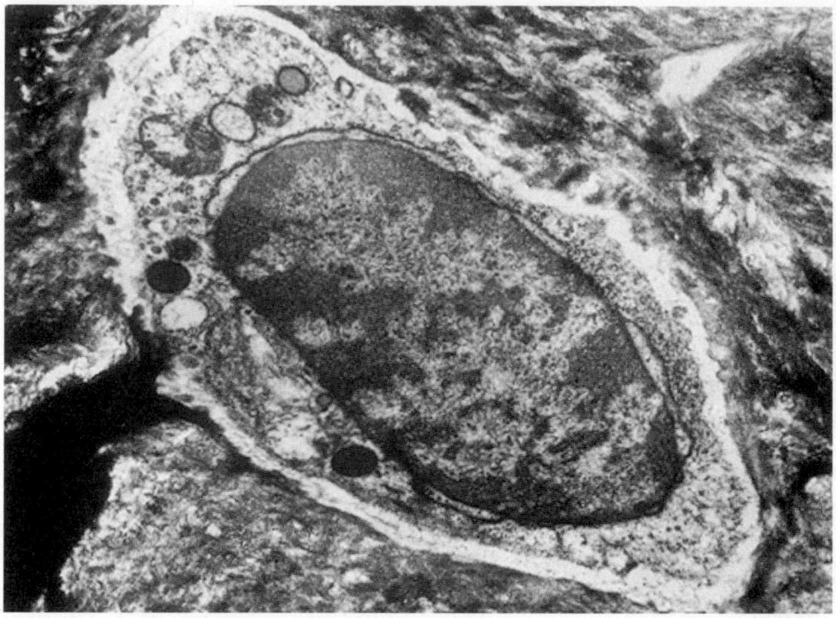

(a)

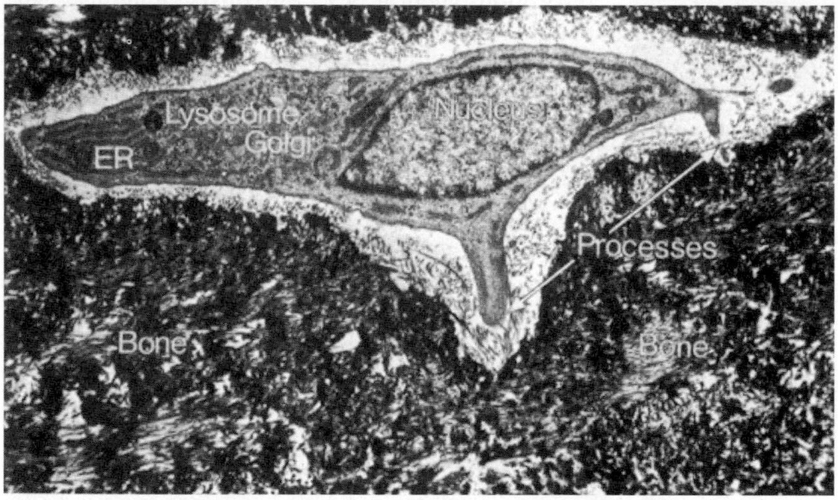

(b)

Figure 2.10 (a) An electron micrograph from adult rabbit bone, showing an osteocyte surrounded by mineralized collagen which is separated by a zone of unmineralized intralacunar matrix (× 24 300). (b) Electron micrograph of an osteocyte lying within bone. To the left of the nucleus, Golgi apparatus separates it from lysosome particles and reticulum (× 9720).

ces which include polypeptides and prostaglandins which activate or inhibit osteoclastic activity. The osteoblasts may also cause a conformational change in the lining cells which cover the whole bone surface which makes the bone physically available to the osteoclast for resorption. Collagenase secreted from the osteoblast may also play a role either by physically preparing the bone surface for attachment of the osteoclast or by allowing release of an osteoclastic activating or chemotactic factor which is secreted within the bone, such as transforming growth factor *β*. Since the coupling of osteoblastic and osteoclastic activity is of fundamental importance to the survival of the organism, it would not be surprising if it was mediated by more than one mechanism.

THE LINING CELL AND THE OSTEOCYTE

Some active osteoblasts are incarcerated in the matrix which they secrete and become buried deep within the bone. These osteocytes have long processes through which they maintain contact with each other and with the superficial bone-lining cells. This layer of flattened, inactive cells, which are probably also derived from osteoblasts, covers the whole of the bone surface, functionally isolating it from the exterior. It is thought that this cell system may mediate a rapid calcium flux between bone and extracellular fluid, although the precise role of this in bone mineral homeostasis is unclear (Figure 2.10).

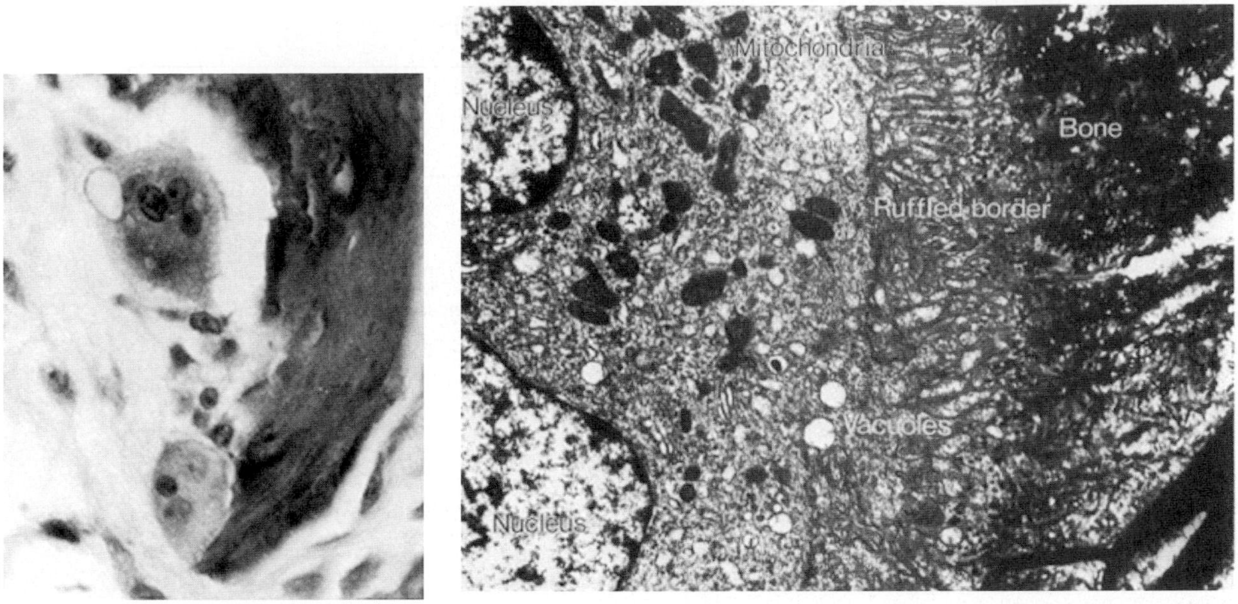

(a) (b)

Figure 2.11 (a) Photomicrograph showing a multinucleated osteoclast lying within a Howship's lacuna, in which bone resorption is occurring (× 365). (b) Electron micrograph of an osteoclast, on the left, with two nuclei, and a large number of mitochondria, with the ruffled border separating the cell from bone on the right (× 8640).

THE OSTEOCLAST

The osteoclast is a very large multinucleate giant cell attached to the bone surface (Figure 2.11). It has 15–20 nuclei and may measure several hundreds of micrometres across. It is the cell responsible for the resorption of living bone and it is formed by fusion of mononuclear cells. Osteoclasts are derived from haemopoietic precursor cells, probably a circulating monocyte of the macrophage type. Evidence for this lineage has come from a variety of sources including studies on osteopetrosis, which is characterized by defective osteoclastic bone resorption.

Morphologically the nuclei are frequently indented with prominent nucleoli. Mitochondria are numerous, there is little rough endoplasmic reticulum and many lysosomes. An important feature is the area of infolded plasma membrane, termed the ruffled border, which is surrounded by an organelle-free clear zone through which the osteoclast attaches to bone and which is the site of bone resorption. Osteoclasts contain the characteristic enzymes tartrate-resistant acid phosphatase (TRAP) and carbonic anhydrase.

The biochemical mechanisms involved in osteoclastic bone resorption have not been fully elucidated but it occurs in the enclosed space beneath the ruffled border enclosed by the clear zone. In order to create this enclosed space, the osteoclast attaches to bone firmly through special attachment proteins called 'integrins'. Carbonic anhydrase catalyses the hydration of dissolved carbon dioxide and the carbonic acid so formed dissociates into bicarbonate and hydrogen ions, which are pumped through the ruffled border, so lowering the pH of the extracellular region within the clear zone. The bone mineral is probably dissolved in the acid environment. Osteoclasts do not produce collagenase (which is, in fact, synthesized by osteoblasts). They probably break down bone matrix by release of lysosomal proteases.

OTHER CELLS

Other cells are described, including reticular cells which are found within the mesh-like stroma of the bone marrow, and possess both osteogenic and haemopoietic potencies; endosteal cells which may be connected tissue cells or resting osteoblasts and fibroblasts with a basophilic cytoplasm and round nucleus.

Chemistry of bone

Bone is made up of organic and inorganic materials and water.

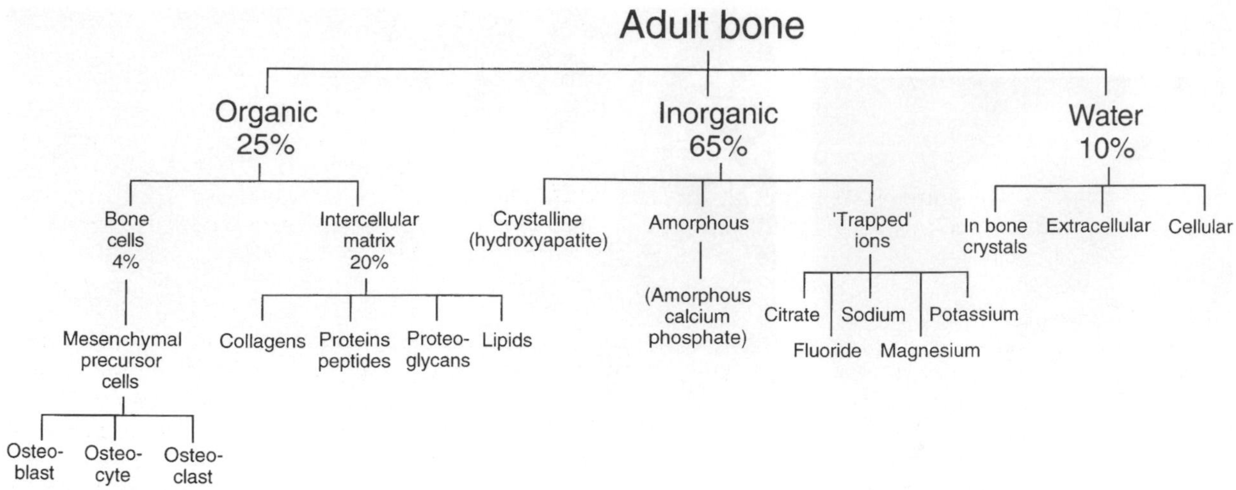

Figure 2.12 The composition of bone. Showing the relative proportions of organic (25%) to inorganic (65%), to water (10%), making up adult bone.

THE ORGANIC PHASE

The organic phase is made up of osteogenic cells as described above, the intercellular matrix of bone which consists of approximately 93% collagen and 7% non-callagenous proteins (Figure 2.12).

Collagen

Collagen is in the form of a crystalline fibroprotein fibril with characteristic x-ray diffraction and electron microscopic pattern, having a periodicity of about 6400 nm, although its length, diameter and density vary with age. In very old bone its diameter may be over 1000 nm (Figure 2.13).

Collagen is the major extracellular protein of the body and comprises some 30% total body protein. Knowledge of its biosynthesis and metabolism generally has increased rapidly since Ramachandran's thesis (1977). Important advances have been made in the elucidation of the structure of the precursors, or procollagens, of tissue collagen, in the discovery of new types of collagen and in the mechanisms of collagen degradation. However, though much is known of the intermediary metabolism of collagen,

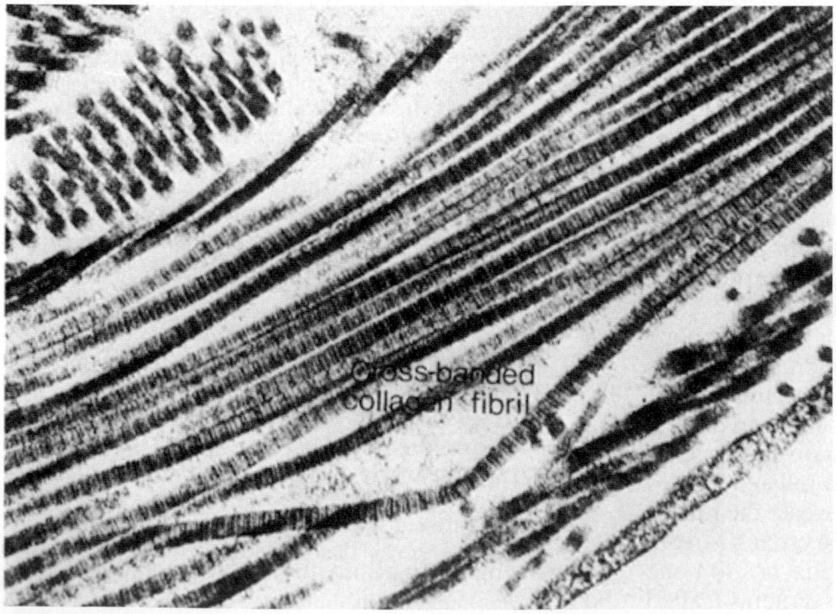

Figure 2.13 Electron micrograph of collagen fibrils, showing the cross-banding (× 4700).

little is known of what controls the deposition and orientation of collagen fibres in the tissues or the quantity of collagen that is formed.

Collagen structures

A collagen molecule is composed of three, distinct, polypeptide chains wound round each other to form a triple helix. The collagen helix will form spontaneously from individual polypeptide chains, or alpha (α) chains, when they are incubated under the appropriate conditions of salt concentration, pH and temperature. This triple helical structure results in a long rigid molecule some 300 nm long and 1 nm wide. The triple helix of human collagen can be dissociated at temperatures above 40°C.

The amino acid composition of the α chains is unusual. One-third of the total number of amino acid residues is glycine, and one-fifth proline and its derivative, hydroxyproline. Hydroxyproline is almost solely confined to collagen. In addition, collagen contains hydroxylysine and several oxidized derivatives of lysine (and hydroxylysine); these derivatives are involved in the chemical links which join together the individual collagen molecules within a collagen fibre. Amino acid sequence analysis has shown that the α chains have the general composition (glycine X–Y) with Y often hydroxyproline. It is this repeating sequence which allows the three α chains to form the triple helix of the collagen molecule.

The collagen molecule is first synthesized as a precursor, procollagen, which consists of three pro-α chains (Figure 2.13). Each pro-α chain contains several distinct regions. The N-terminal region has the structure of a typical globular protein which is maintained by internal —S—S— links. Next there is a short region with composition $(Gly–X–Y)_n$ which can interact with two other pro-α chains to form the typical collagen triple helix. This is followed by a short non-collagenous sequence and then the main length of repeating $(Gly–X–Y)_n$ triplets. The carboxyl terminal region which joins this collagenous sequence is joined by external —S— S— links to the two other pro-α chains which form a procollagen molecule. During biosynthesis the long terminal regions are cleaved by specific proteases to form a collagen molecule consisting of the central $(Gly–X–Y)_n$ region and flanked by two non-collagenous sequences, or telopeptides, of some 10–30 amino acid residues.

The assembly of the molecules appears to be determined chiefly by distribution of charged amino acids along the sequence of the three α chains, but can be influenced by various substances, as for example, the proteoglycans with which collagen is associated *in vivo*. The collagen fibrils show an asymmetric cross-striation pattern with a periodicity of 68 nm with each molecule being 4.4 times this repeat period. The fibres themselves may be formed from bundles of microfibrils, each of which consists of five collagen molecules lying side by side but displaced by the repeat pattern and rolled together to form a long fibril, which in cross-section contains different parts of five collagen molecules (or four molecules and a gap) at any specific level. The physiological control of microfibril formation or of the lateral aggregation of these microfibrils remains unknown.

In vivo and *in vitro* chemical cross-links form between the individual collagen molecules that together make a collagen fibre. These links originate predominantly from the short telopeptide, non-helical regions of the molecule. It is the formation of these cross-links that renders a collagen fibre resistant to tensile forces. In practice, then, a solution of collagen will contain not only individual collagen molecules but also polymers of cross-linked molecules. As a result, if the solution is heated to denature the collagen triple helix, not only individual α chains are released but also units of twice and thrice with the size of α chains consisting of two, three α chains joined together by cross-links. These polypeptides are known as β, γ units and can be distinguished from α chains on gel chromatography or electrophoresis.

Collagen biosynthesis

A summary of the many steps in collagen biosynthesis is given in Tables 2.1 and 2.2, and Figure 2.14.

Table 2.1 Sequence of intracellular collagen biosynthesis

1. Assembly pro-α chains (directed by specific mRNAs)
2. Proline hydroxylation } (Fe^{2+}, O_2, α-ketoglutarate,
3. Lysine hydroxylation } vitamin C enzymes)
4. Hydroxylysine glycosylation
5. Disulphide bond formation
6. Triple helix formation
7. Secretion

The exact order of steps 2–6 is uncertain.

Table 2.2 Sequence of extracellular collagen biosynthesis

1. Amino terminal extension cleavage
2. Carboxyl terminal extension cleavage
3. Microfibril formation
4. Lysine hydroxylysine terminal NH_2 oxidation (Cu-containing lysyl oxidase)
5. Fibril formation
6. Reducible cross-link formation
7. Maturation of cross-links. growth and reorganization of fibres

The exact order of these steps is uncertain, and steps 3, 4 and 6 could be intracellular.

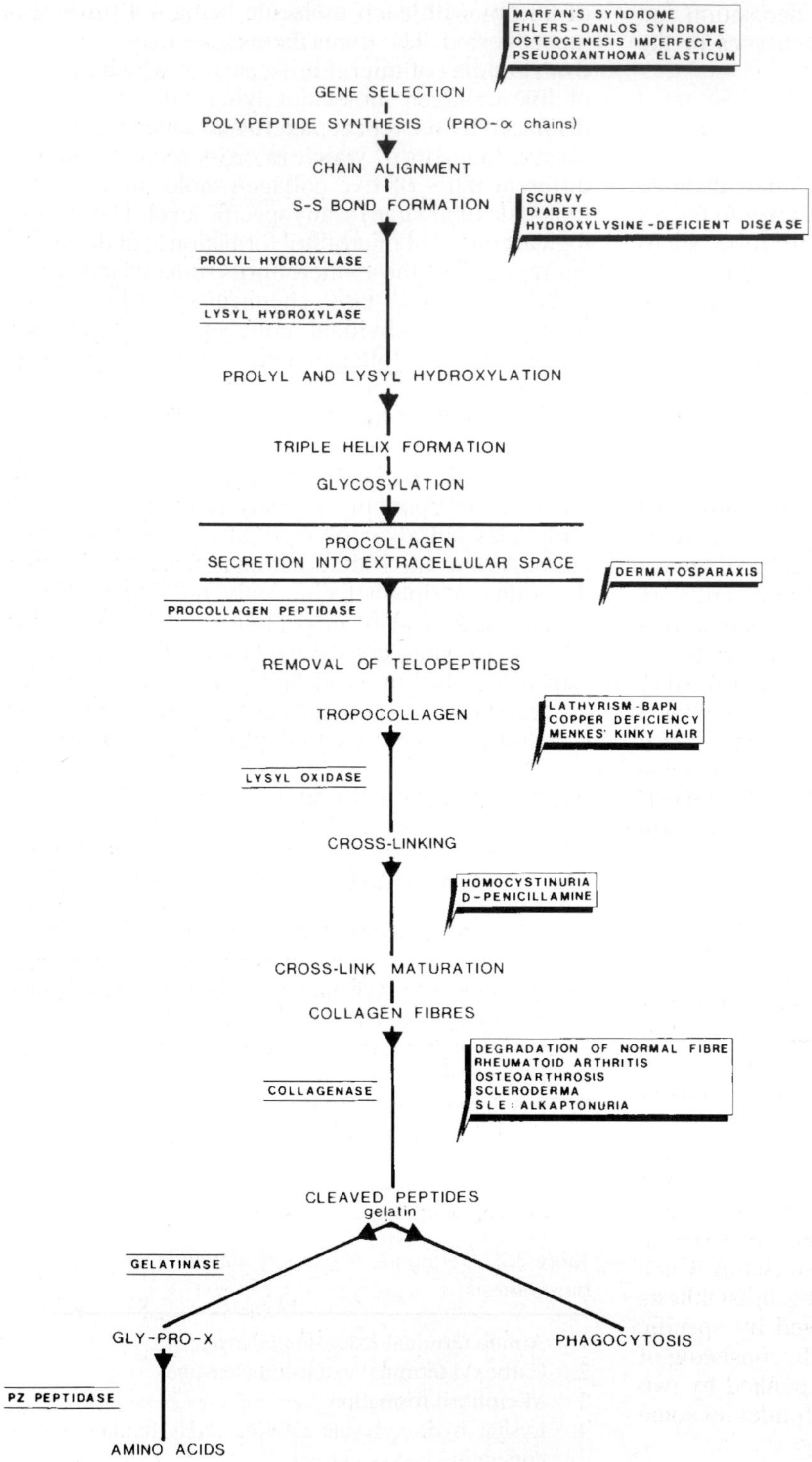

Figure 2.14 The many steps of collagen biosynthesis, and the various clinical abnormalities on the right. BAPN, β-aminopropionitrile; PZ, pancreozymin. (By courtesy of Dr M. Francis)

Specific enzymes are required for the hydroxylation of certain of the prolines and lysines present in the forming collagen peptide α chain. These ferrous iron-containing enzymes require molecular oxygen and α-ketoglutarate as additional substrates, and *in vitro* (and probably *in vivo* as well) vitamin C as a cofactor. Hydroxyproline is thus not incorporated directly into the forming collagen amino acid sequence, and free hydroxyproline will not usually be incorporated into collagen; hydroxyproline is thus a specific marker for collagen. Measurement of hydroxyproline levels provides a marker for estimation of collagen or its breakdown products. It is the introduction of hydroxyproline which leads to an amino acid sequence that can form a triple helix at normal body temperature (37°C). There is fine control of collagen biosynthesis at the hydroxylation stage, as the hydroxylase cannot hydroxylate proline residues in triple helical conformation while some hydroxyproline is required for the triple helix to form.

Galactose and glucose are then added to some of the hydroxylysine residues, so collagen is a glycoprotein. The formation of —S—S— links between the three carboxyl regions of the pro-α chains of a collagen molecule probably occurs before the triple helix is formed and may indeed be essential for this process to occur rapidly and efficiently *in vivo*. The collagen molecule is then secreted, probably via the Golgi apparatus of the forming cell.

Extracellularly, several specific proteases cleave the procollagen molecules to collagen which, in contrast to procollagen, is virtually insoluble in physiological fluids. The levels of these proteases must therefore be important in the spatial control of collagen fibril and fibre formation. The collagen molecules are then chemically cross-linked.

The chemistry of cross-linking is not yet fully understood. It is based, however, on the reaction of the lysine and hydroxylysine residues of two collagen molecules lying side by side in a fibril. The terminal additional, amino group of one lysine residue is oxidized by a specific copper-containing amino acid oxidase to yield a reactive aldehyde grouping at the end of the lysine carbon chain. This active group can then react with the amino group of neighbouring unoxidized lysines, to form a chemical cross-link between two collagen molecules. This link is transformed during the maturation of collagen fibres to unknown, or perhaps new peptide, bonds. Recent evidence suggests that some cross-linking may even occur intracellularly and that collagen is secreted as packets of 10 or so procollagen molecules. In any event, the order of the various extracellular steps of collagen biosynthesis remains uncertain.

Various chemicals can prevent collagen cross-linking and thus lead to a weak connective tissue. These include the lathyrogens (β-amino propionitrile), penicillamine and homocysteine accounting for the connecting tissue defects seen in some penicillamine-treated patients or those with homocystinuria.

Distribution of collagens and musculoskeletal disorders

Miller (1984) reviewed the chemistry of the collagens, emphasizing that there are over 11 types of collagen characterized by having 19 unique chains. He divided them into three general classes:

1. A molecule containing a length greater than 30 nm in uninterrupted helical chain.
2. 301 nm molecules in which the helical chain is interrupted.
3. Relatively short molecules in which the helical region may be continuous and uninterrupted.

In group 1, which includes types 1, 2, 3 and 5, type 2 was most commonly found in the musculoskeletal system, in arteries, in cornea, in neuroretinal tissues, in uterus and in placental membranes. As well as different structural appearances, they have varying amounts of hydroxylysine, glycosylated hydroxylysine, hydroxyproline, etc. Type 1 collagen fibrils serve as a substrate for the deposition of the mineral component. Any alteration in this will produce weakening of the skeleton. This is particularly seen in osteogenesis imperfecta, which can be divided into four clinical groups as regards the expressivity and inheritance. In group 1 there is a 50% reduction in type 1 procollagen, whereas in group 2, there is a reduction to 25%, which may well result in death. In Ehlers–Danlos syndrome, there appears to be disorganization of the cross-linkages due to reduction of the enzyme lysyl hydroxylase. Marfan's syndrome and homocystinuria have protein collagen defects which may also be seen in scurvy, lathyrism, etc.

Eyre (1990) more recently has described extensively that there are 13 types of collagen molecules, based on the products of more than 20 distinct genes consisting of a structural protein in the extracellular matrix with a triple helix structure. The most common, class 1, consists of those molecules that can form the typical banded fibrils seen in virtually all connective tissues with five molecular types (types I, II, III, V and XI) and all having triple helix

Table 2.3 Types of collagen

Type	Tissue
Class 1 (300 nm triple helix)	
Type I	Skin, bone, ligament
Type II	Cartilage, disc, eye
Type III	Skin, blood vessels, ligament
Type V	With type I
Type XI (1α, 2α, 3α)	With type II
Class 2 (basement membranes)	
Type IV	Basal lamina
Type VII	Epithelial basement membrane
Type VIII	Endothelial basement membrane
Class 3 (short-chain <300 nm molecules)	
Type VI	Widespread
Type IX	Cartilage (with type II)
Type X	Hypertrophic cartilage
Type XII	Tendon, other?
Type XIII	Endothelial cells

structure composed of about 1014 amino acid residues in each of the three polypeptide chains. Types I, II and III make up the bulk of the collagen in the body. Type II is restricted to hyaline cartilage, the intervertebral disc, and the vitreous humour of the eye. Types V and XI are fibrillar collagens. Type V is also distributed in small amounts (about 3% of type I) wherever type I collagen appears, and type XI is similarly distributed with type II collagen. Hybrid molecules containing chains of both types V and XI collagens may also occur in bone and cartilage. The remaining collagens can be in the second and third classes, as shown in Table 2.3 Type IV collagen is the major structural component of basement membranes. Some types are localized, e.g. type X collagen appears exclusively in the calcified cartilage zones of the epiphyseal plate, articular cartilage and bone fracture callus. Other types are more widely distributed; for example, type VI collagen appears in small amounts as filamentous material around cells and between the banded collagen fibrils of most soft connective tissues. Type VI collagen is enriched in certain tissues, including the intervertebral disc and the cornea. It appears to act as a structural element between the cells and the matrix of soft connective tissues which can deform. Increased amounts of type VI collagen have been noted in inflamed skin, in skin with certain forms of Ehlers–Danlos syndrome, and in the articular cartilage of patients with osteoarthrosis.

The mechanical strength of the common collagens arises from the formation of two or three covalent intermolecular bonds (cross-links) per collagen molecule. Even though type I collagen predominates in all the musculoskeletal soft tissues (synovium, muscle, tendon, ligament except cartilage), its intermolecular cross-linking varies among tissues. Skin, cornea and rat-tail tendon have collagens that are largely cross-linked by lysine-derived aldehydes. Cross-links based on other pathways can be seen in some connective tissues, such as tendon and muscle. Similarly, ligaments that bear high loads, such as the anterior cruciate ligament of the knee, contain the highest levels of such cross-links in type I collagen (Eyre). Other tissues that dissipate or transmit high mechanical forces, such as fibrocartilages (knee meniscus, intervertebral disc) are also rich in mature hydroxypyridium, a cross-linking amino acid.

Synovial membrane is rich in type II collagen. Nearly equal amounts of types I and II collagens have been found in normal and rheumatoid human synovial-lining tissue.

Although turnover rates of collagen in adult connective tissues are poorly documented, it is said that bone turns over rapidly, articular cartilage collagen more slowly.

Neutral metalloproteinases are now known to be responsible for the degradation of extracellular collagens, proteoglycans, and associated matrix proteins during normal tissue growth and remodelling and during inflammatory responses to injury. These enzymes include tissue collagenase, stromelysin (identical to transin expressed by transformed fibroblasts), and gelatinase.

A variety of cytokines and growth factors are known (see 'Fracture healing') to affect the expression of these enzymes by fibroblasts, macrophages, polymorphonuclear leucocytes, and tumour cells. The major collagenolytic cathepsin, cathepsin L, is another secreted protease that may be responsible for connective tissue degradation and remodelling in inflammation sites.

Collagen in ligaments

Ligaments are composed of a complex macromolecular network with water making up about two-thirds of the weight and the fibrillar protein collagen making up the majority of the remaining dry weight.

A normal ligament consists of about 90% fibrillar type I collagen with less than 10% being type III collagen. Other collagen types are present in smaller quantities.

The collagen is synthesized in connective tissues by fibroblasts, during both intracellular and extracellular stages. Specific hydroxylases, which require iron, ascorbate, and α-ketoglutarate for activity, alter the amino acids proline and lysine to their hydroxylated forms (see Figure 2.14). After hydroxylation, some residues are further glycosylated in the rough endoplasmic reticulum. Glycosylation of these residues is thought to be important in the subsequent regulation of collagen synthesis, the proteoglycan–collagen interaction with fibre size.

Another important process in the formation of ligament microfibrils is the formation of collagen cross-links. During the formation of ligament microfibrils, the enzyme lysyl oxidase acts on peptide-bound lysines and hydroxylysines to form aldehydes. The formation of aldehydes is an important preliminary step in the formation of covalent intramolecular (aldol) and intermolecular (Schiff base) cross-links. It is these Schiff-base cross-links that are thought to have the greatest functional significance.

Collagen in growth plate structure

Trippel (1990) in reviewing growth plate structure of collagen described five types (II, VI, IX, X and XI) which have been identified in epiphyseal cartilage, the most prevalent collagen being type II. This fibrillar collagen takes the form of a classic triple helix composed of three identical α-1(II) chains derived from a procollagen precursor also present for mineralizing cartilage. Type X collagen is a short-chain triple helix composed of three apparently identical α chains.

Although type X collagen is thought to be required in cartilage calcification, its relation to other matrix constituents remains unclear.

For more information, see 'Structure of the joints and the tissues', p. 102.

Collagen in articular cartilage

Mitrovic (1993) has recently described the collagen of articular cartilage. Articular cartilage contains at least five genetically distinct types of collagen, types II, VI, XI, X and XI, which cross-link in a polymeric network to form a fibrillar framework of tissue. Type II collagen is a major component of this framework and represents more than 95% of all cartilage collagens. Type X collagen is a minor fibril-forming collagen. It is only present in the hypertrophic zone of growth plate and basal calcified zone of articular cartilage. Type IX collagen is a minor fibril-nor-forming collagen, covalently linked to the surface of type II collagen fibrils.

In 1992, Hwang *et al.* studied the collagen architecture in normal and degenerate human articular cartilage using a new silver staining technique. They identified, in the superficial zone, three types of early degenerative lesions involving the collagen network, the cause of which was unknown. Type VI collagen was found in the pericellular capsule and matrix around the chondrocytes. Electron microscopy also showed type VI collagen anchored to the chondrocyte membrane at the articular pole, suggesting a dual role of this collagen in the maintenance of chondrocyte integrity and as part of a cell-matrix signalling system.

In normal articular cartilage, matrix molecules are constantly synthesized and degraded by chondrocytes. The rates of synthesis and degradation for different types of molecules varies with ageing and exercise.

The skeleton, the vertebral column and the pelvis are formed by endochondral ossification. Endochondral bone development begins as a condensation of mesenchymal cells derived from mesoderm, which form extracellular matrix. The mesenchymal cells surrounding the cartilage become the periosteum. These cartilage cells go through a maturation process that can be visualized in the area of the developing long bone called the growth plate. Growth plates consist of zones of rapidly proliferating chondrocytes secreting collagens II, IX and XI, maturing and hypertrophic chondrocytes secreting predominantly collagen X. Collagen I is the major extracellular matrix (ECM) molecule of bone. Recent immunolocalization in developing mouse embryos demonstrated that collagen XII is present in intramembranous bone, but this action in bone structure and development is yet unknown.

Other molecules also may be important in bone development. Tenascin, a glycoprotein, is seen in both osteogenic and chondrogenic areas of developing endochondral bone. These data imply that tenascin variants are important is osteogenesis. However, the recent demonstration that mice with a disrupted tenascin gene developed normally in all respects suggests that the role of tenascin in bone development is not yet understood.

Aggrecan core protein, previously considered to be specific to cartilage ECM, in which it interacts with hyaluronate and link protein, is also expressed in chicken calvaria and osteoblasts. Cartilage-specific proteoglycan, aggrecan, has been demonstrated to be present in membranous bone, having dramatic implications for the role of proteoglycans in bone and cartilage formation.

Non-collagenous proteins of bone

Non-collagenous proteins of bone are a heterogeneous group which vary from entrapped serum protein to glycoproteins, which are unique to bone and which probably play a role in mineralization.

Osteocalcin

Osteocalcin or bone Gla protein (BGP) is the best characterized of the non-collagenous proteins of bone and it makes up between 10 and 20% of them. Its amino acid sequence is very well preserved across the vertebrate phylogenetic tree, suggesting that it plays an important role but this is as yet unelucidated. It is synthesized by the osteoblast as a 99 amino acid propeptide which is then cleaved to leave a 50 amino acid protein which is secreted. This has a molecular weight of approximately 6000 Da. Following cleavage and before secretion, three glutamic acid residues are carboxylated by a vitamin K dependent process. Mature carboxylated osteocalcin binds ionic calcium and hydroxyapatite.

Osteocalcin is produced only by osteoblasts and a proportion of the newly synthesized protein escapes into the serum. Raised serum levels of osteocalcin have been reported in diseases which are associated with increased bone turnover such as Paget's disease, renal osteodystrophy and primary hyperparathyroidism. This has led to interest in the measurement of osteocalcin as a biochemical marker of bone formation (Price *et al.*, 1980). However, due partly to difficulty with osteocalcin assays, the exact significance of serum measurements has yet to be elucidated.

Matrix Gla protein

As much as 50% of the total glutamic acid containing proteins of bone are distinct from osteocalcin. The best characterized of these is matrix Gla protein

(MGP), a 10 000 Da protein found in association with bone morphogenetic protein (BMP).

Osteonectin

A number of phosphoproteins and glycoproteins are found in bone. The phosphate is bound to the protein backbone through serine or threonine amino acid residues. The best characterized of these bone proteins is osteonectin. It binds collagen and hydroxyapatite through separate areas of its molecule, is found in relatively large amounts in immature bone and promotes mineralization of collagen (Termine *et al.*, 1981). Thus it is possible that osteonectin plays a crucial role in mineralization.

Proteoglycans

Bone proteoglycan has a small protein core with up to two chondroitin sulphate chains attached. They constitute approximately 10% of the non-collagenous proteins of bone. Their role is unclear.

The sulphated glycosaminoglycans in connective tissue are chondroitin sulphate, keratan sulphate and dermatan sulphate. They are bound at one end to a protein core (Figure 2.15); e.g. 50–100 chondroitin sulphate chains are attached laterally by the saccharide sequence of neutral sugars to the core protein, giving a molecular weight of about $1–3 \times 10^6$. Proteoglycans are particularly vulnerable to proteolytic enzymes, with the whole molecule breaking up when a few peptide bonds are split off (reviewed by Muir, 1978).

Some keratan sulphate chains are also attached to the same protein core. It should be noted that in cartilage the proteoglycan population is heterogeneous, varying in chemical composition and size of their molecules.

Chondroitin sulphate consists of disaccharide units of glucuronic acid and *N*-acetylgalactosamines with sulphate residues. Keratan sulphate has in its structure galactose instead of glucuronic acid, with varying amounts of sulphate.

The elasticity and resilience of cartilage results from this matrix of proteoglycans, collagen and water (Kempson *et al.*, 1973). They have demonstrated how the compressive stiffness of cartilage over short intervals directly correlates to the presence of proteoglycans when measured as glycosaminoglycans.

Because of this, as a load is applied to cartilage there is an increase in the fluid pressure and water is driven out, but the cartilage deforms only slowly. Maroudas (1975) described the internal osmotic pressure of human femoral cartilage as being about 3.4–3.6 atmospheres (343.4–363.6 kPa).

The proteoglycans have a very significant role in controlling swelling, pressure and the movement of water molecules when cartilage is placed under load.

In cartilage, most proteoglycans are in the form of large (200 000 kDa or more) aggregates that provide the tissue with its resilience under compressive loads. The basic structure of the cartilage proteoglycan aggregate has been well established by biochemical methods and molecular biological techniques. It is constructed from glycosaminoglycan chains attached to core protein molecules which are themselves attached to hyaluronic acid under the stabilizing influence of link protein. Although most recent studies of cartilage proteoglycan have dealt with articular cartilage, such data are not uniformly transposable to the growth plate.

The interaction of link protein with proteoglycan monomer and hyaluronic acid from bovine fetal epiphyseal cartilage was recently characterized by Tang *et al.* (1989). These authors demonstrated that the proteoglycan monomers from this cartilage are

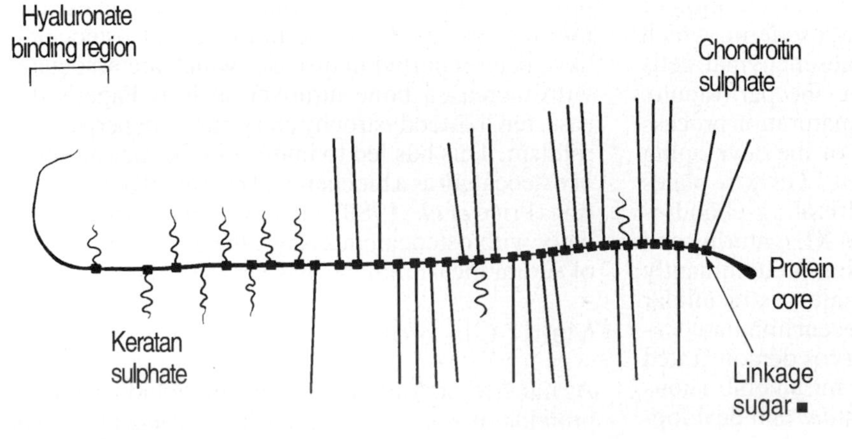

Figure 2.15 The binding of the sulphated glycosaminoglycans to protein core. (By courtesy of Dr M. Francis)

almost entirely aggregating monomers. As expected, link protein substantially increased the percentage of aggregating monomers.

Proteoglycan aggregate stability was found to be highly pH-dependent: decreasing the pH from 5 to 4 in the absence of link protein resulted in essentially complete aggregate dissociation. Link protein was protective against much of the pH-induced instability. These authors further showed that optimization of both pH and link protein increased not only the stability of the aggregate but also its size.

In addition to their contribution to matrix structure, proteoglycans in the growth plate may play a role in mineralization. Focal concentrations of proteoglycan at the sites of mineralization are well documented. Because the chondroitin sulphate chains of proteoglycans bind calcium and because phosphate can displace this calcium from the proteoglycans (Hunter, 1987), proteoglycan may serve as the medium within which calcium release by ion exchange could raise the $Ca \times PO_4$ product above the threshold for hydroxyapatite precipitation (Hunter, 1987).

For a full discussion see under 'Cartilage', p. 76.

Sialoprotein

These are glycoproteins containing the sugar *N*-acetylneuraminic acid (sialic acid). They make up approximately 7.5% of the total non-collagenous protein of bone and their function is unclear.

Serum proteins

These constitute the largest number of non-collagenous proteins in bone. They include serum albumin and some immunoglobulins. They constitute approximately a quarter of the total non-collagenous protein and their function is unknown.

THE INORGANIC PHASE

The inorganic or mineral phase of bone serves two basic functions. First, it determines the mechanical properties of bone. The strength of bone depends on the exact chemical composition, nature and three-dimensional disposition of the mineral phase, while its ability to resist cyclical loading and to

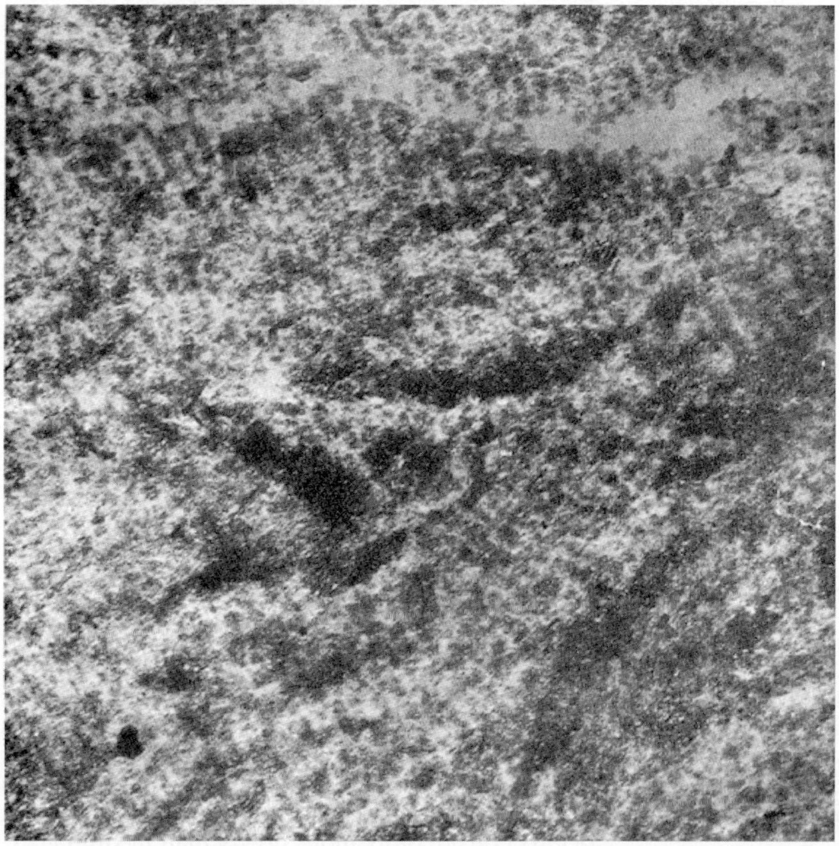

Figure 2.16 Electron micrograph of undecalcified, unstained, bone. The electron dense particles of mineral are located within the collagen fibrils.

regenerate is due to continuous turnover of skeletal elements.

Second, bone mineral functions as a reservoir of ions, particularly calcium and phosphate. In order to perform this function, ions must be able to be sequestered or removed from the bone mineral phase by physiological processes, which implies that the energy changes in these processes are within the narrow range available to biological processes.

Chemical nature

The mineral of bone is a poorly crystalline, imperfect hydroxyapatite ($Ca_{10}(PO_4)_6(OH_2)$), which contains a variety of substituted ions, including carbonate, HPO_4^{2-} sodium, magnesium, citrate and potassium, depending on the diet and other factors. However, the exact chemical composition and structure is not yet clear, since its poorly crystalline structure means the x-ray diffraction patterns which are generated are not sufficiently exact to allow precise resolution and included ions complicate the picture. Furthermore, the ideal stoichiometry, which is a Ca/P ratio of 1.67, is rarely seen, the ratio normally being somewhat lower. Electron micrography reveals bone crystals to be very small and elongated. They measure approximately 15–35 Å (1.5–3.5 nm) by 50–100 Å (5–10 nm) by 400–500 Å (40–50 nm) (Glimcher, 1959; Landis and Glimcher, 1978).

Bone mineral is initially deposited as a very poorly crystallized hydroxyapatite containing carbonate ions. The newly deposited crystals are highly hydrated and have many ion spaces within the crystal unfilled. For this reason they are relatively reactive, the ions being capable of being displaced easily. With ageing, the crystal becomes larger, less hydrated and more perfect, with water being displaced by mineral, and this produces a reduction in the rate and extent of diffusional exchange of ions and of crystallization. It must be appreciated that the age of a bone crystal is not the same as the biological age of the organism, since the age of the mineral also varies with the local rate of bone turnover.

Location of the mineral phase of bone

Electron microscopy, x-ray and neutron diffraction have demonstrated that the overwhelming majority of bone mineral lies within the collagen fibrils (Figure 2.16). The mineral crystals are distributed regularly within the collagen, being deposited first within the hole zone region (spaces between the triple helices) with their long axes aligned with the collagen fibril giving it a 70 nm cross-banding. As mineralization proceeds, this striation disappears (Glimcher, 1990).

Mechanism of calcification

Type 1 collagen is found widely throughout the body. The unique property of bone is its association with the mineral phase. When bone is newly formed, collagen is laid down before inorganic salts. The precise mechanism of bone mineralization is unclear and several hypotheses exist. The mechanism must account for a number of known facts. Mineralization begins, as outlined above, in a precise location related to the whole zone region of collagen. It begins independently at a number of different sites separated by unmineralized regions and starts at some distance (2–10 μm) from the osteoblast. It begins between 1 and 10 days after deposition of non-mineralized osteoid. The region in which mineralization occurs is supersaturated with calcium and phosphate ions so that mineralization does not represent a chemical reaction but a *phase change* from dissolved ions to solid hydroxyapatite. Since the concentrations of calcium and phosphate are sufficient to maintain this phase change once begun, it is the initiator of mineralization which is obscure.

Small plasma membrane vesicles have been described in the extracellular matrices of both bone and cartilage, which contain crystals of hydroxyapatite. Since calcification of these vesicles occurs before calcification of the collagen fibrils, it has been suggested that the presence of solid-phase calcium phosphate in the vesicles directly causes mineralization of the collagen fibrils. It is, however, unclear how a phase change occurring within the membrane vesicle which is a compartment separate from the area of collagen which mineralizes, can affect mineralization of the collagen itself. Thus it seems unlikely that matrix vesicles play a part in the mineralization of collagen which accompanies bone turnover. They may, however, have a role in the calcification of growth plate cartilage which precedes ossification.

Pyrophosphate is an inhibitor of crystallization of hydroxyapatite which is present in bone and other tissues and Russell *et al.* (1969) have suggested that this compound is an important controlling element in calcification. They suggest that the whole bone is coated with pyrophosphate and that calcification is initiated by pyrophosphatases which remove inhibiting pyrophosphate by splitting it into two molecules of phosphate (Figure 2.17). However, this theory does not account for the unique association of the initiation of mineralization with the hole zone of collagen and the finding that if metastable solutions of calcium and phosphate are exposed to pure reconstituted soft tissue collagen, although calcification occurs in a similar manner to that seen *in vivo*, it occurs considerably more slowly than in similar ex-

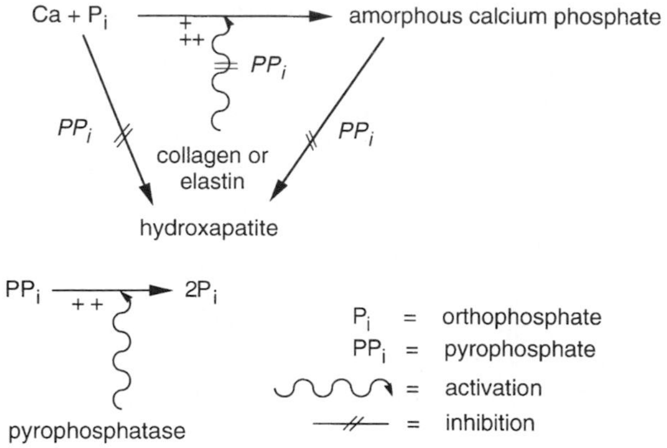

Figure 2.17 Possible role of pyrophosphate (PP_i) in calcification. (Reproduced from Russell *et al.*, 1969)

periments using decalcified bone collagen (Glimcher, 1990). This suggests that there is something unique about bone collagen which encourages mineralization.

There are a number of non-collagenous proteins in bone which are able to bind calcium. It is important to appreciate that although an affinity for hydroxyapatite is an inevitable property of the nucleator of mineralization *per se*, the ability to bind calcium may inhibit mineralization by removing the ion from solution.

Glimcher and his co-workers (Glimcher and Krane, 1968; Glimcher, 1990) have suggested that non-collagenous proteins containing phosphoserine and phosphothreonine residue act as the nucleator of mineralization. These proteins have been shown to be synthesized by osteoblasts and to be found specifically *in vivo* at sites where calcification is initiated. They suggest that these proteins are bound within the whole region of collagen and present a series of phosphate residues specifically orientated in space which then bind calcium (Figure 2.18).

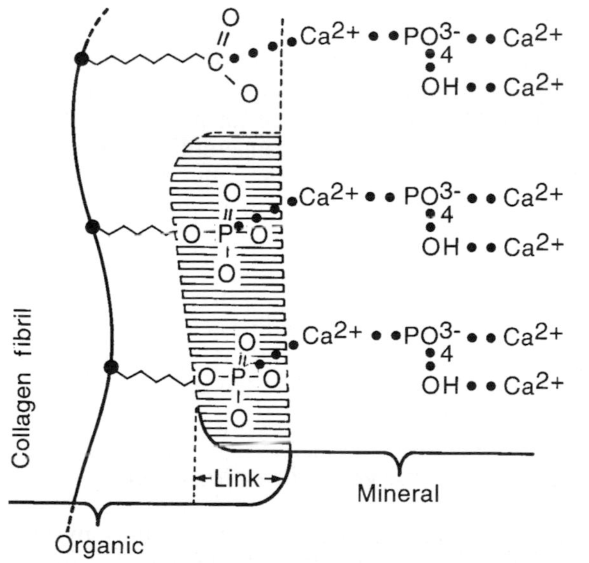

Figure 2.18 The mechanism by which phosphate groups bound to phosphoproteins may initiate mineralization. (From Glimcher, M. J. (1984) *Philosophical Transactions of the Royal Society of London [Biology]* **304**, 479)

WATER OF BONE

Water of bone is seen in the form of interstitial or extracellular fluid, as well as within the hydration shell of the apatite crystals. The total content in bone may decrease from 60% during ossification to 10% in senile cortical bone, becoming all bound water. Robinson (1960) defined more accurately the total content of bone water. There is always a constant supply of active exchangeable bone-mineral constituents throughout life. This is essential to maintain life by providing mineral and alkaline reserves for buffering in most body tissues. There is much water in the organic phase of mucopolysaccharide complexes and collagen, as well as in the inorganic component of bone or in the marrow and osteocytic spaces of bone. Robinson postulated that, as calcification of osteoid tissue takes place, water is the substance displaced from the matrix, with reduction in the space between the crystals and other solids.

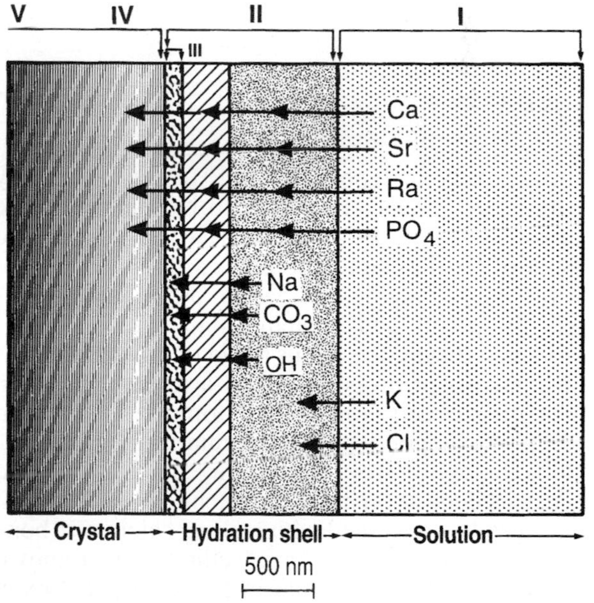

Figure 2.19 Illustrating the concepts of the crystal, its lattice layer, hydration shell and its solution of intracellular fluid. The penetration of various chemical ions is shown. (Reproduced with permission from W. F. Neuman and M. W. Neuman (1957) *Amer. J. Medicine* **22**, 123–131)

Water has also great importance in that most of the ions, such as calcium, sodium, phosphate, potassium, chloride, etc., require hydration for their movement or diffusion, and as the matrix calcifies, the rate of diffusion or exchange of calcium ions is slowed with slowing of crystallization. This calcification of matrix with reduction in diffusion is also seen in the zone of the mature chondroblasts in phase IV of the epiphyseal plate, where calcium is deposited with death of the chondroblasts and their disintegration into calcifying trabeculae.

Robinson suggested that osteoid tissue just before calcification holds relatively large amounts of water, and such water is in two forms:

1. When it is free to hydrate and transport inorganic ions, it is called the 'free water of potentially calcifiable osteoid space'.
2. 'Bound water' when it is made up of:
   (a) *Water of constitution* in which the water may be joined to the —H— bands in the collagen fibril or as part of the water of the apatite crystal.
   (b) *Bound water of the potentially calcifiable osteoid space.* This form, although 'free' at the beginning of calcification, becomes bound or 'caught up' by the reduction in the spaces between the various solids of crystals, ions, collagen fibrils, and mucopolysaccharides, etc., by the laying down of $CaPO_4$ complexes. This Robinson likens to the hydration shell of Neuman and Neuman (1957, 1958) around the crystal (Figure 2.19).

CITRATE

Citrate in bone represents 70% of the total body citrate in animals. It appears to be mainly on the surface of the apatite crystal, but may be bound primarily to the calcium ion. It is actively concerned with the metabolic, oxidative processes of carbohydrate, fat and protein in mammals, and is produced during the Krebs cycle to provide energy, but much of it probably forms a reserve. Its main purpose appears to be in forming soluble but complex compounds with calcium to facilitate calcium absorption from the intestine, its diffusion and hence its deposition into bone (Heintz *et al.*, 1947). It may also be concerned with making calcium in bone more soluble and, therefore, facilitating its removal without significant change in the local pH (Dixon and Perkins, 1956).

One citrate calcium compound is soluble but non-dissociable and is thought to be the bulk of the ultrafilterable non-dissociated serum calcium. The other salt, tricalcium dicitrate, will dissociate completely.

Not only does the citrate content of the serum parallel the calcium content (Freeman, 1960), but there is also a transport function performed by citrate in the cell membrane. This latter function has only been partially investigated, but may have some function in calcium absorption from the intestine, as vitamin D in therapeutic doses causes a rise in serum citrate levels, which is also seen in hyperparathyroidism, and in hypercalcaemic states. Normal serum citrate levels are decreased in conditions of hypoparathyroidism, rickets and osteomalacia. Harrison and Harrison (1952) showed that administration of citrates in the treatment of rickets has a beneficial effect, most probably by increasing the absorption of calcium as well as by producing a shift of calcium phosphates into osteoid tissue. Ordinarily excretion of citrate varies between 200 and 1000 mg/day, and reflects accurately the serum citrate levels.

In vitamin D deficiency rickets, the serum citrate is low even when the calcium remains normal (Harrison, 1956), and the administration of citrate as the sodium salt is followed by healing of the rachitic lesion of bone without affecting the Ca/P product. This implies that citrate makes calcium more available to the growing bone.

Calcium is not permeable to cell membranes except in minute amounts, and a citrate–magnesium–calcium association may regulate this permeability (Freeman, 1960).

BONE ENZYMES

The bone cells contain the normal complement of enzymes similar, for example, to those found in liver cells. Bone cells have an active metabolism and their rate of oxygen consumption can reach at least 50% of that of liver cells. However, as a tissue, bone differs from other tissues in relying largely on glycolysis for energy production. Some enzymes may also be excreted into the organic matrix and there modify the organic constituents; viz. in those reactions preceding calcification. Certain enzymes and enzyme systems appear to assume special importance in bone tissue, however; these include the following.

Glycolytic enzymes in osteoclasts

These enzymes transform glucose into pyruvate together with the formation of ATP, which is used by the cell in various synthetic reactions. The pyruvate can then be metabolized further to lactate or to citrate. Lactic acid formed from pyruvic acid under the influence of lactic acid dehydrogenase is the end product of glycolysis in bone and is produced about 50 times more abundantly than citrate.

Acid hydrolases

These enzymes are catabolic enzymes responsible for cellular digestion. A typical member is cathepsin D, a protease with a pH optimum of about 3.6. Such acid hydrolases are normally found within a distinct intracellular organelle within the lysosome. The extrusion or breakdown of the lysosomes present in cells leads therefore to the digestion of cells and their surrounding matrix. Weis (1967) presented evidence which suggests that there is a release of lysosomal acid hydrolases from osteoclasts when bone is resorbed.

Collagenases

Bone contains enzymes which will specifically degrade collagen, a property that few proteases exhibit.

Alkaline phosphatase

This is a phosphomonoesterase which is:

1. 'Non-specific' and catalyses orthophosphoric monoesters of phenol, alcohol, sugars.
2. With optimum activity about pH 9 (acid phosphatase with optimum about pH 5).
3. Detectable in blood plasma of humans with normal levels of:
   (a) King-Armstrong units 3–14 (21–100 IU/l).
   (b) Bodansky units, 1–5 (8–27 IU/l).
4. In bone, calcifying cartilage, intestinal mucosa, liver and kidney.
5. Role uncertain but serum alkaline phosphatase level is altered in certain disorders of skeletal and hepatobiliary systems (Table 2.4).

Gutman and Yu considered that the enzyme alkaline phosphatase acts in some way during glycogenolysis on the phosphopyruvate compounds to produce an increased concentration of phosphate ions. Siffert (1951) showed histochemically that it is also present in large amounts where organic matrix is being laid down. In general, it is considered to be concerned with preosseous cellular metabolism, with the subsequent elaboration of bone matrix before the crystallization of calcium and phosphate ions.

Serum alkaline phosphatase is increased in conditions in which there is marked osteoblastic activity; e.g. during infancy (two to three times the adult level) and during various growth spurts. Its serial measurement is of help in Paget's disease by a gradual rise indicating extension and a sharp rise in the development of a sarcoma. In carcinoma dissemination there may be an elevated alkaline phosphatase due to spread either to bone or to liver or both. Measurement of 5′-nucleotidase or γ-glutamyltransferase will help to differentiate the spread site.

Table 2.4 Alteration in serum alkaline phosphatase levels

Skeleton			Hepatobiliary
Increased in	rickets and osteomalacia	In calcifying cartilage	
	Paget's disease osteosarcoma carcinoma, osteoblastic metastases	At site of disease	Intra- and extrahepatobiliary obstructions Metastases Thorazine toxicity
Normal in	osteoporosis osteopetrosis		
	healing fracture	Increase in phosphatase locally	
	osteosclerosis		
	fibrous dysplasia	Variable level	
Decreased in	achondroplasia deposition of radioactive substances in bone		
	hypophosphatasia	Arrest of skeletal growth with decreased osteoblasic activity	
	cretinism scurvy		

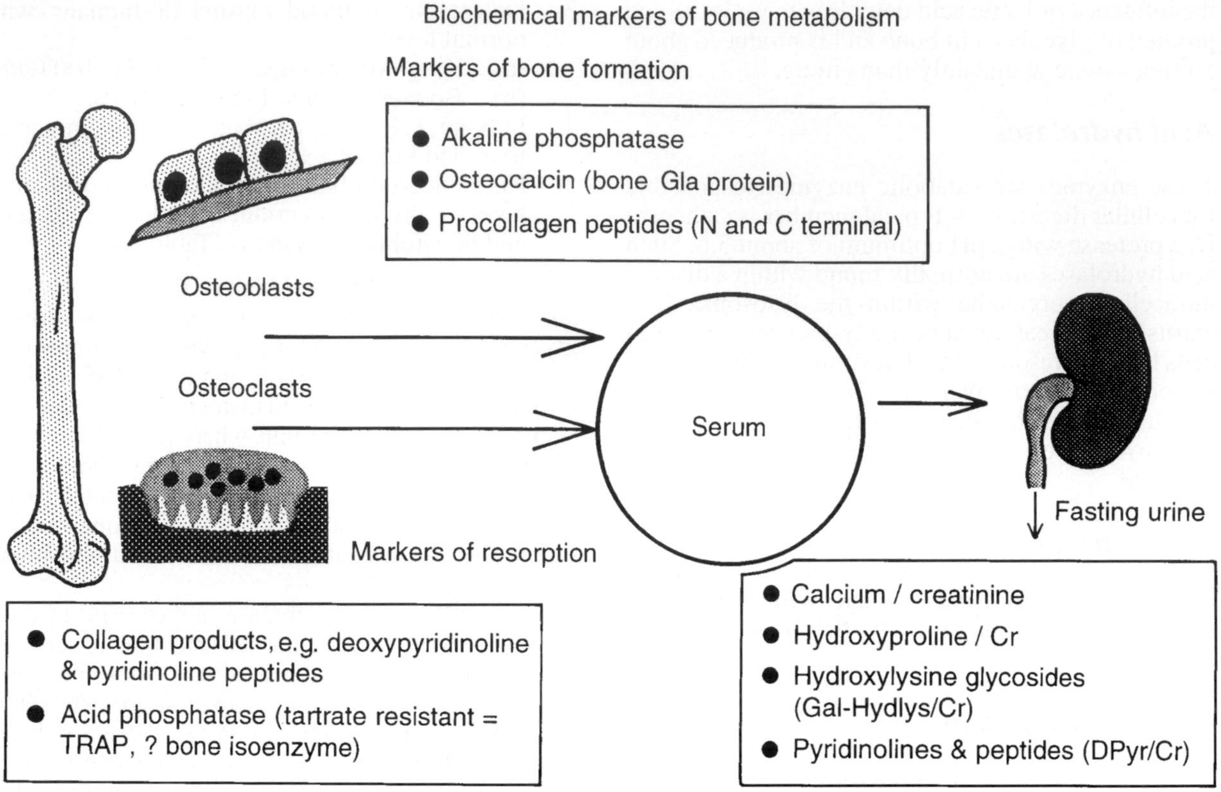

Figure 2.20 Biochemical markers of bone formation and resorption. (Kindly supplied by Professor R. G. G. Russell)

For example, if these two enzymes are normal the raised alkaline phosphatase is probably due to osteoblastic metastases in bone; however, if they are raised in the presence of a raised alkaline phosphatase, liver involvement is indicated (Wilkinson, 1977).

Metastasizing carcinoma of the prostate gives rise to a marked elevation of this enzyme, which can be differentiated in its origin by its being inhibited by L-tartrate (Wilkinson, 1977).

Phosphorylase and glycolytic enzyme systems are particularly concerned with converting glycogen via the hexophosphopyruvates into excess phosphate ions.

Cells of the prostate and seminal fluid have been shown to contain high levels of acid phosphatase. Serum levels in both sexes are very low under normal conditions. However, it is elevated in bony metastases and in Paget's disease.

Azrai and Russell (personal communication, 1992) have recently reviewed how bone formation and bone resorption can be studied *in vivo* by measuring specific enzymes and certain proteins released by osteoblasts and osteoclasts (Figure 2.20). Markers of bone formation are the bone isoenzyme of alkaline phosphatase, osteocalcin (also known as bone Gla protein) and propeptides freed from the N or C terminal ends of the type I procollagen molecule. Markers of bone resorption are also products from collagen breakdown, e.g. deoxypyridinoline and pyridinoline peptides and tartrate-resistant acid phosphatase or TRAP. In the urine the established measurements of hydroxyproline, calcium and creatinine are well known for their lack of specificity. Pyridinolines and deoxypyridinoline – from collagen cross-links – appear to be much more specific.

Metabolism of calcium, phosphate and magnesium

Calcium metabolism should not be considered in isolation from the metabolism of phosphate and magnesium and a brief account of these essential elements will be included in this chapter.

CALCIUM METABOLISM

Calcium is the second messenger in almost every cell system in the body. Control of the extracellular calcium concentration is critical to the maintenance of normal neuromuscular activity and a significant fall leads to convulsions and tetany while a rise is associated with impaired neuromuscular transmission. Skeletal calcium provides a buffer which allows the body to defend normal plasma levels but in addition calcium salts provide much of the strength of the skeleton. Furthermore, the ability of the skeleton to turn over calcium and phosphate is vital to the preservation of skeletal architecture and the prevention and healing of fractures.

Distribution of calcium

The average 70 kg adult male body contains between 1 and 1.1 kg of calcium, 99% of which is found in bone. The soft tissues contain about 10 g and less than 1 g is found in the blood and extracellular fluids. in bone.

Dietary intake

An adequate adult diet contains 1 g (50 mmol) of elemental calcium. Dietary requirements are increased in the young, in pregnancy and lactation and in the elderly. During these times the recommended daily intake is increased to 1.5 g. With an adequate dietary intake, the average adult will absorb approximately 10 mmol (400 mg) of elemental calcium of which 5 mmol (200 mg) will be resecreted back into the gut lumen (Figure 2.21).

Plasma calcium

The plasma calcium concentration in health is maintained within a tight range (2.5–2.7 mmol/l), varying by less than 10%, despite large fluxes between gut, bone and kidney. The large reserve in bone turns over relatively slowly as bone is remodelled, a process which is thought to result in renewal of approximately 10% of the total skeleton each year. Approximately 10 mmol is released from the bone each day due to osteoclastic resorption. Osteoblastic bone formation causes a similar amount to be laid down in newly formed bone. This close association of the amount of bone resorption and accumulation is termed 'coupling' and although the precise cellular mechanisms involved are unclear, it is of extreme importance in the maintainance of skeletal homeostasis. In the growing child, bone formation will exceed resorption, while in the perimenopausal woman, there is a net loss of calcium from the skeleton.

The exchange of calcium as a result of mineralization and bone resorption described above must be differentiated from the large and rapid flux between

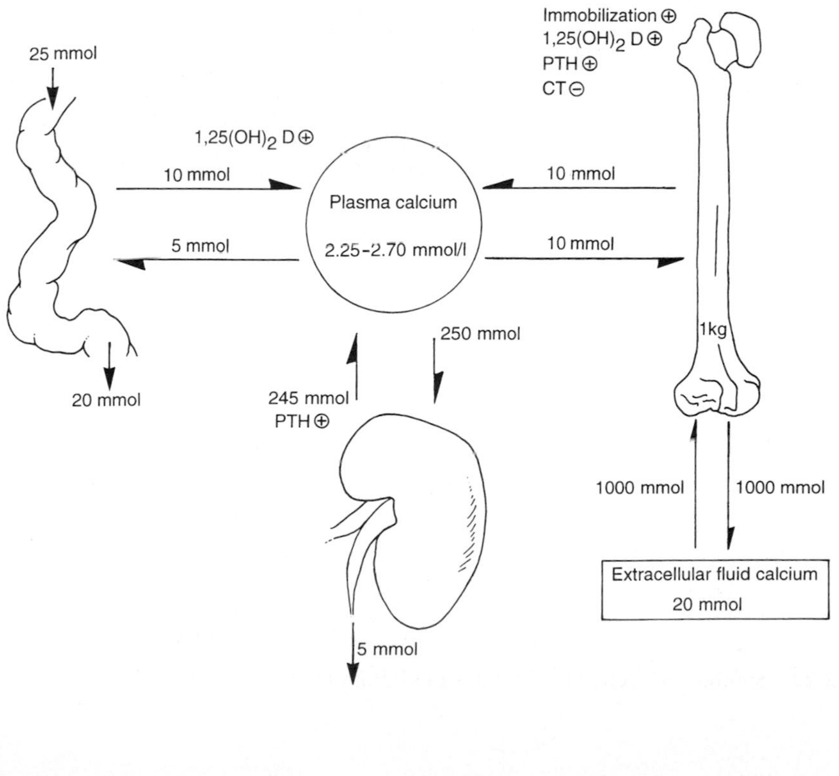

Figure 2.21 Diagram illustrating calcium homoeostasis within the body. PT, parathyroid hormone; CT, calcitonin.

bone and extracellular fluid, which may amount to 1000–2000 mmol/day. This rapidly exchanging pool may be very important in calcium homeostasis but its regulation is poorly understood.

In the intestine calcium is absorbed actively in the duodenum by an active carrier-mediated, energy-dependent process using a calcium binding protein, whose synthesis is dependent on 1,25-dihydroxy-vitamin D_3. Distal to the duodenum in the small bowel and possibly in the large intestine, absorption also occurs either by passive or facilitated diffusion. The relative importance of these different mechanisms and sites of absorption is unclear and is likely to depend on the abundance of dietary calcium since although the duodenum has the greatest capacity for calcium in the entire gut, the relative transit times make it likely that the remainder of the gut makes a contribution to absorption.

The kidney will filter 250 mmol (10 g) of calcium per day, of which all but 245 mmol (9.8 g) will be reabsorbed by a parathyroid hormone-sensitive process.

PHOSPHATE METABOLISM

The majority of the body phosphate is found in the skeleton with approximately 15% being in the intracellular tissues and blood. Less than 1 g/day intake is required by an adult, although more is needed by growing children and pregnant women. Absorption is favoured by the presence of calcium and nearly 60% of the intake is excreted in the urine. Plasma levels are controlled by parathyroid hormone and the range in young children is 1.25–1.5 mmol/litre and in adults 0.75–1 mmol/litre.

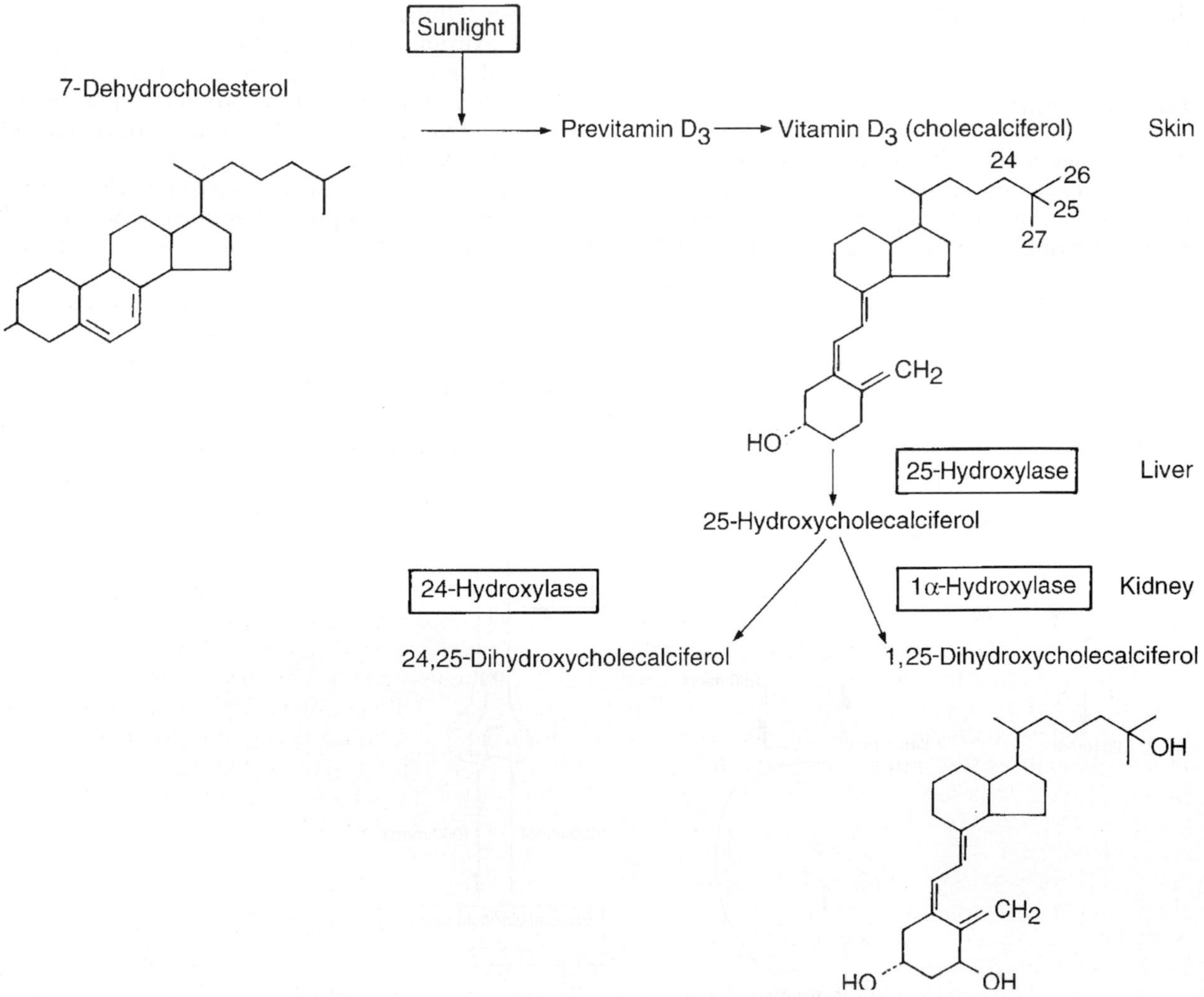

Figure 2.22 Synthesis of active metabolites of vitamin D.

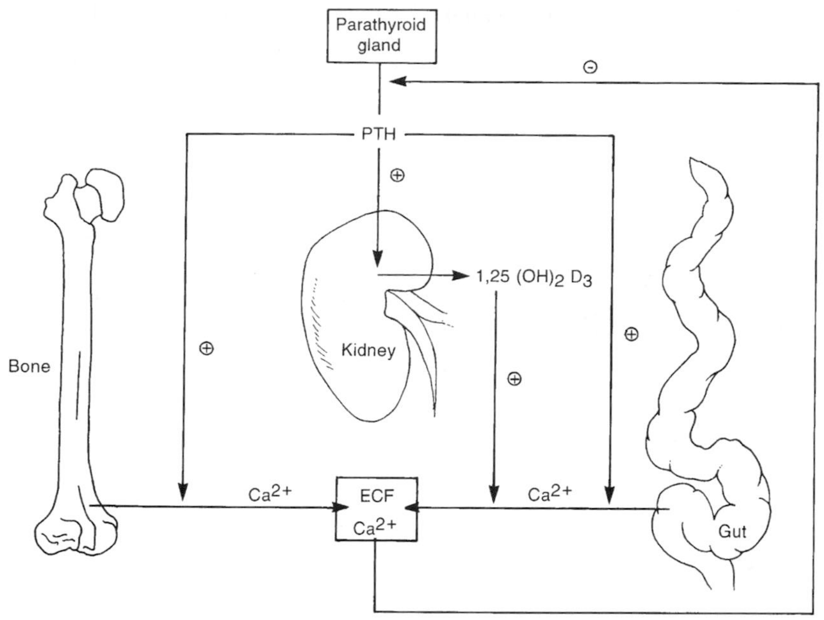

Figure 2.23 The major actions of 1,25-dihydroxyvitamin D_3.

MAGNESIUM METABOLISM

The skeleton of an adult male contains approximately 20 g of magnesium (approximately 0.7%). Two-thirds of the total body magnesium is found in the bone. Approximately 35% of plasma magnesium is protein bound and the mechanism of control of the plasma magnesium levels is poorly understood. Aldosterone increases its renal excretion and PTH may also affect absorption and excretion.

MAJOR CALCIUM REGULATING HORMONES

Vitamin D

In the majority of humans, vitamin D is synthesized in the skin by the action of sunlight on 7-dehydrocholesterol (Figure 2.22). The exceptions are inhabitants of the polar extremities, where there is insufficient light energy. Few foods contain vitamin D, those that do include liver, egg yolks and fish liver oils. In some countries foods are fortified with vitamin. In the USA, milk is fortified but in other countries, vitamin D is added to cereals, margarine or bread. Ingested vitamin D is fat soluble and is absorbed primarily from the duodenum and jejunum via the chylomicron fraction into the lymphatic system and is transported in the plasma bound to a specific binding protein.

Before becoming biologically active, vitamin D is hydroxylated, first in the liver to 25-hydroxyvitamin D_3, which is the major circulating form, and then in the kidney to 1,25-dihydroxyvitamin D_3 (calcitriol), which is the active vitamin. This latter 1-hydroxylation step is the rate-limiting step in calcitriol production and is deficient in severe renal disease. The kidney is the sole site of 1-hydroxylation, apart from the placenta and decidua and the renal conversion is closely regulated, the enzyme being activated by parathyroid hormone. Under conditions where the kidney is not producing 1,25-dihydroxyvitamin D_3, an alternative hydroxylation pathway to 24,25-dihydroxyvitamin D_3 occurs. This compound has in the past been thought of as an inactive waste product, but there is some evidence that it may have a role in normal bone homeostasis.

The major target tissues for calcitriol relevant to calcium metabolism are the intestine and bone (Figures 2.23, 2.24). In the former, synthesis of a specific binding protein leads to an increase in calcium and phosphate absorption. In the latter the effects are less well understood. In pharmacological doses, accelerated bone resorption occurs due to an increase in the number and activity of osteoclasts; however, although vitamin D deficiency is associated with a defect in mineralization, there is little evidence that physiological levels of calcitriol increase bone resorption.

Vitamin D deficiency is accompanied by muscle weakness, which is most marked in the shoulder and pelvic girdles. The aetiology is obscure but the rapid resolution following administration of vitamin D raises the possibility of a direct effect on calcium transport in the sarcoplasmic reticulum.

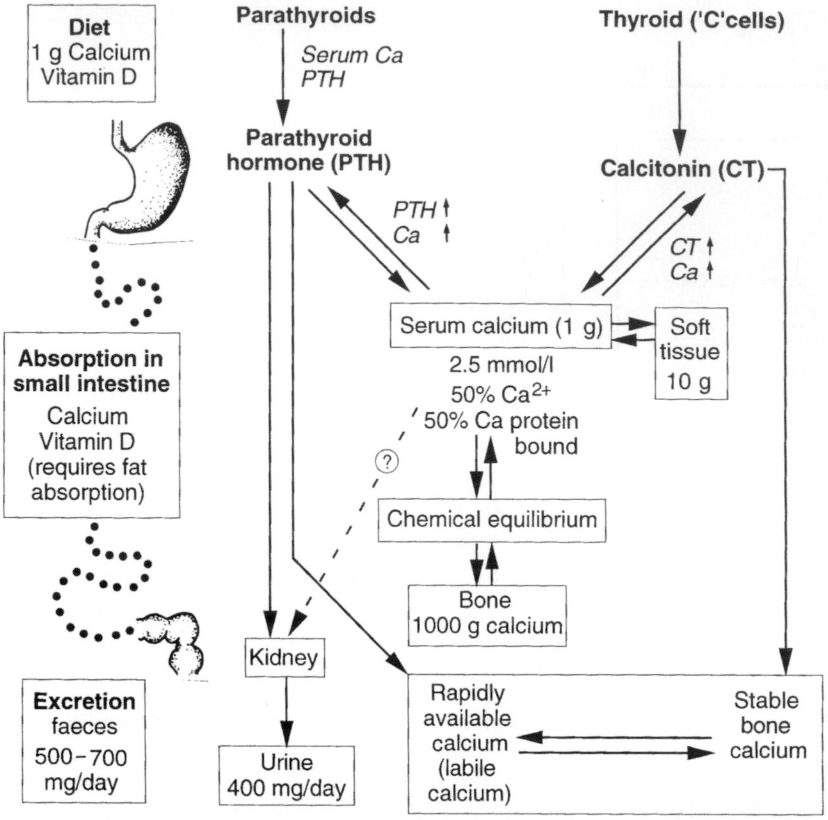

Figure 2.24 The effects of parathyroid hormone on calcium homeostasis and feedback mechanisms which regulate its secretion.

Receptors for calcitriol have been found in other tissues, including brain, gonad, skin, breast and parathyroid tissue. Their function is obscure; however, the demonstration that 1,25-dihydroxyvitamin D_3 can inhibit proliferation and induce differentiation of receptor positive cells and can regulate the secretion of a variety of growth factors has raised the possibility of a more general role in cellular differentiation and maturation in these tissues.

Parathyroid hormone (PTH)

There are normally four parathyroid glands, one in each superior and inferior pole of the thyroid, but there is considerable variation in both the site and number.

PTH consists of a single chain amino acid 84 residues in length. It is synthesized in the parathyroid gland in response to a lowered serum calcium, as a six residue longer proenzyme which is cleaved prior to release. Further cleavage of the molecule occurs in the liver and kidney, to an active amino terminal portion and a larger inactive carboxy terminal molecule. This cleavage may be essential for the hormone to act on bone. Particularly in renal disease, where excretion of the carboxy terminal portion is impaired, the existence of inactive fragments can lead to a false assessment of the plasma level of the active hormone on radioimmunoassay.

A number of factors can modulate the secretion of PTH in response to a fall in the plasma calcium. These include 1,25-dihydroxyvitamin D_3, which inhibits transcription of the hormone. Other factors which influence PTH secretion include hormones such as growth hormone and divalent cations, for example, magnesium (Figure 2.24).

The principal target organs for PTH are bone and kidney, with an additional indirect effect on the gut via calcitriol. In the kidney, PTH stimulates adenylate cyclase along the entire length of the renal tubule. Proximally phosphate reabsorption is reduced, while distally reabsorption of calcium is increased. A second effect is the activation of the 1-hydroxylase enzyme which is responsible for the synthesis of the calcitriol form from calcifediol. Since calcitriol inhibits PTH secretion, there exists a tight feedback loop controlling the level of these calcium regulatory factors. It is now known that the kidney functions as an endocrine organ and produces erythropoietin in response to hypoxia in the interstitial cells of the inner cortex. Erythropoietin is necessary for the proliferation and differentiation of the erythroid precursors of red blood cells. It is now available by recombinant technology for improving haemoglobin levels and the exercise tolerance of patients with severe anaemia.

In bone the major effect of PTH is to increase osteoclastic bone resorption, by increasing both the numbers and activity of osteoclasts. The osteoclast has no PTH receptor, unlike the osteoblast, so that the bone target cell for PTH is probably the osteoblast but the signal mechanism between the osteoblast and the osteoclast is unknown. The increase in osteoclast numbers which follows PTH stimulation is long lasting.

Bone metabolism is severely deranged in patients with renal failure. The complete picture of renal bone disease is extremely complex. Simplistically, in patients with renal failure, production of 1,25-dihydroxyvitamin D_3 is deficient leading to a failure of mineralization of bone osteoid, clinical osteomalacia and a lowered serum calcium and phosphate. The latter causes increased activity of the parathyroid gland and eventually parathyroid gland hyperplasia becomes independent of homeostatic stimulation. In relatively early and simple cases, significant improvement in bone metabolism and calcium homeostasis occurs following administration of oral 1,25-dihydroxyvitamin D_3 and calcium supplementation although in cases where the excessive parathyroid hormone secretion has become independent of the original stimulation by lowered serum calcium due to parathyroid hyperplasia, parathyroidectomy may also be necessary.

In a significant proportion of patients who are on maintenance renal dialysis, excessive aluminium absorption is via the gut which may be enhanced by parathyroid hormone activity or vitamin D analogues. Aluminium has a number of effects on bone homeostasis, particularly the production of profound osteomalacia when it is deposited in bone. This osteomalacia is resistant to treatment with 1,25-dihydroxyvitamin D_3 and calcium supplementation. Thus aluminium bone disease has come to represent a particularly severe subtype of renal bone disease which is indistinguishable from simple renal bone disease without specific bone histology with stains for aluminium.

Calcitonin (CT)

Calcitonin is a peptide hormone 32 amino acids long which is produced by the parafollicular cells (C cells) of the thyroid gland in response to a rise in the serum calcium concentration. Its action is to inhibit bone resorption by a direct effect on the osteoclast, which possesses a receptor for the hormone. Following pharmacological administration, the inhibition of osteoclastic bone resorption leads to a temporary uncoupling of bone resorption from formation, with formation exceeding breakdown. This in turn causes a transient fall in serum calcium. The ability of calci tonin to inhibit bone resorption is exploited in the treatment of diseases in which there is excessive osteoclastic activity, such as Paget's disease of bone.

The physiological importance of calcitonin is unclear, particularly since patients with medullary carcinoma of the thyroid, in which calcitonin levels may be increased vastly above the physiological range, demonstrate little or no alteration in bone homeostasis.

Bone remodelling

Bone is not a dead, inert tissue; instead, the constituent parts are constantly being renewed, with a whole body turnover rate of approximately 10% per year (4% in cortical bone and 25% in trabecular bone; Parfitt, 1983). This process allows the removal of fatigue damage and maintenance of relatively young skeletal tissue by the process of 'remodelling' and the bone is able to adapt to changing mechanical stresses imposed on it by the process of 'modelling'. Modelling and remodelling are both expressions of bone turnover, in which bone is serially removed by osteoclasts and laid down by osteoblasts in a closely coupled fashion.

The term 'remodelling' is used by bone biologists to imply a cycle during which bone is first removed and then new bone laid down at a particular site. This meaning is different from 'remodelling' as used by orthopaedic surgeons to describe the process which occurs when bone is modified to meet structural demands following, for example, a fracture. This process more resembles what bone biologists refer to as 'modelling'. Modelling refers to the overall consequences for the whole bone of the sum of all the units of remodelling activity which are occurring throughout the bone. By progressive bone accretion onto one surface and resorption from another, it is responsible for the gross changes in the shape of bones which occur during development and the adaptation of bone to applied loads which is illustrated by Wolff's law. Although the majority of modelling activity ceases with skeletal maturity, progressive modelling throughout adult life is responsible for the gradual widening of the femoral diaphysis with age and modelling activity can be stimulated by pathological processes.

Bone remodelling occurs at discrete anatomical sites and it follows an orderly cycle (Figure 2.25). First precursor cells differentiate into osteoclasts which erode a cavity on the bone surface. The osteoclasts then disappear and there is a quiescent interval during which the irregular cavity is smoothed off and lined by a layer of 'cement substance' which is of similar composition to bone but is mineral rich and collagen poor. A set of osteoblasts are next recruited which refill the excavated cavity with new

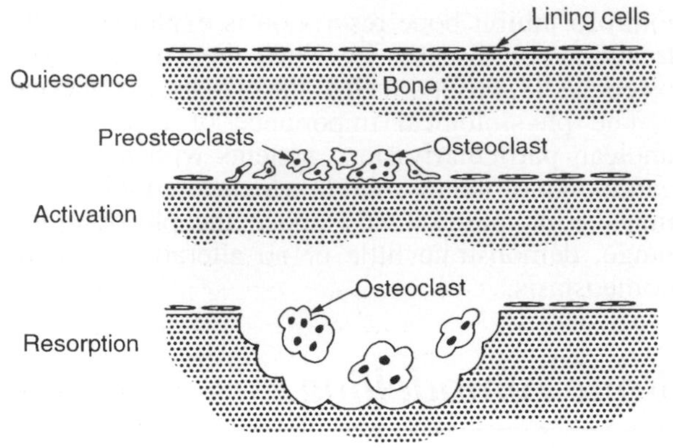

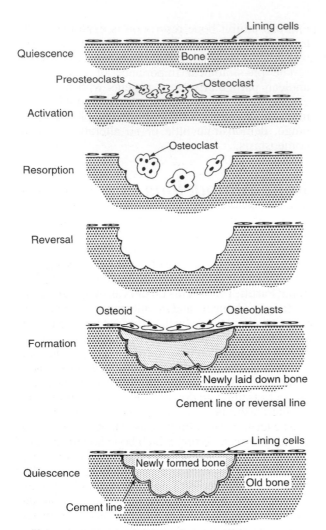

Figure 2.25 A diagrammatic representation of the normal remodelling sequence in adult bone. (After Riggs and Melton, 1988)

bone. Alterations in the dynamics of different parts of the remodelling processes account for the wide variety of age-related changes which occur in the skeleton.

The remodelling cycle is divided into four discrete phases: quiescence, activation, resorption, reversal and formation.

QUIESCENCE

In adult man approximately 90% of the free bone surface is inactive with respect to bone remodelling (Parfitt, 1984). This contrasts to young growing animals in which the majority of free bone surface is involved either in formation or resorption.

During the quiescent phase, the bone surface is covered by a layer of thin flattened lining cells which arise by terminal transformation of osteoblasts. These cells retain their hormonal receptors, but have lost the ability to synthesize collagen (Baron *et al.*, 1984). Between the lining cells and the bone is a thin layer of unmineralized connective tissue which closely resembles osteoid (Van der Weil, 1980) on light microscopy; however, it has fewer collagen fibres than normal bone matrix and these are more randomly orientated. Its function appears to be protection of the bone surface from osteoclastic resorption (Chambers *et al.*, 1985a,b).

ACTIVATION

This is the conversion of a small area of bone surface from quiescence to bone resorbing activity. In an average adult human skeleton, activation will occur somewhere approximately every 10 seconds (Parfitt, 1983). The rate of activation varies with age, sex, race, metabolic state and the particular site and bone involved. It also varies in response to biomechanical requirements.

The precise mechanism by which activation occurs is still unclear; however, it is thought that the lining cells of a quiescent area are stimulated to digest the unmineralized connective tissue overlying the bone. They then retract to expose the mineralized bone surface which is chemotactic for osteoclast precursor cells which undergo fusion into osteoclasts when they reach the bone surface.

RESORPTION

Once assembled on the mineralized bone, the osteoclasts begin to resorb it, producing a Howship's lacuna in trabecular bone or a cutting cone in cortical bone. When the cavity has reached a depth of between 50 and 100 μm, local resorption ceases. The mechanism of cessation of resorption is unclear as is the fate of the osteoclast.

REVERSAL

This is the period between completion of resorption and the start of formation at a particular location. During this period the osteoclastic resorption surface is smoothed out by mononuclear cells and a thin layer of mineral rich cement substance is deposited. The osteoblast precursors are also assembled prior to bone formation. The mechanism coupling bone formation to bone resorption is unclear; however, the phase of bone formation is an inevitable consequence of the preceding bone resorption.

FORMATION

Bone formation occurs in two stages. Soon after the cement substance has been deposited, the newly formed osteoblasts begin to deposit a layer of unmineralized bone matrix, which is referred to as the osteoid seam. After deposition, the collagen fibrils making up the matrix aggregate and cross-link before they become mineralized (Kahn *et al.*, 1984). The new matrix begins to mineralize after approximately 1 week.

IMPLICATIONS OF BONE REMODELLING FOR OVERALL SKELETAL HOMEOSTASIS

The concept that bone remodelling takes place in small coherent packets of resorption followed by formation has a number of very important consequences for the understanding of bone haemostasis (Parfitt, 1988). These derive from the notion that in the adult skeleton after the cessation of skeletal growth, no new lamellar bone formation occurs without a preceding episode of bone resorption. This constraint applies within the cortex, where the physical lack of space for new bone necessitates preceding resorption, and it also seems to apply to periosteal and endosteal surfaces. There is, however, debate as to whether periosteal accretion can occur in adults without preceding bone resorption. There are two definite, pathological exceptions to the rule. One is during the production of callus in a healing fracture, where woven bone will form *de novo*, and the other is after cancellous autografting, where new bone will form directly onto the cancellous graft. However, the contribution of these circumstances to overall bone homeostasis is likely to be very small.

The total body rate of resorption is the product of the number of new resorption cavities eroded in a defined time period and the average volume of each cavity. Since the amount of bone eroded in each resorption cavity is roughly constant, the rate of activation (that is the rate at which new osteoclastic erosion cavities are begun) determines the total body bone resorption. By an extension of this logic, since skeletal homeostasis is maintained over time, the rate of activation also determines the rate of total body bone formation.

During adult life, bone is lost from the skeleton at a rate of approximately 1% of its peak mass per year (Garn, 1981). This overall bone loss is due to a small imbalance between the amount of bone resorbed and the subsequent amount formed in each episode of bone remodelling (Parfitt, 1981). If one were to examine an adult at the time of their peak bone mass, in each bone remodelling unit, an exactly similar amount of bone would be removed by the osteoclasts as was subsequently replaced by the osteoblasts. Later in life, when that individual begins to lose bone, loss may either occur due to the osteoclasts resorbing slightly more bone while the osteoblasts replace the same amount (osteoclastic overactivity, or osteoclast-mediated bone loss) or the osteoblasts may reduce the amount of bone which they replace in each bone remodelling unit (osteoblastic failure, or osteoblast-mediated bone loss). This difference between the amount of bone removed by the osteoclasts and that replaced by the osteoblasts in a single bone remodelling unit is

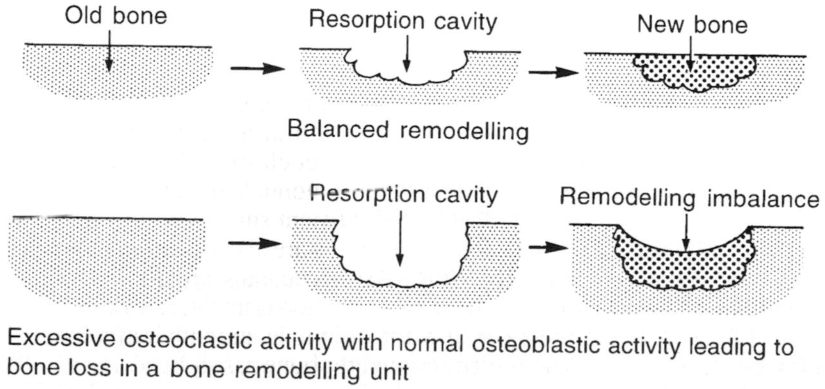

Figure 2.26 Possible mechanisms of focal remodelling imbalance.

referred to as the remodelling imbalance (Figure 2.26).

The balance between formation and resorption varies between different bone surfaces. The average bone remodelling unit will add a small volume on the periosteal surface and subtract a small volume at the endosteal surface (Parfitt, 1988). This is responsible, for example, for the widening of the femoral medullary canal which occurs along with thinning of the femoral cortex with ageing.

For a given difference between the amount of bone resorption and bone formation at any individual bone remodelling unit, the rate of change of total skeletal mass will depend on the number of bone remodelling units taking place at any one time, that is the rate of bone turnover. This acceleration in the rate of bone loss may be caused simply by an increase in the rate of bone turnover. To some extent this explains the rapid phase of postmenopausal osteoporosis.

The concept of the bone remodelling unit as the basic element of skeletal homeostasis implies that after any manipulation of bone turnover, there will be a significant delay before a new steady state is reached. For example, administration of an agent which inhibits osteoclastic bone resorption (such as calcitonin or a diphosphonate) will reduce the rate of activation of new bone remodelling units. Since resorption and formation are occurring at separate sites at any one time, an imbalance will develop while those bone remodelling units which are in a phase of formation complete this phase, but those units which were resorbing are inhibited. There will, therefore, be a temporary excess of bone formation over bone resorption, but as the bone formation in individual remodelling units ceases, bone formation will diminish due to the inhibition of activation. It may take up to three times the normal remodelling period (approximately 1 year) to attain a new steady state after any perturbation (Parfitt, 1988).

Regulation of bone cell function

The regulation of bone cell function during remodelling has been reviewed by MacDonald and Gowan (1992).

Bone remodelling is regulated by systemic hormones (which are discussed elsewhere) and locally by growth factors or cytokines, proteins which regulate the function of differentiated cells at very low concentrations. These factors may be classified according to their effects: *transforming* growth factors, which have the ability to initiate proliferation in anchorage-dependent cells (so causing them to act like transformed cells); *inducing*, which cause cell differentiation and *competency* and *progression*. Competency implies stimulation of a resting cell into a state of proliferation but without the ability to cause the cell to go through a complete cell cycle, for which a progression factor is required. Individual growth factors are widely synthesized through the body and may act on cells of the same class (*autocrine* factors) or on different cells (*paracrine* factors). There is, however, no systematic nomenclature and the cytokines are often referred to by a name which describes their first noted action. As further effects are uncovered, these names may become confusing (Table 2.5).

Bone cells synthesize a number of growth factors and bone matrix itself is a rich source of these polypeptides (Centrella and Cannalis, 1985; Hauschka *et al.*, 1986). The effect of growth factors has been studied primarily *in vitro* and so their exact *in vivo* role is as yet unclear.

Peptide growth factors, in addition to regulating cell migration, proliferation and differentiation, play an important role in morphogenesis, and in particular angiogenesis. For example, angiogenesis results from two signals – an initial chemotactic signal setting up endothelial cell migration and then a cell proliferation signal resulting in cell growth – all important in tumour growth.

Transforming growth factor alpha (TGFα)

TGFα is a 50 amino acid polypeptide which mimics the skeletal effects of EGF. It is produced by tumour cell cultures (Roberts *et al.*, 1983) and it may be a mediator of the excessive bone resorption seen in humeral hypercalcaemia of malignancy (Mundy *et al.*, 1985).

Transforming growth factor beta (TGFβ)

TGFβ is a 24 kDa dimer which is synthesized by many tissues, although bone and platelets are the major sources. It has not been isolated from bone tissue, although *in vitro* it is mitogenic for bone cells and stimulates bone resorption. It exists in three forms all of which stimulate bone DNA and collagen synthesis and cell replication.

Insulin-like growth factor (IGF)

IGF1 (or somatomedin C) is a member of a family of low molecular weight (about 7–8 kDa) insulin-like polypeptides which are widely synthesized. IGF1 is

Table 2.5 Cytokines with actions on bone

	Abbreviaton	Full and alternative names
Stimulators of bone resorption	IL-1α and β	Interleukin 1α and 1β lymphocyte activating factor, catabalin, endogenous paragin
	TNFα and β	Tumour necrosis factor α and β, cachectin, lymphotoxin
	EGF/TGFα	Epidermal growth factor, transforming growth factor α
	PDGF	Platelet-derived growth factor
	FGF	Fibroblast growth factor
Permissive effects on bone resorption	M-CSF	Macrophage colony stimulating factor
	GM-CSF	Granulocyte/macrophage colony stimulating factor
	IL-3	Interleukin 3
	IL-6	Interleukin 6
	LIF	Leukaemia inhibitory factor, I IL-9
Stimulators of bone formation	TGFβ	Transforming growth factor β
	IGF1 and 2	Insulin-like growth factors 1 and 2, somatomedin
	BMPs	Bone morphogenetic proteins
Inhibitors of bone resorption	IFNγ	Interferon gamma
	IL-4	Interleukin 4

synthesized principally in the liver, by a growth hormone dependent process, and is responsible for the effects of growth hormone on bone. It stimulates the proliferation of osteoblastic cells and has a direct stimulatory affect on mature osteoblast collagen synthesis (Cannalis *et al.*, 1971; Cannalis, 1980) but it has no effect on bone resorption (Cannalis *et al.*, 1988). It is possible that bone cells can themselves produce IGF1 in response to growth hormone stimulation (Stracke *et al.*, 1984).

Platelet-derived growth factor (PDGF)

PDGF is a two chain polypeptide with molecular weight of 27–30 kDa. Although PDGF was originally isolated from platelets, it has been isolated from a variety of tissues including bone matrix. It enhances bone resorption by a prostaglandin-mediated mechanism (Tashjian *et al.*, 1982) and stimulates bone DNA and protein synthesis.

Fibroblast growth factor (FGF)

FGF exists in both acidic and basic form. bFGF is a 146 amino acid protein with a molecular weight of 16 kDa and is similar to aFGF although the two factors are produced by different genes (Cannalis *et al.*, 1988). In bone culture, both forms of FGF stimulate DNA synthesis and cell replication but they have no direct stimulatory effect on osteoblast collagen synthesis (Cannalis *et al.*, 1987a,b). FGFs do not affect bone resorption.

Epidermal growth factors (EGF)

EGF, a 6 kDa polypeptide, increases bone resorption, causes proliferation of osteoblasts, but decreases the activity of differentiated osteoblasts, reducing alkaline phosphatase activity and collagen synthesis (Cannalis and Raisz, 1979). The bone resorbing effect may be mediated by local release of prostaglandins (Tashjian and Levine, 1978).

Interleukin 1 (IL-1)

IL-1 exists in two forms, IL-1α and IL-1β, with different isoelectric points but very similar structures. It has a molecular weight of between 17 and 18 kDa. It was originally described as lymphocyte activiting factor (LAF) because it was found to be secreted by macrophages and monocytes and caused proliferation of T cells by inducing the production of interleukin 2 (O'Garra, 1989). It has an important role in the inflammatory response. It is, however, produced by bone tissue (Hanazawa *et al.*, 1987) and accounted in part for the activity originally termed osteoclast activating factor (Dewhirst *et al.*, 1985).

IL-1 has complex effects on bone remodelling (Cannalis *et al.*, 1988). It stimulates cell replication in bone culture and in low doses it stimulates bone collagen synthesis (Cannalis, 1986). Interleukin 1 also stimulates bone resorption (Gowan *et al.*, 1983). However, this is an indirect affect which requires the presence of osteoblasts (Thompson *et al.*, 1986).

CYTOKINE EFFECTS ON BONE RESORPTION

The first cytokine to be shown to stimulate bone resorption was IL-1 and this remains the most potent. Similar activities have now been demonstrated for TNFα. Both of the agents appear to work by stimulating osteoclast precursors to divide and differentiate to mature osteoclasts.

Both GM-CSF and M-CSF have also been shown to stimulate osteoclastic activity and the defect in bone resorption in osteoporotic mice has recently been demonstrated to be due to a failure of M-CSF production.

It is unclear whether termination of osteoclastic activity is due to cytokine action. However, IFNγ and IL-4 both inhibit bone resorption.

CYTOKINES AND BONE FORMATION

Bone formation may be divided into an initial phase of recruitment and differentiation of osteoblast precursors followed by mature osteoblast function in the form of matrix production and mineralization. Cytokines have effects on both of these phases. The majority of stimulants of bone resorption also stimulate osteoblast precursor proliferation while inhibiting mature osteoblast activity. Stimulators of mature osteoblastic action include members of the TGFβ superfamily which includes TGFβ, IGF and BMP. These agents often stimulate precursor proliferation in addition. Since many cytokines of this group are secreted in bone matrix when it is formed by osteoblasts, it is possible that subsequent release by osteoclastic bone resorption allows them to act as site-specific controllers of bone remodelling.

PROSTAGLANDINS

The prostaglandins (PGs) are a family of molecules which are universally distributed in the body and have a bewildering array of actions in very low doses. For example, they may assist in regulation of red blood cell deformation; some decrease gastric acid secretion and inhibit peptic ulceration in experimental models. They modify pituitary responses to hypothalamic hormones and may play a role in the regulation of the female reproductive cycle. They induce abortion when injected intra-amniotically during pregnancy and induce labour when injected

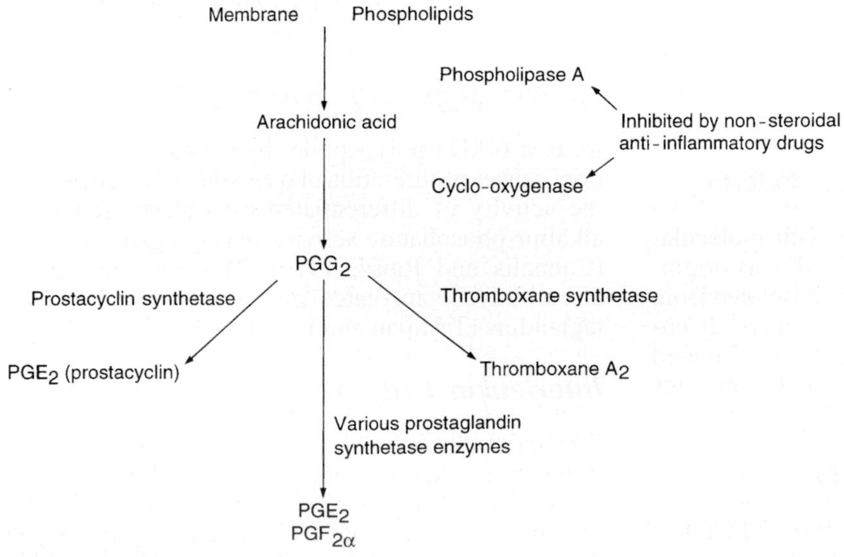

Figure 2.27 The synthesis of prostaglandins and other prostanoids.

near term. They can mimic the effects of a number of hormones and are released from inflamed tissue. They are found in the brain and may have a role in modulation of the effects of neurotransmitters. They have a short half-life and are released and act locally in response to a specific stimulus.

Prostaglandins were first described by Von Euler who noted the ability of semen to cause alteration in uterine muscle tone, the terminology relating to the original belief that they were secreted by the prostate gland. They are 20 carbon fatty acids which contain a pentose ring. The major classes are designated PGA, PGB, PGE and PGF followed by a subscript (1, 2, 3) which denotes the number of double bonds outside the pentose ring.

Prostaglandins are synthesized from arachidonic acid by the action of cyclo-oxygenase (prostaglandin synthetase and other enzymes). The arachidonic acid itself is produced by the action of phospholipase A_2 on phospholipids from cell membranes (Figure 2.27).

The effects of prostaglandins on bone are confusing and it is difficult to come to a synthesis of the wide variety of differing actions which are being reported. It is clear, however, that prostaglandins are important local regulators of bone cell behaviour.

Effects on bone resorption

Prostaglandins are powerful stimulators of bone resorption when added to organ cultured bones (Dietrich *et al.*, 1975; Tashjian *et al.*, 1977), PGE_2 being particularly active. These effects are seen in very low doses. However, when PGI_2, PGE_1 or PGE_2 were added to isolated osteoclasts *in vitro*, they were found to strongly inhibit osteoclastic motility and bone resorption at very low doses and this effect appears to be mediated via cyclic AMP (Chambers *et al.*, 1985b). Hence the stimulatory effect on bone resorption would appear to be indirect and probably mediated by an effect on osteoblasts (Chambers, 1990). Since cytokines can cause osteoblasts to release PGs, this may provide the basis for some of their direct actions on osteoclasts (Gowan, 1988). Chambers has also described an as yet uncharacterized agent which is secreted by osteoblasts and inhibits bone resorption.

Prostaglandins appear to have a role in mediating the basal level of bone resorption, that is the cell-mediated bone resorption which occurs *in vitro* in the absence of added stimulators (Katz *et al.*, 1983) and in addition PGs may mediate the resorption promoting effects of EGF, PGF and TGFα. They are produced in large quantities following fracture (Dekel *et al.*, 1981) and may be responsible for abnormal bone remodelling and sequestrum formation in osteomyelitis (Dekel and Francis, 1981).

PGs replicate the actions of PTH and 1α,25-dihydroxyvitamin D_3 in promoting osteoclast-mediated bone resorption (Holtrop and Raisz, 1979). Finally, the bone resorptive response to mechanical stimulation is coupled with an increase in PGE production (Somjen *et al.*, 1980).

Effects on bone formation

The effects of PGs on bone formation are also confused. They may promote differentiation of preosteoblast into osteoblast (Chyun and Raisz, 1984) and they seem to stimulate periosteal new bone formation preferentially, both *in vitro* (Nefussi and Baron, 1985) and *in vivo* (Ueda *et al.*, 1980). In contrast, in rats PG administration leads to increased trabecular metaphyseal and cortical endosteal bone formation (Jew *et al.*, 1985).

Administered PGs accumulate in osteoblasts, leading to an increase in cAMP (Dziak *et al.*, 1982), increased cAMP-dependent protein kinase activity (Partridge *et al.*, 1981) and collagenase secretion.

ELECTRICAL PHENOMENA AND THEIR EFFECT ON BONE CELL FUNCTION

It is well established that electrical potentials occur in bone. Of most importance to the discussion of bone remodelling are the electrical potentials which are generated when external stresses are applied to bone. Under these conditions an area of bone under compression exhibits a negative potential, while a region under tension becomes relatively electropositive.

Two mechanisms have been proposed for the generation of stress-induced potential: *piezoelectrical* effects which are due directly to deformation of the molecules of bone (Fukada and Yasuda, 1957) and *streaming potentials* which are caused by stress-induced changes in fluid fluxes through the bone. It is probable that in fluid-filled bone, at least for deformations occurring at relatively low frequencies, the latter mechanism is the more important (Pienkowski and Pollack, 1983).

The demonstration that more electronegative areas of bone are associated with net osteogenesis while in positively charged areas there was a tendency for bone resorption, has led to the suggestion that Wolff's law is mediated through stress-induced potentials. While this is an attractive and elegant theory, it is unproven. There is, however, a large amount of experimental work indicating that electricity can promote bone formation both in fracture repair and in epiphyseal bone growth. Effects of electricity have been demonstrated on a wide variety of bone cell functions including matrix formation, calcification and cell proliferation (Pollack, 1990). The demonstration that both stress and applied external electrical fields can cause alteration in cAMP and cGMP levels in bone suggests a possible link between electrical and biochemical events (Rodam *et al.*, 1975).

These demonstrations have led to clinical application of electricity in union of difficult fractures. Experimental studies have demonstrated that stress potentials have a value in the range of 0.05–0.5 V/cm (Pienkowski and Pollack, 1983). This is similar to the values measured in callus during electrical stimulation of tibial non-unions in humans (Vreslovic *et al.*, 1986). Although this suggests that it should be possible to influence union using externally applied electrical fields, definitive scientific evidence for this is still lacking.

Cartilage

Like bone, cartilage is a specialized form of connective tissue characterized by varying amounts of intercellular matrix. Cartilage is seen in four main types: hyaline (Figure 2.28a), fibrocartilage (Figure

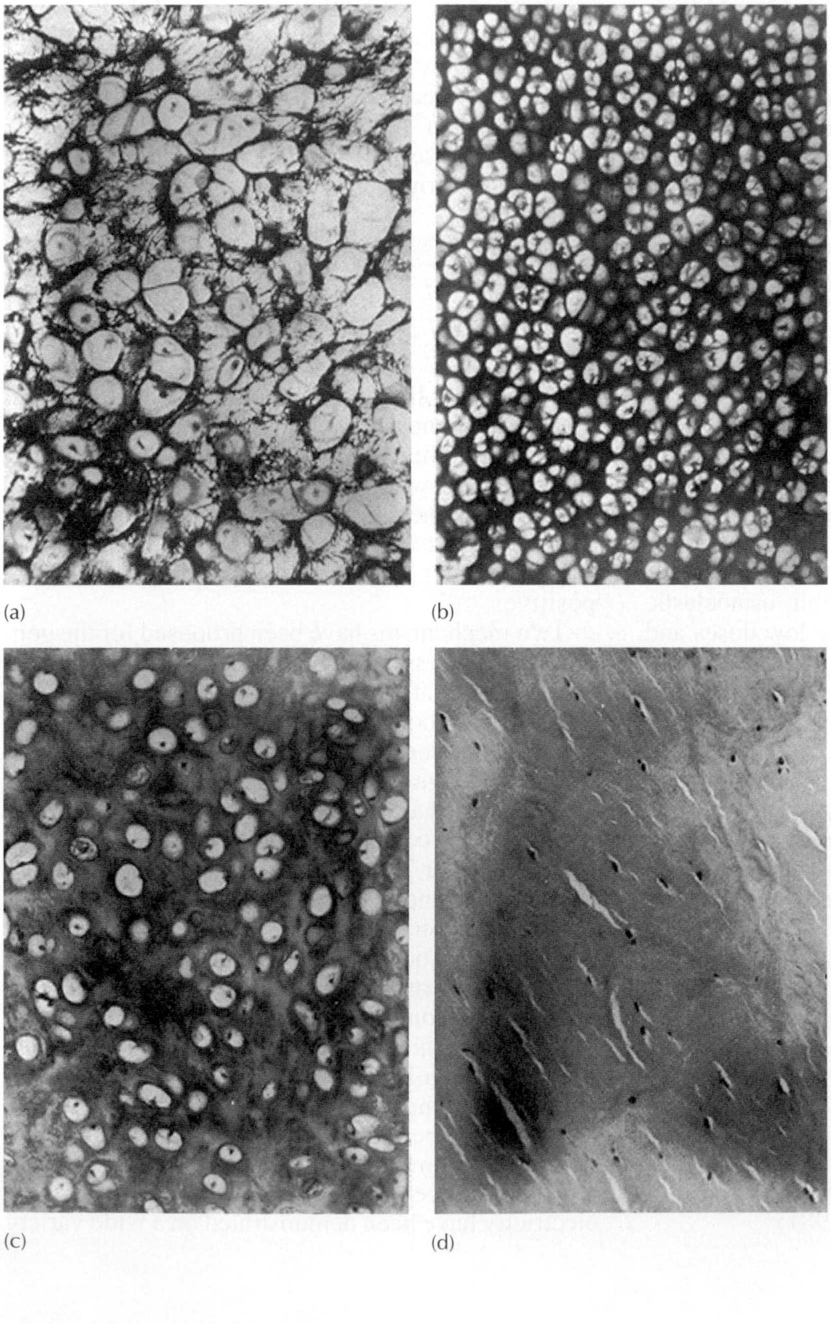

Figure 2.28 (a) Photomicrograph of rat hyaline cartilage stained with toluidine blue solution (× 118). (b) Photomicrograph stained with haematoxylin and eosin to show human fibrocartilage (× 118). (c) Photomicrograph of elastic cartilage stained with a silver stain for its elastic fibre content (× 118). (d) Photomicrograph showing a haematoxylin and eosin preparation of human elastic cartilage (× 118).

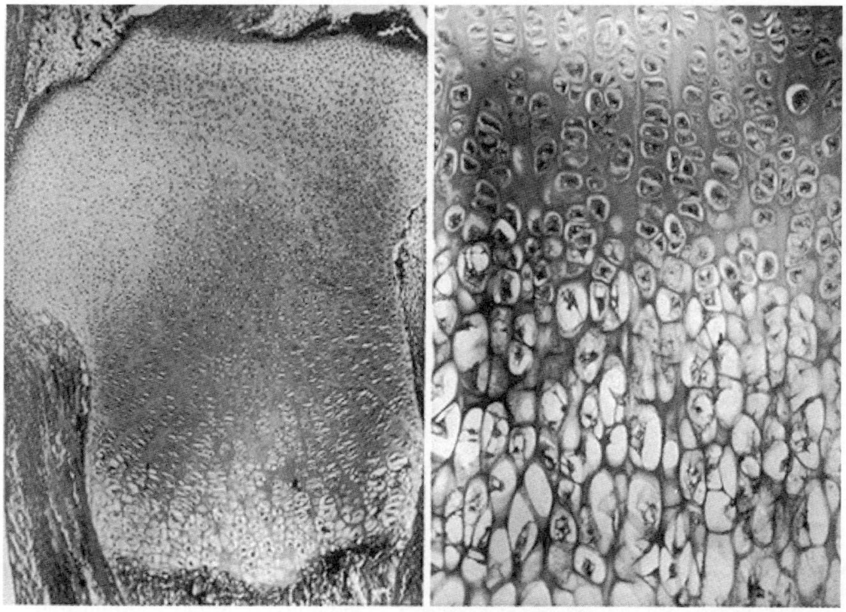

(a) (b)

Figure 2.29 (a) Photomicrograph of growing rat's bone showing endochondral ossification at the lower aspect, with hyaline cartilage at the upper (× 58). (b) Photomicrograph of epiphyseal cartilage of a rat (× 120).

2.28b), elastic (Figures 2.28c,d) and what might be termed endochondral cartilage (Figure 2.29), which subsequently goes on to bone formation. These four main types differ, depending upon the density of the intercellular matrix and its content of fibrous or elastic fibres. All forms originate from differentiation of mesenchymatous tissue in the embryo.

The chondroblast is a large cell with a basophilic nucleus and contains, like osteoblasts, a large amount of rough endoplasmic reticulum and prominent Golgi apparatus (Figures 2.30, 2.31). The cytoplasm stains metachromatically with basic aniline dyes such as toluidine blue. The degree of metachromasia depends on the molecular size of the chondroitin sulphate molecules. The cytoplasm also contains much glycogen and large cytoplasmic lakes which may contain secretory material. The degree of metachromasia depends upon the state of depolymerization

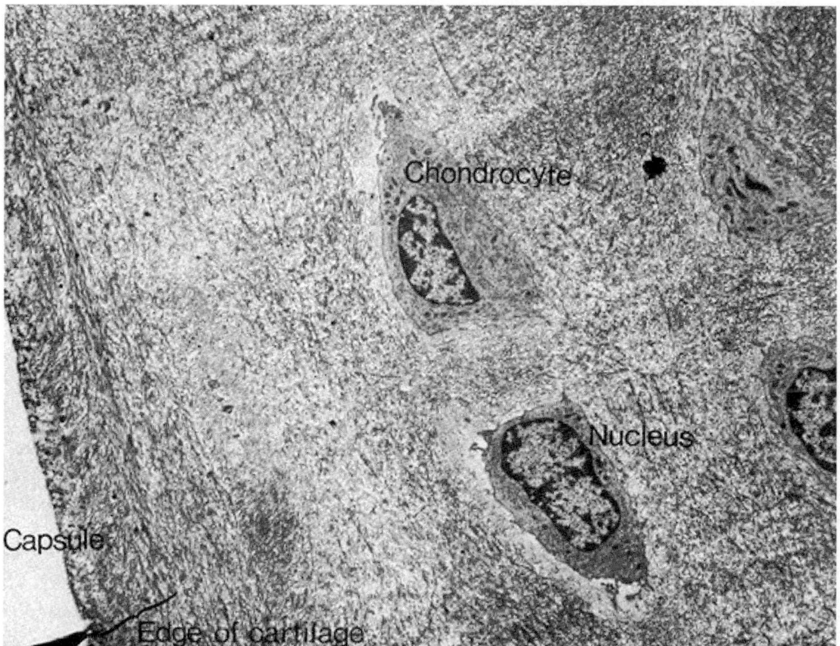

Figure 2.30 Electron micrograph showing two chondrocytes, with a large nucleus lying in condensed proteoglyvan material, with thc edge of the cartilage to the left and the collagen of the capsule covering the surface (× 4860).

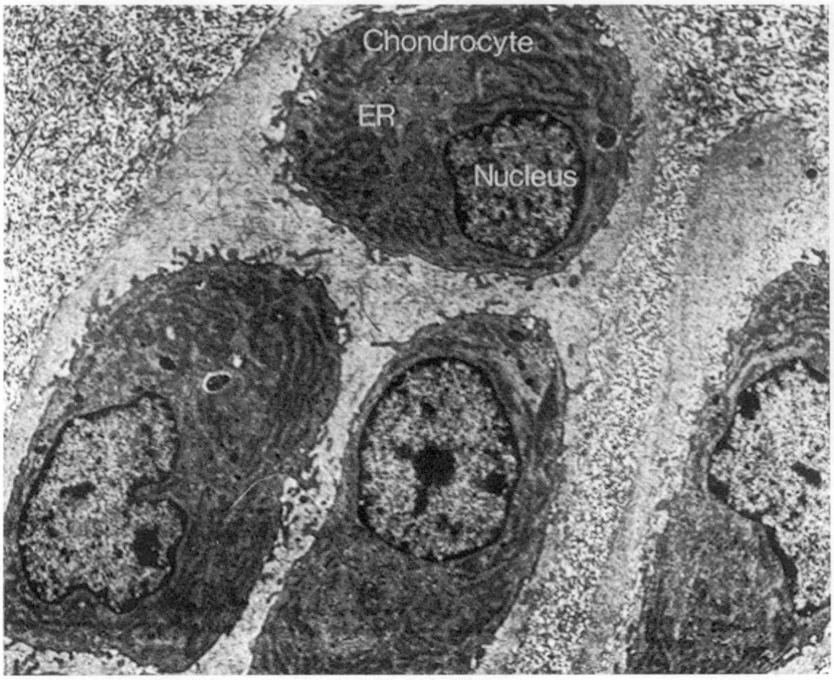

Figure 2.31 Electron micrograph of four large chondrocytes with large nuclei, rough endoplasmic reticulum in the cytoplasm and Golgi aparatus (× 9720).

of the chondroitin sulphates. Robinson showed by electron microscopy that the cytoplasmic walls of the chondroblasts are produced by a thickening or homogeneous condensation of the matrix and is not a true membrane (Figure 2.32). Cartilage is relatively avascular, and when permeated by blood vessels, calcification or ossification usually occurs. The nutrition of the cartilage tissue is usually by diffusion and osmosis.

The chemistry of articular cartilage consists of the matrix which is made up of the chondroitin sulphates A and C, and fibrils of collagen which are 2500–5000 nm in diameter (Cameron and Robinson, 1958). In the femoral epiphyseal cartilage of new-

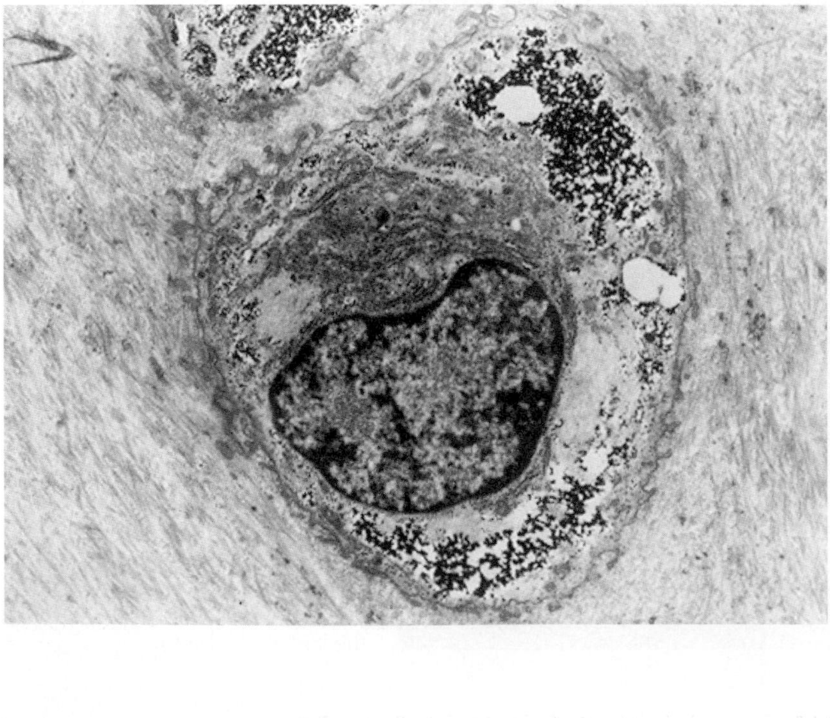

Figure 2.32 Electron micrograph of a chondrocyte, showing the black-stained areas of glycogen in the cytoplasm (× 6750).

born infants, these workers have demonstrated that the fibrils are less dense with poor bundle formation and are about 2500 nm in diameter. The water, content is high, varying from 75% in children to 60% in older age groups. Chondroblasts contain lipids, cholesterol and glycogen within the cytoplasm, which decreases with ageing, as well as precursor chondroitin substances. Deoxyribonucleic acid is present in the coarser granules of the nucleus which gradually become finer during ageing.

Enzymes such as dehydrogenase and lipase have been described and identified in cartilage. Kuhlman (1960), by microchemical techniques in phase III of the epiphyseal plate, demonstrated enzymes which mediate carbohydrate metabolism through the anaerobic Embden–Meyerhof pathway, the citric acid cycle and the direct oxidative pathways. The isotope, sulphur-35 – which labels both the sulphated mucopolysaccharides complex chondroitin and, to a lesser extent, the inorganic sulphate – has been used to demonstrate the diffusion of sulphur from the nucleus and cytoplasm out into the matrix. It is of interest that as the radioactive sulphate label decreases, in the intracellular matrix, radioactive phosphorus-32 and calcium-45 isotopes then appear, during calcification.

Bone growth and development

Bone develops by transformation of pre-existing connective tissue. When bone formation occurs directly in primitive connective tissue it is called *intramembranous ossification*. When it takes place in pre-existing cartilage it is called *endochondral ossification*. The bones with the vault of the skull, the maxilla, the majority of the mandible and the clavicle, are formed by intramembranous ossification, whereas the long bones, vertebrae, pelvis and bones of the base of the skull are formed by endochondral ossification. The skeleton extremities, the vertebral column and the pelvis are formed by endochondral ossification. Endochondral bone development begins as a condensation of mesenchymal cells derived from mesoderm, which form extracellular matrix. The mesenchymal cells surrounding the cartilage become the periosteum. These cartilage cells go through a maturation process, which can be visualized in the area of the developing long bone, called the growth plate. Growth plates consist of zones of rapidly proliferating chondrocytes secreting collagens II, IX and XI, maturing and hypertrophic chondrocytes secreting predominantly collagen X (Lu Valle, 1993).

EXTRACELLULAR MATRIX MOLECULES AND BONE DEVELOPMENT

Collagen I is the major extracellular matrix (ECM) molecule of bone. Recent immunolocalization developing mouse embryos demonstrated that collagen XII is present in intramembranous bone. Its role in bone structure and development is yet unknown.

Other molecules may also be important in bone development. Tenascin, a glycoprotein, is seen in both osteogenic and chondrogenic areas of developing endochondral bone. These data imply that tenascin variants are important in osteogenesis. However, the recent demonstration that mice with a disrupted tenascin gene developed normally in all respects suggests that the role of tenascin in bone development may be delicate.

Aggrecan core protein, previously considered to be specific to cartilage ECM, in which it interacts with hyaluronate and link protein, is also expressed in chicken calvaria and osteoblasts. That cartilage-specific proteoglycan, aggrecan, has been demonstrated to be present in membranous bone has dramatic implications for the role of proteoglycans in bone and cartilage formation.

INTRAMEMBRANOUS OSSIFICATION

Intramembranous bone formation occurs within a primitive vascularized layer of connective tissue consisting of a randomly orientated meshwork of collagen fibrils in which are found cells in contact with each other through long tapering processes. At a certain stage of differentiation, cells begin to proliferate in the area where bone will be formed. The cells hypertrophy and transform into osteoblasts. Progressive bone formation results in the fusion of adjacent bony areas within the membrane to form spongy bone. This is then remodelled into its mature form.

ENDOCHONDRAL OSSIFICATION

The essential difference between this type of ossification and intramembranous ossification is the existence of a cartilage model or anlage formed from mesenchymal tissue which acts as a scaffold for ossification but does not itself become bone. The process is best illustrated by studying the sequence of events in a long bone. Within the cartilage model at a stage of embryonic development, depending on the cellular age and mass of the model, the cells of the region which will form the primary centre of ossification undergo hypertrophy and accumulate

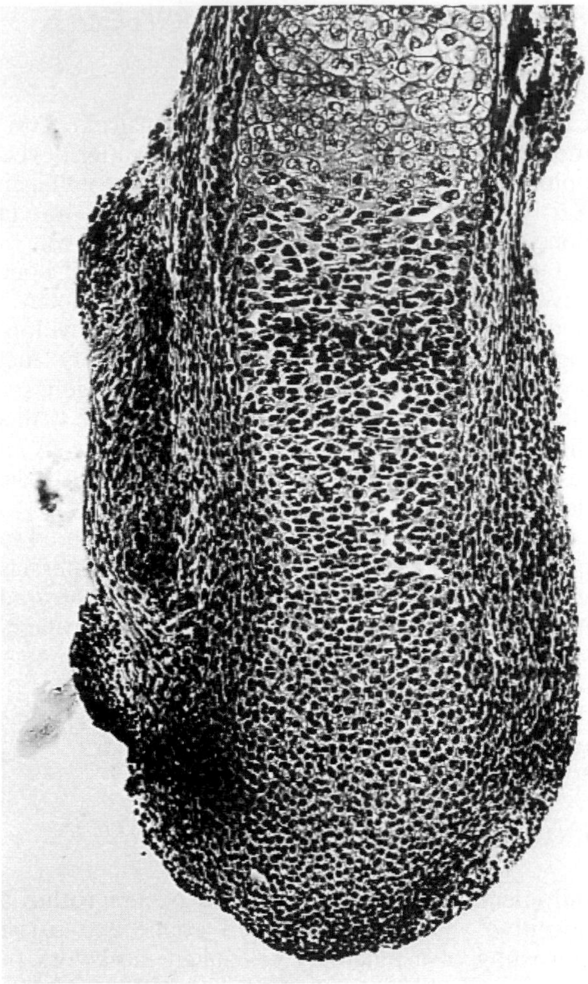

Figure 2.33 The mechanism of ossification of a long bone from a photomicrograph of a limb bud. A condensation of mesenchymal cells occurs which matures into cartilage. A collar of trabecular bone then forms around the centre of the bone (primary osseous collar) and then spreads through the future diaphysis.

glycogen (Figure 2.33). The hyaline matrix remaining in the region of the hypertrophic cartilage cells begins to calcify and simultaneously ossification occurs in the perichondral ring in the region of the midshaft, forming a periosteal band of bone. Blood vessels from the investing connective tissue grow into the diaphysis through the newly formed periosteal shell of bone and invade the region around the hypertrophied cartilage cells. Osteoblasts derived from this connective tissue then begin to lay down osteoid and fetal bone on the cartilage matrix. Haemopoietic cells appear from the invading tissue and red marrow is soon identified.

This process extends up and down the shaft in an orderly fashion until the level of the future growth plate is reached. Here the replacement of the cartilage model ceases and the cartilage organizes into the proliferative epiphyseal growth plate.

The vascular supply of fetal bone is initially through multiple perforating arteries throughout the length of the bone. As growth progresses, these arteries gradually lessen in number until only one persists as the adult nutrient artery which is usually found at the site of the primary invasion of the cartilage model.

The bone initially formed where the primary ossification centre has replaced the cartilage model by endochondral ossification is a loose trabecular network. As it enlarges laterally it fuses with the periosteal collar of bone which is in the form of a multilayered shell and is a product of membranous ossification. Thus even in those long bones which are formed primarily by endochondral ossification, membranous ossification plays a large role.

At the same time as the primary ossification centre has progressed towards the cartilage ends, the primary periosteal collar has also extended towards these regions, being always slightly ahead of the central endochondral ossification process. Once the physis is established, the periosteal ring ceases further extension towards the epiphyses and remains level with the zone of hypertrophic cartilage of the physis. This peripheral ring of bone is also referred to as the ring of Lacroix. Closely related to the ring of Lacroix is found a region of relatively primitive mesenchymal cells which are important to lateral growth of the physis. The association of the osseous ring of Lacroix, the mesenchymal cells and the lateral part of the physis is referred to as the zone of Ranvier (Figure 2.34a).

During fetal and childhood osteogenesis, the endochondral growth of bone continues in the area of the growth plate and within the epiphysis. Growth in length occurs by addition of cells at the physis. In contrast, growth in width is more complex. At the physis a small contribution is by interstitial growth but the majority is by lateral apposition by differentiation of mesenchymal cells within the zone of Ranvier. At the level of the diaphysis lateral growth is accomplished by apposition of bone subperiosteally. All this bone will eventually be remodelled to create the metaphysis and diaphyseal cortex.

The interaction of endochondral and intramembranous ossification in a long bone has led to the concept of the 'endochondral cone'. In certain sea mammals the process of bone remodelling to create a medullary canal and the long bones does not occur and the relative contributions of endochondral and membranous ossification to the long bone structure can clearly be seen.

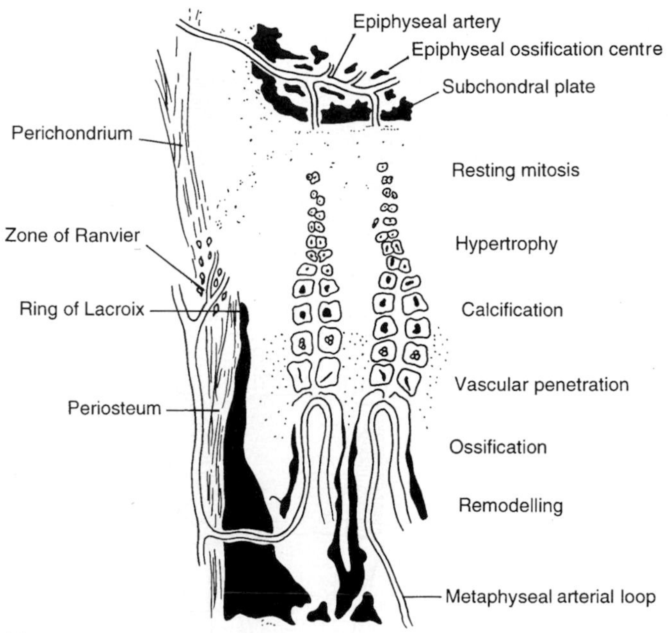

(a)

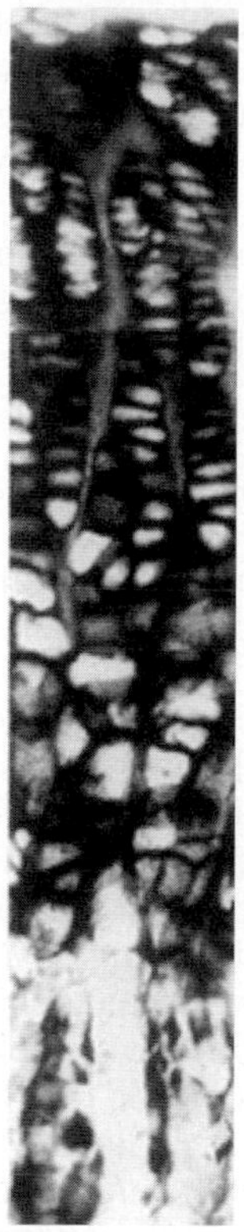

(b)

Figure 2.34 (a) A diagram of the physis showing the stages in longitudinal bone growth and the edge structures of the ring of Lacroix and the zone of Ranvier. (b) Photomicrograph of the epiphyseal plate. The histology of the five phases of cartilage maturation during endochondral ossification. (Reproduced, with permission, from Duthie, R. B. and Barker, A. N. (1955) *Journal of Bone and Joint Surgery* **37B**, 309)

At birth the epiphysis of each long bone is purely cartilaginous with the exception of the distal femur. At a time unique to each site, a secondary centre of ossification develops within the epiphysis and expands by endochondral ossification. As it approaches the physis it forms a dense subchondral plate parallel to it. Externally the growth of the secondary centre of ossification and the adjacent epiphyseal cartilage is modified by forces applied to it through attached muscle fibres, tendons and ligaments and possibly also by intrinsic factors, to produce the characteristic shape of the epiphysis of the long bone. When the hyaline cartilage of the chondral epiphysis first forms, there are no discernible histological differences between the cells which will eventually form the joint surface and those which will take part in the secondary ossification centre. However, at some point differentiation occurs so that the articular hyaline cartilage is unable to ossify (McKibbin and Holdsworth, 1967).

EPIPHYSEAL GROWTH

Since bone itself is a hard and unyielding structure, it can only increase in size by the relatively slow process of *appositional* growth. From infancy until maturity, however, long bones increase in length much more rapidly than this subsequent endochondral ossification process will permit. This comes about by cell division within the cartilaginous physis or growth plate, situated at the junction of the epiphysis and metaphysis at the ends of the long bones. The growth plate is composed of cartilage cells which are arranged in well ordered long columns separated from each other by an intercellular matrix of loosely packed collagen fibres containing proteoglycans (Figure 2.34b). The columns are parallel to each other and to the axis of growth of each particular bone end. Disorganization of this orderly structure is seen in conditions such as achondroplasia, where growth is markedly deficient.

The growth plate cartilage is divided into a series of morphological zones. On the epiphyseal side of each column, the cartilage cells are small and flat in the resting zone. Immediately on the metaphyseal side of this is the layer of active cell division. Mitoses occur mainly longitudinally providing growth in length. Occasional transverse mitoses are seen which contribute to widthwise growth of the physis. Cells of this layer are also responsible for secreting matrix. The blood supply of the peripheral and resting zones is from the adjacent epiphyseal arteries.

Approximately half-way down the cell columns towards the metaphysis, rapid cell division ceases as the hypertrophic zone is entered. This region is distant from both the epiphyseal and metaphyseal blood supplies and is relatively avascular. The chondrocytes mature and hypertrophy, becoming up to five times larger than in the proliferating zone. Type X collagen is found in the hypertrophic cells in this region and may well have a function in provisional calcification.

Within the zone of hypertrophy, calcification begins in the matrix between the cell columns. The last hypertrophic cartilage cell of each column is immediately adjacent to an invading capillary tuft from the metaphysis. Capillary endothelial cells proliferate and, breaking through into the lacuna of this last cell, the proliferating capillary uses its space as a template upon which endothelial cells proliferate and finally form a new extension to the capillary tuft. Thus as new cells form at the epiphyseal side of the growth plate, cells are constantly being lost and replaced by capillary invasion on the metaphyseal side. Osteoblasts are carried in from the metaphysis with this process of capillary invasion and thus come to surround the bars of calcified cartilage matrix between the columns at the base of the growth plate. Duthie and Barker (1955) have shown experimentally during bone growth in the epiphyseal area that, as ^{35}S-labelled mucopolysaccharide complex is released by the disintegrating cartilage cells, radioactive phosphate complexes appear between them and around these masses. There appears to be some quantitative balance between the amount of sulphated chondroitin disappearing and the amount of phosphate being deposited. In the formation of new osteons, during the osteogenesis, Lacroix (1954) demonstrated a similar relationship of radioactive sulphur to radioactive calcium in the formation of concentric lamellae. This accounts for the presence of calcified cartilage within the newly formed trabeculae of the zone of *primary ossification* which lies adjacent to the base of the growth plate in the metaphysis.

REMODELLING OF THE STRUCTURE OF BONE

This consists of extensive but constructive resorption and deposition of new bone, which is most marked during growth and development and continues throughout life in the mature skeleton. During growth at the epiphyseal plate area the remodelling process is essential to change the shape and function of the bones, both in the longitudinal and in the circumferential planes (Keith, 1918), and within the spongiosa of the medullary cavity (Figure 2.35), in order to produce the normal tubular shape of the shaft. There is a morphological remodelling process in the periosteal area, adjacent to the juxtaepiphyseal area or the perichondral ring of Lacroix, which contains large numbers of osteoclasts.

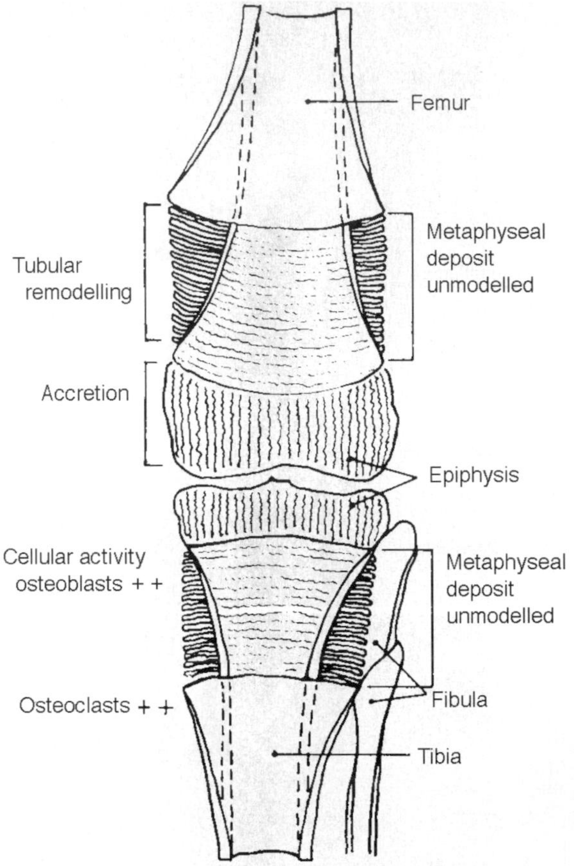

Figure 2.35 Showing tubular and accretion remodelling by osteoblastic and osteoclastic function to give the normal shape of a long bone.

The marrow cavity is also widened during remodelling by osteoclastic activity on the endosteal surfaces of cortex and spongiosa.

Following pathological states, such as fracture repair (Figure 2.36), bony ankylosis of a joint and in response to increased mechanical stresses, etc., there is also remodelling to restore the original morphological identity and purpose of bone.

The association or presence of osteoclasts wherever bone resorption is taking place is obvious, and electron microscopy has shown the passage of bone crystals from the host into these cells (Robinson, 1952; Fitten Jackson, 1957).

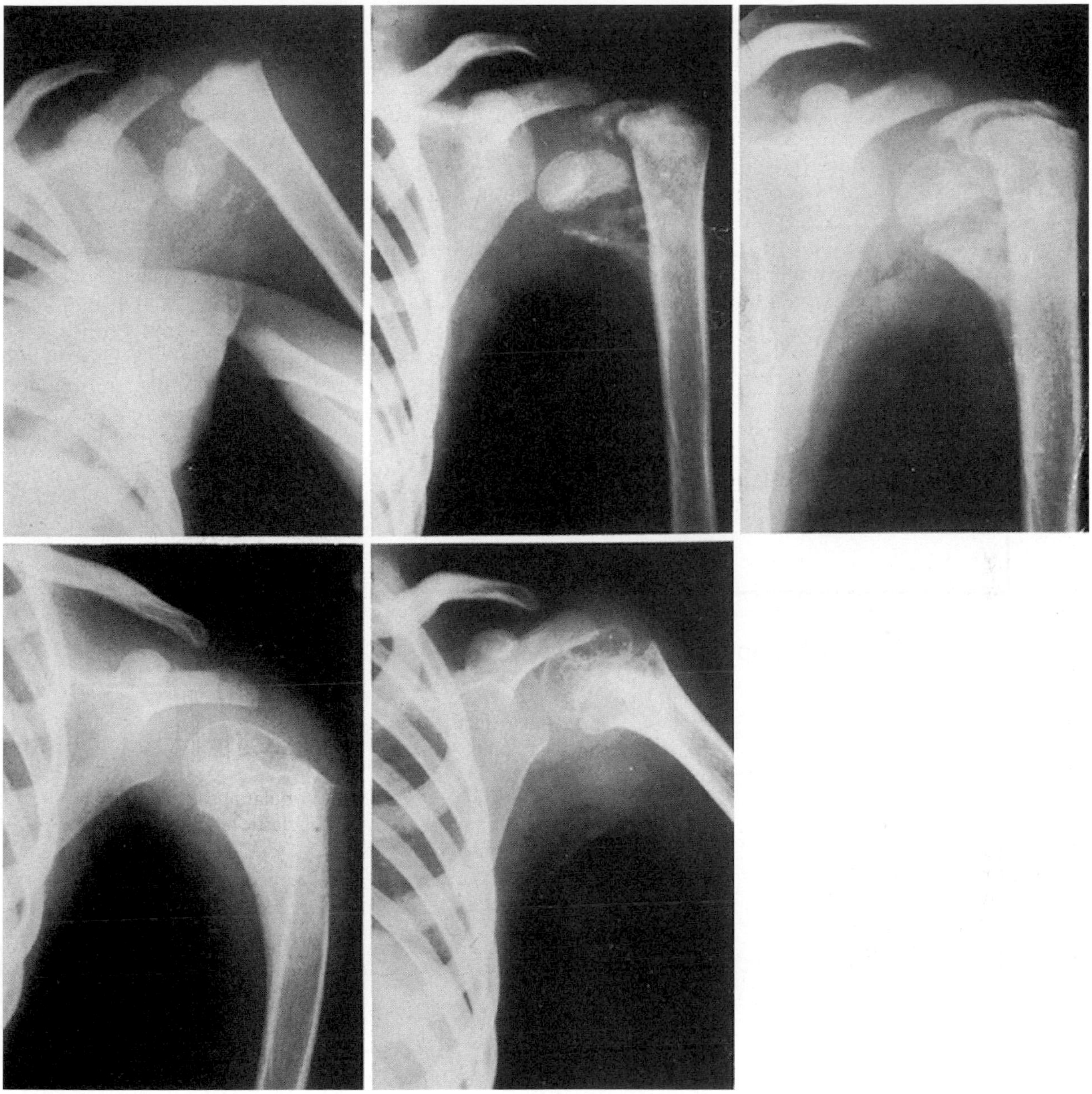

Figure 2.36 Serial radiographs to show the repair and remodelling of an epiphyseal fracture with dislocation of the left humerus over a period of 18 months.

Skeletal growth and development

Growth is defined as an increase in the total mass and size of a body (Weiss, 1939). This must be differentiated from development in which there is maturation and differentiation of tissues and organs necessary to form and complete the whole individual. Whereas longitudinal bone growth is relatively simple to assess by measurement, determination of skeletal maturity depends on the rate and duration of osteogenesis as observed radiographically. However, it is the balance between growth and development which determines the ultimate stature of the individual. For example, if growth and skeletal maturation are both slowed, the ultimate height will be unchanged. However, if growth is slowed while maturation is undisturbed the ultimate stature attained is smaller.

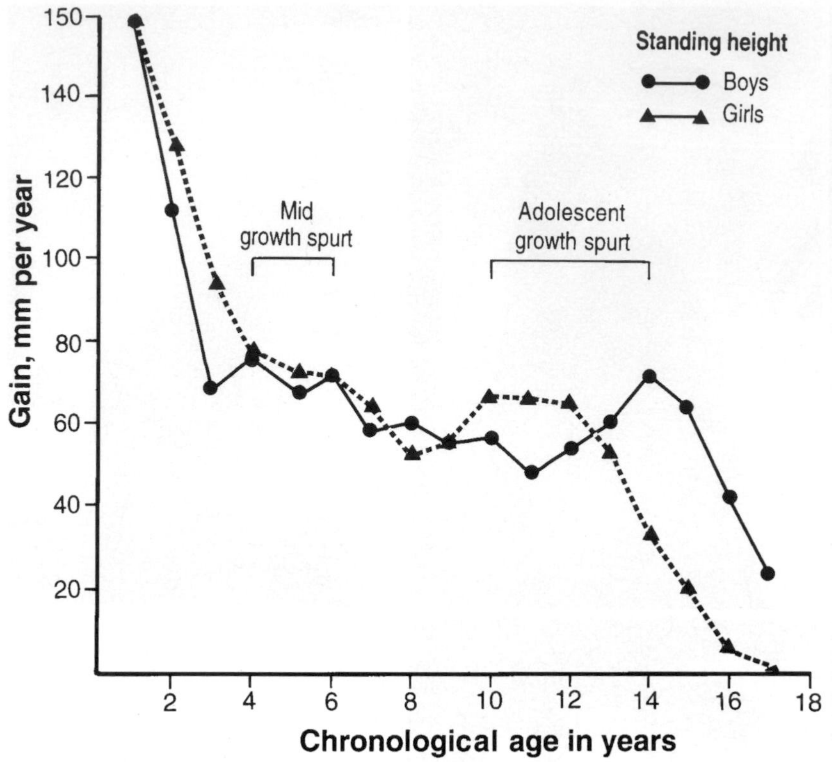

Figure 2.37 Change in height of boys and girls with age in the normal population. (Duthie, R. B. (1958) *Clinical Orthopaedics*, 14.8, with permission)

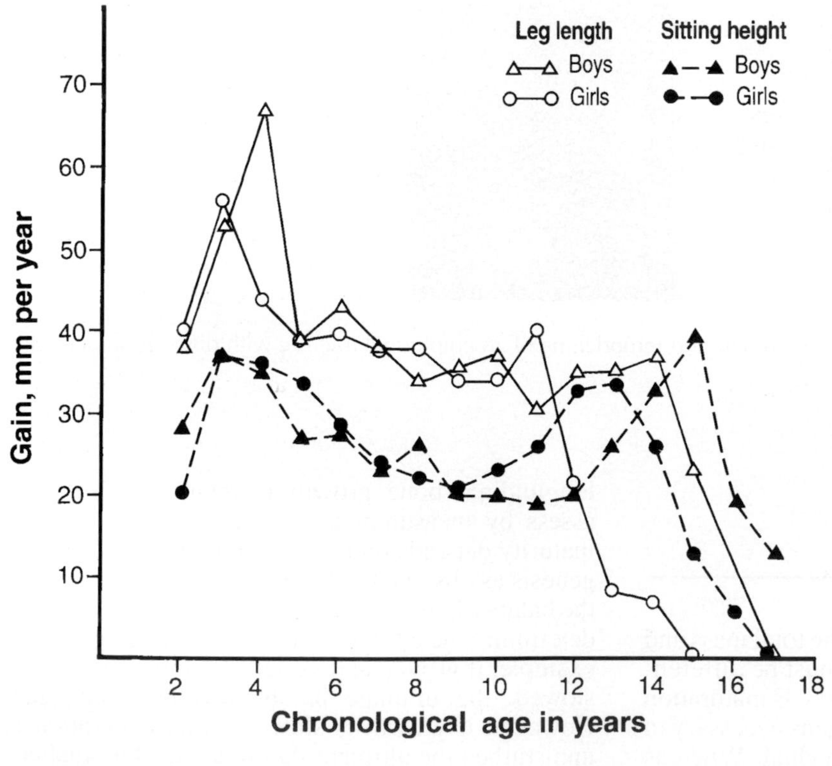

Figure 2.38 Alteration of growth velocity with age – leg length and sitting height. (Duthie, R. B. (1958) *Clinical Orthopaedics*, 14.9, with permission)

The earliest longitudinal study of skeletal growth was carried out by Count Philibert de Montbeillard, who measured the height of his son from 1759 to 1777. Since that time charts have been constructed from measurements of a large number of children of the relationship of height to age in a normal population (Figures 2.37 and 2.38) (Tanner, 1955, 1972). Because of individual variation there is a considerable spread in the figures for a given age and these are normally represented by centile lines. The limits of normality are usually considered as the 97% and 3% centiles, but by definition 6% of normal children will lie outside these lines. Furthermore, the growth of an individual child may follow a curve of substantially different shape and even in healthy children the growth curve often crosses centile lines, particularly early in life. After the age of 2 years, however, each child tends to follow the same centile growth curve, so that deviation may signal a pathological process. Deviation may occur again, however, at puberty since the onset of the pubital growth spurt occurs at differing ages in differing children.

Growth velocity curves may also be plotted (see Chapter 5). In the first year after birth body length increases by approximately 50% and this rapid increase continues to a lesser extent in the second year of life. Thereafter growth settles to approximately 5–6 cm/year until the 'adolescent growth spurt' which begins at between 10 and 11 years in girls and between 12 and 13 years in boys. The spurt lasts for between 2 and 2.5 years.

Height age equals the age at which the child's height falls on the 50th percentile – a useful value when correlated with skeletal maturation. Growth velocity is height increment over 1 year, and can vary considerably from year to year due to measuring artefacts (measuring only a small figure), illness or catch-up growth.

Anthropometric measurements are:

1. Sitting height – can be measured more accurately than head and trunk height, but requires standard equipment.
2. Upper and lower limb segment ratios (US/IS). IS = symphysis pubis to the floor inside the heel. US = total height × IS. For example, in caucasians, the US/IS is:
   (a) infant 1.7
   (b) aged 7–10 years 1.0
   (c) adult 0.95
3. Arm span equals the total height ± a few centimetres; it is useful to determine if short stature is proportionate or not (e.g. short-limbed dwarf has a high US/IS and an arm span less than total height).

Skeletal maturity is determined by:

1. The Greulich–Pyle method is most popular in the USA: a radiograph of the hand is compared with a set of standard films at different ages – different for boys and girls; different bones of the hand may mature at different rates, so greatest reliance is placed on metacarpal and phalangeal centres.
2. Tanner's method gives each bone a maturity rating, and the scores are weighted and combined to give an index of skeletal maturity.

Appearance of epiphyses is delayed in cretinism and epiphyseal dysplasias, and in these cases give no indication of bone age. Height age and bone age are useful in investigating short stature.

SEX DIFFERENCES

It is commonly recognized that boys may be slightly larger at birth and grow slightly faster than girls during the first year, but between the ages of 1 and 9 years the growth velocities in both sexes are about the same. However, the girl starts her adolescent growth spurt 2 years earlier than the boy and grows faster and longer before slowing up in every direction except pelvic growth. During the first 3 years there is increase in leg length in boys which levels off until the adolescent growth spurt, which allows an extended time for growing by boys; therefore their legs once again become longer (Figure 2.38). At this time there is an increased pelvic width in girls and an increased shoulder width in boys. In considering the sitting height as an indicator of the adolescent growth spurt, this occurs earlier in girls and is followed by a more prolonged one in boys.

PREDICTION OF ADULT HEIGHT

By the second birthday, the child should have joined his/her genetic curve which is the basic determinant of height and it becomes possible to predict adult height. A single measurement of height is of little use and the child should be measured serially over a per-iod of time because of alterations of the growth rate with the seasons. The prediction of adult height can be improved if the parents' heights are taken into consideration. Weech has produced the following equation:

$$H_n = 0.545\,H_2 + 0.544\,A + \text{either } 14.84 \text{ (for boys) or } 10.09 \text{ (for girls)}$$

where H_n is height in inches at maturity, H_2 is height in inches at age 2 years, and A is mean height in inches of the parents.

The bone age is also important in this assessment and for girls there is the age at menarche.

ASSESSMENT OF BONE AGE

Skeletal maturity and growth curves be determined either by the Greulich–Pyle method or Tanner's method.

Atlases have been constructed from radiographs of the hand and wrist of children of differing ages, ethnic groups and socioeconomic background. There is a different set for girls and boys. The bones in the hand mature at different rates, so greater reliance is placed on the metacarpal and phalangeal ossification centres.

Tanner's method, based upon a European well nourished Caucasian population, gives each bone a maturity rating and the scores are weighted and combined to give an index of skeletal maturity.

FACTORS AFFECTING SKELETAL GROWTH

Genetic factors

Total stature synaptotype and age of onset of puberty are genetically determined. So too is the sequence of ossification although the timing of ossification may be modified by environmental factors.

Maternal factors

Maternal nutrition, vitamin deficiencies, toxaemia or smoking will affect the embryo directly by changing the environment in which the fetus is growing, or by changing the metabolic or endocrine background. This is well illustrated by the cretin of a hypothyroid mother with marked abnormality in both osseous growth and development.

Children born to alcoholic mothers may have features characteristic of the 'fetal alcoholic syndrome' in which there are facial and other abnormalities and subsequent growth and development are retarded.

Environmental factors

Longitudinal growth is faster in spring than in autumn whereas growth in weight is faster in the autumn than in the spring.

Sociological factors

Children in the top socioeconomic group in England are taller than the children of unskilled labourers. There is a similar but less marked difference in weight in the early years. However, after the onset of puberty an inverse relationship exists between social class and obesity.

Emotional factors

Emotional disturbances are not an uncommon cause of failure to grow normally and this effect may be mediated hormonally.

Nutritional factors

Sufficient food is essential for normal growth. Human malnutrition involves not only a deficiency of calories but a lack of specific foodstuffs and it is impossible to separate the two. Nutritional dietary deficiencies of calcium, phosphorus and vitamins A, C and D are well known disorders which produce disturbance of calcification, ossification and hence total growth. Alterations of skeletal growth closely follow changes in the increase of total body weight. A significant period of skeletal growth arrest causes the formation of transverse lines which is seen radiographically at the ends of long bones. These lines usually indicate periods of prolonged illness or nutritional deprivation affecting the developing bone.

Hormonal factors

The influence of hormonal factors on the growth plate has been outlined above. As a result of these effects and general actions on the body, hormonal dysfunction has profound effects on skeletal growth and maturation (Table 2.6). See also Chapter 5.

Growth hormone

Growth hormone or somatotrophin is a polypeptide hormone secreted by the anterior lobe of the pituitary gland. It is released episodically from the anterior pituitary in response to a variety of stimuli, most physiological of which are stress, exercise and sleep. It has widespread effects throughout the body, the majority of which are mediated by one of three secondary polypeptides termed the somatomedins which are synthesized in the liver. Growth hormone (GH) acts to maintain protein synthesis and inhibit synthesis of fat and oxidation of carbohydrate. $^{35}SO_4$ incorporation into costal, tibial, nasal or xiphoid cartilage and ^{3}H thymidine incorporation into chondrocyte nuclei are increased by GH administration to

Table 2.6 Hormones known to be concerned with growth and development of the skeleton

Growth hormone	Time of max. effect: 5–15 years	Longitudinal growth as a result of: Increased rate of division / Increased in size } of cells of the proliferating and hypertrophic zones of the epiphysial cartilage plate; Increase in amount of matrix: 1. Collagen synthesis (experimentally increased proline → hydroxyline) 2. Synthesis of carbohydrate protein complexes (sulphation factor → ^{35}S uptake)
Thyroid hormone		Appearance at normal age of secondary ossification centres Controls form and shape of ossification centres and the maturation of the epiphyseal cartilage plate
Androgens	Time of max. effect: prepuberty	Limited stimulation of linear growth (due to increased nitrogen retention effect) Marked acceleration of maturation of epiphyseal cartilage plate, resulting in cessation of growth and epiphyseal closure
Oestrogens	Time of max. effect: prepuberty	Inhibition of linear growth Acceleration of maturation of epiphyseal cartilage plate, cessation of growth and epiphyseal closure
Glucocorticoids	Inhibit longitudinal growth (physiological significance unknown)	Retards cellular proliferation and hypertrophy of epiphyseal cartilage plate. Inhibits collagen synthesis Inhibits synthesis of carbohydrate–protein complexes
Insulin		Is essential to proper action of growth hormone Stimulates incorporation of sulphate into protein–polysaccharide complexes ([^{3}H]-uridine into RNA, [^{3}H]-thymidine into DNA) } Similar to action of sulphation factor

hypophysectomized rats but not to normal rats (Denko and Bergenstahl, 1955; Murphy *et al.*, 1956; Kember, 1971). From this work, GH is seen to stimulate chondrocyte proliferation and matrix production, but has no effect on the maturation process that causes cartilage to be replaced by bone. Growth hormone is without effect on isolated chick, rabbit or human chondrocytes (Ashton and Francis, 1977).

These observations led to the proposal that GH has no direct effect on skeletal tissues but mediates its effect *in vivo* via the somatomedin group of peptides which are released by the liver. However, human growth hormone is reported to enhance proliferation of isolated human articular chondrocytes by 97% in the presence of normal human but not fetal calf serum (Scranton *et al.*, 1975).

The group of plasma peptides known as the somatomedins are believed to mediate the *in vivo* effects of growth hormone on the skeleton. Bioassays, radioreceptor and radioimmunoassays have been used to quantify somatomedin activity in plasma as a result of which the somatomedins have been implicated in various growth disturbances as well as in the control of normal development both in childhood and adolescence as well as during fetal life. The last-mentioned situation may be one in which hormones other than GH can promote somatomedin production.

At least eight somatomedin peptides have been isolated and characterized to some extent. In general, they enhance cell replication, and proteoglycan, collagen and RNA synthesis in cartilage, most of these studies having used rat, rabbit, chick or porcine tissue.

Changes in plasma somatomedin activity have been correlated with growth in the human fetus, during childhood and adolescence, and also with growth disorders in both man and experimental animals. However, insufficient suitable preparations of the somatomedins have so far been available to test conclusively their *in vivo* effects on skeletal development (Lebovitz and Eisenbarth, 1975).

Typically, the effects of somatomedins on cartilage *in vitro* include an increase in chondroitin sulphate synthesis, protein and RNA synthesis, chondrocyte proliferation and collagen synthesis – i.e. all the effects which can be produced *in vivo* on skeletal tissue by growth hormone administration.

Somatomedin action in cartilage *in vitro* is sensitive to specific inhibitory factors and also to modulation by other hormones, notably the corticosteroids. Somatomedin peptides may thus offer a fine control mechanism for normal skeletal growth.

The most dramatic effects of growth hormone in the intact animal are on growth. Growth hormone appears to be unnecessary for interuterine growth since achondroplastic infants, in whom there is a failure of pituitary development, are of normal size. It may be that the fetus is dependent on the maternal hormone or on placental lactogen which may stimulate somatomedin production in the infant. At or soon after birth the animal becomes dependent on its own growth hormone for further growth and growth hormone deficient infants have a lower than normal growth velocity. Apart from reduced linear growth of skeletal bones, growth hormone deficiency also leads to delayed maturation of the skeleton and reduced bone and muscle bulk. Adipose tissue is increased.

In contrast, pituitary overfunction results in increased chondrogenesis and longitudinal growth of the skeleton with resultant gigantism or acromegaly. The administration of human growth hormone to growth hormone deficient children results in an advance in bone maturation and a correction of the impaired growth velocity caused by the growth hormone lack. However, administration of growth hormone to non-growth hormone deficient children of short stature or to children whose poor growth is not primarily due to isolated growth hormone deficiency does not improve the growth rate.

Sex hormones

Girls aged 8–10 years mature skeletally more quickly than boys but in girls of 10–15 years the process is slower relative to boys of the same age. These differences in skeletal maturation are probably related to differences in the levels of gonadal hormones.

Testicular deficiency delays epiphyseal growth plate closure which would normally occur at or after puberty, resulting in an extended period of growth with disproportionate overgrowth of the long bones.

Both bone growth and maturation are increased during androgen treatment. However, bone maturation may exceed growth in height and premature growth plate closure may result in a decreased ultimate height.

The level of oestrogen in the blood influences the timing of closure of the epiphyses.

Thyroid hormone

Thyroid hormone deficiency in man results in impaired linear growth and delayed ossification of the skeleton, while hyperthyroidism can cause a short-term increase in the linear growth rate but also accelerate skeletal ossification.

Thyroxine administration does not affect the neogrowth in normal animals although it enhances osseous maturation. Growth hormone and thyroxine have a synergistic effect in increasing bone length *in vivo* although thyroxine alone or in combination with growth hormone has no effect on epiphyseal plate width.

Excessive glucocorticoid treatment in children retards both linear growth and osseous maturation and also prevents the improved growth normally seen with growth hormone treatment in hypopituitary children.

Local factors on bone growth

General skeletal development cannot progress normally without a well regulated metabolic environment. In addition, mechanisms acting locally may alter the rate of growth of individual long bones by their influence on the growth plate cartilage. These local factors (extensively reviewed and referenced by Houghton; see Houghton and Dekel, 1979; Houghton and Rooker, 1979) are particularly important for the understanding of the effects on growth, of pathological processes and surgical procedures in skeletally immature individuals.

Intramedullary trauma

In 1867, Ollier was the first to demonstrate that any intramedullary trauma could give rise to slight long bone overgrowth. The effect was attributed to an interruption of the medullary vascular supply, with increased periosteal vascularity at the ends of the diaphysis. Later experiments in growing rabbits failed to show consistent growth stimulation because trauma which was sufficient only to interrupt the medullary blood vessels and not produce hyperaemia failed to stimulate growth.

Foreign materials in the medullary cavity

Von Langenbeck in 1869 noted a stimulation of growth after the insertion of an ivory plug into the medullary cavity of the dog. Since this time, many substances (e.g. metals and chemicals) have been used with positive results.

It is well known that infective processes adjacent to the growth plate may stimulate growth. If the infection is confined to the medullary bone then this stimulation may be marked. Indeed, von Langenbeck noted that if his intramedullary ivory pegs became infected, growth stimulation was increased.

Despite the uncertainties of experimental results, attempts have been made to stimulate long bone growth in treating leg length inequality, by the insertion of foreign materials into children's long bones, but with little success.

Obstruction of the medullary cavity by tumour (e.g. neurofibromatosis) has been considered to cause increased bone growth and fibrous dysplasia.

Arteriovenous fistulae

Broca first reported, in 1856, increased growth of both femur and tibia in a child with arteriovenous aneurysm immediately distal to the inguinal ligament; other cases have been described since.

Following these clinical reports there followed experimental and clinical attempts to stimulate long bone growth by creating arteriovenous fistulae (e.g. Janes and Jennings, 1961). Their studies showed that growth stimulation was generally achieved, but the amount was variable and not related to age or size of vessels anastomosed. Unfortunately, the method has the severe complication of cardiac failure and it has been largely abandoned.

Distal to the arteriovenous fistula, there was venous hypertension and venous stasis, often with the formation of varicose veins and ulcers.

Venous stasis with a fall in $P\text{O}_2$ and pH is thought to be the feature of arteriovenous fistulae which stimulates the growth plate, and has been tried in many experiments, with changes in oxygen tensions in the different zones of the growth plate (Brighton and Heppenstall, 1971).

Nutrient artery occlusion

The nutrient artery is responsible for about 80% of the bone blood supply; when it is occluded, metaphyseal vessels become the major source with a redistribution of bone blood vessels. It is the redistribution which is thought to be responsible for the overgrowth, although this has not been a constant finding.

More extensive disturbance of bone vascularity may be achieved by extensive stripping of the periosteum from the underlying cortex with stimulation of the growth plate.

Periosteal stripping

Successful growth stimulation after periosteal stripping was first described in 1867 by Ollier, who produced an increase in growth of 2–5 mm in rabbit tibiae. Many experimental and clinical reports have confirmed this finding but the stripping must be confined to the shaft, as permanent growth arrest will result from stripping of the perichondrium.

The entire shaft should be stripped, as a much smaller increase in growth is produced when only one surface of the bone is stripped. The widely accepted view is that growth stimulation is due to changes in vascularity, especially the delay in venous drainage.

It has been suggested that release of the periosteum may mechanically take a restraining force away from the growth plate and thus allow increased growth (Crilly, 1972). Further evidence has shown that the periosteum and the tension within it may have a strong mechanical influence on the growth plate (Houghton and Rooker, 1979). A recent study has shown that longitudinal bone growth is increased after circumferential periosteal division even in the absence of a blood supply (Houghton and Dekel, 1979).

Diversion of blood to bones

Since the pioneering work of Ollier, who tried arterial diversion to rabbit bones with negative results, subsequent workers have had little success with this method. Although patent arteriomedullary anastomoses have been created, the vascular arrangement within the bones rapidly returns to normal after the anastomosis has been established (Dickerson and Duthie, 1963).

Poliomyelitis

Shortening of the limb affected by poliomyelitis usually occurs. Initial stimulation in the early stages of the disease may continue for the first year of paralysis, but subsequent slowing of the growth is inevitable. The initial growth stimulation may be due to bone hyperaemia present in the early stages of the disease. It is known that neurons of the sympathetic nervous system are frequently affected in the disease and this has been held responsible for the observed vascular changes. The other theory is that paralysis reduces pressure on the growth plates and allows an accelerated rate of growth. The later slowing of growth may then be due to a reduction of bone nutrition or an increased pressure across the growth plate after the development of contractures.

In a study of 550 children, Ring (1957) noted that shortening was proportional to reduced muscle bulk, which resulted in reduced vascularity of the bone. He concluded that a mechanical effect was an unlikely cause of shortening.

Sympathectomy

That sympathectomy may result in increased growth has been known for over a century. But many studies of sympathectomy carried out in various animals have failed to show any growth stimulation.

Clinical data have been equally variable; moreover, in the earlier cases the limbs were measured clinically, and so recorded leg length differences are unreliable.

Despite these uncertain results it can be said that sympathectomy is more likely to be effective in stimulating growth in humans than in experimental animals. This perhaps merely reflects a better understanding of the anatomy of the sympathetic nervous system in the human.

The growth effects of sympathectomy are probably secondary to vasomotor changes of reduced vasoconstriction with increased blood flow around the growth plate.

Sympathetic denervation gives rise to hyperaemia of the skeleton, as well as the well known vasodilatory effects on peripheral tissues.

Peripheral nerve section

In 1860, Milne Edwards divided the mandibular nerve of a puppy and noted hypertrophy of the mandible. Other early workers showed that there was a stimulation of bone growth in the leg but that the width was reduced after division of the peripheral nerves. Further studies in different animals have shown no effect on growth in length.

Any observed growth stimulation following motor nerve division has been attributed to either altered mechanics or disturbances in the bone blood supply. Decreased muscle tension may give rise to less compression across the growth plates, with consequent stimulation of growth.

Motor denervation results in decreased limb circulation, and many authors believe this is responsible for growth retardation (Geiser and Trueta, 1958).

Heat

Heating animal skeletons by an electric wire or short-wave diathermy has been shown to give growth increase.

The positive effect on growth of heating the epiphyseal region is believed to be due to secondary hyperaemia, and it was suggested (Ring, 1961) that the growth changes in polio are due to changes in temperature secondary to hyperaemia about the growth plate.

x-Irradiation

In the rabbit, Baunach reported that a small dose of x-rays leads to a brief growth stimulation, but larger doses result in growth retardation which is more pronounced in younger animals. This finding has been confirmed by other investigators in other animal species.

Immobilization

Temporary increased growth has been noted following plastering, tendon division, etc., and it is believed that these effects are secondary to immobilization. However, sustained immobilization in either man or experimental animals results in reduced growth and atrophy. It has been noted that the muscle atrophy of disuse is proportional to the observed growth retardation (Ring, 1957, 1961). Normal muscle function is therefore essential for normal bone development.

Plastering a child's lower extremity, when prolonged, leads to premature closure of the growth plate.

From the evidence available it seems that the growth changes noted during immobilization are due mainly to changes in bone blood supply. Altered mechanical forces probably exert a minor influence at the beginning of the period of immobilization, but despite the reduction of muscular compressive forces across the growth plate, bone growth becomes retarded during prolonged immobilization.

Mechanical forces

Although the general shape and development of a long bone will appear relatively normal in the absence of mechanical forces, the rate of growth and the finer details of the bone require finely balanced mechanical forces if a normal limb is to develop. Persistent postural deformities are well known to cause structural change in clinical practice (e.g. a long-standing compensatory curve associated with structural scoliosis, or secondary tibial torsion associated with excessive femoral neck anteversion), and the phenomenon has been further studied in experimental animals.

The mode of action of the altered mechanics is explained by the 'loi de Delpech' (Delpech in 1829), and the 'Heuter–Volkmann law' (Heuter in 1862; Volkmann in 1862). These state that a compressive force acting on the growth plate slows growth, whereas a tensile force stimulates growth. This is the principle behind the cast treatment of infant skeletal deformity and gives the illusion of plasticity of the immature skeleton.

The force exerted at the growth plate is very high, although it can be modified by abnormal stresses of low intensity in the vicinity of the epiphysis. It has been calculated that the force exerted at the proximal tibial growth plate in man is about 400 kg – that being the force needed to break a Blount staple (Blount and Zeier, 1952). These relatively large forces have led to the failure of epiphyseal stapling in many instances. Inhibition of growth appears to be proportional to the duration of pressure applied to the growth plate. The constant (except during recumbency) force of gravity probably has an important effect on the growth plates of the weight-bearing joints.

The growth plate responds to pressure by narrowing; then there is progressive distortion of the cartilage columns, with horizontal fissures, vascular invasion and eventual bony fusion between the epiphysis and metaphysis (Siffert, 1956; Amako and Honda, 1957).

The effects of tensile forces across the growth plate have received much less attention than the effects of compressive forces.

Distraction applied to the epiphyses has led to increased growth with a noted increase in the width of the growth plate. The technique of epiphysiolysis or callostosis is being used for leg-length discrepancy and will be described in detail later (see Chapter 6).

Fracture

Although Truesdell is attributed as being the first to describe longitudinal bone growth stimulation after fracture, the phenomenon was know to Ollier and von Langenbeck. Many experiments and clinical studies have confirmed these earlier findings. Authors noted growth stimulation of the fractured bone. In addition, there is some evidence that there is an increase in growth of all the long bones of the injured limb.

Clinical series have been studied to ascertain the features which predispose to the variable stimulation seen after fracture. It seems that maximal stimulation occurs at about 8 years of age, and in diaphyseal fractures with overlap.

The cause of the long bone overgrowth is not known, but there are numerous factors operating simultaneously and each of these may contribute to the stimulation. Changes in the blood supply during the fracture repair may well be the most important growth stimulus. In addition, it is well known that maximal stimulation occurs after rigid osteosynthesis when little or no callus is present. This finding supports the idea that blocking of the medullary canal (by callus, screws or rods) activates the periosteal circulation so that blood is forced into the juxtaepiphyseal circulation (Trueta and Cavadias, 1964). The change of periosteal circulation has long been considered to be an important factor.

The mode of action of altered vascularization can simply be that if there is an increased blood supply, there is a concomitant increase in nutrients and thus a stimulation of growth. A reduction in blood supply would have the reverse effect.

For further discussion of skeletal growth and development see Chapter 5.

Fracture healing

Healing of a fracture is a remarkable process since it results not in a scar but in reconstitution of the injured tissue into something resembling its original form. The changes associated with fracture healing may be considered as a series of phases which overlap but occur sequentially. These are the phase of what is loosely called inflammation. Inflammation is defined as being a localized response of vascularized tissues to injury (chemical, physical or biological) with cardinal signs of redness, swelling, heat and pain. This is better described using biological terms as a phase of immediate injury and of defence and demolition (Duthie, 1967) and the phases of healing and regeneration which are concerned with the development of osteogenic repair tissue and the phase of remodelling.

IMMEDIATE INJURY

The immediate injury (Figure 2.43) results in structural and chemical changes in cells and of tissues, which may or may not die; vascular changes (haemorrhage, clotting and exudation); and neurogenic changes. The immediate injury reaction of bone to fracture is similar to that seen in other injuries. Platelets, injured cells, blood vessel and epithelial

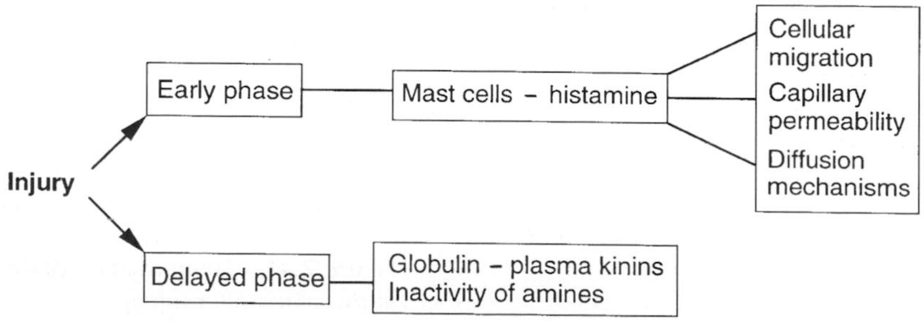

Figure 2.39 The two phases of chemical changes after injury.

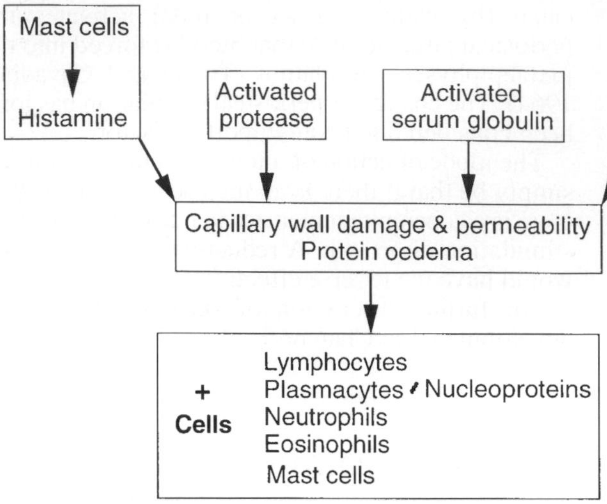

Figure 2.40 The 'agents' affecting the capillary wall after injury, to produce the cellular migration.

cells and macrophages release vasoactive mediators including serotonin, histamine and thromboxane A_2 and growth factors, specifically PDGF and TGFβ. These small proteins influence cell function and matrix synthesis. Miles (1961) described two early phases: an early phase mediated by the local release of histamine from mast cells, platelets and other blood cells; and a delayed phase in which there is activation of peptide systems to form plasma kinins, as well as the globulin permeability factor of Spector and Willoughby (1964) (Figure 2.39). The vasoconstrictor amine, adrenaline, may also be inactivated locally.

Wilhelm (1965) characterized permeability factors into three main groups:

1. the proteases – e.g. plasmin (fibrolytic), kallikrein (vasodepressor) and the globulin permeability factor;
2. the polypeptides – e.g. leucotaxine, bradykinin and kallidin; and
3. the amines – e.g. histamine, 5-hydroxytryptamine, adrenaline and noradrenaline.

These substances are believed to produce increased capillary permeability, cellular migration, small-vessel dilation (similar to the triple response of Lewis) and alteration in the diffusion mechanisms of the intercellular matrix or ground substance (Figure 2.40).

From damaged capillaries or from increased capillary permeability, protein-rich plasma and numerous cells – lymphocytes, neutrophils and eosinophils – leak out. Plasmacytes are thought to be derived from these lymphocytes and are believed to hold or synthesize within their cytoplasm nucleoproteins liberated by the autolysis of cells, the necrosis of tissues and protein leak.

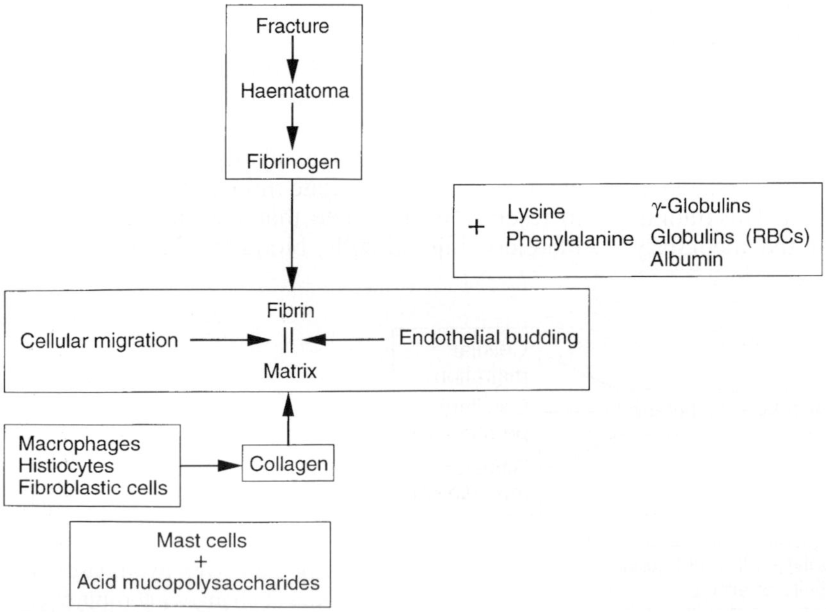

Figure 2.41 The formation of the fibrin matrix after injury.

Following this, a clot of insoluble fibrin forms. This protein is derived from the circulating but soluble fibrinogen by the addition of two amino acids – phenylalanine and lysine – in the presence of thrombin, calcium, platelets and other clotting factors (Figure 2.41). The amino acids are derived from serum albumin, γ-globulin and the globulin of red blood cells from the extravasated blood. Fibrinogenesis provides a screen or framework of fibrin fibres to collect plasma proteins and extravasated cells. This framework is invaded by reticuloendothelial cells (e.g. macrophages, round cells and histiocytes); by endothelial cells, which undergo mitosis to form capillaries; and finally by fibroblasts. The fibrin filaments are orientated to provide a framework for the fibroblasts and capillaries to follow along definite patterns. The fibroblasts arise from undifferentiated mesenchymal cells, and synthesize acid mucopolysaccharides. Although mast cells contain acid mucopolysaccharides in their cytoplasmic granules, they are not the direct source of this material for collagen synthesis.

DEFENCE AND DEMOLITION

In the defence and demolition stage there are significant vascular reactions that affect inflow of tissue fluids and cellular infiltration. The arterioles and efferent veins are particularly involved. There is redistribution of blood flow through capillary channels by shunt mechanisms under ill-understood neurogenic reflexes.

Wray and Lynch (1959) have shown a quantitative increase in vascular volume of fractures by enlargement of existing vessels, as well as formation of new ones. Fibroblastic growth factors may be important for new vessel formation in fracture healing (Simmonds, 1985). Rhinelander and Baragry (1962), in bone microangiographic studies, saw a marked opening of the existing medullary arterial tree within the first day, but it was not until the fourth day that periosteal vessels were seen entering the fracture site. Accompanying these changes, there is a marked cellular infiltration of polymorphonuclear leucocytes, lymphocytes and monocytes. This infiltration alters the physical state of the ground substance from a sol to a gel, as well as producing autolysis, phagocytosis and digestion of debris. Plasmin, with its fibrinolytic and permeability effects, is formed from the circulating but inactive serum protein plasminogen. Plasmin is considered to be able to digest necrotic mesodermal tissues and to release further active substances, and Lack (1962) demonstrated its autolytic digestion of articular cartilage.

HEALING AND REGENERATION

It is at the phase of formation of an osteogenic repair tissue that bone healing begins to differ from other wound healing and the triggering mechanism for this response is unclear.

Blastema formation results from hyperplasia and proliferation of undifferentiated mesenchymal cells, from monocytes, from lymphocytes, and from pseudolymphocytes, which form fibroblasts. The phylogenic characterization or specific naming of cells

Table 2.7 Expression of growth factors in different cell types in fracture healing

Cytokine	Clot	Granulation tissue	Cartilage in #	Osteoblasts in #	Comment
Platelet-derived growth factor (PDGF)	+++	+++	++	+++	Very important in soft tissue healing. Role in bone less clear
Fibroblast growth factor (FGF)	+/–	++	+++	+/–	Important in angiogenesis and cartilage formation
Transforming growth factor β (TGFβ)	++	+++	++	+++	Widely distributed, both in normal bone and fracture repair
Insulin-like growth factor (IGF)	0	++	++	+++	May be important in causing differentiation of bone cells. Osteoblast proliferation *in vitro*
Bone morphogenetic protein (BMP)	0	+	+/–	++	Morphogen (guides stem cells into a bone forming line). May prove therapeutically powerful

+, ++, +++ refers to demonstrated expression on a mRNA or protein basis in fractures. All of these growth factors have effects on bone and cartilage cells, and all have been demonstrated in normal bone matrix. All except PDGF and BMP have effects on endothelial cells and angiogenesis.

Reproduced from Glynne Andrew (1993), p. 538, by kind permission of the Medicine Group (Journals) Ltd.

is much more certain in this stage because their functions and environments are more clearly understood; e.g. fibroblasts form collagen, myxoblasts form ground substance, chondroblasts form cartilage and osteoblasts form bone. Such changes are very rapid. Tonna and Cronkite (1961) demonstrated, within 16 hours of wounding, marked proliferation of local mesenchymal cells making up the periosteum. Within 3 days the proliferative reaction spreads some distance along the shaft away from the fracture site.

There have been many attempts to determine the stimulus for such proliferation. Abercrombie (1964) reviewed various 'wound hormones' and suggested that increased mitosis and increased migration of cells are produced by one chemical stimulus. Neuman demonstrated a possible factor in cell-free extract of human granulation tissue, which accelerated the healing of skin wounds. Needham believed that there was a wound factor in amphibian tissues produced by damaged tissue at the time and site of wounding. Menkin demonstrated that injured cells liberated a growth-promoting factor in the inflammatory exudate.

In bone repair, Bier (1917) thought that the stimulation factor was present in the organized blood clot of the fracture haematoma, and that it promoted new bone formation by the 'chronic irritation of the necrosis and hemorrhage'. It was believed that the stimulation for new bone formation in cranial fractures of rats resided in the inflammatory exudate. However, it was present only after the initial leucocyte invasion had ceased, and was related to the amount of inflammatory reaction after damage to the surrounding muscles.

In 1955, during a study of fracture repair in rats, Duthie and Barker noted the accumulation of mast cells in greater number than those seen in the opposite (control) leg within 48 hours of infliction of the fracture which persisted for the next 7 days. Because of this, it was suggested that their appearance was related to the trauma, and that they might function in the subsequent regeneration processes, especially because of their cytoplasmic content of histamine, heparin and 5-hydroxytryptamine. In a continuation of this study (Duthie, 1962), mast cells were observed during the response of standard fractures to various systemic and hormonal states, as well as to locally applied drugs (Figure 2.42).

Mechanical factors, such as pressure and shearing stresses, were suggested by Glucksman (1939) as possible stimuli, especially since he demonstrated how fibrous tissue was induced to undergo chondrification by such stresses. Experimentally the amount of callus formation can be altered by changing such factors.

Bone-inducing growth factors are found within bone matrix (Hauschka *et al.*, 1986) and release of these from the broken bone ends may contribute to new bone formation. FGF and TGFβ stimulate chondrocyte proliferation, cartilage formation, osteoblast proliferation and bone synthesis (Muthukumaran and Reddi, 1984; Memmeth *et al.*, 1988; Noda and Camillier, 1989; Jingushi *et al.*, 1990) so that TGFβ released by platelets immediately following the injury may play a role in bone induction. Glynne Andrew (1993) has recently reviewed the role of the growth factors throughout the phases of fracture repair (Table 2.7).

Prostaglandins, which are important mediators of inflammation as well as potent stimulators of bone resorption, may play a role in osteogenesis. They have been shown to be produced in high levels from the injured bone and muscle (Dekel *et al.*, 1981). Furthermore, fracture healing in rats is delayed by the administration of indomethacin which is a potent inhibitor of prostaglandin synthesis (Rowe *et al.*, 1976) and the healing of mid-diaphyseal osteotomies in rabbit tibia is accelerated by local infusion of prostaglandins (Voegeli and Chapman, 1985).

The role of local oxygen tension in determining whether bone or cartilage is formed has already been mentioned. In addition, the fracture site is initially acidic, becoming alkaline later. Newman *et al.*, 1985, 1987) have described the use of magnetic resonance spectroscopy *in vivo* technique in studying experimental fractures, to demonstrate the intracallus and intramyocellular pH changes from acidity to alkalinity during the normal progression of healing at the fracture site. The rise in pH may aid the function of alkaline phosphatase, permitting calcification to occur. Finally, the region of a fresh fracture is electronegative, a phenomenon which is independent of applied mechanical stress and this may stimulate osteogenesis (Brighton *et al.*, 1985). Since Urist's original pioneering discovery of bone morphogenetic protein in the 1900s and later, other osteogenic proteins, osteogenin and osteoinductive factors have been isolated and shown to induce bone formation – ectopic sites in animals and now in humans. Amino acid sequences have been analysed for relatively pure source so that human C DNAs have been cloned after isolation. Recombinant human osteogenic protein 1 (also known as bone morphogenetic protein 7) has been combined with an allogenic bone collagen carrier by Cook *et al.* (1994) for restoring defects in the rabbit ulnar diaphysis. In this unique experiment they showed that within 8 weeks there was complete radiographic osseous union with new cortex bone remodelling and marrow elements present. This also was found with an implant of bovine osteogenic protein. Those implanted with collagen carrier alone or with no implant

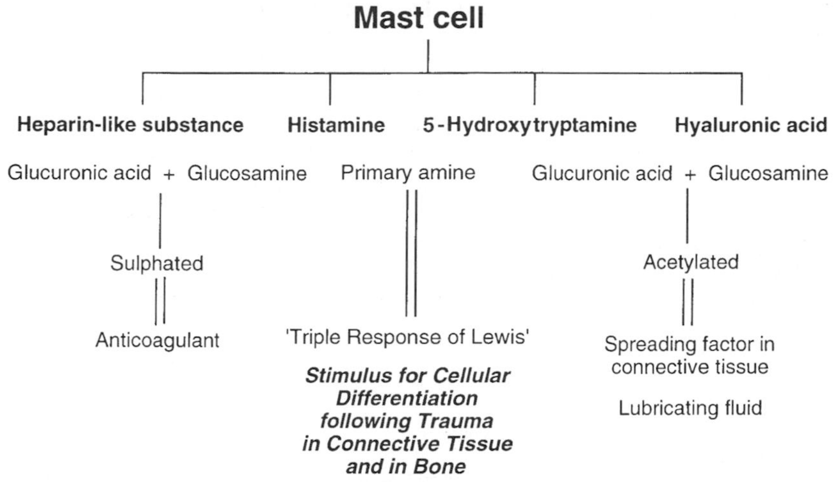

Figure 2.42 Illustrating the chemical substances which have been associated with the mast cell and their possible physiological effects.

showed no bridging of the defect. This may well lead to providing materials for replacing bony defects rather than autogenous, autologous bone grafts.

Dekel and Francis (1981) have demonstrated high concentrations of PGE and F in rabbit experimental fractures and in the surrounding muscle.

Following such cellular differentiation, there is the formation of two regenerative blastemata from the cells possessing osteogenetic activity. From cells in the marrow as well as from the endosteum, there is differentiation of osteoblasts to form osteoid tissue, trabeculae of calcified tissue and finally cancellous bone by intramembranous ossification. Accompanying this there is differentiation of the periosteal cells to form a cartilage blastema which then undergoes the process of endochondral ossification. Chemically, there are two main phases which are so closely intermingled, both spatially as well as in time, that they cannot be differentiated from each other. First, there is the organic phase for healing, which is chiefly concerned with the formation of an intercellular matrix containing chondroitin and the collagen fibrils possibly formed by fibroblasts as well as osteoblasts. Second, there is the mineral phase which is concerned with calcification and ossification both by endochondral and by intramembranous mechanisms. The calcium ion is humeral in origin, whereas the phosphate has to be liberated locally, usually from glycogen of cartilage or other phosphate precursors. It is of interest that the organic phase can only be altered experimentally by such systemic stimuli as cortisone (retarded) or thyroxine (accelerated) and is more sensitive to the local application of the enzyme hyaluronidase, whereas the inorganic and mineral phase of bone repair is much more sensitive to humoral or systemic stimuli of various hormonal, nutritional or vascular factors (Duthie, 1962).

Factors affecting the development of osteogenic repair tissue

The amount and composition of repair tissue varies with the site, type and severity of the fracture, the type of bone involved, the state of the soft tissues surrounding the fracture and whether the fragments are permitted any movement in relation to each other during healing. The following description refers principally to a simple fracture of a long bone in which the fragments are not rigidly immobilized.

There are two sources of repair tissue, medullary and periosteal. The former is most marked in cancellous bone, while the latter predominates in a diaphyseal facture.

Periosteal callus

The potential of periosteum for repair is demonstrated by regeneration of subperiosteally resected bone. Cellular proliferation and hypertrophy begins away from the fracture, often over viable cortex. Repair tissue becomes invaded by osteogenic cells derived from the cambrium (inner) layer of periosteum. If the periosteum is intact, a bridge of callus readily forms, arching over the dead bone ends. If, however, the periosteum is ruptured, cuffs of callus grow outwards from the living bone, eventually joining together (Figure 2.43) (McKibbin, 1978).

In some areas, particularly at the periphery of the callus, a variety of hyaline cartilage forms which becomes converted to bone by endochondral ossification. The amount of cartilage formed is very variable. This may represent a response to low oxygen tension (Ham, 1930; Girgis and Pritchard, 1958), the concept being that if callus outgrows its blood

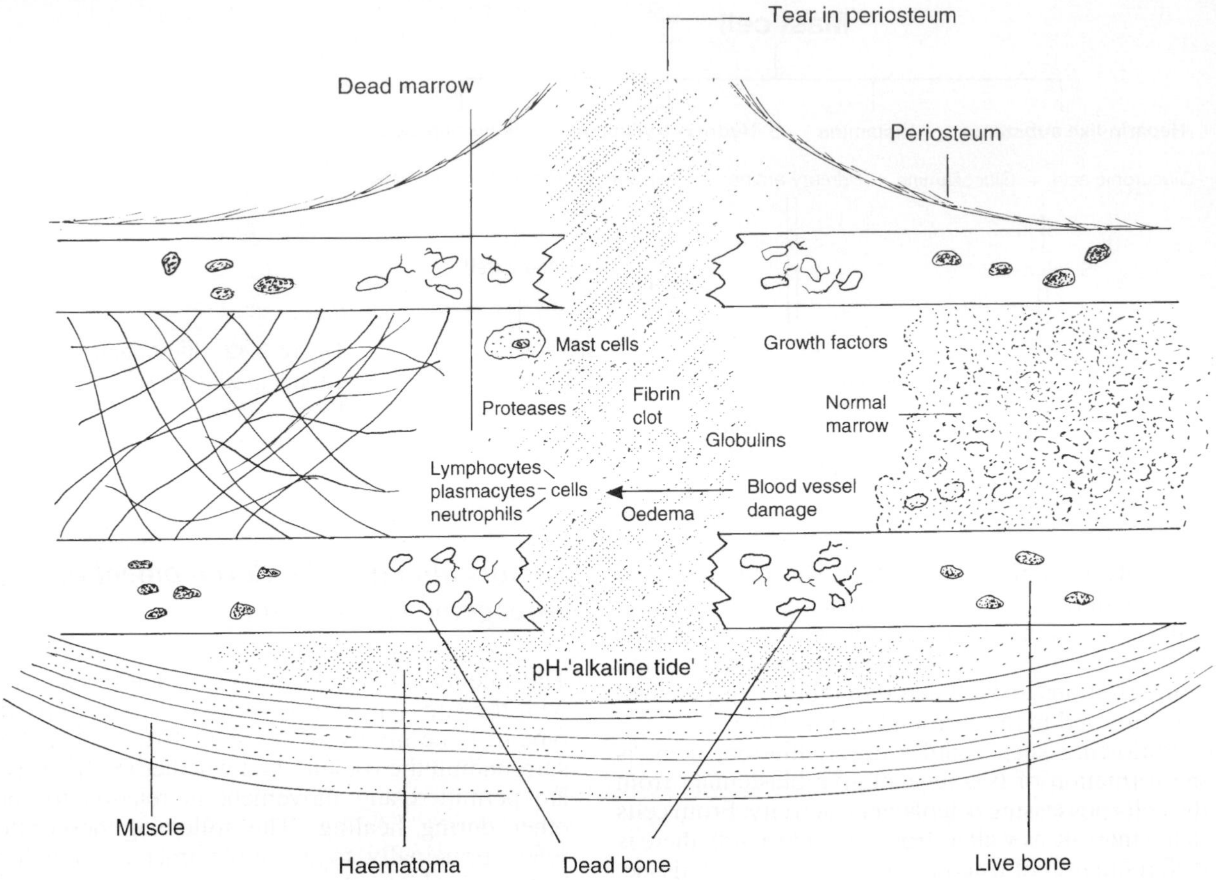

Figure 2.43 Initial events following diaphyseal fracture of the long bone. The periosteum is torn adjacent to the fracture and is stripped from the periosteal surface of the bone, the ends of which become necrotic. Haematoma accumulates around the fracture site, with marked biochemical changes.

supply, cartilage provides a suitable material less demanding of oxygen to bridge the gap until vascularity is re-established (McKibbin, 1978). This view has been challenged by Hulth (1989) who suggests that cartilage is laid down in response to movement of the fracture fragments (Anderson, 1965) and that interfragmentary movement will also inhibit vascular invasion mechanically. This hypothesis is supported by finite element analysis of healing fractures (Blenman *et al.*, 1989).

The blood supply of the periosteal callus comes initially from the periosteal vessels and extraperiosteal soft tissues, including muscle (Gothman, 1961) and only later does the medullary blood supply make a contribution (Rhinelander and Baragry, 1962; Rhinelander *et al.*, 1968). The neovasculature regresses as union occurs and eventually disappears.

Medullary callus

Vascular proliferation in the medullary region is the principal method of union in cancellous bone, for example in a fracture of the tibial plateau, and plays a part in union of the tubular bone, where medullary activity will be particularly marked if the fracture is offset (McKibbin, 1978). The vascular response is slower than that seen in the periosteum (Gothman, 1961).

PHASE OF REMODELLING

Once the fracture has been satisfactorily bridged by callus the newly formed bone is adapted to its new function by the process of remodelling (Figure 2.45). It should be noted that the word 'remodelling' in this context does not refer to the same process as that implied in the 'remodelling cycle'. Indeed, the process which orthopaedic surgeons have for many years been calling 'remodelling' of a fracture corresponds more closely to the 'modelling' which bone biologists describe.

In the context of fracture repair, remodelling refers to the process of readaptation of the skeleton to the loads which will be applied to it. It includes the revascularization and modification of dead bone at the fracture site. In qualitative terms the remodelling process is no different from the process of replacement and repair which is occurring continually within the normal skeleton. However, the activation frequency of bone remodelling units following a fracture is greatly increased. In the dog radius the number is increased from a baseline value of 2.5% of the total number of osteons in a cross-section to over 60% within 8 weeks. This acceleration of remodelling activity does not occur until the third week after fracture and peaks 8 weeks following fracture.

New blood vessels can invade the trabeculae of cancellous bone and bone apposition may take place directly onto the surface of the trabeculum. Once this has happened, the bone may take part in the normal remodelling cycle. This phenomenon is referred to as 'creeping substitution'. In contrast, in cortical bone, although apposition onto the surface of the bone may occur, there will be areas in which the bone cells are dead. In order for these regions to take part in normal bone remodelling, the osteoclastic 'cutter head' must ream out a tunnel down which the new blood supply can enter the bone. The process of revascularization is relatively slow and small areas of dead bone may remain for a considerable length of time following normal fracture union.

SOURCE OF OSTEOGENIC CELLS

There are two possible sources. The cells may arise by differentiation of previously determined osteogenic progenitor cells (DOPC) which are found in the inner layer of the periosteum and within the bone marrow (Owen, 1970) or from previously uncommitted, pluripotent cells from the surrounding soft tissues. These cells are termed inducible osteoprogenitor cells (IOPC; Owen, 1980). The modification of previously undifferentiated soft tissue cells into osteogenic cells is termed bone induction. Although it is not clear to what extent it is important in the healing of a fracture, it is well established that non-specialized cells in extraskeletal sites may be stimulated to form bone (Chalmers *et al.*, 1975).

TYPES OF FRACTURE REPAIR

McKibbin (1978) suggested that fracture repair may be divided into four types with differing time courses and physical requirements. It must be emphasized that these divisions are arbitrary and in a normal fracture it is not possible completely to separate them. They do, however, provide a useful basis for discussion.

Primary callus response

This commences within 2 weeks of injury, forming exuberant external callus, particularly beneath intact periosteum. The callus spreads from the fractured bone end, but if it does not cause union of the bone, it will undergo involution. The primary callus response is relatively independent of environmental and hormonal influences, being an intrinsic property of the fracture and probably involving DOPCs present in the cambium layer of the periosteum.

External bridging callus

If the primary callus response does not result in bone continuity, external bridging callus forms. This stage of callus is under the control of humeral and mechanical influences and probably involves IOPCs from the surrounding soft tissues. The external bridging callus appears rapidly and bridges gaps readily. Its formation depends on the presence of viable external soft tissues which provide the blood vessels for the repair tissue and its appearance is inhibited by rigid fixation. It is, therefore, the predominant form of healing when a simple fracture is treated by cast immobilization or intramedullary nailing (Lane and Werntz, 1987).

Late medullary callus

This often occurs in combination with external bridging callus but is slower in appearance. It is relatively independent of intact external soft tissues, being more dependent on the intramedullary vascularity. It is able to bridge gaps between bone ends and will tolerate a small amount of interfragmentary movement. It is not inhibited by rigid immobilization of the bone ends and it is important in fractures immobilized by rigid plating (see below) (Olerud and Dankwardt-Lilliesterom, 1971). This form of callus is relatively independent of the external soft tissues relying on the medullary blood supply. Bone forming under these circumstances frequently does not show an intermediate stage of fibrocartilage.

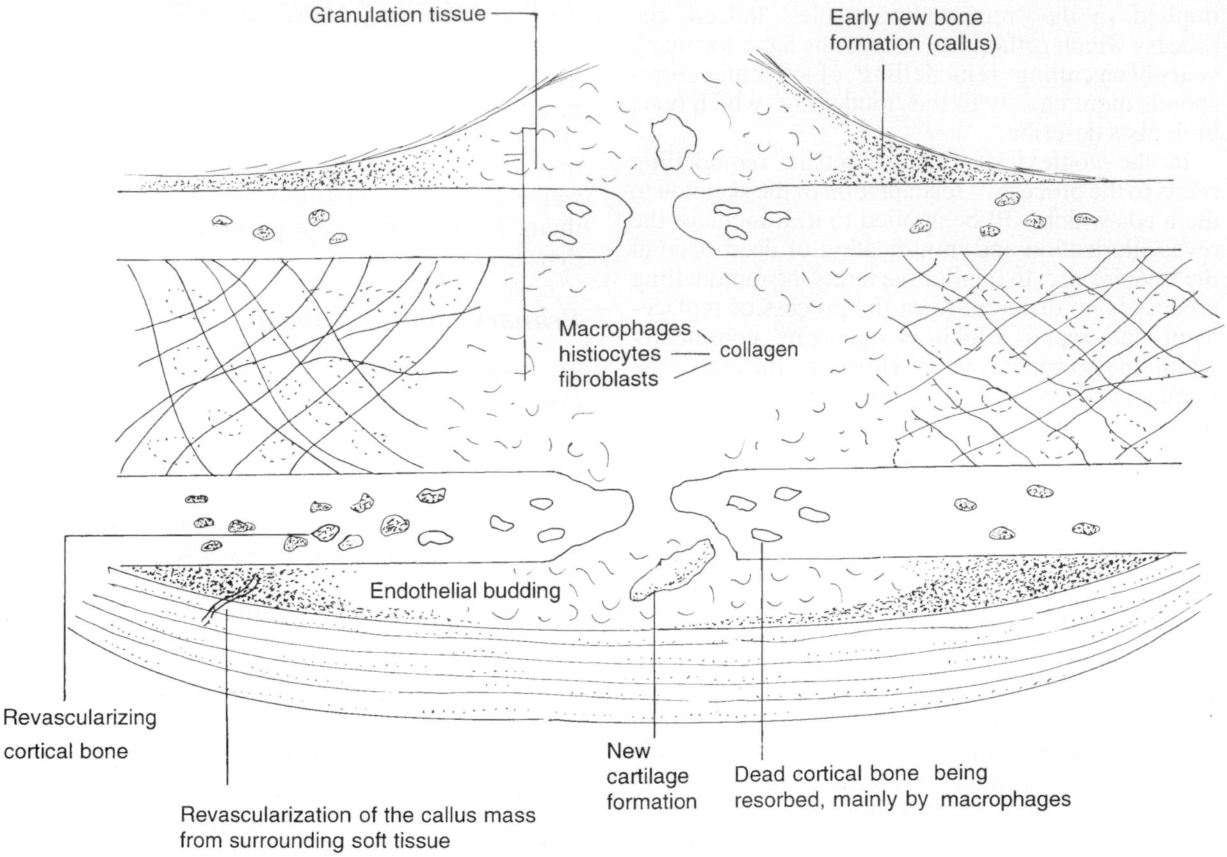

Figure 2.44 Situation some weeks following a diaphyseal fracture in a long bone. The haematoma has organized and early woven bone formation has occurred subperiosteally. Cartilage formation is seen in areas of relative apoxia.

Primary bone union

Primary bone repair is the term given to fracture repair where the fracture ends have been rigidly immobilized by a plate. In the original concept of Lane (1914) and Danis (1949), primary bone healing referred to fractures that healed without radiographically visible callus formation. Schenk and Willinegger (1967) found that when an osteotomy was performed in a dog radius which had been rigidly fixed by a plate, bone deposition occurred on the divided bone ends within a few days, often without preceding osteoclastic resorption. The structure of the newly formed bone depended on the width of the gap; where it was less than 200 μm, the gap was filled by true lamellar bone, whereas larger gaps showed a more irregular pattern. Where the gap exceeded a millimetre, it was not bridged 'in a single jump' by woven bone and complete filling in was considerably delayed (Schenk, 1987). The bone filling the intrafragmentary gap appears *de novo* without intermediate formation of connective tissue or fibrocartilage and it is this absence of an intermediate tissue which distinguishes primary bone repair from that seen under other circumstances. If the interfragmentary gap is small, the lamellae are aligned at right angles to the gap and because woven bone is being laid down *de novo*, the rate of filling of the gap is considerably faster than the normal mineral appositional rate of 0.8–2.5 μm/day.

Gap healing as outlined above is completely intolerant of any movement and will only fill very small gaps (less than 1mm).

Under conditions of rigid fixation, where the two ends of the fracture are in intimate contact, and in the interfragmentary gap once it has been filled in by lamellar bone, normal bone remodelling occurs as outlined above (Figure 2.45).

Distraction osteogenesis

This is not strictly a method of fracture healing. However, it is considered here for completeness. The

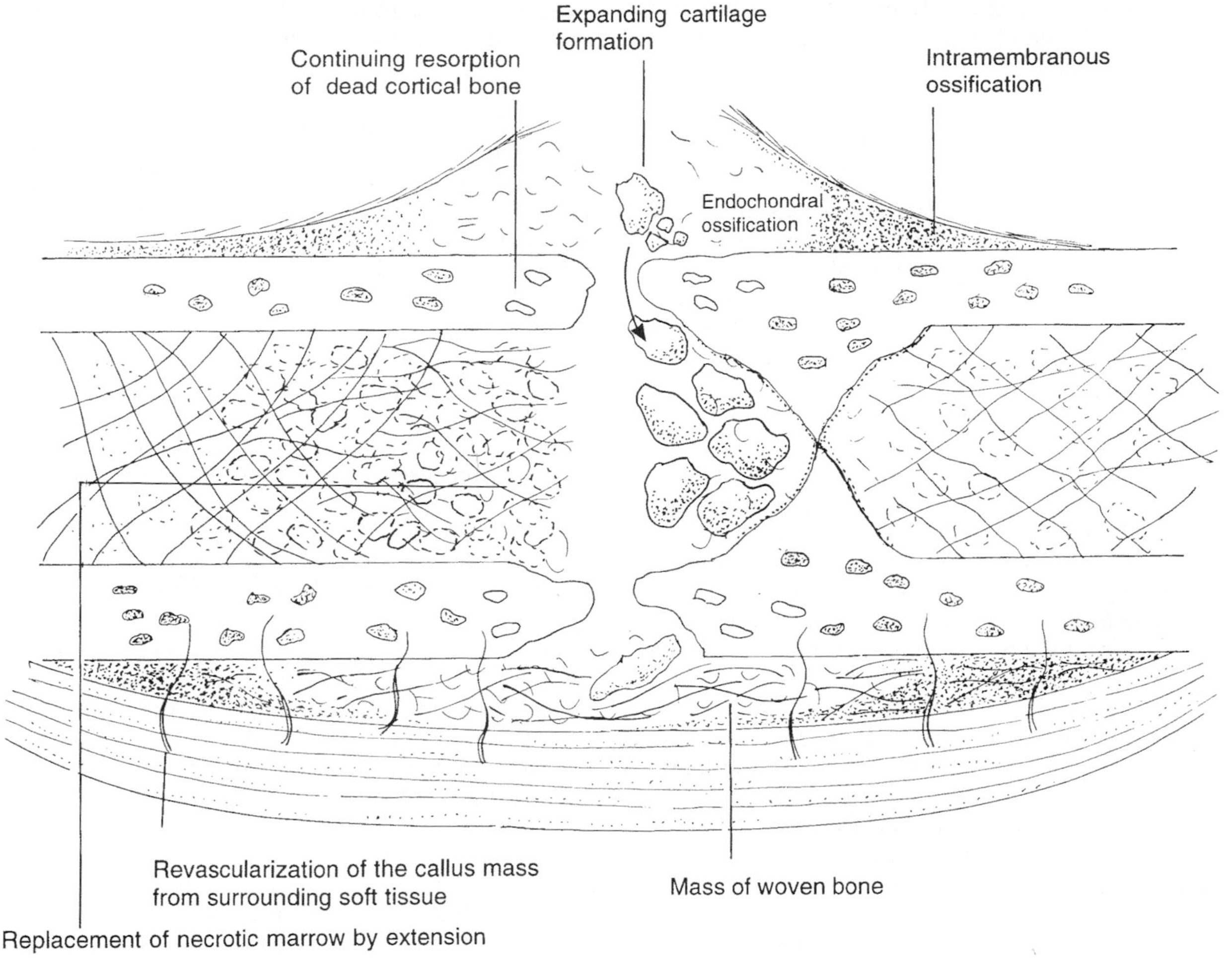

Figure 2.45 A late stage of healing of a diaphyseal fracture. The callus bridge is now complete and the 'dead' bone ends are becoming revascularized, resorbed and intramembranous and endochondral ossification is occurring.

majority of the basic research into this phenomenon was undertaken by Ilizarov (Ilizarov, 1975, 1990). The classic descriptions of bone formation by the AO Group and others rely on compression in order to induce fracture union. Ilizarov demonstrated that mechanical induction of new bone between bony surfaces could occur during gradual distraction. A biological bridge between the surfaces arises from local new blood vessel formation and spans the entire cross-section of the cut surfaces. During distraction, a fibrovascular interface is aligned parallel to the direction of the distraction gap while new bone columns form. New blood vessel formation extends from each medullary surface towards a central fibrous interzone in the distraction gap which remains relatively avascular. Early bone formation occurs by intramembranous ossification and mineralization occurs close to the blood vessels. Bone formation is limited to columns approximately 200 μm long. If mechanical conditions are not optimal, islands of endochondral ossification are seen and the columns of intramembranous ossification become irregular (Aronson *et al.*, 1990; Aronson, 1991).

Transplantation of bone

Bone grafting procedures are frequently required for delayed or non-union of fracture, for stabilization of flail or painful joints, for the correction of bony defects, to fill in cavities caused by tumour, cyst or infection, to aid in the correction of severe deformities and to bridge defects or close epiphyses. Clinical demand for bone grafts is increasing because of improved techniques for limb salvage following tumour resection or severe fracture and because of an increase in the number of failed total joint replacements (Friedlaender and Goldberg, 1991).

HISTORICAL PERSPECTIVE

Wagner reported that in 1867 Ollier was investigating bone grafting in rabbits, cats, dogs and birds. MacEwan in 1881 presented a paper on the transplantation and replacement of a humerus in a patient and followed this by extensive experimental and clinical observations which were published in 'Growth of Bone' in 1912. Between 1909 and 1911 Achausen studied the osteogenic activity of periosteum and concluded that it was highest in autografts and lowest in heterografts. In 1911 Albee established the cortical bone graft and 20 years later Phemister described the use of cancellous graft material.

An autograft is a transfer of tissue into a new site within the same individual. It has the greatest osteogenetic potency, with longest survival of the graft cells and the most rapid revascularization. An isograft is a transplant made from one individual to another genetically identical individual (for example from one identical twin to another, or from one experimental animal to another of the same inbred strain).

An allograft is a transfer made from one individual of the same species. Its antigenicity leads to the rejection phenomenon although the actual site of production is still conjecture.

A heterograft or xenograft is a transfer between individuals of different species. It has a high antigen component which is mainly found in the serum and red cell content of the graft.

If the host site is of the same tissue as that from which the graft was donated, it is called an orthotopic transfer, whereas if it is transferred to a new environment (for example in experimental transplantation of fragments of bone into the anterior chamber of the eye), the term heterotopic transplant is employed.

Duthie (1958) has shown that osteocytes within cortical autografts in tissue culture *in vitro* millipore diffusion chamber systems do not survive longer than 7 days when revascularization is prevented. Also transmission of any osteoinductor substance occurred only when there was physical continuity across the millipore membrane by cell particles. There appears to be an optimum time for transplanting bone into fresh areas of fracture (Siffert, 1961) with more rapid vascularization and greater survival of osteocytes, when carried out 7–10 days after fracture. Urist since 1976 (Urist and Mikulski, 1979; Urist *et al.*, 1982) has prepared allogenic graft material without any hypersensitivity reaction and preserving the morphogenetic osteoinductive potency – a collagenous protein bone morphogenetic protein (BMP).

Transplantation may be further divided according to whether the transplant is living or has been preserved, for example by freeze drying. The transplant may be free or joined to a pedicle containing a blood supply, when it is termed a vascularized transplant.

Preparation of human graft material from one individual to another now includes methods of sterilization against the HIV virus by either antiseptics such as hypochlorite solutions or heat treatment or irradiation by gamma rays. This is in addition to testing the host for the virus and holding and testing the graft material for 90 days before its implantation after retesting the host (see Chapter 11).

BIOLOGY OF BONE GRAFTING

Bone grafts are used for two reasons, to provide structural support or to stimulate osteogenesis, although in many circumstances a combination of these two functions is required.

Stimulation of osteogenesis occurs by a combination of three mechanisms. First, bone cells within the graft may survive the transplantation procedure and synthesize new bone. This can only occur in the case of fresh autograft and has been demonstrated experimentally. Cancellous bone has a greater surface area than cortical bone and more osteocytes are present, so that it has a greater osteogenic potential. In order for the cells from the graft to produce bone, a vascular supply must be present. This can be provided most efficiently by the use of a vascularized graft; alternatively, a new blood supply must be supplied from the local host tissues. This process of *incorporation* will be discussed in more detail below but if the revascularization process is delayed by more than a few days, the majority of graft osteocytes are likely to be non-viable. Since cancellous bone is revascularized more rapidly than cortical bone, this provides a further reason for the greater osteogenicity of cancellous compared to cortical graft material.

Second, the bone graft may induce bone formation by causing a local host cell response which produces bone; this is termed *osteoinduction*. Osteoinduction occurs with both autografts and allografts and is mediated by small polypeptide molecules including the bone morphogenetic proteins. However, bone morphogens are relatively unstable and are likely to be rendered inactive by sterilization procedures such as autoclaving or irradiation.

The third mechanism by which bone graft enhances

bone formation is termed *osteoconduction*. This is a passive phenomenon whereby the graft material acts as a scaffold into which new host bone can grow. It is mainly a property of the physical state of the graft and inorganic lattices with an adequate pore size show it. Mechanical stability of the graft within the host bed is a prerequisite for osteoconduction to occur.

The three mechanisms are not mutually exclusive and, for example, in the case of a cortical autograft, some osteocytes from near the graft surface will become rapidly revascularized and will form new bone. As the revascularized graft bone is remodelled, matrix bound osteogenins will be released, which will lead to an osteoinductive host response. Finally, degradation of the graft surface will lead to a suitable lattice for osteoconduction.

As invasion of the graft by host bone proceeds, the graft is partially or completely replaced by the host in a process termed *incorporation*. This term is used loosely in clinical practice but it is fundamental to the mechanical integrity of the graft. If the graft bone is not replaced by host tissue, it is unable to take part in the normal process of bone remodelling which repairs fatigue damage and in the long term it must fail. Similarly, as the graft is replaced by host bone, it may pass through a phase of mechanical weakness due to the resorption which precedes osteoblastic remodelling and this may lead to graft failure.

Bone graft incorporation occurs in defined stages; inflammation, specific immune response, revascularization, osteogenesis and remodelling. Although described as separate stages, the processes represent a continuum.

In the optimal case of a fresh cancellous autograft, the immediate acute inflammatory response is relatively minor and there is no specific immune response. Revascularization may occur as early as 2 days post-transplantation, allowing survival of the surface osteocytes which produce new bone. Morphogens from within the bone induce host cells to differentiate into osteoblasts and themselves form new bone and osteoconduction proceeds rapidly as capillaries invade the matrix. Dead trabeculae from within the graft become lined with new osteoblasts and seams of osteoid are deposited. Often these will completely surround the dead graft bone, resulting in increased radiographic density and a transient increase in strength (Enneking and Horowitz, 1972). As remodelling occurs, the dead bone may be removed; however, this process may take years and may never be completed in larger grafts.

In contrast, in a fresh cancellous allograft, a vigorous immune response is seen which may be sufficiently severe to delay or even prevent osteoinduction. In this case, new blood vessels from the host become occluded, resulting in graft necrosis. Thus allograft bone functions poorly as a graft compared to autograft. The allograft immune response may be minimized by histocompatibility matching the donor and host or by modifying the allograft antigens by preservation techniques such as freezing.

Fresh cortical autograft incorporates in a similar manner to cancellous autograft, except that the rate of revascularization is slower so that significantly fewer graft cells remain viable and the initial stage of incorporation is marked by a phase of osteoclastic bone resorption which leads to loss of mechanical strength for some time following transplantation (Enneking and Horowitz, 1972). The initial osteoclastic response leads to graft osteoporosis which may be persistent if the remodelling process is interrupted. It is rare for all of the graft to be replaced by new host bone and remodelling occurs only in osteonal systems and not in interstitial lamellae.

Cortical allografts behave similarly to cancellous allograft, except that the specific immune response is delayed for a period while initial revascularization occurs. The immune response results in graft cell necrosis and an inflammatory infiltrate invades the marrow space. If the immunogenicity of the allograft is modified by preservation, its immunogenicity may be reduced, although freeze dried bone retains some immunogenicity (Muscolo *et al.*, 1987). The purpose of a preserved cortical allograft is normally to provide mechanical integrity, as opposed to enhancing osteogenicity and it is therefore important that the mechanical strength of the graft should be optimized. Unfortunately, most preservation techniques reduce the mechanical strength of the bone.

After transplantation of preserved cortical allogenic bone, there is a variable specific immune response. Initially, resorption of the graft predominates; however, appositional new bone formation does occur slowly and this is enhanced if the graft is rigidly fixed with compression. In clinical practice, the extent of revascularization, its time course and the degree to which the graft bone is replaced are all variable (Mankin, personal communication, 1991) and not completely elucidated.

In contrast to the slow and uncertain incorporation of devascularized cortical bone, vascularized cortical autograft incorporates rapidly because its cells retain their viability and the bone rapidly readapts to its new strain environment.

Bulk allografting

In cases of bone tumour where it is considered that local resection may be curative, such as a recurrent osteoclastoma, parosteal osteosarcoma or chondrosarcoma, it is attractive to replace the segment of bone which must be removed by a bulk allograft. The immunogenicity of the bulk allograft is reduced by deep freezing. Infection is excluded by culture at the time of harvesting and immediately prior to insertion and the host allograft junction is stabilized by plates or intramedullary rods as appropriate.

In the short term there is approximately a 30% failure rate due to infection, rejection or fracture of the allograft but once these short-term problems are past, the long-term outcome appears to be favourable.

Biologically at the host allograft junction there is invasion of the allograft by blood vessels and creeping substitution with apposition of new bone onto the scaffold of the allograft dead bone occurs. It is not clear whether this apposition is preceded by a phase of osteoclastic resorption (Mankin, personal communication, 1991). With time, blood vessels also grow in from the periosteal surface from the surrounding host muscle and fibrous tissue. This revascularizes the outer part of the cortex and once again there is a creeping apposition of new bone on to the dead allograft scaffold. This creeping apposition is a very slow process and it appears to continue for the life of the allograft. Continuing creeping apposition has been observed radiographically for up to 20 years by the radiographic observation of increasing sclerosis of the allograft. It is probable that the allograft bone scaffold is never fully replaced by new bone.

STRUCTURE OF THE JOINTS AND THE TISSUES

During embryonic growth, all skeletal tissues are joined by mesenchyme. During development some parts of the mesenchymal tissue become compressed into a compact plate or articular disc due to the pressure of the developing cartilage and bone. This disc is continuous at the circumference with the perichondrium and periosteum which develop into the fibrous capsule of the joint. In some joints a cleft appears in the articular disc which enlarges to form the joint cavity. The mesenchymal cells lining the cavity differentiate to form mesothelial cells which give rise to the synovial membrane. Remnants of the articular disc may persist, becoming organized into compact cartilaginous and fibrous tissue which, for example, in the knee form the meniscii. By the tenth week of embryonic development, most joint cavities in the human body are recognizable.

There are three main types of joint in the human body:

1. *Synarthrosis*. Movement does not occur at these joints and the articular disc remains solid, becoming hyaline cartilage or fibrous tissue. The sutures of the skull are of this type.
2. *Amphiarthrosis*. There is a small amount of movement and the bony surfaces are bound together by fibrous tissue. Examples are the intervertebral disc, symphysis pubis or the inferior tibiofibular joint.
3. *Diarthrosis*. This constitutes the majority of peripheral joints. The articular disc has completely disappeared or is represented only by remnants such as the menisci and the parts of the joint are freely movable. There is a definite joint cavity lined by synovial membrane.

Articular cartilage

Articular hyaline cartilage covers the bone ends and makes smooth movements of the joints possible. It is relatively acellular and has no vascular, neural or lymphatic supply. It has little capacity for repair after injury (Figure 2.46).

Articular cartilage distributes load across joints, minimizing the peak stresses on subchondral bone. It may be deformed and regain its original shape and provides a low friction bearing surface. Structurally it is a fibre reinforced gel (Maroudas *et al.*, 1980). The gel is formed of mutually repellent macromolecules which bind water within their domains. The osmotic pressure so generated produces a swelling pressure which gives hyaline cartilage its resistance to compression. The gel is not contained within cellular membranes but is restrained by fibres of collagen.

Cell shape and size, collagen fibril diameter and orientation matrix water content and proteoglycan content of articular cartilage all change with depth from the articular surface. This has led to the division of articular hyaline cartilage into layers or zones referred to as *superficial* (zone 1), *transitional* (zone 2), *radial* (zone 3) and the zone of *calcified cartilage* (Figure 2.46b). There are differences in chondrocyte morphology between the different zones and within each zone there are variations in the matrix which depend on the proximity of the matrix to the chondrocyte. The regions of the matrix are described as pericellular, territorial or interterritorial.

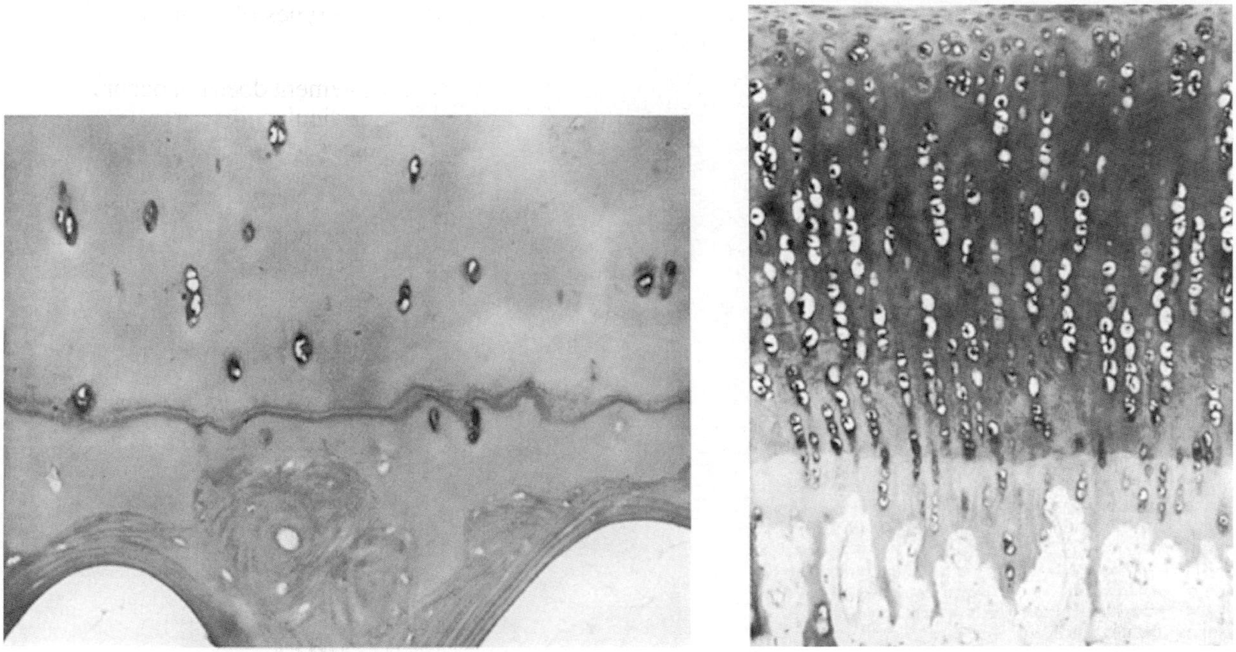

(a) (b)

Figure 2.46 (a) Photomicrograph of articular hyaline cartilage. There are no vessels or nerves and cells are sparse (H & E × 108). (b) Photomicrograph of articular hyaline cartilage, showing the different zones. Note the 'tide' mark separating the zone of calcified cartilage from the deep zone (H & E × 108).

ZONES OF ARTICULAR CARTILAGE

Superficial zone

The surface of articular cartilage is not smooth and the scanning electron microscope has demonstrated broad undulations approximately 400 μm wide with finer 25 μm depressions superimposed. The depressions are up to 2.5 μm deep. The surface is covered with an adsorbed layer of hyaluronic acid which is essential for joint surface lubrication.

The most superficial layer of the cartilage is made up of a narrow zone approximately 3 μm in depth which consists of a mat of fine fibres without cells. This layer corresponds to the 'laminar splendens'.

Beneath this most superficial layer lie elongated chondrocytes aligned with their long axis parallel to the articular surface. These cells are relatively inactive with poorly developed endoplasmic reticulum, few mitochondria and a small Golgi apparatus.

There is little hyaluronic acid present in zone 1 but proteoglycan monomer and link protein are present bound strongly to the collagen fibrils (Poole *et al.*, 1982).

Transitional zone

Several times thicker than the superficial zone, the cells are more rounded and larger than in the superficial zone and are frequently arranged in pairs. The cytoplasm is full of rough endoplasmic reticulum and the Golgi apparatus is well developed with many cytoplasmic vesicles, suggesting cells actively engaged in matrix component synthesis. The collagen fibrils are larger than those in the superficial zone and arranged irregularly (Figure 2.47).

Deep zone

This is normally the largest zone. The cells show similar appearances to those found in the transitional zone but the endoplasmic reticulum, Golgi apparatus and mitochondria are slightly less prominent. The cells typically contain large amounts of intermediate filaments and glycogen granules. Occasional degenerative cells are found. The matrix in the deep zone contains the largest collagen fibrils, has the highest proteoglycan content and the lowest water content. Thus from the superficial zone to the deep zone water content decreases and proteoglycan content increases. The collagen fibrils are thicker and are orientated normally to the joint surface.

The phenotypic differences between the chondrocytes in different zones raises the possibility that they may consist of different populations which have different functions. Alternatively the superficial zone may be a germinal area from which replacement of deep cells occurs slowly throughout life.

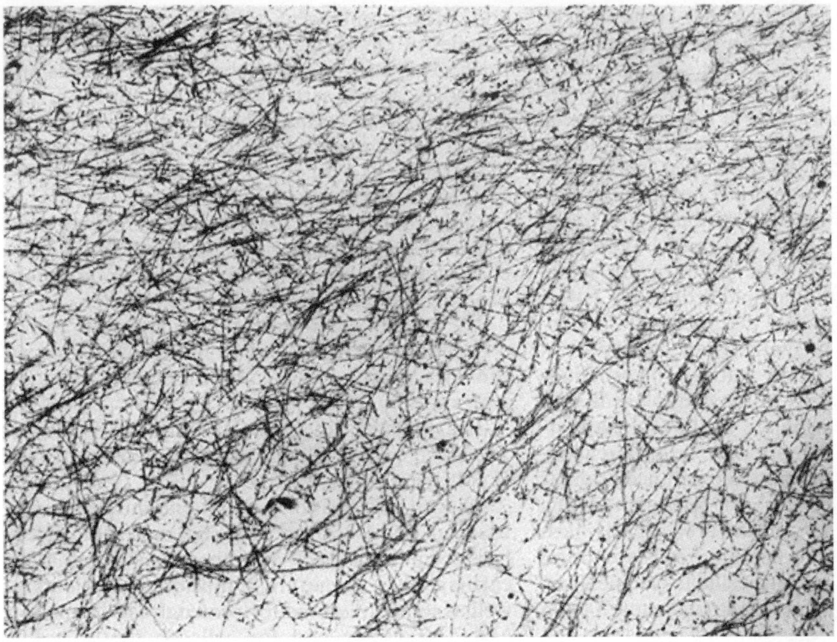

Figure 2.47 Electron micrograph of 'woven cartilage' matrix, made up of collagen in oblique cross-cross patterns (× 4715).

Zone of calcified cartilage

This zone lies immediately beneath the deep zone. It contains small irregular cells with pyknotic nuclei in lacunar spaces surrounded by calcium salts probably in the form of hydroxyapatite. On haematoxylin and eosin staining the calcified zone is separated from the deep zone by a thin wavy basophilic line named the 'tide mark'. The calcified zone is continuous with the subchondral bone plate and the two together are important in maintaining the stability of the cartilage against shearing stresses.

MATRIX REGIONS OF ARTICULAR CARTILAGE

Pericellular matrix

Within the deeper layers of articular cartilage, the chondrocytes lie together in pairs, triplets or quadruplets. Each cell or cell group is protected within a distinctive layer of specialized, pericellular matrix, sometimes referred to as the 'chondron', the margin of which is defined microscopically by a condensed lamina of circumferentially orientated collagen fibrils forming a 'lacuna'. The lacuna was thought until recently to be an artefact due to staining but transmission electron microscopic evidence (Poole *et al.*, 1984) suggests that the lacuna has a definite three-dimensional form. The pericellular matrix contains little or no fibrillar collagen although it may contain some minor collagen types (particularly types VI and IX). The predominant macromolecules are proteoglycans, non-collagenous proteins and glycoproteins. The matrix appears to attach directly to the chondrocyte cell membrane (Poole *et al.*, 1987).

The pericellular matrix may function to modulate pressure transmission to the chondrocyte, preventing squashing during weight bearing, and may have a role in the regulation of chondrocyte responses to pressure.

Territorial matrix

This region surrounds the pericellular matrix and contains thin collagen fibrils, forming a fibrillar basket around the cells (Poole *et al.*, 1984).

Interterritorial matrix

This forms the largest matrix compartment. The boundary between the territorial and interterritorial matrix is marked by an abrupt increase in collagen fibril diameter and a transition from the basket-like fibril orientation found in the territorial matrix to a more parallel arrangement. It is responsible for the mechanical properties of articular cartilage.

Until recently, Benninghoff's original description in 1925 that the collagen fibres of hyaline articular cartilage were arranged in intermingling arcades with each fibre passing up from the underlying bony end plate to the articular surface, arching across and downwards to rejoin the bone, was accepted. Studies with the scanning electron microscope have failed to confirm this arcade structure. There is, however, general agreement that the principal interterritorial matrix collagen fibres in the superficial zone lie parallel to the joint surface forming a dense meshwork (O'Connell *et al.*, 1980), while in the deep zone they are perpendicular to the joint surface (Clark, 1985).

CELLS OF ARTICULAR CARTILAGE: THE CHONDROCTYE

In mature cartilage the cells account for less than 1% of the tissue volume, but their viability is essential for tissue maintenance as they synthesize matrix components continually. Collagen turnover is relatively slow but proteoglycans are constantly being renewed.

Chondrocytes surround themselves with extracellular matrix and do not form cell-to-cell contacts. They contain organelles responsible for matrix synthesis, endoplasmic reticulum and Golgi apparatus and may also contain intracytoplasmic filaments and glycogen. Most articular chondrocytes have a cilium which may be involved in the regulation of matrix turnover.

The mechanisms which influence chondrocyte function are poorly defined. Changes in matrix composition such as decrease in proteoglycan content affect chondrocyte function and the cells also respond to alterations in pressure by changes in macromolecule synthesis.

During embryogenesis and the formation of articular cartilage, chondrocytes proliferate rapidly and synthesize large volumes of matrix. After maturation these processes slow and under normal circumstances mature chondrocytes rarely divide. The cell density within articular cartilage declines with age. The reduction in cell density and synthetic function may limit cartilage reparative ability.

BIOCHEMISTRY OF ARTICULAR CARTILAGE

Collagen

The major collagen of cartilage is type II and this forms the characteristic cross-banded fibrils seen by electron microscopy. It accounts for approximately 90% of the total cartilage collagen and is found only in cartilage and the vitreous humour of the eye. Three minor collagens (type IX, X, XI) which are also unique to cartilage and type VI collagen, which is distributed in other tissues, are also found. Types VI and IX collagen are found in the pericellular matrix and are probably involved in the organization and stabilization of the collagen fibril meshwork.

Type XI collagen is associated with type II collagen fibrils and may have a role in determining their diameter.

Type II collagen is a fibrillar collagen formed of three identical alpha chains providing a continuous triple helix 287 mm long with C terminal and N terminal globular domains which are cleaved prior to fibril formation. The molecules are covalently bonded together and these bonds are essential for the tensile properties of the collagen fibrils and the network they form. Compared to the other common fibrillar collagen (type I) the fibrils are smaller, contain more hydroxylysine residues and are more glycosylated. Type II collagen is normally found in tissues with higher proteoglycan and water content.

Non-collagenous proteins

At least three non-collagenous proteins are found in articular cartilage. Link protein is involved in the binding of glycosaminoglycans to hyaluronic acid whereas the other two proteins, chondronectin (150 kDa) and anchorin CII (34 kDa) appear to have a role in chondrocyte adherence to the matrix.

Proteoglycans

The proteoglycans are a family of glycoproteins in which a large protein core of molecular weight 225 000 Da which has attached glycosaminoglycan side chains (Figure 2.48). The glycosaminoglycans are long chain polysaccharides with a repeating disaccharide structure (Figure 2.49). They are linked to a protein core via a characteristic short sequence of sugar residues and approximately 50 keratan sulphate chains each of molecular weight 5–10 kDa and up to 100 chondroitin sulphate chains of molecular weight 15–20 kDa are attached to each core protein. The proteoglycans in articular cartilage are predominantly of a high molecular weight (124 $\times 10^6$ Da) aggregating type which implies that a number of the monomers shown in Figure 2.48 bind to a central backbone of hyaluronate (Figure 2.49).

The proteoglycan aggregate components are synthesized continuously by chondrocytes and the carbohydrate side chains are synthesized on the protein during intracellular post-translational processing. The proteoglycan core protein contains domains rich in serine–glycine sequences that form glycosaminoglycan attachment regions. There are also three globular domains, one of which contains a specific site for hyaluronate. Proteoglycans aggregate by binding to hyaluronate via this binding region, which

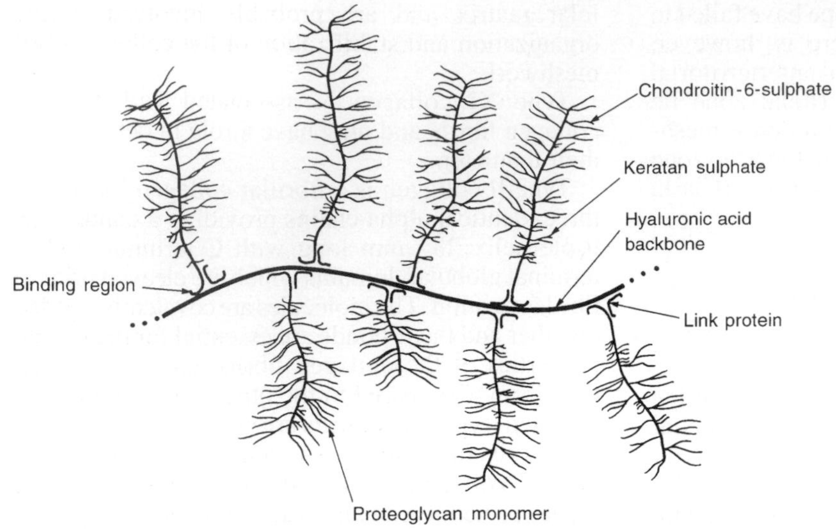

Figure 2.48 Schematic representation of a proteoglycan monomer. The molecule consists of a number of chondroitin sulphate and keratan sulphate chains covalently bonded to a central protein core.

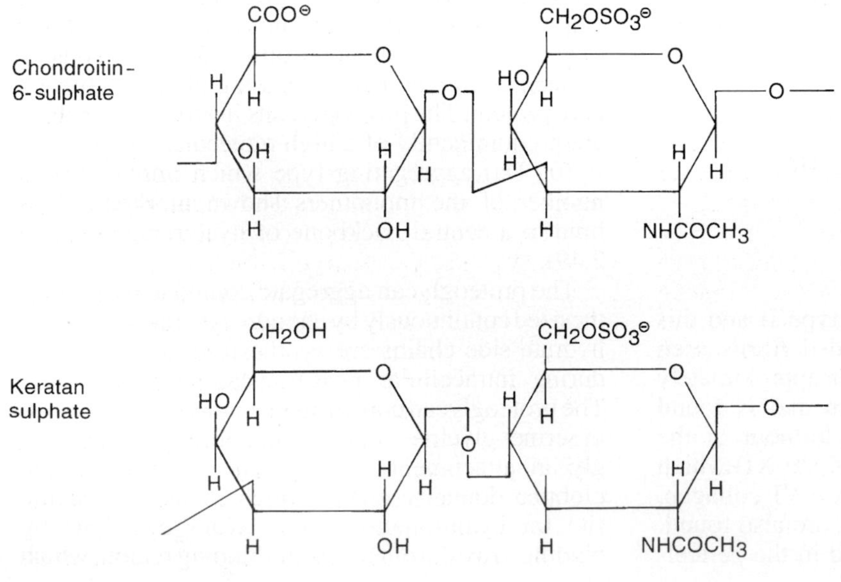

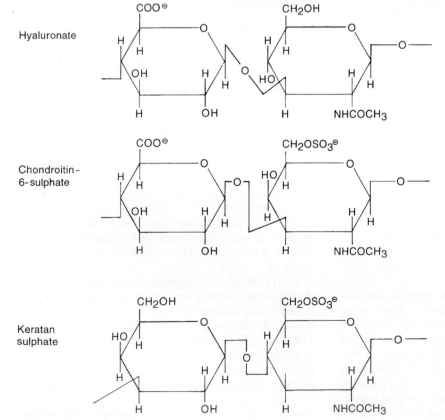

Figure 2.49 Structure of the disaccharide units which make up the proteoglycan, hyaluronate, keratan sulphate and chondroitin-6-sulphate. Repeating polymers of these disaccharide subunits make up the glycosaminoglycans.

is stabilized by a specific link protein. The long, unbranched hyaluronate chains can bind up to several hundred proteoglycan molecules.

Synthesis of glycosaminoglycans

The proteoglycans in cartilage are not homogeneous. The considerable variation in structure and composition is due both to variations in biosynthesis and to degradation. The glycosaminoglycans are synthesized in a series of reactions in which acetylgalactosamine is bonded to glucuronic acid to form chondroitin:

1. *N*-Ac-glucosamine-1-P + UTP
   → UDP-*N*-Ac-glucosamine + UDP
2. UDP-*N*-Ac-glucosamine
   → *UDP-N-*Ac-*galactosamine*
3. Glucose-1-P + UTP
   → UDP-glucose + UDP
4. UDP-glucose
   → *UDP-glucuronic acid*
5. UDP-*N*-Ac-galactosamine
   + UDP-glucuronic acid
   → *Chondroitin + UDP*
   UDP-*N*-Ac-galactosamine

The glycosaminoglycans are sulphated after synthesis. Autoradiography employing systemically administered isotopic sulphate shows that it is first located within the chondrocyte and within 24 hours migrates to the extracellular matrix. The enzymatic pathways are:

1. ATP + sulphate = AMP-sulphate + phosphoprotein
2. AMP-sulphate + ATP
   → Phospho-AMP-sulphate
   (PAPS, 'active sulphate') + ADP
3. PAPS + chondroitin
   → Chondroitin sulphate + Phospho-AMP

There is a combination of ATP and free sulphate to form 3-phosphoadenosine, 5-phosphosulphate known as 'active sulphate'. The sulphate molecule from this high energy material is then linked to *N*-acetylgalactosamine at the C4 or C6 position, to form chondroitin-4-sulphate or chondroitin-6-sulphate. It has been demonstrated that radiosulphate is bound and concentrated in the vesicles of the juxtanuclear Golgi apparatus of the chondrocyte within 3 minutes of its presentation to the cell. Concurrent with the vigorous uptake of $^{35}SO_4$ by cartilage, elimination of sulphated compounds proceeds and the net result may be a negative sulphate balance. Sulphate is fixed in all but zone I cells of the articular cartilage, and the deeper cells continue to be active into old age.

Hyaluronate is synthesized within the chondrocyte by a mechanism entirely different from other glycosaminoglycans (Prehm, 1983). Aggregation of the proteoglycan monomers by linkage with hyaluronate is an extracellular process and the monomers and hyaluronate are secreted separately by the chondrocyte. Although most recent studies of cartilage proteoglycan have dealt with articular cartilage, such data are not uniformly transposable to the growth plate (Trippel, 1990).

The interaction of link protein with proteoglycan monomer and hyaluronic acid from bovine fetal epiphyseal cartilage was characterized by Tang *et al.* (1989). These authors demonstrated that the proteoglycan monomers from this cartilage are almost entirely aggregating monomers. As expected, link protein substantially increased the percentage of the aggregating monomers. Proteoglycan aggregate stability was found to be highly pH-dependent: decreasing the pH from 5 to 4 in the absence of link protein resulted in essentially complete aggregate dissociation. Link protein was protective against much of the pH-induced instability. The authors further showed that optimization of both pH and link protein increased not only the stability of the aggregate but also its size.

Function of proteoglycans

In cartilage, most proteoglycans are in the form of large (200 000 kDa or more) aggregates that provide the tissue with its resilience under compressive loads. The glycosaminoglycan side chains are heavily negatively charged and repel each other, holding the monomers extended. Because of their ionic nature they interact with tissue fluid, attracting water. Comparison of the maximal volume that proteoglycans could occupy in solution with their concentration in articular cartilage shows that they are normally only partially hydrated and exert a constant pressure to expand which is restrained by the collagen fibril mesh (Buckwalter *et al.*, 1985, 1988) (Figure 2.50).

The structure of aggregating cartilage proteoglycans changes with age. With increasing age the keratan sulphate and protein content of the monomer increases, the chondroitin sulphate content decreases, the chondroitin sulphate chains become shorter and the average monomer size decreases. In addition, link protein may fragment and the aggregates become smaller (Buckwalter *et al.*, 1985). These changes are presumably caused by age-related alterations in chondrocyte synthesis and degradation. Although their functional significance is unclear, they demonstrate that alterations of cartilage matrix occur with ageing.

In addition to their contribution to matrix struc-

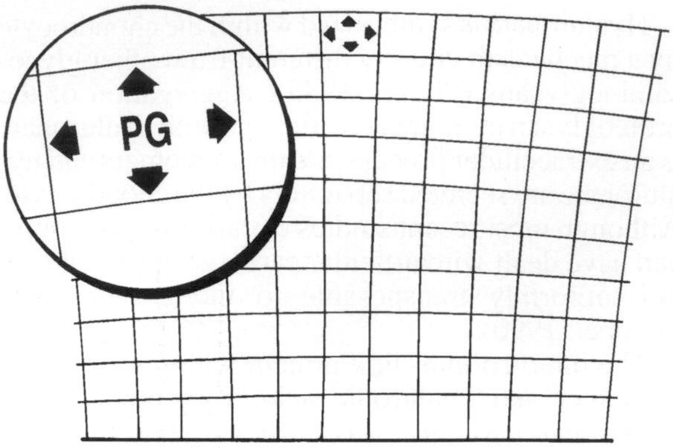

Figure 2.50 How the proteoglycan (PG) pressure draws water into the articular cartilage to maintain its turgor.

ture, proteoglycans in the growth plate may play a role in mineralization. Focal concentrations of proteoglycan at the sites of mineralization are well documented. Because the chondroitin sulphate chains of proteoglycans bind calcium and because phosphate can displace this calcium from the proteoglycans, proteoglycans may serve as the medium within which calcium release by ion exchange could raise the $Ca \times PO_4$ product above the threshold for hydroxyapatite precipitation (Hunter, 1987).

NUTRITION OF ARTICULAR CARTILAGE

Nutrients reach immature articular cartilage via vascular channels in the subchondral bone and the base of the cartilage and also via the synovial fluid. Mature articular cartilage is avascular and is nourished totally by diffusion. The majority of nutrients enter the synovial fluid as a transudate of plasma from synovial vessels with probably a minor con-tribution through the subchondral bone plate. Because of this reliance on diffusion, the microenvironment of chondrocytes is different from that of the majority of cells in the body, with a high level of carbon dioxide and poorer oxygenation. As a result of this relative resistance to hypoxia, chondrocytes survive for two days or more after the death of the organism.

SYNTHESIS AND DEGRADATION RATES OF CARTILAGE MATRIX

Protein synthesis may be measured by the rate of uptake of tritiated proline or glycine and glycosaminoglycan synthesis by uptake of radio-labelled sulphate. The rates of synthesis are more rapid in immature animals and after the initial decline at skeletal maturity they are unaffected by ageing. Synthesis is slowed by cortisol, nitrogen mustard and antimetabolites and is moderately increased for a short period by a laceration of the cartilage or matrix degradation by papain. The rate of synthesis of all matrix constituents is variably increased in cartilage from osteoarthritic joints. The fibrillar collagen network is synthesized slowly and is more

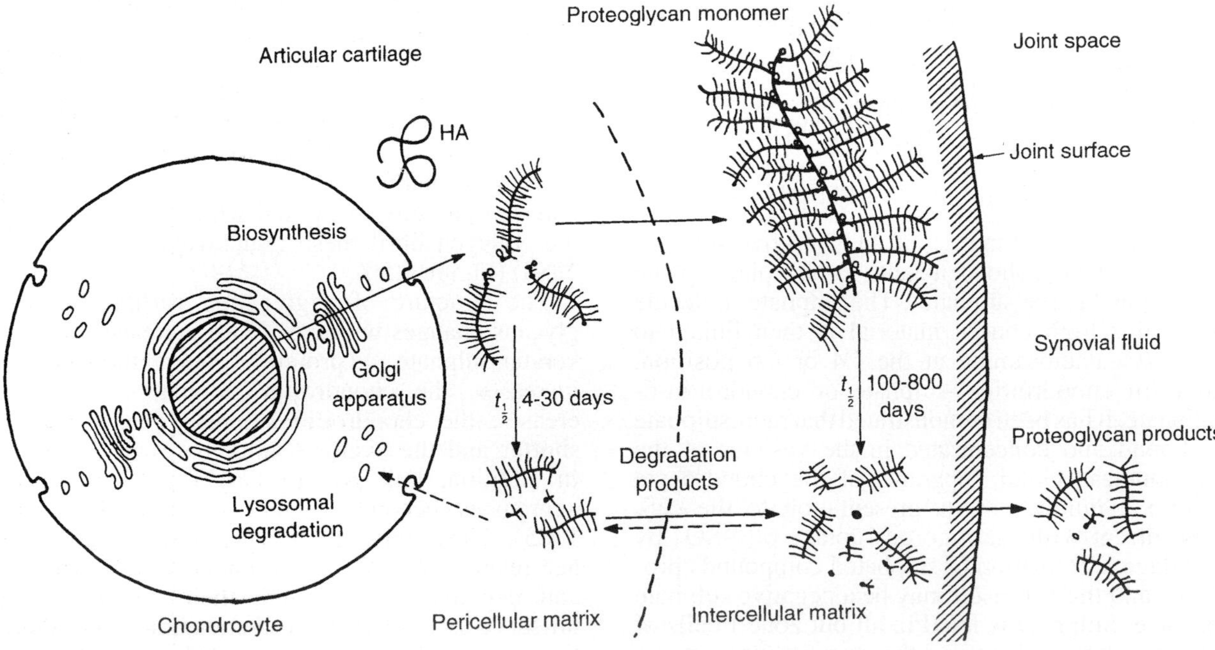

Figure 2.51 The life cycle of a proteoglycan molecule in articular cartilage.

resistant to proteolytic attack than the proteoglycans which are continuously being degraded and replaced by new synthesis.

PROTEOGLYCAN TURNOVER

The rapid turnover of proteoglycan implies that degradation during normal turnover occurs without significant disruption of the matrix. Degradation is by proteinases secreted by chondrocytes which attack the protein core at specific sites, resulting in a large proteoglycan fragment which contains almost the entire monomer intact but which cannot aggregate (Tyler, 1985a,b) (Figure 2.51). Since the residual monomer is unable to aggregate, because it has lost the hyaluronate binding region, it is free to diffuse out of the cartilage (Figure 2.52). However, since the monomer itself is virtually undamaged by degradation, its osmotic properties remain. Furthermore, the binding site on the hyaluronate macromolecule is now available for a newly synthesized monomer molecule.

There are four classes of proteinase, produced by the chondrocyte, which may be involved in matrix degradation (Murphy, 1991). These are classified according to their mechanism of action into metalloproteinases, serine proteinases, cysteine proteinases and aspartic proteinases. The initial step in proteoglycan degradation is an extracellular process often involving metalloproteinases derived from chondrocytes. Mechanical disruption and the presence of free radicals may augment the process of degradation. Matrix fragments are subsequently phagocytosed for processing intracellularly by lysosomes.

Most connective tissue cells secrete three types of metalloproteinase. They are all Zn^{2+} and Ca^{2+} dependent and are secreted in a latent form which requires activation through loss of a peptide fragment. The active enzyme is specifically inhibited by a tissue inhibitor of metalloproteinase (TIMP) as well as the ubiquitous proteinase inhibitor, α_2-macroglobulin. TIMP is a glycoprotein with a molecular weight of 29 000 which is normally present within cartilage in excess. Therefore degradation of cartilage matrix can only occur where locally active metalloproteinase levels exceed those of TIMP. Detailed study of normal wound healing suggests that close regulation of the distribution of TIMP relative to metalloproteinases is necessary for normal repair processes (Chowcat *et al.*, 1988).

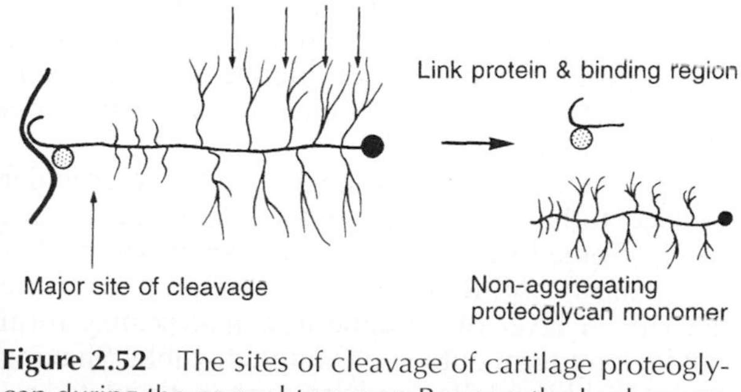

Figure 2.52 The sites of cleavage of cartilage proteoglycan during the normal turnover. Because the hyaluronate binding region has been split from the proteoglycan monomer, the latter is unable to aggregate.

Cytokine effects on proteoglycan turnover

Cytokines are cellular messengers produced locally in tissues in response to various biological stimuli such as inflammation and wound healing. Chondrocytes in young articular cartilage explants have been shown to be susceptible to interleukin 1 which increases the rate of proteoglycan loss from the matrix (Tyler, 1985b) and also inhibits its biosynthesis (Tyler, 1985a). The proteoglycan fragments released by this process are very similar to those produced by the normal turnover of cartilage matrix. The *in vivo* increase in matrix degradation appears to be due to a direct stimulation of chondrocyte-mediated matrix degradation rather than an indirect action on polymorphs or monocoytes.

The local release of cytokines may therefore be a major factor in the initial attack on cartilage in inflammatory joint disease, which leads to a rapid depletion of cartilage proteoglycan. However, experimentally considerable loss of proteoglycan may occur acutely and reversibly provided the collagen and cellular network remains undamaged. Thus the cartilage damage occurring, for example, in a transient acute episode of infective arthritis, may not lead to long-term joint damage.

ROLE OF KININS IN ARTHRITIS

The kallikreins are a group of serine proteases which are widely distributed. They are divided into two main groups, tissue and plasma kallikrein, and they act enzymically on plasma substrates (kininogens) to produce kinins which are vasoactive peptides that increase vascular permeability and cause cell proliferation. When applied to a skin blister base or injected intradermally, they produce pain which lasts for some minutes. Kallikrein inhibitors and kininases exist and there is considerable evidence that the kallikrein–kinin system is active in the rheumatoid joint. There is also some evidence for the involvement of this system in gout and possibly

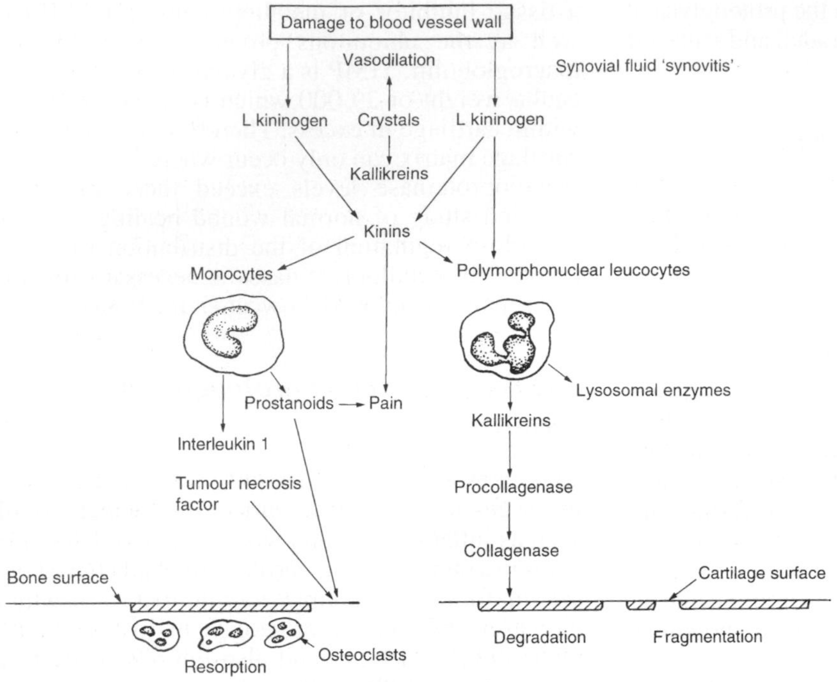

Figure 2.53 Possible role of kinins in cartilage disruption in arthritis.

in osteoarthritis. Kallikreins and kinins may be involved in the destruction of tissue integrity and may contribute to the generation of pain and inflammation in the joints (Worthy *et al.*, 1990; Figure 2.53).

REPAIR OF ARTICULAR CARTILAGE

Since articular cartilage cells synthesize matrix at a rate comparable with other connective tissue, it might be expected that the repair of damaged cartilage would also be comparable. However, tissue healing requires cell multiplication as well as new matrix production and mature chondrocytes divide infrequently, if at all. Although mitosis may be induced by laceration, compression, exposure to papain or osteoarthrosis, the effect appears to be too small and ill sustained to repair any but the smallest defect. Repair capacity is therefore limited even following simple incisions.

Cartilage exposure, infection and prolonged joint immobilization all stimulate proteoglycan degradation or suppress synthesis. They may have other effects on cells and matrix, but the loss of matrix proteoglycan is the most significant initial change. If the insult is transient the cartilage may regain its normal composition. However, if the process is prolonged the damage becomes irreversible. It is not, however, clear at what point this occurs (Reimann *et al.*, 1982).

Blunt trauma which causes supraphysiological loads, but which is not sufficiently severe to cause fracture, leads to cartilage swelling with increased collagen fibril diameter and alteration in proteoglycan content (Donohue *et al.*, 1983).

Repair of penetrating injuries to cartilage depends on whether the injury involves the subchondral bone and on the area involved in the damage, with larger defects healing less satisfactorily than smaller ones.

A laceration of articular cartilage perpendicular to the surface kills the local chondrocytes and creates a wedge-shaped matrix defect. If the injury does not involve the subchondral bone, it will not illicit an inflammatory response and reparative granulation tissue does not appear. Chondrocytes near to the lesion proliferate but do not migrate into the lesion. The defect does not fill in but neither does it progress (Buckwalter *et al.*, 1988).

Superficial lacerations tangential to the articular surface follow a similar course (Ghadially *et al.*, 1977). Some local cell death may occur while other cells show proliferation and increased synthetic activity. A layer of unstable new matrix may form but its long-term outcome is unpredictable. Shaving normal rabbit patella cartilage neither stimulated repair nor caused degeneration (Mitchell and Shepherd,

1987) and a similar observation has been made in human knees (Schmid and Schmid, 1987). These data throw doubt on the mechanism whereby shaving of fibrillated human articular cartilage may improve joint function.

Healing of cartilage matrix has been shown in experimental animals receiving salicylates (Simmonds and Chrisman, 1965). However, articular cartilage defects in humans such as occur in chondromalacia patellae do not heal within a period of 3 months of observation under these circumstances (Bentley *et al.*, 1981).

If cartilage damage is deep enough to involve the subchondral bone then repair may occur by filling of the defect with repair granulation tissue derived from the subchondral marrow which then undergoes metaplasia to fibrocartilage. Compared to normal hyaline articular cartilage this repair cartilage has poor biomechanical properties (Furukawa *et al.*, 1980) and there is a considerable amount of type I collagen. Although in the early phase following injury some proteoglycan may be found in the repair cartilage, this rapidly disappears and undergoes degradative changes (Buckwalter *et al.*, 1988).

Clinically, redirection of the forces across a joint affected by early osteoarthrosis may lead to replacement of damaged hyaline cartilage with fibrocartilage. The mechanism appears to be an augmentation of the normal repair processes and under the influence of an increased blood supply stimulated by the osteotomy, tufts of repair granulation tissue may become a continuous fibrocartilaginous surface which forms an adequate weight-bearing material (Bentley, 1971; Radin and Burr, 1984).

ARTICULAR CARTILAGE AND OSTEOCHONDRAL GRAFTING

Because of the poor ability of damaged articular cartilage to repair and the dubious long-term results of total hip replacements in young patients, it is attractive to attempt to replace damaged cartilage in very young patients using allografted articular cartilage. Resection of bone tumours in young patients may also necessitate sacrificing one side of a joint and in these cases, too, cartilage allografting may be considered. The problems with bone allografting have already been addressed. Grafting of cartilage brings with it certain more specific problems.

First of all, there are mechanical problems of fixation of the cartilage into the host. Secure fixation normally requires bone and therefore at a minimum the cartilage is taken with its underlying subchondral bone. If the underlying bone is not sufficiently stiff the cartilage will be deformed by the stresses placed on the joint in normal function and this will lead to early breakdown. Furthermore, it is necessary that the grafted cartilage fits very accurately into the host joint, otherwise abnormal mechanical forces will again lead to rapid breakdown.

Cartilage itself is highly immunogenic and, as in bone, this may be substantially reduced by freezing. Furthermore, if the cartilage is intact, few of the antigens within it are presented to the host so that the immune response is minimized.

Unlike allografted bone, allografted cartilage is not replaced by the host and its continued function depends on long-term survival of its own chondrocytes. Freezing bone or cartilage for the purposes of preservation and reducing its immunogenicity normally kills all the cells. Death is primarily due to disruption of cell membranes and organelles by ice crystals which form at the moment of freezing. The size of the ice crystals can be minimized by freezing extremely slowly and use of a solvent such as ethylene glycol or dimethyl sulphoxide. Using these techniques up to 40% of the chondrocytes retain their viability despite freezing.

In practice two different techniques have been employed. First, fresh shell allografts, employed within approximately 12 hours of harvest from a donor, have been implanted into the hips and knees of experimental animals and humans. The implantation into human hips has given poor results due in part to the difficulties of providing a truly congruous donor cartilage. The implantation into knees has given slightly better results; however, the long-term outcome is not encouraging.

Second, deep frozen cartilage attached to large segments of bone has been used to bridge defects left by tumour resection. In these cases long-term survival of the cartilage radiographically has been reported in up to 50% of cases.

The difficulties of obtaining either fresh donors or bank bulk allograft limit general clinical use of these techniques at present.

An alternative strategy is transplantation of a chondrocyte containing matrix which has been generated *in vitro*. The early results of experimental animal work of this sort are encouraging (Bentley and Aston, 1985). However, although the chondrocytes can be shown to synthesize type II collagen and a structure closely resembling hyaline cartilage in the experimental animals, considerable further work is required before this can be used in the human (Bentley, 1989).

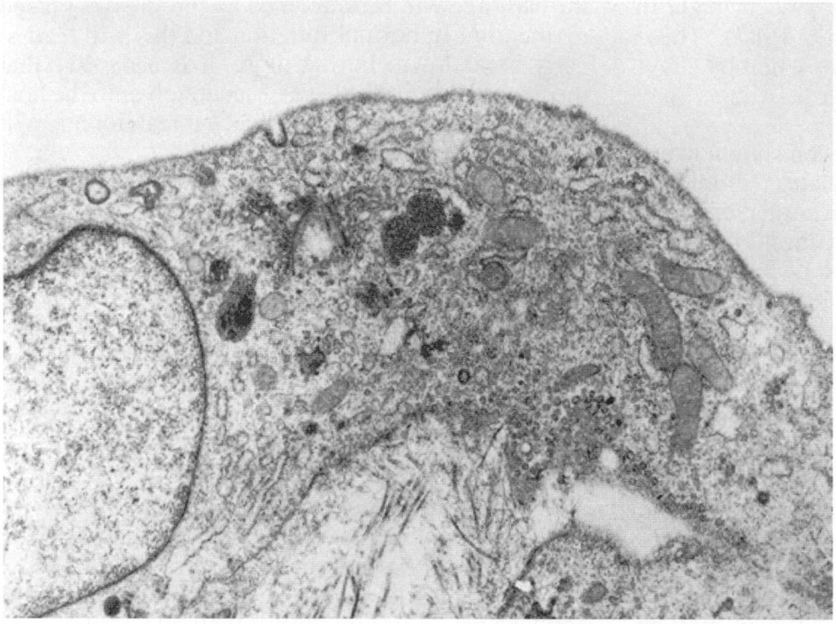

(a)

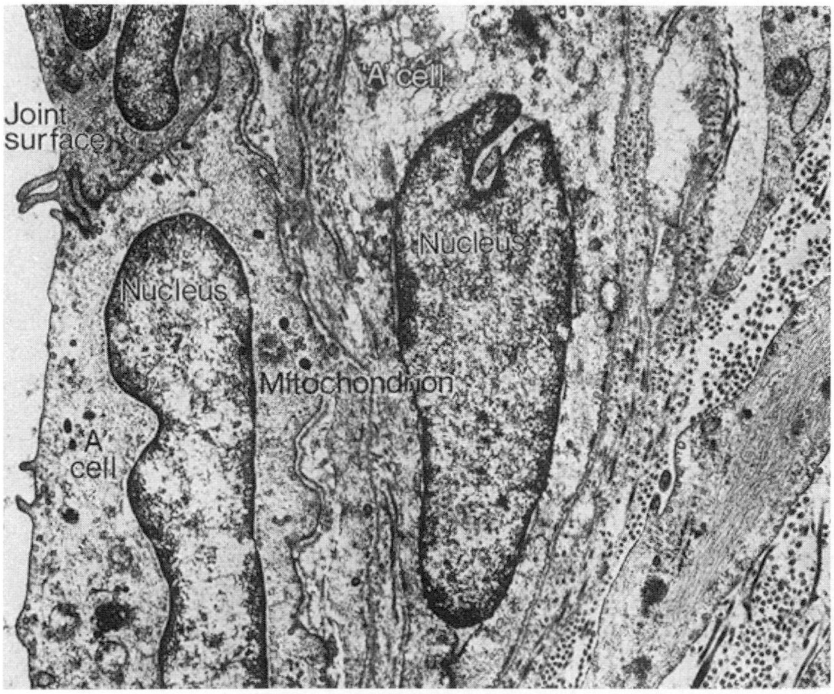

(b)

Figure 2.54 (a) Electron micrograph of adult rabbit synovium, showing the A type cell which is characterized by numerous mitochondria in the cytoplasm (× 13 500). (b) Electron micrograph showing two A cells on the right of the joint surface (× 14 580).

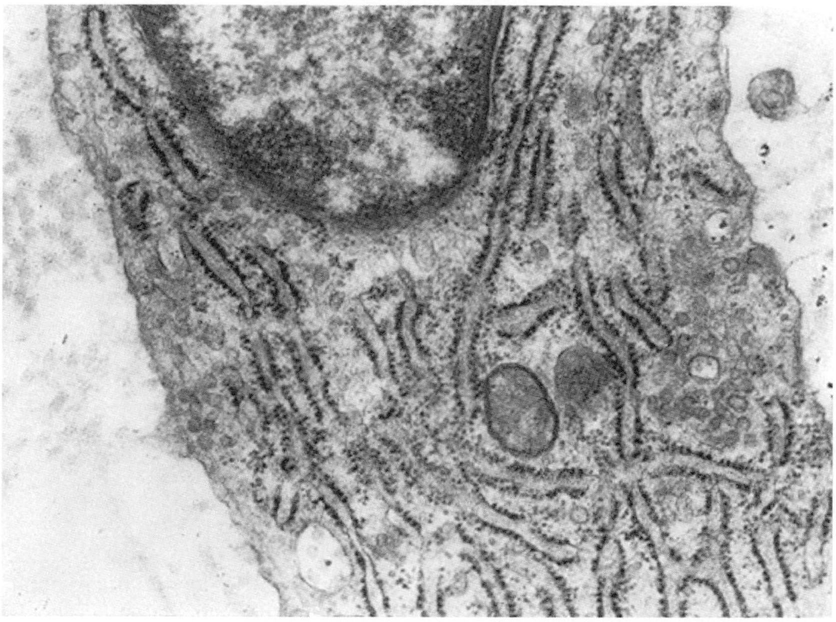

Figure 2.55 Electron micrograph of rabbit synovium, showing the B type cell with its endoplasmic reticulum (× 14 510).

Synovium

SYNOVIAL MEMBRANE

Synovial membrane differentiates from the mesenchymal tissue around the articular disc, clearing the articular surface by the fifth month *in utero*.

Histologically synovial tissue may be fatty, fibrofatty or fibrous and contains types I and III collagen. Two types of cell are found, type A (Figure 2.54), which are macrophage-like phagocytic cells, and type B (Figure 2.55), which resemble fibroblasts and are responsible for the secretion of hyaluronic acid and protein. The subsynovial tissue contains macrophages and fibroblasts and the precursors of the synovial cells, which give rise to the new membrane after synovectomy. A small number of mast cells whose function are unknown are also found.

There is a rich vascular plexus accompanied by lymphatic channels extending up to the synovial membrane itself which is formed by a layer two to three cells thick with no basement membrane (Figure 2.56). This arrangement is presumably to allow ready passage of fluid from the capillaries through the synovial membrane into the cavity. However, the combined effect of the overlapping processes, the hyaluronate in the intercellular matrix and the capillary wall, restricts entry or exit to substances with a molecular weight above 150 000. The surface area of the membrane is increased by numerous villous folds which increase the area for secretion and resorption.

SYNOVIAL FLUID

Synovial fluid is an ultradialysate of blood plasma to which proteoglycan has been added by local synthesis by the joint tissues. Synovial fluid is a clear viscous yellow fluid which does not clot on standing since it contains no fibrinogen. A normal knee joint contains approximately 0.5 ml of fluid. The viscosity of synovial fluid depends on the concentration of hyaluronic acid and is lowered in ageing, osteoarthritis and following trauma. Synovial fluid contains 96% water and 4% solutes with a specific gravity of 1.010 and a pH of 7.3–7.6 which is reduced in osteoarthritis and after trauma. Normal synovial fluid contains very few cells but the numbers are increased markedly in various diseases.

Proteins are present in lower concentration than in plasma and transfer of plasma proteins to synovial fluid in an uninflamed joint is related to the size and shape of the particular molecule. Thus the majority of the protein in synovial fluid is albumin (approximately two-thirds) and large molecules such as α_2-macroglobulin, lipoproteins, fibrinogen and IgM are present in small amounts in normal fluid.

In contrast, when the synovium becomes inflamed, the protein content of the inflammatory synovial fluid increases and the quantity of large molecular

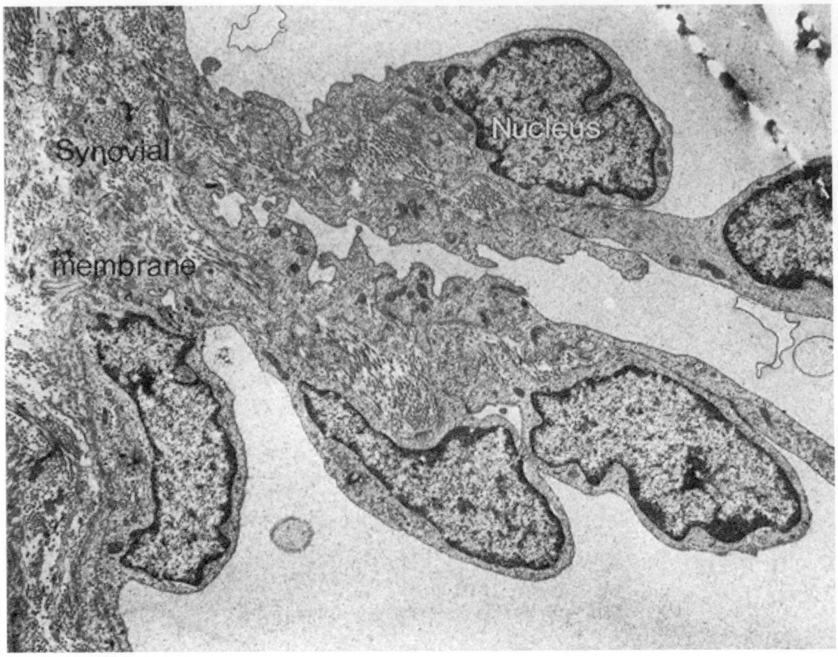

Figure 2.56 Electron micrograph showing the surface of the synovial membrane (× 9720).

weight proteins is greater than in normal fluid. The synovial fluid may clot due to the presence of significant amounts of fibrinogen. In severely inflamed joints, the concentration of protein is similar to that in serum and in classic rheumatoid arthritis IgM and IgG concentrations are higher than would be predicted on the basis of diffusion (Kushner and Somerville, 1971) (see Chapter 13).

Joint lubrication

From an engineering point of view there are two types of lubrication, boundary lubrication in which a monolayer of lubricant is adsorbed onto each bearing surface and fluid film lubrication in which a thin fluid film separates the bearing surfaces. Both types of lubrication occur in diarthrodial joints.

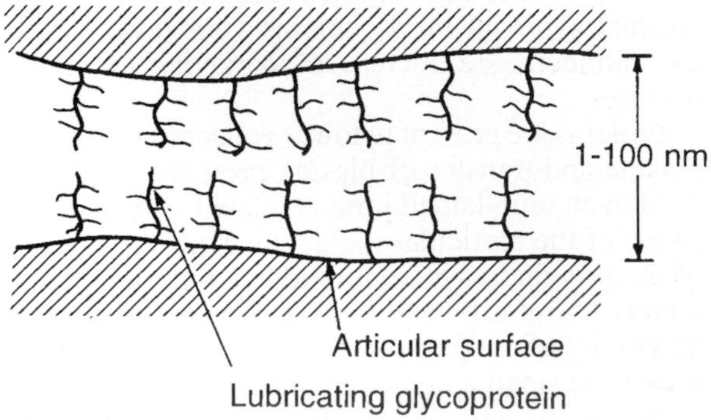

Figure 2.57 A diagram of the role of adsorbed glycoprotein in boundary layer lubrication.

BOUNDARY LUBRICATION

In synovial joints a specific glycoprotein 'lubricin' appears to be adsorbed to each articulating surface and prevents direct surface-to-surface contact, significantly reducing surface wear (Swann *et al.*, 1985). Boundary lubrication depends almost exclusively on the chemical properties of the lubricant (Figure 2.57).

FLUID FILM LUBRICATION

Bearing surfaces including human joints can be lubricated by a layer of fluid between the sliding bearing surfaces (Figure 2.58). The efficiency of the lubricant film depends on its viscosity which is the resistance to the flow and is defined as the sheer stress in the fluid divided by the rate of sheer strain. Viscosity is constant for ideal Newtonian fluids but in most biological fluids it varies with flow rate.

A lubricant with low viscosity produces less viscous drag in the bearing, but is more likely to be expelled from the joint to allow the articulating surfaces to come into direct contact. In human joints

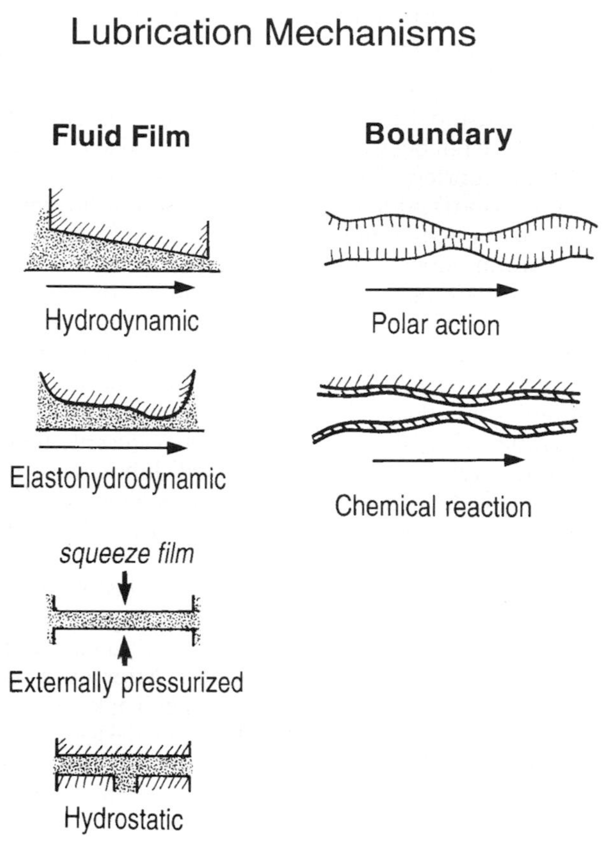

Figure 2.58 A schematic illustration of all lubrications.

the oscillating nature of the joint movements, the flow of synovial fluid into and out of the articulating region and the local deformation of articular cartilage under load contribute to a variety of mechanisms by which the fluid separates and lubricates the articular surfaces.

Hyaluronate is essential for the lubrication of articular surfaces, and its removal by hyaluronidase leads to erosion of the surfaces. The mode of action of hyaluronate is complex and the mode of joint lubrication varies according to the conditions of movement and load. Human joints differ from mechanical bearings in the physical properties of the moving surfaces and also in that they undergo reciprocating and rotating movements at varying velocities with varying loads. The lubricating action of synovial fluids is not viscosity dependent and the hyaluronate undergoes depolymerization into smaller molecules during movements without loss of its lubricating properties. Hyaluronate binds to the surface of articular cartilage as shown on scanning electron microscopy.

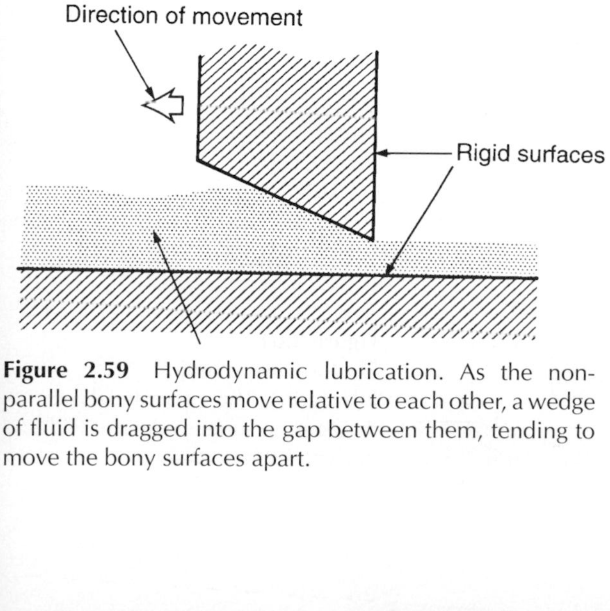

Figure 2.59 Hydrodynamic lubrication. As the non-parallel bony surfaces move relative to each other, a wedge of fluid is dragged into the gap between them, tending to move the bony surfaces apart.

Two classic forms of fluid film lubrication are seen in engineering practice with rigid bearings. These are hydrodynamic and squeeze film lubrication.

HYDRODYNAMIC LUBRICATION

Hydrodynamic lubrication takes place by virtue of the relative motion of the bearing surfaces. When two non-parallel rigid bearing surfaces lubricated by a thin film move tangentially on one another, a converging wedge of fluid is formed which tends to lift the bearing surfaces apart as the motion of the surfaces drags the fluid into the gap between the surfaces (Figure 2.59).

SQUEEZE FILM LUBRICATION

Squeeze film lubrication occurs when the rigid bearing surfaces move perpendicularly towards each other. There is a tendency for the fluid to squeeze out from between the surfaces which is resisted by the viscous forces. Very high fluid pressures are generated which can support heavy loads transiently. However, eventually the fluid film becomes so thin that contact between the bearing surfaces occurs (Figure 2.60).

ELASTOHYDRODYNAMIC LUBRICATION

A variation of fluid film lubrication occurs when the bearing materials are not rigid as is the case in human joints. The soft material deforms under load and the deformations tend to increase the bearing contact area and prevent escape of lubricant fluid. This modification can occur in either hydrodynamic or squeeze film lubrication (Figure 2.61).

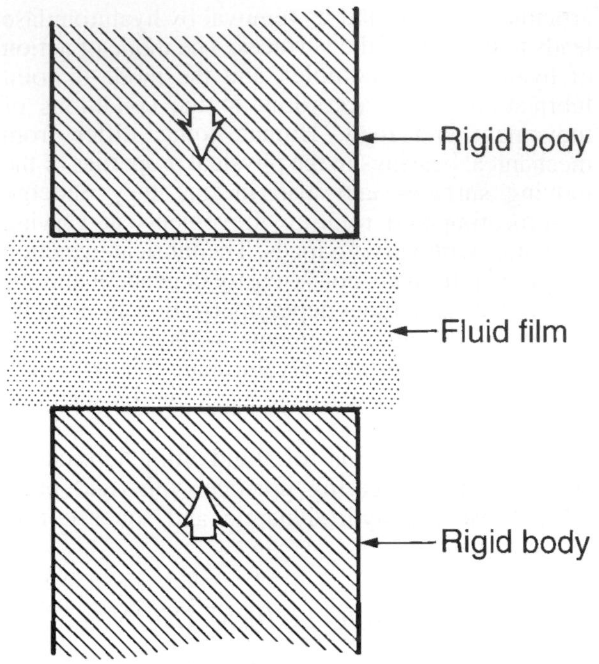

Figure 2.60 Squeeze film lubrication.

BOOSTED LUBRICATION

This form of lubrication, proposed by Walker *et al.* (1968, 1969, 1970) depends on the ability of the solvent component of synovial fluid to pass into the articular cartilage during squeeze film action, leaving behind it a concentrated pool of hyaluronic acid protein complex to lubricate the surfaces. As the two articular surfaces approach each other, pools of lubricating fluid are trapped between asperaties on the surface of the articular cartilage. The trapped pool of fluid becomes progressively more viscous, so boosting the lubrication. This mechanism may also operate in the presence of a sliding load (Figure 2.62).

ACTUAL MECHANISM OF JOINT LUBRICATION

The lubrication mechanisms operating in animal joints have not been completely elucidated and some of the reported findings are contradictory. The precise contribution of each of the types of lubrication mentioned is not fully understood. Boundary lubrication appears to be most important when the joint is stationary and under conditions of severe loading. As movement commences and loading is reduced there is a transition to a mixture of boundary and fluid film lubrication. Under these conditions boundary lubrication occurs between asperaties while fluid film lubrication occurs at other regions (Figure 2.63). In this 'mixed' lubrication, it is probable that most of the friction is generated in the boundary lubricated areas while most of the load is carried by the fluid film.

As speed increases, a conversion to elastohydrodynamic lubrication occurs. During slowing, squeeze film lubrication begins to operate once again and this continues until the limb is at rest. After a period of immobility, boundary lubrication again takes over. Between the extremes of boundary and elastohydrodynamic lubrication, the 'weeping' and the trapped pools systems are operating to an extent as yet undetermined (Figure 2.64).

MUSCLE

There are approximately 434 muscles in the human body with the muscle mass making up 25% of the body weight at birth and 40–45% in the adult. In embryonic life, muscle can act as a source of extramedullary haematopoeisis. At 12 weeks of fetal life, the embryonic muscle fibres split longitudinally and the earliest fetal movements occur, coinciding with the appearance of innervation to the muscles.

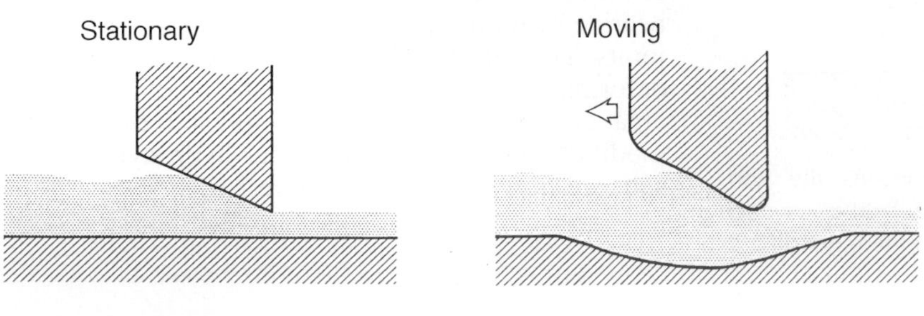

Figure 2.61 Elastohydrodynamic lubrication. The soft materials of the bearing surfaces deform with bearing surface area.

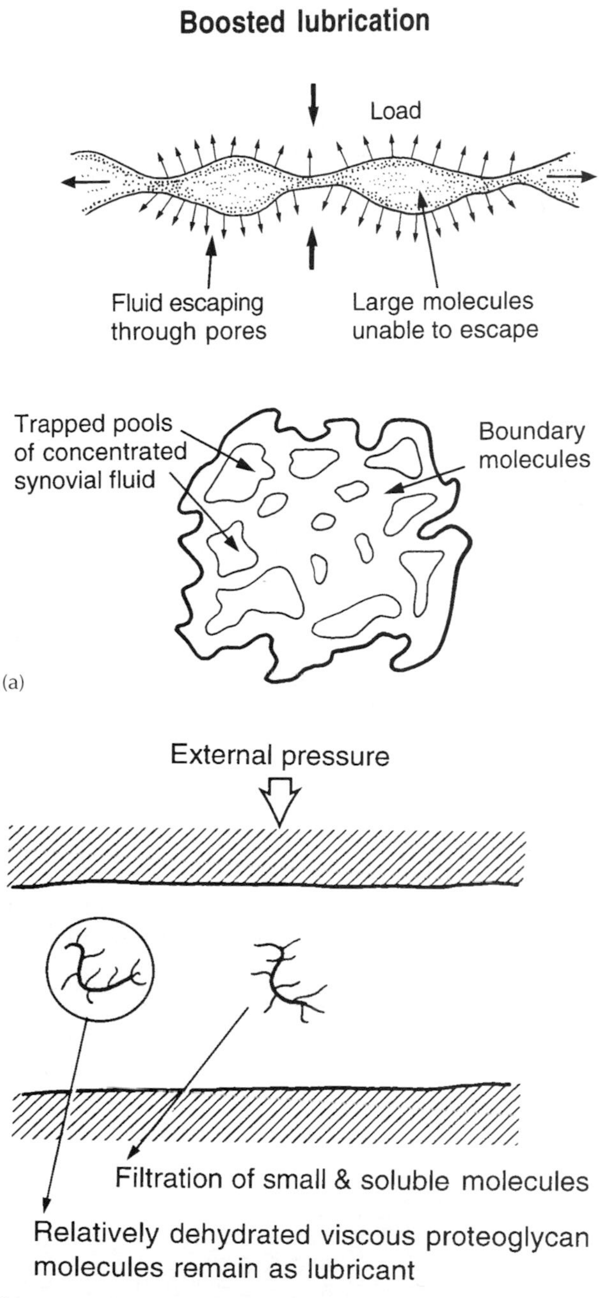

Figure 2.62 Boosted lubrication. (a) Ultrafiltration of the synovial fluid occurs at the articular surfaces. (b) This leaves behind proteoglycan molecules which are relatively dehydrated and which are, therefore, better able to resist the applied loads.

Muscle is made up of bundles of fibres surrounded by fibrous connective tissue sheaths. Different types of muscles have different arrangements of this connective tissue. There are three gross arrangements of muscle fibres:

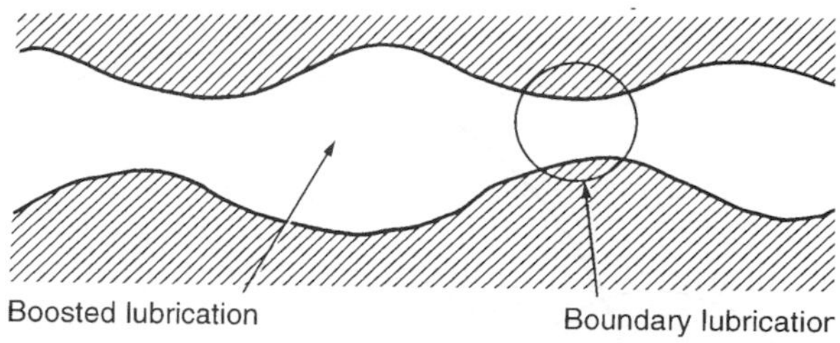

Figure 2.63 The mixed lubrication which occurs in a human joint.

1. Fusiform in which the fibres are parallel to the long axis of the muscle;
2. Pennate muscles where the fibres are oblique to a long axis of the muscle;
3. Radial or fan shape muscles in which the fleshy fibres converge from a wide origin or base to the apex.

In fusiform muscles the connective tissue sheaths run parallel to the long axis of the muscle; however, in all other muscles the sheaths run in more than one direction.

Structure of muscle

The fundamental cellular unit of skeletal muscle is the myofibril, which is a multinucleated syncytium. Clusters of myofibril are grouped together into fascicles which aggregate to form the complete muscle (Figure 2.65). Each myofibril is surrounded by endomysium, a basement membrane which merges into irregularly organized collagen fibrils. These fine collagen fibrils coalesce to form larger fibres which intermingle with elastic fibres to produce a denser connective tissue sheath which covers the fasciculi, termed the perimysium. The whole muscle is enclosed in a sheath of connective tissue, the epimysium of which is directly continuous with the deep fascia of the body.

THE MYOFIBRIL

The basic unit of the muscle fibre is the myofibril which has a diameter of approximately 1μm and may be many centimetres long. Myofibrils are ensheathed by membranes of the sarcoplasmic reticulum and transverse tubules which also contain glycogen granules, mytochondrial lysosomes and the ribosomes of the sarcoplasmic reticulum. Each myofibril is organized into sarcomeres and it is the transverse alignment of sarcomeres in adjacent parallel myofibrils which creates the characteristic striated

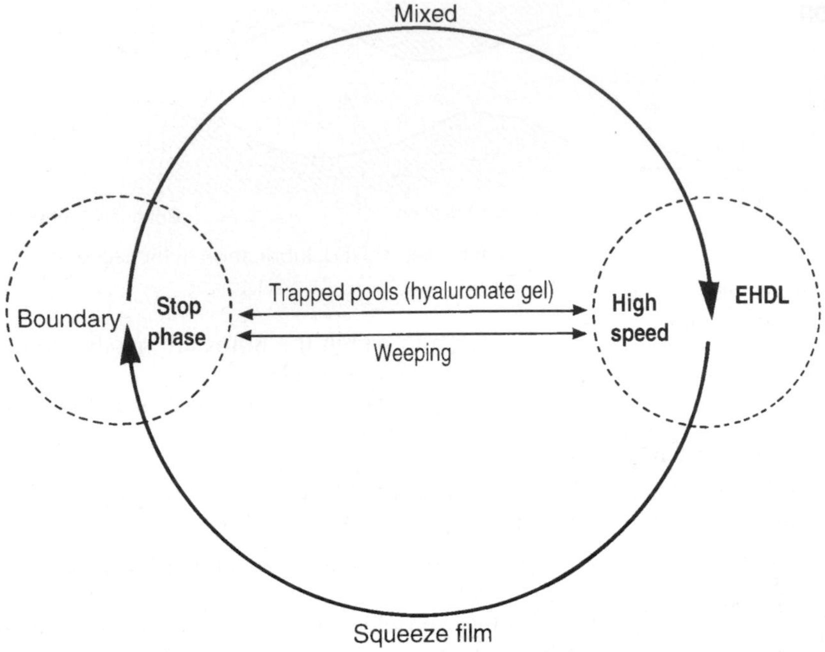

Figure 2.64 Mixed lubrication including stopping and starting. EHDL, elastohydrodynamic lubrication.

appearance of muscle. These striations result from the repetitive transverse bands in each sarcomere and are given the names, the Z, A and I bands. The distance between two Z bands is defined as the unit length of each sarcomere and varies with the state of contraction of the cell. The A band contains thick myofilaments and its length does not change during contraction. The I band contains thin myofilaments. Its length decreases during muscle contraction (Figures 2.66, 2.67).

BLOOD SUPPLY

The blood vessels supplying skeletal muscle run in the connective tissue sector between muscle bundles,

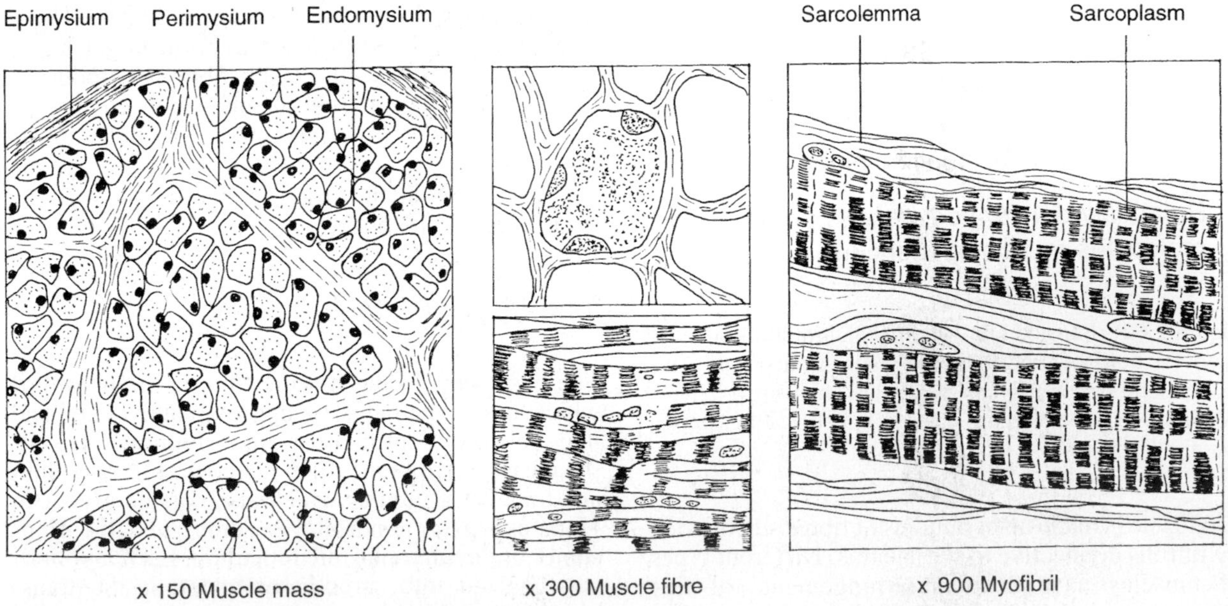

Figure 2.65 A diagram of mammalian skeletal muscle at varying magnifications.

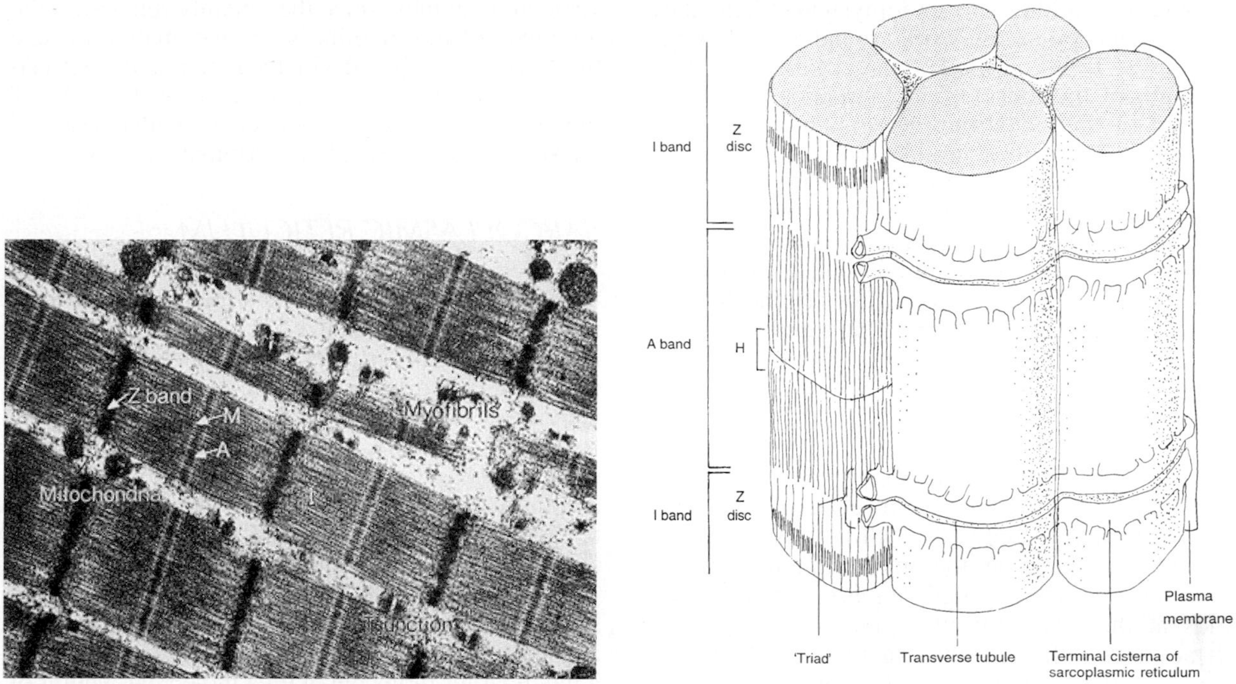

(a) (b)

Figure 2.66 (a) Electron micrograph (× 6912) of striated muscle fibre to show the darkened Z bands of sarcomeres separated by a central light strip of the A band containing the myosin filaments and actin. Mitochondrial particles lie between the filaments. (b) A diagram to show the banding, the plasma membrane, cistern and transverse tubule.

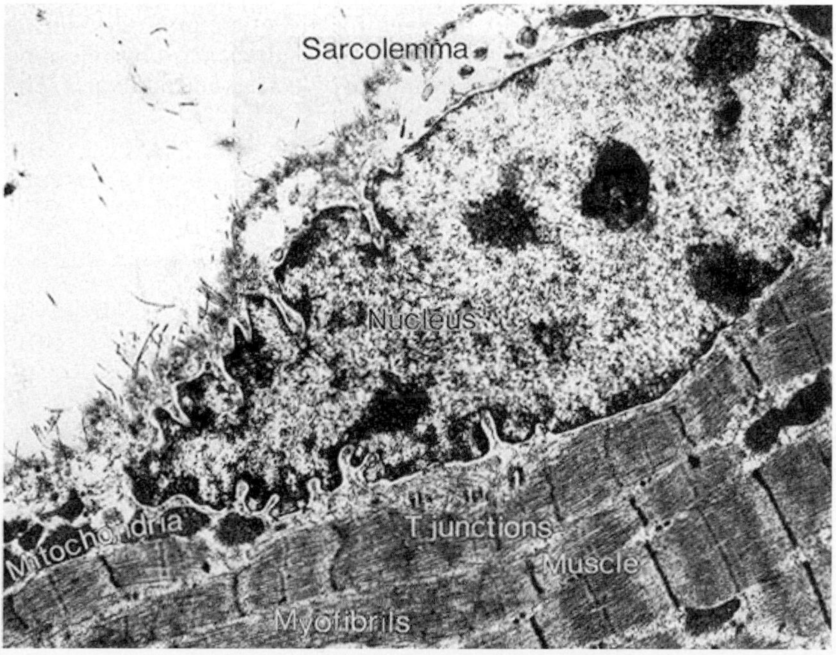

Figure 2.67 Electron micrograph showing the relationship of the myofibrils to the sarcolemma and muscle cell nucleus (× 9720).

eventually reaching the endomysium where they form a rich capillary network around the individual myofibrils. To accommodate the extensive changes in length of the muscle, the capillaries tend to be tortuous in contracted muscle, straightening during extension. Blood flow around the muscle fibres is regulated by terminal arterioles that can either shunt blood through arteriovenous anastomoses or direct it through the capillaries. The arterioles are richlysupplied by vasomotor sympathetic fibres, stimulation of which shuts off the arteriovenous shunts leading to a greater blood flow through the capillary bed.

SARCOLEMMA

The muscle cell plasma membrane (sarcolemma) is similar to that seen in other cells of the body (Horowitz and Schotland, 1986). It is, however, extensively folded at the myotendinous junction which increases the strength of this region. Complex folds at the neuromuscular junction increase the surface area of the myofibril, facilitate acetylcholine reception and invaginations of the membrane form the T system which expedites excitation contraction coupling. The T system and the adjacent cisterns of the sarcoplasmic reticulum are referred to as a triad. During myogenesis, myotubules are coupled together by low resistance gap junctions. These disappear after innervation so that muscle fibres are not directly coupled to other muscle fibres or to neurons.

TRANSVERSE TUBULES

The sarcolemma is invaginated to form an extensive anastomotic network around the myofibrils. These invaginations form tubules which are termed transverse or T tubules, since they mainly run across the long axis of the myofibrils. In mammalian muscle the T system is aligned with the junction of the A and I bands. Where they reach the myofibril, the T tubules are intimately associated with dilated sacs of the sarcoplasmic reticulum (terminal cisterns).

SARCOPLASMIC RETICULUM

The sarcoplasmic reticulum which surrounds the myofibrils is a specialized form of endoplasmic reticulum. It plays an essential role in the storage and release of calcium ions and its extent varies with the activity of the muscle, the largest quantities being found in constantly active muscle, whereas slowly contracting tonic muscles have relatively small amounts. Release of calcium ions from the sarcoplasmic reticulum is the final signal which causes the contractile proteins of muscle to shorten.

Myoglobin is the iron pigment present in the sarcoplasm of striated muscle fibres. Its properties are similar to those of haemoglobin. Haemoglobin is a much larger molecule, with a molecular weight of 68 000 and four iron atoms per molecule, as compared with myoglobin which has a molecular weight of about 17 500 and contains only one iron atom. Both substances have the common properties of combining in a reversible manner with oxygen and carbon dioxide; of being oxidizable to 'met compounds'; and both show similar absorption spectra. Myoglobin has a greater affinity for oxygen than has haemoglobin, although it has less affinity than the cytochromes. It is found in greater concentration in the red or dark muscles than in pale or light muscles. It reduces the need for glycolytic processes during the relative circulatory insufficiencies by releasing oxygen for breakdown of lactates and pyruvates. The

Table 2.8 How the three main types of myofibre motor unit differ in their content of cytochemical enzymes, glycogen and capillary network

Histochemical profile	Physiological type of motor unit FF	FR	S
Myofibrillar adenotriphosphatase	High	High	Low
ATPase activity – preincubation at pH 4.65	Intermediate	Low	High
DPNH succinate dehydrogenase	Low	Intermediate	High
PAS staining (presumed glycogen content)	High	Intermediate to high	Low
Phosphorylase	High	Intermediate to high	Low
Capillary network	Scant	Rich	Rich

FF, fast-contracting fatigue-sensitive; FR, intermediate; S, slow-contracting.
Reproduced, with permission from Burke, R. E.and Tsairis, P. (1973) *Journal of Physiology* **234**, 749–765.

more rapidly contracting flexor muscles in most animals tend to be paler than the extensors. Myoglobin is present in largest quantities in the muscles used for prolonged effort. Diving mammals, which can remain submerged for long periods, have about ten times the concentration of myoglobin as do other mammals, suggesting again that the myoglobin is a source of available oxygen.

Enzymes are now frequently studied by histochemical techniques, and over 50 have been identified and measured in serum; e.g. aldolases, aspartate transaminase and creatine kinase are often raised in primary myopathies (Table 2.8).

MYOFILAMENT PROTEINS

Huxley (1983) demonstrated that the thick myofilaments, which are made up of myosin, are arranged in a hexagonal lattice and that thin filaments, which contain actin, tropomyosin and troponin, interdigitate with them at each trigonal point (Figure 2.68).

Myosin is a complex actin-binding protein. It is made up of two heavy chains and four light chains. The light chains and N terminal portions of the heavy chains form globular heads which contain an actin-binding site and a catalytic site which incorporates an ATPase. Myosin has a total mass of approximately 480 kDa and there are approximately 300 myosin molecules per thick filament (Craig, 1986). In addition to myosin, the thick filaments contain at least six other proteins: C protein, M protein, myomesin, end protein, creatine kinase and titin. Radiating out from each thick filament is a series of cross-bridges interconnecting the thick and thin filaments in the zone of filament overlap.

The thin filament contains actin, tropomysin and troponin. *Actin* is a globular protein of approximately 42 kDa that polymerizes to form a double chain helical polymer. Each thin filament contains approximately 360 actin molecules. Troponin is a complex of three subunits, troponin I, troponin T and troponin C, which together weigh approximately 80 kDa. Troponin binds to F actin, inhibiting the actin–myosin interaction. Troponin C is the calcium-binding subunit. In the presence of calcium it relieves the troponin I induced inhibition of the actin-myosin interaction. Troponin T binds to tropomyosin. It facilitates the binding of troponin C to the actin–tropomyosin complex.

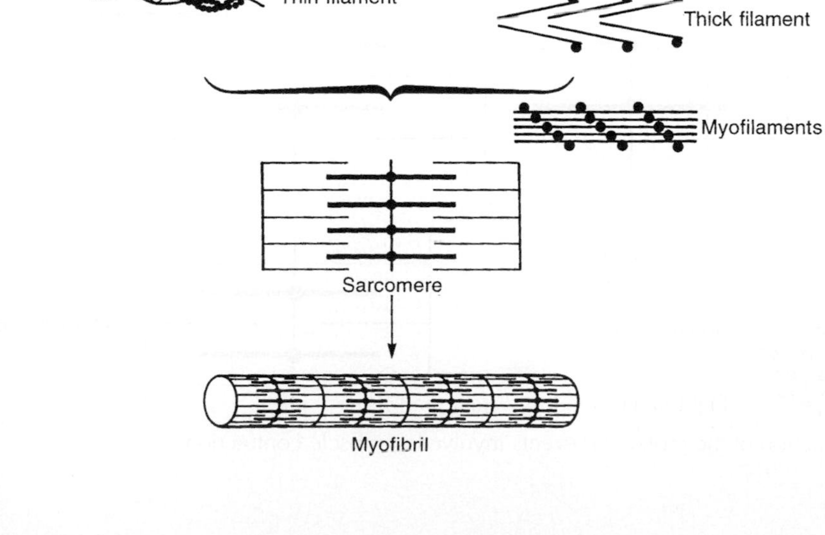

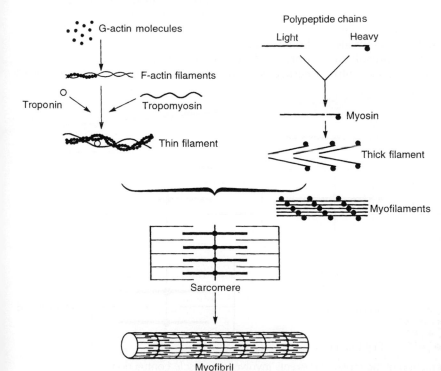

Figure 2.68 Schematic representation of the myosin (thick) and actin (thin) filaments in skeletal muscle, making up the myofilament proteins.

Electrical properties of the muscle cell membrane

The electrical properties of the skeletal muscle are qualitatively similar to those in nerve although there are quantitative differences.

The primary task of the skeletal muscle membrane is the activation of the contractile proteins in response to a received action potential from the motor nerve. In order to provide synchronization of contraction in sarcomeres throughout the length and thickness of the fibre, electrical activity is carried rapidly from its origin at the neuromuscular junction over the entire surface of the muscle fibre and into the interior of the fibre by propagation of the action potential along the surface membrane and the transverse tubular membranes (Horowitz and Spalding, 1986).

As in nerve the initial depolarization is due to the transient increase in permeability to sodium, leading to a passive influx of sodium ions and the subsequent repolarization is due to an increase in the passive efflux of potassium.

EXCITATION CONTRACTION COUPLING

The depolarization of the membrane induced by the action potential triggers the release of calcium ions from the terminal systems, the lateral sites of the sarcoplasmic reticulum next to the T system. The precise mechanism linking T tubule membrane depolarization with calcium release is unresolved (Horowitz, 1986), but the influx of calcium into the muscle fibril from the sarcoplasmic reticulum is mediated via a calcium channel which may be blocked by dihydropyridine.

In resting muscle, troponin I is closely bound through actin and tropomyosin, inhibiting the binding of actin to myosin. When calcium released by the action potential binds to troponin C, a confirmational change ensues, uncovering the actin–myosin binding site. As myosin binds to actin, the myosin ATPase is activated and contraction occurs. Seven myosin binding sites are made available for each molecule of calcium bound to troponin (Figure 2.69).

After the initial release of calcium from the sarcoplasmic reticulum, it begins to reaccumulate calcium by active transport. As the concentration of calcium in contact with the muscle fibrils decreases, the calcium is released from troponin C and the actin–myosin bond is broken (Figure 2.70).

The response of a muscle fibre to neuronal stimulation is not an instantaneous one. Muscle reaction must await transmitter release and diffusion across the synaptic gap from a binding alteration of membrane conduction generation of the end plate potential, generation of the action potential in the muscle fibre, depolarization of the muscle fibre, release and binding of calcium and, finally, the actual contraction of the muscle fibre proteins. There is therefore a definite lag between electrical stimulation and mechanical contraction. The interval between the electrical impulse and the beginning of the muscular contraction is known as the *activation period*. The twitch response begins approximately 2 ms after the start of depolarization of the membrane and its duration varies with the type of muscle fibre. In fast muscle fibres which are mainly concerned with fine, precise movement, the duration of

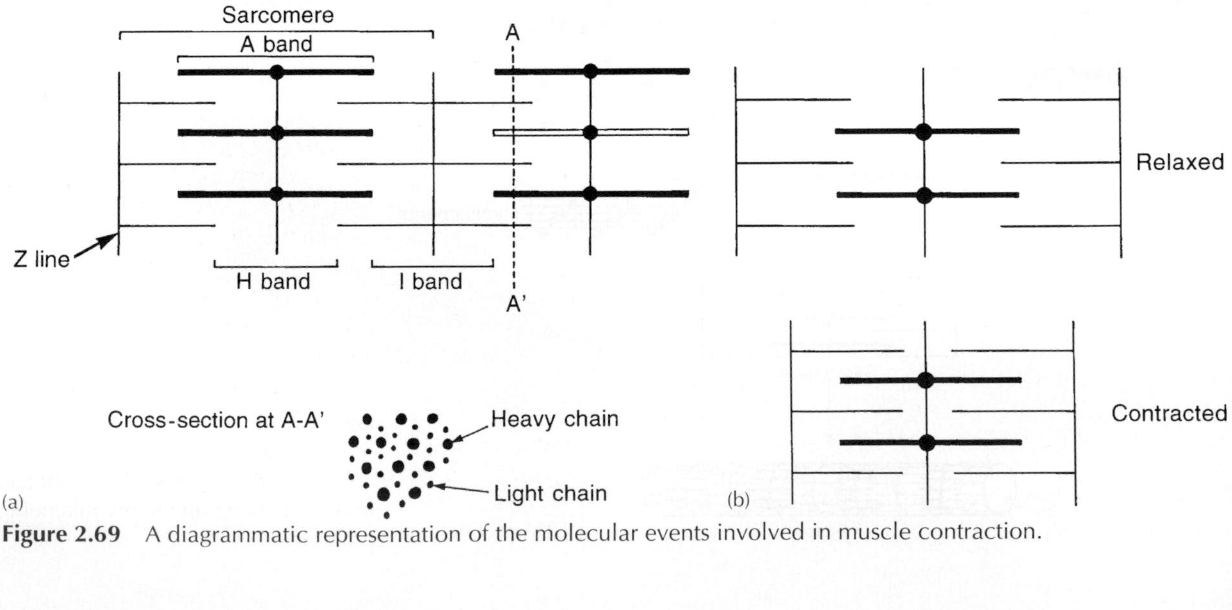

Figure 2.69 A diagrammatic representation of the molecular events involved in muscle contraction.

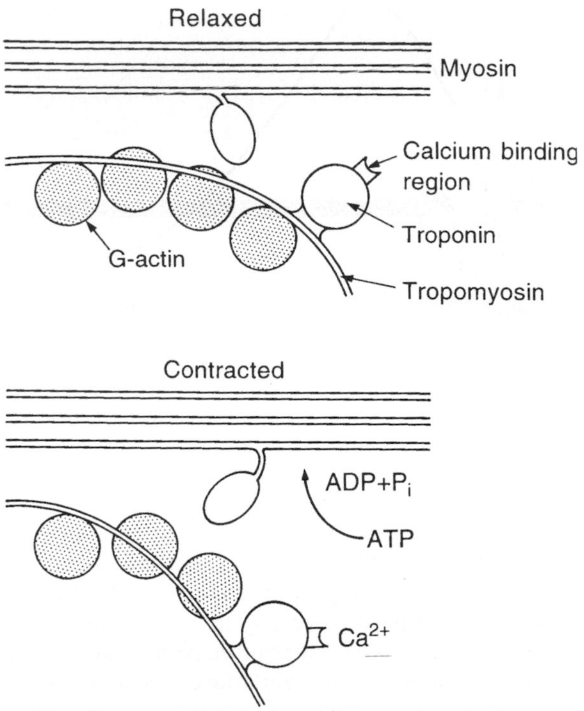

Figure 2.70 A diagram showing binding and release of Ca^{2+} during relaxation and contraction of muscle.

a twitch response may be as short as 8 ms. In slow muscle fibres which are primarily concerned with tonic movements the duration may be as long as 100 ms.

Reactions of muscle

The 'all-or-none' law must be included in any discussion of the conductile and contractile systems of muscle, and with the relationship between stimulation and contraction it is necessary to specify accurately the structure or structures involved. Certain properties must be present to qualify within this, law:

1. absence of graduated responses to graduated stimuli;
2. existence of a threshold;
3. absence of summation;
4. refractory period; and
5. a propagation of response.

It is obvious that a whole muscle does not qualify, for it will respond in greater contractions with graduated stimuli. It also displays summation (twitch to tetani) without a refractory period. The muscle fibre also displays similar properties. If a stimulus is strong enough to set up an impulse, the fibre shows its maximum response to that stimulus, but, with repeated stimuli, more tension is developed. This means that shortening of the contractile system goes on to completion with summation resulting. In this state there is maximum overlap of actin and myosin filament with no refractory period and, therefore, the contractile system cannot be considered as obeying the 'all-or-none' law. However, the conductile system is an all-or-nothing mechanism with a refractory period which is quite short, and roughly equal to the duration of the spike potential which is in turn followed by a negative phase. During this time, which is approximately equal to the twitch contraction phase, no repeated stimuli can be delivered.

PHYSIOLOGY OF MUSCLE CONTRACTION

Contraction of muscle refers to a series of internal events producing either shortening or development of tension. The muscle may shorten and produce movement, or it may perform work (isotonic), or it may partly contract and produce tension (isometric).

Types of muscle contraction

Two different sorts of muscle contraction are commonly described. In *isometric* contraction, the muscle is maintained at a constant length irrespective of the force generated within it. In *isotonic* contraction a constant load is applied and the muscle is allowed to shorten.

Muscle contraction may be sustained or transient. A single nerve impulse will result in a brief phasic contraction of the muscle fibre which is termed a *twitch response*. If a series of impulses stimulate the muscle then each impulse will generate its own twitch response. If the contraction initiated by the first impulse is not over by the time that initiated by the second impulse begins, *summation of contractions* will occur. The tension developed during the sum contraction is greater than during the single muscle twitch. When summation of contractions is maximal, the response is described as *tetany*.

Both the tension exerted by a muscle when it contracts and the resting tension within the uncontracted muscle vary with the length of the muscle (Figure 2.71). The passive tension (curve 1) is the tension within the resting muscle when it is passively stretched. The minimal tension which is present when the muscle is barely stretched is termed the resting tension.

The developed tension resulting from a twitch response is maximal at between 105 and 110% of the resting length and maximal tetanic contraction is

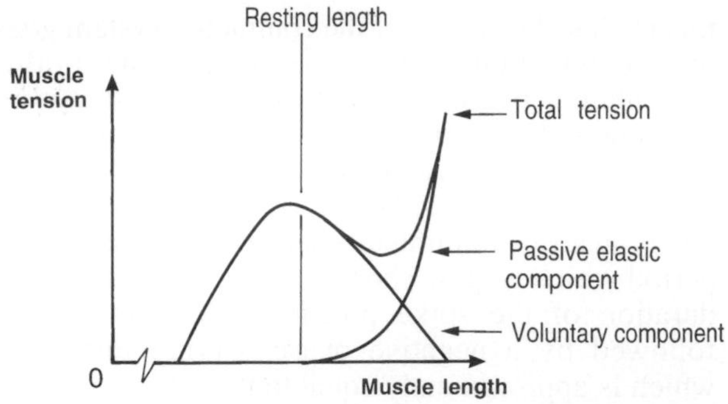

Figure 2.71 The relationship between the length of a muscle fibre and tension: curve 1 (passive elastic component) shows the result of applying passive stretch to a resting muscle until a peak tension develops; curve 2 (voluntary component) shows the tension which is produced by contraction of a muscle after it has been stretched; curve 3 (total tension) brings the summation of these two curves.

obtained at between 100 and 105% of resting length (curve 2).

MYOSTATIC CONTRACTURE

That a muscle as a total functioning unit can adapt to a new functional length is of great clinical importance. This situation obtains when the limb has been fixed by cast immobilization. When the cast is removed the joint motion is impaired. This limitation of the motion of an otherwise healthy joint is due to the development of a myostatic contracture.

By definition, a myostatic contracture is the adaptation of an innervated muscle to a new functional length. The cure of this contracture is effected by active exercises of the muscles involved. Stretching by external force at this stage may lead to tearing of muscle fibres and the development of pain. If the muscle has not been damaged by trauma or disease, it can regain its full function.

The sum of these two curves is the total tension (curve 3, Figure 2.71) and is maximum at resting length. There is a maximum length to which muscle can be passively stretched and activated before tension becomes zero. In these maximally stretched fibres, the tension rises quite slowly.

A variant to the basic tension/length curve pattern can be made by adding the entity of an intact tendon, with the appearance of 'stress relaxation' and 'creep'. Different isometric tensions are developed with and without intact tendons. As a tendon slowly lengthens (stress relaxation and creep), it allows a slight increase in the overlap of filaments and shows an earlier fall than noted without tension.

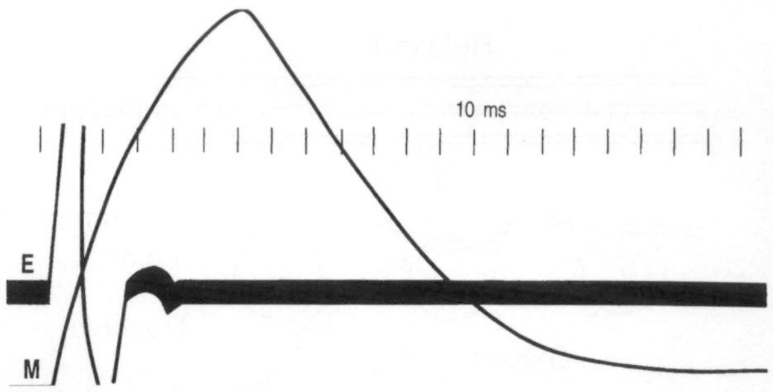

Figure 2.72 Showing the delay in muscle contraction (M) after an electrical stimulus (E).

The response of a muscle fibre to neuronal stimulation is not an instantaneous one. There is a definite lag between electrical stimulation or impulse and mechanical contraction, M (Figure 2.72), which varies with the type and size of the muscle. As already stated, there is an electric potential of +20 to 40 mV which is propagated along the fibre. This sharp wave is followed by a slow restitution of the original negative polarization. Neuromuscular transmission in both nerve and muscle is dependent upon the living membranes, which have a high resistance to direct current as well as excluding sodium ions so as to maintain a high intracellular concentration of potassium, and finally to transmit the excitatory process along the surface of the fibre. At the axon ending, acetylcholine is released which depolarizes the motor end plate as well as the muscle membrane. This renders the membrane more permeable to sodium and potassium ions, with the establishment of an end plate potential by this ion exchange. Near its peak, the end plate potential falls because of hydrolysis of the acetylcholine by cholinesterase and there is a resultant repolarization of all membranes. Deficiency in the amount of ionized calcium depresses the release of acetylcholine and potassium is needed for membrane propagation. The interval between electrical impulse and beginning of contraction is known as the *activation period*, and contains latency relaxation. The greater the activation period, the greater the initial length, with this period being directly related to the contractile elements. Mechanically, there is a greater resistance to stretch due to the formation of cross-bridges, and, thermodynamically, there is heat production. Microscopically, the muscle is seen to have an increased transparency.

Absolute muscle force is a method of comparing muscles of different sizes. It is the total amount of tension a muscle can exert under optimal conditions proportional to the total muscle fibres present. It is expressed as kg/cm^2 of cross-section in a plane at right angles to the force of the muscle fibres. In man it amounts to 3–4 kg/cm^2. It should be noted that for different types of muscles, by virtue of their fibre arrangement, the physiological cross-section will differ.

Two additional entities to be correlated with tension and shortening are speed and load. Load can be compared to the tension of an isometric contraction – the relations of force and speed of shortening being an exponential one. With a greater load, the muscle shortens less and more slowly. In the body, speed is also limited by mechanical inertia. Ramsey and Street (1940) felt that in isotonic conditions, muscles shorten exponentially, with their velocity being proportional to the distance they still have to shorten. Hill (1950) summed it up by stating that under isotonic conditions, with increased load there is:

1. an increased latent period which is equal to the time taken for a muscle to develop isometric tension equal to the isotonic load;
2. a decrease in maximum shortening; and
3. a decrease in initial velocity of shortening.

Tension is also affected by temperature changes. It is known that an increase in temperature decreases the magnitude of twitch tension and increases the magnitude of tetanic tension, whereas with cooler temperatures these are very much less efficient under varying loads and stretch. Since tension is generated by chemical reaction rather than any particular accumulation of the elastic elements the rate of this reaction is a limiting factor in tension development.

HEAT AND ENERGY RELATIONSHIPS

A common factor in all these relationships is heat and/or energy. Muscle in the resting state has a maintenance heat which is above that of its environment and obtained most probably from the lipid content. According to Hill there is, in the basal state, a constant rate of liberation of energy which will increase or decrease proportionately about 2.5 times by an increase or decrease of 10°C. When oxygen is added, there is increased liberation of heat. Maintenance heat can also be raised by increasing potassium ion concentration in the external solution, and by keeping the muscle under the same tension. Conversely, after a resting muscle has been stretched and then released, there is cooling, due to a reversal of chemical reactions. With activation, there is heat production once again, but usually before isometric or isotonic contractions are developed. It is associated with that period of extreme excitation and rapid chemical change. The heat of tetany or maintenance is equal to the sum of the heat of activation and of stimulus. It is that energy which is expressed as heat when maximum tension is attained with a constant length and the speed of shortening is zero. Muscle will liberate a constant amount of heat per unit of shortening, which is independent of load and velocity, but is dependent on distance and is related to isotonic contraction. When contracting muscle has stretch applied, there is less heat produced.

Work of muscle

A muscle lifting a heavy load obviously does more work than one lifting a light load, and therefore total energy developed by a muscle contracting over a given distance increases with the load. Total energy expenditure is equal to heat plus work performed and, therefore, increases with increases in load. Chemical reactions which provide energy for contraction are therefore controlled by the length of muscle and by tension applied. Energy is varied according to the external work done. The final formula is E (energy total) = A (activation heat) + AX (shortening heat) + W (mechanical work) for a twitch response:

$$E = A + AX + W$$

The heat produced is related to the speed of a muscle, the rapid muscles having a larger amount of heat production, whereas the slow have a smaller amount.

The final type of heat production is that of recovery. With the oxidation of carbohydrates or aerobic metabolism, there is a slow rise in temperature. With rapid production, the reactions of adenosine triphosphate and creatine phosphate are involved.

The role of oxygen in relation to energy production is of great significance, because it is needed for oxidation of carbohydrates. During a submaximal contraction, glucose is oxidized to CO_2 and water. Under these circumstances there is also enough energy to recharge the phosphorylated compounds. In the anaerobic state, energy is obtained by hydrolysing glycogen into lactic acid – this being called the *oxygen debt*. In the anaerobic state one also finds an increase in the osmotic pressure and in the molar concentration of water, in muscle with breakdown of phosphate compounds, ATP and creatine phosphate. There is a decrease in vapour pressure and a distillation of water into muscle. The heat of condensation increases the apparent rate of heat production. The oxygen debt of exercise, therefore, results in an apparent increased heat of recovery.

There are additional factors concerned with the function of muscle. The *designed* muscle varies with its role. Muscle is designed either for speed of movement or for economy of energy (e.g. concerned with posture and maintenance of forces). The *size* of muscle is important for maximum power output, but any maintained effort is proportional to the body surface of the muscle mass. Wilkie determined the effective mechanical work to be 3 hp/kg muscle weight, Fenn (1923–4) having established the efficiency of muscle to be 0–25%. The strength of muscle is then determined by the number of fibres, the direction of action, and the manner of origin and insertion. In humans, the two optimum speeds of a muscle, one of maximum efficiency and the other of maximum power output, are usually about the same for any one muscle.

The neuromuscular junction

The neuromuscular junction is a chemical synapse which transmits a signal from a nerve fibre to a well defined post-synaptic region of a muscle fibre. A motor unit has been defined by Liddell and Sherrington (1925) as a single motor neuron and all the fibres which it innervates. The number of muscle fibres per muscle unit depends on the species and the individual muscle, and ranges from approximately 10 in extraocular muscles to over 1000 in human gastrocnemius muscles. The majority of motor units, however, have several hundred fibres. All the muscle fibres of a single motor unit have the same physiological and histochemical characteristics (Salpeter, 1987), raising the question of the extent to which the nature of a muscle fibre is determined by its neural connection.

ANATOMY

As the terminal part of the axon of the motor neuron nears the muscle which it supplies, it divides into branches, each terminating at a motor end plate on a different muscle fibre, usually near to its midpoint. The terminal branch then looses its myelin sheath and divides into a number of small bulbous swellings or end feet which contain multiple clear vesicles containing acetylcholine. The end feet fit into depressions in the motor end plate which itself occupies a recess in the muscle cell surface, described as the sole plate. The post-synaptic membrane of the neuromuscular junction is deeply folded (Engel, 1986), presumably to increase the area of membrane which can be depolarized as a result of acetylcholine release (Figures 2.73, 2.74).

NEUROMUSCULAR TRANSMISSION

Acetylcholine-containing vesicles undergo random exocytosis from the end feet in the absence of an action potential. Each time this occurs, approximately 10 000 molecules of acetycholine are released. These bind to the motor end plate acetycholine receptors and produce a temporary depolarization which is referred to as a miniature end plate potential.

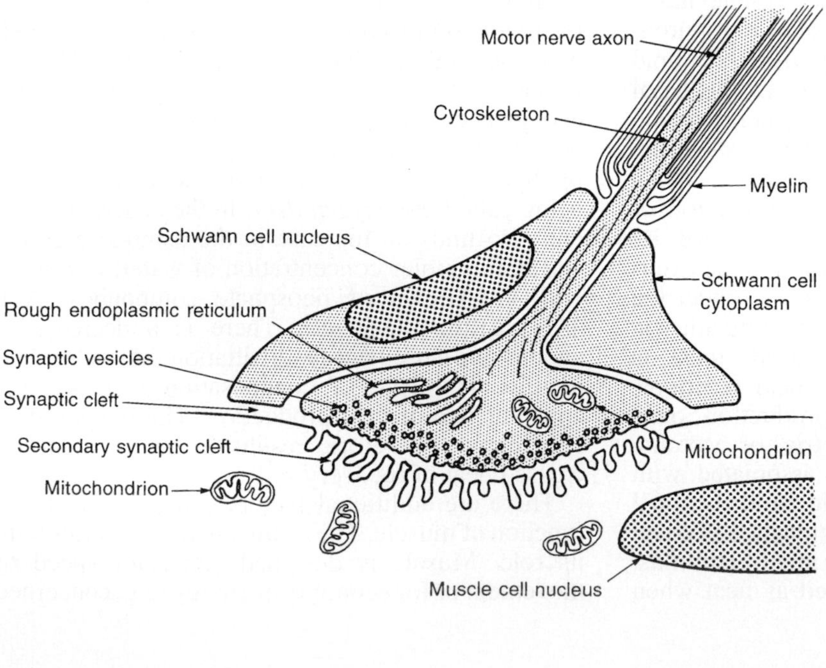

Figure 2.73 A diagram of the neuromuscular junction.

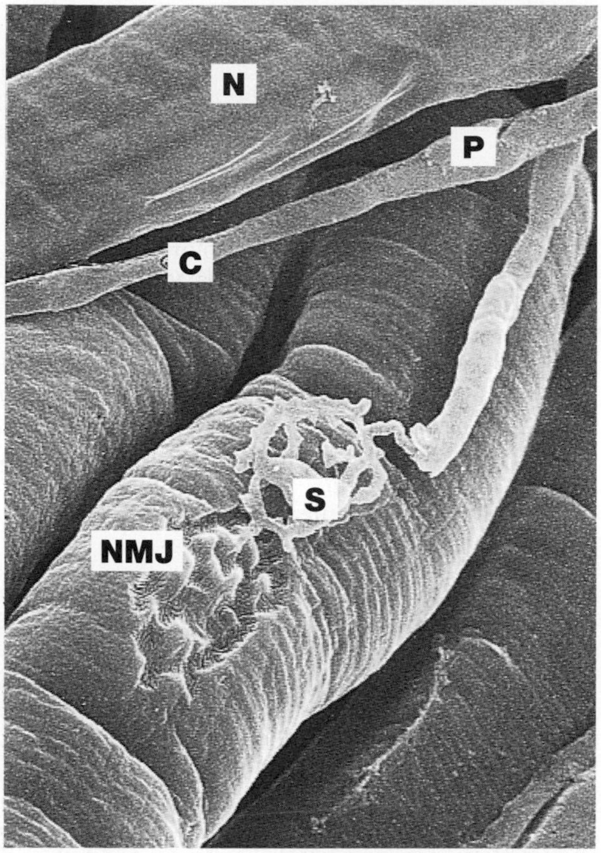

Figure 2.74 Scanning electron micrograph showing a neurovascular junction with nerve fibre leaving the main trunk proximally and running down into the middle of muscle fibres (NMJ). One Schwann cell can be seen (S). Just below the main nerve (N) there is a capillary (C) with a pericyte (P) on its wall. (Reprinted from Matsuda, Y. *et al.* (1988) *Muscle and Nerve* **11**, 1267 with permission of the authors and John Wiley & Sons Inc.)

The nerve impulse arriving at the distal end of the motor neuron increases the permeability of the membrane of the end feet to calcium which results in a transient marked increase in exocytosis of the acetylcholine-containing vesicles. The released acetylcholine diffuses across the synaptic gap and binds to acetylcholine receptors which are concentrated in the folds of the membrane of the motor end plate. Acetylcholine binding increases the permeability of the membrane to sodium and potassium and the resultant influx of sodium depolarizes the motor end plate. If sufficient acetylcholine binds to the motor end plate, the local membrane is depolarized to its firing level and action potentials are generated on either side of the end plating and are conducted away in both directions along the muscle fibre.

The acetylcholine is broken down by acetycholine esterase located in the motor end plate.

NERVE

The human nervous system contains approximately 1 million million nerve cells or neurons and between 10 and 100 times this number of supporting or glia cells. Nerve cells are of many different sorts. They may be motor or sensory, autonomic or somatic and central or peripheral; however, the majority have similar parts to a motor neuron (Figure 2.75). There is a cell body containing a nucleus and a number of processes termed dendrites which extend from the cell body and have multiple branches. A single axon originates from a thickened area of the cell body, the axon hillock, and distally divides into terminal branches, each ending in terminal buttons or synaptic knobs which demonstrate vesicles containing synaptic transmitters.

The axon of the motor neuron is myelinated, that is, it is surrounded by many layers of the cell membrane of a Schwann cell. The myelin sheath surrounds the axon except at its two ends and at nodes of Ranvier which are gaps of approximately

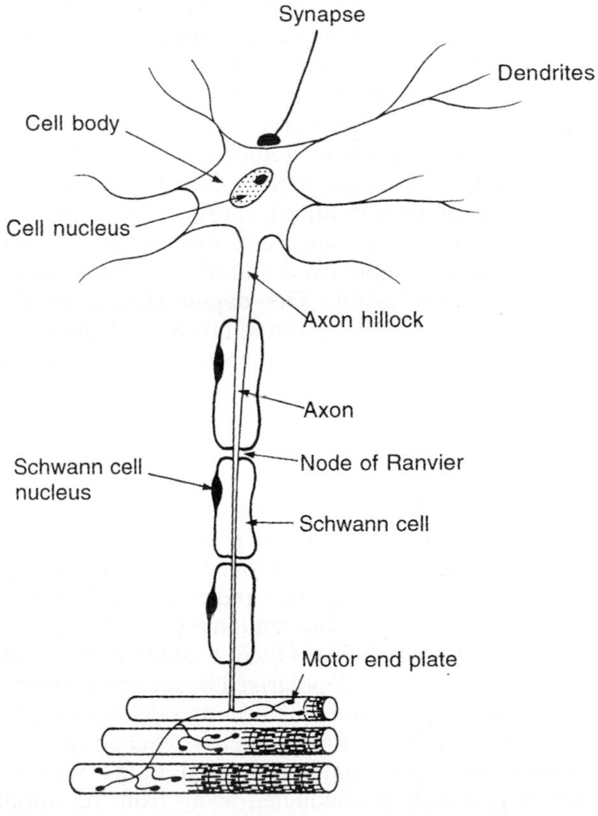

Figure 2.75 A diagrammatic representation of a motor neuron.

1 μm in the myelin sheath which occur roughly every millimetre. The myelin sheath serves to insulate the axon so that the excitatory impulse can jump from one node of Ranvier to the next. Not all the mammalian neurons are myelinated. Unmyelinated nerve fibres have a single covering layer from the Schwann cell. In these, the lack of insulation means that the nerve impulse must be regenerated at more frequent intervals so that conduction is slower and less energy efficient.

If a small alteration in the membrane potential occurs, it will cause slight alterations in the ionic fluxes across the membrane which tend to restore the membrane potential to its resting value.

A potential difference exists across the membrane of a nerve cell, which is found in almost all cells. In a nerve cell it is approximately –70 mV and it is due to active pumping of sodium out of the cell and potassium into the cell by an ATP-linked sodium potassium pump. In the resting state potassium is gradually leaking out of the membrane and sodium leaking in through specific channels which allow the passage of one or other ion. In excitable tissues (that is, tissues which are capable of producing an action potential), these channels are provided with 'gates' which open or close the channel and which are sensitive to alterations in the cell membrane potential.

If a small alteration in the membrane potential occurs, it will cause slight alterations in the ionic fluxes across the membrane which tend to restore the membrane potential to its resting value. However, depolarization of the nerve cell membrane to a threshold level leads to a sudden reduction in the resistance of the cell membrane to sodium ions (sodium channel activation), causing rapid depolarization of the membrane. The increase in sodium conductance is short lived and the sodium channel quickly closes again. The depolarization of the membrane also opens a potassium channel, although this happens more slowly than the opening of the sodium channel and the consequent increase in potassium flux out of the cell causes repolarization of the membrane. As the membrane repolarizes the potassium channel shuts slowly so that there is an initial hyperpolarization which gradually returns to the normal resting membrane potential.

This sequence of local minor depolarization of the cell membrane leading to a rapid complete depolarization followed by repolarization is termed an action potential (Figure 2.76). Once a small part of the membrane has been depolarized by an action potential, the adjacent membrane becomes depolarized by ionic flow until the firing level is reached and the further action potential is generated. In this way the action potential is conducted away from its initial site of insection. In a myelinated fibre, the nerve between the nodes of Ranvier is effectively insulated and the depolarization is able to jump from one node to the next, increasing the speed of conduction of the nervous impulse and reducing the energy requirement by limiting the area of membrane which requires depolarization.

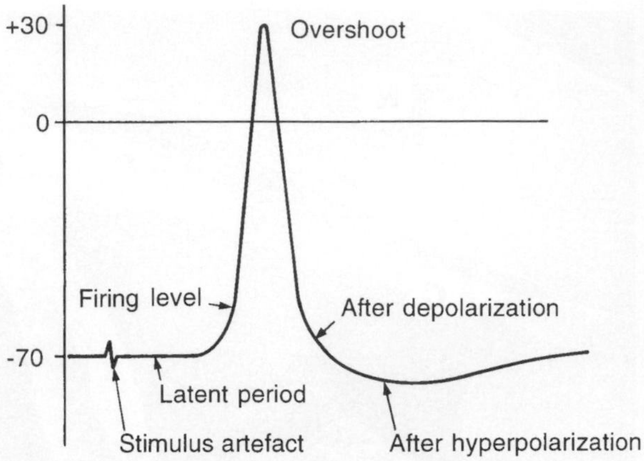

Figure 2.76 A diagrammatic representation of an action potential which can be recorded by placing an electrode within a nerve cell.

The mechanism of generation of an action potential implies that it is an 'all or nothing' phenomenon. If the initial depolarization is not sufficient to overcome the tendency of the resting membrane potential to restore itself, no action potential will be generated; however, if a 'threshold level' of depolarization is reached, then no further depolarization is necessary to initiate an action potential and an increase in the amount of depolarization will not generate a larger action potential.

Immediately following the passage of an action potential the membrane is insensitive to a further depolarization. This period is known as the 'refractory period'.

For further discussion of nerves, see Chapter 13.

BIOMECHANICS

Biomechanics is the application of the principles of engineering and physics to the behaviour of biological materials and in particular for the orthopaedic surgeon, to the human body. It aims to quantify the forces acting on components of the body and the movements that occur between them. Practical applications of biomechanics extend from the forces experienced by the body in everyday living through sporting training to mechanisms of injury and degenerative change. In addition, the majority of orthopaedic treatments, whether surgical or conservative, aim to alter biomechanical forces, emphasizing the central role of this field (Cochrane, 1980; Frankel and Nordin, 1980).

The mechanical principles used to analyse these functional processes are relatively simple; it is the anatomical and morphological complexity of the human body which restricts their utility.

Units of measurement

The currently accepted units of measurement are defined by the metric based 'Système International d'Unités' (SI). This system takes as its basis arbitrary definitions of units of length, mass, time and temperature (as well as several quantities of less interest to orthopaedic surgeons).

Quantities to be measured may be divided into scalar or vector. *Scalar* quantities (such as mass or length) have magnitude but no direction, whereas *vector* quantities such as velocity, force or acceleration must be defined in terms of both magnitude and direction.

Rigid body mechanics

The basic substance which makes up all physical objects is termed matter which is composed of atoms and molecules and occupies space. *Mass* is a property of matter which imparts to it a tendency to resist changes in its movement, which is termed *inertia*. Objects on earth are acted upon by a gravitational force which causes the object to accelerate towards the centre of the earth. The action of the gravitational force is proportional to the mass of the object and is called its *weight*.

The rate of movement of a body is described by its velocity. This is a precise term used to describe magnitude and direction of movement. The units of velocity are metres per second (m/s), and the direction must be defined in terms of a reference such as a horizontal surface, with some direction marker on it.

When a *force* acts on a mass it produces a change in the velocity of the mass in the direction in which the force acts. The rate of change of the velocity is termed *acceleration*, whose magnitude is expressed in metres per second per second (m/s^2). The acceleration of a body is proportional to the applied force, inversely proportional to the mass of the body and in the same direction as the applied force. Thus:

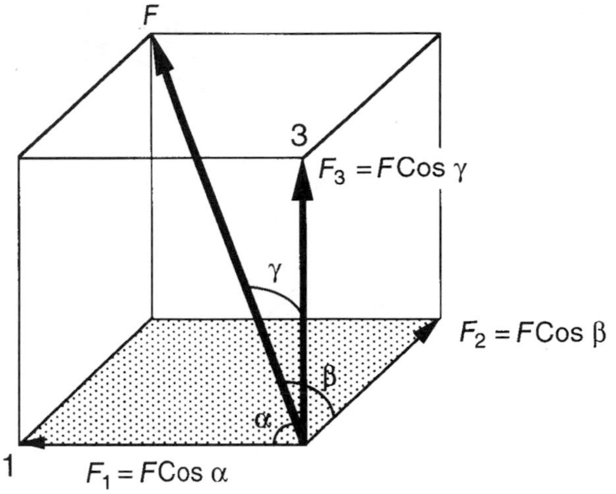

Figure 2.77 Three-dimensional space relationships of forces acting in three principal directions.

$$\text{Force} = \text{mass} \times \text{acceleration}.$$

Scalar quantities may be added and subtracted simply. Thus if a mass of 1 kg is added to a 2 kg mass, the resulting mass is 3 kg. However, where more than one vector quantity is to be considered, the direction in which the vector is acting is crucial.

When considering a vector quantity in three-dimensional space, it is convenient to relate the direction of action of the vector to three perpendicular directions, e.g. two horizontal and one vertical. The vector quantity can be *resolved* or divided into three components, one in each of the principal directions. The magnitude of each component is proportional to the total magnitude of the force and the cosine of the angle between the total force and the principal direction (Figure 2.77).

When adding vector quantities the quantities must first be resolved into components in the principal directions and these components can then be added. This is called *resolution of forces*. The reverse method can be used to find the *resultant* of the components. The magnitude of the resultant is given by:

$$F=\sqrt{(F_1^2+F_2^2+F_3^2)}$$

where F_1, F_2 and F_3 are the magnitudes of the vector quantity in the three principal directions.

The angles of the resultant to the three principal directions are given by

$$\text{Cos}\alpha = \frac{F}{F_1} \qquad \text{Cos}\beta = \frac{F}{F_2} \qquad \text{Cos}\gamma = \frac{F}{F_3}$$

Addition of only two vector quantities is a special case as the addition can be done in the plane in which

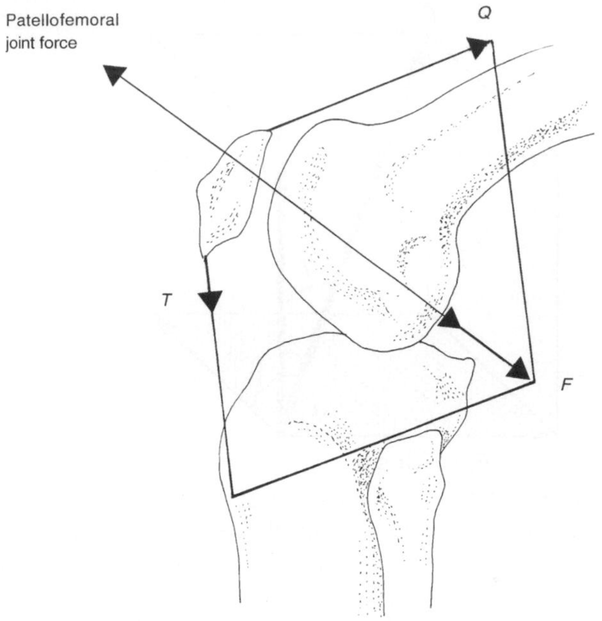

Figure 2.78 Patellofemoral joint force as a parallelogram of forces with *F* as the resultant of the quadriceps force (*Q*) and *T* the infrapatellar ligament tension.

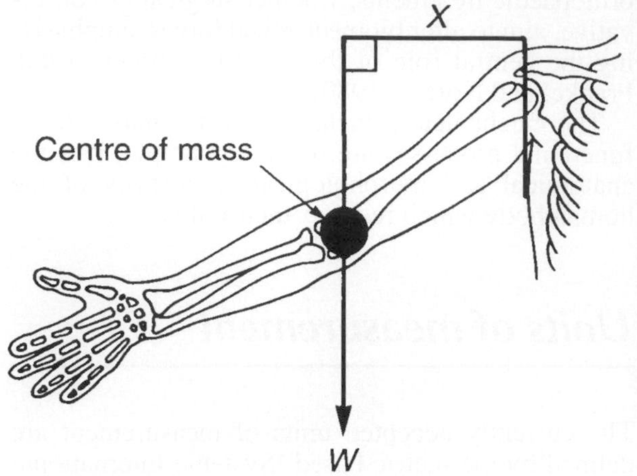

Figure 2.79 Showing the moment of force arising from the magnitude (W) times the perpendicular distance (X).

both the forces act. The parallelogram of forces is a geometric analogy used to describe the resultant two forces. If the two forces are represented by two adjacent sides of a parallelogram, their total can be represented by the diagonal of the parallelogram.

Using the forces on the patella as an example, the resultant of the quadriceps muscle pull (*Q*) and the infrapatellar ligament tension (*T*) is the force *F* (Figure 2.78). If the patella is not accelerating there must be an equal and opposite force in the patellofemoral joint resisting the force *F*. The magnitude and direction of this force can be calculated provided the other two forces are known.

Just as linear movement can be defined by the magnitude and direction of its velocity and acceleration, rotation can be defined by *angular velocity* and *angular acceleration*. The angle may be measured in degrees, radians or revolutions and the movement is defined by the *axis of rotation* about which it occurs. The angular acceleration of a body is proportional to the movements of the applied forces about the axis of rotation.

An example of linear movement is the movement of a fixed point on a motor car driving along a straight road, whereas an example of angular movement is rotation about the axis of the elbow joint in flexion and extension of the forearm (Figure 2.79). It should be noted, however, that movements of the limbs are complicated by the joints having axes of rotation which are not fixed or constant.

The *moment of a force* is the magnitude of the force multiplied by the perpendicular distance from its line of action to the axis of rotation. In the case of a pendulum where the mass is concentrated in a small region which is a relatively large distance away from the centre of rotation, it is easy to calculate the distance of the mass away from the axis of rotation. However, in biomechanics the majority of objects to be considered are irregular and the mass of the object is spread throughout space. It is, therefore, difficult to calculate, for example, the moment of the mass of the forearm about the elbow joint. To overcome this difficulty the concept of *centre of mass* has been introduced. This is an imaginary point of balance through which all the mass of an object may be said to act.

Angular acceleration of a body is proportional to the applied moments of forces and inversely proportional to the *moment of inertia* of the body about the axis of rotation. Moment of inertia is a complex property which is concerned with the distribution of the mass of the body about the axis of rotation. Thus:

Moment of force about axis of rotation =
moment of inertia about axis of rotation
× angular acceleration of body

The equilibrium of a joint depends upon the external loading and the forces in the muscles and ligaments which cross the joint. The absence of rotation in the joint depends on the total of the moments of forces about the joint being zero. The moments of these forces are difficult to estimate because the axis of rotation of a joint is not fixed and the distances of the ligaments and tendons around the joint may vary with its movement. The tension which can be developed in the muscle varies with the degree of stretch (Figure 2.80). Thus the leverages of muscles about a joint are difficult to estimate from

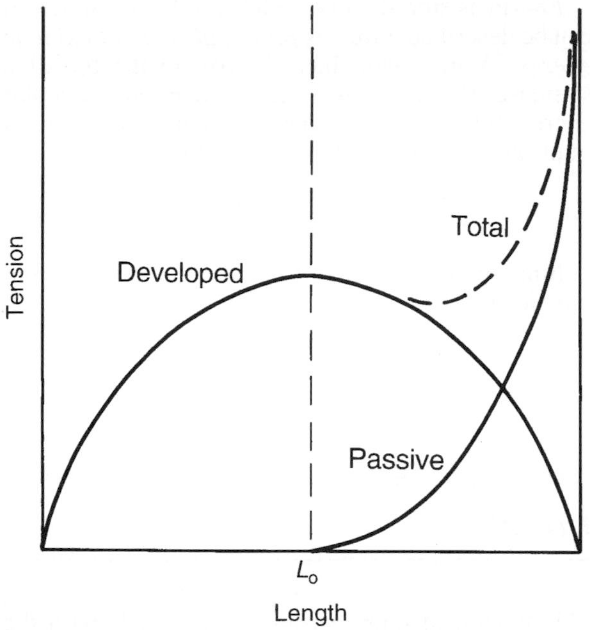

Figure 2.80 Illustrating the amount of tension developing in relationship to muscle length or stretch.

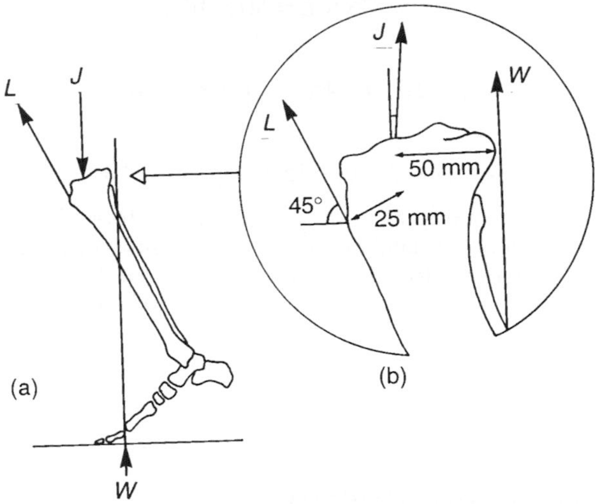

Figure 2.81 The equations for equilibrium in the three directions for the knee joint of a man standing on one leg. *L*, load; *J*, median force; *W*, weight.

consideration of muscle force and anatomical dimensions and conversely it is difficult to deduce the tensions in muscles and ligaments from measurements of externally applied forces. To estimate the forces acting on a joint, the following data must be available:

1. The external forces (including the forces of gravity on part of the body).
2. The positions of areas of contact in the joint.
3. The distances of the external forces from the areas of contact (from which the external moments about the joint can be calculated).
4. The distribution of the forces in ligaments and muscles which cross the joint.
5. The distances of these structures from the joint contact.

This sort of analysis has been undertaken to estimate the forces in most of the major joints of the body. Such analyses depend upon simplifying assumptions about the distribution of tension between the various ligaments and muscle and the structure of the joint in question.

In order to deduce the magnitude, direction and point of application of a force acting on any part of the body in equilibrium, the forces acting in each of the three principal directions are considered and their moments taken about an arbitrary point. Since the body is in equilibrium, the sum of the forces acting in each of the three directions and the sum of the moments about any arbitrary point must be zero (otherwise the body would accelerate in proportion to the force acting, until equilibrium was established) and so four equations of motion can be written.

Consider the case illustrated in Figure 2.81. A man is standing on one leg with the knee flexed and only the magnitude and direction of the force from the floor is known immediately, since this is equivalent to the body weight (*W*). The following simplifications and assumptions can be used to obtain an approximate solution for the forces in the knee joint:

1. All forces act in the central plane.
2. The only ligament force (*L*) is that of the infrapatellar ligament, which acts here at 45° to the vertical.
3. The resultant joint force acts through a point 25 mm from the infrapatellar ligament and 50 mm anterior to the line of the vertical force acting from the floor. (These dimensions could be estimated from a lateral radiograph).

The equations of motion would be:

1. In the mediolateral direction 0 = 0 (no forces act)
2. In the vertical direction:

$$W + L\cos 45^\circ = J_V$$

(vertical component of joint force)

3. In the horizontal direction:

$$L\cos 45^\circ = J_H$$

(horizontal component of joint force)

4. Taking moments about the point where the resultant joint force acts upon the patella:

$$25 \times L = 50 \times W$$

Thus:

$$J_H = 2W \cos 45 = \text{approx. } 1.4W$$

and

$$J_V = W + 2 \times \cos 45 = \text{approx. } 2.4W$$

Thus the total joint force J = the square root $(J_V^2 + J_H^2)$ is approximately equal to $2.5W$. This force acts in a direction α to the vertical where $\cos \alpha = J_V$ which is approximately 2.4 divided by 2.8. So α is approximately 30°.

This sort of analysis for the knee joint has been developed extensively by Maquet (1984).

Work and energy

In a mechanical sense, *work* is done when a force moves its point of application. Thus no work is done by a muscle which contracts isometrically. The work done by a muscle is the tension in it multiplied by the distance it contracts. Since the tension in a muscle may vary during the contraction, numerical integration (summation of small increments of activity) may be needed to find the work done.

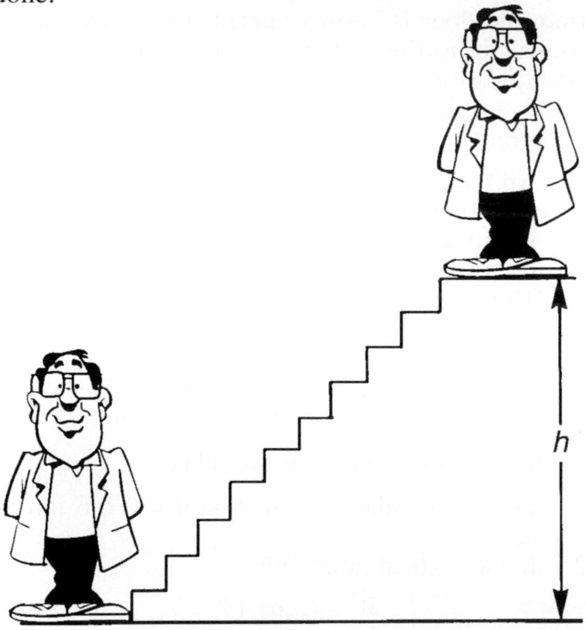

Figure 2.82 Muscle energy, potential energy and kinetic energy. In climbing the stairs the man will develop potential energy equal to his mass times the acceleration due to gravity (= weight) times the height of the stairs. If he falls from the top of the stairs, the potential energy will be converted into kinetic energy (equal to half his mass times his velocity squared).

Energy is stored work which can be reclaimed. It can be described either as *potential energy* or *kinetic energy*. A man who has climbed to the top of a staircase (Figure 2.82) has converted muscular energy into potential energy equal to his weight multiplied by the height of the stairs. Thus:

$$\text{Potential energy} = \text{mass} \times \text{gravitational force} \times \text{height.}$$

Falling involves converting potential energy into kinetic energy:

$$\text{Kinetic energy} = {}^1\!/_2 \text{ mass} \times \text{velocity}^2.$$

Mechanics of deformable bodies

This branch of engineering science deals with the strength of material and with the events within a material as it deforms under an applied load.

Any force which is applied to a body will change the shape of the body, either temporarily or permanently and the effect may range from gross to infinitely small. Change in shape is called *deformation*. *Strain* is the term used to express deformation. It is the overall change in a given direction. For example, if an elastic band 5 cm long is stretched to 6 cm the strain is 1 cm. Alternatively strain may be expressed as *unit strain* or *percentage strain*. In this case a ratio is used expressing the change in dimension as a fraction of the original dimension. Thus in the above example the unit strain is 0.2 and the percentage strain 20%.

In examining the strength of materials, very small strains may be encountered. For example, under biological loading a 10 cm plate may stretch as much as one hundred thousandth of a centimetre. In this case the unit strain is 1×10^6. A unit strain of this order is referred to as 1 *microstrain*.

Strain within a material is the result of a force applied. *Stress* is the force applied divided by the area over which it acts.

Although it is common practice in engineering terms to consider stress before strain since the strain within a material is produced by the stress applied to it, it is probable that in biological systems the more important consideration is the strain experienced by a material and evidence is accumulating that, particularly in bone, the strength of the material is adjusted by the organism in response to applied loads in order to maintain the strain within a constant biologically acceptable range.

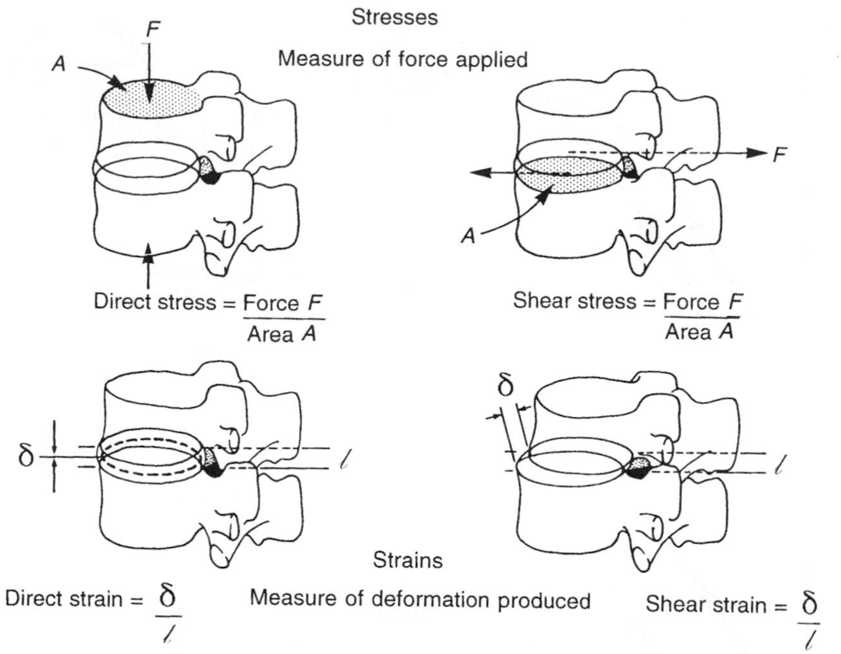

Figure 2.83 Showing the differences between stresses and strains when applied to the lumbar vertebrae.

Stresses and strains may act either perpendicular to a plane (*normal* stress or *compressive* or *tensile* strain) or parallel to a gven plane (*shear* stress or strain). Stress is measured in newtons per square metre (N/m^2). Bending moments produce tension stress on one side of a structure and compressive stress on the opposite side. Torques in a slender structure produce tension and compressive stresses at 45° to the axis of application, so long bones fractured by torques often display a spiral form of fracture.

Strain is the standardized measure of deformation in material. Direct strain is the change in the perpendicular distance between two planes in the material (δ) divided by the unstressed distance between them l). Shear strain is the amount of parallel movement between two planes divided by the distance between them (Figure 2.83). Because strain is a distance divided by a length, it is dimensionless.

Since stresses and strains are never uniform throughout a sample of material, they are only correctly definable at any given point and only for infinitesimally small areas and distances between planes.

In terms of its response to applied stresses, an *elastic* material returns to its original shape when the applied stress is removed. The simplest form of elastic deformation is one where the strain induced is directly proportional to the applied stress over a wide range of stress. Such a material is said to show *linear elastic* behaviour. The *elastic modulus* is given by the stress divided by the strain. For simple mechanical materials, the elastic modulus is independent of the actual strain and the rate of straining. However, in biological materials the elastic modulus changes with the strain and rate of straining and, furthermore, it will vary with the direction of application of strain and with time.

A material which fails to return to its original shape following removal of an applied stress is defined as *plastic*.

Elastic modulus and shear modulus

A homogeneous, isotropic material with linear elastic properties (Figure 2.84) has properties described by two parameters. They relate the direct strain and direct stress to the shear strain and the shear stress. These parameters are the elastic modulus and the shear modulus, which relate strains to stresses acting in the same direction (units are newtons per square metre).

$$\text{Elastic modulus} = \frac{\text{Direct stress}}{\text{Direct strain}}$$

$$\text{Shear modulus} = \frac{\text{Shear stress}}{\text{Shear strain}}$$

Structures made of materials whose elastic properties can be described in this way can be analysed relatively easily, provided the applied stresses are predominantly in one direction. This is often the case for slender structures of materials such as steel. Biological structures are more difficult to analyse accurately because of their complex forms and

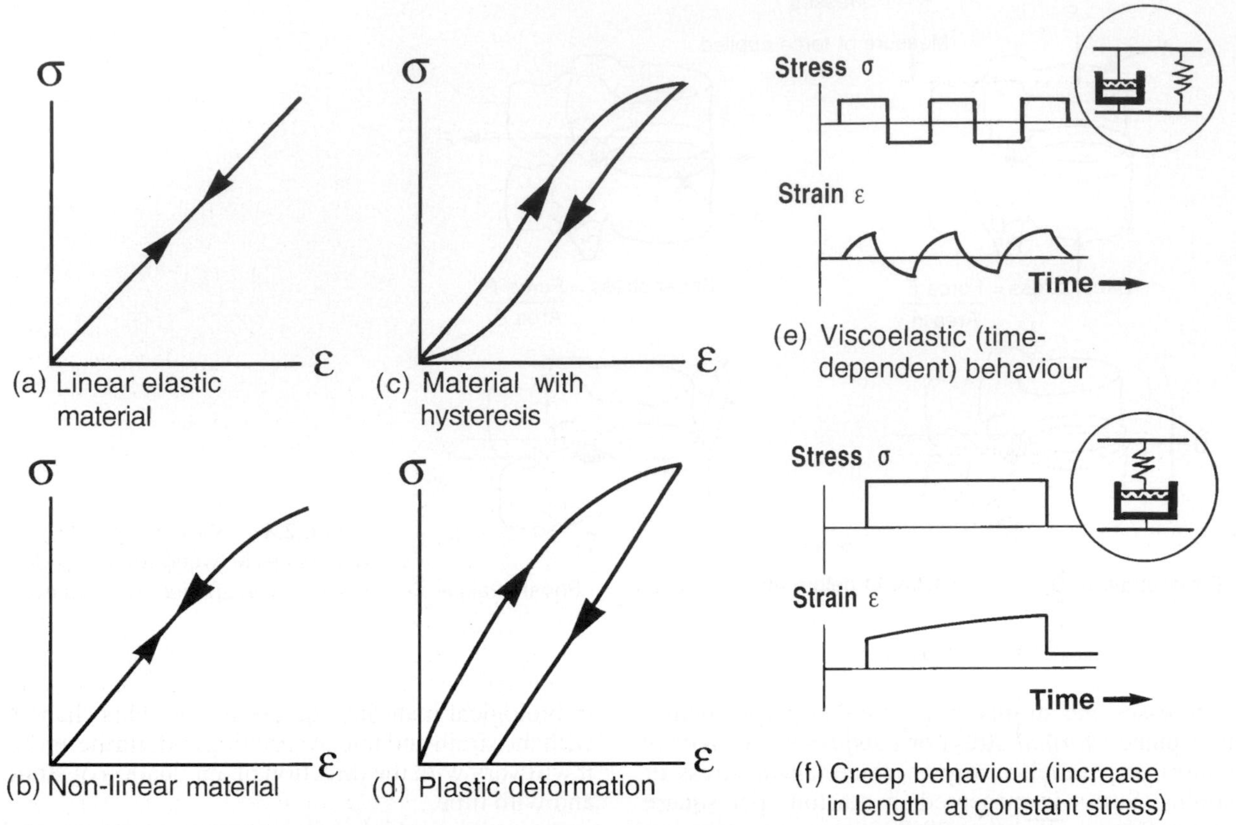

Figure 2.84 Illustrating the elastic modulus and shear modulus of biological materials which display non-elastic behaviour, hysteresis, plastic deformation, viscoelasticity and creep.

because biological tissues display non-linear elastic behaviour, hysteresis, plastic deformation, viscoelasticity and creep. Their response is time dependent and stress dependent. It is difficult to define the properties of biological tissues, as they do not consist of materials which are uniform. Cortical bone has been described as a composite material with mineral crystals lying in a matrix of collagen-based material, with properties which vary with age and mineral content (Currey, 1959, 1969).

A material which undergoes elastic deformation in response to an instantaneously applied stress but when the stress is continued for a period of time demonstrates plastic behaviour is described as showing *creep*.

Hysteresis is a term used to describe the behaviour of material where the stress–strain relationship is different for the loading and unloading phases.

Stuctures may be loaded eccentrically. For example, the load exerted by the body on the femur passes through the femoral head and therefore it is applied eccentrically to the long axis of the femur. This eccentric or *bending* load produces compressive stresses and strains on the medial (concave) femoral cortex and tensile strain at the lateral (convex) surface. These stresses are maximum at each surface and diminish towards the centre of the bone where there is transition from one to the other in a *neutral plane* at which the stresses are zero (Figures 2.85, 2.86).

When a person stands from the sitting position, the body weight passing through the femoral head tends to twist the horizontal femur. This is described as *torsion* and the stresses developed are torsional stresses.

Failure and strength of tissue

The definition of failure depends on the function expected of the structure. A bone plate has failed when it is bent or deformed plastically. Fracture of a bone is its usual mode of failure, since plastic deformation and microfracture cracking may not produce any noticeable loss of function.

Fracture is encouraged by small cracks and discontinuities, since these produce stress concentrations. In brittle materials there is a susceptibility to

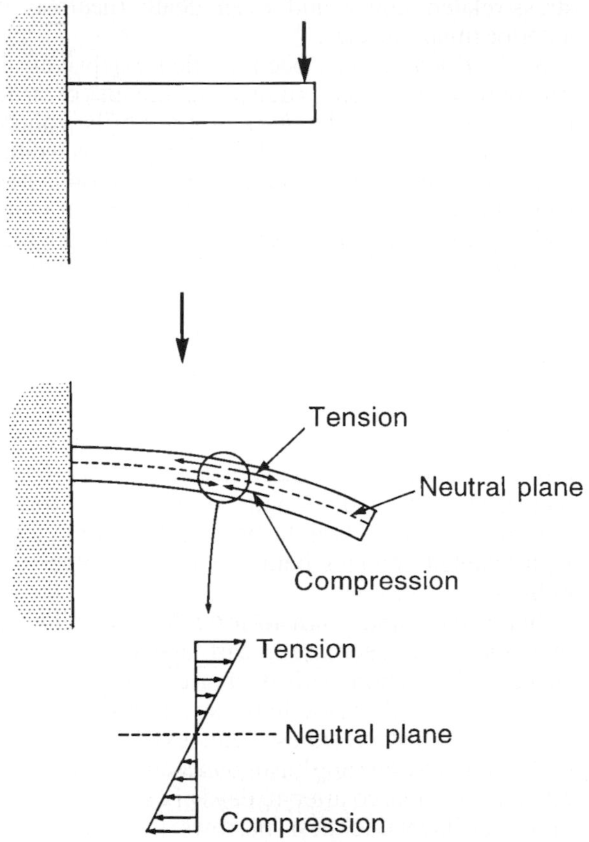

Figure 2.85 Eccentric or bending loading produces compressive and tension stresses and strains.

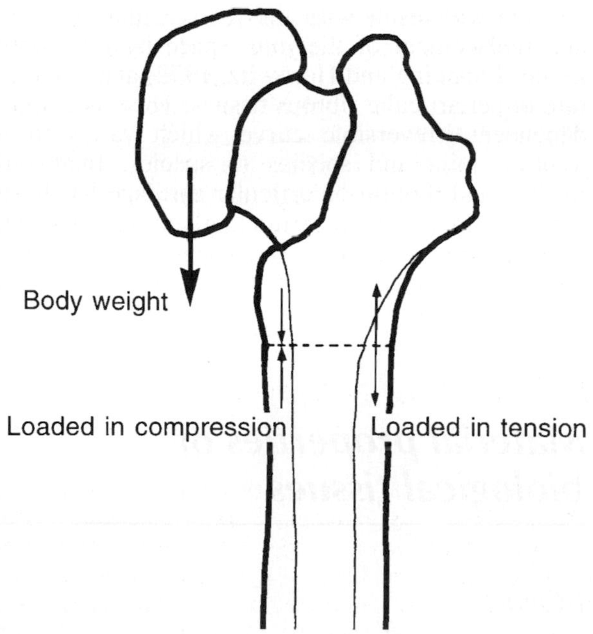

Figure 2.86 Loading of femoral head to produce tension and compression.

fracture by impact loading because such materials allow high local stresses to develop during impacts. Bone becomes more brittle with age (Burstein *et al.*, 1976) so older patients can be susceptible to impact fracture of bones, even before there are significant age-related changes in mineral content.

Repeated force applications can cause a fracture in many materials which would survive the single application of a greater force. This behaviour is called fatigue in metals and has caused aircraft and shipping disasters. At any level of repetitive stress, it is possible to define a 'fatigue life' which is the number of cycles of loading and unloading which produce fracture. This kind of behaviour is responsible for 'march' fractures (Devas, 1975).

The ability of bone to renew itself by the normal process of bone turnover tends to prevent the accumulation of injuries due to cyclical loading. In very old patients the reduction in the rate of bone turnover may allow the accumulation of relatively older mineral which is more susceptible to damage by cyclical loading.

The material properties of cortical bone show it to be weakest in shear and strongest in compression and fractures may be classified according to the nature of the stress which causes them. Fractures caused by tension are normally avulsions of muscle origins or insertions. Compression fractures include crush fractures of the vertebrae and tibial plateau fractures. Pure bending fractures may occur due to a direct blow such as the 'nightstick' fracture of the ulna while excessive torsional loading produces spiral or butterfly fractures of long bones. The majority of fractures are, however, the result of a complex combination of loads.

Small defects in a structure may dramatically alter its strength. A hole drilled at the junction of the mid and distal third of the tibia reduces the strength of the tibia to 50% of normal. A cortical defect created by removal of a cortical strut graft from the tibia reduces the angular deformation to failure to 30% of normal and the energy absorption capacity of the bone to 10% of normal (Frankel and Burstein, 1970). It is likely that bone remodelling would restore the strength of the bone towards normal by realignment of collagen and mineral long before the defect was filled in by new bone.

The rate of loading strongly effects the characteristics of failure of biological structures. Under conditions of constant load, collagenous structures tend to creep, while under higher loads, stiffness, strength and energy absorption to failure all increase. These properties account for the difference between high and low velocity fractures.

Under slow loading conditions, fractures tend to be simple and non-comminuted while under rapid loading, the added energy stored in the bone during loading is released at the moment of fracture and dissipated into the bone fragments and soft tissues causing comminution and added soft tissue damage. Since in older patients the bone is more brittle and weaker, there is less tendency to store energy during the loading phase of fractures which tend to be of the low energy type.

Organic responses of tissues to mechanical stress

Biological tissues have the ability to develop a strength and form according to the mechanical stresses imposed upon them. Cortical thickening is observed in athletes and others who stress their bones heavily whereas immobilization in space flight results in loss of bone mineral. The reshaping of fractured bones which are set in a misaligned position is further evidence of a gross shape adaptation.

The orientation of trabeculae was thought by Von Meyer (1867) to follow lines of maximal stress in the bone. This is well demonstrated in the femoral head and neck and in the calcaneum. Wolff (1882) followed this theory with his 'law of bone transformation' now referred to as Wolff's law. This law may be stated in modern terms in the form that bone adapts itself to the stresses imposed on it. Areas which experience high strains hypertrophy, whereas regions which are not subjected to stress become relatively weaker. The physiochemical mechanisms underlying Wolff's law are not fully understood, but electrical effects may be involved.

Biological tissues of the musculoskeletal system require repetitive loading and motion to maintain their structural integrity, biochemistry and function. Buckwalter (1991) has reviewed extensively these forms of mechanical stress both in health and after injury.

Stresses and strains affect both cells and tissues, e.g. cells change shape, the alignment of the matrix macromolecules, the tissue organization – all in response to repetitive loading. This mechanical force is also responsible for the rate of tissue turnover and its composition, structure and resultant mechanical properties. If physiological stresses and strains are reduced, in general there is a decrease in cell function and vice versa. Included in this general picture there is the property of adaptation of tissues to stresses and strains which can be physiological, e.g. Wolff's law, or pathological, e.g. a stress fracture, will result when tissues fail to adapt, a disruption of tendo Achillis to rupture, degeneration stress-related injury and even death (necrosis of anterior tibial muscle).

Skeletal muscle has been studied extensively in immobilization which produces severe loss of structure in muscle fibre size, loss of myofibrils, volume and power. If the blood and nerve supply as well as cell membranes remains intact, regeneration is possible. Increased use of muscle by various training and physiotherapy modalities, e.g. low tension, high repetition endurance, high tension, low repetition (strength) and stretching (strength), can increase the size and number of muscle cells, the mitochondria, glycogen content, etc.

In bone decreased loading, particularly when cyclic, produces excess bone resorption over bone formation, for example, during immobilization. On the other hand, increased cyclic loading can produce increase in bone and strength, as shown experimentally by excising a weight-bearing bone (e.g. ulna) with adapted changes being seen in the other (the radius).

In cartilage and synovial joint when loading and movement are decreased, cartilage cells alter in shape and function with decrease in proteoglycan synthesis, with decrease in tissue amount and resultant mechanical weakness, e.g. experimentally in dogs the glycosaminoglycan concentrations are significantly decreased after 40 days of cast immobilization. Cartilage thickness narrows (Behrens *et al.*, 1989). More rigid immobilization by external fixators produces greater changes in cartilage, water and hexuronate concentrations, and proteoglycan loss, etc. If the immobilization is continued, irreversible damage will result with loss of articular cartilage and replacement of the joint space by fibro-fatty tissue (Enneking and Horowitz, 1972) and contracture of periarticular fibrous tissues. There is a time-dependent irreversible curve which varies from joint to joint and species to species. Increased loading and motion on articular cartilage has been shown to increase the cartilage glycosaminoglycan concentration as well as its thickness but only at a physiological level – above this there may well be adverse effects.

Material properties of biological tissues

BONE

Bone is a mixture of collagen and mineral. Collagen is a low modulus of elasticity fibre with poor resistance to compression and high tensile strength. Bone mineral is stiff and brittle with high resistance to compression. Because of its structure, bone is *anisotropic*, that is its mechanical properties depend on the direction in which they are measured.

Bone also demonstrates *viscoelasticity*. This implies that the modulus of elasticity increases with increasing rate of strain so that the faster the load is supplied the stiffer the material behaves. As bone ages it becomes stiffer and the maximum strain to failure is reduced. These effects on bone itself are independent of the tendency of the amount of bone mass in the skeleton to reduce with ageing.

TENDON

Like other soft tissues, tendon provides strong resistance to deformation only under tension. It is more flexible than bone with a modulus of elasticity of 5–10% of that of bone. In addition, when initially loaded, the modulus of elasticity is very low due to straightening of the wavy fibres.

Tendon also exhibits *creep* in that after an initial elastic deformation a further slow plastic deformation will occur.

CARTILAGE

Cartilage is considerably weaker than bone with an ultimate tensile strength approximately 5% of it. It is also about 1000 times less stiff; however, the elastic properties are highly dependent on the loading rate. At high loading rates cartilage behaves almost elastically whereas at lower rates creep is far more apparent. This is due to the large amount of water trapped within the proteoglycan matrix of the cartilage which is able to move through the matrix at slow rates of loading.

References

Abercrombie, M. (1964) Behaviour of cells towards one another. In: *Advances in Biology of Skin*, vol. 5, *Wound Healing*, pp. 95–112. Edited by W. Montagna and R. E. Billingham. Pergamon Press: Oxford

Amako, T. and Honda, K. (1957) An experimental study of epiphyseal stapling. *Kyushu Journal of Medical Science* **131**, 138

Anderson, L. D. (1965) Compression plate fixation and the effect of different types of internal fixation on fracture healing. *Journal of Bone and Joint Surgery* **47A**, 191–208

Aronson, J. (1991) The biology of distraction osteogenesis. In: *Operative Principles of Ilizarov*, pp. 42–52. Edited by A. Bianchi, M. E. Maiocchi and J. Aronson. Williams and Wilkins: Baltimore

Aronson, J., Good, B., Stewart, C., Harrison, B. and Hart, J. (1990) Preliminary studies of mineralisation during distraction osteogenesis. *Clinical Orthopaedics and Related Research* **250**, 43–49

Ashton, I. K. and Francis, M. J. O. (1977) An assay for plasma somatomedin: [^{3}H] thymidine incorporation by isolated rabbit chondrocytes. *Journal of Endocrinology* **74**, 205–212

Baron, R., Vignery, A. and Horowitz, M. (1984) Lymphocytes, macrophages and the regulation of bone remodelling. In: *Bone and Mineral Research* **2**, pp. 175–245. Edited by W. Peck. Elsevier: Amsterdam

Behrens, F., Kraft, E. L. and Oegema, T. R. (1989) Biochemical changes in articular cartilage after joint immobilisation by casting or external fixation. *Journal of Orthopaedic Research* **7**, 335–343

Benninghoff, A. (1925) Bau der Gelenkknorpel in ihren Beziehungen zur Funktion: Zweiter Teil. Der aufbau des Gelenkknorpels in seinen Beziehungen zur Funktion. *Zeitschrift fur Mikroskopisch-Anatomische Forschung* **2**, 783–862

Bentley, G. (1971) The effect of 'biological' femoral osteotomy on papaine-induced degenerative arthritis of the hip joint in rabbits. *Journal of Bone and Joint Surgery* **54B**, 173

Bentley, G. (1989) Grafts and implants for cartilage repair and replacement. *CRC Critical Reviews in Biocompatibility* **5**, 245–267

Bentley, G. and Aston, J. E. (1985) Repair of normal and arthritic articular and epiphysial cartilage. *Journal of Bone and Joint Surgery* **67B**, 317

Bentley, G., Leslie, I. J. and Fischer, D. (1981) A study of the effect of aspirin treatment in chondromalacia patellae. *Annals of the Rheumatic Diseases* **40**, 37

Bier, A. (1917) Beobachtungen über Regeneration beim Menschen. *Deutsche Medizinische Wochenschrift* **43**, 705

Blenman, P. R., Carter, D. R. and Beaupre, G. S. (1989) Fracture healing patterns calculated from stress analyses of bone loading histories. *Transactions of the Orthopaedic Research Society* **14**, 469

Blount, W. P. and Zeier, F. (1952) Control of bone length. *Journal of the American Medical Association* **148**, 451–457

Brighton, C. T. and Heppenstall, R. B. (1971) Oxygen tension in zones of the epiphyseal plate, the metaphysis and diaphysis: an *in vitro* and *in vivo* study in rats and rabbits. *Journal of Bone and Joint Surgery* **53A**, 710–728

Brighton, T. C., Hozach, W. J., Brager, M. D. *et al.* (1985) Fracture healing in the rabbit fibula – when subjected to various capacitively coupled electrical fields. *Journal of Orthopaedic Research* **3**, 331–340

Brinker, M. R., Lipton, H. L., Cook, S. D. and Hyman, A. L. (1990) Pharmacological regulation of the circulation of bone. *Journal of Bone and Joint Surgery* **72A**, 964–975

Brookes, M. (1971) *The Blood Supply of Bone*. Butterworths: London.

Brookes, M. (1986) The blood supply of bone. *Bone* **3**, 32–34

Brookes, M. (1987a) Bone blood flow measurement: Part 1. *Bone* **4**, 22–24

Brookes, M. (1987b) Bone blood flow measurement: Part 2. *Bone* **4**, 33–36

Buckwalter, J. A. (1991) Effects of repetitive loading and motion on the musculoskeletal tissues. In: *Orthopaedic Sports Medicine: Principles and Practice*. Edited by J. C. Delee and D. Drez. W. B. Saunders: London

Buckwalter, J. A., Kuettner, K. E. and Thonar, E. J. M. (1985) Age related changes in articular cartilage proteoglycans: electron microscopic studies. *Journal of Orthopaedic Research* **3**, 251–257

Buckwalter, J. A., Rosenberg, L., Coutts, R., Kunzike, R. E., Reddi, A. H. and Mow, V. (1988) Articular cartilage injury and repair. In: *Injury and Repair of the Musculoskeletal Soft Tissues*, pp. 465–482. Edited by SL-Y. Woo and J. A. Buckwalter. American Academy of Orthopaedic Surgeons: Park Ridge, IL

Burke, R. E. and Tsairis, P. (1973) Anatomy and innervation ratios in motor units of cat gastrocnemius. *Journal of Physiology* **234**, 749–765

Burstein, A. H., Reilly, D. T. and Martens, M. (1976) Aging in bone tissue: mechanical properties. *Journal of Bone and Joint Surgery* **58A**, 82–86

Cameron, D. A. and Robinson, R. A. (1958) *Journal of Bone and Joint Surgery* **40A**. 414

Cannalis, E. (1980) Effect of insulin like growth factor 1 on DNA and protein synthesis in cultured rat calvaria. *Journal of Clinical Investigation* **66**, 709–719

Cannalis, E. (1986) Interleukin-1 has independent effects on DNA and collagen synthesis in cultures of rat calvaria. *Endocrinology* **118**, 74–81

Cannalis, E. and Raisz, L. G. (1979) Effect of epidermal growth factor on bone formation *in vitro*. *Endocrinology* **104**, 862–869

Cannalis, E. M., Hintz, R. L., Dietrich, J. W., Maina, D. N. and Raisz, L. G. (1971) Effect of somatomedin and growth hormone on bone collagen synthesis *in vitro*. *Metabolism* **26**, 1079–1087

Cannalis, E. J., Lorenzo, W. H., Burgess, W. H. and Machiag, T. J. (1987a) Effect of endothelial cell growth factor on bone remodelling *in vitro*. *Journal of Clinical Investigation* **79**, 52–58

Cannalis, E., McCarthy, T. and Centrella, M. (1987b) A bone derived growth factor isolated from rat calvaria is $\beta 2$ microglobulin. *Endocrinology* **121**, 1198–1200

Cannalis, E., McCarthy, T. and Centrella, M. (1988) Growth factors and the regulation of bone remodelling. *Journal of Clinical Investigation* **81**, 277–281

Centrella, M. and Cannalis, E. (1985) Transforming and nontransforming growth factors are present in medium condition by fetal rat calvaria. *Proceedings of the National Academy of Sciences of the USA* **82**, 7335–7339

Chalmers, J., Gray, D. H. and Rush, J. (1975) Observations on the induction of bone and soft tissues. *Journal of Bone and Joint Surgery* **57B**, 36–45

Chambers, T. J. (1990) Cellular and hormonal regulations of osteoclastic bone resorption. In: *Bone Morphometry*, pp. 21–28. Edited by H. E. Takahashi. Smith Gordon: London

Chambers, T. J., Darby, J. A. and Fuller, K. (1985a) Mammalian collagenase predisposes bone surfaces to osteoclastic resorption. *Cell and Tissue Research* **241**, 671–675

Chambers, T. J., McSheehy, P. M. J., Thompson, B. M. and Fuller, K. (1985b) The effect of calcium regulating hormones and prostaglandins on bone resorption by osteoclasts disaggregated from neonatal rabbit bones. *Endocrinology* **116**, 234–239

Chowcat, N. L., Savage, F. J., Hembry, R. M. and Boulos, P. B. (1988) Role of collagenase in colonic anastomosis: a reappraisal. *British Journal of Surgery* **75**, 330–334

Chyun, Y. S. and Raisz, L. G. (1984) Stimulation of bone formation by prostaglandin E_2. *Prostaglandins* **27**, 97–103

Clark, J. M. (1985) The organisation of collagen in cryofractured rabbit articular cartilage: a scanning electronmicroscope study. *Journal of Orthopaedic Research* **3**, 17–29

Cochrane, G. V. B. (1980) *A Primer of Orthopaedic Biomechanics*. Churchill Livingstone: New York

Cohen, J. and Harris, W. H. (1958) *Journal of Bone and Joint Surgery* **40A**, 419

Cook, S. D., Baffes, G. C., Wolfe, M. W. *et al.* (1994) The effect of recombinant human osteogenic protein-1 on healing of large segmental bone defects. *Journal of Bone and Joint Surgery* **76A**, 827–838

Craig, R. (1986) The structure of the contractile filaments. In: *Myology*, vol. 1, pp. 79–124. Edited by A. G. Engel and B. Q. Banker. McGraw Hill: New York

Crilly, R. G. (1972) Longitudinal overgrowth of chicken radius. *Journal of Anatomy* **112**, 11–18

Currey, J. D. (1959) Differences in the tensile strength of bone of different histological types. *Journal of Anatomy* **93**, 87

Currey, J. D. (1969) The mechanical consequences of variation of the mineral content of bone. *Journal of Biochemistry* **2**, 1

Cuthbertson, E. N., Sirus, E. and Gilfillan, R. S. (1965) The femoral diaphyseal medullary venous system as a venous collateral channel in the dog. *Journal of Bone and Joint Surgery* **47A**, 965–974

Danis, R. (1949) *Theorie et Pratique de l'Osteosynthèse*. Masson: Paris

Dekel, S. and Francis, M. J. O. (1981) The treatment of osteomyelitis of the tibia with sodium salicylate. *Journal of Bone and Joint Surgery* **63B**, 178–184

Dekel, S., Lenthall, G. and Francis, M. J. O. (1981) Release of prostaglandins from bone and muscle after tibial fracture. *Journal of Bone and Joint Surgery* **63B**, 185–189

Denko, C. W. and Bergenstahl, D. M. (1955) *Endocrinology* **57**, 76

Devas, M. (1975) *Stress Fractures*. Churchill Livingstone: Edinburgh and London

Dewhirst, F. E., Stashenko, P. P., Mole, J. E. and Tsurumachi, T. (1985) Purification and partial sequence of human osteoclast activating factor, identity with interleukin-1. *Journal of Immunology* **135**, 2562–2568

Dickerson, R. C. and Duthie, R. B. (1963) *Journal of Bone and Joint Surgery* **45A**, 356–364

Dietrich, J. W., Goodson, J. N. and Raisz, L. G. (1975) Stimulation of bone resorption by various prostaglandins in organ culture. *Prostaglandins* **10**, 231–240

Dixon, T. F. and Perkins, H. R. (1956) In: *The Biochemistry and Physiology of Bone*, vol. 1. Edited by G. H. Bourne. Academic Press: New York

Donohue, J. M., Buss, D., Oegema, T. R. Jr and Thompson, J. C. Jr (1983) The effects of indirect blunt trauma on adult canine articular cartilage. *Journal of Bone and Joint Surgery* **65A**, 948–957

Drinker, C. K. and Drinker, K. R. (1916) A method for maintaining an artificial circulation through the tibia of the dog with a demonstration of the vasomotor control of the marrow muscles. *American Journal of Physiology* **40**, 512–521

Duthie, R. B. (1958) *British Journal of Plastic Surgery* **11**, 30

Duthie, R. B. (1962) ^{35}S-sulphate in bone repair of rats. In: *Radioisotopes and Bone*, pp. 293–316. Edited by P. Lacroix and A. M. Budy. Blackwell Scientific: Oxford

Duthie, R. B. (1967) Possible role of mast cells in tissue injury and their presence in fracture sites. In: *The Healing of Osseous Tissue*, pp. 195–208. National Academy of Sciences, National Research Council: Washington DC

Duthie, R. B. and Barker, A. N. (1955) *Journal of Bone and Joint Surgery* **37B**, 304

Dziak, R. M., Heard, D., Miyasaki, K., Brown, M., Weinfeld, H. and Hausmann, E. (1982) Prostaglandin E_2 binding and cyclic AMP production in isolated bone cells. *Calcified Tissue International* **35**, 243–249

Engel, A. G. (1986) The neuromuscular junction. In: *Myology*, pp. 209–253. Edited by A. G. Engel and B. Q. Banker. McGraw Hill: New York

Enneking, W. F. and Horowitz, M. (1972) The intra-articular effects of immobilization on the human knee. *Journal of Bone and Joint Surgery* **54A**, 973–985

Eyre, D. R. (1990) The collagens of musculoskeletal soft tissues. In: *Sports-induced Inflammation*, pp. 161–171. Edited by W. B. Leadbetter, J. A. Buckwalter and S. L. Gordon. American Academy of Orthopaedic Surgeons: Park Ridge, IL

Fenn, W. O. (1923–24) *Journal of Physiology* **58**, 175, 375

Fitten Jackson, J. (1957) *Proceedings of the Royal Society, B* **146**, 270

Frankel, V. H. and Burstein, A. H. (1970) *Orthopaedic Biomechanics*. Lee and Febiger: Philadelphia

Frankel, V. H. and Nordin, M. (1980) *Basic Biomechanics of the Skeletal System*. Lee and Febiger: Philadelphia

Freeman, S. (1960) In: *Bone as a Tissue*. Edited by K. Rodahl, J. T. Nicholson and E. M. Brown. Blakiston: New York

Friedlaender, G. E. and Goldberg, V. M. (1991) *Bone and Cartilage Allografts: Biology and Clinical Applications: Workshop; Airlie House, Warrenton, Virginia, October 29–November 1, 1989*. American Academy of Orthopaedic Surgeons: Parkridge, IL

Fukada, E. and Yasuda, I. (1957) On the piezoelectric effect of bone. *Journal of the Physiological Society of Japan* **10**, 1158–1169

Furukawa, A. T., Eyer, D. R., Koide, S. and Glimcher, M. J. (1980) Biochemical studies on repair cartilage resurfacing experimental defects in the rabbit knee. *Journal of Bone and Joint Surgery* **62A**, 79–89

Garn, S. M. (1981) The phenomenon of bone formation and bone loss. In: *Osteoporosis, Recent Advances in Pathogenesis and Treatment*, pp. 3–16. Edited by H. F. De Luca, H. M. Frost, W. S. S. Jee, C. C. Johnston Jr and A. M. Parfitt. University Park Press: Baltimore

Geiser, M. and Trueta, J. (1958) Muscle action, bone rarefaction and bone formation: an experimental study. *Journal of Bone and Joint Surgery* **40B**, 282–311

Ghadially, F. M., Thomas, I., Oryschak, A. F. and Lalonde, J. M. (1977) Long term results of superficial defects in articular cartilage: a scanning electron microscopy study. *Journal of Pathology* **121**, 213–217

Girgis, F. G. and Pritchard, J. J. (1958) Experimental production of cartilage during the repair of fractures of the skull vault in rats. *Journal of Bone and Joint Surgery* **40B**, 274–281

Glimcher, M. J. (1959) Molecular biology of mineralized tissue with particular reference to bone. *Review of Modern Physics* **31** 359–393

Glimcher, M. J. (1984) Recent studies of the mineral phase in bone and its possible linkage to the organic matrix by protein-bound phosphate bonds. *Philosophical Transactions of the Royal Society of London [Biology]* **304**, 479–508

Glimcher, M. J. (1990) The nature of the mineral component of bone and the mechanism of calcification. In: *Metabolic Bone Disease*, pp. 42–68. Edited by L. V. Avioli and S. M. Krant. W. B. Saunders: Philadelphia

Glimcher, M. J. and Krane, S. M. (1968) The organisation and structure of bone and the mechanism of calcification. In: *Treatise on Collagen*, vol. 2B, p.67. Edited by B. F. Scould. Academic Press: London and New York.

Glucksman, A. (1939) *Anatomical Record* **73**, 39

Glynne Andrew, J. (1993) New concepts in fracture healing. *Surgery* **11**, 538

Gothman, L. (1961) Vascular reactions in experimental fractures. *Acta Orthopaedica Scandinavica Supplementum* **284**

Gowan, M. (1988) Actions of IL1 and TNF on human osteoblast-like cells. In: *Monokines and Other Non-lymphocytic Cytokines*, pp. 261–266. Edited by M. Kluger, J. J. Oppenheim, C. A. Dinarello and M. Pavanda. Alan R. Liss Inc.: New York

Gowan, M., Wood, D. D., Ihra, E. J., Maguire, M. K. B. and Russell, R. G. G. (1983) An interleukin-1 like factor stimulates bone resorption *in vitro*. *Nature* **306**, 378–380

Ham, A. W. (1930) Histological study of the early phase of bone repair. *Journal of Bone and Joint Surgery* **12**, 825–844

Hanazawa, A. S., Amamo, S., Mackada, K. *et al.* (1987) Biological characterisation of interleukin-1 like cytokine produced by cultured bone cells from new born mouse calvaria. *Calcified Tissue International* **41**, 31–37

Harrison, H. E. (1956) *American Journal of Medicine* **20**, 1

Harrison, H. E. and Harrison, H. C. (1952) *Journal of Pediatrics* **41**, 756

Hauschka, P. V., Mavrakos, A. E., Iafrati, M. D., Doleman, S. E. and Klagsbrun, M. (1986) Growth factors in bone matrix. *Journal of Biological Chemistry* **261**, 12665–12674

Heintz, E., Muller, E. and Romiger, U. E. (1947) *Zeitschrift für Kinderheilkunde* **65**, 101

Holtrop, M. E. and Raisz, L. G. (1979) Comparison of the effects of 1,25 dihydroxycholecalciferol, prostaglandin E_2 and osteoclast activating factor with parathyroid hormone on the ultrastructure of osteoclasts in cultured long bones of fetal rats. *Calcified Tissue International* **29**, 201–205

Horowitz, A. F. and Schotland, D. L. (1986) The plasma membrane of the muscle fibre. In: *Myology*, vol. 1, pp. 177–207. Edited by A. G. Engel and B. Q. Banker. McGraw Hill: New York

Horowitz, P. (1986) Excitation contraction coupling in skeletal muscle. In: *Myology*, vol. 1, pp. 471–495. Edited by A. G. Engel and B. Q. Banker. McGraw Hill: New York

Horowitz, P. and Spalding, B. C. (1986) Electrical and ionic properties of the muscle cell membrane. In: *Myology*, vol. 1, pp. 445–469. Edited by A. G. Engel and B. Q. Banker. McGraw Hill: New York

Houghton, G. R. and Dekel, S. (1979) The periosteal control of long bone growth. *Acta Orthopaedica Scandinavica* **50**, 635–637

Houghton, G. R. and Rooker, G. D. (1979) The role of the periosteum in the growth of long bones. *Journal of Bone and Joint Surgery* **61B**, 218–220

Hulth, A. (1989) Current concept of fracture healing. *Clinical Orthopaedics and Related Research* **249**, 265–284

Hunter, C. (1987) Proteoglycans and calcification. *Connective Tissue Research* **16**, 111–120

Huxley, H. E. (1983) Molecular basis of contraction in cross-striated muscles and relevance to motility systems in other cells. In: *Muscle and Non-muscle Motility*, pp. 1–104. Edited by A. Stracher. Academic Press: New York

Hwang, W. S., Li, B., Jin, L. H. *et al.* (1992) Collagen fibril structure of normal, ageing and osteoarthritic cartilage. *Journal of Pathology* 167, 425–433

Ilizarov, G. A. (1975) Basic principles of transosseous compression and distraction osteosynthesis (translated from Russian). *Ortopediia Travmatologiia i Protezirovanie* **10**, 7–15

Ilizarov, G. A. (1990) Clinical implication of the tension stress effect for limb lengthening. *Clinical Orthopaedics and Related Research* **258**, 226

Janes, J. M. and Jennings, J. R. (1961) *Proceedings of the Mayo Clinic* **36**, 1

Jew, S. S., Ueno, K., Dane, Y. P. and Woodberry, D. M. (1985) The effects of prostaglandin E_2 in growing rats: increased metaphyseal hard tissue and corticoendosteal bone formation. *Calcified Tissue International* **37**, 148–157

Jingushi, S., Heydeman, N. A., Kana, S. K., Macy, L. R. and Bolander, M. E. (1990) Acidic FGF injection stimulates cartilage enlargement and inhibits cartilage gene expression in rat fracture healing. *Journal of Orthopaedic Research* **8**, 364–371

Kahn, A. J., Fallon, M. D. and Teitelbaum, S. L. (1984) Structure – the function relationships in bone: an examination of events at the cellular level. In: *Bone and Mineral Research*, 2nd edn, pp. 125–174. Edited by W. Peck. Elsevier: Amsterdam

Katz, J. M., Skinner, S. J. M., Wilson, T. and Gray, D. H. (1983) The *in vitro* effect of indomethacin on basal bone resorption, on prostaglandin production and on the response to added prostaglandins. *Prostaglandins* **26**, 545–555

Keith, A. (1918) *British Journal of Surgery* **5**, 685

Kember, N. F. (1971) *Cell and Tissue Kinetics* **4**, 193

Kempson, G. E., Muir, H., Pollard, C. and Tuke, M. (1973) *Biochimica et Biophysica Acta* **297**, 456–472

Kuhlman, R. E. (1960) *Journal of Bone and Joint Surgery* **42A**, 457

Kushner, I. and Somerville, J. A. (1971) Permeability of human synovial membrane to plasma proteins. *Arthritis and Rheumatism* **14**, 560–570

Lack, C. H. (1962) Aetiological factors in the collagen diseases. Increased vascular permeability chondrolysis and cortisone. *Proceedings of the Royal Society of Medicine* **55**, 113–116

Lacroix, P. (1954) *Proceedings of the Second Radioisotope Conference*, vol. 1, p.134. Butterworths: London

Landis, W. J. and Glimcher, M. J. (1978) Electron diffraction and electron proble microanalysis of the mineral phase of bone tissue prepared by anhydrous techniques. *Journal of Ulstrastructural Research* **63**, 188–223

Lane, J. M. and Werntz, J. R. (1987) The biology of fracture healing. In: *Fracture Healing*, pp. 49–60. Edited by J. M. Lane. Churchill Livingstone: New York

Lane, W. A. (1914) *The Operative Treatment of Fractures*, 2nd edn. Medical Publishing Co.: London

Lebovitz, H. E. and Eisenbarth, G. S. (1975) Hormone regulation of cartilage growth and metabolism. *Vitamins and Hormones* **33**, 575–648

Liddell, E. G. T. and Sherrington, C. S. (1925) Recruitment and some other factors of reflex inhibition. *Proceedings of the Royal Society of London, Series B [Biology]* **97**, 488–518

Lu Valle, P. A. (1993) Intramembranous and endochondral bone development. *Current Science and Opinion in Orthopaedics* **4**(5), 85–89

Maquet, P. G. J. (1984) *Biomechanics of the Knee with Application to the Pathogenesis and the Surgical Treatment of Arthritis*, 2nd edn. Springer Verlag: Berlin

Maroudas, A. (1975) Biophysical chemistry of cartilaginous tissues with special reference to solute and fluid transport. *Biorheology* **12**, 233–248

Maroudas, A., Bayliss, M. T. and Venn, M. F. (1980) Further studies on the composition of human femoral head cartilage. *Annals of the Rheumatic Diseases* **39**, 514–523

Matsuda, Y., Oki, S., Kitaoka, K., Nagano, Y., Nojima, M. and Desaki, J. (1988) Scanning electron microscope study of denervated and reinnervated neuromuscular junction. *Muscle and Nerve* **11**, 1266–1271

MacDonald, B. R. and Gowan, F. (1992) Cytokines and bone. *British Journal of Rheumatology* **31**, 149–155

McKibbin, B. (1978) The biology of fracture healing in long bones. *Journal of Bone and Joint Surgery* **60B**, 150–162

McKibbin, B. and Holdsworth, F. (1967) The dual nature of epiphyseal cartilage. *Journal of Bone and Joint Surgery* **49B**, 351–361

Memmeth, G. G., Bolander, M. E. and Martin, M. R. (1988) Growth factors in their role in wound and fracture healing. In: *Growth Factors and Other Aspects of Wound Healing: Biological and Clinical Implications*, pp. 1–17. Edited by A. Barbul, E. Pines, M. D. Caldwell and T. K. Hunt. Alan R. Liss: New York

Miles, A. A. (1961) Local and systemic factors in shock. *Federation Proceedings* **20**, Suppl. 9, 141–157

Miller, E. J. (1984) Chemistry of the collagens and their distribution. In: *Extracellular Matrix Biochemistry*, pp. 41–81. Edited by I. S. Pilz and A. H. Reddifas. Elsevier: New York

Mitchell, M. and Shepherd, M. (1987) Effects of patella shaving on the rabbit. *Journal of Orthopaedic Research* **5**, 388–392

Mitrovic, D. R. (1993) Articular cartilage: composition and metabolism in health and disease. *Current Science and Opinion in Orthopaedics* **4**(5), 69–80

Muir, H. (1978) Proteoglycans of cartilage. *Journal of Clinical Pathology* **31**, Suppl. 12, 67–81

Mundy, G. R., Ibbotson, K. J. and D'Souza, S. M. (1985) Tumour products and hypercalcemia of malignancy. *Journal of Clinical Investigation* **76**, 391–394

Murphy, G. (1991) Current views on proteolytic events in matrix degradation. In: *Osteoarthritis Current Research and Prospects for Pharmacological Intervention*. Edited by R. G. G. Russell and P. A. Dieppe. IBC Technical Services: London

Murphy, W. R., Daughaday, W. H. and Hartnett, C. (1956) *Journal of Laboratory and Clinical Medicine* **47**, 715

Muscolo, D. L., Caletti, E., Schajowicz, F., Araujo, E. S. and Makino, A. (1987) Tissue-typing in human massive allografts of frozen bone. *Journal of Bone and Joint Surgery* **69A**, 585–595

Muthukumaran, N. and Reddi, A. H. (1984) Bone matrix induced local bone induction. *Clinical Orthopaedics and Related Research* **220**, 159–164

Nefussi, J. R. and Baron, R. (1985) PGE_2 stimulates both resorption and formation of bone *in vitro*: differential responses of the periosteum and endosteum in fetal rat long bone cultures. *Anatomical Record* **211**, 9–16

Neuman, W. F. and Neuman, M. W. (1957) *American Journal of Medicine* **22**, 123–131

Neuman, W. F. and Neuman, M. W. (1958) *The Chemical Dynamics of Bone Mineral*. University of Chicago Press: Chicago

Newman, R. J., Duthie, R. B. and Francis, M. J. O. (1985) Nuclear magnetic resonance studies of fracture repair. *Clinical Orthopaedics and Related Research* **198**, 297–304

Newman, R. J., Duthie, R. B. and Francis, M. J. O. (1987) Nuclear magnetic resonance studies of experimentally induced delayed fracture union. *Clinical Orthopaedics and Related Research* **216**, 253–261

Noda, M. and Camillier, J. J. (1989) *In vivo* stimulation of bone formation by transforming growth factor β. *Endocrinology* **124**(6), 2991–2994

O'Connell, P., Bland, C. and Gardner, D. L. (1980) Fine structure of artificial splits in femoral condyle cartilage of the rat. A scanning electronmicroscope study. *Journal of Pathology* **132**, 169–179

O'Garra, A. (1989) Interleukins and the immune system 2. *Lancet* **1**, 1003–1005

Olerud, S. and Dankwardt-Lilliesterom, G. (1971) Fracture healing in compression osteosynthesis. *Acta Orthopaedica Scandinavica Supplementum* **137**

Oni, O. O. A. and Gregg, P. J. (1990) The roots of venous escape from the marrow of the diaphysis of long bones. In: *Bone Circulation and Bone Necrosis. Proceedings of the 4th International Symposium on Bone Circulation, Toulouse, 17–19 September 1987*, pp. 7–10. Edited by J. Arlet and B. Mazieres. Springer Verlag: Berlin

Owen, M. (1970) The origin of bone cells. International Review of Cytology **28**, 213–238

Owen, M. (1977) Paper to the Thirteenth European Symposium on Calcified Tissue, Noordwijkerhout, Holland (September)

Owen, M. (1978) Editorial: Histogenesis of bone cells. *Calcified Tissue Research* **25**, 205–207

Owen, M. (1980) The origin of bone cells in the postnatal organism. *Arthritis and Rheumatism* **23**, 1073

Parfitt, A. M. (1981) Bone remodelling in the pathogenesis of osteoporosis. *Medical Times* **109**, 80–92

Parfitt, A. M. (1983) The physiological and clerical significance of bone histomorphometric data. In: *Bone Histomorphometry. Techniques and Interpretations*, pp. 143–223. Edited by R. Recker. CRC Press: Boca Raton, FL

Parfitt, A. M. (1984) The cellular basis of bone remodelling. The quantum concept re-examined in the light of recent advances in cell biology of bone. *Calcified Tissue International* **36**(suppl.), S37–S45

Parfitt, A. M. (1988) Bone remodelling: relationship to the amount and structure of bone and the pathogenesis and prevention of fractures. In: *Osteoporosis, Aetiology, Diagnosis and Management*. Edited by B. L. Riggs and L. J. Melton III. Raven Press: New York

Partridge, N. C., Kemp, B. E., Veroni, M. C. and Martin, T. J. (1981) Activation of adenosine 3',5' monophosphate-dependent protein kinase in normal and malignant bone cells by parathyroid hormone, prostaglandin E_2 and prostacyclin. *Endocrinology* **108**, 220–225

Pienkowski, D. and Pollack, S. R. (1983) The origin of stress generated potentials in fluid saturated bone. *Journal of Orthopaedic Research* **1**, 30–41

Pollack, S. R. (1990) Electrical effects in bone: relationship to bone remodelling. In: *Bone Morphometry*. Edited by A. G. Takahashi. Smith Gordon and Co.: London

Poole, A. C., Flint, M. H. and Beaumont, B. W. (1987) Chondrons in cartilage: ultrastructural analysis of the pericellular microenvironment in adult human articular cartilage. *Journal of Orthopaedic Research* **5**, 509–522

Poole, A. R., Pidoux, I., Reiner, A. and Rosenberg, L. (1982) An immunoelectron microscope study of the organization of proteoglycan monomer, link protein and collagen in the matrix of articular cartilage. *Journal of Cell Biology* **93**, 921–937

Poole, C. A., Flint, M. H. and Beaumont, B. W. (1984) Morphological and functional relationships of articular cartilage matrices. *Journal of Anatomy* **138**, 113–138

Pooley, J., Pooley, J. E. and Montgomery, R. J. (1990) The central venous sinus of long bones – its role in relation to exercise. In: *Bone Circulation and Bone Necrosis*, pp. 35–39. Edited by J. Arlet and B. Mazieres. Springer Verlag: Berlin

Prehm, P. (1983) Synthesis of hyaluronate in differentiated territocarcinoma cells. *Biochemical Journal* **211**, 181–198

Price, P. A., Parthemore, J. G. and Deftos, L. J. (1980) A new biochemical marker for bone metabolism. *Journal of Clinical Investigation* **66**, 878–883

Radin, E. L. and Burr, D. B. (1984) Hypothesis joints can heal. *Seminars in Arthritis and Rheumatism* **13**, 293–302

Ramachandran, G. N. (editor) (1977) *Treatise on Collagen*. Plenum Press: London

Ramsey, R. W. and Street, S. (1940) *Journal of Cellular and Comparative Physiology* **15**, 11

Reimann, I., Christensen, S. B. and Deimer, M. H. (1982) Observations of the reversibility of glycosaminoglycan depletion in articular cartilage. *Clinical Orthopaedics and Related Research* **168**, 258–264

Rhinelander, F. W. (1980) In: *Internal Fixation of Fractures*, pp. 9–14. Springer Verlag: Berlin

Rhinelander, F. W. and Baragry, R. A. (1962) Microangiography in bone healing. 1. Undisplaced closed fractures. *Journal of Bone and Joint Surgery* **44A**, 1273–1298.

Rhinelander, F. W., Philips, R. S., Steel, W. M. and Beer, J. C. (1968) Microangiography in bone healing. 2. Displaced closed fractures. *Journal of Bone and Joint Surgery* **50A**, 643–662

Riggs, B. L. and Melton, L. J. III (editors) (1988) *Osteoporosis: Aetiology, Diagnosis and Management*. Raven Press: New York

Ring, P. A. (1957) *Lancet* **1**, 980

Ring, P. A. (1961) The influence of the nervous system upon the growth of bones. *Journal of Bone and Joint Surgery* **43B**, 121–140

Roberts, A. B., Frolik, C. A., Anzano, M. A. and Sporn, M. B. (1983) Transforming growth factor from neoplastic and non-neoplastic tissues. *Federation Proceedings* **42**, 2612–2615

Robinson, R. A. (1952) *Journal of Bone and Joint Surgery* **34A**, 389–435

Robinson, R. A. (1960) *Clinical Orthopaedics* **17**, 69

Rodam, G. A., Bourret, L. A., Harvey, A. *et al.* (1975) Cyclic AMP and cyclic GMP: mediators of the mechanical effects on bone remodelling. *Science* **189**, 467–469

Rowe, J., Sudman, E. and Martin, P. F. (1976) Effects of indomethacin on fracture healing in rats. *Acta Orthopaedica Scandinavica* **47**, 588–599

Russell, R. G. G., Raisz, S. and Fleisch, H. (1969) *Archives of Internal Medicine* **124**, 571–577

Salpeter, M. M. (1987) Vertebrate neuromuscular junctions; general morphology, molecular organisation, and functional consequences. In: *The Vertebrate Neuromuscular Junction*. Edited by M. M. Salpeter. *Neurology and Neurobiology* **23**, 1–54

Schenk, R. K. (1987) Cytodynamics and histodynamics of primary bone repair. In: *Fracture Healing*, pp. 23–32. Edited by J. M. Lane. Churchill Livingstone: New York

Schenk, R. and Willinegger, H. (1967) Morphological findings in primary fracture healing. *Symposium Biologica Hungarica* **8**, 75–86

Schmid, A. and Schmid, M. (1987) Results after cartilage shaving study by electron microscopy. *American Journal of Sports Medicine* **15**, 386–387

Scranton, P. E., McMaster, J. H. and Diamond, P. E. (1975) Hormone suppression of DNA synthesis in cultured chondrocyte and osteosarcoma cell line. *Clinical Orthopaedics and Related Research* **112**, 340–348

Shim, S. S. (1968) Physiology of blood circulation of bone. *Journal of Bone and Joint Surgery* **50A**, 812–824

Shim, S. S. and Patterson, F. P. (1967) A direct method of qualitative bone circulation. *Surgery, Gynecology and Obstetrics* **125**, 261–268

Siffert, R. S. (1951) *Journal of Experimental Medicine* **93**, 415

Siffert. R. S. (1956) The effect of staples and longitudinal wires on epiphyseal growth. An experimental study. *Journal of Bone and Joint Surgery* **38A**, 1077–1088.

Siffert, R. S. (1961) *Journal of Bone and Joint Surgery* **43A**, 407

Simmonds, D. J. (1985) Fracture healing perspectives. *Clinical Orthopaedics and Related Research* **200**, 100–113

Simmonds, D. P. and Chrisman, O. D. (1965) Salicylate inhibition of cartilage degradation. *Arthritis and Rheumatism* **8**, 960

Somjen, D., Binderman, I., Berger, E. and Harell, A. (1980) Bone remodelling induced by physical stress is prostaglandin E_2 mediated. *Biochimica et Biophysica Acta* **627**, 91–100

Spector, W. G. and Willoughby, D. A. (1964) Endogenous mechanisms of injury in relation to inflammation. In: *Cellular Injury*. Ciba Foundation symposium. Edited by A. V. de Reuck and J. Knight. Churchill: London; Little, Brown: Boston, MA

Stracke, H., Shulz, A., Moeller, D., Rossol, S. and Schatz, H. (1984) The effect of growth hormone on osteoblasts and demonstration of somatomedin C/IGF1 in bone organ culture. *Acta Endocrinologica* **107**, 16–24

Swann, D. A., Silver, F. H., Slayter, H. S. *et al.* (1985) The molecular structure and lubricating activity of lubricin isolated from bovine and human synovial fluids. *Biochemical Journal* **225**, 195–201

Tang, L. H., Rosenberg, L. C., Rehanian, H. *et al.* (1989) Proteoglycans from bovine fetal epiphyseal cartilage. *Connective Tissue Research* **19**, 177–193

Tanner, J. M. (1955) *Growth at Adolescence*. Blackwell Scientific: Oxford

Tanner, J. M. (1972) *Nature* **237**, 433–439

Tashjian, A. H. Jr and Levine, L. (1978) Epidermal growth factor stimulates prostaglandin production and bone resorption in cultured mouse calvaria. *Biochemical and Biophysical Research Communications* **107**, 1738–1746

Tashjian, A. H. Jr, Tice, J. E. and Sides, K. (1977) Biological activities of prostaglandin analogues and metabolites on bone in organ culture. *Nature* **266**, 645–646

Tashjian, A. H. Jr, Hohlmann, E. L., Antoniades, H. M. and Levine, L. (1982) Platelet derived growth factor stimulates bone resorption via prostaglandin mediated mechanism. *Endocrinology* **111**, 118–124

Termine, J. D., Kleinman, H. K., Whitson, S. W., Conn, K. M., McGarvey, M. L. and Martin, G. R. (1981) Osteonectin, a bone–specific protein linking mineral collagen. *Cell* **26**, 99–105

Thompson, B. M., Saklatvala, J. and Chambers, T. J. (1986) Osteoblast mediates interleukin-1 responsiveness of bone resorption by rat osteoclasts. *Journal of Experimental Medicine* **164**, 104–112

Tonna, E. A. and Cronkite, E. P. (1961) Cellular response to fracture studies with tritiated thymidine. *Journal of Bone and Joint Surgery* **43A**, 352–362

Trippel, S. B. (1990) Articular cartilage research. *Current Opinion in Rheumatology* **2**, 777–782

Trottman, N. M. and Kelly, W. D. (1963) The effect of sympathectomy on blood flow to bone. *Journal of the American Medical Association* **183**, 121–122

Trueta, J. and Cavadias, A. X. (1964) *Surgery, Gynecology and Obstetrics* **118**, 485–498

Tyler, J. A. (1985a) Chondrocyte mediated depletion of articular cartilage proteoglycans *in vitro*. *Biochemical Journal* **225**, 493–507

Tyler, J. A. (1985b) Articular cartilage cultured with kabold (PIG interleukin-1) synthesizes a decreased number of normal proteoglycan molecules. *Biochemical Journal* **227**, 869–878

Ueda, K., Saito, A., Nakamo, H. *et al.* (1980) Cortical hyperostosis following long term administration of prostaglandin E_1 in infants with cyanotic congenital heart disease. *Journal of Pediatrics* **97**, 834–836

Urist, M. R. and Mikulksi, A. J. (1979) A soluble bone morphogenetic protein extracted from bone matrix with a mixed aqueous and non–aqueous solvent. *Proceedings of the Society for Experimental Biology and Medicine* **142**, 48

Urist, M. R., Lietze, A., Mizutani, H. *et al.* (1982) A bovine low molecular weight bone morphogenetic protein (DMP) fracture. *Clinical Orthopaedics and Related Research* **162**, 219

Van der Weil, C. J. (1980) An ultrastructural study of the components which make up the resting surface of bone. In: *Bone Histomorphology. Third International Workshop*, pp. 109–116. Edited by W. S. S. Jee and A. M. Parfitt. Amour Montague: Paris

Voegeli, T. L. and Chapman, M. W. (1985) Utilization of prostaglandins in fracture healing. *Transactions of the Orthopaedic Research Society* **10**, 134

Von Meyer, H. (1867) Die Architektur des Spongiosa. *Archiv für Anatomie und Physiologie* **44**, 615–628

Vreslovic, E. J., Pollack, S. R. and Brighton, C. T. (1986) Considerations for 'electrical dose' *in vivo* during electrically stimulated osteogenesis with external electrodes. *Transactions of the Orthopaedic Research Society* **11**, 249

Walker, P. S., Dowson, D., Longfield, M. D. *et al.* (1968) 'Boosted lubrication' in synovial joints by fluid entrapment and enrichment. *Annals of the Rheumatic Diseases* **27**, 512–520

Walker, P. S., Sikorski, D., Dowson, D., Longfield, M. D., Wright, V. and Buckley, T. (1969) Behaviour of synovial fluid on surfaces of articular cartilage. A scanning electron microscope study. *Annals of the Rheumatic Diseases* **28**, 1–14

Walker, P. S., Unsworth, A., Dowson, D. *et al.* (1970) Mode of aggregation of hyaluronic acid protein complex on the surface of articular cartilage. *Annals of the Rheumatic Diseases* **29**, 591–602

Weis, K. (1967) Intact collagen. In: *Treatise on Collagen*, vol. 1, p.367. Edited by G. N. Ramachandran. Academic Press: London and New York

Weiss, L. (1976) *Histology*, p. 394. Edited by R. O. Greep. McGraw Hill: New York and Maidenhead

Weiss, P. (1939) *Principles of Development*. Holt: New York

Wilhelm, D. L. (1965) Chemical mediators, I. In: *The Inflammatory Process*. Edited by B. W. Zweifach, L. Grant and R. T. McCluskey. Academic Press: New York

Wilkinson, J. H. (1977) The use of enzymes in osteogenesis. *British Journal of Hospital Medicine* **18**, 343–351

Wolff, J. (1882) *Das Gesetz der Transformation der Knochen*. Berlin

Worthy, K. Figueroa, C. D., Dieppe, P. A. and Bhoola, K. D. (1990) Kallikreins and kinins: mediators in inflammatory joint disease? *International Journal of Experimental Pathology* **71**, 587–601

Wray, J. B. and Lynch, C. J. (1959) The vascular response to fracture of the tibia in the rat. *Journal of Bone and Joint Surgery* **41A**, 1143–1148

CHAPTER 3

Congenital Malformations

ROBERT B. DUTHIE

Congenital malformation or anomalies are produced by pathological changes in the normal development processes of the embryo (up to the eighth post-ovulatory week) or of the fetus. The macroscopic abnormalities are usually observable at birth but may well appear only later in life as limitation of some function or deformity.

Fuller and Duthie (1974) have reviewed how, after fertilization of the ovum (i.e. the formation of the zygote), there is a process of cleavage to produce a number of cells or blastomeres. These are hollowed out to form the blastocyst, which contains the presumptive organ regions. These then alter in position, size and shape to form the gastrula, with invagination of certain surface regions to give three primary germ layers – endoderm, mesoderm and ectoderm. Waddington (1964) emphasized that, in trying to understand teratology, one must distinguish between:

1. the primary lesion in which the developmental processes are first deviated from their usual course; and
2. secondary lesions resulting from the primary lesion and perhaps affecting the primitive germ layers.

Waddington also pointed out that up to and including the period of gastrulation there is little evidence of gene activity, such as the formation of such proteins as myosin or actin. Until this time, cells are unresponsive to embryonic inducer substances and therefore are relatively immune to teratogenesis (Wilson, 1961). After this, the neural plate and axial structures are created, together with the mesodermal somites. Organs and tissues then differentiate to develop specific functions; for example, the heart, muscle and glands (Hamilton *et al.*, 1962).

At this time these developmental processes are influenced by DNA, RNA, other activating enzyme systems, ribosomes, complex proteins, lipids, and carbohydrates. They all have important control over the processes by which the embryonic cells mould themselves into characteristic shapes. Further embryonic development is a combination of growth and differentiation. Growth can be: *multiplicative*, involving an increase in the number of cells; *auxetic*, implying an increase in the size of the individual cells; or *accretionary*, with an accumulation of intracellular material. Differentiation can be said to have occurred when cells with the same genome synthesize different proteins (Jacob and Monod, 1963). Early limb budding through an outgrowth of mesenchyme and bulging into the covering ectoderm results from activity of the lateral plate mesoderm. A mesodermal maintenance factor has been described which influences the interaction between the ectoderm and mesoderm of the developing limb (Gruneberg, 1964). The apical ectodermal ridge controls the outgrowth of limb buds, the orientation of pre-axial and post-axial borders, and the differentiation of distal parts of the limb. This ridge arises by the thickening of the epidermis along the outer and peripheral margin of the limb bud.

The mesoderm gives rise to various tissues, including the sclerotomes, dermomyotomes and lateral plate, to make the axial and appendicular skeletons. The lateral plate first appears distinctly in the embryo of about 5 mm crown–rump length, when paired arm and leg limb buds appear on its surface. By 9.6 mm crown–rump length the upper limb shows primary differentiation into arm, forearm and hand, but the hind limb bud retains its primitive paddle shape until the embryo is 12 mm long. By day 40, human form is recognizable and the internal structures are differentiated. By the end of month 3 the upper limb has grown to a relatively normal length proportionate to trunk length, and the smaller hind limb contains toes and other parts. The formation of the joints is first defined as an interzone area (week 7); cavitation occurs by week 8 and rapid limb growth with free joint movement begins at week 20. The development and differentiation from mesenchyme of muscles, blood cells and nerve plexus are all important landmarks.

At week 12, innervation of muscles and the development of spinal anterior horn cells are seen, and reflex movements then occur. By week 15 there is maturation of 'adult' muscle from the primitive myoblast stage.

Fuller and Duthie (1974) have correlated the timing of the normal developmental landmarks to those found in the development of congenital limb anomalies (see Figure 3.50). However, it is often difficult to differentiate whether it is truly of a genetic) or an environmental (intrauterine) origin.

Carter (1976) has pointed out (from family studies) that it is only a minority of congenital malformations which result from chromosomal or monogenetic cases: for example achondroplasia (dominant) or Morquio's disease (recessive). When one malformation is not combined with others, it is likely to be due to polygenic factors (e.g. congenital dislocation of the hip). Environmental factors alone such as seen in cretinism are quite rare in producing malformations except from teratological agents such as the drug thalidomide, the rubella virus, steroid hormones and the folate antagonists of anticonvulsant drugs. It should be recognized that genes can produce their effect either by influencing primarily the essential metabolic processes, such as in ochronosis, or secondarily through affecting the endocrine system, such as the hypopituitary dwarf; but these might not become manifest until well into the postnatal period and as such are not truly 'congenital'.

Determining inheritance

The methods of determining inheritance in genetically determined disorders have been described by Duthie and Townes (1967):

1. Family history and clinical examination.
2. Twin studies.
3. Genetic analysis for pedigree and population frequencies.

FAMILY HISTORY

Enquiry should be made for disorders in relatives of the patient under study to obtain any familial tendency which might show a genetic basis. Further analysis may reveal the occurrence of two distinct clinical entities having some aetiological association; for example, there is an increased incidence of anencephaly and/or spina bifida aperta in siblings of involved children. The patient's siblings and parents should be listed, stating sex, age and the state of health (both past and present) as well as the total number of both the affected and unaffected siblings. The sex is also important to suggest the presence of any form of sex-linked recessive inheritance. Blood relatives are much more likely to have children exhibiting a rare recessive disorder; therefore any parental consanguinity (i.e. first cousins) must be examined. The rarer the recessive trait, the higher the proportion of consanguineous matings which has occurred.

TWIN STUDIES

The twin study method was developed by Galton in 1875, who stated that any difference between monozygotic twins must result from environmental effects, whereas any differences in dizygotic twins can result from both environmental and genetic influences. These studies can give the information to differentiate inherited and environmental factors, but for determining genetic influences alone family studies are required. The zygosity of like-appearing individuals is usually determined by carrying out tests to show similarities in the blood group systems – i.e. A, B and O; Mn, and cDe groups and by the successful acceptance of skin grafts one to each other and fingerprinting. The presence of a single amnion on examining the fetal membrane is presumptive evidence of monozygosity, but this is not entirely true.

One of the major biases to be overcome in using the twin form of study is to ensure against including affected twins in the series more often than one should see as regards their frequency in the population.

Malformations do not seem to be increased much, if at all, in twins even though an unfavourable prenatal environment occurs more frequently in twins. This in itself should lead to malformation.

PEDIGREE CHARTS

Analysis of a pedigree chart with its patterns will provide information on the Mendelian principles of segregation of alleles, as well as the independent and dependent assortment of non-alleles. It provides information on allelism and linkage, as well as single gene mutations. This form of study is usually retrospective, beginning with the diagnosis of a particular disturbance in a person who is called the 'proband' or 'propositus' or the 'index case'. Certain codings or symbols are used in preparing pedigree charts.

Autosomal dominant inheritance

This is a manifestation of a gene on the autosome in a heterozygous state with only one parent of an affected individual carrying the gene. This gene can also be transmitted by the parents of either sex to children of either sex. Dominant inheritance (Figure 3.1a) can be identified by the following:

1. An affected offspring has one or both parents affected.
2. The marriage of an affected person to a normal person results in an equal proportion of affected to normal children.
3. A normal child of an affected person produces normal offspring.
4. The phenotype characteristics occur in both males and females with equal frequency.
5. The pedigree chart shows vertical as well as horizontal patterns of involvement.
6. Dominant traits tend to exhibit varying expressivity; i.e. there is a wide variety in the severity of the phenotype presentation. Orthopaedic examples of this form of inheritance are seen in:
   - Achondroplasia
   - Nail–patella syndrome – osteo-onychondysplasia
   - Brachydactyly
   - Lobster clawing of hands and/or feet (if only one side of the body is affected this is less likely to be inherited than the bilateral cases)
   - Myositis ossificans progressiva
   - Diaphyseal aclasis
   - Ehlers–Danlos syndrome
   - Osteogenesis imperfecta
   - Marfan's syndrome
   - Osteopoikilosis
   - Neurofibromatosis
   - Facioscapulohumeral muscular dystrophy

Osteo-onychondysplasia – nail–patella syndrome

Although first recognized by Little in 1897, this syndrome of a generalized osseous dysplasia was described in detail by Turner in 1933 who noted that it was inherited as a Mendelian dominant – and called 'Turner's syndrome'. Duthie and Hecht (1963) from a single Amish family study of 70 members, showed that the disorder was determined by a simple dominant autosomal gene with complete penetrance, but displaying variable expressivity. In the family of all affected individuals, their blood group was O, demonstrating the chromosomal position of the nail–patella gene and the ABO blood group locus on the same chromosome.

The child can exhibit hypoplasia of the nails with the thumb always affected, but the second to fifth fingers being affected less severely or frequently. The elbow joints showed cubitus valgus with limitation in extension and supination. Bony prominences are seen radiographically arising from lateral surfaces of the ilium – the so-called 'iliac horns'. There

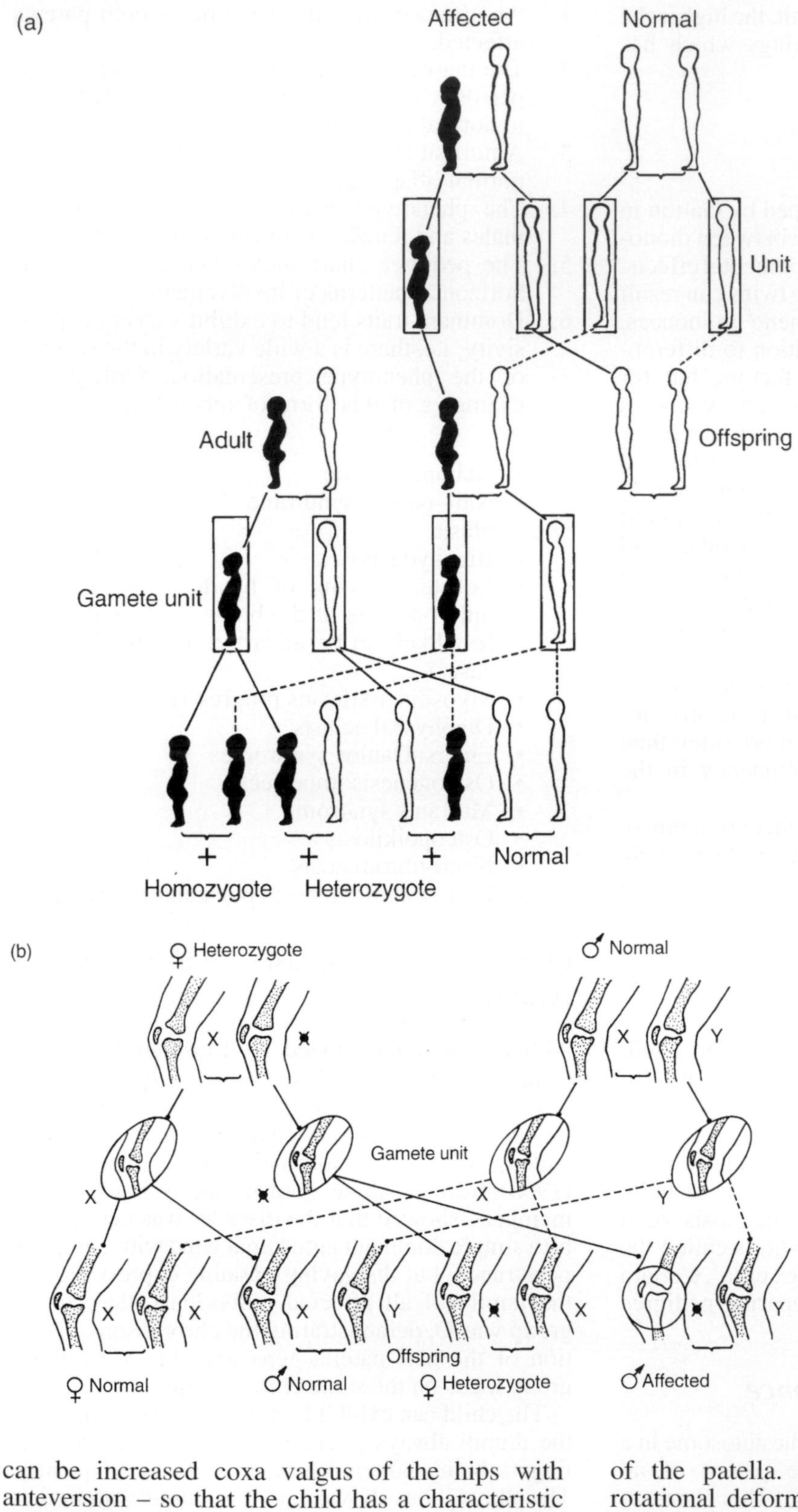

Figure 3.1 (a) The autosomal dominant inheritance of achondroplasia. (b) X-linked recessive inheritance of haemophilia.

can be increased coxa valgus of the hips with anteversion – so that the child has a characteristic gait pattern. When the patella was involved they were hypoplastic, wedge shaped and displaced laterally and could present as a recurrent dislocation of the patella. There is rarely seen externally rotational deformities of the tibiae because of the abnormal positioning of the patella. Duthie and Hecht ascribed the skeletal changes to an abnormal development of the traction epiphysis with an hypoplastic element, rather than to a primary teratogenic effect.

Recessive inheritance

A heterozygote carrying an abnormal gene meets another heterozygote, and from this mating there results a homozygote with the abnormal gene. Usually this can be identified by:

1. The chart showing a horizontal pattern of involvement, with the phenotypic expression necessarily appearing in siblings of the same family – i.e. the affected index case usually has unaffected parents and siblings.
2. It occurs with equal frequency in males and females – i.e. not sex-linked.
3. The individual exhibiting this characteristic must be a homozygote with a one in four subsequent chance of his or her offspring having the same disease.
4. Heterozygous characteristics are produced in children of an individual with a recessive trait and a normal person, the child being a carrier who is usually unaffected by the recessive trait. One-half of the offspring will be affected, giving a pedigree similar to that of a dominant trait.

This form of inheritance is seen in several orthopaedic conditions:

- Chondrodystrophia calcificans
- A severe form of gargoylism – Hurler's syndrome with corneal clouding
- Osteopetrosis – Albers–Schönberg disease
- Brailsford–Morquio syndrome
- Limb-girdle form of muscle dystrophy

Defects resulting from autosomal recessive single gene mutants with a low gene frequency would become increasingly rare in the absence of consanguineous marriages.

X-linked recessive inheritance

This occurs when a recessive gene is on the X chromosome of the female (Figure 3.1b).

When a female heterozygote marries a normal male there are four types of offspring likely to be produced:

1. A normal female having two normal X chromosomes.
2. A normal-appearing female carrier having one normal X chromosome, and one X chromosome with an affected gene on it.
3. A normal male having the mother's normal X chromosome.
4. An affected male having the mother's abnormal X chromosome.

The clinical entity appears almost always in males with unaffected mothers who are carriers – i.e. brothers of the patient, sons of the mother's sisters and the mother's father. Each son of a carrier has a one in two chance of being affected; affected males never transmit the gene to their sons but transmit it to all their daughters, who will be carriers. Unaffected males never transmit the gene to their descendants.

This form of inheritance is seen in classic haemophilia, colour-blindness, the pseudohypertrophic muscular dystrophy of Duchenne, and the Hunter syndrome without corneal clouding.

X-linked dominant inheritance

This is similar to autosomal dominant inheritance except that only daughters of an affected male will exhibit the disease. It is seen in vitamin D resistant rickets and Morquio's osteochondro-dystrophy.

Stevenson (1961) described three categories of congenital and/or hereditary disorders:

1. those malformations which are seen at birth, having arisen during intrauterine life and, therefore, are true congenital malformations;
2. disorders or diseases determined by a single gene substitution or mutation;
3. diseases in which the genetic contribution is made more complex by the presence of environmental factors or prenatal influences.

Malformations due solely to environmental causes are infrequent, but such conditions as viral infection of rubella in the mother and the use of aminopterin drugs and the drug thalidomide are capable of producing marked teratogenic changes in the fetus, particularly when occurring or given during the first 4 weeks of pregnancy. This occurs particularly at this time because the fetus is undergoing marked cellular differentiation and the mother's hormonal and nutritional milieu is also changing markedly. It is of interest that one-third of such cases arise in pregnancies associated with hydramnios, indicating some degree of maternal–fetal incompatibility.

It is difficult to describe accurately the total incidence of congenital deformities because of the marked variation in reporting. McKeown and Record (1960), in an attempt to overcome such inaccuracies, defined a congenital malformation as being 'a macroscopic abnormality of structure attributable to faulty development and present at birth'. In an incidence survey of 1000 live births, using such a definition, they found 23.08% exhibited malformations; 4.44% talipes, 3% spina bifida, etc., and 0.67% dislocation of the hip. Gentry *et al.* (1959) reported that in a population of over 1 million children born alive between 1948 and 1955, 22.8% were found to have skeletal or bone and joint anomalies. Association of malformations with each other was recorded by Record and Edwards (1958). In congenital dislocation of the hip there were 16% and in talipes equinovarus 11.6% other deformities (Crabbe, 1960), although in the latter study the incidence of maternal disease was 21.4% and may influence the association of these conditions.

The diagnosis of fetal abnormality has become most important, especially in mothers whose babies are at risk (e.g. central nervous system and neural tube abnormalities and mongolism), in order to decide on terminations by less hazardous methods – e.g. the use of prostaglandin between weeks 12 and 20 of pregnancy.

In the last trimester of pregnancy, radiology is of the greatest value in distinguishing skeletal abnormalities such as hydrocephaly, anencephaly or limb malformations. Ultrasonics has added further definition of CNS abnormalities at an earlier stage. Amniocentesis, which carries a 1–2% risk of abortion, is indicated when either parent has an abnormal genetic pattern and when the mother is older than 35 years. The amniotic fluid is examined for α-fetoproteins and the exfoliate cells are cultured both for the squames and for macrophages – Down's syndrome, spina bifida, anencephaly and nephrosis can now be diagnosed.

Congenital postural deformities associated with in utero positions

Macroscopic abnormalities observable at birth have been divided by Dunn (1976) into '*malformation* arising from primary disorders of morphogenesis in the embryo, or *deformities* arising in the fetus from alteration in the form or structure of a previously normally formed part'. It is these latter deformities which are believed to be caused by intrauterine mechanical factors. These may be *intrinsic* in nature (e.g. during muscle imbalance because of neuromuscular disease or when the limbs are unable to change the position *in utero*) or *extrinsic*, when there is an imbalance between the amount of amniotic fluid and the uterine wall (e.g. oligohydramnios with bilateral renal anomalies, uteroplacental insufficiency, premature rupture of the membranes or chronic leak of amniotic fluid – all result commonly in the production of Potter's facies, dislocated hip and talipes, etc.).

Dunn (1976), in a personal study of 4486 infants born in Birmingham, found 94.4% to be normal, 3.6% malformed and 2% had simple postural deformities. Obviously the severity varied, this being characteristic of postural deformities. He also described and emphasized how fetal plasticity which is dependent upon the rigidity of the skeleton is gradually lost with increasing ossification; this is accompanied by a fall in amniotic fluid volume. On the other hand, increased fetal plasticity may result from increased joint laxity, a condition commonly associated with girl fetuses or in families. Dunn's study showed an increased ratio of girls to boys with such deformities as congenitally dislocated hips.

Two other factors contribute to congenital postural deformities:

1. The importance of fetal kicking to obtain the subsequent position of presentation or the retention of the legs in the breech position with risk to the hips; the folding across of the legs may result in their becoming trapped, with the formation of club feet, dislocation of the hip, dislocation of the knee, etc.
2. The shape of the amniotic cavity – natural or abnormal: for example unicornous uterus, uterine fibroids, presence of more than one fetus have all been described and analysed in detail by Dunn. It has commonly been observed that congenital dislocation of the hip is twice as common on the left side as it is on the right, and Dunn has observed that such a fetus tends to lie with its back towards the mother's left side (twice as often as the other way) and that the posterior leg against the mother's vertebral column is likely to be adducted and hence dislocatable.

Since the days of Hippocrates, the '*in utero* position' has often been blamed and emphasized as a deforming force in producing several conditions, particularly of the lower extremities (Norton, 1953; Browne, 1956; Gould, 1962). Certain moderately severe postural conditions seen shortly after birth and which can be treated by simple conservative measures are:

1. A metatarsus adductus of one or other foot.
2. An everted or valgus foot.
3. A talipes equinovarus deformity with one or more of the four characteristics: forefoot adduction; hindfoot inversion; equinus of whole foot at the ankle joint; and torsion of the tibia.

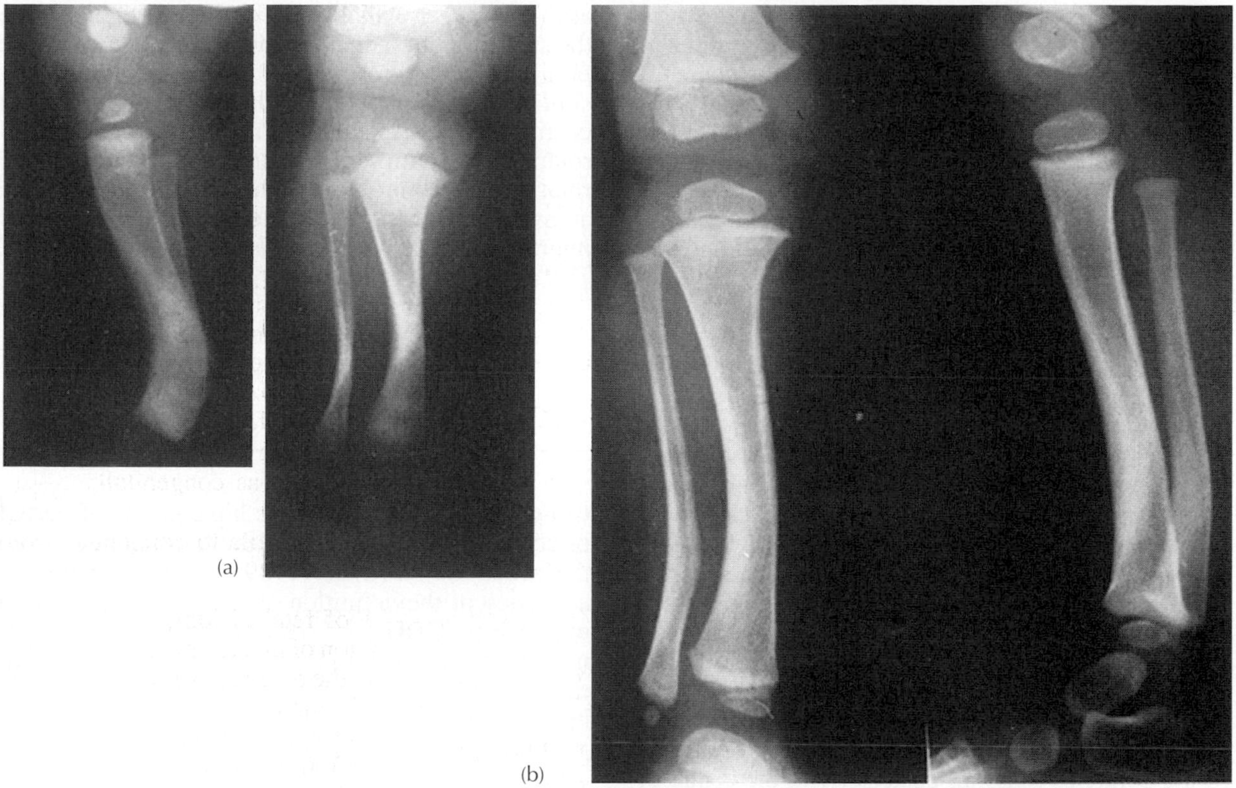

Figure 3.2 Positional bowing due to intrauterine compression syndrome, at 4 months (a). It is important to avoid bracing or casts. Physiological exercise results in gradual straightening with growth as seen in (b).

4. A unilateral externally rotated leg with an everted foot, the other leg either being in a neutral position or in internal rotation (Figure 3.2).
5. Bilateral externally rotated legs, which are aggravated by the prone position.
6. An adducted thigh and hip with some external rotation of the leg as a whole. This latter type of deformity must be closely examined for the probability and exclusion of a congenital dysplasia or dislocation of the hip. These conditions are often aggravated by the sleeping or lying position of the child (e.g. the internally rotated leg and varus foot).

Resistance to achieving the full range of passive movements of the hip, knee, ankle or mid-tarsal joints must be corrected by passive stretching exercises, the use of corrective appliances such as reversed shoes, Denis Browne splints with adjustable footpieces, the wearing of a pillow splint or double diapers, etc.

The child must be examined frequently to be sure that the postural deformity is being overcome and no static deformity due to an underlying structural disorder is becoming manifest. If soft-tissue contractures develop and passive stretching cannot produce an anatomical position after about 6 weeks of such treatment, corrective plaster-of-Paris casting may be necessary and the diagnosis of *in utero* postural deformities may require revision.

Kite (1961) described the torsional deformities of the lower extremities which are postural in nature and produced by positional forces, i.e. in a child sitting with the knees flexed and the feet folded back: in a W or sitting tailor position to produce a marked tibial torsion as well as an adductus deformity of the forefoot, or the child who sleeps in the frog position with the legs externally rotated and flexed at the hips. Kite emphasized that the first step was to break the child of the particular postural habit, either by devices such as shoes with cross-bars to turn the feet outwards or inwards, or by the wearing of soft shoes which can be tied together at the heel.

Bick (1960) made an interesting survey of examining 5000 newborns out of which 430 showed some form of musculoskeletal malformation. Tibial torsion was seen in 30 children per 1000 live births, subluxation of the hip in 17, metatarsus varus in 14, club feet in 8, deformity of the toes in 3, 'bow legs' in 2, and other conditions such as polydactylism, birth fractures, birth palsy and frank dislocation of the hip. He concluded that the optimum time for a detailed musculoskeletal examination was between the third and fourth week, since immediately after birth there are many interpretative difficulties even in congenital dysplasia of the hip.

TORSIONAL DEFORMITY

Torsional deformity of the lower limb occurs when rotational problems of the lower limb exceed the normal range which can be very broad. Most resolve spontaneously but when they persist, disability can occur. Operative correction is rare and only indicated when there is persistent deformity and disability. Tibial torsion occurs when the angle between the axis of rotation of the knee and the trimalleolar axis, when marked, will decrease the range of movement of the knee and talar joints. It can be measured more accurately by fluoroscopy than by CT or ultrasound (Joseph *et al.*, 1987). Femoral torsion of the neck of femur normally varies from 11.9° to 25° and is difficult to measure accurately. The angle of anteversion of the femoral neck is the angle between two planes that intersect the longitudinal axis of the femoral shaft, one passing through the neck and the centre of the head and the other parallel to the transverse axis of the condyles (passing posteriorly to the centre of the head of the femur). Routine AP and lateral views of the hip are taken with very careful positioning of the patient as well as a gonadal shield.

Indications for treatment (Staheli, 1989)

Metatarsus adductus

When flexible, these will resolve in over 90% of cases (the intrauterine positional type). If this deformity becomes rigid and fails to resolve within the first 6 months, attempts should be made by long leg casts within a flexed knee so that the foot may be laterally rotated and abducted more effectively. This can be repeated before surgery is considered after the age of 2–3 years. Surgery involves carrying out a Z-plasty of abductor hallucis tendon with or without mobilization of the internal tarsal joints.

Tibial torsion

If severe medial (over 15°) or lateral (over 30°) torsion persists after the age of 8 years, correction should be obtained by a supramalleolar tibial rotational osteotomy. Lesser deformities will usually resolve.

Femoral antetorsion

Intoeing is the presenting sign and persists up to the age of 5–6 years. Shoe modifications rarely improve the situation but they maintain the confidence of the family. If at the age of 8 years the deformity continues to present a significant functional and cosmetic handicap, with marked reduction in lateral rotation of the hip (<10%) and increase in medical rotation of about 85° and on measurement an anteversion of over 50°, correction by a rotational intertrochanteric osteotomy is considered.

Developmental dysplasia of the hip

Congenital dislocation of the hip consists of partial or complete displacement of the femoral head from the acetabulum. Klisic (1989), because of the inadequacy of the definition of congenital dislocation of the hip (CDH), introduced the term 'developmental dysplasia' (DDH) which covers more accurately the various abnormalities around the hip joint, before, during and after birth.

He subgrouped DDH into:

1. DDH 'at risk' – the 'at risk' factors, e.g. family history, breech presentation, female child, oligohydraminos, associated deformities of torticollis, talipes and genu recurvatum.
2. DDH – hypoplastic with a limited abduction.
3. DDH – reducible displacement with a jerk/click on entry.
4. DDH – reducible displacement with a jerk/click on exit.
5. DDH – subluxation and limited abduction.
6. DDH – dislocation with limited abduction, femoral shortening and telescoping.

It should be noted that this is unusual in newborns and usually associated with arthrogryplasia or myelodysplasia (about 2%).

It is one of the commonest of the congenital deformities and is particularly prevalent in certain areas. The population incidence of this disorder in the Birmingham series was 0.7 per 1000 live children (McKeown and Record, 1960) with a higher incidence in Sweden (2%), in Japan and in certain American Indian tribes (2–5%). Artz *et al.* (1975) in New York city found an incidence of CDH in 15.5 per thousand in Caucasians and 4.9 per thousand in Negroes. Prone sleeping in the knee–chest position or with extended hips can produce torsional deformities opposite to each other. Sitting with crossed legs produces an externally rotated femur, a medial rotated tibia and a varus foot. This may lead to an intoeing gait without metatarsus adductus and/or excessive medial femoral torsion. Bleck and Minaire (1983) have described the cause as being a persistent medial deviation of the talus and not medial tibial torsion.

Although the deformities are described as *in utero* position/postural in cause, they may also result following paralytic conditions, e.g. poliomyelitis and myelomeningocele. Brookes and Wardle (1962) studied the deformity in the femoral neck of polio patients. Paralysis of iliopsoas produced lateral torsion, and glutei increased femoral anteversion. Dias *et al.* (1984) noted that differing muscle and soft tissue contractures and imbalances produce medial tibial torsion (in lateral hamstring weakness) etc. and other femoral and ankle deformities.

The higher incidence in Sweden and in American Indians may well be related to the tight swaddling in which the babies are carried. A. R. Hodgson (1959, personal communication) believed that the lower incidence of hip dislocation in the Orient results from the method of carrying babies with the hips held in wide abduction. Since the introduction of postnatal and neonatal screening by trained staff using either Ortolani or Barlow's manoeuvres, these incidences have increased greatly but with improvement in the diagnosis and utilizing the DDH criteria, the world figures will be revised.

In most series there are 5–8 girls to every boy affected. Chapple and Davidson (1941) suggested that there was a temporary generalized joint laxity in the fetal female because of the placental passage of progesterone and oestrogen hormones. The first born is also more likely to exhibit this malformation.

The fetal position of the baby may be implicated since 16% of the London series were breech born (Muller and Seddon, 1953). Dunn (1976), from his survey, has shown that infants presenting by the breech are about ten times more likely to be deformed than those presenting by the vertex. The incidence of breech delivery and associated deformity was: mandibular deformity 22%, torticollis 20%, postural scoliosis 42%, congenital dislocation of the hip 50%, genu recurvatum 100% and talipes 22%. The breech of the baby with its hips continuing to grow in an abnormal position within the mother's unyielding, rigid bony pelvis will produce these types of deformities, i.e. the crowding phenomenon.

Experimentally, Wilkinson (1963) was able to produce this malformation in rabbits by splinting the hip in flexion and lateral rotation with the knee extended, and then giving oestrogen and progesterone. Carter and Wilkinson (1964) showed that in boys there is persistent joint laxity – often familial – predisposing to congenital dislocation of the hip, whereas in girls there may well be a hormonal basis for such joint laxity.

Joint laxity and femoral neck anteversion have long been thought to be two of the main causes of congenital dislocation of the hip. Carr *et al.* (1993), in measuring the range of motion in both hips of normal children and in the unaffected hip of children with unilateral CDH, as well as a joint laxity, found that joint laxity was more common in the normal group with an internally centred arc of hip rotation than in normal children with a neutral or externally centred arc of hip rotation. In the CDH group there was significantly more joint laxity than in the normal group and more of them had an internally centred arc of hip rotation. They suggested that the lax joint capsule fails to mould or improve the neonatal anteversion of the femoral neck during the first few months of life. Indeed, they considered that it produced the persistent fetal anteversion of the femur.

Genetic factors remain difficult to establish. In Muller and Seddon's series 2.2% of all siblings and 1.3% of parents were affected. In the Carter and Wilkinson series 5.7% of all siblings were involved, and they believe that the genetic effect is probably through two independent mechanisms – one producing a shallow acetabulum and the other a generalized laxity of the articular ligaments. Wynne-Davies (1970) agrees with there being these two genetic influences and has described how identical twins are not equally affected and that only 20% of siblings are involved with a family history. However, it is believed that the factors behind the development of dislocated hips arise in late pregnancy – i.e. after week 20 of gestation (Barlow, 1966).

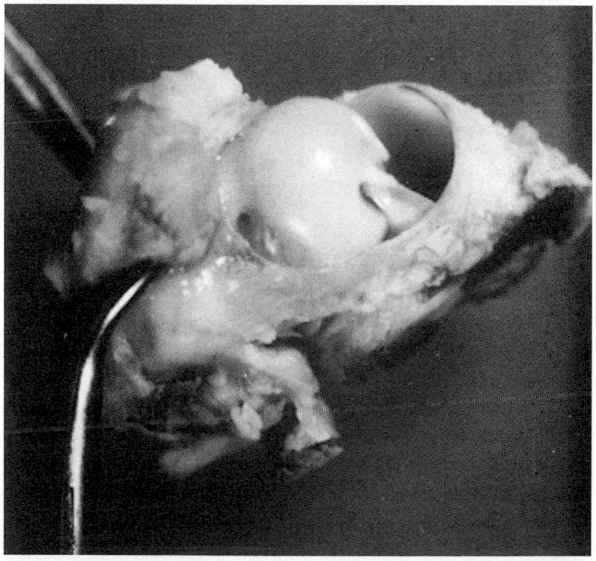

Figure 3.3 Anatomical specimen of the normal infant hip joint showing the cartilaginous acetabulum and concentric head with the ligamentum teres leading from the head into the acetabular floor.

AETIOLOGY

The acetabulum appears as a condensation of mesoderm about the end of the fourth week of intrauterine life, but at first it constitutes only a shallow socket on the outer aspect of the developing innominate bone. Later the socket is deepened by the progressive development of the original depression and in particular that part of the socket which lies in the axis of the transference of weight – the posterosuperior rim or buttress (Figure 3.3). The concavity of the acetabulum results from this pressure of the spherical femoral cartilaginous head.

The cartilage of the acetabulum is triradiate with an anterior/superior segment, a posterior/horizontal segment and a vertical segment. With ossification it develops into the ilium, the ischium and the pubis. The labrum lies at the margin of the acetabular cartilage, with the capsule inserting above its rim. The constant defect in congenital dislocation of the hip is an aplastic development of this osseous buttress, and it is of interest to note that this characteristic is apparent in the acetabulum of the lower forms where the hind limb has no postural function and is not concerned with the transference of weight (e.g. Reptilia).

Post-mortem reports on newborn infants in the predislocation stage are naturally rare. Hass found that the socket was only slightly reduced in circumference but corresponded in shape and depth to normal. The soft parts showed no abnormal change except for slight laxity of the capsule and iliofemoral ligament.

PATHOLOGY OF THE FULLY ESTABLISHED CASE

The pathology can be discussed under two main headings: changes in the bones (Figure 3.4) and changes in the soft parts (Figure 3.5).

Changes in the bones

The acetabulum

The acetabulum is shallower than normal, and at birth the only other error apparent is a gap or groove at its posterosuperior part. Later, its rounded shape disappears, the cavity usually being converted into a triangular depression, with its base in front and below, and its apex above and behind. X-ray examination shows that the outer surface of the ilium and the floor of the acetabulum lie practically in a straight line, owing to the absence of the usual projecting rim at the upper part of the cavity. Instead of containing the head of the femur, the acetabulum becomes occupied by an overgrowth of fibrocartilage, the remains of the ligamentum teres, and is covered over by the anterior portion of the capsule which is usually to some extent adherent to the floor. Above the acetabulum there is a depression on the dorsum ilium, lined with periosteum, in which the head of the femur rests insecurely, a fold of the capsule intervening between the ilium and the head.

Primary acetabular dysplasia, apart from a few established antenatal dislocations, is rare (Stanisavlevic and Mitchell, 1963). McKibbin (1970), in measuring acetabular direction with difficulty because of having to make measurements without standard anatomical orientation, found only a slight increase in anteversion in congenitally dislocated hip from the normal and adults were more anteverted than infants. Uhthoff (1990) from serial sectioning of the fetal CDH hips found that the acetabular roof was well developed but the posterior wall was made up of only a little cartilage, but mainly a fibrous labrum. With increased flexion of the femur and adduction, the head lies against this weakened wall of fibrous tissue.

Clinical risk factors were found during newborn screening in 13% of these joints but only 20% of these presented pathological findings on ultrasonography (Tonnis, 1992).

The head of the femur

The femoral head is at first normal, although ossification of it is often delayed and there is a marked discrepancy between the size of the cartilage head and the reduced acetabulum. Later it becomes flattened on its medial and posterior aspects. If the head rests on the dorsum ilium it becomes buffer-shaped, otherwise it is conical. The cartilage portion is usually large in comparison with the acetabulum.

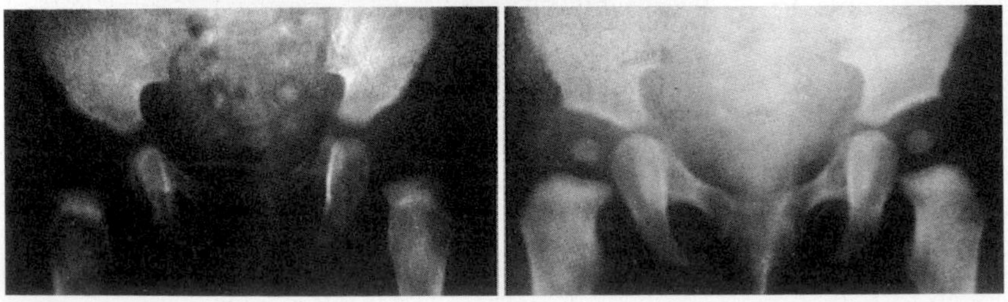

(a) (b)

Figure 3.4 (a) Dysplasia of the left hip, in a child aged 2 months. (b) Same patient treated by simple abduction for 6 months. NB. Mother and sister suffered from congenitally dislocated hip. Infant presented with alteration of buttock creases and limitation of hip movement.

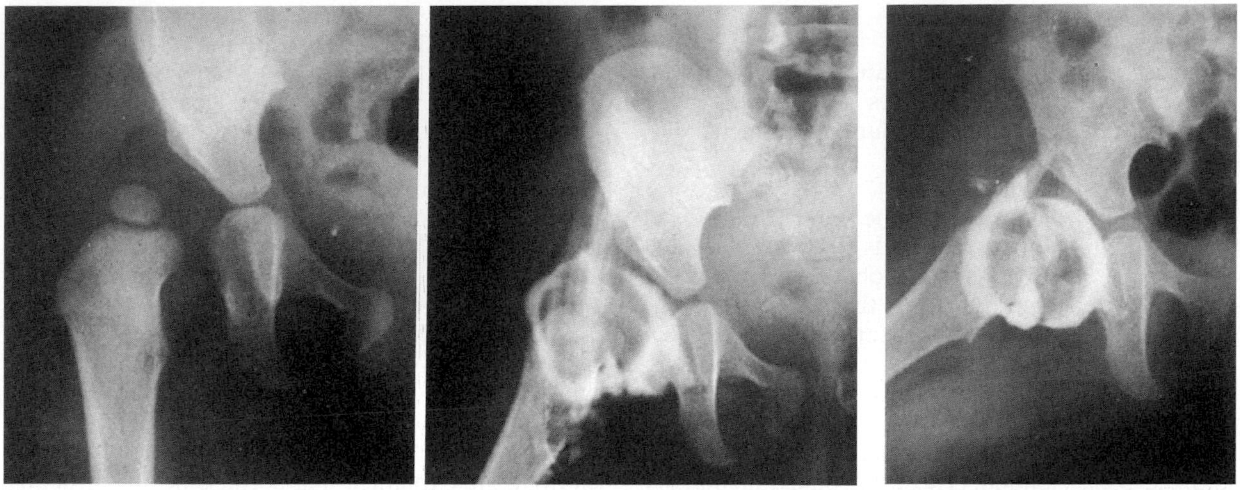

(a) (b) (c)

Figure 3.5 (a) Dislocation of the right hip, with arthrograms (b) before and (c) after reduction.

The neck of the femur

There is marked shortening of the neck of the femur, which increases the shortening of the limb. The neck is also anteverted, so that the normal anteversion of 12° is increased until it may be almost 90°, i.e. the neck appears to project straight forward from the shaft. As a result of this, when the dislocation is reduced, the limb is rotated internally and the patella looks directly medially.

The pelvis

When there is a bilateral dislocation, the pelvis is tilted forwards and the normal lumbosacral lordosis increased. The whole innominate bone may be small and atrophied, and lies more vertically than normal, so that the iliac crests are approximated and the ischia more widely separated.

In unilateral dislocation, the corresponding pelvic bone is imperfectly developed, and the whole pelvis has a lateral inclination, while the shape of the inlet is obliquely ovoid.

Changes in the soft parts

The capsule

The capsule can assume an hourglass shape, one cavity containing the head, the other covering the acetabulum, and the constriction between them being produced by the iliopsoas tendon which crosses the capsule at this level. Through this narrow isthmus, the ligamentum teres passes. The lower part of the capsule is stretched across the entrance to the acetabulum, and, in some cases, is adherent to its contents (Figure 3.6). It will thus be seen that the capsule becomes a suspensory ligament for the pelvis, and, indeed, supports most of the weight of the body. It accordingly undergoes hypertrophy, particularly at its anterior and lower portions. The ligamentum teres is usually attenuated, and may be altogether absent, although in certain cases hypertrophy of the ligamentum teres occurs with a fibro-fatty pad and is said to block reduction.

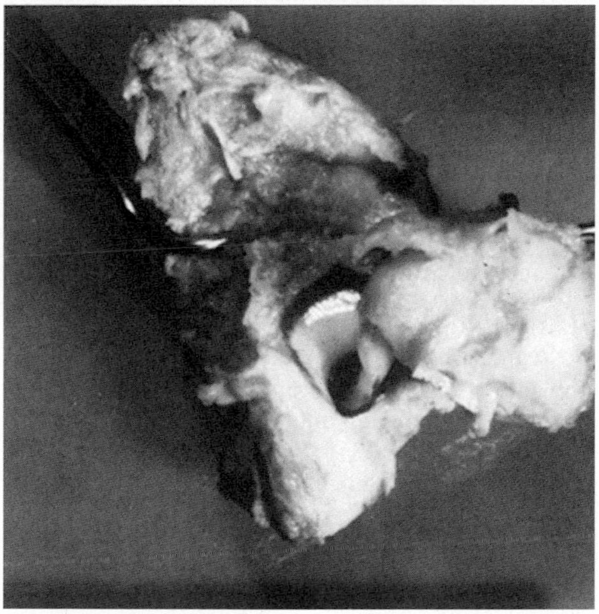

Figure 3.6 Teratogenic hip dislocation noted at birth in an infant with multiple congenital urinary anomalies. The outer edge of the acetabulum has been pushed upwards and medially into the ilium. The capsule clearly tents across the inferior border of the acetabulum, representing an obstacle to reduction. The cartilage of the misshapen femoral head is already striated due to pressure.

The muscles

There is considerable alteration in the muscles; indeed, this is one of the causes of failure to reduce the head into the acetabulum during treatment.

The pelvifemoral group
This runs in the same axis as the femur. As the head of the femur migrates upwards, they shorten, and thus form the most formidable obstacle to reduction. These shortened muscles are the adductors, hamstrings, gracilis, sartorius, tensor fasciae latae, pectineus and rectus femoris.

The pelvitrochanteric group
This consists of the obturators, quadratus femoris and the psoas tendon. These become functionally incompetent, since they are stretched and elongated. The psoas tendon, in addition, is displaced outwards, winds round the capsule and acts as a suspensory ligament which supports the body weight. In addition the iliopsoas, when contracted, forms a block to reduction and also acts as a fulcrum to produce subluxation if not dislocation on adduction. It may well compress the femoral head after reduction.

The gluteal group
These show little organic change but because they are without their fulcrum their power is considerably diminished, while the displacement of the head leads to an alteration in their axis of movement.

Dunn (1972) reported on the *post mortem* appearance of 48 hips and divided them into three groups:

1. Hips which were dislocatable in a posterolateral direction with stretched soft tissues and a slightly everted limbus.
2. Hips as in group 1 but with a greater eversion and stretching of the limbus, a long ligamentous teres and capsule, and the femoral head slightly deformed.
3. The deformed femoral head was fully dislocated with greater soft tissue changes – these presumably being an antenatal dislocation.

NORMAL DEVELOPMENT OF THE HIP IN INFANCY

At birth it is normal for the infant to have a hip flexion contracture bilaterally of 15–20°. This may also be true of the knees. These contractures are normally overcome by the infant's activity in the first 6 weeks.

A trunk contracture results in a gentle curve of the spine, and elevation of the pelvis on one side is also common. This can be overcome passively if it is physiological but the infant tends to lie in this position. This results in an adducted position of the hip on one side, and there may be a contracture which is usually overcome by the manipulation of diapering.

The general incidence of dislocation of the hip is time dependent. Barlow (1962) demonstrated how, if the examination was carried out on the newborn's first day, positive evidence of subluxation was achieved in 1 out of every 60 examined; 68% of these became normal within 7 days, 88% within 2 months and only 1.5 per 1000 live births after this period had frank dislocation. In a similar study, MacKenzie (1972) found that in the newborn there were 4.5 per 1000, with 68% being unstable and 22% having limited abduction. In the neonatal period (i.e. 28 days and onwards), 50% became normal without any treatment and at 9 weeks there were over 66% normal. He explained that because of this difficulty even in a large central maternity unit there was an incidence of 1.12 per 1000 births of 'missed' cases.

SUBLUXATION STAGE

Subluxation is regarded as an intermediate stage in the development from primary dysplasia to complete dislocation and is frequently associated with either predislocation or dislocation of the other hip (Figure 3.7). Subluxation, however, does not always proceed to dislocation and may be observed in adults who have had no previous treatment.

The exact features responsible for migration of the femoral head from the predislocation stage to subluxation and dislocation are not known. The degree of primary hypoplasia affecting the cartilaginous roof of the acetabulum is probably the most important aetiological factor. Its ability to contain the head and to ossify in response to a correctly reduced head will determine the final result.

Le Damany in 1908 suggested that congenital dis-

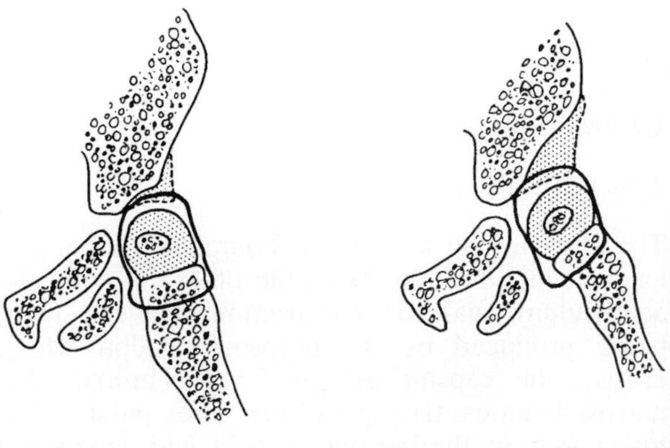

Figure 3.7 Arthrogram tracing of (a) a normal hip and (b) predislocation stage. In the early stages of dysplasia the osseous roof is deficient but the cartilaginous roof (as indicated by the dotted line) approximates normal.

location of the hip was directly attributable to increased anteversion of the femoral neck, although it was not found in all cases. Badgley (1949) considered that the primary dysplasia was produced by increased anteversion with an anterior primary position of the head and subsequent development of a flat socket.

Significant increase in the anteversion of the neck must, however, decrease the concentric pressure stimulus of the head in the acetabulum, and should be regarded as a contributory factor in the persistence of ossific hypoplasia and migration of the head.

In the early subluxated position the anteverted head can be palpated anteriorly when the legs are extended. The extension thrusts of the limb from the flexed position, which are a feature in the normal development of the growing infant, augment the pressure effect of the anteverted head.

In the initial stage of subluxation where only the fibrocartilaginous limbus has been subject to pressure by the migrating head, a normal anatomical outline can be restored by concentric reduction of the head which will then provide the necessary stimulus to ossification.

In more advanced stages of subluxation, the head flattens the limbus and exerts a deforming pressure on the cartilaginous roof, causing further inhibition of ossification and actual flattening of the socket. The response to reduction at this stage cannot be predicted and will depend on the extent to which these changes are reversible (Figure 3.8).

Dislocation occurs when the femoral head loses contact with the original acetabulum and rides up over the fibrocartilaginous rim. Arthrography demonstrates that in complete dislocation the fibrocartilaginous lip or limbus is inverted compared with the eversion which accompanies subluxation.

If dislocation is preceded by subluxation, inversion of the limbus must take place after the head leaves the socket. At operation it is usually the posterior and superior quadrants which are found to be inverted. Haas attributes the inversion to increased elasticity as the head slips out of the elastic loop of the limbus.

Reduction of a dislocation is complicated by secondary changes in the socket, the nature and significance of which remain the subject of much controversy. The secondary changes reported at operation will depend not only on individual interpretation but also on the age of the patient, the duration of the dislocation, and the influence of preoperative attempts at closed reduction. Scaglietti and Calendriello (1960) found one or more of the following factors which prevented reduction of dislocated hips:

- a pericephalic insertion of the capsule: 33%
- the ligamentum teres: 32%
- an inverted limbus: 31%
- the iliopsoas muscle: 25%
- capsular adhesions: 16%

CLINICAL EXAMINATION OF THE HIP IN THE NEONATAL PERIOD

The teratogenic hip dislocation present at birth is usually associated with other anomalies in the infant. It is usually readily appreciated since normal hip joint development has not occurred and the acetabulum is not distorted. More difficult is the apparently normal infant whose hip is not developing normally.

If actually dislocated, the trochanter is riding proximally and can be palpated above Nélaton's line drawn from the anterior-superior spine to the tuberosity of the ischium.

An adduction contracture is usually present. Pal-

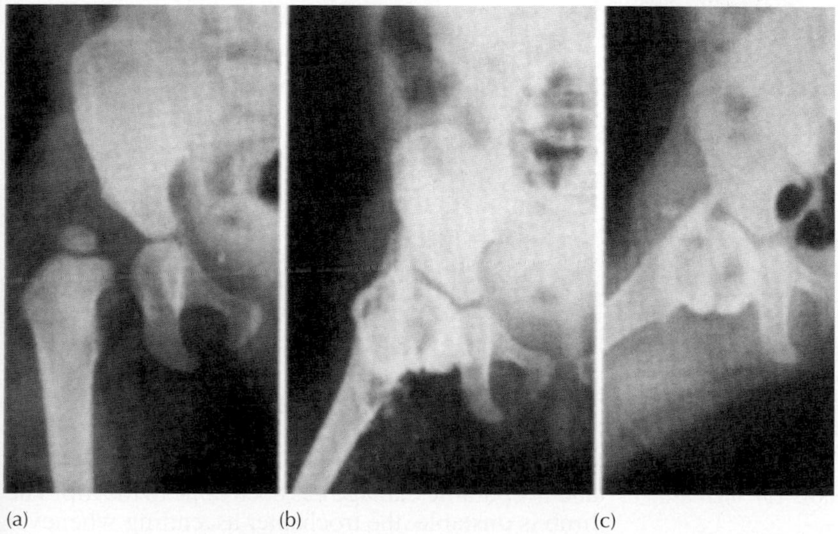
(a) (b) (c)

Figure 3.8 (a) Subluxation of right hip. (b) Arthrogram before reduction, showing flattening of limbus. (c) Arthrogram after frame reduction, showing normal outline of limbus.

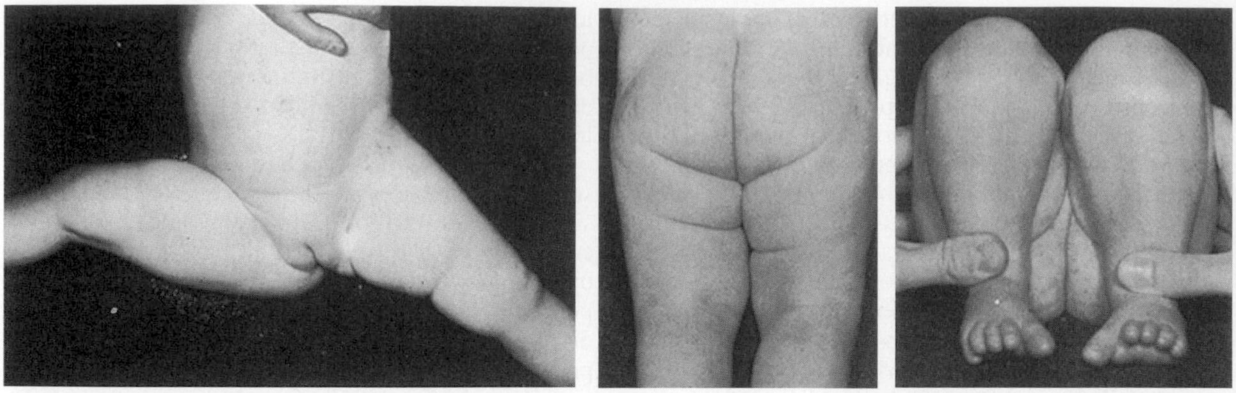

(a) (b) (c)

Figure 3.9 Clinical signs of congenitally dislocated hip: (a) limitation of hip abduction; (b) alteration of skin creases; (c) shortening of thigh.

pation for the femoral head is done one finger's breadth below the inguinal ligament, where the femoral artery pulse can be felt. If dislocation exists, the examining finger fails to meet resistance in this area.

The thigh folds may be asymmetrical and the soft tissues of the thigh overlie the labia eccentrically on one side (Figure 3.9a). When dislocation is bilateral the perineum is widened. Flexing both hips with the pelvis flat on the table permits the examiner to estimate the height of the knees. If the femur has ridden proximally on one side, the lowered height of the knee brings this out (Galeazzi's sign; Figure 3.9c).

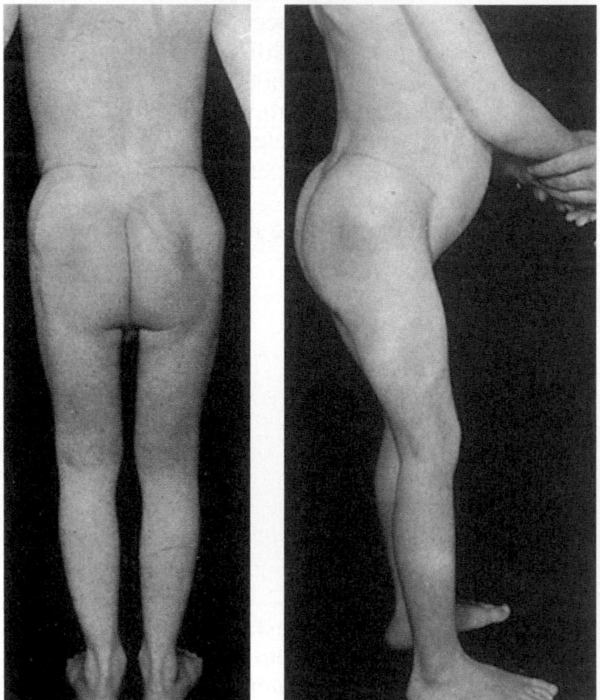

(a) (b)

Figure 3.10 (a) Widening of perineum. (b) Increased lumbar lordosis.

Turning the infant face down, the buttock fold may be higher on the affected side and may be underdeveloped (Figure 3.9b).

Motions of the hip are not limited except for abduction, and even the adduction contracture may not exist. Internal rotation may be increased. Barlow's sign especially for the congenitally unstable hip is also very helpful and consists of slipping the femoral head out of the acetabulum by exerting pressure backwards in full flexion and rotation.

It should be the duty of the doctor and the nurse to examine all neonatal infants for abnormality of the hip joint. It should be emphasized that the success of treatment depends upon diagnosis in the postnatal period or in early infancy. The condition might then be suspected from the marked broadening of the perineum, or the swelling in the gluteal region due to displacement of the head of the femur or an unduly prominent thigh (Figure 3.10). Hart emphasized that the classic signs of hip dysplasia are:

1. Limitation of hip abduction with the knees flexed to 90° and the child on his/her back.
2. A snap or click (Ortolani's sign) elicited when the head rides over the acetabular rim by externally rotating the flexed limb in gradual abduction. This sign may be found only in the first 3 months and may be absent when there is marked ligamentous laxity, or in a fixed, unilateral dislocation or in bilateral dislocations.
3. Apparent shortening of the thigh with the hip and knees flexed to 90°.

EXAMINATION OF A YOUNG CHILD

When the child begins to walk, the gait is abnormal and irreparable damage has been done to the hip. The limb is unstable, the trochanter ascending whenever the body weight is transmitted through the leg of the affected side.

The gait

In a bilateral dislocation the gait has been described as a 'duck-like waddle' or a 'sailor's gait', and consists of an inclination to the side on which the weight is borne.

In a unilateral case, the child lurches towards the affected side. The gait is the result of the inefficiency of the gluteal muscles, the shortening of the neck of the femur, and the displacement of the head, combined with the lordosis and the abnormal lateral mobility of the lumbar spine.

The lordosis

This is particularly noticeable in bilateral cases, but is present in lesser degree in unilateral cases, and is accompanied by a corresponding protrusion of the abdomen.

The deformity

Unilateral cases

There is marked shortening of the leg, which, on measurement, is found to be in the region above the greater trochanter.

Bilateral cases

The legs appear too short for the body, the perineal space is broadened, the trochanters are unduly prominent, and the buttocks broad and flat.

Palpation

On palpating the groins, it will be noticed that on the affected side the pulsation of the femoral vessels is difficult to feel ('vascular sign'). This is due to the displacement of the femoral head which normally supports the femoral artery.

Movements

Movements can be carried out painlessly and freely, except for some limitation of abduction and lateral rotation. In early cases, a distinct telescoping can be elicited when the femur is moved up and down in its long axis, as this produces upward and downward movement of the head on the dorsum ilium.

Measurements

In unilateral cases the affected leg will be found to be shorter than the other, and even in bilateral dislocations there is usually some difference in length. The actual discrepancy varies with the amount of telescoping of the femur that takes place. On closer examination it will be seen that the shortening is above the level of the trochanter.

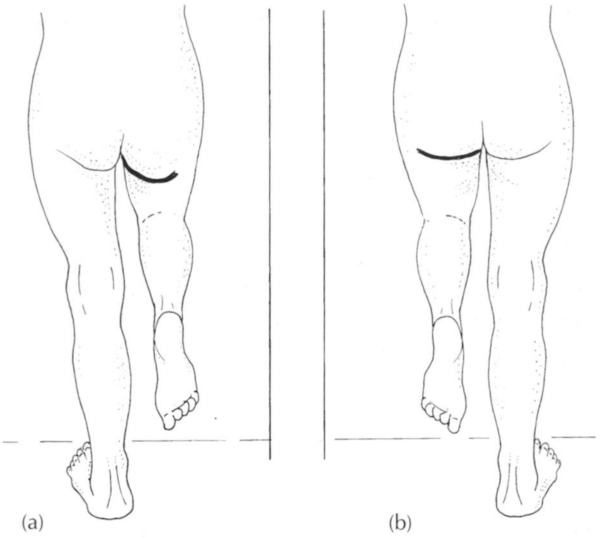

Figure 3.11 Trendelenburg's sign. Congenital dislocation left hip: (a) on lifting sound leg, buttock on lifted side drops; (b) on lifting dislocated leg, buttock rises slightly, i.e. the hip joint is stable.

Trendelenburg's sign

This is elicited by asking the child to stand first on one foot and then on the other. In unilateral cases, when she stands on the sound side, the buttock of the opposite side rises slightly, for the gluteus medius contracts in order to raise the pelvis and bring the trunk more directly above the limb which is sustaining the body weight. When she stands on the dislocated side, the opposite buttock now drops, for the gluteus medius is relatively inefficient and the pelvis cannot therefore be raised or even be kept horizontal (Figure 3.11). The amount of drop depends on the degree of displacement, and continues until the femur and the side wall of the pelvis of the side on which the child is standing are brought into contact. Stability is then attained. In bilateral cases the phenomenon is present on both sides.

The Trendelenburg test is not pathognomonic of congenital dislocation of the hip, but occurs whenever the action of the gluteus medius is interfered with – as for example in poliomyelitis and in coxa vara. In congenital dislocation the inefficiency of the gluteus medius is due to two factors:

1. Its axis – normally vertical – is now altered to a more nearly horizontal direction.

2. Its fulcrum – the head of the femur – is now unstable.

RADIOGRAPHIC EXAMINATION OF THE HIP IN INFANCY

The mere presence of a high acetabular angle when measured does not mean either dislocation or impending poor development even though a high acetabular angle is associated with dislocated hips. Caffey (Caffey *et al.*, 1950) pointed this out in his study of a normal population sample that had serial pelvic x-rays; acetabular angles of 35/40° in children who went on to normal hip development were seen. Also reliance on radiography alone before the fourth month was not high (Smaill, 1968) in a series of 6000 babies.

The obliquity of the acetabulum will vary with the extent of ossification of the outer third and with the position of the infant on the x-ray cassettes.

The ossification centre of the proximal femoral epiphysis appears normally at from 4 to 6 months of age. The development is bilaterally symmetrical and begins in the central portion of the epiphysis.

Prior to its appearance the position of the femoral head relative to the acetabulum must be estimated by the position of the femoral shaft and by a line drawn centrally up the femoral neck. This line should transect the radiolucent shadow of the triradiate cartilage. This should be true no matter what the position of the thigh when the x-ray is taken, but obliquity (fixed or rotational) of the pelvis should be noted.

Adduction contractures are brought out by taking films in abduction in addition to the usual anatomical alignment. The position of the ossified femur should remain related to the depth of the acetabulum, allowing an estimated distance for the cartilaginous epiphysis (Figure 3.12).

The relation of the head to the acetabulum can be established by Hilgenreiner's lines; the epiphyseal nucleus should be inside a vertical line drawn from the acetabular margin and below the horizontal line drawn through the 'Y' cartilages (Figure 3.13).

The development of the osseous roof may be measured from the acetabular angle, and this is of some value in prognosis and in recording the degree of primary dysplasia.

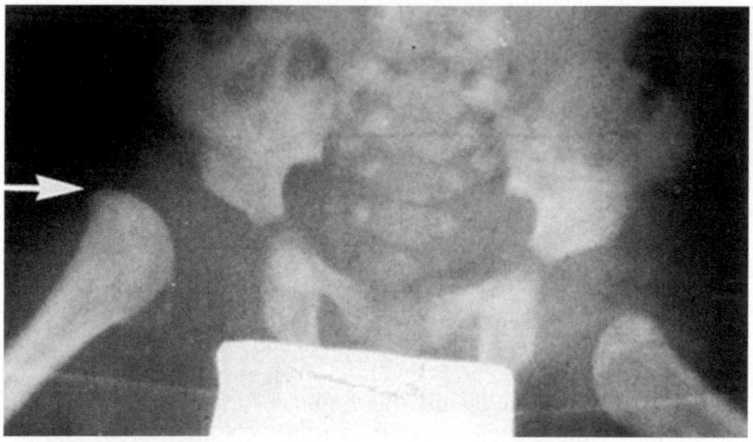

(a)

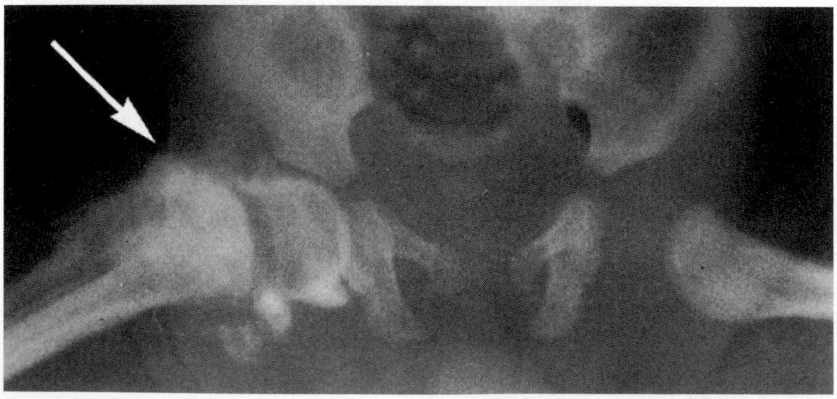

(b)

Figure 3.12 The radiographic examination of the hip in infancy can be misleading. In (a) the relationship of the fumur to the acetabulum indicates dislocation. In (b) an arthrogram of the same infant shows the femoral head located normally but a fracture callus outlined. Actual diagnosis – epiphyseal fracture of the proximal femoral epiphysis.

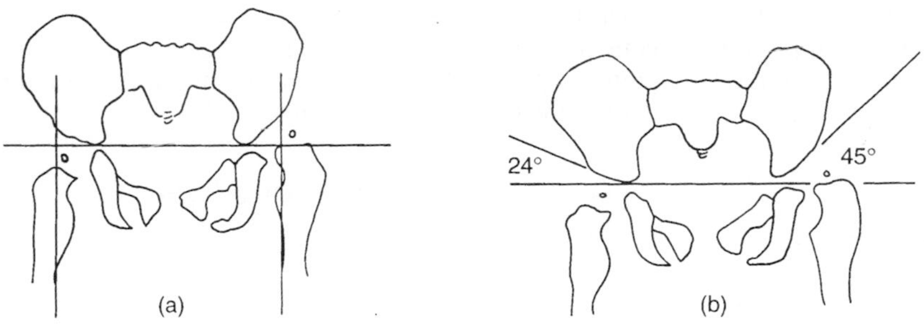

Figure 3.13 x-Ray signs of congenital dislocated hip. (a) Hilgenreiner's lines. Epiphysis in superior outer quadrant. (b) Acetabular angle. Note shallow osseous roof.

Diagnostic imaging

Diagnostic imaging radiography images bone structures and therefore is of least value in the neonatal hip which is mainly cartilaginous up to 6–8 months of age. However, it has been used extensively for classification and diagnosis (Tonnis, 1992). Tonnis has described its use in defining hip dysplasia (disturbance in the ossification of the acetabulum), acetabular dysplasia, subluxation (partial dislocation of the head), etc. but emphasizes the correct positioning of the pelvis as well as the femur in an absolutely neutral position.

Therefore, *arthrography* was developed with the introduction of either air or 1–5 ml of hydrosoluble contrast medium by the anterior route, lateral or inferior under general anaesthesia (see Figure 3.7). It defines causes of instability, of failed reduction by closed methods, prior to open reduction and ascertains whether a congruous reduction has been obtained, when there is delay in appearance of the secondary osseous centres, and helps in determining therapeutic measures. The limbus is clearly shown with its relationship to the subluxation or a dislocation, the ligamentous tear, the transverse acetabular ligament – the capsular outline and condition as well as the articular surfaces. Like all invasive techniques it has had reported complications of femoral artery puncture, septic arthritis, etc.

Ultrasonography has now become established in the static and dynamic analysis of early hip problems, before the age of 6 months, by experienced examiners. The position of the femoral epiphysis and metaphysis can be seen, the labrum, both its size, shape and position are visualized and the covering by the acetabulum cartilaginous roof is outlined. Dynamically the structures are studied when attempting to dislocate the hip under the monitor, for stability and/or instability. Horche and Kumar (1991) have reviewed the accuracy or otherwise of this technique in relationship to its differing use in the USA and Europe.

Engesaeter *et al.* (1990) studied prospectively 100 newborn children with high risk of hip instability, both clinically and by ultrasound. The children were examined at 3 months. None of the standard ultrasound measurements of acetabular depths and femoral head curves correlated with the outcome. Dynamic assessment of the stability was the only ultrasound technique that was significant in defining outcome.

Magnetic resonance imaging

Because of this technique's ability to show up cortical bone marrow, cartilage, both fibro and hyaline, tendons, muscle and fat, it provides very detailed and interesting pathologies, i.e. obstructing soft tissues for reduction, as well as the degree of acetabular and femoral anteversion. However, it is not widely practised because of its cost, its availability and so far it lacks any dynamic testing for stability.

Computerized tomography

Computerized tomography (CT) is particularly useful in demonstrating the femoral head and acetabular relationships when more bone has been formed, i.e. after 6 months. It is helpful to determine accurate reduction, lateral dislocation, subluxation of small degrees that cannot be reduced because of intra-articular bony masses, hypertrophied ligaments, labrum, increased anteversion of the femoral neck as well as small posterior dislocation and acetabular dysplasia with reduced coverage. It is indicated when there is any asymmetry suggesting non-concentric reduction, and bilateral hip dislocation with difficulty in reduction.

DIFFERENTIAL DIAGNOSIS

1. *Coxa vara.* Here the limp is less severe, the head is not palpable in an abnormal position, nor is there any 'telescoping'. The shortening is constant, and the x-ray appearance is quite characteristic.

2. *Pathological dislocation*. In these cases there is usually a history of some previous hip joint trouble developing after birth. There is general limitation of hip movements. The x-ray examination shows greater deformity and absorption of the head, while the acetabulum is usually well developed.
3. *Paralytic dislocation of poliomyelitis*. This condition simulates congenital dislocation in its waddling gait and the shortness of the limb, but the hip joints are normal. There is obvious muscular paralysis.
4. *Cerebral palsy*.
5. *Septic arthritis*.

Screening

Screening for detection of developmental dysplasia of the hip has now become established with national and other bodies, e.g. Department of Health and Social Security, UK who have developed fixed policies and instructions.

It is recognized that at birth there are about 20 per live 1000 births in which hip instability is found. The majority will resolve without treatment but about 10% unstable hips will persist as subluxation or dysplasic hips with an equal number dislocated. Therefore screening within 24 hours of birth, on discharge from hospital, at 6 weeks, between 6 and 9 months and between 15 and 21 months to determine the gait pattern is now strongly recommended. These should be carried out by trained and experienced examiners, using the modified Ortolani/Barlow manoeuvre, any 'at risk' factor noted and recorded, and any instability signs discussed with the parents. Treatment is started with triple diapering, a von Rosen splint or Pavlik harness which requires constant surveillance. The position of ultrasound examination at the very early stage following birth is still being evaluated but certainly it is of help if the clinical signs are positive at the 6 weeks examination. This technique is essential in following the results of early preventive treatment.

In spite of efficient and intensive programmes, late established dislocation of the hip patients are being diagnosed and it is still uncertain whether they have been missed because of failure of clinical screening tests. Sandridson *et al.* (1991) reviewed the results of screening of more than 96 000 infants in Sweden and noted an increase from 0.07 per thousand to 0.6 per thousand over a 31-year period.

PROGNOSIS

Although the condition is never a fatal one, and in some cases, in its early stages, not even a seriously disabling one, symptoms increase during the adolescent period and, with increase of age and weight, painful spasm and rigidity ensue and, at a still later date, arthritis in the false joint.

Natural history of the completely dislocated hip

Weinstein (1992), on extensive reviewing of the world literature, emphasized that the outcome varies with time and various social and psychological circumstances. In some societies a limp is acceptable whereas in others it is unacceptable. The two factors of importance which he found are first, whether a well developed false acetabulum has been formed with degenerative joint disease resulting or, second, whether there is bilateral dislocation in which low back pain results from the increased hyperlordosis position of the lumbar spine.

With unilateral complete dislocation, secondary problems can arise in the back such as a scoliosis, leg length problems with gait disturbances, due to the flexed adduction position of the involved hip and valgus deformity of the ipsilateral knee, followed by degenerative arthritis.

Natural history of subluxation and/or dysplasia

Weinstein (1992) defined subluxation as an abnormal development of both acetabulum and the femoral head, but Shenton's line is 'broken' whereas in the dysplastic hip joint, Shenton's line is intact. He pointed out that as no previous early diagnosis had usually been made, it was often noted on radiographs taken for other reasons or on developing symptoms, particularly with dysplasia being found in the contralateral hip. Many studies have related the onset of degenerative arthritis with pain in dysplastic and subluxed hips with shallow acetabulum, especially in patients older than 6 years and in females. On the other hand, Hoaglund *et al.* (1973) have clearly demonstrated the low incidence of secondary osteoarthritis in the Chinese population of Hong Kong where the incidence of developmental dysplasia of the hip is also very low.

The late results of closed reduction will vary according to the age when treatment is started, the degree of dysplasia and the criteria by which results are judged. Muller and Seddon (1953) reported only 57% of excellent late results following closed reduction in children under 3 years of age. The assessment was made on combined clinical and radiographic criteria.

TREATMENT OF THE HIP IN THE INFANT

Up to 3 months of age

Acetabular dysplasia as shown by an ultrasound positive examination, without a positive Ortolani sign, may be treated prophylactically by triple diapering rather than femoral abduction splintage. This will reduce the overtreatment group and the risk of avascular necrosis, but careful follow-up is essential (Figure 3.14).

Subluxable dislocating hips with a positive Ortolani sign and a positive ultrasound assessment, especially over the age of 3–6 weeks, should be treated with a single abduction splint – a von Rosen splint (Figure 3.15) or a Pavlik harness (Figure 3.15) (although it is now recognized that if the femurs are allowed to adduct a redislocation can occur). Because of this a new flexion, abduction splint, to allow slow extension, was designed by Bernau (1990) – like the Tubigen splint – hopefully to reduce the risk of avascular necrosis.

Continued reassessment of the reduced position by ultrasound examination is imperative up to 6 weeks.

Unreducible dislocations are unusual and are usually associated with neuromuscular disorders when initial treatment is held over for about 3 months until ossification has advanced.

Over the age of 3 months

Over the age of 3 months, on diagnosis, if the hip is reducible then abduction/flexion splintage is carried

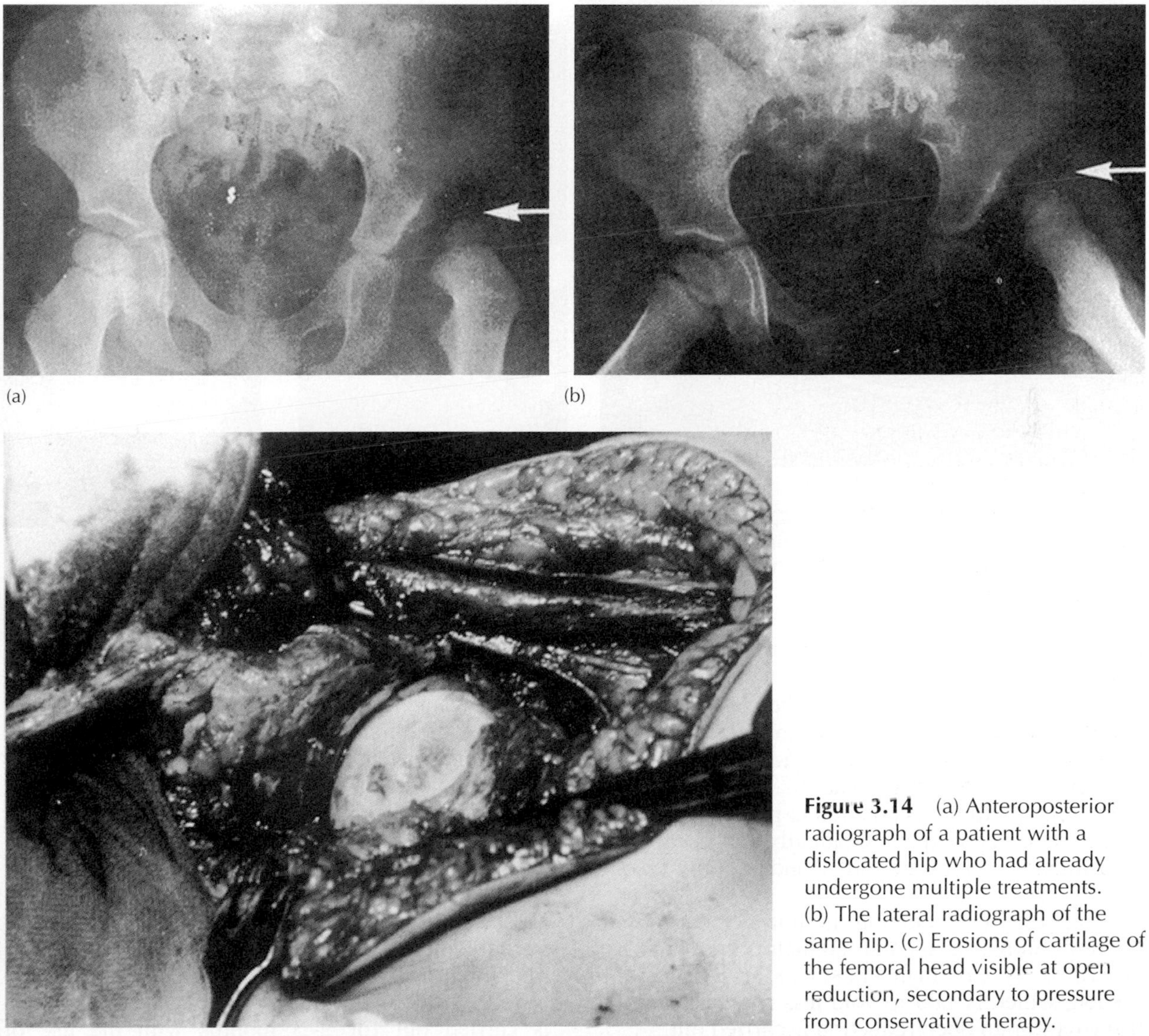

(a) (b) (c)

Figure 3.14 (a) Anteroposterior radiograph of a patient with a dislocated hip who had already undergone multiple treatments. (b) The lateral radiograph of the same hip. (c) Erosions of cartilage of the femoral head visible at open reduction, secondary to pressure from conservative therapy.

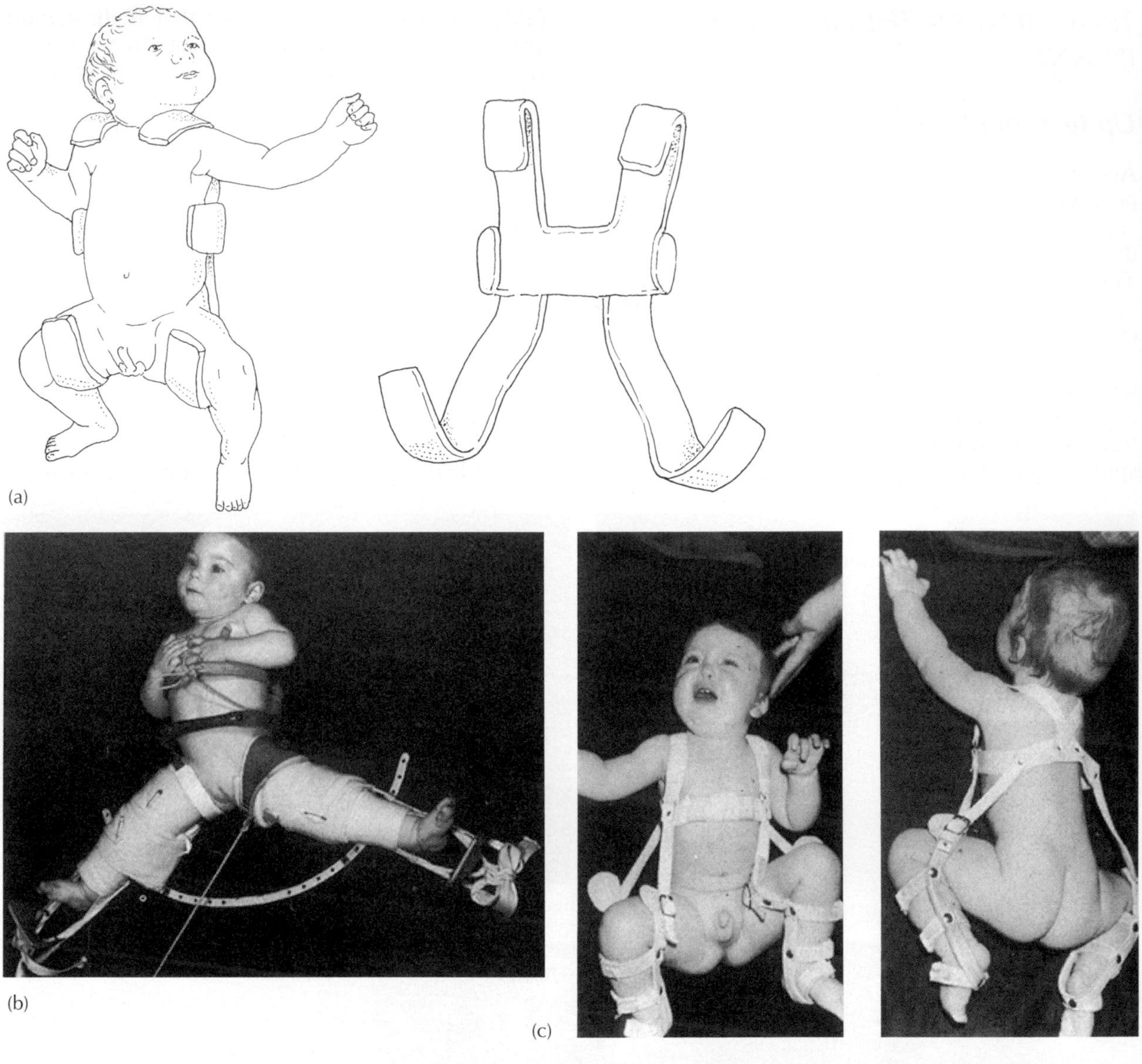

Figure 3.15 (a) Von Rosen splint. (b) 'Wingfield pattern' abduction frame with cross-pull on left thigh. (c) Pavlik harness, front and back views.

out for the next 3–6 months, recognizing that the complication of avascular necrosis is higher.

If the hip cannot be reduced, the child should be admitted for traction – either by an abduction frame or by 'gallows' – after an arthrogram under general anaesthesia or CT examination. With successful reduction, holding this position in plaster for up to 8 weeks is then carried out. Gradually, mobilization in an abduction splint is permitted and a follow-up of 2 years is essential.

If concentric reduction is not achieved with traction, either a medial adductor approach, as described by Coleman (1992) or an anterior approach, which is said to hold less risk of avascular necrosis, for an open reduction is carried out.

Whether traction has any effect upon the increased risk of avascular necrosis in the group is still very controversial. Kahle *et al.* (1990) had a 4% incidence without preliminary traction in both closed and open reduction procedures. Brougham *et al.* (1990) have reported an even greater incidence by including minor ischaemic changes, of 48% osteonecrosis after traction and 45% without traction.

From the medial approach, the adductor longus and iliopsoas muscles are tenotomized, the joint capsule is incised, especially the obstructing anteromedial component, and the ligamentous teres removed. The limbus is rarely an obstruction requiring excision. Immobilization in a plaster-of-Paris cast is carried out for 2–3 months with the use of an abduction brace for at least another 6 weeks to 3 months. The anterior approach is particularly indicated when the hip is highly dislocated, when it is difficult to reduce manually and where there is any significant growth differential. This approach will allow a pelvic osteotomy to be carried if required to stabilize the femoral head within the acetabulum and a strong capsular reefing repair.

Dysplasia

A recent CDH study by Lennox *et al.* (1993) demonstrated that neonatal screening is not totally effective throughout a region. More dislocations had been missed at neonatal examination during the last decade, i.e. 0.13% of live births, and operative treatment was required in 54 of these children, i.e. 0.08% of live births, some of whom had been diagnosed at birth. They noted that 33 such children who had been considered normal at the CDH clinic presented later with a dislocation, i.e. due to *acetabular dysplasia* or what is termed developmental dislocation. These patients are important to follow up until the capital femoral epiphyses are correctly located within a well formed acetabulum. These authors described their operative treatment as closed reduction under anaesthesia with or without an adductor tenotomy (78% of cases) – if this failed open reduction in 6%, pelvic or femoral osteotomy or combined in 15%. Of all the children undergoing operative intervention, 21% developed some degree of avascular necrosis. There was a consistent group of patients who were resistant to treatment which differed from those making up the failure of neonatal screening group, by being breech delivered and having a significantly greater number of open operations.

Subluxation

Subluxation implies incomplete dislocation. The femoral head remains in partial contact with the cartilaginous acetabulum and there is therefore no interposition of soft tissue. Arthrography may reveal eversion of the fibrocartilaginous limbus but after reduction, in the early case, the limbus descends to provide good cover for the head.

This condition has serious implications for the development of the hip joint and mirrors the effect of the iliopsoas tightly pulling in the hip joint capsule medial to the bulk of the femoral head. Pressure laterally may have deformed the outer third of the acetabulum of the femoral head itself. There has not, however, been any proximal progression of the femur to the point of frank dislocation.

Traction is often necessary to overcome the iliopsoas tightness. Traction is put on in line with the trunk without abducting the hip at the beginning. In order to maintain countertraction it is necessary to place the normal side in a hip spica or to use the Wingfield splint (Figure 3.15b) or a Gallows splint.

Traction has been sufficient when 20–30° abduction and 15–20° of internal rotation of the femur leads to perfect positioning of the femur in the hip joint.

If perfect position is not obtained, it will not improve in the future. This leads, on occasion, to the necessity for open reduction with division of the iliopsoas tendon, opening of the capsule to divide its tight band beneath the iliopsoas and possible pulling up of the limbus from its pressed-down position. The capsule is repaired with the hip joint accurately aligned, and hip motion is started after 3 weeks with weight-bearing at least 6 weeks away. A removable plaster spica or a simple abduction device is used during this period.

Prolonged fixation in plaster is avoided, both when closed and when open treatment has been used. Such fixation beyond 3–4 months is relying on pressure to overcome defects which were not corrected.

Batchelor's plaster

Following successful reduction on the frame the hips must be protected until ossification of the acetabular roof provides a more stable socket. The Batchelor plaster position corrects anteversion by internal rotation and allows mobility of the concentrically reduced head, which theoretically should encourage development of the socket (Figure 3.16).

The plaster is applied under general anaesthesia and the legs are internally rotated to compensate for the estimated anteversion angle. The degree of abduction should be sufficient to place the head centrally in the acetabulum. The cross-bar is attached and the position of the femoral head verified by x-rays. The plaster requires renewal approximately every 3 months, and, as the acetabulum develops, the degree of abduction is gradually reduced to produce more stimulus to the roof of the socket.

The duration of treatment depends on the development of the acetabulum but is usually about 6 months. When the plaster is removed, the child should be admitted to hospital for mobilization and supervision of the initial weight-bearing. This period of treatment can often be reduced, especially in the older infant, by a subtrochanteric derotational osteotomy performed 1 month after reduction in order to correct any anteversion deformity. Some degree of varus correction may be added to the osteotomy.

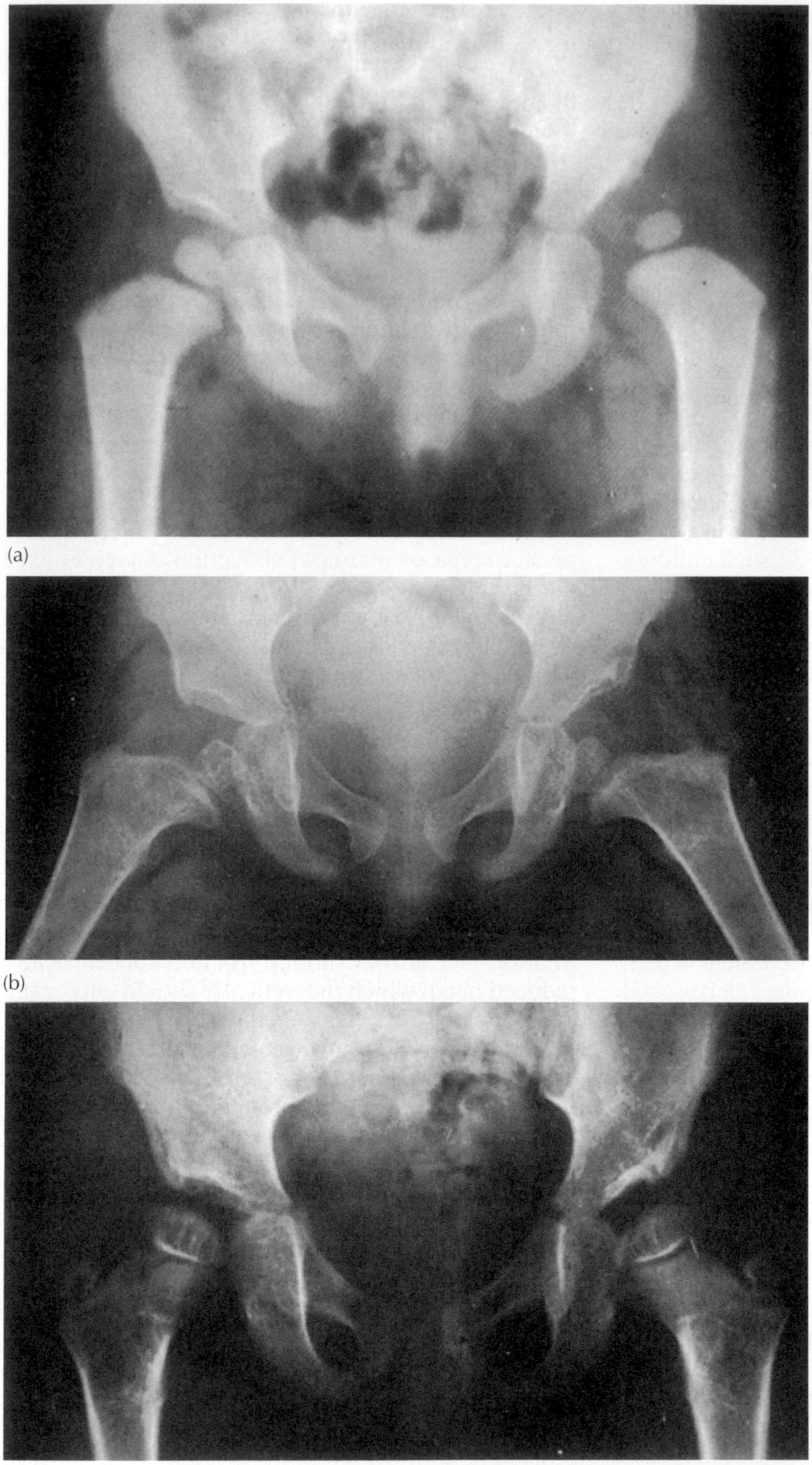
(a)
(b)
(c)

Figure 3.16 (a) Subluxation of left hip. (b) Correction of anteversion in Batchelor's plaster. Note improved ossification of roof after 9 months. (c) Hip remains stable after 18 months of freedom.

Dislocation

Dislocation implies complete displacement of the head and loss of contact with the articular surface of the original cartilaginous acetabulum. Differentiation between subluxation and dislocation may prove difficult in some cases without the aid of arthrography.

Treatment even in the young child is difficult because in complete dislocation interposition of soft tissue may complicate reduction and subsequent joint development.

If an inverted limbus is small, it may be so compressed during reduction and application of abduction plaster that the head appears to be accurately reduced on an anteroposterior radiograph. Under these circumstances the limbus may in some cases be successfully accommodated in the joint.

The underlying principle is perfect location of the hip achieved by closed methods without pressure whether from traction, manipulation or plaster immobilization. If this cannot be achieved, open reduction is used to achieve proper location of the hip. Somerville (1978) has reported, from his vast series, that in children under 2 years of age, traction with progressive abduction and internal rotation with adductor tenotomy gives a 50% chance of reduction, with 10% incidence of ischaemia in the femoral head. Radiographs taken after 4 weeks of such treatment showed one of the following:

1. The hip remained dislocated, and if a single attempt at manipulative reduction under general anaesthesia failed, open reduction was indicated.
2. The hip remained subluxed, but reduction was possible with prolonged immobilization; if not, arthrography was indicated and open reduction was performed.
3. The hip was reduced by traction and held in the reduced position for 6–8 weeks – then operative stabilization was considered.

Over the age of 3 years

Over the age of 3 years, as already described, because of the soft tissue and bony deformities, open reduction is essential. A pelvic osteotomy is performed, either a Salter type for rotational stabilization with capsular reefing or a Pemberton type when there is acetabular dysplasia. On the femoral side either a varus rotational subtrochanteric osteotomy may be sufficient or if reduction cannot be achieved, then femoral shortening with internal fixation should be added to the femoral derotation to reduce the incidence of avascular necrosis, chondrolysis or redislocation.

Coleman (1992) has described in detail the differences between the Salter redirectional osteotomy and the Pemberton pericapsular incomplete osteotomy with their indications. These include failure to achieve a stable reduction at the time of open reduction because of acetabular incongruity or deficiency; progressive subluxation of the hip after either conservative or operative treatment; and failure of the acetabulum to remodel. Before deciding upon which osteotomy to use, concentric reduction must be seen on radiography, abduction and internal movement should almost be normal and flexibility of the triradiate cartilage or symphysis pubis should be present. If there is a shallow or abnormally shaped acetabulum Pemberton should be performed; if the acetabulum has an abnormal direction, a Salter osteotomy should be carried out.

Shelf operations have long been practised as a method to increase the acetabular cover, for persistent acetabular dysplasia, over a well shaped femoral head in good position (Summers *et al.*, 1988). It should be carried out extracapsularly in order to allow the superior capsule to dedifferentiate into fibrocartilage. It is usually carried out in the young adolescent with mild symptoms and can be regarded as a preventative procedure and can be

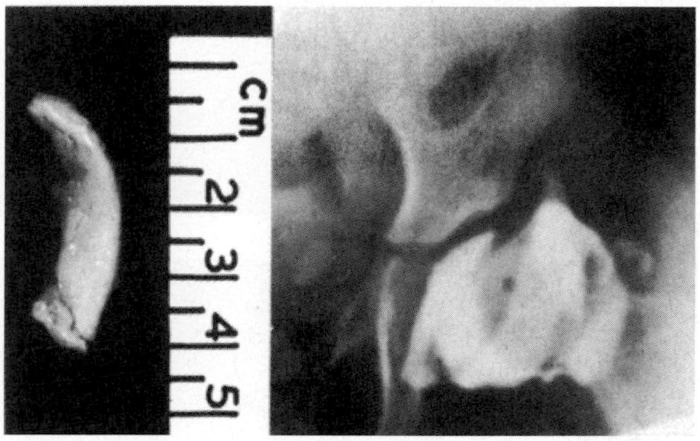

(a)

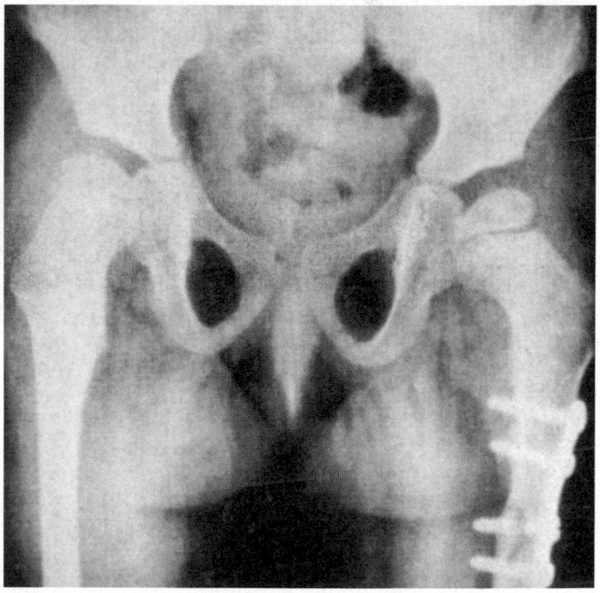

(b)

Figure 3.17 (a) Arthrogram shows inversion of limbus. Specimen removed from posterosuperior aspects of acetabulum. (b) Reduction remaining stable 2 years after excision of limbus and derotation osteotomy. (Case of the late Mr G. P. Mitchell)

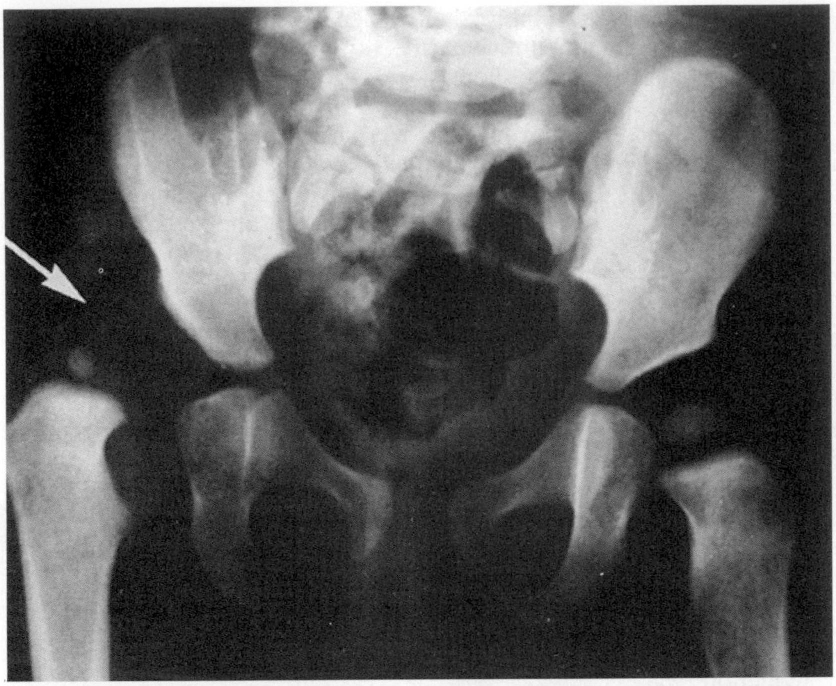

(a)

Figure 3.18(a) Dislocated femur in an infant, which persisted in spite of conservative therapy.

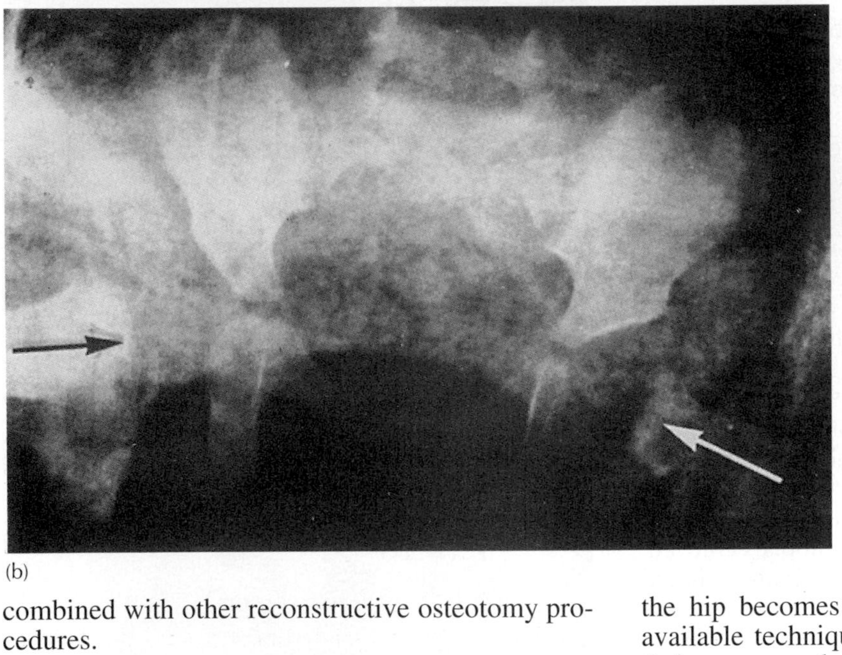

(b)

Figure 3.18(b) Open reduction with the head not located.

combined with other reconstructive osteotomy procedures.

Chiari osteotomy

This osteotomy was originally described for use in the older dislocated hip, i.e. over 4 years of age, as a salvage procedure. It is now reserved for the adolescent or older patient up to middle age when the femoral head has little or no support but the false acetabulum is not too high and there are symptoms. It can also be used as part of a redirectional femoral osteotomy.

It is obvious that as a developmental dysplasia of the hip becomes older into skeletal maturity the available techniques become more numerous with their own complexities.

OPEN REDUCTION OF A DISLOCATED HIP

When open reduction of the hip is carried out early in the course of treatment in a child not previously immobilized for any considerable period of time, atrophy of muscle, contractures and pressure effects on the cartilage of both the femoral head and

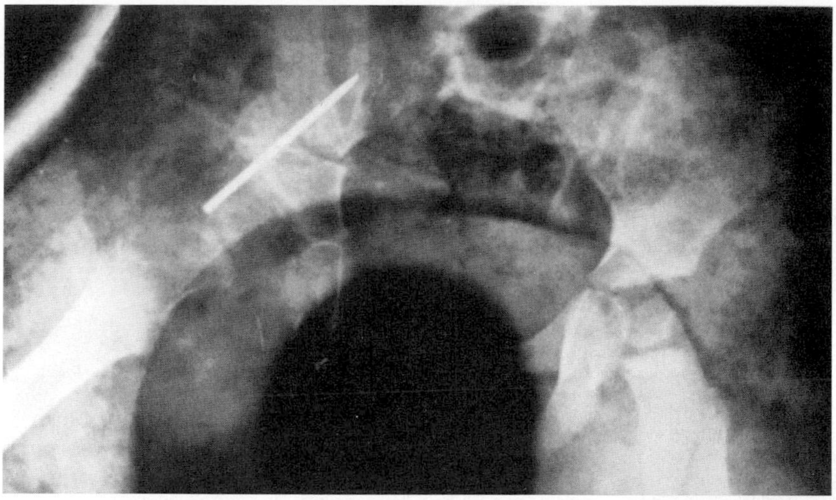

(c)

Figure 3.18(c) A Salter osteotomy with the femoral head still riding laterally.

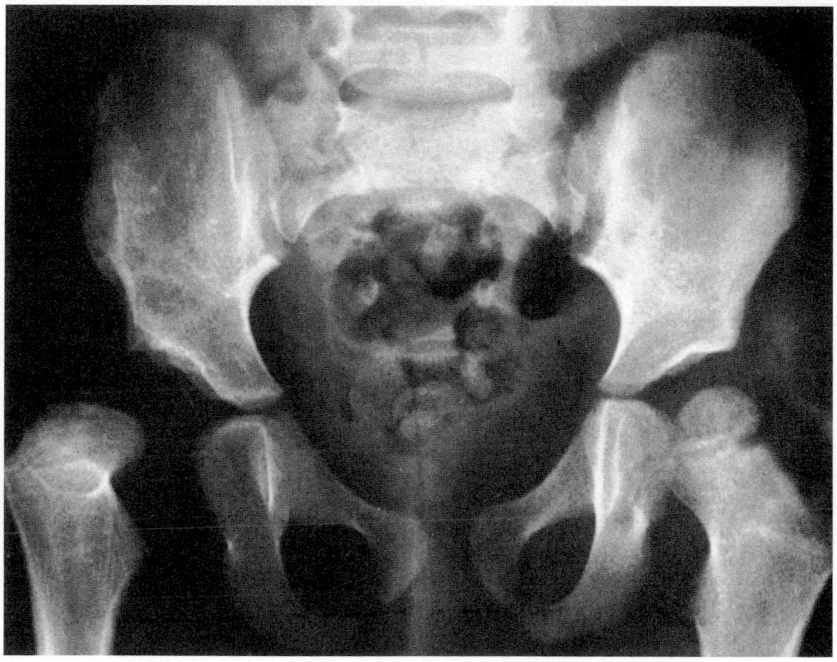

(d)

Figure 3.18(d) Follow-up radiograph with persistence of the dislocation, and irregular ossification of the capital femoral epiphysis. If an open reduction is to succeed, the femoral head must be located within the acetabulum, and this is an essential prerequisite for a Salter innominate osteotomy.

acetabulum can be avoided. When myostatic contractures exist, preliminary traction and exercises should be used to avoid operating on a stiff hip.

In children whose hips cannot be satisfactorily seated in the acetabulum by conservative means, the tendon of the iliopsoas appears as one of the obstructions to reduction. In this case the dissection must be carried sufficiently medial to mobilize the iliopsoas with localization of the femoral nerve by dissection. The usual anterior iliofemoral approach is made between sartorius and tensor fasciae latae. The iliac apophysis is removed as a cap and packed medially. The rectus femoris is divided from its origin from the anterior inferior iliac spine. The femoral nerve will be found at its medial edge and should be carefully separated from it. The insertion of the iliopsoas can then be divided and the muscle retracted superiorly. The indentation left by the tight iliopsoas can now be identified. The capsule is divided proximally and carried anteriorly and then inferiorly to open fully the acetabulum to view the femoral head which can easily be reduced once this is done and the surgeon is not at a loss to identify the true acetabulum. The distal capsule can then be

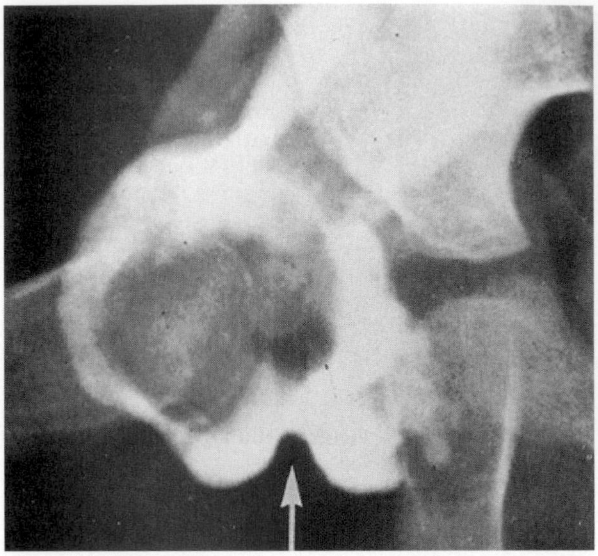

(e)

Figure 3.18(e) The arthrogram shows the reason for the persistent lateral subluxation within the acetabulum. The notch (marked by the arrow) is caused by the hour-glass constriction of the capsule secondary to pressure from the iliopsoas tendon.

brought up over the remaining proximal portion to get rid of the redundancy characteristic of chronic dislocation. Sometimes it has not been found necessary to carry out any removal of acetabular contents, limbus or ligamentum teres once the capsule has been opened to expose fully the acetabulum (Figures 3.17, 3.18).

OPEN REDUCTION OF THE HIP THROUGH A MEDIAN ADDUCTOR APPROACH

Open reduction can be performed through a median adduction approach, as described by Ferguson (1968) or by Mau *et al.* (1971), which allows the excision of the capsule, release of the iliopsoas and easy reduction of the hip with little morbidity. These authors have not found it necessary to release the adductor muscles or to excise the limbus.

The incision was originally described by Ludloff in 1908. It begins just below the pubic tubercle and extends along the medial aspect of the thigh. The adductor longus is found and dissection is carried on beneath it, carrying both the adductor longus and brevis superiorly and anteriorly, with the adductor magnus and gracilis being retracted posteriorly and inferiorly. The operation is done with the patient's thigh flexed, abducted and externally rotated. By finger dissection the interval can readily be split and the lesser trochanter easily palpated. The posterior segment of the obturator nerve can be seen lying on the adductor magnus and need not be disturbed. The sciatic nerve can be palpated posteriorly, and on retraction the iliopsoas can be seen inserting into the lesser trochanter. A small fat pad overlies the hip capsule. The capsule is opened, and the iliopsoas tendon released especially when an hour-glass constriction is present. The femoral head can be readily relocated by pulling it forwards. No extensive filling of the acetabulum with tissue debris has been found.

Derotation osteotomy of the femur

Opinions differ on the significance of anteversion of the femoral neck and the necessity for surgical correction. Muller and Seddon (1953), reviewing the late results of congenital dislocation of the hip, found that 83% of hips which showed a notable degree of anteversion were associated with subluxation or dislocation of the head. They concluded that anteversion is a factor in causing subluxation after reduction, although Salter (1968) believes that femoral anteversion is the result of the dislocation rather than the cause.

Anteversion is reduced while in the Batchelor position and may correct spontaneously during treatment. The exact indications for derotation osteotomy of the femur vary from case to case but as a rule only anteversion exceeding 60° need be considered. It may be stated that the earlier the mobilization, the greater the need for surgical correction. Weight-bearing may be permitted despite residual anteversion in cases where the original displacement has been minimal and the subsequent development of the osseous roof satisfactory. Surgical correction of persistent, marked anteversion is advisable before weight-bearing when displacement has been more advanced and development of the osseous roof less satisfactory.

x-Rays taken at 45° and 65° of internal hip rotation are of value and the impression gained while screening at arthrography is reliable. Clinical estimation of anteversion is regarded as a useful method. With the child supine and the knees flexed over the end of a table, the prominence of the greater trochanter is palpated and the hips are internally rotated until the prominence is maximal. The angle of deviation of the tibia from the midline equals the anteversion angle.

The most suitable site for osteotomy is the subtrochanteric region. The bone is exposed with the hip in the internally rotated position. Two Steinmann pins are inserted as markers and the femur is divided between them by a saw. The lower fragment is externally rotated to the required angle as judged by the markers and rotation maintained by a four-hole vitallium plate and screws.

The femur is immobilized in a hip spica for approximately 6 weeks.

Derotation osteotomy is also indicated if displacement occurs following closed reduction.

Innominate osteotomy

Innominate osteotomy is indicated in the treatment of subluxation or dislocation of the hip, from whatever cause, which either is discovered late or has failed to respond to other methods of treatment.

There are three types of innominate osteotomy which are designed to provide a cover of the femoral head, in order to maintain a stable reduction in the position of function. This is achieved either by altering the orientation of the acetabulum in order to cover the anterolateral defect present in these cases (Salter and Pemberton), or by forming a new lateral extension to the existing acetabular roof (Chiari).

The Salter osteotomy (Figure 3.19)

This was first introduced in 1961 for children from the age of 18 months to 7 years for unilateral cases and up to 5 years for bilateral cases. Its aim was to redirect the entire acetabular roof forwards and downwards to stabilize the reduced hip in the functional position of weight-bearing. It is indicated when the acetabular dysplasia is mild to moderate with reasonable congruity of the hip joint surfaces and any soft tissue contractures, particularly of the adductors and the iliopsoas, have been released. Following open reduction and innominate osteotomy for dislocation in the age group 18 months to 4 years (Salter, 1966), results were over 90% good or excellent, and between 4 and 10 years 56%. For subluxation by innominate osteotomy alone, both groups were over 90%. When carried out for dislocation after failure of other treatments, the results were very poor.

The disadvantages of this osteotomy are that it is unstable, requiring internal fixation; the amount of correction is limited by the size of the graft and the length of the pubic ramus; a 'defect' is created in the posterior acetabulum with some narrowing of the joint space over the femoral head, and some remodelling.

The osteotomy is made just above the acetabulum, running transversely from the anterior inferior iliac spine subperiosteally to the greater sciatic notch. The lower fragment is displaced downwards, outwards and forwards, hinging at the pubic symphysis. A wedge-shaped graft from the anterior part of the iliac blade is inserted into the osteotomy to maintain the position. Reefing of the anterior capsule is essential. Postoperative immobilization in a hip spica for 6 weeks is recommended, with an additional 4 weeks in long leg plasters if the osteotomy was combined with open reduction. Full weight-bearing is then permitted.

The Pemberton osteotomy (Figure 3.20)

This acetabuloplasty was first described by Pemberton in 1955 (1965) and achieves stabilization of a reduced hip by rotating the anterosuperior portion of the acetabulum forwards, laterally and downwards. The posterior portion of the acetabulum remains undisturbed. The degree of acetabular dysplasia can be moderate to severe but requires considering remodelling ability of the acetabulum; it therefore is indicated for children aged between 18 months and 6–7 years. The osteotomy uses the triradiate cartilage as a fulcrum, allowing a good degree of correction but changing the configuration of acetabulum.

The osteotomy extends in a curve from just above the acetabulum at the anterior inferior iliac spine, downwards and backwards to the triradiate cartilage. It is important that the osteotomy does not extend into the greater sciatic notch. The lower fragment is flexed downwards and outwards, hinging at the triradiate cartilage until a gap of 1–10 cm is produced anteriorly. This is maintained by a bone graft from the anterior part of the ilium.

In addition to correcting the acetabular alignment, this osteotomy also reduces the size of the acetabulum, which Pemberton claims is important to

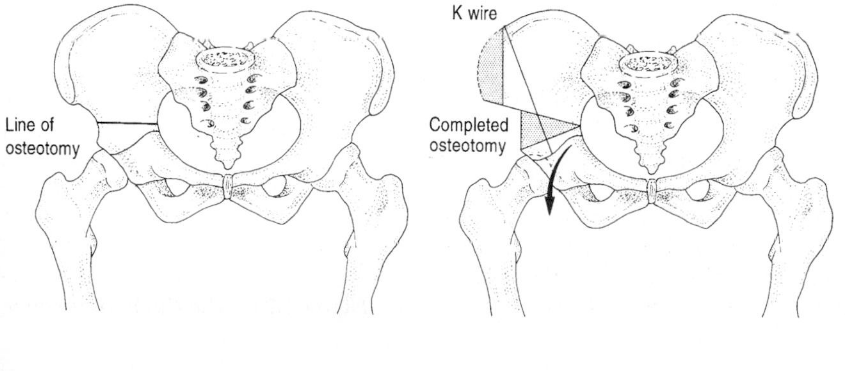

Figure 3.19 A Salter osteotomy, showing the passage of the Gigli saw through the sciatic notch. The cut is then being brought forwards superior to the acetabulum as the distal segment is displaced downwards, outwards and forwards. A bone block graft is placed to hold the fragment in this new position and is transfixed with two Kirschner wires.

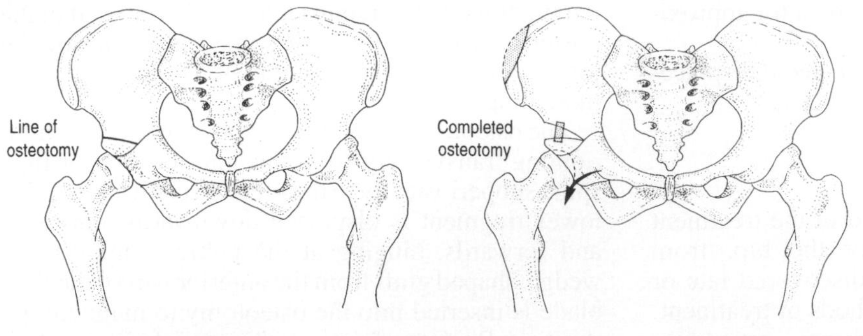

Figure 3.20 The Pemberton osteotomy.

obtain greater conformity of size between femoral head and acetabulum.

Immobilization in a hip spica is recommended for 2 months followed by full weight-bearing.

Faciszewski *et al.* (1993) have reviewed the results in patients of about 4 years of age who had received a Pemberton osteotomy for residual acetabular dysplasia of the hip. After 10 years over 80% of the hips had developed into a normal hip. However, the poorer results were found when there had been femoral head necrosis. Open or closed reduction attempts before or after the osteotomy did not affect the outcome. Controversy remains as to whether adequate correction can be achieved by correcting the proximal femur or by correcting the acetabular side. The basic response to either, or to a combined procedure, results from the remodelling potential of either side which will give rise to a stable hip and normal function. It is accepted that the acetabulum can remodel up to the age of 8 years because of the intermediate cartilage contribution.

TREATMENT OF CONGENITAL DISLOCATION OF HIP OVER THE AGE OF 6 YEARS

A specific outline of treatment is difficult to describe because of the lack of any well documented, well controlled long-term series. Indeed, some believe that the dislocated head should be left until symptoms occur in young middle age, when a total hip replacement can be performed. It may be possible, after a prolonged period of strong skeletal traction, to perform an open reduction with some type of osteotomy (Salter or Pemberton), femoral shortening of Klisic or radical muscle release procedure as described by Arzimanoglu (1976).

The Chiari osteotomy (Figure 3.21)

This operation was introduced in 1950 for children from the age of 4 years up to theoretically any age group (Chiari, 1970). (Chiari used this operation in a 69-year-old with osteoarthritis and subluxation.)

The aim of the operation is to make a deeper acetabulum and displace the femoral head medially to reduce the stresses when concentric reduction is not possible and to cover an irreducible femoral head – i.e. a subluxed head but not a dislocated one.

The osteotomy is made just above the capsule at the anterior inferior iliac spine and extends transversely and upwards to the greater sciatic notch. The lower fragment is moved medially as far as bony contact will allow, the cut edge of the proximal side of the osteotomy forming the extended roof. This is lined by the hip joint capsule, which must not be opened during this operation.

The osteotomy is stable in abduction, with no internal fixation; postoperatively a hip spica is used for 4 weeks, after which weight-bearing can commence.

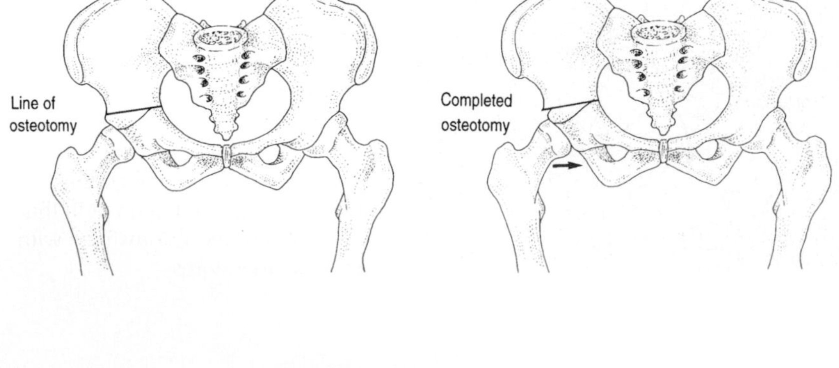

Figure 3.21 The Chiari osteotomy.

PALLIATIVE OPERATIONS

These operations are reserved for cases in which reduction is no longer possible by either closed or open methods. They are designed to improve stability, decrease lordosis, and control pain arising from the hip or lower back. The advisability of palliative procedures in the young patient with symptomless displacement to the hip is doubtful and they should not be lightly undertaken.

Palliative procedures fall into three categories: arthrodesis, osteotomy and arthroplasty.

Arthrodesis

Hip fusion is a satisfactory procedure for relief of arthritic pain in the older patient with unilateral displacement. Arthritic pain occurs more commonly in subluxation than dislocation unless there is a well formed acetabulum.

Osteotomy

The primary object of osteotomy is deflection of weight-bearing by angulation of the femur to bring the axis of the femoral shaft more in line with the direction of weight transmission.

Angulation osteotomy of the Schanz type is preferred to the bifurcation osteotomy of Lorenz in which the upper end of the lower fragment is abducted and inserted into the acetabulum. The Lorenz procedure has the relative disadvantages of increased shortening, less mobility and a greater likelihood of arthritic pain.

Schanz osteotomy

Schanz pointed out that in congenital dislocation of the hip the pelvis tilts on weight-bearing until the femur on the dislocated side impinges on the lower border of the pelvis. If the femur is angled to align the upper fragment with the side wall of the pelvis and the lower fragment parallel with the axis of weight-bearing, the lurching gait will be diminished because the stable position is reached earlier. The depression of the trochanter also improves the leverage of the glutei. The lower femoral fragment should also be extended backwards at the osteotomy site to decrease the pelvic tilt and diminish the lumbar lordosis.

Prior to operation an x-ray is taken with the femur in full adduction, and from the point of bone section a line is drawn vertically to correspond with the normal position of a femur. The correct abduction angle is ascertained by measurement. A strong vitallium plate is angled laterally to this degree; to compensate for the posterior displacement of the head, the plate is angled in extension to approximately 30–40°.

The Schanz osteotomy is a useful palliative procedure in the irreducible case where pain or severe deformity warrants surgical correction (Figures 3.22 and 3.23).

Arthroplasty

Arthroplasty by a total hip replacement procedure can now be considered to produce pain relief, stability and some mobility. However, this can be very difficult to carry out, unless special prostheses are available.

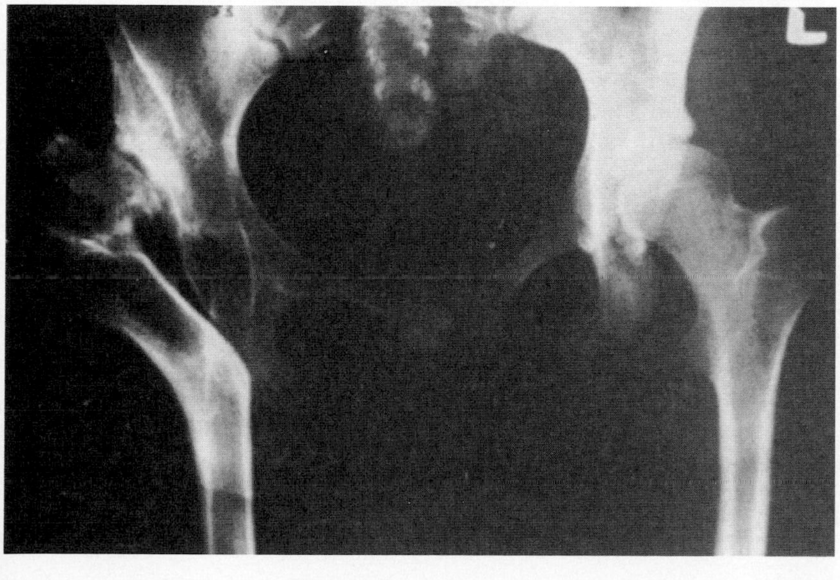

Figure 3.22 Schanz osteotomy of the right femur. Pelvis is balanced by shortening and angulation of right femur.

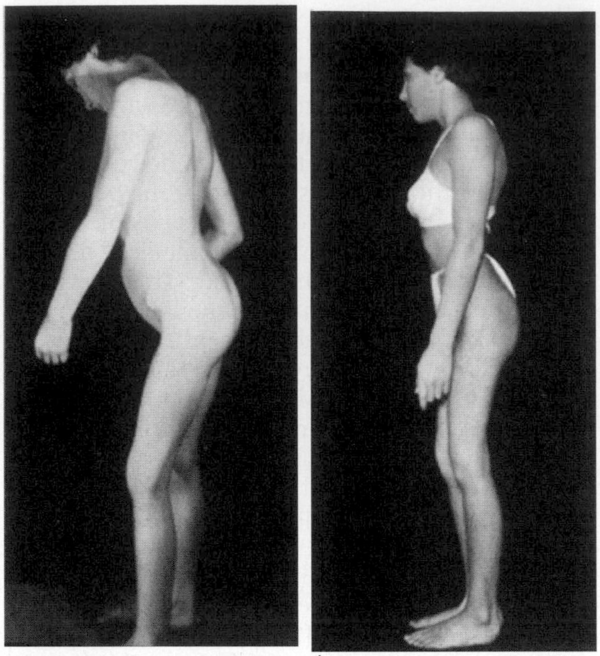

(a) (b)

Figure 3.23 (a) Before and (b) improved posture following bilateral abduction and extension osteotomies in girl of 16 years.

Congenital dislocation of the knee (congenital genu recurvatum)

The rare condition, known since the time of its first description by Chatelain as congenital dislocation of the knee, is also known as congenital genu recurvatum. There are three types:

1. The traumatic developmental type. This is the most common and is considered to be due to malposition *in utero*: the legs may be caught by the chin or axilla with the knees extended and uterine compression may prevent them from assuming the usual flexed position.
2. A primary embryonic defect. This type is usually accompanied by other defects, such as hare-lip, cardiac defects, spina bifida and congenital dislocation of the hip (McFarland, 1951). It is fortunate that this type is uncommon since it is much more difficult to treat and usually requires operation.
3. The third theory is that of contracture of the quadriceps extensor muscle dragging the knee into a deformed position. It is suggested that this contracture is similar to that found in arthrogryposis.

CLINICAL FEATURES

The knee is fixed in hyperextension with a varying degree of subluxation or dislocation forwards of the tibia on the femoral condyles (Figure 3.24), and the skin over the anterior aspect of the joint shows several transverse creases. The patella is small or absent. On the posterior aspect of the joint, the hamstring muscles are palpable as tense cords, and the femoral condyles are felt projecting in the popliteal fossa. The joint is relatively fixed. When attempts are made to flex it, an elastic resistance is appreciated – this is the quadriceps tendon, although if the anterior displacement is severe enough, the hamstring muscles may be the significant resisting factor.

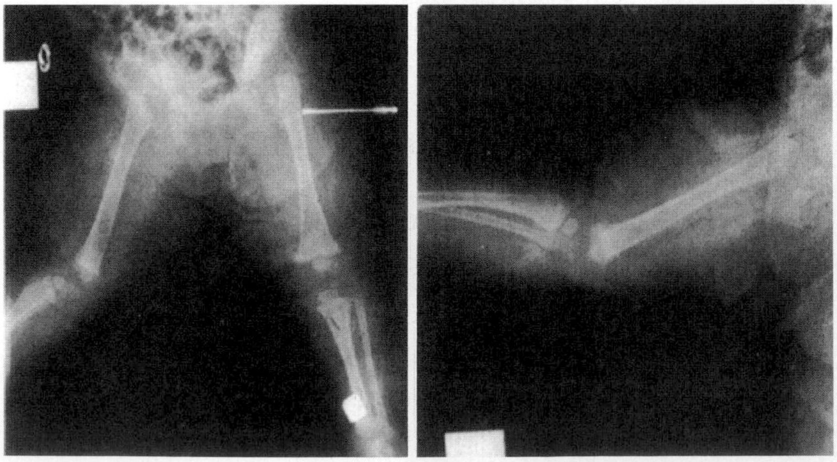

(a) (b)

Figure 3.24 (a) Radiograph of a 3-month-old baby with a bilateral congenital dislocation of hips and dislocation of the right knee joint. (b) Radiograph of the right leg of the same child.

TREATMENT

There are two types which can give an initial clinical picture which may be very similar.

Proximal tibia related to distal femur, but the knee is markedly hyperextended

In this type early and rapid restoration of flexion with maintenance thereafter for a period of 3 months is necessary. Plaster casts are applied, flexing the knee in as much correction as can easily be obtained. Treatment is begun at birth or shortly thereafter and the casts are repeated at 2- to 3-day intervals until flexion beyond 90° is obtained. Thereafter a bivalved cast is used for 3 months. The limb is removed twice a day for 30-minute intervals and active flexion and extension is carried out. An x-ray check-up is obtained during correction to make certain that the proximal tibia is maintaining a normal anatomical relationship to the distal femur. Ordinarily a 3-month period in a removable cast or brace is sufficient in this rapid-growth age group to obviate any tendency to return to a hyperextended position.

Proximal tibia dislocated forwards in relation to the distal femur

This may be due to adherence of the posterior capsule and hamstrings over the anterior aspect of the distal femur onto a short, fibrous lower portion of the quadriceps. If reduction is not accomplished by manipulation and casting, surgical intervention is indicated as soon as the difficulty is recognized at 3–6 months. Once a stable reduction is obtained, further casting into flexion followed by guided activity of the patient is done as in the milder case (Bensahel *et al.*, 1989).

Congenital angulation of the tibia (congenital tibial kyphosis)

In this condition, the tibial diaphysis on one or both sides shows marked anterior angulation. Middleton commented upon other concomitant anomalies, viz. a persistent pes equinus, some apparent atrophy of the affected limb or limbs, absence of the fibula or congenital hip dislocation.

AETIOLOGY

It is believed to be a result of failure in growth in length of the calf muscles, which remain short, pull on the heel and produce a rigid equinus deformity. When the ankle joint is plantar flexed to its farthest limit, the strain falls on the cartilaginous tibial diaphysis, which becomes angled at its weakest point – i.e. the junction of its lower and middle thirds. As soon as the tibia becomes ossified, the angulation ceases.

Congenital angulation of the tibia has also been attributed to intrauterine pressure, constriction by amniotic bands, and to the healing of an intrauterine fracture (Figures 3.25, 3.26). It has even been thought to be related to the condition of congenital pseudarthrosis of the tibia, but the errors have nothing in common save their site. If seen in adulthood, this deformity of 'sabre' tibia has to be

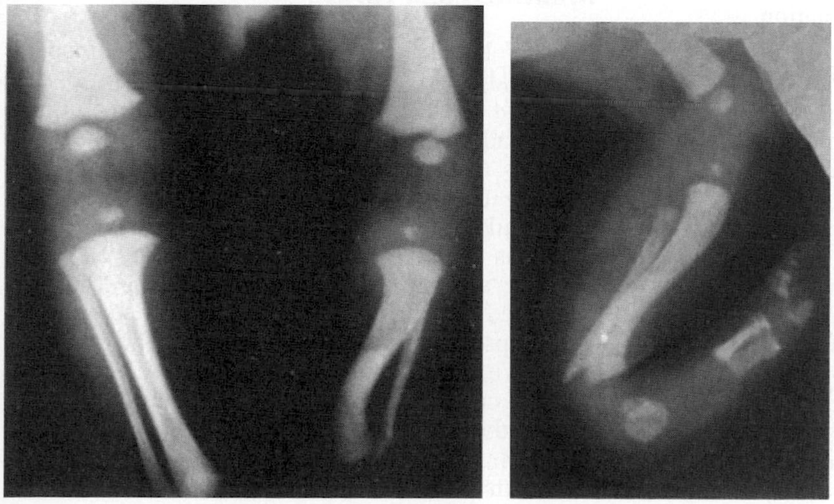

(a) (b)

Figure 3.25 Radiographs showing (a) the lower extremities of a newborn child with an abnormal bowing deformity of the left tibia, and (b) the lateral view of the left tibia and fibula, which was diagnosed as an intrauterine fracture.

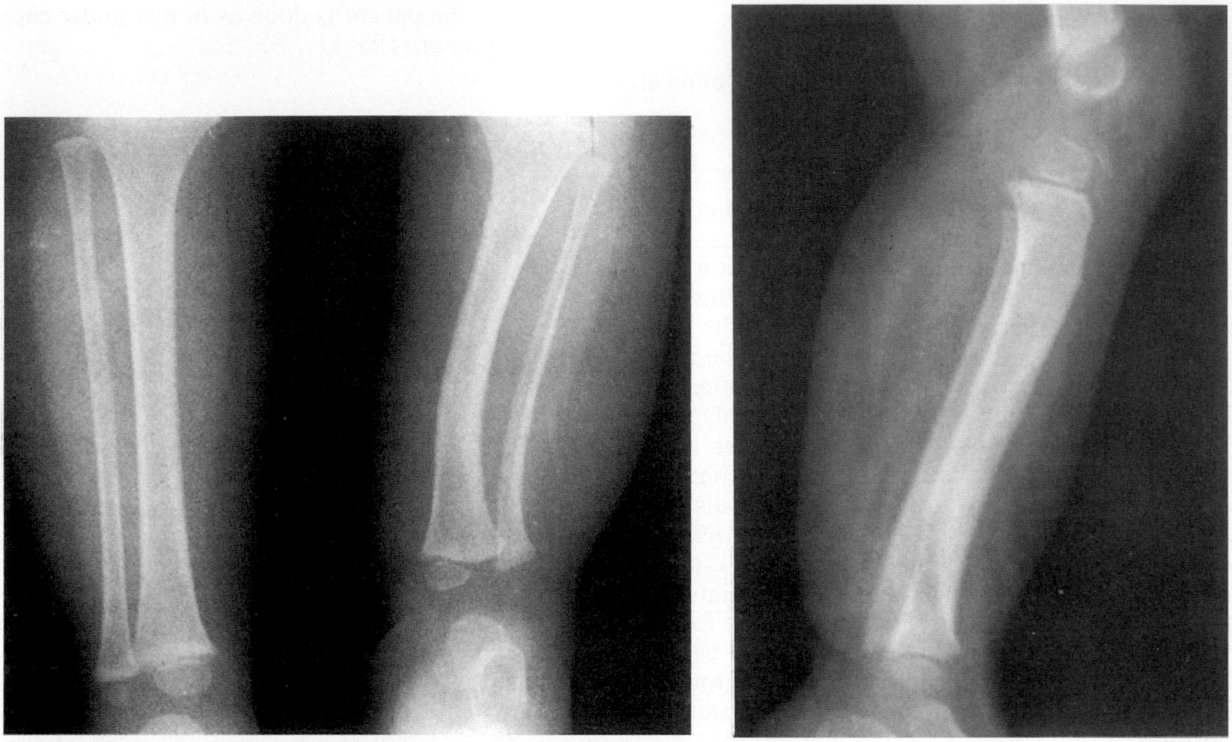

(a) (b)

Figure 3.26 (a) Radiograph of the child in Figure 3.25, 2 years later, showing development and growth of the left tibia – which still appears markedly shortened and bowed in contrast to that of the right. (b) Lateral view, showing the abnormal thickening of the anterior cortex of the tibia at the site of the original 'fracture'.

differentiated from Paget's disease, or the deformity resulting from childhood rickets or syphilis or haemangiomatous formation.

TREATMENT

The distinction between the serious problem and the self-correcting anterior angulation is made by the clinical and the radiographic examination.

Positional bowing due to intrauterine compression syndrome

There is no skin dimple over the apex of the anterior bow. There is a rounded indentation posteriorly on the calf. The opposite leg can readily be positioned in this defect.

On x-ray examination there is an open medullary cavity in the tibia without sclerosis and the gentle rounded bowing of the tibia is followed by the fibula, which is otherwise unaffected.

In this type it is important that restrictive devices to correct the bowing are not used. Normal activity of the baby is necessary for correction. Repeated x-ray examination can be done to follow the spontaneous correction.

Acute traumatic bowing of the tibia without fracture has been reported by Orenstein *et al.* (1985) in a child after a compression injury to the leg. They explain this as the plastic deformation following a three-point pattern of bending stress which was applied to the two bones of the leg of which the fibula sustained a greenstick fracture.

Infantile coxa vara

In 1937 Blount first described this developmental abnormality involving the medial aspect of the proximal tibial epiphysis and physis in both infants and in adolescents. In the infantile type the child presents at the age of 14–16 months – soon after walking unsupported – up to about 3 years. It is commonly seen in the obese, black female child who has walked early or with excessive use of walking aids in infants. Langenskiold (1989) has described the histological changes as being due to compression, reduced growth of the cartilage cells, with abnormal capillary circulation, and in certain cases there may be premature bridging across the medial epiphysis and physis. Greene (1993) in reviewing this disorder has emphasized that with persistent medial rotation, tibial torsion occurs due to relative overgrowth of the fibula, blocking the normal development of external tibial torsion.

Greene carried out radiographs on these children when:

1. the abnormality was severe for the child's age;
2. the abnormality had progressed;
3. excessive internal tibial torsion was present;
4. a height/total stature was less than 25%;
5. there was positive family history;
6. there was marked asymmetry of limb alignment.

The differential diagnosis is physiological bow legs (which resolves), hypophosphataemic rickets, metaphyseal chondrodysplasia and focal fibrocartilagenous dysplasia.

The metaphyseal–epiphyseal angle of a line drawn through the epiphyseal line against the horizontal line is normally less than 11° in physiological bow legs and becomes infantile coxa vara over 12–14°. The medial physeal slope angle may be more reproducible and of value pre- and postoperatively. This consists of an angle formed by two lines – one along the epiphyseal line and the other along the inner side of the tibial epiphyseal/metaphysis area. This angle can be regarded as normal up to 30° but at 50° the child requires orthotic support and bracing. Above this angle Greene recommended a Chevron tibial osteotomy with fibular osteotomy – especially for those over the age of 3 years who have failed bracing. Recurrent varus deformity has been commonly reported following tibial osteotomy especially when it has been carried out in older children, e.g. between 30 and 76%. Epiphysiodesis of the lateral aspect of the tibial epiphysis may be required and any metaphyseal bridge excised, so it becomes a very major operation.

Greene emphasized the high risk of neurovascular complications, e.g. involvement of the anterior tibial artery as it goes through the interosseous membrane with a compartment syndrome; therefore some carry out a subcutaneous release of the anterior compartment fascia. Peroneal nerve problems are also described.

Congenital angulation of the tibia leading to pseudarthrosis

A dimple is often present over the angulation. Considerable shortening may be evident and associated anomalies (e.g. a ray defect of the foot and hypoplasia of the ipsilateral limb) are clearly evident. The radiograph reveals minimal to complete obliteration of the medullary cavity and a tendency to narrowing of the tibia as the height of the angulation is reached. The fibula is frequently affected and may also be narrowed.

Andersen *et al.* (1968) reviewed data on 40 cases of this deformity. Fractures were numerous (15 cases) and, out of these, 11 developed pseudarthroses. All corrective osteotomies healed normally. Obliteration of the medullary canal appeared to predispose to pseudarthrosis development.

The natural history is usually for the deformity to progress and even lead to pseudarthrosis over the next 18 months.

Bracing or casting is necessary to try to direct growth. One must have radiographic evidence of progress to continue on this course.

Operative treatment has two phases. One involves the release of posterior and lateral structures with lengthening to prevent them acting as a deforming force with growth; the second is a direct attack on the angulation itself, which must be done with caution if a fracture or a pseudarthrosis is not to result. One half of the tibia at the apex can be cleared and left in place – as this becomes an adequate callus, the correction can be completed by osteoclasis or osteotomy of the remaining portion of the tibia, as described by Ferguson (1968). The fibula should be corrected at the same time.

Once healed, bracing is frequently necessary to avoid recurrence with growth.

Congenital pseudarthrosis of the tibia

This is a fairly common congenital error which is notable for its resistance to all treatment. The child is born with what appears to be a fracture of the tibia which fails to unite (Figure 3.27).

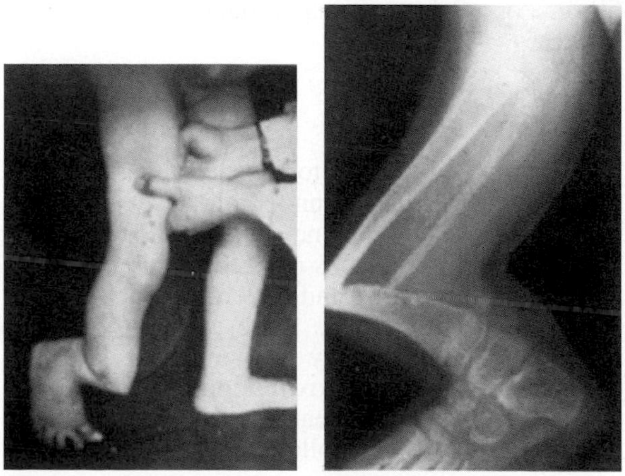

(a) (b)

Figure 3.27 (a) Clinical appearance and (b) x-ray of an untreated congenital pseudarthrosis of the tibia.

PATHOLOGY

The pseudarthrosis is usually situated at the junction of the middle and lower thirds of the tibia. The ends of the bone are sclerosed, and there is a considerable gap between the fragments occupied by fibrous tissue. The leg is therefore much shorter than its neighbour. As in ordinary transverse fractures of this region, there may be considerable overlapping which may mask the extensive loss of tibial substance.

AETIOLOGY

The essential nature of the error is the aplasia of a portion of the tibial shaft, which most likely arises as a sequel to a nutritional disturbance. It has also been suggested that it results from intrauterine pressure or from constriction by amniotic bands.

Association between congenital pseudoarthrosis and neurofibromatosis is now well established having first been described in 1937 by Ducroquet. Paterson and Simonis (1985) have described from their large series of 25 patients (with 27 pseudarthroses) that 48% had one or more of the stigmata of neurofibromatosis but that this did not necessarily point to a bad prognosis. Using Boyd's classification of 1982 they found the highest number (7) of Boyd's type II in which the child was born with an anterior bowing and an hour-glass constriction and spontaneous fracturing before the age of 2 years, fewer (4) of type IV in which there is a sclerotic segment with minimal medullary cavity and a late stress fracture and only one in type V which as well as the tibial lesion, has a dysplasia of the fibula with late development of the pseudarthrosis. It should be noted in Boyd's type VI the very rare discovery of an intraosseous neurofibroma or a Schwannoma is found.

TREATMENT

This is usually unsatisfactory, especially as the child may present after having undergone several attempts to obtain union and has never walked on the limb. Leg length discrepancy is marked and the bones are markedly osteoporotic and underdeveloped.

Short of amputation, there are two possible methods of treatment: by shortening the leg sufficiently to get good approximation and side-to-side apposition of the fragments; and by some method of bone grafting. The following procedures are in use.

1. The massive inlay method of Albee. Socur believed that the intact fibula is the obstacle which prevents the consolidation of the tibia after the bone graft. This method has about a 12–20% success rate. The tibia is useless physiologically, as the axial pressure is transmitted by the fibula only and therefore no callus is formed after the grafting. A simple osteotomy does not help, as it heals too quickly. Socur performed a resection of the greater part of the fibular shaft and uses this as a graft on the tibia.
2. The McFarland method of grafting. McFarland (1951) suggested ignoring the zone of absorption of the pseudarthrosis and placing a strong bone graft behind the tibia, implanting the graft into the back of the bone well above and below the site of non-union. It is a sort of 'bony bypass' and carries the weight directly from the upper part of the bone to the lower. Good results are reported of about 7%.
3. Paterson and Simonis (1985) have described their much improved results of almost 80% union by their technique of correction of the tibial deformity, intramedullary fixation, cancellous bone grafting, augmented by an implanted cathode bone growth electrical stimulator. Their failures in five patients were due to inadequate correction of the anterior bowing deformity, poor internal fixation, incorrect implantation of the stimulator and extensive disease.
4. Pho *et al.* (1985) have described in detail the efficacy of a free vascularized fibular graft, after radical excision of diseased bone and soft tissue. This procedure also permits primary bone lengthening as well as correction of the deformity in a single operation.

Congenital talipes equinovarus (club foot)

Congenital talipes equinovarus is a deformity in which the foot is turned inwards to a varying degree. In its most characteristic form there are usually said to be four elements of deformity – flexion of the ankle, inversion of the foot, adduction of the forefoot and medial rotation of the tibia (Figure 3.28). Slighter degrees of deformity are met with, however, and to these the name of congenital club foot is equally applicable.

The condition was recognized in very early times and like so many medical conditions well described by Hippocrates (400 BC). There are numerous references to it in Ancient Greek and Old Testament

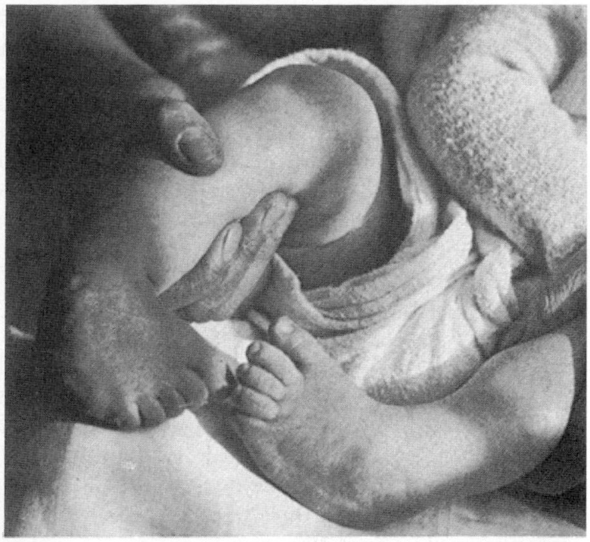

Figure 3.28 Bilateral congenital talipes equinovarus of a baby aged 3 months.

writings. Nicholas Andre laid down the principles of conservative management. Treatment came into the surgeon's domain when Little, himself afflicted by the condition, introduced tenotomies (Strach, 1986).

The incidence of club foot is about 1:1000 live births in Caucasians. Skeletal disorders along with meningomyelocele and congenital dislocation of the hip are common. Geographically, it is reduced in Orientals and substantially increased in Polynesians and Maoris (Drvaric *et al.*, 1989). Fifty per cent of all cases are bilateral.

AETIOLOGY

Club foot may result from an osseous, a muscular or a neuropathic error, or may be termed idiopathic. Of these, the last is by far the most frequent and will be discussed first.

Environmental factors such as intrauterine compression through change in the size of the uterus or reduction in the amount of amniotic fluid has been described over many years, but surprisingly little is known about intrauterine biomechanics to substantiate such observations. Such anatomical disturbances as seen in the talocalcaneal joint, in the innervation of the peroneal muscles and in the insertion of the tibialis posterior muscle tendon have also been described (Figure 3.29).

As regards the genetic factors, Wynne-Davies (1964) studied over 100 patients with their first degree relatives and found that 2.9% of siblings had this deformity although in the general population there were only 1.2 per 1000 cases. No significance in such features as consanguinity, age of parents, birth order, etc. was seen. Palmer (1964) in studying

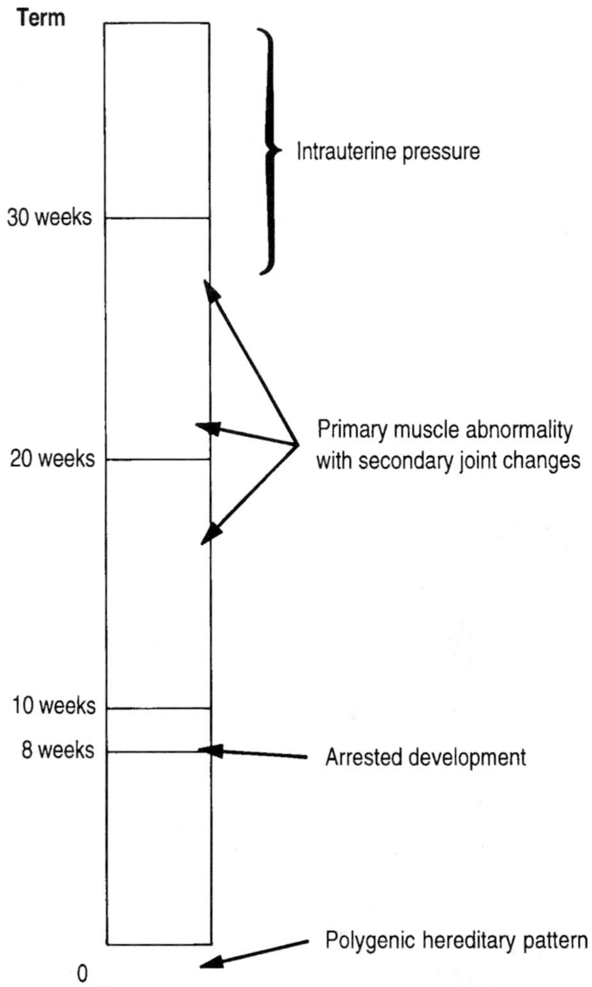

Figure 3.29 The four major factors which may produce a club foot deformity. (Reproduced, with permission, from Fuller, D. J. and Duthie, R. B. (1974) *AAOS Instructional Course Lectures* **23**, 53–61)

110 families, found that 43 had one or more affected relatives, whereas 67 had no affected relatives. From these studies it was suggested that polygenetic factors, probably in the form of an autosomal dominant inheritance with reduced penetrance, were present in the positive family group.

In the classic twin studies of Idelberger (1939) there was a 32.5% concordance (i.e. both twin members were affected by the same disorder) in monozygous twins, but only 2.9% in the dizygotes – the latter having the same incidence as found by Wynne-Davies in non-twin siblings. This reduced, but highly significant concordance rate in monozygotic twins suggested a markedly reduced penetrance with a number of possible genetic mechanisms.

In spite of such studies, there is really no recognizable or acceptable pattern of inheritance of this condition as yet. However, there is a 1:800 chance of any individual having this deformity, 1:35 chance of having it if any sibling has the deformity, and a 1:3 chance if an identical twin is involved.

In general, two varieties of talipes equinovarus may be present at birth: *primary*, idiopathic or *secondary* to a systemic condition such as arthrogyposis multiplex, muscular dystrophies or distant lesions like meningomyelocele or cerebral palsy. The condition is idiopathic when a diametrically opposed deformity exists on the opposite side (Turco, 1979). Delayed and progressive 'club foot' may result from other neuromuscular conditions, including cerebral palsy, muscular dystrophies and poliomyelitis.

PATHOLOGICAL ANATOMY

The typical congenital club foot is at first a deformity of soft tissue only. The essential features are plantar flexion of the talus, inversion of the calcaneus (and with it the other tarsal bones) and adduction of the forefoot. At birth the bones of the foot are normal in shape but altered in position. Over the skin on the outer part of the foot there are usually dimples which may be so marked as to resemble scars. The lateral malleolus is prominent; the medial appears flattened and poorly developed.

The muscles and tendons

The muscles are poorly developed and the tendons attenuated. The tendo calcaneus passes downwards and inwards to its insertion into the calcaneus, while the plantar muscles, especially on the medial side, are tensely contracted. The anterior muscles of the leg are elongated.

The ligaments

The ligaments on the medial and inferior surfaces of the talocalcaneonavicular joints are contracted, the plantar calcaneonavicular ligament being very small and short. The deltoid ligament of the ankle joint is similarly affected.

The bones

Bony changes appear as a result of the long-continued contraction of the soft parts. They are at first confined to the talus, but subsequently the calcaneus, the navicular and the cuboid become appreciably altered.

The talus

The head of this bone in normal alignment with the leg can be felt as a prominence on the dorsum of the foot. Later a large portion of the upper surface of the talus escapes from between the malleoli and becomes prominent on the dorsum of the foot. This portion, now free from pressure, becomes broadened, and, in severe cases, is an obstacle to passive dorsiflexion of the foot even after the soft structures have been stretched or divided. The head and neck of the talus are deflected downwards and medially, carrying the navicular and the forefoot with them.

The calcaneus

The calcaneus becomes tilted and so its medial tuberosity approaches the medial malleolus. Its vertical height is less on the medial side, and the anterior part of the bone is deflected medially, following the direction of the neck of the talus.

The navicular and the cuboid

These are displaced inwards. The phalanges are plantar flexed.

It has been the usual convention to suppose that the tibia was medially rotated. This, however, has been challenged by Swann *et al.* (1969), who demonstrated lateral rotation of the tibia which indicated the need for a rotational osteotomy in some cases.

CLINICAL FEATURES

In a small proportion of cases, structural bone changes are present at birth. This type is distinguished by the presence of a small inverted heel and hard stringy shrunken calf muscles, the condition of which suggests a primary myodysplasia. This type is difficult to correct and to maintain in correction.

In unilateral cases the deformity is never very severe, but the leg is obviously smaller and less well developed than on the healthy side. The skin of the foot may be normal, though stretched and thin on the dorsum and thrown into creases along the medial border and on the sole. In addition, there may be signs of external pressure on the dorsum in the shape of scars. The head of the talus can be felt on the dorsum of the foot. The lateral border of the foot is convex and the medial concave. The forefoot is plantar flexed upon the hindfoot. The heel is rotated medially and may be drawn upwards, throwing the whole foot into equinus. In many cases a well marked genu valgum is present. The patient walks with a stumbling gait, which lacks elasticity. Bursae and callosities develop over the weight-bearing areas. By pretreatment assessment one can grade the severity of the deformity. Kawashima and Uhthoff

Table 3.1 Soft tissue contractures

	Type 1 Extrinsic/non-rigid	Type 2 Intrinsic/rigid
Foot	Normal size, mild varus	Smaller, marked varus
Heel	Normal size, can be brought down with ease	Small, elevated, cannot be brought down with ease
	Minimal varus	Marked varus
Creases	More or less normal	Deep medial, posterior and plantar creases, reduced creases laterally
Telescoping	Negative	Positive

Adapted from Kawashima and Uhthoff (1990).

(1990) divided idiopathic club foot into two types (Table 3.1):

1. Extrinsic: flexible with abnormal bone relationship but without marked fibrosis, most can be managed conservatively.
2. Intrinsic: rigid with marked fibrosis and abnormal relations of bones. This comprises the largest group, most of whom will require an operation.

The navicular and calcaneum are displaced medially around the talus. The talus is the least displaced bone but is the most deformed. There is marked lack of development of the trochlea causing flattening and failure of the ankle mortise. The talar neck is often shortened and reduction of the amount of constriction of bone may prevent dorsiflexion. The head and neck relative to the axis of the body is reduced from the normal 150°. There is also plantigrade deformity of that axis. The articular surfaces of the talar head are wedges and displaced medially so that the talar navicular joint line lies out of the coronal plane and towards the sagittal. The navicular is medially displaced, even dislocated, from its position in front of an abnormally directed talar head. With the calcaneum the posterior tubercle (an important landmark in club foot) is displaced under the talus (Figure 3.30). The sustentaculum tali is often poorly developed.

Bansal *et al.* (1988) used Kawashima and Uhthoff's clinical method on 47 club feet to see if it would help with decision regarding early surgery. They were unable to classify 14 (29%) into either of these two groups.

Radiology using plain films only shows the bone, not the cartilage or soft tissues. At birth ossification centres of the calcaneus, talus and metatarsals are

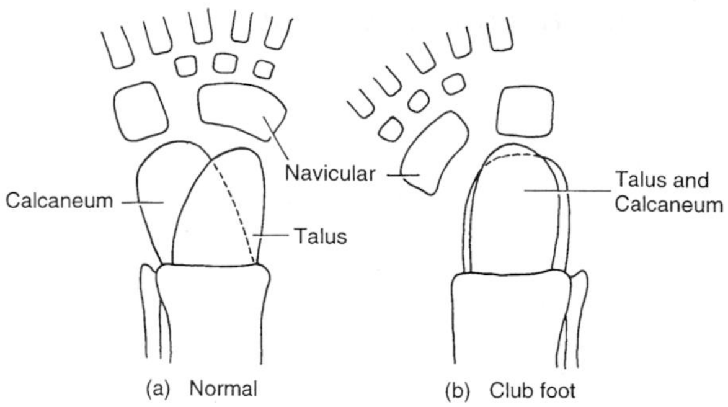

Figure 3.30 (a) The normal separation and divergence of the talus and calcaneum. The talus is fixed within the ankle joint and the calcaneum is linked to the remaining bones in the foot through joint capsules and ligaments as one separate unit. (b) If the calcaneum passes underneath the talus (and this is what happens in hindfoot varus), all the remaining unit of the foot moves with it. It can be seen that when the talus and calcaneum are superimposed, the navicular bone has displaced medially from the head of the talus and the bones of the foot now lie in a club foot relationship.

present and usually in the cuboid. The cuneiforms appear later and the navicular last. Ossification is often delayed in club foot and affects the radiographic sensitivity.

The two standard views of the club foot are the anteroposterior projection taken with the foot plantar flexed 30° and the tube angled 30° anteriorly in the sagittal plane, the 'Kite (1939) view' and a lateral view at the limit of passive dorsiflexion. The tube is centred on the ankle. From these films the angles between the calcaneum and talus in two planes can be measured. To do this the lines must be drawn through the ossification centres to represent the axes of these bones. It is known that the ossification centres do not develop in the centres of the bones and that true axis may not be drawn until the age of 2 or 3 (Turco, 1979). Herzenberg *et al.* (1988) have demonstrated the variation of the radiological axes from the true axes. They point out that the talus is a complex-shaped bone and should be considered to have at least two axes in each plane: the axis of the body and a second axis through the neck and head.

Tomography

Tomography suffers from the same problems with the presence of cartilage on plain radiography and is thus of limited value in the newborn. It has been used in follow-up work when more complete ossification has occurred. It shows the talus and calcaneum in malalignment and confirms their irregularity but is of little value in assessment (Ono and Hayashi, 1974).

Computerized tomography

CT scanning has the same restrictions with cartilage. Its use has been reported as helpful in defining the abnormalities in resistant feet. Fahrenbach *et al.* (1986) describe that it enabled them to visualize the difficult posterior aspect of the hindfoot especially the horizontal rotation of the calcaneum. They found a high incidence of lateral subluxation of the calcaneum in these resistant feet even in the presence of acceptable plain radiological analysis using Simons' method with T–C angles of >15° in the AP and >25° in the lateral being regarded as acceptable.

Arthrography

Arthrography of the ankle, subtalar and talonavicular joints has been used. It is extremely difficult to carry out (Turco, 1979). It undoubtedly displays the dysplasia of the talus by outlining the cartilage margins, an advantage over plain films.

Magnetic resonance imaging

There is no literature on the use of this technique. To obtain satisfactory images general anaesthesia is required in babies and infants.

Laaveg and Ponsetti developed a functional system in 1980 that put great emphasis on function and pain rather than anatomy. Results from this scoring method were well correlated with the talocalcaneal angle on the lateral plain radiograph. Green and Lloyd-Roberts (1985) confirmed that function and anatomy do not always go hand in hand.

With the ossification developing in the foot bones, complex parameters can be measured. Indicators of talar distortion, with the flattening of the talar dome, can be calculated as the R/L ratio. Many of these fall into the 'so what' category with poor correlation with function such as the heel–toe angle between perpendicular lines at the level of the second web space and the mid-heel (Levin *et al.*, 1989).

PROGNOSIS

Without treatment, the deformity increases, the gait becomes more unsightly and the foot permanently deformed, with callosities and ulceration. With early, effective and continued treatment, cases of club foot should be cured, and a useful and properly shaped foot obtained. In older children the condition can be improved, although delay in treatment gives the worst results.

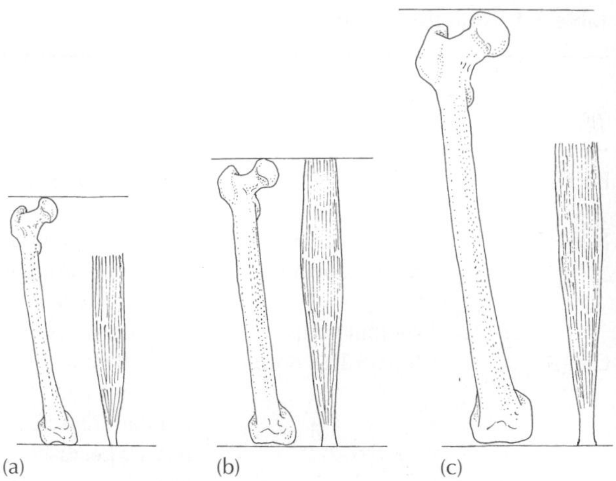

Figure 3.31 (a) Congenital contractures relative to the physiological length of the bone and muscle. (b) With treatment the soft tissue bone length is equalized. (c) In a growing child, continued enlargement of the bone can result, with recurrence of the original relationship unless treatment is continued. (Reproduced, with permission, from *Orthopaedic Surgery in Infancy and Childhood*, 3rd edn, Williams & Wilkins, 1968)

TREATMENT

The objectives of successful treatment are two in number: the deformity must be corrected, and the muscular power of the limb developed to a sufficient extent to maintain the correction (Figure 3.31). This implies constant supervision until the period of growth is over, as there is a distinct tendency to retrogression. The mode of treatment varies with the age and the extent of the deformity. The important point is to get the forefoot deformity corrected so that it points outwards 20°. Following this, the hindfoot deformity, which is the keystone to the function of such a deformed foot, must be brought into a vertical plane before the equinus deformity is corrected.

Treatment in an early case

The treatment should be begun as early as possible.

Manipulation, frequently repeated, but gently, is the method of treating the deformity in an infant. The infant lies supine on its mother's lap, while she protects the knee, and prevents any strain from falling on the ligaments, by grasping the upper end of the tibia. While one hand fixes the heel, the other reduces the adduction of the forefoot. To do this, the thumb of one hand rests on the talus and acts as a fulcrum, while the other hand presses the forefoot into abduction. The maximum result is maintained for a few seconds at each sitting, and should be repeated six times at each 'nappy' change.

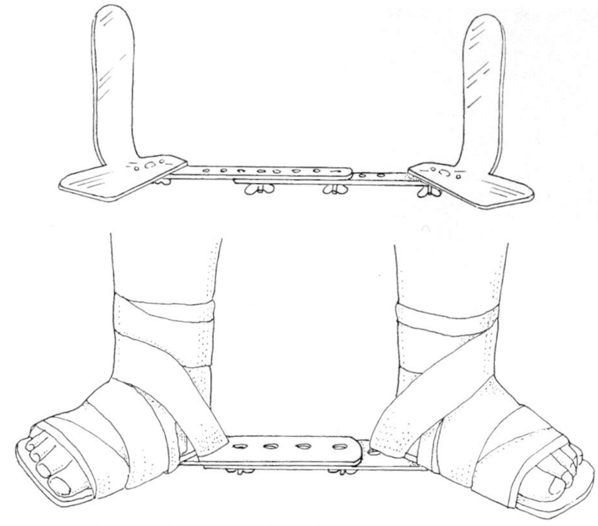

Figure 3.32 Denis Browne's splint.

Splintage and plaster immobilization

After manipulation some form of splint must be used.

Splints

Denis Browne designed a splint (Figure 3.32) which promotes correction of the deformity and at the same time encourages the activity which is so important for muscular development. The essential of the method is that the feet are connected horizontally at any desired angle to the sagittal plane of the body. To hold the feet, an L-shaped piece of aluminium is cut and bent up one side. This is put on so that the bent part is applied to the outer side of the leg, while the remaining limb of the L lies against the sole of the foot. After the manipulation the splint is applied and kept in place by a few turns of adhesive tape, while each foot splint is fixed by a friction-joint at a satisfactory angle to an aluminium cross-bar. If the club foot is unilateral, the normal foot should be fixed to the cross-bar so that it is turned outwards at an angle of 20°; that is, at its natural inclination. In the case of the club foot the splint is fixed so that the toes are directed outwards at an angle of 90° from the sagittal plane. The splints should be removed each week and an opportunity taken then to manipulate the foot. Browne advised treatment by this splint for about 6 months. The child is encouraged to kick and to stand up as much as possible in the splint. When he is capable of holding the feet naturally in the corrected position and the feet have the full range of movement, the sticking plaster and the aluminium splint are discarded and replaced by a pair of boots (worn only at night) riveted to the aluminium cross-piece to hold the feet in the same position as they occupied in the splint. These boots have open toes and unlace completely from one end to the other. It is often helpful in retaining the correction to reverse the boots, wearing the right boot on the left foot.

The complication of a 'rocker-bottom' foot, which is produced by the overcorrection of a fixed equinus deformity and holding such a position in a cast, must be avoided (Figure 3.33). Therefore, it is important to correct the forefoot deformity first so that no 'break' occurs at the mid-tarsal joint on bringing the whole foot up in the neutral position.

If it becomes apparent after a period of 2–3 months that the equinus deformity has not been completely overcome, it is necessary to carry out surgery.

The deformity may be considered cured when there is no adduction or inversion deformity, when there is a hollow on the dorsum of the foot in the position previously occupied by the head of the talus, passive movement to the full calcaneovalgus position, and when the child is able to evert and dorsiflex the foot voluntarily to about a right angle.

Casts

Other workers have greater success in maintaining and progressively correcting the deformities by plaster-of-Paris casts. Although Kite (1961) obtained most of his initial correction by wedging at the mid-tarsal and ankle-joint levels, the cast applied to the foot and leg after manipulation, most prefer to change the cast frequently, manipulate the foot and ankle into a better position and reapply a more corrective and moulded cast. Such treatment may well have to be continued up to 1 year of age until all soft tissue contractures are overcome.

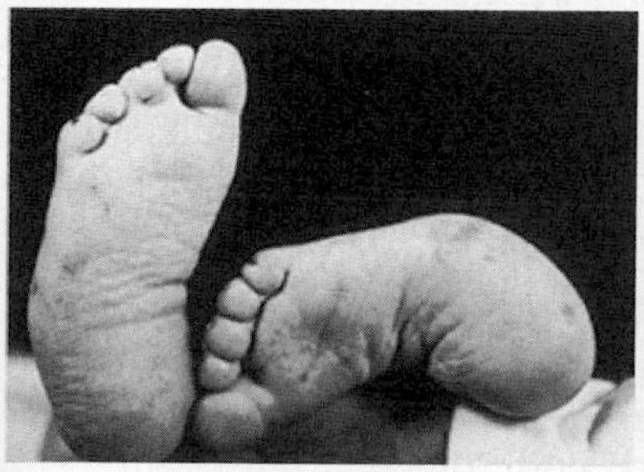

(a)

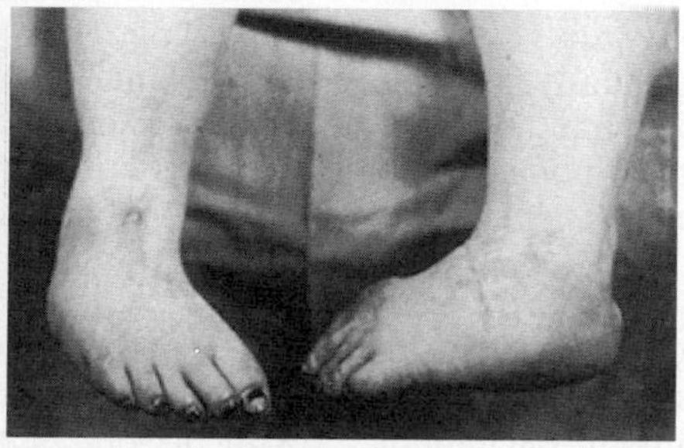

(b)

Figure 3.33 (a) The plantar surface of a resistant club foot which has gone on to develop a typical 'rocker-bottom' foot. (b) The same patient, showing the very marked internal rotation deformity of the tibia and metatarsus varus, particularly of the left foot.

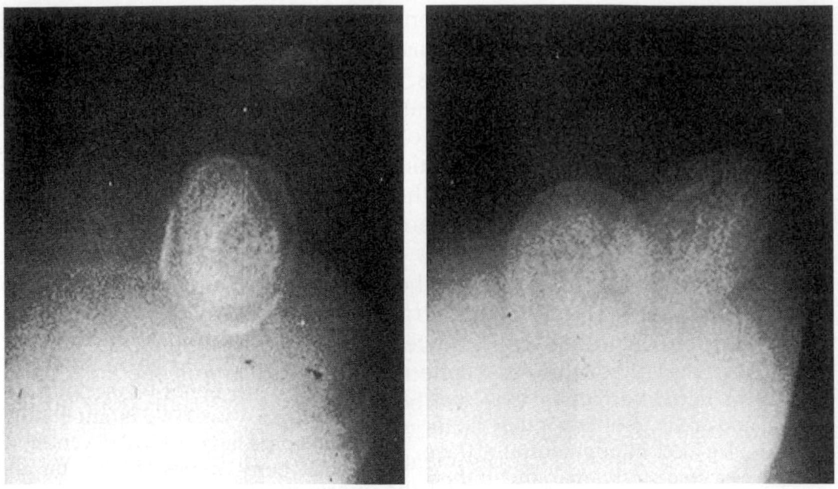

(a) (b)

Figure 3.34 (a) Left-sided talipes equinovarus deformity in a 4-week-old child with the ossific centres of talus and calcaneus superimposed. (b) The normal foot in which they are separate and diverging.

Turco (1979) has described how his management was based on the following principles:

1. The abnormal tarsal relationship is maintained by pathological contractures of the soft tissues.
2. Soft tissue contractures must be overcome to restore the normal relationship.
3. Once correction is attained, it must be held until maturity.
4. Recurrence occurs from failure to achieve or maintain correction.

Treatment begins with diagnosis at birth (Figure 3.34). Gentle manipulation is performed. As complete a correction as possible is obtained without undue force, and this is held by splintage either by adhesive strapping or in plaster. Alternatively, manipulation and physiotherapy can be performed on a daily basis, initially requiring less use of splintage. All three methods have their advocates, but there appears to be little to choose between them. In the European Paediatric Orthopaedic Society (EPOS) study (Bensahel *et al.*, 1990) most surgeons preferred the use of plaster.

The principle of the strapping is to produce an eversion force at the ankle from active knee movement. The manipulation, prior to application of plaster, is the same as followed by the application of a well padded and moulded, above-knee plaster. The process should be repeated at weekly intervals until 6–8 weeks, and then fortnightly, gradually increasing the correction. If full correction has not been achieved by 3 months, conservative management has failed and interventional methods must be considered.

When full correction has not been achieved, operative intervention is considered. While awaiting surgery, splintage will be continued to maintain any incomplete correction. The Denis Browne bar cannot be used if the deformity is too severe, as the foot cannot be placed accurately in the boot. Some advocate an early tendo Achillis lengthening at the musculotendinous junction at this stage to gain sufficient preliminary correction to allow splintage, prior to definitive surgery at a later date.

Soft tissue releases

The rationale for soft tissue release is that realignment of the talus, calcaneum and navicular allows remodelling of the articular surfaces to occur. The earlier the intervention the greater the remodelling potential, but surgery before 3 months is not generally practised. Turco (1979) claimed his best results were achieved by operating between 1 and 2 years of age. Simons (personal communication, 1993) who advocates the complete subtalar release, suggests that size and not age should be the limiting factor – the foot should be at least 8 cm long.

Posterior release

If the forefoot adduction and heel varus are virtually corrected after conservative treatment, a posterior release can be performed. Attenborough (1972) described lengthening of the tendo Achillis (TA) and posterior capsulotomy of the tibiotalar and subtalar joints. Fuller (1984) stressed the tethering of the fibula, preventing its forward movement that accompanies ankle dorsiflexion, and added release of the posterior talofibular and calcaneofibular ligaments to this procedure. Transfer of the tibialis posterior tendon to the peronei has been used in conjunction with posterior release.

Posteromedial release

Turco presented his results of 15 years of experience with his one stage posteromedial release in 1979.

This procedure consists of lengthening of TA and tibialis posterior, posterior ankle capsulotomy, posteromedial release of the subtalar joint with division of the interosseous talocalcaneal ligament and plantar release of abductor hallucis and the plantar fascia. Division of flexor hallucis longus and flexor digitorum longus is performed if easy reduction cannot be obtained without it. The reduction is then held with a Kirschner wire across the talonavicular joint. Of his results, 83.8% were claimed to be good or excellent.

Turco's method is favoured by many surgeons. Levin *et al.* (1989) published a long-term follow-up study of the posteromedial release with an average follow-up of 8.2 years.

Circumferential release
McKay (1983) based this procedure on the belief that abnormal rotation of the talus must be corrected. In effect this is a complete subtalar release. Brougham and Nicol (1988) supported the use of the Cincinatti incision, claiming 75% good or excellent results with minimum 2-year follow-up. There were no problems with wound healing in their series.

Tendon transfer
A passively correctable deformity resulting from muscle imbalance may be restored by transferring tendons such that muscle pull acts to correct rather than produce deformity. Tendon transfer is never indicated as primary treatment. Transfer of the tibialis anterior to the more lateral cuneiforms or fifth metatarsal may correct some of the deformity.

Osteotomy

In general these procedures are carried out on residual deformities in older children. Metatarsal osteotomy to correct the forefoot is described and should be reserved for children over 6 years old. In 1963, Dwyer described an opening wedge osteotomy of the calcaneus to correct residual varus deformity. The Dillwyn–Evans procedure consists of a closing wedge resection of the calcaneocuboid joint after release of the talonavicular capsule, division of the tibialis posterior and release of the plantar fascia. The shortening of the lateral side of the foot thus achieved is usually held by a staple. Addision *et al.*(1983) reviewed this procedure and found it useful when carried out at around 6 years of age for correction of a 'bean-shaped' foot.

Arthrodesis

Triple arthrodesis is a salvage procedure for the stiff and painful foot. It is carried out when the skeletal age is at least 12 years. At this stage the rate of pseudarthrosis is reduced and undue shortening of the foot is avoided. These patients have almost always had previous surgery unsuccessfully.

Treatment of old and relapsed cases

The Dillwyn–Evans operation

Evans described his procedure of soft tissue release and calcaneocuboid fusion in 1961. The operation is in four stages: the first three consist of an extensive soft tissue release which enables the whole hindfoot to be realigned; finally, a calcaneocuboid wedge is excised, so removing a deformed joint and shortening the lateral border of the foot.

Stage I
A closed tenotomy of the plantar fascia is performed and the plantaris (cavus) deformity can then be corrected with a Thomas's wrench (Figure 3.35a).

Stage II
A medial skin incision is made from just in front of the tubercle of the navicular, back to a point beneath the medial malleolus. Tibialis posterior tendon is identified and divided in Z fashion. The soft tissue between tibialis posterior and the neurovascular bundle is then excised. The talonavicular joint is identified, this joint being very oblique in a varus foot, and the capsule is divided using a tenotome slid into the joint to cut the superior and inferior components. Next the anterior talocalcaneal joint is identified and its capsule also divided with a tenotome. Similarly, the capsule of the posterior talocalcaneal joint is divided as completely as possible. The tibialis posterior is then sutured in an elongated position (Figure 3.35b).

Stage III
The calcaneal tendon is exposed through a posterior medial incision approximately 7 cm long and extending down to the insertion. The tendon is divided in Z fashion. Next the sural and posterior tibial nerves and vessels are identified laterally and medially, respectively. All deep fascia between them is excised.

The posterior capsule of the ankle joint and the posterior tibiotalar ligament are divided with a tenotome. Then capsulotomy of the posterior talocalcaneal joint is completed, the tibiocalcaneal fibres of the deltoid ligament being included in the division. Both the ankle and subtalar joints are often visible only as thin fissures posteriorly if severe equinus deformity is present. Lastly, the posterior talofibular and calcaneofibular ligaments are divided (Figure 3.35c,d).

Powerful manual dorsiflexion of the foot now achieves full correction of the equinus and mobility

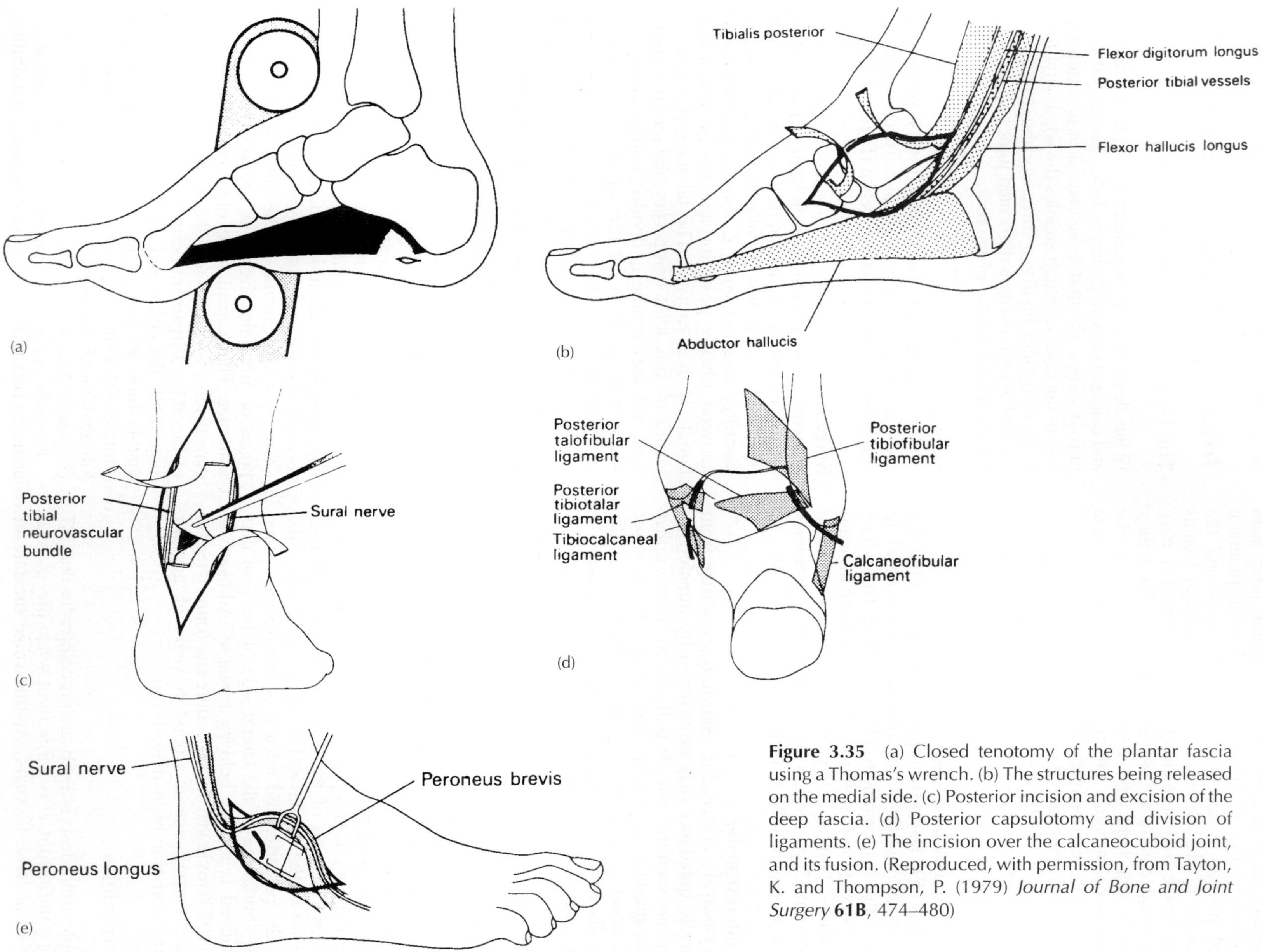

Figure 3.35 (a) Closed tenotomy of the plantar fascia using a Thomas's wrench. (b) The structures being released on the medial side. (c) Posterior incision and excision of the deep fascia. (d) Posterior capsulotomy and division of ligaments. (e) The incision over the calcaneocuboid joint, and its fusion. (Reproduced, with permission, from Tayton, K. and Thompson, P. (1979) *Journal of Bone and Joint Surgery* **61B**, 474–480)

of the entire hindfoot. The calcaneal tendon is now sutured in the elongated position.

Stage IV
A short incision is made over the calcaneocuboid joint parallel with peroneal tendons (Figure 3.35e). The sural nerve is identified and retracted, and extensor digitorum brevis is partially divided and stripped up to expose the calcaneocuboid joint. This joint is then excised with a knife, if cartilaginous, or with an osteotome. The amount excised is usually less than anticipated and is wedge shaped to correct the varus deformity. If the foot is cavus then the wedge needs to be wider dorsally as well as laterally. If a rocker-bottom foot has been produced before operation, the wedge can be made wider inferiorly. Next, supination of the forefoot is corrected by rotating the forefoot on the capsulotomized talonavicular joint. The calcaneal and cuboid surfaces are apposed and are held with two staples which maintain the correction. The amount of correction needed was judged by Evans by the external appearance of the foot.

Following operation, the foot is immobilized in a below-knee plaster cast for 4 months. Weight-bearing is not permitted for the first 6 weeks. When the plaster is removed, normal shoes are worn and no further treatment is necessary. The staples remain in position until union is sound or until growth is finished.

The results of this procedure were reported by Tayton and Thompson (1979), and although bony deformity remained in a considerable number of feet, their long-term survey showed that 78% had an acceptable functional result.

Treatment in the adult patient

In the adult, no manipulation, tenotomy or muscle operation is likely to be of benefit; operation on the bone is necessary. Cuneiform tarsectomy is satisfactory (Figure 3.36).

Cuneiform tarsectomy

A vertical wedge of bone, with its base laterally, is removed from the calcaneus, behind the mid-tarsal joint; a similar wedge is removed from the cuboid in front of the joint; and finally a curved wedge with its base upwards and laterally, from the head and neck of the talus. An incision is then made on the medial side of the foot and the talonavicular capsule and the deltoid ligament divided. It should then be possible to manipulate the foot into the correct position without undue force.

The foot is encased in plaster, which should reach the knee. This is applied for 6 weeks, although it may be necessary to change the plaster at the end of 2 weeks in order to overcorrect the deformity, as in the treatment of the relapsed case.

In most cases, the best result will be obtained by stabilizing the foot as in the operation of Naughton Dunn. Here the mid-tarsal and subtaloid joints are arthrodesed as in some forms of flail foot.

The long-term results, following a triple arthrodesis of the talocalcaneal and mid-tarsal joints, or a Lambrinudi or a Hoke in 37 children or young adults for permanent fixed deformities of the foot after poliomyelitis, cerebral palsy, club foot, etc., have been reported by Monson and Gibson (1978). Functional results were good or excellent in 91%,

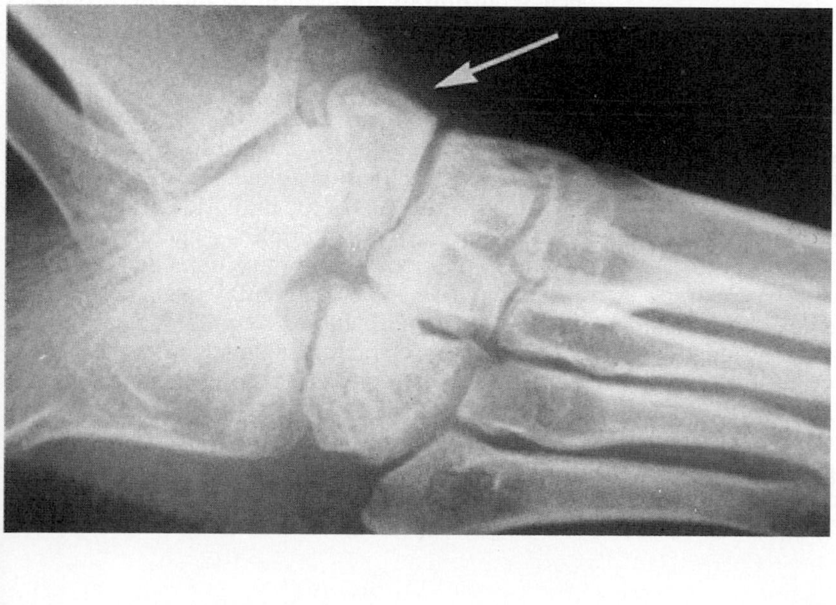

Figure 3.36 An osteotomy through the neck of the talus may leave the body of the talus without a circulation. This patient has been walking on the dense body of the talus since childhood.

and overall good objective results were obtained in 70% of the cases. The two most serious complications of triple arthrodesis were persistent varus of the hindfoot and non-union of one or more of the tarsal joints.

Other types of club foot

THE MUSCULAR TYPE

This type of club foot occurs in arthrogryposis multiplex congenita. The foot deformity is extreme, the foot as a whole being more rigid than in the ordinary type of congenital club foot. The toes are flexed into the sole and can only be straightened with great force. Recurrence of the deformity takes place whenever the force is released. The leg and thigh are thin and the amount of muscle tissue is diminished. There is usually a fixed flexion-deformity of the knee and of the hip.

THE OSSEOUS TYPE

This type is associated with partial or complete absence of the tibia, the loss of support of the tibia resulting in an inversion deformity of the foot. Frequently this coexists with other abnormalities, such as absence of the toes, and failure of development of some of the bones of the tarsus.

Examination of the bones of the foot shows that, in addition to alterations in position, structural abnormalities are present, the talus and the calcaneus being either completely or partially fused together to form a single bony mass.

Arthrogryposis multiplex congenita (amyoplasia congenita)

This is a congenital deformity affecting the extremities, characterized by marked muscular wasting with loss of mass, increased fibrous tissue around the joints, and therefore disturbance of mobility and various characteristic deformities. Bone changes are usually secondary to the overlying soft tissue changes, as well as to the changes which have taken place within the joint. In its usual form, there is unilateral or bilateral club foot and club hand, and these constitute the most obvious of the deformities with the rigidity of the parts, it being impossible often to obtain any degree of movement at the affected joints.

When the condition affects the lower limbs, there are also present contractures of the knee and the hip, which are often the site of a congenital dislocation. As in the foot and hand, the hip deformity is gross and intractable, and the muscular activity of the limb is restricted completely or to a minimum.

AETIOLOGY

Middleton drew attention to the importance of muscular derangement in the mechanism of congenital deformity, the errors of the bones being in the nature of structural adaptations to the primary error of the muscle. He believed that the pathology of the muscular derangement may be of three types:

1. There may be an arrest of development at the myoblastic stage.
2. The muscles may develop normally but fail to elongate.
3. The muscles, fully formed, may be the site of intrauterine degeneration, with progressive conversion into scar tissue (amyoplasia congenita).

He attributed these changes to a process of intrauterine muscular degeneration – myodystrophy – allied, at least in its pathological effects, to the muscular dystrophies of a later age period. Many theories have been suggested, such as amyoplasia, abnormal intrauterine conditions, virus infection, developmental disturbance of the embryonic nervous system. There have been no strong familial instances described as yet. In the pathology there has been seen fibrous infiltration of the nerve bundles and peripheral nerves. Microscopically the muscle is variable in appearance with greatly hypertrophied muscle fibres lying adjacent to hypoplastic fibres and infiltrated by fat. There is no systemic disturbance in biochemistry or other tests and no genetic factors have been demonstrated.

The characteristics of the individual lesions which arise in arthrogryposis multiplex congenita have been recounted previously (see developmental dysplasia of the hip (p. 152), congenital genu recurvatum (p. 174), congenital club foot (p. 178), etc.).

The work of Drachman and Coulombe (1962) opened up a new concept of experimental club foot and arthrogryposis. They have produced limb deformities at the time of hatching in chick embryos by the infusion of curare. These deformities result from ankylosis of the limb joints because of contractures involving the periarticular and intra-articular soft

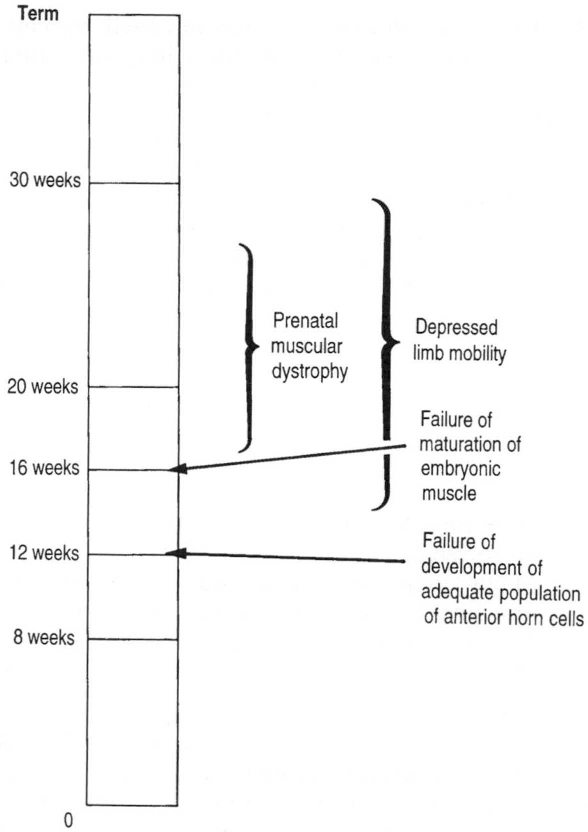

Figure 3.37 The possible factors which may produce arthrogryposis. (Reproduced, with permission, from Fuller, D. J. and Duthie, R. B. (1974) *AAOS Instructional Course Lectures* **23**, 53–61)

tissues. Even a brief period of immobilization due to paralysis will disturb the mechanism of joint cleavage (Figure 3.37).

CLINICAL FEATURES

The classical case is seen in a child born to an older than average mother who had noticed reduced fetal movements during pregnancy. The skin is smooth, with loss of the normal contours around the joints and there would be some abnormal dimpling, and possibly skin webbing. The shoulders are internally rotated and adducted, with elbows flexed, and wrists pronated and flexed, metacarpophalangeal (MCP) joints flexed and fingers extended. The hips are externally rotated and abducted, with knees flexed and bilateral talipes equinovarus. The child is of normal, or greater than normal intelligence (Lloyd-Roberts and Lettin, 1970).

Skin

The precise incidence of abnormality of the skin is not known, but common features are a smooth shiny skin with loss of normal skin creases and frequently webbing. There may be abnormal dimpling. The subcutaneous tissue is very thin, which in conjunction with the loss of muscle gives rise to loss of normal contours and the fusiform or apparently swollen appearance of the joints.

Muscle

There is a patchy and variable atrophy of muscle tissue. Individual muscles have been reported as being completely absent – especially around the elbow (Williams, 1973).

Joints

The characteristic feature of the joint is that it usually has only a small arc of movement, either actively or passively. At the end of this arc there is a firm mechanical block to further movement which is painless. The most frequent distribution is involvement of all four limbs (usually over 50%). In general, the more distal joints are involved marginally more commonly than the proximal, with the ankle being the most frequently involved. The deformity in the shoulder is nearly always adduction and medial rotation. The elbow may be fixed in either flexion or extension. When flexed there is usually a reasonable range of motion about a right angle. An extension rigidity appears more common than flexion with a small range of motion; this deformity is usually associated with a strong triceps and the wrist is usually rigidly flexed and the forearm pronated.

Wrist and hand

Smith (1973) in studying 39 patients with hand deformities divided his cases into three groups:

1. Limited motion in all joints, forearm pronated, wrist flexed and in ulnar deviation, interphalangeal points flexed (also extended elbow).
2. Ample subcutaneous tissue, thumb and finger MCP joints flexed.
3. Joints rigid with bizarre hand deformities such as polydactyly.

The most common deformity generally reported at the wrist is flexion and ulnar deviation – sometimes associated with proximal extension of the hypothenar eminence (Daniel's sign).

Hips

Although the classical description is of flexion, abduction and external rotation, in most of the larger series, flexion without abduction or external rotation occurs rather more commonly. It has been pointed out by Lloyd-Roberts that the hips must abduct and externally rotate, in a baby, if the knees are fixed in flexion.

Knees

The most common problem is fixed flexion, but in between a quarter and a third of affected knees the problem is of extension; this does not delay walking.

Foot and ankle

By far the most common problem is equinovarus; however, all the other foot and ankle problems have been reported in small numbers, particularly calcaneovalgus, and congenital rocker-bottom foot.

PATHOLOGY

Joints and periarticular tissue

Macroscopically the joints are usually normally formed, apart from the ankle joint. Intra-articular adhesions are not usually found, but the periarticular tissues are greatly thickened and fibrosed.

Muscles

A fairly constant finding is of greater or lesser degree of muscle atrophy with either fatty or fibrous replacement of muscle bulk. Where no autopsy has been done EMG studies confirm a neurogenic atrophy. Further evidence is provided by the usually normal muscle enzymes (Bigelow, 1969). Drachman and Banker felt that the deformity bore a direct relationship to the muscles most affected and if the muscle causing the contracture was divided the joint moved freely.

MANAGEMENT

Principles of management have been described by Drummond *et al.* (1974):

1. Muscle balance should be established – it is usually easier than in other paralytic conditions.
2. Deformity will recur even when muscle balance has been established. This results chiefly from soft structures about the joint that fail to elongate as the limb grows.
3. The further from a joint that any surgery is performed the more likely is the deformity to recur.
4. Unless tenotomies are accompanied by capsulotomies and splinting for a long time after surgery, the deformity will recur.
5. Osteotomy cannot prevent recurrence of deformity if the tight and thick capsule of the joint is left, and this type of procedure is contraindicated before maturity.
6. Even though the range of motion of the joint is usually not increased significantly, the arc of motion can usually be changed to a more functional position.
7. Because the deformities are more severe distally and the proximal joints are less involved, tendons suitable for transfer are more likely to be found proximally.

The principles behind surgical procedures are:

1. Disabling deformities and contractures should be corrected.
2. Major joints should be put in an axis of movement most useful for the patient's needs.
3. Tendon transfers are occasionally required to bring more efficient motor power (particularly around the elbow).

When arthrogryposis is diagnosed at birth, and other paralytic disorders ruled out, a general examination should be performed to rule out congenital abnormalities involving other organ systems, since they are much commoner in arthrogryposis than in the general population. Contractures in the feet, knees, hands and elbows should undergo serial manipulation and casting. This may allow temporary correction but more important, allows time for a more complete assessment.

Lower extremities

In the management of the lower limb problems, the principal aim is independent walking. If many joints are involved a system of priority should be drawn up, and as a guideline it is considered that the feet should be operated upon at about 4 weeks of age, the knee 4 months, and the hip between 6 and 8 months of age.

The foot

The severest deformities occur in the foot and despite the best surgical procedure deformities tend to recur. Equinovarus deformity is most commonly found and usually associates with stiffness at the ankle and tarsal joint. The aim of treatment is to convert the rigid deformed foot to a rigid plantigrade foot.

At about the fourth week a radical posterior release is carried out, in which a segment of the tendo Achillis is removed to prevent a return of continuity which may cause a recurrence of equinus. Some feet are so rigid that astragalectomy is indicated. In such feet it is usually found that the subtalar and mid-tarsal joint are poorly differentiated and articular cartilage may be almost absent (2° exception after square condyles). When astragalectomy has to be performed in the growing child, the following must be taken into consideration:

1. Excision of the talus must be complete. Small cartilagenous fragments left behind grow and reproduce the original deformity.
2. The calcaneus must be placed under the tibia and fixed with a K-wire for 3 weeks.
3. Astragalectomy should be followed by at least 3 months in plaster. If unacceptable residual deformity is present at maturity, triple fusion should be indicated.

The knee

In the knee the deformity is either stiff in flexion (most common) or stiff in extension.

1. In flexed knees the hamstrings and posterior capsule are contracted. In infancy, manipulations and plaster casts have been successful, but only in changing the arc of movement to a more extended position without increasing the range of movement. Even if full extension cannot be obtained, small flexion deformities are compatible with a good gait. In growing children, posterior soft tissue release should be done.

   In skeletally mature patients a supracondylar osteotomy is the best form of correcting the deformity. In some of these flexed knees, exploration anteriorly reveals a plug of undifferentiated fibro-fatty tissue filling the joint and blocking movement. This can be excised.
2. In extended knees operative treatment is not so often indicated because this deformity does not delay walking. However, when increased range of movement has to be obtained, serial splinting can be tried in the first few months of life. If that fails, the rectus femoris (which gives rise to the main contracture) may be transected highly at the musculotendinous junction, the patella released from the front of the femur and the mechanism repaired with the knee held at 90°.

The hip

In the hip without dislocation

A fixed flexion deformity is often associated with abduction and with lateral rotation. In these cases a double hip spica has been found to be the best method and knees and feet may also be corrected at the same time. When deformity is persistent in the young, neither osteotomy nor soft tissue release can achieve full correction and persistent deformity must be accepted and osteotomy should be performed (subtrochanteric osteotomy) at the end of growth.

When the hip is dislocated

This deformity is not as disabling as a hip contracture and the patients are able to walk.

An open reduction of the hip should not be done if the knee previously deformed in flexion has not been treated. The first plaster after the open reduction should be changed after a month and converted to a broomstick type for long periods of time.

Upper extremities

Contrary to the usual concepts in reconstructive surgery on the upper extremities, the presence of a functional hand is unnecessary before surgery on the shoulder and elbow. The minimum requirements for the patient are the ability to feed him/herself and to attend to personal hygiene.

In the shoulder joint the deformity is usually adduction and internal rotation. The presence of one shoulder with an adduction and internal rotation contracture where the elbow is extended does not in itself require surgery. When the deformity is severe and bilateral, an osteotomy distal third of humerus, plated or nailed, with release of pectoralis major and subscapularis is indicated for the older children. Soft tissue release does not seem to give good results.

In the elbow joint two different types of deformities are seen:

1. Stiff in flexion and usually with a useful range of movement around 90°. The biceps are strong, but the triceps often weak or absent. In these cases nothing should be done.
2. Stiff in extension in which occasionally they have about 30° of flexion available, the triceps are strong; biceps and brachialis are usually absent, but forearm flexors may be present. These cases require surgery.

At the wrist joint capsulotomy and proximal row carpectomy are available because this shortens the wrist, giving a relative lengthening of the flexor tendon of the fingers. As the wrist extensor are absent, some form of bracing must be used continuously. Arthrodesis may be considered at maturity because at this stage most of the carpal bones will have formed a conglomerate mass so that a simple wedge osteotomy through the radiocarpal joint is all that is required.

In the fingers the commonest deformity is proximal interphalangeal joint flexion and the MCP joints are flexed or extended. If the hand has some pinch and some grasp, it is often best left alone. In hands which have stiff interphalangeal joints in extension and flexed MCP, the deformity appears to come from a contracture of the interosseous muscles. The long tendons have little or no function and some improvement can be gained in the earlier age by dorsal release of the interphalangeal joints, continued if necessary with shortening of the flexor tendons. Later multiple interphalangeal fusions are indicated and the fingers should be set in sufficient flexion to provide hook function.

In the thumb the clinical features are adduction of the thumb due to lack of abductor pollicis brevis, laxity of ulnar collateral ligament of the MCP joint. Their procedure is Z-plasty in the web or local transplantation flap.

Congenital high scapula

Congenital high scapula (Sprengel's shoulder) is a deformity which has aroused much interest since its first description in 1863 by Eulenberg. It consists of an abnormally high and permanent elevation of the shoulder, and is frequently associated with other deformities such as congenital scoliosis, absence of vertebrae, fusion of ribs or cervical rib – i.e. errors in segmentation or position of the cervical spine. There is often also a midline cleft between the two occipital bones.

AETIOLOGY

This deformity is the result of imperfect descent of the shoulder girdle, which first appears as a cervical appendage, but which should descend by the end of the third month to the level of the upper part of the thorax. The proper designation, therefore, should be undescended, or high, scapula. Various explanations of this permanent arrest in the descent of the shoulder girdle have been suggested, but hitherto none has accounted satisfactorily for the gross abnormalities of vertebrae and ribs, nor for the development of a bridge of bone anchoring the scapula to the spine, all of which frequently coexist.

The muscles which suffer in their normal development will not fulfil their later function. In this respect the complete or partial defect of the muscles, their fibrous appearance and the interruption of the normal differentiation of muscle fibres at the myoblastic stage are most significant. They represent the end results of muscles which have undergone degeneration and necrosis at an early embryonic stage, and account for secondary contractions.

PATHOLOGY

Changes are found in the bones and in the muscles.

The bones

The scapula may be of normal shape, or may be broadened at the expense of its length. It lies at an unusually high level, and may be attached to the vertebral column or the occipital bone by a band of imperfect muscle tissue, or by fibrous tissue, or even by a bar of cartilage called the omovertebral mass. This mass is analogous to the suprascapular bone of the lower vertebrates, between the fourth cervical and the third dorsal vertebrae. Among the associated errors in segmentation of the cervical spine are included hemivertebrae and wedging of the vertebrae, both of which produce congenital scoliosis. The atlas may be in two halves, one or both of which may be fused to the occipital condyles.

The muscles

Constant alterations in the musculature of the shoulder girdle are found. The trapezius may be largely absent, the rhomboid and the levator scapulae muscles being represented by the muscular fibrosis or cartilaginous band which passes up to the ver-

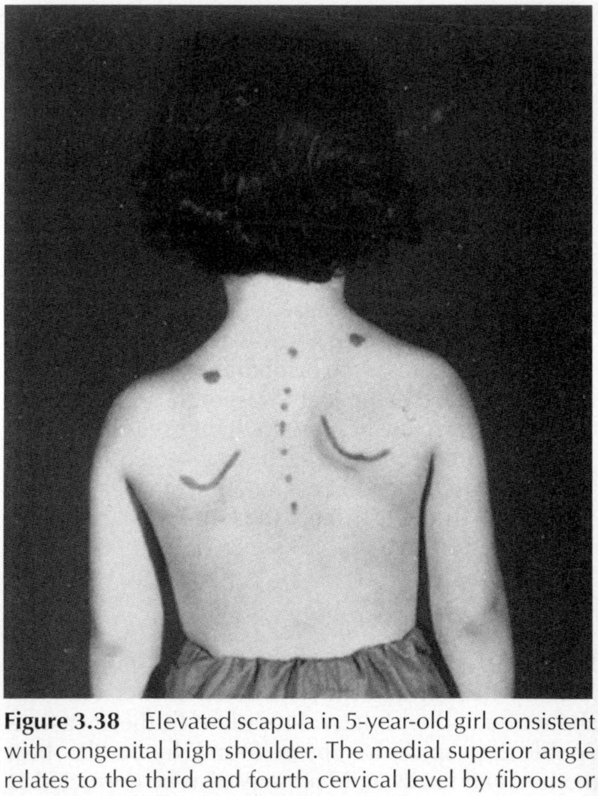

Figure 3.38 Elevated scapula in 5-year-old girl consistent with congenital high shoulder. The medial superior angle relates to the third and fourth cervical level by fibrous or bony attachment in the true deformity.

tebral column or the occipital bone. Occasionally this anomalous band of tissue may be ossified in whole or in part.

CLINICAL FEATURES

The scapula on one or both sides is 2–10 cm higher than usual. It is also tilted forwards so that the shoulder appears to be displaced upwards and forwards (Figure 3.38). When the arm is raised the scapula does not move laterally, nor does its lower angle rotate when the arm is raised above the horizontal.

The deformity of the shoulders rather than any functional disability of the arm attracts the notice of parents, and only occasionally is there weakness of, or disinclination to use, the limb. All movements of the arm are complete except abduction and elevation to the vertical position. The neck is frequently short in appearance, though the shortness is often more apparent than real, being caused or accentuated by the high position of the shoulder girdle. Torticollis is present in about 10% of cases. Cranium bifidum and spina bifida are often present. The skull may show the type of cranium bifidum which is caused by an unclosed tectal plate and consequent prolongation of the foramen magnum backwards between the two halves of the squamous occiput. Congenital kyphosis affecting the thoracic region is an almost invariable accompaniment of the deformity, whilst scoliosis is quite frequently present as well. This deformity causes cosmetic disturbance, functional impairment, and it can cause pain.

Clinically the severity of the elevation of scapula has been described by Cavendish (1972) as:

- Group 1 – very mild, with the deformity almost unobservable and the shoulder joints level.
- Group 2 – mild, with the shoulder joints slightly unaligned.
- Group 3 – moderate, with the shoulder joint obviously higher.
- Group 4 – severe, with the superior angle of the scapula near the occiput, and webbing may be present.

DIAGNOSIS

The x-ray appearances are characteristic, the films showing the unduly high situation of the scapula. Other congenital defects in the neighbourhood may also be apparent (Figure 3.39).

PROGNOSIS

Even if operation is undertaken, the prognosis is not very favourable. Published results indicate that while the mobility of the shoulder may be improved, asymmetry almost always persists.

TREATMENT

Many operations have been performed – the omovertebral bone has been removed, the band of fascia has been tenotomized or excised, and a portion of the scapula has been excised – but usually without great improvement. McFarland suggested that nothing less than the removal of the whole of the scapula, with the exception of the portion of the glenoid and coracoid process, should be carried out. The author doubted, however, the advisability of suggesting operation in this deformity, especially if the functional and cosmetic defect is slight, as the results are disappointing for improving the function of the shoulder joint. However, Green (1957) described 'satisfying' results by dissecting all the muscles attaching the scapula to the spine and trunk –

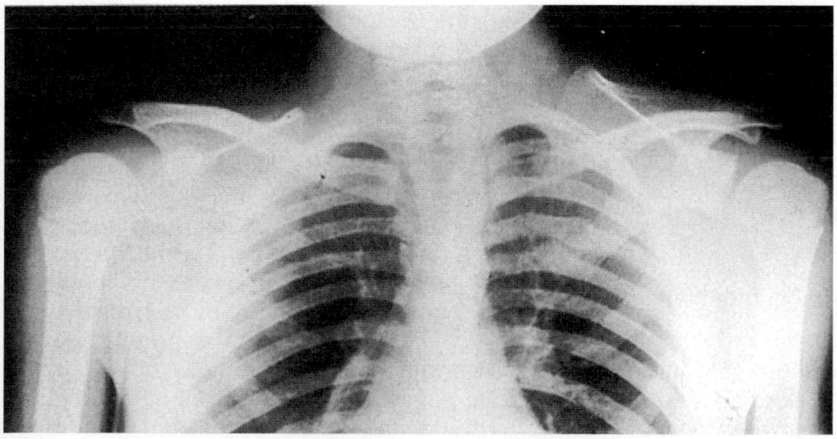

Figure 3.39 A high left scapula.

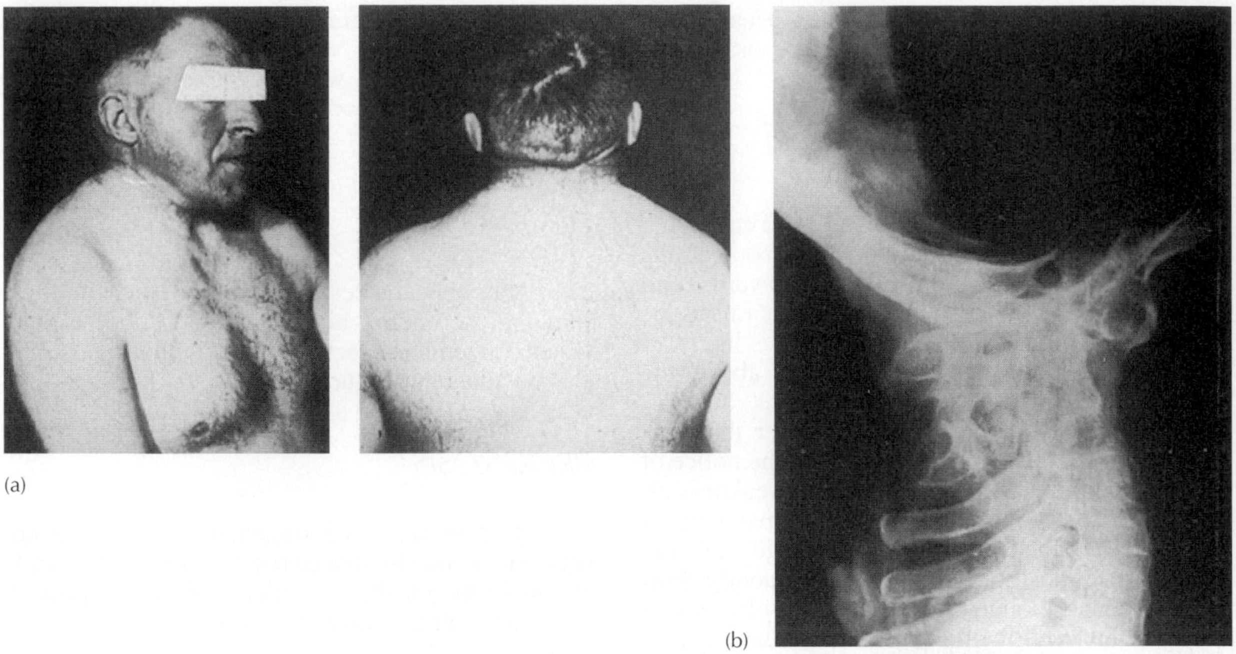

(a)

(b)

Figure 3.40 (a) Klippel–Feil syndrome. (b) x-Ray of case of Klippel–Feil syndrome, showing abnormality of the C1 and 2 vertebrae.

including the omovertebral muscle if present – and reattaching them at a lower level. The supraclavicular portion of the scapula can be excised and the realigned scapula is held in position by wires within a body cast for 3 weeks. Obviously, traction lesions on the brachial plexus – by mobilizing the middle third of the clavicle (after Robinson) – and on the accessory nerve must be avoided.

Congenital short neck (Klippel–Feil syndrome; brevicollis)

Klippel in 1912 described a case which has formed the basis of all subsequent work on this subject. It would appear to be an advanced stage of high scapula. The prominent features which are emphasized as being the essentials of this syndrome are:

1. Short neck or absence of neck (Figure 3.40a).
2. Absence, or limitation, of movement of the head.
3. Lowered hair line.
4. Often there is an expressionless mongoloid type of face.

The neck is frog-like and so short that the individual may appear to have no neck at all – the type called by the French *les hommes sans cou.* Movement of the head is very slight or is practically absent, and movement of the facial muscles is sometimes limited as well. The trapezii are tense and produce a wing-like appearance which has given rise to the name 'congenital webbed neck'. There may be an added torticollis of muscular or bony origin. The posterior hair line of the scalp is so low that it reaches the upper part of the thoracic wall. Scoliosis, elevation of the scapula and other congenital anomalies may be present.

Varying degrees of the deformity occur. In the slighter cases the cervical shortening is not marked to any great extent. The conditions found on x-ray examination vary in an extraordinary way. In the typical extreme case there is fusion of the lower cervical vertebrae and usually the thoracic vertebrae into a solid mass. Less extreme cases vary from simple atlanto-occipital fusion to all possible combinations of fusions of different vertebrae (Figure 3.40b). There is thus evident a considerable deformity of the cervical spine and usually numerical reduction of its component elements. Cervical spina bifida is usually present. As in other congenital defects, there are frequently associated defects in other parts of the body. Thus one case showed a supernumerary lobe of the lung, while in another there was a patent foramen ovale, in another a cleft palate, and several involving the renal tract. Occasionally mental retardation is present. A few have shown functional impairment of the upper extremities suggestive of a common neurogenic origin. This is the result of morbid conditions

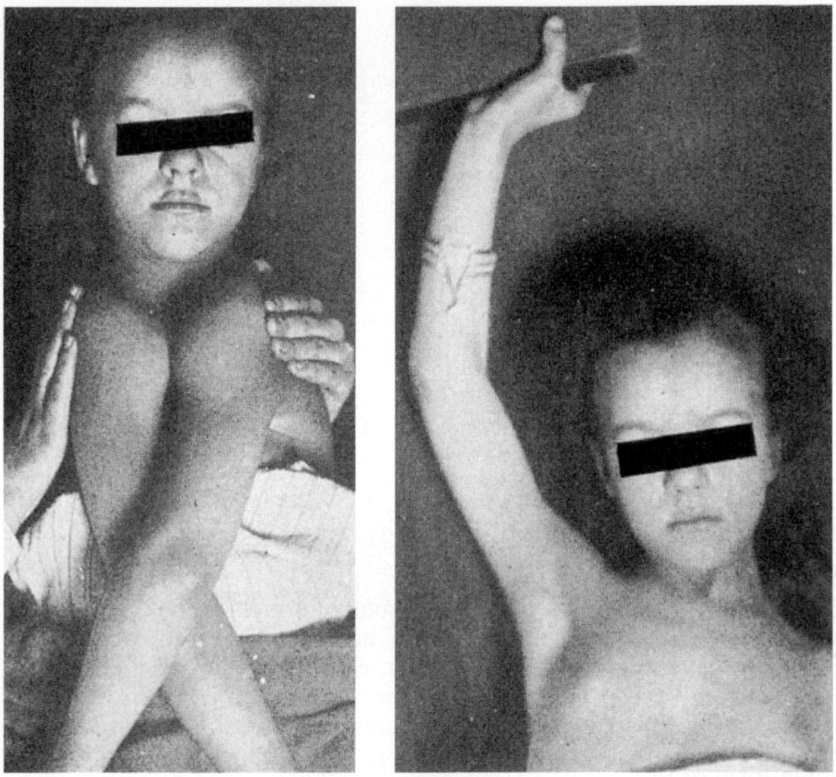

(a) (b)

Figure 3.41 Cleidocranial dysostosis. Note (a) the approximation of the shoulders but (b) the excellent function of the limb.

in the parent interfering with the normal fetal development.

The importance of recognizing the condition lies, not in any hope of remedying the deformity, but in its differentiation from other conditions which present a somewhat similar appearance and are to some extent amenable to surgical treatment, namely, congenital torticollis and Pott's disease. The simpler congenital deformity of elevation of the scapula has also to be considered.

It is desirable to investigate the cervical spine in all patients presenting with Sprengel's deformity, since it is invariably one of the elements of the more severe Klippel–Feil syndrome. Basilar impression – which is a deformity at the base of the skull around the foramen magnum – is often found in association with Klippel–Feil syndrome, odontoid abnormalities. There is an increased risk of neurological damage as well as obstruction to vascular or cerebrospinal fluid flow. Symptoms usually present in the second or third decade of life.

TREATMENT

Treatment as a general rule is not indicated, but in cases where there is an extensive fold of skin a plastic operation may produce marked improvement.

Cleidocranial dysostosis

The syndrome known as cleidocranial dysostosis, and described by Marie and Fenton in 1897, is a relatively rare condition, of which the leading features are:

1. aplasia of the clavicles;
2. exaggerated development of the transverse diameter of the cranium;
3. delay in closure of the fontanelles (Figure 3.41).

Hereditary transmission is the rule. The condition affects both sexes equally, and may be transmitted by either father or mother, to either sons or daughters. Several cases are reported, however, in which neither a familial nor a hereditary history was discoverable.

The following varieties of congenital defect of the clavicle may be distinguished.

1. Where the ends of the bone are normal, but a pseudarthrotic gap filled with connective tissue exists between them.
2. Where there is a partial defect of one end, usually the acromial, its place being taken by fibrous tissue.
3. Where the whole clavicle is absent (Figure 3.42).

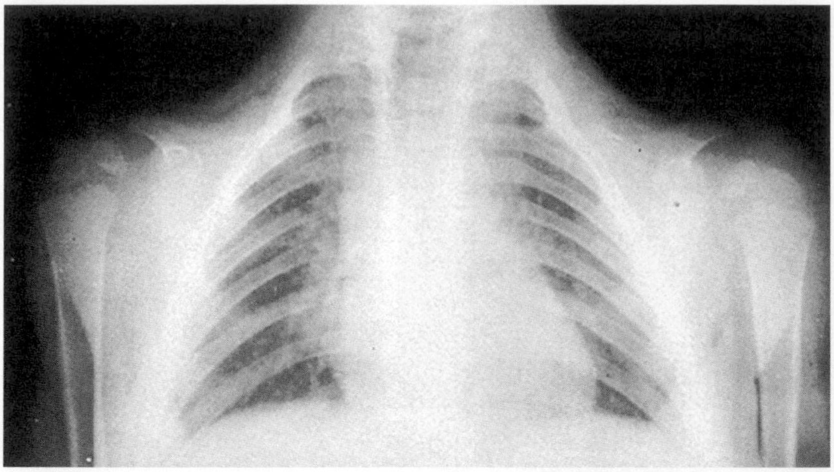

Figure 3.42 The absent clavicle of cleidocranial dysostosis.

Where the scapula is absent in addition, the deformity must be regarded as an aplasia of the whole shoulder girdle rather than a dysostosis.

The deformities of the clavicles are always accompanied by variations in the muscles. The clavicular portion of the trapezius may be absent; there may be maldevelopment of the pectoralis major; the clavicular portion of the deltoid may be deficient; or there may be a wide variation in the form of the sternomastoid.

Many other malformations have been reported in association with defective clavicles. Some of these are: brachycephaly and dolichocephaly; malformations of the various sutures, fontanelles and bones of the skull and face; disturbances of dentition; achondroplasia; variations in the small bones of the hands and feet; deformities of the thorax, spine and pelvis; prolapse of the virginal uterus; inguinal hernia; and spina bifida.

AETIOLOGY

Little or nothing is known of the aetiology of this condition. Steindler in 1940 thought it belonged to the class of intrinsic systemic deformities, arising during the first week of embryonic life. The condition affects the bones which are formed in membrane. Thus the vault of the skull may show membranous areas which persist throughout life (Figure 3.43). The clavicle itself is mainly formed in membrane. Its ends, however, are ossified from cartilage, and in this deformity the ossification of the ends usually proceeds as in the normal condition, so the clavicle is represented as a flexible membranous rod with a portion of bone at either end. In Heineke's other types, the error is evidently more extensive, and the normal ossification of the parts derived from cartilage is also interfered with.

CLINICAL FEATURES

The patient is usually brought to the surgeon on account of some accidentally discovered trouble with the shoulder. Sometimes an indefinite injury precedes, but more frequently no such history is obtained. Examination usually shows an apparently un-united fracture, or complete absence, of the clavicle, and the patient can usually approximate the tips of his shoulders to each other below the chin.

TREATMENT

If pain is present from the pressure of one or other of the ends, then removal of the part is indicated. As a rule there is little or no disability or discomfort and the abnormal mobility is not usually a hindrance.

Congenital anomalies of the odontoid

Congenital anomalies of the odontoid are more commonly associated with Down's syndrome, Klippel–Feil syndrome, and Morquio's syndrome. There is often atlantoaxial instability, but rarely spinal cord compression due to extradural soft tissue enlargement. Atlantoaxial arthrodesis is indicated if there is a 'shift' or stability of more than 10 mm between C1 and C2, but complications are frequent (Smith *et al.*, 1991).

Atlantoaxial instability has a significant risk of insidious myelopathy or cervical cord injury and is seen in the mucopolysaccharidoses. In achondro-

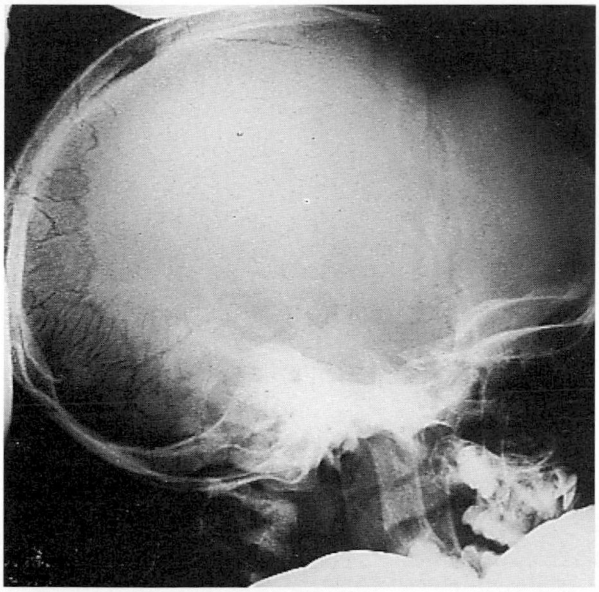

(a)

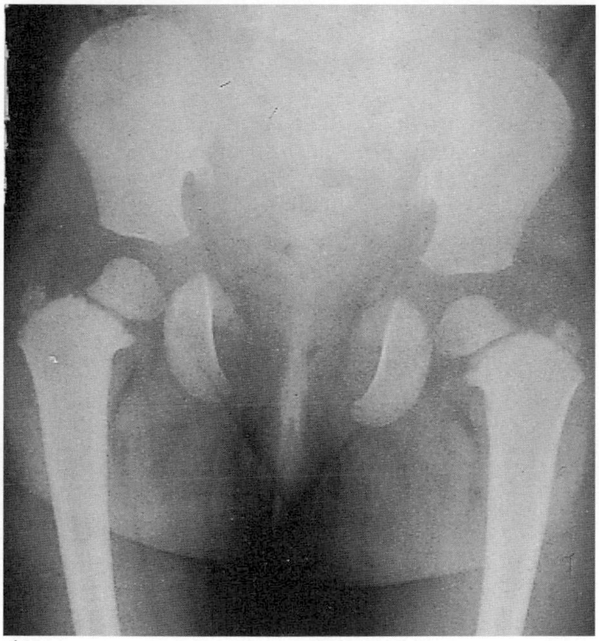

(b)

Figure 3.43 (a) A young female child with cleidocranial dysostosis, a dolichocephalic skull – i.e. long-headed where the breadth is less than four-fifths of the length and is the opposite of brachycephaly. (b) The radiograph of the same child showing abnormality of the femoral head and epiphyseal line as well as the upper femoral configuration.

plasia with increased growth around the foramen magnum, it can give rise to stenosis with impingement of the brain stem.

A safe technique using onlay grafts with wiring of the spinous processes and hole fixation has been described by Letts and Slutsky (1990).

Congenital dislocation of the shoulder

True congenital dislocation of the shoulder is very rare, but the term is, wrongly, applied to acquired dislocations occurring at or shortly after birth, which are not so uncommon. The commonest forms of acquired dislocation are those arising from trauma at birth, or developing as a sequel to birth palsy. Dunkerton (1989) has described four cases of posterior dislocation of the shoulder in association with obstetric brachial plexus, and a late diagnosis. The true congenital form is not associated with difficult labour, and there is therefore no evidence of bruising at birth. It is often not discovered for some time.

The dislocation is invariably posterior, and subspinous.

Congenital dislocation of the shoulder has been described in association with congenital dislocation of the hip. In cases operated upon, the head of the humerus has been found to be small and atrophied and resting on a facet on the posterior aspect of the glenoid fossa. Greig (1923) stated 'that muscular action alone hardly seems a likely possibility. Uterine pressure alone seems equally unlikely, but the two together, accompanied or not by some spasmodic contraction of a muscle or group of muscles, seems to give a possible explanation.' It seems not unlikely, however, that, as in congenital dislocation of the hip, an aplasia of the glenoid fossa may be the most potent factor in producing such a lesion. Those who have operated on the condition appear to have found no great difficulty in reducing the dislocation. Some cases have been reduced by manipulation alone. If this is successful, then the arm must be splinted for a few weeks to keep it in position.

Congenital torticollis (wry-neck)

This is a deformity characterized by lateral inclination of the head towards the shoulder, accompanied by torsion of the neck and deviation of the face. It is caused by unilateral contracture of the sternomastoid, with secondary shortening of the fasciae and the other muscles of that side of the neck (Figure 3.44a).

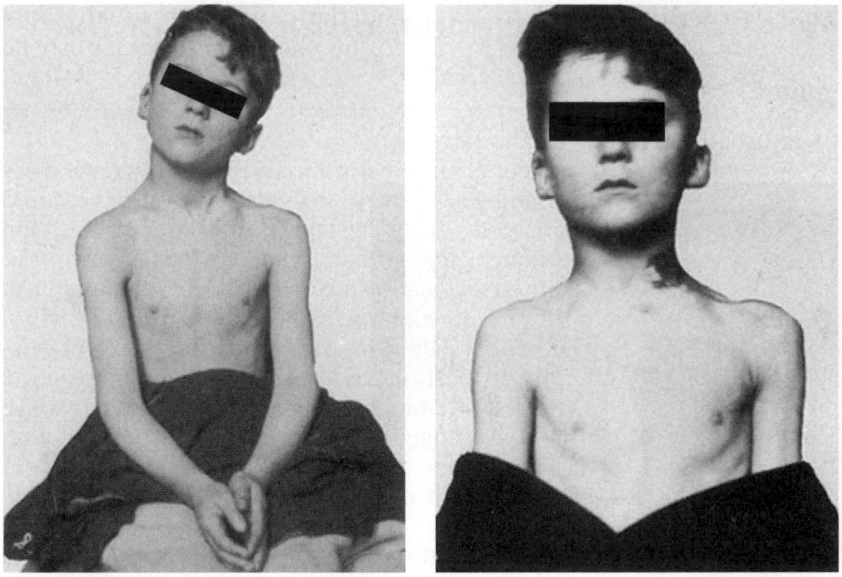

(a) (b)

Figure 3.44 Congenital torticollis: (a) before and (b) after open division of the shortened structure. Note the associated facial asymmetry.

AETIOLOGY

Nové-Josserand and Vianny thought it was ischaemic in origin. They stated that the middle part of the sternomastoid muscle is supplied by an 'end artery' – branch of the superior thyroid – and they noted that in every case of torticollis the lumen of the sternomastoid artery had been obliterated at the anterior border of the muscle.

It is generally held that the primary cause of this deformity is trauma, such as a breech, forceps or a difficult delivery (i.e. 0.4% of all live births). The usual belief is that during labour a temporary acute obstruction of the veins of the muscle occurs, and that this is rendered permanent by patchy intravascular clotting in the obstructed venous tree. In the early months of life this clotting is evidenced by the development of the sternomastoid tumour of infancy. The tumour eventually disappears, its place being taken by fibrous tissue which later contracts. The mechanism, therefore, is very similar to that which produces ischaemic contracture of the flexor muscles of the forearm (Volkmann's contracture).

PATHOLOGY

A sternomastoid tumour appears about 2 or 3 weeks after birth, as a spindle-shaped swelling occupying the position of one sternomastoid muscle. It may affect only the sternal head, but frequently both heads are implicated. The tumour gradually becomes absorbed and finally disappears in from 4 to 6 months after birth. On microscopical examination it is found to consist of young cellular fibrous tissue, containing, here and there, remnants of the original muscle fibres, which are seen to be undergoing degeneration.

At the end of about a year, changes, hitherto confined to the sternomastoid muscle, become evident in other structures in the neck. The muscle has now been reduced to fibrous tissue which has contracted, and there is also some thickening and contraction of the deep cervical fascia and of the scalenus anterior and medius. The vessels on this side of the neck likewise become shortened in the later stages of the condition, and are smaller in calibre.

The majority of cases show, in their later stages, a well marked asymmetry of the face, which on the affected side becomes shorter from above downwards, and wider from side to side. In addition, on the affected side the frontal eminence is flattened, while there is a well marked protrusion of the occipital region on that side. The vault of the skull is thrown backwards on the affected side and forwards on the opposite side, giving rise to a deformity which is comparable to that seen in the thorax in cases of thoracic scoliosis and hence the name scoliosis capitis is sometimes, and quite accurately, applied to it. Occasionally an exostosis appears on the clavicle at the site of attachment of the clavicular head of the sternomastoid.

CLINICAL FEATURES

The condition first becomes evident in the first few months of life when the mother notices an elongated swelling in the lower half of the sternomastoid muscle. This swelling is at first tender, and the child cries bitterly if it is palpated or if the muscle is stretched in any way. Gradually the swelling and the tenderness subside, but by the end of the first year of life it is noticed that the muscle is tense. This tenseness is due to the development in the substance of the muscle of a band of fibrous tissue which, by a slow but progressive contraction, pulls the head into the characteristic attitude, so that the ear on the affected side appears to be pulled down towards the sternoclavicular joint of the same side, while the face is rotated towards the opposite side. If the deformity is not corrected, a gradual atrophy of the face on the affected side develops and becomes increasingly evident with the growth of the child. As growth continues, changes take place in other tissues: all the soft parts on the affected side undergo adaptive shortening, while the bones of the cervical and upper thoracic acquire a fixed scoliotic deformity.

DIAGNOSIS

The recognition of congenital torticollis should, theoretically, present no difficulty, but some cases are obscure. Every case should be x-rayed to exclude any vertebral anomaly which may be the primary error. Brougham *et al.* (1989) has reported the combination of sternomastoid contracture with congenital vertebral anomalies in four patients. These authors emphasize the difficulty of identifying accurately the malformation in the spine by radiography and therefore in patients failing to respond to division of the muscular contracture, a continuing search must be maintained for the spinal abnormality.

Because of the decreasing incidence of true birth injury torticollis, congenital anomalies are becoming more important to diagnose early and treat in order to prevent increasing deformity with serious illness. Hensinger (1991) has described in detail the radiographic measurements required to assess atlanto-instability and basilar impressions with their outcome and Saltzman *et al.* (1991) have emphasized that such cervical spinal anomalies are inherited and therefore families should also be examined.

There is often a history of difficult birth, although cases have been reported after a Caesarean section. The early fusiform swelling may have escaped notice, but the later cord-like contraction of the sternomastoid is characteristic.

TREATMENT

The treatment should be begun at an early stage, as the development of the deformity may thus be arrested in mild cases. It is unwise to manipulate and stretch the sternomastoid muscle while the tumour is tender.

In mild cases, however, manipulation and exercises are sufficient. The head, having been grasped by the hand, is moved into a position in which the deformity is overcorrected, the object being to stretch the affected sternomastoid. The manipulation must be performed gently. If this is carried out daily there will probably be little or no evidence of

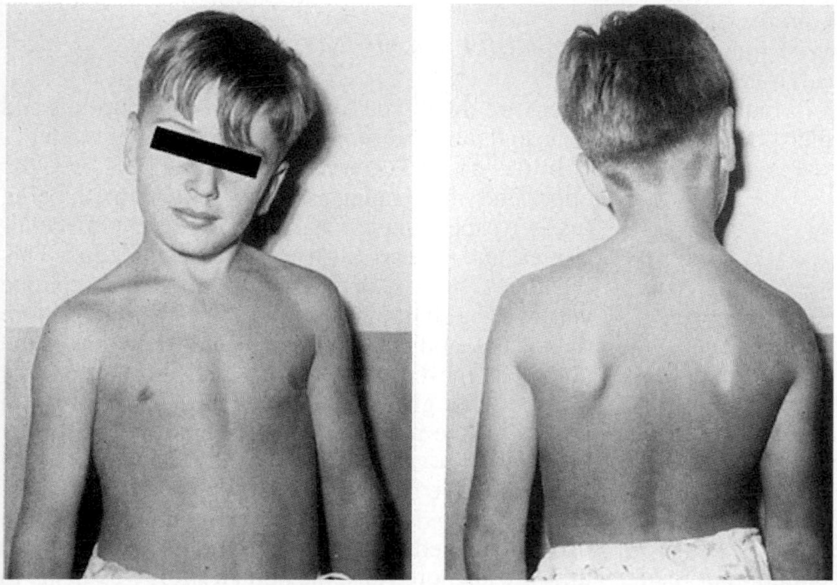

(a) (b)

Figure 3.45 Recurrence of relative shortening of the sternocleidomastoid muscle in an older child as the result of cervical spinal growth.

contracture at the end of a few months.

When the child is not seen until the age of 2 or 3 years, operation is usually indicated, for at that date manipulation is not likely to stretch the fibrous cord which replaces the muscle. Subcutaneous tenotomy is not advised, as it is impossible to ensure that all the shortened structures will be divided, and there is a danger of injuring the great vessels at the root of the neck.

An open operation can be performed through a comparatively short incision so that the scar is insignificant. The operation is carried out under general anaesthesia, the head being laid over a sandbag so that the shortened muscle is rendered prominent. An incision 4 cm in length is made 1 cm above and parallel to the clavicle, with its centre over the attachment of the affected muscle. In making the incision the skin is pulled down over the clavicle so that there is no risk of injuring the vessels at the root of the neck. The muscular heads are defined and, a flat dissector having been slipped beneath their deep surfaces, each head is divided. When the muscle has retracted, the deep cervical fascia is divided, and, if necessary, the carotid sheath and the scalenus anterior. During the operation the head is gradually manipulated into the correct position, in order to bring any shortened structures into prominence (Figure 3.44b).

The after-treatment, which is of great importance, should be continued for about 6 months. It consists of active and passive movements to prevent any recurrence of the deformity (Figure 3.45).

When it is desired to avoid a visible scar, a muscle-slide operation may be carried out. An incision is made over the origin of the sternomastoid from the mastoid process; this lies entirely in the hairy scalp. The muscle is erased from the mastoid process and from the superior curved line of the occipital bone. The operation is inadvisable where more than 2.5 cm of lengthening is required, as greater mobilization may damage the spinal accessory nerve.

Dystonia

Dystonia is a condition in which there are repetitive, jerking twisting movements, or abnormal postures due to sustained muscle contraction. Most commonly it is seen as a focal disorder, e.g. torticollis, which may be held in one position tonically or may occur with jerking or tremor (i.e. chronic spasms). It can affect the arm involving one specific skilled movement, e.g. simple writer's cramp, but can spread to other hand movements when it is a true dystonic writer's cramp. The eye (blepharospasm), the jaw and the trunk have all been described particularly in the adult. Generalized dystonias have been described rarely in children or as a toxic reaction to neuroleptic drugs or levodopa drugs in Parkinson's disease. The abnormality lies in the extrapyramidal system of controlling movement and posture, e.g. in athetoid cerebral palsy.

Clinically, the abnormal movements or postural appearance may be absent at rest, aggravated by physical or mental effort. It is often misdiagnosed as being hysterical or functional or even maligning, especially when secondary psychological problems supervene.

Treatment is directed towards reassurance, education as 5% of dystonias, e.g. torticollis, remit spontaneously and drugs like benzhexol (an anticholinergic drug used in Parkinson's disease) have all been used successfully. For spasmodic torticollis, a posterior primary laminectomy can be carried out by a neurosurgeon.

Congenital radioulnar synostosis

In congenital radioulnar synostosis one or both forearms are fixed at birth in a position midway between pronation and supination as a result of fusion of the proximal ends of the radius and ulna. In some cases the condition is hereditary, and it is equally common in both sexes.

MORBID ANATOMY

There are three types of synostosis of the radius and ulna, and the condition may be unilateral or bilateral.

In the *true congenital radioulnar synostosis*, the upper end of the radius is imperfectly formed, being fused to the ulna for a distance of several centimetres, and appears to grow from its upper end. This 'headless' type is sometimes classified as a separate variety. The shaft of the radius arches forwards more than usual, and is longer and stouter than that of the ulna – suggesting that there has been either some arrest in the growth of the ulna or stimulation in growth of the radius. Primary synostosis is usually bilateral; in over 80% of the recorded cases both forearms have been affected.

In the *second type*, there is a congenital dislocation of an ill-formed head of the radius, and the radius and ulna are anchored at some point a short way distal to their upper extremities, usually in the region of the coronoid, by a short, thick, interosseous ligament. The radius is relatively longer and stouter than the ulna, but shows the same curvature as in the primary type. Though not a true synostosis, there is no trace of movement.

In the *third type*, the head of the radius is present but is malformed and, together with the upper part of the shaft, is fused with the upper end of the ulna.

AETIOLOGY

Congenital radioulnar synostosis is essentially an arrest of development. The radius and ulna develop from a single mass of mesoderm as a pair of separate cartilaginous rods. From about the fifth week, the volar aspect of the developing arm is applied to the trunk, so that the radial and ulnar cartilaginous rods are in a position midway between pronation and supination. If the normal separation into distinct rods does not occur at the upper part of the developing bones, or if chondrification and, later, ossification extend across the mesoderm filled interval between their upper ends, a congenital radioulnar synostosis develops.

CLINICAL FEATURES

The main feature is fixation of the forearm in a position of mid-pronation. Movements of the elbow joint are usually free, although extension may be limited. Wrist movements are often unduly free. There is no movement of the radius on the ulna, however, and there appears to be firm osseous union between the bones (Figure 3.46).

In a unilateral case the affected forearm is thinner, and has a curious twisted appearance due to an alteration in the axis of the principal groups of muscles. At the point normally occupied by the head of the radius there may be a well marked sulcus, owing to the head being displaced backwards or forwards, or being imperfectly developed. The limitation of movement in the forearm is to some extent compensated for by rotation of the humerus, but the palm can never be fully supinated (Figure 3.47). The functional disability is therefore considerable, although there may be little or no complaint, since the normal use of the hand has never been experienced.

DIFFERENTIAL DIAGNOSIS

'Pulled elbow'

A small child or infant may present with an arm held in the mid-pronation flexed position, with some pain on attempting to straighten the elbow. Usually the parent can remember the child stumbling or being swung round with the hand being held. On examination there may be tenderness over the radial head, which is aggravated by attempting to supinate the forearm. Radiographs of both elbow joints are

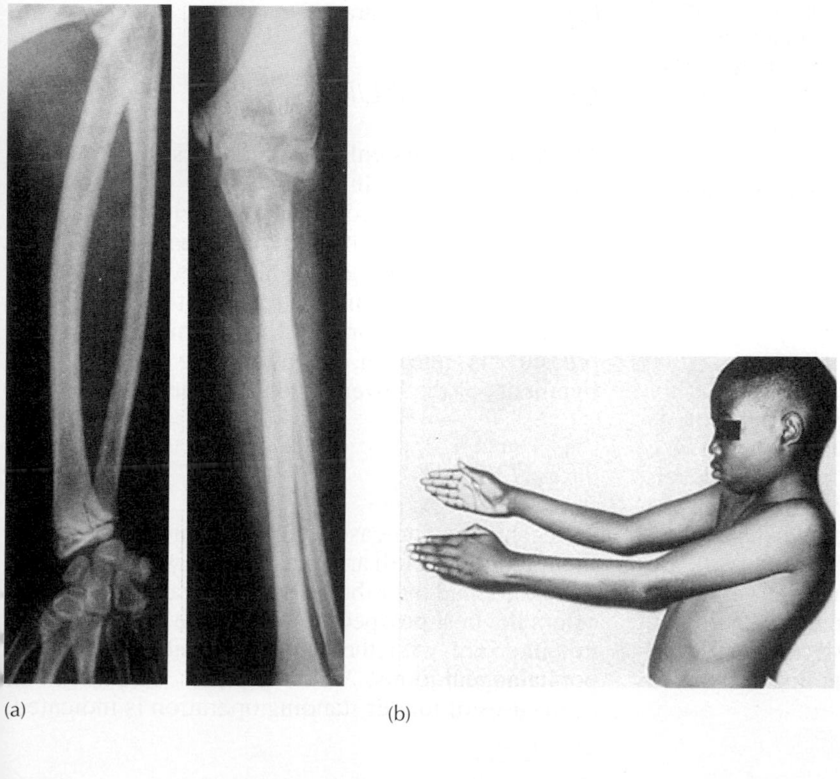

(a) (b)

Figure 3.46 (a) Congenital radioulnar synostosis with bowing of the radius and ulna with growth. (b) Attempting pronation and supination of the forearm. The functional limitation is real despite some substitution by rotation at the shoulder.

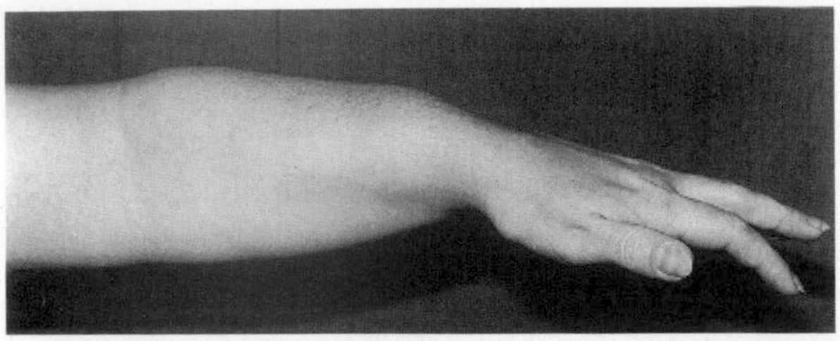

(a)

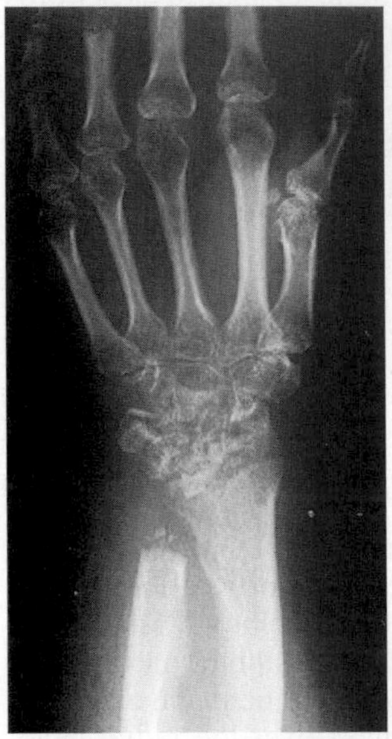

(b)

Figure 3.47 (a) A congenital radioulnar synostosis showing the characteristic 'dropped' wrist appearance. (b) A radiograph showing the postoperative position after excision of the lower end of the ulna and an arthrodesis of the proximal radiocarpal joint.

necessary to delineate the abnormal axial position of the involved radial head. Reduction is usually easy, by a full pronation of the forearm and compression of the radial head posteriorly.

TREATMENT

Although it seems obvious that an operation is indicated, the bony bridge is only part of the deformity; the soft tissues are not normally developed and the recorded results of operation are disappointing. In the type associated with dislocation of the head of the radius, where the soft parts are more normal, the prospect of helpful intervention is more hopeful, but, in any case, prognosis should be guarded. If the pronation is extreme it can be reduced by osteotomy, but in most cases the disability does not warrant operation.

Congenital subluxation of the wrist (Madelung's deformity)

Despite its name this deformity is probably not a true congenital one. Gibson (1923) classified inferior ulnar dislocations, of which Madelung's deformity is a type, as follows:

1. With fracture.
2. Without fracture:
   (a) Congenital (Madelung's);
   (b) Acquired – traumatic, pathological.

The deformity described by Madelung in 1879 is associated, Brailsford pointed out, with a defective development of the inner third of the growth cartilage at the lower end of the radius. This results in stunted growth of the epiphysis and diaphysis on the inner side. Growth of the outer two-thirds continues and, as a result, the radial shaft is bowed backwards, the interosseous space is increased, and the lower end of the ulna is subluxated backwards while the radial epiphysis appears to peter out towards the inner third where early fusion with the diaphysis is suggested (Figures 3.48 and 3.49).

The deformity is often bilateral, most common in females, and appears frequently for the first time in adolescence. The hand and wrist are weak, and while flexion may be increased other movements are restricted and may be painful. Brailsford suggested that it is a localized chondro-osteodystrophy resembling that of coxa vara.

CLINICAL FEATURES

The wrist appears enlarged, and dorsiflexion of the hand is impaired. In severe cases pronation and supination are limited. The wrist is loose, insecure and irritable. In long-standing cases the lower extremity of the radius is bent or curved forwards.

Pressure on the ulna reduces it into line with the radius, but the deformity recurs immediately the pressure is released, owing to the laxity of the ligaments of the lower radioulnar joint.

TREATMENT

In recent or acute cases, dorsiflexion of the wrist – maintained by a full arm plaster for 4 weeks and with a pressure pad over the prominent head of the ulna – offers the best prospect of relief. The plaster should not interfere with the movements at the metacarpophalangeal joints.

In cases of longer standing operation is indicated,

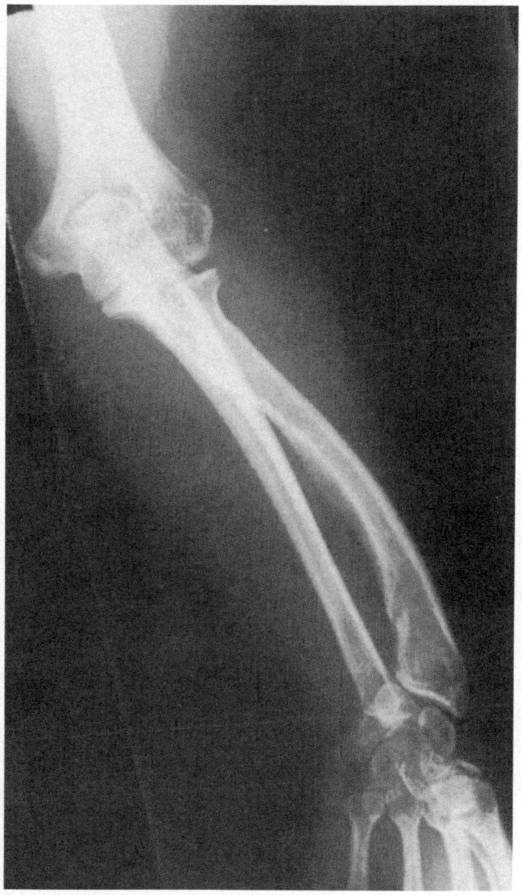

(a)

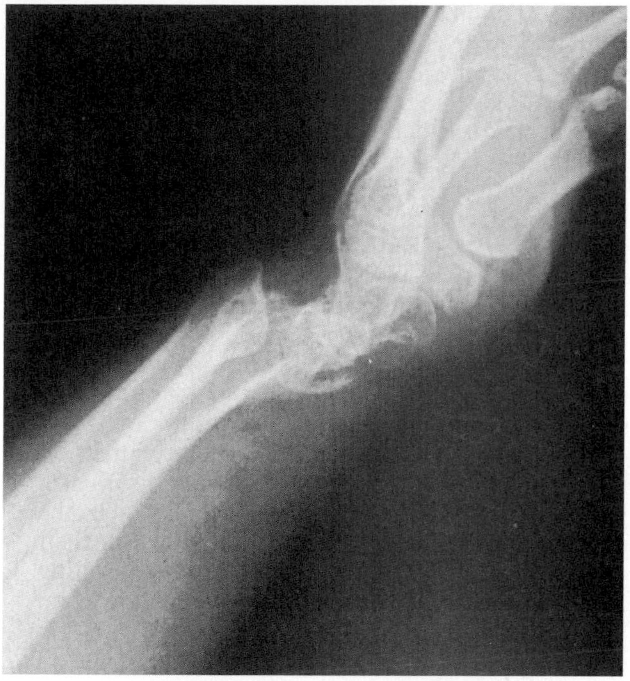

(b)

Figure 3.48 Madelung's deformity: (a) anteroposterior and (b) lateral views, showing the bowing of the radius and the abnormal wrist joint.

and may be directed either to the ligaments or to the bones.

Osteotomy of the lower end of the radius is recommended by some, the articular surface being rotated backwards into its normal position and the correction maintained by a plaster cast.

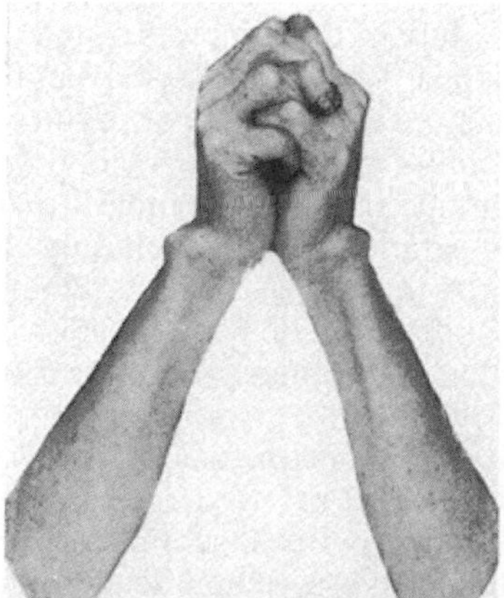

Figure 3.49 Bilateral congenital dislocation of the ulnae.

Darrach advocated the simpler operation of subperiosteal resection of the lower end of the ulna, and this gives as satisfactory a result as the more elaborate procedures. These operations may need to be combined for older cases, and include an arthrodesis of the radiocarpal joint for a painful restriction of motion (see Figure 3.47b).

Congenital malformations of the extremities

Congenital malformations or anomalies are produced by pathological changes in the normal developmental processes of the embryo or fetus. These macroscopic abnormalities of form and function are usually observable at birth.

In development after fertilization of the ovum (i.e. the formation of the zygote) there is a process of cleavage to produce a number of cells or blastomeres. These are hollowed out to form the blastocyst which contains the presumptive organ regions which then alter in position, size and shape to form the gastrula, with invagination of certain surface regions to give the three primary germ layers of endoderm, mesoderm and ectoderm. Waddington (1964) pointed out that during gastrulation there is little evidence of gene activity – i.e. to produce proteins which characterize adult tissues (e.g. the myosin or actin of muscle). At this time cells are unresponsive to embryonic inducer substances and therefore these tissues are relatively immune to teratogenesis (Wilson, 1961). Following this the neural plate and axial structures are created together with the mesodermal somites.

Waddington (1964) also emphasized that, in trying to understand teratology, one must distinguish between (1) the primary lesion in which the developmental processes are first deviated from their usual course, and (2) secondary lesions resulting from (1) and perhaps affecting the primitive germ layers.

The mesoderm gives rise to various tissues including the sclerotomes and the dermomyotomes to make up the axial and appendicular skeletons. The latter first appears distinctly in the embryo of about 5 mm CR length (or 35th day) when paired arm and leg limb buds appear on its surface. By the 9.6 mm CR stage the upper limb shows primary differentiation into arm, forearm and hand but the hind limb bud still retains its primitive paddle shape until the 12 mm stage. By the 47th day the digits of the hands separate but the feet are later again. By the end of the third month the upper limb has grown to a relatively normal length to that of trunk length and the smaller hind limb contains toes.

In achieving appendicular development, Gruneberg (1964) described the interaction between the mesoderm and ectoderm by the 'maintenance' factor and the 'apical ectodermal ridge' which controls the outgrowth of limb buds. This ridge arises by thickening of the epidermis along the outer margin of the limb bud and disappears in mice by the 13th day (Saunders *et al.*, 1957). Zwilling and Hansborough (1956), by transplantation and other reorientation experiments with the ridge, produced reduplication, turning, etc. They also described the various processes which are disturbed during the progression of limb budding and in the regression process with selective cell death to provide physiological cleavage planes in digits and in joints.

Classifications of congenital limb deficiencies have gradually evolved, becoming much more specific as the result of grouping patients for treatment and from their increasing numbers:

1. Descriptive
2. Embryological
3. Aetiological
4. Topographical
5. Morphogenetic (geny – indicating mode of progression.

DESCRIPTIVE CLASSIFICATION

Such groupings as deficiencies, additions, cleavage, pseudarthrosis, dislocation, have long been used, especially in the absence of knowledge concerning aetiology. Terms such as adactyly, arachnodactyly, brachydactyly, polydactyly, cleft hand, lobster-claw hand, club hand, etc., have all been used in various hand anomalies but are purely descriptive, giving no information about their origin or the amount of tissue involved, or subsequent changes during development. These were adequate when the numbers of limb anomalies were rare and spread throughout the patient population without grouping in centres. However, for studying epidemiological and management problems on a national or international basis, such terms are too ill-defined.

EMBRYOLOGICAL CLASSIFICATION

This was based upon attempts to describe or locate the stage of development in which the deviation from normal first occurred. Teratogenesis or abnormal development has long been studied by embryologists and experimental zoologists, etc., especially to differentiate genetic and environmental factors.

An early classification (Hamilton *et al.*, 1962) was based upon abnormalities of:

1. *Size:*
   (a) Of the whole organism, to give generaized gigantism or dwarfism (e.g. achondroplasia).
   (b) Of individual organs.
2. *Differentiation:*
   (a) Failure of certain parts of the primordia to appear because of lack of an inducer substance (e.g. absence of digit or limb).
   (b) Failure of tissue or blood supply (e.g. uterine fractures, pseudarthrosis).
   (c) Separation of inducer substance within growing spaces which would result in subdivision or reduplication into supernumerary organs (e.g. hyperdactylism).
3. *Development:*
   (a) By arrest or non-fusion of embryonic parts.
   (b) By failure of tissue movements, as described by Beechschmidt, of selective cellular repression and death (e.g. congenital dislocation of hip or knee).

The anatomist Arey (1965) used the following terminology:

- Amelia Limbs either fail to develop or remain as buds.
- Hemimelia Proximal segments of limb are normal but distal segments are deficient and taper to a stump.
- Phocomelia Reverse of above, with expansion of distal segments into a 'seal flipper'.
- Sympodia Varying degrees of union of legs, due to developmental failure of a median, wedge-shaped mass of trunk mesenchyma.
- 'Lobster-claw' Fusion of fingers separated by a long cleft.
- Dichiria Partial duplication.
- Polydactyly Presence of supernumerary digit.
- Brachydactyly Abnormal shortness of digits.
- Club hand/club foot Primary defect in the differentiation of the limb buds with retention of a transitory condition normal to fetus.
- Congenital elevation of shoulder Arrested descent of the upper limb from a cervical embryonic position.
- Congenital dislocation of hip Failure of the outgrowth to produce acetabular rim and socket of appropriate shape.
- Intrauterine amputation Focal deterioration of tissues – not umbilical or amniotic cords, etc.

AETIOLOGICAL CLASSIFICATION

Although a few anomalies can be specifically identified as genetic in origin (e.g. achondroplasia) or due to chemical embryopathy, the majority are still unknown even though teratology has long been studied. Indeed in 1832 Geoffrey Saint-Hilaire described teratological evolution as being an arrest of development. He also introduced the term 'phocomelia' to describe the seal-like appearance of the hand. Wolff (1937) confirmed this by using x-rays to arrest development and described other teratological properties such as monsters which can be produced by x-irradiation without any hereditary basis, and x-irradiation acting upon the anlage between the time of determination and differentiation of tissues.

Embryopathy may be induced by physical, chemical and viral agents in certain dosages, vitamin imbalance, nutritional deficiencies – all modifying the uterine environment, or acting perhaps on the embryo directly (Nishimura, 1964).

However, with the thalidomide tragedy, a great deal more work is going into studying specific effects of drugs and chemicals. Various agents such as trypan blue can produce spina bifida, club foot and axial torsion; hypervitaminosis A – anencephaly, absence or dysplasia (these are also produced by thalidomide in certain species of animals); and nitrogen mustard producing polydactyly, etc.

In 1966, Lenz reviewed the malformations produced by drugs in human pregnancy. From exact morphological studies of phocomelia and aplasia, etc., he described certain patterns of malformations which were more typical of thalidomide embryopathy than the excessively rare ones of mutation. He emphasized the association of these anomalies with lesions of the ear, of paralysis of nerves, of the heart and other viscera. Such studies are vital because they will provide important data about how, when and where the primary deviation first occurred and provide the ultimate in any classification. Further work revealed that the primary cause of thalidomide abnormalities may result from injury to the endothelial lining of the limb bud axial artery (Jurand, 1966) (see Figure 3.50).

TOPOGRAPHICAL CLASSIFICATIONS

These are based upon detailed descriptions of surface appearances with reference to the underlying

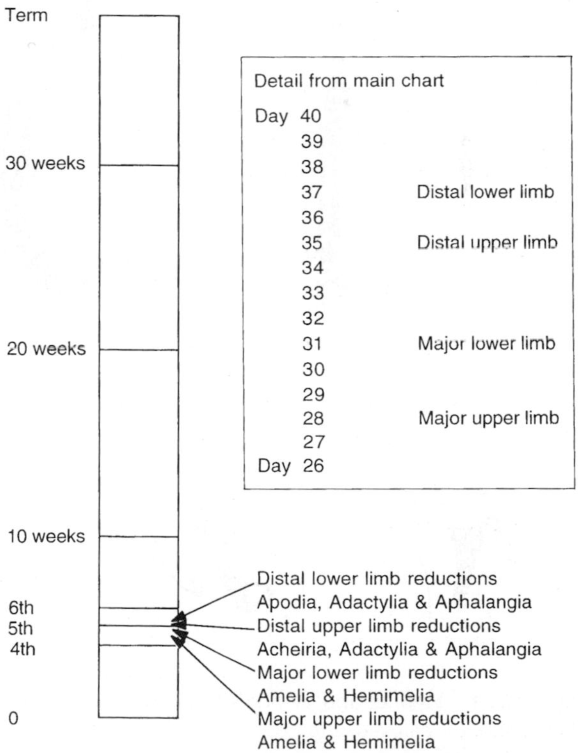

Figure 3.50 The timing of development of the limbs and the timing of the various limb reduction deformities. (Reproduced, with permission, from Fuller, D. J. and Duthie, R. B. (1974) AAOS Instructional Course Lectures **23**, 53–61)

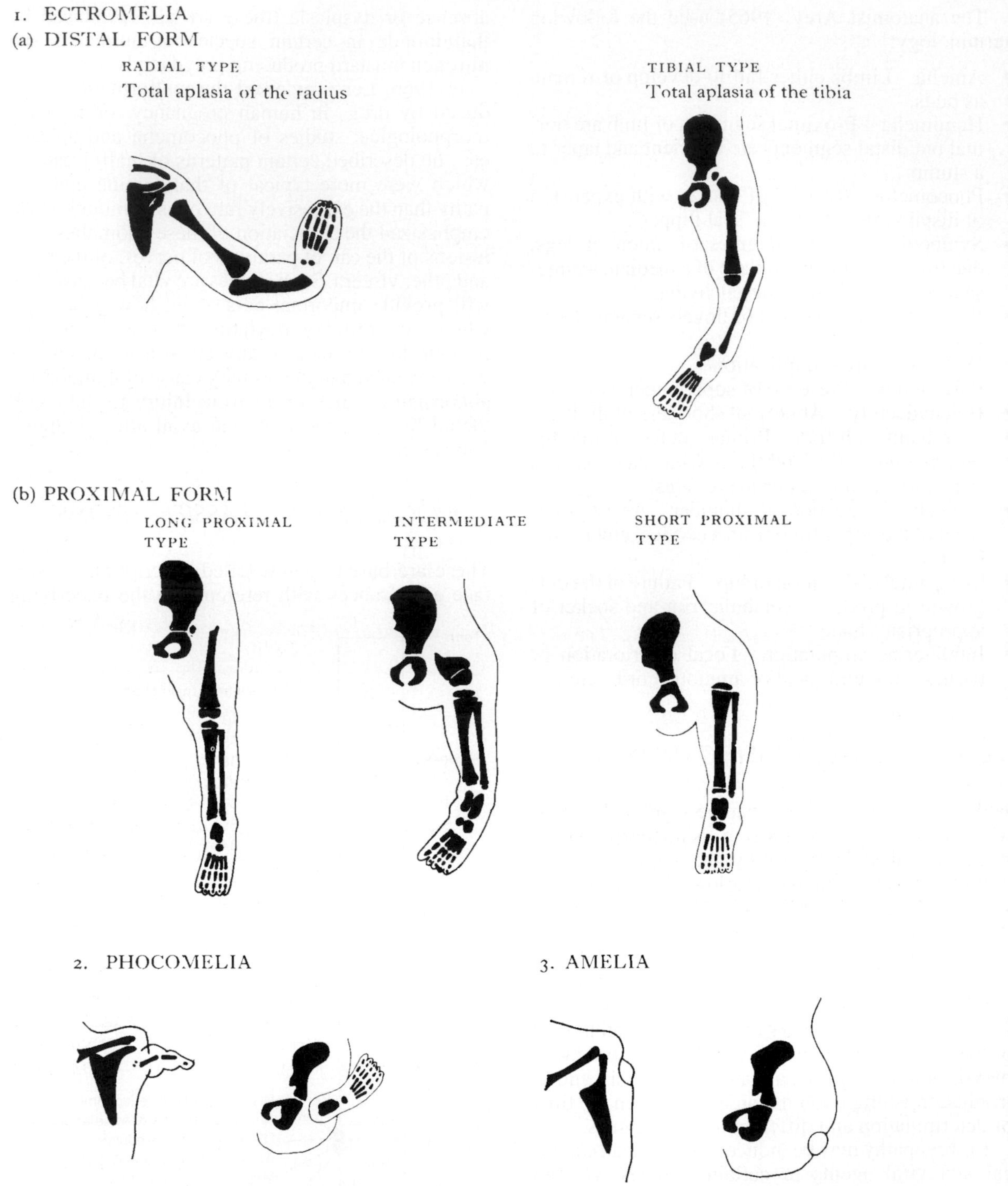

Figure 3.51 Henkel and Willert's three forms of dysmelia: (1) ectromelia (distal and proximal forms), (2) phocomelia, (3) amelia.

parts or lack of them. They were devised in order to group clinical entities with a minimum of confusion (Swanson, 1966) but broad enough to accommodate complex cases.

In 1951 O'Rahilly, by publishing his work on the morphological patterns in limb deficiencies and duplications, gave rise to classifications by Frantz and by Hall. The classification of Frantz and O'Rahilly (1961) has become the standard one. These authors used seven descriptive terms:

- Amelia Absence of whole limb
- Hemimelia Absence of large part of limb
- Phocomelia Absence of adjoining segment of limb
- Acheria Absence of hand
- Apodia Absence of foot
- Adactylia Absence of digit, including metacarpal, metatarsal
- Aphalangia Absence of phalanges.

To include the segmentation of duplication defects they used the terms:

- para-axial/pre-axial: border of a limb on which the thumb or big toe arises, either radial or tibial.
- post-axial: the opposite border, either ulnar or fibular.

These are based upon the arrangements seen in a $5^{1}/_{2}$-week-old embryo in which both the thumbs and big toes are on the cephalic borders of the limbs. The defects may be terminal, in which there are affected parts distal to the lesion, or intercalary, in which the middle parts of the limb are deficient but tissues above and below are normal. Finally, the defects may be longitudinal or transverse.

The Frantz–O'Rahilly classification system was applied to 577 limb-deficient conditions and 85% were classifiable within this system (Burtch, 1963). However, in order to improve this system still further, a revision was carried out in 1966 by a committee (Burtch). In this, the basic principles of Frantz and O'Rahilly were used – i.e. the description is that of the absent skeletal parts with two main divisions:

1. terminal and intercalary and subgroupings;
2. transverse and longitudinal.

Anatomical terms (e.g. radial, fibular) were substituted for the more classical descriptive terms (e.g. hemimelia, dysmelia, phocomelia), with only two being retained: amelia – complete absence of free limb; and meromelia – partial absence of a free limb.

CLASSIFICATION BASED UPON MORPHOGENETIC PATTERNS

A classification based upon the changing and maturing of the skeleton and its possible malformations was evolved by Willert and Henkel (1968). This classification deals with morphological patterns and sequential changes of congenital defects of dysmelia in the upper and lower extremities (Henkel, 1968; Henkel and Willert, 1969) (Figure 3.51).

These authors, by analysing a large number of limb deficiencies, have shown certain morphological patterns which can be arranged in a teratological sequence, particularly in a group of malformations called 'dysmelia'. This is defined as a group of defects of the long bones of the arm and/or leg (e.g. the radius or tibia) with involvement of the hand or foot rays. These deficiencies can be grouped into:

1. A distal form with varying degrees of hypoplasia, partial or total aplasia with or without synostosis (Figure 3.52).
2. A proximal form – long, intermediate or short in position.
3. An axial form – long, intermediate or short in position (Figure 3.53) with varying degrees of hypoplasia or aplasia.
4. Phocomelia and amelia are the most severe stages. There are several main groups:

   (a) In which there was frank loss of skeletal mass with the remaining parts showing a disturbance of maturation and ossification. This reduction of skeletal mass followed certain rules called reduction tendency, i.e. individual bones (in the thumb, big toe, radius, tibia, humerus, femur) were not reduced in an irregular fashion. This reduction in a series of cases affected by differing degrees of severity (i.e. from hypoplasia, to partial aplasia, to total aplasia), followed a distinct sequence in direction (proximo-distal or distal-proximal) and in amount; e.g. the humerus showed deficiencies only in those cases where the radius was already either totally absent or its remnants fused to the ulna.

   The impairment of the pelvic and shoulder girdles followed closely the severity of the reduction of the limb parts. In certain cases the degree of involvement of the shoulder or hip joints could not be determined initially. Reduction of the number of finger and hand rays was frequent and mirrored the severity of the malformation of the arm. The reduction of the foot components was less common and was not marked; e.g. normal feet were found in severely deformed legs. In teratology it has been shown

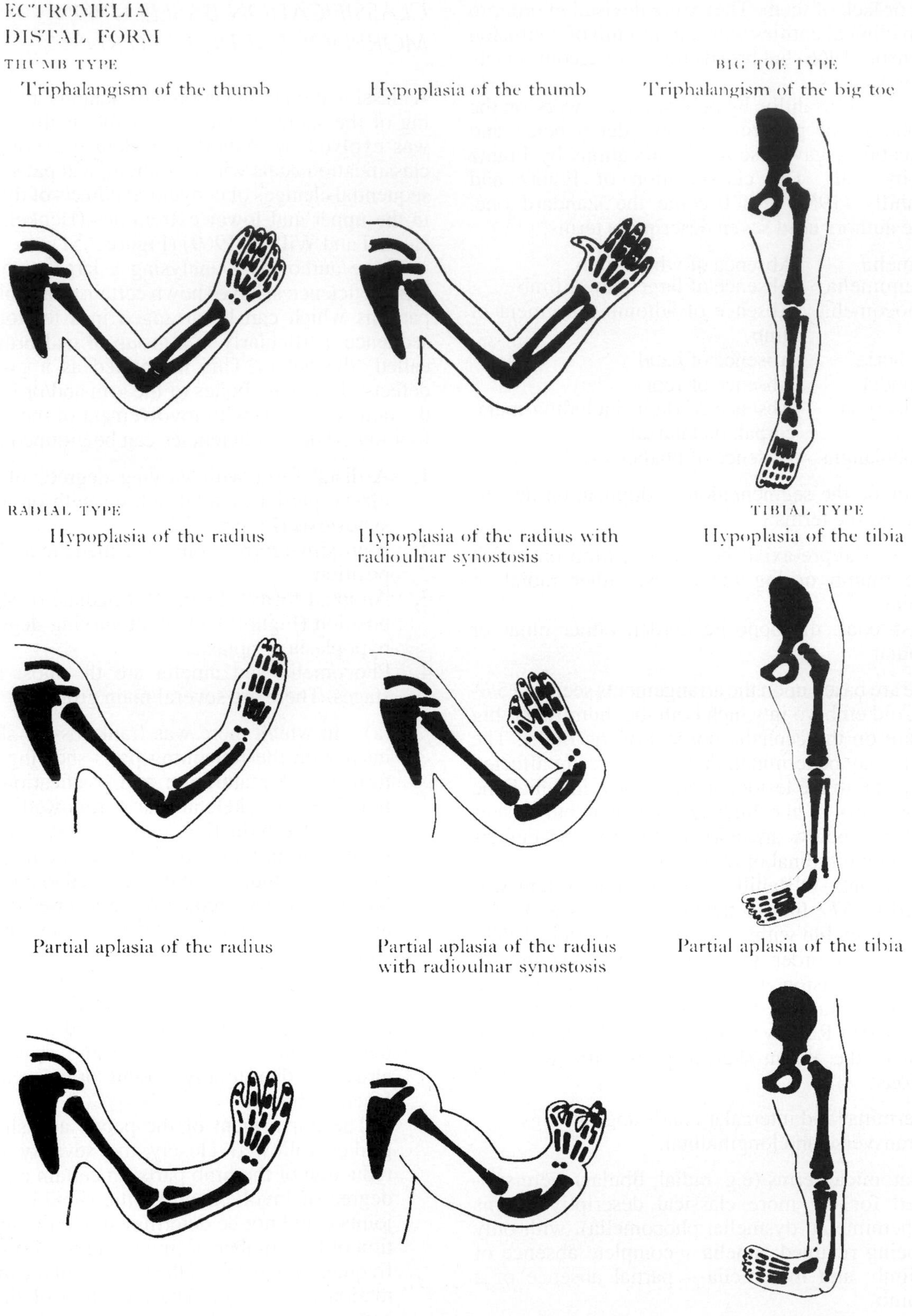

Figure 3.52 Distal form of ectromelia: thumb and big toe type, radial and tibial types.

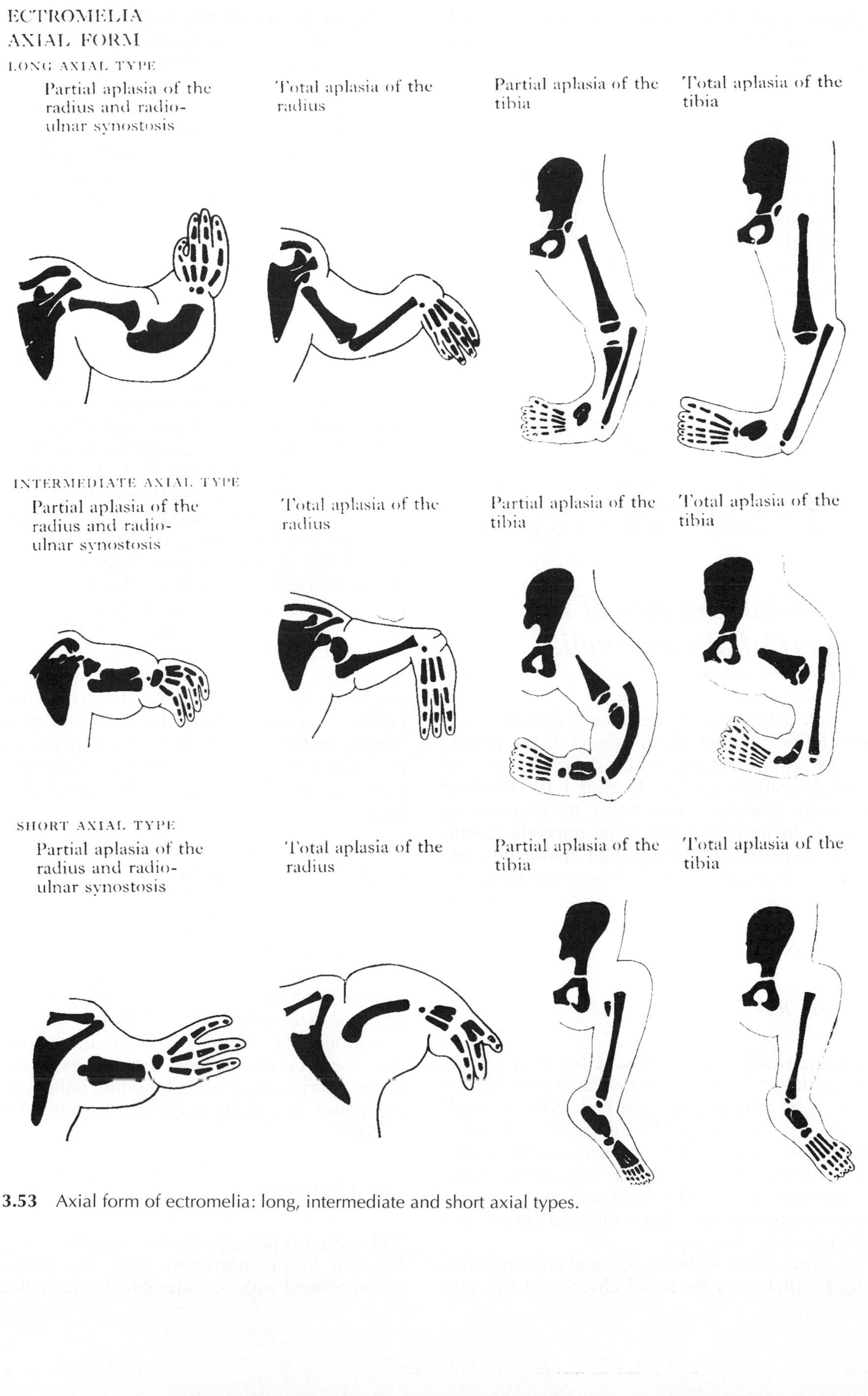

Figure 3.53 Axial form of ectromelia: long, intermediate and short axial types.

that experimentally produced peripheral defects in the leg buds can be 'repaired' much more easily by the surrounding blastema than in the arms (Rickenbacher); i.e. the upper limbs – especially the fingers – are much more vulnerable than the toes to permanent embryopathic changes.

(b) In which there were axial types of malformation – e.g. the radial rays of the hand, the radius and the humerus were affected – and in the leg the tibial ray of the foot, the tibia and the femur were affected. This combination of affected parts was called the axis of malformation.

(c) In which certain patterns and sequences of fusion of affected skeletal elements or lack of them were seen; e.g. coxa vara and proximal femoral defects.

(d) In which there was disturbance of ossification; e.g. seen as delay in epiphyses of parts far away from the defect itself.

In addition, they have described in the vicinity of defects, cartilage centres which ossify and appear on radiography in later years of life (e.g. coxa vara).

Congenital absence of the radius (radial meromelia)

This is an intercalary, longitudinal defect which clearly defines hypoplasia or aplasia of the radius. There are varying degrees of the deformity with or without synostosis. The incidence is 1:100 000 live births with bilateral cases being as frequent as unilateral. In unilateral cases the opposite thumb may be hyperplastic. Associated anomalies are common, e.g. cardiac septal defects in the Holt–Oram syndrome; blood cell changes in Fanconi syndrome; trisomy 17; and thrombocytopenia (in the first 2 years).

PATHOLOGY

Usually the whole radius is absent, but occasionally when the defect is only partial, a small portion of it remains, generally at the upper end. When a small fragment of radius is present the ulna may be fused to it, giving rise to a form of radioulnar synostosis. The ulna, which may attain a considerable size in many cases, is short, thick and curved, and the concavity of its curvature is nearly always directed towards the radial side of the forearm.

The carpus often shows associated abnormalities amongst which may be noted absence of the scaphoid, or fusion of that bone with neighbouring carpal bones. More rarely, the lunate is absent.

When the radius is totally absent, the biceps is usually inserted into the lacertus fibrosus, though in some cases the muscle is either completely absent, or fused with the brachialis anterior or the coracobrachialis. The brachialis is absent in about half the number of cases, and when it is present it is usually short and stout, and appears to be a continuation of the short head of the biceps. Occasionally it is continuous with the extensor carpi radialis longus, and the two may be inserted into the ulna. The extensor carpi radialis longus and brevis are frequently absent, or fused with the extensor digitorum communis, while the extensor pollicis longus may also be lacking, or fused with neighbouring tissues. The flexor pollicis longus and the pronator quadratus are rarely present. The radial nerve usually terminates at the elbow, and there is often no radial artery.

In 1980 Marquardt described how the 'radial hand' is positioned towards the body, the little finger compensates for the absent thumb and closing of the hand is achieved by marked radial abduction and acute flexion. This gives good functional response, much better than the cosmetic appearance. Because of this, he recommends that early operation must be avoided until the end of the growth period. At birth, physiotherapy is begun to reduce the all too common contracture and to maintain an increasing range of movement. Passive stretching by the mother is taught to bring the club hand into as normal a position as possible, with the distal end of the ulna serving as the fulcrum. This is then held by plaster and plastic splints. Marquardt's operation is to fuse the distal end of the ulna to the lunate and triquetrum bones.

CLINICAL FEATURES

The affected arm shows some degree of atrophy, but this is most marked in the forearm which is invariably short, stubby and bowed with a posterior convexity. The hand is small and atrophic. Further, it is deviated to the radial side, and slightly palmar flexed – 'radiopalmar club hand'. The thumb is occasionally absent, but despite these deformities the limb may retain a surprisingly good function, although grasping power is usually impaired (Figures 3.54 and 3.55).

TREATMENT

Although it is possible to see a surprising degree of function in the untreated case, this function is accomplished with considerable cosmetic disability

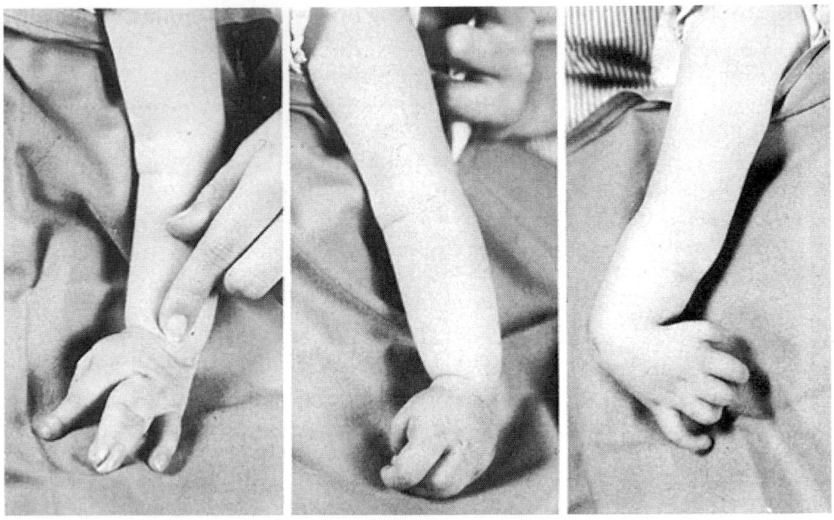

(a) (b) (c)

Figure 3.54 (a) The left upper extremity of a 2-year-old boy, showing abnormality of the left thumb and index finger, and syndactylism of the middle two fingers. (b) The same child attempting to make a fist. (c) Showing an attempt to move his wrist. x-Rays show that he had a congenital absence of the radius.

and can be improved upon. Grasp is often accomplished by using the hand against the upper arm. Whatever growth might have been obtained is negated by the excessive curvature of the ulna.

Riordan (1955) pointed out that the aim should be to overcome the radial deviation and proximal progression of the carpus as soon as the deformity s recognized. This is accomplished by progressive casting to push the hand over the distal ulnar styloid. This normally takes about 6 weeks. At this point the carpus can be brought in line or slightly beyond the ulna but when not passively held tends to drop back to its former position. A holding splint can then be used moulded along the ulna with. Velcro straps pulling the hand into the corrected position.

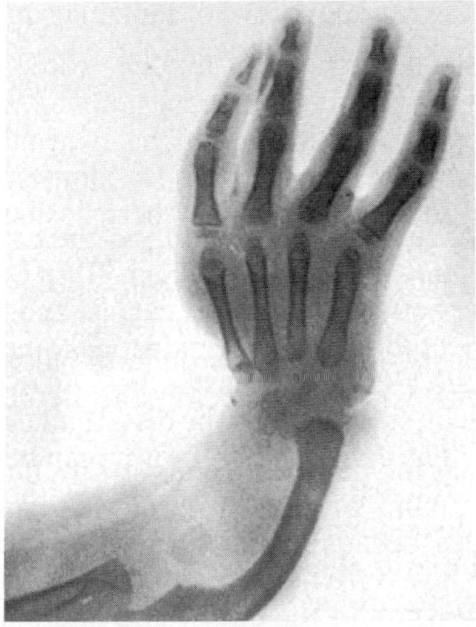

Figure 3.55 Congenital absence of radius, right side. (Both thumbs were absent.)

The best results in terms of permanently maintaining the carpus over the ulna requires operation below the age of 1 year.

Operation

The carpus must be brought directly over and at right angles to the distal epiphyseal line of the ulna rather than into axial alignment with the forearm. The importance of this is realized when one examines the residual curve of the ulna which is still present. This curve is corrected later by osteotomy if necessary. The distal ulna is the part which must now be centred in the carpus.

By far the most successful cosmetic and functional result in treatment of this deformity is found only in infancy. In later childhood the patient has developed motor patterns in which grasp essentially takes place between the entire carpus and forearm. Development of more normal appearance and a greater degree of function can be obtained if the carpus can be stabilized on the distal end of the ulna in infancy. The distal end of the ulna can be released from the attached carpal ligaments without damaging the distal ulna epiphysis. The carpus can then be brought over the distal ulna. A socket is now needed to secure a stable relationship. This is formed by excision of the lunate. The distal ulna is reduced into this space and maintained by a Kirschner wire running down the third metacarpal and engaging the ulna. The ulna is frequently bowed. It is important that the carpal be placed as a continuation of the distal end of the ulna rather than in relationship to the long axis of the forearm.

The pin fixation with external plaster support is continued for 6 weeks. Thereafter continued external support with a plaster splint or laced cuff is continued for approximately 1 year or until the position of the carpus is maintained without a tendency to recurrence. If the bowing of the ulna fails to straighten with growth it can be osteotomized at a later date.

In summary, in adult cases with mild deformities, lethal associated anomalies, severe neurovascular and soft tissue contractures and with elbow flexion, no treatment is indicated. At birth, mild cases should be splinted. When radial contractures are resistant to splintage and radial deviation progresses, centralization procedures should be carried out with pollicization of a functioning index finger, especially in bilateral cases.

Congenital absence of the ulna (post-axial ulnar hemimelia)

This is a much more uncommon lesion than the absence of the radius and is most difficult to differentiate from the latter lesion. In contrast to the radial club hand, the hand in the ulnar club hand deformity usually is stable with an unstable elbow joint and the associated anomalies tend to be musculoskeletal in site.

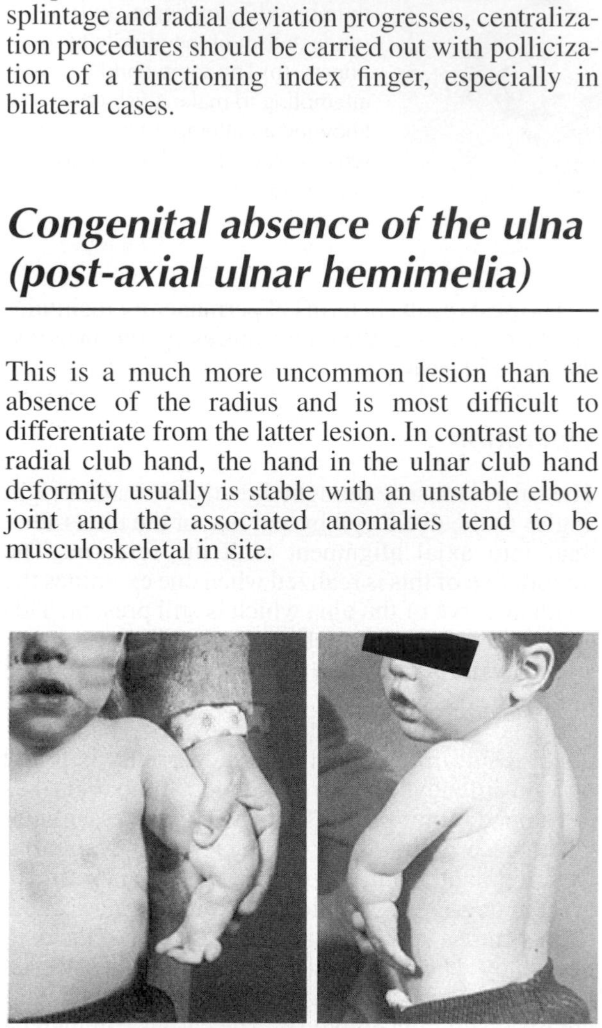

(a) (b)

Figure 3.56 (a) A 3-year-old boy with a left upper extemity which is markedly foreshortened without obvious elbow or wrist joints. The hand consists of two main digits and a soft tissue appendage. (b) The same child from the back, showing two creases, one where the elbow joint should be, and the other where the wrist joint was. This was a case of congenital absence of the ulna, in which at operation the cartilaginous ulnar anlage was removed, and an arthroplasty attempted between the lower end of the humerus and the radius.

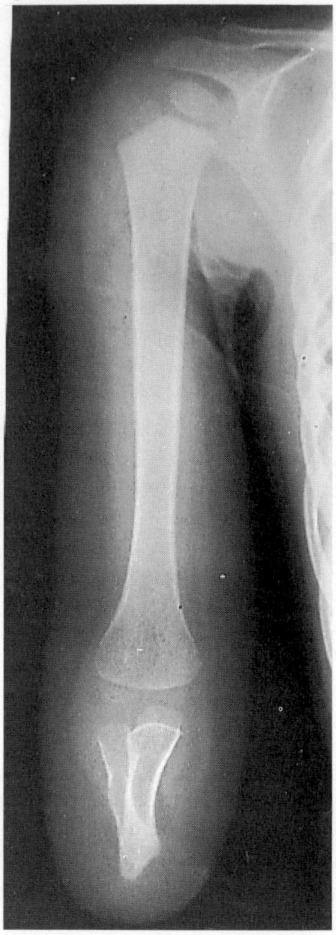

Figure 3.57 A radiograph showing a unilateral transverse melia of the forearm with a normal elbow joint and humerus above.

CLINICAL FEATURES

The overall deformity is milder, with the hand slightly deviated, but the radius is bowed, shortened and thickened with the radial head usually dislocated. This interferes with elbow joint flexion and supination. In a personal case, there has been union of the 'radius' to the humerus with marked bowing deformity of the radius. At operation, the osseous-cartilaginous anlage of the ulna was removed and an arthroplasty attempted through the lower end of the humerus with a sheet of soft tissue (Figure 3.56).

The ulnar club hand deformity means that it is the back of the hand which lies downwards and on the work surface because of the usual fixed supination deformity and even a humeroradial synostosis. There is hyperextension of the elbow and internal rotation at the shoulder – all producing a severe functional deformity.

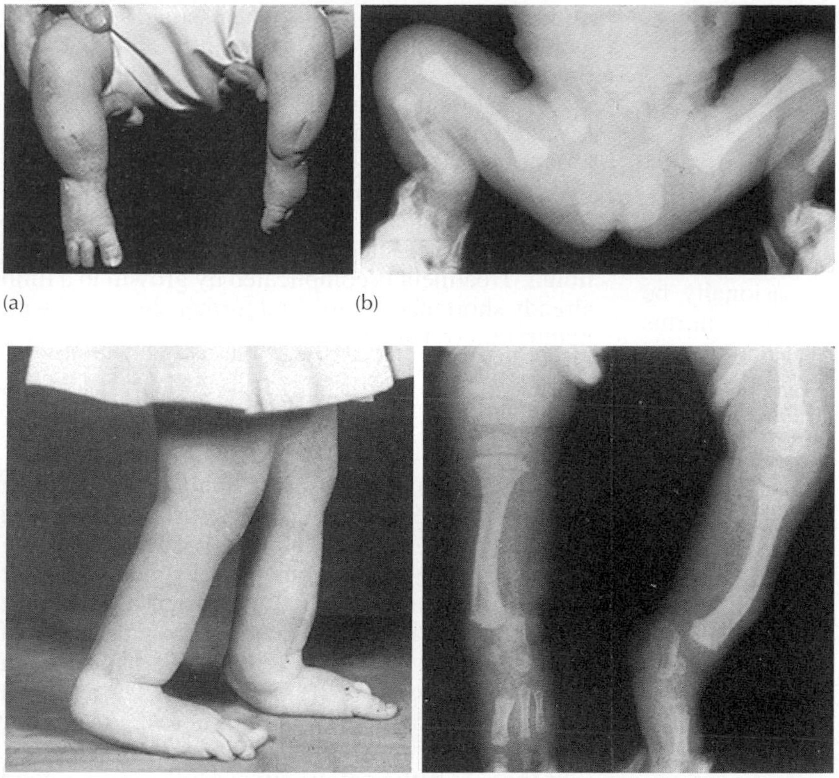

(a) (b) (c) (d)

Figure 3.58 (a,b) The lower extremities of an 8-month-old child, showing normal knee joints with abnormal-appearing ankle joints, with only three digits being present, and the absence of the fibula bilaterally. (c,d) The same child at the age of 3 years. There is marked instability and giving way of both ankle joints, so the child was unable to walk without crutches in the absence of the normal ankle mortice.

Therefore, Marquardt (1980) recommends a rotational osteotomy of the humerus on one side and a flexion osteotomy in the area of synostosis to provide a hand-to-hand activity.

At a later time, consideration should be given to construct a 'one bone' forearm and then operate upon the hand deformities.

Transverse melia

For the transverse deficiencies (Figure 3.57) orthotic end-appliances (with cosmetic gloves) are required for grasp, so that the patient may be encouraged to take part in everyday activities. The appliances are modified during growth but fitted by 6 months.

The Krukenberg operation of separating the radius and ulna in the presence of good skin and sensation is particularly indicated on one side in a bilateral transverse lesion.

Congenital absence of the fibula (paraxial fibular hemimelia)

The types of congenital absence of the fibula have been described by Coventry and Johnson. Such a classification leads to an understanding of prognosis and early definitive treatment where indicated. This particularly relates to expected length.

In type I there is a partial absence of the fibula. Minimal leg length discrepancy is expected and there are no associated anomalies. Type II is the usual anomaly. There is dysplasia of the entire limb, including complete absence of the fibula. The tibia is bowed anteromedially and short. The growth of the femur is frequently hypoplastic. The foot without lateral support goes into an equinovalgus position. There are various tarsal bone fusions and the fourth and fifth rays are frequently absent. The skin may be dimpled over the anterior aspect of the tibia. There is at least 8 cm of expected overall shortening in the affected limb and it may reach

13 cm. Bilateral deformities and unilateral anomalies with associated other deformities are grouped as type III. (See Figure 3.58.)

TREATMENT

When the foot is intact, treatment is directed towards achieving a normal weight-bearing position for the foot. Heel cord lengthening may occasionally be indicated. Bowing of the tibia is not severe in this group and may show improvement if full activity and normal weight-bearing are achieved. Leg length discrepancy is less than 8 cm and is subject to correction by lengthening procedures and later epiphyseodesis as indicated. Excision of the fibular remnant may occasionally result in better foot position and improvement in the deformity of the bowed tibia.

In type II the dysplasia involves shortening of the femur as well as severe involvement of the foot and tibia. When the poorly formed foot cannot be maintained in good position, the shortening accompanying this anomaly (8–13 cm) leads to consideration of a Syme-type amputation. The shortening is severe enough that girls as well as boys tolerate this type of amputation well since the bulky ankle of the conventional Syme prosthesis is avoided. The weight-bearing tissue of the heel is preserved by subperiosteal dissection and this flap is brought under the tibia and carefully maintained.

Kruger and Talbott (1961) outlined the expected shortening in this anomaly when the fibula is completely absent. In a study of 62 patients, shortening of over 7.5 cm was found in the majority of cases, with 5 cm usually occurring by the age of 1 year.

Congenital absence of the tibia (pre-axial tibial hemimelia; hypoplasia or aplasia of the tibia)

This is an unusual deformity occurring in 1:1 000 000 live births with a family incidence being reported. There is a high-risk association of CDH; aphalangism of upper and lower limbs; proximal femoral focal deficiency and hypoplasia of the femoral condyles.

There are varying degrees of tibial absence but it is usual for at least some of the proximal segment to remain. At birth this may not be ossified sufficiently to recognize the extent of the limb, and there are times when so little remains that possibilities for the knee as a functioning joint no longer exist. The limb is not angulated anteriorly as often as seen with an absent fibula. Tarsal anomalies in various combinations are the rule rather than the exception. The fibula lies more proximally at the knee than normal and the foot is subluxed medially on the distal end of the fibula. Treatment is complicated by growth in a limb already shortened at birth and further shortened with maturation of the child.

TREATMENT

The temptation to rush into amputation in view of all these problems is a real one, particularly in the unilateral case. It should be recognized that the fibula has great possibilities for hypertrophy if it can be united at either end to the remnants of the tibia. If there is a good bony fragment of fibula present, a Brown procedure can be performed, in which the transposed head of fibula is stabilized into the intracondylar femoral notch. At a later stage a Syme's amputation can be performed.

If there is sufficient proximal tibia so that a good functional knee is possible, the initial stages of treatment should certainly involve union of the fibula to this remnant even if later amputation is to be considered. This should be done as early as sufficient ossification has occurred to ensure union.

The ankle may be similarly stabilized by union of the distal fibular segment to the tibia. Once this is obtained, active use of the limb with weight-bearing is encouraged often supported by a leather or plastic orthotic brace during the period of fibular hypertrophy.

In later years one can evaluate the growth that has occurred and come to an intelligent decision regarding the possibilities for an active usable extremity with the shortening being over-come by lengthening procedures or by epiphyseal arrest on the other side. If little function is present, amputation or knee disarticulation may be the procedure of choice.

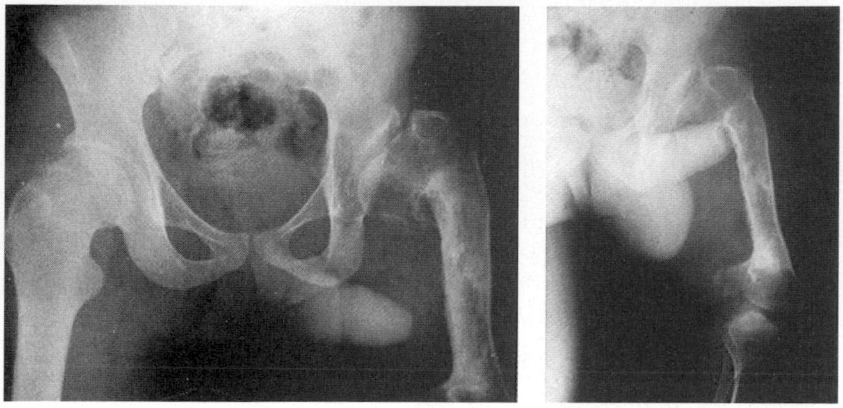

(a) (b)

Figure 3.59 (a) Radiograph of pelvis and upper femora of a young man showing the very rudimentary development of the upper third of the femur and a marked coxa vara. (b) lateral view of the same patient to show the abnormal articulation at the hip joint with a severe rotational deformity at the knee as well as the foreshortening of the total length of the femur.

Proximal femoral focal deficiency (congenital shortening of the femur)

Unlike the fibula, the dysplasia appears to affect mainly the proximal end of the femur rather than its centre aspect. In severe cases there may be only remnants of the neck and trochanteric area with any bony continuity. Boden *et al.* (1989) have reported from a study of a 21-week-old fetus with unilateral proximal femoral focal deficiency that the proximal growth plate was markedly abnormal. There was failure of this plate to migrate proximally as well as in its formation. The longitudinal columns of proliferative and hypertrophic cartilage cells were disrupted and the pattern of vascular invasion grossly disorganized. In contrast, the distal growth plates of femur and other bones were normal. Steindler (1940) divided this type of dysplasia into:

1. Those with only rudimentary development of the upper third of femur and marked coxa vara (Figure 3.59).
2. Coxa vara with a normal shaft.
3. Overall shortening of shaft, but a normal upper third component (Figure 3.60).
4. Dysplasia of lower third with synostosis at the knee.

As growth proceeds, the deformity becomes more severe, with marked leg length discrepancy due to disturbance in all bones of the lower extremity. Often these children never bear weight through the involved limb.

Henkel and Willert (1969), from Blauth's work showed that it is most difficult to describe from the first 6 months' appearance of defects involving the upper femoral components how much and to what extent the cartilage will develop (Figure 3.61). These workers also described the radiographic typing of this lesion.

Aitken and Frantz (1953), in their study on proximal femoral focal deficiency, described the surgical treatment – particularly in those patients who have an adequate acetabulum, varying amounts of the head of the femur but a very short femoral segment. A pseudarthrosis may be present. These, usually with delayed ossification, give rise to a marked coxa vara, subtrochanteric pseudarthrosis and marked femoral shortening. They carried out an excision of the pseudarthrosis and a subtrochanteric valgus osteotomy. Some patients had the proximal end of the femur implanted into the femoral head with or without bone grafting. Fixation was by pins and a POP cast. Later knee fusion and terminal amputation was carried out. Early prosthetic fitting was essential around the age of 5 years.

Treatment is directed towards providing some means of ambulation, through an ischial-bearing, weight-relieving brace. Gillespie and Torode (1983) classified this complex deformity particularly from the point of view of shortening into:

- *Group 1* – in which the foot is at the mid-tibial level, the hip is abducted and laterally rotated and the knee flexed but lax. Radiology shows up to 60% of the femur but a normal hip with a stable coxa vara, a hypoplastic knee and lateral bowing of the femoral shaft. The estimated leg length discrepancy will be about 20%. Treatment in this group is directed towards physiotherapy for knee and hip contractures, an extension prosthesis, surgical correcting of the coxa vara deformity and plan for a femoral lengthening procedure.
- *Group 2* – the foot is at the knee level, with severe fixed flexion of hip and knee. Radiology shows a

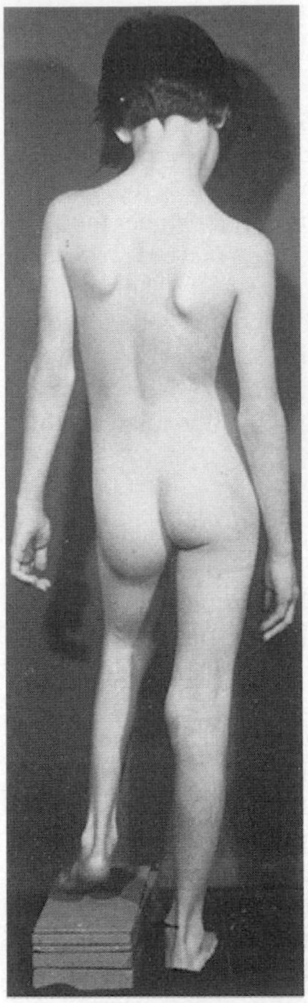

(a)

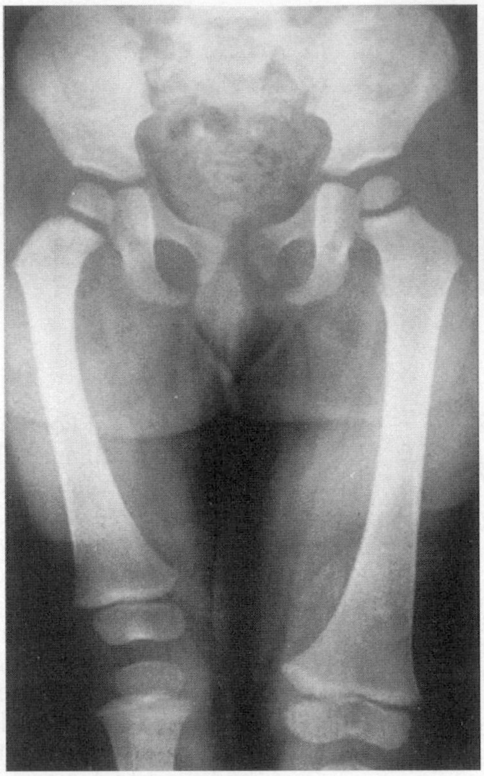

(b)

Figure 3.60 (a) Congenital short femur leading to marked disfigurement in a girl. (b) Mild degree of congenital short femur with great possibilities for reconstruction – lengthening, etc.

very short femur, a defect deficiency of the proximal femur, and head and neck, a hypoplastic knee and marked distal deficiencies. The estimated leg length discrepancy is over 40–50% (Figures 3.62 and 3.63).

Because the hip and knee joints are useless, one has to decide by the age of 3 years to carry out a Van Nes procedure with its better functional result although poorer psychologically; a Syme's amputation for a unilateral foot abnormality and/or a knee fusion to increase the skeletal lever arm.

Although bracing allows ambulation, it does not provide for the normal stimulation to growth by weight-bearing and, therefore, as well as the aplastic or dysplastic element, the remaining 'normal' components of bone fail to grow and develop. Therefore, if the main disturbance is in the more distal components, knee fusion and early amputation with a prosthesis is indicated. Such a procedure may well be considered even in the presence of a coxa vara deformity which can be corrected by an angulation osteotomy. Van Nes (1950) described a rotationplasty of the leg through an arc of 180° with fusion of the knee and then fitting an above-knee prosthesis. The ankle joint acts as the knee but this procedure is not satisfactory for function or even cosmetically. Indeed. rotational correction is difficult to achieve (Figure 3.63a,b).

Congenital asymmetry

This term is preferred to that of hemiatrophy or hemihypertrophy because of frequent difficulty in determining whether it is an abnormality of growth or development of one limb (Smithells, 1965). The human form has long been recognized as being asymmetrical and this is seen in Greek and Roman sculpture. In 1822 the first case on human asymmetry was presented by Meckel and in 1908 Liebreich published his treatise on asymmetry in normals.

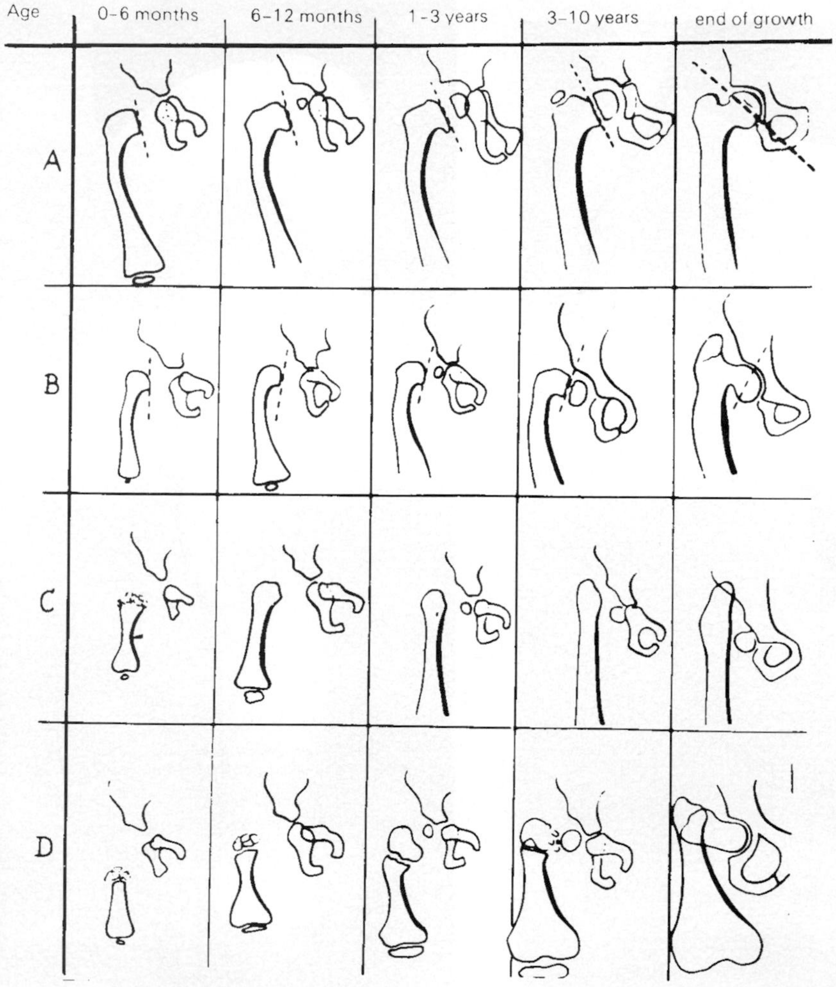

Figure 3.61 Diagrams of radiographic outlines from four cases of femoral dysplasia, as they developed over the months and years to skeletal maturity in the right column. (Reproduced, with permission, from Willert, H. G. and Henkel, H. L. (1968) *Dysmelia of the Extremities*. Springer-Verlag, Heidelberg)

It may be associated with haemangiomatous and/or lymphatic changes or neurological disorders (e.g. neurofibromatosis).

The skin, hair, nails and bone length of the involved limb must be carefully examined. A systematic inspection of the face for the typical appearance of Silver's disease, sexual development and secondary deformities such as scoliosis must be carried out (Figures 3.64, 3.65). Palpation of the abdomen for a Wilms' tumour of the kidney, or adrenal or liver neoplasm, which have been associated with hemihypertrophy of a limb, is necessary and requires a long follow-up of these patients.

An old but very useful classification was described by Ward and Lerner (1947):

1. *Congenital*
   (a) Total hypertrophy involving all systems can be segmental, crossed or hemihypertrophy.
   (b) Limited hypertrophy involving one or more systems; muscular, vascular, skeletal, neurological.
2. *Acquired*
   (a) Total hypertrophy, e.g. gigantism resulting from hyperpituitarism or neurofibromatosis or Silver's syndrome (Silver, 1964).
   (b) Limited, e.g. elephantiasis: Milroy's disease, lipomatosis, neurofibromatosis, arteriovenous aneurysms.

Vascular anomalies, e.g. haemangiomata, telangiectasis and varices (in Milroy's disease) are frequently associated with asymmetry, especially when the lesions are deep, extensive, multiple or diffuse. The condition of infantile angioectatic hyperplasia when associated with Klippel–Trenaunay–Weber syndrome (Figure 3.66; nerves, bone and soft tissue hypertrophy and venous varicosities) and Parker–Weber syndrome can present with significant

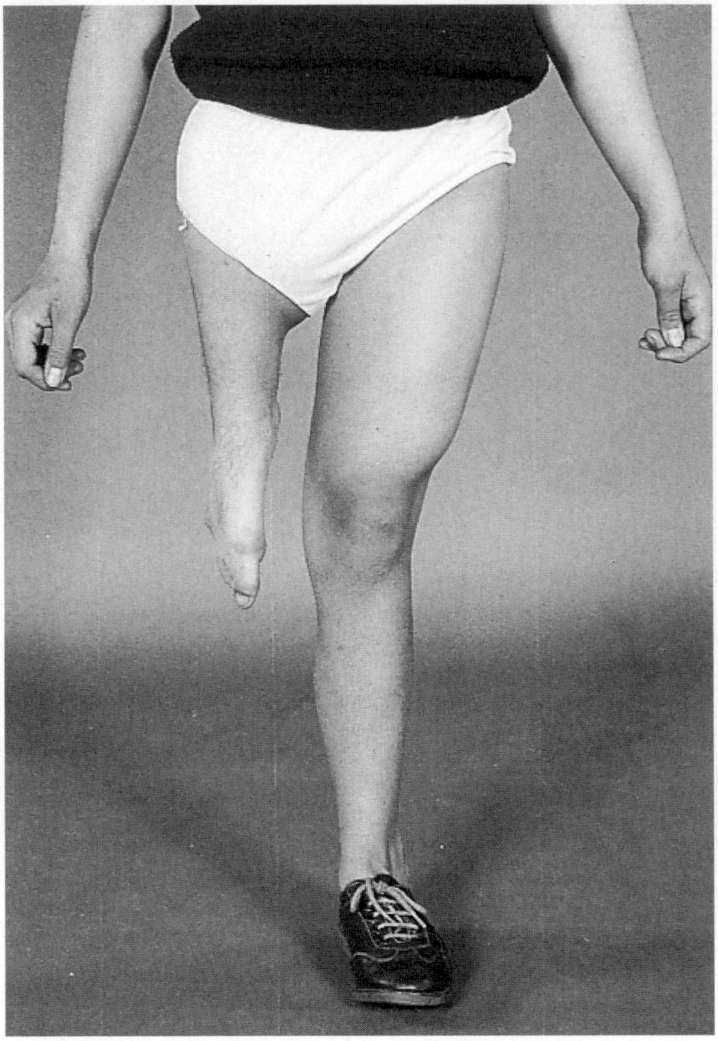

(a)

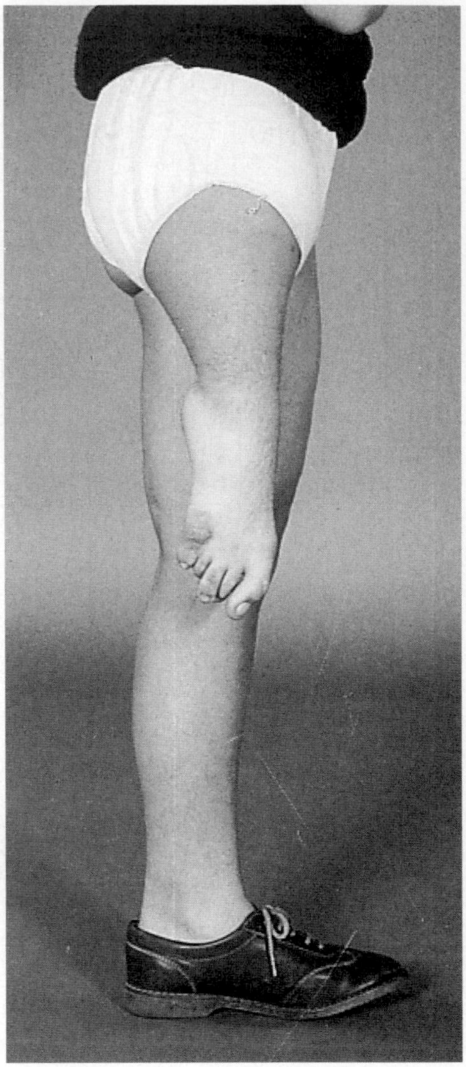

(b)

Figure 3.62 (a,b) Photographs, anteroposterior and lateral, to show a deformity of the foot and knee level without any angular deformity above – due to marked deficiency of femur, tibia and a hypoplastic knee.

asymmetry. Shapiro (1982) found that in 83% of his series overgrowth had occurred with vascular anomalies.

McCullough and Kenwright (1979) have classified patients with generalized lower limb hypertrophy and leg length discrepancy into two main groups:

1. *Congenital total hypertrophy*
   (a) Segmental type, in which there was involvement of other structures on that side of the body.
   (b) Crossed type, with overgrowth of one-half of the body and segmental hypertrophy of the other side.
   (c) Hemihypertrophy, with overgrowth of the entire one side of the body.

   In these groups there was hypertrophy of all tissues of the involved limb, without neurological deficit. (There is often difficulty in deciding whether one limb or side of the body is hypertrophied or the other atrophied.) Muscle power was normal. Leg length discrepancy ranged from 2.6 cm in one group at the end of growth, to more extensive discrepancies in another group who required surgical corrective methods of epiphyseodesis, subtrochanteric osteotomy with segment removal, etc.

2. *Lower limb hypertrophy with congenital vascular abnormality*. This group comprised the Klippel–Trenaunay syndrome – the triad of congenital limb hypertrophy associated with varicose veins and cutaneous haemangiomata.

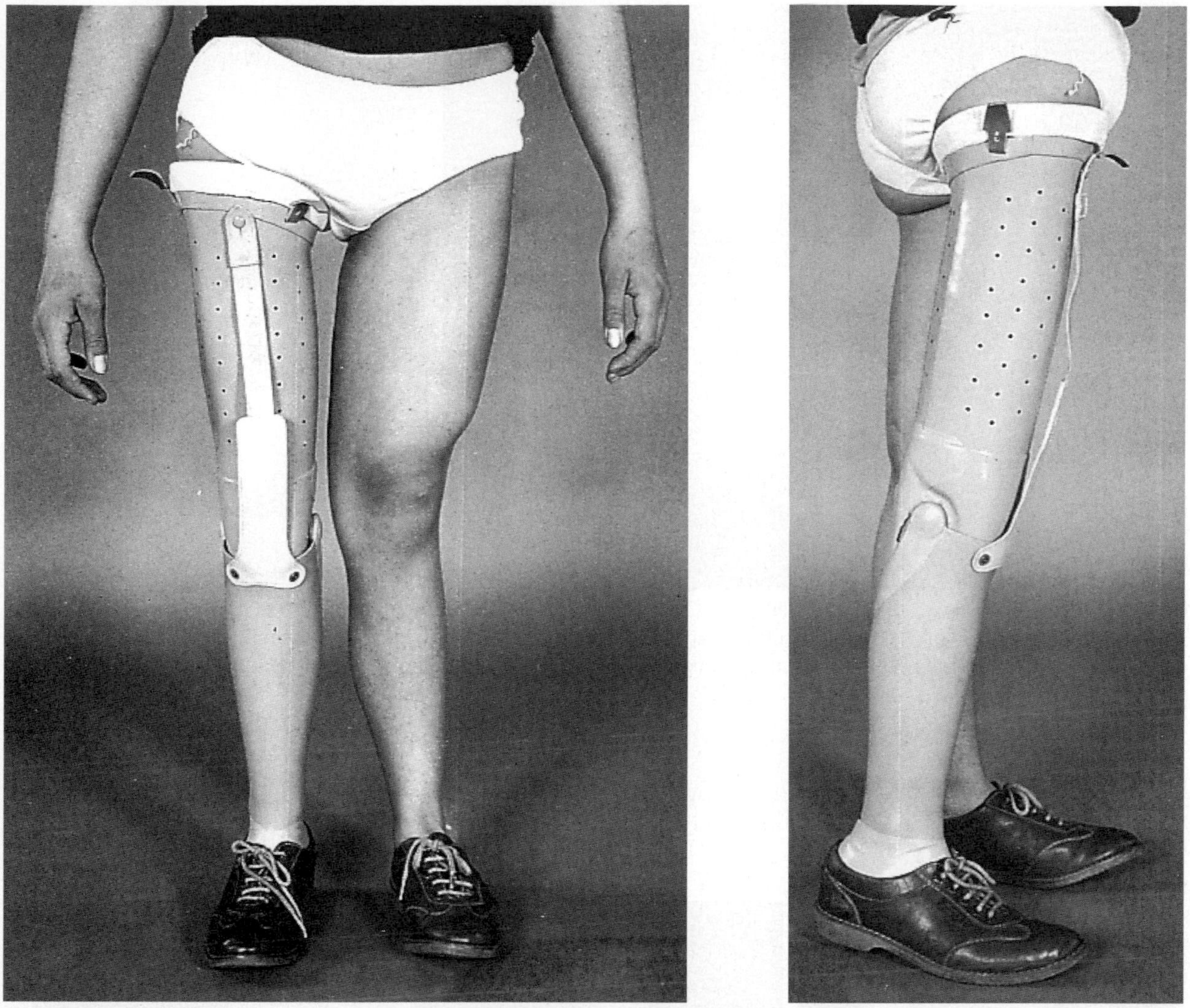

(a) (b)

Figure 3.63 (a,b) An ischial-bearing arthrosis for weight-bearing and walking with knee and ankle joints.

Gigantism of the toes was also seen with congenital diffuse arteriovenous fistulae, with a bruit as well as ulceration and pain.

Angiography is a most helpful procedure for differentiating between the lesions of normal or diffusely dilated veins, those with intramuscular cavernous angiomata and those with true fistulae formation requiring surgical correction.

It is very important to be able to predict at an early stage the expected leg length discrepancy when growth has ceased so that appropriate and timely regimens can be carried out. Also, the parents need to know an accurate prognosis, particularly for the cosmetic appearance of the limb as well as its function.

TREATMENT

Treatment of the primary cause, e.g. vascular haemangioma, arteriovenous fistula, lymphangioma, is usually undertaken by vascular surgeons, Wilms tumour (nephroblastoma) by urologists, etc. However, for congenital segmental or crossed hemihypertrophy, leg shortening by epiphyseodesis, resection osteotomy, or more recently leg lengthening can be performed.

In planning for surgery full leg length radiographs are taken on the same plate side by side with an engraved length marker. Shapiro (1982) has defined five abnormal patterns of growth with their growth potential of the bad leg. Bone age assessment using the Greulich and Pyle's atlas (1959) or more recently Tanner and Whitehouse's atlas (1982), is carried out and from this, growth potential and even velocity can

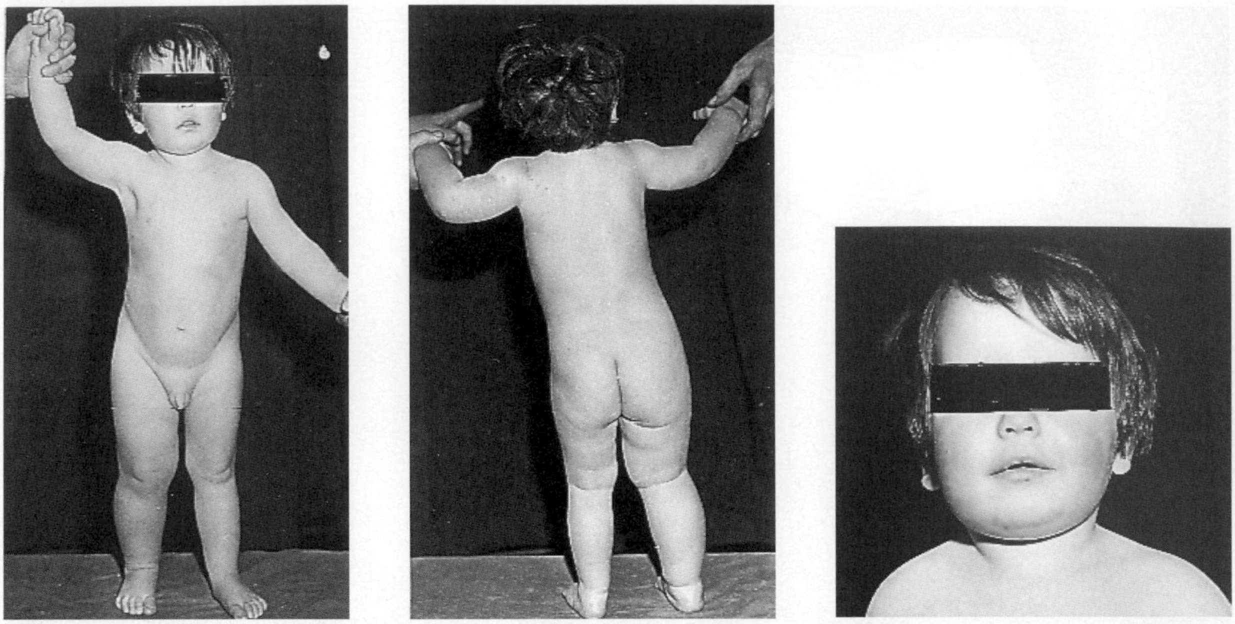

(a) (b) (c)

Figure 3.64 (a,b) Frontal and posterior photographs of a 2-year-old boy showing the idiopathic congenital hypertrophy of the right lower extremity with its effects upon the posture of standing. (c) Photograph of face to show the hypertrophy of the right side.

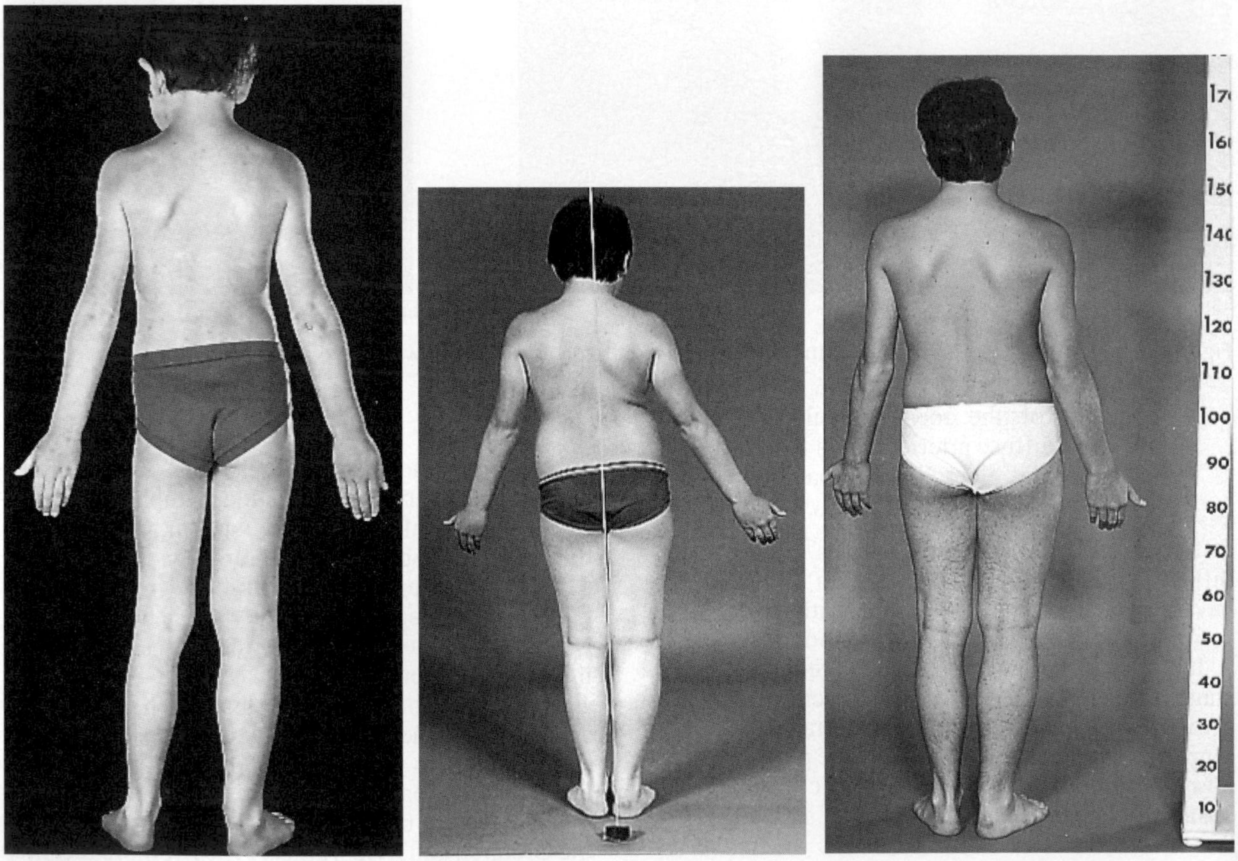

(a) (b) (c)

Figure 3.65 (a) Posterior photograph of the same boy as in Figure 3.64 at the age of 7 years, with the idiopathic congenital deformity persisting and now a scoliosis. (b) Same boy at age 13 years with a scoliosis deformity. (c) Same boy at age 17 years without the scoliosis deformity.

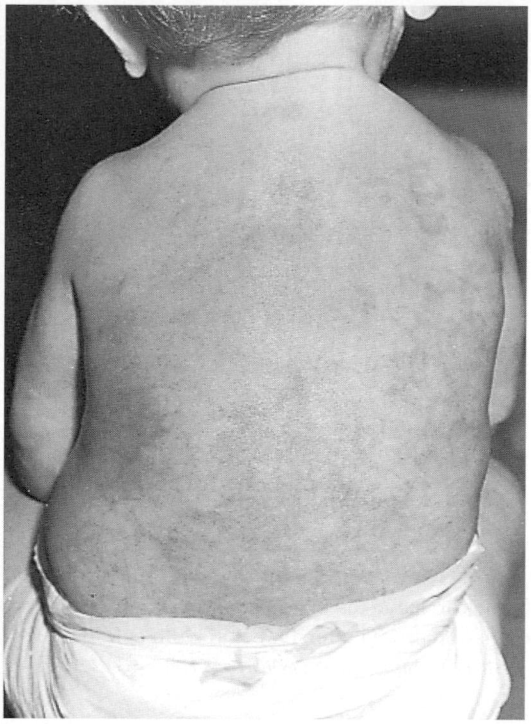

(a)

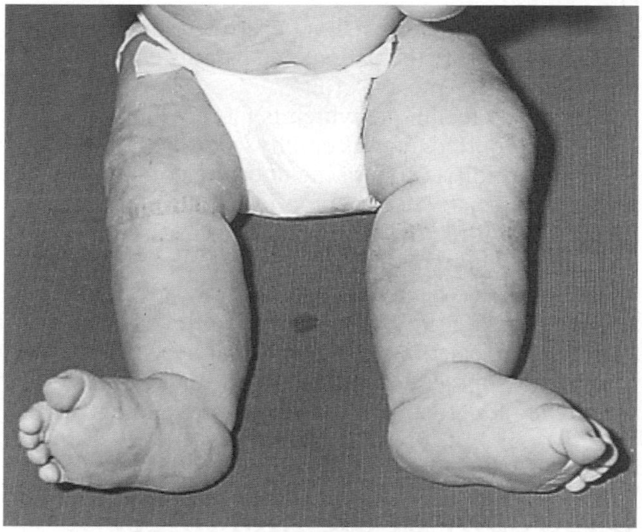

(b)

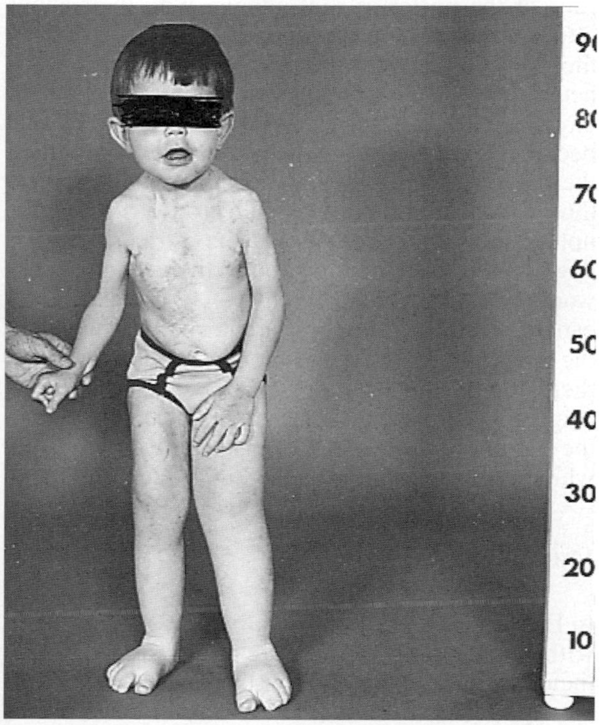

(c)

Figure 3.66 (a,b) A child with Klippel–Trenaunay–Weber syndrome at the age of 1 year showing the port wine stain of the trunk and the hemihypertrophy of the left lower extremity. (c) The same child at age 4 years, showing the increasing hypertrophy of the left lower extremity and the trunk port wine staining.

be worked out. Specifically, when the actual pattern of growth is found by serial measurements, 'growth' charts are available but there are difficulties in determining accurately skeletal age or velocity in the dysplasias, in different races, in circumstances of illness or inactivity, and at different times of growth, etc.

When making the decision to perform surgery and in discussing with the patient and parents composite photographs are most useful.

The oldest technique which is more widely practised and reported upon is epiphyseodesis. It has the lowest morbidity, is operating upon the non-affected leg and is relatively uncomplicated, but accurate prediction with knowledge of growth is essential.

Femoral shortening, particularly for up to 5 cm discrepancy, has been recommended by McCullough and Kenwright (1979). This can be achieved by subtrochanteric osteotomy, or mid-diaphyseal osteotomy, or a supracondylar osteotomy, etc. Equalization by leg lengthening is still being developed.

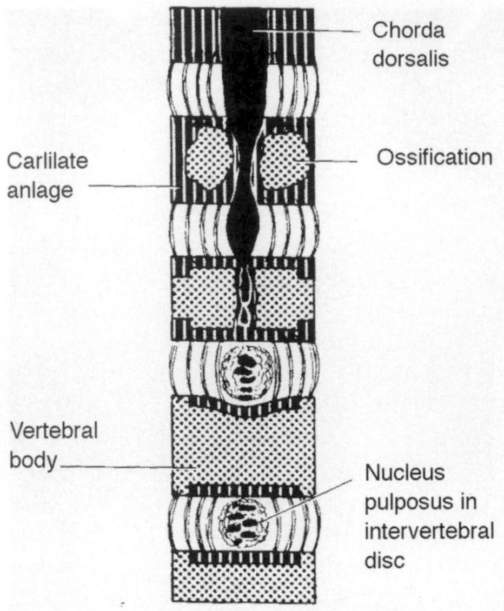

Figure 3.67 The development and closure of the vertebral bodies, to leave the nucleus pulposus. (Reproduced, with permission, from Fuller, D. J. and Duthie, R. B. (1974) *AAOS Instructional Course Lectures* **23**, 53–61)

Dystrophy of the fifth finger

A curious dystrophy of the fifth finger, where there is a lateral curve of the distal phalanx, was described by Kirner (1927). The condition is often bilateral, is more common in females, and occurs round about the age of 10. The finger appears to be short and the tip curves outwards. There is no pain or tenderness, and, in fact, beyond the deformity, there are no symptoms. No cause is known.

Spina bifida

DEVELOPMENT OF THE SPINAL CORD

In the third and fourth weeks of intrauterine life the neural groove appears on the dorsum of the embryo. This deepens into a furrow and finally closes off to form the neural canal which then develops into the whole central nervous system. The lumen persists as the central neural canal. Closure starts in the cervical region and proceeds caudally and cranially, the cranium closing last at about 26 days. After the neural tube has been formed, proliferating cells of the neuroepithelium differentiate to form neuroblasts or neurons of the spinal cord. Processes of these grow out from the cord as the motor axons of the peripheral nerves. The neural crest, after the enfolding between the ectoderm and the posterior surface of the neural tube, forms the sensory neurons of the posterior root ganglia with their axons into the peripheral nerves. The meninges arise from the loose mesenchymal tissues surrounding the neural tube. The pia mater differentiates at about 40 days, and the dura slightly later. The neural canal becomes separated from the ectodermal covering of the body by an ingrowth of mesoderm. Anterior to the neural canal there is a solid rod of cells – the notochord – and around this the vertebral bodies develop. From each of the bodies there extend backwards two projections which grow round the neural canal to form the vertebral arch. The two halves of the arch fuse behind in the thoracic region and from there the fusion extends up and down the spine (Figure 3.67). When this fusion fails there is a gap in the vertebral neural arch, constituting spina bifida which is most common in the lumbosacral region.

INCIDENCE

In England and Wales approximately 2500 children with spina bifida cystica are born each year, an incidence of 2.5 per 1000 live births. However, there are significant differences between England, Wales and Northern Ireland – the latter two being 4.5 per 1000 live births. The world-wide incidence is about 1 per 1000 live births, being much lower in Japan, North America (Negroes having a lower incidence than Caucasians) and Australia.

If the anencephaly and encephalocele types are added to spina bifida – i.e. the neural tube defects – the prevalence in England and Wales is doubled. Antenatal screening of the α-fetoprotein (AFP), when performed between the 15th and 18th weeks of pregnancy, is now most important to identify the population of women at risk of having such an affected infant. If α-fetoprotein is raised, an amniocentesis should be performed, as well as ultrasonography of the fetus. AFP is an α-globulin with about the same molecular weight as albumin, and is synthesized by the fetal liver and the lining of the yolk sac. A woman having had a fetus with a neural tube defect has a 10-fold increased risk of the next child being similarly affected, and 50-fold with a third child. There appears to be a genetic predisposition to this condition, with some environmental factors determining the first child's affection.

The actual cause is not known, although contaminated potatoes have been blamed in humans. In animals, experimental defects have been produced by vitamin A deficiency, azodyes, x-irradiation, hyperthermia and disturbed zinc metabolism.

Genetic factors have been considered because of the higher frequency of diagnosis in monozygote twins, in girls and siblings. There are seasonal and geographic variations, e.g. in Ireland. A recent report from the Medical Research Council (MRC) Vitamin Study Research Group of Great Britain (1991) now recommend folic acid supplementation in early pregnancy of all high-risk mothers who have a prior history of delivering babies with neural tube defects.

PATHOGENESIS

Although spina bifida was first described in 1652 by Turl, with Morsagri in 1761 observing the association of spina bifida and hydrocephalus, it was von Recklinghausen in 1886 who suggested it was due to a failure of the posterior mass of the neural tube. Patten (1952) described it as an overgrowth of neural tissues, or failure of the pontine flexure around the site of the posterior closure defect – especially in myelomeningocele. Gordon in 1960 believed that if the opening of the IVth ventricle roof was delayed or never took place, overdistension of the neural canal occurred with encephalocele, anencephaly and spina bifida resulting. Kallen (1968) described, from a series of experiments, the inductive stimulus of the mesodermal tissue on the formation of the neural tube and its differentiating structures.

MORBID ANATOMY

This can be considered under the two headings of spina bifida cystica and spina bifida occulta (Figure 3.68).

Spina bifida cystica

Meningocele

In this type there is a saccular trusion of only the meninges – pia and arachnoid. The dura mater stops at the margin of the bony defect. The spinal cord is not involved, so there is no paralysis and the sac contains only cerebrospinal fluid. This makes up 5% of spina bifida cystica. Surgical closure is required in order to prevent rupture of the sac with the likelihood of meningitis. Associated lesions such as lipomata, cyst formation or dilation of the spinal canal – hydromyelin – may be found.

Myelomeningocele

The majority of cases of spina bifida cystica are of this type or variants of it. There is a gap in the posterior wall of the spinal column through which protrudes a flat plaque of neural tissue surrounded by meninges. The spinal cord is open on the surface of the back for a distance of three to four segments usually. The plaque and meninges are enlarged into a sac, by accumulation of cerebrospinal fluid, within a few hours of birth. The sac may be burst during or just after birth, to leak cerebrospinal fluid, and therefore infection may supervene. Infection of the exposed plaque may cause some necrosis of neural tissue unless the defect is closed, or even death which frequently follows from meningitis. There are three zones on the surface (Figure 3.69a):

1. Central neural plaque (vasculosa).
2. The meninges (serosa).
3. The surrounding hairy skin which is often thickened (dermatica).

In addition to failure of fusion of the bony arches, vertebral body deformity and absence of intervertebral discs may lead to spinal deformity, and a diastematomyelia may be present.

Syringomyelocele

In this type the spinal cord is spread out to form the lining of the sac and is thinned into a cyst by distension of the central canal of the cord.

Myelocele

This variant is characterized by the presence of gross spinal cord deformity and an elongated fissure

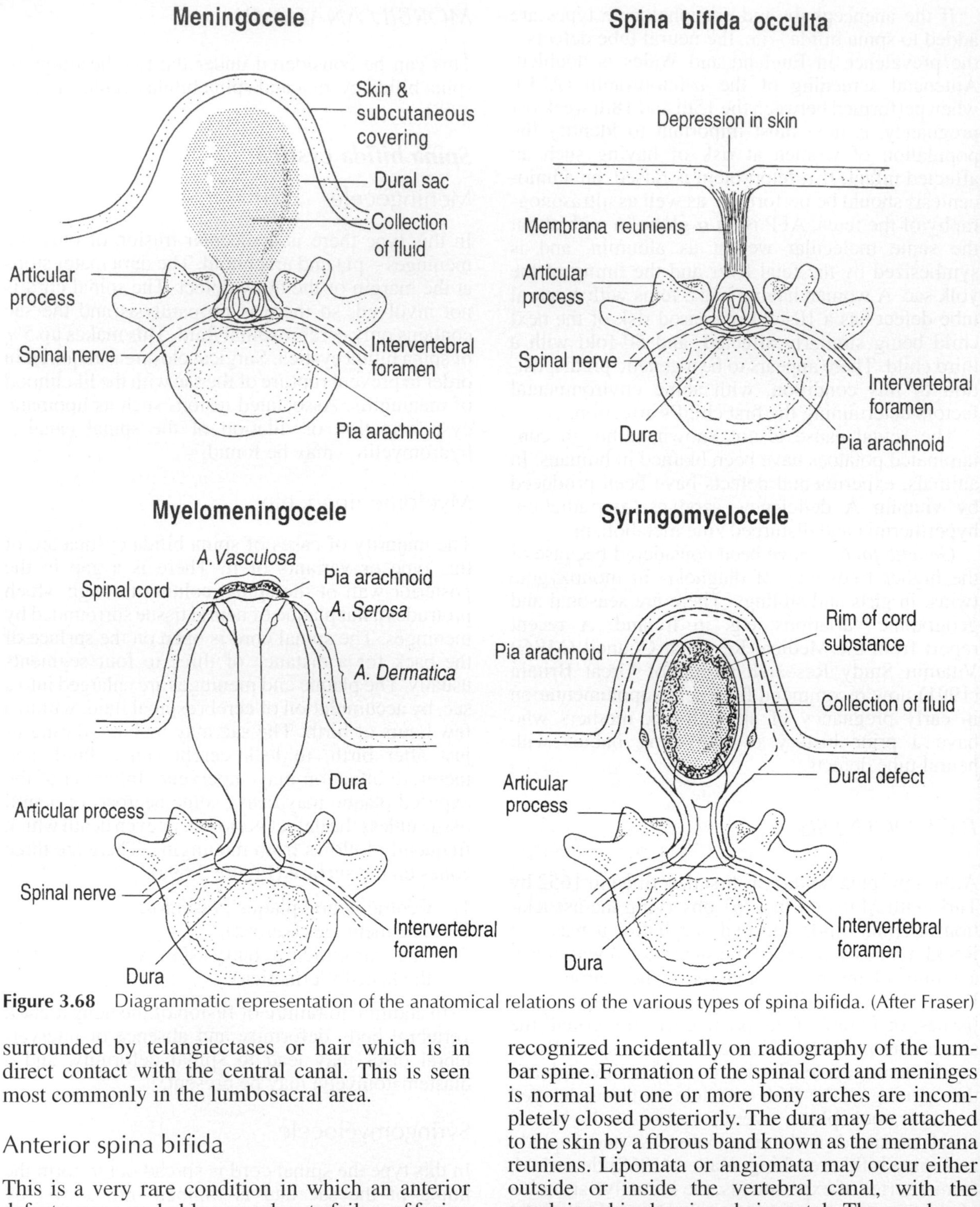

Figure 3.68 Diagrammatic representation of the anatomical relations of the various types of spina bifida. (After Fraser)

surrounded by telangiectases or hair which is in direct contact with the central canal. This is seen most commonly in the lumbosacral area.

Anterior spina bifida

This is a very rare condition in which an anterior defect occurs, probably secondary to failure of fusion of the two segments of the vertebral body.

Spina bifida occulta

This mild defect often passes unnoticed except when recognized incidentally on radiography of the lumbar spine. Formation of the spinal cord and meninges is normal but one or more bony arches are incompletely closed posteriorly. The dura may be attached to the skin by a fibrous band known as the membrana reuniens. Lipomata or angiomata may occur either outside or inside the vertebral canal, with the overlying skin showing a hairy patch. The membrana reuniens does not appear to increase in size with the growth of the child, so a traction lesion of the cord may occur around the age of 10 years, causing paralytic deformity of the lower limb or bladder.

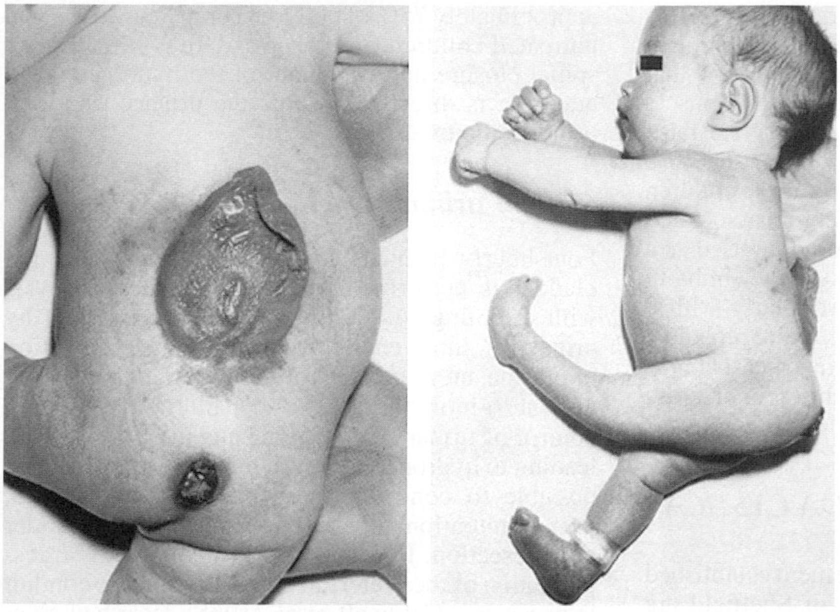

(a) (b)

Figure 3.69 A 2-month-old child with myelomeningocele, showing (a) the three zones and the frequently patulous anus, and (b) the appearance of dislocated hips, hyperextension of the left lower extremity, club foot, etc. (Patient of Mr Malcolm Gough)

There may be an associated intraspinal lesion – called by Till an occult spinal dysraphism:

1. diplomyelia or duplication of the spinal cord but within the same dural tube;
2. diastematomyelia, in which the spinal cord structures have been bivalved by a septum of bony, cartilaginous or even fibrous tissue between the lamina and vertebral body;
3. others – intraspinal lipomata or a hydromyelia of the central canal.

Urinary incontinence, neurological abnormalities (particularly in the lower extremities) or a meningitis resulting from an infection of a dermal sinus – all warrant radiography, myelography, etc., before any surgical exploration.

The American Academy of Orthopedic Surgeons Committee for the Care of the Handicapped Child (Donaldson, 1974) brought out the following useful classification of the open and closed defects making up neural spinal dysraphism.

Open defects

1. Myelomeningocele (hydromyelia, dysraphism rachischisis)
2. Meningocele.
3. Dermal sinus.

Closed defects

1. Spina bifida occulta:
   (a) diastematomyelia;
   (b) intraspinal tumour (lipoma, chondroangioma, dermoid).
2. Myelodysplasia:
   (a) aplasia or hypoplasia of nerve roots, or cord;
   (b) absent anterior horn cells (arthrogryposis);
   (c) diplomyelia (double cord).
3. Errors in skeletal segmentation:
   (a) absence of sacrum;
   (b) absent lumbar vertebrae;
   (c) hemivertebrae;
   (d) congenital segmental fusion;
   (e) failure of fusion or absence of odontoid process;
   (f) others.

At birth – selection for closure

Although the orthopaedic surgeon may not be actively involved in determining a policy of selection for closure, he may well be involved in evaluating the orthopaedic deformity. Stark and Baker (1967) described two main types:

- Type I (about 33%), in which there is complete loss of all spinal cord function below the level of the lesion with flaccid paralysis, sensory deficiency and absent reflexes.
- Type II (the remainder), in which there is preservation of reflex activities from the isolated and intact distal segment but with interruption of the corticospinal tracts with paralysis. In this large group there are three subgroups in which segments of flaccid paralysis, sensory and reflex losses vary in severity and in distribution.

When early operation at 48 hours without selection was carried out because of the initial optimism based upon the observation by Sharrard (1964) that there was likely to be some improved muscle function, it was found that although survival rates were improved (e.g. 60% alive at 3 years and 40% alive at 11 years), the quality of life for these children was pitiful. Lorber (1971) defined factors associated with a bad prognosis, and these should be used as a basis for selection: gross paralysis of the limbs in the thoracolumbosacral lesion, particularly with a scoliosis or kyphosis; an enlarging hydrocephalus; any evidence of an intracerebral injury; heart abnormality; and those who develop meningitis or gross mental disturbance.

TREATMENT OF SPINA BIFIDA CYSTICA

The principles of combined management established by Sharrard, Zachary and Lorber in Sheffield are directed towards the five major problems found with these children:

1. Myelomeningocele.
2. Hydrocephalus.
3. Urinary tract paralysis.
4. Locomotor system.
5. Education.

The aim of treatment, as with traumatic paraplegics, is to achieve independence as far as possible.

Surgical closure of the myelomeningocele defect is performed, when indicated, within the first 48 hours after birth, under general anaesthesia. Baseline neurological examination, measurement of head circumference and assessment of any hip dislocation are made before closure of the spine. The neural plaque, cord and nerve roots are isolated and the plaque is covered by suturing the dura over its surface in the form of a tube. The skin is then mobilized to cover the defect, which should be closed without fashioning flaps where possible. When the wound has healed (after 2–3 weeks), air ventriculography is performed to assess the presence and severity of hydrocephalus and the thickness of the compressed cerebral cortices. *Hydrocephalus* is treated by drainage of cerebrospinal fluid from the dilated lateral ventricles through a one-way ventriculoatrial Spitz–Holter type of silicone-rubber valve which is implanted subcutaneously behind the ear and drains via the internal jugular vein into the right atrium. Since the hydrocephalus arrests spontaneously by the age of 5 or 6 years, the valve is required to function only for this length of time; if it blocks or becomes infected, it can be replaced. Prompt recognition and treatment of hydrocephalus has resulted in a normal range of intelligence in approximately 75% of children compared with 2% in untreated children (Laurence and Tew, 1968). After spinal closure and treatment of the hydrocephalus, attention is directed towards the urinary tract and orthopaedic treatment.

Care of urinary tract

Four-hourly manual expression of urine from the bladder is performed if there is bladder paralysis with dribbling. Assessment of the urinary tract by urinalysis, intravenous pyelography and estimation of plasma, urea and electrolytes is necessary initially and at 6-monthly intervals. Failure to maintain control of urinary drainage results in back pressure leading to hydronephrosis. In most male patients it is possible to control urinary drainage. In females, urinary retention with overflow may require bladder neck resection. In some, urinary diversion by transplantation of the ureters to an ileal or colonic conduit is necessary. Caldwell *et al.* (1965) described electronic pacemakers which may make incontinence controllable in future. Control of continence has been improved by the use of drugs such as imipramine and propantheline (which inhibits detrusor contractions or hyperactivity).

Orthopaedic management of myelomeningocele

Unbalanced paralysis caused by spina bifida at different levels leads to paralytic deformities in the lower limbs, and Sharrard (1964) classified the neurological defects in patients with myelomeningocele into six groups according to the neurological level of the paralysis. He also correlated the radiological state of the hips and the deformities of knees and feet with the lower limit of innervation (Table 3.2).

However, the initial understanding and optimism by these earlier workers, that these were simple lower motor neuron lesions similar to poliomyelitis and to traumatic paraplegia and therefore could be operated upon by aggressive surgical techniques, subsequently proved to be a total failure and unacceptable. Indeed, it is not until the age of 3–4 years that an accurate muscle and neurological examination can be made and this requires to be performed accurately and serially.

It is now recognized that, in addition to the distal neurosegmental lesion, there are significant upper motor neuron lesions and distal reflex movements, as well as brain changes primary or secondary to the hydrocephalus, which alter all forms of coordination in the upper extremities, balance of the trunk, cognitive and visual efficiency, intelligence and

Table 3.2

Group	Neurological level	Sequelae
I	T12	Total flaccidity. Postural deformities only
II	L1 or L2	Moderate hip flexors and adductors. Hip subluxation. Occasional dislocation
III	L3 or L4	Hip flexors and adductors normal. Quadriceps normal Hip extensors and abductors paralysed; disclocation of hips recurvatum of knee
IV	L5	Hip flexors, adductors and quadriceps normal Hip extensors paralysed, abductors moderate – 50% have hip subluxation
V	S1 or S2	Hip extensors weak. Other groups normal – hips stable
VI	Normal	No deformity

therefore ability to respond and contribute to rehabilitative measures. More recently greater emphasis has been given to developing the intellectual capacity of these children, with very active rehabilitation programmes aimed at the upper extremities and at trunk support, to improve and maintain as much independence as possible.

The role of the orthopaedic surgeon, therefore, is to provide, by non-surgical or surgical means, the ability to sit and to stand as well as effective but not excessively demanding walking. To achieve this, the patient's centre of gravity must be over his feet and there should not be excessive flexion deformities of hips or knees.

Early management of the infant

Careful neurological examination should be carried out, together with a muscle power chart. Note is made of flexion deformities and contractures. Radiographs of hips are obtained to detect any subluxation or dislocation (Figure 3.70), and also of the spine – not only for the maldevelopment of the posterior elements but also for providing a baseline in the subsequent development of kyphosis or scoliosis.

Beaty and Canale (1990) in reviewing the orthopaedic aspects of myelomeningocele have pointed out that only 30% of these patients will function independently and only 30% have gainful employment. All will use a wheelchair when the lesion is at the level of L1 or higher, and when the lesion is lower

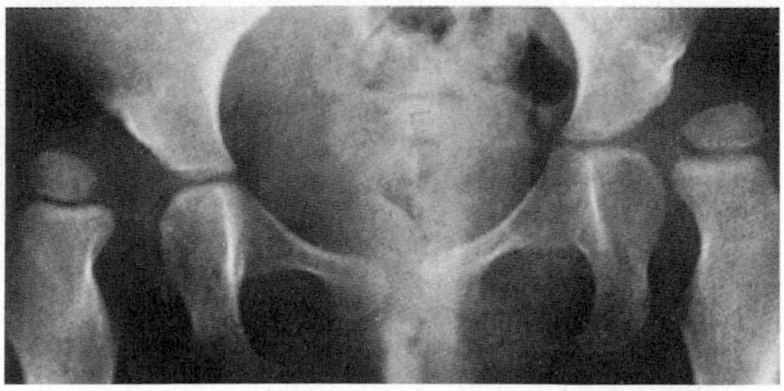

Figure 3.70 Radiograph of a patient with spina bifida and bilateral dislocation of the hips.

78% will use a wheelchair some of the time. They emphasize that a child who has not been able to stand independently by the age of 6 years is most unlikely to be able to walk, requiring a wheelchair or extensive orthotic support.

Obviously the upright posture with weight-bearing decreases the incidence of decubitus ulcer (about 17%), the risk of osteoporosis and improving the urological problems. But for this the child has to wear heavy braces with gross energy and time expenditures, motivation for much disappointment and this must be considered carefully. Roach (1990) has pointed out that every child around the age of 12 months should have the opportunity to try to stand and walk using standing tables and light and simplified braces. If the child and parents become more interested and committed, more advanced bracing can be tried. Light reciprocating braces for a four-point walking gait can be used by thin people with good control of head and trunk, without significant muscle contractures, and with a highly motivated family.

However, most children with a lesion above L1 will discontinue bracing and use a wheelchair. This should be properly prescribed and fitted for proper support for the buttocks and trunk as well as being able to fit axillary devices for independent function at home and school.

Mazur *et al.* (1989) have compared a matched group of patients with a high spina bifida who walked at an early age with those who used a wheelchair early in life. Only 30% who had walked were still able to do so effectively at the time of the study, e.g. 12–20 years of age. These had fewer fractures and pressure sores and were more independent than those who had used a wheelchair early, but the latter had spent fewer days in hospital. There were no differences in skills or in severity of obesity.

Some deformities respond to passive stretching and exercises taught to and practised by the parents. Splintage can be used, noting the degree of anaesthesia and its distribution; however, night splintage can often produce ulceration and, indeed, because the muscle imbalance is often excessive, splintage will fail. Immobilization should be limited because of the risk of pathological fracture, which may be as high as 20%. Menelaus (1980), in an excellent and authoritative monograph, has summarized the functional expectations, the aims of treatment to the level of the neurosegmental lesion:

1. Children with *upper thoracic lesions* lack sitting stability and require spinal support to enable them to sit with their hands free; 85% will develop scoliosis requiring surgical correction and fusion. The goals to be achieved are good sitting balance, walking ability until age 15 if upper limb function is good and the ability to transfer from a chair.
2. Children with *lower thoracic regions* are usually good sitters with independent transfer. They usually walk in childhood but require a wheelchair around the age of 15. They have a high risk of trophic ulceration.
3. Children with *upper lumbar lesions* have activity in the hip flexors and adductors, weak quadriceps, flexion deformity of the hip and knee which requires surgical correction. They become household walkers in long braces but always require crutches, and some take to a wheelchair in adolescence.
4. Children with *lower lumbar lesions* have variable weakness around the hip and knee but usually have strong quadriceps. They are usually committed walkers with or without crutches, and surgical treatment is required only for muscle imbalance below the knee.
5. Children with *sacral lesions* require surgery only for foot deformities. Their goal is community walking without braces.

Banta and Lubicky (1990) pointed out that these children have often a combined local, cutaneous, neural and osseous complex pathology. In addition, 90% have hydrocephalus with or without an Arnold–Chiari syndrome. Hydromyelia occurs in over 50% and often there is scarring adhesions around the spinal cord following any repairs which can produce tethering of the cord. The clinical picture of local pain, progressive spinal deformity with increasing spasticity and weakness of muscles in the legs demands myelography and CT examination followed by operative release of the tethered cord.

From experience they describe the goal of treating any spinal deformity which can be either congenital or paralytic or a mixture, in myelomeningocele patients, to obtain a compensated spine of normal height with preservation of normal sagittal alignment. Orthotic bracing of a total contact thoracolumbar type is useful in the paralytic curve until puberty. It will promote growth and a better sitting posture, but eventually these patients will require surgery. Even patients with osseous dysraphism at the level of the 12th thoracic vertebra or above are at great risk of a progressive severe scoliosis deformity and require arthrodesis (Piggott, 1980).

However, it should be appreciated that the risk of complications, e.g. sepsis, pseudarthrosis and loss of correction, is high. Combined anterior and posterior fusions with resection and internal instrumentation are required to achieve a major correction and stabilization. Improved posterior instrumentation, e.g. the Luque of Mexico or the Cotrel-Duboussett system of France, has in many cases reduced the necessity for anterior instrumentation. Similarly, better fixation to the pelvis of the posterior instrumentation has improved the pelvic obliquity deformity.

Kyphotic deformity is often associated with a marked gibbus, breakdown of the overlying soft tissues and progression leading to respiratory compromise, poor and fatiguing sitting posture, etc. Vertebral resection and short arthrodesis has been performed at birth (Letherman and Dickson, 1978) in order to achieve closure of the overlying soft tissues. During growth, recurrence with loss of correction can occur and this will require a refusion operation but of the whole spine (see Chapter 8).

Hip deformity and dislocation

The two common hip deformities are flexion and abduction.

Flexion deformity requires extensive anterior release, including sartorius, rectus femoris, iliacus, anterior hip capsule and other tight structures. Tension in the femoral nerve and vessels may prevent correction of more than 45° fixed flexion deformities; any additional correction can be obtained by subtrochanteric extension osteotomy. Early tenotomy of the psoas may prevent the development of severe flexion deformity.

Abduction deformity results from contracture of anterolateral structures, so abduction deformity is present while the hips are in extension and a flexion deformity develops when the hip is adducted to neutral. The deformity tends to be progressive and severe, and requires division of tensor fascia lata at its origin together with release of any other tight structures on the anterolateral aspect of the hip. It may also be necessary to divide the iliotibial band and lateral intramuscular septum as described by Yount (see Poliomyelitis, Chapter 7).

Obviously these are major surgical procedures demanding much from the patient. An early and sensible decision has to he made whether the child is going to be an active walker or will live within the confines of a wheelchair. The latter should not be submitted to major procedures.

Barden *et al.* (1975) found no correlation between walking ability and the dislocated or reduced state of the hips. All patients with deficit below L3 and bilateral hip dislocation were walking and pain free (Feiwell, 1980). Treatment of a paralytic dislocation is not as important as correcting any fixed deformity so that the child can stand with a stable posture. The strength and lack of any spasticity should be carefully noted because it has now been shown that iliopsoas transplantation and reduction of hip dislocation should be reserved for children who have strong quadriceps and weak glutei – i.e. those who will be walkers with below-knee braces. These patients have most to gain from radical hip surgery and the majority are severely handicapped if it is not carried out, whereas children with weak quadriceps should have simple tendon division or excision to correct any fixed deformity and recurrence prevented. Unilateral hip dislocation will cause leg length discrepancy with poor sitting balance and pelvic obliquity. Therefore, it should be treated unless contraindicated by late diagnosis, obesity, previous hip surgery or stiff hips. Menelaus (1980) has described how dislocation is generally due to active hip flexors (especially iliopsoas) with or without active adductors in the absence of abductors and extensors. Many present at birth but usually become obvious during the first 4 years. Later dislocation is commonly associated with pelvic obliquity secondary to a lumbar scoliosis. Carroll and Lindseth (1990) have divided the children into two groups:

1. The dislocation is found at birth and therefore congenital or teratological. If bilateral, no operation is indicated and the goal is to prevent contractures which can interfere with walking within an orthotic support, until the child uses a wheelchair, usually by the age of 10 years.
2. The dislocation results from muscle imbalance due to paralysis. If the child has a low lumbar lesion, reduction of the hips is indicated to prevent progressive deformity which would interfere with walking. Operation is particularly indicated in the unilateral dislocation between the ages of 1 and 3 years and has a stable neurological status. It can also be indicated in the older child with bilateral dislocation which has progressed from a subluxation and who has been walking with a lower lumbar lesion.

Treatment of hip dislocation

Correction of flexion/adduction deformity is by radical adductor release, plus iliopsoas division. There is usually no difficulty in reducing the hip at

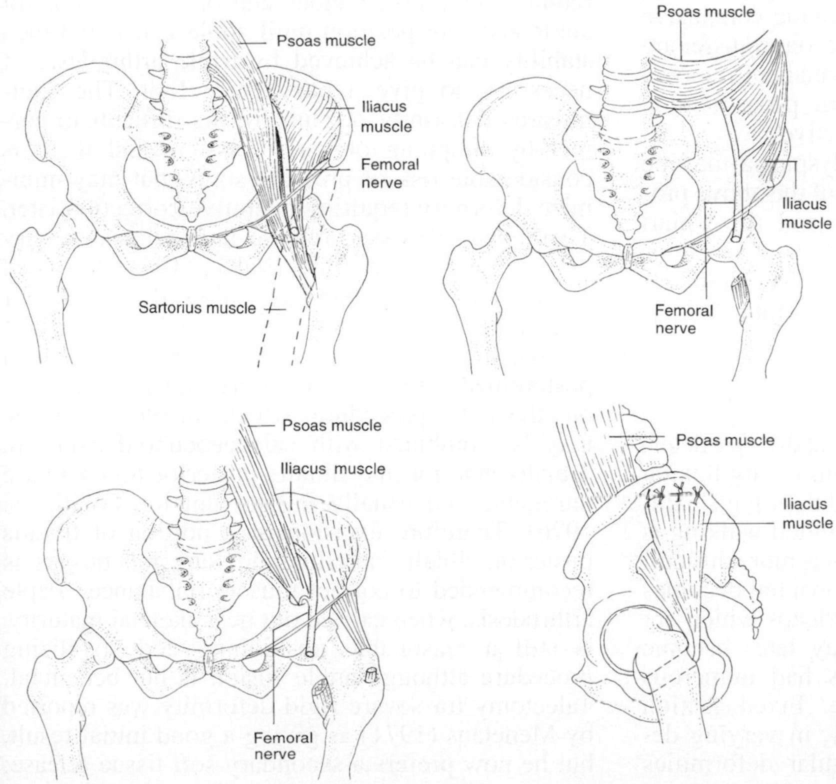

Figure 3.71 The various steps in a psoas muscle transfer operation.

this stage and holding it for a short period in an abduction plaster.

Correction of muscle imbalance is imperative, when present, by:

1. Mustard procedure (Mustard, 1959) – transferring the iliopsoas laterally into greater trochanter (Figure 3.71). This usually prevents dislocation but without any functional improvement (Cruess and Turner, 1970). This transfer tends to act as flexor abductor, whereas extension is required and later it causes a troublesome flexion/abduction deformity.
2. Posterolateral iliopsoas transfer as described by Sharrard (1964). It has been shown to be generally successful in preventing dislocation, although other series report higher incidences of redislocation and only variable functional improvement (Cruess and Turner, 1970; Carroll and Sharrard, 1972; Parker and Walker, 1975). Although electrical activity can be demonstrated in the muscle during hip flexion, the procedure rarely confers significant power of abduction or extension; indeed, some regard it purely as tenodesis. Some patients lose the ability to climb stairs because of weakened hip flexion, and abduction deformity occasionally occurs.
3. Psoas tendon excision. Despite the good results reported above, Menelaus (1980) has expressed doubt concerning the efficacy of iliopsoas transfer. The literature does not provide conclusive evidence that the results of iliopsoas transfer are due to anything more than permanent removal of psoas action and therefore psoas tendon excision might be equally effective.

   Correction of acetabular dysplasia may be necessary, combined with any of the above procedures; both the Pemberton and the Chiari osteotomy have been described, as well as a femoral osteotomy to correct rotational or angular deformities of the upper femur.

Knee deformities

Obviously the absence of strong quadriceps determines the walking ability of the child. Any flexion deformity implies quadriceps weakness with hamstring contracture, and therefore limited walking is likely in adult life. Hamstring spasm is more difficult to elicit when the patient is lying down but becomes apparent on weight-bearing. Quadriceps which are recorded as strong in infancy may later become weak, especially if the child has had numerous operations or has become obese. Fixed flexion deformities occur most commonly, in varying degrees of severity, with other angular deformities being quite rare. Until the age of 10 years or more, knee–ankle–foot arthoses are required for quadriceps weakness, as well as for preventing hyperextension or flexion deformities of the knee.

Management of quadriceps weakness without deformity can be improved by a hamstring transfer to quadriceps. However, when there is a fixed flexion deformity, an Egger procedure with hamstring lengthening and/or division, or transfer to distal femur will give a 50% decrease in fixed flexion deformity to less than 20% (Abraham *et al.*, 1977). Hamstring transfer to patella is probably more effective, but can lead to stiffness in extension which may be painful and a great handicap in sitting (Frank and Fixsen, 1980). Wound closure difficulties may not allow full correction initially but can be accomplished with a change of cast after an interval of 1–2 weeks. Incomplete correction usually carries a high risk of recurrence. A supracondylar osteotomy is not suitable for older children with gross deformity. If performed at a younger age, it may need to be repeated and can cause awkward anterior angulation of the femoral condyles.

Foot and leg deformities

Almost every fixed foot deformity which can occur does so in spina bifida, and almost invariably leads to pressure areas requiring complete operative correction. However, a flail foot with mobility above requires appropriate shoes and orthoses to control ankle and foot position until adolescence and then stability can be achieved by triple arthrodesis, if necessary, to give a plantigrade foot. The equinovarus deformity or club foot is difficult to correct by strapping or serial plasters and there is considerable risk of pressure sores, but may minimize deformity requiring operative correction later. Therefore, soft tissue release is usually necessary during the first year of life. Walker (1971) described good results from strapping followed by posterior release. However, Menelaus showed that one-half of his patients required further surgery after radical posteromedial release. Therefore, most authors favour the latter procedure, which, in older patients, may be combined with calcaneocuboid excision. Tibialis anterior and tibialis posterior transfers are unreliable and usually fail to function (Williams, 1976). Therefore excision of a portion of tibialis posterior, tibialis anterior and long toe flexors is recommended to correct muscle imbalance. Triple arthrodesis, when carried out near skeletal maturity, is still a reasonable positioning and stabilizing procedure although ankle fusion is not beneficial. Talectomy for severe rigid deformity was reported by Menelaus (1971) as giving a good initial result, but he now prefers a secondary soft tissue release;

feet that develop recurrent deformity after talectomy are very difficult to manage (Menelaus, 1980). Persistent varus deformity can be corrected by a closing wedge osteotomy of the calcaneus – after Dwyer (1963).

The equinus deformity is common. Caused either by the effect of gravity on flail foot with contracture of the tendo Achillis or by spastic calf and toe flexors, it gives rise to a severe deformity of the hindfoot. Dias and Drennan (1990) have described the operations required for correcting a persistent valgus deformity of the ankle. A fibular tenodesis with the tendo Achillis can be carried out for mild deformity in children with a low lumbar lesion between the ages of 6 and 10 years with a medial tibial epiphyseodesis; in an older child a supramalleolar osteotomy is performed.

The calcaneus deformity with the prominent heel is prone to ulceration and difficult to accommodate in shoes. There a tibialis anterior transfer has been reported as giving good results (Turner and Cooper, 1971), the tibialis anterior being transferred through the interosseous membrane into the lateral aspect of os calcis, provided tibialis anterior has a power of 3. Transfer of other anterior muscles may lead to equinus deformity, and strongly active toe extensors and peronei should be tenotomized, but revision rates are often too high. A subtalar arthrodesis for valgus deformity at 4–10 years is also recommended. A triple arthrodesis is also of use in varus deformity, when (unlike valgus deformity) bony excision is required. Menelaus (1980) has described a lateral inlay fusion, excising a rectangle of bone from the junction of talus, navicular, cuboid and calcaneum, replacing it with a corticocancellous graft and inserting a cancellous graft into the subtalar joint.

A vertical talus deformity has been described by Sharrard and Grosfield (1968) resulting from a sacral lesion and therefore has good walking potential. At 12–18 months of age, they recommend a soft tissue release with transfer of peroneus brevis behind the tibia to navicular, or of tibialis anterior into the neck of talus (Walker and Cheong-Leen, 1973) or an extra-articular subtalar arthrodesis of Grice-Green (if unsuitable for tendon transfer). In older children, the above procedures can be carried out, but with excision of the navicular in order to correct the deformity.

References

Abraham, E., Verinder, D.G.R. and Sharrard, W.J.W. (1977) The treatment of flexion contracture of the knee in myelomeningocele. *Journal of Bone and Joint Surgery* **59B**, 433

Addison, A., Fixsen, J.A. and Lloyd-Roberts, G.C. (1983) A review of the Dillwyn–Evans type collateral operation in severe clubfeet. *Journal of Bone and Joint Surgery* **65B**, 12–14

Aitken, G.T. and Frantz, C.H. (1953) The juvenile amputee. *Journal of Bone and Joint Surgery* **35A**, 659

Andersen, K.S., Bohr, J. and Sneppen, O. (1968) Congenital angulation of bow legs; cross-curvature congenitum. *Acta Orthopaedica Scandinavica* **39**, 387–397

Arey, L.B. (1965) *Developmental Anatomy: a Textbook and Laboratory Manual of Embryology*, pp. 210–212. Saunders: Philadelphia and London

Artz, T.D., Levine, D.B., Lim, W.N., Salvatie, E.A. and Wilson, P.D. (1975) Neonatal diagnosis, treatment and related factors of congenital dislocation of the hip. *Clinical Orthopaedics and Related Research* **110**, 112–116

Arzimanoglu, A. (1976) Treatment of congenital hip dislocation by muscle release, skeletal traction and closed reduction in children. *Clinical Orthopaedics and Related Research* **119**, 70–75

Attenborough, C.G. (1972) Early posterior soft tissue release in severe congenital talipes equinovarus. *Clinical Orthopaedics* **84**, 71–78

Badgley, C.E. (1949) *Journal of Bone and Joint Surgery* **31A**, 341

Bansal, V.P., Daniel, J. and Rai, J. (1988) Radiological score in the assessment of clubfoot. *International Orthopaedics* **12**, 181–185

Banta, J.V. and Lubicky, J.P. (1990) Spinal deformities. In: Beaty, J.H. and Canale, S.T. (1990) Orthopaedic aspects of myelomeningocele. *Journal of Bone and Joint Surgery* **72A**, 628–629

Barden, G.A., Mayer, L.C. and Stelling, F.H. (1975) Myelodysplastics. Fate of those followed for 20 years or more. *Journal of Bone and Joint Surgery* **57A**, 643

Barlow, T.G. (1962) Early diagnosis and treatment of congenital dislocation of the hip. *Journal of Bone and Joint Surgery* **44B**, 292

Barlow, T.G. (1966) *Proceedings of the Royal Society of Medicine* **59**, 1103–1106

Beaty, J.H. and Canale, J.T. (1990) Current concepts review. Orthopedic aspects of myelomeningocele. *Journal of Bone and Joint Surgery* **72A**, 626–630

Bensahel, H., Dal Monte, A., Hjelmstedt, A. *et al.* (1989) Congenital dislocation of the knee. *Journal of Pediatric Orthopedics* **9**, 174–177

Bensahel, H., Catterall, A. and Dimeglio, A. (1990) Practical applications in idiopathic clubfoot: a retrospective multicentric study in EPOS. *Journal of Pediatric Orthopedics* **10**, 186–188

Bernau, A. (1990) The Tubigen hip flexion splint for treatment of congenital hip dysplasia (in femurs). *Zeitschrift fur Orthopädie und ihre Grenzgebiete* **128**, 432–435

Bick, E.B. (1960) *American Journal of Diseases in Children* **100**, 861

Bigelow, D.R. (1969) Arthrogryposis. Proceedings. *Journal of Bone and Joint Surgery* **51B**, 191

Bleck, E.E. and Minaire, P. (1983) Persistent medial deviation of the neck of the talus: a common cause of in-toeing in children. *Journal of Pediatric Orthopedics* **3**, 149–159

Boden, S.D., Fallon, M.D., Davidson, R., Mennuti, M.T. and Kaplan, F.S. (1989) Proximal femoral focal deficiency. *Journal of Bone and Joint Surgery* **71A**, 1119–1129

Boyd, H.B. (1982) Pathology and natural history of congenital pseudarthrosis of the tibia. *Clinical Orthopaedics and Related Research* **166**, 5–13

Brookes, M. and Wardle, E.N. (1962) Muscle action and the shape of the femur. *Journal of Bone and Joint Surgery* **44B**, 398–411

Brougham, D.I. and Nicol, R.O. (1988) Use of the Cincinatti incision in congenital talipes equinovarus. *Journal of Pediatric Orthopedics* **8**, 696–698

Brougham, D.I., Cole, W.G., Dickens, D.R.V. and Menelaus, M.B. (1989) Torticollis due to a combination of sterno-mastoid contracture and congenital vertebral anomalies. *Journal of Bone and Joint Surgery* **71B**, 404–407

Brougham, D.I., Brougham, N.S., Cole, W.B. and Menelaus, M.B. (1990) Avascular necrosis following closed reduction of congenital dislocation of the hip. *Journal of Bone and Joint Surgery* **72B**, 557–562

Browne, Denis (1956) *Proceedings of the Royal Society of Medicine* **49**, 395

Burtch, R.L. (1963) The classification of congenital limb deficiency: a preliminary report. *Inter-Clinic Information Bulletin* 4–9

Caldwell, K.P.S., Flack, F.C. and Broad, A.P. (1965) *Lancet* **1**, 846

Carr, A.J., Jefferson, R.J. and Benson, M.K. (1993) Joint laxity and hip rotation in normal children and in those with congenital dislocation of the hip. *Journal of Bone and Joint Surgery* **75B**, 76–78

Carroll, N.C. and Lindseth, R.E. (1990) Dislocation of the hip. In: Beaty, J.H. and Canale, S.T. (1990) Orthopedic aspects of myelomeningocele. *Journal of Bone and Joint Surgery* **72A**, 629–630

Carroll, N.C. and Sharrard, W.J.W. (1972) Long-term follow-up of posterior iliopsoas transplantation for paralytic dislocation of the hip. *Journal of Bone and Joint Surgery* **54A**, 551

Carter, C.O. (1976) Genetics of common single malformations. *British Medical Bulletin* **32**, 21–27

Carter, C. and Wilkinson, J. (1964) Persistent joint laxity and congenital dislocation of the hip. *Journal of Bone and Joint Surgery* **46B**, 40

Cavendish M.F. (1972) Congenital elevation of the shoulder. *Journal of Bone and Joint Surgery* **54B**, 395

Chapple, C.C. and Davidson, C.T. (1941) A study of the relationship between fetal position and certain congenital deformities. *Journal of Pediatrics* **18**, 483

Chiari, K. (1970) *Journal of Bone and Joint Surgery* **52B**, 174

Coleman, S.S. (1992) The pericapsular (Pemberton) pelvic osteotomy and the redirectional (Salter) pelvic osteotomy. *Mapfre Medicina* **3**, Suppl. 1, 124–127

Crabbe, W.A. (1960) *British Medical Journal* **2**, 1060

Cruess, R.L. and Turner, N.S. (1970) Paralysis of hip abductor muscles in spina bifida. Results of treatment by the Mustard procedure. *Journal of Bone and Joint Surgery* **52A**, 1364

Dias, L.S. and Drennan, J.C. (1990) Spinal deformities. In: Beaty J.H. and Canale, S.T. (1990) The foot. Orthopedic aspects of myelomeningocele. *Journal of Bone and Joint Surgery* **72A**, 627–628

Dias, L.S., Jasty, M.J. and Collins, P. (1984) Rotational deformities of the lower limb in myelomeningocele. *Journal of Bone and Joint Surgery* **66A**, 215–223

Donaldson, W.F. (1974) Neural spine dysraphism. In: *Spinal Deformity in Neurological and Muscular Disorders*, p. 140. C.V. Mosby: St Louis, MO

Drachman, D.B. and Coulombe, A.J. (1962) Experimental club foot and arthrogryposis multiplex congenita. *Lancet* **1**, 523–526

Drummond, A.C., Siller, T. and Cruess, R. (1974) Management of AMC. *AAOS Instructional Course Lectures* **23**, 79–95

Drvaric, D.M., Kuivila, T.E. and Roberts, J.M. (1989) Congenital clubfoot, etiology, pathoanatomy, pathogenesis and the changing spectrum of early management. *Orthopedic Clinics of North America* **20**, 641–647

Dunkerton, M.C. (1989) Posterior dislocation of the shoulder associated with obstetric brachial plexus palsey. *Journal of Bone and Joint Surgery* **71B**, 764-766

Dunn, P.M. (1972) The anatomy of congenital dislocation of the hip. *Journal of Bone and Joint Surgery* **54B**, 174

Dunn, P.M. (1976) Congenital postural deformities. *British Medical Bulletin* **32**, 71–76

Duthie, R.B. and Hecht, F. (1963) The inheritance and development of the nail-patella syndrome. *Journal of Bone and Joint Surgery* **45B**, 259–267

Duthie, R.B. and Townes, P.J. (1967) The genetics of orthopaedic conditions. *Journal of Bone and Joint Surgery* **49B**, 229–248

Dwyer, F.C. (1963) The treatment of relapsed clubfoot by the insertion of a wedge into the calcaneum. *Journal of Bone and Joint Surgery* **45B**, 67–75

Engesaeter, L.B., Wilson D.J., Nag, D. *et al.* (1990) Ultrasound and congenital dislocation of the hip. *Journal of Bone and Joint Surgery* **72B** 197–201

Evans, D. (1961) The relapsed club foot. *Journal of Bone and Joint Surgery* **43B**, 722

Faciszewski, T., Kiefer, G.N. and Coleman, S.S. (1993) Pemberton osteotomy for residual acetabular dysplasia in children who have congenital dislocation of the hip. *Journal of Bone and Joint Surgery* **75A**, 643–649

Fahrenbach, G.J., Kuehn, D.N. and Tachdjian, M.O. (1986) Occult subluxation of the subtalar joint in clubfoot (using computerised tomography). *Journal of Pediatric Orthopedics* **6**, 334–339

Feiwell, E. (1980) Surgery of the hip in myelomeningocele as related to adult goals. *Clinical Orthopaedics and Related Research* **148**, 87

Ferguson, A.B. Jr (1968) *Orthopedic Surgery in Infancy and Childhood*. Williams and Wilkins: Baltimore, MD

Frank, J.D. and Fixsen, J.A. (1980) Spina bifida. *British Journal of Hospital Medicine* **24**, 422

Frantz, C.H. and O'Rahilly, R. (1961) Congenital skeletal limb deficiencies. *Journal of Bone and Joint Surgery* **43A**, 1204–1224

Fuller, D.J. (1984) Oxford Clubfoot Programme. Proceedings. *Journal of Bone and Joint Surgery* **66B**, 142–143

Fuller, D.J. and Duthie, R.B. (1974) The timed appearance of some congenital malformations and orthopedic abnormalities. *AAOS Instructional Course Lectures* **23**, 53–61

Gentry, J.Y., Parkhurst, E. and Rulin, G.V. Jr (1959) *American Journal of Public Health* **49**, 497

Gibson, A. (1923) A critical consideration of congenital radio-ulnar synostosis, with special reference to treatment. *Journal of Bone and Joint Surgery* **5**, 299

Gillespie, R. and Torode, I. (1983) Classification and management of congenital abnormalities of the femur. *Journal of Bone and Joint Surgery* **65B**, 557–568

Gould, N. (1962) *American Journal of Orthopedic Surgery* **4**, 2, 46, 1–2

Green, A.D. and Lloyd-Roberts, G.C. (1985) The results of early posterior release in resistant clubfoot. A long-term review. *Journal of Bone and Joint Surgery* **67B**, 588–593

Green, W.T. (1957) *Journal of Bone and Joint Surgery* **39A**, 1439

Greene, W.B. (1993) Infantile tibia varus. AAOS Instructional Course Lectures, vol. 42. *Journal of Bone and Joint Surgery* **75A**, 130–143

Greig, D.M. (1923) True congenital dislocation of the shoulder. *Edinburgh Medical Journal* **30**, 157

Greulich, W.W. and Pyle, S.I. (1959) *Radiographic Atlas of Skeletal Development of the Hand and Wrist*, 2nd edn. Stanford University: Stanford/Oxford University Press: Oxford

Gruneberg, H. (1964) The genesis of skeletal abnormalities. In: *Proceedings of the 2nd International Conference on Congenital Malformation*, 1963, pp. 219–223. International Medical Congress: New York

Hamilton, W.J., Boyd, J.D. and Mossman, H.W. (1962) *Human Embryology*. Heffer: Cambridge

Harrison, M.H. (1962) *Journal of Bone and Joint Surgery* **44B**, 858–868

Henkel, L. (1968) Das Fehebildungsmuster der Dysmelia (The pattern of malformation of dysmelia). *Beitrage zur Orthopädie und Traumatologie* **16**, 369–376

Henkel, L. and Willert, H.G. (1969) Dysmelia – a pattern of malformation and a classification of a new entity of congenital limb deformities. *Journal of Bone and Joint Surgery* **51B**, 399–414

Hensinger, R.N. (1991) Congenital anomalies of the cervical spine. *Clinical Orthopaedics and Related Research* **264**, 16–38

Herzenberg, J.E., Carroll, N.C., Christofersen, M.R., Lee, E.H, White, S. and Munroe, R. (1988) Clubfoot analysis with three-dimensional computer modelling. *Journal of Pediatric Orthopedics* **8**, 257–262

Hoaglund, F.T., Yau, A.C. and Wong, W.L. (1973) Osteoarthritis of the hip and other joints in Southern Chinese in Hong Kong. *Journal of Bone and Joint Surgery* **55A**, 545–548

Horche, H.T. and Kumar, J.J. (1991) The role of ultrasound in the diagnosis and treatment of congenital dislocation and dysplasia of the hip. *Journal of Bone and Joint Surgery* **73A**, 622–628

Idelberger, K. (1939) Die Ergebnisse der Zwillingsforschung beim angeboren Klumpfuss. *Verhandlung der Deutschen Orthopädischen Gesellschaft* **33**, 272

Jacob, F. and Monod, J. (1963) *Cytodifferentiation and Macromolecular Synthesis*. Academic Press: New York

Joseph, B., Carver, R.A., Bell, M.J. *et al.* (1987) Measurement of tibial torsion by ultrasound. *Journal of Pediatric Orthopedics* **7**, 317–323

Jurand, A. (1966) *Journal of Embryology and Experimental Morphology* **16**, 289–300

Kahle, W.K., Anderson, M.B., Alpert, J., Stevens, P.M. and Coleman, S.S. (1990) Value of preliminary traction in the treatment of congenital dislocation of the hip. *Journal of Bone and Joint Surgery* **72A**, 1043–1047

Kallen, B. (1968) Early embryogenesis of the central nervous system, with special reference to closure defects. *Developmental Medicine and Child Neurology* Suppl. 16

Kawashima, T. and Uhthoff, H.K. (1990) Development of the foot in prenatal life in relation to idiopathic clubfoot. *Journal of Pediatric Orthopedics* **10**, 232–237

Kite, H.J. (1961) *West Virginia Medical Journal* **57**, 92

Klisic, P. (1989) Congenital dislocation of the hip – a misleading term. *Journal of Bone and Joint Surgery* **71B**, 136

Kruger, L.A. and Talbott, R.D. (1961) Amputation and prosthesis as definitive treatment in congenital absence of the fibula. *Journal of Bone and Joint Surgery* **43A**, 625–642

Laaveg, J. and Ponsetti, I.V. (1980) Long-term results of treatment of congenital clubfoot. *Journal of Bone and Joint Surgery* **62A**, 23–31

Langenskiold, A. (1989) Tibia vara – a critical review. *Clinical Orthopaedics* **246**, 195–207

Laurence, K.M. and Tew, B.J. (1968) *Developmental Medicine and Child Neurology* Suppl. 11, 10

Lennox, I.A.C., McLauchlan, J. and Murali, R. (1993) Failure of screening and management of CDH. *Journal of Bone and Joint Surgery* **75B**, 72–75

Lenz, W. (1966) Malformations caused by drugs in pregnancy. *American Journal of Diseases in Children* **112**, 99–106

Letherman, K.D. and Dickson, R.A. (1978) Congenital kyphosis in myelomeningocele. Vertebral body resection and posterior spinal fusion. *Spine* **3**, 222–226

Letts, M. and Slutsky, D. (1990) Occipitocervical arthrodesis in children. *Journal of Bone and Joint Surgery* **72A**, 1166–1170

Levin, M.N., Kuo, K.N., Harris, G.F. and Matesi, D.V. (1989) Posteromedial release for idiopathic talipes equinovarus. A long term follow-up study. *Clinical Orthopaedics* **242**, 518–520

Lloyd-Roberts, G. and Lettin, A. (1970) AMC. *Journal of Bone and Joint Surgery* **52B**, 494–508

Lorber, J. (1971) Results of treatment of myelomeningocele. *Developmental Medicine and Child Neurology* **13**, 279

Marquardt, E. (1980) The operative treatment of congenital limb malformation, part 1. *Prosthetics and Orthotics International* **4**, 135–145

Mau, H., Dörr, W.M., Henkel, L. and Lutsche, J. (1971) Open reduction of congenital dislocation of the hip by Ludloff's method. *Journal of Bone and Joint Surgery* **53B**, 238

Mazur, J.M., Shurtliff, D., Menelaus, M. and Colliver, J. (1989) Orthopedic management of high level spina bifida. *Journal of Bone and Joint Surgery* **71A**, 56–61

McCullough, C.J. and Kenwright, J. (1979) The prognosis in congenital lower limb hypertrophy. *Acta Orthopaedica Scandinavica* **50**, 307–313

McFarland, B.L. (1951) *Journal of Bone and Joint Surgery* **33B**, 36

McKay, D.W. (1983) New concepts of and approach to clubfoot treatment: Section II – correction of clubfoot. *Journal of Pediatric Orthopedics* **3**, 10–21

MacKenzie, I.G. (1972) Congenital dislocation of the hip. The development of a regional service. *Journal of Bone and Joint Surgery* **54B**, 18

McKeown, J. and Record, R.G. (1960) In: *Congenital Malformations*. Ciba Foundation symposium. Edited by G.E.W. Wolstenholme and C.M. O'Connor. Churchill: London; Little, Brown: Boston, MA

McKibbin, B. (1970) Anatomical factors in the stability of the hip joint in the newborn. *Journal of Bone and Joint Surgery* **52B**, 148

Menelaus, M.B. (1971) Talectomy for equinovarus deformation in arthrogryposis and spina bifida. *Journal of Bone and Joint Surgery* **53B**, 238

Menelaus, M.B. (1980) *The Orthopaedic Management of Spina Bifida Cystica*. Churchill Livingstone: Edinburgh and London

Monson, R. and Gibson, D.A. (1978) Long-term follow-up of triple arthrodesis. *Canadian Journal of Surgery* **21**, 249–251

MRC Vitamin Study Research Group (1991) Prevention of neural tube defects. *Lancet* **338**, 131–137

Muller, G.M. and Seddon, H.J. (1953) Late results of treatment of congenital dislocation of the hip. *Journal of Bone and Joint Surgery* **35B**, 342

Mustard, W.T. (1959) A follow-up study of iliopsoas transfer for hip instability. *Journal of Bone and Joint Surgery* **41B**, 289

Nishimura, H. (1964) *Chemistry and Prevention of Congenital Anomalies*. Charles C Thomas: Springfield, IL

Norton, P.L. (1953) *Pediatric Clinics of North America* **3**, 1427

Ono, K. and Hayashi, H. (1974) Residual deformity of treated congenital clubfoot. A clinical study employing frontal tomography of the hind part of the foot. *Journal of Bone and Joint Surgery* **56A**, 1577–1585

O'Rahilly, R. (1951) Morphological patterns in limb deficiencies and duplifications. *American Journal of Anatomy* **89**, 155–187

Orenstein, E., Duonch, V. and Demos, T. (1985) Acute traumatic bowing of the tibia without fracture. *Journal of Bone and Joint Surgery* **67A**, 965–967

Palmer, R.M. (l964) Hereditary club foot. *Clinical Orthopaedics and Related Research* **33**, 138

Parker, B. and Walker, G. (1975) Posterior psoas transfer and hip instability in lumbar myelomeningocele. *Journal of Bone and Joint Surgery* **57B**, 53

Paterson, D.C. and Simonis, R.B. (1985) Electrical stimulation in the treatment of congenital pseudarthrosis. *Journal of Bone and Joint Surgery* **67B**, 454–462

Patten, B.M. (1952) Overgrowth of the neural tube in young human embryos. *Anatomical Record* **113**, 351

Pemberton, P.A. (1965) *Journal of Bone and Joint Surgery* **47A**, 65

Pho, R.W.H., Levack, B., Satku, K. and Patradul, A. (1985) Free vascularised fibula graft in the treatment of congenital pseudarthrosis of the tibia. *Journal of Bone and Joint Surgery* **67B**, 64–70

Piggott, H. (1980) The natural history of scoliosis in myelodysplasia. *Journal of Bone and Joint Surgery* **62B**, 54–58

Record, R.G. and Edwards, J.H. (1958) *British Journal of Preventive and Social Medicine* **12**, 8

Riordan, D.C. (1955) *Journal of Bone and Joint Surgery* **37A**, 1129

Roach, J.W. (1990) Orthoses. In: Beaty, J.H. and Canale, S.T. (1990) Orthopaedic aspects of myelomeningocele. *Journal of Bone and Joint Surgery* **72A**, 626–627

Saint-Hilaire, G. (1832) *A General or Particular History of Anomalies of Giantism, or A Textbook of Teratology*. Baillière: Paris

Salter, R.B. (1966) Role of innominate osteotomy in the treatment of congenital dislocation and subluxation of the hip. *Journal of Bone and Joint Surgery* **48A**, 1413

Salter, R.B. (1968) Etiology, pathogenesis and possible prevention of congenital diseases of the hip. *Canadian Medical Association Journal* **98**, 933–945

Saltzman, C.L., Hensinger, R.N., Blane, C.E. and Phillips, W.A. (1991) Familiar cervical dysplasia. *Journal of Bone and Joint Surgery* **73A**, 163–171

Sandridson, J., Redlundjohnell, I. and Uden, A. (1991) Why is congenital dislocation of the hip still missed: analysis of 96891 infants screened in Malmo 1956–1987. *Acta Orthopaedica Scandinavica* **62**, 87–91

Saunders, J.W. Jr, Cairns, J.M. and Gasseling, N.T. (1957) The role of the apical ridge of ectoderm in the differentiation of the morphological structure and inductive specificity of limb parts in the chick. *Journal of Morphology* **101**, 57–87

Scaglietti, C. and Calendriello, B. (1960) *International Orthopaedics* **43**

Shapiro, F. (1982) Developmental patterns in lower extremity length discrepancies. *Journal of Bone and Joint Surgery* **64A**, 639–651

Sharrard, W.J.W. (1964) *Journal of Bone and Joint Surgery* **46B**, 426

Sharrard, W.J.W. and Grosfield, I. (1968) The management of deformity and paralysis of the foot in myelomeningocele. *Journal of Bone and Joint Surgery* **50B**, 456

Silver, H.K. (1964) Asymmetry, short stature and variations in sexual development. *American Journal of Diseases of Children* **107**, 495–515

Smaill, G.B. (1968) Congenital diseases of the hip in the newborn. *Journal of Bone and Joint Surgery* **50B**, 453–454

Smith, M.D., Philips, W.A. and Hensinger, R.N. (1991) Complications of fusion to the upper cervical spine. *Spine* **16**, 702–705

Smith, R.J. (1973) Hand deformities in arthrogryposis multiplex congenita. *Journal of Bone and Joint Surgery* **55A**, 883

Smithells, R.W. (1965) Congenital asymmetry. *Developmental Medicine and Child Neurology* **7**, 698–700

Somerville, E.W. (1978) A long-term follow-up of congenital dislocation of the hip. *Journal of Bone and Joint Surgery* **60B**, 25

Staheli, L.T. (1989) Torsion – treatment indications. *Clinical Orthopaedics and Related Research* **247**, 61–66

Stanisavlevic, S. and Mitchell, C.L. (1963) Congenital dysplasia, subluxation and dislocation of the hip in stillborn and newborn infants. An anatomical pathological study. *Journal of Bone and Joint Surgery* **45A**, 1147

Stark, G.D. and Baker, G.C. (1967) The neurological involvement of the lower limb in myelomeningocele. *Developmental Medicine and Child Neurology* **9**, 732

Steindler, A. (1940) *Orthopedic Operations: Indications, Techniques and End Results*. Charles C Thomas: Springfield, IL

Stevenson, A.C. (1961) *British Medical Bulletin* **17**, 254

Strach, E.H. (1986) Clubfoot through the centuries. *Progress in Pediatric Surgery* **20**, 215–237

Summers, B.N., Turner, A. and Wynn-Jones, C.H. (1988) The Shelf operation in the management of late presentation in congenital dislocation of the hip. *Journal of Bone and Joint Surgery* **70B**, 63–68

Swann, M., Lloyd-Roberts, G.C. and Catterall, A. (1969) Anatomy of uncorrected club feet: study of rotation deformity. *Journal of Bone and Joint Surgery* **51B**, 263–269

Swanson, A.B. (1966) Classification of limb malformation on the basis of embryological failure. A preliminary report. *Inter-Clinic Information Bulletin* **6**, 1–15

Tanner, J.M. and Whitehouse, R.H. (1982) *Atlas of Children's Growth: Normal Variation and Growth Disorders*. Academic Press: London

Tayton, K.J.J. and Thompson, P. (1979) Relapsing club feet. *Journal of Bone and Joint Surgery* **61B**, 474

Tonnis, D. (1992) Radiological classification and diagnosis. *Mapfre Medicina* **3**, Suppl. 1, 42–45

Turco, V.J. (1979) Resistant congenital clubfoot – one stage posteromedial release with internal fixation. A follow-up report of a fifteen year experience. *Journal of Bone and Joint Surgery* **61A**, 805–814

Turner, J.W. and Cooper, R.R. (1971) Posterior transposition of tibialis anterior through the interosseous membrane. *Clinical Orthopaedics and Related Research* **79**, 71

Uhthoff, H.K. (1990) Die Embryologie der menschlichen Hufte unter besonderer Beruchsichtiging der Entwichling der Labra. *Zeitschrift fur Orthopädie und ihre Grenzgebiete* **128**, 341–343

Van Nes, C. (1950) *Journal of Bone and Joint Surgery* **32B**, 12

Waddington, C.H. (1964) Developmental mechanisms – introduction. In: *Proceedings of the 2nd International Conference on Congenital Malformation*. International Medical Congress: New York

Walker, G. (1971) The early management of varus feet in myelomeningocele. *Journal of Bone and Joint Surgery* **53B**, 462

Walker, G. and Cheong-Leen, P. (1973) Surgical management of paralytic vertical talus in myelomeningocele. *Developmental Medicine and Child Neurology* **15**, Suppl. 29, 112

Ward, J. and Lerner, H.H. (1947) A review of the subject of congenital hypertrophy and a complete case report. *Journal of Pediatrics* **31**, 403–414

Weinstein, S.L. (1992) Natural history of congenital hip dislocation (CDH) and hip dysplasia. *Mapfre Medicina* **3**, Suppl. 1, 65–74

Wilkinson, J.A. (1963) *Journal of Bone and Joint Surgery* **45B**, 268–283

Willert, H.G. and Henkel, L. (1968) *Die Dysmelie der oberen Extremitäten (Dysmelia of the Upper Extremities)*. Springer: Heidelberg

Williams, P. (1973) The elbow in AMC. *Journal of Bone and Joint Surgery* **55B**, 834

Williams, P.F. (1976) Restoration of muscle balance of the foot by transfer of the tibialis posterior. *Journal of Bone and Joint Surgery* **58B**, 217

Wilson, J.G. (1961) General principles in experimental teratology. In: *Proceedings of the 1st Conference on Congenital Malformation*, pp. 187–194. Edited by M. Fishbein. Lippincott: Philadelphia

Wolff, E. (1937) *Appointments, Distinction and Scientific Works*, p. 20

Wynne-Davies, R. (1964) *Journal of Bone and Joint Surgery* **46B**, 445–463

Wynne-Davies, R. (1970) *Journal of Bone and Joint Surgery* **52B**, 704

Zwilling, E. and Hansborough, L.A. (1956) Interaction between limb bud ectoderm and mesoderm in the chick embryo. III. Experiments with polydactylous limbs. *Journal of Experimental Zoology* **132**, 219–239

CHAPTER 4

Developmental Diseases of the Skeleton

ROBERT B. DUTHIE AND ROGER SMITH

Classification

Classification of skeletal dysplasias is changing as more syndromes are described and different syndromes are recognized as variants within a group. The following is based on the pathological classification of Aegerter and Kirkpatrick (1975).

I. Dysplasias due to disturbances in chondroid production

A. Abnormal maturation of growth plate chondroblasts
   1. The mucopolysaccharidoses (chondro-osteodystrophy).
   2. Idiopathic.
      (a) Achondroplasia.
      (b) Cartilage-hair hypoplasia.
      (c) Metaphyseal dysostosis.

B. Heterotopic proliferation of epiphyseal chondroblasts
   1. Enchondromatosis (dyschondroplasia; Olliers disease).
   2. Osteochondromatosis (hereditary multiple exostoses).
   3. Epiphyseal hyperplasia (dysplasia epiphysealis hemimelia).

II. Dysplasia due to disturbances in osteoid production

A. Abnormal epiphyseal ossification.

1. Diastrophic dwarfism.
2. Spondyloepiphyseal dysplasia.
3. Multiple epiphyseal dysplasia (Fairbank) – including Blount's and pseudoachondroplasia.
4. Stippled epiphyses.

B. Abnormal metaphyseal and periosteal ossification
1. Deficient osteoid production.
   (a) Osteogenesis imperfecta.
2. Excessive osteoid production or deficient osteolysis.
   (a) Osteopetrosis (Albers-Schönberg).
   (b) Pyknodysostosis.
   (c) Metaphyseal dysplasia (Pyle).
   (d) Diaphyseal sclerosis.
   (e) Melorheostosis.
   (f) Osteopathia striata.
   (g) Osteopoikilosis.
3. Abnormal osteoid production.
   (a) Polyostotic fibrous dysplasia.
   (b) Neurofibromatosis (p. 894).
   (c) Congenital pseudarthrosis (Chapter 3, p. 177).

III. Miscellaneous dysplasias

A. Dyschondrosteosis (Madelung).
B. Marfan's syndrome.
C. Apert's syndrome.
D. Cleidocranial dysostosis.
E. Chondroectodermal dysplasia.
F. Asphyxiating thoracic dysplasia.

The epiphyseal cartilage proliferates normally in columnar fashion and in due course undergoes maturation, degeneration and calcification in its conversion to bone. If the chondroblast is defective, multiple pathology may occur as a result of the failure or an irregularity in the maturation and calcification of the cartilage cell.

If the failure of maturation and calcification is diffuse, the lack of the zone of preliminary calcification will result in a widespread retardation of epiphyseal ossification and, therefore, dwarfism.

If the failure is irregular throughout the skeleton, multiple pathological pictures will appear, depending on the site of the abnormal chondroblasts.

A central immature chondroblast, If it continues to proliferate, will form an enchondroma, which gives the bone an apparent cystic appearance, and, if peripheral, this proliferating chondroblast will produce an enchondroma. If ossification occurs in relation to this peripheral group of cartilage cells, exostosis results. The primitive connective tissue cells may continue to proliferate when there is an absence of calcium in the adjacent zone of preliminary calcification, and as a result fibrous tissue masses will occur. The resultant picture is a conglomeration of stunted growth, exostoses, enchondromata, ecchondromata and cysts; when one of these predominates, names have been applied to the clinical appearances.

The mucopolysaccharidoses – 'dysostosis multiplex' (chondro-osteodystrophy) (by Roger Smith)

INTRODUCTION

The mucopolysaccharidoses (MPS) are a group of recessive disorders caused by a deficiency of lysosomal enzymes necessary for the stepwise degradation of the mucopolysaccharidoses (glycosaminoglycans). There are many other lysosomal storage disorders which include the mucolipidoses, sphingolipidoses and Gaucher's disease (LeRoy and Wiesmann, 1993).

The glycosaminoglycans, which include dermatan sulphate, heparan sulphate, keratan sulphate and chondroitin sulphate, are normally degraded by specific enzymes. When these enzymes are lacking or ineffective, the large complex glycosaminoglycans accumulate in the lysosomes with impaired function of cells, tissues and organs and are found in excessive amounts in the urine.

The type of mucopolysaccharidosis depends on the enzyme defect and on tissue expression. Common features include a chronic progressive cause, involvement of many systems, enlargement of organs, widely variable bone disease and an abnormal appearance. Hearing, vision, cardiovascular function and joint mobility may be limited. Mental retardation, which may be profound, is limited to the Hurler and severe Hunter syndromes and all subtypes of the San Filippo disorder (Neufeld, 1989).

DIAGNOSIS

The diagnosis is made from the clinical features and the results of enzyme assays from fibroblasts, leucocytes and serum. So far as the skeleton is concerned the most characteristic features are found in the Hurler (MPS IH) and Morquio (MPS IV) syndromes. MPS IH shows all the changes of 'dysostosis multiplex', which is common to all MPSs.

In MPS IV (Morquio) there are additional diagnostic skeletal changes.

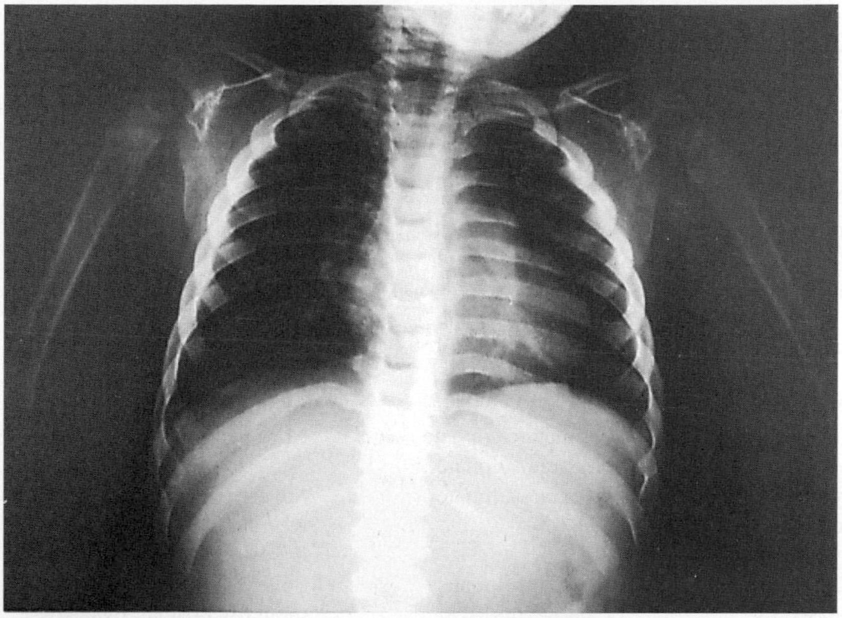

Figure 4.1 Hurler syndrome (MPS IH). The ribs are 'paddle'-shaped, being broad anteriorly and narrow at their posterior ends; the medial ends of the clavicles are broad; and the humeral heads are small with poorly formed glenoid fossa.

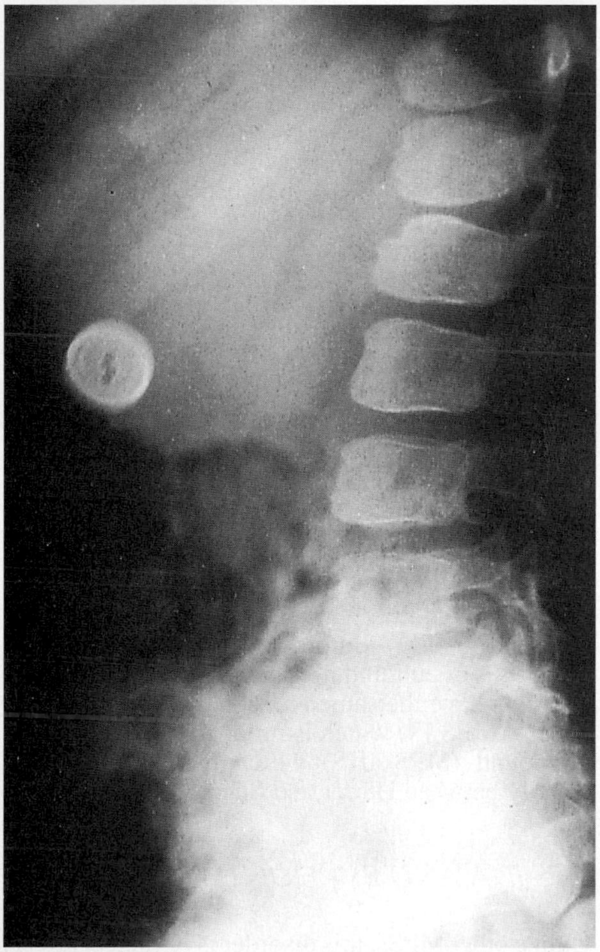

Figure 4.2 Hurler syndrome (MPS IH). There are inferior hooks on the vertebral bodies in the upper lumbar region, at the site of the kyphosis.

The major features of 'dysostosis multiplex' are:

1. Skull – macrocephaly, abnormal shape (dyscephaly) J-shaped sella, thick calvarium.
2. Chest – wide oar-shaped ribs, wide clavicles, plump scapula (Figure 4.1).
3. Spine – oval (immature) and hook-shaped vertebrae in lateral views of the spine (Figure 4.2).
4. Pelvis – overconstriction of the iliac bodies: wide iliac flare; dysplasia of capital femoral epiphyses; coxa valga.
5. Long tubular bones – irregular diaphyseal modelling; submetaphyseal overconstriction; shortening; (periosteal cloaking in infants with gangliosidosis type I and mucolipidosis II).
6. Short tubular bones – shortening; metaphyseal widening; epiphyseal dysplasia; proximal tapering of the second to fifth metacarpals.
7. Bone structure – osteopenic with a coarsely laced trabeculum.

CLASSIFICATION

The features of the different types of mucopolysaccharidoses and their defective enzyme defect are shown in Table 4.1. Because lack of the same enzyme can cause different types of MPS, correct diagnosis requires a combination of clinical and biochemical features. MPS IH (Hurler syndrome), MPS II (A and B) (Hunter syndrome) and MPS IV (Morquio syndrome), all of which affect the skeleton, are sufficiently distinct to merit further description.

Table 4.1

Name		Defective enzyme	Main metabolites affected	Main clinical features
MPS-IH	Hurler	α_1-Iduronidase	Dermatan sulphate Heparan sulphate	Severe short stature, progressive mental retardation; grotesque
MPS-IS	Scheie	α_1-Iduronidase	Dermatan sulphate Heparan sulphate	Nearly normal
MPS-IHS	Compound	α_1-Iduronidase	Dermatan sulphate Heparan sulphate	Reduced stature, dysostosis
MPS-IIA	Hunter	Iduronate sulphatase	Dermatan sulphate Heparan sulphate	Short stature, severe mental retardation; destructive, severe dysostosis
MPS-IIB		Iduronate sulphatase	Dermatan sulphate Heparan sulphate	Mild variant
MPS-III (A, B & C)	Sanfilippo	Different enzymes for each type	Heparan sulphate	Severe psychomotor retardation; insignificant dysostosis
MPS-IVA	Morquio A	Gal NAc-6-sulphate sulphatase	Keratan sulphate	Severe short stature, mentally normal; dysostosis plus other features
MPS-IVB	Morquio B	β-D-galactosidase	Keratin sulphate	Mild form
MPS-VIA	Maroteaux–Lamy	Gal NAc-4-sulphate sulphatase	Dermatan sulphate	Appearance, stature and radiographs may be as abnormal as MPS-IH, but intelligence normal
MPS-VIB	Maroteaux–Lamy	Gal NAc-4-sulphate sulphatase	Dermatan sulphate	Mild variant

Maroteaux–Lamy disease (MPS VI) which also affects the skeleton is very variable in its expression.

MPS IH (HURLER SYNDROME) – 'GARGOYLISM'

This is the prototype mucopolysaccharidosis described by Hunter in 1917. It can be recognized within the first 6 months of life and slowly progresses to cardiorespiratory death about 10 years later. The neonate shows noisy breathing, hypotonia and inguinal herniae. In infancy features include an enlarging scaphocephalic head, restricted joint movements (especially shoulders), corneal clouding, enlargement of the abdomen and hepatosplenomegaly. Height and weight may be temporarily excessive.

By about 18 months the growth rate falls and the head stops enlarging. Psychomotor development is slow; there is considerable physical disability and conductive hearing loss. Repeated respiratory infections occur. There is increasing grotesqueness (hence the previous term 'gargoylism') with thickening of the facial features. Independent walking is delayed, and speech rudimentary and hoarse.Thoracolumbar kyphosis and umbilical herniae develop. Mental function and social contact later decline. Radio-graphs show all the features of dysostosis multiplex. These include 'breaking' of the vertebrae in kyphosis, most common in the lumbar region, irregular thickening of the diploë of the skull, delay of ossification of the carpus and shortening and thickening of the long vertebrae in kyphosis, most bones of the upper limb. The long bones of the lower limb are un-affected but the femoral necks are valgoid and the acetabular shallow with flared ilia (Figures 4.3, 4.4 and 4.5).

The lack of α_1-iduronidase can be detected in white cells or cultured fibroblasts; two other clinical disorders have the same enzyme deficiency, Scheie disease (MPS IS) which is mild, and Hurler–Scheie compound (MPS IHS) which is intermediate in severity between Hurler and Scheie.

MPS II (A AND B) – HUNTER SYNDROME

Unlike other MPSs, this disorder is X-linked, affecting males only. Although normally milder than the Hurler syndrome, the severe MPS IIA closely resembles Hurler syndrome.

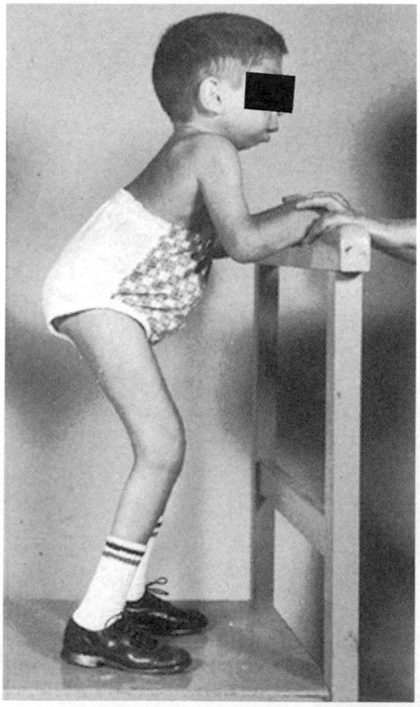

Figure 4.3 A small child, showing deformities resulting from Hunter-Hurler's disease, or gargoylism, with flexion contractures of both hips and knees, spinal deformity and inability to stand unsupported.

MPS IIA may be suspected from about the age of 3 by slow speech, short attention span, noisy breathing with recurrent respiratory infections and inguinal hernia. Growth may be temporarily excessive, only to slow and halt at about 7 years. The head is large, the cornea clear, the hands and fingers stiff (Figure 4.6), the movement of shoulders reduced and the abdomen enlarged by hepatosplenomegaly. Progressive deafness occurs. Later the facial features coarsen, there is mental and motor deterioration and cardiorespiratory or neurological death by the age of 10–15 years. In the mild form (MPS IIB) attendance at normal school is sometimes possible though death may occur in early adult life from cardiac valve disease.

MPS IV – MORQUIO'S DISEASE

Skeletal abnormalities are prominent, with characteristic short trunk, short stature. Walking is delayed but intelligence is normal. By the age of 3 years pectus carinatum, thoracolumbar kyphosis and genu valgum are present and by 6 fully developed. Large head, normal facial appearance, cloudy cornea, widely spaced teeth with hypoplastic enamel, short neck, protruding sternum, prominent and very lax joints and conductive hearing loss complete the clinical picture (Figure 4.7) Physical disability and early fatigue are progressive and later the signs of spinal cord compression due to odontoid hypoplasia and atlanto-axial instability appear.

The growth in length of shafts of long bones is slowed with irregularity of the metaphysis and increase in thickness of epiphyseal and articular cartilage. The epiphyseal centres appear as multiple foci and distortion and fragmentation occur. The diaphyses are unaffected (see Figure 4.8). The upper limb shows radial club hand with carpal irregularities and the hips show coxa vara and epiphyseal irregularity which may mimic Perthes' disease (Figure 4.9a).

The spinal changes are very obvious, showing flattening and anterior 'breaking' of the vertebral bodies due to irregular ossification as well as defects in the neural arches (Figure 4.10). Kyphosis results (Figure 4.9b). The odontoid process may be hypoplastic or absent and the body of C2 so large that it encroaches on the spinal canal, producing myelopathy. These radiological appearances are more those of spondylo-epiphyseal dysplasia than dysostosis multiplex.

PROGNOSIS

Disability and life expectancy depend on skeletal complications of which cervical myelopathy is most important. This may be prevented by early and appropriate spinal fusion. Genu valgum may require treatment by bracing or realignment osteotomy in childhood and secondary osteoarthritis of the hips is treatable by total hip replacement. Upper limb abnormalities can be controlled to some extent by judicious control of bone length and osteotomies during growth. A milder form of Morquio disease exits (MPS IV) (see Table 4.1).

MPS VI (A AND B) – MAROTEAUX–LAMY DISEASE

MPS V does not exist. In MPS VI the short stature, grotesque appearance and radiographic changes may be as severe as in MPS IH but intelligence is normal.

MANAGEMENT OF MUCOPOLYSACCHARIDOSES

Knowledge of the biochemical cause of the MPSs has made prenatal diagnosis and genetic advice possible. Various procedures to supply the missing enzyme have been largely unsuccessful and gene replacement remains in the future. For the moment

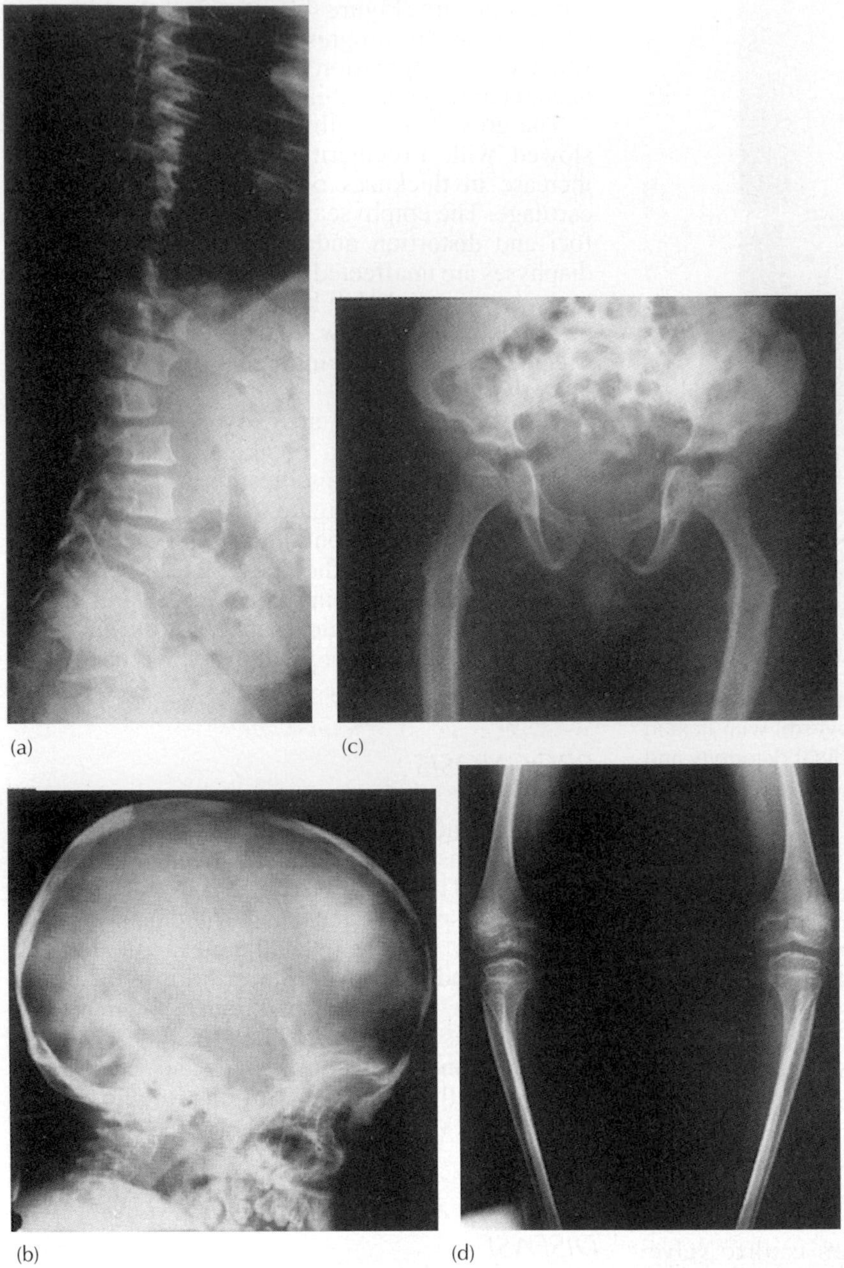

Figure 4.4 (a) Radiograph of the boy's spine with Hurler's syndrome (MPS IH) of Figure 4.3, showing the subluxation forward of L2 with wedging and beak formation of the third vertebral body which has produced an angular kyphosis, and loss of the normal lumbar lordosis. (b) Radiograph of the skull in this child to show widening of the sella turcica and abnormality in ossification. (c) Radiograph of the femora and pelvis with a marked coxa valgus deformity, narrowing of the long bones with abnormal cortical thickness of the outer femoral shafts. (d) Radiograph of the knee joints, showing the marked coxa vara deformity and thinned, attenuated shafts of bone but normal-appearing epiphyses.

the patient with an MPS requires symptomatic treatment, the correction of limb deformity, and in MPS IV (Morquio's disease) orthopaedic stabilization of the spine (see Chapter 8).

Achondroplasia (chondrodystrophia fetalis)

In the disturbance known as achondroplasia, the development of the bones laid down in cartilage is at fault. The membranous bones are formed, and continue to develop, normally. The disease has been known since the earliest times, for achondroplasts are dwarfs with easily recognizable features. Their intelligence is often above average, and their physical strength great. The Egyptian goddess Ptah was an achondroplast, and achondroplasts were regularly installed as court jesters in the Middle Ages. There are different degrees of the disorder, and in very severe cases the fetus dies *in utero* and is aborted. An example of this disease in an animal is the dachshund dog.

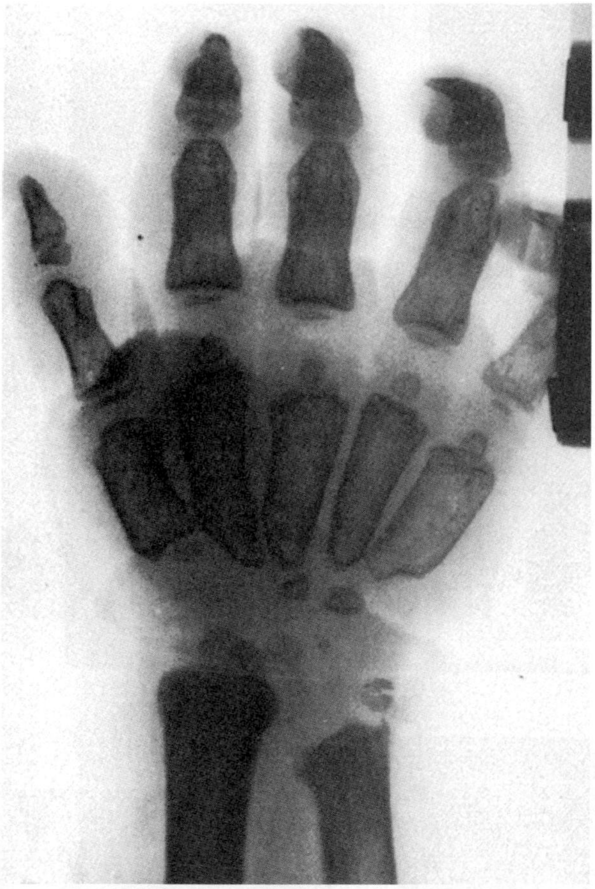

Figure 4.5 Radiograph of the hands, showing the pointing of the bases of the metacarpals and the marked broadening of the shafts of the short miniature bones.

CLINICAL FEATURES

At birth, a typical achondroplast has a normal-sized body, very short, fat, flabby limbs, and a large head, with a characteristic depression at the root of the nose (Figure 4.11). The small stature is largely due to the absence of growth of the lower extremities, and becomes increasingly evident during childhood. The child walks at the usual age, teeth, appear at the normal times, and the rolls of fat which disfigure the limbs slowly disappear. Growth is permanently retarded, however, and the child is recognized as of unmistakable short stature long before adult life is reached.

Standing erect, the tips of the fingers may only reach the greater trochanter or the iliac crest, whereas in the normal person they extend to the lower part of the thigh. The central point of the body, normally at the umbilicus, is situated much higher, sometimes as high as the xiphoid process. While the proximal segment of the limbs is most affected, the achondroplastic hand is also short and broad, with the fingers of equal length. With the hand outstretched, the fingers diverge in a characteristic fashion, to which Marie applied the term *main en trident* (Figure 4.12).

The short limbs, especially the lower, are often curved. This is due to an angular displacement of the two components of the knee, the articular surface of the tibia looking slightly outwards.

The trunk is practically normal, and the impression conveyed is of the body of an adult to which are fitted four child-like limbs.

The head is both absolutely and relatively enlarged. Its shape is rounded and markedly brachycephalic. The face is broad, and at the root of the short nose is

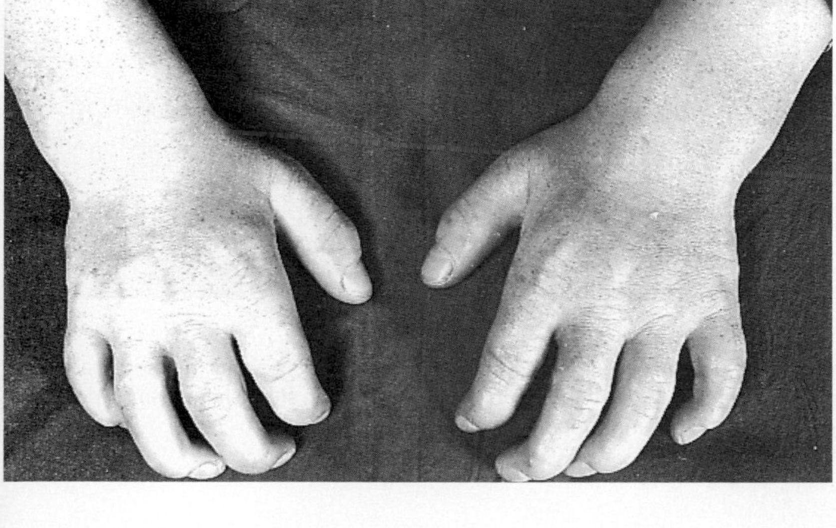

Figure 4.6 A 7-year-old child with a mild variant of Hunter's syndrome of mucopolysaccharidosis type MPS IIA, showing the nodular skin lesions over the hands and forearms. The fingers are abnormally shaped in flexion, particularly at the distal interphalangeal joints.

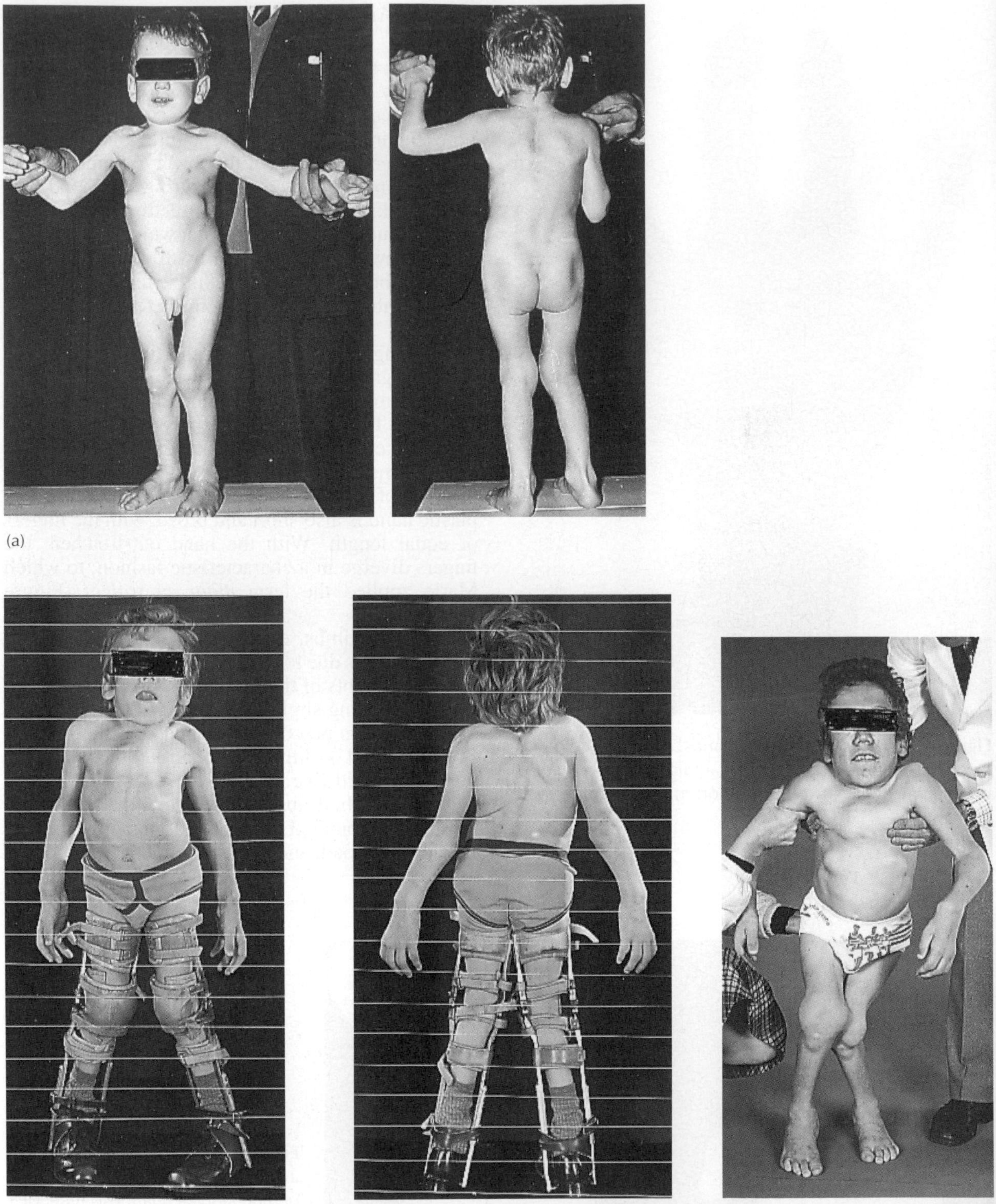

Figure 4.7 (a) A child of 2 years, exhibiting early features of Morquio's type A. (b) At the age of 6 years, requiring calipers to stand and walk, and showing fast and severe progression. (c) At the age of 7 years, showing short stature, small deformed trunk, head large and sunk between the shoulders, requiring support to stand.

a characteristic depression or indentation. The upper alveolar processes protrude, and prominence of the lower jaw results in prognathism. The sacrum is tilted and in consequence contracture of the pelvic inlet follows, while the outlet is correspondingly increased.

Intellect

Achondroplastics are usually of normal intelligence, and frequently they are lively and amusing. In some cases, however, the intellect is impaired and they are backward for their age.

Because of their deformed bodies they have strong feelings of inferiority and are emotionally immature, and are often vain, boastful, excitable, fond of drink, and sometimes lascivious. Sexual development is usually normal, but may be retarded.

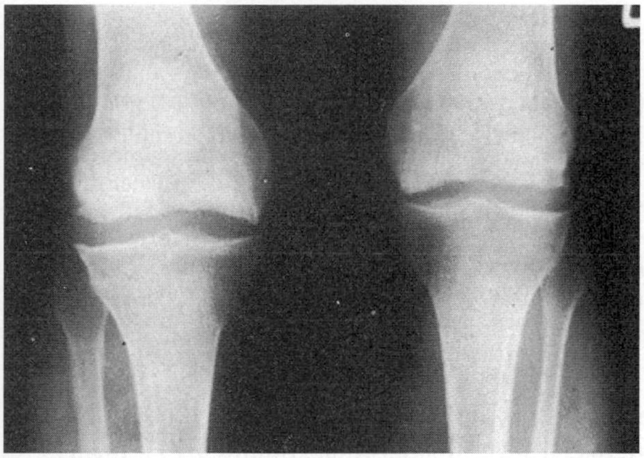

Figure 4.8 Mucopolysaccharidosis of Morquio B type, showing the apparent increase in joint space by thickening of the articular cartilage surrounded by sclerosis and distortion of the tibial plateau with spur formation.

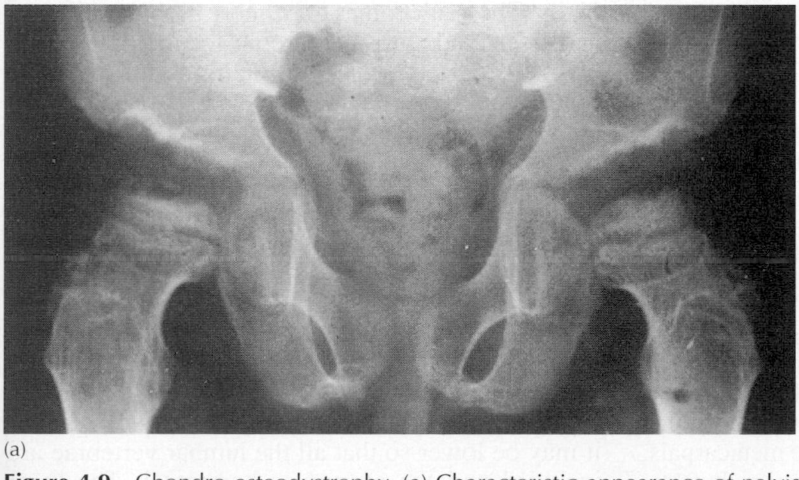

(a)

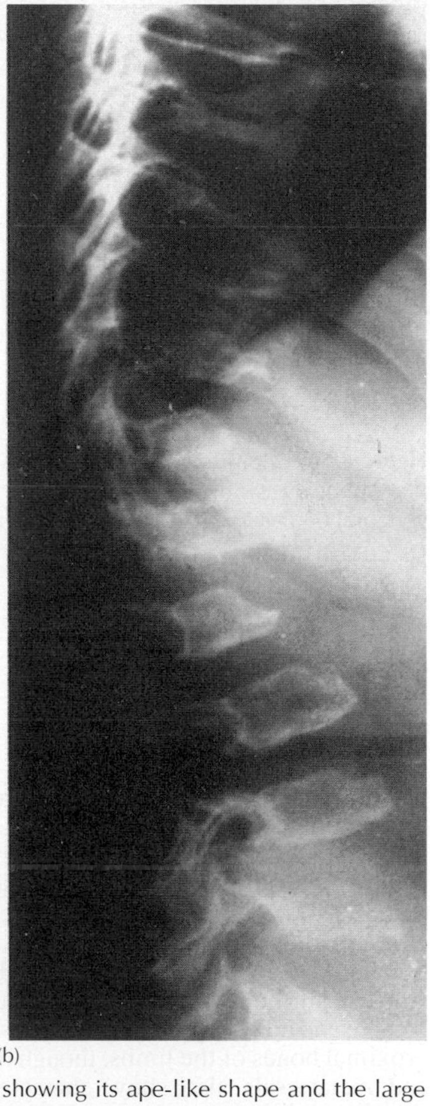

(b)

Figure 4.9 Chondro-osteodystrophy. (a) Characteristic appearance of pelvis, showing its ape-like shape and the large irregular acetabula and deformed femoral heads with a marked coxa valgus. (b) The appearance of the spine, showing tongued vertebral bodies.

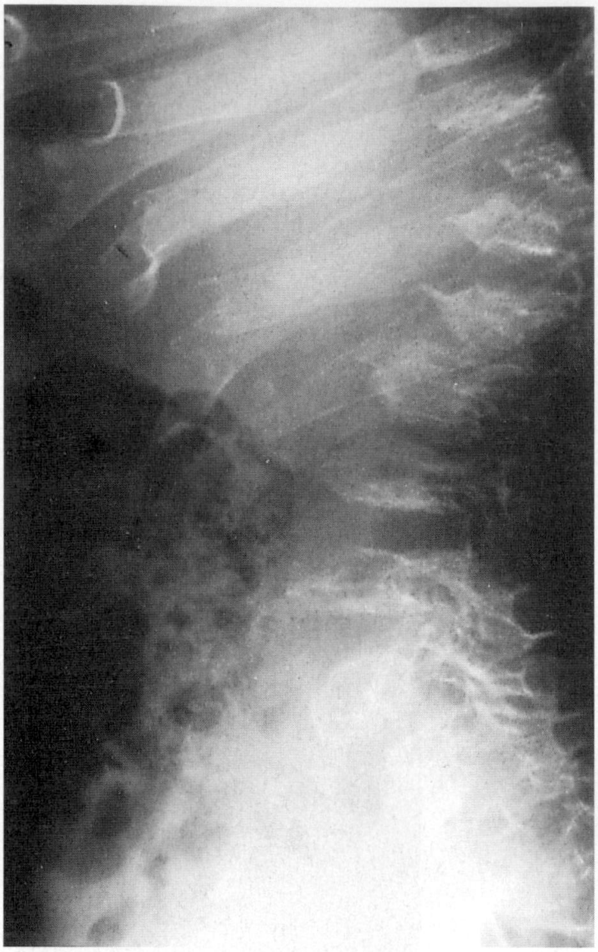

Figure 4.10 Morquio syndrome (MPS IV). Characteristic platyspondyly with a central anterior tongue of the vertebral bodies and a thoracolumbar gibbus.

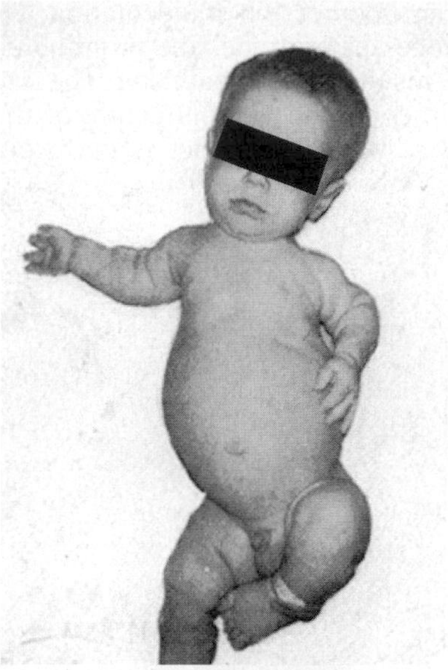

Figure 4.11 A 7-month-old achondroplastic boy, showing normal trunk size, but markedly reduced limb lengths, with multiple creasing of the soft tissues. The large head and the depression at the root of the nose are obvious.

PATHOLOGY

The long bones of the limbs

These bones are exceedingly short (Figure 4.14). In other respects the shaft is normal; the muscular prominences are pronounced, and the thickness of the shaft is often equal to that of the normal bone (Figure 4.13). The ends of the bones roughly preserve their usual form. It would seem, however, that this is not invariably the case, and Knaggs (1926) believed that the epiphyses are disproportionately large, and roughly shaped (Figure 4.15).

The long bones are often abnormally curved or bowed, and all changes tend to be most marked in the proximal bones of the limbs, though the metacarpals and metatarsals also show characteristic changes (Figure 4.16).

The short bones of the limbs – the carpus, tarsus, os calcis, etc. – are usually remarkably normal in architecture.

The skull

The portion of the skull developed in cartilage–the base – is grossly abnormal (Figure 4.17). Instead of the usual centres of ossification for the pre- and post-sphenoid and the basiocciput, there is an irregular single mass of bone formed by synostosis of the individual centres. In consequence of this synostosis, the growth of the skull base is retarded – it remains short while the remainder of the skull grows normally. The vault comes to be more globular in form, and is expanded to make room for the developing brain since little or no contribution to the available intracranial space is made by the base. The fontanelles are correspondingly enlarged. Hydrocephalus occurs. The smallness of the base of the skull is responsible for the marked depression at the root of the nose and for the flattening of the face.

The vertebral column

The vertebral column is of normal length, but the centres of ossification of the bodies may be smaller than normal, with excessive cartilage. Often there is a long regular kyphosis at the lumbodorsal region or it may be lower so that all the lumbar vertebrae are included and the sacrum is horizontal. The most striking feature is the early synostosis between the body and the arch, which in some cases is so severe

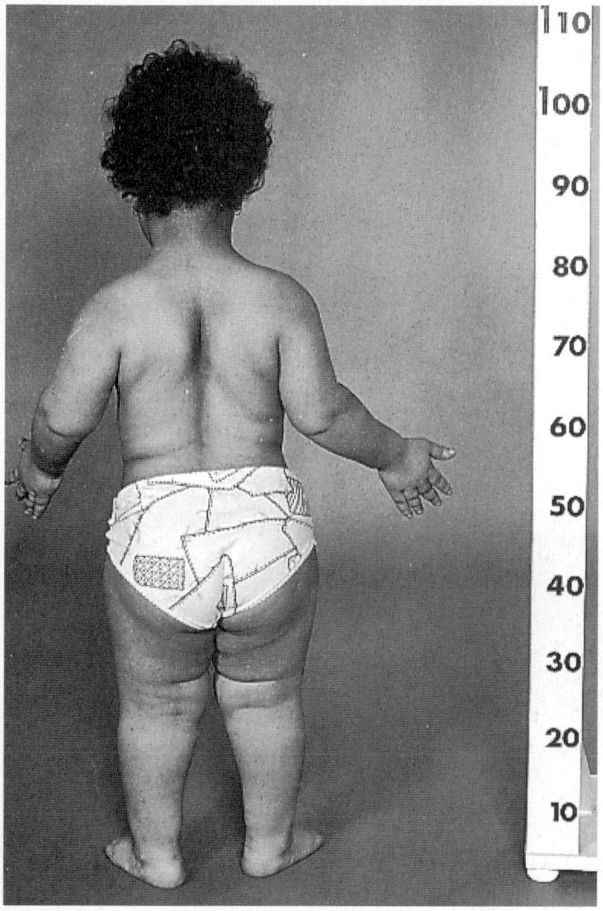

Figure 4.12 A posterior photograph of an 11-year-old girl with achondroplasia to show her markedly reduced stature – less than 110 cm – her divergent fingers (*main en trident*) and a lordosis.

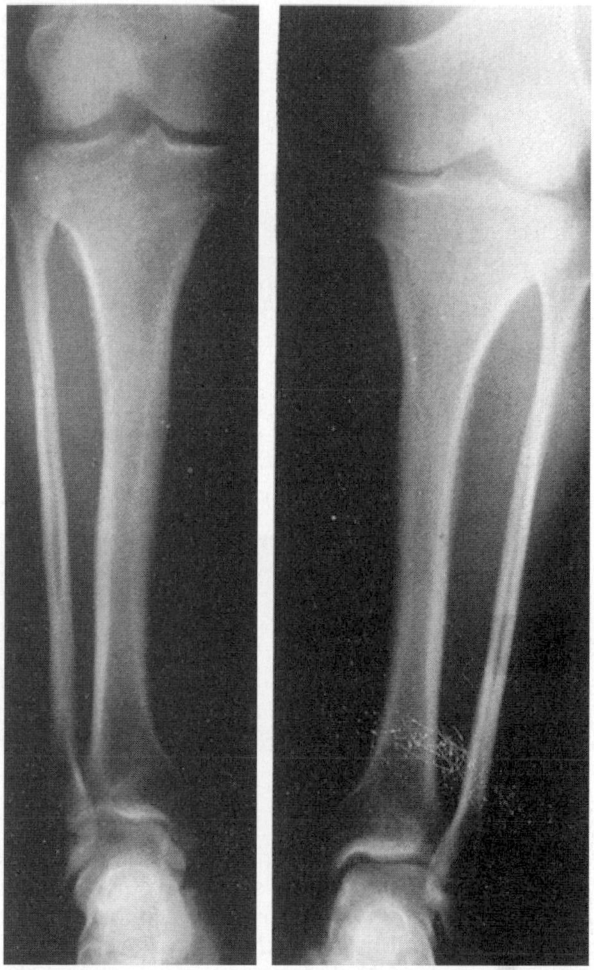

Figure 4.13 In achondroplasia the bone has marked alteration in shape and length but bone that exists has normal histology and radiodensity.

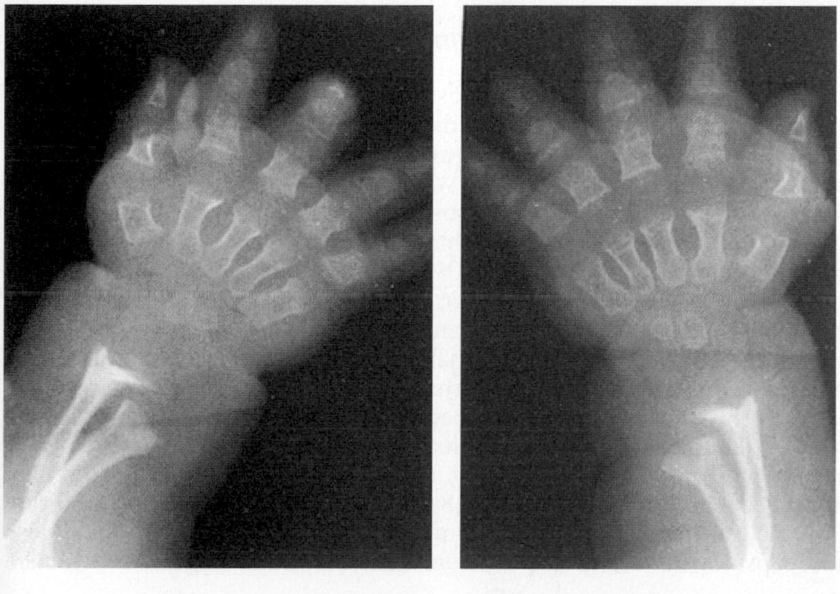

Figure 4.14 A radiograph of the boy shown in Figure 4.11. The stunting effect on the short miniature bones and forearm bones, with broadening and cupping of the epiphyses which appear sclerotic.

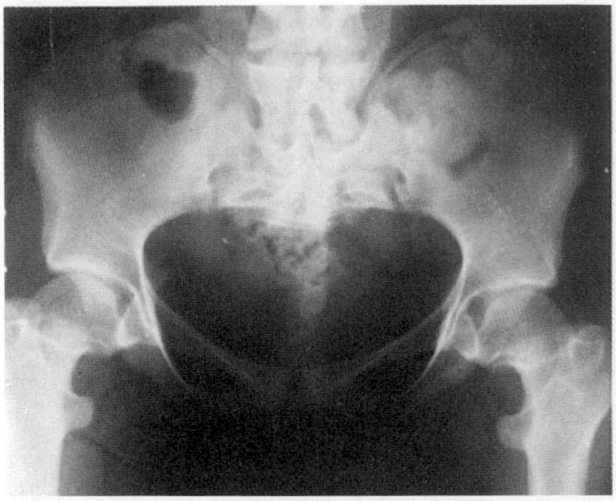

(a)

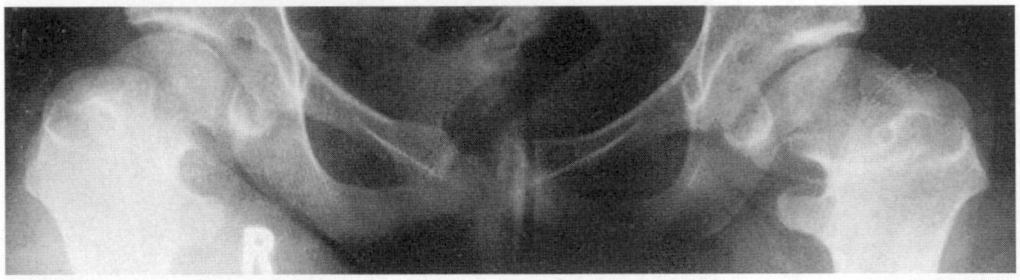

(b)

Figure 4.15 Achondroplasia. (a) The ilia are broad and the acetabula flat, and the proximal long bones are shortened relative to those distal to them. (b) The femoral neck area is disproportionate in length to the growth of the trochauteric areas.

as to lead to marked diminution in the calibre of the vertebral canal. Spinal stenosis can occur with both upper and lower motor neuron signs depending upon the level. Monitoring for this is required by CT scanning and MRI for any cord changes. The membranous bones, the ribs and sternum, are of normal adult development.

HISTOLOGICAL FEATURES

The most striking feature of the histology of the growth area of the achondroplastic long bone is the great absence of cartilage proliferation, so that the normal – and necessary – palisade arrangement is absent. Ossification does take place – and the achondroplastic bone grows in length – but the process is very slow. The deposition of subperiosteal bone, on the other hand, proceeds at a normal pace, so the diameter of the bone is maintained. The retardation at the growth line may lead to an indragging of the periosteum which is attached to the growth cartilage, and the osteogenic layer of the infolded periosteal shelf may deposit a layer of compact bone over the peripheral part of the metaphysis. This is a secondary phenomenon.

Harris (1933) drew attention to another feature – a widespread mucoid degeneration of the cartilage cells; the cells become swollen, the capsules distended, and the matrix of semi-fluid consistency. The mucoid change is patchy, and intervening between the mucoid areas may be areas of normal cartilage proliferation, and of ossification, but the presence of the mucoid areas renders the normal growth in length and the maintenance of the exact form of the bone impossible.

Explanation of the process

Achondroplasia appears sporadically, but there is a distinct hereditary tendency. There appear to be two different types of achondroplastic child. First, there is the child who survives infancy and has resulted from an autosomal dominant gene mutation, with normal parents and siblings i.e. heterozygous. However, over 80% are new mutations. Second, there is the baby who, at birth, is recognized achondroplastic and dies during infancy i.e. usually homozygous or double-dormant. In 1941, Mörch pointed out that in this type perhaps only 1 in 5 survive the first year, and it has been recorded that the pregnancies are often complicated by hydramnios.

The exact nature of the process is not known. Jansen (1928) attributed it to increased amniotic pressure, from either hydramnios or undue smallness of the amnion. There is some suggestive evidence

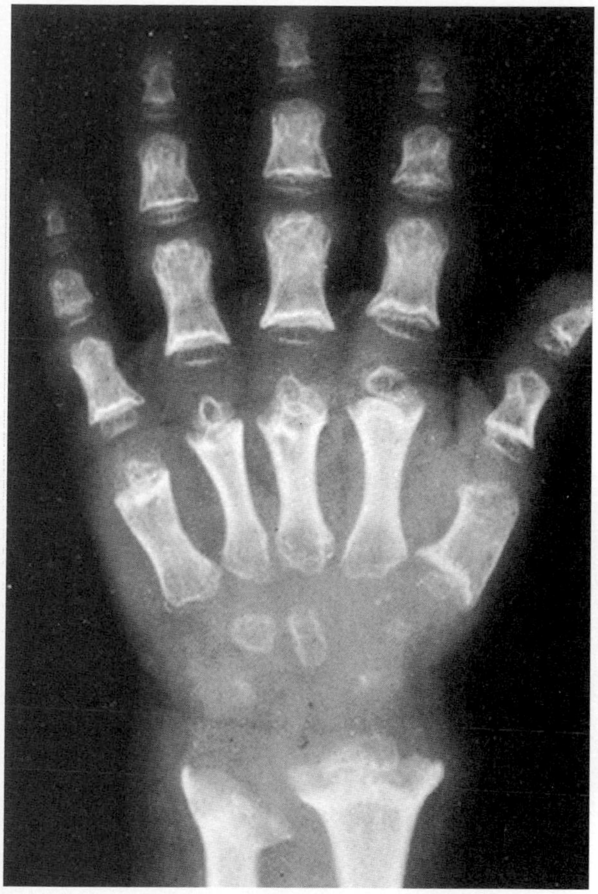

Figure 4.16 Radiograph of an achondroplastic hand, showing the sclerotic irregularities of the wrist and other epiphyses which have all ossified in proper sequence.

that a like condition in animals is associated with an error in development of the pituitary gland, and it may well be that there is an endocrine disturbance undiagnosed as yet.

DIAGNOSIS

With such a very striking clinical picture, there should be little difficulty in diagnosis. The disease has to be differentiated from rickets, and this can be done by an x-ray examination of the epiphyses. The epiphyseal outline is distinct, as ossification in the epiphyses is normal; in rickets, on the other hand, the epiphyseal outline is blurred and ossification delayed.

Achondroplasia may be confused with cretinism, but in the latter there may be mental deficiency and stupidity. In cretinism the essential feature is delay in ossification. In some cases it is associated with stippling of the epiphyses and calcium deposits.

The achondroplastic is a 'dwarfed' individual in whom:

1. Trunk length (crown to pubis) is normal.
2. Leg length (pubis to heel) is reduced.
3. Span length (fingertip to thumbtip) is reduced.

This form of dwarfism has to be differentiated from other forms of stunting in which there is a decrease in the trunk length with both the leg and span lengths possibly being normal (Table 4.2).

TREATMENT

No known therapy has any effect on the course of the disease, but the structural complications in achondroplasia requiring treatment are:

1. Thoracolumbar kyphosis, in which the majority progress with ambulation. However, if the cord becomes compressed, decompression with spinal fusion is required.
2. Spinal stenosis is most pronounced in areas of lumbar hyperlordosis and affects 40% of adult achondroplastics. It may well occur in the thoracic and cervical spine. Decompression may be needed with stabilization.

Table 4.2 Dwarfism – short stature

	With bony deformities	
Spine	Spine and limbs	Limbs
Mucopolysaccharidoses	Congenital syphilis	Cretinism
Scheuermann's disease	Hand–Schüller–Christian disease	Achondroplasia
Tuberculosis	Diastrophic dwarfism	Metaphyseal dysostosis
Spondylolisthesis	Spondyloepiphyseal dysplasia	Pyknodysostosis
Osteoporosis	Paget's disease	Metaphyseal dysplasia
		Rickets

	Without bony deformities		
Genetic	Endocrine	Calorie deficiency	Chronic disease
Familial	Hypopituitary syndromes	Malnutrition	Congenital heart disease
Racial	Hypothyroidism	Malabsorption syndromes	Nephritis
	Ovarian agenesis		Juvenile rheumatoid arthritis
			Diabetes
			Hepatitis
			Malaria

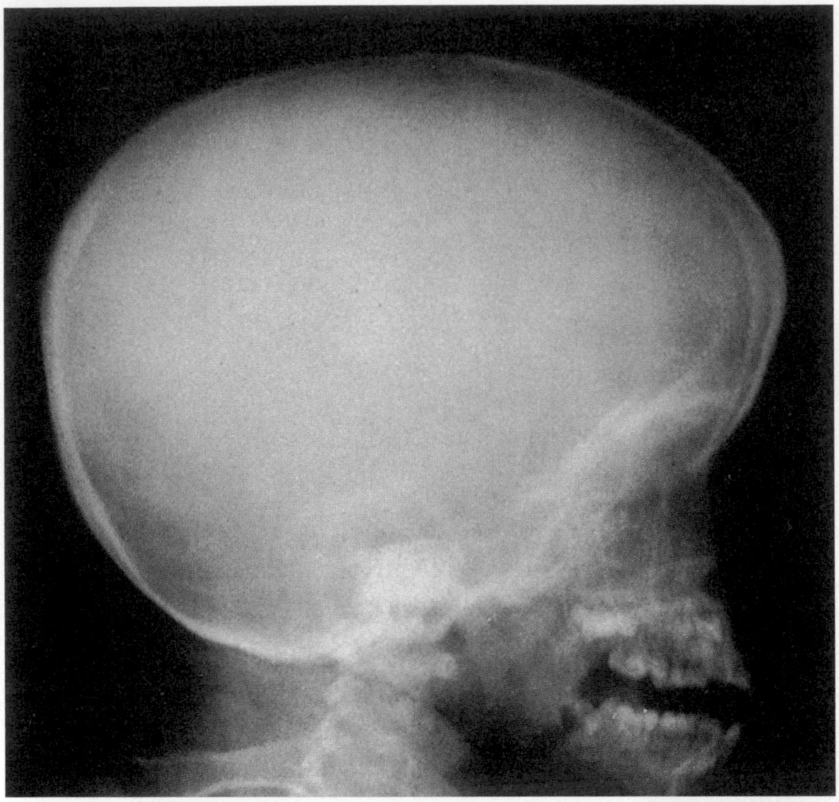

Figure 4.17 Radiograph of the child in Figures 4.11 and 4.14, showing the globular shape of the vault with a reduced skull base. The fontanelles are still patent, with flattening of the face and depression of the root of the nose.

3. Failure of posterior occipitoatlanto segmentation is present in a majority of cases. These have been reviewed by Kopits (1976) and stabilization is sometimes required.
4. Laxity of knee joints which seldom interferes with gait because of muscle stabilization. Bow leg deformities occur frequently, and may well require tibial and/or femoral osteotomies if joints are misaligned.
5. Leg lengthening – with improved instrumentation and techniques, lengthening of the femoral and tibial shafts can now be carried out, with fewer complications. However, it is important for the patient and the parents to be given exact treatment details – extended periods in hospital, complications of nerve, blood vessel injury, bone grafting for pseudoarthrosis, fracture, etc. Also, it is helpful to use standing photographs to indicate where lengths will be achieved and particularly point out the continuing shortening of the upper extremities as a deformity.

Aldegheri *et al.* (1988) have described their results of lengthening in 117 lower limbs over 30% of which were in achondroplastic patients. They compared four methods – transverse osteotomy: oblique osteotomy, callotasis of the shaft and chondrodiastasis of the epiphysis. The latter two gave far fewer complications. They also emphasized that major lengthening of one limb at a time allows greater independent mobility during treatment, earlier progress, in the event of any complications the patient can walk and weight-bear on the unoperated limb, etc. They recommend operating between the ages of 9 and 12 years. This form of treatment requires longer-term evaluation regarding its overall benefit to the patients.

Cartilage-hair hypoplasia

This syndrome was intensively studied by McKusick and his colleagues (1978) amongst Amish sects in Pennsylvania and Canada. It had previously been described as achondroplasia or metaphyseal dysostosis, but is now considered to be a distinct entity. It is an autosomal recessive and 77 cases were found amongst 45 000 older Amish, i.e. 1–2 per 1000 live births.

At birth the short length of the limbs is noted, and as development proceeds dwarfing is marked. Most patients reach not more than 1.22 m (4 feet) in height

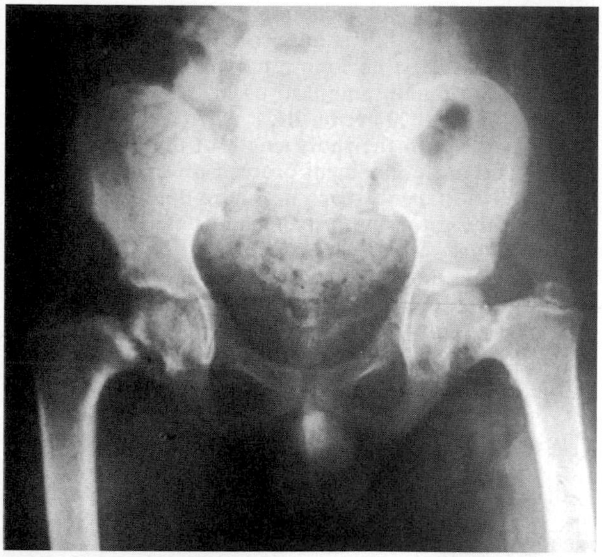

Figure 4.18 Metaphyseal dysostosis. Anteroposterior radiograph of both hips and pelvis, showing the coxa vara with irregularity of the metaphyses but normal epiphyses and diaphyses of the femora.

at maturity. There is a characteristic deformity of excessive length of the fibula at the ankle and a loose-jointed flat foot. There is inability to fully extend the elbows and hyperextensibility of the wrists and fingers. The digits are extremely short. The overall appearances are similar to those in achondroplasia but the head in cartilage-hair syndrome is always normal and the epiphyses are radiologically normal. The hair is fine, sparse, short and brittle.

Intelligence is normal. Histologically there is a deficiency of chondroblastic proliferation and of normal columnation similar to that found in achondroplasia.

Metaphyseal dysostosis

This covers a range of disorders which McKusick (1966) divided into three types:

1. The Jansen – which is rare but most severe, shows no hereditary pattern.
2. The Schmid – milder but more common, with autosomal dominant pattern.
3. The Spahr – Fwhich shows only bowing, and is autosomal recessive.

Typical cases of the Schmid type of metaphyseal dysostosis show inhibition of growth of all cylindrical bones, particularly the large long bones, bilateral coxa vara and a tendency for slipping of the epiphyses. There is normal development of the osseous nucleus of the epiphyses and lack of involvement of the head, trunk, and carpal and tarsal bones. Kidney function and serum chemistry are normal. As a result moderate dwarfing, marked bowing and a waddling gait are the main clinical features. Eventually the lesions heal with epiphyseal fusion.

There has been dispute as to whether some cases of metaphyseal dysostosis are atypical examples of hypophosphataemic rickets.

Characteristically, the radiographs show involvement of the metaphysis with normal diaphysis. The zone of provisional calcification is irregular because of radiolucent masses of what has been reported as cartilage; the metaphyses are broad and at times cup-shaped. The epiphyseal centres are normal (Figure 4.18).

Histologically, Aegerter and Kirkpatrick (1975) reported that there was a mass of unidentifiable amorphous material replacing the cancellous tissue immediately beneath the enchondral plate, but whether this was degenerating collagen or osteoid was uncertain.

Enchondromatosis (dyschondroplasia; Ollier's disease)

There has been a tendency in the past to regard this condition (which Ollier described in 1899) as identical with the condition variously known as metaphyseal aclasis or hereditary deforming chondrodysplasia. There are good reasons for separating the two lesions, but it is nevertheless certain that cases intermediate between them occur.

Dyschondroplasia may be unilateral or bilateral; it is perhaps more common as a unilateral affection and occasionally it may be confined to a single bone (Figure 4.19). There is no evidence of any genetic basis.

PATHOLOGY

The disease is one affecting proliferating cartilage in the metaphyseal region so that cartilage persists abnormally. Six different processes have to cooperate harmoniously in order that the bones shall attain proper size, structure and composition when

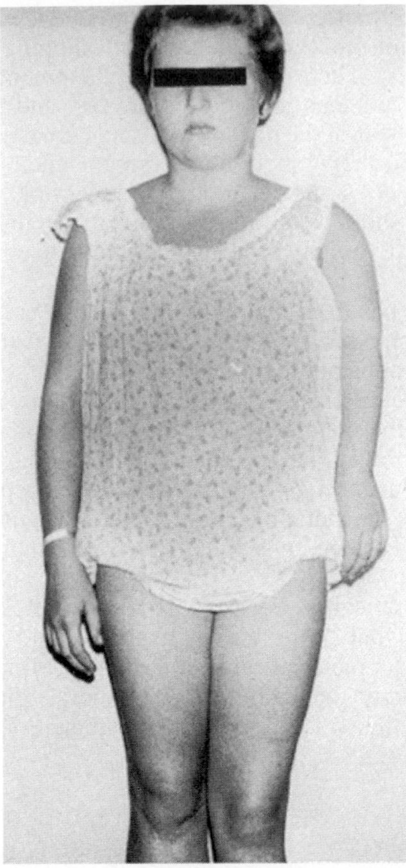

Figure 4.19 Enchondromatosis (Ollier's disease) with obvious shortening of the left upper limb.

completing their growth: resorption, tubulation, cancellation, cell division, cell enlargement, as well as differentiation. Sometimes one or more of these processes will be delayed and the dissociation of each evokes its own characteristic changes such as masses or columns of uncalcified or even disintegrating cartilage cells extending down into the metaphysis and diaphysis (Figure 4.20).

RADIOLOGICAL APPEARANCES

The typical appearances may be seen near the ends of the diaphyses in the long bones – humerus, femur, radius, etc. – or in the short long bones of the hands and feet (Figures 4.21 to 4.23). Usually the more rapidly growing ends of the bone are involved.

The metaphysis is usually broadened and its texture poor. It presents a cystic appearance bridged across by a series of fine septa which tend to run in parallel lines or stripes in the long axis of the bone. Occasionally, small exostoses project from the surface. These are less well formed than in metaphyseal aclasis, and are usually taken to represent

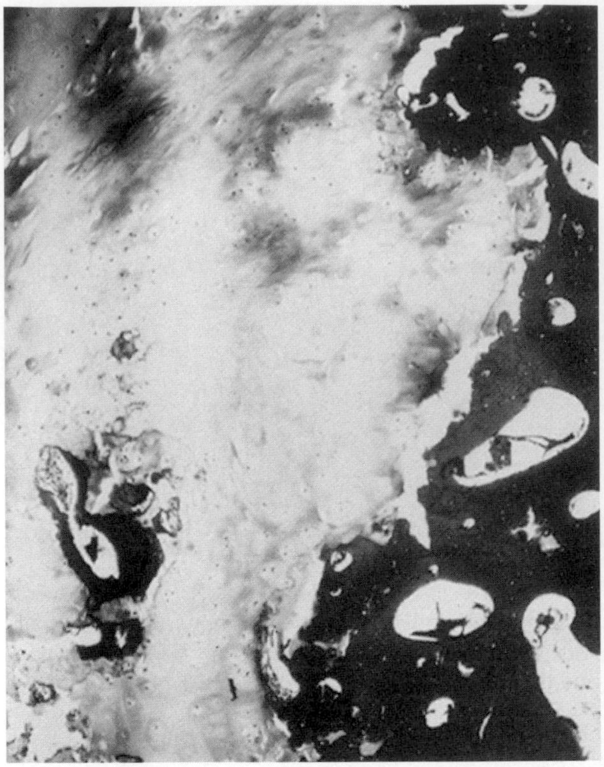

Figure 4.20 Biopsy at the site of the deformity reveals broad irregular sheets of cartilage matrix with scattered chondrocytes.

the diaphyseal limit of the affected area of the bone.

In the short bones the appearances may be very similar, or there may be multiple enchondromata.

In the ilium, Hunter and Wiles (1935) pointed out that the disease affects a fan-shaped area, with the apex at the nutrient artery; a characteristic appearance of striping is again produced.

The ischium and the pubis may appear fluffy and stippled, due to the presence of small rounded areas of cartilage.

The epiphyses are unaffected at birth (Hunter and Wiles, 1935) but later may also appear speckled.

As the child grows, the striping of the bones is replaced by irregular mottling and speckling, and the affected bones are stunted.

CLINICAL FEATURES

The clinical picture is characterized by its extreme polymorphism. In some cases only a single bone is affected, while in others the condition presents itself on both sides. It is a hereditary retardation phenomenon transmitted without regard to sex.

The disease usually becomes apparent during the

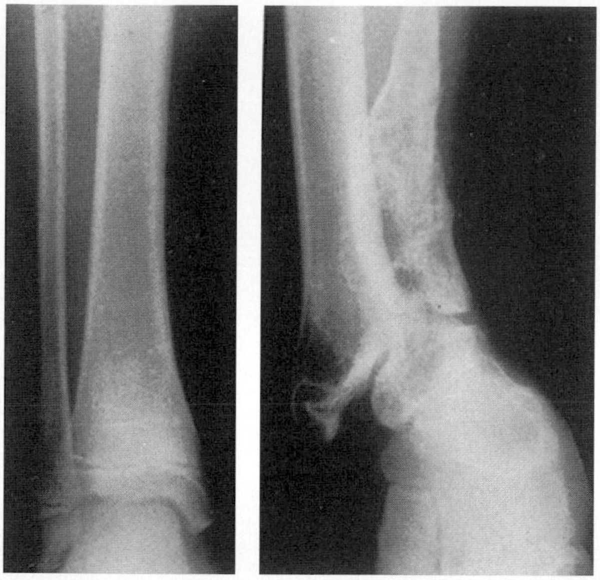

Figure 4.21 Involvement of distal tibia and fibula in enchondromatosis.

first few years of life. When unilateral, it is seen that one limb is not growing at the same rate as its fellow. When bilateral, the general growth appears to lag. Sometimes the enlargement of the affected hand bones is the earliest feature to attract attention.

Later, deformity may appear. It is due to weight-bearing, or to unequal affection of the metaphysis, and a consequent difference in the growth rate between the affected and unaffected parts.

DIFFERENTIAL DIAGNOSIS

Hunter and Wiles in 1935 pointed out that a positive diagnosis can be made on three main points:

1. The onset is in early childhood.
2. The changes are limited to the ends of long bone (see Figure 4.22).
3. Biopsy reveals that the clear areas in the radiograph are composed of cartilage.

Metaphyseal aclasis

Metaphyseal aclasis can be excluded by its striking hereditary tendency, by the invariable presence of

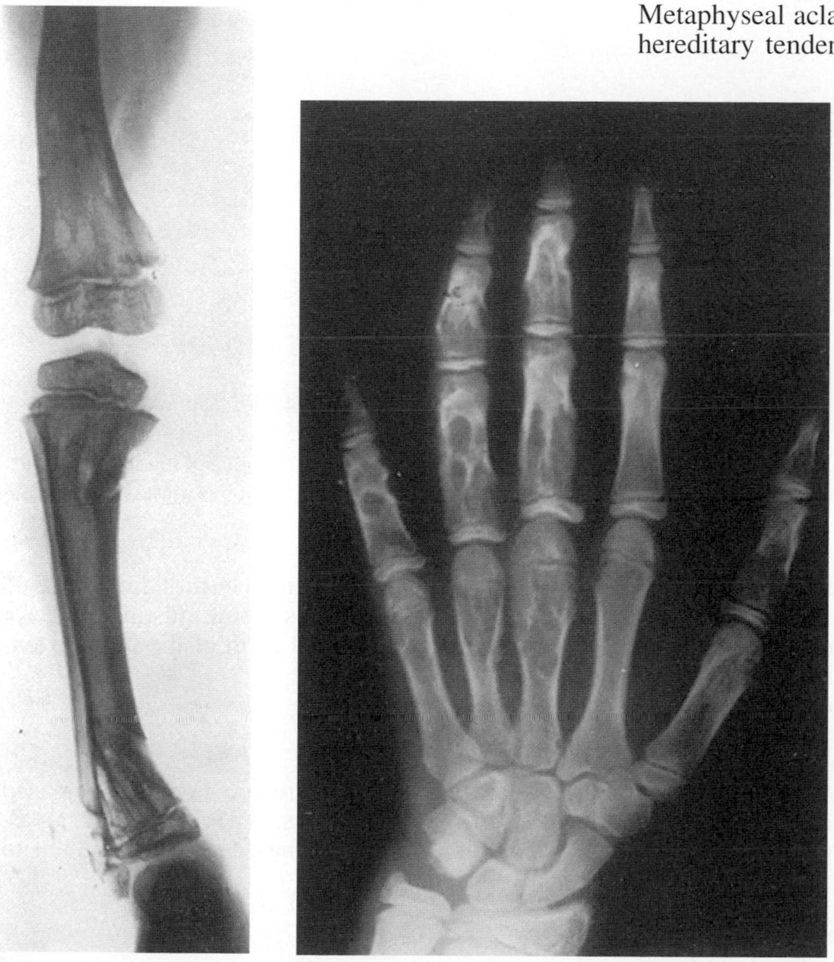

(a) (b)

Figure 4.22 Dyschondroplasia. Radiographs showing both metaphyseal and diaphyseal lesions of (a) the right tibia, and (b) the hand with involvement of the short bones, widening of the shafts by large cyst-like areas and thinning of the cortex. There is a pathological fracture of the ring middle phalanx.

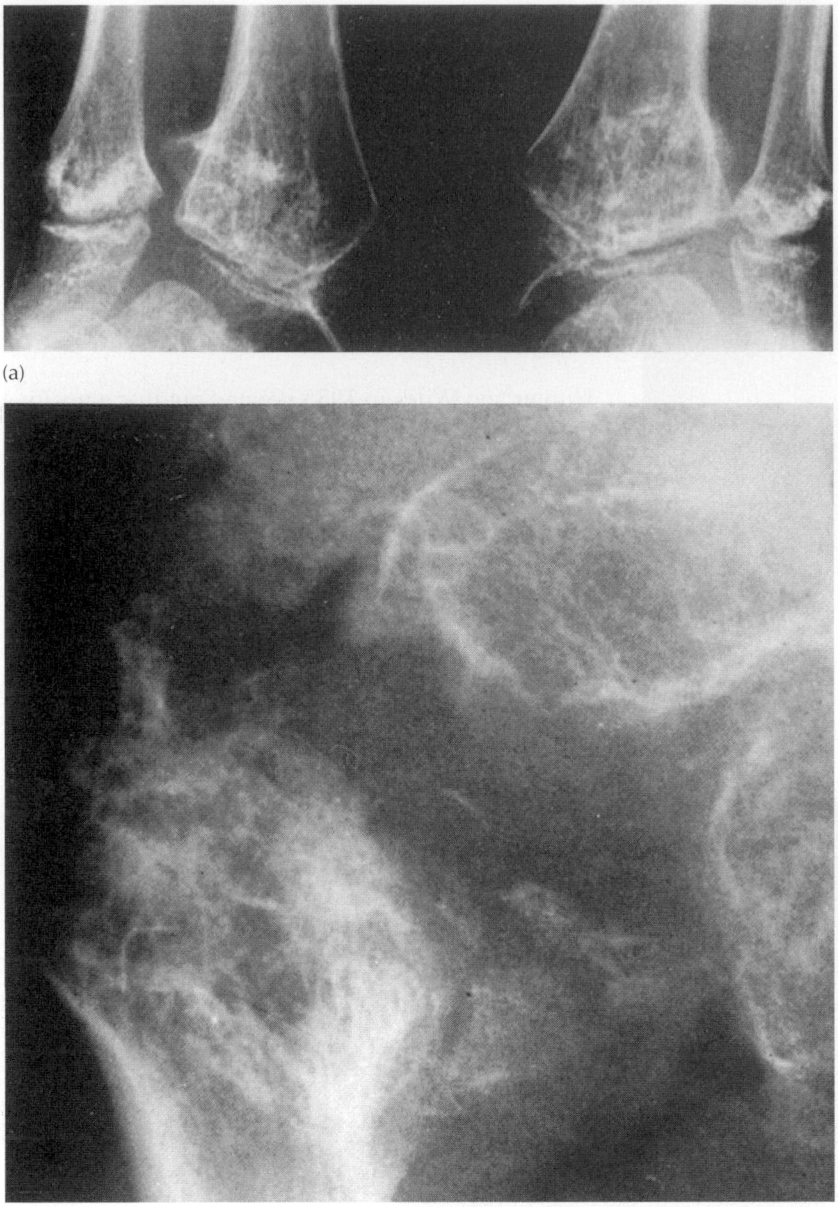

(a)

(b)

Figure 4.23 Young girl with radiographic changes of dyschondroplasia involving (a) the wrist and (b) hip joints.

multiple exostoses which are pedunculated and usually point away from the end of the bones. In metaphyseal aclasis, the metaphysis is always expanded and the sides of the broadened area are usually parallel; there is a sharp line of demarcation between the expanded area and the normal shaft – an appearance well described by Keith as 'trumpeting'. In dyschondroplasia the metaphyseal expansion, when present, is fusiform in outline.

Multiple enchondromata

The appearance of multiple enchondromata may be present in radiological studies of the hands and feet in dyschondroplasia. When an enchondroma occurs alone, therefore, there is some justification for regarding it as a localized form of the more extensive disease.

Osteopathia striata

In osteopathia striata there are lines of increased density in the metaphysis. The less dense areas, however, are not due to masses of cartilage but to bones of normal texture.

Osteopoikilosis

In osteopoikilosis there are again rounded or elongated areas of increased density, but these are scattered throughout the entire bone, and are often arranged in the long axis of the bone.

The age of onset, the number of bones affected and the characteristic metaphyseal change are sufficient to exclude the generalized fibrocystic diseases.

PROGNOSIS

Thc prognosis as regards life appears to be good. In some cases quoted by Hunter and Wiles (1935), death occurred from the supervention of sarcoma; in others anaemia resulted, apparently from the restriction of the available marrow space.

Deformity and secondary arthritis are constant sequelae.

TREATMENT OF DEFORMITIES

There is a tendency to growth variation of one side of the epiphyseal line as compared to the other. When this occurs at the ends of long bones, the deformity produced leads to secondary complications. This is evident with medial facing of the ankle producing secondary pronation of the feet, for example. Pressure localized to one side of the joint may produce flattening of the epiphysis and of the joint cartilage. For this reason, real deformity cannot be left unattended even if more than one correction may be required in the growth cycle.

Osteotomy to realign joints in an anatomical relationship to the weight-bearing line or anatomical line in the upper extremity is frequently necessary. Occasionally, near the end of the growth period unilateral stapling of an epiphyseal line or epiphyseodesis may be necessary. Diminished growth of the ulna and fibula may occur, leading to secondary deformation of the distal joint at wrist and ankle. Release of this tethering effect, restoration of normal alignment by lengthening procedures and osteotomy may be indicated before the deformity becomes so severe that anatomical restoration is impossible.

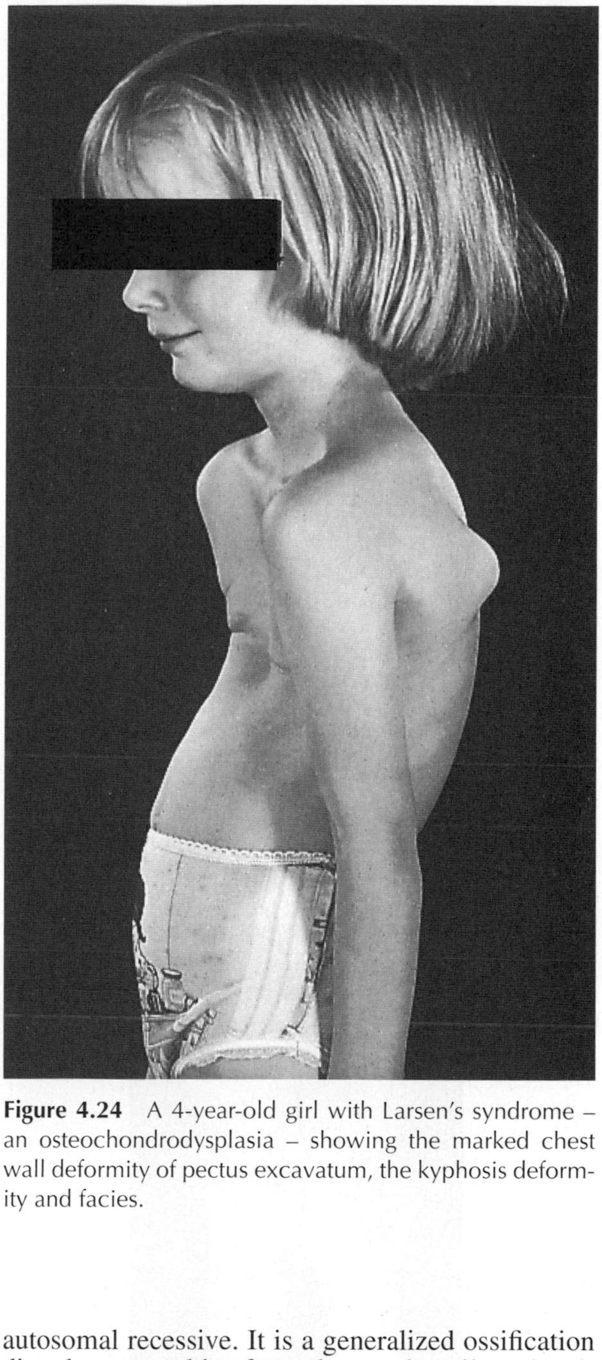

Figure 4.24 A 4-year-old girl with Larsen's syndrome – an osteochondrodysplasia – showing the marked chest wall deformity of pectus excavatum, the kyphosis deformity and facies.

Osteochondrodysplasia – Larsen's disease

This is a heterogeneous disease with a varying inheritance pattern of autosomal dominance and of autosomal recessive. It is a generalized ossification disturbance resulting from abnormal cartilage development, affecting all the spine (kyphosis), chest wall with pectus excavatum (Figure 4.24), limbs, fingers and toes with shortening of the metacarpals and lengthening of digits (Figure 4.25), various weight-bearing joint deformities, especially the knees and feet due to marked joint laxity (Figure 4.26). The facies are abnormal with a forward thrust of the head. However, these abnormalities do not usually progress and the various deformities can be corrected (Figure 4.27).

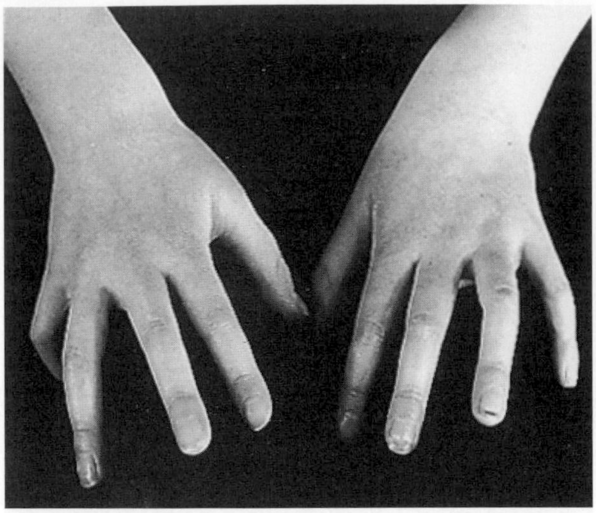

Figure 4.25 The hands of the patient in Figure 4.24, showing foreshortening of the metacarpal lengths and lengthening of the 4th and 5th digits.

Maffucci's syndrome

Maffucci's syndrome is a combination of multiple enchondromata and cavernous haemangiomata, and can be severely disabling in terms of dwarfing.

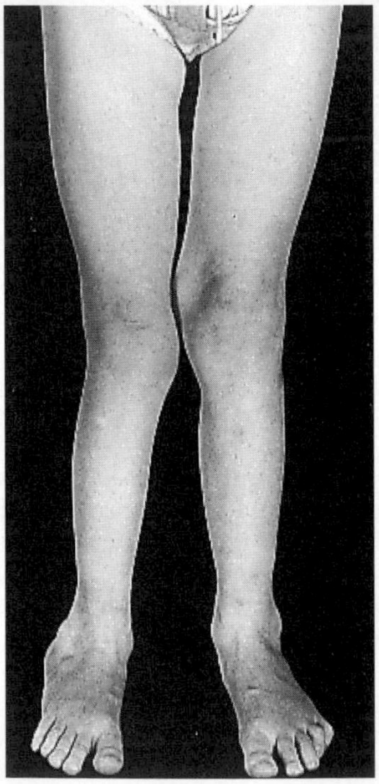

Figure 4.26 The same patient as in Figure 4.24, showing the genu valgum deformity of the knees and ankles.

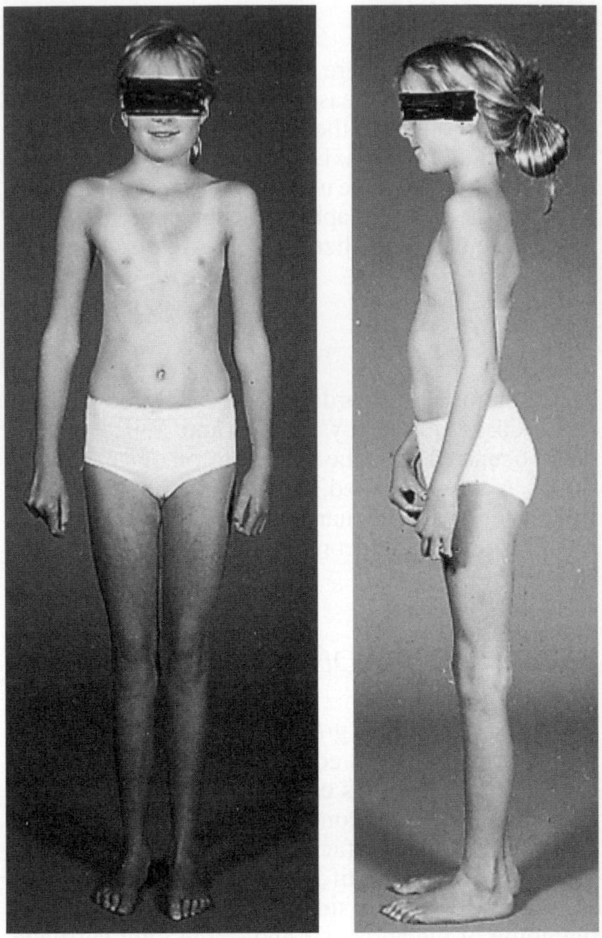

Figure 4.27 The patient in Figure 4.24, at the age of 11 years, with surgical correction of the pectus excavatum deformity and improvement in posture.

Affected persons are of normal intelligence and normal at birth but nodules begin to appear on fingers or toes, followed by other tumours of the long bone. Distribution is asymmetrical but may tend to be unilateral. Dilated veins and soft bluish haemangiomata occur in the subcutaneous and soft tissues, often in conjunction with these areas. In the second decade tumour growth usually ceases and the disease becomes quiescent. There is no visceral involvement and no pain. Circulatory phenomena may occur due to pooling of blood in the dependent haemangioma, and the excessive size of the tumours may interfere with normal function and lead to consideration of amputation. The vascular component is a diffuse cavernous haemangioma with phlebectasia, with frequent thrombi and phleboliths. The affected long bones are usually shortened and bowed, and the metaphyseal regions are widened. Marrow spaces may be filled with confluent cartilage masses separated by bony septa. Bone contour may be distorted and distinct bumps apparent. Normal epiphyseal closure occurs at the proper age. On microscopic examination there is a very cellular disorganized type of cartilage seen, cell nuclei are larger than normal and occasionally doubled. There is some evidence of cartilage proliferation. Chondrosarcomata were found in 7 of 42 cases of Maffucci's syndrome when reviewed by Johnson *et al.* (1960); i.e. a malignancy rate of 16.7%.

Osteochondromatosis (multiple exostoses; diaphyseal aclasis; metaphyseal aclasis)

This is one of the most interesting of the developmental growth disturbances, and may well prove important as an intermediate condition between achondroplasia and the other disturbances of enchondral ossification.

The disease affects only those bones, or portions of bones, which are developed both from cartilage and from membrane, and it has a marked hereditary tendency.

The most characteristic features of metaphyseal aclasis are a failure of remodelling of the metaphysis and the occurrence of multiple outgrowths or exostoses from the surface of the shaft of many of the long bones. In addition, there is often some stunting of skeletal growth. Originally known as multiple exostoses, the disease was renamed diaphyseal aclasis by Sir Arthur Keith, but later Greig pointed out that it was really a metaphyseal affection and suggested the title of metaphyseal aclasis. Inheritance is by an autosomal dominant gene.

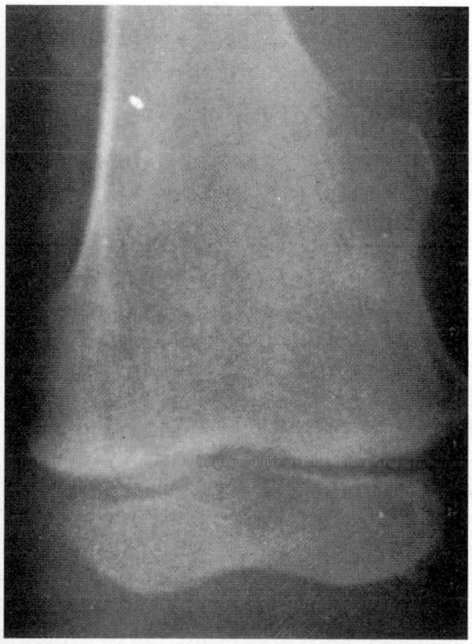

(a)

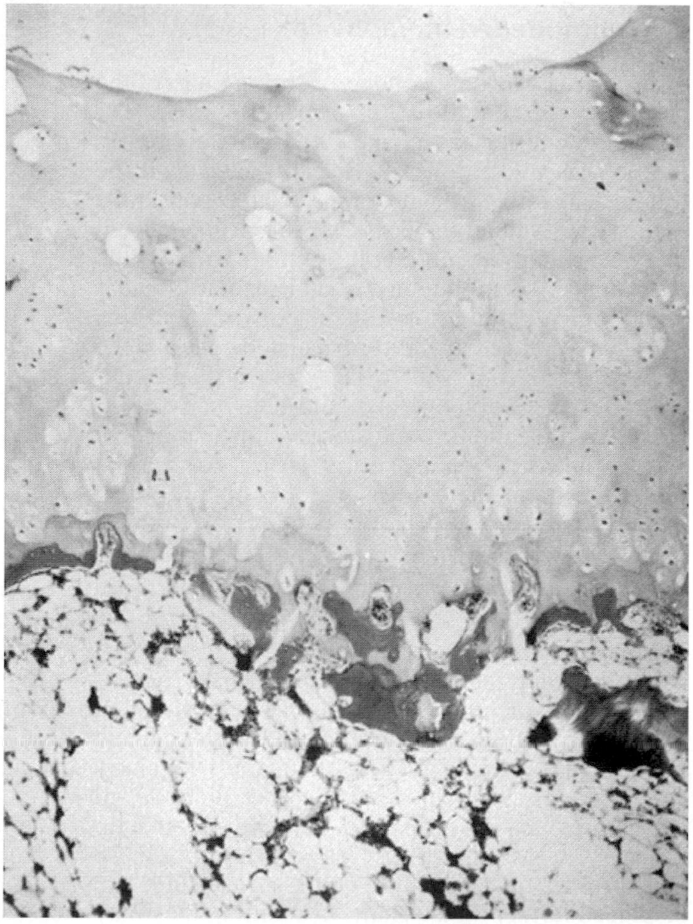

(b)

Figure 4.28 (a) Osteochondroma of the distal femur at both sides of the metaphysis. (b) Cartilage from the growing cap of the osteochondroma.

PATHOLOGY

The membranous bones of the skeleton are immune, as are those developed entirely within cartilage, such as the tarsal and carpal bones and the epiphyses of the long bones. The condition affects those parts of the skeleton where bone arising in cartilage comes to be surrounded by a sheath of subperiosteal bone – hence it is found at the growing ends of the long and the short long bones. It is most marked where growth is most extensive and most prolonged, i.e. the distal end of the femur (Figure 4.28), the proximal ends of the tibia and fibula, the distal ends of the radius and ulna, and the proximal end of the humerus. It is also well seen at the medial and lateral ends of the clavicle, at the cristal border of the ilium, the vertebral border of the scapula, and occasionally at the neurocentral synchondroses of the vertebrae.

The two principal features of the disease are: the unmodelled metaphysis, and the exostoses.

The unmodelled metaphysis

This may or may not be the most striking part of the anomaly. The central part of the shaft is usually of normal cylindrical form, and of normal calibre. As the bone is traced towards its extremity it will be found that, instead of the calibre of the bony tube increasing gradually, there is an abrupt increase in diameter, and the extremity of the bone – the metaphysis – is in the form of an irregular cylinder with roughly parallel sides. In the growing bone this cylinder is composed of ill-trabeculated bone and the surface is covered with a layer of cartilage continuous with the epiphyseal cartilage. In many cases, irregular projections – exostoses – appear on the surface, and occasionally surface projections may be present without increase in the size of the parent bone (Figure 4.29).

The exostoses

Normally most marked at the extremities of the bone, they may be found at practically any part of the shaft. Frequently an exostosis marks the junction of the normally calibrated shaft and the expanded extremity. At this situation they are irregularly spiky. Others occur in relation to the unmodelled extremities and these tend to be more globular in shape. As the shaft increases in length, those exostoses at first near the epiphyseal cartilage are displaced farther up the shaft. In addition, they may become obliquely disposed to the shaft, with their extremity directed away from the extremity of the bone.

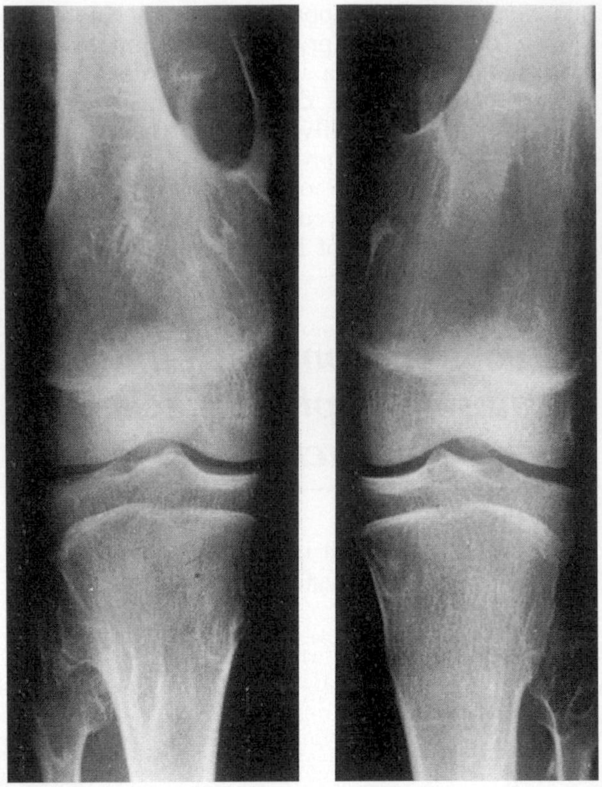

Figure 4.29 Metaphyseal aclasis of the femora and tibiae.

The exostoses are composed of poorly trabeculated bone in direct continuity with the bone of the shaft. During the years of growth the exostosis is surmounted by a cap of cartilage, from which progressive growth in size of the exostosis may take place.

In association with the above features there is usually marked interference with growth in length of the affected bones. From irregularity of the ossification at the epiphyseal line some cartilage cells are not ossified. Those that are central, if they continue to grow, form enchondromas while the peripheral ones form exostoses. It is essentially a failure of maturation of the cartilage cells. In the forearm the growth of the ulna is more interfered with than that of the radius, and perhaps in consequence the radius becomes curved, or dislocation occurs at its proximal extremity. In the leg the fibula lags behind the tibia. In the forearm and the leg an exostosis from one of the bones may cause pressure absorption of the adjacent surface of the neighbouring bone.

The changes in the short long bones are essentially similar and are not to be confused with multiple enchondromata, which is part of the disturbance of *dyschondroplasia*.

Two occasional complications of metaphyseal aclasis must be mentioned:

1. The occasional growth of a *chondroma*, which projects from the surface of the bone near the epiphyseal cartilage. Such a tumour may attain great proportions and is liable to become chondrosarcomatous.
2. *Osteosarcoma* or *chondrosarcoma* may arise in one of the exostoses, sometimes following, but occasionally in the absence of, operative removal. This leads to rapid increase in size of the exostosis. The tendency to malignancy is most marked in exostoses of the pelvis and spine.

Nature of the process

Keith (1920) originally showed that the essential factor in the disease is a failure of the normal remodelling process which trims the metaphysis down to the calibre of the remainder of the bone. To this normal remodelling and adapting process Jansen applied the term 'tubulation'. In addition to the failure of normal tubulation, however, the exostosis possesses a power of continued growth equal to that of the parent bone. Keith accordingly supposed that the growth of the sheath of subperiosteal bone did not keep pace with the growth of bone from the growth cartilage, and the absence of the normal bony ferrule left the cartilage of the growth disc uncovered on the surface, and free to give rise to irregular excrescences (Figure 4.30).

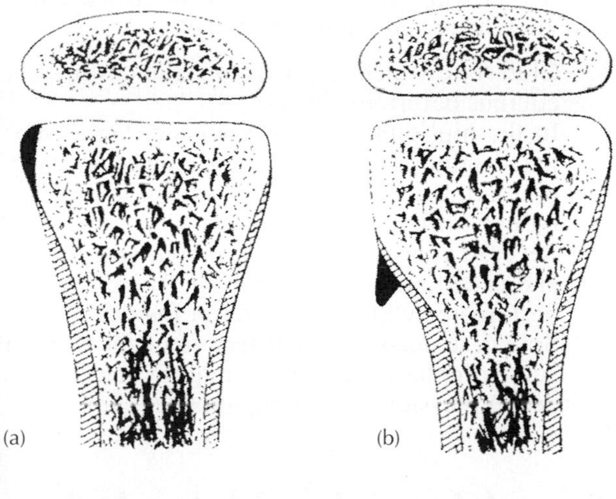

Figure 4.30 Development of an osteochondroma from the periphery of the epiphyseal cartilage. (a) Areas of chondrodysplasia such as this are not subject to remodelling. (b) The bone which does not support the cartilage cap is subject to remodelling, leaving the osteochondroma projecting from the cortex.

Time factor in osteochondromatosis

Though the tendency to the disease is usually inherited and present at birth, obvious evidence of its presence appears only after 7 or 8 years, when growth is speeded up and the exostoses become apparent. Exostoses situated towards the mid-shaft have commenced to grow at an early age, and been gradually displaced to their mid-shaft position by subsequent growth in length of the bone.

CLINICAL FEATURES

The process may be local or diffuse. When local, one of the extremities is involved, while the remainder of the skeleton is normal. In the diffuse type there may be extensive distortion and deformity of the whole skeleton.

The stature is short or even dwarfed. In addition, the limbs may show deformities of the nature of bowing, or knock-knee. Fracture from slight trauma is common, but the fragments unite as readily as in normal individuals.

The most typical feature is the presence of numerous exostoses. These are most common at sites of active growth, such as the knee and shoulder. The projections are hard, the skin overlying them is normal, and the soft tissues move easily on them. They may be associated with pain if the tumour presses on a peripheral nerve or a nerve root, or if the process is inadvertently fractured. They are also liable to interfere with the free play of associated tendons, or may even act as a mechanical obstruction to joint movement, in which event they may give rise to considerable disability. A bursa may form over the projection and become, from time to time, inflamed.

RADIOLOGICAL APPEARANCES

The radiological examination shows an irregularly expanded metaphyseal mass, with little or no compact cortical bone. The architecture of the interior is altered The normal cancellous tissue is replaced by a mass of less dense tissue, in which islands of normal ossification may be observed.

The exostoses appear as definite projections from that metaphyseal region. Their structure is similar to that of the metaphysis – clear interior, with a thick shell of cortical bone.

PROGNOSIS AND TREATMENT

The disease has no effect on the general health, but there may be disability as a result of nerve pressure or interference with joint or tendon movement. Malignant change with formation of osteogenic and chondrosarcomata has been recorded.

The only treatment indicated is the symptomatic one of removing exostoses which are increasing in size rapidly or giving rise to trouble by pressure or malignant change.

Epiphyseal hyperplasia (dysplasia epiphysealis hemimelia)

This unusual growth disturbance produces overgrowth of long bone epiphyses, forming an anterior, posterior or side projection. It has been described as an osteochondroma which affects the epiphysis instead of the diaphysis. It affects a single epiphysis, the great majority being of the talus, the distal femur or the proximal tibia.

The lesion presents during childhood and is asymptomatic until the protruding epiphyseal mass interferes with joint function. The disturbance of the epiphyseal osseous nucleus results in an excessive growth anterior, posterior or to one side, or a separate osseous nucleus may be established with hyperplasia of the overlying cartilage zone (Figure 4.31).

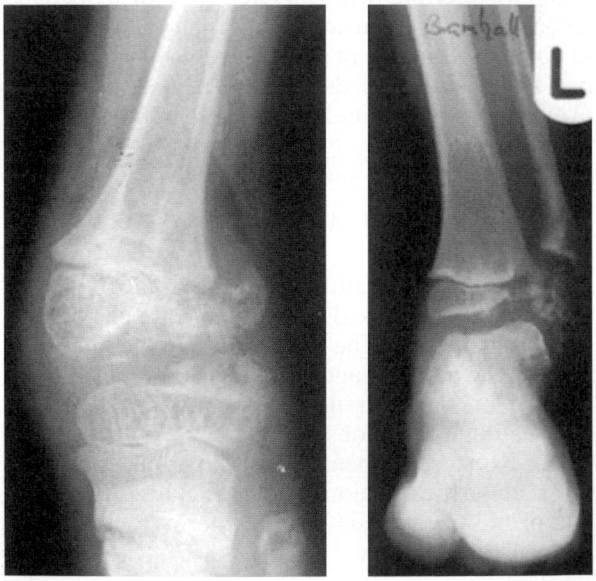

(a) (b)

Figure 4.31 Dysplasia epiphysealis hemimelia. Radiographs of (a) the knee and (b) the ankle, with lateral overgrowth of the lower femoral and lower fibular epiphysis affecting only the left leg.

Diastrophic dwarfism

This autosomal recessive disease was described in 1960 by Lamy and Maroteaux. There is micromelic dwarfism with little disturbance in the axial skeleton except for occasional cleft palate and lumbar scoliosis. It does not cause death but will cause severe loss of function such that some patients may never be able to walk. In the majority of cases there is a laxity of the tendons and ligaments so that the joints are hyperextensile. Aegerter and Kirkpatrick (1975) regarded this as a result of an inability to produce normal chondroid but there is also a defect in collagen formation which produces the ligament laxity.

The child may present at birth with dislocation of the hip though at that stage the spine will be straight. Hyperplasia of cervical vertebral bodies has been reported. Of particular diagnostic significance are the deformities of the hands and feet, which show the short metacarpal and metatarsal bones with a rectangular configuration, causing a so-called 'hitch-hiker thumb' and talipes equinovarus. Scoliosis develops as time goes by, and the long bones become short and broad with flat epiphyseal centres and distorted shapes. The epiphyseal centres of the tubular bones of the hands and feet are delayed, and the centres for the carpus and tarsus are accelerated.

Deficiency of tracheal cartilage formation may result in lack of rigidity which causes respiratory distress and may precipitate early death.

The following deformities are common in diastrophic dwarfism, and require treatment.

1. Club foot, which responds to serial casting but equinus deformity recurs.
2. In the hip joint one sees flattened, large, subluxed femoral heads which are prone to early osteoarthritis; total hip replacement is possible though difficult to perform.
3. Severe kyphoscoliosis is common, progressive and usually resistant to bracing. Therefore it is best treated with early posterior fusion.
4. Spinal stenosis is much less frequent than in achondroplasia, and may require multi-level decompression when symptomatic.

Spondyloepiphyseal dysplasia

Whereas dwarfing in Morquio's disease is due largely to failure of trunk growth and in achondroplasia is due to deficiency of limb growth, in spon-

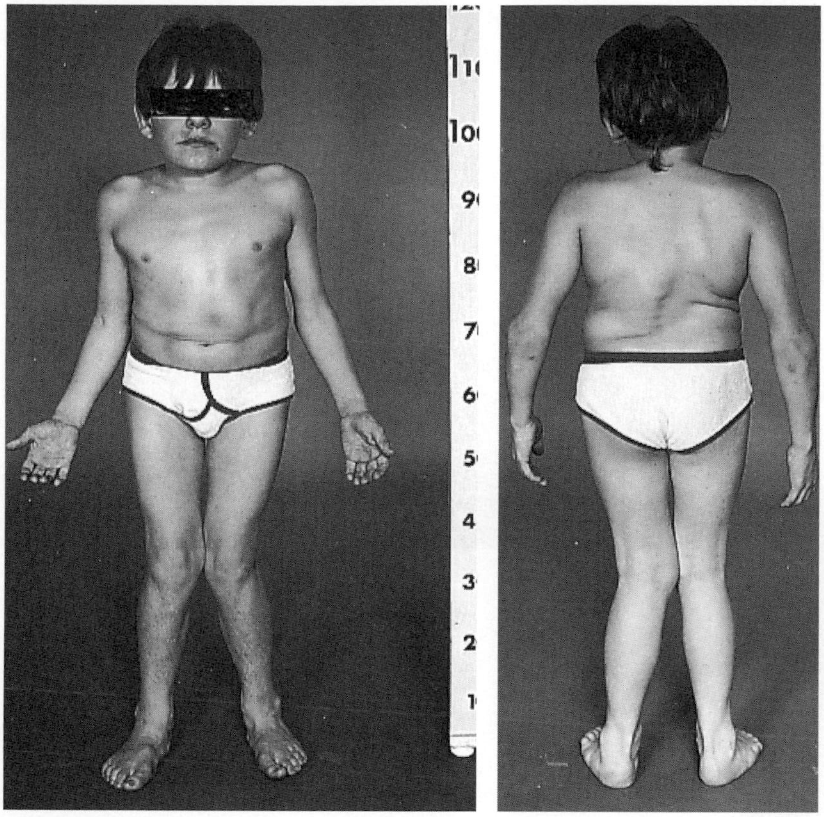

Figure 4.32 A 14-year-old boy with spondyloepiphyseal dysplasia showing the severe dwarfing of both trunk and all extremities. The hands are short and stubby; cubitus valgus as well as genu valgus deformities.

dyloepiphyseal dysplasia deficient growth occurs in both the vertebrae and the extremities. The principal metabolic fault appears to be inability to ossify epiphyseal centres. This causes failure of support to the articular cartilage, which leads to early osteoarthritis in adults. This condition presents at birth but without the saddle nose and prognathism present in achondroplasia, and the epiphyseal centres are much more irregular and often multiple. McKusick has suggested two forms of this condition, one being autosomal dominant and the other X-linked recessive. The dwarfing of the trunk and extremities is severe, with short stubby hands and vertebra plana (Figure 4.32). Occasionally the condition is overlooked until adulthood and presents with early osteoarthrosis of the hips.

The radiographs show thickening and irregularity of the vertebral bodies, narrowing of the intervertebral discs with enlargement of the posterior portions of the bodies. Hypoplasia of the odontoid has been described. The epiphyseal centres – especially of the long bones – are fragmented, and ossification is defective with secondary alterations in the epiphyseal line and in some instances in the metaphysis (Figure 4.33).

Spondyloepiphyseal dysplasia is commonly accompanied by odontoid aplasia, which may require fusion. An exaggerated lumbar lordosis with hip flexion contracture is seen, and may be treated by psoas lengthening.

Coxa vara deformity of the hips is progressive and requires a valgus osteotomy to prevent further subluxation.

Multiple epiphyseal dysplasia

This condition (first described by Fairbank in 1935) is a congenital disturbance in the ossification of the epiphyses. It is usually first seen when the child begins to walk with a waddling gait and is noted to have short stubby digits of the hands and feet. Later it is manifested particularly by early development of osteoarthrosis of the hips. Multiple irregular ossification centres cause enlargement of the epiphyses and sometimes flaring of the diaphyseal ends. The tibiae are usually curved with knock-knee or bowleg deformity and some flexion deformity. The

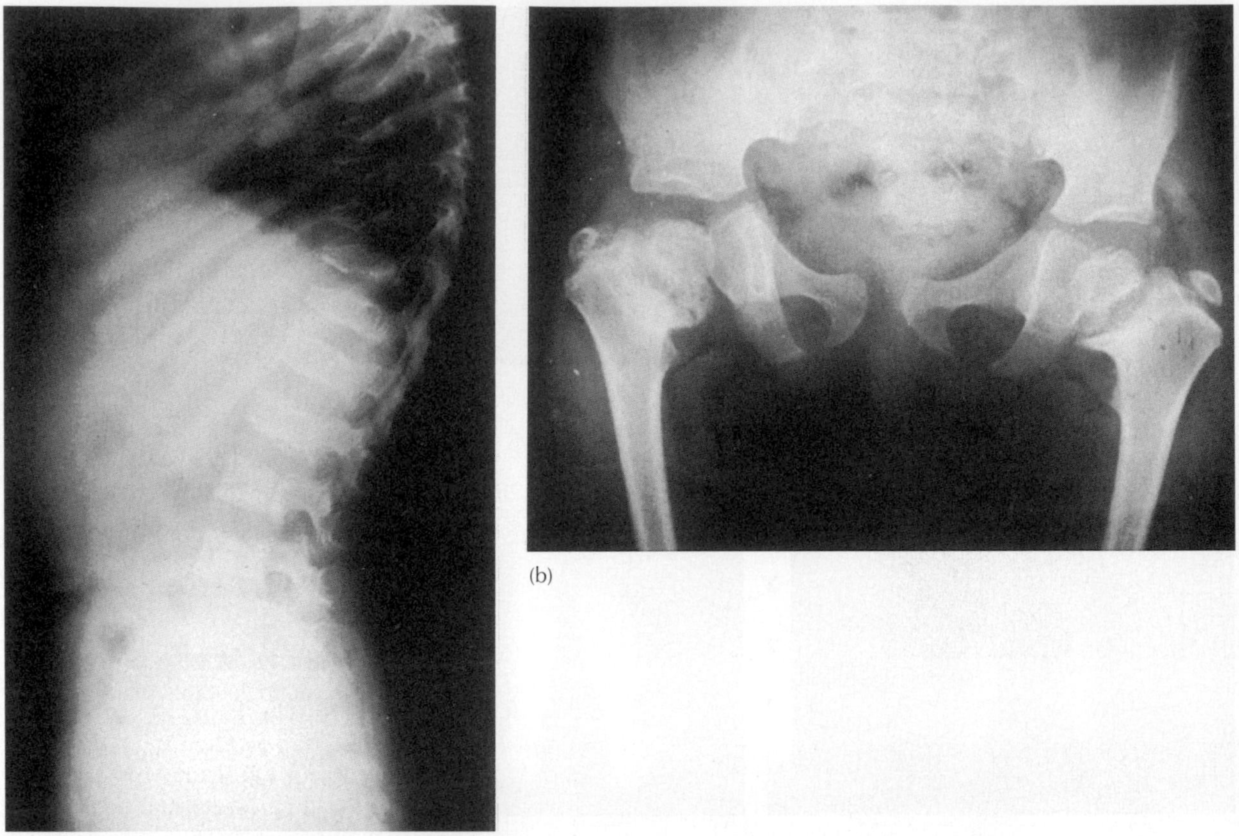

(b)

(a)

Figure 4.33 Spondyloepiphyseal dysplasia. (a) Lateral radiograph of the spine, showing vertebra plana, thoracic kyphosis and deficiency of anterior vertebral bodies. (b) Hip radiograph, showing the shortening of the femoral necks, imperfect ossification of the femoral heads and resultant coxa vara.

vertebrae are usually minimally affected, so the appearances are like that of achondroplasia. The fusion of the epiphyses is irregular, leading to joint surface irregularities and thus early osteoarthrosis. The prognosis is good in general, the limitations being due to the early development of degenerative joint disease (Figure 4.34).

Blount's disease

Blount's disease or osteochondrosis deformans tibiae is probably a clinical subvariety of multiple epiphyseal dysplasia. It has been suggested that it could be analogous to the ischaemic necrosis of the head of the femur seen in Perthes' disease (Figures 4.35 and 4.36).

See Chapter 3 for further information.

Stippled epiphyses (punctate epiphyseal dysplasia)

This rare condition is characterized by multiple punctate opacities appearing in the unossified epiphyseal cartilage at birth. Infants are frequently stillborn or die of associated anomalies within the first year. There is a milder form which is not noted at birth. Dwarfism is absent, and the stippled areas merge into normal-appearing epiphyseal osseous centres.

Osteogenesis imperfecta

This condition – variously named osteitis fragilitans, fragilitas ossium congenita, osteopsathyrosis idiopathica and brittle bones – is a hereditary, often congenital and familial disease. The incidence is

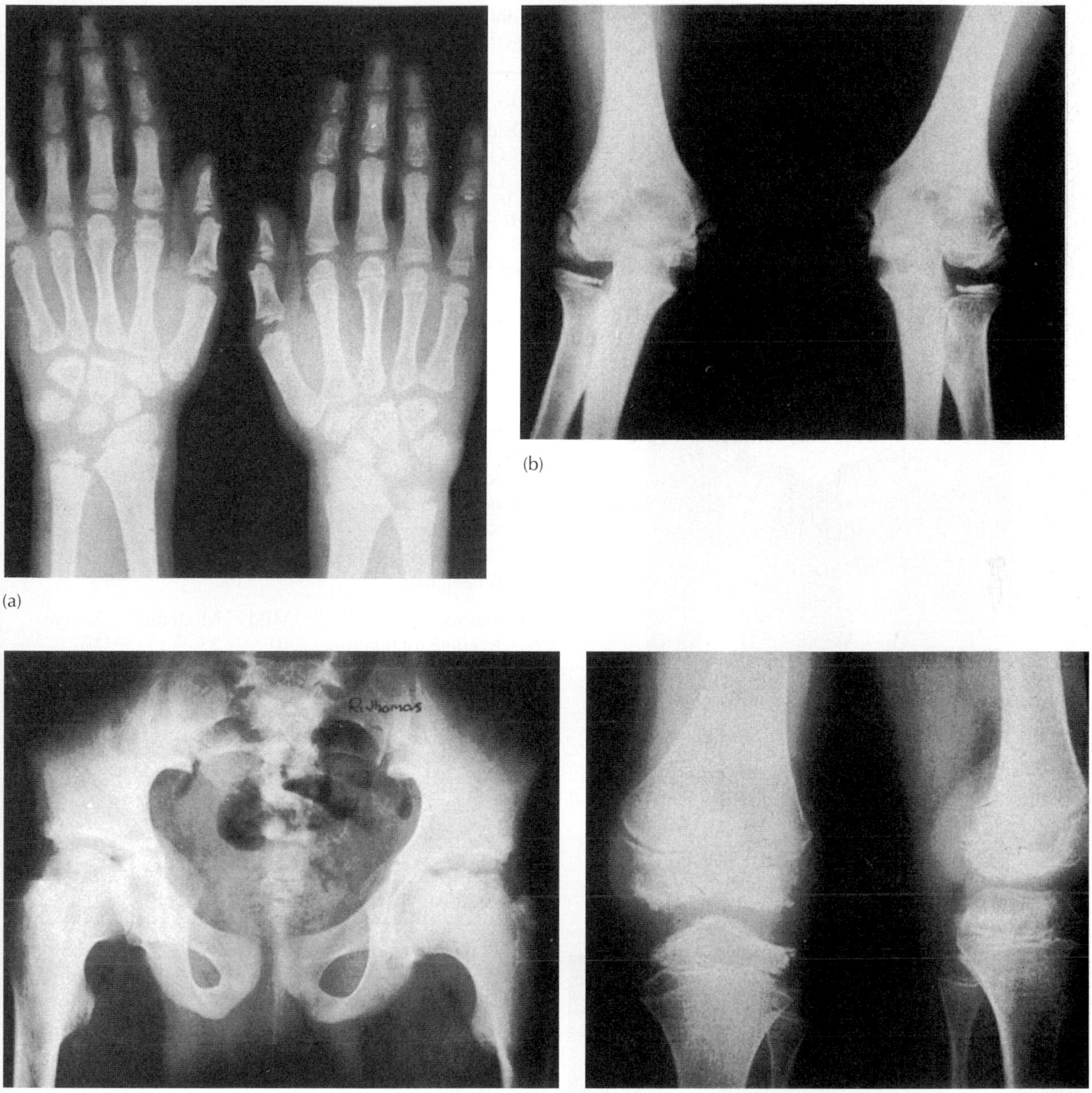

(a) (b) (c) (d)

Figure 4.34 Multiple epiphyseal dysplasia. Radiographs of (a, b) the upper and (c, d) the lower limb joints, showing the irregularity of epiphyses and articular surfaces, which will lead eventually to osteoarthrosis. The metaphyses and diaphyses are normal.

1:20 000–50 000 live births and about 36 per million of population.

Classifications have been numerous but fraught with difficulties due to difficulty differentiating between types II and III. A clinical classification has been described by Bauze *et al.* (1975a,b) and is shown in Table 4.3.

Sillence *et al.* (1979) have also classified osteogenesis imperfecta into:

- OI type I – dominant inherited with blue sclerae. There is a defective formation type I collagen, half normal amounts of $\alpha 1(I)$ chains.
- OI type II – new mutations being lethal perinatal, with radiographically crumpled femora and headed ribs. Thc biochemistry is variable, probably many mutations causing delayed helix formation and overmodification of the collagen.

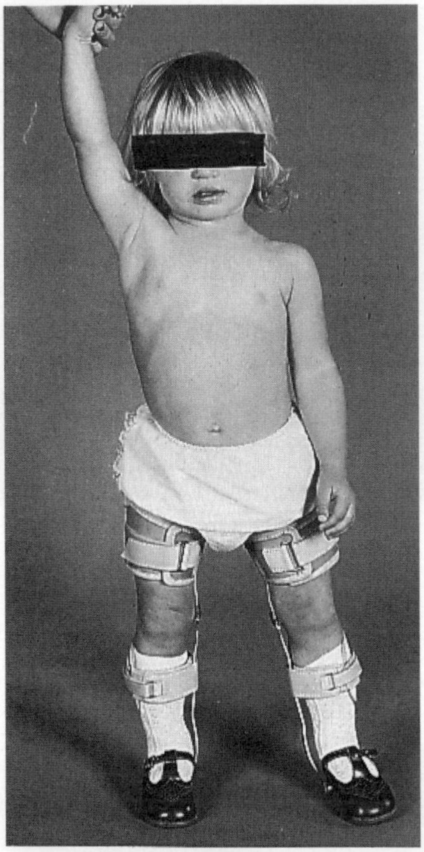

Figure 4.35 Two-year-old child with bilateral orthotic supports for correcting Blount's disease with bilateral tibial varus.

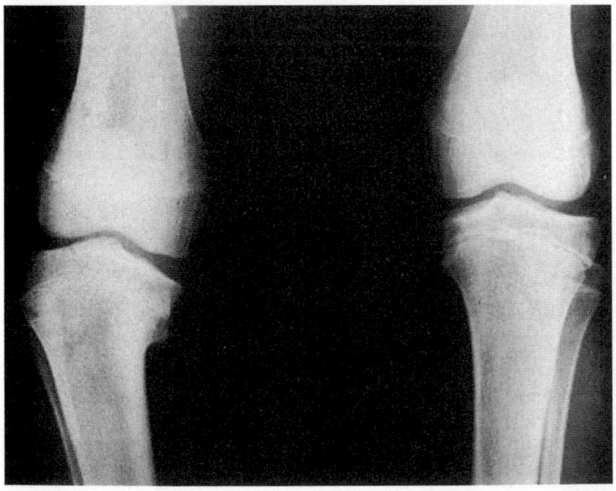

Figure 4.36 Blount's disease. Anteroposterior view of both knees, demonstrating the typical growth abnormality of the right medial upper tibial epiphysis which will produce gross genu varum.

Table 4.3 Clinical classification of osteogenesis imperfecta

Osteogenesis imperfecta congenita			
Osteogenesis imperfecta tarda			
Gravis < 1 year			
Levis > 1 year			
Mild and severe osteogenesis imperfecta			
	Mild		Severe
Scleral colour			
Blue	161		62
White (normal)	7		54
Unknown	3		9
Deafness	19/36		5/90
Dentinogenesis imperfecta	12/103		45/97
Heart disease	6		2
Bruising/bleeding	13		2
Keloid/wide scars	8		0
Disability			
None	86%		13%
Crutches/stick	12.5%		29%
Wheelchair	1%		58%
Fractures	Mild	Moderate	Severe
Average total number	10	23	36
Age of onset			
Average	3.5 years	20 months	12 months
Range	Birth–24 years	Birth–12 years	Birth–13 years
Fractures present at birth (%)	1.5	22	51
Scoliosis	11%	19%	73%
Hyperplastic callus	0	0	5
'Cystic' epiphyses	0	0	12

After Bauze *et al.* (1975a,b).

- OI type III – some are progressive with progressive deformation but normal sclerae. The biochemistry is unknown.
- OI type IV – dominantly inherited with normal sclerae. There is some evidence of link to $\alpha 2$(I) gene.

The classical clinical features are:

1. *Skeletal*
   (a) Deformity and short stature in severer forms.
   (b) Osteoporosis proportional to severity.
   (c) Long bones
   Diaphysis: width may be normal, or narrow in infants, or wide in children.
   Metaphysis: usually very thin or even an absent cortex.
   Epiphysis: usually normal, but may be cystic.

(d) Skull – wormian bones ('Tam O'Shanter') skull.
(e) Spine – prominent vertebral trabeculae. ? biconcave. Usually kyphoscoliosis in severer forms.
(f) Pelvis – triradiate in severe forms.
(g) Ribs – irregular thickness in severe forms.

2. *Extraskeletal*
Blue sclerae, 80–90%
Deafness, 40%
Dentinogenesis, 10–50%
Ligamentous laxity, 50–70%
Cardiac abnormalities, 10%
Other ocular abnormalities (arcus juvenilis and senilis, hypermetropia, myopia, keratoconus), 5%

AETIOLOGY

The abnormal biochemistry has been described by Smith (1994) and Byers (1993). Osteogenesis Imperfecta is caused by mutations in the genes for type I collagen (the major fibrillar collagen). Type I collagen consists of three chains that combine to form a triple helical molecule; the association of these molecules forms the collagen fibre. The considerable strength of collagen depends on its absolute structural integrity and exact intramolecular and intermolecular cross-linking. A single nucleotide mutation in a collagen gene may be sufficient to cause lethal OI. This is particularly so where the mutation results in the replacement of glycine, which lies in the centre of the helix, by an amino acid with a large side chain:

- In type I OI there is a 50% reduction in type I collagen, apparently because of a non-functional allele.
- In type II, the most common change is a single base mutation leading to the replacement of glycine by a larger amino acid, so that the tissues contain an excess of abnormal collagen and a markedly reduced amount of normal collagen.
- Similar mutations occur in type III OI, but with less severe effects. Occasionally, one of the constituent chains ($\alpha 2$) of the triple helix of type I may be absent.
- Family studies have shown that type IV OI is also often linked to mutations in the $\alpha 2$ chain.

HISTOPATHOLOGY

Knaggs in 1926 made a comprehensive contribution to the pathology of this condition. He showed that in osteogenesis imperfecta the epiphyseal cartilage is

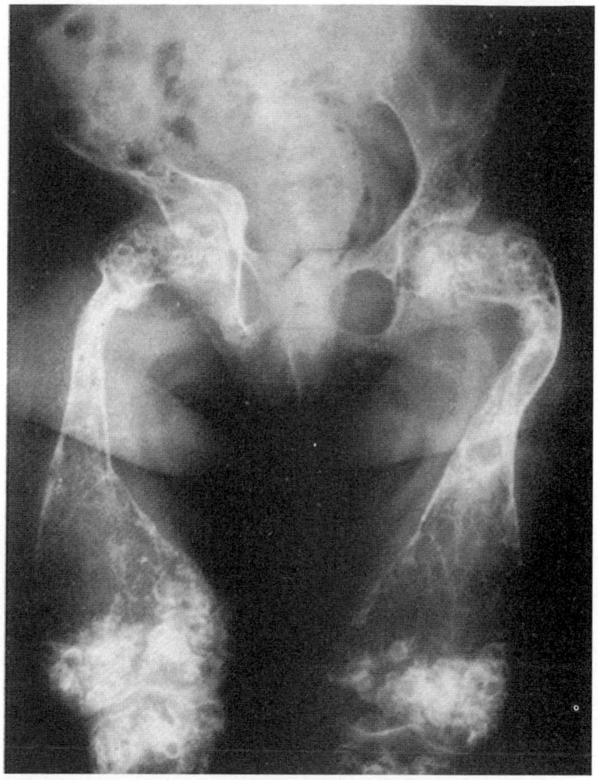

Figure 4.37 Osteogenesis imperfecta cystica.

of normal extent and the zone of calcified cartilage is normal in appearance; but that in the zone of ossification – the metaphysis – the trabeculae are slender and delicate, and widely separated by interstices filled with cellular connective tissue or fibrous marrow. No cross-trabeculae are present as a general rule. The periosteum is thick, and there is no compact cortical layer of bone, but delicate and discrete subperiosteal trabeculae.

The bones as a general rule are shorter, smaller and thinner than corresponding bones of normal individuals at a comparable age, so the general skeletal development tends to be stunted (Figure 4.37).

In most cases there have been many healed fractures, many in bad position. The consequent deformity, producing as it does shortening of the affected bones, adds to the dwarfing.

The essential feature of the histopathology of fragilitas ossium is a scattered defect of the primitive mesenchymal cells in which there is a failure of maturation and calcification. These abnormal cells enlarge to resemble in appearance cartilage cells. Normally, at the epiphyseal line the primitive mesenchymal cells should arrange themselves in an orderly manner about the invading capillaries of the metaphysis. The arrangement is irregular and, as bone is

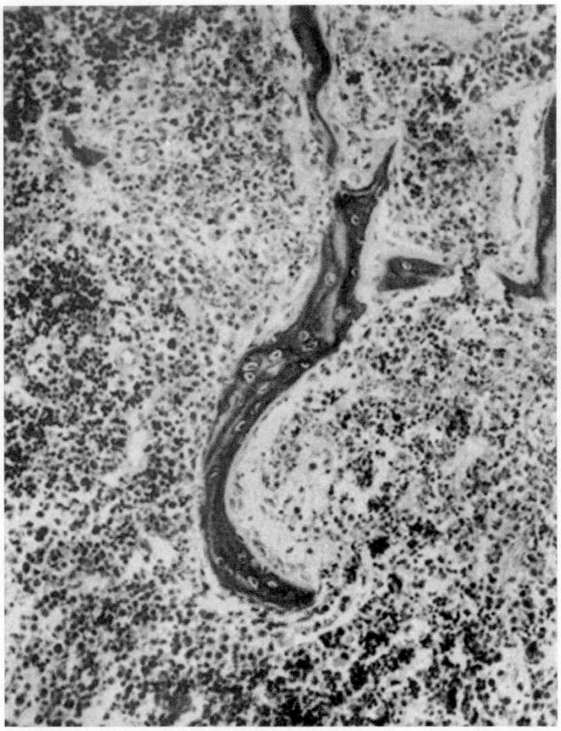

(a)

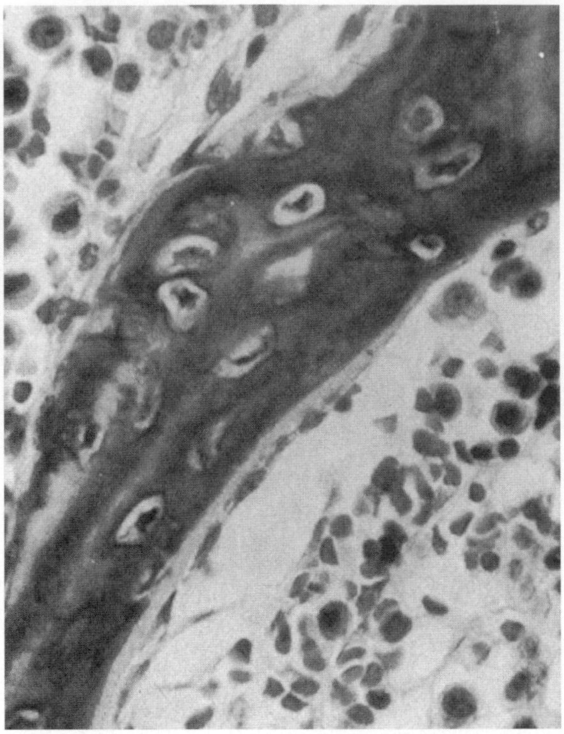

(b)

(c)

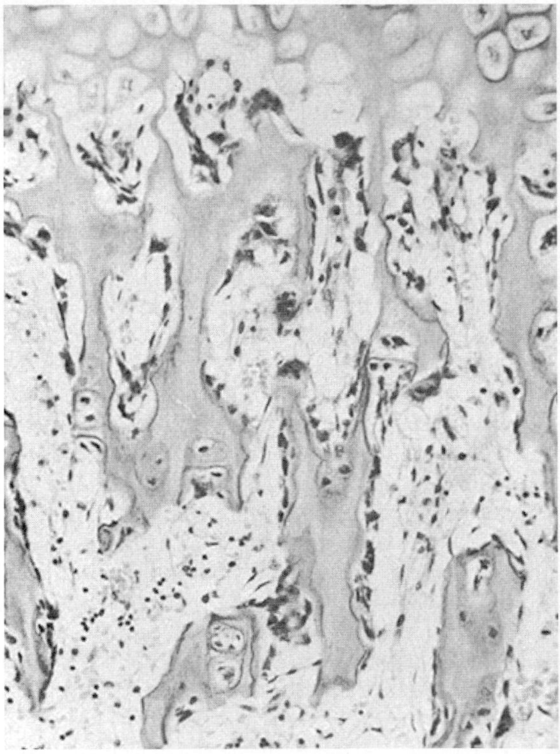

(d)

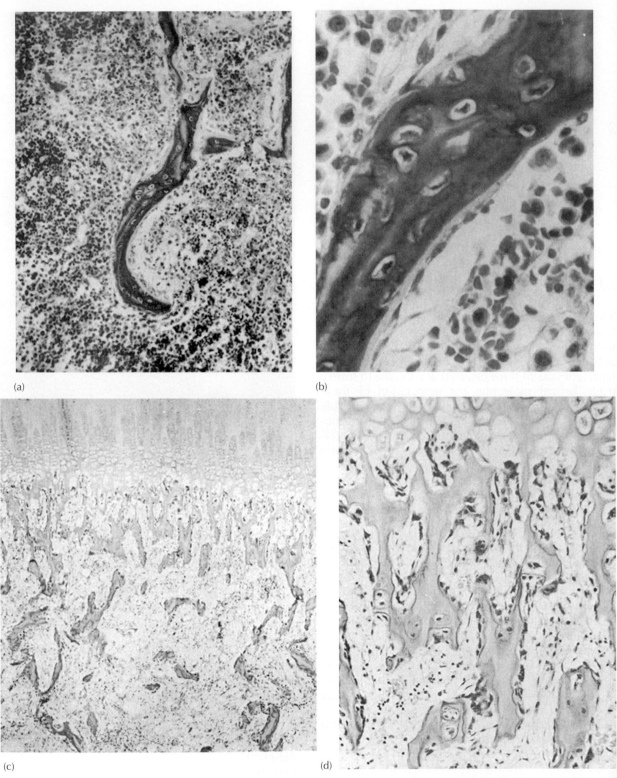

Figure 4.38 (a) Photomicrograph of osteogenesis imperfecta, showing an attenuated and narrowed trabecula within a very cellular stroma. (× 156). (b) Photomicrograph showing the greater detail of the trabecula containing osteocytes in an irregular way and the cells around it. (× 465). (c) Photomicrograph of an epiphysis in osteogenesis imperfecta, showing the normal-appearing epiphyseal zone down to the level of calcified cartilage which appears fragmented and irregular, extending far down into the metaphysis. (× 42, H & E). (d) Photomicrograph showing the irregular cartilage and spicules of primitive bone and relatively few osteoblasts. (× 162, H & E).

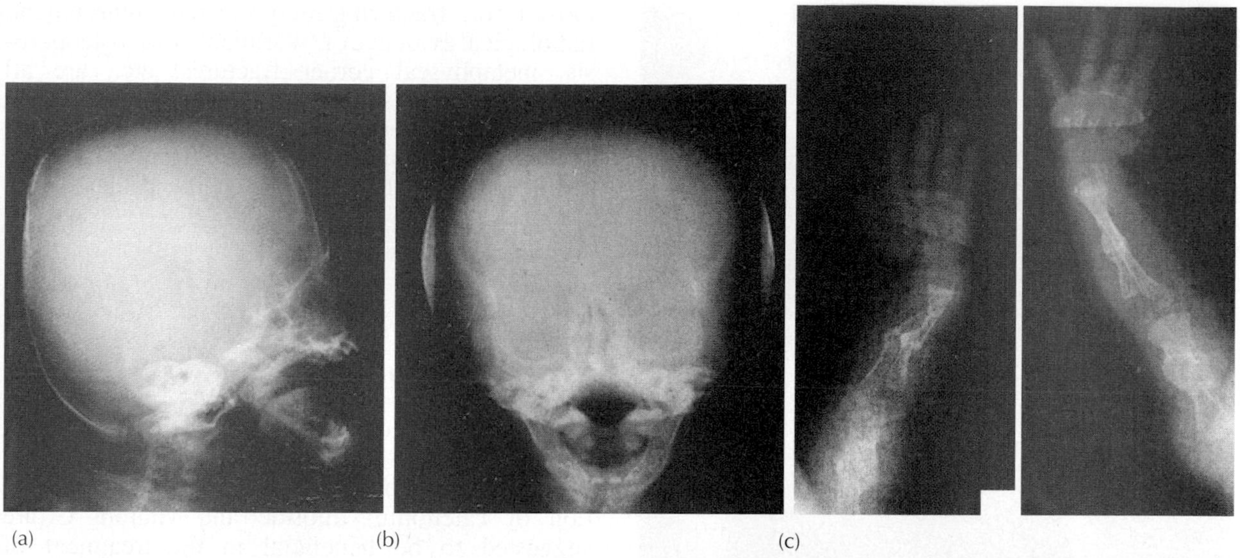

Figure 4.39 (a) Lateral view of skull of child with osteogenesis imperfecta, to show the marked globular shape and reduction in size of the base. (b) Anterior view of the skull, with distension and thinness of the diploe and the hydrocephalic shape. (c) Radiographs of the same child, showing bilateral healing fractures of both bones of the forearm and humeri. There is abnormality of the widened epiphyseal lines, and stunting of longitudinal growth — sometimes a micromelia (tiny extremities).

elaborated, the swollen defective primitive mesenchymal cells are enclosed within the irregular Haversian systems (Figure 4.38). A similar pathological differentiation of the primitive mesenchymal cells occurs in the subperiosteal region where there is no normal compact bone.

Nature of the bone formed

The bones are extremely fragile and difficult to interpret from biopsy samples. Robichon and Germain (1968), from a detailed examination of 29 specimens, described how this condition is associated with a marked increase in osteocytes, in intratrabecular resorption and in much immature bone architecture leading to the fragility. It is a disease of bone matrix with an abnormal secretion of amino acids and hence synthesis of collagen. The blue coloration of the sclera results from thinning of the sclera allowing the choroid to show through more clearly. Knaggs suggested that, since the outstanding feature of the disease is a failure to produce osteoblasts, there is an inherent and hereditary inability on the part of the mesoderm to produce this highly specialized cell.

Francis *et al.* (1974) identified abnormalities in cross-linking of skin collagen in severe disease indicating the nature of the cellular abnormality.

The raised serum alkaline phosphatase which is a frequent finding is probably due to the increased osteoblastic response to injury.

CLINICAL FEATURES

The skull with minimal trauma may assume a globular shape and may appear large in proportion to the rest of the body. True hydrocephalus may develop, and this again may be related to intracranial damage at birth (Figure 4.39).

RADIOLOGICAL APPEARANCES

These depend on the age of the patient and the severity of the condition. The bones in severe types may show practically complete absence of cancellous texture, the cortex appearing as a faintly pencilled line. The bones are shorter than normal, and occasionally broader. In less severe types the long bones are stunted, diffusely rarefied, and may have expanded club-shaped extremities. Fractures, or old deformity following fractures, are often apparent. In adult cases the shafts of the bones appear to shrink, and show a dense, relatively thick cortex with no medulla. In sharp contrast to the slender and often deformed shafts, the ends of the bones are expanded and show coarse cancellation with poor density. Ultimately the long bones may appear as two poorly calcified end bulbs joined by a slender rod of denser bone (Figure 4.40).

The ribs are usually bent sharply downwards at their angles, and the thorax is therefore greatly

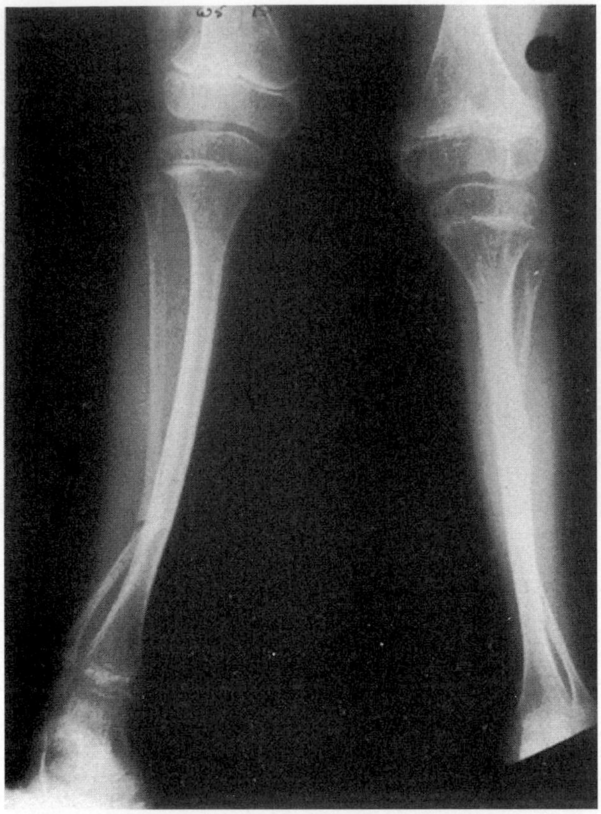

Figure 4.40 Osteogenesis imperfecta. Thin bone type of deformity of the femora, tibiae and fibulae with healing fractures and residual deformities.

deformed (Figure 4.41). This may be accentuated by the occurrence of scoliosis. The pelvis shows asymmetrical and irregular deformity. The skull shows irregular ossification, with islands of denser bone in a poorly calcified matrix – the so-called wormian bones.

DIAGNOSIS

The diagnosis is usually evident, but occasionally rickets may afford some difficulty, especially since fractures are common. In rickets, however, the radiological picture is characteristic – the epiphyseal cartilage is broad and fuzzy, the junction of the metaphysis with the zone of calcified cartilage is irregular and poorly defined, and the metaphysis itself is cup-shaped and expanded. On the other hand, the rarefaction of the rest of the bone is considerably less than in osteogenesis imperfecta.

An increasing but important differential diagnosis is now suspected child abuse patients (Ablin *et al.*, 1990). Details of the clinical and family history must be obtained, blue sclera, deafness and abnormal teeth looked for, fracturing in protected environment, radiological evidence of 'wormian' bone, osteoporosis, metaphyseal corner fractures, etc., are all required to be present to exclude child abuse. Ablin and colleagues recommend a punch biopsy of the skin for collagen analysis of the production of pro-$\alpha 1$ chains or pro-$\alpha 2$ chains as a biochemical diagnosis in doubtful cases.

TREATMENT

Systemic treatment

Multiple treatments were suggested in the past including: cod liver oil, fresh air, exercise, various diets, x-ray therapy, etc. More recently, administration of calcitonin, fluoride and vitamin C are suggested to be beneficial in the treatment of osteogenesis imperfecta. So far none of these treatments has been proven to be conclusively beneficial. At present there is no agreed medical treatment.

Conservative local treatment

This consists of:

1. Splinting fractures – to keep bone alignment at the fracture site, although long periods of immobilization are to be avoided and early mobility is initiated.
2. Prophylactic bracing of long bones by very light orthoses is recommended to prevent recurring fractures. When a femur is braced, a pelvic band and external hip articulation joint should be added to the brace to avoid any stress riser effect on the femoral shaft.
3. Anaesthetic considerations are important because these patients are quite fragile. Even application of a blood pressure cuff may cause a fracture. It is very difficult to intubate these patients because of a narrow airway. Perioperative hyperthermia probably causes secondary calcium metabolism disturbance, but can be lessened with preoperative administration of dantrolene. Increased capillary and cortical fragility results in increased blood loss.
4. In closed operative treatment manual closed osteoclasis is used on the fractures, with realigned long bones being splinted or braced.

Operative treatment

In the open operative treatment of long bone deformities and fractures the general goal is to minimize the extent of immobilization and the amount of external support required.

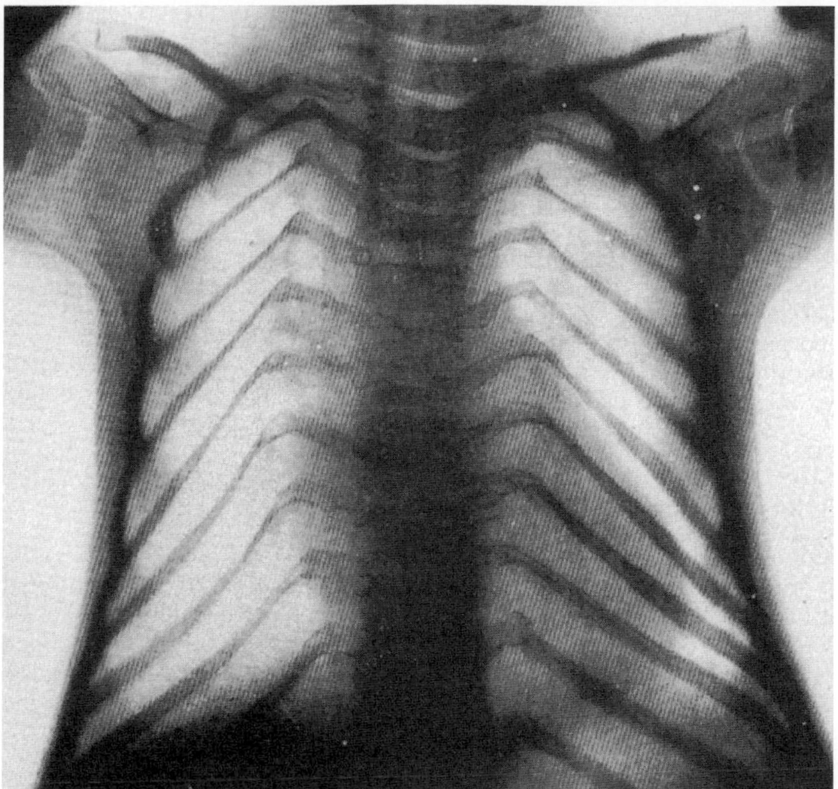

Figure 4.41 Radiograph of the chest of a child suffering from osteogenesis imperfecta. Note the delicate outline of the ribs and the existence of fracture at the angle of practically every rib.

The Sofield method of fragmentation was reported in 1959 by Sofield and Miller. This method involved subperiosteal removal of the long bone shaft from its periosteal and muscle bed, division of the shaft into as many fragments as necessary to allow the correction of deformity, individual reaming of the fragments, then threading these fragments back on a rigid rod. The method proved to be quite successful. But there was a problem with the bone overgrowth the length of the rod, resulting in bone deformity or fracture at that region.

In 1963 Baily *et al.* introduced the extending rod. This rod ensured a reduced frequency of the implant replacement, and became a more popular treatment for OI fractures. The major disadvantages of this method are the more extensive procedure requiring an articular exposure, an increased rate of infection and often implant failure.

In 1984 Middleton reported a method involving percutaneous rodding of the femur and tibia. Solid Sofield rods were used combined with closed osteoclasis in the treatment of the long bone deformities. He was able to perform this procedure in very young infants (8–14 weeks of age), to improve the care for severely affected infants.

Nicholas and James (1990) have reported on their results of using intramedullary telescoping nails in 16 patients with osteogenesis imperfecta. Over half these patients were able to walk again wearing braces. The most common complication found in 20% of patients was mechanical with loosening and disengagement of the holding cap.

Treatment of spinal deformity

Progressive lordo- and kyphoscoliosis secondary to ligamentous laxity and repeated micro-fractures is quite common in patients with osteogenesis imperfecta. Brace treatment has proved to be ineffective and produced potentially harmful rib deformities. Harrington instrumentation has been used supplemented with cement to reduce hook site failure. However, Luque-type instrumentation with fusion was found to be more successful in arresting the progression of the curves, but it was only able to correct curvatures averaging 17%. With further experience of this spinal deformity it is now recommended that early instrumentation should be performed (if the curve becomes more than 40°), and more than average blood loss should be anticipated (studies report up to 70% of estimated blood volume of the patients was lost during these stabilization procedures (Yung Hing and McEwen, 1982)).

PROGNOSIS

Bone morphology

Thompson *et al.* (1987) have studied patients with OI types II, III and IV and concluded from their observations that poor bone morphology at birth predicted poor survival and better morphology predicted better survival. From their study recurrence risk of types III and IV was overall 6.9%. In type II it was 7.7%.

Parental age

Thompson *et al.* (1987) also noticed in type III and IV cases, the mean age of the fathers was somewhat increased, when compared with controls, but the age of mothers was not different from controls.

Fracture frequency

Even though frequency of fractures decreases with the onset of adolescence, the severity of fractures increases. Despite ligamentous laxity, joint dislocations are not common. Intra-articular fractures are also very rare. Five per cent of the surviving patients with osteogenesis imperfecta have a mitral valve prolapse.

Biochemical abnormality

There is no consistent biochemical abnormality in serum or urine.

Relationship between fracture and walking age

Correlation between the timing of the first fracture and ambulation prognosis was established and showed that:

- Children with a fracture prior to beginning of walking results in 33% being wheelchair bound and 67% able to ambulate.
- If children sustained fractures after initiation of walking, 100% maintained independent ambulation.

Recently Oohira and Nokomi (1989) have discovered an elevated collection of above-normal levels of hyaluronate in involved tubular bones of imperfecta. This followed the work of Turakainen (1983) who had found that cultured skin fibroblasts of patients with OI synthesized hyalronate above the levels secreted by normal skin fibroblasts.

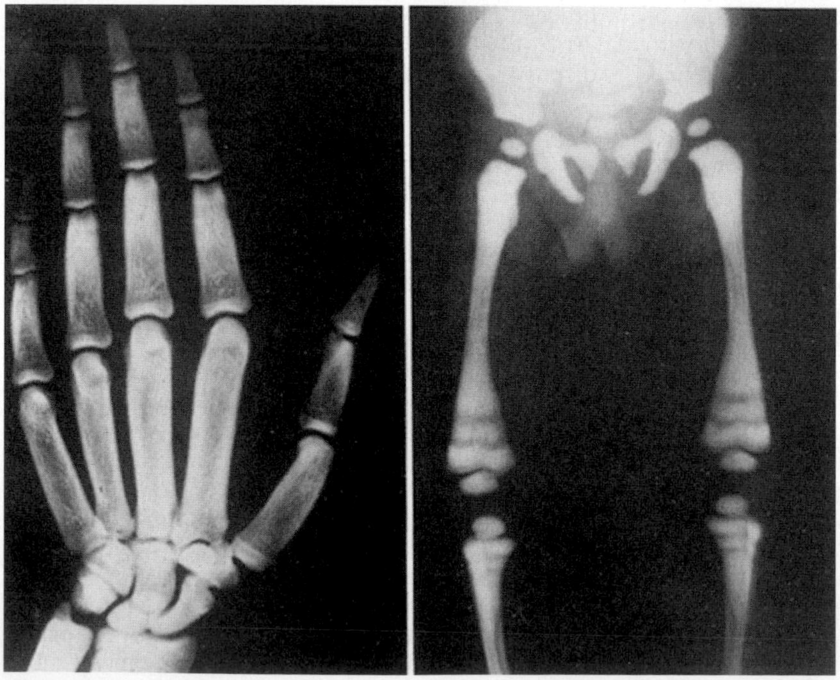

Figure 4.42 Radiographs of a case of osteopetrosis, showing the marked increase in bone density, the obliteration of the normal epiphyseal lines (particularly of the digits) and of the medullary cavity. The transverse banding effect of the femora and tibiae suggests periods of relative remission of the disease process.

Osteopetrosis (Albers-Schönberg disease; marble bone disease)

Albers-Schönberg, in 1904, was the first to describe a rare bone disease associated with increased density of the skeleton. The condition has not infrequently affected several members of a family, and there have been minor differences in the pathology of the disease in individual families, though it tends to be true to type in the members of any particular group.

PATHOLOGY

Both the membrane and cartilage bones are involved. The characteristic change is the increased density and thickness, and complete loss of trabeculation of the affected bone. Any or all of the bones may be affected, and the condition is usually symmetrical.In the case of the long bones, the usual differentiation into cortex and medulla is lost, and the change may affect any part of the bone but is most common at the metaphysis. In the growing long bone, there is no alteration in the size or appearance of the epiphyseal cartilage, but the bony nucleus of the epiphysis may show similar changes. In addition to the loss of architecture, the bone density is grossly increased and the texture appears closely granular. The increased thickness of the bone indicates that the condition affects not only the bone developed from the epiphyseal cartilage, but also that growing from the subperiosteal osteogenic layer (Figures 4.42 and 4.43).

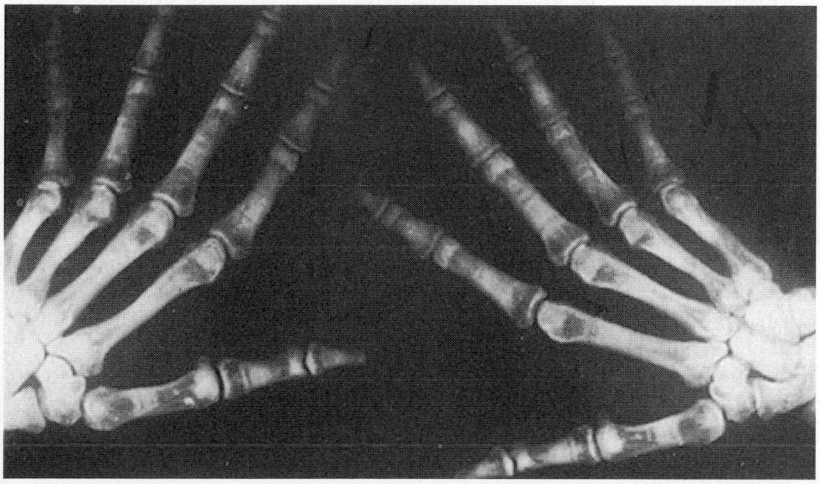
(a)

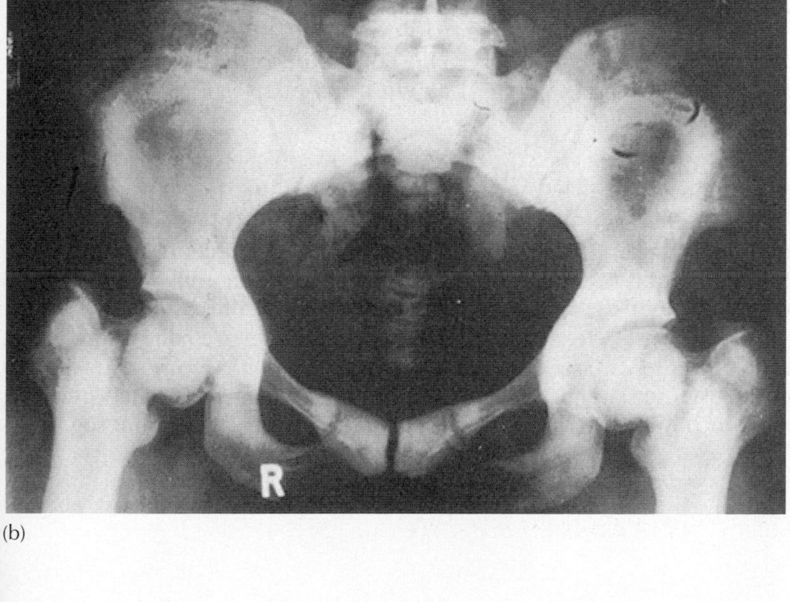

(b)

Figure 4.43 Radiographs of (a) the hands of a woman with the mild dominantly inherited form of osteopetrosis, and (b) the pelvis in the same patient. Note again the alternation of dense unmodelled bone with less dense bone.

The most marked changes are found in the most rapidly growing extremities of the long bones – the lower end of the femur and radius, and the upper end of the tibia and the humerus.

The ribs are similarly affected – thick, dense and apparently structureless. The vertebrae may be uniformly dense, or a dense zone at the upper and lower thirds of the body may be separated by a zone of normal density in the middle, indicating that the process is affecting the bone laid down from the cartilage end plates of the body. The skull may be so dense that no detail of its architecture can be made out. The bones of the carpus and tarsus are ringed by layers of dense bone, the result of peripheral accretions.

The extent of the change depends on the age at which the disturbance begins. If it does not commence till after birth, the first indication is a dense streak at the extreme limit of the metaphysis, but if it has commenced *in utero*, even at birth a considerable part of the diaphysis may show the change. The disease progresses during the growth period by the addition of further dense accretions, both subperiosteally and from the epiphyseal cartilage, so that in the adult the bones still show the characteristic changes.

Relation of increased density to bone strength

It is well known that so-called marble bones are liable to fractures, especially in the adolescent. It was for this reason that it was originally grouped with fragilitas ossium. It is generally accepted that the increased bone density in osteopetrosis is not an index of increased strength. Thus it is said to be possible to cut a so-called 'marble' bone with a knife, the sensation experienced being similar to that on cutting chalk, so that Pirie suggested the name 'chalky bones' for the condition.

HISTOPATHOLOGY

Microscopically the affected areas are seen to consist of calcified cartilage masses, bone, necrotic bone and sclerotic fibrous tissue. It is noticeable that the tissues are hypovascular, the marrow spaces being filled with sclerotic tissue with very few capillaries. There is absence of true ossification or any lamellar system by osteoblastic activity and much of the sclerosis is due to excessive calcification of osteoid tissue (Figure 4.44) and a defect in bone resorption with few osteoclasts being seen.

Secondary pathological changes

Two sets of symptoms secondary to the bone changes are of importance, as it is usually for these that the patient seeks advice. They are due to the involvement of the haemopoietic and nervous systems by encroachment of the thickened bone.

The progressive sclerosis of the long bones gradually reduces the medullary cavity and the bone marrow to a degree incompatible with normal blood formation associated with failure of bone resorption. At first, overactivity of the residual marrow results in an increase of recticulocytes and nucleated red cells but later a true aplastic anaemia develops followed by extramedullary haematopoeisis with hypersplenism and death. In attempted compensation there is enlargement of the liver, spleen and lymphatic glands of the body.

In the skull the thickening is apt to restrict the size of the foramina, leading to pressure on, and paralysis of, the cranial nerves. Thus blindness, nystagmusand ocular palsies may arise and deafness (Figure 4.45). Occasionally the density of the bones of the skull may lead to hydrocephalus, and when the clinoid processes are grossly increased there may be injurious pressure on the pituitary, with signs of hypopituitarism. The teeth are late in erupting and extensive caries lead to osteomyelitis and necrosis of the mandible.

The radiological appearances are due to the failure of resorption of the osteochondroid of the metaphysis, producing an 'elongated metaphysis' of equal diameter so that the shaft is thickened except for the middle third.

In considering the diagnosis it is to be noted that a condition closely resembling 'marble bones' was found in those working with cryolite, a compound of fluorine, sodium and aluminium, while Speder (1936) found the same condition in the phosphatic zones of Morocco in the local inhabitants as well as in animals. The condition is said to be due to the ingestion of calcium fluoride.

AETIOLOGY

Osteopetrosis is a hereditary and often congenital disease. It is inherited as an autosomal recessive gene and frequently blood relatives of both parents manifest the disease. A more benign surviving form, associated with fractures and osteomyelitis of the mandible, is inherited as an autosomal dominant; involvement of the cranial nerves, producing deafness and facial paralysis, is sometimes seen.

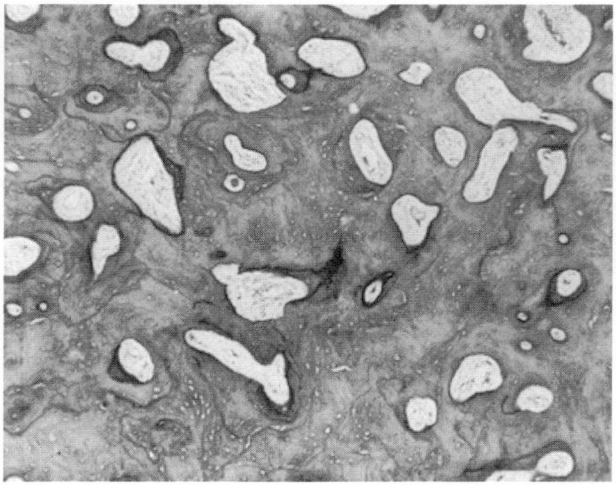

(a)

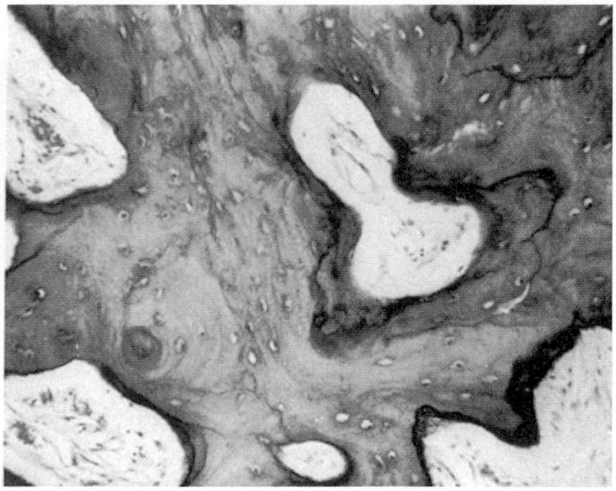

(b)

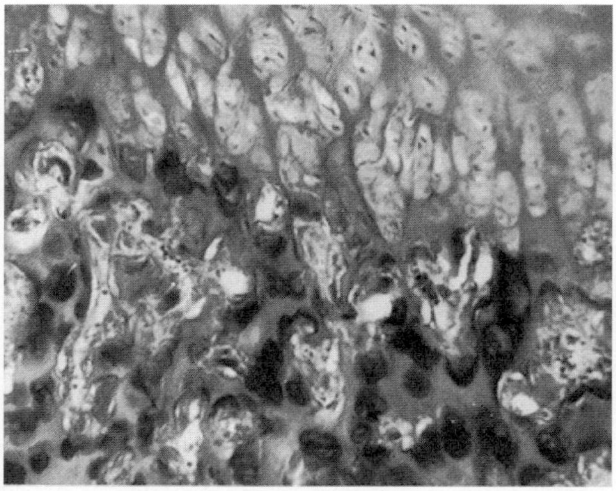

(c)

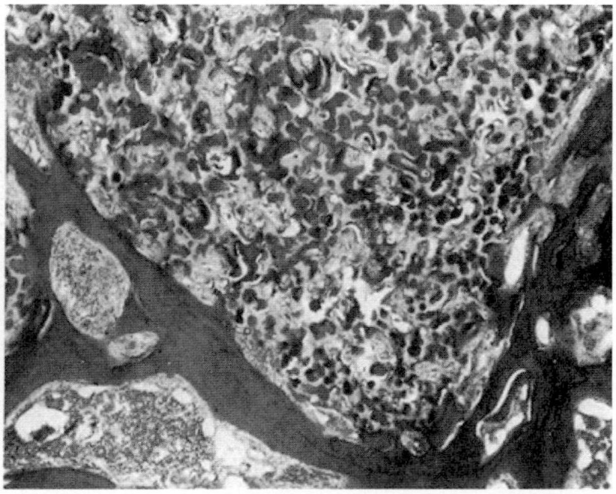

(d)

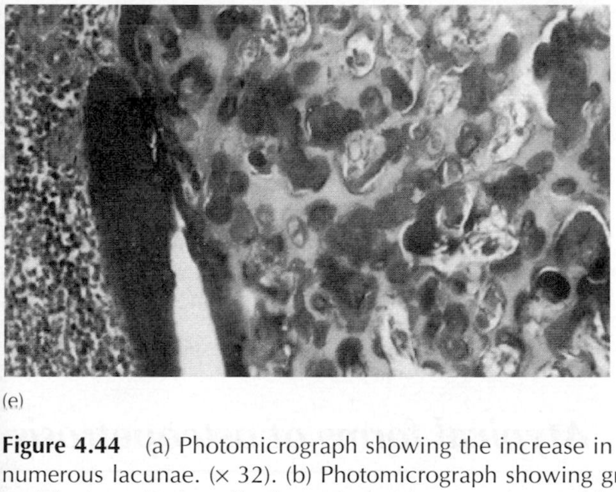

(e)

Figure 4.44 (a) Photomicrograph showing the increase in abnormal ossification without real osteoblastic activity and numerous lacunae. (× 32). (b) Photomicrograph showing greater detail of the osteocytes contained within the lacunae and the irregular lamellar formation without much osteoblastic activity. There is excessive calcification of osteoid tissue taking place rather than true ossification. (× 112). (c) Photomicrograph showing the epiphyseal plate area of osteopetrosis with abnormality in the zones of calcification, the invasion by blood vessels, and the final phase of disintegration of the cartilage cells. There are abnormal areas of increased osseous density alternating with less dense areas made up of calcified osteoid tissue. Osteoblastic activity is markedly reduced. (× 168). (d) Photomicrograph showing alternating areas of increased and decreased density with trabeculae of bone in the marrow but little osteoblastic activity present. Much of the medullary space and content has been replaced by abnormal calcification. (× 32). (e) Photomicrograph showing a trabeculum of bone with small round cells on one side and the varying osseous densities on the other, but no organized ossification. (× 112).

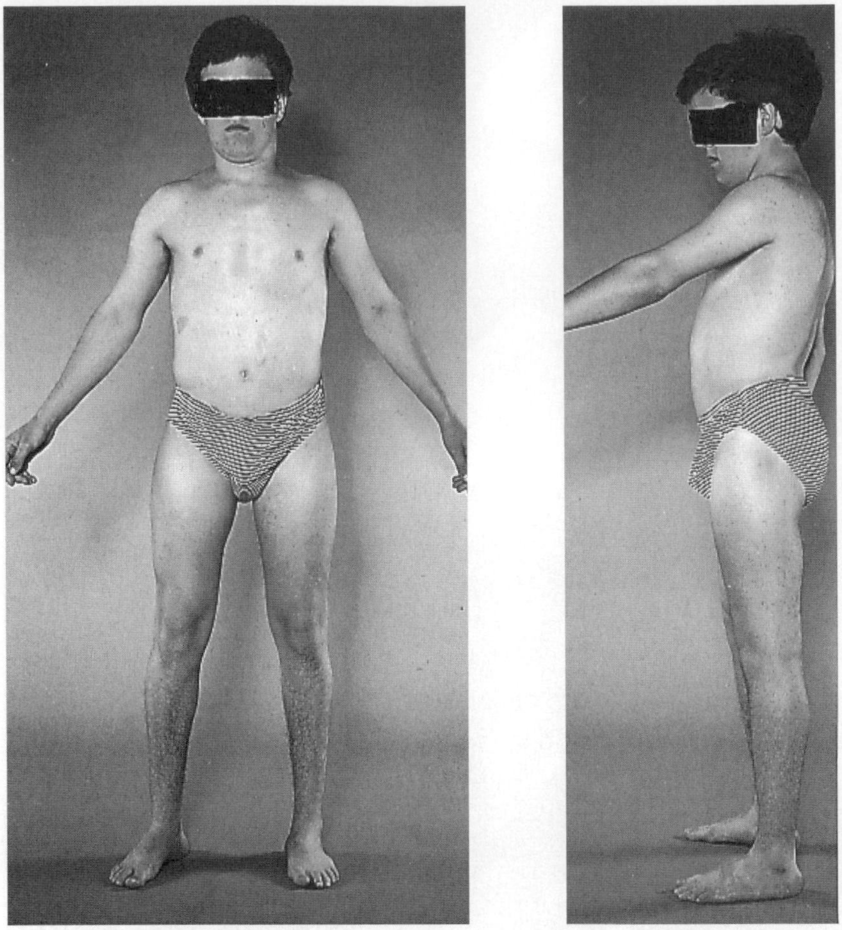

(a) (b)

Figure 4.45 An 18-year-old patient of short stature, increasing blindness and deafness with osteopetrosis.

Dupont's theory that the primary factor was parathyroid overactivity was founded on the discovery of parathyroid adenoma in a case of his own. There is some experimental evidence to support this, as it seems that while daily injections of parathyroid hormone in animals leads to mobilization of skeletal calcium, the reverse is obtained if the injections are prolonged, for the osteoblasts are stimulated to deposit bone.

Ellis suggested that while it is difficult to credit the theory of a continued hyperparathyroidism, it may be that periods of parathyroid activity alternate with periods of normality.

TREATMENT

Cournot *et al.* (1989) have reviewed the role of transplantation of bone marrow cells in malignant osteopetrosis as well as the place of vitamin D metabolism in the pathogenesis. They describe the success in some patients with disease – free survival after the age of 4 years. In young age groups, death occurred because of infection, graft immunological response and failure of the haemopoietic cells to survive. They emphasize that this disease exhibits a wide spectrum of phenotypic expression. Elevated $1,25\ (OH_2)D$ plasma concentrations have been found in a few of these patients but this had no correlation with the success or failure of bone marrow transplantation.

Atypical forms of osteopetrosis

This group, discussed below, comprises the conditions pyknodysostosis, metaphyseal dysplasia, diaphyseal sclerosis, melorheostosis, osteopathia striata, osteopoikilosis, Engelmann's disease and infantile cortical hyperostosis.

Pyknodysostosis

This condition is distinguished by the fact that it is considered to be the dysplasia that affected Henri Toulouse-Lautrec. It appears to be autosomal recessive, the abnormal chromosome being a member of the G22 pair. Dwarfing occurs with a total height of not more than 1.5 m (5 feet) but this may be due to the numerous fractures which occur during life.

There is a failure of closure of the cranial sutures with the appearance of numerous wormian bones. Thc mandibular ramus is hyperplastic, resulting in a receding jaw. The hands are short and stubby with spoon-nail deformity. The deciduous teeth are malformed and the clavicles are incompletely formed, with hypoplasia of the acromial ends. The entire skeleton displays an increased bone density.

Metaphyseal dysplasia (Pyle)

Metaphyseal dysplasia, sometimes known as craniometaphyseal dysplasia, is a disturbance of enchondral bone growth, in which there is a failure of modelling of cylindrical bones so that the ends of the shafts remain larger than normal in circumference. The amount of cancellous tissue, however, is increased and it impinges upon and reduces the extent of the medullary cavity. Thus it appears that there is a lack of osteoblastic activity in the metaphyses and diaphyses, affecting the periosteum as in osteopetrosis, but there is osteoblastic activity for enchondral bone formation which is unlike osteopetrosis. The disease is familial but its hereditary pattern is uncertain due to its rarity. The stature is normal and general health is not affected except for a tendency for pathological fracture during life. The distal femora and proximal tibiae are particularly

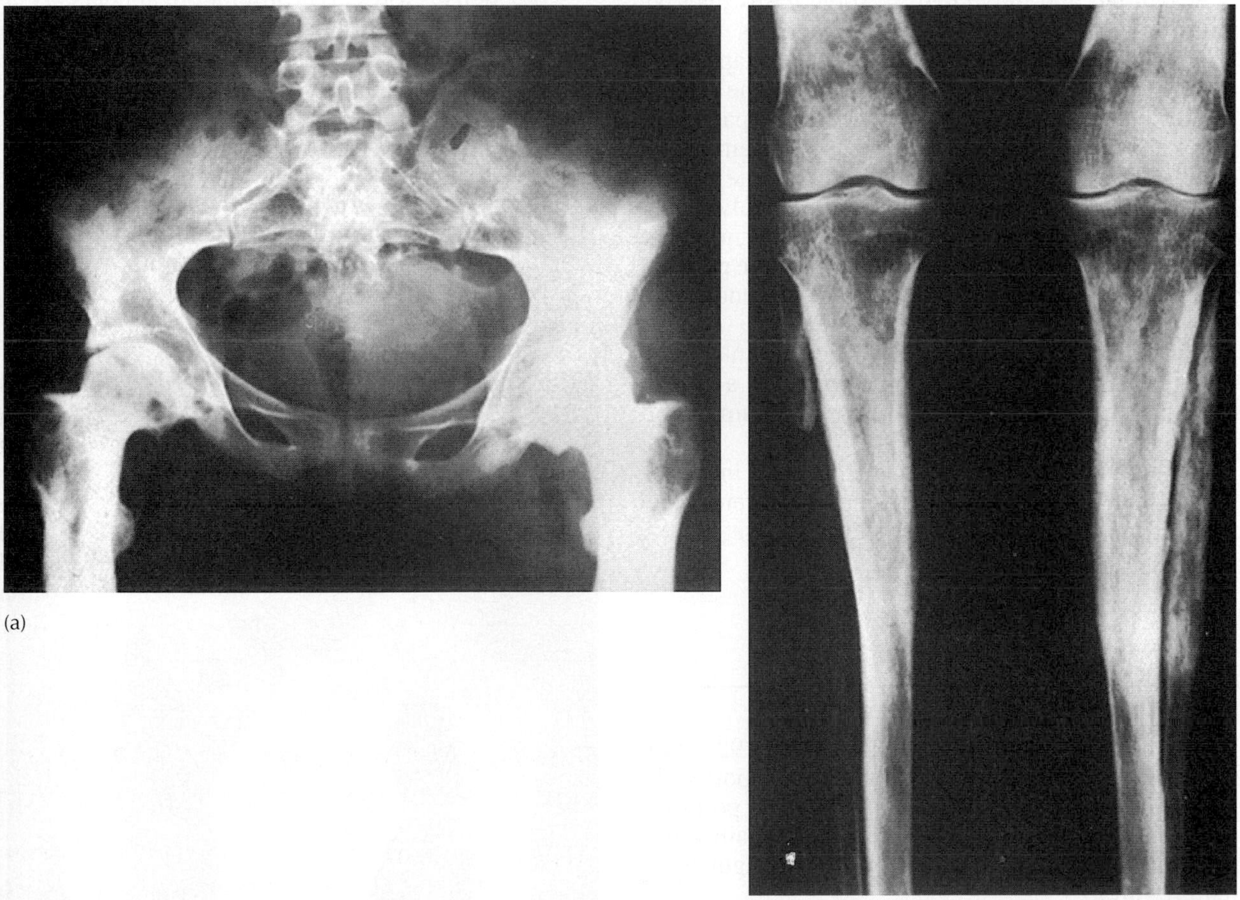

(a)

(b)

Figure 4.46 Diaphyseal sclerosis. Radiographs (a) the hips and (b) the tibiae, showing the excessive bone deposition in the diaphyseal cortices.

affected. There is often overgrowth of the head bones, producing leontiasis ossea with overgrowth of the bridge of the nose. Bone overgrowth at nerve foramina may lead to neurological symptoms, blindness and impairment of hearing.

Diaphyseal sclerosis (Camurati–Engelmann–Ribbing disease)

This appears to be a group of conditions characterized by diaphyseal sclerosis, which was reviewed by Lennon *et al.* in 1961.

The severity of the condition varies from the florid cases beginning early in childhood to the mild cases which may be undiscovered until adult life. The condition is frequently familial and probably hereditary. The gait is described as shuffling or waddling, and movement in some cases may be painful and restricted due to tenderness of the bones. There is thickening of the mid-diaphyseal cortex which affects mainly the tibia and the femur. There may eventually be inadequate space for haematopoeisis, with development of anaemia and enlargement of the spleen and liver. As time passes most bones of the skeleton become involved. In late cases neurological symptoms may occur, producing deafness, optic atrophy and cranial nerve palsies. In addition, the muscles are small, flabby and weak (Figure 4.46).

The pathogenesis of this condition is unknown, though histologically it is characterized by a dearth of Haversian canals and a subnormal number of blood vessels.

In the cases which do not have muscular involvement it may be exceedingly difficult to differentiate from the childhood form of Caffey's disease.

Melorheostosis (Leri)

The condition was first reported by Leri in 1922, and since then more than 30 cases have been reported. It is a rare condition in which certain bones, or portions of a bone, are petrosed but different in certain ways from ordinary 'marble bones'. The distinguishing features are:

1. The changes are confined to one limb.
2. The outline of an affected bone is definitely distorted.
3. The presence of pain, often severe.
4. Limitation of movement in the joints formed by the affected bone.

PATHOLOGY

A portion of the cortex of one of the limb bones is irregularly enlarged, sufficiently to give rise to a swelling with an undulating surface. Between one undulation and another, a linear band of increased density may extend, which has been likened to a 'flow' of hyperostosis. The condition is sometimes known as 'monomelic flowing hyperostosis'. Leri employed this original title because the hyperostotic areas in appearance resemble 'candle drippings' (Figure 4.47).

Sometimes the lesion is associated with deformity of the affected bone. Thus in the lower limb, bowing of the femur and of the tibia is common. Kraft (1933) distinguished three types of the disease:

1. Where a whole extremity is affected – in this the dense cortical proliferation appears as a regular and continuous flow from shoulder to fingers, or hip to foot. Usually it is limited to one side of the bone, and in some cases appears to occupy the distribution of a nerve or vessel without having any apparent relationship to them.
2. In the second group, only half the extremity – the proximal half – is involved.
3. In the third group, a whole extremity is irregularly involved and there are multiple interruptions of the flow.

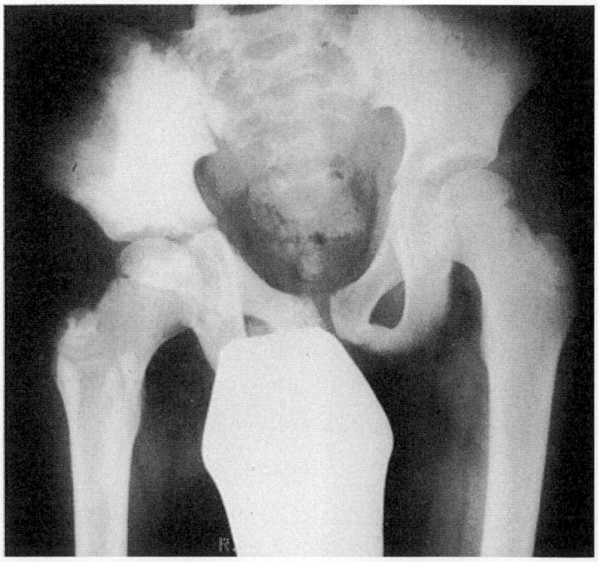

Figure 4.47 Melorheostosis. Radiograph showing how the dense, wavy cortex encroaches on the bone cavity of the pelvis and femur on the right side.

AETIOLOGY

Nothing is known of the aetiology of the condition, but it was suggested by Moore and DeLorimler (1933) that the deformity associated with it is the result of overloading a bone less well adapted to withstand strain, or to the mechanical leverage effect exercised by the hyperostotic processes. Fairbank (1951) suggested that fibrosis of the marrow may be the fundamental change present. Hall (1943) considered that the local disorder of osteogenesis occurred because of some periosteal disturbance with extension of the ossification into adjacent soft tissues such as connective or fibrous tissue, muscle and even skin.

CLINICAL FEATURES

Apart from the deformities or the swellings resulting from the local lesion, there may be 'rheumaticky pains' in the affected extremities. It is usually accepted that the pain is a sequel to chronic arthritis of the joints of the limb, with which the condition is usually associated. There is usually limitation of movement at the affected joints. Occasionally, there is an indefinite complaint of progressive muscular weakness.

During growth the deformities usually progress rapidly, but in adult life progression is slow.

There is no specific treatment for this condition.

Osteopathia striata

This condition was described in 1924 by Voorhoeve and is characterized by multiple condensations of cancellous bone tissue which begin at the epiphyseal line and extend into the diaphysis. In the ilium the striae form a sunburst about the acetabulum and fan out towards the iliac crest. Any or all of the long bones may be involved, and the end of greatest growth is said to be more obviously involved. The condition differs from osteopetrosis, melorheostosis, Camurati–Engelmann–Ribbing disease in that only cancellous bone is affected. It has occasionally been described in association with osteopetrosis in other bones. It is usually an incidental finding on radiographs.

Osteopoikilosis (osteopathia condensans disseminata; spotted bones)

This condition was described by Albers-Schönberg in 1904. It is characterized by the presence of dense spots in large numbers in the long and short bones. The skull, vertebrae and ribs seem to be exempt. The spots, which may be very numerous, are round, oval or lanceolate, with their long axes parallel to the long axis of the bone. They are usually uniformly dense, but may have clear centres, and are grouped towards the end of the bone in the epiphysis (Figure 4.48). They give rise to no symptoms and are usually discovered by chance. Schmorl found that they consisted of numerous closely packed trabeculae in the lamellae lying mostly in a longitudinal direction.

Various skin lesions – dermatofibrosis lenticularis disseminata and sclerodermal – have been found in a number of cases of osteopoikilosis overlying the bony lesions.

Its cause is unknown. Zimmer attributed the bone condition to maldevelopment in a limb bud.

Engelmann's disease

This unusual condition is characterized by symmetrical fusiform enlargement and sclerosis of the shaft of the long bones, associated with changes in the skull. The condition is seen most commonly in males and usually in childhood. Pains in the legs and head may be complained of; weakness and difficulty in walking, sometimes with a waddling gait, are common. The essential feature is the bilateral hyperostosis of the shafts of the long bones. This may be palpable. The epiphyses are not involved. The bones affected, in order of frequency, are the femur, tibia, humerus and fibula. In the skull, increased density of the base and frontal region has been found.

Biopsy shows nothing but sclerosis. The only disorder resembling this condition is infantile cortical hyperostosis. This occurs during the first year of life and tends to recover within a few months. The bone changes can extend and other bones become involved.

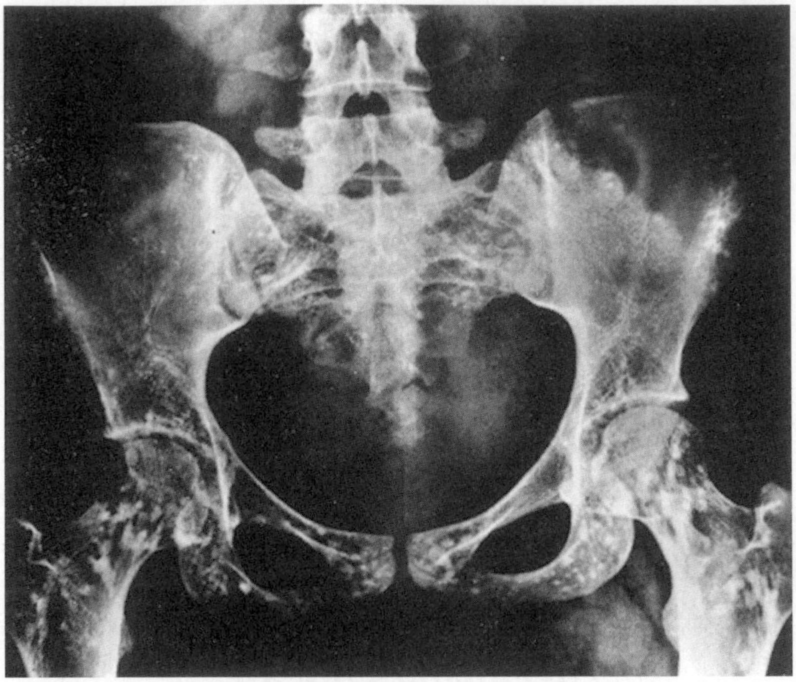

(a)

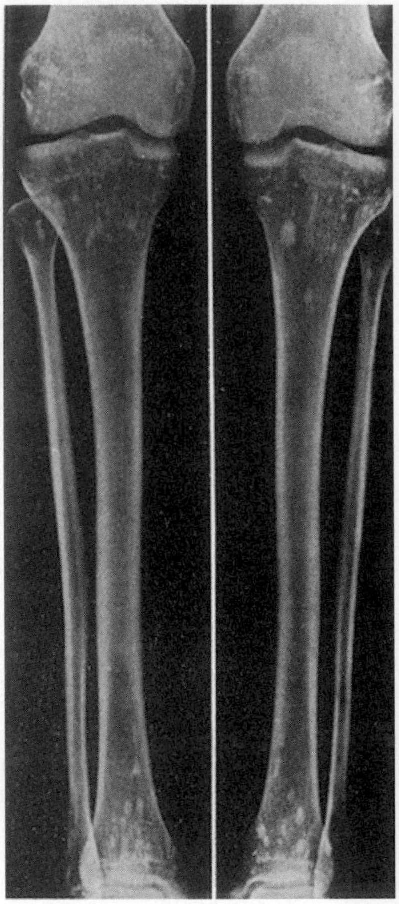

(b)

Figure 4.48 The distribution of dense irregular calcific densities in both metaphyseal and epiphyseal areas is seen in (a) the femora and (b) the tibiae of this individual in whom osteopoikilosis was found.

Infantile cortical hyperostosis (Caffey's disease)

This disease was probably a new entity, since prior to 1930 there are no recorded descriptions, either clinical or radiographic, of a syndrome similar to infantile cortical hyperostosis. It is unlikely that earlier clinicians would have overlooked its striking and distinctive clinical and radiographic manifestations.

The condition starts in the early weeks of life and is characterized by the formation of subperiosteal bone on the shafts of long bones and on the mandible. Males are affected in the proportion of 3 to 1 female. Van Zeben (1948) reported a brother, sister and cousin all with definite signs of the disease.

The postnatal disease commonly begins suddenly, with swelling of the face and jaw without premonitory signs. The infant usually becomes feverish and hyperirritable. In a few cases swellings have first appeared in the legs and arms, and the face becomes swollen 3 or 4 days later. There is limitation of movement of the limbs and tenderness, but no discoloration, oedema or increased heat. The swellings are wood-hard, deeply situated and fixed to bone. Pallor and anaemia develop. The ESR is increased.

RADIOLOGICAL APPEARANCES

The cortical walls of the bones which underlie the swellings thicken externally. The subperiosteal shadow encloses a varying length of the shaft or the whole of it. The mandible is thickened. In time the enlarged porotic bone gradually shrinks away and the shaft resumes its normal appearance, and if this has been curved it is slowly or spontaneously corrected (Figure 4.49).

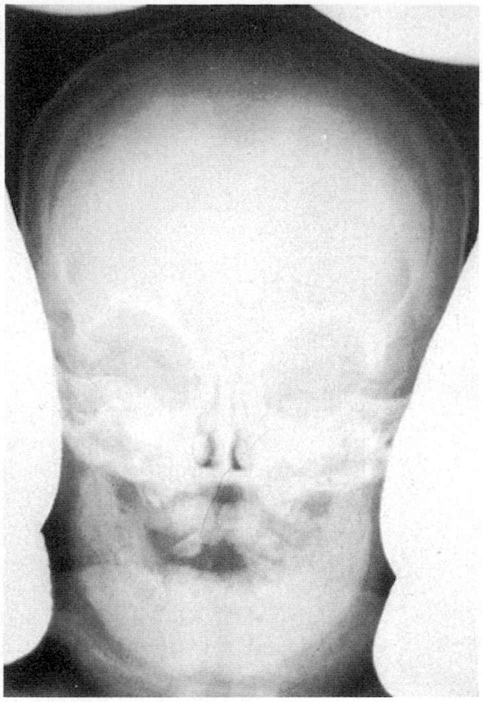

(a)

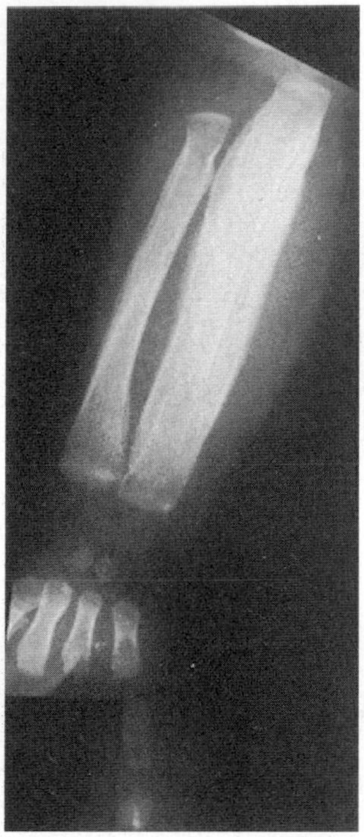

(b)

Figure 4.49 Infantile cortical hyperostosis. Caffey's disease affecting (a) the skull and (b) the forearm bones.

Prognosis

Recovery sets in in a few months and is usually complete within 8–12 months.

Simple bone cysts

Simple bone cysts can be relatively asymptomatic or produce real problems. The anatomical location affects this situation. Thus a location in the femoral neck can readily lead to severe coxa vara deformity with repeated fractures. In this site, treatment may be demanded at any stage of development. Simple bone cysts are always metaphyseal in location and always occupy the full width of the bone (Figures 4.50 to 4.52). An eccentric location should raise a suspicion of the diagnosis.

Simple cysts appear to be the product of an epiphyseal line aberration. The cartilage growth is no longer converted to bone. As a form of chondrodysplasia it is not subject to remodelling. Because the bone proximal and distal to it is remodelled, a false appearance of expansion is produced. It is not wider than the epiphyseal line and this is a diagnostic feature (Figure 4.53).

The cyst is occupied by fluid and is lined by a

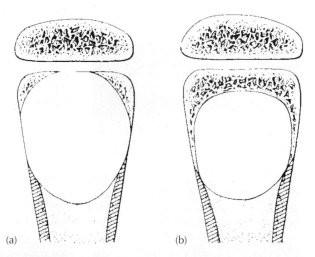

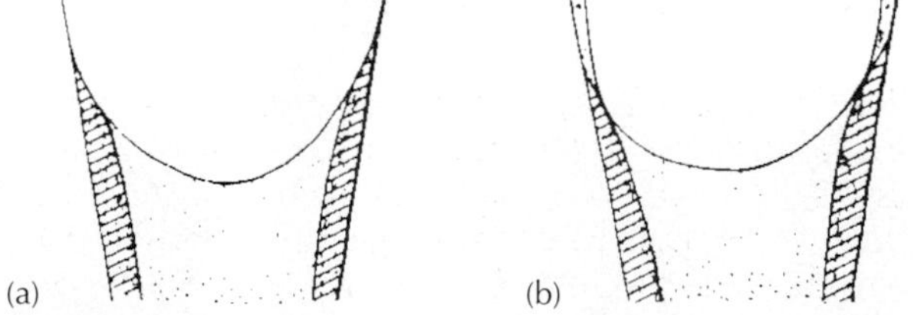

Figure 4.50 (a) The development of the simple bone cyst is an abnormality of the epiphyseal line. Bone is not produced, the area occupied by the cyst is not subject to remodelling and an apparent expansile lesion is produced. It is not wider than the original epiphyseal line. New metaphyseal bone is laid down as the child matures and the cyst then occupies an area towards the diaphysis. (b) In the adult state many cysts are obliterated radiographically by new bone deposition on the overlying cortex. It becomes smaller than the width of the adult bone.

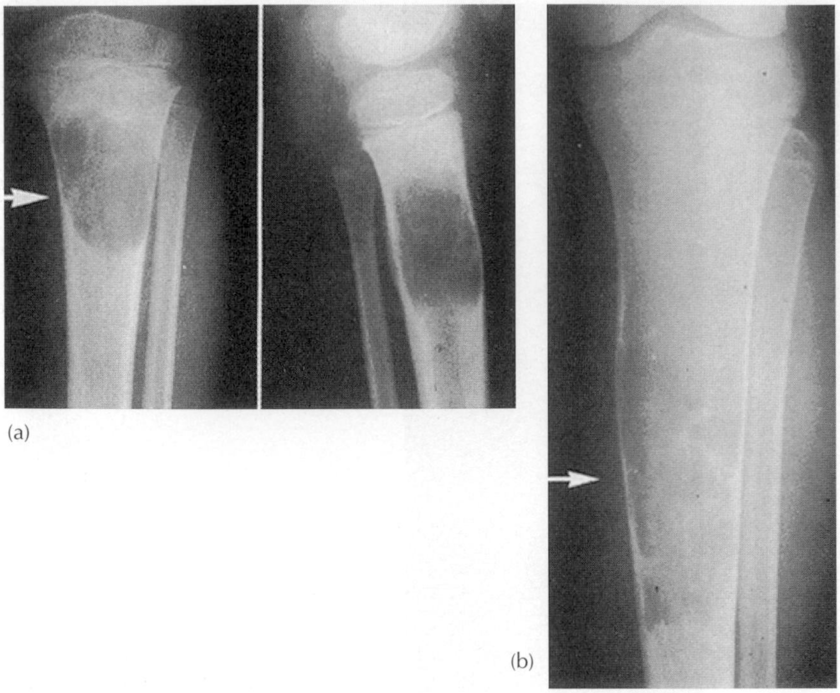

Figure 4.51 Follow-up of simple bone cyst over 7-year period. Bone laid down in the metaphysis leads to a more diaphyseal location of the cyst. At (a) the cyst is radiolucent due to thinness of the overlying cortex. At (b) the cyst has not been remodelled but more bone has been laid down over the cortex and it becomes less visible.

membrane (Figure 4.54). Recent haemorrhage from trauma will stain the fluid reddish brown, but it is normally pale yellow in colour.

As metaphyseal bone is laid down once again the cyst occupies a position further down towards the diaphysis. Towards adult life more bone is laid down about it and may finally obscure the lesion from the radiographic point of view.

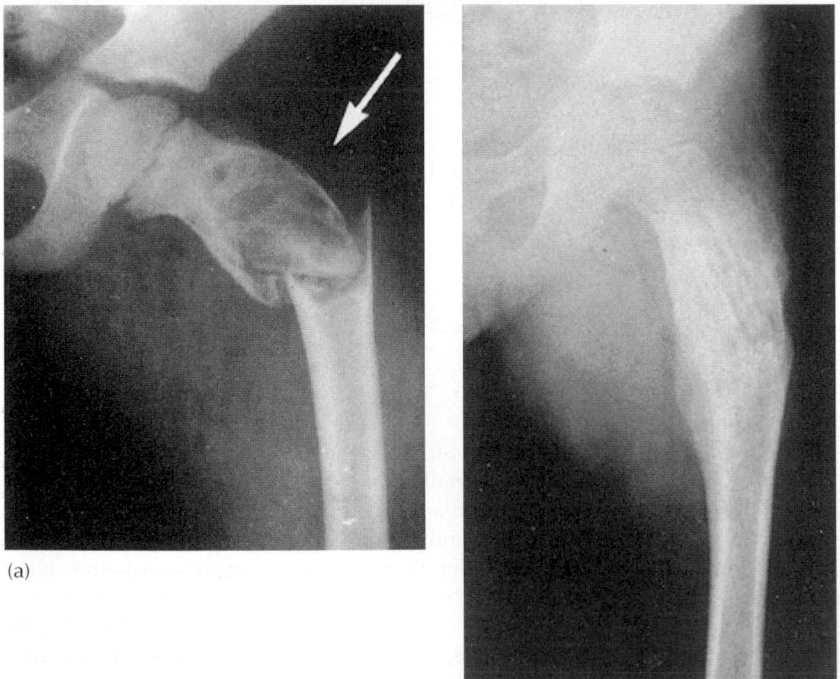

Figure 4.52 (a) Fracture through a unicameral cyst, (b) showing healing.

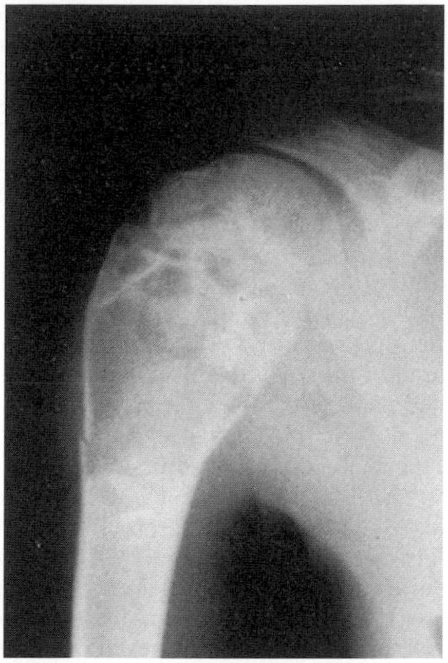

Figure 4.53 Radiograph of a right shoulder joint of a young girl, showing a solitary bone cyst involving the upper humerus. There is expansion with thinning of the cortex and a pathological fracture is present. Its smooth, oval-shaped lower surface, with normal adjacent bone, is characteristic.

In the childhood years the cyst tends to be found against the epiphyseal line. Over the age of 9, bone may be produced again, isolating the cyst from the epiphyseal line.

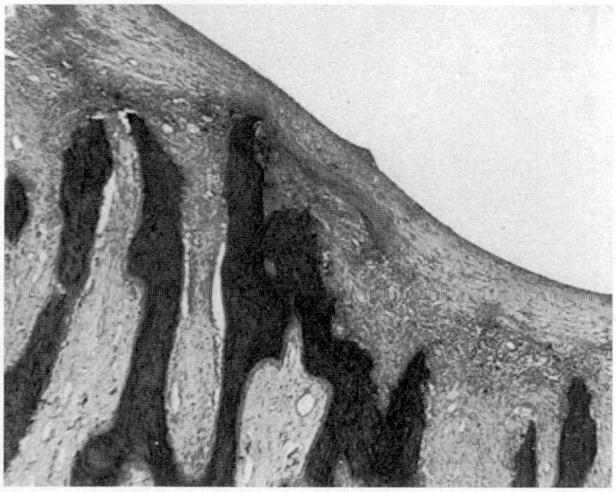

Figure 4.54 Photomicrograph showing the thick, densely fibrous cyst wall and the underlying normal trabecular bone with a fibrous marrow. (× 47).

TREATMENT

The results from cartilage bone grafting and attempting to obliterate the cyst are better in the older age groups. Treatment is required in the younger age group, when a coxa vara deformity is produced in the femoral neck or when the extent of the cyst results in fracture or deformity in any location (i.e. in the proximal humerus or femur).

A wide segment of cortex is removed in order to pack the cyst with autogenous bone chips. The cortical segment removed can be placed against the cortex to aid in obliterating the cyst cavity.

In troublesome recurrent cysts, Fahey and O'Brien (1973) left only a strut of cortex filling in the rest of the area with cancellous bone to maintain the periosteum widely open.

Fracture through a cyst exerts a healing influence, through the callus of repair, for about 0.3 cm on either side of the fracture line. This effect can be negligible in larger cysts.

In a series reported by Neer *et al.* (1966), of 129 primary operations for unicameral bone cysts, recurrences after surgical treatment were significantly more frequent in patients under the age of 10 years. Unicameral bone cysts were most common in the humerus, even in this non-weight-bearing bone, 92% of the cases, after being treated by immobilization and observation, eventually came to operation. One or two refractures occurred in 80% of these patients during the period of watchful waiting. Growth disturbance and deformities occurred in 4 of these 41 patients. It was felt that a second operation was indicated only for any enlarging cyst with the threat of fracture. The thickness of the cortex in adulthood frequently masked the presence of the symptoms Scaglietti *et al.* (1979) successfully treated a series of 72 patients by injection of the cysts with methylprednisolone acetate. A more recent series by Malawer (1986) described that 5% eventually healed after one or more aspirations with injections with methyprednisolone acetate. He recommended that if the diagnosis was in doubt, a Craig needle or small incisional biopsy be carried out to obtain the cyst lining cells. These characteristically are chronic inflammatory cells, haemosiderin-laden macrophage and a few giant cells.

Polyostotic fibrous dysplasia

This condition is also known as osteitis fibrosa juvenilis, osteodystrophia fibrosa, osteitis fibrosa disseminata and Albright's disease. Although the aetiology of the disease is unknown, the essential lesion is a developmental disorder of the bone-forming mesenchyme. Other theories presented are those of a neurological lesion stimulating the pituitary to abnormal secretion, and of a hypophosphataemia stimulating the parathyroids to give a chronic hyperparathyroidism. The latter was the basis of aluminium acetate treatment where one attempts to fix the phosphates of the bowel as an insoluble aluminium phosphate and thus reduce the hyperphosphataemia.

The disease usually appears in childhood or puberty with cyst formation in the diaphysis or metaphysis, but rarely in the epiphysis, of long bones. The bones most frequently involved are the femur, tibia, humerus and radius, with bending deformities of the weight-bearing bones and pathological fractures. Involvement of the skull or jaw may be indicated by pain and swelling. On biopsy, there is usually a distinctive appearance of bony trabeculae formation in a stroma of fibrous tissue. Giant cells are not a usual feature except following an injury (Figure 4.55). Blood calcium and phosphates are usually normal and occasionally the alkaline phosphatase is raised, probably denoting compensatory osteogenesis. The parathyroids are normal.

The radiograph shows expansion of the bone and thinning of the cortex, with numerous trabeculated cystic areas which contain giant cell collections, fibrous tissue and collections of cartilaginous tissue (Figure 4.56). It is usually a disease affecting multiple long bones. When it affects only one bone it is known as monostotic fibrous dysplasia, and when restricted to one limb as monomelic fibrous dysplasia.

In differential diagnosis from hyperparathyroidism, this latter disease rarely occurs in the adolescent. The blood calcium and phosphate changes of hyperparathyroidism are absent and on x-ray the unaffected parts of the bones have a normal appearance and do not present the diffuse osteomalacic appearance of hyperparathyroidism.

The treatment is that of the deformities; the prognosis is good, as it is a self-limiting disease, usually at skeletal maturity. However, certain lesions may require curettage and autogenous bone grafting, or even wide block excision with prosthetic replacement. Sarcoma has been reported a rare, late, complication.

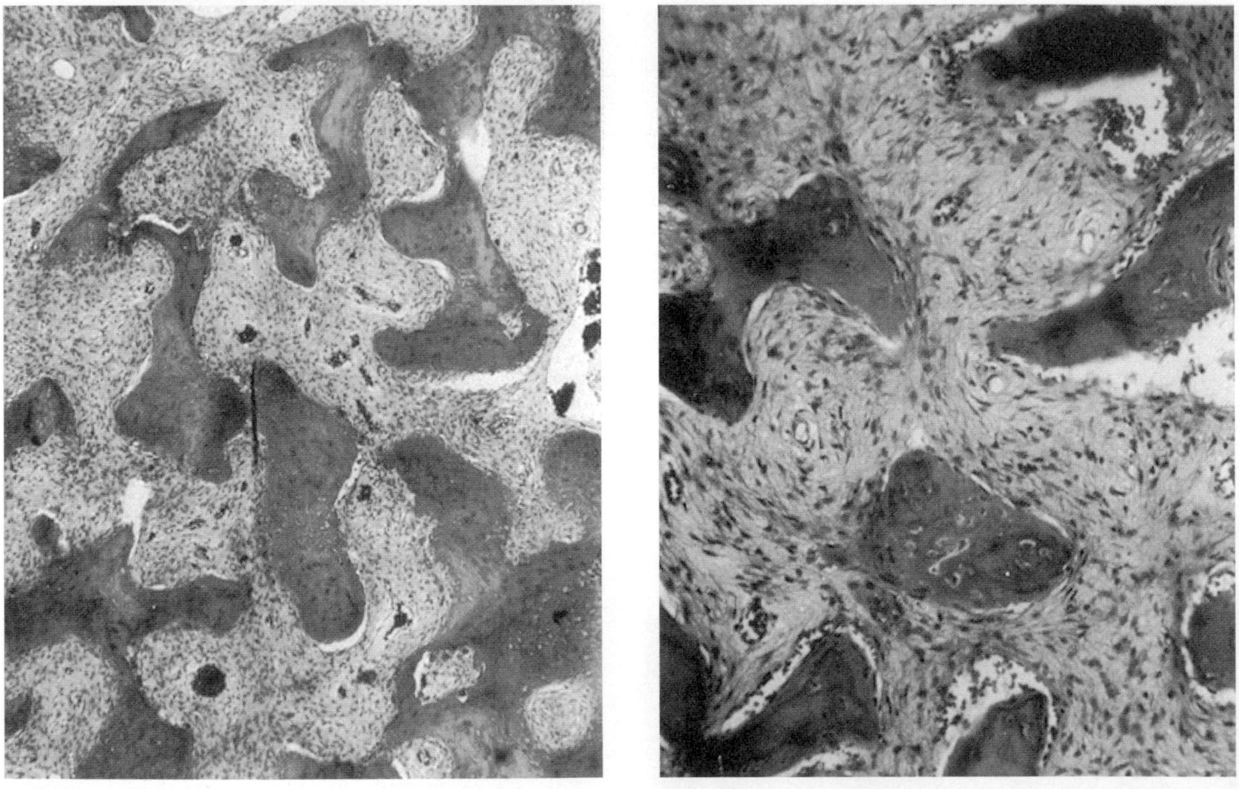

(a) (b)

Figure 4.55 (a) Photomicrograph of fibrous dysplasia, showing the numerous fine bony trabeculae and marked fibrous tissue stroma containing some giant cells. (× 40). (b) Photomicrograph showing greater detail of the bone trabeculae, osteoblastic activity and the cellular content of the fibrous stroma. (× 210).

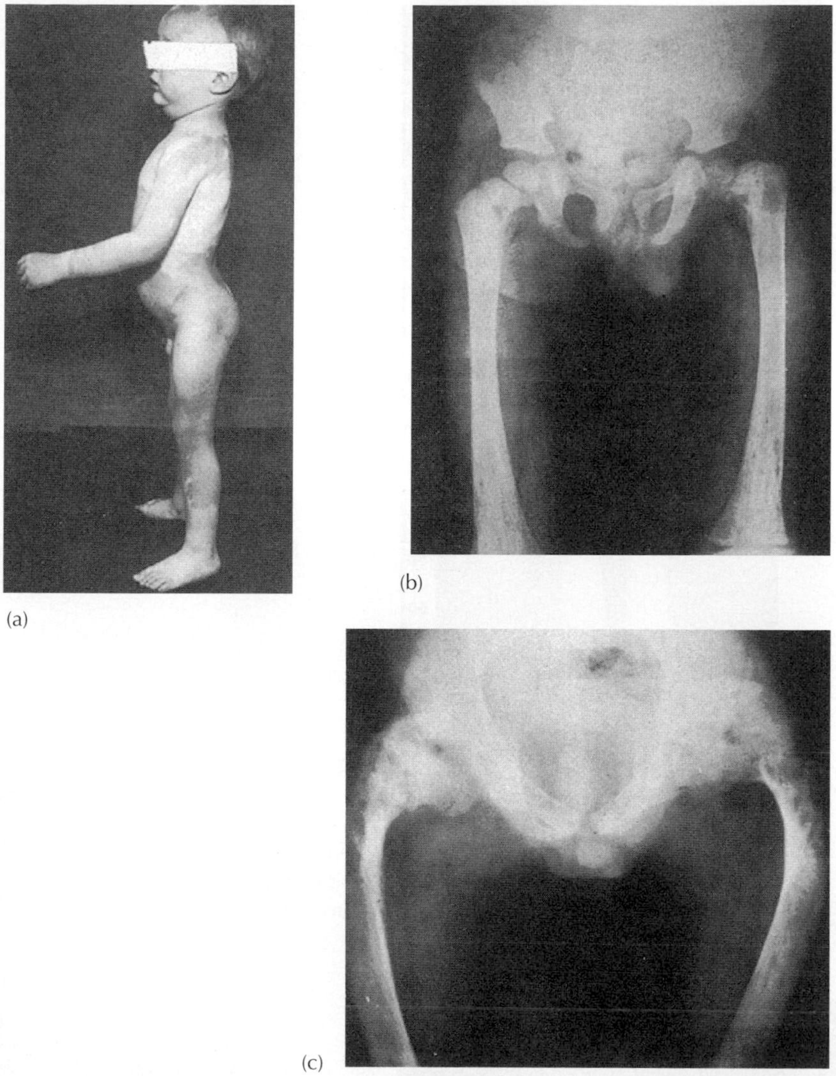

(a)

(b)

(c)

Figure 4.56 (a) Polyostotic fibrous dysplasia showing pigmentation. (b) Polyostotic fibrous dysplasia. (c) The same patient 8 years later. (By courtesy of Dr W. McLeod)

Monostotic fibrous dysplasia

In this condition a single bone is the site of partial replacement of its substance by fibrous tissue, with or without the additional presence of osteoid. If present, osteoid is occasionally calcified and cysts are sometimes formed. Any bone may be involved. The blood chemistry is within normal limits. The clinical findings are local swelling where the bone is superficial, and pain if the lesion is near a joint. Schlumberger (1946) suggested that the condition may represent a disturbance of the normal bone reparative process following trauma.

Dyschondrosteosis (Madelung's deformity)

This autosomal dominant condition, which is four times more common in males than females, is characterized by moderate shortness of stature due to failure of length of growth of the tibia and a short radius which produces the particular wrist deformity. This condition is described in Chapter 3.

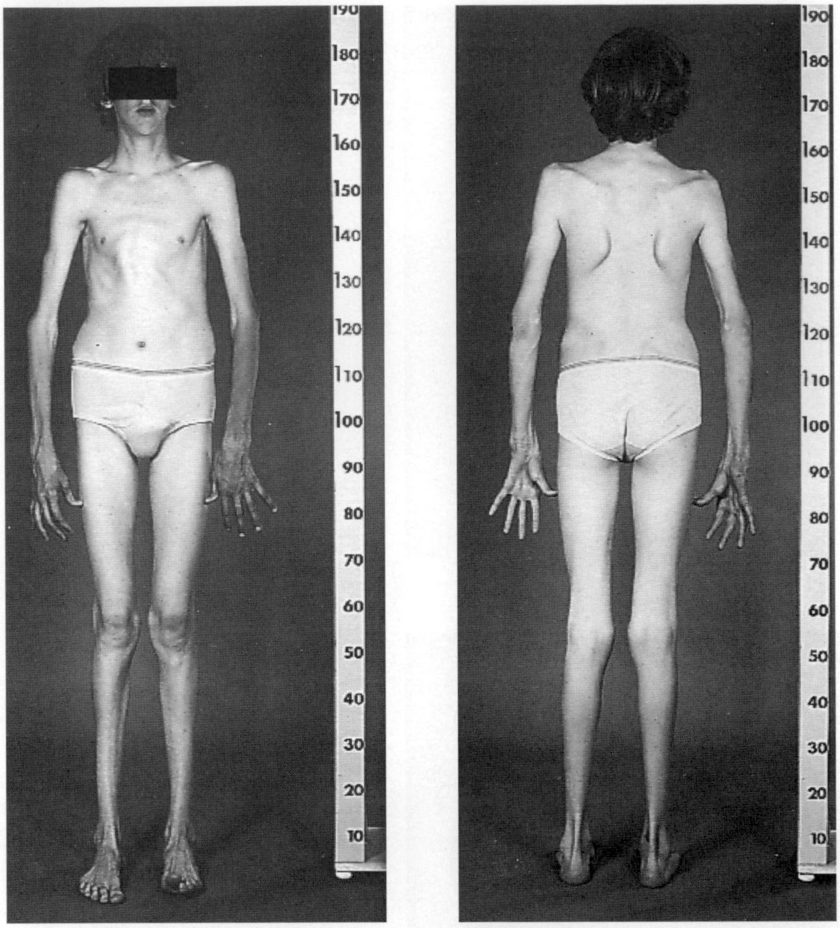

(a) (b)

Figure 4.57 Photograph of a boy of 15 years with Marfan's syndrome – very tall, slender stature; long slender digits, spider hand; without body fat, but with chest wall deformities.

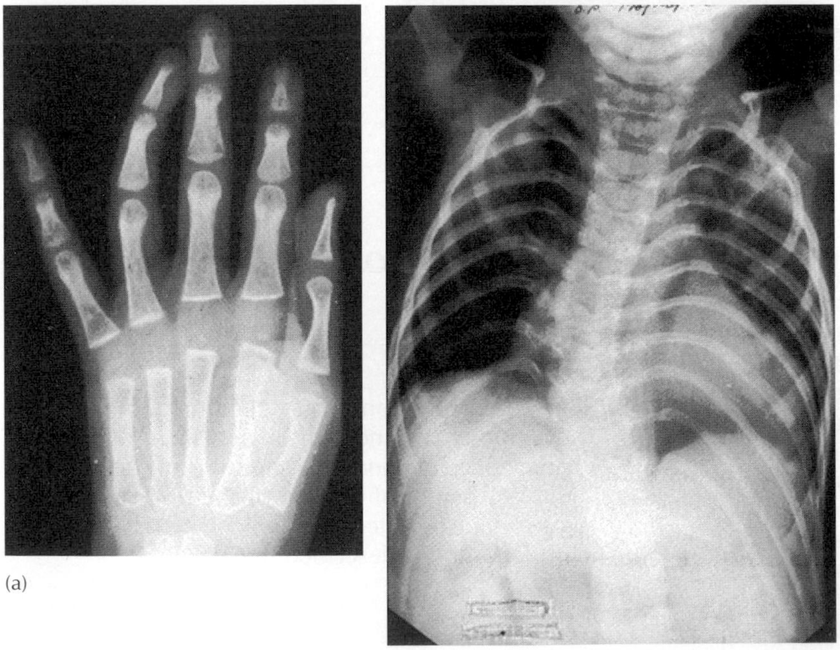

(a) (b)

Figure 4.58 Marfan's syndrome. Radiographs of (a) the hand with arachnodactyly, and (b) the spine showing early scoliosis.

Marfan's syndrome (arachnodactyly)

Marfan's syndrome is characterized by a growth disturbance affecting the musculoskeletal, cardiovascular and ocular systems. It was described by Marfan in 1896 and named arachnodactyly by Achard in 1902 due to the long slender digits resembling the limbs of a spider. This is a relatively common condition which is a simple Mendelian autosomal dominant, and may present with a congenital heart lesion or later in childhood as the characteristic musculoskeletal deformities appear.

All of the cylindrical bones are abnormally long and slender and the patient is tall, the adult usually attaining a height of over 6 feet (Figures 4.57 and 4.58). The arch of the palate is unusually high and there may be a double row of teeth. There is associated dolichocephaly. The thorax may be funnelled and pectus excavatum is common.

The muscles are poorly developed and show poor tone. The hypotonicity together with laxity of tendons and ligaments results in hypermobile joints, particularly of the fingers, wrists, knees and elbows. Dislocation of the hips, genu recurvatum, dislocating patellae and pes planus result. Inguinal and diaphragmatic hernia are common.

The most important cardiovascular abnormality is dilatation of the ascending aortic segment, leading to aneurysm formation of a dissecting type which may result in early death.

Poor vision is a common accompaniment of this condition. It is usually due to dislocation of the lens because of lax or torn suspensory ligaments. The voice is described as high pitched. Frequently the patient develops a severe scoliosis. Sections of bone have revealed no abnormality in the histological appearances. It now appears that there is a defect in the cross-linking of collagen and this is manifested by an excess urinary excretion of hydroxyproline.

Although Marfan's syndrome is expressed as an abnormal autosomal dominant gene, it contains

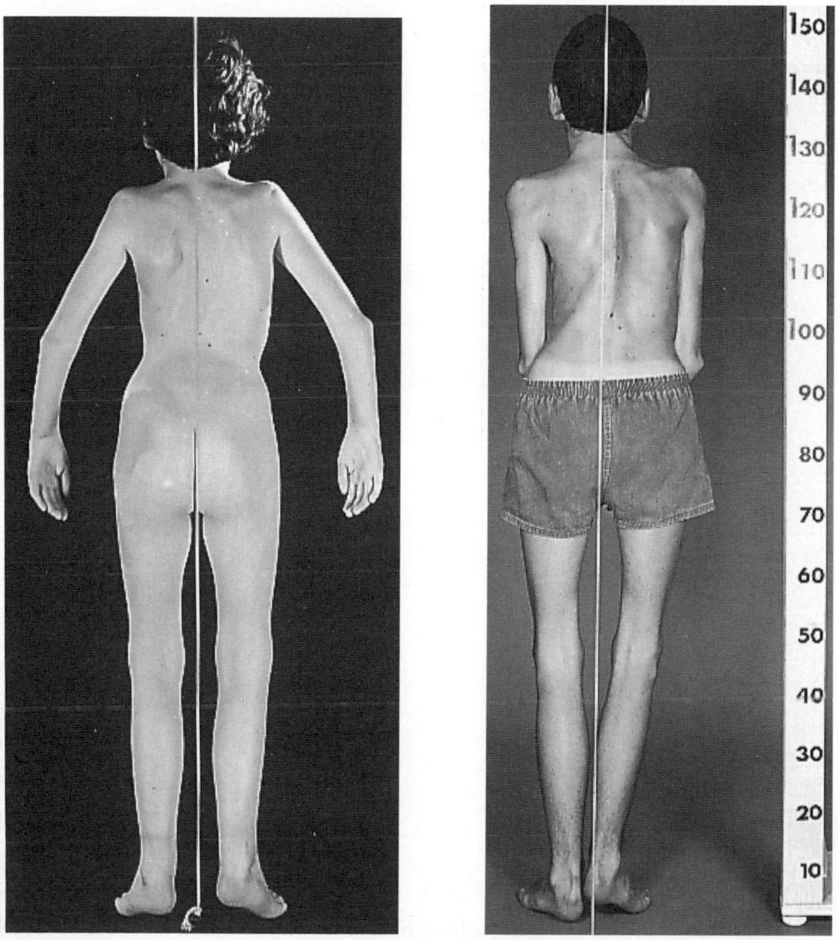

(a) (b)

Figure 4.59 (a) Photograph of a boy aged 6 years with congenital contractual arachnodactyly – showing spider-like but rigid digits, fixed flexion deformities of both ankles. (b) Same boy now aged 16 years with a marked right-sided rigid scoliosis.

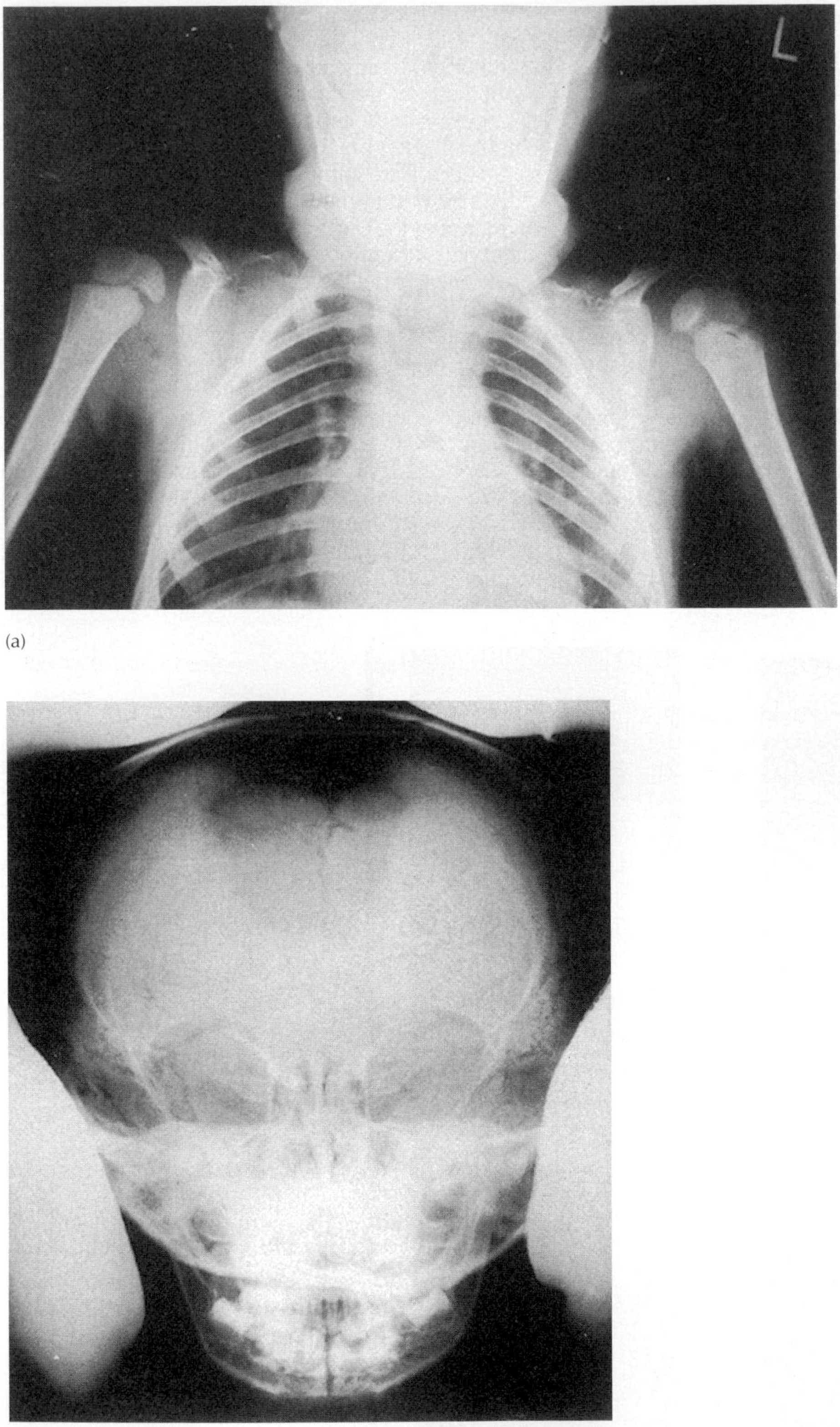

(a)

(b)

Figure 4.60 Cleidocranial dysostosis. Anteroposterior radiographs of (a) the chest showing complete absence of both clavicles, and (b) the skull.

much heterogeneity and variable expressivity. At one end of the scale is the classical Marfan's with very tall stature and involvement of all connective tissue in muscle, skeleton, heart and eye; at the other end there is short stature without generalized connective tissue or neurological disorder, involving the hands which dominate the picture when young, i.e. arachnodactyly. The hands show marked periarticular fibrosis with loss of flexion and extension of the interphalangeal joints of the hand and of the foot and ankle. This condition is called congenital contractural arachnodactyly. In one particular family, one of the two sons went on to develop a severe progressive scoliosis requiring surgical correction (Figure 4.59).

The bones are of normal density and architecture but all the long bones are elongated, especially those of the hands and lower limbs. The condition may be confused with homocystinuria but the different clinical features and the presence of homocystine in the urine distinguish the two.

Prognosis for life is restricted by the cardiovascular complications of the disease and by the scoliosis which may precipitate respiratory failure in early adult life. There is no effective treatment for the condition, though scoliosis can be controlled by spinal fusion. It has been suggested that induction of early skeletal maturity by hormonal means may arrest some of the skeletal manifestations of the disease.

Cleidocranial dysostosis

This developmental disturbance of the skeleton is characterized by involvement of the skull and the clavicles, the striking feature being the absence or gross dysplasia of the clavicles. The typical case is a patient with a large head, a small face, drooping shoulders and a narrow chest. There is delay in closure of the sutures of the skull, so the frontal and parietal bones are prominent and the head is described as having a 'hot-cross bun' appearance. The clavicles are incompletely developed from the three ossification centres and may be completely absent so that the patient may be able to approximate the shoulders until the tips of the acromion processes touch beneath his chin (Figure 4.60). There may also be associated abnormalities of the hips with delayed ossification of the heads of the femora, the pelvis and the spine, leading to lordosis, scoliosis or kyphosis. In addition, the deciduous teeth are usually normal though often delayed and the growth of the permanent teeth is markedly impaired. The child usually presents with difficulties in gait due to femoral neck deformity or disturbances in dentition.

It appears that the basis for this disturbance is a failure of the normal development of the midline junctions between bones. The condition is relatively benign (see Chapter 3).

References

Ablin, D. S., Greenspan, A., Reinhart, M. and Grix, A. (1990) Differentiation of child abuse from osteogenesis imperfecta: a review article. *American Journal of Roentgenology* **154**, 1035–1046

Aegerter, F. and Kirkpatrick, J. A. (1975) *Orthopaedic Diseases*. W. B. Saunders: Philadelphia, London, Toronto

Albers-Schönberg, H. (1904) *Münchener Medizinische Wochenschrift* **51**, 365

Aldegheri, R., Trivella, G., Renzi-Brivio, L. *et al.* (1988) Lengthening of the lower limbs in achondroplastic patients. *Journal of Bone and Joint Surgery* **70B**, 69–73

Baily, R. W. *et al.* (1963) Studies of longitudinal bone growth resulting in extensible nailing. *Surgical Forum* **14**, 455

Bauze, R. J., Smith, R. and Francis, M. J. O. (1975a) A new look at osteogenesis imperfecta. *Journal of Bone and Joint Surgery* **57B**, 2

Bauze, R. J., Smith, R. and Francis, M. J. O. (1975b) Osteogenesis imperfecta; a new classification of birth defects. *Original Article Series* **11**, 99–102

Byers, P. H. (1993) Osteogenesis imperfecta. In: *Connective Tissue and its Heritable Disorders*, pp. 317–350. Edited by P. M. Royce and B. Steinmann. Wiley-Liss: New York

Cournot, G., Thil, C. L., Fischer, A. and Garabedran, M. (1989) Osteopetrosis: the role of transplantation in marble bone disease. *Bone* **6**, No. 2, 15–18

Fahey, J. J. and O'Brien, E. T. (1973) Subtotal resection and grafting in selected cases of solitary unicameral bone cyst. *Journal of Bone and Joint Surgery* **55A**, 59–68

Fairbank, T. (1935) *Proceedings of the Royal Society of Medicine* **268**, 1611

Fairbank, T. (1951) *Atlas of General Affections of the Skeleton*. Livingstone: Edinburgh

Francis, M. J. O., Smith, R. and Bauze, R. J. (1974) Instability of polymeric skin collagen in osteogenesis imperfecta. *British Medical Journal* **1**, 421–424

Hall, G. S. (1943) *Quarterly Journal of Medicine* **36**, 77

Harris, H. A. (1933) *Bone Growth in Health and Disease*. Oxford University Press: London

Hunter, C. (1917) *Proceedings of the Royal Society of Medicine* **10**, 104

Hunter, D. and Wiles, B. (1935) *British Journal of Surgery* **22**, 507

Jansen, M. (1928) Dissociation of bone growth. In: *The Robert Jones Birthday Volume*. Oxford University Press: London

Johnson, J. L., Webster, J. R. and Sippy, H. I. (1960) Maffucci's syndrome. *American Journal of Medicine* **28**, 864–866

Keith, A. (1920) *British Journal of Surgery* **22**, 507

Knaggs, R. L. (1926) *Inflammatory and Toxic Diseases of Bone*. Wright: Bristol

Kopits, S. E. (1976) Orthopedic complications of dwarfism. *Clinical Orthopaedics and Related Disease* **114**, 153–179

Kraft, E. (1933) *Radiology* **20**, 47

Lennon, E., Schecter, M. and Hornabrook, R. (1961) *Journal of Bone and Joint Surgery* **43B**, 273

Leroy, J. G. and Wiesmann, U. (1993) Disorders of lysosomal enzymes. In: *Connective Tissue and its Heritable Disorders*, 1st edn, pp. 613–639. Edited by P. Royce and B. Steinmann. Wiley-Liss: New York

McKusick, V. A. (1966) *Hereditable Disorders of Connective Tissue*, 3rd edn. Mosby: St Louis, IL

McKusick, V. A., Neufeld, E. F. and Kelly, T. E. (1978) The mucopolysaccharide storage diseases. In: *The Metabolic Basis of Inherited Disease*, 4th edn. Edited by J. B. Stanbury, J. B. Wyngaarden and D. S. Fredrickson. McGraw-Hill: New York

Malawer, M. M. (1986) The diagnosis, treatment and management of unicameral bone cysts by percutaneous aspiration haemodynamic evaluation and intracavity methyl-prednisolone acetate. *Orthopaedic Update Series IV* **26**, 1–7

Middleton, R. W. D. (1984) Closed intrameduular rerodding in osteogenesis imperfecta. *Journal of Bone and Joint Surgery* **66B**, 652–655

Moore, J. J. and DeLorimler, A. A. (1933) *American Journal of Roentgenology* **29**, 161

Mörch, E. T. (1941) *Chondrodystrophic Dwarfs in Denmark*. Munksgaard: Copenhagen

Neer, C. S., Francis, K. C., Markof, R. C., Terz, J. and Carbonera, P. N. (1966) Treatment of unicameral bone cysts. *Journal of Bone and Joint Surgery* **48A**, 731–745

Neufeld, E. F. (1989) The mucopolysaccharidoses. In: *The Metabolic Basis of Inherited Disease*, 6th edn, pp. 1565–1587. Edited by C. R. Scriver, A. L. Beaudet, W. S. Sly and D. Valle. McGraw Hill Co.: New York

Nicholas, R. W. and James, P. (1990) Telescoping intramedullary stabilization of the lower extremities for severe osteogenesis imperfecta. *Journal of Pediatric Orthopedics* **10**, 219–223

Oohira, A. and Nokomi, H. (1989) Elevated occumulation by hyaluronate in the tubular bone of osteogenesis imperfecta. *Bone* **10**, 409–413

Robichon, J. and Germain, B. (1968) Orthogenesis of osteogenesis imperfecta. *Canadian Medical Association Journal* **99**, 975–979

Scaglietti, O., Marchetti, P. G. and Bartolozzi, P. (1979) The effects of methylprednisolone acetate in the treatment of bone cysts. *Journal of Bone and Joint Surgery* **61B**, 200

Schlumberger, H. G. (1946) *Military Surgeon* **99**, 504

Sillence, D. O., Senn, A. and Danks, D. M. (1979) Genetic heterogeneity in osteogenesis imperfecta. *Journal of Medical Genetics* **16**, 101–116

Smith, R. (1994) Osteogenesis imperfecta. *Surgery (Oxford)* **12**, 44–47

Sofield, H. A. and Miller, E. A. (1959) Fragmentation realignment and intramedullary rod fixation of deformity of long bones in children. *Journal of Bone and Joint Surgery* **41A**. 1371–1391

Speder, E. (1936) *Journal de Radiologie et d'Electrologie* **20**, 116–122

Thompson, E. M., Young, I. D., Hall, C. M. and Pembrey, M. E. (1987) Recurrent risk and prognosis in severe sporadic osteogenesis imperfecta. *Journal of Medical Genetics* **24**, 390–405

Turakainen, H. (1983) Altered glycosaminoglycen production – cultured osteogenesis imperfecta skin fibroblast.*Biochemical Journal* **213**, 171–178

Van Zeben, W. (1948) *Acta Paediatrica* **35**, 10

Voorhoeve, T. (1924) *Acta Radiologica* **3**, 407

Yung Hing, K. and McEwen, G. D. (1982) Scoliosis associated with osteogenesis imperfecta: results of treatment. *Journal of Bone and Joint Surgery* **64B**, 36

CHAPTER 5

Metabolic, Hormonal and Bone Marrow Diseases

ROBERT B. DUTHIE AND ROGER M. ATKINS

Classification

Our knowledge of bone diseases and their origin is still too incomplete to permit a classification at the same time comprehensive and scientifically accurate. Table 5.1 is given only as a convenient one for discussion.

In the examination and diagnosis of these conditions Shearer (1954) said: 'If a bone lesion as seen radiographically does not show reactive change in the adjacent bone or periosteum, which suggests an inflammatory process or the invasive character of a neoplastic process, you should then have in mind the possibility of a dysplasia. Study then the localization; is it involving primarily metaphyseal bone or does it, in some conditions, involve only the epiphyses or only the small bones? Study then the nature of the abnormal process. Is it merely an arrest of growth; does the appearance suggest a cartilage dysplasia or a fibrous dysplasia? Then proceed to carry out a survey of the skeleton to show the distribution of the abnormal bone. Do not forget to note whether the condition is associated with a generalized osteoporosis or whether bone, apart from the involved area, is normal. Then consider the findings in relation to the full history and clinical examination as well as blood biochemical analysis.'

A radiographic classification is shown in Table 5.2.

Table 5.1 Classification of generalized bone disease

Developmental	Achondroplasia Chondro-osteodystrophy Dyschondroplasia Multiple enchondromata Metaphyseal aclasis Osteogenesis imperfecta Polyostotic fibrous dysplasia Osteopetrosis
Metabolic	*Defect of mineralization* Due to a deficiency of vitamin D or a disturbance of its metabolism: 1. Vitamin D deficiency: 'Nutritional rickets' Osteomalacia 2. Malabsorption: Gluten-sensitive enteropathy (coeliac disease) Post gastrectomy Pancreatic disease liver disease, small bowel resection – rare 3. Renal disease: Renal glomerular failure 'Renal osteodystrophy' Renal tubular disorders: Inherited hypophosphataemic rickets (type I Dent) Adult-onset hypophosphataemic osteomalacia Renal tubular acidosis Fanconi's syndrome (inherited and acquired) Wilson's disease Rarely with neurofibromatosis Rarely due to an anticonvulsant *Defect of bone matrix* Osteoporosis (also osteogenesis imperfecta) Cause unknown: 1. Idiopathic 2. Juvenile 3. Postmenopausal 4. Senile Cause known: 1. Hyperadrenocorticism (spontaneous and iatrogenic) 2. Hyperthyroidism 3. Hypogonadism 4. Immobilization *Excessive bone resorption* Hyperparathyroidism *Paget's disease*
Hormonal	Normal, excessive or deficient secretion from the: 1. Pituitary 2. Sex glands 3. Thyroid 4. Adrenals 5. Parathyroids with the effect being seen in: a *child* as altered rate of epiphyseal growth and skeletal maturation: an *adult* as alteration in the balance of osteolytic activity and osteoblastic activity

Table 5.1—*continued*

Reticulosis	Disease of bone marrow constituents, such as:
	Reticuloendothelial system
	Histiocytic granulomatosis:
	1. Letterer–Siwe disease
	2. Eosinophilic granuloma
	3. Hand–Schüller–Christian disease
	Lipoid granulomatosis:
	1. Gaucher's disease
	2. Niemann–Pick disease
	3. Xanthomatosis with hypercholesterolaemia
	Lymphatic system
	Hodgkin's disease
	Lymphosarcoma
	Haemopoietic system
	Leukaemia:
	1. Lymphoblastic
	2. Myeloblastic
	Multiple myeloma
	Haemolytic anaemia:
	1. Mediterranean or Cooley's anaemia
	2. Sickle cell anaemia
	3. Erythroblastosis fetalis
Vascular	Osteodystrophy or Sudeck's atrophy
	Massive osteolysis or 'disappearing bones'

Osteomalacia and rickets

Osteomalacia and rickets are conditions which are characterized by defective mineralization of bone matrix which is seen histologically as excessive unmineralized osteoid. However, an increase in the proportion of bone covered by unmineralized osteoid or in the osteoid seam width is seen in a number of conditions other than osteomalacia, such as Paget's disease of bone. The term osteomalacia is therefore conveniently restricted to conditions where defective mineralization arises as a result of abnormalities of vitamin D metabolism. The majority of these conditions have similar clinical, histological, biochemical and radiographic features with the exception of type I hypophosphataemic rickets.

The majority of causes of rickets are similar to those of osteomalacia. Rickets refers to the condition where it occurs before closure of the growth plates so that abnormalities of skeletal growth are superimposed.

PATHOPHYSIOLOGY

Defective vitamin D metabolism leads to lowering of the serum 1,2-dihydroxyvitamin D $(OH)_2$ D (calcitriol), which in turn causes intestinal malabsorption of calcium. The normal calcium homoeostatic mechanisms initially defend the serum level of calcium so that urinary excretion is reduced. The serum calcium falls despite the reduction in excretion and this stimulates the parathyroid glands to produce parathyroid hormone (PTH) which tends to normalize serum calcium at the expense of reducing serum phosphate. Since phosphate absorption is often also defective, hypophosphataemia may be marked.

Osteoblastic activity is increased in osteomalacia for complex reasons which probably include raised serum activity of parathyroid hormone and the mechanical and biological effects of defective osteoid mineralization. This leads to a rise in serum alkaline phosphatase activity.

The defective osteoid mineralization is seen radiographically as widening and cupping of the growth plate, while histological examination of undecalcified bone sections confirms widened osteoid seams and tetracycline labelling reveals defective mineralization.

Osteomalacia is commonly associated with proximal muscle weakness. The cause of this and the reason for its distribution are unclear. It is probably due to abnormalities of calcium and phosphate metabolism within muscle but it is possible that vitamin D directly effects muscle biochemistry.

Table 5.2 Radiographic features of generalized bone disease

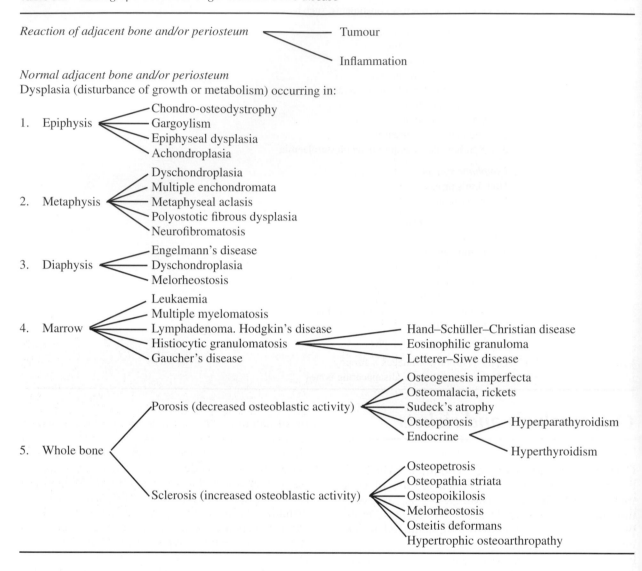

Reaction of adjacent bone and/or periosteum
- Tumour
- Inflammation

Normal adjacent bone and/or periosteum
Dysplasia (disturbance of growth or metabolism) occurring in:

1. Epiphysis
   - Chondro-osteodystrophy
   - Gargoylism
   - Epiphyseal dysplasia
   - Achondroplasia
2. Metaphysis
   - Dyschondroplasia
   - Multiple enchondromata
   - Metaphyseal aclasis
   - Polyostotic fibrous dysplasia
   - Neurofibromatosis
3. Diaphysis
   - Engelmann's disease
   - Dyschondroplasia
   - Melorheostosis
4. Marrow
   - Leukaemia
   - Multiple myelomatosis
   - Lymphadenoma. Hodgkin's disease
   - Histiocytic granulomatosis
     - Hand–Schüller–Christian disease
     - Eosinophilic granuloma
     - Letterer–Siwe disease
   - Gaucher's disease
5. Whole bone
   - Porosis (decreased osteoblastic activity)
     - Osteogenesis imperfecta
     - Osteomalacia, rickets
     - Sudeck's atrophy
     - Osteoporosis
     - Endocrine
       - Hyperparathyroidism
       - Hyperthyroidism
   - Sclerosis (increased osteoblastic activity)
     - Osteopetrosis
     - Osteopathia striata
     - Osteopoikilosis
     - Melorheostosis
     - Osteitis deformans
     - Hypertrophic osteoarthropathy

AETIOLOGY

The causes of osteomalacia are legion and often multifactorial. For example, in an elderly person an abnormal diet may lead to poor vitamin D and calcium intake, disability may lead to lack of exposure to sunlight and there may be impaired renal function. The causes of osteomalacia (and rickets) may be divided into nutritional, absorptive, renal and others (see Table 5.1). The mechanism by which an abnormality causes osteomalacia is readily understood by consideration of normal vitamin D metabolism.

Synthesis of vitamin D in the skin depends on direct exposure to sunlight. It is reduced in latitudes distant from the equator, by atmospheric pollution and by increased skin pigmentation. The duration of exposure to direct sunlight depends on the patient's lifestyle and mobility and the dermal production of vitamin D is also reduced in winter compared with summer. Few normally consumed foods contain high levels of vitamin D. However, it is found in fish and eggs. A number of countries routinely fortify foodstuffs with vitamin D, for example margarine in the United Kingdom and milk in the USA. The dietary requirement of vitamin D is increased in the elderly (Parfitt *et al.*, 1982) and in pregnancy because of fetal requirements for vitamin D.

Breads which are rich in phytate, such as chapatties, bind dietary calcium and reduce absorption and although calcium deficiency alone does not cause osteomalacia in adults, it can do so in growing children (Marie *et al.*, 1982). A high intake of wheat fibre increases faecal excretion of bile acids which may impair vitamin D absorption.

In practice in Great Britain today, two groups of patients are particularly at risk of vitamin D deficiency due to failure of intake or skin production: the very elderly and young ethnic Indian emigrants to the UK. Vitamin D absorption may also be defective in coeliac disease or biliary obstruction. The production of active metabolites from vitamin D may be inhibited at the 25-hydroxylation stage in the liver, for example, by anticonvulsant therapy, and at the renal 1-hydroxylation stage by nephrectomy, renal failure, hypoparathyroidism or hypophosphataemia.

Like osteomalacia, in adults, rickets arises from a defect in mineralization of the organic matrix, during growth, and is caused by:

1. Deficiency in vitamin D or its metabolism – associated with poor dietary intake of calcium and vitamin D; decrease in the effect and amount of sunlight (e.g. in northern climates); pigmented skin in the Asian immigrant and in the elderly.
2. Malabsorption (e.g. gluten-sensitive enteropathy of coeliac disease, hepatic osteodystrophy, etc.).
3. Renal disease (e.g. glomerular failure or renal osteodystrophy) – this has to be distinguished from the more common renal tubular disorder or X-linked inherited hypophosphataemia as described by Dent as type I vitamin D resistant rickets (see Table 5.1).

Vitamin D_3 (cholecalciferol) is made in the dermis by the action of ultraviolet light on 7-dihydrocholesterol. Vitamin D_2 is absorbed from the diet through the small intestine. Transport in the serum is by binding with an X-globulin which has been synthesized in the liver. 25-Hydroxylation of the vitamin Ds also occurs in the liver, and in patients with normal renal function this level of serum 25-hydroxycholecalciferol reflects the total body state. The active dihydroxylated hormone of 1,25 $(OH)_2D$ is then produced in the kidney. It is this hormone which is directly (but not solely) concerned with bone mineralization and formation as well as calcium absorption (Dekel *et al*., 1979).

PATHOLOGY

The main interest of the orthopaedic surgeon is in the bony and muscle manifestations of the disease as well as the metabolic disturbance.

Skeletal changes

The bones of the skeleton are soft and porotic, and bend easily from the weight of the body or from other external causes. Normally the epiphyseal line of the long bones is a well defined narrow strip of cartilage 2 mm deep, but in rickets it forms a wide irregular band and the metaphysis is broad and irregular from excessive proliferation of the cells of the epiphyseal line (Figure 5.1).

The cartilage in the proliferating zone is hyperplastic, but instead of the normal palisade arrangement of the cells, the proliferating cells are arranged more haphazardly. The extent of the zone is increased.

In the zone of calcified cartilage the deposit of calcium salts in the intercellular matrix is greatly deficient, or even absent.

In the zone of ossification the bone deposited by the osteogenic cells from the diaphysis is poor in quality, deficient in calcium and of patchy distribution. Associated with this is a poor development of the bone marrow (Figure 5.2). The osteoid zone is increased greatly and covers most surfaces undergoing mineralization (Figure 5.3). Bone resorption may be increased and replaced by fibrous tissue.

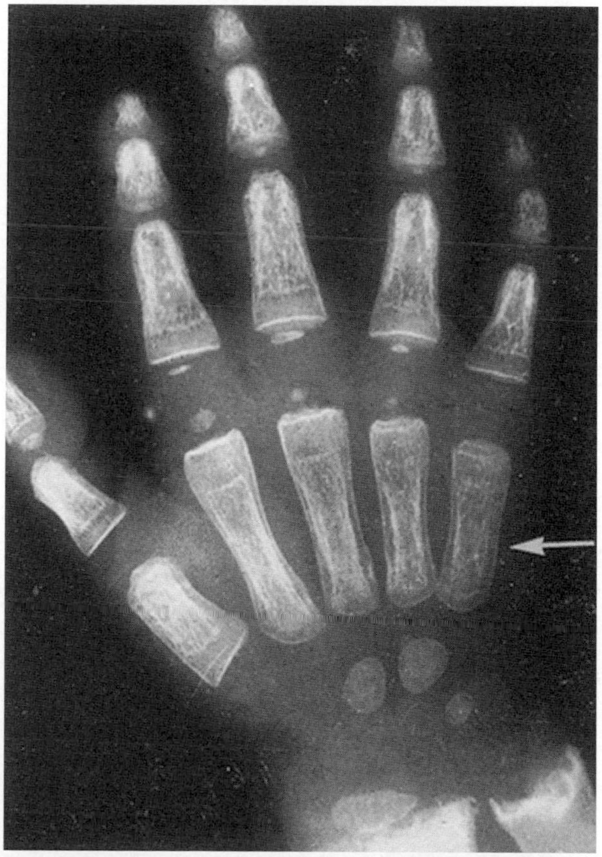

Figure 5.1 The hand of a small boy with vitamin D resistant rickets, showing the marked cupping effect at the wrist epiphyses, the reduced number of carpal ossification centres, and the bone within bone effect in the metacarpals.

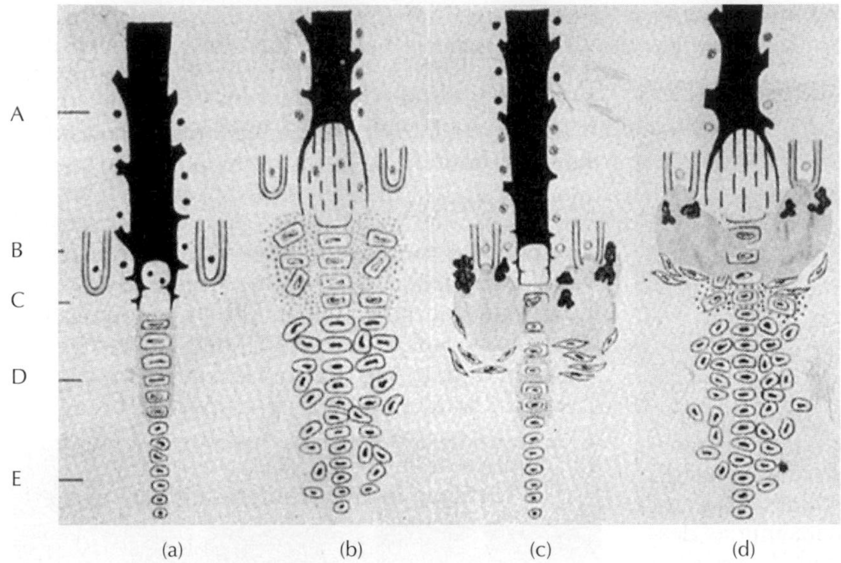

Figure 5.2 Showing the characteristics of the growth area in various conditions. (a) A normal bone: note the regular column of proliferating cartilage and of calcified cartilage cells. A, diaphysis; B, capillary with accompanying osteoblastic invasion; C, zone of ossification; D, zone of calcified cartilage; E, zone of proliferating cartilage. (b) Rickets: note the irregular and excessive proliferation of cartilage cells, the poor calcium deposit in the zone of calcified cartilage, and the scanty bone formation in the ossification zone. The whole growth area shows greatly increased thickness. (c) Simple scurvy: there are intra-metaphyseal haemorrhages and a fibroblastic reaction. New bone, as it is formed, is broken up by the haemorrhage. (d) Scurvy rickets: in addition to the changes in rickets (as in (b) above) there is evidence of scorbutic capillary haemorrhage. (After H. A. Harris)

In the metaphysis the bony trabeculae are weakened by lack of calcium, the continued strain stimulates connective tissue hyperplasia so that the extremity of the bone appears mis-shapen and unmodelled.

These changes are most marked at the most actively growing part of the bones, and only affect the bone being deposited during the active phase of the disease. Bone formed before that is for the most part normal, while bone formed after

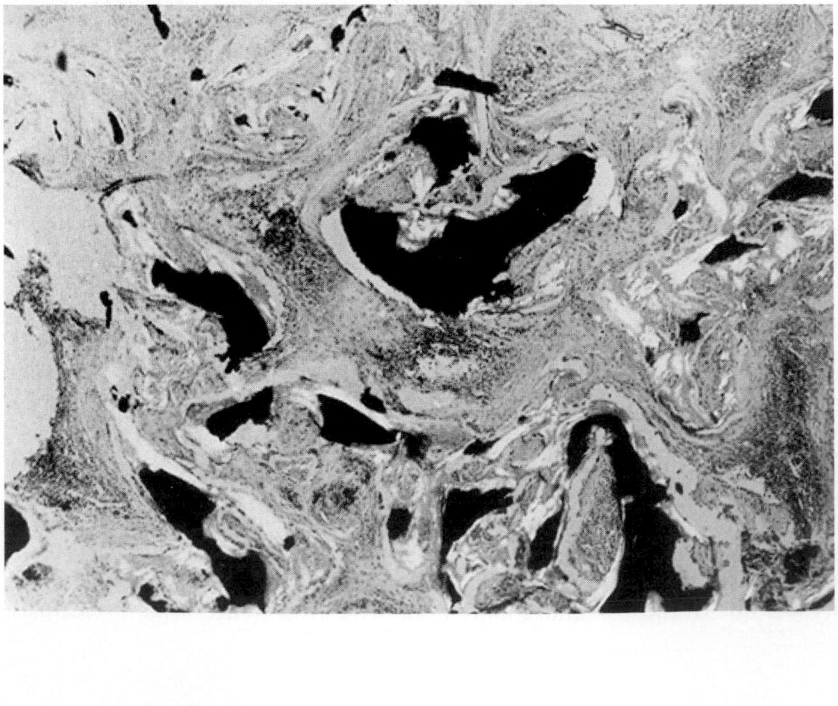

Figure 5.3 Photomicrograph of 'osteomalacia' bone taken from an iliac bone biopsy. Von Kossa stained to show calcium as black surrounded by non-calcified birefringent osteoid; interspersed between these areas are cellular regions of vascular connective tissue. (x 32).

the active phase of the disease is passed is also normal.

The deformities of rickets

During the active phase of the disease, enlargement of the metaphyseal segments of the long bones gives rise to obvious swellings at the bone ends. These are especially prominent at the costochondral junctions, and at the lower ends of the radius and tibia.

When the child is able to crawl or to walk, the long bones of the lower limb may become bent. The femur becomes bowed anteriorly and to the lateral side. The neck-shaft angle of the femur may be diminished (coxa vara), the tibia, bowed, or the knee may assume a valgus attitude (Figure 5.4).

The pelvic deformities are of most importance to the obstetrician. The whole pelvis may be flattened, or it may assume a trefoil shape as in osteomalacia (p. 291).

The skull is broadened, the forehead square, and bosses of new bone may form in the parietal and frontal regions.

The vertebral column may come to assume exaggerated curvatures.

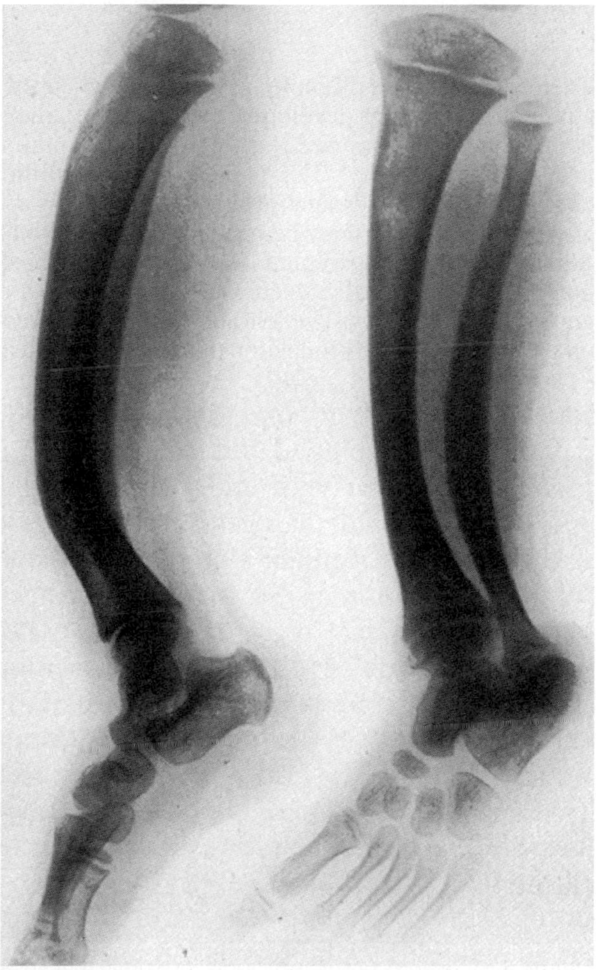

Figure 5.4 Rachitic deformity of the tibiae and fibulae after the condition has healed – the 'sabre' shin.

CLINICAL FEATURES

There are certain features of osteomalacia or rickets which are due to the metabolic abnormality of bone rather than the underlying disease. These are common to the condition whatever its aetiology. The major symptoms are bone pain and tenderness with skeletal deformity and proximal muscle weakness. Features of hypocalclemia may also be seen. Tenderness of all the bones occurs, but may be most marked in the ribs and over Looser's zones. It may be severe enough to keep the patient awake at night.

In a typical case of rickets, the clinical picture is very characteristic and the prominent features may be tabulated as follows.

1. Large head, open fontanelles and craniotabes.
2. Prominent abdomen.
3. Separation of the recti muscles over the protuberant abdomen.
4. Narrow chest.
5. Enlarged epiphyses.
6. Beaded ribs – the rickety rosary.
7. Bowing of the long bones with genu valgum.
8. Delayed dentition, with irregular soft, decaying teeth.
9. Pale skin, flabby subcutaneous tissue and typical wizened look.

RADIOLOGICAL APPEARANCES

The radiographic changes are characteristic and important. Four stages are described.

1. The *acute stage*. The normal rounded appearance of the epiphysis is replaced by a cloudy area containing one or more indistinct centres of ossification. The metaphysis is splayed out, and deficient in calcium shadow. There may also be evidence of a thickened periosteum, while fractures of the long bones are frequently seen.

2. In the *second stage*, the epiphysis appears as a mottled, irregular, ill-defined shadow. The metaphysis is ragged, but is now broader than normal, running out from the side where the pressure is greatest. Periosteal thickening has

disappeared, but, if bowing has occurred, the cortical part of the affected bone will be thickened on the side of the concavity of the curve.

3. In the *third stage* the shadow becomes denser, and at the end of the metaphysis a dense line appears. This is due to the deposition of calcium, and, while it is often considered characteristic of scurvy, it also occurs quite frequently in rickets. The epiphyseal shadow is more clearly outlined, but is still inclined to be mottled rather than clean-cut. This is essentially the stage of repair. The most characteristic feature is the marked difference in size between the end of the shaft and the epiphysis.
4. In the *fourth stage* the characteristic increase in breadth of the metaphysis is still present, but the bone is now clearly defined, and shows a normal content of calcium salts. This stage marks the end of the process, the bone being now completely repaired.

BIOCHEMISTRY

The total calcium levels are normal or low, with low phosphates. Alkaline phosphatase levels are increased. It should be noted that the normal levels in the child, the young adult and in the elderly do differ.

Urinary calcium levels are lowered. The importance of biochemical values in these conditions is their return to normal upon correct therapy. The 24-hydroxylase assay is of help in the diagnosis of vitamin D dependency rickets, specially for any carrier status or relationship. Serum 25-hydroxyvitamin levels are monitored before and after commencement of treatment to indicate the lowered vitamin D Storage levels or their build-up (normal range of 25-hydroxyvitamin D levels is 3–30 μg/l). These serum blood chemistries can he correlated to bone biopsy in the elderly which will show excessive osteoid formation.

Levels of 25-oxyhydroxyl-D are low compared with the normal values for the particular age group and will indicate the effectiveness or otherwise of the administration of oral or injected compound as part of treatment.

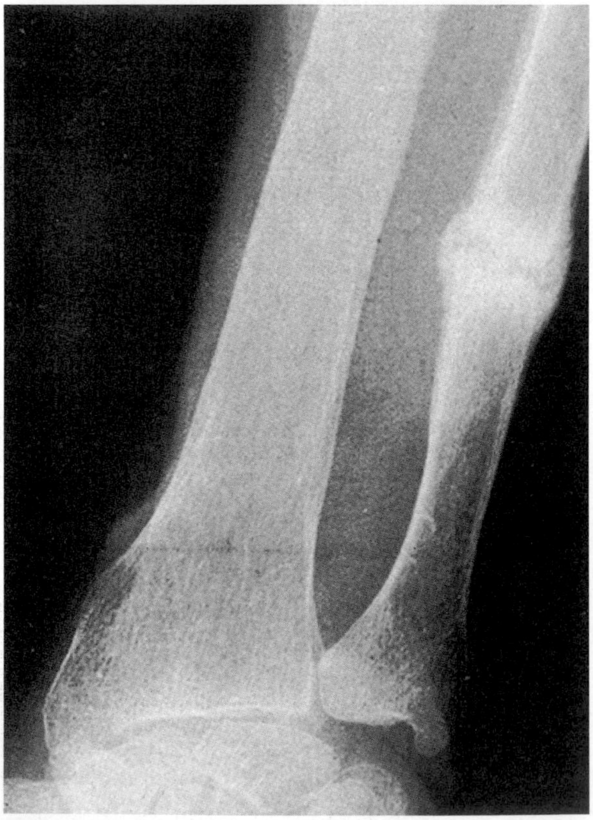

Figure 5.5 A Looser zone in the forearm of an elderly woman with nutritional osteomalacia.

DIAGNOSIS

There should be no difficulty in diagnosis when the complete picture has developed, but the disease may occasionally be confused with congenital syphilis and infantile scurvy. The congenitally syphilitic child usually has other signs of syphilis, but occasionally the chief lesion may be a syphilitic osteochondritis. The epiphyseal region is tender, oedematous, hot, painful and swollen; there is loosening and separation of the epiphysis, which can usually be moved on the shaft, with the production of muffled crepitus.

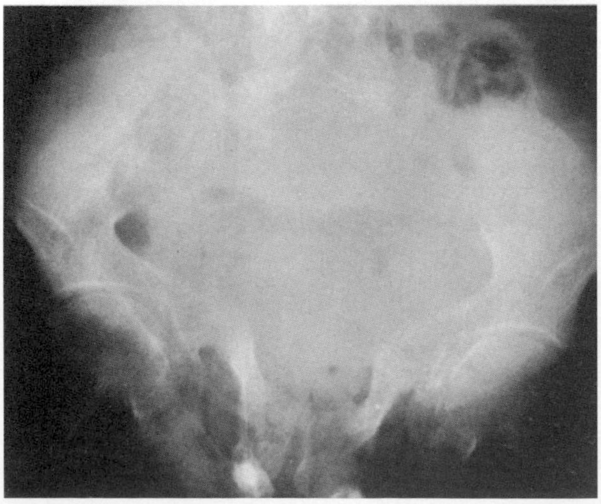

Figure 5.6 Severe post-gastrectomy osteomalacia in a woman of 69 years. Note the deformity of the pelvis and the healing Looser zones in the inferior pubic rami.

There is usually a history of parental syphilis, and the child responds to antiluetic treatment.

In infantile scurvy, swelling also occurs, it is not limited to the region of the epiphysis but encroaches on the shaft. There are usually haemorrhages in other situations, and the general signs of scurvy are present. Tender Looser zones are frequently present (Figures 5.5, 5.6 and 5.7).

TREATMENT OF RICKETS

The treatment may be considered under three headings – medical treatment, prevention of deformity and treatment of existing deformity.

Medical treatment

A milk-and-cheese diet should be given, with a reduction in the amount of cereals – some of which contain phytates, which reduce the absorption of calcium. A calcium preparation can be used initially, but the most important preparation to give is vitamin D (e.g. calciferol. 3000 i.u. per day) (Figure 5.8). Failure to respond to these measures suggests that the condition is not due to a vitamin D deficiency state and that other causes should be sought.

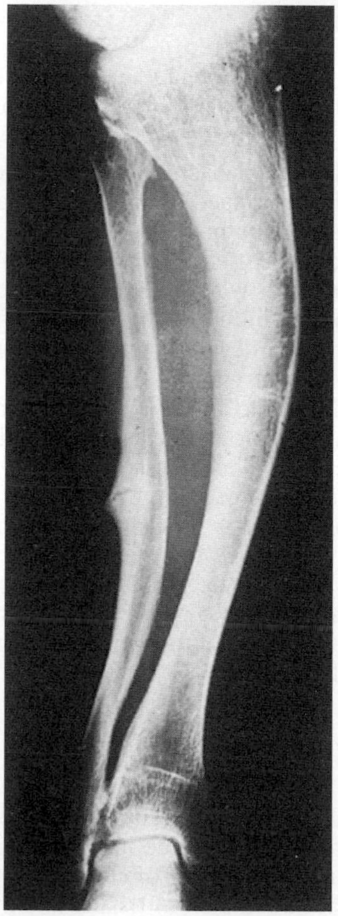

Figure 5.7 A Looser zone in a patient with X-linked renal tubular osteomalacia. Note also the deformity and characteristically dense bones.

Prevention of deformity

When the bones are so soft that they are easily bent by pressure, or muscle strain, the child's movements should be so controlled that little or no pressure is exerted upon his limbs. In difficult children it is often advisable to fit 'rickets' splints.

Treatment of the established deformity

Deformity is usually corrected by splints or by osteotomy.

Correction by splinting

This method is used where the deformity is slight and the disease still active. It is employed particularly in young children, especially in those below the age of 4, and is most useful in deformities of the lower limb.

The method is slow and requires continual supervision to ensure a good result and to prevent the formation of sores.

Correction by osteotomy

This method is used when the deformity is in the neighbourhood of a joint

Osteotomies should never be carried out until the radiograph indicates that at least the third stage of rickets has been reached. There is then eburnation, clearness and regularity of outline. If corrective operations are attempted before this period non-union is apt to follow.

TREATMENT OF OSTEOMALACIA

The treatment depends on the cause of the osteomalacia. Nutritional osteomalacia will respond to less than 1000 i.u. of vitamin D_2 daily. Osteomalacia due to gluten-sensitive enteropathy requires larger doses, especially if the gluten-free diet is not adhered to. The renal tubular forms of osteomalacia are 'resistant' to vitamin D and may require up to 1.25 mg daily.

With a growing ageing population there is a real increase in the incidence of osteomalacia due to poor dietary intake, reduced sunlight exposure, use of drugs, etc. Numerous publications have correlated

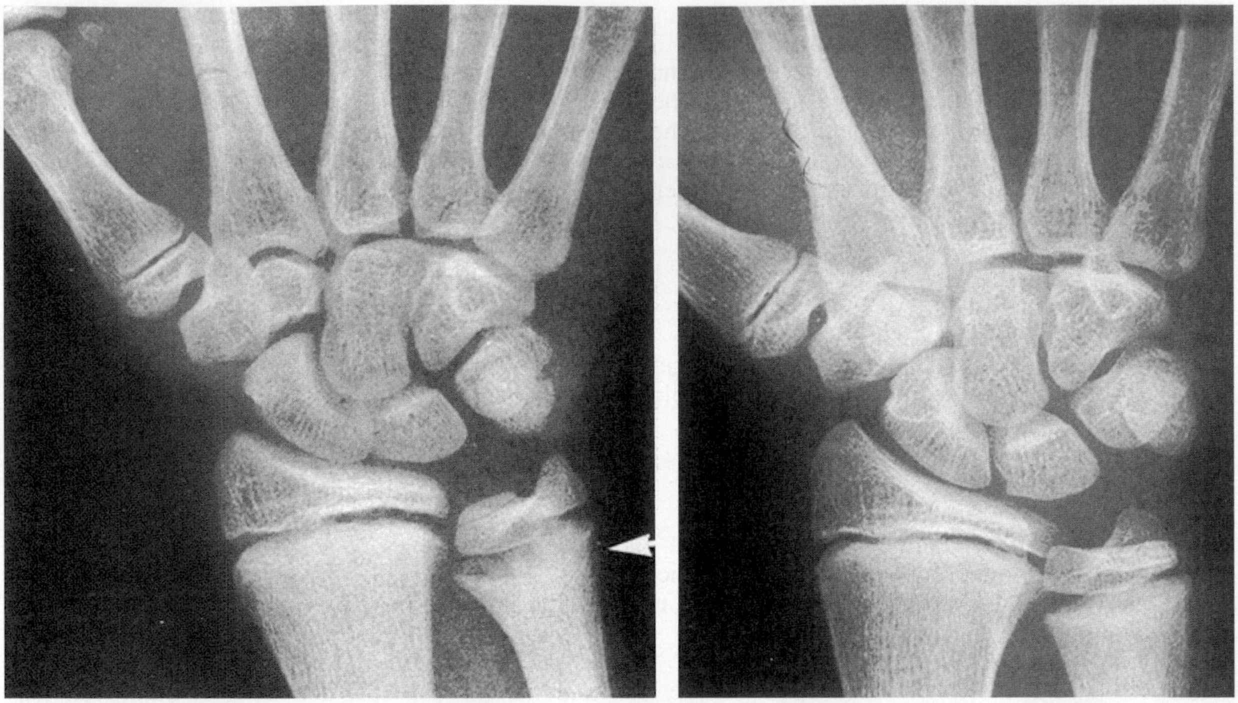

(a) (b)

Figure 5.8 Mild nutritional rickets in an adolescent immigrant (a) before, and (b) 2 months after, treatment with small doses of vitamin D; note the widened epiphyseal lines and the cupped and widened metaphysis before treatment.

this condition with the increased incidence of fractured femoral neck. Obviously in this age group there is more osteoporosis due to immobility, which also contributes to increased fracturing.

Some workers have suggested a vitamin D deficiency state as well, but direct measurements of 25(OH)D levels have failed to substantiate this concept. However, if osteomalacia is diagnosed, treatment with oral vitamin D 1.25 mg daily should be given for a short period of time. As yet, evidence is not good enough to warrant prophylactic administration of calcium compounds or vitamin D metabolite to this group of the population. (More specialized works should be consulted for details on the use of vitamin D.)

Scurvy

The anti-scorbutic vitamin C is found in the majority of fresh foods – fruit juices, green vegetables and to a lesser extent in potatoes, milk and raw meat. Because it is destroyed by heating at 100°C, it is absent in dried, canned and preserved foods, and in vegetables subjected to prolonged boiling.

The absence of vitamin C from the diet gives rise to the clinical condition of scurvy, the characteristic symptom of which is haemorrhage in various parts of the body. The orthopaedic surgeon is concerned with its manifestations in bone.

The disease most commonly occurs in infants of from 6 to 8 months who have been fed exclusively on artificial food which has had its vitamin content destroyed in the process of manufacture or which has never possessed a vitamin C content at all. It also occurs in adults who are deprived, for a time, of fresh food – as in old people living alone and subsisting on an inadequate diet of bread and tea.

A diet deficient in vitamin C is not necessarily deficient in the other vitamins. Nevertheless, it is frequently so and if there is, in particular, a deficiency in vitamin D, a rachitic element may be added to the scorbutic in the case of the growing child, while in the adult there may be some evidence of osteomalacia.

PATHOLOGY

The cardinal feature of scurvy is a defect in the formation of certain intercellular substances which results in haemorrhage – from the gums, the alimentary tract, the subcutaneous tissues and in bone. The haemorrhage is capillary in origin and occurs at sites at which new capillaries are sprouting – bone, for example, at the most actively growing metaphyses

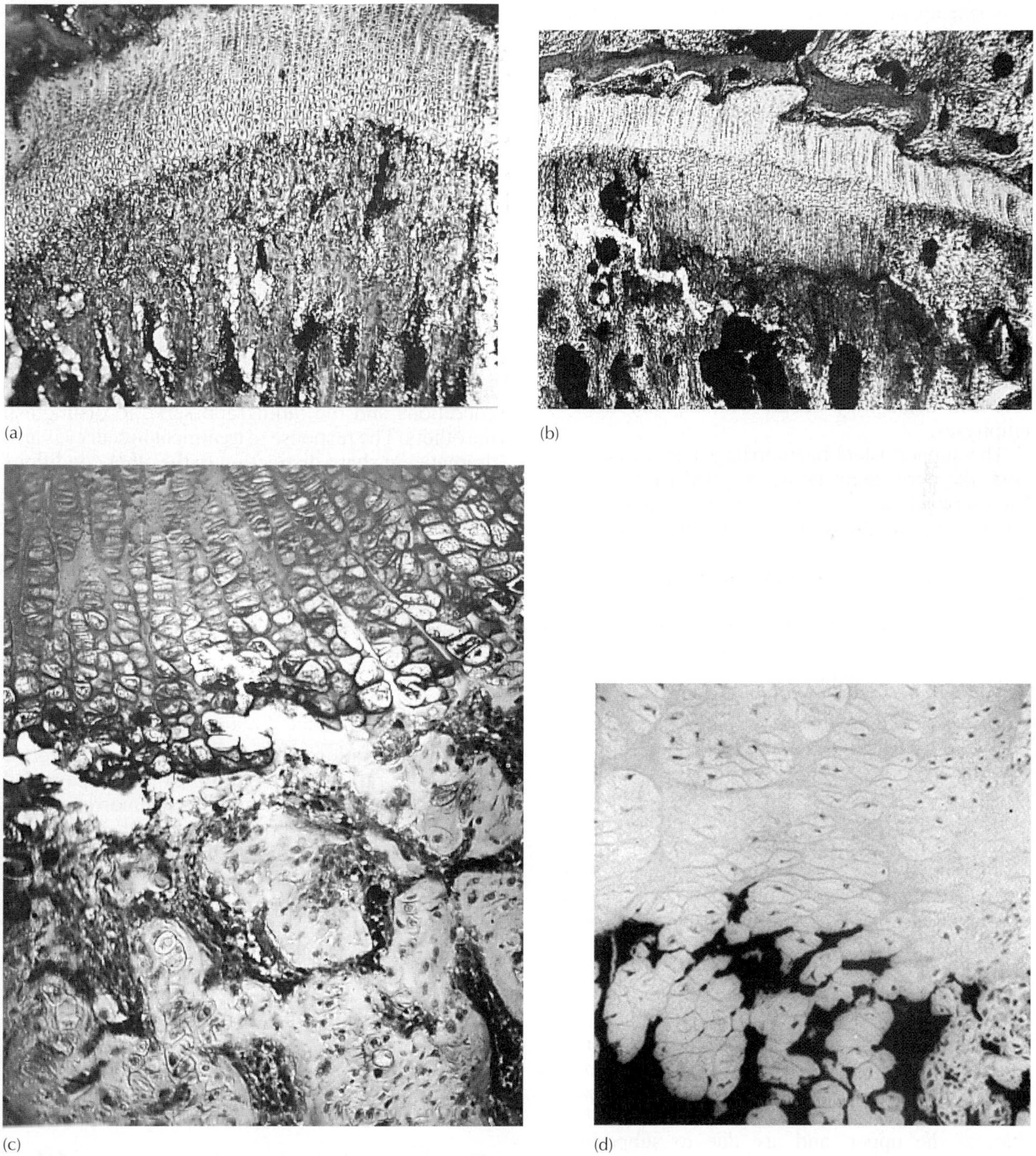

Figure 5.9 (a) Photomicrograph of a normal epiphyseal plate with trabecular formation, invasion of blood vessels and ossification taking place. (× 17). (b) Photomicrograph of scorbutic epiphyseal plate showing the decrease in depth of the physis with loss of the normal columnal appearance, irregular trabeculae and ossification zones. (× 17) (c) Photomicrograph of the irregular trabecular formation, containing islands of chondroid tissues, osteoid and osteoblasts – all without pattern or organization. (× 180). (d) Photomicrograph of a human scorbutic epiphysis, showing the disturbance of phases 4 and 5 of epiphyseal cartilage cell maturation in which there should be cartilage cell disruption and trabecular formation with invasion by blood vessels and osteoblasts. This is occurring in only one small area, and abnormal calcium deposition is seen. (× 35).

and beneath the periosteum. It is thought that vitamin C controls the nutrition of capillary endothelium, and the amount of intercellular cement which binds the endothelial cells together.

The pathological change in the affected bone was well described by H.A. Harris many years ago.

From the capillary loops growing up into the zone of ossification from the diaphysis, there occurs an irregular and patchy oozing of blood so that small pools of blood collect and disrupt the newly forming bone, the calcified cartilaginous strata and even the proliferating cartilaginous palisades. The blood clots and contracts, and is replaced by fibrous tissue or, in favourable circumstances, by bone.

In very extreme cases, the haemorrhage may be sufficient to disrupt the growing area, so that massive cell death may occur, with separation of the epiphyses.

The subperiosteal haemorrhages are often extensive, the periosteum being stripped from the shaft for a considerable distance. They organize or are replaced by bone exactly as in the intrametaphyseal haemorrhages.

In *true scurvy*, there is in addition to the features outlined above some irregular proliferation of the cartilage columns; otherwise the effects are similar. In all forms of scurvy there is an important secondary effect, for the metaphyseal disturbance is also responsible for failure of differentiation of the bone marrow, and this, with the repeated haemorrhages, may lead to a degree of anaemia (Figure 5.9).

CLINICAL FEATURES

The child may or may not appear ill-nourished. The earliest features are restlessness and fretfulness, and it is apparent that one or more of the extremities is not being used. Handling of the parts produces pain, and ultimately the child screams whenever he is turned over or moved. Systemic reaction (fever) is absent in the initial stages.

When the limbs are examined, the observer may find obvious swelling, in relation to the shaft of one or more of the long bones. Such swellings are said to be ten times more common in the lower limb bones than in the upper, and are due to subperiosteal haemorrhages. The joints may appear swollen, and are exquisitely sensitive to touch – so much so that an infective condition may be stimulated. On the other hand, the immobility of the parts may simulate paralysis, and this feature is known as the 'pseudoparalysis of scurvy'. Haemorrhages may also occur into and beneath the skin, and the gums may be swollen and spongy.

DIFFERENTIAL DIAGNOSIS

In the absence of visible or palpable haemorrhage, there may be difficulty in the diagnosis of scurvy. The conditions most liable to confusion in the early stages are anterior poliomyelitis, injury to joint, bone and nerve, osteomyelitis, arthritis and syphilitic osteochondritis.

According to Harris the syphilitic lesion, in contrast to scurvy, affects the more slowly growing end of a bone; as for example the elbow. It is also common in the short long bones of hand and foot, the proximal end of the femur, and the distal end of the tibia.

The absence of fever serves to rule out the inflammatory conditions, and the history, the dietetic conditions and the radiograph serve to distinguish the others. The response to treatment in scurvy is also dramatic, in sharp distinction to the other conditions enumerated.

The typical x-ray appearance is seen in Figure 5.10. Fairbank (1951) described, as a sign of diagnostic value, a clear line in the bone parallel to the growth disc and separated from it by a clear zone – very wide and often associated with subperiosteal haemorrhages.

TREATMENT

The administration of vitamin C in any of its forms leads to a rapid cure. Within 24 hours pain and crying cease, and in a few days haemorrhages are beginning to heal. It is some months, however, before the bone texture returns to normal. The easiest way to exhibit vitamin C is as fresh orange, or lemon, juice or by the synthetic vitamin product – ascorbic acid.

Rest in bed is indicated in the early stages; later, massage and exercises may be usefully employed to augment muscle tone. Unprotected weight-bearing should be forbidden until there is radiographic evidence of a return of structure to the metaphysis, as otherwise deformities may arise.

Coeliac rickets (gluten-sensitive enteropathy)

The frequent occurrence of skeletal changes as in association with coeliac disease can escape recognition in early childhood, while the bone changes do not appear till the age of 7, when they are often attributed to late rickets.

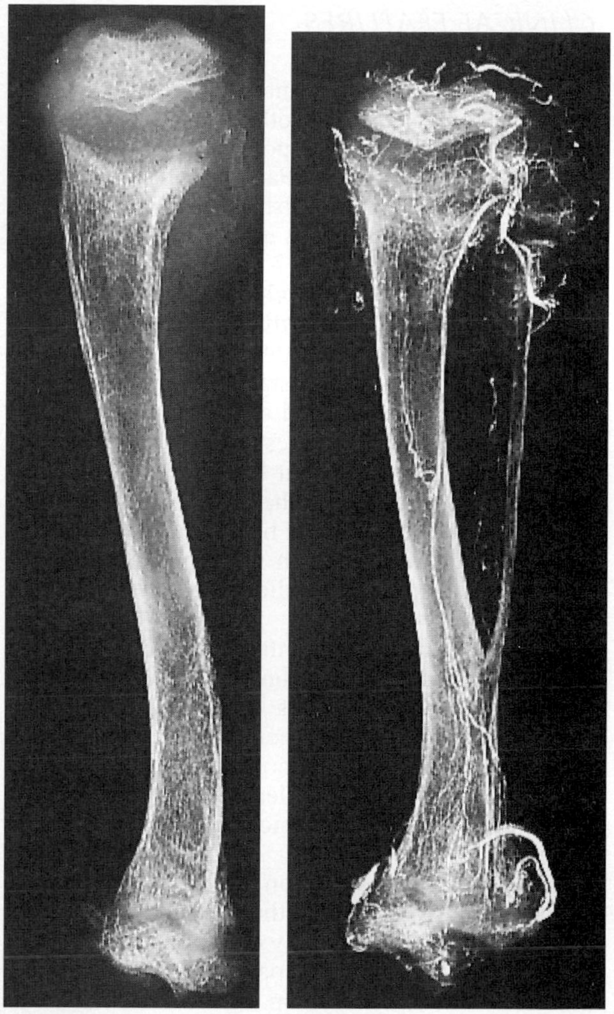

(a) (b)

Figure 5.10 (a) Radiograph of a scorbutic tibia animal specimen exhibiting the gross epiphyseal plate disruption with marked subperiosteal soft tissue shadow of haemorrhage laterally. (b) Same specimen after arterial injection of radiopaque material to show the abnormal circulation pattern around the haematoma mass laterally and into the epiphyseal area.

PATHOLOGY

The bone changes appear only in late and long-established cases, and are similar to those of rickets. The metaphysis is broad and irregular, the palisade arrangement of cartilage cells is lost and instead there is an irregular hypertrophy of the cells. The zone of calcified cartilage is narrow and its calcium content is poor or absent, while the osteogenic process is retarded or arrested, and instead of bone there is deposited an imperfect type of osteoid tissue.

AETIOLOGY

Coeliac disease (gluten-sensitive enteropathy) is due to sensitivity to the gluten of wheat. The small intestine shows subtotal or total villous atrophy. There is probably malabsorption of vitamin D, and a resistance to its action. The bone disease will not heal with physiological doses of vitamin D unless the diet is free of gluten.

CLINICAL FEATURES

In association with the characteristic appearance of coeliac disease – pallor, cachexia, muscular hypotonicity and abdominal swelling – there is lack of body development (stunting). In addition, there may be skeletal deformity. Genu valgum in particular is a common feature. Enlargement of the distal ends of the radius and ulna are also frequent signs (Figure 5.11), but occasionally still more extensive deformation may be present – enlarged costochondral junctions, Harrison's sulcus, kyphosis. coxa vara, bow leg, etc. Fractures may occur with mild trauma.

There may be recurring attacks of tetany.

RADIOLOGICAL APPEARANCES

The x-ray appearances are very variable, but the whole bone is usually fragile and porotic. Parsons (1932) believed that the other changes were similar to those of rickets; i.e. the metaphysis was swollen and its extremity uneven. The epiphyseal cartilage was broad and fuzzy. In most cases transverse striations of denser bone may be detected in the neighbourhood of the metaphysis. Harris believed

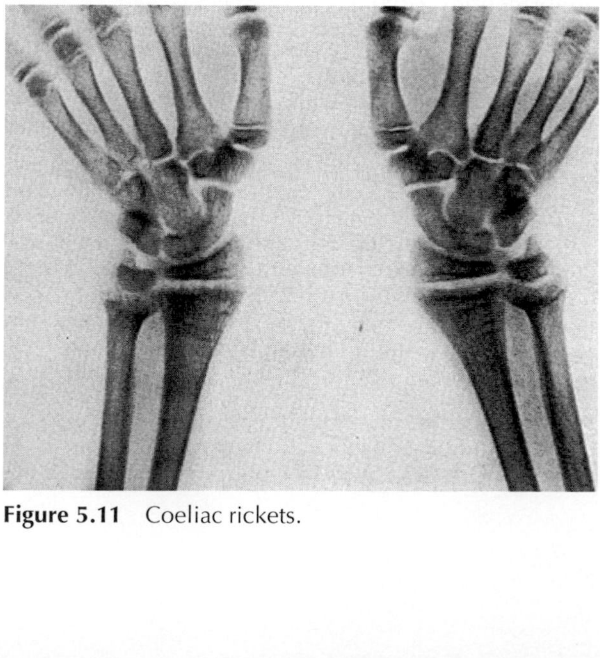

Figure 5.11 Coeliac rickets.

that these striations were indicative of periodic arrests of growth, but most people regard them as indicating bands of more perfect bone deposited during periods of temporary improvement in the disease.

BLOOD CHEMISTRY IN COELIAC DISEASE

In coeliac rickets there is a lowered serum calcium content and a very high alkaline phosphatase. Impaired fat digestion results in insoluble calcium soaps with decreased calcium absorption. The occurrence of tetany is the result of the low serum calcium.

TREATMENT

The great majority of cases respond rapidly to vitamin D and a gluten-free diet. It has been reported that in previously untreated disease there is no improvement with the administration of $1,25(0H)_2D_3$ because of the damage to the intestinal cells and hence to their ability to form calcium in binding protein.

RENAL BONE DISEASE

Patients with chronic renal failure develop abnormalities of skeletal homoeostasis, termed renal osteodystrophy, which are not cured and may even be compounded by dialysis treatment. In addition, chronic dialysis treatment is associated with joint abnormalities (dialysis arthropathy) and systemic amyloidosis.

Renal osteodystrophy

This is the term given to the bone changes which accompany chronic renal failure. The changes are due to a combination of hyperparathyroidism and osteitis fibrosa, osteomalacia, osteosclerosis and periosteal new bone formation, osteoporosis and growth disturbances in children. The bone changes are associated with extraskeletal calcification.

CLINICAL FEATURES

The children are always stunted in growth, often to a degree not equalled by any other form of infantilism. The body weight is correspondingly small, though malnutrition is not present. Patients surviving beyond puberty may show infantilism as well as dwarfism. The mental development is normal up to the age of puberty

Although by the time chronic renal failure is severe enough to warrant dialysis, the majority of patients have histological evidence of bone abnormalities, symptoms at this stage are rare.

Both osteitis fibrosa and osteomalacia may produce bone pain and tenderness, which may be severe enough to make the patient bedridden. The pain is usually vague and often in the lower back, pelvis and legs, it may be exacerbated by exercise.

Muscle weakness, which is usually proximal, is common. The onset is insidious and it is frequently progressive.

The incidence of osteomalacia varies between dialysis units. In those units where aluminium toxicity is a problem, it is common and indolent fractures occur. These are seen most frequently in the spine, ribs, pelvis and femoral neck. Softening of bone due to osteomalacia leads to marked skeletal deformity including thoracic kyphosis and lumbar scoliosis.

Extraskeletal calcification in the skin may contribute to pruritis, while in the eye it may be seen as a band keratopathy and may cause conjunctivitis.

Renal bone disease is particularly common in children, who may develop deformities similar to those in rickets combined with growth retardation due to toxic inhibition of the growth plates and poor nutrition. Slip of the capital femoral epiphysis also occurs.

RADIOLOGY

Early in the condition radiographic changes may be absent. The characteristic feature of hyperparathyroidism is bony erosion which commonly affects the tufts of the femoral phalanges, where collapse of the overlying soft tissues may cause clubbing. Periarticular phalangeal erosions are also common and erosions may also involve the proximal tibia, neck of femur or humerus and the outer end of the clavicle (Figure 5.12).

Increased bone resorption may produce osteoporosis with a widened medullary canal and intracortical porosis. Osteosclerosis is due to increased numbers and thickness of trabeculae and produces a 'rugby jersey' spine.

The radiographic changes of osteomalacia may

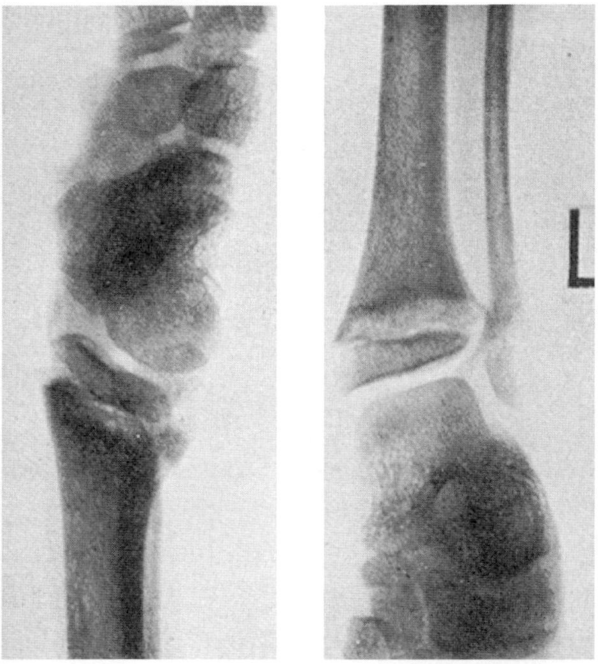

Figure 5.12 Renal rickets at the lower ends of radius and tibia. Note the 'cupping' of the diaphyseal end, but no gross changes in the shaft. The epiphyses at the lower end of both femora and at the upper ends of both humeri were separated.

not occur and bone biopsy is necessary to exclude the condition. Looser's zones may occur and may give rise to indolent stress fractures, particularly in the presence of aluminium toxicity. In children, features suggestive of rickets are seen.

BIOCHEMISTRY

The biochemical abnormalities of renal failure include raised serum urea and creatinine and oxidosis. Hyperphosphataemia is normal combined with a low serum calcium due to poor calcium absorption secondary to low levels of $1,25(OH)_2D$. Serum activity of alkaline phosphatase is raised as is the PTH level. More rarely, in tertiary hyperparathy roidism, hypercalcaemia occurs.

BONE HISTOLOGY

In patients with osteitis fibrosa due to high circulating levels of PTH increased numbers of osteoclasts and resorption surfaces are seen (Figure 5.13). There is also evidence of increased bone turnover and excessive woven osteoid with a random collagen fibre arrangement. The excessive osteoid may be due to increased bone turnover rather than defective mineralization, which can be assessed by double tetracycline labelling. Evidence of aluminium deposition can be sought by appropriate staining.

PATHOPHYSIOLOGY

The kidneys' central role in calcium homoeostasis is important in the pathogenesis of renal osteodystrophy.

Abnormal vitamin D metabolism

The major active metabolite of vitamin D is $1,25(OH)_2D_3$ (calcitriol) which is produced by 1α-hydroxylation within the kidney. Serum levels of calcitriol are decreased when the glomerular filtration rate drops below 40 ml/min and are very low in end-stage renal failure.

The lack of calcitriol leads to diminished intestinal calcium absorption, retardation of skeletal growth and defective mineralization.

A further vitamin D metabolite, $24,25(OH)_2D_3$, is also produced by the kidney. Low levels of this compound in renal failure may contribute to abnormalities of bone homoeostasis.

Abnormal calcium and phosphate metabolism

As renal tissue is lost during chronic renal failure, the ability of the body to excrete phosphate is diminished. The rise in serum phosphate so caused lowers the ionized serum calcium and tends to cause extraskeletal calcification by raising the calcium × phosphate product. The reduction in ionized calcium contributes to increased parathyroid hormone levels.

Abnormal PTH metabolism

The kidney, in addition to being a site of PTH action, is also a principal site of degradation, so that in renal failure, PTH action may be enhanced. Pure hyperparathyroidism or 'fibro-osteoclasis' is still the most common form of renal bone disease. In addition, excretion of PTH degradation products is reduced in renal impairment. These metabolically inactive polypeptides may interfere with PTH assays, giving a falsely high value for the serum parathyroid hormone level.

Aluminium toxicity

Patients on dialysis accumulate a number of trace elements from the dialysis fluid. Of these, aluminium has been shown to be important in the pathogenesis

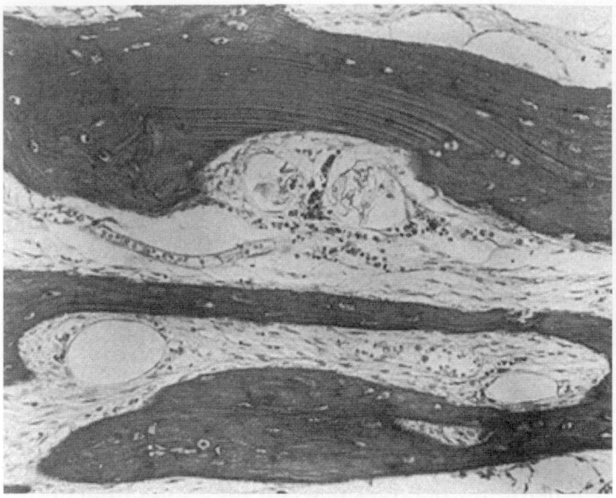

(a)

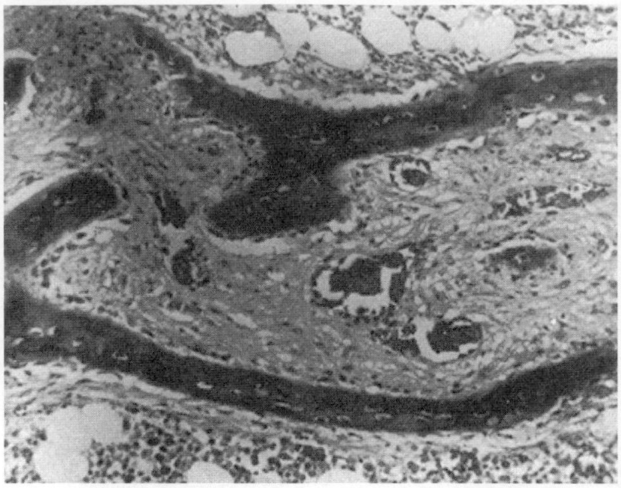

(b)

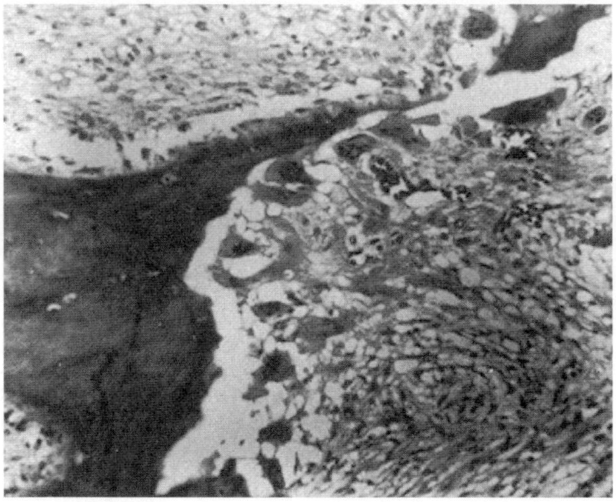

(c)

Figure 5.13 (a) Photomicrograph of human adult cortical bone, showing the altered lamellar bone patterns resulting from many episodes of reabsorption and deposition during hyperparathyroidism. (× 170). (b) Photomicrograph of human trabecular bone, showing reabsorption and replacement by cellular fibrous tissue. (× 400). (c) Photomicrograph of a trabecula of bone which is undergoing absorption of its margin by numerous osteoclasts, behind which is fibrous tissue. (× 455).

of osteomalacia. Aluminium may also be ingested due to excessive use of aluminium-containing phosphate binding compounds.

PATHOLOGICAL CHANGES IN THE KIDNEYS

The radiological examination of a patient with renal osteodystrophy is directed to the demonstration of calcification in the kidneys, irregularities of the renal pelves and ureters by pyelography and changes in the skeleton. Calcium deposits in the kidney, with or without calculus formation, may be found in hyperparathyroidism but are not common in chronic nephritis.

Kidney lesions

1. *Total renal insufficiency*, as found in chronic glomerulonephritis, focal nephritis, congenital cystic disease where there is reduced glomerular function with failure to excrete phosphorus, as well as general uraemia and acidosis. The main skeletal change is an osteitis fibrosa, with little osteoid formation, either as rickets or as osteomalacia.
2. *Tubular insufficiency*. The reabsorption of phosphorus, amino acids, glucose, electrolytes and water is impaired, particularly from the proximal convoluted tubules. If there is disease of the distal tubules, there is disturbance of potassium and creatinine secretion into the urine. As well as these defects of reabsorption or secretion, there is marked disturbance in the general

acid–base regulation of the body by alteration in the bicarbonate, ammonium and hydrogen ion concentrations which are usually added to the urine to achieve the acid–base equilibrium.

Snapper and Nathan (1957) reviewed the renal lesions which can give rise to the following syndromes.

The Lignac–Fanconi syndrome

In this, there is a proximal tubular deficiency, with polydipsia, polyuria, anorexia and vomiting. The children exhibit rickets as well as dwarfism and usually die before puberty. There is hyperphosphaturia with a low serum phosphate level, but a normal calcium level, a glucosuria which is sometimes accompanied by a mild ketonuria, as well as marked aminoaciduria. The primary lesion appears to be an impaired reabsorption of glucose and phosphate because of some failure of phosphorylation in the tubules. Massive dosages of vitamin D may improve the skeletal disorder. Abnormal deposition of cystine crystals in the cornea, spleen and lymph nodes gives the syndrome the name 'cystinosis' and is the underlying cause of this disorder.

Renal or hyperchloraemic acidosis

In this contdition, the primary defect is in the distal tubules, which fail to reabsorb water and to secrete ammonium As well as excreting large amounts of water containing sodium, potassium and calcium, there is a marked disturbance in the acid–base mechanism of the body with severe loss of bicarbonate and a corresponding retention of chlorides. The skeletal changes of either osteitis fibrosa or rickets are caused by the excessive mobilization of calcium from bone in response to the acidosis. This condition can be improved by administering excessive alkalizing salts, such as ammonium or calcium chlorides, and vitamin D.

Vitamin D resistant rickets

In this there is failure of phosphate reabsorption with marked hyperphosphaturia and hypophosphataemia. Accompanying this, there is also excessive faecal loss of calcium leading to the typical changes of rickets in children or osteomalacia in adults. Unlike avitaminosis D rickets, this form requires massive dosages of vitamin D (i.e. 50 000–100 000 units) daily. This can now be explained as a defect in the formation of $1{,}25(OH)_2D$ by the kidney. Indeed, very small doses of this metabolite can improve dramatically the skeletal changes of renal rickets. These children tend to survive into adulthood, when they can present features of osteomalacia (Dent and Harris, 1956) with reduction in the intestinal absorption of calcium and phosphates. The number of renal tubular lesions which may be associated with rickets or osteomalacia is large, and many clinical syndromes have now been described.

PROGNOSIS

Complete cure of the skeletal dystrophy may occur if the individual survives, for after the age of 16 or 17 there is much less liability to tetany, and the demand for calcium to ossify the bones is reduced. During the course of the disease there may be remissions associated with improvement in kidney function and better excretion of phosphate.

Nevertheless, the ultimate prognosis as to life depends on the renal pathology. The renal dwarf is especially liable to intercurrent infection which is apt to prove fatal. The occurrence of bone deformities is itself a grave omen, and the average duration of life after their appearance is said to be less than 2 years if the kidney lesion is not treated.

TREATMENT

Details of medical treatment is beyond the scope of this book. In summary the ingested phosphate load is reduced by administration of oral phosphate-binding compounds and if possible by reducing the dietary phosphate load, by giving aluminium hydroxide orally although a low phosphate diet is unpalatable and this may lead to aluminium overload.

Vitamin D compounds, e.g. alfacalcidol, which bypass the renal 1α-hydroxylation step are effective in augmenting calcium absorption and dietary calcium supplementation ensures adequate intake. These should be introduced as soon as the serum calcium decreases or the alkaline phosphatase increases.

Aluminium toxicity may be prevented by avoidance of aluminium-containing phosphate-binding compounds and by excluding aluminium from dialysis fluids. Parathyroidectomy is effective in treating parathyroid bone disease, particularly in cases of tertiary hyperparathyroidism, when a raised serum calcium coexists with osteitis fibrosa, bone pain and pruritis.

Renal transplantation restores normal vitamin D and phosphate metabolism and leads to an improvement in renal bone disease, which may be slow, especially in the presence of aluminium toxicity. If the transplantation does not suppress the excess parathyroid activity, parathyroidectomy may be indicated if there is progressive hypercalcaemia.

Transplantation in the presence of aluminium-related osteomalacia is usually very successful as long as there is not aluminium overload with encephalopathy. This may well require chelation therapy with desferrioxamine for up to a year within the dialysis regimen.

Treatment of orthopaedic complications

Patients suffering from renal failure may have impaired coagulation and are more susceptible than unaffected people to infection. Fluid replacement and electrolyte imbalance require careful monitoring.

The common complication of avascular necrosis of bone, particularly in the hip, and dialysis arthropathy/amyloidosis are described in Chapter 11.

Hypophosphatasia

This is an inherited rachitic disease of bone, first described by Rathbun in 1948 as a marked mineralization disturbance with bony changes in the long bones and skull. The blood shows an increased or normal calcium, phosphate and non-protein nitrogen level, but a very low alkaline phosphatase level (if any).

Radiographically and pathologically the lesion suggests severe rickets (Figure 5.14) with dwarfism.

McCance *et al.* (1955) and Fraser *et al.* (1959) have shown that there is a large urinary excretion of phosphoethanolamine without the other amino acids commonly seen in other forms of 'renal rickets'. The actual cause of the hypophosphatasia is not known but is not thought to be due to hyperparathyroidism, nor to any true resistance to vitamin D. However, large doses of vitamin D will improve the radiographic appearances, with a fall in the alkaline phosphatase levels.

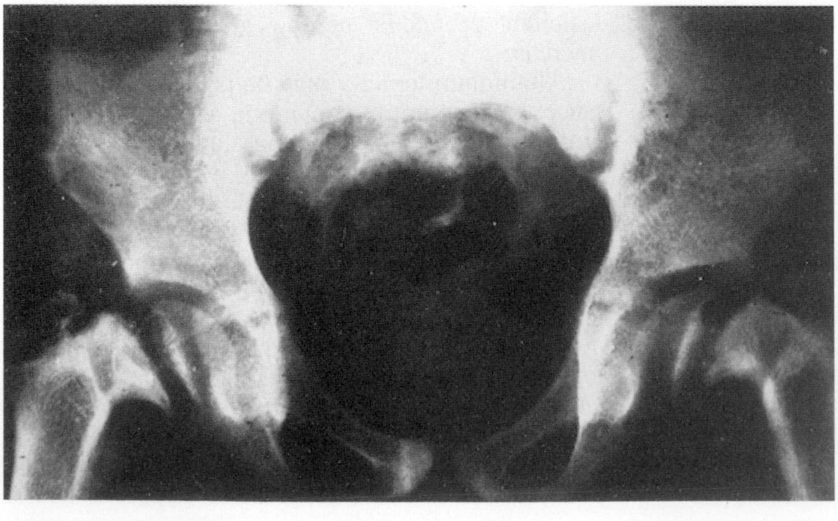

Figure 5.14 The rachitic-like lesion in hypophosphasia leads to weakening of the epiphyseal line and varus deformity of the hips.

PARATHYROID BONE DISEASE

Parathyroid hormone is an 84 aminoacid polypeptide which is secreted by the parathyroid gland in response to a lowered ionized serum calcium. The physiology of parathyroid hormone is discussed fully in Chapter 2. Hyperparathyroidism is normally the result of a parathyroid adenoma (88%); however, it may be due to hyperplasia of the chief cells or clear cells of the parathyroid gland which may be primary or secondary to prolonged hypocalcaemia. Rarely, carcinoma of the parathyroid gland may secrete functional parathyroid hormone. Hypoparathyroidism may also occur as part of the syndrome of multiple endocrine adenomata where tumours are also found in the pituitary, the pancreas and the thyroid.

The clinical effects of hyperparathyroidism are due to its function in mobilizing calcium from bone and inhibiting renal secretion.

CLINICAL FEATURES

Primary hyperparathyroidism may effect either sex but is more common in women. The majority of cases occur in the third, fourth and fifth decades. However, it has been reported in a child aged 14 years. Today many cases are discovered incidentally by the finding of an abnormally raised serum calcium on multichannel serum analysis. Clinical features include pain from renal stones and nephrocalcinosis or polyuria and nocturia due to hypercalcaemia. Gastrointestinal symptoms include anorexia, nausea, vomiting and constipation and psychotic disturbances may occur.

Bone pain is diffuse and is associated with generalized muscle weakness. In the advanced disease fractures may occur from trivial injury and are difficult to unite.

RADIOGRAPHIC APPEARANCES

The severe changes described as osteitis fibrosa cystica occur in less than half of patients with hyperparathyroidism (Figure 5.16). More mild changes, particularly phalangeal subperiosteal resorption, are more common.

The radiographic appearance consists chiefly of irregular diffuse rarefaction with resorption of the compact bone and cyst-like degeneration. In the skull the bones show well marked stippling with pinhead-sized opaque areas which differentiate them from the grosser mottling of Paget's disease. The vertebrae are porotic and show central collapse with concave upper and lower surfaces. The pelvis shows course striations amongst which large clear cyst-like spaces are often visible.

The femur and long bones show loss of trabeculation (Figure 5.15). Deformity is common with coxa vara and bowing. Cyst-like spaces may be present at the extremities and in the midshaft. Over the cysts the bone may show a slight fusiform enlargement only.

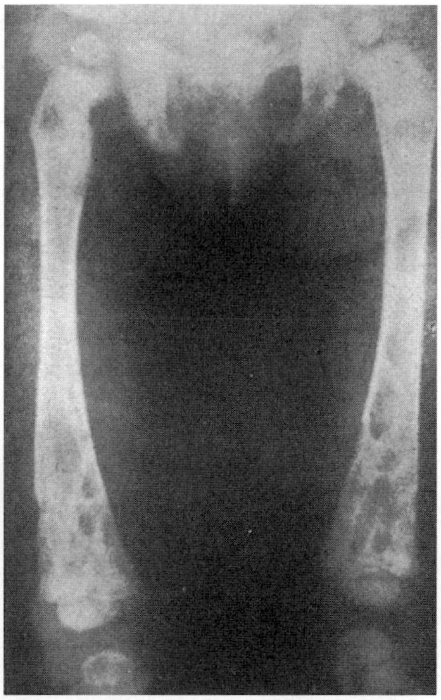

Figure 5.15 Osteitis fibrosa cystica of the femur.

The diagnostic feature of parathyroid bone disease is subperiosteal resorption of the phalanges (Figure 5.17). This is almost invariably present in generalized osteitis fibrosis cystica but may be absent in the localized form. Erosion of the tufts of the phalanges is also seen but this sign is more difficult to diagnose.

Extraosseous calcium deposits are frequently seen, often as calci.

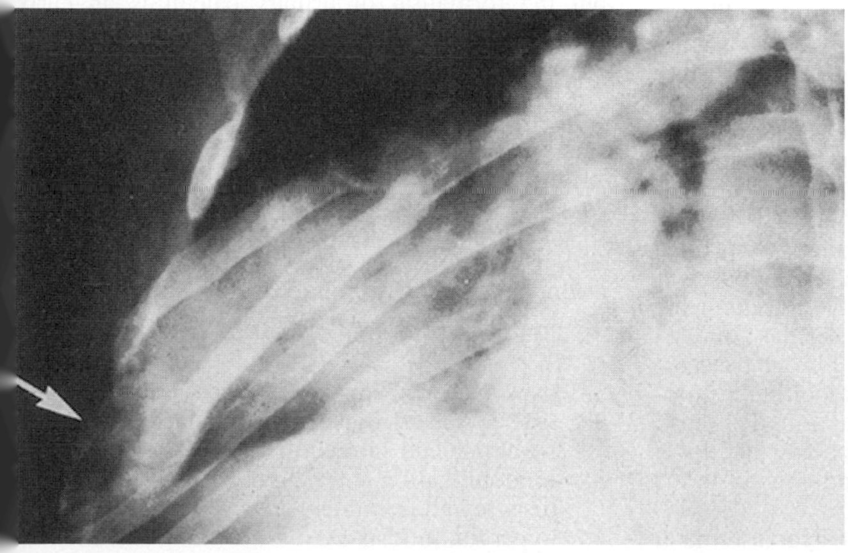

Figure 5.16 Tomogram showing osteoclastomata in the ribs in a patient with primary hyperparathyroidism.

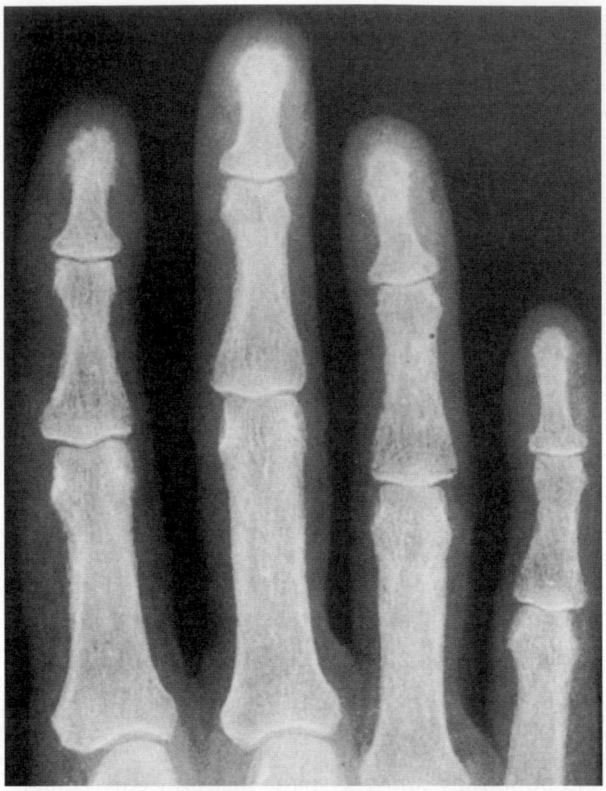

Figure 5.17 Subperiosteal resorption of the phalanges in a patient with primary hyperparathyroidism.

BONE PATHOLOGY

The bone changes consist of progressive rapid resorption and softening of the bones with deformity together with some new bone formation. Cysts and collections of giant cells are also seen.

The rapid osteoclastic resorption may proceed until the bone is virtually converted into a fibrous tissue cylinder. The width of the bone is usually increased but the periosteum is normal. Deformity occurs due to the effect of gravity, weight-bearing or muscle action on the softened bone. Histologically vascular granulation tissue is seen to occupy the bone with a thin, spongey cortex. There is widespread increase in osteoclastic activity with Haversian canals enlarged into large irregular spaces lined by zones of osteoclasts and filled with vascular tissue. Adjacent spaces eventually communicate with each other as the bone between them is removed and these spaces slowly fill in with fibrous tissue.

Associated with the increased osteoclastic resorption, there is some new bone formation. This may result in spicules of laminated bone being laid down but often mineralization is poor and osteoid tissue only is seen.

Accumulation of giant cells (osteoclastomata) vary macroscopically from large reddish brown masses to minute spheres. Microscopically they are composed of masses of osteoclasts in a matrix of connective tissue.

The cysts vary in size but may be several centimetres across. They contain a thin brownish fluid and are found in relation to areas of giant cells.

BIOCHEMISTRY

The essential features of primary or tertiary hyperthyroidism is a persistent and significant elevation of the plasma calcium concentration. The measurements should be done on at least two occasions, with the patient fasted and the measurement should be corrected for the plasma albumin level.

Parathyroid hormone levels can be measured by radioimmunoassay. However, current assays are inaccurate since inactive fragments of parathyroid hormone will react positively with the assay. For this reason these measurements must be interpreted with caution.

Serum activity of alkaline phosphatase will be raised depending on the extent of the bone disease and urinary calcium excretion may be increased.

The formation of urinary calculi

This is due to the increased excretion of calcium and phosphate in the urine. The calculi may be formed in the pelvis, in the collecting tubules, or actually in the parenchyma. They lead to sclerotic changes in the kidney. F. Albright pointed out many years ago that if the disease is of short duration and the amount of calcium in the diet is high, the bone changes may be late in appearing, but the formation of urinary calculi is an early feature. In long-standing diseases, with low dietary calcium, the reverse obtains.

Hypercalciuria

This is an excess excretion of calcium in the urine in amounts above 200 mg/day when the dietary intake is less than 500 mg. This can be determined by adding the Sulkowitch reagent to the urine when a whitish clouding is produced, or by direct measurement.

The condition is seen in:

1. hyperparathyroidism;
2. osteolysis of bone in malignancy, multiple myeloma and sarcoidosis;
3. immobilization – for chronic diseases, Paget's disease and fractures;
4. hypervitaminosis D.

DIAGNOSIS

The diagnosis of parathyroid osteodystrophy depends on the demonstration of the hypercalcaemia and hypophosphataemia in association with the characteristic bone changes. Differential diagnosis of hypercalcaemia is critical because this state is produced by numerous other conditions – e.g. metastases (from lungs, prostate, breast, etc.) to bone, multiple bone lesions of myeloma, sarcoidosis, immobilization, hyperthyroidism, acute renal failure and Addison's disease (Table 5.3).

There is a second form of parathyroid enlargement which occurs in chronic renal disease and is due to persistent raised phosphates in the blood with a concomitant depression of the blood calcium. This low blood calcium stimulates the activity of the parathyroids to futile attempts of compensation to lower the renal threshold for phosphates.

In late hyperparathyroidism, renal damage due to renolithiasis may result in a rise of the phosphate renal threshold with a rise in the blood phosphate. This can cause a depression of blood calcium and may confuse the diagnostician. It can be seen that at times it is well nigh impossible to differentiate the primary lesion when hyperparathyroidism and chronic renal disease exist together.

Renal disease in calcium and phosphate metabolism

In uraemia, osteodystrophy such as osteomalacia or secondary hyperparathyroidism may be found due to abnormal absorption of calcium because of resistance to vitamin D in the gut, or even to an accelerated destruction of vitamin D by a defect in its conversion to its active form 25-hydroxycholecalciferol (Avioli *et al.*, 1968). In some, in spite of renal dialysis, these changes remain. In others, the administration of vitamin D, or giving large amounts of oral calcium or phosphates with haemodialysis, does improve the calcium–phosphate balance although maybe not in the bones (Curtis *et al.*, 1970).

Metatastic calcification is always a risk in arteries, eyes and joints (Stanbury, 1962).

DIFFERENTIAL DIAGNOSIS

The conditions affording most difficulty are those where – focally or generally – there is radiological and histological similarity to osteitis fibrosa, but without the disturbance in the plasma calcium and the plasma phosphate.

Many conditions reproduce certain of the clinical features of parathyroid osteodystrophy, but the majority of these – gout, low back pain – have no radiological evidence of bone disturbance. Certain general bone diseases also bear an occasional or a superficial resemblance to fibrocystic disease. Some of these are considered below. However, where there are characteristic subperiosteal resorptions of the phalanges, the diagnosis of parathyroid bone disease is definite.

Osteoporosis

In this condition the blood calcium is normal, and the age of onset is late, in contradistinction to fibrocystic disease. Nevertheless, the tendency to fracture, deformity and bone pain may lead to some confusion, and the radiographic bone changes are not markedly dissimilar to the changes of the milder forms of hyperparathyroidism.

Osteitis deformans – Paget's disease

Here the occasional occurrence of cysts, the histological resemblance and the occasional occurrence of hypercalcaemia may render it difficult to distinguish from parathyroid osteodystrophy. The radiological appearances, the age of onset and the absence of characteristic blood changes will lead to a correct diagnosis in the majority of cases. Where there is alteration in the blood chemistry, it is likely, as Albright suggested, that there is a superadded element of disuse atrophy from recumbency, and the two are not to be regarded as cause and effect. In Paget's disease there is usually a marked rise in blood alkaline phosphatase.

Osteomalacia

In this disease the characteristic circumstances – starvation, poverty, diet, pregnancy – together with the fact that there is bending of the bones rather than fracture, that the blood calcium is low and that there is a rapid response to vitamin D therapy should make the diagnosis clear.

Osteogenesis imperfecta

In the so-called adult form of fragilitas ossium there should be no difficulty in diagnosis. The disease has persisted from childhood, there is a history of multiple fractures, the sclerotics are usually blue and the individual is dwarfed. The blood chemistry is normal and the radiological picture characteristic.

Multiple myeloma

The radiological appearance of multiple myeloma

Table 5.3 Points in differential diagnosis between hyperparathyroidism and other bone diseases

Disease	Differential points as regards			Serum		Alkaline phosphatase	Miscellaneous
	Symptoms	x-Ray appearance	Biopsy	Calcium	Phosphorus		
Hyperparathyroidism with bone involvement	Bone: pain, deformity, fracture, tumour; polyuria; those related to stones	Increased radiability; generalized deformity; cysts; tumours; fractures; stones	Rarefied bone; fibrosis of marrow; osteoclasts +++; osteoid tissue only slightly increased; osteoblasts + + +	High	Low	High	All age groups
'Senile' osteoporosis	No bone tumour, polyuria or stones	No cysts, tumours or stones	No fibrosis of marrow; osteoclasts normal; osteoid tissue normal or decreased; osteoblasts decreased	Normal	Normal or low	Normal	Old age
Paget's disease	Bones enlarged; no polyuria; stones infrequent	Polostotic but not generalized; bones hypertrophied (e.g. thickened skull)	May occasionally be difficult or impossible to differentiate	Normal or slightly high	Normal or slightly high	Very high	Runs in families; predilection for weight-bearing bones; seldom seen under 40; arteriosclerosis + + +
Osteomalacia	No bone tumour, polyuria or stones	No tumours or stones; bending deformities + + +	Osteoid tissue + + +; Osteoblasts + +; osteoclasts increased	Normal or Low	Low	High	Practically absent in the West except with fatty diarrhoea
'Solitary' cysts	Confined to cysts	No generalized changes; cysts may be multiple	Cannot differentiate if taken from lesion	Normal	Normal	Normal	
Solitary benign giant cell tumour	Confined to tumour	No generalized changes	Cannot differentiate if taken from lesion	Normal	Normal	Normal	
Osteogenesis imperfecta	Fractures + + +; no bone tumour, polyuria or stones	Cysts rare; no tumours or stones	No fibrosis of marrow; osteoclasts normal	Normal	Normal	Normal or very slightly elevated	Hereditary, often coupled with blue sclerae and deafness; improves after cessation of growth
Multiple myeloma	Can cause some bone symptoms and renal symptoms	Can be almost indistinguishable	Tumour tissue	Normal or high	Normal or high	Normal	Bence Jones proteinuria

Normal values for: calcium 2.2–2.6 mmol/l (9–11 mg/100 ml); phosphorus 0.8–1.6 mmol/l (2.5–5 mg/100 ml); alkaline phosphatase 21–92 i.u./l (3–13 King–Armstrong units/100 ml).

After F. Albright, J. C. Aub and W. Bauer, 1934. *Journal of the American Medical Association* **102**, 1276.

may simulate closely the appearance of parathyroid osteodystrophy, especially in the collapse of the vertebrae, the occurrence of punctate areas of diminished density in the skull and long bones, and fine mottling of the pelvic bones. The blood calcium/phosphate ratio is as a rule normal, while an abnormal protein – the Bence Jones protein – may appear in the urine. Raised blood protein frequently results in raised total blood calcium but the diffusible fraction remains normal. Biopsy may be demanded.

TREATMENT

In the presence of generalized osteitis fibrosa, the neck should be explored for parathyroid adenoma, even in the absence of a palpable swelling. A wide exposure should be aimed at, as it may be necessary to continue the search behind the trachea, or down into the mediastinum.

Normally, there are at least two parathyroid bodies on each side, and in some individuals there may be three or four. The superior bodies, though variable in their lateral and vertical position, are usually situated between the pretracheal fascia and the posterior part of the capsule of the thyroid gland, and may be found around the veins at the root of the neck and in the thymic region.

The inferior bodies, although usually described as also lying between the fascia and the thyroid capsule, may lie below the inferior thyroid artery, and beneath the pretracheal fascia; in this case they are visible only from the posterior surface or after division of the fascia. When misplaced they should be sought in the region of the oesophagus and in the superior mediastinum. The enlarged parathyroid has a characteristic yellowish-brown appearance which renders it distinctive to the naked eye. In patients with extensive bone disease, there is often prolonged hypocalcaemia with tetany. Large doses of vitamin D are needed – especially the quick-acting metabolite 1α(OH)D – together with intravenous calcium gluconate and a high calcium intake. Aluminium hydroxide has been used, and hypomagnesaemia may need correction. There still remains controversy about how much (or many) of the parathyroids should be removed. Some recommend the transplantation of some of the parathyroid tissue into the forearm musculature where further removal for secondary hyperparathyroid tissue can be more readily accessed.

Orthopaedic treatment is directed merely towards the adequate protection of the softened bones from all deforming stresses and strains. Urological treatment is directed towards removal of calculi and maintenance of renal function. After the disease has been arrested and recalcification of bone occurs, the established deformity may be corrected by the usual means – e.g. osteotomy.

In patients who refuse operation or who have mild hyperparathyroidism, in postmenopausal women, or in whom an unsuccessful neck exploration has been done, the hypercalcaemia can be controlled by oral phosphate.

PROGNOSIS AFTER OPERATION

After parathyroidectomy, the prognosis is good. The bone pains are immediately abolished. There is usually a marked gain in weight, and crippled individuals are able to dispense with sticks and crutches.

Removal of the parathyroid tumour is followed by rapid and progressive healing of the bones.

Osteoporosis

Osteoporosis is a condition which is difficult to define accurately. A simple definition is that it is an abnormal reduction in bone tissue mass per unit volume of anatomical bone. In other words the total quantity of bone is diminished but the bone present is qualitatively normal (Solomon, 1978). This definition begs the question what is 'an abnormal reduction'. Many would accept that it is present in a patient whose bone mass is two standard deviations below the mean for that age and sex. However, this is a purely arbitrary level to take. Neither is it a simple matter to measure bone mass, and measurements made at one site, for example the distal radius or metacarpal bone, may have a poor correlation with the relative amount of bone mass compared to the total population present at another site, for example within the vertebral body. In addition, it is far from certain that the bone which remains in an osteoporotic patient is qualitatively the same as the bone present in a young fit patient.

The final shortcoming of the definition given above is that the importance of osteoporosis is not the osteoporosis itself but the reduction in bone strength which is an association of bone thinning. However, bone strength is not precisely correlated with bone mass since it will depend on the disposition of the bone in space and the strength of the individual units of bone. Despite these shortcomings, for practical purposes, the definition given above is satisfactory.

The importance of osteoporosis is in its predisposition to fracture following relatively minor trauma.

PATHOPHYSIOLOGY

The pathophysiology of skeletal failure includes a course of osteoporosis and bone weakness and the trauma which is the direct cause of a fracture. There is reduction in the thickness of the cortex, especially from the endosteal surfaces with the intramedullary contents being made up of a yellow and fatty cancellous bone tissue. In this on microscopy, and on microradiography of undecalcified bone specimens, there is a reduction in the number and size of the trabeculae and in the number of osteoblasts present. This results in a marked reduction in the mechanical strength of the involved bone which therefore fractures or crushes with minor trauma.

TYPES OF OSTEOPOROSIS

Primary osteoporosis is mainly a disease of the elderly. Idiopathic osteoporosis in young adults is, however, an occasional finding. The disease occurs more commonly in women than in men and is generally relatively mild. There is also a very rare form of idiopathic juvenile osteoporosis which occurs in young children and adolescents, who have bone pain, fractures of weight-bearing long bones, and vertebral collapse. Systemic disease and disorders of mineralization must be excluded. Then the main finding is of demineralized skeleton and a continuous urinary calcium loss. Saggese *et al.* (1991) have reported on the successful use of 1,25(0H)$_2$ vitamin D$_3$.

Primary osteoporosis of old age may be either postmenopausal (type I) or senile (type II) osteoporosis. These differ in their age, sex ratio, type of bone loss and in the sort of fractures which they cause.

Postmenopausal osteoporosis (type I)

This disease was characterized by Albright and colleagues in 1941. The condition characteristically affects women, between 10 and 20 years following the menopause. Men may rarely be affected. These

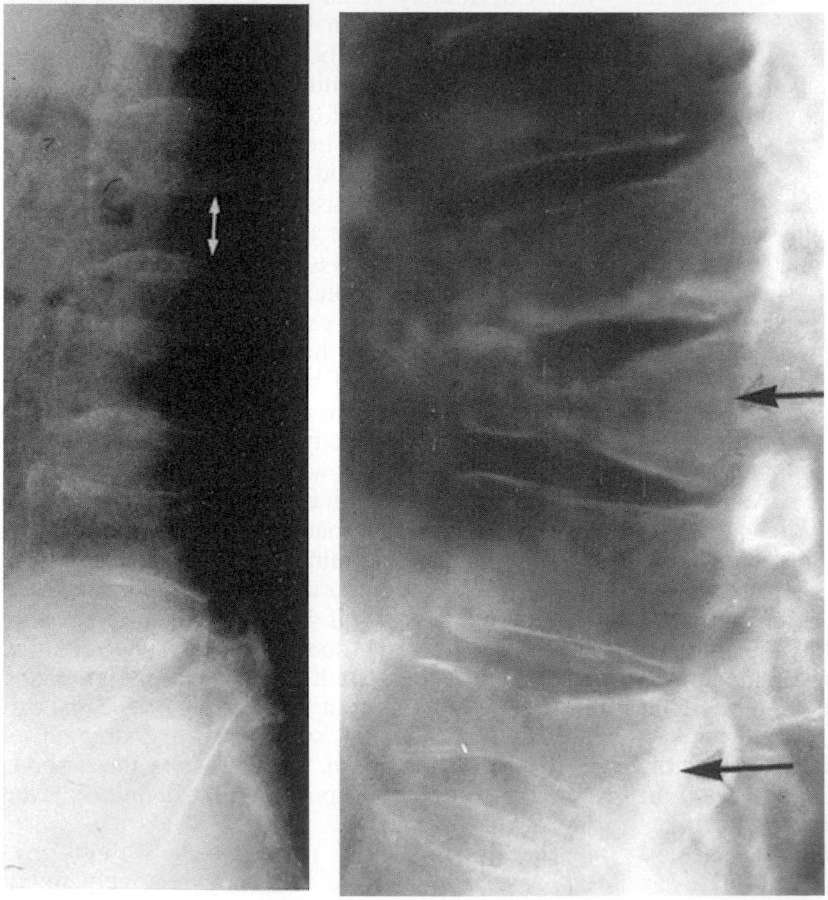

(a) (b)

Figure 5.18 (a) Severe osteoporosis in a young man. (b) The characteristic wedge-shaped vertebrae collapse in osteoporosis.

patients are characterized by high bone turnover and rapid loss of trabecular bone. They suffer acutely painful crushing fractures of the vertebrae (Figure 5.18) and Colles' fractures of the distal radius.

Senile osteoporosis (type II)

This syndrome affects men and women aged over 70 years. It is due to the chronic effect of bone loss since peak bone mass was attained in the fourth decade with a superimposed senile lowering of the rate of bone turnover. This leads to accumulation of fatigue damage throughout the skeleton. It is characterized by multiple wedge fractures of the vertebrae which are often pain free and fractures of the femoral neck.

Because women have a lower peak bone density than men and also suffer the increased bone loss at the time of the menopause, this form of osteoporosis is more common in women than men. However, this preponderance is not as great as for type I osteoporosis.

Secondary osteoporosis

There are a number of associated causes of osteoporosis. These may be broadly divided into endocrine causes including Cushing's disease, hyperthyroidism, hypopituitarism, hypogonadism, diabetes mellitus in pregnancy; other causes of osteoporosis are associated with chronic disease such as rheumatoid arthritis, liver disease, chronic lung disease, skin discase or neurological disorder and drug administration including corticosteroid, heparin, alcohol abuse, smoking, post-gastrectomy syndrome and, rarely, osteoporosis of pregnancy.

Hypothyroidism may lead to osteoporosis, because thyroxine directly stimulates bone resorption, leading to an increase in bone turnover which, particularly in the more elderly where there may be a greater remodelling gap, predisposes to bone loss. The osteoporosis occurs throughout the skeleton. However, there may be more severe axial and appendicular skeletal involvement.

Osteoporosis is a common complication in Cushing's syndrome resulting from a basophil adenoma of the pituitary, or from disease of the adrenal cortex. These give rise to an excess of glucocorticoid hormone. The adrenal corticoids are considered to withdraw amino acids from protein synthesis, during glyconeogenesis, with disturbance in *matrix formation*. Accompanying the generalized osteoporosis, there are other endocrine disorders, of sexual characteristics, of obesity and of diabetes mellitus. Similar changes, especially in the vertebral column, are seen in patients who have rheumatoid arthritis and who have been given prolonged cortisone therapy.

In von Recklinghausen's disease of bone, with hyperparathyroidism resulting from an adenoma, there may be osteoporosis of the skull and spine, before the appearance of the fibrocystic lesions, osteoclastomata and stone formation.

In other endocrine diseases such as in acromegaly and giantism, resulting from pituitary dysfunction, or in hvpothyroidism of cretinism or myxoedema or thyrotoxicosis, in which there is excessive utilization of nitrogen-containing substances, with reduction in matrix formation, osteoporosis has been recorded.

CLINICAL FEATURES

Pain is in the nature of a lumbar backache which radiates around the trunk or down the lower limbs. It is aggravated by movement or jarring, and although suggestive of a nerve root compression, this is rarely seen. Acute sudden onset of pain with localized tenderness in the chest or back is most suggestive of a pathological fracture of a rib or vertebral body.

Loss of height may have been noted by the patient, and the appearance of a thoracic kyphosis and an approximation of the rib margin to the iliac crests. The patient usually seems older than his or her years.

Elderly people fall more frequently than young adults due to unsteadiness, blackouts and possibly drowsiness from multiple drug ingestion. These same factors tend to slow their protective reflexes so that when they fall they may damage themselves more severely.

A final possible contributory factor is alteration in environment and this plus the increasing medication of elderly patients may explain in part why the rate of osteoporotic neck of femur is increasing even when corrected for age and bonc density.

A number of fractures are specifically associated with osteoporosis. Noteworthy amongst these are fracture of the neck of femur, suprachondylar fracture of the femur, fracture of the distal tibial metaphysis, Colles' fracture, fracture of the neck of the radius, subcapital fracture of the humerus and vertebral body fracture. In the majority of these the presentation is of an acute fracture following a fall, and particularly in the case of fracture neck of femur but with vertebral fractures the patient may not recall a traumatic incident.

Grisso *et al.* (1991) have found that over 90% of fractures are the result of a fall, in elderly women whose proximal femoral bone density is well below the fracture threshold. They recommend aggressive diagnosis and treatment of visual disorders, physical therapy for impaired mobility, stopping of drugs affecting cognitive function and improving the home circumstances.

Fractures of the vertebrae probably occur in stages, with the initial change being intrusion of the vertebral discs into the bone leading to a biconcave vertebra followed by a progressive loss of height. Osteoporotic vertebral crush fractures may cause only minimal symptoms. However sometimes the pain is very severe with a band-like dermatomal radiation. The most commonly affected vertebrae are in the lower thoracic and upper lumbar region with the first crush normally affecting T12. Progressive vertebral fractures lead to an increase in the thoracic kyphosis with secondary postural problems in the cervical spine. Investigations for patients presenting with vertebral fractures are ESR, full blood count, serum protein electrophoresis, serum calcium, phosphate, thyroxine and alkaline phosphatase. Bone biopsy may well be indicated as well as 25-hydroxyvitamin D levels.

Reduction in lung capacity may be due to exacerbation of pre-existing chronic lung disease while decreased abdominal capacity may lead to hiatus hernia.

RADIOGRAPHIC APPEARANCES

The involved osteoporotic bone may have a ground-glass appearance because of the loss of definition of the trabeculae. Cortical thinning is normally obvious. In the spine the vertebral bodies may become concave and flattened with collapse and wedging.

Assessment of bone density is now being routinely performed by either dual photon absorptiometry or dual energy x-ray absorptiometry. Any single bone density measurement cannot determine any future fracture rate but is of use in determining treatment patterns.

LABORATORY INVESTIGATIONS

Investigation of osteoporosis is directed towards exclusion of underlying abnormalities which account for the osteoporosis.

Serum, calcium and phosphate are invariably within the normal range. Serum alkaline phosphatase may be raised following a fracture. However, this increase will be slight unless the patient is suffering from Paget's disease of bone. Urinary calcium excretion and hydroxyproline excretion may be slightly increased in cases of rapid bone loss.

Measurement of bone mass

Measurement of bone mass is indicated for:

1. Patients who are post-hysterectomy with primary oestrogen deficiency.
2. Patients with premature menopause.
3. Diagnosis in patients with radiographic osteopenia.
4. Diagnosis in young patients with radial or hip fractures.
5. Patients with a history of prolonged corticosteroid therapy in rheumatoid patients or renal dialysis patients.

However, once again this is poorly correlated with bone mineral density in the hip and spine.

More accurate estimation of bone mineral and density of the lumbar spine, femoral neck, whole body, may be obtained by quantitative computerized tomographic scanning. This has a high radiation dose and indeed the highest of all techniques except ordinary radiography. But it is excellent for separating cortical bone from trabecular bone. Photon absorptiometry may be used directly to measure the bone density of the forearm and of the wrist (single photon absorptiometry) or in the vertebral column or proximal femur or even whole body (dual photon scanning) – with good precision and small radiation dose but the presence of fat can produce large errors.

More recently, dual energy x-ray absorptiometry (DEXA) has been introduced as a reliable and accurate method for bone density determination with very little radiation. Ultrasound with no ionizing radiation can be used for the calcaneus or the patella especially in 'at risk' populations studies.

Protein electrophoresis will reveal the presence of a monoclone indicating myloma.

Measurement of bone metabolism in vivo by bone markers

Azria and Russell (1992) have recently reviewed this important subject (Figure 5.19).

DIFFERENTIAL DIAGNOSIS

There are a number of causes of bone pain which may mimic osteoporotic fracture. These include osteomalacia, myeloma, secondary tumours, Paget's disease of bone, osteogenesis imperfecta, monostotic fibrous dysplasia, hypophosphatasia and osteomyelitis.

TREATMENT

Once established, osteoporosis is extremely difficult to reverse. The mainstay of clinical management is therefore directed at its prevention.

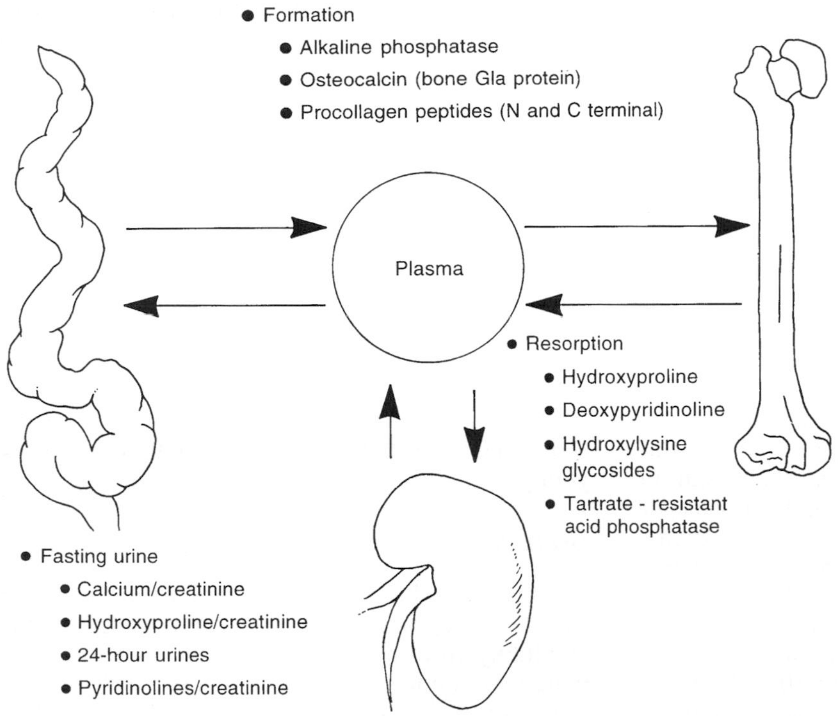

Figure 5.19 Markers for biochemical measurement of bone formation and resorption. (Reproduced with kind permission of the authors and publishers from Azria, M. and Russell, R. G. G. (1992) *Current Opinion in Orthopedics* **3**, 103–109)

Ambulation must be encouraged, and support given to relieve the pain of the diseased spine in the form of a light plaster jacket or a Taylor brace, or to the pathological fracture of the femur by a walking non-weight-bearing caliper. Internal fixation is sound in principle because of the loss in mechanical strength of the surrounding bone.

Maximization of peak skeletal mass is encouraged by exercise, diet and possibly calcium supplementation. In the perimenopausal period, hormone replacement therapy may be employed.

The evidence strongly suggests at patients in whom a premature menopause is induced by bilateral oophorectomy are protected from excessive rapid bone loss by the administration of oestrogens (Lindsay *et al.*, 1976) but even so only about 30% of women in the UK do so. A similar protection against rapid bone loss has been shown in the distal radius in patients following a natural menopause treated with oestrogen replacement therapy (Christiansen *et al.*, 1981). However, after cessation of hormone replacement therapy bone loss occurred at the same rate as in the original placebo treated group. It has been shown that HRT does reduce the risk of osteoporotic fracture, but also the risk of cerebrovascular accident and ischaemic heart disease. Even so, it is not widely accepted.

These results imply that in order to preserve bone mass long-term hormone replacement therapy may be necessary. This may carry with it side effects. It is therefore necessary to select those patients most likely to suffer from osteoporotic fractures. Most usually identifiable risk groups are slender with low body mass, blonde caucasian women with a late menarche, early menopause, who smoke or drink. They may have a history of low calcium intake in childhood or have a sedentary lifestyle. An alternative approach is that adopted by Christiansen and Rodborough (1985) who has attempted to identify those women at risk of osteoporotic fractures by selecting a group of patients losing bone rapidly ('fast losers').

In contrast to preventative treatment, reversal of established osteoporosis is less certain. Treatment by exercise, calcitonin therapy, hormone replacement therapy, fluoride therapy and calcium and vitamin D and diphosphonate have all been examined. Although some of these treatment regimens show short-term promise in terms of increased bone mineral content, their benefits for preventing fracture are yet to be determined. Law *et al.* (1991) have shown the benefits of regular physical activity in reducing the risk of hip fractures across the whole of the population by almost a half.

Possibly the most interesting method of treatment is so-called 'coherence treatment or ADFR (activate depress free repeat)'. This form of treatment is directed particularly at type II osteoporosis where there is a low rate of bone turnover in conjunction with severe loss of bone mineral. Treatment begins with an agent that activates bone remodelling such as phosphates (which induce a state of hyperparathyroidism), parathyroid hormone or fluoride. As soon as bone remodelling is activated, the resorptive phase is transiently suppressed using an inhibitor of bone resorption which is normally calcitonin. This is given for a short period so that a secondary effect on bone formation will not occur. The patient is then left free of treatment for the formational part of the newly activated bone remodelling units to work before the treatment cycle is repeated. This form of treatment is still at the experimental stage; however, early results are encouraging.

In the treatment of established vertebral fractures in postmenopausal women, prophylaxis against further fractures, i.e. HRT, is rarely successful or indicated because of vaginal bleeding. Etidronate – a bisphosphonate which binds to the hydroxyapatite crystal and inhibits bone resorption – with calcium and exercise can be given intermittently.

Rico *et al.* (1992) in a randomized prospective study compared the effects of salmon calcitonin with calcium supplements given for 10 consecutive days each month with calcium supplements alone. Both groups had the same number of vertebral fractures and mean values of spinal deformity index. At 2 years the new vertebral fracture rate was significantly lower in the calcitonin/calcium group.

BONE MASS AND THE FRACTURE THRESHOLD

If bone mass were simply related to bone strength, one would predict that there would be a threshold bone density below which fracture became extremely common. While this is true that elderly patients who fall and suffer a fracture are in general more osteoporotic than those who fall and do not suffer a fracture, there is a considerable overlap (Cooper *et al.*, 1987). Two explanations offer themselves for this observation, the first is that the nature of the fall differs in different people and the second that bone strength is not the same thing as bone mass.

The resistance of bone to a particular fracture will depend first on its orientation in space compared to the forces which are being placed across it. Therefore the pattern of bone loss may be more important than the absolute loss of bone mass. Postmenopausal osteoporosis is associated with a relatively greater loss of the horizontal trabeculae of the vertebrae than the vertical trabeculae and this loss of cross-strutting may weaken the vertebra more than would be anticipated on the basis of a simple bone mass measurement.

Bone is constantly being subjected to trauma and individual trabeculae within a bone are subject to microfractures which normally heal. If, however, bone turnover is very slow, trabecular microfracture healing may be impaired so that the bone is weaker than a bone mass measurement would suggest.

Bone strength

It is possible that the collagen which makes up the organic matrix of bone is itself subject to fatigue damage which leads to a weakening of the bone or indeed that the collagen laid down in the elderly may be less strong than that seen in younger, fitter individuals. A similar effect to this is seen in the skin which is thinner in older patients than in the young.

Bone mass

The mass of a bone increases until about the fourth decade. After that bone is lost remorselessly and inevitably from every region of the skeleton. This bone loss is not a result of unopposed bone resorption but it is due to an imbalance of bone formation and bone resorption within bone remodelling units. In a long bone there is periosteal bone deposition and endosteal bone resorption. The latter is greater than the former so that the result is a net loss of bone mass. This bone loss occurs in both men and women. However, in women there is an acceleration of bone loss at the time of the menopause.

Peak bone mass appears to be determined by a combination of genetic, environmental, nutritional and hormonal factors. Thus there is a strong racial association of osteoporosis with negro races, having a very low incidence of osteoporotic fracture compared to caucasians. Athletes tend to have relatively high bone mass; however, this effect is negated in women athletes who become amenorrhoeic. In contrast bed rest, space flight and misuse due to quadraplegia are all associated with loss of bone mineral.

Whether or not high calcium diet is associated with an increase in bone mass is controversial. In women, lactation and the use of the oral contraceptive pill all tend to increase peak bone mass.

Bone loss with ageing is increased in women who have an iatrogenic early loss of ovarian function and this may be reversed by oestrogen therapy. Exercise reduces the rate of bone loss as does calcium supplementation. Smoking and alcohol or caffeine consumption are all associated with decreased bone mass in the elderly.

Thyrotoxic osteoporosis

In thyrotoxicosis there is a marked increase in the general metabolism with a marked nitrogen loss producing a secondary rarefaction of bone. Krane *et al.* (1956), by radioactive calcium-45 studies, showed that there is increased bone resorption and formation in this state. Biochemically there is a hypercalciuria with a negative calcium balance and increased serum phosphate and alkaline phosphatase.

In association with this, the bones undergo very marked rarefaction, through the agency of increased osteoclastic activity, and eventually become so weak that spontaneous fractures occur. Apart from definite fractures, deformities may arise from weight-bearing or from muscular action. Thus kyphosis or scoliosis, and pelvic asymmetry, may be present. Deformity is less common in the long bones (Figure 5.20).

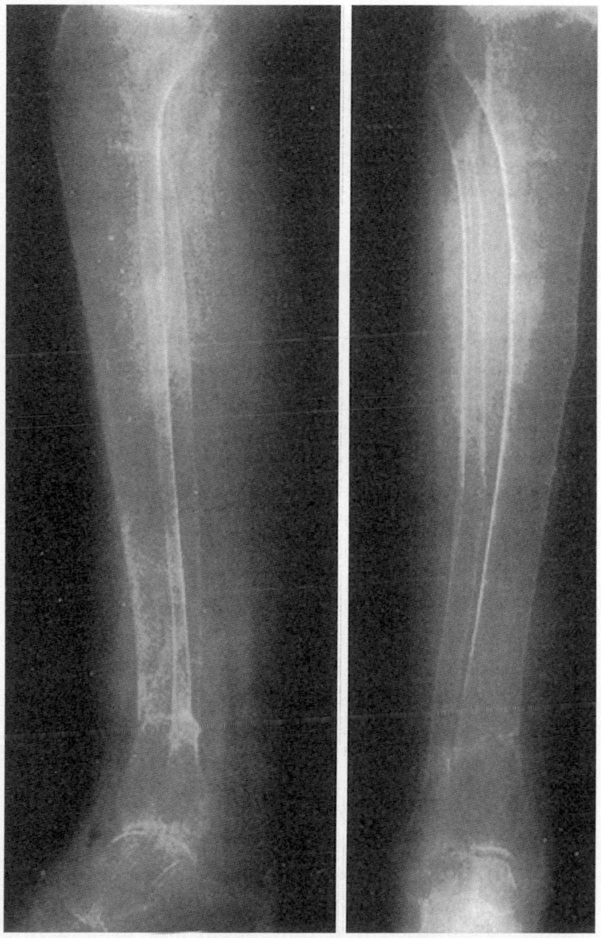

Figure 5.20 Radiograph of the leg, showing the extreme degree of thyrotoxic osteoporosis with narrowing of the cortex and a healing fracture in the lower diaphyseal area.

The cause of the increased excretion of calcium is not known, but Hertz has shown that, in animals, the calcium excretion and skeletal rarefaction are greater after the administration of the thyrotropic factor of pituitary secretion than after equal amounts of parathyroid hormone. It may be that the effects on calcium metabolism are due to simultaneous stimulation of the thyroid glands by this pituitary hormone.

In addition to the above, increased protein metabolism may result in a deficiency of the connective tissue elements of the bone. This occurs only when the limit of body tolerance is exceeded. A milder degree of hyperthyroidism through stimulation of the eosinophilic cells of the pituitary will result in an increased skeletal growth.

Homocystinuria

This condition was identified in 1969 by Cusworth and Dent, and is now known to be autosomal recessively inherited. This metabolic error of development can resemble Marfan's syndrome in that the infant, appearing normal at birth, develops mental retardation, skeletal abnormalities including scoliosis, dislocation of the eye lenses, etc. The defect is found in the failure of homocysteine to be converted into cystathionine – with the former amino acid flooding over into the urine, where it can be detected by the nitroprusside test. The amino acid methionine also accumulates in the plasma. This condition can be differentiated from Marfan's syndrome by the greater widening of the epiphyses and metaphyses of the long bones, and its earlier presentation of osteoporosis – particularly of the vertebrae (Brenton *et al.*, 1972).

Large dosages of pyridoxine (vitamin B_6) may correct the chemical defect but it still awaits proof of any effect upon the skeleton. An additional effect of this agent is to reduce the platelet stickiness and hence post-operative thromboses.

Algodystrophy (reflex sympathetic dystrophy or Sudeck's atrophy)

Algodystrophy is not a general affection of the skeleton. However, in view of its association with severe osteoporosis it is convenient to discuss it here.

The syndrome consists of excessive pain and tenderness, vasomotor instability and abnormalities of sweating, swelling and joint stiffness. It is associated with regional osteoporosis.

Although the syndrome was known to Hunter and there were sporadic reports in mediaeval literature of cases which almost certainly represented examples of it, the first systematic treatment of the condition was by Mitchell dealing with victims of gunshot wounds from the American Civil War. Sudeck was the first to apply radiographs to the condition and noted that it was associated with severe osteoporosis. However, some of his original cases were, in fact, tuberculous affections of limbs.

The condition has protean clinical manifestation, which to some extent reflect the site affected and occurs after a variety of precipitating causes and for these reasons it goes under a number of different names. Mitchell originally called the condition causalgia because in his cases, which were associated with major nerve trauma, the pain was often of a peculiar burning quality. The term Sudeck's atrophy was applied to the condition by Nonne, one of Sudeck's co-workers, because of the severity of the osteoporosis. The term reflex sympathetic dystrophy owed its origin to the French school following Leriche's demonstration that sympathectomy might improve the condition. The term is unfortunate since the association of the condition with a reflex arch in the sympathetic nervous system is controversial. More recently the term 'sympathetically mediated pain' has been introduced to denote syndromes in which pain, with or without other features of algodystrophy, may be relieved by sympathetic manipulation. The name algodystrophy was introduced in the early 1970s by Doury who studied the condition extensively.

The aetiology of the condition is unclear. It has long been assumed that there is an abnormal autonomic reflex arch which is initiated by trauma or a noxious stimulus. An autonomic reflex is of course an invariable accompaniment of injury and indeed it is the factor that initiates healing. What is unclear is why it should become prolonged and why it is associated with such excessive pain.

The condition may occur at almost any site but most commonly affects the peripheral parts of the limb and it is in these cases that the classic changes of vasomotor instability and swelling are most prominent. When it affects more proximal joints such as the knee and hip in isolation, pain and osteoporosis may frequently be found without concomitant swelling or vasomotor instability.

The most common precipitating factor is trauma which may range from a knock or sprain to a fracture. However, almost any painful stimulus can cause the condition and Steinbrocker emphasized the occurrence of the 'shoulder hand syndrome' following myocardial infarction. There appears to be an increased incidence in epileptic patients, particularly when taking phenytoin, and there is probably an association with diabetes mellitus. The condition is well described in pregnant women when it has been termed 'painful osteoporosis of pregnancy'.

The incidence of the condition following trauma has in the past been considered to be very low. Thus Plewes (1956) reported an incidence of one in 2000 trauma cases in a District General Hospital population and Bacorn and Kurtzke (1953) in a retrospective study of 2000 cases of Colles' fracture reported an incidence of 1%. In contrast a number of prospective studies (Atkins *et al.*, 1990) have demonstrated an incidence soon after trauma of approximately 30%. This apparent discrepancy is most easily explained if the majority of cases are transient, and this would indeed appear to be the case (Bickerstaff, 1991). However, it seems likely that even in those cases where the overt symptoms resolve there may be significant subclinical sequelae.

No age is exempt from the condition, but it appears to be relatively rare in children and the very old. The sex incidence is probably equal although most series show some bias normally due to the sorts of patient they were examining.

CLINICAL FEATURES

The description which follows is of the condition as it occurs classically affecting the peripheral part of a limb. The natural history is conveniently described in two phases, early and late.

Some weeks following a precipitating trauma and often after the initial severe pain of the trauma has passed, the patient becomes aware of a new pain affecting the traumatized region. The pain is of a different quality from that originally caused by the trauma. It is more diffuse, unpleasant in nature and may be associated with allodynia, hyperpathia and trigger zones. At first the pain may only be brought on by movement but as time passes if the condition is not treated, particularly in severe cases, it will become more severe, occur at rest and radiate proximally.

Hallmarks of the early phases of the condition are vasomotor instability with abnormalities of sweating and swelling. The vasomotor phenomena vary. It is classically described that initially the affected part is warm, vasodilated and dry, becoming after a few days or a week cold, blue, mottled cyanotic and sweaty. Although this classic pattern is seen in more severe cases, particularly in milder cases, the vaso-

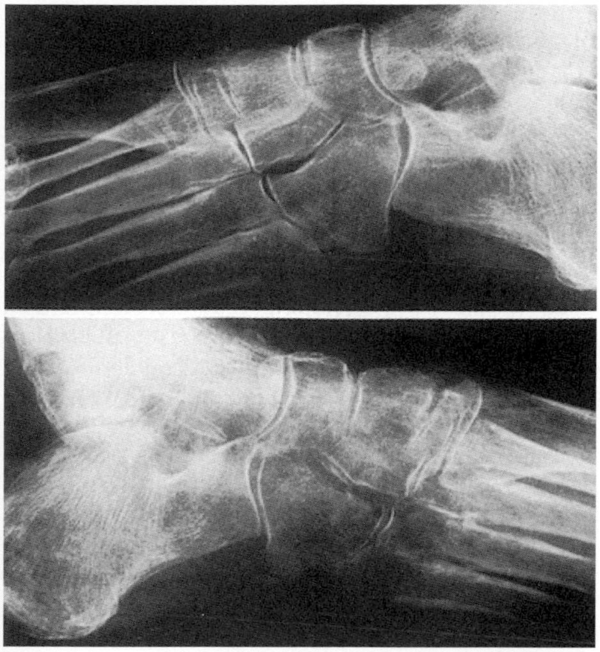

Figure 5.21 Lateral radiographs of right and left hindfeet, showing the spotty decalcification and osteoporosis of the left foot which had sustained a mild twisting injury.

motor instability more frequently takes the form of an abnormal temperature sensitivity with invariably increased sweating. Where the latter is severe, the perspiration sometimes has a pungent and offensive odour.

Swelling early in the condition takes the form of a pitting oedema. However, it rapidly becomes more fixed and brawny. Limitation of joint movement initially appears to be due to the combination of the pain, which is produced by joint movement, and the swelling.

In the late stage of the condition, the vasomotor instability normally disappears, as does the increased sweating. The pain becomes more severe and constant but curiously the patient's sleep is often undisturbed.

The swelling subsides and as it does so, the limb is seen to be contracted. The skin becomes thin and shiny with an almost glass-like appearance, the subcutaneous fat disappears and collateral ligament and tendinous retraction lead to fixed deformities of joints.

Serial radiographs show evidence of rapid osteoporosis (Figure 5.21). This normally appears within 3 months of the onset of the condition with accentuated metaphyseal bone loss, intracortical erosion and patchy osteoporosis. Later in the condition there is almost complete loss of trabecular bone with profound cortical thinning. When only one site is affected, for example the knee, the osteoporosis may be remarkably localized.

The delayed phase of the technetium-99 methylene diphosphonate bone scan shows increased uptake throughout the bones in the affected area early in the condition and this returns to normal, usually within 6 months from onset of the condition.

In severe cases a particular psychological effect has frequently been noted with the patient apparently being neurotic and dependent. This does not appear to occur in the mild cases and it is not clear whether it is the result of the severe chronic pain which attends the condition or a pre-existing abnormality.

PROGNOSIS

The majority of cases are mild or even subclinical and resolve with little or no residual disturbance of function. Recovery may, however, be protracted. It seems likely that even in mild cases there is often some minor permanent limitation of joint function and, although in very mild cases, the osteoporosis is probably reversible, it is probable that in the majority there is some permanent loss of bone density.

When the foot is affected, recovery tends to be more complete than when the upper limb is involved and fixed flexion contracture of the proximal interphalangeal joints and extension contractures of the metacarpophalangeal joints are very common. When the condition affects the shoulder there is often a permanent limitation of abduction and external rotation. When the knee is affected in isolation permanent stiffness is frequently seen. However, this is in part due to the difficulty in diagnosis at this site.

DIAGNOSIS

A classic case of algodystrophy affecting the distal part of a limb is almost impossible to miss. Unfortunately the majority of cases are not classical and particularly when the condition affects a proximal joint such as the knee or hip it may be months or even years before the diagnosis is made. This is especially unfortunate since the most important predictor of a good outcome of the condition is early aggressive treatment.

In atypical cases it is important to bear the possibility of the diagnosis in mind, particularly in patients with resistant non-specific knee pain.

The best diagnostic examination is a combination of delayed bone scintigraphy and serial radiography, with comparative exposure controlled views of the contralateral part. The condition is almost excluded by the finding of normal bone density and a normal delayed bone scan since in the first few months of the condition the bone scan may be expected to show increased uptake and by 3 or 4 months comparative radiographs should demonstrate osteoporosis. Children represent an exception to this since they may present with a normal or even cold bone scan.

TREATMENT

The majority of mild cases will respond to non-steroidal anti-inflammatory drugs and gentle, understanding physiotherapy. It is important not to worsen the pain by overmobilizing affected joints. Local application of heat may improve the pain. Night splintage can be useful but if employed it must be in a position of safety rather than of comfort. In the treatment of hand affectations, high elevation has been reported to be useful.

Sympathetic manipulation has been the mainstay of treatment for many years, although its efficacy is currently in dispute. Guanethidine blockade is a simple and often effective method of temporary sympathetic manipulation and it may be repeated as necessary. Stellate or lumbar sympathetic blockage with local anaesthetic or epidural blockade is also used. Caution should be exercised before performing a surgical or chemical sympathectomy.

A number of other forms of treatment have been used in the past, including oral steroid therapy, calcitonin, diphosphonate therapy. The efficacy of these treatments are unclear.

The effect of operating on somebody with algodystrophy is uncertain. It seems logical to defer operations which are not strictly necessary until satisfactory treatment of the condition. If an operation needs to be performed, for example to remove painful stimulus which may be causing the condition, some would advocate covering the operative

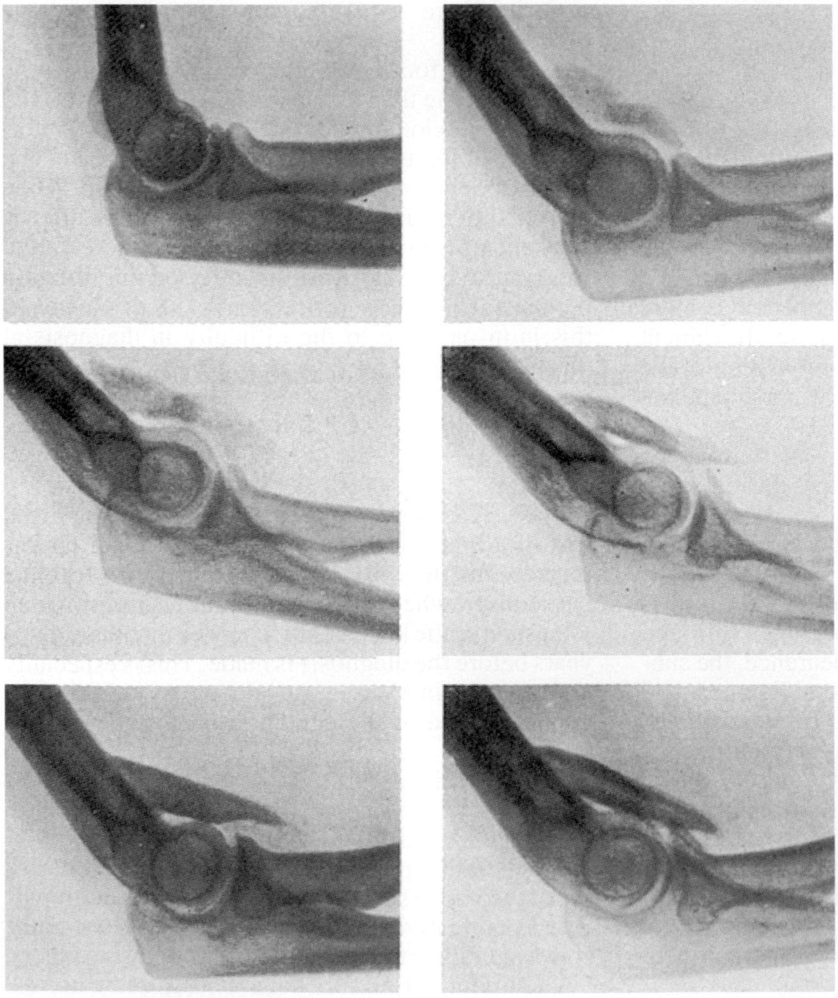

Figure 5.22 Radiographs taken over a period of 5 months of an elbow joint after dislocation to show the gradual development of ossification in the brachialis and capsular tissues overlying the anterior aspect of this joint.

period with sympathetic blockade, although the efficacy of this is uncertain. It is essential, if operating on a patient with algodystrophy, to be prepared to provide long-term postoperative analgesia and in the lower limb this may be conveniently undertaken using an epidural. Urgent postoperative mobilization with continuous passive motion and analgesia cover is probably the safest option.

Heterotopic ossification

Heterotopic ossification is the formation of true bone outside the skeleton, often within the connective tissue of muscles. It must be distinguished from ectopic calcification in which radiodense calcium phosphate deposits are laid down. However, the mineral phase differs from that in bone and no true bone matrix is formed.

Ectopic calcification as opposed to ossification affects tissue including blood vessels, cornea, skin, brain, kidneys and conjunctiva and may occur where there is an increase in the level of serum calcium. Thus it is seen in hyperparathyroidism, renal failure and hypoparathyroidism (due to the high serum phosphate level). It may also occur in certain diseases such as dermatomyositis, scleroderma and following tuberculous infection and it is seen in orthopaedic practice as calcification in supraspinatous tendonitis.

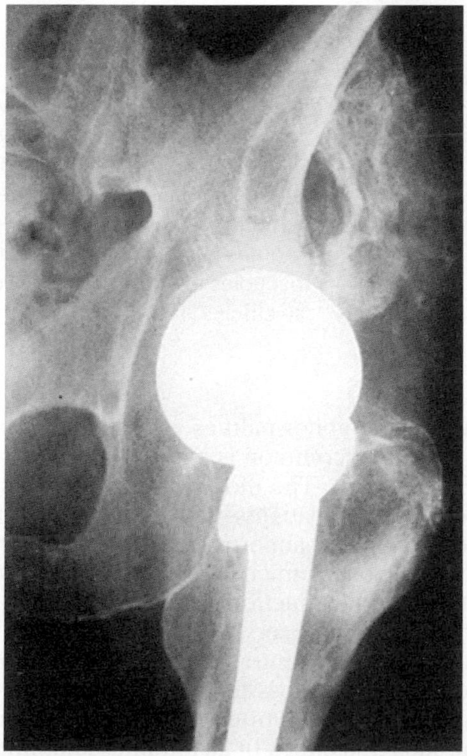

Figure 5.23 Heterotopic ossification occurring in a Smith–Petersen exposure for prosthetic replacement of a fractured neck of femur.

In contrast, true heterotopic ossification is seen following burns, neurological injury (especially spinal cord and head injury), soft tissue trauma and a variety of orthopaedic procedures, most notably total hip replacement (Figure 5.22).

In the post-traumatic situation, local heterotopic ossification occurs most frequently in young adults after direct injury to muscle groups (Figure 5.23). Organization of the haematoma occurs with fibroblastic hypoplasia, osteoid formation and finally radiographic evidence of ossification by 6–8 weeks after the initial injury (Figures 5.24 and 5.25).

Ackerman (1958) emphasized that there are four zones seen in microscopy (Figure 5.25):

1. An innermost zone, containing highly active cells with mitotic figures, varying in size and shape. These cells may be almost impossible to differentiate cytologically from malignant sarcomatous cells. Immediately outside this, there may be dead muscle fibre.
2. An adjacent zone containing cells less 'active' in appearance, but forming osteoid tissue.
3. A zone showing new bone with osteoblasts and fibrous tissue undergoing trabecular organization. If this mass is intimately adjacent to the host bone, there may be evidence of osteoclastic activity and the presence of giant cells. Indeed, some of these lesions have been called a 'subperiosteal giant cell tumour' (Figures 5.26 and 5.27).
4. A peripheral zone of fibrous tissue.

If the biopsy is taken before 4 weeks, or if it is not extensive enough, one may not see organized new bone at the periphery, and therefore the diagnosis will be inaccurate.

The majority of cases of heterotopic ossification are asymptomatic. However, they may cause pain or loss of range of joint movement.

Risk factors for the formation of heterotopic bone following total joint replacement are male sex, hypertrophic osteoarthritis, previous hip surgery, previous formation of heterotopic bone following surgery and youth (see Chapter 11).

Treatment is normally by watchful inactivity. Mature cases may be excised *in toto*. However, there is a risk of recurrence which is particularly high if operation is performed before the osteogenic process has ceased which usually takes at least 2 years.

Formation of heterotopic bone may be prevented by low dose irradiation (Ayers *et al.*, 1991) or by

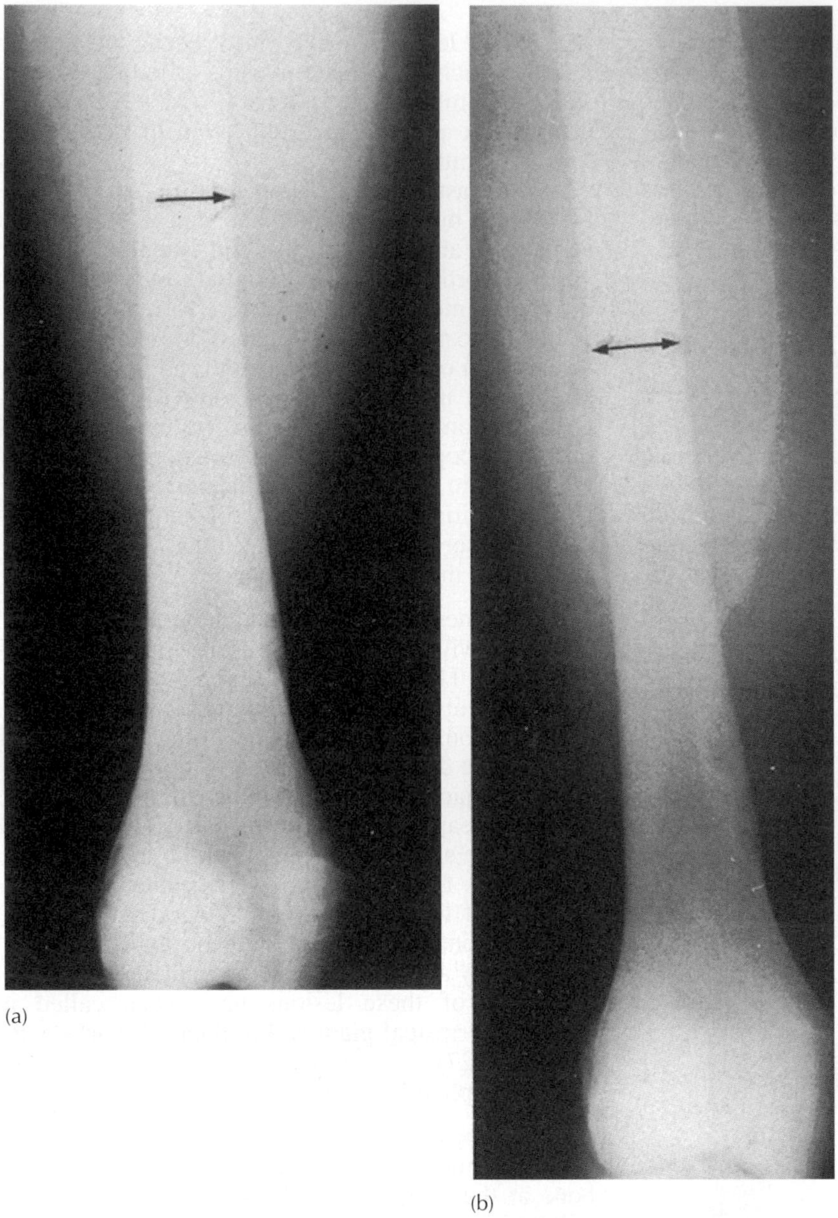

Figure 5.24 (a) Soft tissue swelling from a direct blow on the thigh in a 16-year-old male. Medially there is a benign cortical defect in the femoral metaphysis. (b) Two months later a mature ossification occupies the area of soft tissue swelling.

pretreatment with a non-steroidal anti-inflammatory drug such as indomethacin (Pagnani *et al.*, 1991).

Myositis ossificans progressiva

This is a rare congenital condition (prevalence approximately one per million) which is autosomal dominant with a variable penetrance. It is characterized by progressive ossification within muscles and certain specific skeletal abnormalities (Figures 5.28 and 5.29).

The skeletal abnormalities are usually present at birth. The most common is a monophalangeal great toe (Figure 5.30). The monophalangeic great toe is characteristic of patients with myositis ossificans progressiva. Other abnormalities include short first metacarpal bones, microdactyly, malformation of the little finger, reduction defects of all limbs and abnormalities of the cervical vertebrae.

The ossification centres may also be abnormal.

The progressive ossification occurs in discrete episodes. These are often precipitated by minor trauma such as a knock or an intramuscular injection in the thigh. The region becomes swollen, tender and inflamed. If a large area of muscle is involved the

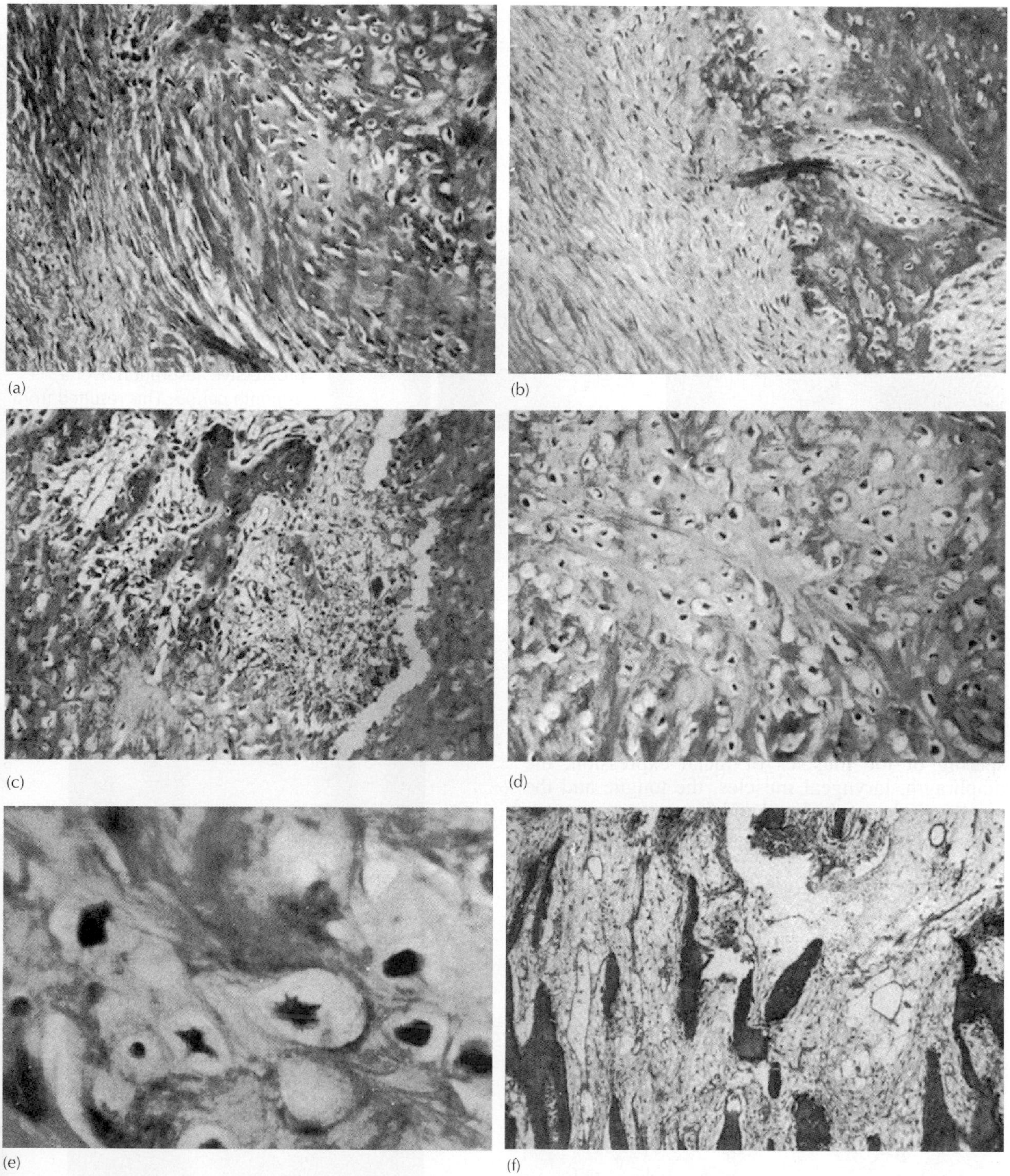

Figure 5.25 (a) Photomicrograph of a myositis ossificans, showing the muscle and fibrous tissue at the bottom left and abnormal osteoblastic activity top right. (× 94). (b) Photomicrograph showing the fibrous tissue of the peripheral zone at the left with the new bone formation and osteoblasts on the right, forming trabeculae. (× 94). (c) Photomicrograph showing a very active cellular zone with trabeculae forming, osteoblastic activity and vascularity. (× 94). (d) Photomicrograph showing the innermost zone which is made up of highly active osteoblasts containing mitotic figures as well as varying in size and shape, and hence suggesting neoplastic change. (× 113). (e) Photomicrograph illustrating the 'neoplastic' appearing cells in the innermost area of myositis ossificans. (× 395). (f) Photomicrograph showing the formation of trabeculae which are surrounded by cellular fibrous tissue. (× 33).

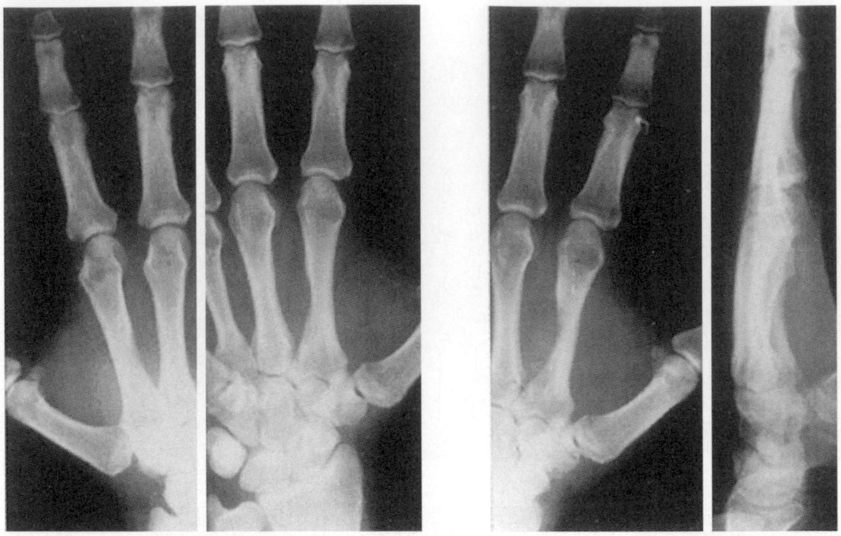

(a) (b)

Figure 5.26 Radiographs showing a subperiosteal giant cell tumour of periosteal myositis ossificans of the second metacarpal bone with progressive absorption over a 2-month period. This resulted from a direct blow to the hand.

patient may be pyrexial and unwell. As the swelling subsides the muscle mass involved is replaced by bone. As the disease progresses there is interference with the function of the affected muscle, leading to progressive immobility. Death is commonly due to respiratory complication.

Ossification characteristically involves the muscles of the head and back in early childhood followed by the shoulders and arms. The muscles around the hips are involved later. There is characteristic sparing of the muscles of facial expression, the diaphragm, laryngeal muscles, the tongue and the small muscles of the hand and feet.

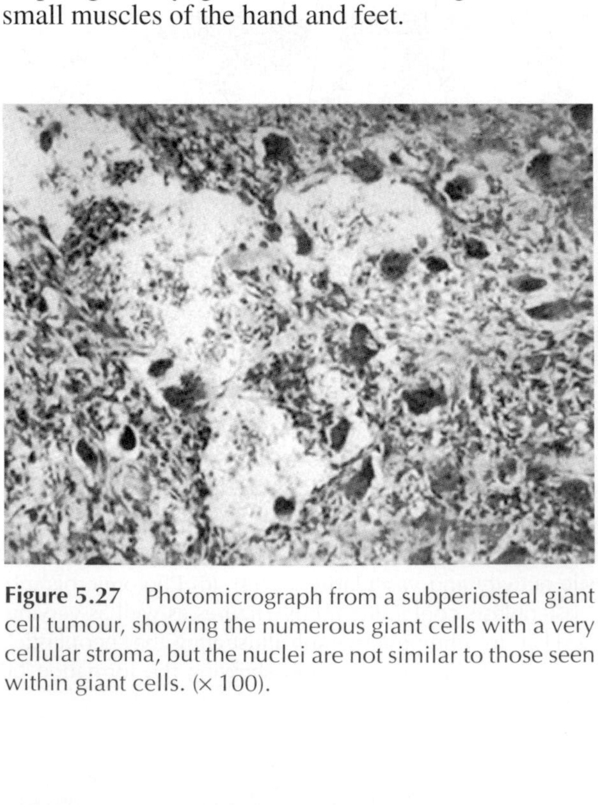

Figure 5.27 Photomicrograph from a subperiosteal giant cell tumour, showing the numerous giant cells with a very cellular stroma, but the nuclei are not similar to those seen within giant cells. (× 100).

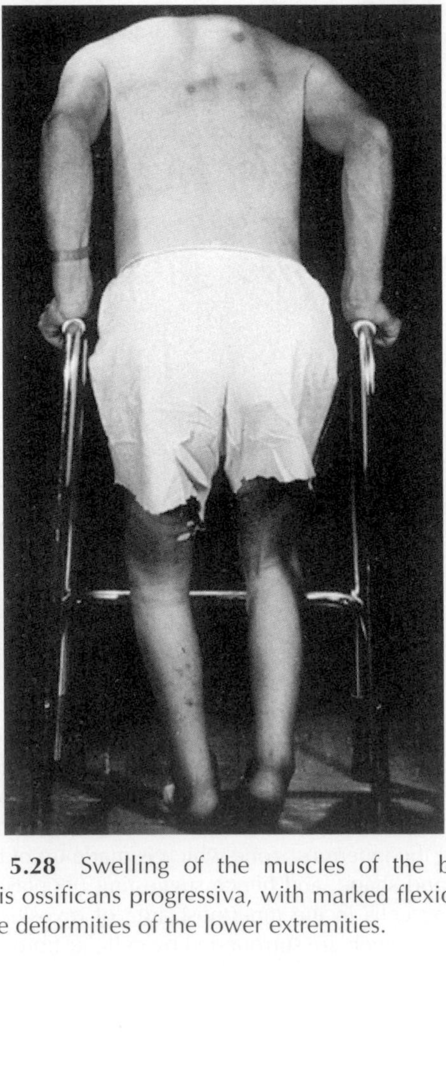

Figure 5.28 Swelling of the muscles of the back in myositis ossificans progressiva, with marked flexion contracture deformities of the lower extremities.

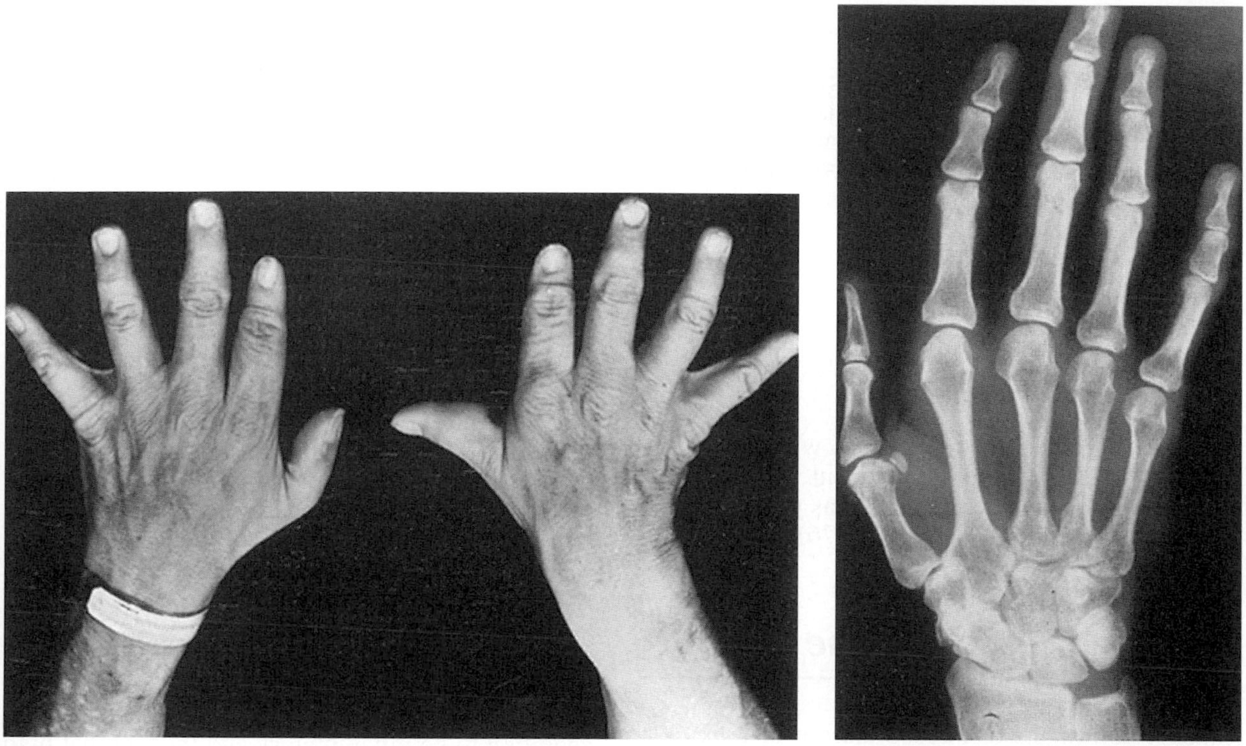

(a) (b)

Figure 5.29 (a) Microdactyly of the index finger in progressive myositis ossificans. (b) Radiograph of the deformity.

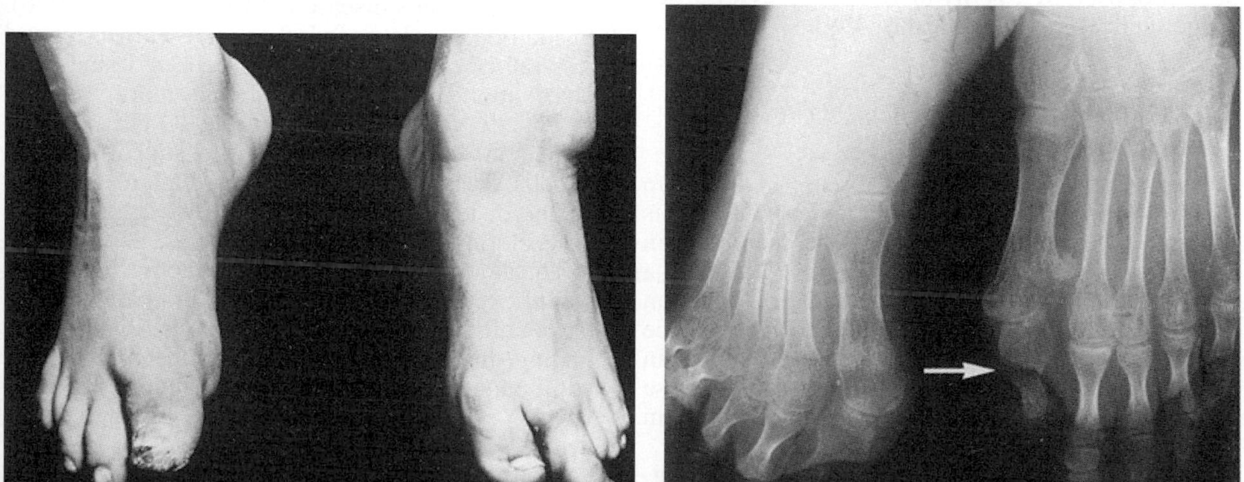

(a) (b)

Figure 5.30 (a) Abnormalities of the toes in the same patient as in Figure 5.29. (b) Radiograph of the deformities showing the monophalangeal big toe.

PATHOLOGY

The striking feature of the disease is the replacement of muscle, tendon and aponeurosis by masses of bone. Study of early lesions reveals that the new bone deposits are not laid down within the actual muscle fibre but in the connective tissue between the fibres. This has led to the alternative name for the condition of fibrodysplasia ossificans progressiva.

TREATMENT

There is no known treatment which will prevent the episodes of ossification. Treatment with diphosphonates has been attempted but has proved generally disappointing (Smith *et al.*, 1976).

Paget's disease of bone

Osteitis deformans or Paget's disease of bone is a disorder characterized by excessive disorganized bone turnover. Initially there is markedly increased osteoclastic bone resorption, leading to an osteolytic lesion which is the site of subsequent increased bone formation producing sclerosis. The condition was first described in detail by Sir James Paget in 1876 although isolated examples had been noted prior to this and the name osteitis deformans had already been proposed by Czerny in 1873. For reviews, see Singer and Krane, 1990; Kanis, 1991.

INCIDENCE AND EPIDEMIOLOGY

The majority cases of Paget's disease of bone are subclinical so that the population prevalence is difficult to estimate accurately. The incidence in England has been assessed by Collins (1956). In a study of 600 autopsies in England he found an incidence of 3.7%. Pygott (1957) found an incidence of 3.5% in a population over 45 years of age in London using radiographic criteria. The disease becomes more common with age, being very rare in patients under 30.

The epidemiology of Paget's disease is fascinating because the prevalence varies widely throughout the world. It is probably most frequently seen in England but is also common in Australia and the United States of America while the disease is very well reported in China, Japan and Scandinavia. Moreover, there is a wide variation in prevalence within one country and Barker *et al.*, (1980) demonstrated that the disease was common in Lancashire compared to the rest of England.

AETIOLOGY

A number of different theories have been proposed concerning the aetiology of the condition.

Genetic

A family history of Paget's disease is found in approximately 15% of cases and when the disease runs in families the site affected and course is often similar in different siblings; consequently, it has been suggested that there is either an autosomal dominant or recessive pattern. However, the condition is rarely found in identical twins (Melick and Martin, 1975) and there is only a weak association with HLA type (Cullen *et al.*, 1976).

Inflammatory disorder

In 1876 Sir James Paget originally believed the condition to be inflammatory and the fact that high doses of corticosteroids or aspirin can suppress disease activity, relieve bone pain and improve the patient's general condition has lent some credence to this theory.

More recently intranuclear inclusion bodies similar to those seen in slow viral infections of the paramyxovirus family have been found within the giant multinucleate osteoclasts which are characteristic of Paget's disease (Mills and Singer, 1976). In addition a variety of viral antigens to measles and respiratory syncytial virus have been found. The observation that dog ownership is more common in Pagetic subjects than controls (O'Driscoll and Anderson, 1986) has led to the suggestion that Paget's disease may be a slow viral response to canine distemper virus which is also a paramyxovirus closely related to measles.

The slow viral hypothesis is attractive because it would explain the wide variation in epidemiology, the familial incidence, the age distribution, the finding, the multisite involvement and it is consistent with a number of the pathological findings. Until a virus is isolated from Pagetic bone, however, this theory will remain speculative.

From a very large series of prior dog and cat owners 433 patients with Paget's disease and an equal number of matched controls living in the USA, Siris *et al.*, (1990) did not find any differences by very careful statistically analysed data. They concluded that previous dog or cat ownership was not a risk factor in the development of Paget's disease.'

Abnormality of collagen

The finding of angioid retinal streaks in approximately 15% of patients, the association with pseudoxanthoma elasticum and the high incidence of vascular and skin calcification have led to the suggestion that Paget's disease is due to an abnormality of collagen metabolism. Moreover, abnormal collagen has been demonstrated in skin from Pagetic patients (Francis *et al*., 1974). However, this concept fails to explain why Paget's disease remains localized and more recent evidence has suggested that the bone collagen in Paget's disease is normal (Krane, 1977).

Endocrine disorder

It has been suggested that Paget's disease may be due to calcitonin deficiency. However, calcitonin concentration has been shown to be within normal limits in patients with Paget's disease (Heyman and Franchimont, 1974), as are other hormone levels.

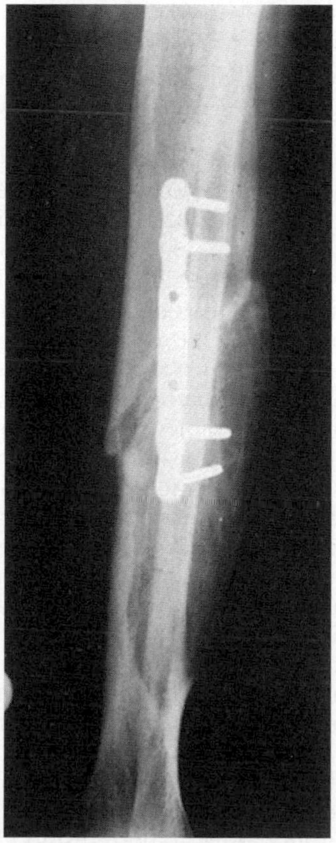

Figure 5.31 The osteoporotic form of Paget's disease in the tibia of a young man, which had undergone a pathological fracture and an internal fixation procedure.

PATHOLOGY

Paget's disease is a focal disorder of bone characterized initially by excessive osteoclastic activity followed by disorganized, excessive new bone formation. This temporal sequence of events leads to three definable phases of the disease, namely lytic (Figure 5.31), mixed and finally, sclerotic.

Initially during the lytic phase, overactive osteoclasts resorb bone at a higher rate than normal. The osteoclasts are large and irregular and appear very active. The cytoplasm contains glycogen particles and may demonstrate fragments of calcified tissue which have been phagocytosed. The number of nuclei is excessive and may be up to 100. Nuclear inclusion bodies are frequent. During this phase, large areas of bone are covered with actively resorbing osteoclasts and fatty tissue adjacent to bone and haemopoietic bone marrow are replaced by ingrowing fibrous tissue.

In contrast to the osteoclasts, the osteoblasts are relatively normal in appearance. However, the new bone formed in Paget's disease is abnormal. It is very vascular and can be physically larger than the preexisting bone which leads to cortical widening and contributes to the deformity. In addition, the bones are soft, due both to the high rate of turnover and to the abnormal formation, and become deformed by muscle action and weight-bearing. The diagnostic histological feature of Paget's disease is irregular areas of lamellar bone fitting together like a jigsaw with randomly distributed cement lines (Figure 5.32).

Later in the sclerotic phase, bone turnover may be reduced and the combination of deformity and abnormalities of bone turnover lead to brittleness and fissure fractures.

In 1925 Knaggs described the classical three stages in the pathology, particularly in the skull:

1. Vascular with porosity of bone.
2. Advancing sclerosis with increasing thickness of skull.
3. Diffuse complete sclerosis with condensation of bone through the skull calvaria.

CLINICAL FEATURES

In the majority of cases Paget's disease of bone is asymptomatic, being found incidentally during investigation of another disorder. For example, in Collins' series only 5% complained of Pagetic symptoms. The most common presenting feature is pain, particularly when weight-bearing bones are involved and although it is often not aggravated by weight-bearing, night pain is frequent. The cause of

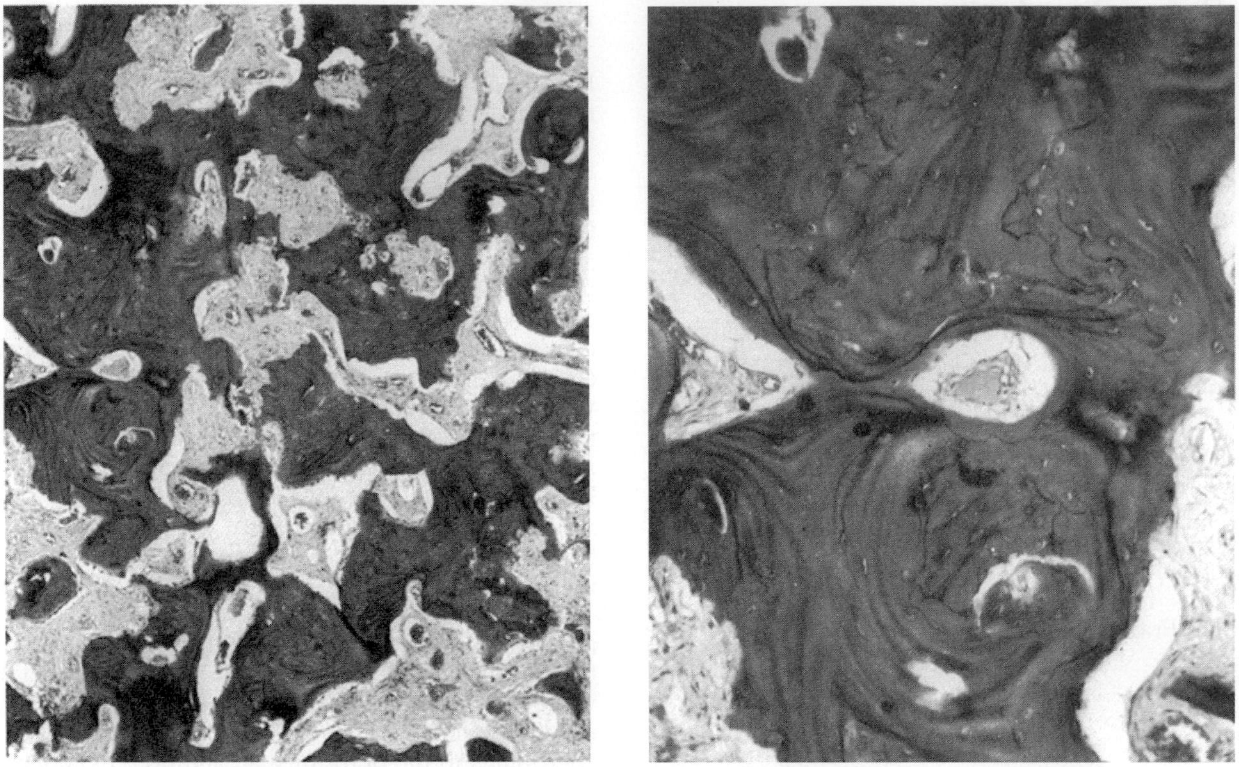

(a) (b)

Figure 5.32 (a) Photomicrograph showing the abnormal bone formation with a mosaic appearance due to an irregular lamellar system. In between these there is a vascular cellular stroma. (× 40). (b) Paget's disease showing the typical irregularity of the lamellar structure and some of the scanty cellular stroma. (× 203).

Pagetic bone pain is not clear. It may be due to vascular hypertension as a result of increased blood flow or to stretching of periosteum overlying an expanding bone. Arthritis of adjacent joints and fissure fractures may also be painful. Headache and vertigo can be found.

The second leading presentation is deformity. Classically, the patient notices that his hat size is becoming larger due to skull involvement, however, the most frequent site of deformity is the lower limb where bowing of the softened femur laterally and tibia anteriorly may be so severe that the legs are crossed even with the hips maximally abducted (Figure 5.33). Characteristic deformities also occur in the forearm, clavicle and face and overgrowth of the jaw may cause dental problems.

Lower limb bowing may be pain free; however, microfractures are common on the convex side of deformed bones, occurring in up to one-third of patients and although the majority are asymptomatic, the onset of pain may presage complete fracture. This may occur with minimal trauma, especially in the deformed femur and tibia, and the fracture line generally runs transversely. Vertebral compression fractures are also characteristic.

Arthritis of joints adjacent to involved bones is frequent and may have two aetiologies (Figure 5.34). Mechanical malalignment due to deformity may overfissure the joint, particularly at the knee or the joint may itself be distorted by expansion of an involved bone.

The spine is a common site of Paget's disease and involvement of the vertebral bodies may lead to nerve entrapment. Paraplegia due to a vascular steal is a rare finding. Occasionally, peripheral nerve entrapment occurs. Skull involvement frequently causes deafness and other cranial nerve lesions, including progressive visual impairment, due to optic nerve compression, and hemifacial pain, due to trigeminal nerve involvement, are rarer. Platybasia (upwards invagination of the base of the skull) may lead to ataxia, long tract signs, lower cranial nerve dysfunction and brain stem lesions, although usually it is asymptomatic. Headaches and confusion are also seen.

Pagetic bone has increased blood flow, particularly in the early stages, and this may be so great that high output cardiac failure results (Mercer and Duthie, 1956). The combination of deformity and increased bone vascularity may compromise skin integrity, leading to indolent ulcers.

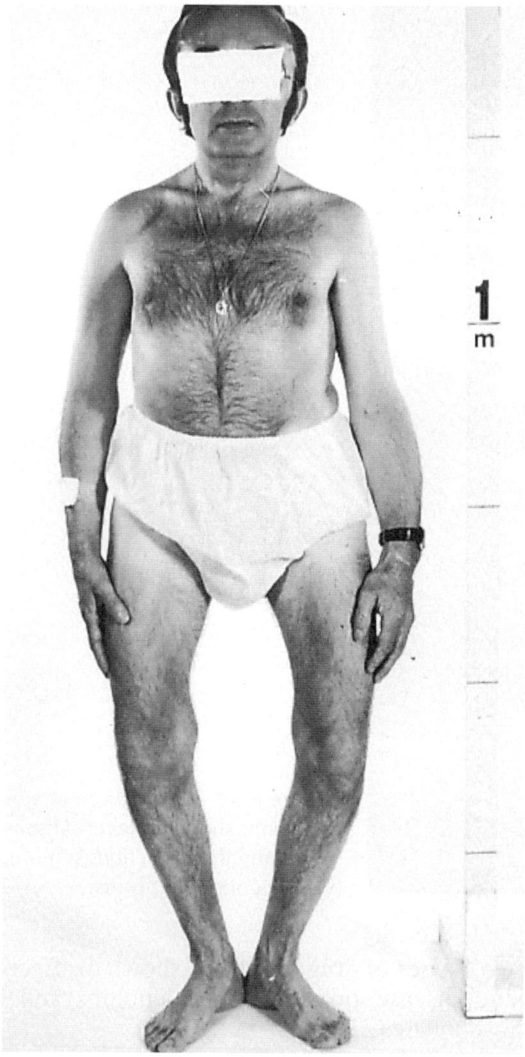

Figure 5.33 An elderly man showing the structural deformities which result from Paget's disease of the skeleton with marked bowing of the femora.

Sarcomatous change in a Pagetic bone is a rare but serious complication.

RADIOLOGICAL FEATURES

General features

The disease is normally polyostotic but monostic and facial forms are reported. The bones most commonly involved in order of frequency are the pelvis, lumbar spine, femur, thoracic spine, sacrum, skull, tibia, humerus and scapula.

Pelvis

The pelvis is involved in approximately two-thirds of cases and the appearance is normally sclerotic. Protrusio acetabuli may occur and if involvement is bilateral, the pelvis assumes a trefoil shape. Alternatively, uniform loss of hip joint space with little osteophyte formation may occur.

Spine

The incidence of spinal involvement increases from the cervical to the lumbar spine. Normally, the vertebra is slightly enlarged with coarse trabeculations and a rim of thickened cortex which has the appearance of a 'rugger jersey' spine. Vertebral wedge fractures are frequent.

Long bones

The affected long bones become wider and bow due to loss of rigidity. The direction of bowing depends on mechanical loading and muscle pull. Typically the femur bows laterally and the tibia anteriorly.

Skull

The disease begins as an area of osteolysis termed osteoporosis circumscripta, most frequently seen in the frontal or occipital regions. Later, patchy sclerosis results in thickening of the skull, with irregular islands of dense bone giving a cotton wool appearance as the distinction between the outer and inner tables is lost.

Fairbank (1951) described four typical radiological appearances which can be seen in most bones:

1. A honeycomb or spongy appearance – which is the commonest and most widespread manifestation.
2. A striated appearance, as seen in the pelvis, sacrum and calcaneum.
3. A uniform and increased density, which is most frequently seen in the vertebrae.
4. The occurrence of true cystic areas, as seen in the pelvis or long bones.

Bone scintigraphy

Due to the increased bone turnover, Pagetic lesions show an increased uptake of technetium-99m labelled methylene diphosphonate, except in the very earliest stages before there is any increase in osteoblastic activity. Scintigraphy with ^{99m}Tc is a useful screening test since it allows visualization of the entire skeleton and may demonstrate lesions before they are radiologically apparent.

Bone scanning by ^{99m}Tc phosphate gives a very varied picture of 'hot' areas due to active bone

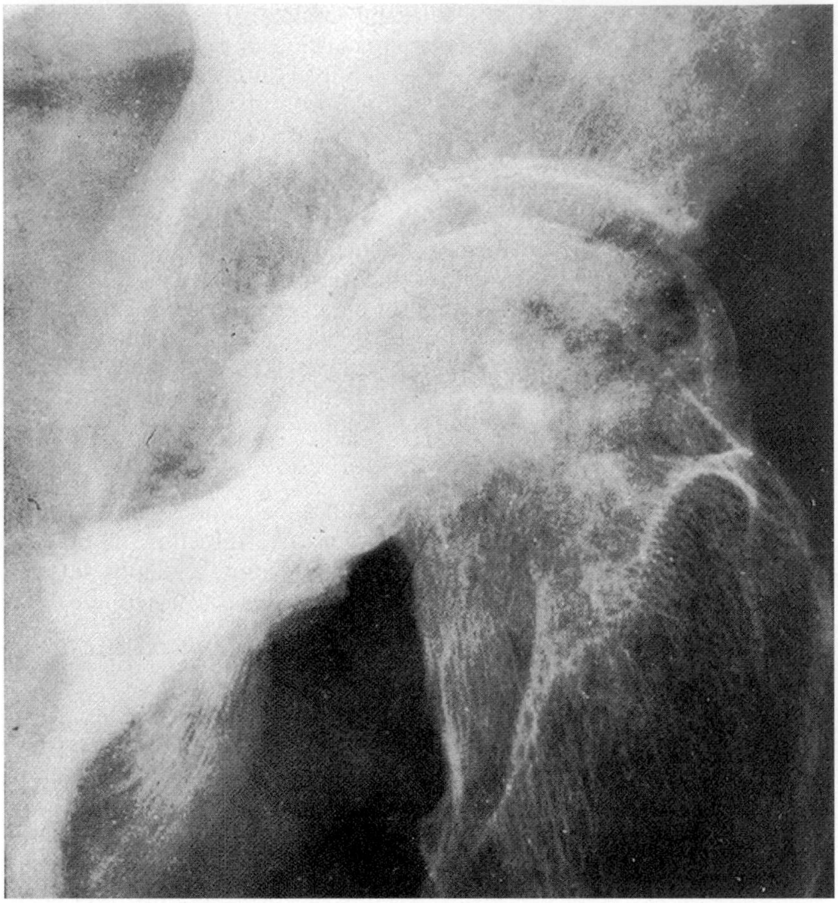

Figure 5.34 Radiograph of a left hip joint, showing Paget's disease involving the ilium and ischium, with secondary arthritis.

formation, 'diffuse' areas, background areas of normal bone, depending upon the geography of the lesion and the timing of the change. Its use even for studying the effects of treatment is uncertain.

BIOCHEMICAL FEATURES

From an early stage in the condition, increased osteoclastic activity leads to excessive excretion of hydroxyproline in the urine and serum alkaline phosphatase activity is increased due to osteoblastic overactivity. Serum calcium and phosphate levels are usually within normal limits, unless the patient has been immobilized, when hypercalcaemia may occur.

MEDICAL TREATMENT

The majority of patients with Paget's disease have no symptoms and treatment is not indicated. In the future it may be that prophylactic treatment of asymptomatic lesions with diphosphonates in order to prevent disease progression will become accepted but this cannot yet be recommended.

Two classes of drug have been shown to affect the Pagetic disease process, the calcitonins and the diphosphonates.

Calcitonin

Calcitonin is a naturally occurring polypeptide secreted by the parafollicular 'C' cells of the parathyroid gland and it acts as a direct inhibitor of osteoclastic bone resorption. Several different preparations are available, including porcine and salmon, the latter resembling human calcitonin more closely. Currently, calcitonin has to be given by subcutaneous injection, which is associated with nausea, flushing and diarrhoea. An intranasal spray is under investigation but is not yet widely available.

Rapidly following calcitonin injection, changes occur in the osteoclasts, which lose their motility and retract from the bone surface. The number attached to the bone surface also decreases. As a result of the sudden reduction in osteoclastic activity, mineral removal from bone is depressed which leads to a temporary reduction of the serum calcium (this is the basis of the calcitonin test for estimating the total body bone resorptive activity).

Long-term regular use of calcitonin leads to normalization of urinary hydroxyproline excretion as bone resorption is reduced and of serum alkaline phosphatase activity as bone formation rates are reduced by the influence of coupling. Thus treatment with calcitonin leads to normalization of bone remodelling; however, after an initial response, resistance to further treatment may occur. In addition, the initial response is variable and may be incomplete.

Diphosphonates

The diphosphonates (or bisphosphonates) are a group of synthetic pyrophosphate analogues, which have a central P–C–P backbone rather than the P–O–P of pyrophosphate. This makes them resistant to chemical and enzymatic hydrolysis and allows them to be administered orally. Like pyrophosphate, they inhibit hydroxyapatite crystal growth and in tissue culture and *in vivo* they inhibit bone resorption probably both by a direct effect on the osteoclast and by reducing precursor recruitment. A wide variety of other metabolic actions have been reported, including effects on glycolysis and fatty acid oxidation as well as alterations in prostaglandin synthesis but the relevance of these actions is unclear.

The diphosphonates are a relatively new class of drug and are still undergoing evaluation. Three drugs have been extensively used in Paget's disease of bone and are commercially available in various countries. These are hydroxyethylidene diphosphonate (etidronate, EHDP), dichloromethylene diphosphonate (clodronate, Cl_2MDP) and aminohydroxypropylidene diphosphonate (pamidronate, APD). Of these only etidronate is currently licensed for Paget's disease. A number of other diphosphonates are currently being tested, including, aminohexane diphosphonate (AHDP) and aminobutane diphosphonate (ABD).

Administration of diphosphonates either orally or intravenously leads to reduction of bone resorption to normal. Approximately one month after the lowering of bone resorptioin, osteoblastic activity also returns to normal due to coupling. The effect is not so rapid as with calcitonin but it is more certain and lasts for some time after the drug has been stopped, so that short courses of diphosphonates evoke a prolonged remission in the Pagetic process and bone remodelling becomes more normal.

Treatment with etidronate is, however, associated with an inhibition of mineralization which causes osteomalacia and may cause fissure lesions to progress to frank fracture. For this reason, widespread use of diphosphonates for Paget's disease must await the licensing of a second generation drug for the disease.

SURGICAL TREATMENT

Indications for surgical treatment include osteotomy for the correction of deformity and treatment of painful fissure fractures; total joint replacement for arthritis; internal fixation of fractures and ablative surgery for Paget's sarcoma. Pagetic bone often bleeds excessively (Dove, 1980) and may either be abnormally soft, making it difficult to obtain a grip with a screw, or unusually hard, so that cutting and drilling it is difficult. Bony landmarks may be difficult to identify and in severe cases the medullary canal may be partially obliterated. Preoperative radiographic investigation will identify these problems and the severity and spread of the disease can be assessed by serum alkaline phosphatase, urinary hydroxyproline excretion and bone scintigraphy. Successful medical treatment of Paget's disease will reduce bone vascularity and limit excessive operative bleeding and, after a period of remission, the bone quality may be improved, rendering operation technically easier. If a rapid reduction in bone blood flow is necessary, pretreatment with calcitonin rather than diphosphonates is preferred because it has a more rapid effect.

Total joint replacement is the procedure of choice for hip or knee pain due Pagetic arthritis. However, the pathological process producing the pain must be accurately identified. For example, hip pain may be due to upper femoral fissure fractures, coxarthrosis or the Paget's disease itself and medical treatment may delay the need for operation. The blood loss during total hip replacement is on average twice that seen in an unaffected hip (Goutallier *et al.*, 1984) and this may be reduced by medical pretreatment. Technically the operation may be difficult due to bone deformity and preoperative assessment must be adequate to ensure that a suitable prosthesis is available. Long-term follow up of cemented total hip replacement in patients with Paget's disease suggests that the prosthesis does not fail more quickly than in the general arthritic population (Ludkowski and Wilson-MacDonald, 1990). Metabolic activity of the disease subsequent to the surgery had no effect upon the outcome nor did the actual location of the disease (acetabulum and/or femur) or the presence of protrusio. There is no evidence that fissure fractures are improved by medical therapy and if they are painful, external splintage may be helpful. Mechanical realignment of a deformed bone to remove the fissure from the concave surface by the use of external fixation is being considered and osteotomy can be strikingly successful, although experience is limited (Kanis, 1991). The osteotomy is fixed with an intramedullary nail.

Pathological long bone fracture is the most common presentation of Paget's disease to an orthopaedic surgeon. The fractures are usually transverse and often the result of completion of a fissure fracture. Fractures may heal with conservative management (Barry, 1980) but there is a high incidence of non-union, especially for fracture of the femoral neck (Dove, 1980). To this must be added the risks of prolonged imobilization which is associated with rapid bone loss in Pagetic patients. Where internal fixation is performed, intramedullary devices are preferred when practical. Long bone deformity may be corrected at the time of fracture stabilization.

SARCOMA IN PAGET'S DISEASE

Although rare (less than 0.1% of all patients), it has been more commonly found in post-mortem material (up to 15% of cadavers). A survey of 22 cases by Moore *et al.* (1991) has emphasized that pain or a swelling is the most common presentation, a pathological fracture or neurological symptoms being less frequent. Their important observations were on the aggressiveness of this tumour with a survival time from 5 days to nearly 3 years, with the pathology being 16 high-grade osteogenic sarcomas, three chondrosarcomas, two fibroblastic sarcomas and one malignant fibrous histiocytoma.

DISORDERS OF GROWTH

Pituitary disturbances

The anterior lobe of the pituitary gland, by its thyrotropic, adrenocorticotropic and gonadotropic secretions, 'controls' the activity of the thyroid, the adrenal cortex and the sex glands. However, there is the reciprocal relationship of 'feedback' or control by the amount of circulatory hormone as well as indirect relationships to each other. Above this endocrine control, there is the integration of the endocrines with the nervous system by the hypothalamus.

The anterior lobe is made up of:

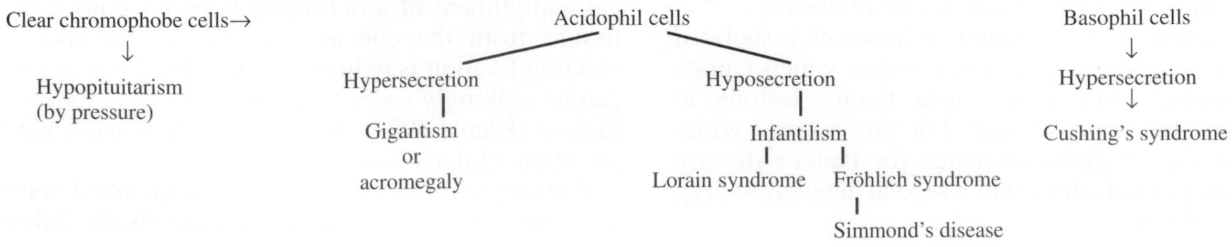

The posterior lobe is made up of neurological cells and fibres which are connected to the supraoptic nuclei of the hypothalamus. Its secretion of oxytocin or vasopressin does not appear to have any direct effect upon osseous tissues.

Short stature (dwarfism)

The term 'dwarf' is applied to an individual whose physical dimensions are considerably beneath those peculiar to his race, whereas 'short stature' usually implies only an unexpected decrease in height. However, both are intermingled and are considered together (Table 5.4).

Table 5.4

Short stature	Tall stature
Constitutional short stature	*Constitutional tall stature*
Genetic short stature	Genetic tall stature
Intrauterine growth retardation	Tall stature syndrome
	Cerebral gigantism
Malnutrition	Marfan's syndrome)
Short stature syndromes (e.g. Turner's syndrome)	Chromosomal abnormalities
Skeletal dysplasia	
Chronic disease	
Endocrine causes	*Endocrine causes*
Growth hormone deficiency	Pituitary gigantism
Hypothyroidism	Sexual precocity
Cushing's syndrome	Homocystinuria
Pseudohypoparathyroidism	
Abnormal diet analysis of vitamin D metabolites	
Hypoxia	
Malabsorption	
Hepatic disease	
Renal disease	
Juvenile rheumatoid arthritis	
Cardiac disease	
Pulmonary disease	
Blood dyscrasias (e.g. sickle cell anaemia)	

Disorders of growth hormone secretion and action are obviously very important. Disorders may occur at all levels of hypothalamic–pituitary–somatomedin–chondro-osseus axis and can be considered as:

1. Acquired pituitary insufficiency in a growing child, due to birth trauma, cranial irradiation for neoplasm, a craniopharyngioma or in histiocytosis X.
2. Multitropic pituitary hormone deficiency or panhypopituitary dwarf, which occurs sporadically and is a rare autosomal or X-linked recessive. The clinical picture depends on which of the hormones is absent. If growth hormone is absent, this produces proportionate dwarfism, high-pitched voice, subcutaneous adipose tissue and wrinkled skin. In gonadotropic deficiency there is sexual infantilism and infertility.
3. Isolated growth hormone deficiency – there is proportionate dwarfism with normal sexual development. The commonest form is inherited with increased subcutaneous fat, characteristic round full face with high-forehead, high-pitched voice and wrinkled skin. There is a tendency to spontaneous hypoglycaemic attacks in infancy.
4. Major developmental malformations or congenital absence of pituitary.

Both short stature and gigantism produce psychosocial problems in proportion to their severity. There is a wide range of adult height and growth during childhood may be affected by accelerated or retarded skeletal maturation without affecting the ultimate stature.

Investigation of disorders of stature depends on the careful clinical history of the child, parents and family for growth data, family stature, gestation period, birth history, birth weight, perinatal history and any familial history of growth disturbance. The child should be examined for height and weight against the normal percentile chart and trunk to height proportion should be measured (Figure 5.35). Skeletal age is assessed from hand radiographs and clinical assessment of the stage of puberty is made (Greulich and Pyle, 1959; Tanner *et al.*, 1975). Chromosomal analysis by buccal smears may be required and radiology will demonstrate characteristic skeletal syndromes.

Plasma assays for the majority of hormones involved in control of growth are now available.

A differential diagnosis for causes of abnormalities of growth is given in Table 5.5.

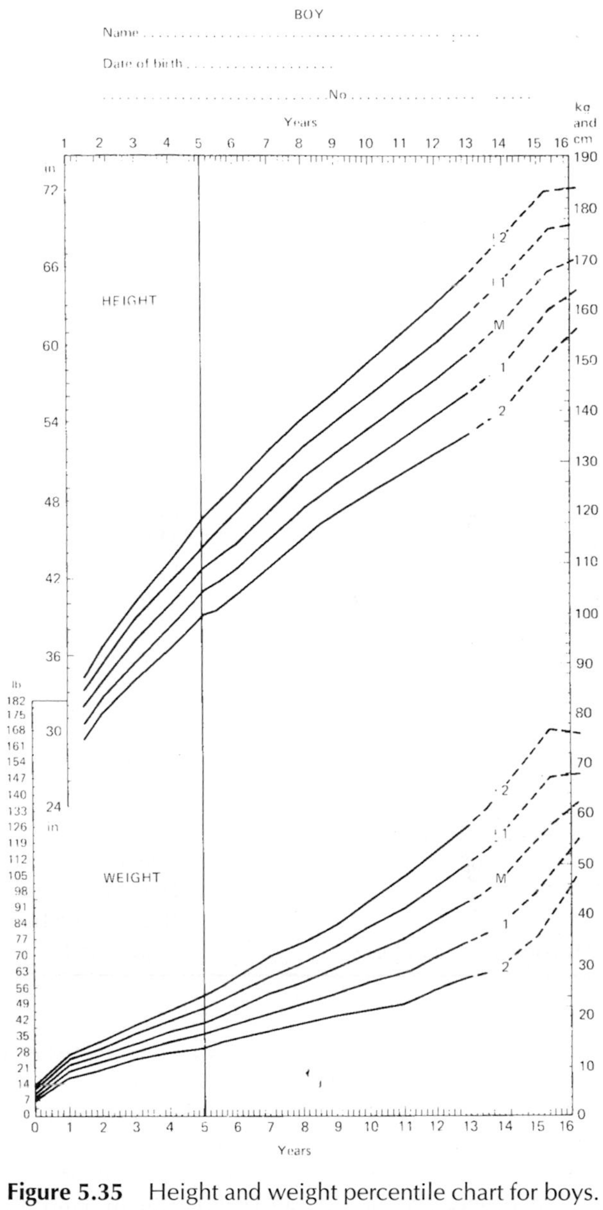

Figure 5.35 Height and weight percentile chart for boys. Each group of five lines shows the mean (M) and values of 1 and 2 standard deviations above (+1 and +2) and below (-1 and -2) the mean. (By courtesy of Dr P.E. Polani and the Paediatric Research Unit, Guy's Hospital Medical School, London)

AETIOLOGY

The usual cause of hypopituitarism is a tumour or cyst (suprasellar cyst) compressing and destroying the gland. In some cases where the dwarfing is already present at birth, there is said to be an aplasia of the gland, or a failure of differentiation of the eosinophil cells.

SKELETAL CHANGES

The growth of all parts of the skeleton is delayed or arrested. The epiphysis remain un-united for a

Table 5.5 Causes of short stature as described by Dr P. H. W. Rayner of Children's Hospital, Birmingham

Familial and congenital dwarfism	Hereditary short stature – commonest cause of referral without symptoms or signs of disease and within the 3rd percentile Syndromes – e.g. achondroplasia, Cushing's syndrome etc., osteogenesis imperfecta, chondro-osteodystrophy Chromosomal disorders – mongolism; Turner's syndrome; gonadal dysgenesis, Bloom's syndrome
Constitutional growth delay	Second most common cause of referral, with a delay of growth or a slow skeletal maturation, but no endocrine disease. Such children tend to enter puberty late but often have a normal pubertal growth spurt and reach a normal adult stature. Height prediction charts are of particular value to reassure the patient and family
Intrauterine growth delay	Low birth weight babies, due to infection (syphilis, toxoplasmosis, cytomegalic inclusion disease), placental abnormality, maternal consumption of alcohol, nicotine or warfarin
Malnutrition	Inadequate calorie intake Malabsorption – coeliac disease. cystic fibrosis of pancreas Specific protein deficiency – kwashiorkor, marasmus, etc.
Hormonal causes	Growth hormone deficiency – hypopituitarism Thyroxine deficiency – cretinism Corticosteroid – drug excess for lung disease Androgen and oestrogen deficiency Psychosocial/emotional deprivation syndrome – the bone age is delayed and some have a transient hypopituitarism with lack of response to growth hormone or adrenocorticosteroid hormone. The drug input presumably has affected the hypothalamus hormone releasing mechanism
Factors disturbing cellular nutrition	Hypoxia (e.g. chronic heart disease) Renal disease Hepatic disease Regional ileitis
Mucopolysaccharidoses	Types I to IV

prolonged period, and the metaphysis terminates in a line of dense bone. The histological change is an absence of division of the cartilage cells in enchondral bone, and absence of division of the primitive connective-tissue cell in the membranous bones.

Histologically there is an absence of division of cartilage cells in endochondral bone and failure of division of the primitive connective tissue cells and membranous bone.

TREATMENT

Once the diagnosis of growth hormone deficiency is established, treatment may be begun by growth hormone replacement therapy. In 1985 three cases of Creutzfeldt–Jakob disease were reported which might have been due to slow virus contamination of the growth hormone preparation. As a result pituitary human growth hormone has been withdrawn. Recombinant growth hormone is now the treatment of choice for these cases.

Human growth hormone has been used since 1958 to treat short stature secondary to hypopituitarism. Such therapy has been steadily developed and with the availability of recombinant human growth hormone (HGH), more short children and Turner's syndrome are being treated.

There is still no long term study showing the efficacy of administering growth hormone is 'normal' short children, nor indeed in non-growth-hormone deficient children. In the latter group there may be a falling away of the initial gain. Side effects, i.e. involving loss of fat mass and increase in lean body – a lipolytic and anabolic effect of recombiant growth hormone – have been observed and are concerning.

However, it is also being used in other conditions of short stature, e.g. bone dysplasia, steroid-induced growth disturbance in juvenile theumatoid arthritis and in chronic renal failure. In adults its ability to convert catabolic states, e.g. after major operations or malnutrition, into anabolic states is proving of benefit although expensive and the effects upon haemostasis, blood pressure and glucose metabolism require careful monitoring. At the dosage of 25–50 μg/kg per day which is markedly below that produced by patients with acromegaly (50–1000 μg/kg per day) it is slightly higher than usual levels produced by normal persons.

Ismail and Scanlon (1993) have described that there it acts as a dual effector, stimulating both the local synthesis of insulin-like growth factors (IGF-1) by the liver as well as the local differentiation of precursor cells to committed IGF sensitive cells. Therefore it is acting as an autocrine or paracrine agent. IGF-1 inhibits growth hormone (GH) secretion at the hypothalamus level by stimulating somatostatin secretion and at the pituitary level. GH function is particularly active during prepubertal years, in gonadal development – both in ovaries and in the testes – thus augmenting the actions of the gonadotrophins as well as effecting the thyroid–pituitary axis. These authors have also described the metabolic effect of GH therapy:

1. On carbohydrate metabolism with insulin antagonistic effects.
2. On lipid metabolism – reducing body fat.
3. On protein metabolism – anabolic with increase in lean mass.
4. On sodium and water metabolism with retention and oedema.
5. On mineral metabolism – causing calcium and phosphorus retention, reduced urinary calcium secretion, increase in osteocalcin, type I procollagen and alkaline phosphatase.

Congenital hypothyroidism (cretinism)

The prominent features are:

1. Signs of mental deficiency.
2. Abnormal genital development.
3. Disturbances in growth.

Thyroid hormone deficiency decreases the rate of longitudinal growth and if the onset is at or before birth this causes mental retardation. The short stature of the cretin is due to delayed ossification and retardation of growth and skeletal maturation (Figure 5.36). The long bones are short, while ossification of the skull is delayed and the fontanelle closes late. The root of the nose is depressed from defective growth of the base of the skull. The vault of the skull may appear large in comparison with the body. The retardation of long bone growth leads to an increased ratio of the upper to lower segment.

The principal skeletal changes are the late appearance of the epiphyses and of bones whose ossific nuclei develop after birth and the delayed union of the epiphyses.

Histologically there is arrest of both enchondral and subperiosteal new bone formation due to failure of cartilage proliferation and of osteoblastic activity.

Tall stature (gigantism)

When growth – both longitudinal as well as by accretion – is increased proportional to that of normal during adolescence and when the epiphyses continue to grow and fail to close, the syndrome of tall stature or gigantism is found.

The common causes are hyperpituitarism, cerebral gigantism, arachnodactyly and Marfan's syndrome, homocystinuria, chromosomal abnormalities of the XXY/XYY types, and the constitutional or familial type in otherwise healthy individuals. It is the last group which produces the most psychosocial problems in both the child and the parents. These are added to sometimes by the serious physical and economic handicaps which these children have to endure.

Hyperpituitarism begins before the epiphyses

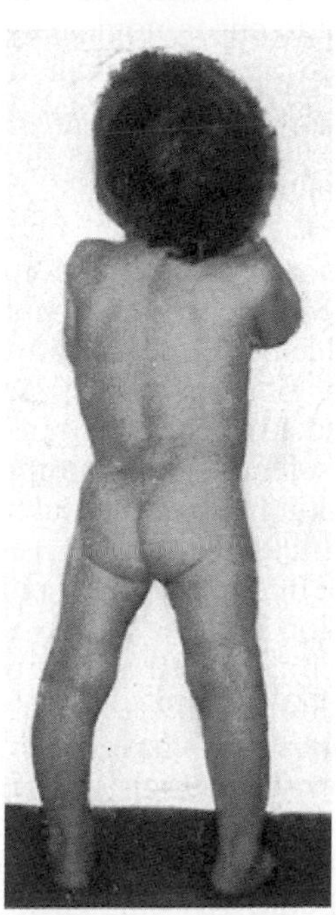

Figure 5.36 The back of a 5-year-old cretin girl who had the general skeletal measurements of a child of 2 years. She had an obvious genu varum deformity and difficulty in walking.

have fused with the shaft, and there is an increase in the rate of epiphyseal growth as well as in the maturation of the skeleton. There is also thickening of the jaw. The mental development is subnormal, and the body strength often surprisingly slight. In the majority of cases some of the features of acromegaly develop later.

PATHOLOGY

The bones of the skeleton show increased thickness and length; the membrane bones are also hypertrophied.

At the epiphyseal cartilage growth of the cartilage cells is active, but the orderly palisade arrangement is lost, the cells being arranged in irregular groups. The amount of matrix is increased. The number of vascular buds and the number of advancing osteogenic mesenchymal cells are increased, so osteogenic activity is maximal.

In the subperiosteal area, as in the membrane bones, the osteogenic cells show increased proliferation, and there is rapid new bone formation. The layers of bone may be more irregular as well as more numerous than normal.

Children of exceptionally tall parents are likely to have an ultimate height above the normal range. Such children will be tall for their age and will exhibit high growth velocity despite their bone age being equivalent to chronological age.

Some children are taller than their peers with advanced bone age and a normal growth velocity. These children will usually have an ultimate height within the normal range.

Accurate prediction of final height based upon estimation of bone age from a hand radiograph using either the Greulich–Pyle radiographic atlas (mainly from black children) or a more recent atlas by Tanner and Whitelaw (derived from Anglo-Saxon stock) and a measurement of standing height is still not a scientific end point. This can be improved by taking serial measurement over 2 or more years. Difficulties are that very rarely is the excessive height due to a disease rather than part of a normal variation and the family's concern especially the mother's, as well as that of the patient, is pre-eminent (Editorial 1992).

Normann *et al.* (1991) have described successful height reduction in 539 girls whose final height prediction was greater than 2.5 standard deviations above the mean (> 181 cm) – the average height in Scandinavians being 164 cm. Their treatment regimen consisted of three different dosages of ethinyloestradiol over 15 years – varying between 0.5 mg, 0.25 mg and 0.1 mg daily. There was no significant difference in gaining reduction by about 3 cm per year with any of the dosages. Treatment was most successful if started before the age of 12 years. Short-term side-effects were described – nausea, increase in weight, pigmentation, leg cramps transient hypertension, hyperlipidaemia, glucose sensitivity. Some of these may give rise to long-term effects but fertility is not believed to be impaired.

Cerebral gigantism (Sotos' syndrome)

Children with this syndrome are usually above the 90th centile for weight and height at birth and grow rapidly for the first few years, after which the rate decreases towards normal, although stature remains tall. Characteristic features include a large head, prominent forehead, large ears and coarse facial features. Skeletal maturation is accelerated and there is usually mental retardation.

See Sotos *et al.* (1977).

Marfan's syndrome

See Chapter 4.

Homocystinuria

This is a rare disorder which is inherited as an autosomal recessive. It is due to a defect in the enzyme cystathionine synthetase which leads to a block in the conversion of homocysteine to cystathionine. Accumulated homocysteine is converted to homocystine and increased amounts may be detected in plasma and urine by the nitroprusside test.

There are a number of different subvarieties of homocystinuria.

The clinical manifestations of the condition include musculoskeletal abnormalities resembling Marfan's syndrome and mental retardation. Dislocation of the lens is characteristic. Skeletal abnormalities include scoliosis, widening of the epiphyses and metaphyses of long bones with flattening of the vertebrae. The femoral head may appear large with an abnormal shaped neck. The skeletal abnormalities are progressive and are not present at birth.

Venous and arterial thromboses are common and the skin may be thin with a malar flush.

The differential diagnosis is from Marfan's syndrome which may be made by the demonstration of homocystine in the urine.

A proportion of cases respond to treatment with piridoxine (vitamin B_6). However, it is not clear whether correction of the biochemical defect in this way will improve or prevent progression of the skeletal manifestations of the condition.

Chromosomal abnormalities

Patients with Klinefelter's syndrome tend towards tall stature, although this is not invariable. Patients with extra Y chromosomes (XYY) have greater than average adult heights. They have normal birth lengths but higher than normal growth rates.

Pituitary gigantism

If a growth hormone-secreting pituitary adenoma occurs before epiphyseal fusion, the result is an increase in the rate of epiphyseal growth with overgrowth of the soft tissue. Mental development is subnormal and in the majority of cases some of the physical features of acromegaly such as enlargement of the jaw and thickening of the hands and feet will develop later in the disease.

Syndromes of sexual procosity

Early onset of secretion of sex hormones will lead to an increase in growth velocity. Bone age will be advanced and puberty will be early. Early closure of growth plates may lead to reduction in the ultimate adult height.

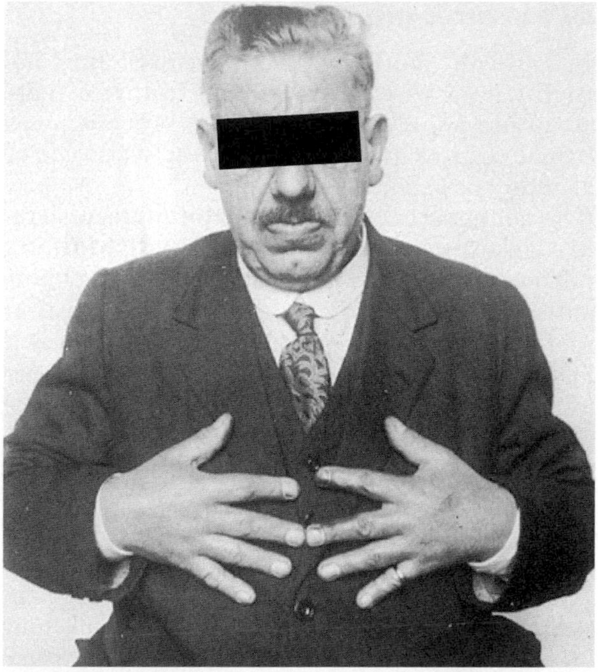

Figure 5.37 An elderly male with acromegaly, showing the increase in skull size and the marked increase in the size of the hands, and very thick lips.

Acromegaly

AETIOLOGY

When excessive growth hormone secretion occurs after the growth plates have fused, gigantism cannot occur. However, features of acromegaly are seen. The commonest cause of excessive growth hormone secretion is a growth hormone secreting eosinophilic adedoma within the anterior pituitary. Occasionally ectopic growth hormone will be produced by a malignant tumour elsewhere, particularly the lung, ovary, breast or pancreas. Growth hormone releasing factor can also be produced by carcinoid tumours or pancreatic islet-cell tumours.

PATHOLOGY

There are deposits of porous bone in the alveolar margins of the jaw, leading to elongation of the face and projection of the chin. The ramus of the jaw is narrow and elongated. Similar deposition occurs in the malar bones and the vault of the skull may be thickened (Figure 5.37). Changes within the skull begin and are most marked in the frontal bone and occasionally osteomata grow from the inner table of the skull. The foramen magnum is normally displaced forward and the pituitary fossa is enlarged from the presence of the adenoma or hyperplastic eosinophilic cells. The thorax is massive due to increased rib length which is partly the result of exaggerated bone growth and partly due to pulmonary hypertrophy.

In the long bones the most obvious changes are found in the extremities which are massive and less well modelled than normal. Muscular insertion in tuberosities is often accentuated and the bone is perhaps longer and thicker than normal.

The short long bones are thick and usually elongated with prominent muscular and tendinous insertions and lipping of the articular ends.

Within the vertebral column deposits of new subperiosteal bone are seen which are thickest on the anterior surface of the body and tail off towards the vertebral canal. Cervicothoracic kyphosis is common.

Increased bone growth only occurs to a large degree in bones subject to repeated stresses and strains so that the cranial vault bones whose growth depends on the size of the brain are little affected. In the late stages of acromegaly bone atrophy may replace the hypertrophy of the earlier phases.

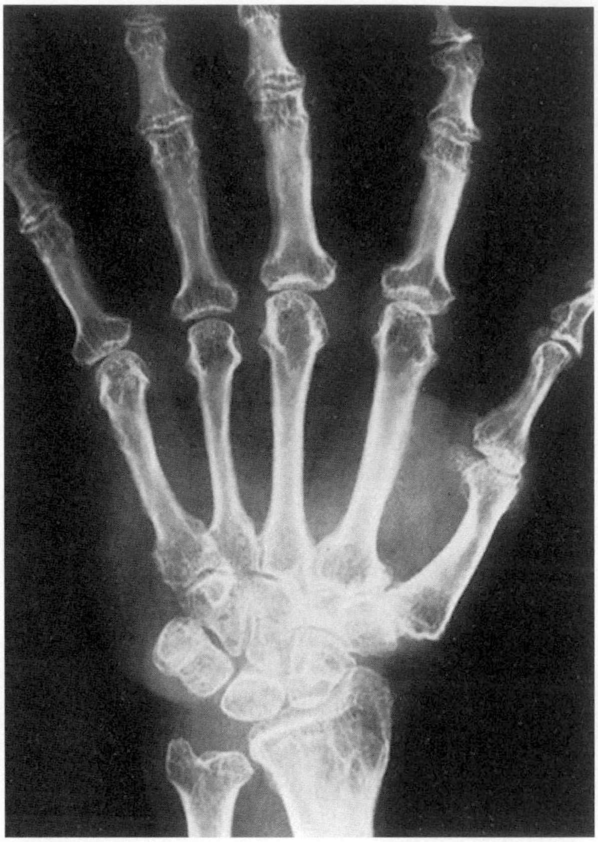

Figure 5.38 Arthritis in a patient with acromegaly. Note also the osteoporosis and bony distortion.

Acromegalic arthritis

This may affect the limb or spinal joints. It is caused by subchondral bone deposition which compresses and progressively thins the articular cartilage, producing the secondary changes of osteoarthrosis (Figure 5.38).

HISTOLOGY

There is excessive periosteal new bone formation and thickening of the trabeculae of cancellous bone. There is particular evidence of new bone formation at the site of muscular or tendinous insertions where traction is applied to the bone.

TREATMENT

The objectives of therapy are to restore growth hormone levels to normal. Local surgical treatment of the adenoma by transsphenoidal hypophysectomy is often effective. An alternative is external irradiation of the pituitary fossa. Yttrium-90 implantation may also be used. In patients where surgical or radiotherapy is inappropriate bromocriptine administration will be effective in approximately 75% of cases.

Orthopaedic treatment may include epiphyseodesis in growing children or predicted tall stature or, rarely, excisional osteotomy in young adults who may be excessively tall.

Leg length discrepancy

There is a physical as well as psychological handicap to the individual or family when there is *excessive tallness*, e.g. acromegaly, or *shortness*, e.g. achondroplasia, or unequal leg lengths of more than 5 cm. This difference can produce marked asymmetry with spinal rotation but there is still no study to prove that leg length discrepancy produces back pain. See Chapter 6.

Short people and/or leg discrepancy

In adults anyone below the height of 1.4 m in women and 1.5 m in men are thought to be abnormal and tend to be treated as if they were children. They tend to become reclusive and withdrawn from most social activities, although in their own circle they are very mobile and appear to be 'normal'. The symmetrical disorder type, e.g. achondroplasia, is now being operated upon using techniques which have proved to be successful in asymmetrical disorders, e.g. congenital hypoplasia of femur or tibia or acquired disorders, i.e. epiphyseal arrest after trauma or after infection, after poliomyelitis or osteomyelitis and after joint infection. Leg lengthening is increasing in popularity.

Lengthening a deformity is correcting it rather than merely compensating (by shortening). It corrects the patient's stature and greater lengths can be achieved than by shortening techniques. However, lengthening still has more complications, it is not as simple and it is lengthy, time consuming and very demanding on the patient as well as his/her family.

Although periosteal division or stripping can lead to increased longitudinal growth with increase in bone length up to 2 cm, it is usually carried out in children with slight discrepancies and usually combined with other orthopaedic procedures, e,g. corrective osteotomies and tenotomies. Open osteotomy with distraction in the early 1900s (Codivilla in 1905, Putti in 1921 and Abbot in 1927) and has steadily been improved by modern technology (see Chapter 6).

The osteotomy through the disphysis is carried out without damaging surrounding tissues, e.g. blood vessels, periosteum, circumferentially by drilling and an external fixator distractor is applied.

Epiphyseolysis or physeal distraction is now used and involves inserting screws on each side of the epiphyseal plate, between which a distraction force is applied, disrupting the plate. Up to 7 cm has been achieved but as in other forms of lengthening very careful assessment of predicted growth is essential because of permanent damage to the growth plate as well as stiffness in knee and ankle joints, sepsis, loss of alignment, etc. which have all been reported.

Callotasis, which is lengthening by distraction of the consolidating callus at the osteotomy site, is also now also being used with some success. A dynamic axial fixator is applied and as the osteotomy heals, distraction is set up about the tenth day.

Tall people and/or leg length discrepancy

Tall people and/or leg discrepancy increase may arise symmetrically from congenital causes, e.g. Marfan's syndrome, or from endocrine conditions, e.g. pituitary adenoma, or asymmetrically involving a single limb, e.g. hyperplasia of femur or tibia or epiphyseal plate disorders.

Leg shortening is by open osteotomy, percutaneous epiphyseodesis in growing children and is the method of choice, where there is 2–5 cm leg length discrepancy in skeletally immature patients. It is reliable, easy to perform with about 10% complications of angulation or abnormal growth.

Open osteotomy with removal of up to 6 cm of femoral bone subtrochanterically, or 2–3 cm of tibial bone, can be carried out in single bone or bilaterally in young adults. Greater shortening will produce bunching of soft tissues, difficulty in closing the wound, infection, non-union or asymmetric fusion with breakage of screws or plate or rod of the internal fixation method. It must be remembered that these are all potential complications involving the good leg. Measurement of quadriceps strength has shown a 90% recovery of quadriceps muscle strength with 5 cm of shortening but less with greater lengths of shortening (see Chapter 6).

HAEMOPOIETIC SYSTEM

Diseases affecting this system have profound effects on bone structure and function.

Leukaemia

The leukaemias are neoplastic disorders characterized by uncontrolled proliferation of haemopoietic cells which result in replacement of normal bone marrow and often infiltration of other organs. The leukaemias are normally divided into acute and chronic by their pattern of behaviour with time and as myeloid or lymphatic according to their pattern of differentiation.

Bony lesions may be found in any part of the skeleton, although they are most commonly seen in the metaphyseal regions around the knee and shoulder. The skull is rarely involved.

On x-rays, the characteristic lesion is a radiolucent zone adjacent to the metaphysis, but there may be a diffuse spotty osteolysis with vertebral collapse and deformity as well as abnormal periosteal ossification. The metaphyseal radiolucent zone is not specific for these diseases, but is seen in numerous unrelated conditions such as prolonged immobilization of the limb or in scurvy.

The main differentiation is from juvenile rheumatism; both may present as a polyarticular 'arthritis' with pain, swelling, and loss of movement.

Treatment with ACTH and antimitotic drugs or with bone marrow transplantation has been successful in these diseases.

Myeloma

Myeloma is a neoplasm of mesenchymal bone marrow cells which differentiate uncontrollably into a plasma cell line. The majority of myelomas therefore secrete a monoclonal paraprotein consisting either of a whole or part of an immunoglobulin. It is possible to classify myelomas according to their secreted paraprotein; however, there is little clinical difference between the subclasses when analysed in this fashion.

The disease most commonly effects the skull and vertebrae, ribs, pelvis, femur and humerus and the bones of peripheral parts of the limbs are relatively spared (Figures 5.39 and 5.40).

Two common types of tumour are found:

1. *Solitary myeloma.* Here the cells frequently resemble plasma cells and produce a localized medullary area of bone destruction. It has been confused with other cystic lesions. Very few cases have been reported in the literature and they usually become multiple with the passage of time. Treatment is by x-irradiation, as surgical curettage may lead to its dissemination.

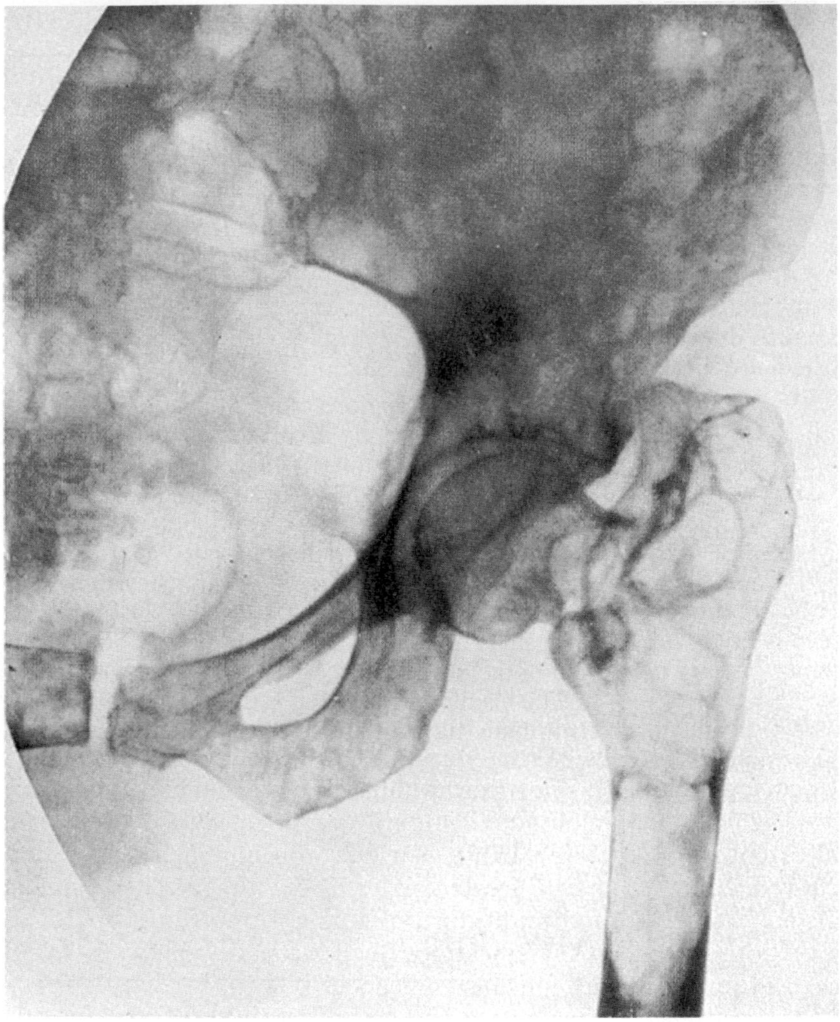

Figure 5.39 Radiograph of the pelvis and upper femora, showing multiple myelomatosis with marked loculated radiolucent areas extending throughout the medulla and cortex but no expansion of the shaft. There is an obvious transcervical fracture through the neck of the femur and the ilium is also involved.

2. *Multiple myeloma.* This is a rare disease characterized by the development – on many parts of the skeleton – of swellings, varying in size from a bean to an orange (Figure 5.39).

PATHOLOGY

The affected bones show replacement of their marrow by grey or reddish-grey tumour masses which tend to be circumscribed and oval in shape. The bone trabeculae and adjacent cortex are completely destroyed, and there is no reactive new bone formation, so the tumours bear a close resemblance – on inspection as well as on radiological examination – to diffuse carcinomatosis. Haemorrhage with cyst formation is common; pathological fracture is frequent and often precedes extension of the tumour to the soft parts overlying it. When the disease is extensive, there may be gross restriction of the absolute amount of red marrow, and so anaemia arises.

Myelogenous tumours are most commonly encountered in the skull and vertebrae (Figure 5.40), ribs, pelvis, femur and humerus, but the bones of the peripheral parts of the limbs are only occasionally the site of disease. In many instances small lesions can only be demonstrated radiologically. The sternum frequently contains tumours, and sternal puncture in consequence may be a valuable diagnostic procedure. It is difficult to be certain whether we are dealing with something which is multicentric in origin, or is evidence of widespread metastases arising early from a single primary focus. The disease is closely related to the leukaemias but a point of distinction is made that in the leukaemias, unlike myelomatosis, the plasma cell is rarely the predominant type.

It is now realized that myelomatosis is a malignant disease – the cells of which produce measurable

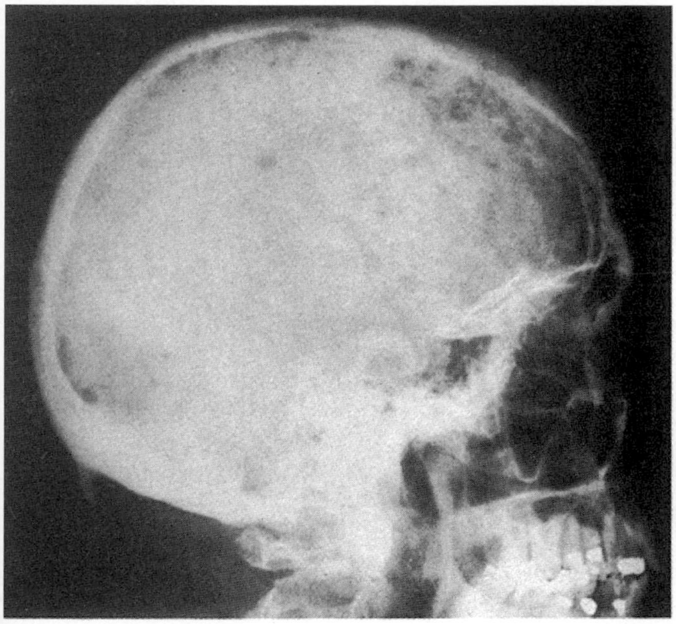

(a)

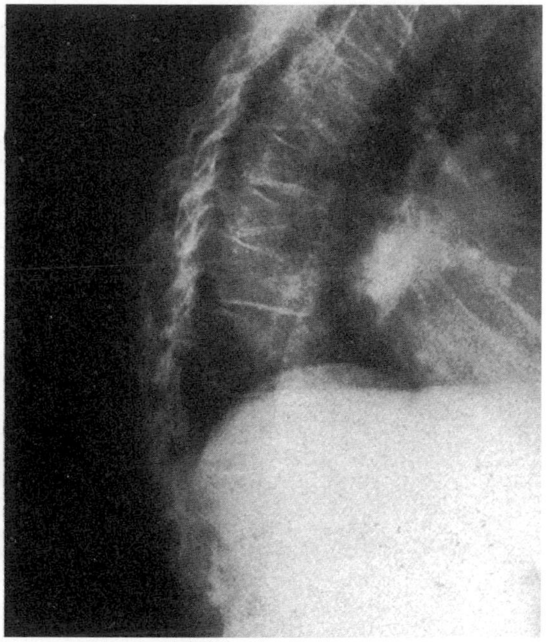

(b)

Figure 5.40 (a) Radiograph of the skull of a patient with numerous translucent areas due to multiple myeloma. (b) Radiograph of the thoracolumbar spine of an elderly individual with diffuse multiple myelomatosis producing several compression fractures of vertebral bodies in the mid-thoracic and thoracolumbar junction.

amounts of metabolites (e.g. serum paraproteins such as IgA, IgG or IgM). This condition can be differentiated from extramedullary plasmacytoma. Wiltshaw (1971) has shown the majority of plasmacytomata present as a tumour of the upper respiratory tract and its spread is more like that of a reticulum cell sarcoma (e.g. early invasion of lymph nodes). That author believes that the solitary myeloma is merely an unusual form of myelomatosis.

HISTOLOGY

The microscopical appearance of the tumour is very variable and the most common cell type seen resembles the plasma cell, but in other cases cells suggestive of myeloblasts, lymphoblasts or, occasionally, fibroblasts have been observed (Figure 5.41).

In myelomatosis metabolic disturbance is common, the blood calcium is raised and there is a hyperproteinaemia, the globulin being raised. In 50% of patients, globulin (Bence Jones protein) is present in the urine, a fact which, however, can also occur in leukaemia, skeletal carcinomatosis and, rarely, in nephritis.

Amyloid deposits in muscles and joints have been described in 10% of cases of myelomatosis and are particularly common when large amounts of globulin are present in the urine. Renal insufficiency is another frequent complication and is believed to be due to plugging of the renal tubules by globulin casts, and the cortex may be eroded from the marrow surface. There is rarely bone reaction or ossification around the osteolytic areas with only a slight amount of callus being seen around a pathological fracture. In the spine, it is difficult to differentiate it from osteoporosis with or without collapse.

In certain myelomata when the tumour is sectioned the cut surface exhibits a bright green colour which is due to a pigment, the character of which is not fully understood. The colour rapidly fades. To this group of tumours the name of chloroma has been given.

Backache as an initial symptom is noteworthy, and the condition should be borne in mind as the cause of such symptoms in the elderly, especially in the presence of osteoporosis and where the pain is not relieved by rest. Fever may be observed in the course of the disease; pathological fracture is not infrequent and egg-shell crackling may be noted on examining the individual lesion. While the lungs are not usually involved, death as a rule occurs from visceral metastases.

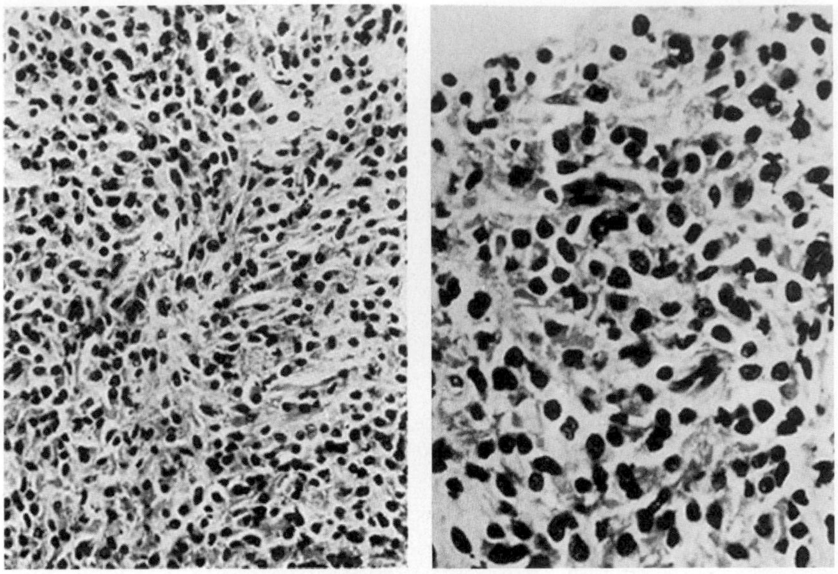

(a) (b)

Figure 5.41 Photomicrographs: (a) of multiple myeloma tissue, showing the uniform cellular appearance but some pleomorphism (× 250, H & E); (b) showing the same cells with a dense nuclear membrane and clumped chromatin material (× 465).

CLINICAL FEATURES

The peak incidence of myeloma is in the seventh decade and it is slightly more frequent in men. The majority of patients will present with skeletal pain commonly affecting the back or ribs and a history of acute pain may indicate a vertebral fracture. Some patients present with a vague history of malaise and occasionally the disease is found incidentally as a result of haematological, renal or radiographic investigation.

Hypercalcaemia is associated with widespread bone disease, particularly if the patient is immobilized due to pain or a fracture.

Approximately 50% of patients show some evidence of renal impairment due to laying down of casts of immunoglobulin-like chains within the glomeruli. The degree of apparent renal insufficiency may be exaggerated at the time of presentation by dehydration and hypercalcaemia. In chronic cases amyloidosis may further impair renal function.

If sufficient paraprotein is present in the blood to raise the plasma viscosity significantly, neurological symptoms may occur.

The presence of the paraprotein may be detected in the urine as 'Bence Jones protein' and in the blood as a monoclone. Because of the large amount of excess protein in the blood, plasma viscosity and erythrocyte sedimentation rate may be markedly elevated.

RADIOGRAPHIC FEATURES

The classic radiographic appearance is of numerous punched-out lytic lesions in the skull, the vertebral column, ribs, pelvis and proximal long bones (Figures 5.39 and 5.40). Characteristically there is no evidence of periosteal reaction to the deposits.

DIAGNOSIS

The diagnosis of myeloma is suspected on the basis of radiographic appearances and markedly elevated plasma viscosity or erythrocyte sedimentation rate and is confirmed by the finding of a monoclone in the blood or the Bence Jones protein in the urine.

TREATMENT

Solitary plasmacytomas may be treated by radiotherapy. Multiple myeloma is treated by chemotherapy with adjunctive local radiotherapy as necessary.

Orthopaedic treatment will consist of supportive measures for bone pain and appropriate treatment of pathological fractures. As far as possible the patient should not be immobilized because of the risk of hypercalcaemia.

PROGNOSIS

Multiple myeloma is a progressive malignant condition. Although chemotherapy may temporarily control the condition, sooner or later it will escape control and death is ultimately due to the complications of the condition.

Solitary myeloma

Rarely, cases have been described of solitary lesions of bone in which, on careful examination, the histological picture has been that of a myeloma typical of the plasmacyte type and in which other lesions have not been demonstrated. Cases of this character in which the local lesion has been resected or treated by irradiation have survived without evidence of recurrence or of other foci developing elsewhere in the skeleton, and accordingly it is now accepted that solitary myeloma constitutes a definite disease entity. The condition is almost invariably found as the result of pathological fracture and the diagnosis made only after histological study.

Haemolytic anaemia

Both Mediterranean (or Cooley's) anaemia and sickle cell anaemia produce bone marrow changes in the vertebral bodies, but most prominently in the bones of the skull and face. The skull shows a striking picture similar to periosteal 'sunray' formation and is called 'brush skull' (Figure 5.42). Lucent areas in the shafts of long bones are also interspersed with areas of increased radiodensity.

It is caused by an abnormality of haemoglobin due to a single amino acid substitution (VALine for GLUtamic acid) at position 6 of the β chain of globin, and is inherited as an autosomal recessive. Above 8–10% of the US black population have sickle trait

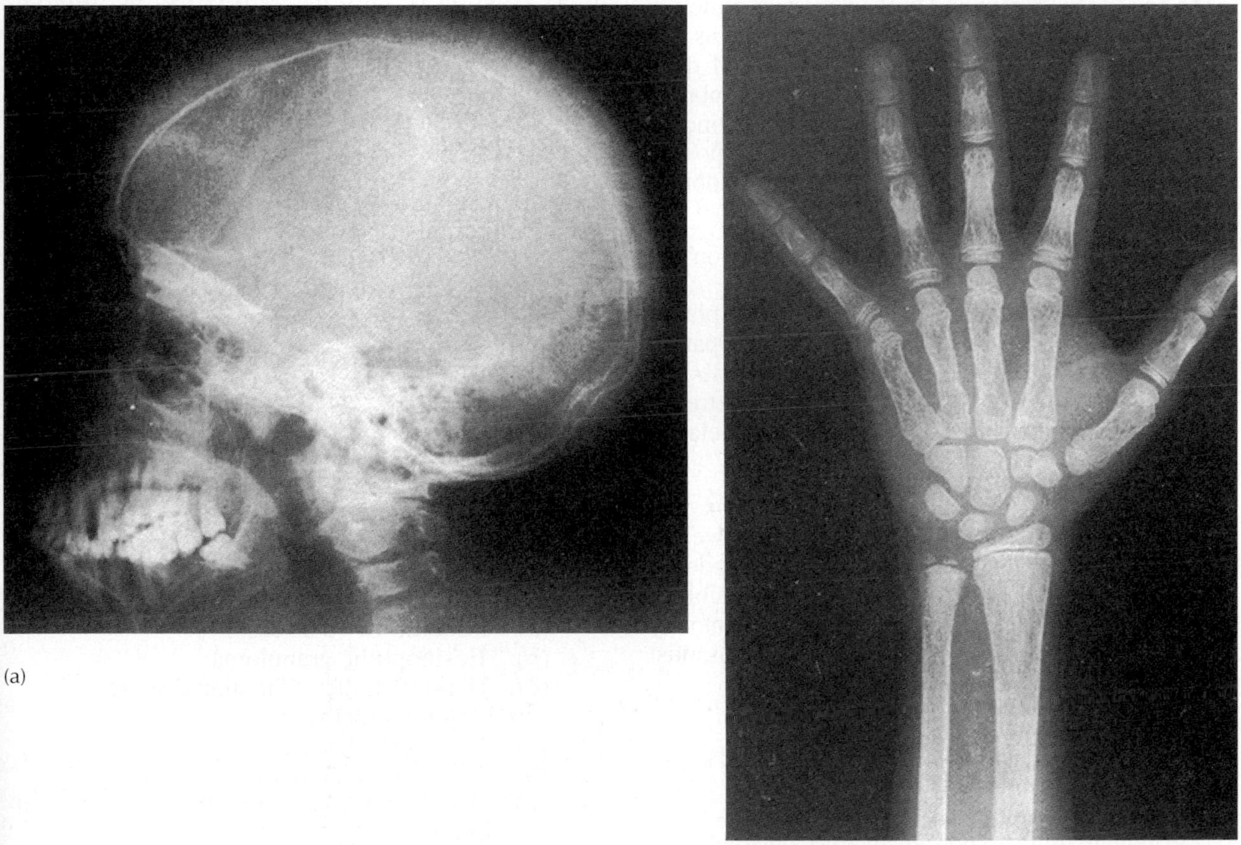

(a) (b)

Figure 5.42 (a) Radiograph of the skull of a child with Cooley's anaemia, showing the marked sunray formation or 'brush' skull, particularly involving the outer diploë. (b) Radiograph of the hand of the same patient, showing a stippling involvement of the short miniature bones, the shafts of the radius and ulna, with thinning of the cortex and some irregularity of outline, particularly in the hand. The epiphyseal lines appear normal.

(i.e. are heterozygotes) and up to 40% of some African populations are heterozygotes – the gene in single dose appears to confer relative protection against falciparum malaria.

The pathological changes are produced by haemoglobins being less soluble than HbA (normal) when in the deoxygenated state. The rigid malformed sickled cells become trapped in small vascular channels and damage cell membranes, leading to decreased red cell survival, increased viscosity and decreased flow (sludging), and hence directly and indirectly causing local anoxia and thus infarcts.

Clinically these patients present with 'crises' – which are acute self-limiting episodes of pain and fever precipitated by infection, cold, altitude, alcohol or any cause of circulatory stasis and tissue hypoxia. 'Hand and foot syndrome' may be the earliest bone lesion: swelling, local pain and tenderness in the marrow of tubular bones most distant from the lungs and hence with lowest Po_2 and also most exposed to cold. This results in 'dactylitis'.

A vascular necrosis of juxta-articular bone occurs in the head of the femur and of the humerus, although the cartilage is usually spared in the humerus as it is non-weight-bearing. In the hip, fragments of dead bone, degenerate cartilage and synovial membrane fill the joint – which may eventually fuse. Secondary infection (often *Salmonella*) may be superimposed.

In general, the bone changes in the haemoglobinopathies are due to:

1. Infarction resulting from vascular occlusion due to sickling.
2. Chronic haemolysis with marrow hyperplasia, hence osteoporosis, cortical thinning and pathological fractures. Characteristically sickle cell patients have disproportionately long extremities (delayed epiphyseal closure) and delayed sexual maturation.

Treatment is, in early crisis, hyperbaric oxygen with the administration of low molecular weight dextran and the reversal of any metabolic acidosis. Infections must be treated (e.g. chloramphenicol for salmonella organisms). Total joint replacement may be considered but certain operative precautions must be taken:

1. Maintain adequate Po_2.
2. Prevention of acidosis with alkaline fluids.
3. Correct blood loss with transfusion.
4. Vasodilator drugs.
5. Adequate fluids to prevent haemoconcentration.
6. Warmth to prevent vasoconstriction.
7. Avoid respiratory depressants and no tourniquet should be used.

This subject has been well reviewed by Sennara and Gorry (1978).

The results of total hip joint replacement in patients with sickle cell disease are relatively poor. There is a high incidence of complication, particularly infection and mechanical and septic loosening (Hanker and Amstutz, 1988).

Massive osteolysis – 'disappearing bones'

This disease was first mentioned in the *Boston Medical and Surgical Journal* in 1872, but became of more recent interest from reviews by Gorham and Stout (1955) and Blundell-Jones *et al.* (1958).

The patient is often a young adult with a history of a minor injury who presents with pain, stiffness and swelling of a large joint. X-rays show varying degrees of absence of the bony structures by adsorption, with extension across joint surfaces without any bony reaction (Figure 5.43). It has to be differentiated from severe Sudeck's dystrophy or disuse atrophy of a joint.

Pathology shows replacement of both bone and marrow by a vascular fibrous tissue containing dilated capillaries and other thin-walled blood vessels. Indeed, the tissue has been described as cavernous or sinusoidal vascular tissue. Osteoblasts are few in number, as are osteoclasts.

Its cause is unknown, although it is regarded by some as a haemangiomatous condition, and therefore based upon some vascular disturbance.

Reticulosis

Reticulosis is a disease of bone marrow constituents such as the reticuloendothelial system:

1. Histiocytic granulomatosis:
   (a) Letterer–Siwe disease;
   (b) Eosinophilic granuloma;
   (c) Hand–Schüller–Christian disease.
2. Lipoid granulomatosis:
   (a) Gaucher's disease;
   (b) Niemann–Pick disease;
   (c) Xanthomatosis with hypercholesterolaemia;
   (d) Tay–Sachs disease.

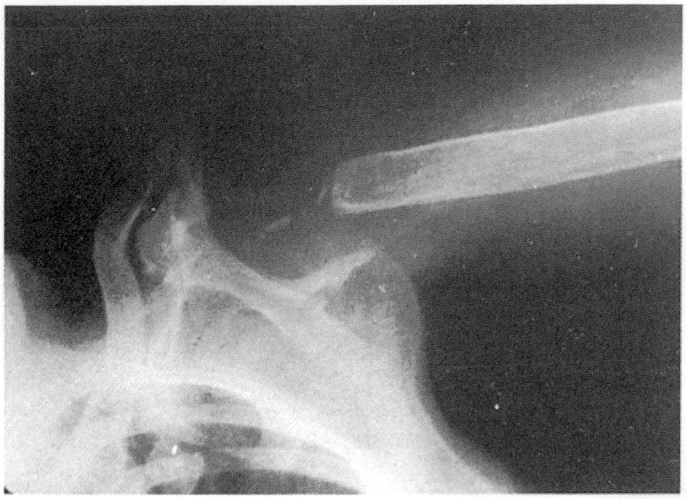

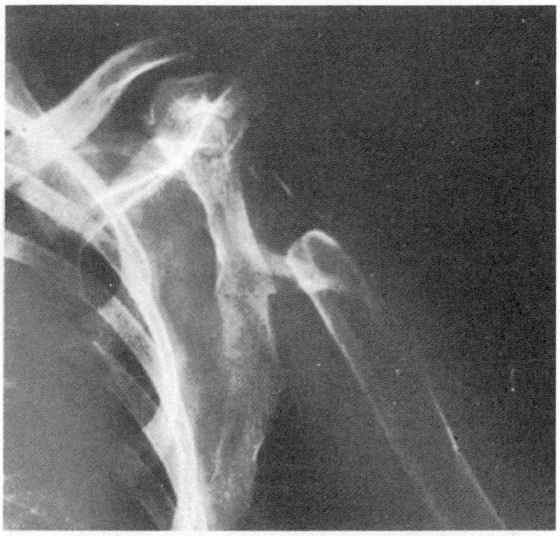

(a) (b)

Figure 5.43 Radiographs of (a) the scapula area and (b) upper left humerus, with complete disappearance of the upper third of the humerus as well as the glenoid area of the scapula. A case of massive osteolysis involving the shoulder joint.

RETICULOENDOTHELIAL DISTURBANCES OF BONE

Among the cells lining the vascular channels of bone marrow are pleuripotent stem cells which have the ability to differentiate into reticuloendothelial cells which possess phagocytic properties. They may also give rise to haemopoietic cells and connective tissue cells, that is fibroblasts, chondroblasts, osteoblasts and synovial cells. While the reticuloendothelial (or mononuclear phagocyte) system is widely dispersed throughout the tissues of the body, most of its content is present in the liver, bone marrow, lymph nodes and spleen.

The functions of the reticuloendothelial system are as yet imperfectly known, but its cells are typically the scavengers of the body, and their activity is concerned mainly with the removal from the circulating fluid of dead and damaged cells, bacteria and other foreign or noxious material. It is also energetic in the disposal of such metabolic substances as haemoglobin and cholesterol.

Red bone marrow consists of blood-forming cells as well as reticuloendothelial ones. Affections of any of these resulting in increased volume or vascularity will result in absorption of the adjacent bony trabeculae. In response to continued strain, new bone is laid down to buttress the weak site. Thus reticuloendotheliosis or diffuse malignant involvement such as Hodgkin's or myeloblastic leukaemia or chloroma will lead to a typical picture. Hodgkin's usually affects the spine, skull and pelvis; leukaemia usually the long bones; and chloroma usually the bones of the orbit.

On the other hand, if the malignant involvement elicits a marked response of mature fibrous tissue, such as scirrhous carcinoma, a sclerosis of bone occurs with a heavier bone formation.

In the adult, the red marrow is confined to irregular or flat bones or to the ends of long bones. It is here that malignant involvement and bony changes first occur.

The reticuloendothelial tissue of bone is – from the nature of it – mainly congregated at the ends of the long bones and in the spongy bone of the flat and short bones, and it most likely shares in the affections to which the system elsewhere is liable.

Histiocytic granulomatosis

The three conditions listed in this section are somewhat rare and obscure but the combined title is preferred because the permanent and constant pathological feature is the presence of numerous histiocytes and granulomatous tissue (Mercer and Duthie, 1956). Farber pointed out in 1941 that an atomically the underlying lesion in eosinophilic granuloma is related to the lesion of Hand–Schüller–Christian disease and that of Letterer–Siwe disease. In the 1970s Jaffe and Lichenstein described these three conditions as different clinicoanatomical expressions of the same disorder.

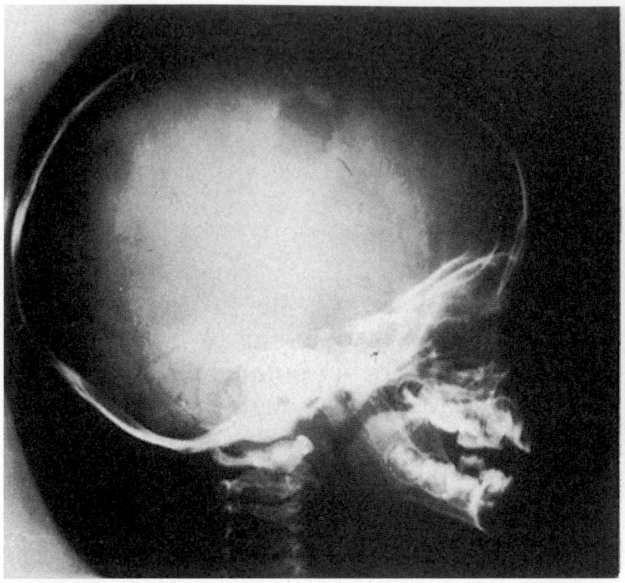

(a)

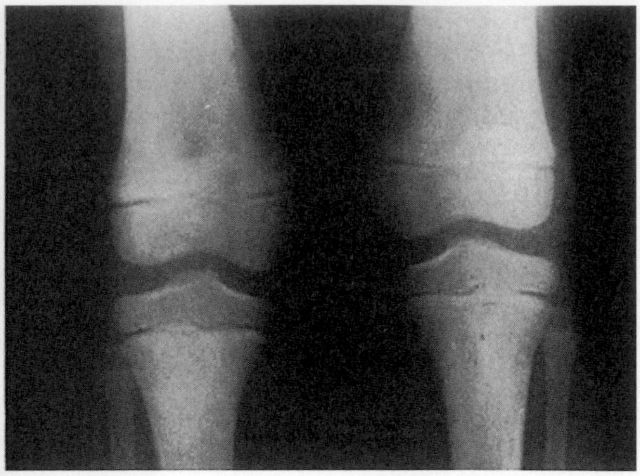

(b)

Figure 5.44 (a) 'Scalloped' skull lesion and (b) failure of tubulation of the long bones in Gaucher's disease in a child.

Lipoid granulomatosis

Disturbances in lipoid metabolism may give rise to a specific pathological change in the reticuloendothelial system in which that part of the system situated in the spongy skeleton may participate. The actual nature of the lipoid whose metabolism is deranged varies, and so a group of different diseases has been described, though in each the underlying mechanism is similar. In Gaucher's disease a lipoprotein of the cerebroside type is at fault (Figures 5.44 and 5.45); in Niemann–Pick disease a phosphatid lipoid; in Tay–Sachs disease a cerebroside protein; and in Hand–Schüller–Christian disease, a cholesterol. In all of these, bone changes have been reported or observed, though the main effects of the disease are wrought on the extra-osseous portions of the reticuloendothelium; but it is only in connection with the Hand–Schüller–Christian disease that the osseous effects have attained a clinical or pathological importance.

PATHOLOGY

Fraser *et al.* (1959) presented a very comprehensive review of the condition, and he suggested that the initial change is one of increased lipoid content in the circulating body fluids. As a result of this increase, and in an attempt to adjust the balance, the reticuloendothelial cells proceed to absorb and deposit the substance, so that accumulation occurs in individual areas. That an excess of cholesterol is the essential

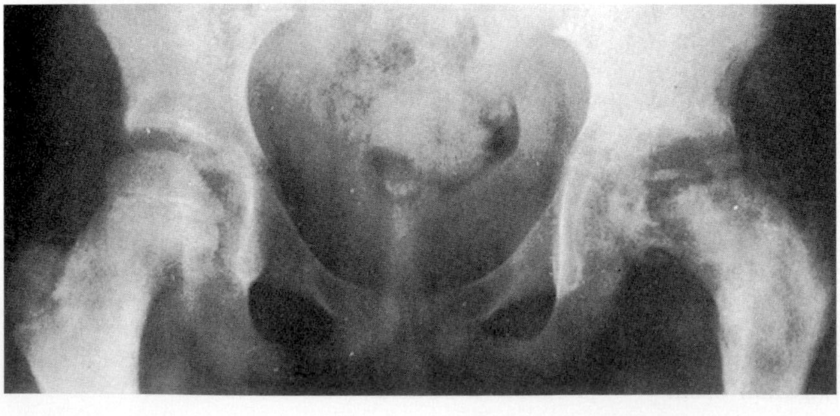

Figure 5.45 Aseptic necrosis of the left capital femoral epiphysis secondary to involvement of the proximal femur in generalized Gaucher's disease.

factor is borne out by the constancy of the hypercholesterolaemia, and Fraser *et al.* suggested that this is the result of a failure on the part of the normal mechanism for maintaining the blood cholesterol content at a constant level. It is surmised that a congenital or acquired deficiency in these tissues throws the onus on the reticuloendothelium elsewhere – especially in bone. In the skeleton, the diploë of the skull, the cancellous tissue of the mandible, clavicle, ribs, pelvis and vertebrae are affected. In addition, the pleura, the lungs, the liver and the cerebellum have been the site of typical deposits. It is apparent that in the skeleton the lesion, though by no means confined to them, tends to favour bones developed in membrane. In this situation, the deposits appear as multiple circumscribed, rounded tumours, which characteristically have a golden-yellow or brownish-yellow colour.

The histology is equally striking. The tumours are composed of large, often multinucleated reticuloendothelial cells, with small nuclei and a finely reticulated cytoplasm. The cytoplasm contains for the most part innumerable globules of lipoid which give the cell a 'foamy' appearance. The largest foam cells are found away from the vessels; round the vessels are arranged smaller reticuloendothelial cells, so that, as Fraser *et al.* demonstrated, the process is evidently one of flow and ebb, the cells congregating round the vessels carrying the excess of lipoid, being charged, and then migrating towards the periphery to make way for others. The presence of the deposits of lipoid excites the production of granulation tissue around the periphery and the granulation tissue may infiltrate widely.

The effect of the granulation tissue on the bones is to cause destruction of the bone without new bone reaction. In the skull this gives rise to large defects with irregular margins, in the midst of which the lipogranulomatous tumours are situated.

The condition in a typical case is well marked on the skull base in the vicinity of the sella turcica. The pituitary gland may be compressed or obliterated and the lipogranulomatous tissue may extend forwards through the superior orbital fissure to collect behind, and protrude, the eyeball. When the collection is marked in the vicinity of the sella, the hypothalamic area of the brain may also be indented. The basisphenoid and the clinoid processes escape.

CLINICAL FEATURES

The disease, as originally described, consisted of a distinctive syndrome – defects in the membranous bones, exophthalmos, and thirst and polyuria (diabetes insipidus). It is to this triad of effects that the term Hand–Schüller–Christian syndrome is applicable. The exophthalmos is the result of the retrobulbar accumulation of lipoid-laden reticuloendothelial cells, while the diabetes insipidus is the sequel to the distortion of the hypothalamus.

In an individual case, however, these striking evidences may be absent until a late stage, while in many cases there are further features. Thus interference with the pituitary may lead to retardation of growth, and the irritation or tension on the dura mater to irritability and restlessness. Should the extraosseous reticuloendothelium be affected, splenomegaly or hepatic enlargement may be present, and in the latter case jaundice may be observed. The blood shows a cholesterol content which may be raised to as much as 7.46 mmol/l (287 mg/100 ml).

DIAGNOSIS

The disease, although at first sight of little more than academic importance, is probably much more common than is realized. The growing number of cases reported in the literature is eloquent witness to this, and Fraser's experience that in two cases an erroneous diagnosis of neoplasm was made, and in one a mutilating and serious operative procedure advised, may well serve to emphasize its clinical significance.

The diagnosis should be based on the age of the child and the characteristic triad of clinical features when present, together with the demonstration of a high cholesterolaemia. In all cases a biopsy should be done to make a definite diagnosis.

PROGNOSIS

The disease tends to be progressive, and in many published cases death has resulted from asthenia, or from the contraction of an intercurrent disease.

TREATMENT

The treatment falls naturally into several distinct parts. An attempt is made to reduce the hypercholesterolaemia by dietetic means. Deep radiotherapy is employed to control the deposits, while in the event of polyuria and thirst from diabetes insipidus, pituitary extract may be exhibited.

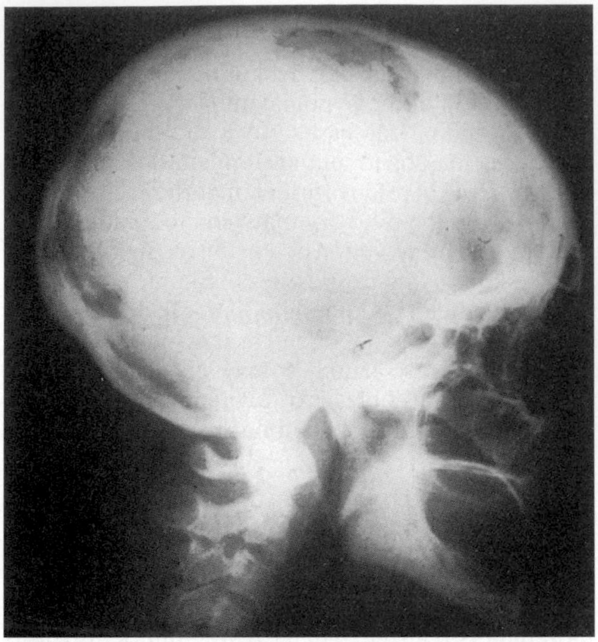

Figure 5.46 Radiograph of a skull of a patient with histiocytic granulomatosis, showing the 'geographical' or scalloped margins of multiple areas of radiolucency involving the outer diploë.

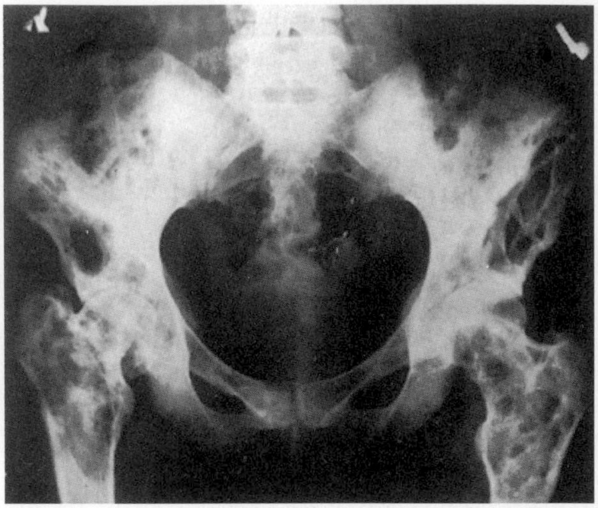

Figure 5.47 Pelvis affected by eosinophilic granulomatosis. The left femoral epiphysis is not involved.

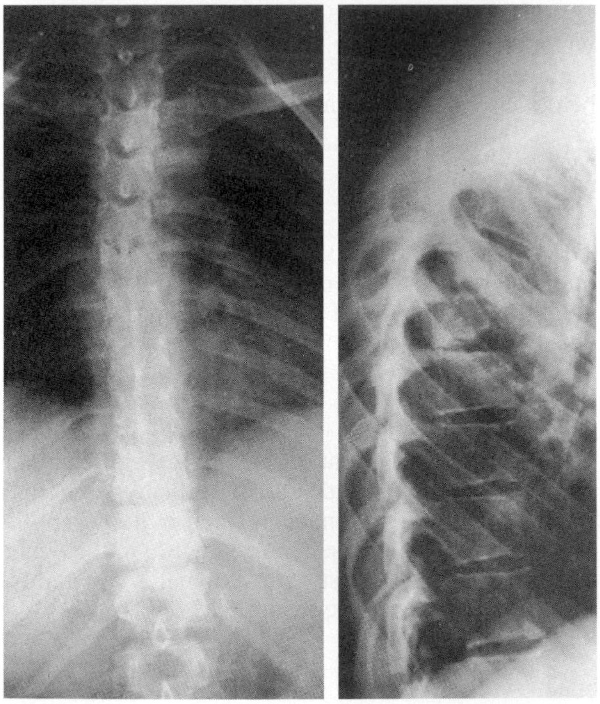

Figure 5.48 Radiographs of a 12-year-old boy, showing the deformed and wedge-shaped body of the sixth thoracic vertebra due to a solitary eosinophilic granuloma with a kyphosis.

Eosinophilic granulomatosis

In this variety a lesion is developed in one or more bones, apparently inflammatory in nature, and closely allied to the lipoid granulomata, though sections reveal an excess of eosinophils and no lipoid deposits.

It is an affection of the young, 64% occurring at under 20 years of age. Its cause is unknown, though it is believed to be an infection or toxin of some sort (Fairbank, 1951). The lesions, usually multiple, affect the skeleton almost exclusively, although in some cases the glands and the lungs may also be involved. The local lesion, though frequently silent, may give rise to local pain and tenderness and even swelling. The illness may be initiated by fever. Where the skull is affected, headache is often a complaint. In such cases a hole in the skull may be felt. Blood examination is not characteristic although eosinophilia may be present with an eosinophil level up to 11%.

The radiological appearance is usually generalized, but varies and may simulate other types of disease. Most commonly the lesion is oval or circular, translucent and cyst-like, as though, indeed, a piece of bone had been removed because of its punched-out and sharply defined appearance. It may be accompanied by some periostitis adjacent to the osteolytic area. The confluences of the translucent areas, particularly in the skull, sometimes give the appearance of the 'geographical' skull (Figure 5.46). In the long bones the lesions are endosteal and usually affect the shafts; only occasionally is one

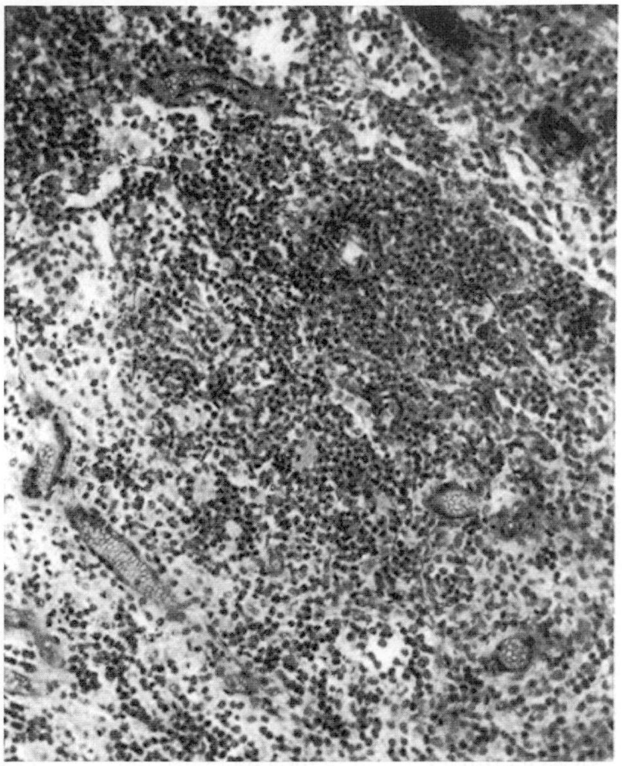

(a)

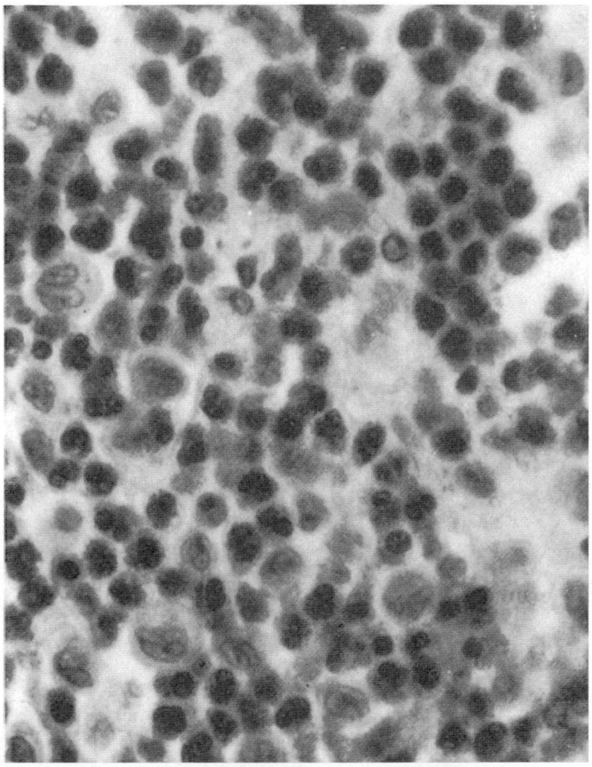

(b)

Figure 5.49 (a) Photomicrograph of an eosinophilic granuloma, showing the marked cellular invasion of small round cells of uniform appearance with numerous vascular spaces. (× 40). (b) Photomicrograph to show the single nucleated but bilobular cells with numerous small particles in the cytoplasm which were brightly eosinophilic. (× 516).

seen in the epiphysis (Figure 5.47). There is nothing characteristic or distinctive and the diagnosis is difficult. Local disease presenting as vertebra plana due to eosinophilic granuloma has been described by Compere *et al.* (1954). Biopsy was carried out in their four cases and demonstrated the typical eosinophilic granulomatous lesion. They emphasized how important it is that an inflammatory lesion must be excluded and that, with rest and splinting, the symptoms may disappear and even the deformed vertebral body may reossify (Figure 5.48). In the Compere *et al.* series only one vertebra was affected and this was completely flattened while the neighbouring discs were of normal appearance. The early x-ray appearance is osteolytic, then the body of the vertebra disappears. Later the body is flattened and dense.

A lesion may resolve spontaneously; it may heal up after curettage without the aid of radiotherapy, or after radiotherapy alone. The experience of those authors is that the affection is very recalcitrant to any form of treatment.

PATHOLOGY

The contents of a relatively early lesion consist of soft brownish granulation tissue which may be streaked with yellow necrotic material. Patches of haemorrhage may be present. Histologically it shows histiocytes, eosinophils in large numbers, leucocytes and large multinuclear giant cells, especially near haemorrhage or necrosis (Figure 5.49). The histiocytes may contain droplets of the neutral fat present in the invaded bone or disintegrated cells.

DIFFERENTIAL DIAGNOSIS

When multiple lesions are present diagnosis from Hand–Schüller–Christian disease is made by the absence of exophthalmos and diabetes insipidus, or on biopsy.

It is distinguished from myelomatosis by the lesions in the skull being larger and less numerous and by the absence of Bence Jones protein in the

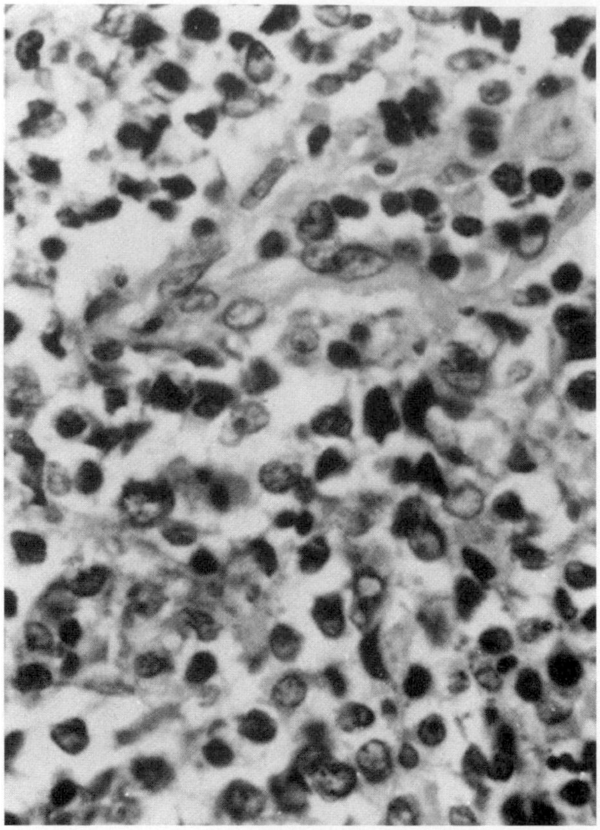

Figure 5.50 Photomicrograph of an H & E preparation from Hodgkin's disease of bone, showing the characteristic Reed–Sternberg cells with overlapping nuclei, 'pencilled' chromatin outline of the nuclear membrane and large nucleoli. Plasmacytes and lymphocytes are also present. (7 × 845).

urine. Polyostotic fibrous dysplasia also has to be excluded.

Letterer–Siwe disease

This very rare condition, a reticuloendotheliosis, is met within infants up to the age of 3 or 4, and is regarded as an acute form of Hand–Schüller–Christian disease. It usually runs a short and rapidly fatal course, without the secondary deposits of cholesterol esters in the cells of the granulomata. The soft tissues, particularly the viscera, are chiefly affected, although in most cases destructive lesions are found in the skeleton. There is a low and progressive anaemia, and lesions are found in the liver and spleen (which are usually enlarged) as well as in glands, lungs, skin and in the bones of the skull. The x-ray picture closely resembles that of Hand–Schüller–Christian disease. If the base of the skull is involved, the characteristic symptoms of this latter disease may develop, although the lesions are without foam cells.

In most cases death ensues within a few weeks. The lesions are of two kinds – nodular and diffuse (Jaffe, 1972). The nodular lesions are found in the lymph glands but also in the spleen, skin and bone marrow. The diffuse lesions are found in the lungs, the dura and in the periosteum overlying a nodular focus. Histologically there is difficulty in distinguishing the condition from the other two forms of histiocytic granulomatosis. The three conditions are compared in Table 5.6.

The bone changes of lymphoma/Hodgkin's disease

Lymphomata may involve the bone either as part of multisystem spread of spleen and lymphatic glands, or as a primary lesion In the latter case the prognosis may be good if the affected part is resected and appropriate adjunctive therapy given. Both sexes are equally involved and age bears no relation to the frequency of the bone changes. Pain is the first indication of osseous spread.

Lesions are most frequently found in the vertebral column and pelvis and within the spine the lumbar vertebrae are most commonly involved. The proximal femur is also a site of predilection while the skull (especially the diploë), distal femur, proximal tibia and the proximal and distal humerus are less commonly affected.

Histologically the lesions are characteristic of lymphomata with variable adjacent bone reaction (Figure 5.50). In the long bones there is often considerable subperiosteal new bone formation but also osteolysis with loss of trabecular pattern leading to fracture of long bones or collapse of adjacent vertebrae. In the ribs complete destruction of the affected segment can be pathognomonic.

TREATMENT

In common with the other lesions of Hodgkin's disease, the bone changes appear to respond to radiotherapy. The pain is relieved and in some cases reparative changes appear in the affected bones. Internal fixation of fractures, or potential fractures, is indicated.

Table 5.6

	Hand–Schüller–Christian Disease	Eosinophilic granuloma	Letterer–Siwe Disease
Age at onset	Early childhood but occasionally in adults	Older children, adolescents and young adults	Infants
Clinical features	Triad of exophthalmos, polyuria + polydipsia, swelling. NB. Other pituitary dysfunction	Pain, swelling and local tenderness. Systemic manifestations of fever; loss in weight	Low fever, pain and swelling. Low-grade anaemia. Short and rapidly fatal course in most cases
Localization	Base of skull, spine, ilium, mandible – most common in 'membranous bones'. Liver and spleen sometimes	72% – solitary lesion involving all bones but mainly ribs, skull, femur, pelvis, humerus. Soft tissues rare	Multiple lesions of liver, spleen, glands, skin, lungs and mainly skull
Pathology	Secondary deposition of cholesterol in 'foam cells' following formation of granulomata. ?Unknown infection	Granulomata formation with histiocytes, eosinophils in large numbers, multinucleated cells and areas of necrosis	Eosinophils + +. Foam cells sometimes present. True reticuloendotheliosis
Radiology	Cannot be differentiated	Cannot be differentiated	Cannot be differentiated
Blood picture	Normal	'Circulating' eosinophilia	Anaemia
Biochemistry	Hypercholesterolaemia in most cases	Normal	Normal
Prognosis	Slow and benign except in 25% of cases	Good but guarded in multiple lesions	Fatal

Sphingolipidoses

These are lysosomal storage diseases in which an enzyme catalysing the intralysosomal breakdown of complex molecules normally derived by endocytosis. The precise abnormality of sphingolipid metabolism differs between the diseases. Table 5.7 shows the names and enzymes defects of some of the better known of these syndromes. It should be noted that they are all rare. In the majority of these conditions bone changes have been reported.

Gaucher's disease

Gaucher's disease presents with skeletal deformities, pathological fractures of the vertebrae or long bone, osteonecrosis of the femoral or humeral head, and an acute, very painful osteonecrosis of the medullary cavity and adjacent cortex of a long bone or the pelvis. Mankin (1993) has reviewed how Brady *et al.* (1965) described that this disease was caused by a specific enzyme deficiency of glucocerebroside hydrolase. The enzyme is responsible for splitting the glycoside bond between a glucose and a ceramide which is usually released from the cell membrane when it dies. The glucocerebroside is not secreted and becomes stored by macrophages or by other reticuloendothelial cells of the spleen, liver, medullary marrow, etc. A significant breakthrough was made by Barton *et al.* (1991) who discovered that when a mannose terminated enzyme Ceredase (Genzyme Corp) was given to Gaucher patients, the glycocerebroside hydrolase enzyme was recognized by a lectin and was transported across the cell membrane to function. Storage of lipid ceased and the amount of lipids in the liver, spleen and marrow significantly decreased with improvement in bone marrow fat and histology, medullary haematopoiesis and increased bone density. With increasing knowl-

Table 5.7

Name	Enzyme deficiency
Farber disease	Ceramidase
Niemann–Pick disease	Sphingomyelinase
Gaucher's disease	Glucocerebroside β-glucosidase
Fabry disease	α-Galactosidase
Tay–Sachs disease	N-β-D-hexosamindase A

edge, gene altering or substitution should be possible.

In Gaucher's disease skeletal symptoms consist of pain and pathological fractures. Bone infarcts are also seen and avascular necrosis of the femoral head may occur. Bone growth and mineralization are deficient and scallop lesions may be seen and there is deficient tubulization of the long bone.

TREATMENT

When only one system is involved spontaneous resolution is usual and supportive therapy may be sufficient. Intralesional steroid injections may control severe pain or prevent loss of function of the vital structure.

In multisystem disease spontaneous resolution can occur. However, if systemic systems are severe or organ failure is present, systemic treatment with corticosteroid is indicated. Antimitotic drugs may also be required.

Intercurrent infection and hormone deficiency will require appropriate therapy.

The skin is frequently affected, producing a maculopapular rash. Involvement of the oral mucosa and the gastrointestinal tract leads to ulceration and may cause malabsorption. Lung function tests are frequently abnormal, although pulmonary symptoms are relatively rare. There is a characteristic honeycomb appearance on chest x-ray which represents lung cysts. These may give rise to spontaneous pneumothoraces if they rupture into the pleura.

The liver and spleen may both be involved by histiocytosis X, resulting in hepatosplenomegaly and regional lymphadenopathy which is normally pain free. Lesions within the brain may involve the pituitary leading to diabetes insipidus with infiltration of the orbital regions leading to exopthalmus.

Any bone may be affected. However, the small bones of the hands and feet are least commonly involved while the skull is the most frequent site (see Figures 5.44 and 5.45). In this situation the deposits appear as multiple circumscribed lucent lesions. They may excite a florid periosteal reaction, particularly in young children, and may heal with a sclerotic margin. Less than half of the bone lesions are painful.

DIAGNOSIS

Clinical diagnosis is difficult due to the wide variety of presentations. An exact diagnosis is normally made by histology.

PROGNOSIS

The prognosis for patients with single system disease is uniformly good. Progression to multisystem disease is rare and mortality extremely uncommon.

In patients with multisystem disease, the prognosis is less good. Approximately 20% or 30% of patients will remit and 10%, particularly those who present with organ failure, will die. The remaining cases enter a chronic course.

References

Ackerman, L.V. (1958) *Journal of Bone and Joint Surgery* **40A**, 279

Albright, F., Smith, P.H. and Richardson, A.N. (1941) Postmenopausal osteoporosis. *Journal of the American Medical Association* **116**, 2465–2474

Atkins, R.M., Duckworth, T. and Kanis, J.A. (1990) Features of algodystrophy after Colles' fracture. *Journal of Bone and Joint Surgery* **72B**, 105–110

Avioli, L.V., Birge, S., Lee, S.W. and Slatopolsky, E. (1968) *Journal of Clinical Investigation* **47**, 2239

Ayers, D.C., Pellegrini, V.D. and Evarts, C. (1991) Prevention of heterotopic ossification in high risk patients by radiation therapy. *Clinical Orthopaedics* **263** 887–8938

Azria, M. and Russell, R.G.G. (1992) Biochemical approaches to the measurement of bone metabolism *in vivo*. *Current Opinion in Orthopedics* **3**, 103–109

Bacorn, R.W. and Kurtzke, J.F. (1953) Colles' fracture: a study of 2000 cases from the New York Compensation Board. *Journal of Bone and Joint Surgery* **35A**, 643–658

Barker, D.J.P., Chamberlain, A.T., Guyer, P.B. and Gardner, M.J. (1980) Paget's disease of bone: the Lancashire focus. *British Medical Journal* **1**, 1107

Barry, H.C. (1980) Orthopaedic aspects of Paget's disease of bone. *Arthritis and Rheumatism* **23**, 1128–1130

Barton, N.W., Brady, R.O., Dambrosia, J.M. *et al.* (1991) Replacement therapy for inherited enzyme deficiency – macrophage-targeted glucocerebroside for Gaucher's disease *New England Journal of Medicine* **324**, 1464–1470

Bickerstaff, D. (1991) Post-traumatic algodystrophy. DM Thesis, University of Sheffield.

Blundell-Jones, G., Midgley, R.L. and Smith, G.S. (1958) Massive osteolysis – disappearing bones. *Journal of Bone and Joint Surgery* **40B**, 494–501

Brenton, D.P., Dow, C.J., James, J.I.P., Hay, R.L. and Wynne-Davies, R. (1972) Homocystinuria and Marfan's syndrome. A comparison. *Journal of Bone and Joint Surgery* **54B**, 277–298

Christiansen, C., Christiansen, M.S. and Transbol, I. (1981) Bone mass in post-menopausal women after withdrawal of oestrogen/gestagen replacement therapy. *Lancet* **1**, 459–461

Christiansen, C. and Rodborough, P. (1985) Does postmenopausal bone loss respond to oestrogen replacement therapy independent of bone loss rate? *Calcified Tissue International* **35**, 720–722

Collins, D.H. (1956) Paget's disease of bone. Incidence and subclinical forms. *Lancet* **2**, 51–57

Compere, E.L., Johnson, W.E. and Coventry, M.B. (1954) *Journal of Bone and Joint Surgery* **36A**, 969

Cooper, C., Barker, D.J.P., Morris, J. and Griggs, R.S.J. (1987) Osteoporosis falls age in fracture of the proximal femur. *British Medical Journal* **295**, 13–15

Cullen, P., Russell, R.G.G., Walton, R.J. and Whitely, J. (1976) Frequencies of HLA-A and HLA-B histocompatability antigens in Paget's disease of bone. *Tissue Antigens* **7**, 55–56

Curtis, J.R., deWardener, H.E., Gower, P.E. and Eastwood, J.B. (1970) *Proceedings of the European Dialysis and Transplant Association* **7**, 141

Cusworth, D.C. and Dent, C.E. (1969) *British Medical Bulletin* **25**, 42

Dekel, S., Ornoy, A., Noff, D. and Edelstein, S. (1979) Contrasting effects on bone formation and on fracture healing of cholecalciferol and of 1α-hydroxycholecalciferol. *Calcified Tissue International* **28**, 245–251

Dent, C.E. and Harris, H. (1956) *Journal of Bone and Joint Surgery* **38B**, 204

Dove, J. (1980) Complete fractures of the femur in Paget's disease of bone. *Journal of Bone and Joint Surgery* **62B**, 12–17

Editorial(1992) Too Tall? *Lancet* **339**, 339–340

Fairbank, T. (1951) *Atlas of General Affections of the Skeleton.* Livingstone: Edinburgh

Francis, M.J.O., Smith, R.N. and Bauze, R.J. (1974) Instability of polymeric skin collagen in osteogenesis imperfecta. *British Medical Journal* **1**, 421–424

Fraser, D., Ceeming, J.M., Cerwerka, E.A. and Keanyers, K. (1959) *American Journal of Diseases of Children* **98**, 586

Gorham, L.W. and Stout, A.P. (1955) *Journal of Bone and Joint Surgery* **37A**, 985

Goutallier, D., Sterkers, Y. and Cadeau, F. (1984) Expérience de la prosthèse totalc au cours de la coxopathie Pagetique. *Rheumatoligie* **36**, 81–82

Greulich, W.W. and Pyle, S.I. (1959) *Radiographic Atlas of Skeletal Development of the Hand and Wrist*, 2nd edn. Stanford University Press: Stanford, CA

Grisso, J.A., Kelsey, J.I., Strom, B.L. and Chio, G.Y. (1991) Risk factors for falls as a cause of hip fractures in women. *New England Journal of Medicine* **324**, 1326–1331

Hanker, G.J. and Amstutz, H.C. (1988) Osteonecrosis of the hip in the sickle cell diseases: treatment and complications. *Journal of Bone and Joint Surgery* **70A**, 499–506

Heyman, G. and Franchimont, P. (1974) Human calcitonin radio immunoacid in normal and pathological conditions. *European Journal of Clinical Investigation* **4**, 213

Ismail, I.S. and Scanlon, M.F. (1993) Endocrine and metabolic effects of growth hormone treatment. *Hospital Update* **19**, 443–448

Jaffe, H.L. (1972) *Metabolic Degenerative and Inflammatory Diseases of Bones and Joints.* Lea and Febiger: Philadelphia

Kanis, J.A. (1991) *Pathophysiology and treatment of Paget's Disease of Bone*. Martin Dunitz: London

Knaggs, R.L. (1925) *British Journal of Surgery* **13**, 206

Krane, S.M. (1977) Paget's disease of bone. *Clinical Orthopaedics* **127**, 24–36

Krane, C., Brownell, G.L., Stanbury, J.R. and Corrigan, H. (1956) *Journal of Clinical Investigation* **35**, 874

Law, M.R., Wald, N.J. and Meade, T.W. (1991) Strategies for prevention of osteoporosis of hip fractures. *British Medical Journal* **303**, 453–459

Lindsay, R., Aitken, J.N. and Anderson, J.B. (1976) Long-term prevention of post-menopausal osteoporosis by oestrogen. *Lancet* **1**, 1038–1040

Ludkowski, P. and Wilson-MacDonald, J. (1990) Total arthroplasty in Paget's Disease of hip. *Clinical Orthopaedics and Related Research* **255**, 160–167

McCance, R.A., Morrison, A.D. and Dent, C.E. (1955) *Lancet* **1**, 131

Mankin, H.J. (1993) Editorial. Gaucher's disease. A novel treatment and important breakthrough. *Journal of Bone and Joint Surgery* **75B**, 2–3

Marie, P.J., Pettifor, J.N., Ross, F.P. and Glorieux, F.H. (1982) Histological osteomalacia due to dietary calcium deficiency in children. *New England Journal of Medicine* **307**, 584–588

Melick, R.A. and Martin, T.J. (1975) Paget's disease in identical twins. *Australian and New Zealand Journal of Medicine 5*, 564–565

Mercer, W. and Duthie, R.B. (1956) *Journal of Bone and Joint Surgery* **38B**, 279–292

Mills, B. and Singer, F. (1976)) Nuclear inclusions in Paget's disease of bone. *Science* **194**, 201–202

Moore, T.E., King, A.R., Kathol, M.M. *et al.* (1991) Sarcoma in Paget's disease of bone; clinical, radiologic and pathologic features in 22 cases. *American Journal of Roentgenology* **156**, 1199–1203

Normann, E.K., Trygstad, O., Larsen, S. and Dahl-Jorgensen, K. (1991) Height reduction in 539 tall girls treated with three different dosages of ethinyloestradiol. *Archives of Disease in Childhood* **66**, 1275–1278

O'Driscoll, J.B. and Anderson, D.C. (1986) Past pets and Paget's disease. *Lancet* **2**, 919–921

Pagnani, M.J., Pellicci, P.F. and Salvati, E.A. (1991) Effect of aspirin on heterotopic ossification after total hip arthroplasty in men who have osteoarthritis. *Journal of Bone and Joint Surgery* **73A**, 924–929

Parfitt, A.M., Gallagher, J.C., Heaney, R.P. *et al.* (1982) Vitamin D and bone health in the elderly. *American Journal of Clinical Nutrition* **36**, 1014–1031

Parsons, I.G. (1932) *American Journal of Diseases of Children* **43**, 1293

Plewes, L.W. (1956) Sudeck's atrophy in the hand. *Journal of Bone and Joint Surgery* **38B**, 195–203

Pygott, F. (1957) Paget's disease of bone. The radiological incidence. *Lancet* **1**, 1170–1171

Rathbun, J.C. (1948) *American Journal of Diseases of Children* **75**, 822

Rico, H., Hernandez, E.R., Revilla, M. *et al.* (1992) Salmon calcitonin reduced vertebral fracture rate in post menopausal crush fracture syndrome. *Bone and Mineral* **16**, 131–138

Saggese, G., Bertelloni, S., Baroncelli, G.I., Perri, G. and Calderazzi, A. (1991) Mineral metabolism and calcitriol therapy in idiopathic juvenile osteoporosis.

American Journal of Diseases of Children **145**, 457–462

Sennara, H. and Gorry, G. (1978) Orthopedic aspects of sickle cell anaemia and allied hemoglobinopathies. *Clinical Orthopaedics and Related Research* **130**, 154–157

Shearer, W.S. (1954) *Edinburgh Medical Journal* **61**, 101

Singer, F.R. and Krane, S.M. (1990) Paget's disease of bone. In: *Metabolic Bone Disease*, pp 546–615. Edited by L.V. Avioli and S.M. Krane. W.B. Saunders: Philadelphia

Siris, E.S., Kelsey, J.L., Flaster, E. and Parker, S. (1990) Paget's disease of bone and previous pet ownership in the United States: dogs exonerated. *International Journal of Epidemiology* **19**, 455–458

Smith, R., Russell, R.G.G. and Woods, C.G. (1976) Myositis ossificans progressiva. Clinical features of eight patients and their response to treatment. *Journal of Bone and Joint Surgery* **58B**, 48–57

Snapper, I. and Nathan, D.J. (1957) *American Journal of Medicine* **22**: 939

Solomon, L. (1978) Bone loss in aging individuals. *Orthopedics* **6**, 121

Sotos, J.F., Cutler, E.A. and Dodge, P. (1977) Cerebral gigantism. *American Journal of Diseases of Children* **131**, 625–627

Stanbury, S.W. (1962) In: *Renal Disease*: p. 537. Edited by D.A.K. Black. Blackwell Scientific: Oxford

Tanner, J.M., Whitehouse, R.H., Marshall, W.A., Healey, M.J.R. and Goldstein, H. (1975) *Assessment of Skeletal Maturity and Prediction of Adult Height: TW2 Method*. Academic Press:London, New York, San Francisco

Wiltshaw, E. (1971) Myeloma Workshop. Extrameduallary plasmacytoma. *British Medical Journal* **2**, 327

CHAPTER 6

Affections of the Epiphyses

GEORGE BENTLEY

The epiphysis is the part of a bone concerned with growth in length; in addition, it takes part in the formation of joints and acts as an attachment for muscles and tendons. Three types of epiphysis have been described:

1. Pressure epiphysis, which transmits weight from one bone to another.
2. Traction epiphysis or apophysis, situated at the point of attachment of muscles or tendons.
3. Atavistic epiphysis, which represents a part of the skeleton that has lost its function.

The epiphysis develops from a secondary centre of ossification and is at first separated from the main bone by an area of unossified cartilage. Later it joins the shaft to make the adult bone. The cartilage lying between the bony tissue of the epiphysis and the diaphysis is known as the epiphyseal cartilage, and it does not ossify nor does the epiphysis become joined to the body of the bone until growth has ceased (Figure 6.1).

Epiphyseal disturbances may be caused by many factors, of which the chief are circulatory changes, trauma, infection, diet, exercise and endocrine disturbances.

Osteochondrosis (osteochondritis)

The term 'osteochondritis' (or 'epiphysitis') is used to signify a derangement of the normal process of bone growth which occurs at the various ossification centres during the period of their greatest activity. The name 'osteochondrosis' has been applied in the standard nomenclature of disease. No epiphysis in the body is immune to the disease, and there is little doubt that the same underlying pathological process is present, no matter where it occurs, though the particular location modifies its features in certain respects. Cases have been recorded in which almost every epiphysis of the body has been simultaneously the site of this condition, though in each situation

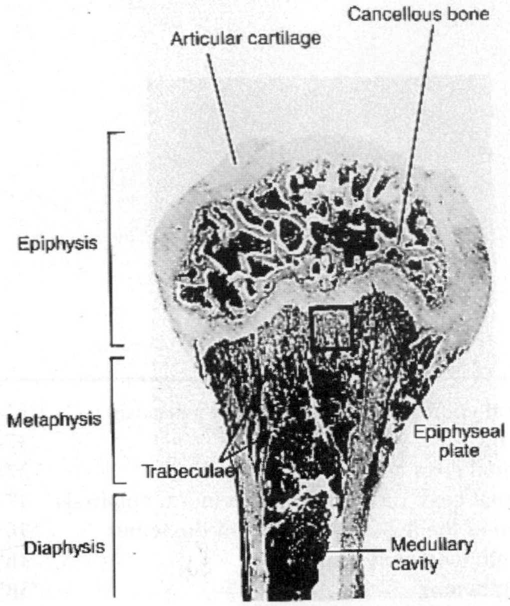

(a)

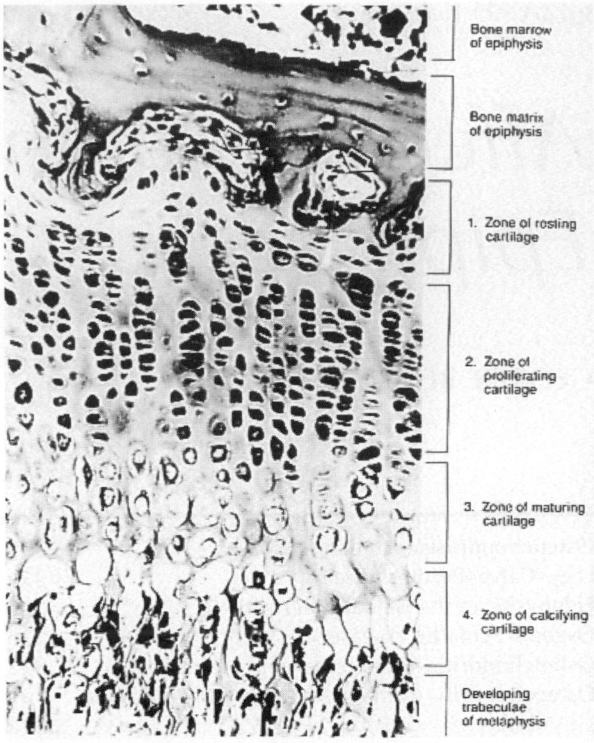

(b)

Figure 6.1 Low power photomicrograph of growing long bone. Osteogenesis has spread from the epiphyseal centre of ossification so that only the articular cartilages and the epiphyseal plate remain cartilaginous. On the diaphyseal side of the epiphyseal plate, bony trabeculae extend down into the epiphysis. (b) The epiphyseal plate (syn. growth plate, physis) showing the zones.

there have been essential differences due to the various stresses and strains to which the various epiphyses have been subjected.

Unfortunately, in most instances the lesion has come to be known by the name of the original observer. This has the disadvantage of giving no hint

Table 6.1 The osteochondroses (original description, date)

Primary centres	Secondary centres
Vertebral body (Calvé, 1925)	Vertebral epiphysis (Scheuermann, 1921)
Carpal scaphoid (Preiser, 1910)	Sternal end of clavicle (Friedrich, 1924)
Lunate, adult (Kienböck, 1910)	Head of humerus (Haas, 1921)
Patella (Köhler, 1908)	Capitellum of humerus (Panner, 1929)
Talus (Mouchet, 1928)	Head of radius (Brailsford, 1935)
Tarsal scaphoid (Köhler, 1908)	Distal ulna (Burns, 1931)
Medial cuneiform (Buschke, 1934)	Heads of metacarpals (Mauclaire, 1927)
	Iliac crest (Buchman, 1925)
	Pubic symphysis (Van Neck, 1924)
	Ischiopubic junction (Oldberg, 1924)
	Head of femur (Legg, 1910)
	Trochanter of femur (Monde Felix, 1922)
	Patella (Sinding-Larsen, 1921)
	Head of tibia (Ritter, 1929)
	Tubercle of tibia (Osgood–Schlatter, 1903)
	Os calcis (Sever, 1912)
	Metatarsal head (Freiberg, 1914)

as to the pathological process and, further, of implying that in each instance we are dealing with an independent disease (Table 6. 1).

There is confusion between irregular ossification in the formation of the ossification centre of an epiphysis and irregular ossification as an ossification centre re-forms after avascular necrosis. In many cases it is evident that a normal stage of development of an epiphysis or an apophysis with increased radiodensity or with separate ossification centres has been implicated as diseased (e.g. in the os calcis).

In any event, inflammation is not a feature of these conditions. Some conditions have been found with a definite aetiology such as eosinophilic granuloma in Calvé's disease. Irregular ossification of the vertebral plates in Scheuermann's disease is obviously associated with adolescent wedging of juvenile kyphosis.

It is evident that the conditions are so diverse that grouping together the group of diseases listed in Table 6.1 as osteochondritis should be abandoned except for its historical interest in terms of association of a specific individual's name with a specific area.

Legg (1910) described the sequence of changes as follows: 'As a result of injury there is an obliteration of a portion of the vascular supply of the epiphysis, which consequently undergoes the atrophy of anaemia. A compensatory hyperaemia of the adjacent portions of the diaphysis is the natural response, and is the starting-point of these hypertrophic changes which have been noted in the occurrence of broadening.'

Duthie and Houghton (1981) believed that some degree of trauma is needed to give rise to the bone compaction, destruction and changed architecture of osteochondrosis. The spine and lower limbs are chiefly affected, from trauma of minor stresses in weight-bearing. Relatively severe trauma is needed for some osteochondritic processes such as osteochondrosis dissecans of the talus but relatively minor trauma in Perthes' disease.

TIMING OF THE OSTEOCHONDROSES

The clinical presentation of the osteochondroses often occurs shortly after the appearance of the bony nucleus, when the epiphysis is mainly cartilaginous and growing rapidly; it therefore is susceptible to the osteochondrotic process (Duthie, 1959) and generalized hormonal or nutritional changes.

Most of the osteochondroses occur in early childhood, around the so-called 'mid-growth spurt' (e.g. Perthes' disease). Others, such as Scheuermann's disease and Osgood–Schlatter's disease, occur at the time of the adolescent growth spurt. The osteochondroses, with the exception of Freiberg's disease, are much more common in boys. This constitutional difference between the sexes is probably due to the later appearance and maturation of secondary growth centres in males. Furthermore, boys are probably subjected to increased trauma and stresses in early childhood.

Many affected individuals are shorter and relatively undersized compared with the average at the end of skeletal growth. 'Standstill growth' has been observed following the development of Perthes' disease, when there may be a cessation of growth for periods of up to 3 years (Harrison *et al.*, 1976). However, early onset of Perthes' disease occurs with little bone/skeletal age discrepancy, whereas the majority of the later onset cases show a distinct lagging of bone age. Delayed skeletal maturity is also found in unaffected siblings of Perthes' patients. Burwell *et al.* (1978), from a cross-sectional anthropometric study in Perthes' patients, described how Nottingham schoolboys had impaired stature of most linear dimensions, and therefore a definite proportionate growth abnormality. However, this was not found in Liverpool boys. Those authors concluded that the growth rates are different, and questioned the significance of environmental factors operating as well.

HEREDITARY AND ENVIRONMENTAL FACTORS

Both osteochondrosis dissecans and the osteochondroses may occur within families. Wansborough *et al.* (1959) reported 12 of 129 Perthes' patients with a positive family history but this was not confirmed by Wynne-Davies and Gormley (1978), who found an extremely low frequency of this disorder among relatives. But this condition occurred particularly in children who were thirdborn or later in the family and had older than average parents from low-income groups. One in 10 had an abnormal intrauterine lie, and they concluded that these children were constitutionally and socially at a disadvantage.

Blount's disease is much more common in negroes (Golding *et al.*, 1959) while Perthes' disease is rare. A family study suggested that a dominant inheritance pattern is present in Blount's disease (Sibert and Bray, 1977).

OSTEOCHONDROSES AND OTHER DISORDERS

Hall and Harrison (1978) showed that, in 90 cases of Perthes' disease, 8 had major congenital defects, 5 of which were multiple. In the remaining 82 patients, there was twice the rate of minor congenital defects when compared with a control group. In a further series, 4.3% of patients with Perthes' disease had major genitourinary disorders and there was eight times the expected incidence of inguinal hernia (Catterall *et al.*, 1971). There was also a high incidence of these defects seen in first- and second-degree relatives. This association has been explained by the fact that the genitourinary system and the hip joint are developed from the same embryonic tissue – the mesonephric ridge. Scheuermann's disease may occur with other conditions. Houghton and Nicolino (1981, personal communication) found 11 of 104 patients with slipped upper femoral epiphysis affected by this condition.

Other metabolic and hormonal conditions give rise to bone changes which show radiological similarities to the osteochondroses. Hypothyroidism predisposes to osteochondrotic lesions indistinguishable from these conditions.

Sickle cell anaemia and juvenile haemochromatosis produce epiphyseal changes similar to Perthes' disease (Golding *et al.*, 1959). Bone infarction has been incriminated in the aetiology of these radiological changes, but bone marrow destruction may also occur. Direct bone marrow infiltration is also present in Gaucher's disease, with appearances identical to Perthes' disease. A similar process occurs in the mucopolysaccharidoses.

VASCULAR CHANGES

Many writings attribute osteochondrosis to circulatory disturbances in growing bone (Editorial, 1978), but without real evidence. Experimental studies which interrupt the capital epiphyseal vessels in animal models, such as the rabbit, do give rise to radiological changes similar to Perthes' disease, but Glimcher and Kenzora (1979) have clearly described that the radiographic picture of ischaemia is often indistinguishable from the appearance of other causes of osteonecrosis. Accordingly, routine radiographs offer no explanation of understanding of the biological status of osteonecrosis. They state that there is no substantial evidence of interruption of the blood supply. In Perthes' disease there is often partial epiphyseal involvement as well as reossification and reconstitution.

In Perthes' disease the radiological observation of lateral, medial or whole head disease corresponds to the blood vessel pattern of the capital femoral epiphysis but it does not follow that deficiencies in the blood supply cause the disease. For example, Herring *et al.* (1980) suggested that an interruption of blood flow occurs by infarction, occlusion or malformation of blood vessels – although these were never demonstrated. Nishio and Yakushiji (1962) found thrombosis in metaphyseal vessels in Perthes' disease, but these changes could be secondary to necrosis occurring in the tissues served by these vessels. A histological study by McKibbin and Ráli˘s (1974) suggested that two ischaemic episodes were more likely in Perthes' disease rather than avascular necroses of the femoral head.

The development of an effusion or haemarthrosis under pressure has been implicated in the aetiology of Perthes' disease by compressing the retinacular vessels. But in over 60 hip bleeds in haemophilia, requiring hospital admission, we have not seen a single case of femoral head osteochondrosis.

TRAUMA

In only a small proportion of cases of osteochondrosis can a history of significant trauma be elicited. The osteochondroses are relatively rare but minor traumatic episodes are an almost daily event in normal growing children. It is difficult to accept that trauma alone can give rise to an osteochondrotic process unless the bone involved is already inadequate. Osteochondrosis of the capitellum usually affects the elbow of the dominant upper limb in males, suggesting a traumatic aetiology.

Osteochondrosis dissecans of the capitellum commonly follows repetitive trauma to the elbow such as is seen in professional baseball pitchers or in schoolboy javelin throwers. The capitellum or the radial head or both may be involved.

Freiberg's disease is more common in girls. Osteochondral fracture is believed by many to be the cause; however, sufficient trauma to cause a fracture is rarely incurred. It is suggested that the affected metatarsal is abnormally long and therefore subjected to abnormal stress.

Osgood–Schlatter's disease can result from trauma to the developing bone by the ligamentum patellae on the tibial tubercle Indeed It has been suggested by Lancourt and Cristini (1975) that a relatively short patellar ligament would put increased stress at its insertion and therefore an increased chance of avulsion.

HORMONAL FEATURES

It has been suggested (Duthie, 1959) that hormone changes during periods of altered growth give rise to increased osteogenic proliferation, and these rapidly dividing cells are more susceptible to trauma or minor ischaemia. The mesenchymal stem cells under such circumstances differentiate into fibroblasts having reduced metabolic requirements. As fibrous tissue has relative mechanical instability compared with bone, the developing bone is subjected to yet further trauma and vascular embarrassment.

Duthie and Houghton (1981) have proposed a model for the development of the osteochondroses. The developing epiphyseal anlage may be normal or may have a constitutional minor or major defect – i.e. may be normal, mildly dyschondrotic or severely dyschondrotic. The developing epiphysis is then subjected to various degrees of mechanical stress and trauma:

1. A normal epiphysis may be exposed to extreme trauma and give rise to an osteochondrotic lesion – usually osteochondrosis dissecans (e.g. 'pitcher's elbow' with osteochondrosis dissecans of the capitellum; at operation in this condition, the appearances are typical of those of an osteochondral fracture, with the remainder of the epiphysis appearing entirely normal).
2. An example of a mildly dyschondrotic epiphysis is often found in osteochondrosis dissecans of the knee which, when it is exposed to excessive mechanical forces, will give rise to clinical osteochondrosis dissecans. At operation, not only is the loose fragment of osteochondrosis dissecans affected but very often the adjacent femoral condyle is abnormal and filled with necrotic bone and fibrous tissues. Perthes' disease probably fits into this mildly dyschondrotic group.
3. A severely affected dyschondrotic epiphysis, such as the capital femoral epiphysis in Gaucher's disease or hypothyroidism, will give rise to osteochondrosis when exposed to the normal mechanical forces of weight-bearing.

Constitutional osteocartilaginous deficiencies may be localized or generalized. The extreme forms of generalized disorder such as chondroectodermal dysplasia and dysplasia epiphysealis multiplex give rise to well recognized multiepiphyseal defects. In these conditions there is no attempt at repair by the affected bones, which remain abnormal throughout growth. However, the resemblance between dysplasia epiphysealis multiplex and bilateral Perthes' disease is so striking that other epiphyses should be radiographed to make the correct diagnosis.

Legg–Calvé–Perthes' disease

Coxa plana, Legg–Perthes' disease, osteochondritis deformans coxa juvenilis and pseudocoxalgia have been used as names for this condition. Legg described the condition in 1910 when it had been formerly confused with conditions such as tuberculosis of the hip in childhood (Waldenström in 1909).

It may be defined as a disease of the hip, limited sharply by age group and largely by sex; it results from changes in the capital femoral epiphysis, apparently secondary to loss of an adequate blood supply for at least a portion of the femoral head. The age group is usually between 3 and 10 years, with 80% of the patients being males. Occasionally cases may be seen as young as the age of 2 years and as old as 12. Bilateral cases are relatively rare (10%).

AETIOLOGY

The anatomy of the vascular supply to the proximal femoral epiphysis at age 3–10 is such that only a rare blood vessel passes through the epiphyseal line to supply the epiphysis. The remainder of the circulation comes via the femoral neck and across the periphery of the epiphyseal line mainly in a lateral location. As such it is obviously at risk to increased intracapsular pressure. This may result from any inflammatory condition of the hip such as synovitis or from septic arthritis or traumatic haemarthrosis, but very rarely secondary to haemophilia, if at all. Medical conditions such as rickettsial infections, Caisson's disease, cretinism and Gaucher's disease (Figure 6.2).

Irregular ossification due to fundamental cartilage defects such as epiphyseal dysplasia can be confused with the condition by x-ray but arc differentiated by the bilateral nature (Figure 6.3) and the involvement of other epiphyses in the knee and ankle.

Legg–Calvé–Perthes' disease is best understood as a disease secondary to soft tissue disease of some unknown cause.

PATHOGENESIS

Elucidation of the pathogenesis of Perthes' disease has been restricted by the lack of availability of material from human hips Therefore, most of the studies and theories of causation are based on animal models simulating Perthes' disease

It is generally agreed that the defect in Perthes' disease is a healing infarct of the capital femoral

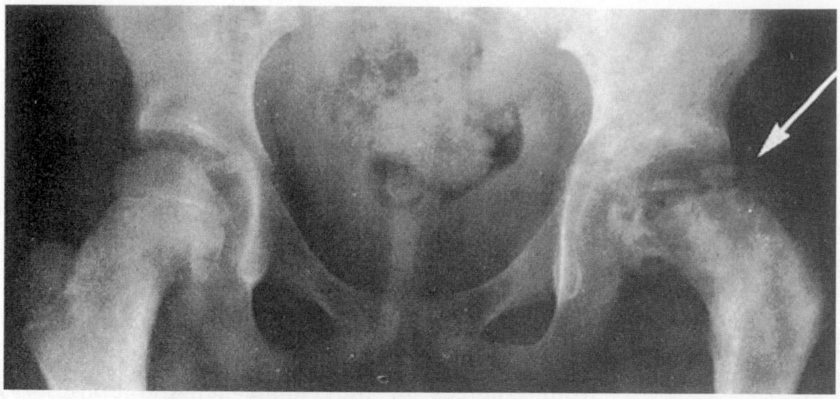

Figure 6.2 Aseptic necrosis of the capital femoral epiphysis secondary to Gaucher's disease. Widespread deposits are seen in the whole of the upper femur.

epiphysis. The histological changes in the femoral heads examined so far have been described as showing three main types of change in the bony nucleus (McKibbin, 1975):

1. The appearances of a healed infarct interspersed with areas of entirely normal bone The inter-trabecular spaces are filled with granulation and fibrous tissue, and there is intense osteoblastic activity so that dead bone trabeculae are covered with new bone, giving an increased radiological density of the area and sometimes the 'head within a head' (Figure 6.4a).
2. At the apex of the head the bone may be dead and blood vessels are absent with fragmentation of the trabeculae (Figure 6.4b).
3. In the junctional zone between dead and living bone, osteoclastic resorption predominates over osteoblastic activity, resulting in complete fibrous replacement of bone, producing radiolucency, while the simultaneous osteoblastic activity in other areas may result in the appearances of fragmentation (Figure 6.4c).

The articular cartilage shows increased thickness early in the disease because the deeper layer which ultimately forms the epiphyseal bone is deprived of its nutrition. The superficial layer, nourished from the synovial fluid, remains alive and thus appears relatively thick. The death of this deepest zone is not usually complete because recovery occurs and the head continues to grow subsequently. It is known that during this time of nutritional impairment the deep zone of the cartilage is dependent on synovial fluid nutrition. This is facilitated by joint movement (Maroudas *et al.*, 1968) which indicates a theoretical basis for treatment by a method involving joint movement.

The growth-plate receives its nutrition from vessels on its epiphyseal side (Trueta and Amato, 1960). Interruption of these vessels causes infarction with necrosis of the proliferative zone of the growth plate. Ossification of the metaphysis is interrupted and so the plate becomes thinner. Vessels may grow across the plate from the metaphysis, and permanent damage to the plate will ensue. Metaphyseal changes of widening and 'cyst' formation are seen commonly, but the histological changes recorded, of accumulation of plasma cells and new bone trabeculae, are not remarkable in the metaphysis (McKibbin and Ráliš, 1974).

Controversy still exists regarding the cause of deformity of the femoral head occurring in Perthes'

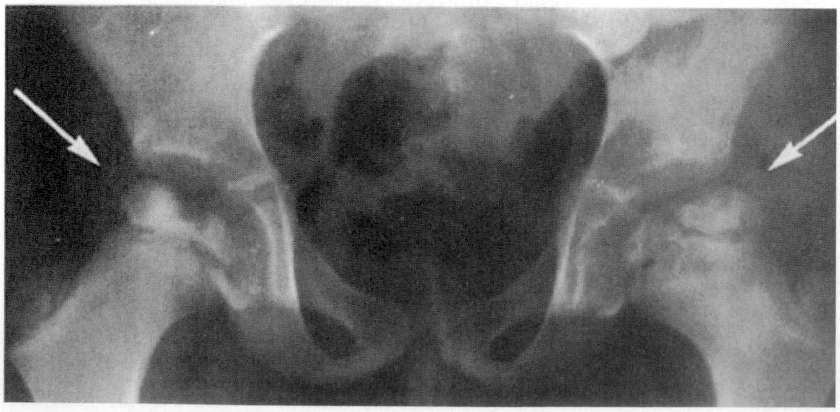

Figure 6.3 Meyer's (epiphyseal) dysplasia with bilateral involvement of the femoral capital epiphysis. The epiphysis is ossifying irregularly. The hip movement range was normal.

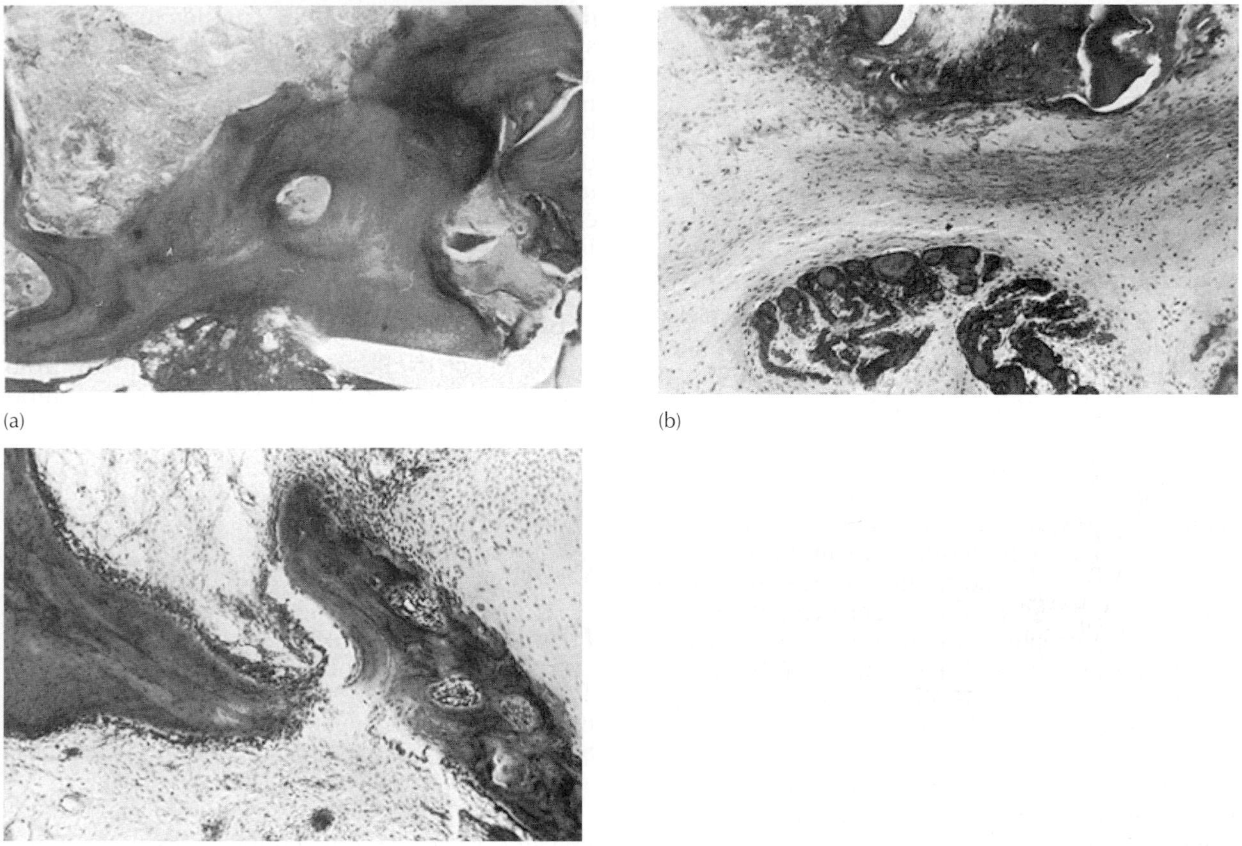

(a) (b) (c)

Figure 6.4 (a) Part of the necrotic trabecula in the superficial portion of the capital nucleus from a patient with Perthes' disease. The trabeculae are dead but the thickness and structure indicate a previous succession of events, i.e. bone necrosis and appositional repair. Throughout the specimen of the dead nucleus many examples of bone death and reossification could be found. The findings indicated that repeated vascular infarction and revascularization play an important part in human Perthes' disease (× 56). (b) Cellular and fibrous granulation tissue (bottom) advancing from the basal lining revascularized part of the capital nucleus into the superficial dead part at the top (× 56). (c) Typical feature from the basal revascularized part of the capital nucleus showing increased osteoblastic activity and accelerated bone building and remodelling (× 56). (From McKibbin, B. and Ráliš, Z.A. (1974) *Journal of Bone and Joint Surgery* **56B**, 438–447, with permission)

disease. Trabecular fragmentation is common in the apex of the head, but how much is due to mechanical collapse and how much due to bone resorption is unknown. Salter (1966) claimed that the femoral head was no more mechanically soft than the control head in experimental Perthes' disease in pigs and that the final distortion of the head was due to failure of remodelling of bone, which could be prevented by placing the femoral head in flexion and abduction. However, this manoeuvre in man results in uncovering of the posterior aspect of the head, so this animal model is not totally relevant in human disease. Experience of treatment of the disease by weight-bearing 'containment' methods and by recumbency suggests little difference in the outcome and no evidence that weight-bearing is harmful unless the head has already subluxed from the acetabulum. It appears much more likely that the primary cause of deformity of the head is impaired and uneven revascularization of the head following infarction, which can be aggravated by mechanical forces if the head is subluxed.

Most recent studies suggest that repeated phenomena occur, causing impairment of nutrition, though the mechanism of the infarction remains unclear. The most popular explanation – that repeated effusion or haemarthrosis in the joint cavity causes a build-up of pressure which occludes the capsular veins – cannot be accepted as the only mechanism.

CLINICAL FEATURES

A limp and pain usually felt around the hips and sometimes down to the knee are the presenting complaint. The limp may be present for several weeks, and there may be a history of several previous episodes of limp in the past which had cleared. There are sometimes cases with no clinical complaints which are discovered incidentally at x-ray examination for some other reason.

Hip motion is, invariably, limited at the extremes or completely, by pain. Limitation of internal rotation is often marked and is accompanied by hip flexion contracture. Failure to find such signs in the face of symptoms necessitates a very careful evaluation of the radiographs to make certain that one is not dealing with an irregular ossification of the proximal femoral epiphysis. There is sometimes tenderness, both anteriorly and posteriorly over the hip joint area.

Measurement of the thigh may reveal atrophy, and buttock atrophy may be apparent. Where not measurable, atrophy is often appreciated by palpation. Children may be seen in acute distress; equally, however, severe disease may on occasion require detailed and accurate examination of the hip joint motion to demonstrate this lesion.

One of the most important conditions to differentiate from Legg–Calvé–Perthes' disease is transient synovitis, which occurs most commonly between the ages of 3 and 8 years against Perthes' occurring at 4–6 years mainly in male children, and more likely to be bilateral in 10% (Gledhill and McIntyre, 1969).

Pain is common in both conditions – one-third present with a limp. About 1% of cases of Perthes' disease begin as a synovitis similar to a transient synovitis before showing radiographic evidence of avascular necrosis. Bone-scanning techniques utilizing technetium-99 have allowed early differentiation because the femoral epiphysis shows reduced uptake of the isotope in early Perthes' disease (Calver *et al*., 1981). Magnetic resonance imaging also detects early Perthes' changes and demonstrates early articular cartilage thickening but false negatives have been described (Elsig *et al*., 1989; Egund and Wingstrand, 1991) (Figure 6.5).

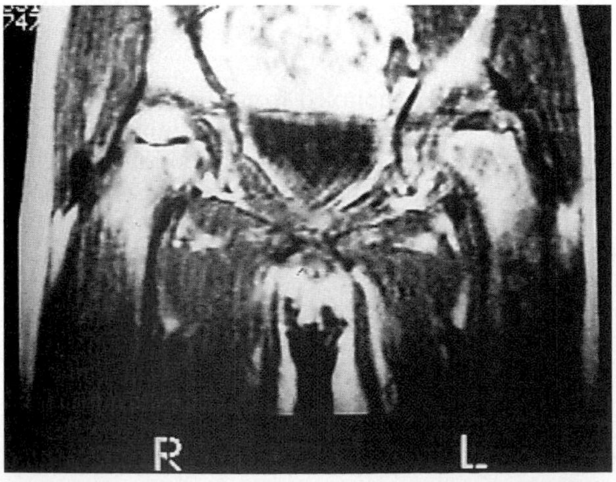

Figure 6.5 Magnetic resonance imaging (MRI) of Perthes' disease showing the angularity and altered signal on the affected left side.

Futami *et al*. (1991) differentiated joint space widening due to effusion in transient synovitis from synovial thickening in Perthes' disease by ultrasonography.

RADIOLOGICAL APPEARANCES

Various stages are evident on this examination.

First stage (incipient)

The capsular shadow may be swollen around the involved hip. Cessation of growth may be indicated by a zone of demineralization of the metaphysis adjacent to the epiphyseal line (Figure 6.6).

Caffey (1968) described how the skeletal maturation in 30 patients with Perthes' disease was significantly reduced, with the bone age being reduced by half or more of the chronological age. He emphasized that the first radiographic changes were segmental fracture, flattening, and sclerosis in the anterosuperior lateral quadrant of the epiphyseal ossification centre. Translucent defects in the metaphyseal area were noted after 4–12 months, directly beneath the cartilage plate with the deformed and flattened anterior segment of the ossification centre being above it. He believed that these changes were more likely to result from a direct segmental compression injury rather than from ischaemic necrosis.

Second stage (aseptic necrosis)

The changes of the first stage are present, and in addition the bony segment of the proximal femoral epiphysis reveals apparently increased density and often flattening and broadening of outline. There may be a sparing of the area supplied by the ligamentum teres. In addition, early in the disease a linear radiolucency from a small segment of head may be present. It may be that this represents a fracture line, as described by Caffey, separating a segment of bone from the parent nucleus in a manner similar to that found in osteochondritis dissecans (Figure 6.7).

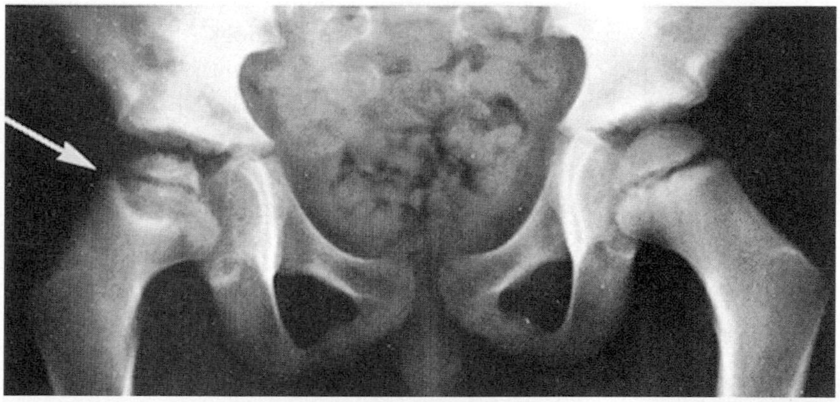

(a)

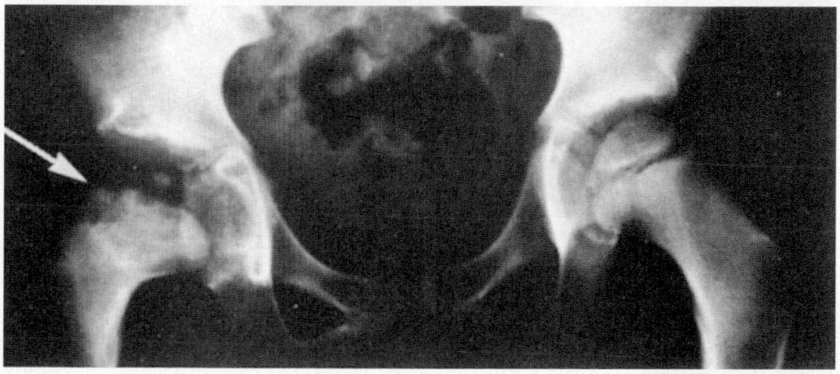

(b)

Figure 6.6 (a) Unilateral Legg–Calvé–Perthes' disease. The medial aspect of the joint space on the right is widened. Growth has stopped in the epiphyseal centre of the head, which is small. There is a radiolucent area extending into the broadened metaphysis. (b) Continuation of the disease as the new blood supply invades the capital femoral epiphysis. The old bone is removed. The acetabulum begins to mirror the head deformity.

Third stage (regenerative)

The dense head is revitalized and the old bone is removed. Flattening has often already taken place if the patient is first seen at this time. The bony segments are irregularly distributed. The neck is widened. Regeneration, as it takes place, will do so in relationship to this widened neck and the flattening already present. This condition may lead to coxa magna as described by Ferguson and Howarth (1935) (Figure 6.8).

Changes in the neck of the femur

Deformity of the neck can develop very early in the disease, even before the head has been deformed. The upper part of the neck is expanded and its metaphyseal end becomes rounded off. At the same time the neck becomes progressively shorter, but it does not usually bend.

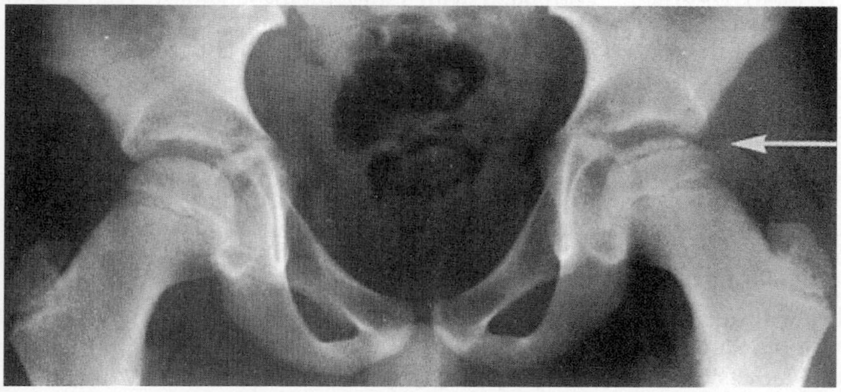

Figure 6.7 Early signs of Legg–Calvé–Perthes' disease. The line visualized in the capital femoral epiphysis represents a division between living and dead bone.

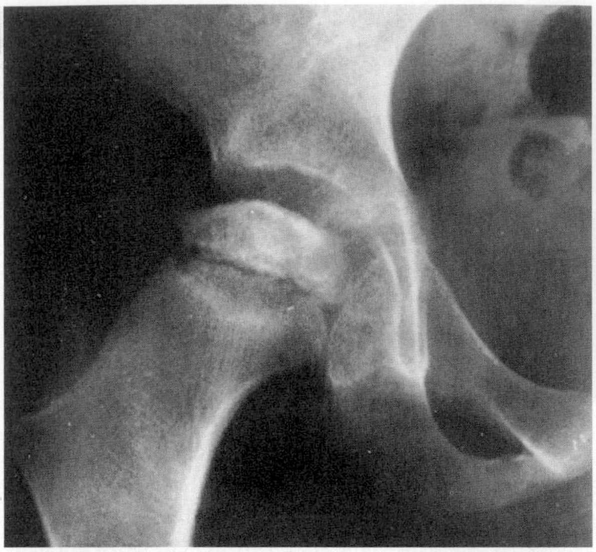

(a)

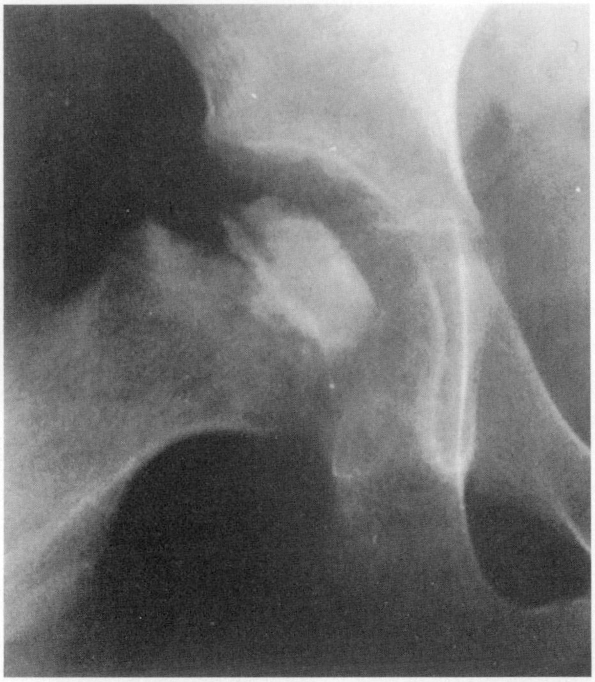

(b)

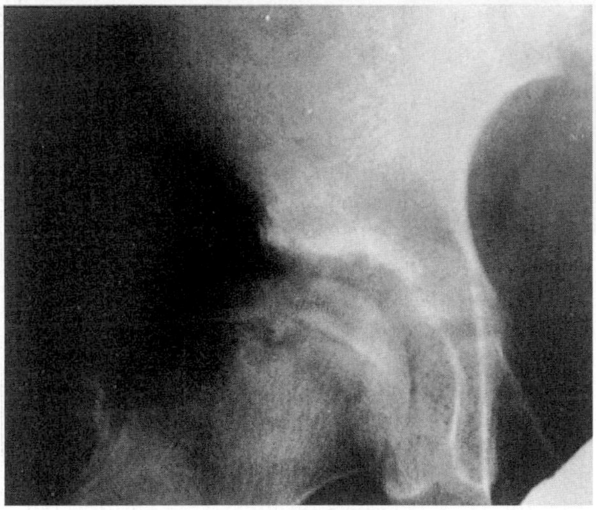

(c)

Figure 6.8 (a) Legg–Calvé–Perthes' disease showing the 'head within a head'. Growth has ceased in the capital femoral epiphysis, allowing a radiographic increase in the cartilage formed joint space. (b) The anterior portion of the head and metaphysis has already been invaded by new blood supply giving rise to radiolucent areas in the lateral view (the positive 'Gage's sign'). (c) In healed Legg–Calvé–Perthes' disease the decreased height of the capital femoral epiphysis and widened neck leads to the coxa magna deformity.

Changes in the acetabular cavity

Waldenström (1938) described as an early sign an increased distance between the medial pole of the head and the floor of the socket. This may reach such a degree that the shadows of the head and the ischial bone no longer overlap but leave a gap between them, with the ligamentum teres being grossly swollen and congested.

Changes in the acetabulum (Figure 6.6b)

The acetabular floor is altered, as it adapts itself to the alteration in the shape of the head. It does not show the usual contour but is hollowed out abruptly. This excavation occurs later than Waldenström's sign but is never seen in the absence of the latter.

Although pathological changes cannot be directly correlated with radiographic changes, Duthie and Houghton (1981) have studied the radiographic appearances in areas other than the capital femoral epiphysis in 68 cases of Perthes' disease; of these, 58 had changes in the acetabulum consisting of irregular ossification, cysts and increased radiodense areas. Perhaps of more significance, in 51 cases there were abnormalities of the triradiate cartilage, consisting of irregular ossification, subchondral cysts and 'beaking'. This aspect, together with investigation of all epiphyses in cases of osteochondrosis, needs further study and may help to elucidate the basic defect in these conditions.

Multiple epiphyseal involvement is common in

Perthes' disease, although frank generalized epiphyseal abnormality is not often recognized clinically or radiologically. This does not mean such abnormalities are not present histologically; they have merely not declared themselves, having not been subjected to the necessary mechanical stresses. Much morbidity of psychological as well as physical type can be produced by unnecessary treatment and Weinstein (1983) pointed out that no study had shown a clear advantage of operative over conservative treatment. Thus the decision to treat with restrictive casts and braces, or to operate must be judged carefully.

Catterall (1971) proposed a classification indicating degrees of involvement of the femoral head and, therefore, severity of the disease, aimed at clarifying prognosis. He emphasized the importance of good quality radiographs and the need for both anteroposterior and 'frog-lateral' views. Four grades were described (see Figure 6.9a–e).

Group I

Only the anterior part of the epiphysis is involved. It differs from other groups in that no collapse occurs and complete absorption of the involved segment occurs without sequestrum formation. Metaphyseal changes are unusual. Radiologically, the course of the disease appears to be absorption of the involved segment followed by complete regeneration.

Group II

In this variety more of the anterior part of the epiphysis is involved. Radiologically, the major difference in the course of the disease is that the involved segment after a phase of absorption undergoes collapse, with the formation of a dense collapsed segment, or sequestrum. This is absorbed before healing commences. In the anteroposterior radiograph the sequestrum appears as a dense oval mass with viable fragments on both medial and lateral sides. When collapse occurs, the viable fragments maintain epiphyseal height. On the lateral radiograph the sequestrum is separated posteriorly from the viable fragments by a V-shaped segment of viable epiphysis. If there is metaphyseal change, this is usually a well defined cyst which is transitory and disappears with healing.

Group III

In this variety only a small part of the epiphysis is not sequestrated. The anteroposterior radiograph shows the appearances of a 'head within a head', while in the later stages there is a collapsed sequestrum centrally placed with very small amounts of normal-appearing bone on the medial and lateral sides (see Figure 6.8a). When collapse occurs, the lateral segment becomes displaced – producing gross broadening of the neck (see Figures 6.6a and 6.8c). The course of the disease is essentially the same as in group II except that the broadening is a more important sequel. Metaphyseal changes are more generalized and, when extensive, are frequently associated with broadening of the neck.

Group IV

In this variety the whole epiphysis is sequestrated. On the anteroposterior radiographs total collapse of the epiphysis may be seen producing a dense line. Displacement of the epiphysis can occur not only anteriorly but posteriorly, producing a mushroom-like appearance of the head. The metaphyseal changes may be extensive.

Catterall also emphasized the concept of the 'head at risk'. He described the following signs of 'head at risk' which indicated a bad radiological prognosis:

1. Gage's sign.
2. Calcification lateral to the epiphysis.
3. Lateral subluxation.
4. Horizontal alignment of the growth plate.

On the basis of his review, Catterall concluded that conventional non-operative treatment did not improve the natural history of group I and group II cases occurring in children below the age of 4 years. It did improve hips in group II children over that age.

This classification has been useful as a guideline to treatment, although it is now realized that in many cases the radiological appearances change during the course of the disease, and the interobserver error is high (Hardcastle *et al.*, 1980). Simmons *et al.* (1990) reported an alternative method of radiological grading described by Salter and Thompson (1984). This is a two-group classification which they showed had less interobserver error and was simpler and more reliable in the early stages of disease when decisions regarding treatment are made.

PROGNOSIS

Legg–Calvé–Perthes' is a self-limiting disease with a strong tendency to spontaneous recovery. The immediate good results have in the past tempted surgeons to be unjustifiably optimistic. In a résumé of the end results, Legg (1927) showed that the final results could be placed in one of two categories, and

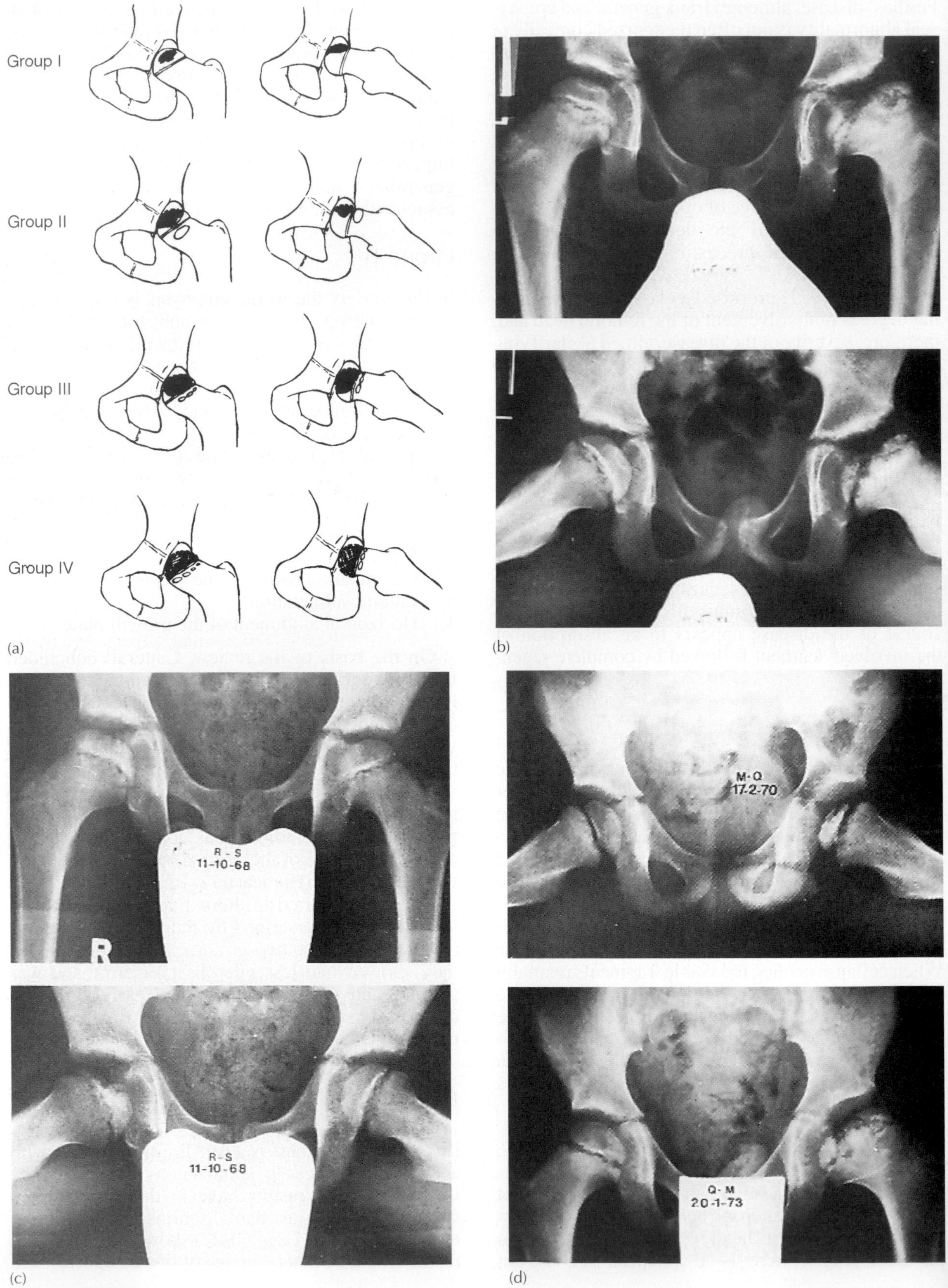
Group I
Group II
Group III
Group IV
(a)
(b)
R - S
11-10-68
R
R - S
11-10-68
(c)
M-Q
17-2-70
Q- M
20-1-73
(d)

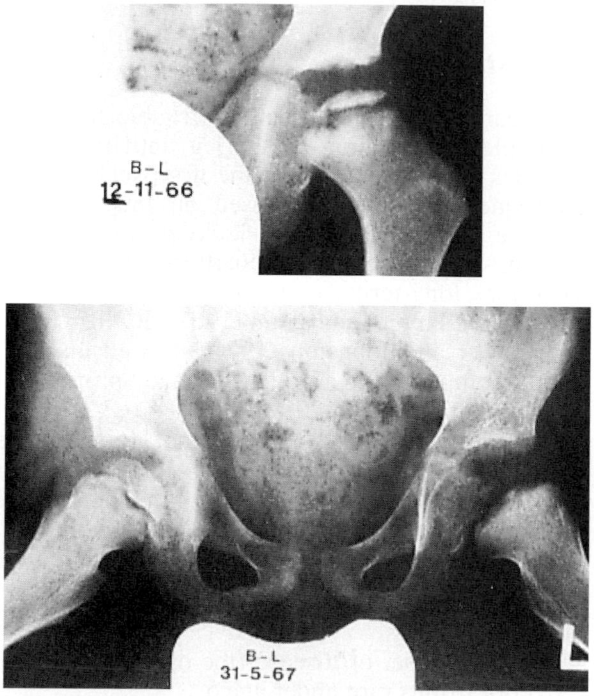

(e)

Figure 6.9 Diagram to illustrate the Catterall grading on the anteroposterior and lateral radiographs. (b) Anteroposterior and lateral radiographs of group I disease in the right hip. (c) Anteroposterior and lateral radiographs of group II disease in the right hip with central lucency and destruction of the anterior half of the head on the lateral view. (d) Anteroposterior and lateral radiograph of group III disease showing the 'head within the head' on the AP and involvement of the anterior three-quarters of the head on the lateral view. (e) Anteroposterior and lateral radiograph showing group IV disease with total head involvement. (From Hughes, S.E.F., Benson, M. and Colton, C.L. *Orthopaedics*. Churchill Livingstone. Edinburgh, London, Melbourne and New York, with kind permission)

that there were distinct differences between the two types of case.

1. The *mushroom type* does not show marked atrophy or fragmentation of the epiphyseal bone centres. In some cases the epiphysis migrates considerably towards the greater trochanter, while in others this displacement is slight. Abduction (and, at times, rotation) is limited when the epiphysis shows marked migration; otherwise, motion at the hip may be restored to normal in adult life. In this there is also less shortening.
2. The *fragmented type* shows marked variation in x-ray density in the epiphyseal centre and the neck, fragmentation of the epiphyseal bone centre, and shortening and rounding off of the upper end of the neck. Indeed, the epiphysis in some cases seems to be obliterated. The ultimate limitation of movement and the permanent shortening of the leg are generally considerable in this variety.

Perfunctory treatment led to poor results. Ratliff (1956) found that the results in those patients followed into adult life were disappointing. He classified his fairly small series as 38% good, 38% fair and 24% poor. A high percentage had no pain and good function, but only 40% had a good hip radiologically, while there was evidence of arthritis in 51%. The end results of those adequately treated were better than those untreated. The inference is drawn that the prognosis of Perthes' disease, although good on the whole, is less certainly favourable than had been supposed, but is definitely improved by early treatment in hips showing signs of 'head at risk'.

Cameron and Isat (1960) reviewed 185 cases, in which the ratio of 4.3 to 1 was in favour of the boys. Further consideration of the sex ratios suggested that the disease was inherited and based upon a sex-influenced autosomal dominant gene with a varying expression. The mean age of first diagnosis in girls was 5.9 years, whereas in boys it was 6.5 years. There was no evidence that the disease was related to any endocrine factor causing any retardation of growth. They concluded that those affected under the age of 7 years of either type had a better radiographic result than the older age groups, irrespective of any form of treatment, but none ended with a completely normal-appearing femoral head. Prognosis depended upon the type, the age at onset, the duration of symptoms prior to receiving treatment and the efficiency of such treatment. In particular, reviews have shown no evidence of long-term bad results when the disease began before the age of 5 years (McKibbin, 1975).

TREATMENT

Early stages

In the early stages when the hip is irritable, treatment is simple skin traction on the leg until irritability subsides over the course of the first week or two. Subsequent treatment is based on the desire to produce a spherical, normal-looking femoral head and thus prevent later osteoarthritis of the hip. Therefore, long-term follow-up is required to justify any method employed. Eaton (1967), Ratliff (1967) and Gower and Johnston (1971) showed that disabling symptoms occurred in a small proportion, amounting to between 20% and 30%.

It is now generally agreed that four factors determine the degree of deformity of the femoral head at maturity and thus, by implication, the prognosis. (It must be noted that most long-term studies show variance between the radiological appearances and the presence of symptoms.) They are:

1. Age of onset of disease (the older the worse). Poor results rare under age 5.
2. Extent of involvement of the femoral head (the greater the worse).
3. Anterolateral subluxation (loss of containment).
4. Persistent loss of hip movement (which inhibits remodelling) and probably hinders cartilage nutrition.

Treatment of established disease

The background to all treatment must be the 59% good radiological results reported by Catterall in untreated cases. In 1936 Eyre-Brook described containment of the femoral head within the acetabulum as the basis of treatment. Since then the dispute has been whether treatment is necessary and, if so, by what method should containment be achieved. Sharrard (1992) summarized the situation by saying that for conservative methods there is a distinct advantage in any method in which abduction is maintained for the hip which is at risk of deformation. However, prolonged bed rest (up to 2 years) in abduction traction reported by McKibbin (1975), although giving excellent radiological results, is unacceptable and treatment is focused on treating the 'head at risk' patient by the most effective and rapid method which carries least risk and interferes least with everyday life and development. Thus, although 'broomstick' plasters achieve containment by abduction, they are inconvenient and require frequent changes.

The child can live a relatively normal life in a weight-relieving caliper or abduction splint but there is evidence to show that these methods affect growth of the femur. The great advantage of operative treatment is that after protection in a hip spica for 6–8 weeks following the operation the child is free of all restrictions and can return to his normal life. Therefore, the following treatment plan is proposed:

1. Children under the age of 5 years: no treatment except for 'irritable' hip by bed rest and bilateral in 10–20° abduction.
2. Children over 5 years:
   group I No treatment.
   group II or group III No treatment unless signs of 'head at risk'.
   group IV No treatment unless signs of 'head at risk'. Careful preoperative radiological evaluation to exclude 'hinged acetabulum' where the femoral head will not reduce into the acetabulum; varus osteotomy in such circumstances will not produce correction and may aggravate the disease (Somerville, 1971).

Where signs of 'head at risk' are present, varus subtrochanteric osteotomy is performed (Lloyd-Roberts *et al.*, 1976) with rotation only where indicated by arthrography or presence of anteversion. The plaster spica is removed at 6–8 weeks depending on age. Following mobilization, full activity is permitted on discharge from hospital.

Innominate osteotomy (Salter, 1984) has been claimed to produce superior results to femoral osteotomy but Sponseller *et al.* (1988) found no difference following 42 femoral osteotomies and 49 innominate osteotomies. Both procedures gave poor results in patients over the age of 10 years. We, therefore, favour the more straightforward femoral osteotomy.

Contraindications to 'containment' treatment

There are those cases which have a good prognosis without treatment or in which treatment will have no effect. They are:

1. Group I cases.
2. Group II and III cases under age 5 with no signs of 'head at risk'.
3. Cases in which severe flattening of the femoral head has occurred as demonstrated by arthrography.
4. Healed cases.
5. Cases with 'hinged acetabulum' (hinge-abduction). Here valgus osteotomy of the femur may be helpful (Figure 6.10) in cases where improved containment of the femoral head can be demonstrated on arthrography by abduction (Salter *et al.*, 1978).

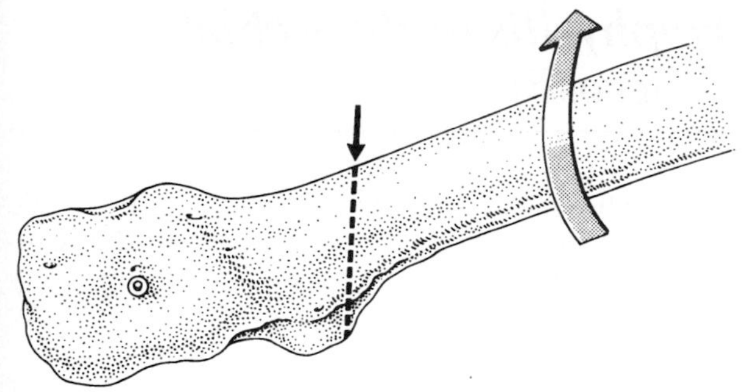

(a)

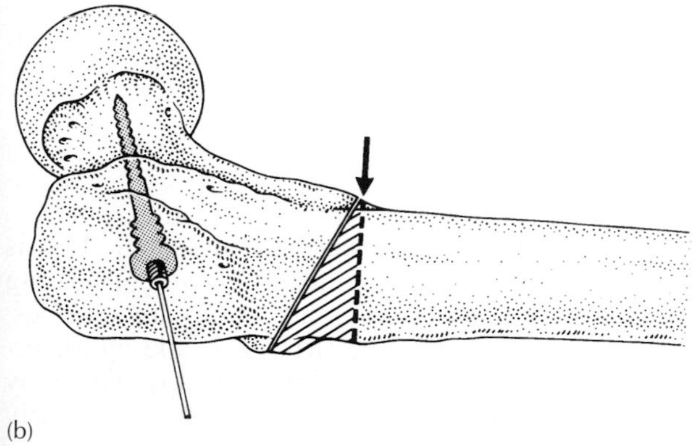

(b)

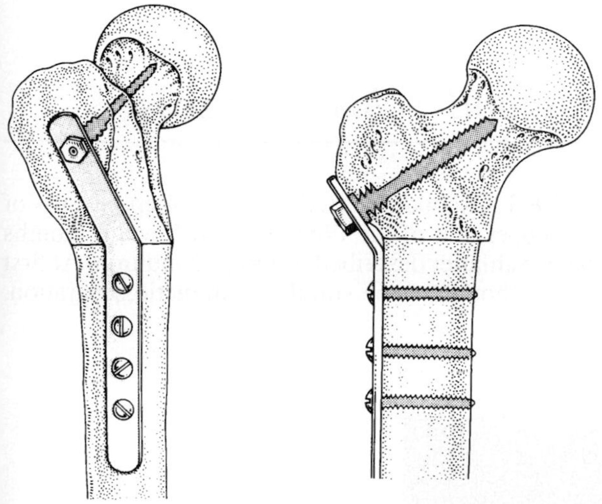

(c)

Figure 6.10 (a–c) Valgus-extension osteotomy of the femur for correction of abduction and flexion deformity. (From Catterall, A. (1991) Operations for congenital dislocation of the hip. In: *Rob & Smith's Operative Surgery: Orthopaedics*. Edited by G. Bentley and R. B. Greer. Butterworth-Heinemann: London, Boston, Sydney, Wellington, Singapore)

Fulford *et al.* (1993) have shown from a prospective, randomized trial that a proximal rotational varus osteotomy did not produce a better result than conservative treatment. Indeed, they also showed that the femoral head shape on first diagnosis was more important for determining the prognosis than Catterall's grading system.

ORTHOSES

The aims of treatment by abduction ambulation are to:

1. Place the head of the femur into the depths of the acetabulum.
2. Avoid pressure from the rim of the acetabulum of the head of the femur.
3. Equalize the pressure over all the femoral head.
4. Diminish the average pressure per unit area of the acetabulum and head.
5. Maintain a good range of motion.
6. Promote as nearly as possible a round head in a normal acetabulum.

Petrie and Bitenc (1971) described their results in 68 children treated by abduction and internal rotation plasters. The hips were fixed in 45° of abduction and 10° of internal rotation. Average time in plaster was 19 months. (The average age of onset was 7 years. Their results showed 60% good, 31% fair and 9% poor.) They concluded therefore:

1. That the duration of the disease seemed to be shortened by this treatment.
2. That the contour of the femoral head was better preserved than with the previous conservative method.

Gunther and Gossling (1973) treated 29 children with a Newington abduction brace between 1965 and 1969. The mean age of onset was 8 years and the mean duration of treatment was 18 months. Their conclusion was that the involved femoral head responds favourably to weight-bearing forces when the extremities are so positioned as to sit the capital epiphysis centrally within the mould of the acetabulum.

Many other authors have described different orthotics which keep the femoral head in a similar fashion into the mould of the acetabulum (e.g. the Toronto brace of Bobechko and the braces of Tachdjian and Harrison).

The advantages of a subtrochanteric osteotomy (Figure 6.10) are:

1. The treatment is complete 6–8 weeks after surgery.
2. No further restrictions after surgery.
3. Osteotomy produces hyperaemia in the upper femur.
4. The treatment does not rely on long-term bracing.

5. The end results seem to be the same as with abduction brace treatment (Axer *et al.*, 1973).

Lloyd-Roberts *et al.* (1976) compared (1) no treatment, (2) conservative treatment with weight-relieving calipers and (3) intertrochanteric osteotomy, and showed that there was no difference between methods (1) and (2). An osteotomy in Catterall group II did not improve the lesion at all, and probably not significantly in group III or IV. Osteotomy gave better results in children over 6. In 'head at risk' cases, osteotomy gave better results.

The complications of osteotomy are shortening, residual coxa vara, non-union and limitation of joint movement. The factors influencing the end result are:

1. Age of onset.
2. Time of diagnosis.
3. Degree of involvement of the capital femoral epiphysis.
4. Radiological signs of 'head at risk'. These signs indicate a bad prognosis – worse in girls than in boys, probably due to more extensive involvement of the epiphysis.

In conclusion, even if it is very difficult to compare different results achieved by different methods of treatment, it is believed that results with intertrochanteric or subtrochanteric osteotomy are at least as good as those results achieved with abduction braces. However, surgery is not indicated in every instance and certainly not in the partial involvement epiphysis. Surgery must be left for 'head at risk' cases provided containment can be demonstrated.

Epiphysitis of the ischial tuberosity

Although called an epiphysitis, this is a traumatic lesion, resulting from an acute injury to the hamstrings origin in the region of the ischial tuberosity (Figure 6.11). There may be tenderness with failure to heal adequately.

The initial lesion is accompanied by a large tender haematoma. If running or other activity which had produced the initial lesion continues, new bone formation may take place in an irregular manner. This mass remains tender for many months.

TREATMENT

Immediate non-weight-bearing is essential. This is followed by crutches with partial weight-bearing after 3 weeks and is necessary until pain subsides. Injections of bupivacaine (Marcain) and hydrocortisone may reduce the pain. Physiotherapy, diathermy and ultrasound aggravate the lesion in its early stages.

Osgood–Schlatter disease

In 1903, Osgood reported 10 cases of epiphysitis of the upper end of the tibia in boys. Several months later, Schlatter described a similar condition. At first it was thought to be simply a traumatic separation,

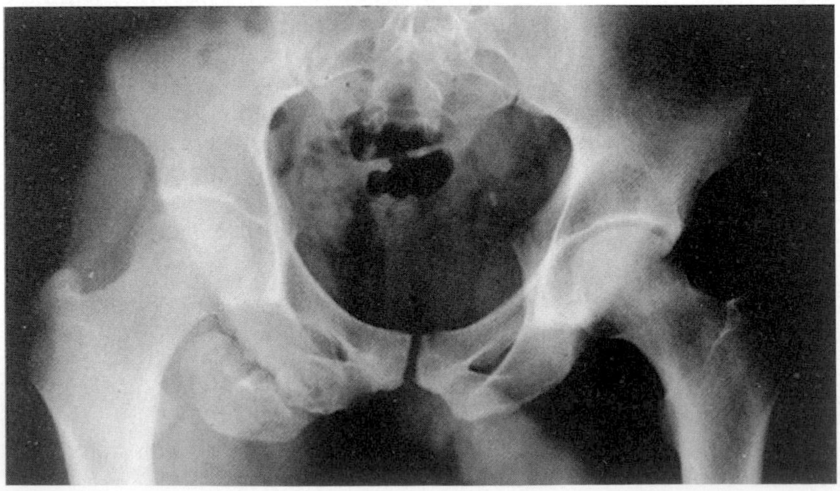

Figure 6.11 Radiograph of the pelvis of a young man showing a large bony fragment in the vicinity of the right ischial area which is irregularly ossified and is separated.

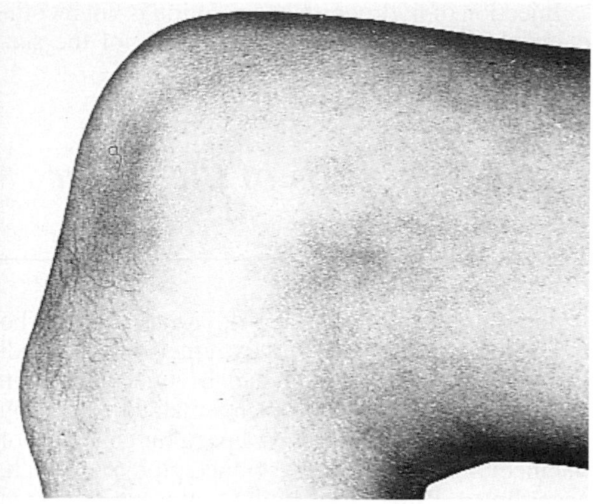

Figure 6.12 Osgood–Schlatter disease of the tibial tuberosity showing the prominent tibial tubercle. (From Aichroth, P. (1992) Disorders of the knee in children. In: *Knee Surgery, Current Practice*. Edited by P. Aichroth, W.D. Cannon and V.K. Patel, Martin Dunitz: London)

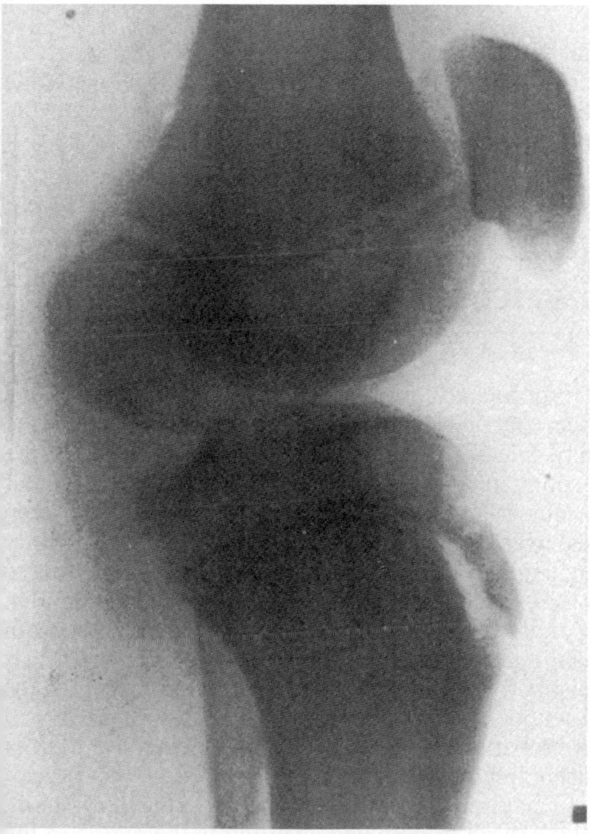

Figure 6.13 Osteochondritis of the anterior part of the upper tibial epiphysis – Osgood–Schlatter disease.

combined sometimes with an actual fracture of the epiphysis. This, of course, does sometimes occur, but the true Osgood–Schlatter disease shows, in addition, characteristic bony changes which stamp it as a definite disease entity.

The tibia is developed from four centres – one for the shaft, one for the lower epiphysis, and two for the upper epiphysis. The tuberosity usually arises as a tongue-like protrusion from the lower end of the upper epiphysis, but it may have two centres of ossification, one extending down from the epiphysis, and one reaching up from the shaft. While the centre of ossification for the head appears first, it unites with the shaft last. There may be earlier points of union in the tuberosity which permits circulation to the fragments.

Partial separation of the tuberosity from trauma, such as violent contraction of the quadriceps muscle, occurs mostly in males between the ages of 16 and 18. There is immediate pain over the affected site, aggravated by any attempt to straighten the knee; the tuberosity is tender and swollen; and radiographs show the detachment of the tongue-like epiphysis.

True Osgood–Schlatter disease occurs at an earlier age, usually from 13 to 15; in most cases injury is to some extent an exciting factor, but it does not play the prominent part that it does in the traumatic separation.

The onset of pain and local tenderness is insidious. The patient first complains of some aching in front of the knee after any exercise, or after a long walk. In many cases such overexertion is the only history of trauma obtained. The pain is increased by full voluntary extension of the joint, since the affected epiphysis is then pulled on by the contracted quadriceps muscle. There is also pain on passive complete flexion, as the epiphysis is then dragged on by the stretched quadriceps. The epiphysis itself is tender, and in many cases there is some localized swelling (Figure 6.12).

The radiographic appearance is characteristic. The texture of the bony nucleus of the epiphysis is altered; it is irregular in contour, or even fragmented (Figure 6.13). There may be localized haziness in the adjacent tibial metaphysis.

Occasionally a similar condition may affect the lower pole of the patella and this may occur together with the Osgood–Schlatter condition described. The patellar epiphysitis is sometimes referred to as a 'reversed Osgood–Schlatter' and was first described in 1921 by Larsen. He presumed an accessory ossifying centre here.

DIAGNOSIS

Osgood–Schlatter disease has to be differentiated

from osteomyelitis, sarcoma of the head of the tibia, bone cysts and infrapatellar bursitis.

The first three occasion little difficulty, but an infrapatellar bursitis may be difficult to distinguish unless fluctuation is present. Aspiration of the bursal fluid usually indicates the source of the trouble.

TREATMENT

In many cases, reduction of activities and the exclusion of violent sport for a few weeks are all that is required. In more severe cases, the condition is treated very much like an epiphyseal separation. First, a plaster cast is applied. Later, physiotherapy is employed. Weight-bearing is permitted from the start, but if there is great tenderness, rest in bed or the use of crutches may be insisted on. Flexion of the knee joint is not allowed for at least 5 weeks, and violent exercises are prohibited for about 4 months.

Complete restitution of the tuberosity to normal is usual, although the tubercle is often prominent. The condition, however, is apt to recur, and the cure is never really complete until the epiphysis joins up with the tibia.

Stirling (1952) described two interesting late complications of the condition. The epiphysis may be pulled upwards, indicating some separation. The consequence of this may be that the patella, displaced proximally from its more irregular contact with the lower end of the femur, is apt to develop osteoarthritis. This is diagnosed by taking lateral radiographs of both knees with the quadriceps muscle fully contracted. If there is displacement, it may be advisable to correct this by operation. The second complication is that the abnormal epiphysis of the tubercle may cause early fusion of the anterior part of the upper tibial epiphysis. With continuing growth of the posterior part a genu recurvatum is a possibility.

Thomson (1956) believed that when there are repeated attacks of pain and disability, or recrudescence after conservative treatment, and when the child is old enough to justify such a procedure, he should be treated by operation. Thomson split the tendon of the patella and, by means of a thin osteotome, opened the tubercle by reflecting the cortical bone on each side of a central incision. With a sharp curette, fragments and debris were removed from within the tubercle. The tendon, with cortex and periosteum attached, was allowed to fall back into place and impacted to minimize bulging. He treated 41 cases in this way. They were from 10 years of age upwards and results were uniformly successful.

Injection of hydrocortisone solution is not recommended because it may cause atrophy of the surrounding tissues.

Osteochondritis of the upper end of the tibia

Ritter reported the case of a girl, 7 years of age, who before the age of 4 years was extremely bow-legged. By the age of 4, one leg had become normal in appearance, whereas the other remained extremely bowed. Radiographs showed a peculiar condition of the medial half of the upper tibial epiphysis, which, according to Ritter, was similar to the appearance in osteochondritis of the hip joint (Ritter and Wilson, 1968).

Osteochondritis of the lower end of the tibia and fibula

In 1922, Sterne demonstrated a case of osteochondritis of the lower ends of the tibia and fibula, while 6 years later Ritter reported a similar condition in the lower end of the tibia.

Köhler's disease of the tarsal navicular

Unfortunately, two quite different conditions have been named Köhler's disease: one affecting the navicular of the foot, and the other the head of the second metatarsal. Köhler's disease of the navicular occurs usually in young children, especially between the ages of 3 and 6. It affects boys more commonly than girls. The navicular is the last bone of the foot to ossify, and, as it forms the keystone of the long arch, it must be subjected to a very considerable strain while yet in the cartilaginous state. The disease is distinctly analogous to the condition known as Kienböck's disease, which will be described later. It is probably an osteochondritis, but its cause has not been definitely established.

The clinical manifestations are often very slight, and consist of pain and swelling in the region of the tarsal navicular. The pain is exaggerated by weight-bearing, and the affected region is sensitive to

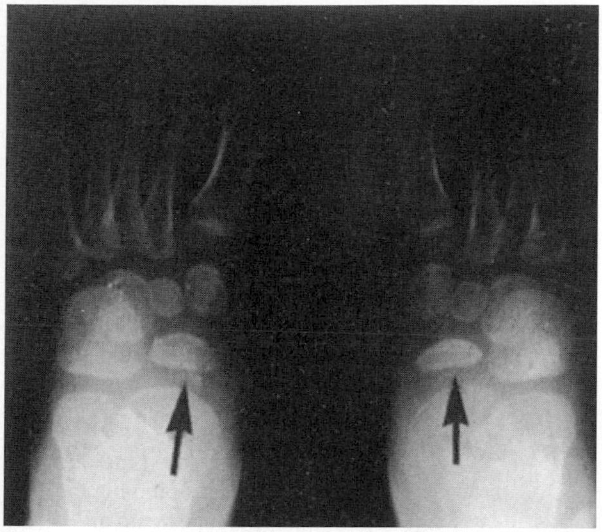

Figure 6.14 Growth cessation shown at right (arrowed). This is an early sign of true Köhler's disease.

movement and tender on pressure. There may, or may not, be reddish discoloration in addition to swelling. The patient limps, and usually walks and bears weight on the lateral border of the foot, to relieve the affected side.

The condition is usually detected from the physical examination in conjunction with the history, and is confirmed by the radiographs which reveal definite changes in the bone. These changes consist of a narrowing of the bone in its anteroposterior diameter, along with a condensation of the bony structure. There is no fragmentation of the bony nucleus. The joint spaces remain clear, and the neighbouring tarsal and metatarsal bones are normal in appearance.

RADIOLOGICAL APPEARANCES

One must be familiar with the appearance of normal ossification centres in the tarsal scaphoid in childhood. It is normal for this bone to ossify from two or three separate centres, thereby giving the appearance of irregular ossification. Diagnosis of circulatory interference is most definite when there is true loss of expected transverse diameter and an increased density is present (Figure 6.14). Later when new blood supply is established, bone develops with an irregular appearance.

TREATMENT

The treatment of this condition is comparatively simple, symptomatic recovery usually occurring in a few months. A plaster cast should be applied to hold the foot in a slight varus position. After a few weeks the plaster is removed and adhesive strapping used to support the ankle and the mid-torsal region. A valgus insole in the shoe may be used if pain persists.

Epiphysitis of the os calcis

There is uncertainty whether there is such an entity as loss of circulation to the apophysis of the os calcis with subsequently increased radiodensity, and later irregular translucent areas when the circulation is regained.

A review of the radiographic appearance of the apophysis of the os calcis as it develops shows that increased radiodensity is normal. The apophysis ossification centre appears at 8 years and completes its development by 14 years. There may normally be several extra ossification centres lying proximally in a chain towards the tendo Achillis.

There is, however, a syndrome of heel pain present, particularly in boys aged 9–15 years. Some of these may be produced by inflammation of the bursa beneath the tendo Achillis. Most, however, appear to be directly related to excessive, repeated trauma or strain of the insertion of the tendo Achillis into the os calcis. The tenderness is not only posteriorly, but lateral over the posterior portion of the os calcis as well.

DIAGNOSIS

In the differential diagnosis the following conditions have to be considered: calcanean bursitis; tuberculous and pyogenic infection of the calcaneum; and tenosynovitis of the tendo calcaneum.

PROGNOSIS

The duration of the acute condition is short, varying from a few weeks to a few months. Under appropriate treatment, the prognosis is excellent, but recurrences are possible until the parent bone and the epiphysis are solidly united. Frequently the condition is transient.

TREATMENT

Pain is relieved by a plaster of Paris cast from toes to just above the knee to hold the foot in a 10–15°

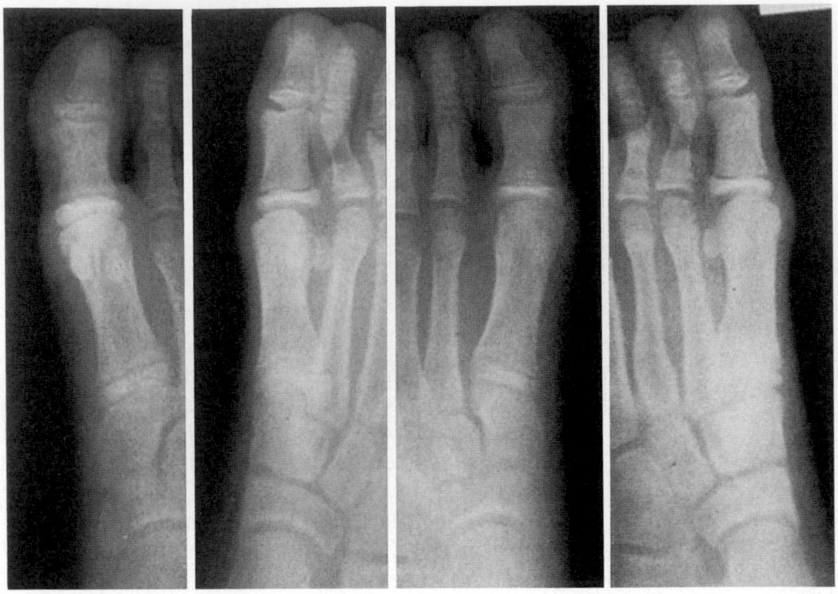

Figure 6.15 Anteroposterior and oblique radiographs of both feet, showing the increased radiodensity on the epiphyses of the big toe proximal phalanges with an overlying soft tissue swelling, but joint space is well maintained.

equinus position and relax the pull on the tendo Achillis. The plaster is retained for 3 weeks and then Tubigrip bandage is applied below the knee until the pain disappears. Occasionally a plaster applied in the neutral position is required for a further 3 weeks to achieve resolution of symptoms.

Epiphysitis of the proximal phalanx of the big toe

The epiphysis of the base of the proximal phalanx usually appears at the age of 2–3 years and fuses with the shaft by the age of 15–18 years. This condition is not well documented in the literature. However, in one case of a young boy aged 9 years, the presenting symptom was of pain and swelling of the first metatarsophalangeal joint of several months' duration which then involved the other foot. There was soft tissue swelling and local tenderness with aggravation by running on tiptoe or body push-up exercises. Radiographs (Figure 6.15) showed increased radiodensity with irregularity of each epiphyseal outline, but the joint space was normal. The symptoms improved with simple stiffening of the shoe.

Vertebral epiphysitis (Scheuermann's disease)

For a full discussion of this disease, see Chapter 8.

Coxa vara

In the adult femur the neck is set on the shaft at an angle which varies from 120° to 140°. A decrease in this normal neck–shaft angle is known as coxa vara, while if the angle is over 140°, coxa valga is said to be present. Coxa vara consists, therefore, of a depression of the neck, and is a feature of many different conditions, although at one time it was thought to be due invariably to active softening and bending of the bone. The depression of the neck results in certain obvious mechanical disadvantages. The normal apposition between the joint surfaces is lost, since the head of the femur no longer accurately fits the acetabulum. The trochanter is displaced upwards, and hence, during abduction, is liable to impinge on the side of the pelvis. The marked shortening of the limb leads to a waddling gait, not unlike that of congenital dislocation of the hip. As coxa vara is a symptom of many diseases, it is usually classified according to the condition which causes it (Figures 6.16 and 6.17).

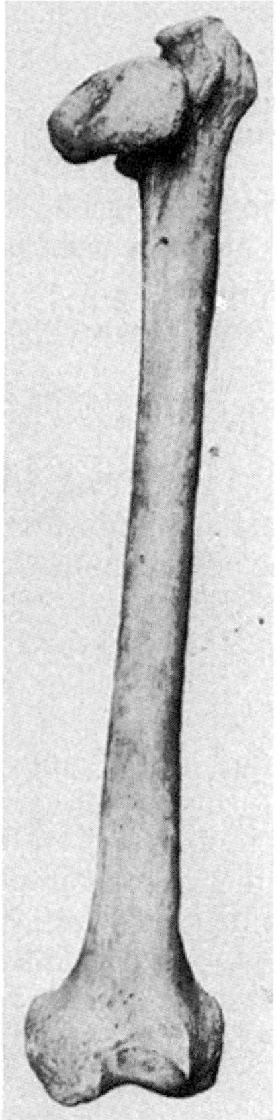

Figure 6.16 Coxa vara from old Perthes' disease.

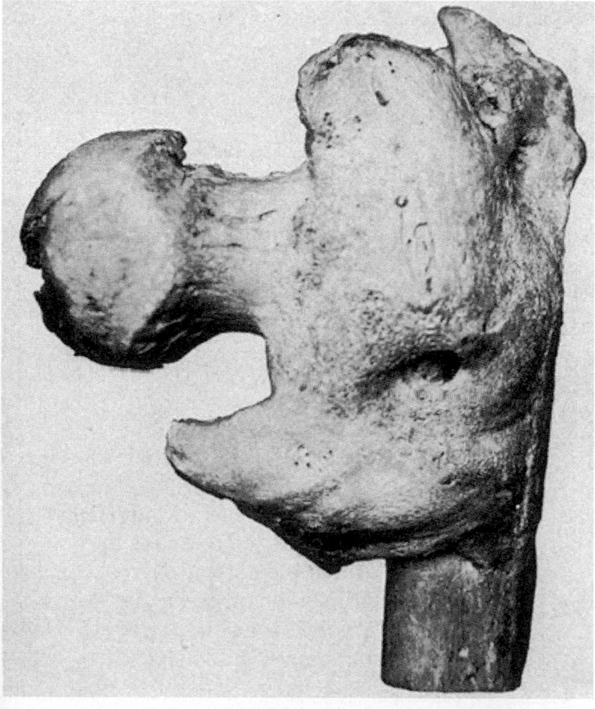

Figure 6.17 Coxa vara following fracture of the base of the neck involving the trochanter.

The deformity may be localized:

1. Congenital coxa vara.
2. Congenital short femur with coxa vara (p. 215).
3. Congenital bowed femur with coxa vara.
4. Secondary, e.g.
   (a) Perthes' disease;
   (b) slipped upper femoral epiphysis;
   (c) septic arthritis of infancy.

or part of a generalized skeletal dysplasia:

1. Mucopolysaccharidoses (e.g. Morquio's disease).
2. Dysplasia epiphysealis multiplex.
3. Achondroplasia.
4. Cleidocranial dysostosis.

Congenital coxa vara

Coxa vara may be a primary congenital deformity, occurring alone, or in association with other congenital defects, especially defective growth of the femur. It may also be a secondary congenital error, when it is associated with some intrauterine affection of bone, such as achondroplasia.

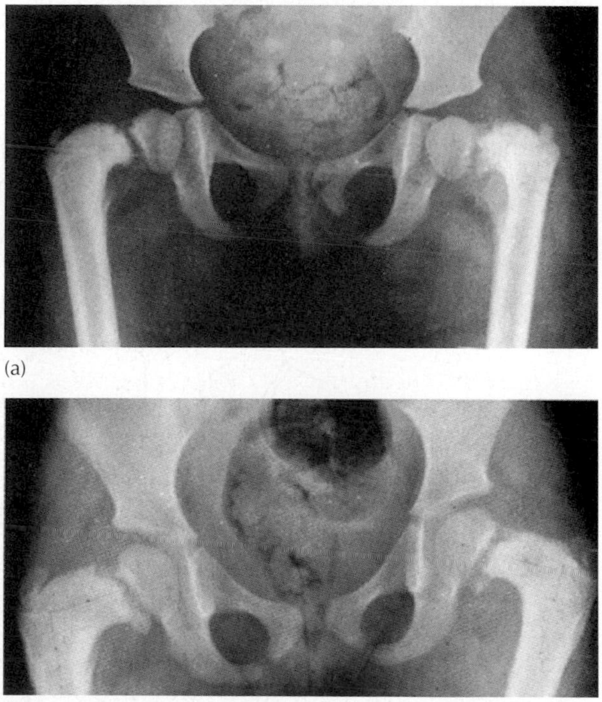

(a)

(b)

Figure 6.18 (a) Bilateral coxa vara – a progressive disease with the mechanical stress on the epiphyseal line to show the development of further deformity. (b) Same patient 18 months later. The triangular fragment at the lower border of the neck is clearly seen.

Congenital coxa vara, also described sometimes as cervical or infantile coxa vara, is characterized according to Fairbank (Wynne-Davies and Fairbank, 1976), by the presence in a radiograph of a triangular piece of the neck adjacent to the head being separate from the rest of the bone. The condition is often bilateral and often symptoms are evident as soon as the child walks, but they may be delayed for some years (Figure 6.18).

The patient is usually small in stature and limps, and, in bilateral cases, rather resembles a patient with congenital dislocation. Often there is pain and stiffness. On examination, the greater trochanter is on a level higher than the normal, with consequent shortening of the limb. Rotation and abduction are limited, while there may be a flexion contracture present.

Zadek (1935) reported the histological findings in four of his own cases. These all showed abnormality of bone trabeculation with alteration of pattern and direction as well as abnormal islands of disintegrating cartilage cells, but, he added: 'The histology was not sufficiently characteristic to permit a definite diagnosis as to the cause of the bone change.'

A typical case shows interesting radiographic features which are tabulated as follows, although all may not be present at one time.

1. The angle of the neck is reduced to something below a right angle.
2. The neck varies in length but is short and may even be non-existent, and may be fragmented through incomplete ossification. Often the neck shows a prolonged lower extremity which forms a down-hanging lip.
3. The head is unusually translucent, situated low in the acetabulum, and may be fluffy in outline.
4. There is a fragment of bone, triangular in shape, occupying the lower part of the neck close to the head. This is bounded by two clear bands traversing the neck and forming an inverted 'V'. The inner band is the epiphyseal line, while the other is part of the epiphysis as the two lines usually disappear at the same time.
5. There is some deformity of the acetabulum due to the malposition of the head.
6. In extreme cases the greater trochanter curves inwards, is beaked, and may articulate with the ilium above the acetabulum.

TREATMENT

Although this is a rare lesion, unless it is corrected, the severe deformity and disability which can result from it are well recognized. Therefore, it is recommended that an angulation osteotomy of the Dickson type, at the intertrochanteric level, should be carried out. In this, by removing a wedge-shaped area of bone with the base on the lateral side, it is possible to abduct the distal femoral shaft and hold the two fragments with screws and a plate. With the limb taking up the neutral plane, the vertical epiphyseal and neck defects become horizontal, thereby relieving much of the shearing stress and the varus deformity (Figures 6.19 and 6.20).

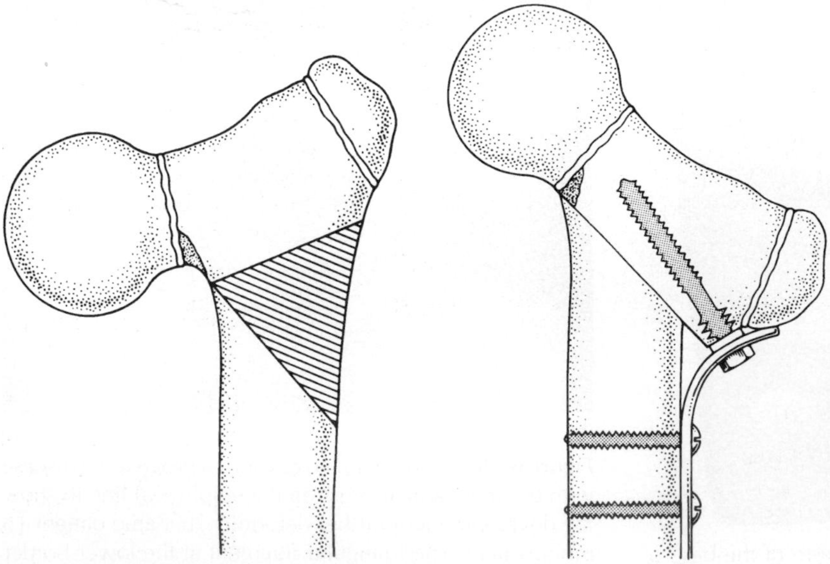

(a) (b)

Figure 6.19 Osteotomy for coxa vara showing excision of large wedge. (b) Fixation with angled nail-plate. (From Catterall, A. (1991) Operations for congenital dislocation of the hip. In: *Rob & Smith's Operative Surgery: Orthopaedics*. Butterworth-Heinemann: London, Boston, Sydney, Wellington, Singapore)

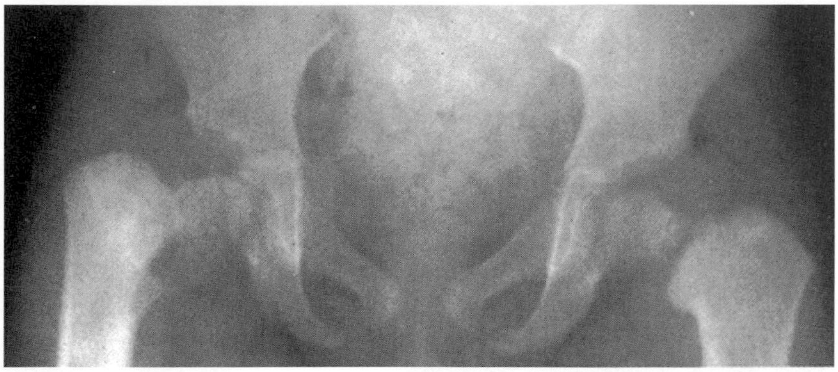

(a)

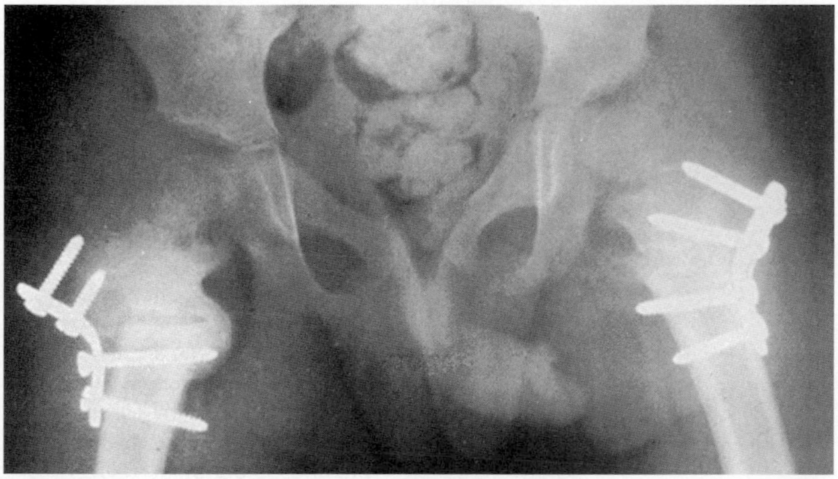

(b)

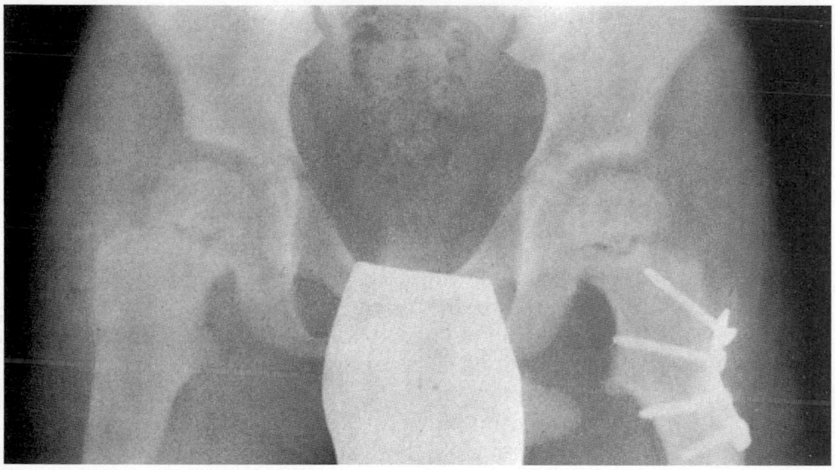

(c)

Figure 6.20 Radiographs of the pelvis of a boy aged 5 years. (a) Severe bilateral deformity of a congenital coxa vara. (b) Same boy 6 months later with bilateral angulation osteotomies and internal fixation. The horizontal nature of the epiphyseal lines should be noted. (c) Two years later with one internal fixation plate removed, showing the irregular appearance of the epiphyseal lines, but good development of the femoral neck in a valgus position.

Epiphyseal coxa vara or slipping femoral epiphysis

The condition occurs more often in males, in the proportion of about 5:2. It commonly occurs between the ages of 10 and 16, when the capital epiphysis of the femur is actively growing, although in females it tends to begin at a rather earlier age than in males. It is not unusual to find the condition bilaterally (25%), and left is more common than right.

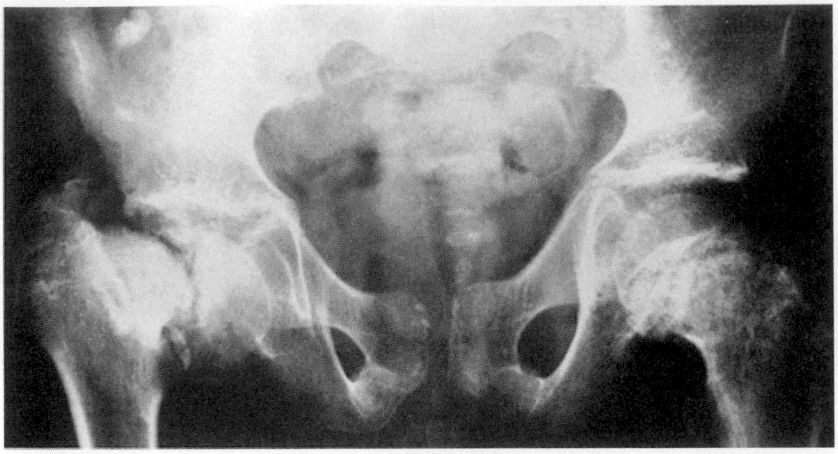

(a)

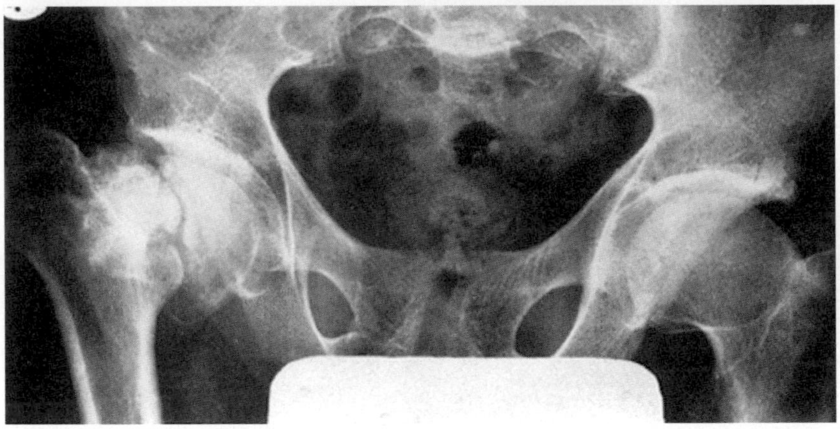

(b)

Figure 6.21 Bilateral slipped femoral epiphysis in a man aged 40 years who was a hypopituitary dwarf with a bone age of $13^1/_2$ years. (b) Same patient after 5 years of hormone replacement treatment, showing fusion of the epiphyseal growth plate on the left and persisting slipped epiphysis on the right. (Reproduced by permission of the editor and authors from Semple, J.C. and Goldschmidt, R.G. (1969) *Orthopaedics, Oxford* 2, 31–43)

AETIOLOGY

The deformity results from a weakening of the union between the epiphysis and the femoral neck and the effect of the normal shearing strain at this site.

Hormonal theory

Although the softening is due to a failure of maturation of cartilage into bone, the reason for this failure remains obscure. The analysis of the evidence seems to suggest that it is the result of a hormonal imbalance. It is well recorded in animals that a variety of agents will weaken or change the histological appearance of the epiphyseal plate in this area – e.g. hyperoestrogen administration, hypophysectomy (Silberberg and Silberberg, 1949) and by cortisone (Duthie and Barker, 1955). Slipping of an epiphysis will occur only while the growth-plate remains open (Figure 6.21). Growth and maturation of the epiphyseal cartilage plate depend on hormonal factors; viz. growth hormone, thyroid hormone and the sex hormones. In connection with this, Harris (1950) observed that epiphyses tend to slip at times of fast growth and in certain types of individuals (e.g. adiposogenital syndrome) or in tall thin children. The former he suggested had a deficiency of sex hormones, and the latter suffered from excess of growth hormone. Experimentally with rats he showed that growth hormone increased the thickness of epiphyseal plates, which required less force to slip; oestrogen treatment led to thinner, more mature, plates, and more force was required to detach them. Unfortunately, there are no human studies to support any theory of a hormonal basis for slipping. Indeed, the majority of biochemical studies, including hydroxyproline, have been normal.

Traumatic theory

Many writers consider the condition to be a purely traumatic separation of a normal femoral epiphysis. The epiphyseal line is said to be the weakest part of the normal adolescent bone.

There is no doubt that trauma and static influences are both important factors in the development of epiphyseal coxa vara, but it is probable that they act upon a femur in which the epiphysis is less firmly attached than normal. The pathological conditions which cause the loosening of the epiphysis are not definitely known, but Key pointed out in the 1930s that they may be neither in the bone nor in the epiphyseal cartilage, but in the periosteum of the femoral neck. In childhood this periosteum is thick, and thrown into folds or ridges known as the retinacula of Weitbrecht; actually it is the chief factor in holding the head in place. In adolescence this periosteum begins to atrophy, and to approach the adult type, thus tending to produce a point of weakness at the epiphyseal line. He also pointed out that most cases of coxa vara give a history of very rapid growth prior to the epiphyseal displacement, and he suggested that during this period the periosteum crossing the epiphyseal line is stretched and thinned, and consequently weakened, thus permitting the epiphysis to be easily separated.

Fairbank described a form to which he gave the name 'infantile coxa vara'. He pointed out that the epiphysis is set obliquely on the neck and faces upwards and medially. This setting, somewhat insecure as a means of supporting the body weight, is strengthened by a spur projecting from the lower half of the metaphysis. Walmsley (1938) showed that this spur provides a natural ledge on which the epiphysis rests. Occasionally the spur ossifies from a separate secondary centre which may remain isolated from the rest of the metaphysis by a strip of cartilage till puberty. This increase in the amount of cartilage weakens the neck in proportion to the body weight, while the inadequacy of the spur, increased occasionally by fragmentation of its centre, allows the epiphysis to slide gradually downwards.

Haas (1948) showed that once the periosteum has been stripped off the humeral epiphysis of rats, the middle zone of the epiphyseal plate will slip when a shearing stress is applied.

PATHOLOGY

The only abnormality in the early stages is in the epiphyseal cartilage. This is immature and forms fibrous tissue instead of bone. This abnormality appears to be the primary factor in the histological picture and it proceeds towards the fragmentation and disappearance of the epiphyseal plate.

Lacroix and Verbrugge (1951) described the pathology seen in a case of slipping femoral epiphysis. They believed that the primary lesion was the replacement of the normal endochondral ossification by fibrous tissues. Also, when the head slipped, it pulled down the periosteum with absorption on its upper surface and new bone was laid down on its lower surface, with remodelling of the trabeculae. Indeed, these workers could find no evidence to show weakening of the periosteum, low-grade infection, circulatory disturbances, rickets or a localized osteomalacia. They believed that such conditions have no relation to the aetiology of the condition.

It is apparent that a balance of growth hormone and sex hormones is required for normal growth and closure of the growth-plates at maturity and a disturbance of the balance produces excessive widening of the hypertrophic zone, predisposing to separation from the metaphysis.

SYMPTOMATOLOGY

Epiphyseal coxa vara or slipped upper femoral epiphyses (SUFE) may be idiopathic (non-traumatic) or traumatic, though this distinction is dubious.

Idiopathic type

There is seldom any history of preceding illness or constitutional disturbance. The onset is gradual, and in many cases the earliest symptom is that the patient gets tired easily after walking or standing. He may then complain of pain, which may be confined to the hip, but usually radiates down to the lower thigh and knee. There may be slight limitation of abduction. These symptoms are evanescent and disappear for a time, only to reappear with increased severity. In the early stages the pain is relieved by rest, and the patient is not troubled at night.

The pain is accompanied by a limp, and, as the error progresses, the limp may be present even when the pain is absent. The affected leg gradually be comes shorter and smaller than its neighbour, and tends to turn laterally, while its movements are restricted. There is often a delay of many weeks between the onset of symptoms and diagnosis.

Traumatic type

In this type the patient has usually had a fall, or received a blow on the hip, some time before. In many cases, however, the trauma is very trivial, and not infrequently the history is elicited that the patient had some disturbance in the affected hip even before the injury. It is unlikely that trauma can displace a normal epiphysis. Following the trauma, there is usually a dull ache, associated with little disability in the hip, although occasionally the pain is so severe that it prevents the patient from being able to walk – i.e. an 'acute' slip.

Loder *et al.* (1993) have introduced a classification of the slipped epiphysis as being either stable or unstable. Slipping or slipped hips were classified as 'unstable' where the patient had severe pain when weight-bearing even using crutches. Slips were 'stable' when the patient could bear weight with or without crutches. On reviewing their 55 hips who were all treated with internal fixation with this classification, reduction occurred in 26 out of 30 'unstable' hips, but only 2 of the 25 'stable' hips. Only 47% of the 'unstable' hips had a satisfactory result against 96% of the 'stable' hips – similarly 47% of the unstable hips developed avascular necrosis and none in the stable hips. There was no association between early reduction and the development of avascular necrosis. This classification appears useful but clinically it is often difficult to differentiate patients so precisely.

PHYSICAL SIGNS

During its early stages the condition is associated with considerable pain, but by the time the patient is seen, the disease is usually well developed and the painful acute stage is passed. He walks with a waddling gait, the body swaying over to the affected side. The pelvis on the sound side tends to drop when weight is borne on the affected extremity.

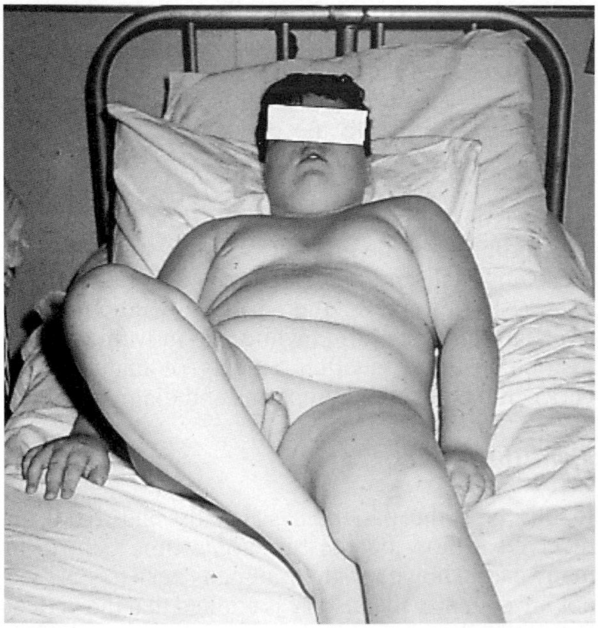

Figure 6.22 Clinical photograph of a male patient with slipped upper left femoral epiphysis showing the classical external rotation with flexion of the hip (with kind permission of Mr J. Wilkinson).

The patient stands with the leg rotated laterally and slightly abducted, while inspection shows the pelvis to be tilted down on the affected side. A slight scoliosis towards the affected side is present in the lumbar region, and towards the sound side in the thoracic. The buttock is atrophied, and the gluteal fold lower than on the normal side.

On palpation of the groin, a hard mass can often be felt, which moves with the femur; it is the thickened head and neck.

Measurement shows the trochanter to be higher than on the sound side, the tip usually being situated about 1 cm above Nélaton's line.

Movement on the affected side is limited. With the patient recumbent on his back, the position of the leg is one of lateral rotation and slight abduction. Flexion is limited to about 80° or 90° and, as the thigh is flexed, it rotates laterally. Adduction and lateral rotation are free, but abduction, medial rotation and extension are greatly restricted (Figure 6.22).

In a recent complete separation, the signs resemble those of recent fracture of the neck of the femur, with great pain, external rotation of the limb being restricted by muscular spasm.

RADIOLOGICAL APPEARANCES

The condition is progressive and the x-ray appearance varies with the stage. Both hips should be x-rayed in such a way that they are shown in exactly comparable positions on the same film with both anteroposterior and lateral views.

Preslipping stage

In early cases the x-ray shows:

1. Minimal slipping, indicated by the absence of the normal 'shoulder' on the upper aspect of the neck and head (i.e. Trethowan's sign, in which a line drawn along the superior surface of the neck will pass above the femoral head rather than through it) (Figure 6.23).
2. The head is more or less sickle-shaped instead of hemispherical and its height is diminished.
3. The epiphyseal plate is widened, and rarefaction or even streaks of sclerosis may be seen underneath it.
4. The lateral view shows the slightest backward displacement better than in the anteroposterior view (Figure 6.24).

These features should be sought in children suffering from discomfort or pain in the hip joint. Their recognition demands measures to prevent slipping

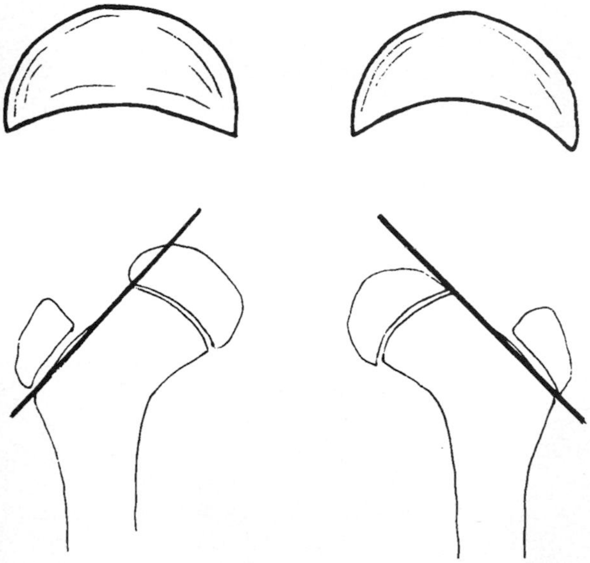

Figure 6.23 Diagram of Trethowan's sign of early slipped upper femoral epiphysis. (From Hughes, S.P.F., Benson, M.K. and Colton, C.L. (1987) *Orthopaedics*. Churchill Livingstone: Edinburgh, London, Melbourne and New York)

(see Figure 6.25). The epiphyseal plate should be at right angles to the axis through the femoral neck.

Early stage

The head of the femur lies in the acetabulum but is rotated so that its lower and posterior borders are displaced downwards and laterally (Griffith, 1991). The head is slightly displaced in relation to the neck, its lower border projecting as a beak-like process below the lower margin of the neck. The upper margin of the head is thinned out and separated by a short distance from the prominence made by the upper angle of the metaphysis. The femoral neck bears its normal relation to the shaft, but its upper border is lengthened and roughly convex upwards, while its lower border is shortened and also appears to be more sharply curved upwards than normally. The lower border of the neck is buried in the concave cervical surface of the epiphysis, and appears to be shortened. In the angle between the lower border of the neck and the underhanging head, new bone is formed.

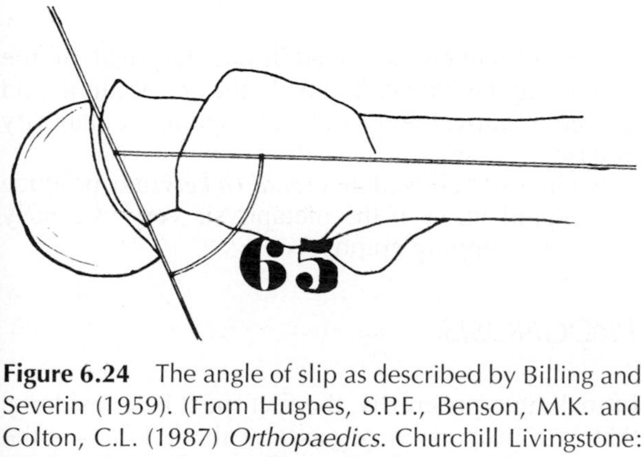

Figure 6.24 The angle of slip as described by Billing and Severin (1959). (From Hughes, S.P.F., Benson, M.K. and Colton, C.L. (1987) *Orthopaedics*. Churchill Livingstone: Edinburgh, London, Melbourne and New York)

Advanced stage

The femoral head is atrophic, especially in its projecting lower half, and it has now become so rotated and displaced that only a small anterior portion is actually in the acetabulum (i.e. the slip is posteromedial). The articular surface is thus directed medially, backwards and downwards. The projecting lower edge of the head is now curved laterally and upwards, and is in contact with the lower border of the neck. The neck is thick and short, and its lower border sharply bowed upwards. The neck–shaft angle appears to be decreased to about 90°. The joint space is clear and there is usually no evidence of arthritis. However, Heyman *et al.* (1957) described how there is new bone formation occurring at the anterosuperior aspect of the neck at its junction with the epiphysis, which may easily produce impingement on the acetabular margin to restrict the movements of abduction and internal rotation.

In cases where displacement has been severe, the head is often completely separated from the neck, and lies loose in the acetabulum. Except for this displacement, the contour of the bones is normal, but the joint margins and the joint space may be hazy from the extravasation of blood.

DIAGNOSIS

Harris (1950) drew attention to the importance of early diagnosis and described a characteristic symptom-complex – a limp of spontaneous onset and pain referred to the knee in an obese adolescent.

Diagnosis is further suggested by the adducted, laterally rotated position of the limb. In addition, the radiographic appearance is characteristic.

DIFFERENTIAL DIAGNOSIS

Slipping femoral epiphysis is to be distinguished from tuberculosis of the hip, Perthes' disease and congenital dislocation.

The *tuberculous hip* is adducted and medially rotated, with movement limited in all directions. The atrophy is greater, and the hip is more sensitive and

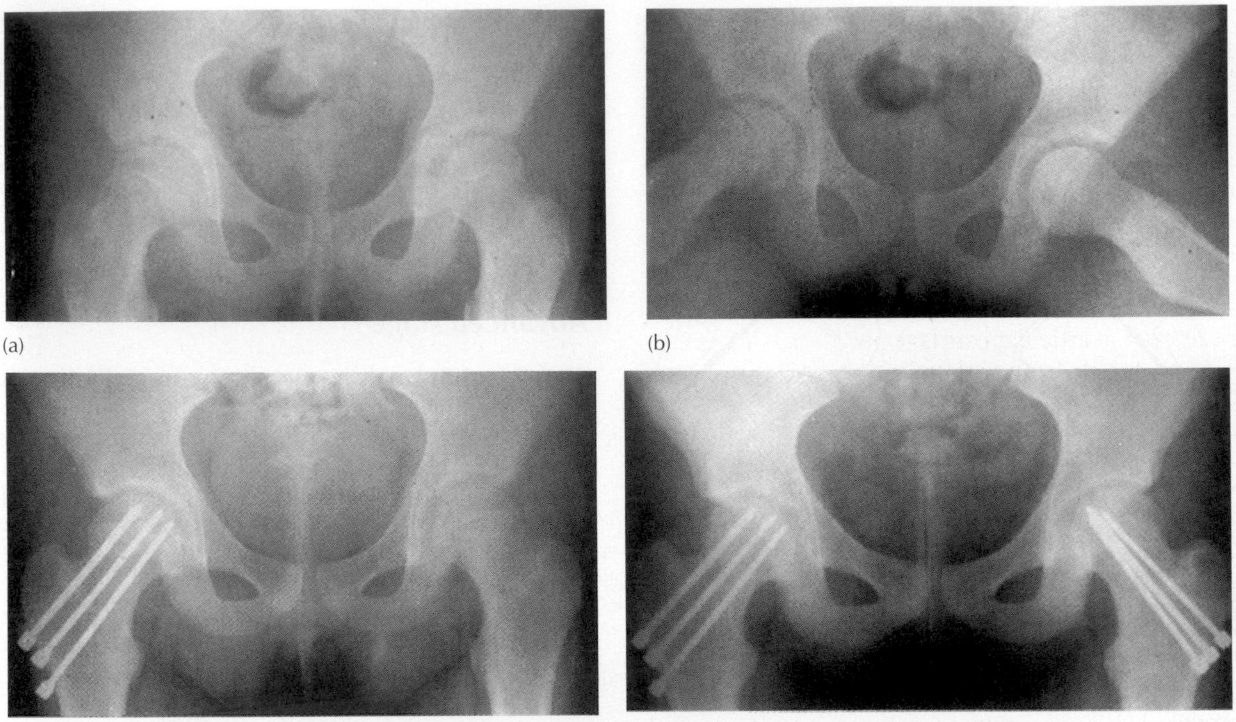

(a) (b) (c) (d)

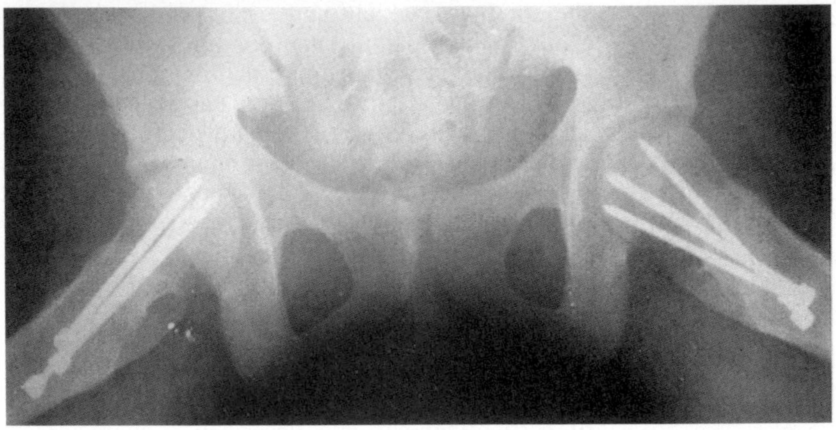

(e)

Figure 6.25 (a–e) Radiographs of a very obese girl aged 10 years who presented with a painful limp of the right hip. (a) The anteroposterior view was suspicious for a slipping femoral epiphysis which is readily seen in (b) the abducted and rotated view. (c) Right femoral epiphysis was fixed *in situ* with three Knowles pins. (d) and (e) Six months later this girl developed a painful limp on the left side and Knowles pins were inserted into this incipient slipping epiphysis. These radiographs were taken just before the removal of the Knowles pins from the right side where the epiphysis had united.

painful even while at rest. Radiographs show extensive demineralization of the femoral head and acetabulum without any epiphyseal displacement.

In *Perthes' disease* the history, the limitation of movement, the slight atrophy and the shortening are identical with those of a mild coxa vara. The chief points of difference are the age of the patient and the x-ray appearance. Perthes' disease rarely begins after the tenth year, while epiphyseal coxa vara seldom begins before it; also, in Perthes' the head is not displaced but actually deformed, and may in the mushroomed type 'overflow' onto the upper border of the neck.

In *congenital dislocation of the hip* there is along history of lameness. In addition, the head of the femur may be palpated outside the acetabulum, and telescopic movement can be elicited in the majority of cases.

Brailsford believed that *renal rickets* may produce a disorganization of the metaphysis very like early cases of a slipping epiphysis.

PROGNOSIS

In making a prognosis, the fact must be considered that in a proportion of cases – about 1 in 4 – the second hip becomes affected.

The end result depends to a certain extent upon the degree of displacement of the head, but it is only in the early cases where there is minimal slipping that the end result is completely satisfactory. Nevertheless very good results can be achieved with good reduction provided avascular necrosis is avoided and even with up to 50% displacement of the head when this is followed by corrective osteotomy. The remodelling capacity of the hip is considerable at this age.

All treatment is aimed at avoiding avascular necrosis and articular cartilage necrosis. A review of the end results from various sources forces the conclusion that, save in the exceptional case, manipulation does more harm than good and should be avoided. Similarly, skeletal traction is associated with an unacceptable incidence of avascular necrosis and is probably ineffective in achieving reduction (Griffith, 1991).

Some patients with a displaced epiphysis despite treatment, develop avascular necrosis, cartilage necrosis and arthritic changes during adult life.

Data on long-term follow-up are sparse but the review by Conybeare and Houghton (1980) of 41 patients with 50 slipping femoral epiphyses (of which all but one had been treated surgically) showed that after 17–30 years, 18 were pain free, and 19 had slight or intermittent pain. Radiological changes often appeared more severe than their clinical symptoms would suggest.

TREATMENT

Adolescent slipping epiphysis should be treated as a surgical emergency no matter the degree of slip or the mildness of the symptoms. The extent of the displacement on the anteroposterior and lateral radiographs must be assessed. Various classifications are employed but if the displacement of the head on the metaphysis of the neck of the femur is less than one-third, acceptable results will be achieved by stabilizing the head with pins to achieve fusion followed by corrective femoral osteotomy. If the displacement is more than 30% then reduction and fixation by a surgeon experienced in the procedure is the best method and can produce excellent results (Dunn and Angel, 1978). A major fixed deformity after growth-plate closure is a reconstructive problem dealt with by osteotomy of the femur and occasionally arthrodesis or arthroplasty.

The early case with minimal deformity > 25% angulation

These cases are usually acute in the onset with severe symptoms of less than 3 weeks' duration. Such cases, unless immobilized and fixed, are apt to continue slipping and pass into the second category. Wilson's criteria for the degree of displacement which could safely be accepted as compatible with normal subsequent function, except for slight limitation of internal rotation, was that clinically there should be free abduction and not more than 10° of fixed external rotation, that the anteroposterior radiograph should show the upper border of the epiphysis well above the surface of the neck, and that in the lateral view the epiphysis should not be displaced posteriorly more than one-third of the diameter of the neck. This is still an acceptable guideline.

No attempt is made to alter this position in such cases and they are pinned by means of the Moore or Knowles type of fixation pins. These are only 2.5 mm in diameter and they do not tend to push the epiphysis away from the metaphysis (Figure 6.25). In 2 weeks the patient is allowed up on crutches but full weight-bearing is not permitted for 3 months. The pins are removed at 12 months, by which time the epiphysis is usually fused.

Cases with unacceptable displacement

The early case – acute-on-chronic slip

These patients present sometimes with a sudden exacerbation of symptoms due to an acute displacement of an already chronically slipped epiphysis. Where the disability has occurred suddenly and acutely the case is treated as an emergency and treatment instituted forthwith since each day that passes makes a successful result less probable. An anaesthetic is given and the hip gently moved under radiological control to ascertain any mobility of the epiphysis. If the epiphysis is mobile, it may be reduced by gentle manipulation or by skeletal traction using a 5 kg long pull on the limb and an internal rotation pull of about 2 kg.

The late case – chronic slip

The operative treatment of this type is controversial. There are three possibilities:

1. *Open anatomical reduction* (Dunn, 1979). With the joint opened and the neck and epiphysis exposed, the epiphysis is freed by dissection from the metaphysis. The neck is then, by abduction and internal rotation of the limb, manipulated into its correct relationship with the epiphysis. Sufficient bone has to be removed from the metaphysis to make reduction possible with out any great force (Figure 6.26). There is a risk of avascular necrosis of 10–20%.

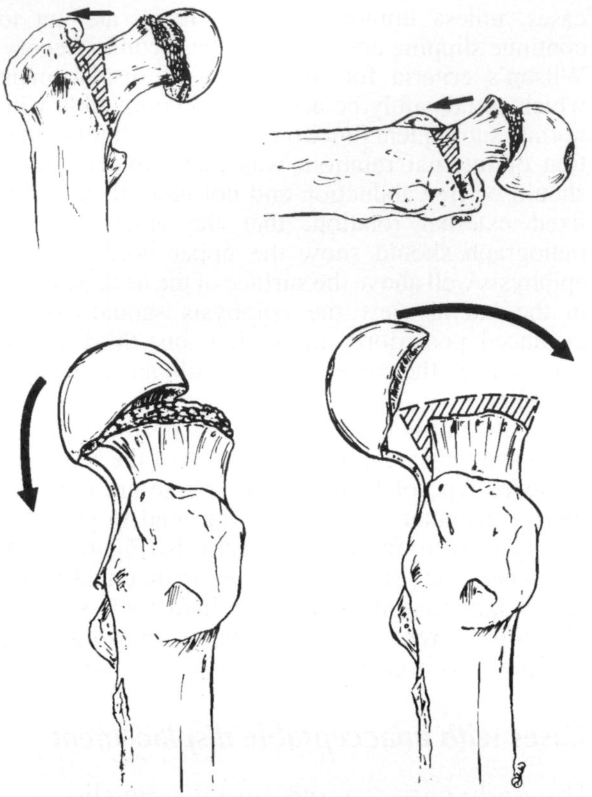

Figure 6.26 Diagram to illustrate the Dunn osteotomy in which the femoral neck is shortened before the capital epiphysis is replaced to avoid tension on the retinacular vessels. (From Hughes, S.P.F., Benson, M.K., Colton, C.L. (1987) *Orthopaedics.* Churchill Livingstone: Edinburgh, London, Melbourne, New York)

2. *Osteotomy of the femoral neck.* By this means the deformity is corrected by removal of a wedge at the base of the neck. The base of the wedge is anterolateral and sufficiently large to compensate for the deformity and allow the gap in the neck to be closed. Avascular necrosis is the complication to be particularly feared in this operation but it is a risk in all degrees of slipping, varying between 25% and 50%. The preferable operation is open reduction, especially in reasonably early cases, before secondary bone remodelling has become fully established.
3. *Subtrochanteric osteotomy.* This is safe but not ideal. The hip left as it is with a severe degree of slip gives a marked limp, permanent disability and the likelihood of early arthritic change. It does, however, compensate to some extent for the deformity and may in the early stages considerably improve the gait and relieve symptoms (Griffith, 1991).

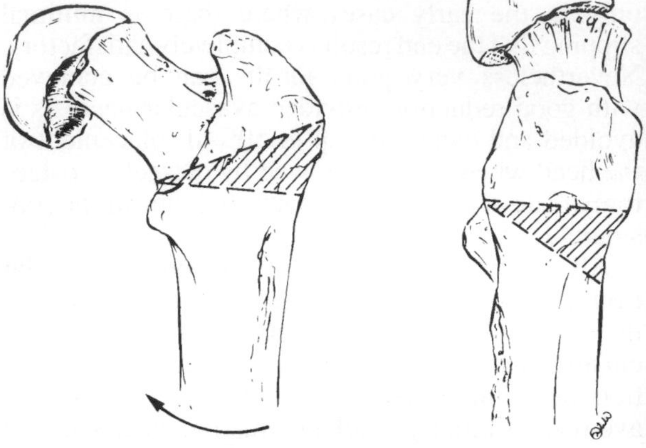

Figure 6.27 Diagram to illustrate the Southwick type of osteotomy through the region of the lesser trochanter which achieves correction of the posterior tilt of the capital epiphyses. (From Hughes, S.P.F., Benson, M.K., Colton, C.L.(1987) *Orthopaedics.* Churchill Livingstone: Edinburgh, London, Melbourne, New York)

Wilson *et al.* (1965), in reviewing their experience, emphasized how avascular necrosis is a disastrous complication of treatment, although cartilage necrosis *per se* was a more frequent and equally serious complication. They found subtrochanteric osteotomy to be the safest method of correction, and wedge osteotomy through the neck remains a difficult and risky procedure.

Southwick (1967) described an accurate biplanar osteotomy at the level of the lesser trochanter to correct the deformity with a very low incidence of avascular necrosis. However, he did not consider the cases which go on to cartilage necrosis and hence joint narrowing. He suggested a very long follow-up for at least 3 years before considering further reconstructive procedures. (Figure 6.27).

Chondrolysis occurs in over 12% of cases, particularly in negroes, in females and with chronic slips which have required open reduction or osteotomies or Smith-Petersen nails. Some do recover good function without symptoms.

It is generally agreed that manipulation and skeletal traction both carry an unacceptable risk of avascular necrosis in cases with acute or chronic severe slip. Therefore open replacement of the femoral epiphysis as described by Dunn and Angel (1978) appears to be the best procedure in experienced hands. Alternatively, the displacement is accepted pinned *in situ* and femoral osteotomy is performed later. This may be trochanteric (Griffith, 1991) or subtrochanteric (Southwick, 1967) but the trochanteric osteotomy, whilst giving more perfect correction, is complicated by a low incidence of avascular necrosis.

Acute chondrolysis

Pain with limitation of movement after operative treatment for slipping femoral epiphysis is of great concern because it may imply postoperative infection, avascular necrosis or acute chondrolysis. Cartilage necrosis is seen radiographically as a concentric narrowing of the 'joint space' with no evidence of bone involvement. It does not appear to be related to the severity of the slip and its cause is unknown. It occurs in approximately 12% of cases and only occurs following treatment. Usually severe pain and stiffness result which require arthrodesis.

Chondrolysis in slipping upper femoral epiphysis is a significant complication particularly after immobilization or multiple pin fixation. Vrettos and Hoffman (1993) have described a series of 44 patients with 55 hips exhibiting slipped femoral epiphysis over a 25-year period. Eight already had evidence of chondrolysis on first presentation in all coloured or black female patients; six had had persistent pin penetration into the joint – but none developed chondrolysis who had had transient intraoperative pin penetration. Removal of the pins improved the symptoms of pain and the range of movement. Maximum joint space narrowing of chondrolysis developed within the first year, but improvement in the narrowed space and range of movement did improve up to three years. At the average follow-up of 13.3, years no patient had pain but 5 (30%) were stiff. The actual cause and pathogenesis of this complication are still unknown, but there is a genetic predisposition.

The healed case in young adults

In this type the head is markedly deformed, the neck is thickened, and its upper surface rests against the upper portion of the acetabulum. No line of demarcation is present between the epiphysis and the neck.

Frequently, the joint, although lacking some movement, is functionally good unless avascular necrosis or cartilage necrosis has occurred. In such cases with severe pain, it should be realized at the outset that even a moderately normal joint is unlikely to result. This being so, the operation of choice will be an arthroplasty by replacement or a realignment femoral osteotomy. Indeed, it may now be looked on as a severe arthritic condition but with the obvious advantage that the patient is young. It is therefore a suitable case for an arthro-osteotomy, and the results of this are good in selected cases with marked pain.

Avulsion of the lesser trochanter of the femur

The lesser trochanter of the femur is the comparatively weak structure into which the iliopsoas tendon is inserted. Its ossification centre appears about the twelfth year and unites with the shaft at the eighteenth; during the intervening years it is liable to be avulsed by undue traction exerted by the ilopsoas.

The cause is usually traumatic and the condition, therefore, occurs more often in boys and athletic girls, who are more subject to injury.

SYMPTOMS

One of the functions of the iliopsoas tendon is to flex the hip joint; therefore, where the trochanter has been avulsed, the patient is unable to perform this movement. In consequence a limp develops, and, at the same time, attempts to carry out the movement are painful.

On examination, tenderness is elicited in the region of the lesser trochanter, and when the patient lies on his back on the examination couch, he is unable to raise his thigh. He is also unable to mount stairs unless he drags the affected limb after the sound one. He cannot bend from the hip, and fails to pick up an object from the floor.

An x-ray examination reveals the separation of the epiphysis.

TREATMENT

Complete immobilization is unnecessary; it is usually sufficient to put the patient to bed until discomfort has settled, then crutch walking. Union usually takes place in about 6 weeks.

The prognosis is good.

Leg length inequality

Minor discrepancies in leg length are very common and, if less than 2 cm, are best treated if required by a small heel or total shoe raise. A difference of 2.5 cm or more will often cause postural imbalance and an uneven gait. Patients usually seek a cosmetic improvement and reject cumbersome shoe-raises. There are also good orthopaedic reasons to equalize limb lengths to prevent osteoarthritis of the hip and knee of the longer leg, fixed scoliosis and backache in later life.

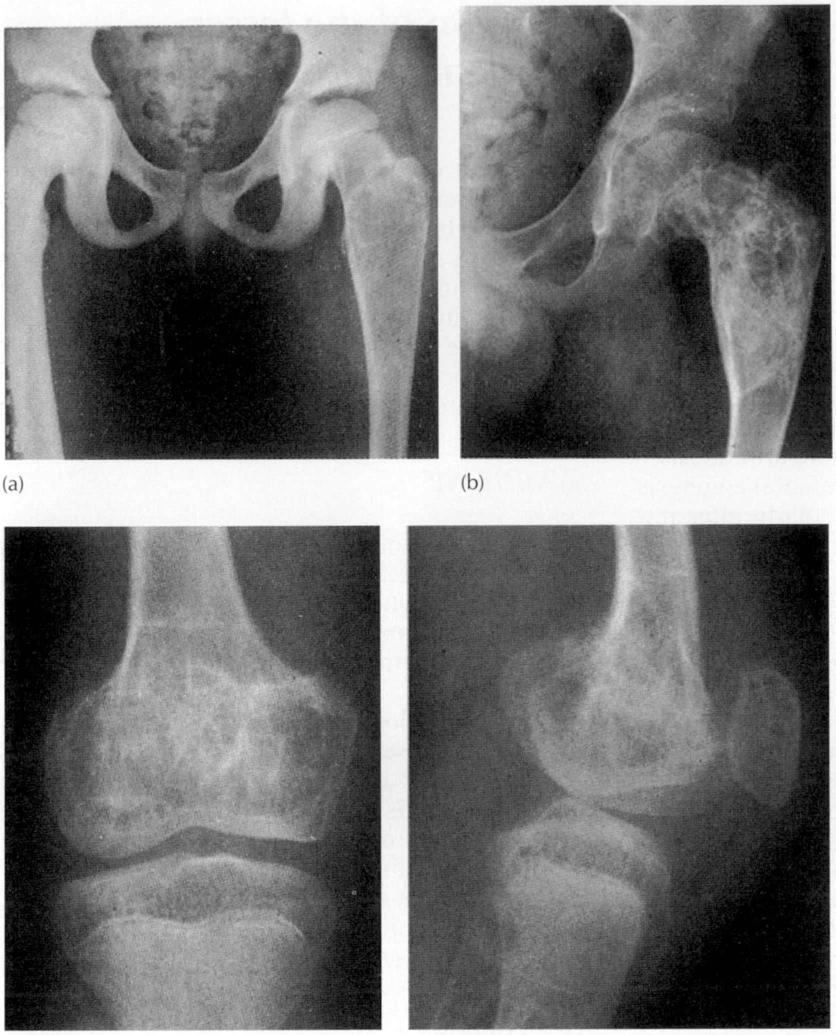

(a) (b) (c) (d)

Figure 6.28 (a) and (b) Radiographs of a 12-year-old boy who had had several episodes of plaster-of-Paris immobilization for a pathological fracture and bone-grafting operations on a bone cyst involving the upper end of the left femur. (c) and (d) Radiographs of the knee joint of the same limb, showing premature closure and deformity of the lower femoral epiphysis. The upper tibial and fibular epiphyses were still open with two transverse lines of growth arrest being seen in the upper aspect of the tibia. The shortening in this case was 4 cm.

The discrepancies that require correction usually have a congenital basis or are caused by premature epiphyseal arrest during growth. *Congenital* causes include a spectrum of lower limb dysplasias, hemiatrophy and hemi-hypertrophy, vascular malformation, congenital pseudarthrosis of the tibia, neurofibromatosis, Ollier's disease, Klippel–Trenaunay syndrome and Silver's syndrome.

Premature growth-plate arrest may be iatrogenic, e.g. following avascular necrosis after treatment of CDH or secondary to trauma, septic arthritis and osteomyelitis, or radiotherapy. Both infection and trauma may also cause overgrowth of a limb.

Malunion of fractures with shortening, malrotation and angulation may need correction.

Neurological disorders such as poliomyelitis, spina bifida, spinal dysraphism, cerebral palsy, produce a large number of limb length discrepancies, some of which are correctable.

Limb lengthening is being performed increasingly for some types of *dwarfism*, e.g. achondroplasia, but such patients require careful evaluation.

The short, paralysed limb secondary to poliomyelitis is now much less common than previously. Two or three centimetres of shortening in a paralysed limb is advantageous if associated with a foot drop or weak hip flexors since it enables the foot to clear the ground more easily. Longer discrepancies can be reduced but never fully. It is well to remember that prolonged immobilization can cause epiphyseal change and shortening as seen in Figure 6.28.

Miscellaneous causes

Other factors such as genetic, dietetic, endocrine, vascular and physical, are well recognized as affecting epiphyseal growth, and have been described earlier. There has been much experimental work carried out to study the vascular factors which may or may not accelerate epiphyseal growth. Methods to improve or alter inequality of leg lengths have been directed towards either changing the rate of growth or surgical correction.

CHANGING THE RATE OF GROWTH

Stimulating the growth of the shortened leg

This has been attempted by:

1. Local stimulation of growth by periosteal stripping with the insertion of bone pegs or dissimilar metals in the vicinity of the epiphyseal line.
2. Lumbar sympathectomy (Barr *et al.*, 1950). Lowenstein *et al.* (1958) studied experimentally the effects of lumbar sympathectomy on muscle and bone blood flow in dogs and demonstrated that the average turnover rate in the sympathectomized limb was only 27% higher than in the normal limb 1 hour after surgery, but 90% higher 1–8 weeks later. The effects of sympathectomy in the 'shrunken' limbs after poliomyelitis have been well recorded, and this work tends to confirm that there may be a definite beneficial effect of augmenting blood flow through bone by such a procedure.
3. Interfering with the intramedullary circulation by mechanical blocking of the medullary cavity (Trueta, 1953).
4. Creation of an artificial arteriovenous fistula. Results of an artificial or induced arteriovenous fistula procedure were described by Janes and Jennings (1961) in 42 patients over a 10-year period. They showed that 72% of the cases had either a decrease or no change in the discrepancy originally present. There were no cardiac complications, but two of the fistulae closed off spontaneously. An increase in the circumference of the leg on the side of the fistula was noted in several cases with prominent veins. Janes and Jennings warned that 'the technical difficulty of closing the fistula may be such as to render the method unjustifiable considering the amount of equalization in leg length that may be achieved'.

In general, none of the above methods has had much success. Their effect has been transitory and the actual increase in longitudinal growth has never been great enough or maintained sufficiently to make them routinely applicable.

Retarding the growth in the normal or longer leg

This may be achieved by placing staples across the epiphysis as a temporary measure, or by an epiphyseodesis for a more permanent closure of the epiphysis.

SURGICAL RECONSTRUCTION

This is performed either to obtain lengthening of the short leg, or to shorten the longer or normal leg.

In the clinical investigation of a patient with leg length inequality one must look for:

1. The precise cause of the discrepancy.
2. The skeletal maturity or 'bone' age of the patient, by comparing the radiographs of the hand and carpal bones with standards established by Greulich and Pyle (1951) or Tanner and Whitehouse (1976).
3. Accurate leg lengths by CT scanograms taken of each joint against a radiopaque marker.
4. The strength of the leg musculature as well as the blood supply and function of the hip, knee and ankle joints.
5. Any disturbance of the lumbar spine (e.g. spina bifida or scoliosis, producing scoliosis with pelvic tilt.

Such an examination should be carried out every six months to obtain and record a longitudinal growth study before planning any specific procedure.

It should be noted that a child with a discrepancy of 1–2 cm will limp only slightly by dropping the pelvis onto the shorter limb. But any discrepancy greater than this will require a greater adaptation; e.g. a talipes equinus deformity at the ankle of the involved leg or else a flexion deformity of the normal knee. Wooden blocks are of help in eliciting the presence of contractures with pelvic obliquity. The patient will present because of fatigue on exertion in relation to this altered gait, or because he has to wear a high boot, or because of the development of pelvic obliquity and a scoliosis

Leg lengthening

Leg lengthening is a procedure which should not be undertaken lightly. The potential complications due to faulty selection of cases or failures in the technique are considerable. There is, however, a definite place for lengthening of the affected limb in suitably chosen cases. The advantages are that the affected deformed leg is being corrected, height is preserved and body proportions are improved. The disadvantages are the numerous procedures required, with a higher complication rate and the stiffening of adjacent joints.

Selection of cases

Patients with 5 cm or more of shortening may be considered for leg lengthening if the leg is flail or the foot already unbalanced. Each case is considered individually and the choice of lengthening the affected limb, or shortening the sound limb, fully discussed with the parents. Female patients in particular are grateful for discarding a cumbersome and unsightly high boot even if they still have to wear a caliper.

Leg lengthening should be performed as early as possible; the younger the patient, the easier the procedure and the better the results. Lengthening should preferably be carried out between the ages of 10 and 14 years. When lengthening is to be limited to 5 cm, the operation can be carried out whenever that disparity is evident rather than waiting for the final growth period.

If shortening exceeds 8 cm, the affected leg may be lengthened by 5 cm and the sound leg subsequently shortened so that a shoe-raise can be abolished without serious loss of the patient's height.

A definite contraindication to tibial lengthening is the patient with a balanced foot despite involvement of the leg muscles. Tibial lengthening in such cases will upset the muscle balance and produce a foot deformity which will require stabilization.

TRUE AND APPARENT SHORTENING

It is important to distinguish between true and apparent shortening and to bear in mind that some patients have both. Fixed deformity of the hip should be corrected before considering other equalization procedures.

A special problem arises in children with a short leg secondary to a poor outcome of treatment for congenital dislocation of the hip. Corrective osteotomies need to be carefully planned since the future of the hip joint is of equal importance to the correction of the leg length discrepancy. A preoperative arthrogram may be helpful. An abduction osteotomy may uncover the femoral head and need to be combined with an acetabular procedure and possibly a trochanteric epiphyseodesis. A Salter innominate osteotomy may improve the cover of the femoral head and add a little to leg length. Rarely a more ambitious transiliac lengthening may be contemplated.

A true leg length discrepancy associated with a fixed pelvic obliquity and scoliosis is a particular problem. It may well be to the patient's advantage to have a short leg on the lower side of the pelvis and correction of true leg length in such a patient may render it difficult for them to compensate for an unbalanced scoliosis.

Table 6.2 Abnormalities to be assessed in the spine and involved leg

Spine	Structural scoliosis
	Mobility
Pelvis	Fixed obliquity
	Asymmetry
Hip	Soft tissue contracture
	Bony deformity
	Dysplasia
	Muscle weakness (+ve Trendelenburg)
Knee	Soft tissue contracture
	Bony deformity
	Dislocation of patella
	Ligamentous instability
Tibia	Deformity (angular or rotational)
Ankle	Soft tissue contracture
	Bony deformity
	Absent fibula
	Ball-and-socket joint
Foot	Soft tissue contracture
	Bony deformity
	Dysplasia
General	Muscle
	wasting
	weakness
	fibrosis
	Neurovascular abnormalities
	Congenital fibrous bands

After Jackson (1991).

ASSESSMENT OF ASSOCIATED ABNORMALITY

Jackson (1991) strongly recommended that a systematic list is made of all the features which adversely affect the patient's stance and gait (Table 6.2). For example, if leg length discrepancy does not stand out as being a major contributor to the problem, then an equalization procedure will not, on its own, result in improvement. It is important to remember that there are contraindications to femoral lengthening, particularly in the case of acetabular dysplasia and instability of the knee due to congenital ligament deficiency since a major joint dislocation may follow distraction.

Patients with severe limb dysplasias will not be candidates for leg equalization procedures. If the foot is useless, an early Syme's amputation may be appropriate. If the length at maturity is out of range of leg lengthening techniques, then there is no alternative but to treat the patient with a suitable orthosis or prosthesis.

ASSESSMENT OF THE PATIENT AND PREDICTING DISCREPANCY

When the patients are referred early then maturation and leg length discrepancy can be monitored on an annual basis. Factors which are important are the parental height and the child's standing height on the normal leg which is recorded on a growth chart. Skeletal age is estimated between the age of 10 and 12 years to rule out any serious abnormality of skeletal development. Predicting the patient's overall height at maturity is necessary in choosing an appropriate course of action. This is also important if epiphyseodesis is to be performed at the correct time, or if leg lengthening is to be performed much before the end of growth. One of the three methods of prediction of growth should be used and charted at the annual attendance (Moseley, 1977).

The annual visit also allows the surgeon to check on the progress of any associated deformities, to try the effect of a shoe-raise as an interim measure, and to assess the patient and the parents. Some assessment of the character and emotional stability and motivation are important because leg lengthening is demanding on the patient and the parents. It is essential to give realistic expectations of surgery and explain the complications that can occur. In some instances if the shortening exceeds 8 cm, the affected leg may be lengthened by 5 cm and the normal leg shortened. In general terms it is better to operate on the abnormal leg than on the normal opposite leg.

Leg lengthening

FEMORAL AND TIBIAL LENGTHENING

The advantage of recent developments in design of distraction apparatus is that lengthening can now be performed on an ambulatory basis. The demonstration that a bone gap can consistently be bridged with callus without the need for bone grafting, and also the development of epiphyseal distraction (De Bastiani *et al*., 1986, 1987) have revolutionized the approach and shortened the duration of treatment. Decisions about the choice of apparatus and the technique are complex and depend on the particular patient.

The apparatus to be used is a choice between a single bar distractor such as the Wagner or Orthofix and a frame with an all-round support such as the Ilizarov or Monticelli. The single bar fixators are sturdy and compact and the minimum of soft tissues are transfixed by the pins. However, they fail to keep perfect alignment during lengthening usually, whereas the frames produce a straight length of segment but are more bulky and difficult to apply, especially to the femur.

Choice of site

Diaphyseal lengthening allows both the upper and lower pins to be placed through solid cortical bone and should internal fixation be necessary at a later date, there is good bone stock on either side of the lengthened segment. Plating can also be used to correct deformity at the end of lengthening. Metaphyseal lengthening has the advantage that the callus response is more readily achieved when the lengthening is made through cancellous bone but the pin fixation can be less reliable. Metaphyseal lengthening is the first method of choice if deformity at this site is to be corrected concurrently with lengthening. Epiphyseal lengthening has the advantage that no osteotomy is required and the lack of incisions is cosmetically attractive. However, the lengthening can be very painful. A strong, wide lengthened segment can be produced which consolidates quickly. However, one has to assume that even if distraction is performed slowly and the growth-plate does not rupture, it may not function normally at the end of the procedure.

Synchronous lengthening of the femur and tibia of the same leg and epiphyseal lengthening synchronously at the upper and lower end of the tibia have been developed but can be difficult procedures. Therefore larger discrepancies are better handled by a combination of lengthening of one leg and shortening of the other.

FEMORAL LENGTHENING

On admission to hospital the patient is assessed by a physiotherapist and taught to shadow walk with crutches without weight-bearing.

Technique

The principles of leg lengthening were evolved by pioneers such as Anderson (1967) and Wagner (1978). De Bastiani *et al*. (1986) and Ilizarov made major advances in introducing chondrodiastasis and the use of a symmetrical frame to control the alignment of the femur and tibia which had previously been big problems. These methods have been reviewed by Jackson (1991).

In general terms lengthening of the tibia is preferred to femoral lengthening which is a more difficult procedure with higher complications and more likely to cause problems with knee joint contracture. However, femoral lengthening is becoming more reliable and therefore the priority is to attempt to achieve lower limbs which are as symmetrical as possible with the knees at the same level.

The preferred method is a mid-shaft lengthening procedure using a single bar lengthening device applied to the lateral aspect of the femur. The method of bone division is an oblique diaphyseal corticotomy. The use of the image intensifier facilitates the insertion of the four pins which are placed in line 1 cm anterior to the mid-lateral line. Large 6 mm cortical threaded pins are required which are self-tapping in the distal cortex. Great care is needed in inserting the pins using a low speed power drill to reduce bone thermal necrosis and to ensure that the pins are at 90° to the long axis of the bone. The pins are then inserted in sequence, the order being upper pin, lower pin, and central two pins and the knee is flexed fully during the insertion of the pins to ensure that there is no tethering of the quadriceps. Trial application of the leg lengthening device is then carried out prior to the division of the bone.

Bone division is carried out in oblique fashion to present a greater surface area for callus formation. Oblique corticotomy is performed and multiple drill holes joined by osteotomy and final division of the bone by gentle flexing of the thigh. The leg lengthening device is then applied and after wound closure over a suction drain, movement of hip and knee are encouraged on the first postoperative day (Figure 6.29). The patient is then allowed to shadow

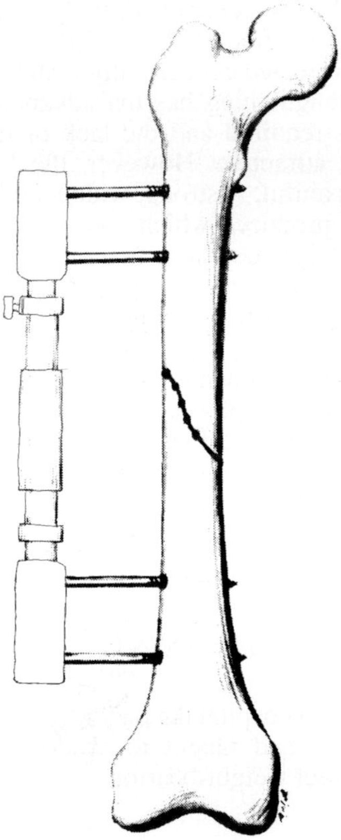

Figure 6.29 Diagram of femoral lengthening employing an oblique, multiple drill-hole corticotomy and distraction by a single external fixator. (From Jackson, A. (1991) Treatment of leg length inequality. In: *Rob & Smith's Operative Surgery: Orthopaedics*. Edited by G. Bentley, and R.B. Greer R.B. Butterworth-Heinemann: London, Boston, Sydney, Wellington, Singapore)

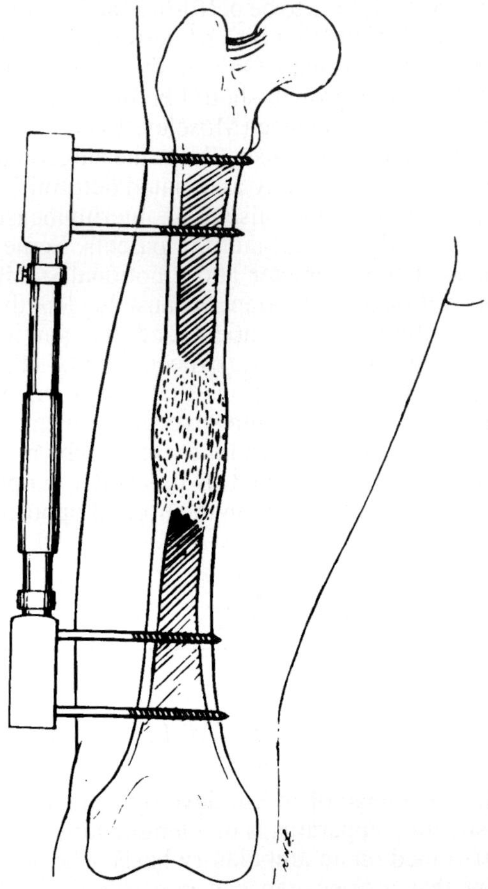

Figure 6.30 Diagram of femoral lengthening at the end of treatment with callus formed in the distracted segment just prior to removal of the external fixator. (From Jackson, A. (1991) Treatment of leg length inequality. In: *Rob & Smith's Operative Surgery: Orthopaedics*. Edited by G. Bentley and R.B. Greer. Butterworth-Heinemann: London, Boston, Sydney, Wellington, Singapore)

walk with crutches. The leg lengthening device is left undisturbed for 2–3 weeks depending on the age of the patient. Lengthening is then commenced at the rate of 0.5 mm twice daily and alignment radiographs are taken at 2-week intervals. These films will show the separation of the corticotomy site and the quality of the callus response. If callus response is poor, then distraction is discontinued for a week.

Careful attention to dressing of the pin sites daily with an alcohol solution is necessary and avoidance of skin tension around the pins.

When the desired length is reached, then provided there are no problems with the fixator, such as loosening of pins or pin tract infection, it may be maintained for a further 6 or 8 weeks before removal (Figure 6.30).

If there is deformity at the end of lengthening the best way of correcting this is by plating the femur through a posterolateral approach. At least four screws are required above and below the lengthened segment and special heavy duty bridging plates, which are not weakened in their central section by screw holes, are employed (Figure 6.31).

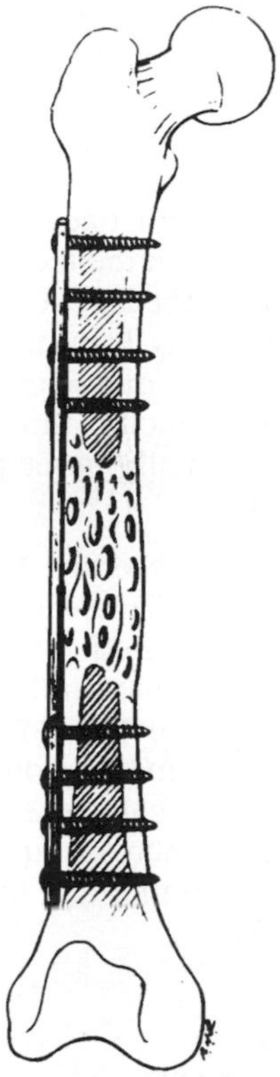

Figure 6.31 Plating of the lengthened femur (From Jackson, A. (1991) Treatment of leg length inequality. In: *Rob & Smith's Operative Surgery: Orthopaedics*. Edited by G. Bentley and R.B. Greer. Butterworth-Heinemann: London, Boston, Sydney, Wellington, Singapore)

The third alternative is to stabilize the bone by means of closed femoral nailing. This can be performed at the stage when the callus is mature enough to resist axial compression forces. Nailing gives immediate whole bone protection and facilitates the recovery of stiff joints as well as allowing early and safe weight-bearing. There is a risk of infection and for this reason the fixator must be removed and the leg maintained on traction for 2 weeks so that the pin tracts are healed before closed nailing is performed.

Tibial technique

The principles of lengthening the tibia are exactly the same as for the femur.

The pins are inserted in the standard way through the subcutaneous border of the tibia under image intensified control. An oblique mid-shaft corticotomy is made and division exactly as for femoral lengthening.

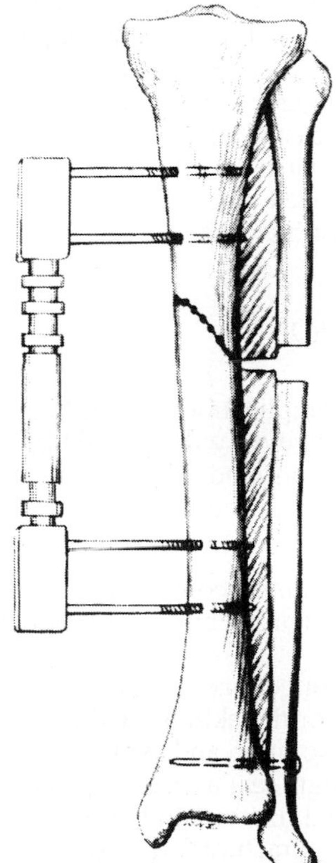

Figure 6.32 Diagram of the technique of tibial lengthening with the external fixator and oblique osteotomy plus the stabilization of the fibula to prevent ankle deformity. (From Jackson, A. (1991) Treatment of leg length inequality. In: *Rob & Smith's Operative Surgery: Orthopaedics*. Edited by G. Bentley and R.B. Greer. Butterworth-Heinemann: London, Boston, Sydney, Wellington, Singapore)

Through a separate lateral incision at the same level, a 1 cm length of fibula is excised and the interosseous membrane is also divided.

A third incision is made 1 cm long over the distal fibula and a diastasis screw inserted to neutralize any distraction forces that may be imposed on the lateral malleolus. If the heel cord is tight preoperatively, it will have to be lengthened and after passage of the diastasis screw, dorsiflexion of the foot is checked again (Figure 6.32).

The limb is elevated postoperatively and physiotherapy commenced on the first postoperative day. In the case of the tibia, a foot-drop spring splint is worn from the beginning and the patient is allowed up shadow walking when the pain and swelling have subsided. Lengthening is commenced usually at 2 weeks and regular radiographs are taken to check alignment and the quality of callus.

As with the femoral lengthening, the rate of lengthening depends on the response of the callus and when the appropriate length has been achieved, the patient may walk retaining the fixator for a further 6–8 weeks. The rule of thumb is that the device is left on for a further one week per centimetre lengthened. Provided the x-ray shows good consolidation, the fixator is removed and a full-length plaster-of-Paris cast is applied.

Full weight-bearing is allowed and 2 weeks later the cast is removed and replaced by a cast brace which is used for 8 weeks.

COMPLICATIONS

The potential complications of leg lengthening are considerable. However, with careful vigilance on the part of the surgeon, and with patient compliance, most of these may be avoided. Complications include:

1. Loss of patient compliance – resulting in over-rapid lengthening and subsequent problems.
2. Pin tract infections – minimized by regular cleansing of the skin around the pins with an alcoholic solution and avoiding skin tension.
3. Loss of alignment avoided by placing a single bar external fixator parallel to the bone.
4. Muscle contractures – mostly occurring in patients with congenital contracture. Slight preoperative contractures will become more pronounced during lengthening and must be anticipated by tenotomies prior to lengthening (e.g. elongation of tendo Achillis). Physiotherapy is vital in minimizing contractures and keeping the joints as mobile as possible during lengthening.
5. Joint damage – dislocation of hip or knee is usually a foreseeable complication and should be avoided with careful lengthening.
6. Pain – this is due to nerve distraction and usually due to too rapid stretching. The cause must always be sought and care exercised in using analgesics. Epiphyseal lengthening is the most painful form of distraction but pain is often encountered towards the end of lengthening and may be a reason to reduce the rate.
7. Neurovascular damage – this is rare provided care is taken in distracting.
8. Tibiofibular joint displacement – downward migration of the head of the fibula will tighten up the lateral collateral ligament of the knee and cause fixed flexion deformity whereas upward migration of the lateral malleolus will destabilize the ankle mortice. A correctly placed osteotomy and a diastasis screw should prevent these complications.
9. All the well known complications of internal fixation – these include infection and failure of fixation and fracture at one or other end of the bone plates due to osteopenia.
10. Delayed union – if there is poor callus response bone grafting is best performed early using cancellous bone from the iliac crest. Non-union after leg lengthening is extremely rare.
11. Fractures – fractures may occur at a variety of sites and times.
    (a) Early fracture at one end of the lengthened segment when the fixator is removed.
    (b) Fracture at the level of the end of a plate.
    (c) Fracture away from the site of lengthening related to disuse osteoporosis.
    (d) Late stress fracture through a length of the segment usually in the presence of slight deformity.

Sofield *et al.* (1958) observed that with any leg-lengthening operation there was evidence of bone stimulation with increased longitudinal growth. Thus lengthening performed early in life may stimulate growth but the effect is not great. They also emphasized that the major complication of leg lengthening is muscle weakness especially in the hip abductors which may increase limp following operation. This is very important in counselling the patients and relatives.

Leg shortening

Shortening is ideal if the long leg is the abnormal one. If the patient stands and walks with the knee of the long leg slightly flexed, then procedures that shorten the long leg will not significantly reduce the effective height of the patient.

EPIPHYSEODESIS

Permanent epiphyseodesis as first suggested by Phemister in the 1930s is preferable to stapling since only one operation is required and the complication rate is lower. Staples can displace or break and the removal of staples is not always followed by the normal resumption of growth (Blount, 1949).

The timing of epiphyseodesis is critical and depends on predictions that the short leg will continue to grow at a specific rate until maturity. Epiphyseodesis requires the shortest possible hospital admission and recovery should be complete within 6 weeks.

The disadvantage of epiphyseodesis is that the predictions are not always realized in practice and therefore it is the least accurate method of correcting a discrepancy. Therefore it is wise to aim at reducing the discrepancy to within 1 cm since the patient is usually displeased if the procedure converts the longer leg into the shorter one.

Haas (1948) pointed out that if the growth of the plate continues, but is prevented from expanding, this factor of compression will produce cessation of growth. Siffert (1956) described the structural changes which occur in compression of the epiphyseal plate, and Strobino *et al.* (1952) showed experimentally that pressures of 40–45 lb/in^2 (2.8–3.2 kg/cm^2) are required to retard epiphyseal growth and these forces have to be markedly increased before growth is stopped. The magnitude of these forces readily explains the difficulties associated with the so-called simple procedure of stapling, both from the mechanical aspects of design and from properties of the metal staples, as well as their exact positioning.

In 1960 Stampe and Lamsche reviewed their very extensive experience with 140 patients; 60% of all cases undergoing epiphyseodesis achieved a satisfactory result which was defined as 'the involved extremity was within 2 cm of the desired length at the end of growth'. Only 11 cases underwent a stapling procedure, but 82% were satisfactory, particularly when the shortening of the leg was due to poliomyelitis.

These workers emphasized the difficult nature of these procedures in avoiding further deformities. For example, after femoral shortening the most common complication was genu valgum at the knee, and with the procedure of epiphyseal arrest there were 11 cases which had some deformity requiring correction. Angular deformities around the knees were very common, and close postoperative follow-up was essential to observe and to prevent the development of such deformities.

In comparing the results of epiphyseodesis by the bone grafting technique of Phemister and by Blount's epiphyseal stapling, Høstrup and Pilgaard (1969) found from their series that there were fewer primary operative complications such as angular deformities – varus, valgus or recurvatum. There were also fewer secondary complications, such as breaking of stapling or insufficient inhibition of longitudinal growth, after the Phemister procedure than after stapling. The results were also better with bony epiphyseodesis.

The indications for epiphyseodesis are:

1. If there is sufficient growth left to effect a correction.
2. If the patient is growing on or above the 50th centile and will be taller than average.
3. If discrepancy is 6 cm or less – with increasing discrepancy the potential for error is magnified.

Technique

A preoperative radiograph is necessary to check the anatomy of the physis to be fused. The growth-plates are usually convex towards the joint. Image intensification enables the surgeon to make small vertical incisions 3.5 cm in length centred at the correct level with certainty. Growth-plates are approached from both the medial and lateral aspects.

Lower femoral physis

The lateral incision splits the fascia lata and the medial incision splits the deep fascia 1 cm in front of the adductor tubercle. On both sides the superior geniculate arteries may have to be divided.

Upper tibial physis

The lateral incision is made just in front of the fibular head and the anterior aspect of this bone is exposed. Care must be taken to avoid the common peroneal nerve immediately posteriorly. The tibia is exposed and the origins of peroneus longus and tibialis anterior are reflected downwards for 1 cm. The anteromedial aspect of the growth plate lies subcutaneously and is easily exposed.

In both femoral and tibial lengthening an 'I' shaped incision is made 2 cm long in the periosteum and then the anterior and posterior flaps are elevated with an osteotome. The physis is clearly seen as a white line traversing the window that has been opened in the periosteum (Figure 6.33). Using a 1.5 cm osteotome, a square block of bone as deep

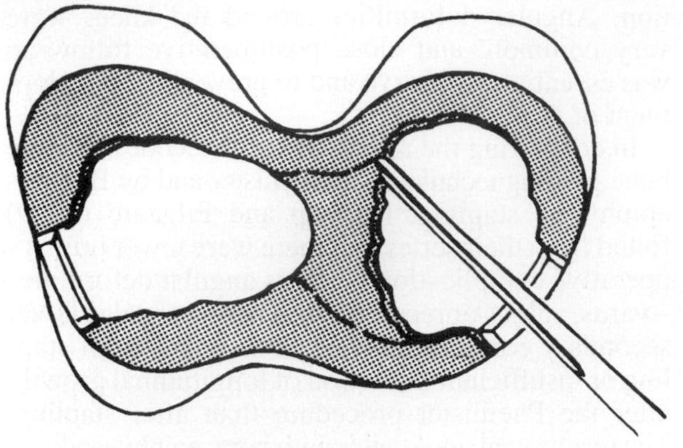

Figure 6.33 Technique of epiphyseodesis. Removal of bone block including epiphysis. (From Jackson, A. (1991) Treatment of leg length inequality. In: *Rob & Smith's Operative Surgery: Orthopaedics.* Edited by G. Bentley and R.B. Greer. Butterworth-Heinemann: London, Boston, Sydney, Wellington, Singapore)

as possible is removed with care. Then as much of the growth plate as possible is removed with a gauge or curette, from the depths of the hole anteriorly and posteriorly towards the centre of the bone. The same procedure is performed on the opposite side. The two excavations on the medial and lateral sides should meet centrally. When this has been achieved the bone blocks are rotated through 90° and punched back into the holes from which they were taken. The osteoperiosteal flaps are then sutured back in position over the blocks. The limb is supported in a plaster-of-Paris cylinder for 2 weeks.

Postoperatively weight-bearing is allowed as soon as possible and physiotherapy is commenced at 2 weeks after removal of the cast. It usually takes 6 weeks for the knee to regain a full range of motion.

FEMORAL AND TIBIAL SHORTENING

These procedures have the advantage of being precise and are applied once skeletal growth has ceased. Good internal fixation allows early mobiliza-

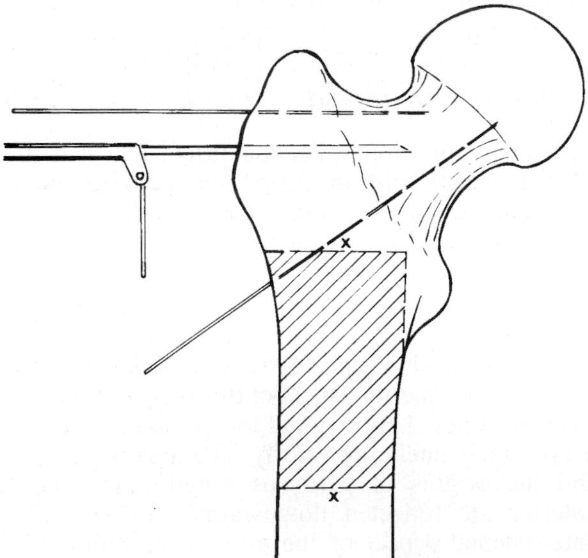

Figure 6.34 Technique of femoral shortening by resection of a 5 cm segment of the upper femoral shaft and fixation with a compression spline; (From Jackson, A. (1991) Treatment of leg length inequality. In: *Rob & Smith's Operative Surgery: Orthopaedics.* Edited by G. Bentley and R.B. Greer. Butterworth-Heinemann: London, Boston, Sydney, Wellington, Singapore)

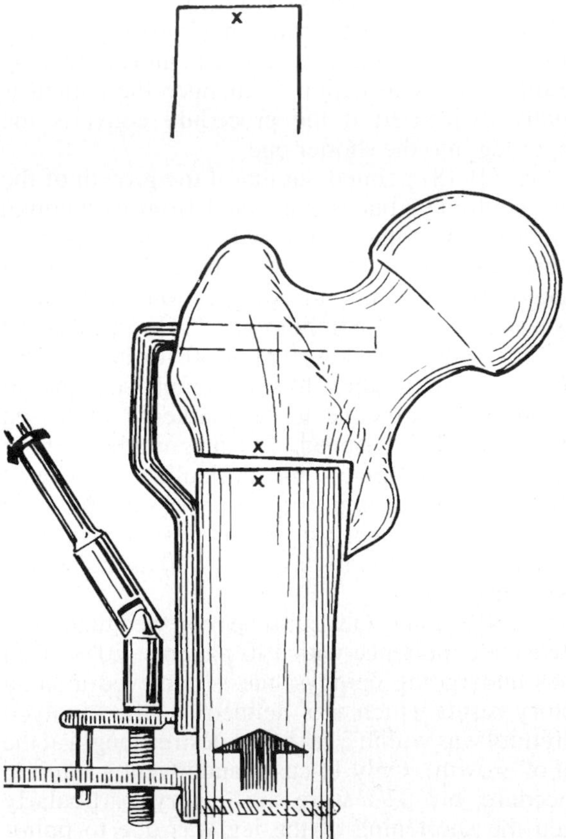

Figure 6.35 Fixation of compression spline. (From Jackson, A. (1991) Treatment of leg length inequality. In: *Rob & Smith's Operative Surgery: Orthopaedics.* Edited by G. Bentley and R.B. Greer. Butterworth-Heinemann: London, Boston, Sydney, Wellington, Singapore)

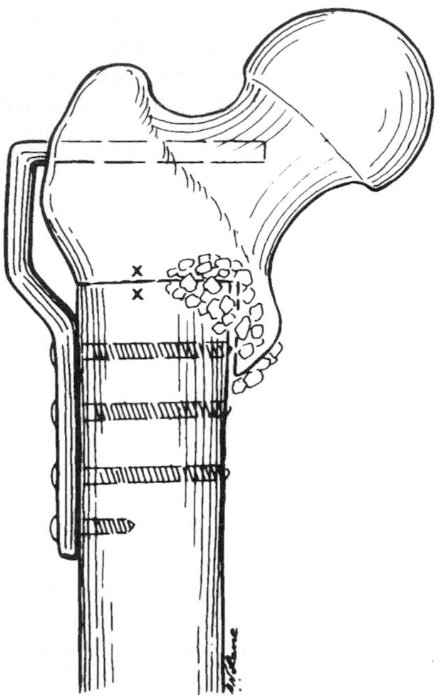

Figure 6.36 Final position supplemented by bone graft. (From Jackson, A. (1991) Treatment of leg length inequality. In: *Rob & Smith's Operative Surgery: Orthopaedics.* Edited by G. Bentley and R.B. Greer. Butterworth-Heinemann: London, Boston, Sydney, Wellington, Singapore)

tion and postoperative muscle weakness and non-union are most unlikely. Shortening of the femur leads to an increase in soft tissue and bulk, but if the shortening is carried out proximally the bulkiness is not obvious.

Tibial shortening gives a poor cosmetic result and the muscles may never take up the slack. If more than 2 or 3 cm are resected there is liable to be a problem with skin closure and the vascularity of the limb may be threatened. There are therefore few indications for this procedure.

The indications for femoral shortening are:

1. If the patient is skeletally mature.
2. If the discrepancy is less than 6 cm.
3. If the discrepancy is principally in the femur.
4. If the patient is on or above the 50th centile.

Whenever possible femoral shortening is preferable by bone resection at the end of the growth phase rather than epiphyseodesis. In general shortening should not exceed 6 cm in the femur, and as indicated above, shortening of the tibia is not recommended. The intertrochanteric region is the preferred site for femoral shortening.

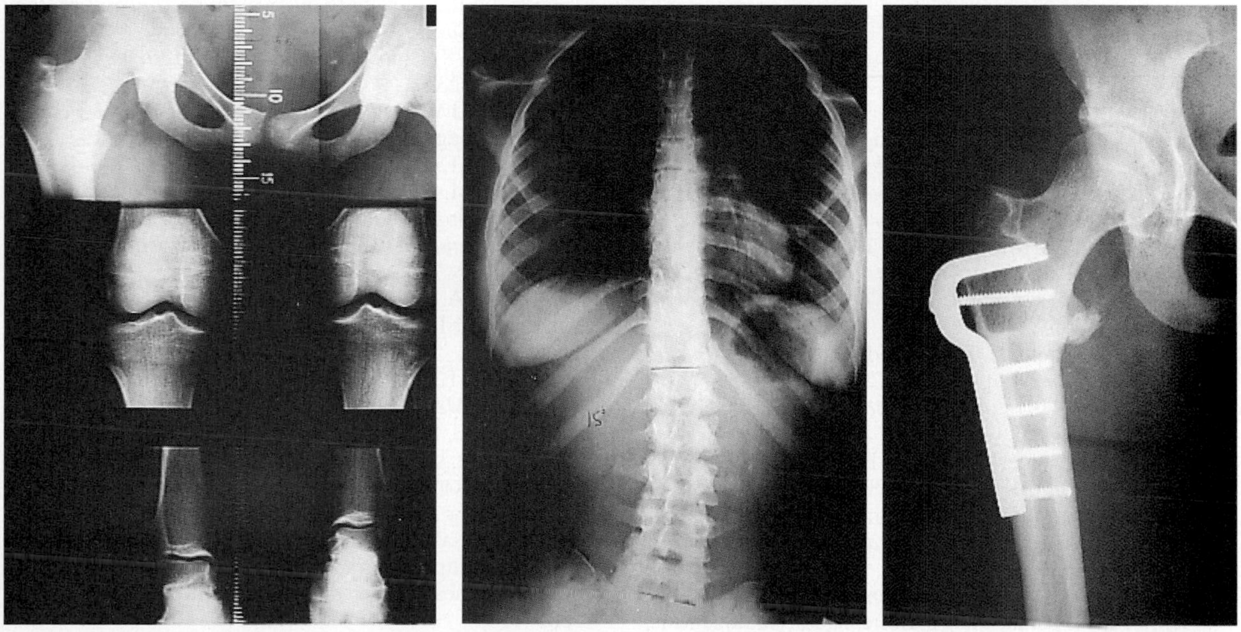

(a) (b) (c)

Figure 6.37 Preoperative radiographs of a 20-year-old woman with 3 cm leg length discrepancy from congenital tibial shortening producing a pelvic tilt and (b) compensatory scoliosis causing backache. (c) An excellent result was achieved with a 3 cm upper femoral resection.

Technique

The patient is positioned on an orthopaedic table and image intensification is employed. A standard lateral approach to the shaft of the femur is carried out and the position of the shortening is checked by the guide wire and by image intensification. The use of the 90° AO spline is preferred since this gives a good internal fixation and allows rapid mobilization. The osteotomy is planned so that the lesser trochanter remains intact. The level of the proximal osteotomy is opposite the upper margin of the lesser trochanter and the length of bone to be resected is measured from this point down the shaft. Longitudinal marks are made above and below the bone resection to maintain the correct rotational alignment (Figures 6.34 and 6.35).

The position of the right-angle spline is assessed and a starting chisel used to make the track in the greater trochanter prior to the removal of the segment of bone. The distal osteotomy is carried out first followed by the proximal osteotomy following which the right-angle spline is inserted and compression applied (Figures 6.36 and 6.37).

Postoperatively the leg is supported in 'slings and springs' for 3–4 days and the patient is then allowed up partial weight-bearing with crutches. Union occurs usually by 12 weeks.

References

Anderson, W. V. (1967) Lengthening of the lower limb: its place in the problem of limb length discrepancy. In: *Modern Trends in Orthopaedics – 5*, p. 1. Edited by J. M. P. Clark. Butterworths: London

Axer, A., Schiller, M. G., Segal, D. *et al.* (1973) Subtrochanteric osteotomy in the treatment of Legg–Calvé–Perthes' syndrome. *Acta Orthopaedica Scandinavica* **44**, 31–59

Barr, J. S., Stinchfield, A. J. and Reidy, J. A. (1950) *Journal of Bone and Joint Surgery* **32A**, 793

Blount, W. P. (1949) *Journal of Bone and Joint Surgery* **31A**, 469

Burwell, R. G., Dangerfield, P. H., Hall, D. H., Vernon, C. L. and Harrison, M. H. M. (1978) Perthes' disease. An anthropometric study revealing impaired and disproportionate growth. *Journal of Bone and Joint Surgery* **60B**, 461–477

Caffey, J. (1968) Early roentgenographic changes in essential coxa plana; their significance in pathogenesis. *American Journal of Roentgenology* **103**, 620–634

Calver, D., Venugopal, V., Dorgan, J., Bentley, G. and Gimlette, T. (1981) Radionuclide scanning of irritable hips in the early diagnosis of Perthes' disease. *Journal of Bone and Joint Surgery* **63B**, 379

Cameron, J. M. and Isat, M. W. (1960) *Scottish Medical Journal* **5**, 148

Catterall, A. (1971) The natural history of Perthes' disease. *Journal of Bone and Joint Surgery* **53B**, 37–53

Catterall, A., Lloyd-Roberts, G. C. and Wynne-Davies, R. (1971) Association of Perthes' disease with congenital anomalies of genito-urinary tract and inguinal region. *Lancet* **1**, 996

Conybeare, M. E. and Houghton, G. R. (1980) Slipping of the upper femoral epiphysis: 41 patients after 24 years. *Journal of Bone and Joint Surgery* **62B**, 527

De Bastiani, G., Aldeghiri, R., Renzi-Brivio, L. and Trivella, G. (1986) Chondrodiastasis – controlled symmetrical distraction of the epiphyseal plate. Limb lengthening in children. *Journal of Bone and Joint Surgery* **68B**, 550–556

De Bastiani, G., Aldegheri, R., Renzi-Brivio, L. and Trivella, G. (1987) Leg lengthening by callus distraction (callotasis). *Journal of Pediatric Orthopaedics* **7**, 129–134

Dunn, D. M. (1979) Slipped upper femoral epiphysis. In: *Operative Surgery*, 3rd edn, *Orthopaedics*, Vol. II. Edited by G. Bentley. Butterworths: London and Boston

Dunn, D. M. and Angel, J. C. (1978) Replacement of the femoral head by an open operation in severe adolescent slipping of the upper femoral epiphysis. *Journal of Bone and Joint Surgery* **60B**, 394–403

Duthie, R. B. (1959) *Clinical Orthopaedics* **11**, 7

Duthie, R. B. and Barker, A. N. (1955) *Journal of Bone and Joint Surgery* **37B**, 691

Duthie, R. B. and Houghton, G. R. (1981) Constitutional aspects of the osteochondroses. *Clinical Orthopaedics and Related Research* **158**, 19–27

Eaton, G. O. (1967) Long-term results of treatment in coxa plana: a follow-up study of 88 patients. *Journal of Bone and Joint Surgery* **49A**, 1031–1042

Editorial (1978) Clues in Perthes' disease. *British Medical Journal* **2**, 231

Egund, N. and Wingstrand, H. (1991) Legg–Calvé–Perthes' disease; imaging with MR. *Radiology* **179**, 89–92

Elsig, J. P., Exner, G. U., Von Schulthess, G. K. and Weitzel, M. (1989) False-negative magnetic resonance imaging in early stages of Legg–Calvé–Perthes' disease. *Journal of Pediatric Orthopedics* **9**, 231–235

Eyre-Brook, A. I. (1936) Osteochondritis deformans coxae juvenalis or Perthes' disease. *British Journal of Surgery* **24**, 166

Ferguson, A. B. and Howard, M. B. (1935) *Journal of the American Medical Association* **104**, 808

Fulford, G. E., Lunn, P. G. and MacNicol, M. F. (1993) A prospective study of nonoperative and operative management for Perthes' disease. *Journal of Pediatric Orthopedics* **13**, 281–285

Futani, T., Kasahara, Y., Seizuki, S., Ushikubo, S., Tsuchiya, T. (1991) Ultrasonography in transient synovitis and early Perthes' disease. *Journal of Bone and Joint Surgery* **73B**, 635–639

Gledhill, R. B. and McIntyre, J. M. (1969) Transient synovitis and Legg–Calvé–Perthes' disease: a comparative study. *Canadian Medical Association Journal* **100**, 311–320

Glimcher, M. J. and Kenzora, J. E. (1979) The biology of

osteonecrosis of the human femoral head and its clinical implications. *Clinical Orthopaedics and Related Research* **138**, 284

Golding, J. S. R., MacIver, J. E. and Went, L. N. (1959) The bone changes in sickle cell anaemia and its genetic variants. *Journal of Bone and Joint Surgery* **41B**, 711

Gower, W. E. and Johnston, R. C. (1971) Legg–Perthes' disease. Long-term follow-up of 36 patients. *Journal of Bone and Joint Surgery* **53A**, 759

Greulich, W. W. and Pyle, S. I. (1951) *Radiographic Atlas of Skeletal Development of the Wrist and Hand.* Stanford University Press: Stanford, CA

Griffith, M. J. (1991) Slipped upper femoral epiphysis. In: *Rob and Smith's Operative Surgery: Orthopaedics*, pp. 909–920 Edited by G. Bentley and R. B. Greer. Butterworth-Heinemann: London

Gunther, S. F. and Gossling, H. R. (1973) Legg–Perthes' disease. IV. Treatment by abduction ambulation. *AAOS Instructional Course Lectures* **22**, 305

Haas, S. L. (1948) *Journal of Bone and Joint Surgery* **30A**, 506

Hall, D. J. and Harrison, M. H. M. (1978) An association between congenital abnormalities and Perthes' disease of the hip. *Journal of Bone and Joint Surgery* **60B**, 138

Hardcastle, P. H., Ross, R., Hamalainen, M. and Mata, A. (1980) Caterall grouping of Perthes' disease. An assessment of observer error and prognosis using the Caterall classification. *Journal of Bone and Joint Surgery* **62B**, 428–431

Harris, W. R. (1950) *Journal of Bone and Joint Surgery* **32B**, 5

Harrison, M. H. M., Turner, M. H. and Jacobs, P. (1976) Skeletal immaturity in Perthes' disease. *Journal of Bone and Joint Surgery* **58B**, 37

Herring, J. A., Lundeen, M. A. and Wenger, D. R. (1980) Minimal Perthes' disease. *Journal of Bone and Joint Surgery* **62B**, 25

Heyman, C. H., Herndon, C. G. and Strong, J. M. (1957) *Journal of Bone and Joint Surgery* **39A**, 293

Høstrup, H. and Pilgaard, S. (1969) Epiphyseodesis and epiphyseal stapling on lower limbs. *Acta Orthopaedica Scandinavica* **40**, 130–136

Jackson, A. M. (1991) Treatment of leg length inequality. In: *Rob and Smith's Operative Surgery: Orthopaedics*, pp. 1152–1168. Edited by G. Bentley and R. B. Greer. Butterworth-Heinemann: London

Janes, J. M. and Jennings, J. R. (1961) *Proceedings of the Mayo Clinic* **36**, 12

Lacroix, P. and Verbrugge, J. (1951) *Journal of Bone and Joint Surgery* **33A**, 371

Lancourt, J. E. and Cristini, J. A. (1975) Patella alta and patella infera. *Journal of Bone and Joint Surgery* **57A**, 1112

Legg, A. T. (1910) *Boston Medical and Surgical Journal* **162**, 202

Legg, A. T. (1927) *Journal of Bone and Joint Surgery* **9**, 26

Lloyd-Roberts, G. C., Catterall, A. and Salamon, P. B. (1976) A control study of the indications for and the results of femoral osteotomy in Perthes' disease. *Journal of Bone and Joint Surgery* **58B**, 31

Loder, R. T., Richards, B. S., Shapiro, P. S. *et al.* (1993) Acute slipped femoral epiphysis: the importance of physeal stability. *Journal of Bone and Joint Surgery* **75A**, 1134–1140

Lowenstein, J. M., Panporte, J., Richards, V. and Davison, R. (1958) *Surgery* **43**, 768

McKibbin, B. (1975) Recent developments in Perthes' disease. In: *Recent Advances in Orthopaedics – 2*, p. 173. Edited by B. McKibbin. Churchill Livingstone: Edinburgh and London

McKibbin, B. and Ráliš, Z. A. (1974) Pathological changes in a case of Perthes' disease. *Journal of Bone and Joint Surgery* **56B**, 438–447

Maroudas, A., Bullough, P., Swanson, S. A. V. and Freeman, M. A. R. (1968) The permeability of articular cartilage. *Journal of Bone and Joint Surgery* **50B**, 166

Moseley, C. F. (1977) A straight line graph for leg length discrepancies. *Journal of Bone and Joint Surgery* **59A**, 174–179

Nishio, A. and Yakushiji, K. (1962) Legg–Calvé–Perthes' disease: histology and treatment. *Yonago Acta Medica* **6**, 1

Petrie, J. G. and Bitenc, I. (1971) The abduction weight-bearing treatment in Legg–Perthes' disease. *Journal of Bone and Joint Surgery* **53B**, 54–62

Ratliff, A. H. C. (1956) *Journal of Bone and Joint Surgery* **38B**, 498

Ratliff, A. H. C. (1967) Perthes' disease. A study of 34 hips observed for 30 years. *Journal of Bone and Joint Surgery* **49B**, 108

Ritter, M. A. and Wilson, P. D. (1968) Colonna capsular arthroplasty – a long-term follow-up of 40 hips. *Journal of Bone and Joint Surgery* **50A**, 1305–1326

Salter, R. B. (1966) Experimental and clinical aspects of Perthes' disease. *Journal of Bone and Joint Surgery* **48B**, 393

Salter, R. B. (1984) The present status of surgical treatment for Legg–Perthes' disease. *Journal of Bone and Joint Surgery* **66A**, 961

Salter, R. B. and Thompson, G. H. (1984) Legg–Calvé–Perthes' disease. The prognostic significance of the subchondral fracture and a 2-group classification of the femoral head involvement. *Journal of Bone and Joint Surgery* **66A**, 479–489

Salter, R. B., Willis, R. B. and Malcolm, R. W. (1978) The treatment of residual subluxation and coxa vara by combined innominate osteotomy and abduction femoral osteotomy. *Annals of the Royal College of Physicians and Surgeons of Canada* **16**, 63

Sharrard, W. J. W. (1993) *Orthopaedics and Fractures*, 3rd edn. Blackwell Scientific Publications: London, Edinburgh

Sibert, J. R. and Bray, P. T. (1977) Probable dominant inheritance in Blount's disease. *Clinical Genetics* **11**, 394

Siffert, R. S. (1956) *Journal of Bone and Joint Surgery* **38A**, 1077

Silberberg, M. and Silberberg, R. (1949) *Growth* **13**, 359

Simmons, E. D., Graham, H. K. and Szalai, J. R. (1990) Interobserver variability in grading Perthes' disease. *Journal of Bone and Joint Surgery* **72B**, 202–204

Sofield, H. A., Blair, S. J. and Millar, E. A. (1958) *Journal of Bone and Joint Surgery* **40A**, 311

Somerville, E. W. (1971) Perthes' disease of the hip. *Journal of Bone and Joint Surgery* **53B**, 639

Southwick, W. O. (1967) Osteotomy through the lesser trochanter for slipped femoral epiphysis. *Journal of Bone and Joint Surgery* **49A**, 807–835

Sponseller, P. D., Desai, S. S. and Millis, M. B. (1988) Comparison of femoral and innominate osteotomies for the treatment of Legg–Calvé–Perthes' disease. *Journal of Bone and Joint Surgery* **70A**, 1131–1139

Stirling, R. I. (1952) *Journal of Bone and Joint Surgery* **34B**, 149

Strobino, L. J., French, E. O. and Colonna, P. C. (1952) *Surgery, Gynecology and Obstetrics* **94**, 694

Tanner, J. M and Whitehouse, R. H. (1976) Clinical longitudinal standards for height, weight, height velocity, weight velocity and stages of puberty. *Archives of Disease in Childhood* **51**(3), 170–179

Thomson, J. E. M. (1956) *Journal of Bone and Joint Surgery* **38A**, 147

Trueta, J. (1953) *Bulletin of the Hospital for Joint Diseases* **14**, 147

Trueta, J. and Amato, V. P. (1960) The vascular contribution to osteogenesis. III. Changes in growth cartilage caused by experimentally induced ischaemia. *Journal of Bone and Joint Surgery* **42B**, 571

Vrettos B. C. and Hoffman E. B. (1993) Chondrolysis in slipped upper femoral epiphysis. *Journal of Bone and Joint Surgery* **75B**, 956–961

Wagner, H. (1978) In: *Progress in Orthopaedic Surgery*, vol. 1, pp. 71–94. Edited by D.S. Hungerford. Springer-Verlag: Berlin, Heidelberg, New York

Waldenström, H. (1938) *Journal of Bone and Joint Surgery* **20**, 559

Walmsley, T. (1938) *Journal of Bone and Joint Surgery* **11**, 40

Wansborough, R. M., Carrie, A. W., Walker, N. F. and Ruckerbauer, G. (1959) Coxa plana: its genetic aspects and results of treatment with the long Taylor walking caliper. *Journal of Bone and Joint Surgery* **41A**, 135

Weinstein, S. L. (1983) Legg–Calvé–Perthes' disease. *American Academy of Orthopaedic Surgery Instructional Course Lectures*, p. 272

Wilson, P. D., Jacobs, B. and Schecter, L. (1965) Slipped capital femoral epiphysis. *Journal of Bone and Joint Surgery* **47A**, 1128–1145

Wynne-Davies, R. and Fairbank, T. J. (eds) (1976) *Fairbank's Atlas of General Affections of the Skeleton*, 2nd edn. Churchill Livingstone: Edinburgh, London, New York

Wynne-Davies, R. and Gormley, J. (1978) The aetiology of Perthes' disease. *Journal of Bone and Joint Surgery* **60B**, 6

Zadek, I. (1935) *Archives of Surgery* **30**, 62

CHAPTER 7

Neuromuscular Affections in Children

ROBERT B. DUTHIE, A. CAMPOS DA PAZ JR, SÁURIA M. BURNETT AND ALVARO M. NOMURA

Examination and classification

Although many types of muscle weakness may be of little surgical significance, they are of considerable importance from the point of view of diagnosis (Table 7.1).

An accurate and detailed neurological examination is essential to determine diagnosis, prognosis and pattern of change in order to outline any management programme for the child. This should consist of the following.

1. *Muscle/motor evaluation.* Careful observation is made of muscle appearances of atrophy, and of contour or surface outlines for abnormal fullness or concavity. The muscle mass may be palpated for abnormal feeling of firmness or rubbery local tenderness. Muscles which should receive particular attention are the gastrocnemius, quadriceps, anterior abdominal wall muscles, deltoid and supraspinatus, the anterolateral muscles of the forearm, and both the thenar and hypothenar groups of the hand. Muscle power measurements should be charted. The limbs are passively moved for tone: if reduced, flaccidity of hypotonia is diagnosed; if increased (i.e. in upper motor neuron lesion) and sustained, it is called spasticity. If the tone is greater at the beginning of the movement (i.e. 'clasp knife' sign) and if it is sustained ('lead pipe' rigidity) or alters during the movement ('cogwheel' rigidity), it represents basal ganglion disease.
2. *Reflexes* of the deep tendons should be checked for being absent, normal, increased or spreading beyond their normal pathway (e.g. to the quadriceps at the knee or to the deltoid and pectoralis from the biceps reflex). This is seen particularly

in an upper motor neuron (UMN) lesion when the alpha motor neuron pool in the spinal cord is lost and the reflex activity is no longer contained at the level stimulated. It may also be seen during a Babinski response when the UMN lesion is massive with the dorsiflexion of the foot, knee and thigh. A positive Babinski response is thought to be a primitive withdrawal reflex by releasing the usual inhibitory controls in a UMN lesion. Myostatic reflexes result from direct striking of the muscle mass and are due to a monosynaptic spinal-cord-mediated reflex, causing a direct contraction of muscle. Hyperactivity is seen in UMN lesions, uraemia, hypocalcaemia and hyperkalaemia. Decreased response is seen in hypothyroidism or myxoedema or in uraemia. Coarse fasciculations can be seen as a normal response in anxious individuals. Fine fasciculations, however, are pathognomonic of denervation or neuromuscular disease such as amyotrophic lateral sclerosis.

3. *Sensory evaluation* for light touch perception, vibration and position senses is vital, particularly for spinal cord or spinocerebellar degeneration diseases.
4. *Cranial nerve evaluation.* Cranial nerve function should be looked for, particularly visual fields for optic nerve, muscle control of eye for nystagmus and strabismus (III and IV). The jaw jerk (V) is elicited and the facial nerve VII assessed by facial expression and mouth control. The cranial nerves IX and X are tested for by looking at speech and swallowing and any gag reflex. The tongue should be carefully examined for atrophy, fasciculations and movements.
5. *Sitting, standing and walking* evaluation should also be recorded. The classic Gowers sign of Duchenne muscular dystrophy (the manoeuvres required to stand up from the lying position) is well known. However, it only indicates any condition involving the motor power control of the pelvis and the trunk. Rhythmic standing (marking time) is a good indication of cerebellar function, as are opening and closing the digits or rapid rotation of the hands. The patient is requested to walk, and is watched for the regular rhythm of arm swinging, heel–toe impact gait patterns – all of which can be exaggerated by light running.
6. *Autonomic* (*sympathetic/parasympathetic systems*) bladder and bowel function, sweating and abnormal capillary appearances should be observed.

From such an examination it should be possible to differentiate between a lower motor neuron (LMN) lesion (infantile spinal muscular atrophy, myasthenia gravis, congenital myotonia, etc.) and an upper motor neuron (UMN) lesion (e.g. one of the spinocerebellar degeneration syndromes such as Friedreich's ataxia or Charcot–Marie–Tooth disease.

In LMN disease the characteristic feature is of motor power weakness with atrophy of muscle groups, leading eventually to loss of movements and severe muscular functional disability. Deep tendon reflexes are lost and evidence of denervation can be seen on electromyography and muscle biopsy. These changes are usually evident in early infancy.

In the UMN lesion, because the disease or disorder is above the anterior horn cell, spasticity, increased deep tendon reflexes with a positive Babinski sign are present, producing gait abnormalities of ataxia, abnormal postures and inability to carry out skilled or rhythmic movements. Weakness of muscles to direct testing may not be an obvious sign because of the spasticity. Cranial nerve abnormalities are frequent and the age at diagnosis is well into childhood and adolescence.

Another important differentiation is between the lesion being a *myopathy* (e.g. Duchenne's muscular dystrophy) – the muscle fibre alone – or a *neuropathy* (e.g. Charcot–Marie–Tooth disease), a denervating disorder of the neuromuscular junction or peripheral nerve.

However, Munsat *et al.* (1974) have pointed out that the changes attributed to a primary disorder of the myofibre may well have arisen by abnormal trophic function of the motor axon on the motor fibre. Changes in the neuronal input into the motor fibre can alter its physiology and biochemistry (e.g UMN lesions can influence motor fibres). On the other hand, with duration of disease, anterior horn cell lesions can produce myopathic changes difficult to differentiate from primary ones including increased serum muscle enzymes. He has also emphasized that in the early stages of myopathic disease, weakness is out of proportion to the amount of atrophy present, whereas in neuropathic disease the converse is true.

The muscular dystrophies

The chief clinical types of myopathy (Table 7.2) which will be described are:

1. The pseudohypertrophic type (Duchenne)
2. The juvenile type (Erb)
3. The facioscapulohumeral type (Landouz–Déjérine)
4. Infantile hypotonia
5. Myotonia atrophica congenita (Oppenheim).

Table 7.1 Childhood neuromuscular diseases

Site of lesion	Disease	Usual age on first symptoms (years)		Creatine phospho-kinase	Needle electro-myography	Nerve conduction velocities	Muscle biopsy
		< 1	<3				
Central nervous system	Cerebral hypotonia	+		N	N	N	Type 2 fibre atrophy
Anterior horn cell	Spinal muscular atrophies: e.g. infantile (Werdnig–Hoffmann)	+		N or ↑	Denervation	N	Diagnostic
Peripheral nerve	Hereditary motor and sensory neuropathies: e.g. Charcot–Marie–Tooth		+	N	Denervation	↓ or N	Denervation
	Acquired neuropathies: traumatic, toxic, metabolic	+	+	N	Denervation		
Neuromuscular junction	Myasthenia gravis	+	+	N	N	Fatigue of evoked response	Type 2 fibre atrophy
Muscle	Dystrophies:						
	Duchenne's			↑ ↑	'Myopathic'	N	Diagnostic
	Facioscapulohumeral	+	+	↑	'Myopathic'	N	Myopathic
	Limb girdle		+	↑	'Myopathic'	N	Myopathic
	Myotonic	+	+	↑	Diagnostic	N	Diagnostic
	'Congenital'	+		↑	Myopathic	N	Myopathic
	Congenital myopathies: central core, nemaline myotubular	+		N or ↑	N or myopathic	N	Diagnostic
	Inflammatory diseases: polymyositis and dermatomyositis		+	↑ or ↑ ↑	Both denervation and 'myopathic'	N	Diagnostic
	'Biochemical' disorders: phosphorylase deficiency, glycogen storage disease		+	↑	N	N	Diagnostic
Unknown	Benign congenital hypotonia	+		N	N	N	N

Reproduced, with permission from Florence, J.M., Brooke, M.H., and Carrol, J.E. (1978), *Orthopedic Clinics of North America*, **9**, 410–411.

Pseudohypertrophic muscular dystrophy (Duchenne type)

In spite of Duchenne having described this condition as long ago as 1868, only recently in 1987 has the gene for this and other similar conditions been located, e.g. the gene for Duchenne muscular dystrophy is localized on the short arm of the X chromosome, the gene in facioscapulohumeral dystrophy on the long arm of the 4 chromosome, the gene for myotonic dystrophy on the long arm of chromosome 19 (Cwik and Brooke, 1992). Cwik and Brooke emphasize that there still remains very little known about the gene structures or gene products in their excellent review of this complex subject.

In 1987, after cloning of the gene, its protein product was identified and named dystrophin by Hoffman *et al.* (1987) and who have given much detail about this protein.

Abnormalities or deletions of this gene result in the absence of detectable dystrophin protein in Duchenne dystrophy and in Becker's muscular dystrophy (a milder form of Duchenne). This is thought to arise either from this protein not being produced or if it is, poor detection of mutant forms or its form is unstable and rapidly degraded.

This protein can be localised to the cytoplasmic surface of the sarcolemma and because of its similarities to 'a' activin and spectrin, it is believed to maintain the structural integrity of the membrane. Indeed, Koenig and Kunkel (1990) have described it as adding to the flexibility of the cytoskeletal membrane when the muscle fibres contract or relax.

It is also found at the myotendinous junctions –

Table 7.2 Muscular dystrophies

	Progressive muscular dystrophy	Facioscapulo-humeral muscular dystrophy	Limb-girdle muscular dystrophy	Dystrophia myotonica
Age of onset	Childhood	Adolescence	Any	Early adult
Sex incidence	Male	Either sex	Either sex	More common in females
Inheritance	Sex-linked recessive	Autosomal dominant with incomplete penetrance	Autosomal dominant or recessive	Autosomal dominant with incomplete penetrance
Initial distribution	Pelvic girdle	Shoulder girdle	Either girdle	No pattern
Involvement of face	Rare	Always	Rare	Always
Rate of progression	Rapid	Slow and abortive	Intermediate	Slow
Pseudohypertrophy	Common	Absent	Very rare	Absent
Serum aldolase	Elevated	Borderline	Slightly elevated	Normal

Reproduced, with permission from Dowben, R.M. (1961), *Archives of Internal Medicine* **107**, 430.

and in its absence, this junction is abnormal and responds poorly to mechanical forces.

It may also have a role in the regulation of intracellular calcium and, when deficient, there is an increase in intracellular calcium which could lead to abnormal protein degradation and fibre necrosis (Turner *et al.*, 1988).

This is a disease of early childhood. Frequently its first symptoms are observed when the child attempts to walk, but sometimes the onset is delayed until the fourth or fifth year, or occasionally until after puberty. In the late cases, previous enlargement of muscles may have escaped notice. Boys are attacked much more frequently than girls. Sometimes several members of a family are affected, and although the females usually escape they may transmit the disease to their sons with 50% of all muscles being involved. However, in about 10% it is inherited as an autosomal recessive and hence some girls can exhibit this disorder. There is an overall incidence of about 1 per 3500 live male births.

CLINICAL FEATURES

Usually the first symptom to attract attention is insecurity in standing or in walking; the child falls easily, gets up clumsily, and in going upstairs has to support himself by the banisters before the age of 6 years.

Enlargement of the muscles is most conspicuous in the calves, which often feel firmer than usual. The infraspinatus often shows enlargement, and is firm as well as bulky and prominent. The biceps is commonly wasted. The muscles of the forearm and hand are rarely involved.

One of the most constant features of the disease is a bilateral atrophy or even an entire absence of the latissimus dorsi and of the lower part of the pectoralis major. In consequence, the axillary folds are thin or practically absent, and it is almost impossible with the hands in the armpits to lift the patient up, for

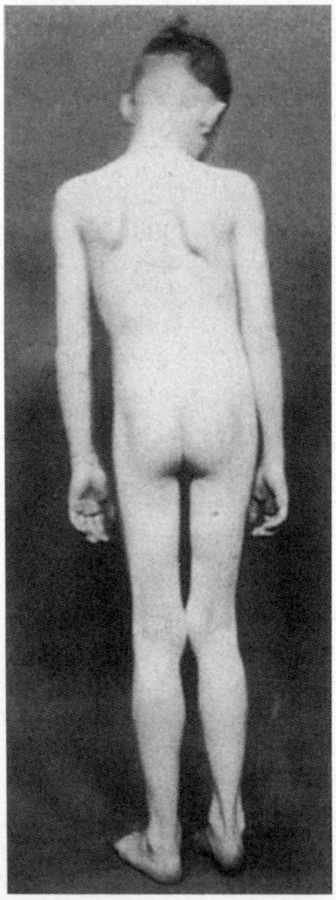

Figure 7.1 A characteristic posture of prominent scapulae mild enlargement of the calves and an equinus deformit of the right foot and ankle in Duchenne muscular dystrophy.

the shoulders offer no downward resistance.

The degree and the distribution of muscular weakness give rise to characteristic defects in the attitude and movements of the body (Figure 7.1). In standing, the child preserves his balance by keeping the feet wide apart and throwing back the shoulders and upper part of the body. In walking, the feet, widely separated, are lifted off the ground with difficulty, and the body is inclined first to one side and then the other. This waddling gait is effected by alternate contractions of the gluteus medius, these are necessary to enable the advancing foot to clear the ground. Occasionally, when the flexors of the hip are not weak, there is a 'high-stepping' gait, and in rising from the supine position on the floor the patient employs the classic method of 'climbing' up his legs.

As time goes on, certain deformities develop. The elbows and knees become flexed and the spine shows lateral curvature. Alternatively, the patient becomes bedridden, and is helpless, except perhaps as regards the movements of his hands. The limbs now become thin, and the muscles – even those of the calf which were formerly enlarged – small and wasted. The electrical irritability of the muscles, normal at first, shows a quantitative decrease to both faradic and galvanic current when the disease is fully developed. The knee jerks gradually disappear as the weakness of the extensors of the knees increases.

Sensation is unaffected; weakness of the sphincters is rare, and the general health is not necessarily interfered with until the final stage of the disease. The mental condition is generally lower than normal, although never at the mental retardation level.

The disease progresses slowly and insidiously, but it is rare for a patient to reach adult life. The usual cause of death is a primary involvement of the cardiac musculature or secondary cardiopulmonary complications.

DIAGNOSIS

The following features should be looked for.

1. Because of the damage to muscle fibres, there is leakage of enzymes into the serum to give an increased level. An elevated serum aldolase level in boys under the age of 15 years is a most significant finding. Thompson and Vignos (1959) showed that 90% of boys with muscular dystrophy have an increase in this serum enzyme. In disturbances of the neuromuscular junction or in secondary diseases of muscle, levels of this enzyme are normal. Serum levels of the enzyme creatine kinase, as first described by Ebashi and his co-workers in Tokyo, have been shown to be greatly raised in the early stages of the disease (Walton, 1964) and are a very sensitive diagnostic indicator. This enzyme is also increased in the female carriers of the sex-linked recessive gene in about 70% of cases.
2. On electromyography there is a typical pattern of a lower potential and polyphasic pattern during voluntary contraction, with an increase in the number of pulses and their rate of firing. Spontaneous fibrillation potentials are seen with reduction in the number of motor unit potentials, but not in amplitude.
3. Biopsy of muscle, when taken from reliable situations such as the rectus abdominis, can provide a definite positive histological diagnosis. Vignos *et al.* (1963) warned against using the gastrocnemius, which, although conveniently situated, is a poor choice since its strength is often well preserved in early muscular dystrophy. Also the pain and weakness following such a biopsy may temporarily impair walking and produce some degree of heel-cord contracture. There is an intermingling of normal and abnormal fibres which show an irregularity in diameter and proliferation of the sarcolemmal nuclei with prominent nucleoli as well as marked variation in size of the fibres. Movement of the nuclei into the centre of the muscle fibres is also seen. Various forms of degeneration and replacement by fat and fibrous tissue are seen (Figure 7.2). The basic deformity appears to be loss of integrity of the muscle-cell membrane. Unfortunately denervated muscle may exhibit these changes secondarily and therefore distinction between this disorder and that of denervation is not absolute.

TREATMENT

There is no curative treatment for Duchenne dystrophy and in the past numerous remedies, i.e. glucose, vitamin E, multiple amino acids, anabolic steroids, etc. have been given without any success. However, recently Dubowitz (1991) has recognized the success of prednisolone in improving muscle strength and function as well as pulmonary function. Indeed De Silva *et al.* (1987) reported that prednisolone slowed the progression of this disease and allowed ambulation until a later age.

Prednisolone does not increase the level of dystrophin in the muscle cells, but appears to decrease the breakdown of muscle protein as well as having an immunosuppressive role on the T cells and monocytes.

Partridge (1991) has recently reviewed the pos-

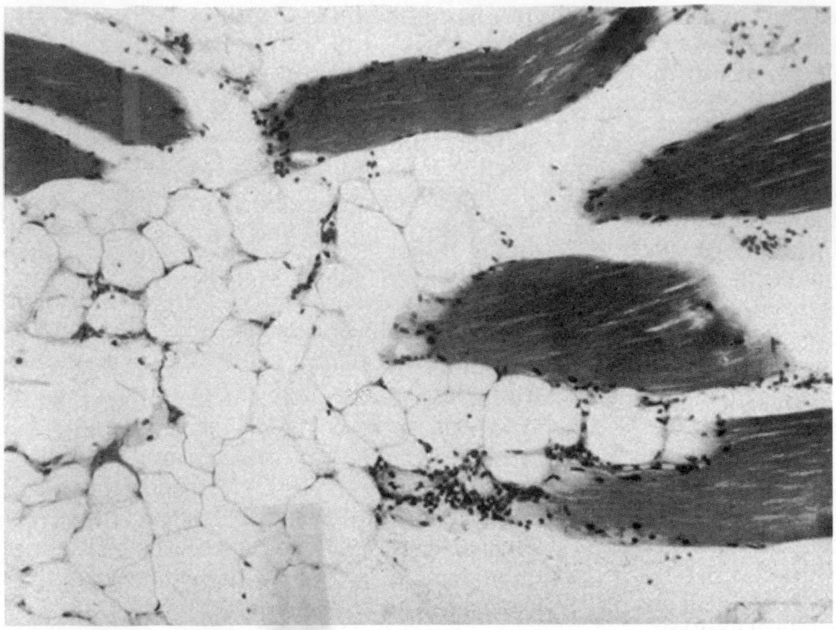

Figure 7.2 Photomicrograph showing the replacement of muscle bundles by fatty tissue, with abnormal nuclei arrangement, in a biopsy from a patient with muscular dystrophy.

sibility of myoblastic transfer of large numbers of normal donor myoblasts and injecting them into human dystrophic muscle. Bone therapy or substitution is also being considered.

Vignos *et al.* (1963) outlined the comprehensive care for these children, warning particularly against a negative type of programme with early confinement to a wheelchair and loss of ambulation prematurely. Paul (1955) reported that, out of 90 patients with muscular dystrophy, one-third had stopped walking or were confined to wheelchairs by the age of 6 years. These workers emphasized a well supervised programme of exercises during the early stage of the disease and eventually the early fitting of long light alloy leg braces to continue independent ambulation as long as possible. They emphasized the multidisciplinary approach for comprehensive care with consideration of the child's entire needs. The family must be instructed that although the natural course of this disease is slowly progressive, there is a variety of measures available to maintain optimum function. With such understanding, better co-operation is achieved by all concerned. Practical aids and equipment are available to solve specific problems for individual patients but require careful selection and supervision. Occupational therapists and others should be involved in planning for optimum access and convenience in the home, school and work place.

These workers emphasized how desirable it is for serial evaluations to be carried out with accurate recording based upon the functional testing of certain activities – those involving walking and climbing stairs with or without assistance, walking unassisted, getting up from a chair, using long leg braces, etc.

In physiotherapy, it should be recognized that it is the imbalance between the synergic and antagonistic muscle groups which insidiously limits the child's total functional capacity. Stretching exercises of the hamstrings, of the iliotibial tracts and the triceps surae groups of muscles both by the physiotherapist and by the parents should be started early. The child should stand for a minimum of 3 hours a day in order to prevent disuse of muscle, to stretch contractures (particularly of the heel cord) and to preserve extension of the knee. The onset of any contractures should be immediately attacked by further and more extensive stretching. Exercises should be either of the active type or of progressive resistance type, particularly of the hip and knee extensors, ankle dorsiflexors and evertors of the foot. In the upper extremities, the extensors, the supinators, the shoulder abductors and the rotators should be exercised.

Spencer and Vignos (1962) described the use of double upright long leg braces before or after the correction of any contractions by stretching or by surgery. After any procedure they should ambulate as soon as possible (i.e. within 2 or 3 days). These workers do not recommend night splints because of the discomfort and interference with change of position and sleep. They believe that it is best to maintain the child in as normal a school environment as possible, for as long as possible, although they are functioning at a lower intellectual level. Their academic achievement is well correlated with their mental age.

Lengthening of the tendo calcaneus by percutaneous tenotomy (Bowker and Halpin, 1978) in the presence of fixed heel-cord contractures should be carried out early, before these deformities can involve the knee, hip and finally the lumbar spine.

Lordosis occurs early in the disease process and is most often due to weakness of the hip-joint extensor muscle group, with a forward pelvic tilt producing a movement posterior to the centre of gravity of the trunk. Anteriorly, there is tightness leading to contractures of the hip flexors and requires treatment only by stretching and lying face down. Surgical correction can be achieved and may have to be resorted to, as any form of orthotic appliance has proved to be ineffective. Scoliosis – a collapsing type – appears slowly either during walking or even when in a wheelchair and can be helped by a body jacket of light plastic material. Miller and Moseley (1985) described that the spinal support systems on wheel-chairs rarely prevented the development or progression of an existing scoliosis. Ninety-three per cent of Duchenne patients develop a significant scoliosis and hence were offered spinal surgery. (See Chapter 8 for its pathogenesis and treatment.)

The juvenile type of Erb

In this type the sexes are more equally affected than in pseudohypertrophic paralysis. It usually begins in the second decade of life, and the muscles of the upper arm and thigh, together with certain muscles of the shoulder and pelvic girdles, are affected; those of the forearm and leg are generally spared. There is therefore a striking contrast between the size of the arm and forearm, and of the thigh and leg, in a typical case.

The biceps, triceps and brachioradialis are the first muscles to show any change. Subsequently the latissimus dorsi, the lower part of the pectoralis major, the trapezius, the serratus anterior and the rhomboids are involved. The deltoid and the spinati usually escape. The atrophy of the serrati leads to bilateral winging of the scapulae. Later in the disease the glutei, the flexors of the hip and the muscles of the thigh, especially the quadriceps extensor, become wasted and weak. The gait and the manner of rising from the ground may be the same as in the pseudohypertrophic form.

The facioscapulohumeral type of Landouzy and Déjérine

This is a type in which weakness of the facial muscles begins to develop in infancy, or is present at birth, and is followed by wasting of the scapulohumeral muscles. In other respects the distribution of the atrophy resembles that of the juvenile form, and the two diseases are in all probability of the same nature.

The hereditary nature of this type is sometimes shown by its presence in successive generations and has been analysed genetically as dominant autosomal in type. In many cases, however, no other members of the family have been affected.

The characteristic feature is the early and marked involvement of the facial muscles. The orbicularis oris and orbicularis palpebrarum are prominently affected, the patient being unable to close the eyes completely, or to whistle or blow. A sphinx-like facies develops: the lips are everted, the lower lip projects and the mouth has, not inaptly, been compared to that of a tapir. The smile is often peculiar, for the mouth forms a straight line, and the angles of the mouth are not drawn upwards and outwards.

After the facial atrophy develops, the muscles of the shoulders and the arms are implicated and subsequently the muscles of the back, hip and thigh, but life expectancy may be normal.

Infantile hypotonia – 'the limp child'

WERDNIG–HOFFMANN DISEASE

It is autosomal recessive with early death by the age of 2 years. The creatine phosphokinase levels may be significantly elevated and muscle biopsy may show secondary myopathic features.

Muscular weakness and hypotonia in infancy and early childhood are important physical signs, often difficult to understand and interpret.

Werdnig and Hoffmann described infantile spinal muscular atrophy. This is one in which the child appears normal during the first few months of its life but then develops a rapidly progressive flaccid paralysis of the limbs and trunk, progressing inexorably to death. It commonly affects more than one member of a sibship.

AMYOTONIA CONGENITA

This is a rare infantile condition characterized by smallness and extreme flaccidity of the voluntary muscles, by loss of the deep reflexes and by a tendency to gradual improvement.

Oppenheim described amyotonia congenita and suggested that the condition was present at birth and, in contrast to the Werdnig–Hoffmann disease, tended to improve slowly but steadily and was not familial.

The condition is usually congenital and is noticed at birth or shortly afterwards. In a few cases it has developed in a previously healthy infant, apparently as a result of diarrhoea or acute bronchitis. There is no evidence of either hereditary or familial tendency, so it is not certain whether this disorder should be included among the myopathies or not. The health of the parents, including that of the mother during pregnancy, has usually been good.

The limbs, especially the lower ones, are the most severely affected; the trunk is often involved, the face but rarely. There is general weakness of the limbs but no actual paralysis, voluntary power in individual muscles, although feeble, being retained. The distribution of the muscular flaccidity is symmetrical. The limbs flail at all their joints, and may assume the most curious positions. Thus the wrist and the ankle may be so overextended that the metacarpus touches the forearm, and the dorsum of the foot the front of the tibia. The hands and feet are often long. Some consider this condition to be the underlying cause of arthrogryposis multiplex.

The children never learn to walk but adopt some strange method of getting about, by rolling over and over or by assuming a squatting attitude, so that the name 'frog-child' or 'the limp floppy baby' may be given to them.

Contractures are apt to occur in the course of time, and the knee and hip may become flexed.

The muscles show a lowered excitability to faradism – indeed, when the amyotonia is severe the current must be very powerful to obtain any response. The strong current is borne without complaint, despite the fact that no loss of sensibility to any other form of stimulation can be detected.

The superficial reflexes are normal; the deep are lost, but may return in cases in which improvement takes place. The sphincters are never affected. The mental condition is normal and the child learns to talk at the ordinary age. The growth of the bones and the general bodily development are not interfered with.

The course of the disease is one of slow and progressive improvement which may be hastened by the persevering use of massage and passive movements, although complete recovery has never been recorded.

OTHERS

1. Benign congenital hypotonia of Oppenheim–Walton.
2. Glycogen storage disease–type 5 and type 6 of McArdle.
3. Central core disease.

Myotonia atrophica

This is a very rare condition characterized by the association of muscular atrophy with a slow relaxation of the muscles of the extremities after voluntary contraction. This myotonic condition is very limited in its distribution. It is most conspicuous in the flexor muscles of the hands, the patient finding it impossible to relax his grasp suddenly.

The atrophic weakness affects the facial muscles, the sternomastoids, the vastus muscles and the dorsiflexors of the ankle, and occasionally the forearm muscles, the masseters and the temporals.

The disease is a familial one and affects males rather than females. Its manifestations usually appear between the ages of 20 and 30. Its course is slow and progressive, and in many cases muscular wasting is present for several years before the myotonic state appears. It may be associated with either gonadal or thyroid hormonal dysfunction as well as cataracts in 90% of patients. Frontal baldness, cardiac condition defects are common, mental retardation or even dementia are documented.

DIAGNOSIS

Well marked types are easy to recognize, but there are many aberrant forms in which it may be difficult to decide whether the muscular atrophy depends on an abnormal condition of muscular tissue or on disease of the spinal cord. In favour of a myopathy would be:

1. The onset of the atrophy at an early age.
2. Its occurrence in more than one member of the family.
3. Its distribution. Progressive wasting of the muscles which do not correspond to destruction of a definite group of cells in the spinal cord.
4. The absence of fibrillary twitchings and of a definite reaction of degeneration.
5. The condition of the tendon reflexes, which are

never exaggerated and disappear as the muscular wasting progresses.
6. Biochemical tests of serum aldolase, creatine phosphokinase levels, etc.
7. Electromyography for the size and frequency of the motor unit potentials during voluntary contractions.
8. Muscle biopsy with special staining techniques.

Volkmann's ischaemic contracture

In 1875 Volkmann described a contracture of the muscles of the wrist and fingers which followed tight bandaging of the arm in the treatment of fractures about the elbow. He believed that it was essentially due to ischaemia of the muscles, and that, as a result of deprivation of arterial blood, the muscles suffered from want of oxygen; the condition, he thought, was thus akin to rigor mortis. He also showed that paralysis occurred simultaneously with the contracture, differing in this respect from the contracture which follows a primary nerve lesion.

INCIDENCE AND AETIOLOGY

The condition occurs most commonly in children in the first 10 years of life, and follows injuries, particularly to the elbow, and especially those associated with pressure, either internal or external.

At one time it was accepted that the condition was caused by the effect of improper application of splints or by acute flexion of the elbow in turn producing a venous obstruction.

Volkmann's contracture is the result of infarction produced by a segmental arterial spasm of the main artery to an extremity with reflex spasm of the collateral circulation. Ischaemia is produced, and the muscle bellies – demanding the greatest amount of blood and therefore the most vulnerable tissue to its loss – are first affected. Possibly gangrene of the fingertips would occur if the spasm continued in sufficiently severe degree, but the usual result of ischaemic contracture implies that some improvement in the collateral circulation intervenes. This vasomotor activity is under the control of the sympathetic nervous system.

The cause is usually a fracture or injury of the upper arm, and in the cases where the injured site is explored, a profound segmental arterial spasm is discovered. Usually at a point about 2 cm above its bifurcation the brachial artery is pulsating normally or even a little dilated, but below that it suddenly becomes narrowed to a string-like size extending down into the radial and ulnar branches. The injury need not directly affect the vessel to produce the spasm. Although there may be a minor injury to the vessel wall, that is not sufficient to occlude the vessel by the damage itself but causes the artery to occlude itself, probably through the sympathetic nerves. A similar spasm is seen following the lodgment of an embolus, and in fact may result from any disturbance of the peripheral circulation. The operation of arteriectomy may reveal an internal torn flap, which is producing the obstruction to the flow. It is evident that a good collateral circulation is capable of supplying all the needs of the peripheral circulation and that the chief danger in cases of main-artery occlusion lies in the degree of constriction or dilatation of the collaterals under sympathetic vasomotor control. Arteriography will outline the narrowed segment as well as the present state of the collaterals.

PATHOLOGY

The gross picture, which is one of central degeneration of the muscle bundle, is duplicated histologically by only one other condition – infarction, Seddon (1956) pointed out that the infarct takes the form of an ellipsoid with its axis in the line of the anterior interosseous artery and with its central point a little above the middle of the forearm. The greatest damage is at the centre and usually falls most heavily on flexor digitorum profundus and flexor pollicis longus, which are often necrotic. Those muscles most superficially placed and sometimes the deep extensors are more likely to exhibit fibrosis. The median nerve runs near the centre of the ellipsoid and may exhibit profound ischaemia. The ulnar nerve tends to be less severely affected. The most extensive degeneration occurs in the centre of the muscle sequestrum, and cellular activity and fibrosis take place only at the periphery, which is surrounded by a sheath of dense fibrous tissue. In the centre of the mass, the muscle fibres lose their nuclei and cross-striations, and fuse into a homogeneous mass. As the periphery is approached, some signs of function are preserved, and there is an area of intense cellular activity, both fibroblastic and phagocytic. This picture is in contrast to muscle degeneration from all other causes, such as denervation and sepsis, in which the appearance is one of diffuse interfibrillar fibrosis.

This entity has also to be differentiated from the compression compartment syndrome of the forearm, due to lying on a limb for a long period of time, poisoning by drugs, e.g. alcohol, etc. (Geary, 1984) or in haemophilia with bleeding into the forearm.

The succeeding phases are those of replacement: fibroblasts appear, and deposit fibrous tissue at first in thin threads and later more densely. The whole process thus seems to be one of absorption and replacement by fibrosis of dead muscular tissue. A similar condition occurs where the anterior leg muscles are chiefly affected because of oedema in the anterior compartment of the leg in a patient taking much unaccustomed exercise.

Seddon pointed out there is reversible damage following vascular ischaemia to muscles. The dead muscle fibres are removed and can be replaced by new ones which grow longitudinally along the surviving sarcolemmal tubes. He emphasized that in Volkmann's ischaemia there is often initially a total paralysis of the forearm, but within 2 or 3 months the extensor muscles recover well, with some recovery of the flexors. There are varying degrees of severity between this and irreversible damage in which little contractile tissue survives. The degree of damage to a nerve also varies from reversible to irreversible; in the latter there is usually complete fibrosis of the muscle mass. It is of interest that peripheral nerve tissue is definitely less susceptible to ischaemia than muscle; therefore, one should wait for at least 3 months for evidence of spontaneous recovery before embarking on operative treatment. During this time, treatment should be aimed at splinting to minimize contractures, as well as to maintain joint function. Careful evaluation of nerve recovery is also important.

CLINICAL FEATURES

The symptoms usually begin within 1–24 hours of the injury. Severe pain, pallor, paralysis and pulselessness are all present in greater or lesser degree. Pallor is usually the first change and it is often striking; pressure on a nail will readily show whether the circulation is impaired. The pulse distal to the obstruction is invariably absent and therefore it is wise whenever possible to leave an accessible pulse uncovered by bandages for regular examination. Often there is intense pain, especially on attempted movement, and numbness in the fingers; ultimately voluntary movement is totally abolished. It is to be noted, however, that pain may be absent in some cases. The complete process is over in the first 2 days, so the necessity for prompt initial treatment is very urgent. After this period the swelling gradually disappears and the muscles become hard, fibrosed and resistant. As the fibrosis increases, deformity becomes obvious – especially flexion of the fingers. The fully developed picture is very characteristic: the wrist is flexed; the fingers are extended at the metacarpophalangeal joints and flexed at the interphalangeal joints; while the forearm is often pronated and the elbow flexed (Figure 7.3).

There are various degrees of the deformity:

1. *Mild degrees* are often first brought to the consultant several years after an injury to the elbow. The patient may be unable to extend the fingers completely but yet may possess a considerable range of movement when the wrist is flexed; indeed, it is usually possible to straighten the fingers completely with the wrist fully flexed (Figure 7.4).
2. The *severe type*, with the fully developed and characteristic attitude described above (Figure 7.5).
3. A *severe type complicated by nerve involvement*. Either the median or the ulnar nerve may be coincidentally involved, but it must be remembered that, where the primary lesion is a supracondylar fracture, these nerves may be

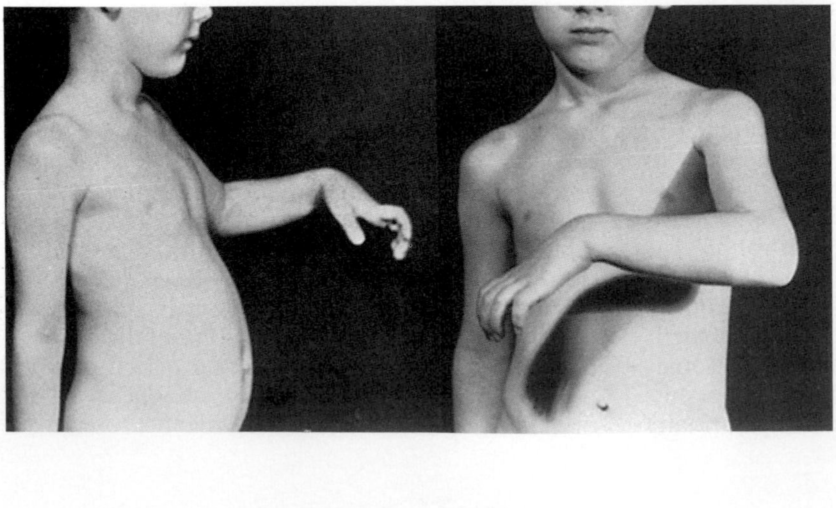

Figure 7.3 Volkmann's contracture resulting in severe loss of hand function.

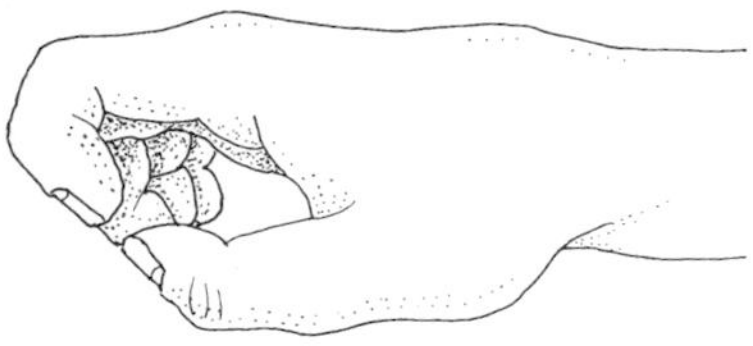
(a)

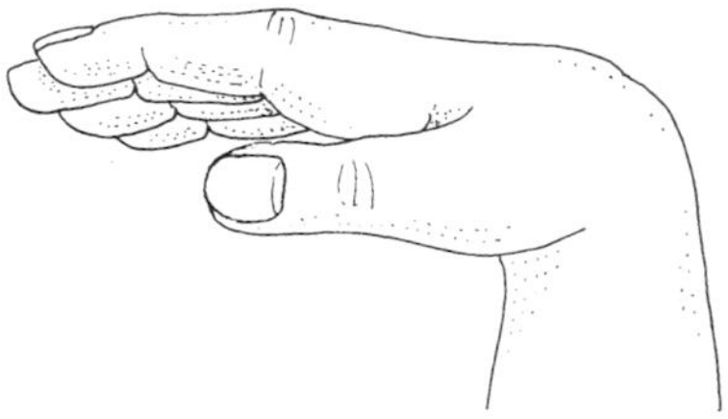
(b)

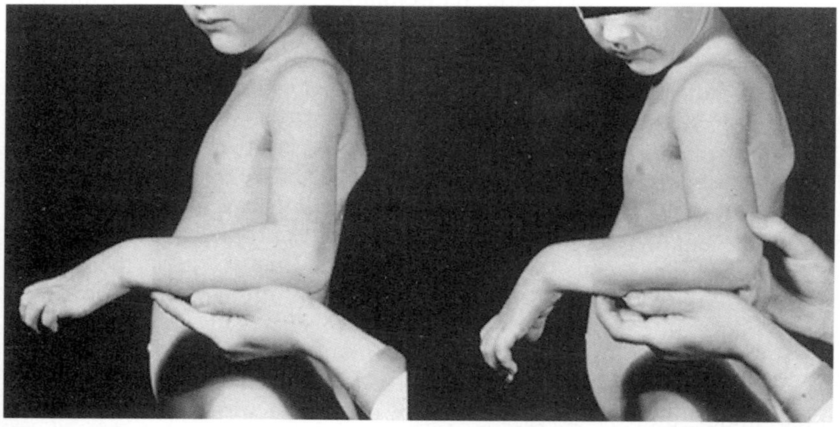
(c)

Figure 7.4 Ischaemic contracture. Extension of the fingers is possible only while the wrist is flexed.

injured – not by the Volkmann's contracture, but by the projecting fragments of bone. In the absence of direct damage, however, either nerve may be implicated in the actual ischaemic contracture. The median nerve is frequently compressed where it passes between the two heads of the pronator teres, and the ulnar nerve may suffer from the contraction of the fibrous tissue which surrounds it; in each case, the signs are those of an incomplete nerve lesion – usually partial anaesthesia, and paralysis of the small muscles of the hand. In addition, the nutrition of the limb is impaired, the hand is cold and blue, and trophic ulceration occurs.

When the damage is reversible, a limited number of muscle fibres die and they are gradually replaced by new ones growing longitudinally along the surviving sarcolemmal tubes. Seddon pointed out that this takes a considerable time, and in one of his cases the intrinsic muscles of the hand showed no improvement until after the 200th day. When there are irreversible changes, all grades of fibrosis are present up to almost complete fibrous replacement.

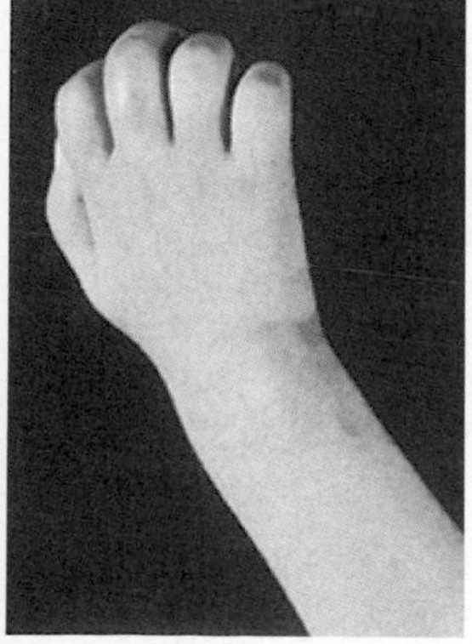
(a)

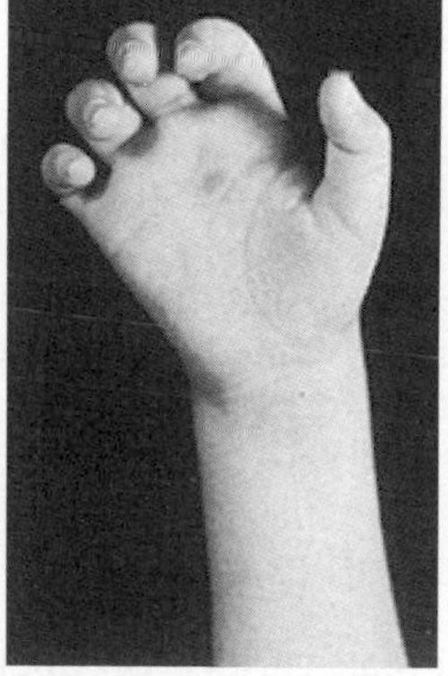
(b)

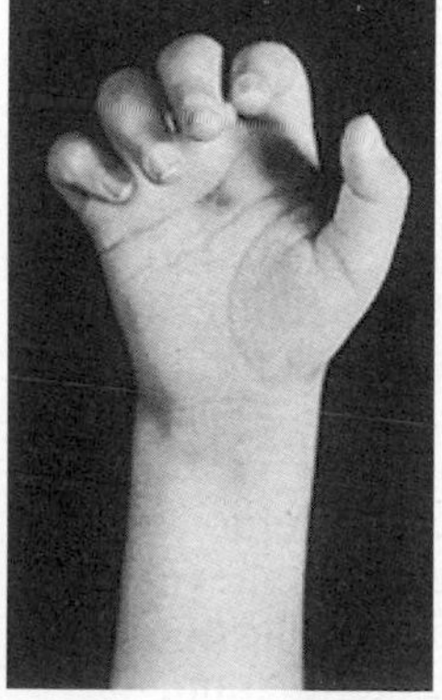
(c)

Figure 7.5 (a) The claw-like position of a child's hand following Volkmann's contracture of the forearm muscles. (b) and (c) The same patient, showing attempts at extension and flexion of the fingers and adduction of the thumb.

PROGNOSIS

The prognosis will depend upon the stage at which treatment is instituted: the earlier it is undertaken, the better the prognosis is likely to be. The outlook is grave in the severe types, and in cases with accompanying nerve involvement, but in the slighter degrees of contracture, without nerve involvement, treatment usually gives a comparatively good result.

PROPHYLAXIS

Many limbs have been lost by adopting an attitude of wishful thinking after some or all of the signs of interference with the arterial circulation have been recognized. Action must be immediate.

The condition of the forearm and hand must be carefully watched in the early stages of treatment of all injuries of the elbow joint; in this connection, supracondylar fracture of the humerus is particularly dangerous. The position of the elbow joint after reduction of these fractures will depend upon the extent of any swelling present.

It is inadvisable to treat fractures about the elbow with plaster-of-Paris splints or bandages, particularly if they are applied in a circular fashion. In all cases of elbow injury a look-out should be kept for pain, stiffness, swelling, cyanosis or lividity of the fingers, or obliteration of the radial pulse. The first step, if the event has followed a fracture, is to see if the fragments are displaced. If they are, a further reduction should be carried out at once; even if they have not moved, it is wise to extend the limb slightly because this is followed occasionally by relief of the spasm. Failure of the pulse to return within a few minutes is an indication for immediate operation.

TREATMENT

The treatment may be divided conveniently into various stages.

The acute stage

The goal of treatment is to restore adequate circulation before irreparable damage is done, and thus to avert contracture deformities. In treatment, time is a major factor. The condition is a progressive one in which more and more damage is done. All measures favouring circulation generally are of the greatest value. These include elevation of the part, removal of any splint or circular bandage, and the application of mild external warmth. The contralateral limb, or other limbs, may be warmed.

The next logical step is the interruption of the sympathetic reflex supply by ganglion injection or arteriectomy. The former is tried first, and if successful its results are at once apparent and an open operation is avoided. The appearance of a Horner's syndrome is evidence of a successful cervical sympathetic block. The local arterial spasm may, however, be the result of a local reflex that does not include the paravertebral ganglions and so the injection cannot be expected to be universally successful; if circulatory improvement is not immediately apparent or maintained, the artery should be exposed. Indeed, this is now the treatment of choice. This at once affords an opportunity of determining any local trauma to the artery. When the contracted artery is exposed, the effect of perfusion by papaverine is tried, especially if the vessel does not appear to be too badly damaged. The whole length of the affected part of the artery is flooded in a 2% solution of papaverine; in very many cases the spasm disappears within 2 or 3 minutes and the pulse returns at the wrist. If this is unsuccessful, complete interruption of the sympathetic arc is achieved by doing an arteriectomy, resecting a section of the artery at the level of the fracture. Arteriectomy, in addition to the complete interruption of the reflex, has the advantage of the removal of a segment of the vessel which possibly contains a small break or intimal tear not grossly visible, yet sufficient to maintain continued abnormal sensory stimuli. Its removal effectively produces vasodilatation of the collaterals.

If the x-ray examination (which should have been completed by this time) does not show perfect reduction, the question of improving the alignment must be considered. It will be better in most cases to complete the reduction by open operation with wire external fixation since additional manipulation will further traumatize the tissues, and so increase the pain and probably the deformity also.

The fully developed stage

Physiotherapy

The first step in treatment is to prevent contractures and maintain a supple joint with a full range of movements, and so a splint is applied which makes use of elastic traction to prevent the muscles contracting while at the same time permitting the joints of the fingers and wrist to be moved, if necessary passively, to prevent them from becoming stiff.

Operative treatment

A great variety of operations have been recommended for this condition, from tenoplasty, bone section and excision of the elbow joint, to the muscle-sliding operation described by Max Page. In every case, operation should be preceded by a course of thorough stretching as described above.

Littlewood recommended lengthening of all the shortened tendons, but this is a serious operation in a young child, and requires great care and neatness if even a moderate result is to be secured, especially as lengthening a tendon may weaken the power of the muscles more than an operation which does not alter the length of the whole contractile unit (Seddon, 1965). It should be attempted only if the contraction is limited to one or two of the forearm muscles.

Shortening of the bones of the forearm by resection of 2–2.5 cm from each is also a severe operation, and (as described by Sir Robert Jones) it is liable to be followed by non-union due to the trophic changes in the arm. The operation was recommended by Garré, but the results are not encouraging.

Max Page described a muscle slide operation in which a straight incision is made from just above the medial epicondyle downward for about 10 cm on the medial aspect of the forearm, and the flexor muscles, arising from the medial epicondyle of the humerus and the upper ends of the radius and ulna, are erased from their origins by a periosteal elevator. The hand and fingers are then hyperextended, and in this way the muscle origin is dragged downward. The muscles obtain, in time, a new origin lower down the forearm. In performing the operation great care must be taken to avoid the ulnar nerve; if the nerve is involved, it should be freed from the surrounding fibrous tissue, and at the same time, the median nerve may be similarly dissected out and freed. The after-treatment consists of careful splinting of the hand and fingers, and physiotherapy.

Seddon achieved good results in severe cases by excising completely the belly (or the scar representing it) of every muscle that has been completely destroyed, except for flexor carpi ulnaris because of danger to the ulnar artery which may be the only remaining blood supply to the hand. Reconstructive procedures are carried out either at the same time or later by transplanting living muscles to replace the dead ones. He emphasized that although all the bone operations described (such as removal of the carpal bones, bone shortening, arthrodesis of the wrist) will leave the soft tissues relatively undisturbed, and therefore little fibrosis results, they do little for the paralysed muscles.

Tendon transfers or tenotomies appear to be the most rational, but they have the risk of recurrence because of contractures. Seddon described total excision of necrotic muscle to prevent deformities with increasing contractures – never before 3 months and he considered it probably wiser to wait 6 months. He followed this procedure by lengthening or transplanting tendons of shortened, but active, muscles. Any median nerve lesion, which frequently accompanies this condition, can be replaced by pedicle grafting. When both the ulnar and median nerves are involved, a free graft can be carried out with some success. In the very severe case, Seddon recommends an arthrodesis of the wrist, particularly where it has been necessary to use extensors for giving flexion to the various digits.

Treatment of the nerve complications

When there is clinical evidence of nerve involvement, which does not show any sign of improving, after a reasonable period of 2 or 3 months' physiotherapy, the nerves should be explored at the sites where they are most likely to be compressed. The median nerve should be free from the callus of the fracture, and also released from compression as it passes under the superficial head of the pronator teres. The ulnar nerve is freed throughout the length of the flexor muscle bellies. If the nerves have suffered irreversible damage, they should be dealt with by one of the several types of graft according to Seddon. General physiotherapy should afterwards be carefully carried out, the muscles at the same time being protected from overstretching by adequate splints.

Poliomyelitis

Poliomyelitis was recognized as a clinical entity in the first half of the nineteenth century. Outbreaks were reported by Badham in England in 1834 and by Colmer in the USA in 1843. Von Heine published his monograph describing the clinical aspects of the disease in Germany in 1840. Larger epidemics appeared at the end of the nineteenth century in Scandinavia and subsequently in North America, Australia and New Zealand. Sporadic outbreaks continued in Great Britain, with the first major epidemic in 1947. In the Scandinavian countries and in the United States large-scale epidemics have occurred, but with the immunization programmes using both the Salk and the Sabin vaccines, these are now prevented. However, epidemics are still seen in developing countries and in travellers to those countries, in whom their vaccination status has broken down. In England and Wales from 1970 to 1984 there were only 70 cases reported (PHLS, 1986) but the WHO, has estimated that there are more than 250 000 fresh cases in the world each year (Hinman *et al*., 1987).

The characteristics of the disease have altered and poliomyelitis can no longer be regarded as truly infantile. The change in the age group of patients is illustrated by statistics in the State of Massachusetts where in 1907 only 7% of the patients were over 15 years of age compared with 25% in 1947. There has also been a great increase in the proportion of non-paralytic cases, which is probably not entirely due to improved diagnosis.

AETIOLOGY

Three serological types (I, II and III) are known to exist with type I being the most common in man. So far no living reservoir other than man has been found. Although isolated from flies during epidemics, there is no proof as yet that the virus multiplies or undergoes part of its life cycle in flies.

The virus gains entrance to man by way of the oropharynx and can be isolated from pharynx and faeces in both the preparalytic and postparalytic phase. The virus can also be isolated from healthy carriers.

There is no agreement as to whether infection is transmitted from the oropharyngeal or faecal source, but both should be considered as possible sources of infection.

The actual invasion of the central nervous system was generally assumed to take place along nerve pathways and it has been demonstrated that the virus can travel proximally along a nerve to the spinal cord.

The virus has been recovered from the blood of abortive cases of poliomyelitis (Horstmann and McCollum, 1953) and in the preparalytic phase in chimpanzees after oral virus feeding (Bodian, 1952; Horstmann, 1952). There is evidence to support the presence of a viraemia in human poliomyelitis and blood stream invasion precedes central nervous system invasion.

The presence of the virus in the central nervous system is usually associated with the onset of meningitic symptoms, but its effect may vary from the slight paresis found clinically without any history of a previous illness to the severe meningitic case which recovers without any demonstrable muscle weakness.

The factors governing the degree of destruction of the motor cells are not fully understood, but clinical observations indicate that certain conditions influence not only the incidence but also the localization of paralysis. Ritchie Russell (1947) drew attention to the fact that physical activity during the preparalytic stage increased the incidence and severity of paralysis. Injections or trauma to the limbs may precipitate paralysis which is often localized to the affected limbs, while recent tonsillectomy appears to increase the frequency of bulbar poliomyelitis.

PATHOGENESIS

The poliomyelitis virus, once established in the central nervous system, has a special affinity for the anterior horn cells of the spinal cord and for certain motor nuclei in the brain stem.

The pathological changes which take place in the spinal cord motor neurons have been clarified by Bodian and are based on evidence obtained both from human autopsies and from experimental work with monkeys.

The earliest visible change is chromatolysis of the Nissl substance in the cytoplasm of the nerve cell; this is followed by inflammatory infiltrations of polymorphonuclear and mononuclear cells, at first in the perivascular regions and then diffusely in the grey matter.

Interference with function of a motor cell in poliomyelitis may be reversible or irreversible, and early recovery of some muscle groups is often a striking feature in the early weeks of the disease. It was previously considered that oedema was responsible for temporary paralysis, but Bodian's experimental work does not support this view. Bodian considers that nerve cells are either destroyed during the early days of the illness or undergo slow recovery leading to morphological recovery within about a month.

In the irreversible case chromatolysis progresses, the cell nucleus shrinks and the necrotic cell is removed by neuronophagia.

Changes in the chronic stage of poliomyelitis

As a result of the destruction of the nerve cells in the anterior horn, the peripheral nerve degenerates and the muscles supplied by it atrophy. The extent of muscle degeneration depends on the amount of nerve involved. The atrophied muscle fibres are recognized by their yellowish-white colour. In some cases complete degeneration is shown by the fatty deposit around the atrophied muscle. Tendons atrophy from disuse and lose their normal glistening appearance. Bones are also involved in the pathological process – they are more attenuated than normal with a considerable degree of osteoporosis. Shortening invariably occurs in paralytic limbs; the exact cause is not known but reduction of the musculo-osseous blood supply from paralysed muscles is probably an important factor. Joint capsules and ligaments when not protected by healthy muscles become stretched, the joints become unduly mobile and occasionally may dislocate if not protected. The skin circulation of the paralysed limb is affected and responds more readily to local temperatures. In cold conditions the cyanotic leg with recurring chilblains may be a source of discomfort to the patient.

CLINICAL FEATURES AND COURSE OF THE DISEASE

In epidemic poliomyelitis it is known that the virus is present in the faeces of 'healthy carriers' and most probably also in the pharynx at the time of infection. In these cases either the virus has not extended beyond the alimentary tract or else the disease has been asymptomatic. 'Silent infection' is probably very common during epidemics and while of no clinical significance it is obviously an important factor in the spread of disease.

The incubation period is difficult to define in many cases. It varies from 3 days to several weeks, with a probable average of 10 days. Direct questioning of close contacts of paralytic patients frequently brings to light minor symptoms such as brief headache, back pain or sore throat.

Poliomyelitis usually presents as an acute illness with symptoms of meningitis followed by paralysis. Different forms of the disease are described, but they refer merely to variations in symptomatology, depending on the differences in the intensity and location of lesions within the central nervous system (Table 7.3).

The clinical course of paralytic poliomyelitis passes from the acute stage to the convalescent or recovery stage and finally to the chronic or residual stage when no further significant recovery in muscle power can be expected.

Minor illness

In approximately one-third of patients admitted to hospital with poliomyelitis there is a definite history of a short prodromal stage with symptoms of slight headache, malaise, fever and sore throat. This minor illness lasts only for 48 hours. The symptoms, while not specific for poliomyelitis, warrant close observation of the patient during localized outbreaks of the disease.

The illness may not proceed beyond the prodromal stage and an abortive form of poliomyelitis is recognized. In less fortunate patients the minor illness is followed by 4 or 5 days of well-being before the onset of the major illness. This apparent recovery frequently encourages the patient to resume work or strenuous holiday activity, which may have some bearing on the eventual severity of the paralysis.

Acute stage (major illness)

This stage describes the main febrile phase of the disease and is regarded as the most dangerous phase of invasion of the motor nerve cell. The major illness, which lasts from 4 to 7 days, occurs in all typical cases of poliomyelitis and includes both the preparalytic and paralytic stages.

Preparalytic stage

The preparalytic stage is characterized in the majority of cases by an abrupt onset of meningeal symptoms accompanied by headache, fever, malaise and nausea or vomiting. The temperature rises, neck stiffness becomes more marked, the patient is often irritable and complains of pain in the trunk or limbs.

The patient does not wish to sit up. On examination there is definite stiffness of the back and neck, and in severe cases retraction of the head and arching

Table 7.3

Stages in development of poliomyelitis			Clinical forms of disease	
(Minor illness)	Prodromal stage		Abortive poliomyelitis	
(Major illness)	Preparalytic stage	→	Non-paralytic poliomyelitis	
	Paralytic stage	→	paralytic poliomyelitis	Bulbar type Spinal type

NB. Recovery at prodromal stage = Abortive poliomyelitis
Recovery at preparalytic stage = Non-paralytic poliomyelitis

Clinical course of paralytic poliomyelitis

Acute stage = Major illness
Convalescent stage = Stage of recovery
Chronic or residual stage = No further significant recovery

of the back are maintained by spasm of the posterior spinal muscles.

It should be recognized that the preparalytic stage may be less dramatic, and patients are sometimes seen in whom muscle weakness is the only evidence of poliomyelitis.

The term 'non-paralytic poliomyelitis' describes the case in which the symptoms and signs of the preparalytic stage subside without clinical evidence of paralysis.

Paralytic stage

Paralysis supervenes usually on the third or fourth day but may appear at any time during the major illness. The onset of paralysis is not marked by any particular change in the signs and symptoms of the preparalytic stage, although diminution or loss of deep reflexes may precede paralysis in the affected muscle groups.

The degree of meningeal symptoms and signs is variable and is not related directly to the severity of the paralysis. The patient complains of headache and pain in the back. Photophobia is marked in some cases, while in others pain and tenderness of the limbs are prominent features.

Spasm of the posterior spinal muscles with neck retraction and a positive Kernig's sign are found in the majority of patients, but true muscle spasm in the extremities is not a feature of poliomyelitis.

Paralytic poliomyelitis presents either as the spinal or bulbar form of the disease. Fortunately, combination of the two forms in the same patient is rare.

The spinal form

This is the more usual type. Partial or complete paralysis affects the muscles of the neck, trunk and extremities. The paralysis is of the flaccid lower motor neuron type, with loss of tendon reflexes. The lower limbs are affected at least twice as frequently as the upper limbs and there appears to be a certain predilection for muscles such as the tibialis anterior and posterior, quadriceps, glutei and deltoid. The bladder is affected in a small percentage of cases and retention of urine may require catheterization.

Paralysis of the diaphragm and intercostal muscles is manifest by rapid shallow respirations. The patient becomes restless, apprehensive and fatigued. The appearance of cyanosis of the lips indicates the need for mechanical respiration.

The bulbar form

This form of poliomyelitis, though less common than the spinal form (about 25% of all cases), is nevertheless of extreme importance as it accounts for a high proportion off deaths attributable to poliomyelitis. The initial symptoms indicating involvement of the cranial nuclei are nasal intonation, difficulty in swallowing and accumulation of saliva in the pharynx. Cyanosis in these cases is an indication of obstruction to the airway. Prompt recognition and treatment will relieve obstruction to the airway, but in severe bulbar cases progressive involvement of the vital centres may rapidly prove fatal.

Muscle spasm

The term 'muscle spasm' is so frequently associated with the early stages of poliomyelitis that consideration of its definition and aetiology is warranted.

Definition of 'muscle spasm'

In the acute and early recovery stages of poliomyelitis passive movement is sometimes limited by pain or resisted by muscle contraction. The muscle contraction usually described as muscle spasm is an involuntary contraction to prevent a potentially painful movement and resembles the muscle spasm associated with fractures.

In the acute febrile stage sustained painful spasm of the posterior spinal muscles is a characteristic feature and resembles the protective spasm of other inflammatory meningitic conditions. This sustained tone disappears, but spasm of the back muscles can be elicited by spinal flexion for a variable period in the recovery stage.

Pain in the limbs not necessarily associated with movement may present as a feature of the preparalytic and paralytic stages. This type of pain is probably referred from lesions in the spinal ganglia.

When the patient has recovered from the acute stage, passive movement of the limbs may be limited by pain or painful muscle contractions which, if treatment is neglected, encourage faulty positioning with possible joint stiffness and deformity.

Passive movement of the limbs in the early stages of poliomyelitis is limited by spasm only when the muscles are active, and by pain alone when muscles are paralysed. The term 'muscle resistance to stretch' is a more accurate description of this guarding action of muscles, but the term 'muscle spasm' is more convenient for clinical description.

Aetiology of muscle spasm

Muscle spasm or muscle resistance to stretch is most

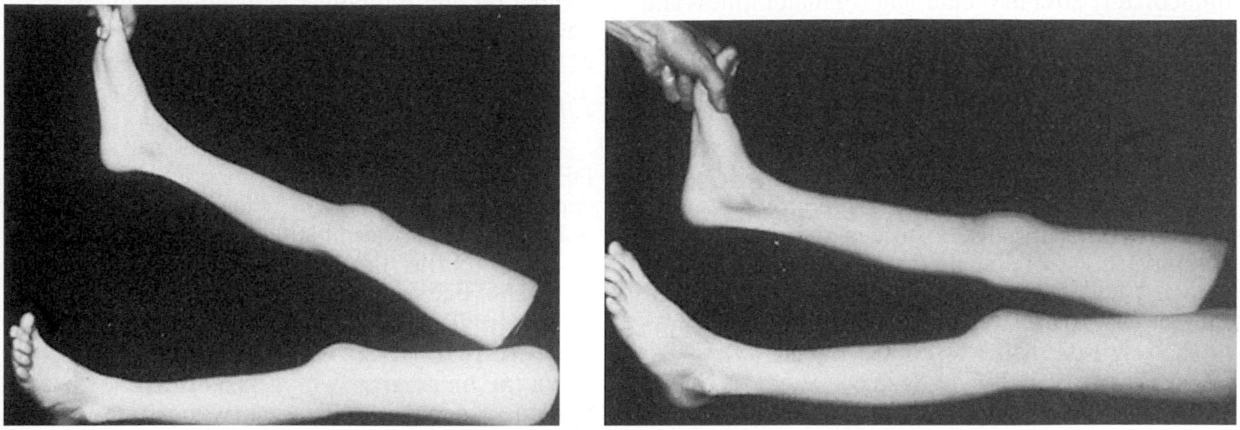

(a) (b)

Figure 7.6 (a) Limitation of straight leg raising in early weeks of poliomyelitis. (b) Limitation increased by dorsiflexion of foot.

frequently manifest as a contraction of the hamstring group which limits straight leg raising to an angle of 30° in a high proportion of patients with lower limb involvement (Figure 7.6). The muscle spasm in these patients can be aggravated by nerve tests; e.g. Lasègue and Kernig (Mitchell, 1952). The limitation of straight leg raising is equal on both sides, irrespective of the degree of paralysis. When muscle resistance is ineffective, the straight leg raising may be limited by pain alone. Schlesinger (1951) found that limitation and pain persisted even with muscles rendered atonic with intravenous mephenesin.

Muscle spasm is less common in the upper limbs and appears usually as a resistance to full abduction of the shoulder or as a temporary limitation of elbow extension. Only approximately 2% of paralytic cases show a significant degree of muscle spasm in the upper limbs. In such patients the muscle spasm is also aggravated by tests which exert a traction effect on the nerve roots; e.g. upper arm traction and contralateral neck flexion (Figure 7.7).

The muscle contraction at first sight appears to resemble true spasticity, but there is no true evidence of an upper arm motor neuron type of lesion and the increased tone subsides rapidly on sedation.

The painful stimuli probably arise from the residual inflammatory changes which have been found at autopsy in the region of the posterior nerve roots and meninges.

Convalescent stage (stage of recovery)

The convalescent stage or stage of recovery is defined as that period of the disease which starts

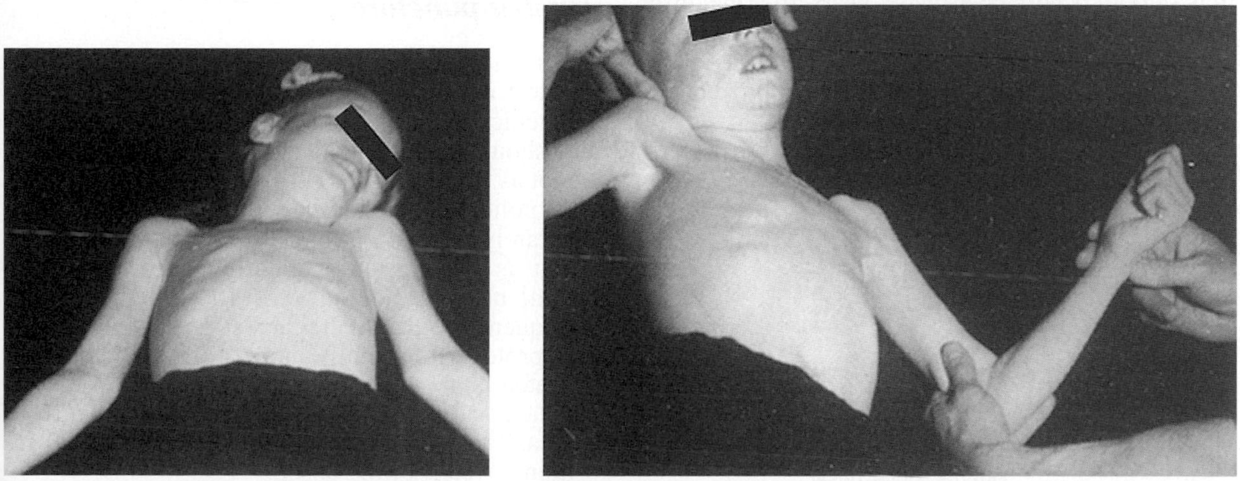

(a) (b)

Figure 7.7 (a) and (b) Protective spasm in biceps limiting extension, produced by contralateral neck flexion and also by traction on upper limb.

immediately after the acute stage of major illness and ends when no further significant recovery in muscle power is anticipated.

Recovery of muscle power depends on the distribution of the destructive lesions in the grey matter of the cord and on the proportion of recoverable to irrecoverable lesions.

According to Bodian (1949), the affected motor cells are either rapidly destroyed during the acute paralytic stage of the disease or undergo gradual recovery changes leading to complete morphological recovery within a month. While Bodian's deductions are based mainly on experimental work with Rhesus monkeys, clinical evidence suggests that in human poliomyelitis the fate of the motor cell is decided in the early weeks of the disease.

Several factors must be considered in attempting to estimate prognosis in the early stage of the illness. Pain, muscle spasm of antagonistic groups, inadequate early treatment and lack of co-ordination in younger children all tend to delay or mask muscle recovery.

In the absence of these factors, complete paralysis of a muscle persisting beyond the third month indicates severe motor-cell destruction and a poor prognosis as regards useful recovery. Where worthwhile return of function is to be anticipated, the muscle will either show evidence of early recovery or the initial paralysis will have been incomplete.

Muscle recovery is most marked in the first 3–6 months but continues to improve up to 18–24 months (Figure 7.8) (Green, 1949).

Residual stage

Significant increase in reliable muscle chart recordings seldom occurs later than 2 years after the onset of poliomyelitis, but functional improvement may continue for several years especially in young children. This can be attributed to improved co-ordination and willpower assisted by general body development.

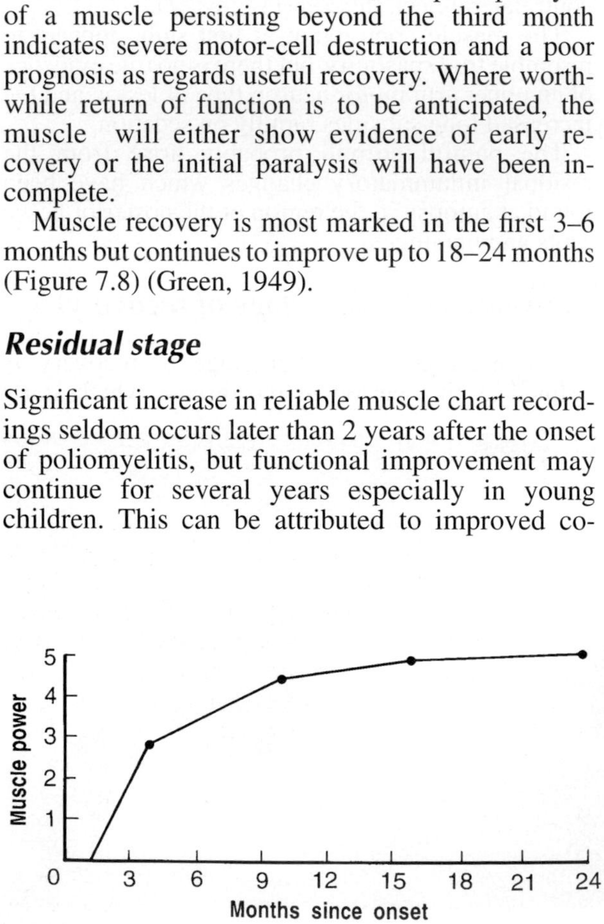

Figure 7.8 Muscle recovery chart, showing rise in total muscle power during first 2 years after onset.

DIAGNOSIS

Diagnosis of the prodromal illness (minor illness) can only be presumed during localized outbreaks of poliomyelitis, as the clinical features are not specific. A brief febrile illness may be associated with headache, malaise, nausea, vomiting or sore throat. Indeed in developed countries these symptoms are more likely to be caused by 'epidemics' of meningococcal meningitis which is characterized by a blotchy skin rash, etc. If contact with poliomyelitis is suspected, these patients should be confined to complete rest at home for about a week.

In the major illness the subjective symptoms are more intense. Headache, nausea and vomiting are common together with pain in the neck, back or limbs. The most important objective findings are nuchal and spinal rigidity. The patient is unable to kiss the knees, and when asked to sit up he frequently supports the stiff spine by placing his hands behind him on the bed–tripod sign. Kernig's sign is positive in a high proportion of cases.

Diminished or absent tendon reflexes may precede actual muscle weakness by 24 hours. Detailed muscle testing is not justified during the acute stage. Main muscle groups can be examined by active movement against the slight resistance of the clinician's hand. In the infant, a paralysed limb does not participate in the general rhythm of body movement and offers no resistance when handled. The tone of the abdominal muscles is evident in crying.

Lumbar puncture

Examination of the cerebrospinal fluid is of the greatest importance in the differential diagnosis of pyogenic and bacterial meningitis, and lumbar puncture should be carried out immediately if there is any doubt as to the diagnosis.

In poliomyelitis the cerebrospinal fluid is variable but rarely normal. During the acute stage the cell count is usually only slightly raised to around 20/ml, but higher counts of 100–200/ml are not infrequently found. In the early stage of poliomyelitis the protein is initially normal or only slightly elevated, but as the paralysis develops, the cell increase subsides whereas the protein tends to increase, reaching a level of 100–300 mg/100 ml within 3 weeks of the onset.

DIFFERENTIAL DIAGNOSIS

1. *Meningitis.*
   (a) Meningoencephalitis due to antigenically untreated viruses; e.g. mumps, Coxsackie virus.
   (b) Pyogenic meningitis; important when clinical picture has been modified by chemotherapy prior to admission.
   (c) Tuberculous meningitis.
2. *Infective polyneuritis* (*Guillain–Barré syndrome*). May closely simulate poliomyelitis but the paralysis is symmetrical, sensory changes can usually be demonstrated, and paraesthesiae are very marked and common. The cell count is within normal limits and the protein is elevated to over 300 mg/100 ml in the CSF.

PROPHYLAXIS OF ACUTE POLIOMYELITIS

Trials of poliomyelitis vaccine in the USA in 1954 showed that a formalin vaccine could protect against paralytic poliomyelitis, and other countries have confirmed the value of vaccination against this disease. In 1957 in the USA a protection rate of about 90% was achieved in children receiving three doses of vaccine. The problem is to determine the most effective way of maintaining immunity. The mechanism of immunity is not fully understood.

A better antibody response in infants and young children is obtained with three doses of inactive virus vaccine rather than with two or one. Salk recommends two primary doses, 4–6 weeks apart, followed by a third dose 7 months later. There is a considerable decline in the antibody level (especially in types I and III) after immunization with two doses of the vaccine, but a substantial antibody response is obtained after the third or 'booster' dose.

The introduction of the Sabin live attenuated vaccine has added much to any mass immunization programme. This virus is no longer capable of producing outward clinical symptoms of poliomyelitis, but it is, however, capable of eliciting an antibody response in the individual. It is described as multiplying in the mucosa of the intestinal tract, where it produces its antibody response as well as developing a relative resistance in the alimentary tract. Antibodies are detected in the serum 7–10 days after taking this oral vaccine.

Type I poliomyelitis is responsible for at least 85% of all paralytic disease during most epidemics. The Sabin vaccine can be used to boost existing antibody titres after Salk vaccine, to fill any immunological gap, and to provide intestinal resistance, thereby limiting the carrier state and their numbers.

Its use, particularly against types I and II, is indicated for rapid mass vaccination in preschool children and in young adults. It should be noted that live virus vaccine type III has been associated with the development of paralytic poliomyelitis in a few instances of young adults or in older age groups.

TREATMENT

The treatment of poliomyelitis is conveniently divided into three stages: the acute stage, the convalescent or recovery stage, and the residual stage.

In the UK the acute stage of poliomyelitis is usually treated in isolation hospitals and the orthopaedic surgeon is principally concerned with recovery of function during the convalescent stage and with the treatment of residual disability when recovery has ceased.

The acute stage

Poliomyelitis patients should initially be admitted to isolation units where the medical and nursing staff are experienced in the differential diagnosis and treatment of acute febrile illnesses. Trained personnel and the necessary facilities must be available to deal adequately with the different problems of respiratory complications which are such an important feature of the acute stage.

No specific treatment is indicated during the acute stage. Detailed recording of muscle power at this stage is both unnecessary and harmful; an approximate estimation of the extent of paralysis can be obtained by gentle handling of the limbs.

The patient should be nursed in a quiet cubicle and is allowed to assume whatever position is most comfortable. The position of severely paralysed patients should be changed for nursing purposes and to ease back pain which is often marked. Anti-inflammatory drugs can be given for their analgesic effects. Retention of urine may require catheterization, which should be intermittent and carried out with the strictest aseptic precautions; normal micturition is usually restored early if infection is avoided.

Respiratory difficulty

Prompt recognition and accurate clinical analysis of the functional defect is necessary for successful treatment of respiratory difficulty. In some cases, however, extensive destruction of the brain stem with its vital centres renders a fatal outcome inevitable.

The two main types of respiratory complications are:

1. intercostal and diaphragmatic paralysis of the spinal form of poliomyelitis and
2. pharyngeal paralysis of the bulbar form.

Intercostal and diaphragmatic paralysis

The signs of progressive respiratory involvement in order of likely sequence as described by Wilson (1953) are:

1. *Increased respiratory effort*
   - Increased rate of breathing
   - Dilation of nostrils
   - Interruption of speech
   - Use of accessory muscles of respiration
2. *Effort and/or failure*
   - Anxiety
   - Restlessness or sleeplessness
   - Disorientation
3. *Respiratory failure*
   - Coma
   - Cyanosis
   - Convulsions

Intercostal and diaphragmatic paralysis of a degree which prevents the maintenance of normal alveolar ventilation, requires the use of artificial aids to respiration. The mechanical respirator of the tank type was commonly used, but with improvement in design, artificial airways have proved to be more efficient and manageable with fewer complications. (For example, cuffed endotracheal tubes, through the nose or mouth, can be used for up to 3 weeks – after which they should be removed because of the risk of infection and scarring, and replaced by Silastic tracheostomy tubes.) Various respirators are now available with either pressure-cycled or volume-controlled mechanisms.

Pharyngeal paralysis

Pharyngeal paralysis is the most important of the bulbar forms, causing respiratory failure on account of its frequency. Prompt treatment is essential and often effective.

The danger of pharyngeal paralysis lies in the constant risk of aspiration of unswallowed secretions. Effective coughing may be impossible and obstruction of the airway causes irregular respiration and fatigue. If the obstruction is not relieved, inadequate respiration or aspiration of accumulated secretions leads to anoxia, coma and ultimately death.

Early signs of bulbar involvement include nasal intonation and difficulty in swallowing. Ritchie Russell (1950) emphasized the importance of a rattling sound with breathing, due to respiration bubbling past mucus. This rarely occurs in a conscious patient except with pharyngeal paralysis; it is therefore an important sign which can be recognized by listening to the patient's breathing.

The essentials of treatment in pharyngeal paralysis are prompt diagnosis, immediate postural drainage and aspiration of the throat. Tracheostomy should seldom be necessary unless bilateral abductor paralysis of the vocal cords develops.

Correct positioning of the patient is important. The patient is nursed in the semi-prone position and turned to the other side every few hours. The foot of the bed should be elevated at least 46 cm.

The respiratory problem usually persists and is the condition which will limit the everyday activity of the patient and add hazard to life with increased risk of infections, particularly after general anaesthesia. Therefore frequent and successive pulmonary function evaluation is necessary. The degree of pulmonary embarrassment should be elicited by enquiring about the frequency of chest infections, dyspnoea at rest and on exercise, coughing or expectoration ability, and any cyanosis or undue fatigue. At examination, the function of the thoracic cage movement and ranges should be charted, as should the efficiency of the diaphragm, abdominal and extra muscles of respiration in the neck and glossopharynx. Pulmonary function studies to measure vital capacity and tidal air flow are essential, as are arterial gas tensions ($Pa\text{O}_2$, $Pa\text{CO}_2$). Radiographs in full inspiration and expiration are helpful, as is the 'sniff' test for diaphragmatic function. Such radiographs may show structural changes in the spine and thoracic wall.

Convalescent or recovery stage

This stage begins with the subsidence of the acute symptoms and continues up to the time when no further significant recovery in individual muscle groups is to be expected (i.e. approximately 18 months).

The aim of treatment in the early stages is to eliminate deforming tendencies, restore joint mobility and to train the co-ordination of recovering muscles. In the later stages the residual muscle power is built up with resistance exercises and the patient is fitted with suitable apparatus to enable treatment to be continued as an outpatient.

Specific treatment is not indicated during the acute stage but may commence 48 hours after the fever has subsided. Treatment must be delayed when encephalitic signs persist and should be subordinated to the care of acute respiratory complications when necessary.

An approximate estimation of paralysis is recorded, and any limitation of passive movement is noted and particularly any tendency to 'muscle spasm'. A comprehensive examination must not be attempted in the early days as it proves exhausting and depressing for patients with severe paralysis. Muscle charts can be completed at subsequent examinations.

The method of muscle strength recordings as advocated by the MRC has certain disadvantages but is sufficiently accurate for treatment purposes.

Grade 0 Complete paralysis
1 Flicker of contraction
2 Movement with gravity eliminated (e.g. in pool)
3 Movement against gravity
4 Movement against resistance
5 Normal muscle power

The psychological aspect of treatment is important and the patient should be as relaxed and confident as possible under the circumstances. Pain is alleviated by codeine, and sedation with small doses of temazepam assists relaxation and allays apprehension. The treatment of muscle spasm presents no major problem except in severe respiratory cases. Because the muscular contraction is purely protective, no vigorous stretching is necessary. Spasm likely to interfere with subsequent joint mobility will respond readily to rest, heat and regular gentle passive movement.

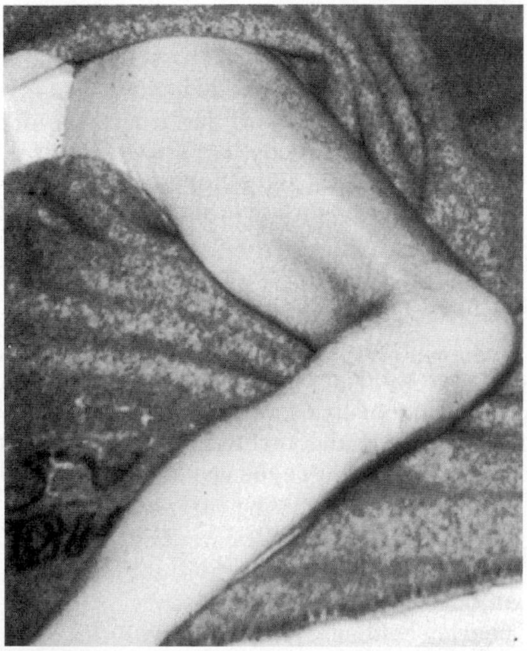

Figure 7.9 Tightening of the iliotibial band in an untreated case.

Hot packs

Hot, moist packs relieve pain and 'muscle spasm' during the early days of treatment but should only be used where indicated as their overzealous application can be tiring to the patient. They have no specific effect on the actual recovery of nerve cell lesions.

Passive movements

All joints are moved through a passive range twice daily. When movement is restricted by pain or muscle spasm, treatment is increased to four times a day but restricted to the pain-free range. The patient should be turned regularly to relieve pain and stiffness, and at least one period a day is spent in the prone position.

Certain patients show a tendency to loss of elasticity of fascial structures, which may lead to contraction if not detected in the early stage. Particular attention must be paid to the iliotibial band and plantar fascia. Regular stretching of tight fascial structures in the early stage is essential if serious contractures are to be eliminated (Figure 7.9).

Positioning

Limbs and spine are so positioned as to prevent the stretching of paralysed muscles and the development of any overacting tendency in active muscles.

Spine

Children are nursed on a firm mattress. Heavy adults with severe spinal paralysis are more comfortable on a 10 cm Dunlopillo mattress supported by fracture boards. Periods in the prone position are important in maintaining tone of the posterior spinal muscles and glutei.

Lower limbs

The knees are maintained in slight flexion on a pillow. The feet are supported by a foot board but felt-padded plaster splints may be applied when indicated to control leg rotation or foot imbalance, or to prevent tightness of the plantar structures developing in the cavus type of foot. In severe paralysis of the calf the foot should be placed in slight equinus and stretching of the calf avoided as overstretching of a paralysed calf accentuates calcaneus deformity of the foot.

Upper limbs

If there is any tendency to muscle spasm when shoulder and arm are involved, position may be maintained by a felt sling under the elbow suspended from an overhead beam. This method is comfortable for the patient, maintains a satisfactory position of all joints and allows passive movement to be carried out with minimal disturbance. Felt slings are also suitable in the later stages when the patient is allowed to sit up for periods – gentle active movement is possible with the support of slings. Felt opponens splints maintain the thumb in opposition and are comfortable for the patient – they are not practical, however, in infants. In maintaining splintage it is emphasized that they should be padded with felt and that regular passive movements of the joints be carried out. Splintage is used only when satisfactory position cannot be achieved or maintained by simpler methods.

Muscle re-education

The re-education of a muscle establishes better co-ordination between the remaining nerve fibres and enables the patient to obtain the maximum possible contraction. When pain and tenderness have subsided, the patient concentrates his attention on the attempt to accomplish the desired movement while it is performed passively. It helps co-ordination to get him to perform the same action on the healthy limb. When the muscle becomes capable of spontaneous action, it is allowed to contract with gravity eliminated – this is best accomplished in a warm-water tank. Underwater therapy is a useful aid to treatment even in the early recovery stage. Residual pain and muscle spasm are relieved and back stiffness is more easily overcome. The patient appreciates the greater mobility of water immersion and benefits both psychologically and physically.

In the early recovery stage muscle fatigue should be avoided. Later the resistance to the muscle is increased depending on the degree of recovery. Movement against gravity is increased to movement against resistance either by the hand or by pulleys and weights.

In the later recovery stages maximum resistance can be applied to the muscle. With maximum resistance the muscle groups should be exercised in rotation to give a rest interval between contractions.

Two sessions of treatment daily are sufficient. One should be carried out in the physiotherapy department and the other one in the pool. This gives variety of surroundings, allows the patient to meet others, and maintains his interest in treatment.

Physiotherapists should use the suspension sling apparatus. This is best constructed by erecting a heavy-gauge wire-mesh overhead screen from which are suspended canvas slings to support the limbs during exercise periods.

Pool therapy

The swimming pool is an invaluable aid to treatment. The small tank is useful in the early weeks of recovery but more freedom is required during the later stages. Walking is commenced in the large pool and swimming is excellent exercise to improve overall body tone.

Apparatus used in convalescent and residual stages

During the ambulatory stage, apparatus may be necessary to protect a weak muscle, to prevent deformity or to support the patient. The apparatus may be permanent in severe cases while in others it may be discarded when the patient gains more control or when stabilization of the part is achieved by surgical means(see Chapter 13).

Abduction shoulder splint

The abduction splint for paralysis of the deltoid muscle is seldom indicated. When worn for long periods it may actually delay the recovery of the deltoid and throw an unnecessary strain on the spine. Adequate support for the shoulder during the ambulatory recovery stage is obtained by wearing a sling supporting the elbow. This allows the patient to use the forearm and hand while protecting the shoulder from the effects of gravity. When it is evident that no significant recovery of the deltoid is likely, complete freedom should be encouraged and exercises concentrated on the development of the scapulothoracic muscles which will later carry the arthrodesed shoulder.

'Cock-up' wrist splint

Light splints to support the wrist are necessary when the extensors are paralysed. 'Lively' splints, as advocated by Capener, leave the palm relatively free; individual finger extensions can be incorporated if necessary.

Weight-bearing caliper

In severe paralysis of the hip muscles the body weight may be taken on a padded metal ring and transmitted down the metal side bars to the shoe into which the ends of the appliance fit. Stability of the hip through the ischii on the caliper ring will enable the patient to bear weight and avoid undue strain on the hip which might otherwise lead to paralytic dislocation.

Below-knee appliances

These are used to control mobile foot deformities which result from muscle imbalance.

In infants the foot is best controlled by double below-knee irons with flat sockets inserted into the heel. In children the irons should have round sockets inserted into the heel. Permanent appliances for adults are made with ankle-joint hinges.

Equinus deformity is prevented by adding a toe-raising spring or drop-foot stops to the heel. Anterior check-stops are used for calcaneus deformity.

A valgus foot due to paralysis of the invertors is corrected by an outside iron and an inside T strap attached to the shoe. An inverted foot due to peroneal paralysis is corrected by an inside iron and an outside T strap (Figure 7.10).

Spinal brace

Adequate support for severe spinal paralysis is difficult to achieve. Paralysis of the abdominal muscles is controlled by an abdominal corset. Mild trunk weakness is treated with a corset.

More extensive trunk weakness with spinal instability or early scoliosis should be supported with a moulded orthotic jacket constructed from a plaster cast taken with the patient standing under slight traction from a head sling.

Advancing scoliosis merits consideration of spinal fusion (see Chapter 8).

Treatment of the residual stage

Treatment of the residual or chronic stage includes regular out-patient supervision of the physical, social and economic problems arising from the disability. Experienced advice is invaluable to the rehabilitation of the patient in suitable employment and in his social environment.

Although recovery of individual muscle power may not show significant increase after 18 months or so, some functional improvement may continue in children as the general musculature and co-ordination improve with growth.

Orthopaedic procedures in the residual stage are indicated:

1. to correct soft tissue contracture,
2. to improve function and to prevent deformity by tendon transfer and stabilization procedures, and
3. to correct inequality of leg length.

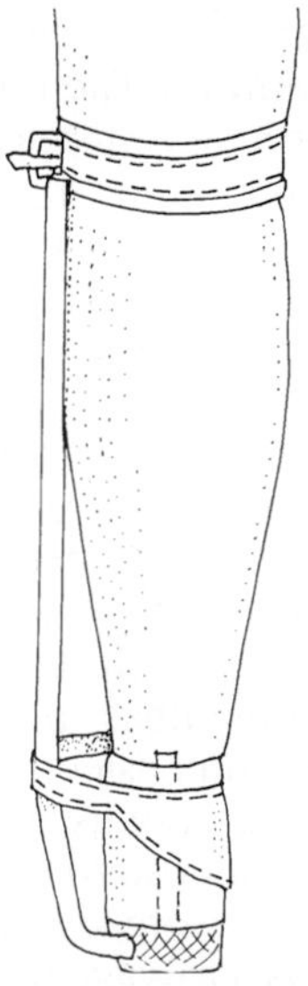

Figure 7.10 Poliomyelitis. Medial iron and lateral T strap for use in peroneal paralysis. The strap and iron may be transposed for use in other deformities.

Treatment of the hip

PARALYTIC INSTABILITY

Paralytic dislocation of the hip is particularly common either acutely or slowly and indeed can be unnoticed. It follows flexion deformity, especially when associated with adduction. The relaxation of the joint capsule facilitates dislocation. The dislocation may be incomplete, giving rise to what is known as a 'snapping hip'. The diagnosis is not difficult, as the head of the femur slips from the socket whenever the leg is adducted. The condition causes great lameness, and occasionally much irritability of the joint.

Flexion and adduction should be prevented by conservative methods and these patients should acquire the habit of sitting and sleeping with their knees separated – the abduction being more important than extension in the prevention. The best splint is made from two half cuffs of metal joined together by a metal rod, about 30–45 cm long, attached to the middle of their convex surfaces. This is bandaged on nightly to the patient's legs just above the knees. This is only of value during the acute phase of the disease.

Somerville (1959) divided these cases into two types: *the first* is a true paralytic dislocation in which the cause of the dislocation lies within the hip, in the paralysis of muscles, in the stretching of ligaments and in the excessive coxa valgus deformity which is present due to a normal iliopsoas muscle acting as an external rotator of the hip. Splintage is of little use. He recommended treating the coxa valgus deformity by an osteotomy at the base of the neck as well as correcting any rotational element of anteversion.

which may be present. This should not be carried out until the deformity of the hip is fully corrected and abduction is obtained by gradual reduction on a frame. Tenotomy of the adductors may be necessary. *The second type* is a postural, paralytic dislocation in which the dislocation results from obliquity of the pelvis, from a structural scoliosis, which is usually progressive. It is better to treat the spinal deformity (see Chapter 8).

The other infrapelvic cause of pelvic obliquity is found when one of the hips has a severe abduction or adduction contracture.

Shelving operation

If there is any difficulty in reducing the hip, the contracture is relieved by fasciotomy. Thereafter the hip is reduced. Through a Smith-Petersen approach, a shelf is turned down from the side of the ilium. The shelf should be accurately placed on the upper and posterior part of the acetabulum and be of a more massive type than in the operation for congenital dislocation. The actual method is described under the treatment of a congenital dislocation of the hip (Chapter 4).

Bosworth *et al.* (1960) reviewed the shelf operation in 82 hips, 12 of which were for poliomyelitis. They believed that this operation is contraindicated in a child who does not have sufficient motor power to control the hip.

Arthrodesis of the hip

This procedure is particularly indicated where dislocation occurs in spite of other forms of management and in those hips which become painful due to degenerative arthritis. It is emphasized that hip fusion should not be carried out if there is any paralysis of the abdominal muscles. Indeed, a test period within a short hip spica on the involved side may be beneficial in determining how much disability will result from fixing the hip. This is especially important in the presence of paralysis elsewhere in the extremity or in the trunk.

FIXED PELVIC OBLIQUITY

This concept was first introduced by Mayer (1931) and later outlined in greater detail by Irwin (1947). A true, fixed pelvic obliquity is when the pelvis is held in a fixed oblique position by contractures, which may be above or below the pelvis or both. Opposite contractures in the hips – one in abduction and the other in adduction – occur, usually, with a scoliosis. This results in a marked disturbance in weight-bearing and in locomotion. The angle of pelvic obliquity can be measured between a line joining the posterior iliac spines and a line through the midline of the body. Weissman *et al.* (1961) described using a weighted goniometer to obtain this angle. Patients may have a fixed flexion deformity of the hip as well as the abduction and adduction contractures, and this adds much to the overall disability.

Irwin (1947) described three major causes for pelvic obliquity: *infrapelvic*, due to fixed contractures of soft tissues involving one or both femoral pelvic articulations; *suprapelvic*, due to fixed contractures at the spinal pelvic junction; or *intrapelvic*, when there is hypoplasia of one or both hemipelves Poliomyelitis scoliosis is often associated with pelvic obliquity and perhaps a short lower extremity.

Weissman *et al.* also described an intertrochanteric osteotomy with realignment in both a coronal plane for the pelvic obliquity and in the sagittal plane for the flexion deformity. The valgus and the anteversion of the femoral neck can be corrected at the same time. Hyperextension of the distal femoral fragment is often required to correct the flexion contracture and therefore a small pelvic support on top of the perineal post may be required. As well as the intertrochanteric osteotomy, these workers found it important to divide the iliotibial band. Review of their results was based upon three features:

1. the walking ability and the need for support;
2. the type of apparatus being used, and
3. the amount of activity possible.

Thirteen cases were reported with all having improved locomotor ability and increased functional activity.

Lau *et al.*, (1986), from a large series of 64 patients, have described their choice of treatment of this complex deformity. Their good results were obtained by correcting the muscle imbalance with an anterolateral transfer of the iliopsoas muscle and tendon (Mustard, 1959) to augment the abductor power by one MRC grade. This improved the gait. The pelvic obliquity if *suprapelvic* can be improved by correcting the scoliosis or when *pelvic* or *infrapelvic* by a femoral osteotomy which corrects the flexion deformity as well as the increased anteversion to produce the necessary femoral neck shaft angle. Because the hip always dislocates posteriorly with a shallow acetabulum, an increased inclination and sometimes a defect posteriorly, which means that a Salter osteotomy is not sufficient, they have carried out various pelvic osteotomies – Chiari, or a Steel, or a posteroacetabuloplasty shelf, etc. – but their results were variable. An arthrodesis may be necessary as a salvage procedure for painful instability but these authors point out the resultant difficulty in dealing with problems of patients with a sedentary job. Also the indications are very rarely met, i.e. good contralateral gluteus and ipsilateral hip flexors, a stable knee without distal foot and ankle deformities, etc.

HIP FLEXION CONTRACTURE

This results from contracture of the tensor fasciae latae, the iliopsoas, the sartorius and the rectus femoris. It rarely occurs alone, being frequently associated with adduction of the hip, flexion deformity of the knee and talipes equinus of the foot. It may be obviated to a certain extent by placing the patient in the prone position for some hours daily during the earlier stages of the disease. Once the deformity has developed, it may be treated in one of two ways – either by stretching the paralysed tissues or by division of these structures by open operation. Each method has its advantages and its advocates. Stretching is said to be unreliable because of the nerve irritation produced, and because of the local pain. Furthermore, it damages other tissues and may interfere with the circulation. On the other hand, division of a shortened muscle or erasion of its normal origin leaves it very much weakened. We use the gradual stretching method in mild contractures; in severe cases and in cases which resist stretching we have performed the Soutter type of operation.

Open division and fasciotomy – Soutter's operation

By this method, the flexors of the hip are stripped subperiosteally from their original position, and allowed to slip down the side of the pelvis. This permits of full extension of the hip.

Technique

A vertical incision is made from 5 cm above the anterior superior spine downwards along the anterior edge of the tensor fasciae latae for about 10 cm. The fascia is exposed and divided in a line from the greater trochanter to a point near to the anterior superior spine. The muscles are then stripped from the spine subperiosteally by an elevator. The thighs are then extended. In most cases the deformity is in this way completely corrected. In more severe cases it may be necessary in addition to divide the iliopsoas muscle. This can be reached in the depth of the wound by following the neck of the femur down to the lesser trochanter after retracting the sartorius medially and the tensor fasciae latae laterally. In still more severe cases, it may be necessary to divide the anterior portion of the capsule of the hip joint.

After-care

The patient is placed in a plaster spica with the hips hyperextended for 2 or 3 weeks until the wound is healed and the muscles have become united to their new attachments.

In the early recovery stage, deforming tendencies should be noted and corrected by regular stretching, supplemented when necessary by padded plaster splints. Early contraction of the iliotibial band and plantar fascia of the foot responds to treatment at this stage.

When treatment in the convalescent stage has been inadequate, patients may present with established soft tissue contractures which must be overcome before joint mobility can be regained and the remaining muscles re-educated. In such cases where conservative methods fail, the deformity must be corrected by operation.

Hip transfer operations

Paralysis of the gluteus maximus and medius muscles give rise to serious disabilities. In paralysis of the gluteus maximus the lumbar lordosis is increased and the body is thrown back with a sudden lurch when weight is borne on the affected side. When the gluteus medius muscle is paralysed, the pelvis cannot be stabilized on weight-bearing and the patient lurches over to that side with consequent upset of balance. Severe gluteal paralysis cannot be satisfactorily corrected by muscle transference but transplantation of the erector spinae (Ober, 1944) may help in severe lordosis due to gluteus maximus paralysis. Gluteus medius limp may occasionally be improved by posterior transference of the tensor fascia lata when some residual power remains in the glutei.

Muscle transference for gluteal paralysis should not, however, be undertaken without considerable deliberation as results are uncertain.

Paralysis of gluteus maximus

Ober's operation

The fascia is incised longitudinally near the spinous processes and cleared from the muscles (Figure 7.11). The lateral half of the sacrospinalis, with its aponeurosis, is separated from the medial half and from the muscles lateral to it, the incisions being carried down to the lower end of the skin incision. An incision is next made on the lateral aspect of the thigh from the tip of the greater trochanter to 2.5 cm above the level of the patella, exposing the fascia lata and its tensor. The tensor is freed, and parallel incisions are made in the fascia to the level of the skin incision in order to form a long flap of fascia 2.5 cm

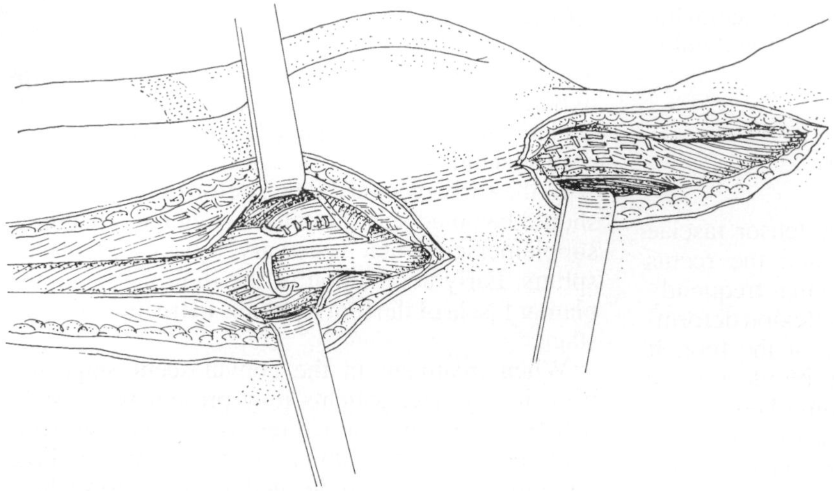

Figure 7.11 Ober's operation. The active erector spinae muscle is used to take the place of the paralysed gluteus maximus by transplantation of a strip of fascia lata.

wide. A hole is drilled through the femur at the level of the gluteus maximus tendon just below the neck, and the long flap of fascia is drawn through the bone from before backwards. At that point, the edges of the fascia are sutured to the gluteus maximus tendon. The free end of the fascial flap is then drawn up under the gluteal fascia to the lower end of the first incision, care being taken to keep the gliding surface of the fascia next to the iliac bone, so that extension of the hip is obtained by the sacrospinalis muscle acting on the femur.

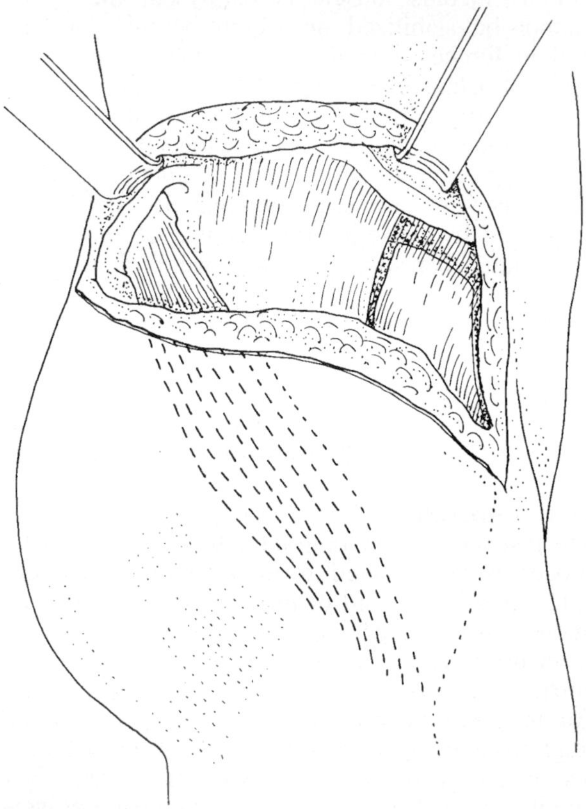

Figure 7.12 Dickson's operation, showing the method of transplantation.

Dickson's operation

The origin of the tensor fascia latae is transplanted with a piece of its bony attachment to a groove on the crest of the ilium near the posterior superior spine, the muscle thus being changed from an abductor and flexor to an abductor and extensor. Postoperatively the limb is maintained in abduction in a plaster cast which is bivalved at 3 weeks to commence muscle training (Figure 7.12).

Paralysis of the gluteus medius muscle

The gluteus medius is frequently affected in poliomyelitis. Its function is to abduct the limb, and, when the weight is borne on one side, to raise the opposite side of the pelvis. When the muscle is paralysed, the resulting gait is characteristic. When, in walking, the weight is borne by the affected side, the patient lurches over to that side, with consequent upset of balance. The limp is often indistinguishable from that produced by a short leg, and it cannot be compensated for by any apparatus or by any building up of the sole of the boot. It can, however, be eliminated to a great extent if the patient carries a weight of about 6–7 kg in the hand of the affected side. This changes the centre of gravity and compensates for the weakness of the muscle.

Legg's operation

The insertion of the tensor fasciae latae is transferred to the posterior surface of the femur (Figure 7.13).

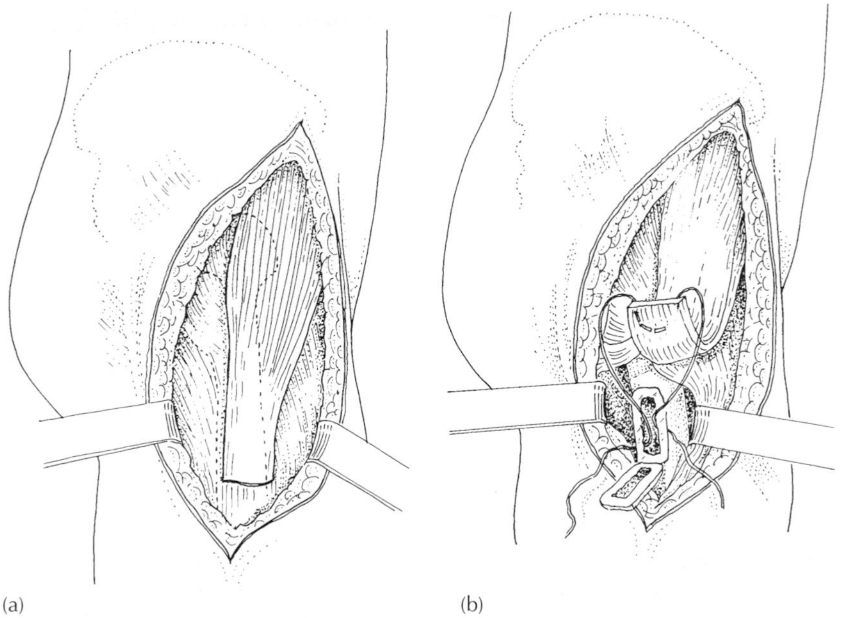

Figure 7.13 Legg's operation for gluteal paralysis. (a) The line of division of tendon of fasciae latae. (b) The fixation of the tendon into the femur.

The operation should not be performed when there is, in addition, marked involvement of the gluteus maximus.

Mustard (1952) described an operation in which a transferred iliopsoas tendon will act as the hip abductor in the presence of a normal gluteus maximus and of a normal sartorius muscle. The rectus femoris muscle will also aid in flexion of the hip joint. In this operation, the iliopsoas tendon, with the lesser trochanter attached, is freed and retracted proximally. A large notch is removed from the iliac surface between the two anterior iliac spines and the iliopsoas pulled out through this area and anchored to the greater trochanter. A plaster-of-Paris hip spica is maintained for 6 weeks before commencing active exercises and full weight-bearing about the eighth week.

Mustard (1959) reviewed 50 cases and described cases in which the transferred iliopsoas was actingas a hip stabilizer, but with no real power of abduction being obtained. The adherence of the iliacus to the bony trough was important. The increased stability of the pelvis will ensure that weight can be taken on the affected leg. The lurching gait was also improved.

Contracture of the iliotibial band

Attention was drawn to the deforming influences of the iliotibial band by Yount (1926) and Irwin (1947). Contractures of this structure are responsible for flexion–abduction deformity of the hip and also for obliquity of the pelvis. Bilateral contractures will produce increased lumbar lordosis.

Kaplan (1958) pointed out that the iliotibial tract is an independent structure acting essentially as a ligament, but not as a tendon, during the maintenance of the erect position. Contractures of the tensor fasciae latae do not transmit any force below the middle of the thigh. The femur is stabilized synergistically by the tensor fasciae latae, and the gluteus maximus in standing and walking. It is a stabilizer of the knee, particularly the part between the lateral femoral condyle and the tibial tubercle of Gerdy. Tensor fasciae latae produce flexion and medial rotation of the thigh.

Contracture and paralysis of tensor fasciae latae are intrinsically bound up with similar diseases of the gluteus medius and minimus, and it only acts as a stabilizer of the pelvis in flexion and not in abduction.

Kaplan did not believe that tensor fasciae latae contribute to flexion–abduction contractures of the hips and flexion contractures of the knee. He believed that these are due to contractures of gluteus minimus and the anterior half of gluteus medius and the short head of the biceps.

Gardner (1958), in discussing Kaplan's paper, pointed out that in order to assess the function of any specific muscle and to determine whether a muscle is inactive, all joints except the one being studied must be stabilized, and the influence of gravity minimized. He doubted whether tensor fasciae latae and gluteus maximus act synergistically during standing and walking.

Established contractures of the iliotibial band will not respond to conservative measures. Early contractures may be satisfactorily corrected by division of the iliotibial band distally as suggested by Yount. In flexion–abduction contracture of the hip of long standing, division of the iliotibial band may be supplemented by Campbell's transference of the crest of the ilium.

Division of the iliotibial band and lateral intermuscular septum (Yount)

Prior to operation a close-fitting single-hip spica is applied to the sound leg under traction. This leaves the affected leg in abduction until the tight iliotibial band has been divided – traction is then applied to the affected leg which is stretched daily to maintain the operative correction. The fascia lata is exposed through a longitudinal incision. The iliotibial band is divided between the biceps tendon and the anterior surface of the thigh at a level 2.5 cm proximal to the patella. A 5 cm section is excised from the iliotibial band and from the lateral intermuscular septum at this level.

Deformities of the knee

FLEXION DEFORMITY

This occurs where there is paresis of the anterior thigh muscles with overaction of the posterior group. The deformity can be prevented by the use of a Thomas's knee splint; and frequently this splint may be used also to correct the condition when applied along with plaster traction on the side of the leg.

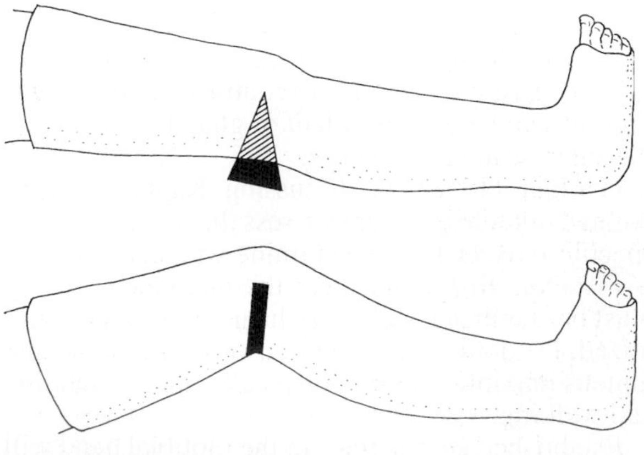

Figure 7.14 The method of correcting flexion deformity of the knee by wedge plasters.

Methods of reduction of the established deformity

Wedge plasters

A circular plaster is applied to the leg from the toes up to the groin in the position of the deformity and allowed to harden. A transverse slit is then made through the posterior three-quarters or the plaster at the level of the knee joint (Figure 7.14). An instrument devised on the lines of a ribspreader is used to force open the divided plaster.

Reversed dynamic traction

This has been most successful in the fixed flexion deformity resulting from haemophilia, trauma and in rheumatoid arthritis. With the simple apparatus described in the section on haemophilia (p. 817), it is possible to apply synchronously a longitudinal force with skin strapping, a forward extension force on the leg component and a downward force on the thigh. Muscle activities can be pursued at the same time with surprisingly little discomfort. Deformities of over 40° can be reduced down to 10° or less within a 10-day period, and then a quadriceps-enhancing splint is applied (see haemophilia section).

Tendon lengthening

This operation may be carried out by a single longitudinal and medial incision in the popliteal space, or by two separate lateral incisions. The semimembranosus, semitendinosus, gracilis and sartorius muscles are lengthened on the medial aspect, and the biceps and tensor fasciae latae on the lateral. Directly in the line of the incision in the fascia of the popliteal space are the popliteal artery and the common peroneal nerve; at a deeper level is the popliteal vein. These structures must be carefully avoided. Each of the tendons is lengthened in the usual Z-shaped fashion, and after closing the wound the leg is put up in a straight back splint.

Wilson (1953) showed that many of the cases which resist correction by other means can be treated satisfactorily by a capsuloplasty of the posterior part of the capsule of the knee joint. This tends to be very short in flexion contracture.

KNOCK KNEE

This deformity is often seen as a result of paralysis of the quadriceps and may be due to the stronger pull of the hamstring muscles, and particularly that of the tensor fasciae latae. Prophylactic measures should be adopted in cases in which the deformity is likely to develop. In these cases the application of a plaster cast may help.

Mild cases may be overcome by manipulation and traction, recurrence being prevented by the application of a caliper splint fitted with a knock-knee strap to secure leverage. If knock knee is greater than 8°, an osteotomy is indicated, and should yield very satisfactory results.

GENU RECURVATUM

In the presence of adequate muscle power, such as 3–5 grading of the hip flexors, the gluteus maximus and the hamstrings, the transfer of biceps femoris into a weakened quadriceps will give good results, seen especially in the ability to go up and come down stairs. However, good hip extensors and flexors must be present. The transfer of semitendinosus and of biceps femoris into the lateral and medial sides respectively of the quadriceps mechanism was described by Schwartzmann and Crego (1948). After such a procedure, the limb is immobilized in a plaster cast for 3 weeks and then physiotherapy is commenced before allowing full weight-bearing in 8 weeks.

The other form of genu recurvatum is where the knee hyperextends because of the relaxation of the posterior capsular structures and weakness in the calf and hamstring muscles (Figure 7.15) This is often accompanied by a calcaneovalgus deformity of the foot. When the child is small, bracing is sufficient and usually acceptable but will be discarded when the bracing becomes painful and the deformity then becomes very disabling. Mehta and Mukerjee (1991) have reported their excellent results from 21 flexion osteotomies of the femur in 18 patients. They emphasize that accompanying the deformity of genu recurvatum there is a secondary flattening of the femoral condyles which then remodelled in a few. In this deformity the hamstring muscles subluxate anterior to the axis of the knee – becoming extensors and with weight bearing. This deformity steadily increases. However, the flexion osteotomy reverses these abnormal lines of forces. They found that the

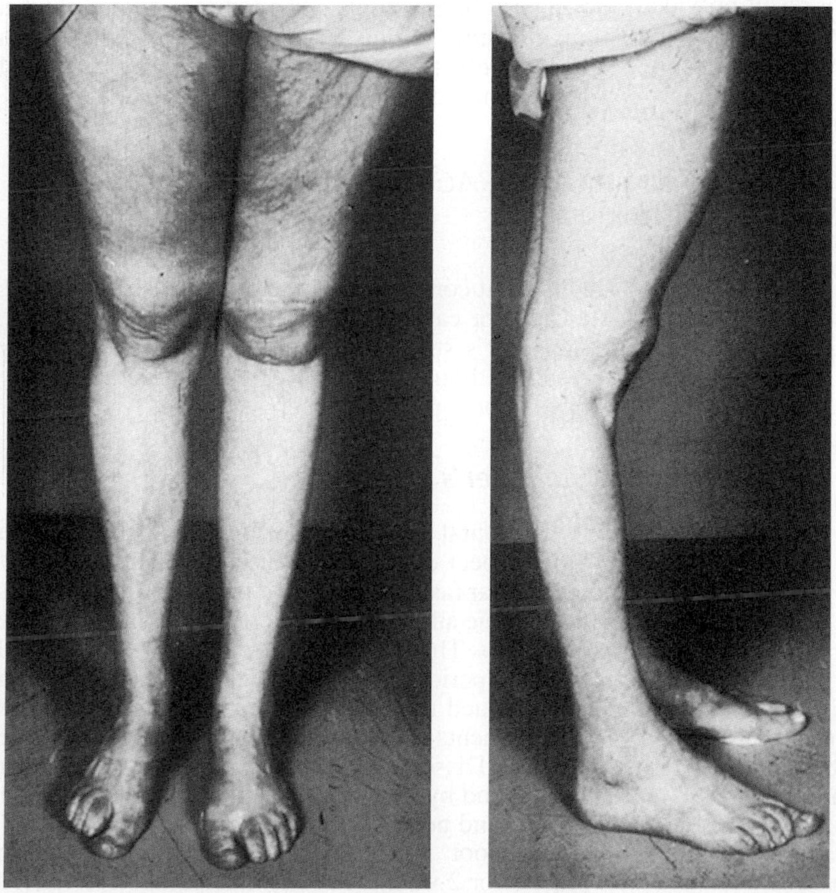

Figure 7.15 Bilateral genu recurvatum with hyperextension of both knee joints. Because of development of osteoarthritis of the left patellofemoral joint, a left patellectomy was carried out with transfer anteriorly of the iliotibial tract and semitendinosus into the quadriceps tendon.

majority were able to discard the use of bracing after 6 months, especially in the younger children under the age of 7–14 years. Over the age of 16 none was stable without the use of an orthosis. However, its use was more comfortable and efficient.

KNEE JOINT

The quadriceps is commonly affected in lower limb paralysis but these patients walk well provided there is adequate power in the hamstring and gastrocnemius muscles to steady the knee in extension. They have, however, difficulty in running or walking over rough ground.

No clear-cut indications can be given for tendon transplantation to improve quadriceps power. Each patient must be judged individually and transplantation advised if instability of the knee interferes with ordinary walking or when transplantation to the quadriceps might enable the patient to dispense with a caliper.

The quadriceps may be strengthened by transplanting one or more of the following muscles – biceps femoris, semitendinosus, sartorius and tensor fasciae latae. Transplantation of a powerful biceps femoris tendon gives a satisfactory result provided the remaining hip and calf muscles are sufficiently strong to support the back of the knee.

Transference of biceps femoris to patella

An incision is made over the lateral aspect of the thigh from the upper third to 5 cm below the head of the fibula. The lateral popliteal nerve is defined and retracted and the biceps tendon is freed from the head of the fibula. The biceps tendon and muscle belly are dissected upwards and the origin of the short head is freed from the femur up to the level of entrance of its nerve and blood supply.

Through a second medial parapatellar incision a subcutaneous tunnel is made to the upper part of the lateral thigh incision and the biceps tendon is drawn down to the patella and attached subperiosteally by sutures inserted through drill holes in the patella.

ARTHRODESIS

Knee arthrodesis may be worthwhile if conservative methods fail to correct knee deformity. The operation is best carried out early, before secondary deformities have become established.

Leg and ankle

CONTRACTURE OF THE HEEL CORD

Shortening of the tendo calcaneus may occur from overaction of the calf muscles unopposed by paralysed extensors. In neglected cases the heel cord may require stretching by manipulation followed by wedging plasters. In severe cases the tendo calcaneus may have to be lengthened by open operation and the posterior capsule of the ankle joint divided if contracted. Before deciding on operative lengthening of the tendo calcaneus, it should be remembered that patients with quadriceps insufficiency may depend on a tight heel cord in the absence of active gastrocnemius contraction to enable the hamstring muscles to lock the knee on a stable foot.

Lateral rotation deformities of the leg are commonly seen due to the muscular imbalance around the knee and ankle joints when either flexion or equinus contractures develop. Asirvatham *et al.* (1990) reviewed 51 patients who had received an O'Donoghue rotational osteotomy of the tibia, fully correcting a lateral rotational deformity of 57° in all patients. Interestingly, 38 of those patients had a simultaneous Grice–Green subtalar arthrodesis in one or both feet – utilizing a piece of the cortical bone remould for the osteotomy.

CONTRACTURE OF THE PLANTAR FASCIA

Persistent contracture of the plantar fascia produces a cavus or cavo-adducted foot. In this type of foot, Steindler's stripping operation gives a satisfactory result, although in some cases the operation may have to be repeated in later years.

Steindler's procedure

A horizontal incision 4 cm long is made over the inner aspect of the calcaneus. The undersurface of the plantar fascia is separated from the subcutaneous fatty tissue and is divided close to its origin from the calcaneus. The short muscles of the foot are stripped from the periosteum of the calcaneus, and dissection is continued to the calcaneocuboid joint to include the ligaments which extend from the calcaneus to the cuboid. Dissection should be carried out under vision, and by keeping close to the bone the plantar vessels and nerves will escape injury.

The foot is manipulated and immobilized in plaster for 2 weeks. Further manipulation is carried out and a second plaster applied for 4 weeks. Aftercare consists of wearing a plaster night splint and ensuring that regular stretching of the foot is carried out at home.

GENERAL PRINCIPLES OF TENDON TRANSFER FOR REGIONAL DEFORMITIES

Tendon transfer to improve muscle balance is most successful in the wrist and hand. In the foot it is more commonly used in conjunction with stabilization operations on the bones.

Certain points in the technique of tendon transfer are of importance:

1. The deformity must be corrected before transplantation is performed. There must be a free-range of passive movement in the joints to be activated by the transplanted muscle.
2. The muscle to be transferred must be sufficiently strong to substitute for the paralysed muscle.
3. The transferred tendon must pass in a direct line through subcutaneous fat or through a tendon sheath to avoid friction.
4. The tendon should be inserted into bone through drill holes or subperiosteally if possible. In the wrist, however, the flexor tendons are transferred directly into the extensors.
5. The tendon should be attached under moderate tension.
6. Muscles which have similar or related actions give better results.
7. The tendon should be protected by splinting in the relaxed position for 3 weeks. Careful re-education of the transplanted muscle is essential.

Deformities of the foot

Transfer of tendons for paralytic foot deformities is usually used in conjunction with stabilizing operations on the bones. Opposing muscle groups must be balanced so that recurrence of deformity can be avoided, or corrected with improvement in function (Figure 7.16).

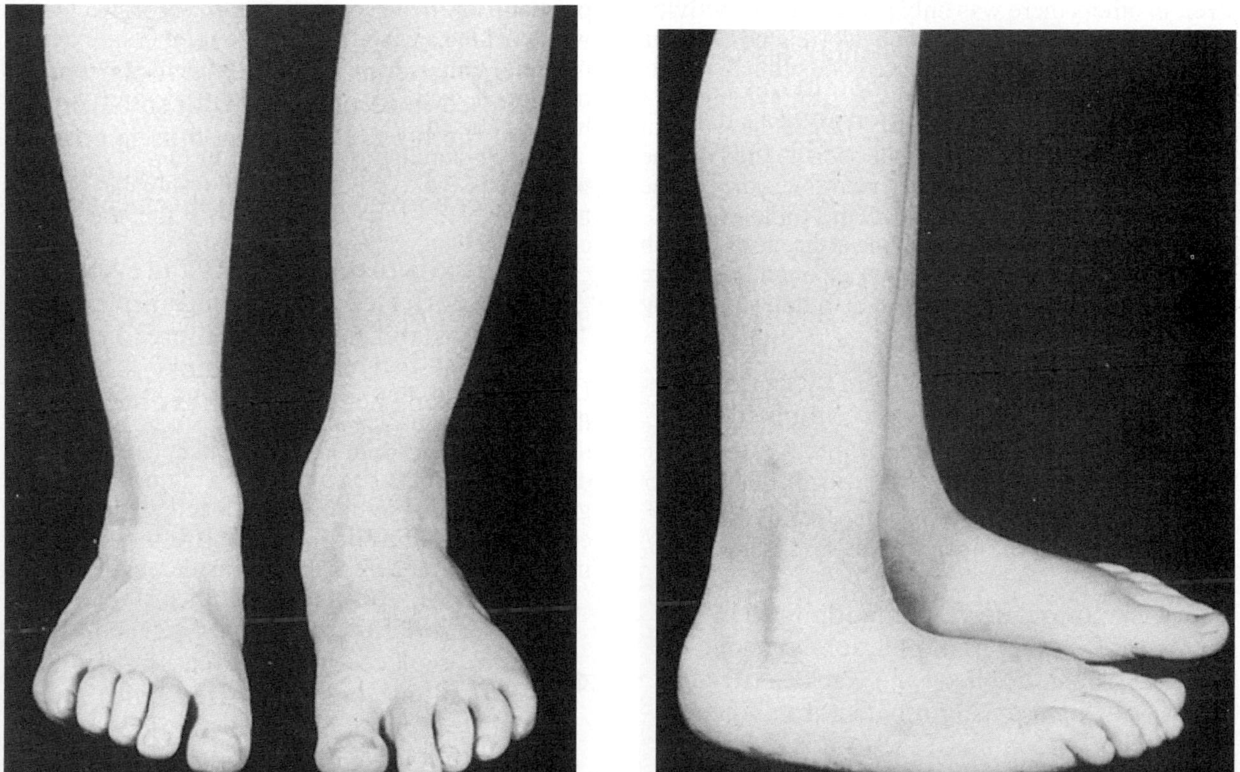

(a) (b)

Figure 7.16 (a) The loss of medial arch secondary to anterior paralysis in poliomyelitis. (b) The lateral view clearly shows the arch depression.

Imbalance between invertors and evertors should always be corrected by tendon transposition following any stabilization procedure. Tendon transfer alone is not satisfactory.

The opposing action of tibialis anterior and peroneus longus should be kept in mind. Tibialis anterior elevates the base of the first metatarsal and supinates the forefoot, while peroneus longus depresses the base of the first metatarsal and pronates the foot (Figure 7.17).

In the foot, the most significant feature is the removal of a deforming force and using the active muscle to replace, in some cases, the paralysed muscle. It should be emphasized that the forces of the body weight aggravate minimal deformities. Full passive correction must always be possible, but it is also important that the tendon transfer itself comes into action at the same phase of walking as the replaced muscle; for example, peroneus longus and the various calf muscles.

Blodgett and Houtz (1960) carried out electromyographic studies in cases in which anterior transfer of peroneus longus was carried out for weakness of the dorsiflexors. These workers showed that the transfer of activity of this muscle from the usual stance phase to the swing phase may occur. However, in others there was only partial shift of activity. The clinical results could not be correlated with the electromyographic results since good clinical results were obtained when there was no evidence of electromyographic transition. They believed that some of the results may have been related to the tendon acting as a tenodesing force or to the elimination of a dynamic deforming force.

Standard procedures involving arthrodesis of both until the age of 10 or 12 years in order to secure sound fusion and avoid growth disturbance. During this period the foot should be protected by a caliper. Marked foot imbalance, however, cannot be completely controlled by a caliper and some structural deformity of the foot is inevitable. While this can be corrected at the definitive procedure it will usually entail some loss of shape and height of the foot following bone resection.

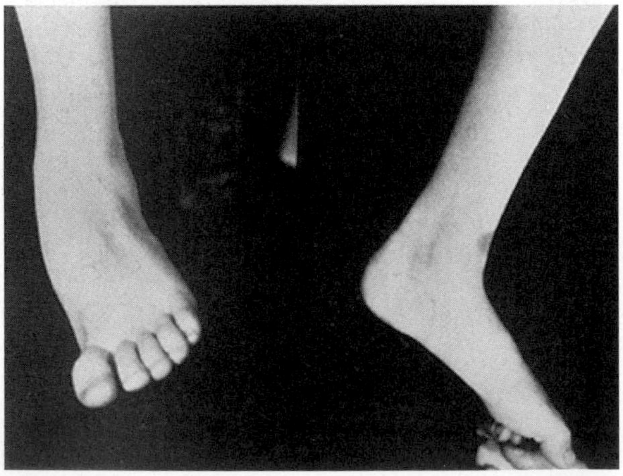

Figure 7.17 The forces developing a valgus foot deformity in poliomyelitis are clearly shown as this child attempts dorsiflexion.

The strut-graft operation described by Grice (1952) has therefore proved of great value in stabilizing the subtalar joint in young children with paralytic flat foot. This procedure, combined with tendon transplantation, will maintain the arch of the foot during the growing years.

TALIPES VALGUS

This results from paralysis of the tibialis muscles. The calcaneum everts and no longer supports the head of the talus, which inclines medially and downwards with depression of the longitudinal arch. In children over the age of 4 the deformity can be corrected by strut-graft stabilization of the talocalcaneal joint in the corrected position. If the peronei are active, the peroneus brevis should be transplanted into the medial cuneiform. In the presence of overactivity of the peroneus longus with cocking of the big toe, the tendon of extensor hallucis longus can be transplanted to the first metatarsal and the interphalangeal joint of the hallux is fused.

In long-standing deformities in the older patient where passive correction of the subtalar joint is not possible, triple arthrodesis is the method of choice.

TALIPES VARUS

Less common, this deformity is due to paralysis of the peroneal muscles, the foot becoming inverted by the action of the tibialis anterior and posterior. It is a difficult deformity to control by a caliper during the growing years. While the foot is still mobile, correction may be obtained by a strut-graft inserted into the sinus tarsi from the inner side, supplemented

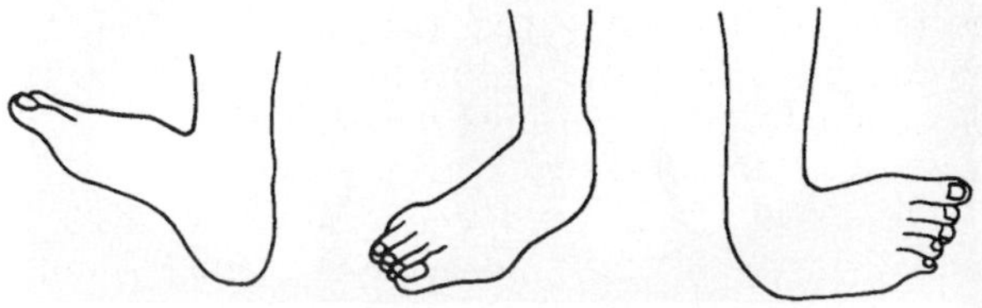

(a) (b) (c)

Figure 7.18 Types of foot deformity: (a) talipes calcaneus; (b) talipes valgus; (c) talipes varus.

by transplantation of the tibialis anterior to the cuboid.

Even lateral transplant of the tibialis anterior alone will allow the foot to be more easily controlled by an inside iron and outside T strap.

TALIPES CALCANEUS

This is an inevitable deformity in isolated paralysis of the gastrocnemius. Active dorsiflexors plus active peronei and tibialis posterior muscles produce a progressive calcaneocavus deformity despite caliper protection.

In the young child the deformity may be minimized by transplantation of the tibialis posterior and peroneal tendons into the heel cord, followed by protection with a caliper.

In the older child, transplantation of tendons into the heel cord should be accompanied by triple arthrodesis.

TALIPES EQUINUS

Paralytic drop-foot is satisfactorily controlled by a caliper with a toe-raising spring or a dorsiflexion spring at the ankle joint. Lambrinudi foot fusion with transplantation of overacting peronei to the dorsum of the foot is reserved for the older patient.

CLAW-TOE DEFORMITY OF THE HALLUX

Claw-toe is frequently found in paralytic feet. The hypertension deformity of the first metatar-sophalangeal joint, which occurs on attempted dorsiflexion of the foot, is caused by unco-ordinated contraction of the extensor hallucis when the tibialis anterior is paralysed. The clawing of the hallux increases the depression of the first metatarsal head produced by unopposed action of the peroneus longus.

Claw-toe deformity occurring in a foot with adequate dorsiflexion power is satisfactorily treated by interphalangeal fusion of the hallux.

Transference of the extensor hallucis tendon to the neck of the first metatarsal accompanied by interphalangeal fusion of the hallux is a satisfactory procedure when the power of dorsiflexion of the foot is only slightly impaired.

Transplantation of the extensor hallucis by itself is not satisfactory when dorsiflexion of the foot is weak or where there is a fixed cavus deformity.

STABILIZING OPERATIONS ON THE FOOT

Various stabilizing operations are carried out with success on the foot. It has already been mentioned that tendon transplantation alone is seldom satisfactory, but when combined with one or other of the stabilizing procedures greatly improved function can be anticipated.

Triple arthrodesis (i.e. operations involving the talocalcanean, talonavicular and calcaneocuboid joints) ensures lateral stability, and with modifications will correct varus, valgus and calcaneocavus deformities. The Lambrinudi triple arthrodesis is designed to limit plantar flexion.

Foot fusion operations should be postponed until the age of 10–12. Fusion at an earlier age may be necessary if deformities are severe, but where possible should be delayed to avoid disturbance of growth and ensure more certain fusion and lasting correction.

Extra-articular arthrodesis was suggested by Grice (1952) to stabilize the talocalcaneal joint in paralytic flat foot in children. It has proved of great value and is successfully carried out in young children where it preserves the architectural shape of the foot through-out the growing years.

Extra-articular arthrodesis of the subtalar joint

Grice (1952) pointed out that in paralytic flat foot the calcaneus is everted and displaced laterally and posteriorly in relation to the talus. As a consequence there is loss of normal support beneath the head of the talus, which drops into equinus and deviates medially in relation to the abducted forefoot. If the deformity persists, secondary adaptive changes take place in the joint capsules, tendo Achillis and in the osseous structure.

It is desirable to correct this deformity in the young child before it has become fixed and the operative technique should not therefore interfere with the subsequent growth of the foot.

Surgical correction entails the reduction and maintenance of the calcaneus in normal relationship to the talus by means of strut bone grafts placed in the sinus tarsi. Muscle balance is restored by tendon transplantation to avoid recurrence.

Operative technique

An osteotome of suitable width is inserted into the sinus tarsi to test stability and to determine the size of the grafts and the most suitable site for their insertion. The sinus tarsi is prepared for the grafts by removal of a thin layer of cortical bone but a rim of intact cortex should be left at the lateral surfaces to hold the notched portions of the grafts when they are countersunk.

Grafts approximately 2–2.5 cm long and 1.5 cm wide are cut from one piece of cortical bone obtained from the iliac crest or the patient's tibia (Figure 7.19).

The grafts are inserted while the foot is overcorrected so that in the corrected position they are firmly held under compression and the foot is stable. An inverted position of the heel must be avoided. Correct compression of the grafts prevents displacement and accelerates healing.

After operation the foot is immobilized in a long-leg plaster. In 3 months the grafts are soundly healed but tendon transplantation may be carried out at 6 weeks if the indications are clear. Either peroneus longus or peroneus brevis can be transplanted to the inner side of the foot. In doubtful cases, tendon transplantation can be postponed until the foot is fully mobilized and a more accurate assessment of function is possible. Residual tightness of the heel cord sometimes gives an awkward gait in the early mobilization phase; if significant, this should be corrected by equinus wedging plasters.

The indications for this procedure have been widened to include flexible flat foot deformity, myelodysplastic feet and hemiplegic deformity resulting from cerebral palsy. However, Ross and Lyne (1980) have recently reviewed 113 feet which had received this operation and found the most satisfactory results when performed for polio and for the mild cerebral palsy foot. The other conditions had not achieved very satisfactory results, because of overcorrection into varus with ankle valgus and instability. They and others have emphasized that the graft must be placed and held correctly, with the talocalcaneal position being in a neutral plane and never overcorrected. Of course, the foot must be in balance as regards the soft tissues (e.g. any equinus corrected).

Triple arthrodesis

Fusion of the subtalar and midtarsal joints is indicated when deformity or instability of the foot is accompanied by lateral stability of the talus in the ankle mortice. Varus or valgus deformities are corrected by excising appropriate wedges of bone from the midtarsal and subtalar joints. A varus heel must be avoided; a slightly valgus heel gives a satisfactory result. At the time of operation the foot should be aligned in relation to the ankle joint. Deformities such as knock knee and tibial torsion should be corrected at the site of deformity.

If the foot is flail, it is desirable to move the fulcrum of the ankle nearer the centre of the foot. This can be accomplished by the technique of Dunn where the foot is moved backwards at the subtalar joint after removal of the navicular (Figure 7.20).

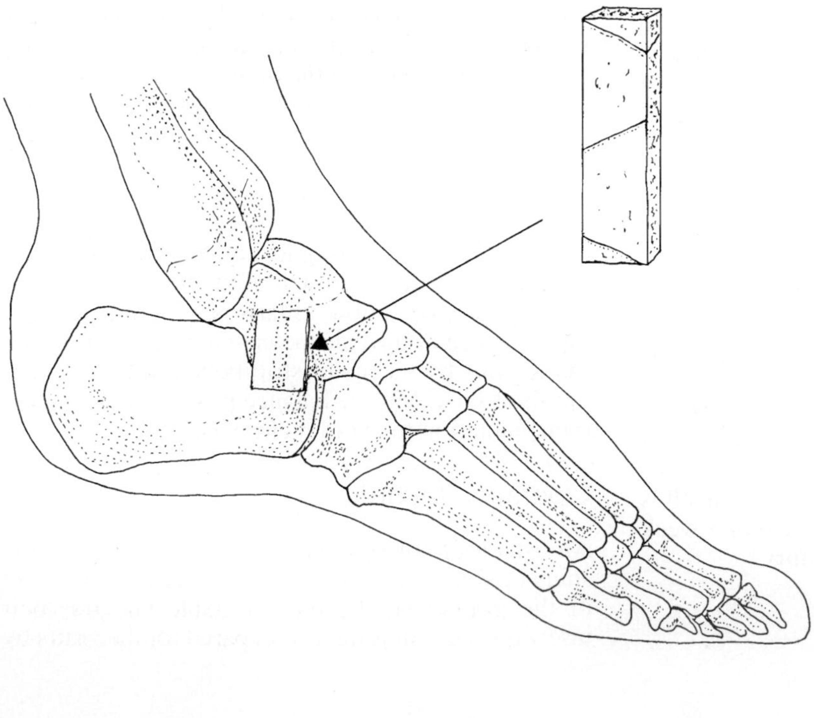

Figure 7.19 The Grice–Green extra-articular operation.

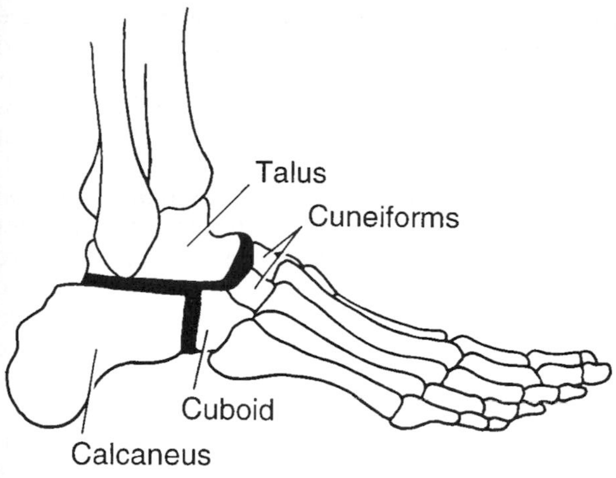

Figure 7.20 Naughton Dunn's operation for stabilization of the flail foot.

In paralytic drop-foot, the Lambrinudi fusion corrects the equinus at the subtalar joint by part excision of the talus and stabilization of the foot in a functional position. Paralytic drop-foot may also be corrected by the Campbell (1923) posterior bone block and foot fusion.

A two-stage fusion at the midtarsal and subtalar joints with transplantation of the peronei and tibialis posterior tendons into the heel (Elmslie, 1934) is a satisfactory procedure and gives a stable foot with some increase in the power of push-off.

Robins (1959) followed the results of a triple arthrodesis for paralysis, with preservation of the ankle joint for several years. There was a striking absence of osteoarthritis in the ankle joint and a very low incidence of lateral instability. However, triple arthrodesis for a completely flail foot, without active muscle control at the knee, was often disappointing because of the persistent flexion deformity in the knee, which necessitated the wearing of an appliance. The results of pantalar arthrodesis for flail foot was satisfactory because it helped to stabilize the knee in walking by encouraging hyperextension.

Factors affecting pseudarthrosis after triple arthrodesis

Factors affecting pseudarthrosis after a triple arthrodesis were analysed by Wilson *et al.* (1965). The primary factors were found to be poor contact between the joint surfaces on early weight-bearing. There was no relation to age or to anatomical deformity, to the type of disease, to the total time in a plaster cast or to the use of associated tendon transplants with the procedure or to the development of infection. Pseudarthrosis occurred usually in the talonavicular joint and most were in patients who had bilateral procedures.

The Naughton Dunn operation

In those deformities of the foot in which, because of severe static deficiencies, it is desirable to secure forward displacement of the talus on the calcaneus, the operation of Naughton Dunn (1922) is indicated. This operation combines a subtalar arthrodesis with a reconstructive shortening of the forefoot. A degree of symmetry between the two halves of the longitudinal arch is thus established, so that the static condition of the foot is improved.

The calcaneocuboid joint is exposed by retracting or dividing the peroneal tendons. The articular surfaces of the calcaneus and cuboid are removed by means of a sharp osteotome. The head of the talus is now divided behind its articular cartilage, and this, along with the proximal surfaces of the cuneiform bones, is removed together with the whole, or a portion, of the navicular. The strong interosseous ligament between the talus and the calcaneus and the lateral ligament of the ankle are divided, and the foot is dislocated medially at the subtalar and midtarsal joints. This exposes the subtalar joint, the cartilaginous opposing surfaces of which are removed by an osteotome.

The foot is displaced backwards at the subtalar joint so that the head of the talus will rest in a cup-shaped depression prepared for it by the removal of bone from the dorsal surface of the cuneiform bones. In some cases a transplantation of tendons or a tenodesis is now carried out. A more secure fixation may be obtained by a stainless steel staple across the calcaneocuboid joint. With the foot held in a good weight-bearing position, and with the cleared bone surfaces adequately opposed, the whole is fixed in plaster. The plaster should be split and the foot elevated for 48 hours, during which period a close watch is maintained for circulatory insufficiency. The position of fixation of the foot is of great importance. The talus and calcaneus are directly centred under the bones of the leg. The relation of the forepart of the foot to the posterior segment allows restoration of the normal arch and weight-bearing with both the first and fifth metatarsal heads. Weight-bearing should be avoided during the first 3 months and then a walking plaster is used for a further 2 months. During the early months of mobilization the foot should be protected by a below-knee caliper.

Lambrinudi's operation

The special indications of this operation are paralysis of the foot dorsiflexors and peronei, but with some muscular control of the knee and preferably with active calf muscles. The aim of the operation is to use the anterior process of the talus to prevent dropping of the foot. The plane of bone section is carefully planned before the operation.

The tarsus is approached through a lateral incision and the foot is dislocated medially below the talus. The talus is then cut by a saw in the desired plane as shown in the line drawing (Figure 7.21a). The upper surface of the calcaneus and the calcaneo-cuboid joint are cut with a sharp osteotome. The navicular is cut so as to make a posteroinferior notch. The bones are now opposed and the beak in the talus fitted into the notch in the navicular, and held in place while the incision is closed and a leg plaster applied.

In estimating the exact line of section of the bones, the surgeon can make paper tracings from the radiographs before operation. The tracing is divided into three components which are then fitted together to give a plantigrade foot. The overlap of the tracings indicates the precise amount of bone to be excised at operation.

The early results of the Lambrinudi operation are very satisfactory but unfortunately the foot tends to drop further in later years. It is therefore preferable to postpone this procedure until the patient is over 18 years of age as the foot can be adequately controlled by an appliance during the earlier years The foot should be fused in only a few degrees of equinus.

Mackenzie (1959) reviewed 100 cases of Lambrinudi's arthrodesis in cases in which the foot had a

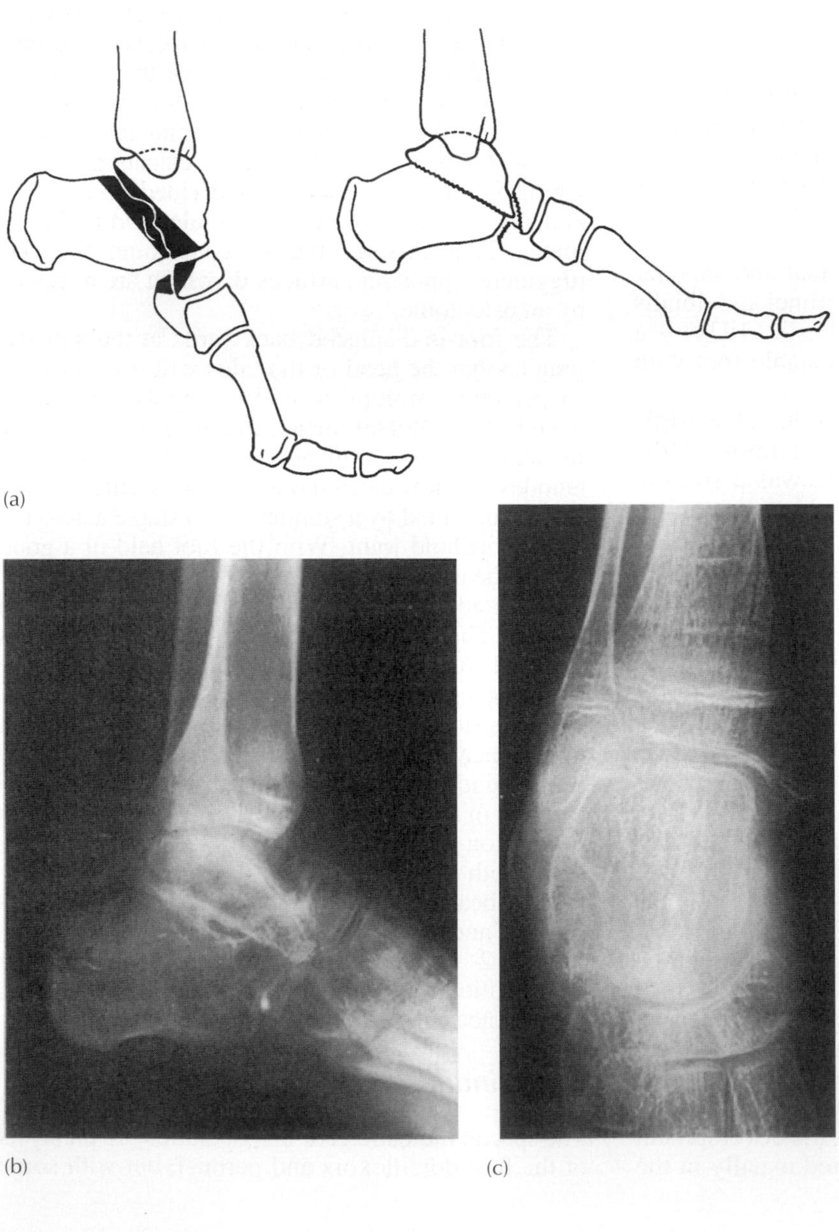

(a)

(b)

(c)

Figure 7.21 (a) Lambrinudi's operation for drop-foot. (b) and (c) Radiographs showing the result, 4 years after a Lambrinudi procedure.

balanced muscle power and those with a fixed equinus deformity. Pseudarthrosis occurred more often in younger patients. It was contraindicated in a flail foot and to a lesser extent in a dynamic drop-foot. Alternative procedures, such as transfer of the tibialis posterior through the interosseus membrane, or, when the knee is unstable, a pantalar arthrodesis as described by Barr and Record (1947), were more useful. Mackenzie pointed out that a common technical error was the removal of too small a wedge which left an excessive equinus and varus deformity to cause painful callosities. There were 37% successful cases, but 19% were failures and were associated with faulty techniques.

Two-stage fusion for calcaneocavus deformity

First stage

Tight structures are released from the heel by a Steindler's stripping. Through a longitudinal incision on the dorsum of the foot, a wedge is excised from the midtarsal joint and the alignment of the forefoot corrected on the hindfoot. The foot is then immobilized in plaster in maximum dorsiflexion for 1 month.

Second stage

The peroneal tendons and the tendon of tibialis posterior are divided on the lateral and medial aspects of the foot and withdrawn through the posterior wound. The long flexors of the toes are also used if they are sufficiently powerful. A wedge of bone is removed from the subtalar joint in order to correct the calcaneus deformity. With the deformity corrected and the foot in equinus the tendons are transplanted into the tendo Achillis, and where possible they are continued through the tendon to be inserted into a large drill hole in the calcaneus. The foot is immobilized in plantar flexion for 3–4 months.

It may assist the surgeon if paper tracings are made from the preoperative radiographs. These are cut into the three components and thus the correct size of the bony wedges to be removed can be ascertained.

Shoulder

Paralysis of the deltoid with adequate power in the scapulothoracic muscles should be treated by arthrodesis of the shoulder joint after the upper humeral epiphysis has closed. In the interval, unrestricted use of the arm is encouraged to maintain tone in the scapular muscles.

Tendon transfer to improve abductor power in childhood should wait until shoulder fusion can be carried out.

Elbow

Surgery should be confined to restoring flexion at the elbow, provided function of the hand is satisfactory. Gravity will extend the elbow once flexion is restored; transposition for paralysis of triceps is unlikely to give sufficient power to enable the patient to push up from a chair or to improve crutch walking materially.

Steindler's operation of proximal transposition of the common flexor origin from the medial epicondyle gives satisfactory results if normal power is present in the flexors of the wrist and fingers. As brachioradialis is normally a supplementary flexor of the elbow, proximal transposition of the extensor origin may also be carried out when the flexor group is below normal strength.

When biceps, brachialis and brachioradialis are completely paralysed, but good power is present in the pectoralis major, Clark (1946) advocated transposition of part of the pectoralis major to the biceps tendon.

FLEXOR TRANSPOSITION AT THE ELBOW

The best results are obtained when the brachioradialis is still functioning. Some loss of full extension of the elbow may occur after successful transplants and this should be explained to the patient before operation. Its other disadvantage is that any relaxation of grip will allow the elbow to extend (Steindler, 1923).

Upper extremity

The common flexor origin is detached close to the bone in one mass. The superficial head of the pronator teres, the flexor carpi radialis, the palmaris longus and the flexor carpi ulnaris are transplanted to the periosteum of the humerus 5 cm above the epicondyle. The muscle mass may be more firmly secured by sutures passing through drill holes in the bone. The arm, acutely flexed, is immobilized in plaster midway between pronation and supination for 3 weeks, after which a back splint is worn in acute flexion for a further 3 weeks to allow muscle training.

TRANSPOSITION OF PECTORALIS MAJOR

The lower third of pectoralis major is separated from the remainder of the muscle and from its origin together with a portion of the sheath of rectus abdominis in continuity with the distal end of the transplant to serve as a tendon. The transplant is stripped proximally off the ribs and the medial anterior thoracic nerve and its accompanying blood vessels are exposed. An L-shaped incision is made on the lateral aspect of the lower third of the arm with the horizontal limb across the front of the elbow joint. A space is opened up beneath the deep fascia for reception of the transplant, with a wide diameter for the proximal part of the tunnel to accommodate a considerable mass of muscle without jeopardizing the blood supply. The elbow is flexed to 30° above the right angle and placed in full supination and the aponeurotic extension of the transplant is sutured to the biceps tendon.

The position of the arm is maintained in a dorsal slab which is removed after 3 weeks but a sling is retained for a further 3 weeks while the re-education of the muscle is started. At first flexion of the elbow is accompanied by contraction of the undisturbed part of the pectoralis major, but after a variable period independence of the transplant is achieved and a good range of supination may also result (Clark, 1946).

Segal *et al.* (1959) reviewed the various forms of treatment for paralysed flexors of the elbow joint in 21 cases after poliomyelitis and in 20 cases after brachial plexus injury. The results of pectoral transplantation were good where there was no significant shoulder paralysis. Pectoral transplants were poor in brachial plexus lesions in which there was simultaneous contracture of triceps, since this muscle then had to be transferred. These workers found that, when a free choice is possible, a Steindler operation is preferable, because the pectoral transplantation usually calls for arthrodesis of the shoulder when there is any appreciable paralysis of the shoulder muscles. They did not believe that the Brooks–Seddon technique of pectoral major transfer should be employed unless the biceps is completely and permanently paralysed.

FOREARM

Loss of pronation of the forearm may be improved by transposing the tendon of flexor carpi ulnaris across the anterior aspect of the forearm to the radial aspect of the distal radius.

Restoration of some degree of supination may be expected if biceps activity is restored as in Clark's transplantation of pectoralis major. Supination may also be improved by transposing the tendon of flexor carpi ulnaris around the ulna and inserting it into the radius just proximal to the wrist.

WRIST AND HAND

The most successful results in tendon transplantation are obtained when the wrist flexors are transferred to the finger extensors, since they normally have a synergic action. If care is taken to ensure that the wrist will be balanced after transplantation, supplementary arthrodesis to ensure wrist stability will only occasionally be necessary.

The operations described in Chapter 12 (p. 859) may be modified to suit the type of paralysis met with in poliomyelitis. It is to be noted that the extensors do not act well when transplanted into the flexors of the forearm.

In complete flexor paralysis, extensor carpi radialis longus and extensor carpi ulnaris may be transplanted to the tendon of flexor pollicis longus and to the deep flexor tendons of the fingers.

In extensor paralysis, the pronator teres is transplanted into the extensor carpi radialis longus and brevis. The flexor carpi radialis is inserted into the abductor pollicis longus and the extensor pollicis brevis. The palmaris longus is transplanted to extensor pollicis longus. The tendon of flexor carpi ulnaris is inserted into the extensor digitorum tendons. Arthrodesis of the wrist will often release good hand function.

Loss of active opposition of the thumb is a common and disabling feature in poliomyelitis. The grasp is weakened and the useful pinch action between thumb and index finger is lost. Restoration of opposition is an important step in the recovery of hand function in poliomyelitis. Satisfactory results from tendon transplantation are possible only when full passive movement of the thumb has been maintained; any tendency to web contracture should be overcome before operation.

Several methods are described to restore opposition. Bunnell (1938) used flexor sublimis but passed the tendon round a pulley at the pisiform. He emphasized two principles:

1. The tendon must pass from its insertion into the thumb subcutaneously in a direct line to the

pisiform bone so that the thumb may be angulated forwards and towards the ulna.
2. The tendon must be attached to the dorsiulnar aspect of the base of the proximal phalanx of the thumb to restore opposition.

Technique

Through a small incision in the metacarpophalangeal crease of the ring finger, the slips of sublimis tendon are divided and the proximal portion is withdrawn from the wrist incision.

A pulley is constructed at the pisiform bone using half the thickness of flexor carpi ulnaris which is sutured to the pisiform bone. The motor sublimis tendon is passed round flexor carpi ulnaris before passing through the pulley, thus utilizing flexor carpi ulnaris to aid the motor tendon.

An incision is made over the metacarpophalangeal joint of the thumb, the motor tendon is passed through a subcutaneous tunnel across the thenar eminence and secured to the ulnar border of the base of the proximal phalanx.

The tendon is sutured under moderate tension with the wrist flexed and the thumb in full abduction. This position is maintained by a plaster splint for 3 weeks, when muscle re-education is commenced.

ARTHRODESIS OF THE SHOULDER

Shoulder fusion is indicated in deltoid paralysis when the trapezius and serratus anterior are sufficiently strong to rotate the scapula and thereby abduct the arm. Operation should be postponed until closure of the upper humeral epiphysis.

The technique of intra-articular fixation is preferred because the joint is often underdeveloped and fixation maintains the desired abduction during the healing phase.

The precise angle of abduction should be determined before operation and secured by the insertion of a Smith-Petersen pin after excision of the articular surfaces. Excessive abduction should be avoided; otherwise, symptoms may arise from scapular contact or shoulder drag, particularly when the trapezius has been slightly affected. Fusion at 60° abduction gives a useful shoulder with strong scapulothoracic muscles (Figure 7.22) fusion between 45° and 60° should be accepted if these muscles are below normal. The shoulder should be fused with the elbow joint on the same plane as the anterior surface of the body and with the forearm slightly above the horizontal, corresponding to slight lateral rotation of the humerus.

The plaster may be changed in 1 month's time and a fresh plaster applied until there is radiographic evidence of fusion. It is wiser to retain plaster protection for at least 4 months as radiographs are difficult to interpret. When considered fused, the shoulder should be protected by an abduction splint during the initial mobilization.

The collapsing spine in poliomyelitis

Spinal deformity commonly follows the involvement of the paravertebral muscle groups required to stabilize the spinal column to the thoracic cage and to the pelvis as well as to maintain the vertical position with the normal thoracic kyphosis and lumbar lordosis. Also, maintaining intra-abdominal pressure, and hence spinal posture, are the muscle groups of abdominals, the diaphragm, quadratus lumborum, psoas, etc. These, too, are commonly involved in poliomyelitis, and imbalance – both by paralysis and contracture formation – does occur and is aggravated by growth in young children. When paralysis predominates, a long C-shaped scoliosis or collapsing spine is seen (Figure 7.23). This retains flexibility and is correctable initially without too much verebral rotation. There still remains controversy about whether the stronger muscle groups are found on the convex or concave sides.

Conservative treatment by physiotherapy, orthotic appliances, Milwaukee braces and surgical release of hip contractures is particularly indicated when the curves are mild or moderate (less than 20–40°) and up to puberty. However, some correction with stabilization using Harrington rod internal fixation must be carried out on severe, unstable scoliosis to improve pulmonary function, to discard a spinal brace, and for relief of fatigue, discomfort and backache. It should be noted that this surgery is not as straightforward as that required for idiopathic scoliosis because often there is severe pulmonary disease, the curves are much longer and therefore require staging, pseudarthrosis incidence is higher with osteoporotic bone producing less hold for the internal fixation devices. Autogenous bone graft material may be limited because of growth abnormalities of the pelvic bones (see Chapter 8).

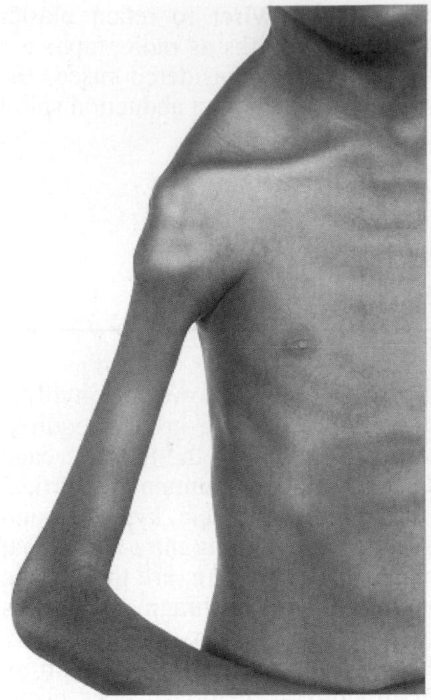
(a)

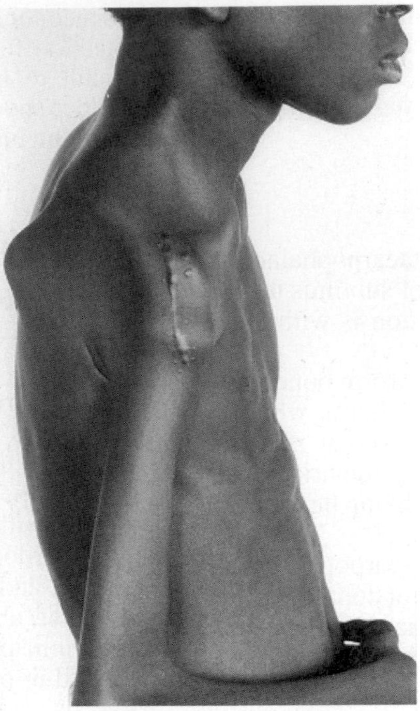
(b)

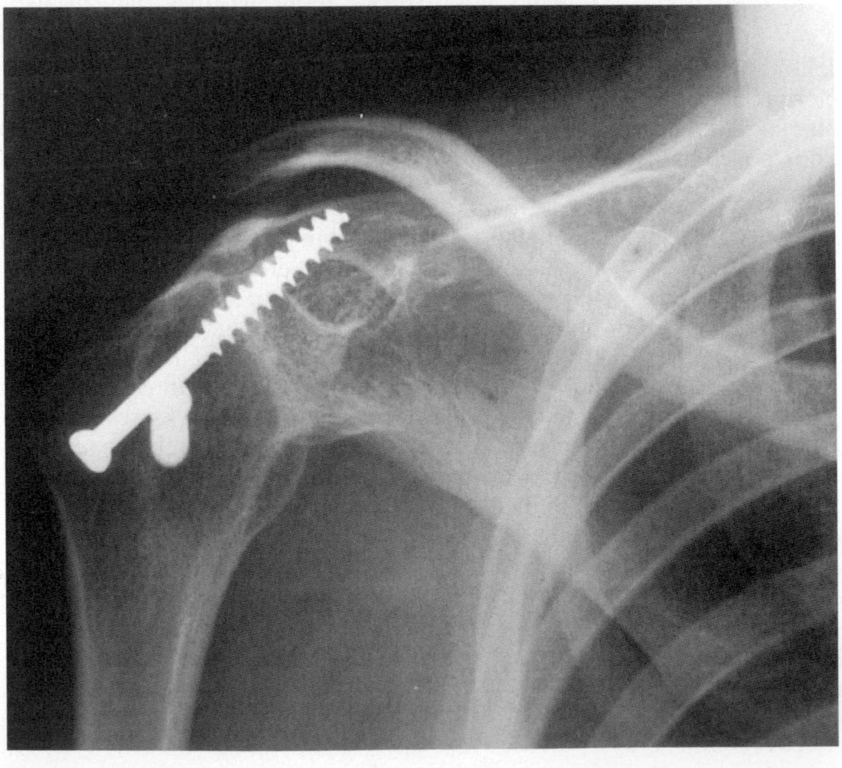
(c)

Figure 7.22 (a) and (b) Photographs to show an arthrodesis of the right shoulder in a 16-year-old boy. His scapulothoracic muscle group is functioning well with some winging of the scapula. (c) Radiograph to show the fusion of the shoulder with two bone screws.

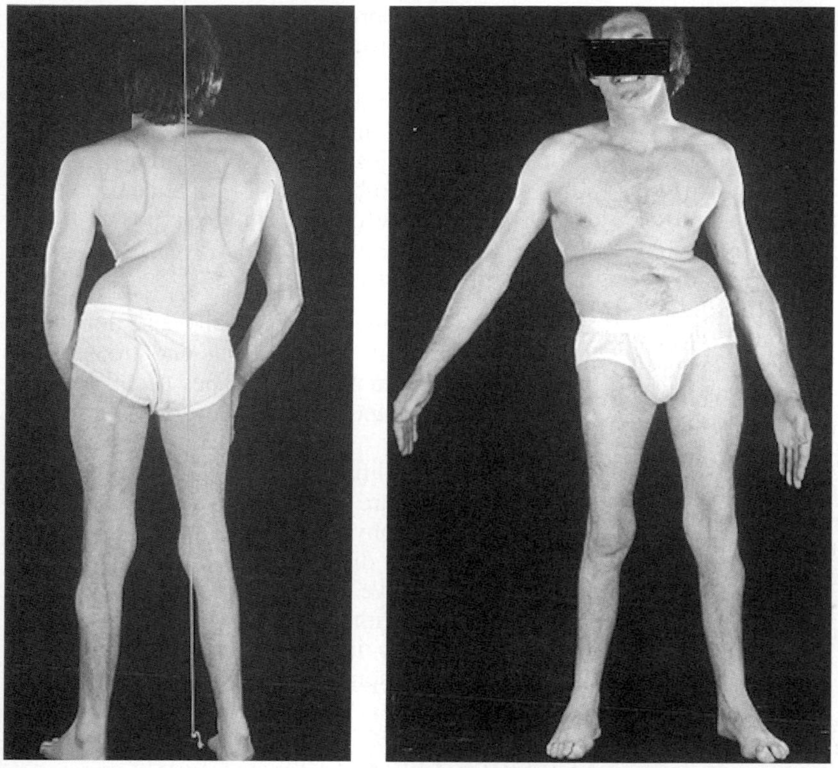

(a) (b)

Figure 7.23 (a) Photograph from the back to show the collapsing C-shaped deformity in a 33-year-old man who had sustained poliomyelitis 10 years before. (b) Same patient from the front, showing the impingement of the left costal margin on to the left iliac crest with pelvic obliquity.

Inequality of length of the lower extremities

Significant muscle paralysis in the lower limb is almost always accompanied by some degree of shortening. The degree of paralysis bears some relationship to the final amount of shortening in that those with severe paralysis are likely to have greater shortening than those with slight paralysis. It is impossible, however, to give an accurate prognosis of the final shortening to be expected in any one patient.

While routine clinical measurement by the same surgeon gives a reasonable idea of the progress of shortening, periodic radiographic measurement is essential for an accurate recording or when contemplating leg equalization procedures.

The following observations are made from radiographic analysis of patients with paralysis confined to one limb (Ratliff, 1957). The greatest shortening is to be expected in patients affected at about the age of 3 years. The maximum shortening is unlikely to exceed 9 cm. Both the tibia and the femur are usually involved and the disparity appears soon after the illness. In general, the shortening in the more severe group tends to be progressive but in the milder group the shortening may progress to 2.5 cm or 4 cm over a few years and then remain constant. Reduction of discrepancy is not to be expected.

Ratliff (1957) reviewed 225 children who had paralysis due to poliomyelitis in one leg. In 97% the paralysed leg became shorter. He found it impossible to predict accurately the degree of shortening, but in general, the more severe the paralysis, the greater the shortening, although this was not related to paralysis of any particular muscle group. Much of the shortening took place in cases in which the muscles were involved above and below the knee. Lengthening of the paralysed leg may occur during the first 2 years after the onset of the disease, but this is always temporary. The cause of leg shortening is unknown (see Chapter 3).

Post-poliomyelitis syndrome

During the past 40 years or more, thousands of patients have continued to require orthotic support, physiotherapy and operative care for the sequelae of their paralytic poliomyelitis deformities. However, a new syndrome – post-poliomyelitis – has recently appeared in which there is new weakness, increased and abnormal fatiguability and pain – 35 years or more after the acute disease (Munsat, 1991). Cashman (1992) has recently reviewed the world literature as well as his own experience to describe in detail this new symptom complex. The new weakness commonly occurs in limbs which had been most severely affected, although sometimes in limbs without such a strong history. It has been well known for many years that there is an average decline of about 1% in muscle power year by year, but this new weakness is much more severe and rapid. It occurs also in muscles involved before, responsible for bulbar and respiratory functions and these too may show this rapid change, e.g. difficulty in swallowing and breathing with dysproea. Although it has been suggested that these changes might be due to reactivation of the virus or autoimmune changes, a more likely cause is thought to be the terminal axonal degeneration which has been ongoing for many years. Continual remodelling of denervation and re-innervation of the post-polio motor units is believed to occur – the latter in response to insulin-like growth factors for both muscle and liver. At the menopause there may be a decrease in these factors as well as the growth hormone resulting in decreased re-innervation.

The other symptoms are of generalized as well as local increased weakness on exertion as well as pain. The latter can result local pathologies in joints and tendons but also the condition of fibromyalgia which has an increased incidence in this syndrome with diffuse chronic muscle pain and trigger point tenderness.

Treatment is directed toward a controlled systematic exercise programme, non-steroidal anti-inflammatory drugs for pain and pyridostigmine or other anticholinsterases for swallowing and breathing difficulties.

Spinocerebellar degenerative diseases

Forgan and Munsat (1974) have described that a broad group of conditions (Friedreich's ataxia, hereditary spastic ataxia of Marie, perhaps Charcot–Marie–Tooth disease without ataxia, etc.) can be considered together because they involve both the central and peripheral nervous systems, are genetically determined (often dominant) and have a high incidence of orthopaedic complications. Clinically, one can elicit:

1. Spasticity, hyper-reflexia and a Babinski sign.
2. Peripheral neuropathy with sensory loss; paraesthesia.
3. Dorsal column dysfunction with loss of vibration and position sense.
4. Cranial nerve lesions in seeing and hearing.
5. Cerebellar inco-ordination – balance problems.
6. Orthopaedic deformities of the spine (scoliosis) and foot (pes cavus).
7. Cardiomyopathy.

Pathological evidence of atrophy and degeneration can be found in various tracts and areas of the brain and brain stem nuclei, etc. They usually appear in early childhood and adolescence and continue into late adulthood.

The three conditions most likely to be seen by orthopaedists are Friedreich's ataxia, Charcot–Marie–Tooth atrophy and hereditary ataxia – polyneuritis (Refsum's disease). The last is a very rare autosomal recessive disease, often called a lipid storage disease, with the serum levels of phytanic acid being greatly increased and found in nerve tissue and cerebrospinal fluid.

FRIEDREICH'S ATAXIA

This is a developmental disease in which there is an ataxic paraplegia as a result of sclerosis of the posterolateral columns of the spinal cord. It occurs in both sexes but males predominating, with all forms of inheritance (e.g. autosomal recessive, dominant or X-linked) being found. The symptoms usually appear during adolescence, and consist of inco-ordination and weakness of the legs, clumsy speech, nystagmus, scoliosis and pes cavus. The deep reflexes are absent but the plantar reflex is of the extensor type. In the later stages there is a profound loss of joint sense in the lower limb, and often diminished tactile sense, although sensibility to pain and temperature remain unimpaired to the end.

The characteristic claw-foot deformity of the well marked case occasionally develops at an early stage, even before the characteristic ataxia. For this reason a neurological examination should be made in cases of adolescent claw-foot before operative correction is undertaken.

The disease is progressive and unremitting and little can be done to arrest it. Death usually occurs in young adulthood by primary cardiomyopathy and failure, or dysphagia with aspiration pneumonia because of brain stem disease.

Few patients live longer than 15–20 years after the onset of recognizable symptoms. However, tendon transfers to relieve muscle imbalances should be performed early to maintain function as long as possible. This also applies to bracing (see Chapter 8).

PERONEAL MUSCULAR ATROPHY (CHARCOT–MARIE–TOOTH)

This is a slowly progressive form of muscular atrophy which presents a clinical affinity with the distal (Gowers') type of myopathy, and a pathological resemblance both to multiple neuritis and anterior poliomyelitis. The pathology of atrophy and reduction in the number of cells is found mainly in the cerebellum, spinal cord (dorsal columns, anterior and posterior spinocerebellar, pyramidal tracts – particularly the anterior horn cells, dorsal root ganglia and horn cells) and in the large myelinated fibres of the peripheral nerves. As a rule the disease begins in childhood, and is seen only rarely after the age of 25. It is genetically heterogeneous, existing in autosomal dominant, recessive and X-linked forms. Males are more severely affected than females.

Differential diagnosis includes such conditions as multiple sclerosis, tabes dorsalis, mucopolysaccharidoses and progressive muscular dystrophy.

The first symptom to attract attention is weakness and wasting of the peroneal muscles; the feet become flexed and inverted, so that the child walks on their outer borders. About the same time, or perhaps earlier, the small muscles of the feet begin to atrophy; subsequently the wasting spreads to the muscles of the front of the leg and later to those of the calf. The next muscles to be affected are those of the lower part of the thigh, especially the vastus medialis; in consequence of the diminution in the circumference above the knee, the thigh is sometimes said to be bottle-shaped, the neck of the bottle being the lowermost part – the 'champagne glass' deformity. The patient is able to walk, for some time at any rate; the gait is high-stepping.

After a period, the small muscles of the hand are gradually involved. Fasciculations can be seen in the wasted muscles, with hyporeflexia and flaccidity of a lower motor neuron type. Vasomotor disturbances of coldness and sweating can be found in the lower limbs.

Scoliosis is quite commonly seen along with pes cavus deformity, which will require surgical correction by a triple arthrodesis.

Laboratory investigations are usually normal except for slowing of conduction speeds. The ankle-jerk is lost, frequently in the initial stage, but the knee-jerk is preserved unless the extensor muscle of the thigh has become involved.

Pains and cramps in the legs are often complained of. In some cases the cutaneous sensibility remains normal, but as a rule patches of anaesthesia are present on the outer aspects of the legs and over the feet. The muscles are not tender. The power of the sphincters is preserved. The disease is not fatal, runs a very chronic course, and sometimes its progress is arrested.

Obstetrical paralysis

Paralysis of one or both upper extremities occasionally follows the birth of a child. This is more common when the labour is complicated by obstetrical difficulties which necessitate forcible manipulation or traction on the baby's arm: the condition is accordingly known as 'obstetrical paralysis'. Brachial plexus injury at birth still remains a significant problem with an incidence of 0.9–2.5 per 1000 live births (see Chapter 12).

AETIOLOGY

The paralysis is the sequel to a lesion of the cords of the brachial plexus whereby they are stretched, and not due to the results of a dislocation of the shoulder. Sever (1916) pointed out that traction on the arm in adduction puts the upper cords of the plexus (which arise from the fifth and sixth cervical roots) under the greatest amount of tension, and causes them to stand out like bowstrings. If the tension is increased, the cords are liable to be injured.

Types

There are three types of obstetrical paralysis:

1. *The upper arm type*, or the Erb-Duchenne paralysis, which results – according to the supporters of the neurogenetic theory – from downward traction exerted on the arm. The shoulder is forcibly separated from the neck, beyond its normal limits, and the fifth and sixth cervical roots are consequently overstretched.
2. *The lower arm*, or the Klumpke type, which is said to result when the arm is pulled upwards above the head and the eighth cervical and first thoracic roots are overstretched.
3. *The whole arm type*, where the exciting cause has been one of unusual severity, and all the cords of the plexus have been to some extent involved.

Sever (1916) found that in his series of cases the incidence of the three types was as follows: upper arm, 400; whole arm, 64; and lower arm type, 9.

CLINICAL FEATURES

Upper arm type

Soon after birth the affected arm is seen to hang loosely at the side of the body; the forearm is pronated and the elbow slightly flexed, while the child is unable to abduct the arm. For the first few days after birth some swelling or tenderness may be observed in the region of the deltoid, but this usually subsides, leaving a paralysis of the deltoid, supraspinatus, biceps, coracobrachialis and brachioradialis. Contractures soon develop from the unopposed action of the adductors and medial rotators of the shoulder.

In many cases the paralysis of the deltoid and supraspinatus is only temporary, and with the repair of the injured nerve these muscles begin to function again. In the early stages, therefore, the greatest care must be taken to prevent the formation of adduction contractures. The cases in which the nerve lesion fails to heal, and in which the muscle paralysis is permanent, form a small minority. The typical course consists of a temporary paralysis, followed by a permanent contracture. In some cases the contracture may even be complicated by subluxation or dislocation of the shoulder joint.

Whole arm type

In a small proportion of cases, the lesion involves all the cords, so that not only are the muscles of the shoulder affected, but also those of the arm, the forearm and the hand. In these cases the paralysis of the intrinsic muscles of the hand, together with that of the muscles of the shoulder, is liable to persist. The lesion involves especially the fifth and sixth cervical roots, and the ulnar and median nerves, which are derived from the eighth cervical and first thoracic roots.

Lower arm type

In this type there may be at first paralysis of the whole arm, followed by a quick recovery of the muscles of the upper arm, those supplied by the lower segment of the plexus remaining more or less permanently paralysed. The resulting paralysis is when of the inferior radicular group of Klumpke type.

In the whole arm and the lower arm types, sensory disturbances are present. The anaesthesia is usually complete in the forearm and on the lateral side of the arm, but the medial aspect of the arm is unaffected, owing to the distribution of the intercostobrachial nerve. Frequently, also, in the inferior radicular type, there are oculopupillary signs – miosis, pupillary contraction and recession of the eyeball.

Sometimes associated are injuries in the region of the shoulder joint: fracture of the clavicle, separation of the upper humeral epiphysis and dislocation of the head of the humerus. Fracture of the clavicle greatly facilitates a rupture or tear of the plexus, especially of the lower cords. The dislocation of the humerus is usually a posterior one, although the anterior form has also been described.

The injury to the nerve roots is usually limited to the sheath, but in some cases the roots may be completely torn across. When the sheath is injured, the paralysis in the early stages is due to the resultant haemorrhage and the oedema, but later the formation of scar tissue may also play a part. The exact situation of the lesion is generally close to the point of exit of the roots from the vertebral column, but in some cases the lesion is stated to have been actually within the canal.

PROGNOSIS

A minority of cases recover completely in 3 months, and it is therefore impossible to determine clinically the exact extent of the lesion at an earlier date. In all cases of the upper arm type, the prognosis is good, but in the lower arm and whole arm forms the restoration of function is unlikely.

TREATMENT

Early diagnosis as soon as possible after birth should be made by looking for failure of the child to move the limb, absence of the Moro embrace reflex, loss of sensation and/or local swelling with tenderness, particularly in the supraclavicular area. On diagnosis the child should have the involved extremity abducted to 90°, flexed at the elbow to 90°, and this position should be maintained by pinning it to the crib surface. Before going home, the child should be fitted with a brace to maintain this position, with the mother being taught to carry out a passive range of full abduction at the shoulder joint, at least three times a day. If recovery fails to take place, transfer of the latissimus dorsi and teres major to the posterior surface of the humerus between the long and lateral heads of the triceps should be carried out. Often it is essential to divide the pectoralis major or even subscapularis, as well

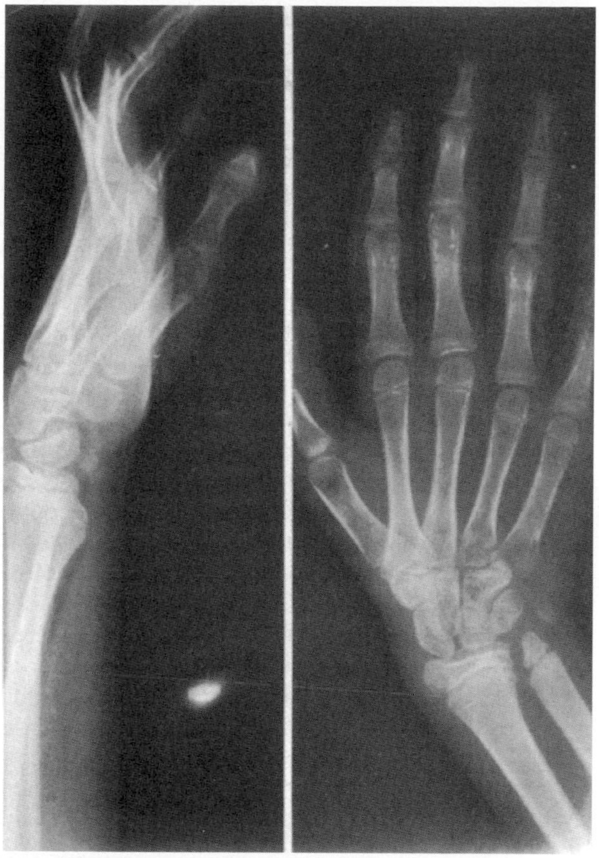

Figure 7.24 Radiographs of the hand and distal forearm of an Erb's palsy, showing the characteristic deformities of the fingers and wrist.

as the anterior capsule, particularly in the presence of contractures. This method was first described by L'Episcopo (1934).

In a few cases, the function in the hand and forearm of the involved limb may not improve. They will take up the position of full pronation with acute flexion deformity of the fingers and hands at the wrist (Figure 7.24). Growth disturbance occurs and the hand loses much of its function. With this type of deformity, reasonable function can be achieved by carrying out an osteotomy through the junction of the upper and middle third of the ulnar bone (which is held by a plate and screws) and placing the hand into a mid-position. The limb is immobilized in a long arm cast until bony union is obtained. Following this, the excision of the proximal row of the carpal bones may give additional length to help in relieving the flexion soft tissue contractures (Figure 7.25).

Sever's operation

An incision is made from the acromion process downwards over the anterior aspect of the shoulder. The interval between the deltoid and the pectoralis major muscle is defined, and these muscles are retracted to either side. The upper part of the pectoral muscle is then divided, at or near its tendinous insertion, in order to give better access to the head of the humerus. The subscapularis tendon is then located as it swings across the head of the humerus to the lesser tuberosity. A blunt disector is passed deep to it, between it and the capsule, and the tendon severed. The arm can now be completely laterally rotated. The muscles are allowed to fall together, the wound is closed, and the arm is put up in plaster in abduction and lateral rotation for 2 weeks, after which a splint is applied as previously described.

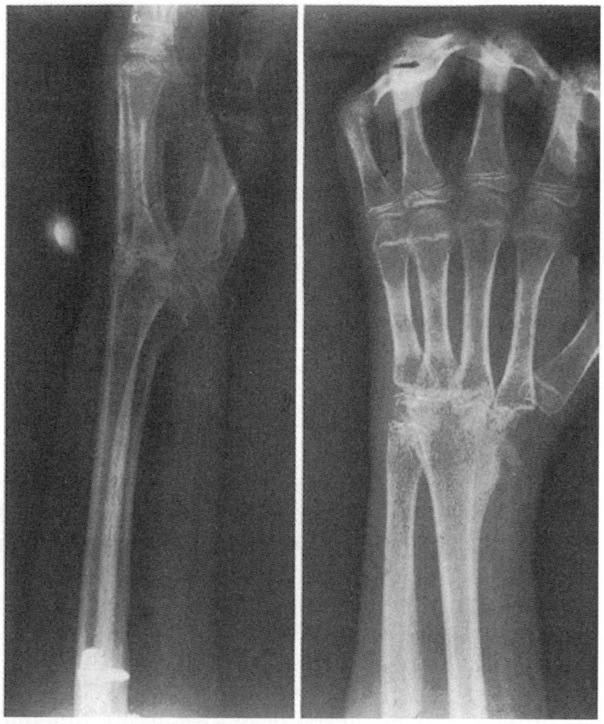

Figure 7.25 Radiographs of the same patient as in Figure 7.24, showing the wrist joint after excision of the proximal row of the carpal bones with improvement in the extensor deformities of the metacarpophalangeal joints and the lower end of the plate for the osteotomy through the ulna.

Some authorities advocate osteotomy of the humerus, with subsequent lateral rotation of the lower fragment. In severe cases the coracohumeral ligament close to the biceps, the short head of the biceps and, if necessary, the coracobrachialis should be divided.

The majority of these recover with physical therapy – between 80 and 95%, up to 92% by 3 months, but only minimal improvement after 6 months. But Jahnke *et al.* (1991), on reviewing a secondary referred series of 66 patients without surgical intervention, found 75% incomplete resolution with significant functional disability, and 15% severely disabled. Tendon transfer and/or humeral osteotomies improved cosmesis but not the overall function of the limb.

Gilbert *et al.* (1991) have developed a surgical indication protocol in which there were three important prognostic factors:

1. Complete recovery occurred only in patients who had some biceps recovery by one month.
2. A good result did not occur if the biceps failed to regain good contractions by 3 months.
3. Poor results occurred if there was late recovery of contractions by the biceps and if they were not normal by 5 months.

They recommended surgical exploration and nerve grafting if the biceps remained paralysed at over 3 months with recovery of normal shoulder function in 50% of C5 and C6 injuries.

In investigating these injuries myelography is still the most sensitive in detecting traumatic meningoceles but has a high false-positive rate. Computed tomography myelography and magnetic resonance imaging are of greatest use in visualizing brachial plexus injury.

Intraspinal tumours in infants and children

Intraspinal tumours in infants and children are often first seen by the orthopaedic surgeon because of musculoskeletal abnormalities. As Tachdjian and Matson (1965) emphasized, prolonged delay may occur in treating a patient with torticollis, scoliosis, unexplained limp or weakness of the extremity unless one is alert to this possibility. Additional presenting complaints include weakness of an extremity, a sphincter disturbance or pain which is located either in the trunk or in the extremity for which no reasonable explanation is found. Tachdjian and Matson pointed out that the highest incidence is in the early childhood age group below 7 years with an exceedingly high incidence in the first 3 years. The principal tumour found is a glioma, with neuroblastomas, metatastic tumours, dermoid cysts, teratomas, lymphomas; neurofibromas being less common.

Of 115 intraspinal tumours, 63 were benign and 52 were malignant (Tachdjian and Matson, 1965). The most common initial complaint was weakness of the legs resulting in a limp, with back pain a close second, followed by torticollis, urinary incontinence, abdominal pain and weakness of the arms. Pathological reflexes with spastic paralysis were most common followed by a flaccid paralysis and sensory loss, development of scoliosis and unexplained muscle spasm in the paravertebral area. Torticollis and kyphosis are surprisingly common but changes seen on radiography are frequently minimal since growth adapts to the intraspinal mass and no bone erosion may be seen. A spinal deformity may develop instead. This includes widening of the canal which, in its early stages, may easily be missed. The interpedicular distance can be accurately charted and measured. A necessity for films of the entire spine is evident even though the presenting complaint may be related to the lower extremities. Any suspicion of course leads to myelography and examination of the spinal fluid. The spinal fluid protein is usually elevated. This finding, together with the detection of abnormal cells, may give a clue to the diagnosis of the type of tumour present.

Cerebral palsy (by A. Campos da Paz Jr, Sáuria M. Burnett and Alvaro M. Nomura)

Cerebral palsy is a disorder of posture and movement secondary to a static lesion of the developing brain (Bax, 1964).

Neurological development begins at conception. The basic mechanisms that regulate the various steps of nervous system development are genetically determined but this regulation may be modulated at any stage by environmental factors (Herschkowitz, 1988). Cerebral growth reaches its highest velocity in the third trimester of pregnancy. By the end of the second postnatal year the brain is three times heavier than at birth (Brody *et al.*, 1987).

Central nervous system (CNS) myelination begins in the fetal period and continues through adult life with important changes in the first two postnatal years. The fastest changes in the degree of myelination occur in the first 8 months after birth. In some areas the process continues more slowly until the end of the second year, and in others goes on even beyond that, but at a much slower rate (Kinney *et al.*, 1988). The period of active myelin synthesis associated with maximal myelination rate is considered to be vulnerable for myelination, that is, more sensitive to external aggressions.

PREVALENCE

In epidemiology, prevalence expresses the number

of cases of a disease or condition present in a population during a certain time period. Incidence is the number of new cases occurring within a certain time period in a population at risk. Incidence is not the more appropriate term for studies in cerebral palsy, given the heterogeneous aetiology, the appearance of the alterations suggesting the diagnosis at different stages, and the relatively high mortality in the neonatal period (Alberman, 1984).

Cerebral palsy prevalence, at school age, is estimated to be approximately two per 1000 live births in the developed countries (Paneth and Kiely, 1984).

CLASSIFICATION

The widely accepted classification of cerebral palsy described by Minear (1956) includes seven major categories, 34 minor categories and numerous subcategories.

A study of 21 children carried out in Australia to test the validity of a classification demonstrated discrepancies in cerebral palsy diagnosis. The clinical diagnoses made by paediatricians and neurologists, trained in the diagnosis of neurological disorders, were compared. Concordance rates were of only 40% on the type of motor involvement, 50% on the topographic determination, and 60% on the severity (Alberman, 1984).

Classification based on motor involvement

Spasticity

There is an increased resistance to passive movement, and after the initial resistance there may be relaxation (as in opening a jack-knife). It is present in pyramidal tracts, usually in the motor cortex (precentral gyrus). Besides spasticity, deep tendon hyper-reflexia, clonus and extensor plantar response are other pyramidal signs. Children affected tend to develop joint deformities, and this is the most frequent type of cerebral palsy.

Involuntary movements

Involuntary motor activity, accentuated by emotional stress, occurs in lesions of the basal ganglia. Normally, these centres inhibit spontaneous rhythmic movements which are initiated by the cerebral cortex. Involuntary movements are usually classified, according to their characteristics, *choreoatetoid* (combination of choreic and athetoid movements) and *dystonic*. Choreic movements are gross, fast, arrhythmic and of sudden beginning. Athetoid are continuous, uniform and slow. Dystonia is characterized by intermittent twisting movements secondary to the simultaneous contraction of agonist and antagonist muscles involving extremities, neck and trunk. Dystonic movements commonly determine bizarre postures, sustained for a variable period of time, followed by relaxation.

Rigidity

This movement disturbance, also a consequence of lesions of the basal ganglia, relates to a generalized hypertonia secondary to a continuous contraction of flexor and extensor muscles.

Ataxia

It is characterized mainly by clumsy gait with broadening of the base secondary to the lack of balance. Ataxia is related to cerebellar or cerebellar tract lesions. Other clinical signs are dysdiadochokinesia, dysmetria, decomposition of movements, nystagmus and 'scanning' dysarthria. Ataxia is frequently associated with cerebellar hypoplasia and is rare in cerebral palsy. The more frequently found is the mixed form: ataxia and spasticity, one or either predominates.

Hypotonia

It means decreased resistance to passive movements and is a rare condition in cerebral palsy. Usually found in children who, after reaching a greater level of cerebral maturity, will present choreoathetosis, ataxia or even spasticity. Hypotonia, commonly accompanied by hyper-reflexia, in a small number of children, persists for life. With some frequency such children have severe cognitive and motor deficiencies (Taft, 1984).

Mixed

This consists of combinations of the movement alterations as described above. The mixed class should not be used often, as the predominant motor symptoms determine the classification.

Classification based on topography

Monoplegia

It is a rare condition, in which only one limb is involved. Spasticity is the usual motor disorder.

Hemiplegia

It involves both upper and lower limb on the same side. A significant number of patients have a cortical sensory deficit with abnormal stereognosis, two point discrimination, and position sense. Hemianopia is also frequently found. This may represent a difficulty for the individual especially when driving a car. Although spasticity is the more frequent motor disorder, children with unilateral involuntary movements are usual (Figure 7.26).

Paraplegia

Alterations observed are restricted to the lower limbs. A precise description is extremely important, because if the child has a true paraplegia, cerebral palsy is not the most likely diagnosis; medullary lesion or hereditary spastic paraplegia must be considered.

Diplegia

Upper and lower extremities are involved, the legs more than the arms. It is commonly related to prematurity.

Triplegia

There is predominant involvement of three limbs, generally both legs and one arm; spasticity is the more frequent motor disorder.

Quadriplegia

It involves all four limbs, trunk, neck and head; the movement disorder can be spasticity, choreoathetosis or a mixed form. The term 'total body involvement' has been accepted as more appropriate because paralysis of four limbs without trunk involvement must be rare (Bleck, 1987). In the underprivileged populations, quadriplegia – frequently associated with severe anoxia or cerebral trauma – is more predominant than diplegia. The likely explanation for this difference may be related to the decrease in neonatal mortality of premature babies with the advent of the intensive care units.

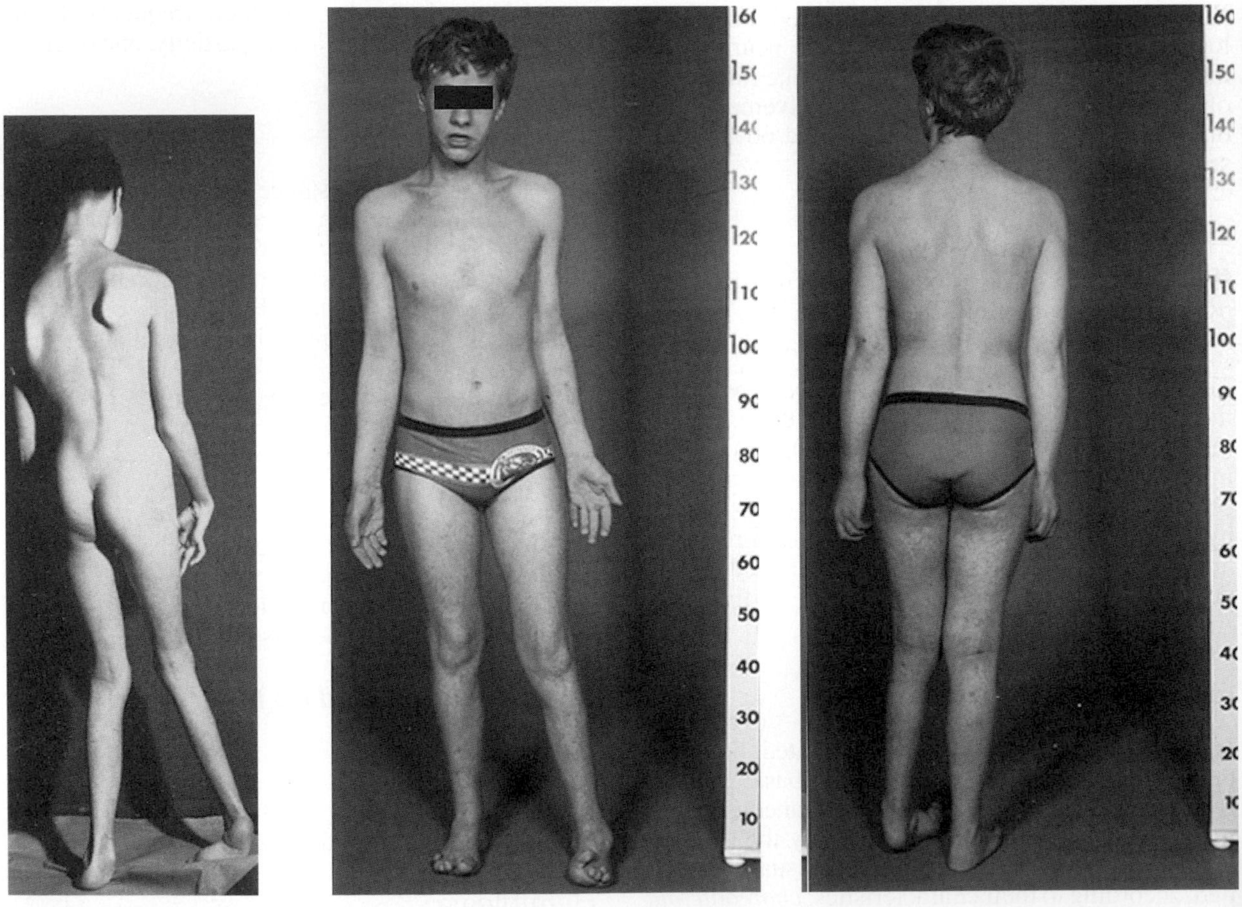

(a) (b) (c)

Figure 7.26 (a) Cerebral palsy can lead to severe deformity, as in this boy with spastic hemiplegia of the right side. (b) Photographs to show a spastic quadriplegic with mental retardation, chromosomal mosaicism.

Classification based on the degree of severity

This depends basically on the perception of the observer. The functional aspect is the most relevant. The degree of motor involvement can be classified as:

1. *mild* – fine movement alterations only;
2. *moderate* – variable difficulty in relation to speech and gross movements, but daily living activity performance is functional;
3. *severe* – inability to walk, use the hands and communicate through speech (Denhoff, 1976).

AETIOLOGY

The causes of cerebral palsy are numerous. They include insults in the *prenatal*, *perinatal* and *postnatal* periods Table 7.4. The aetiological diagnosis is basically made through data elicited by the clinical history. However, the antecedent is not always recognized, with certainty. About 20–30% of the cases do not show any apparent risk factor (Taft, 1984).

Prenatal insults are secondary to complications like congenital infections and fetal distress due to obstetric problems or other influences; all can interfere with normal cerebral development.

In *congenital toxoplasmosis*, clinical manifestations may be present at birth or not be evident for a few days. The detection of a pregnant woman potentially able to infect the fetus is very important because early diagnosis and appropriate treatment of the newborn can decrease the severity of the neurological and ocular complications.

In *congenital rubella*, the infection is chronic, and the child may shed the virus throughout the first year of life. Auditory impairment is an important manifestation and mental retardation, if present, is usually severe. In recent years, immunization with alive virus has produced a decrease in its incidence.

Cytomegalovirus is universally distributed and infects all ethnic and socioeconomic groups. In the United States, United Kingdom and Canada, 0.4–2.5% of newborns are CMV-positive, a figure which makes this to be considered the most common human fetal infection (Spector, 1987). Usually, the encephalitic type causes an injury to the developing central nervous system; late alterations may appear in children who were asymptomatic in the neonatal period.

Nelson and Ellenberg (1985), from a large prospective study, have concluded that *smoking in pregnancy* is not a factor significantly related to cerebral palsy. Tobacco, however, is considered a cause of fetal growth retardation, a factor that may increase the vulnerability.

Alcohol effects on the fetus are now well known; the main alterations include growth retardation beginning *in utero*, microcephaly, short palpebral fissures, decreased intellectual ability and irritability followed by hyperactivity (Jones, 1988). No

Table 7.4 Causative and risk factors

Prenatal
Congenital infections
Toxoplasmosis
Rubella
Cytomegalovirus
Abuse of drugs
Tobacco
Alcohol
Marijuana
Cocaine
Cerebral malformations
Obstetric complications
Pre-eclampsia/eclampsia
Abruptio placentae
Placenta previa
Perinatal
Prematurity
Low birth weight
Complicated delivery (dystocia)
Asphyxia
Cerebral trauma
Infections
Meningitis
Herpes
Hyperbilirubinaemia
Blood incompatibilities
Other haemolytic disorders
Hypoglycaemia
Postnatal
Infections
Meningitis
Encephalitis
Head trauma
Cerebrovascular accident
Cyanotic congenital heart disease
Sickle cell anaemia
Vascular malformations
Cerebral anoxia
Near-drowning
Aspiration asphyxia
Cardiac arrest
Seizures
Malnutrition

teratological effect of *marijuana* has been described as yet but, premature labour, premature rupture of membranes and haemorrhage in pregnancy may be associated with its use.

Cocaine is more important, and the number of pregnant woman who use this drug is growing. A clear causal relationship between cocaine and placentae praevia, secondary to its vasoconstrictive properties, has been observed (Chasnoff *et al.*, 1985); intracranial haemorrhage in the intrauterine-exposed newborn was also described (Spires *et al.*, 1989).

Perinatal injuries are more frequently related to prematurity or to asphyxia secondary to complicated labour and delivery; severe hyperbilirubinaemia when inadequately treated is still relatively common in developing countries.

Severe prolonged hypoxia is generally associated with cortical grey matter lesions in term newborns and with periventricular lesions in the premature. The Apgar score is widely used in neonatology. It basically evaluates the CNS and cardiovascular integrity, through the observation of heart rate, respiratory effort, muscle tone, reflex response to nasal catheter and skin colour. It is generally accepted that low scores at 5 minutes are related to an increased incidence of CNS lesion. However, Nelson and Ellenberg (1981), in a study of 49 000 children, considered low Apgar scores to a risk factor, but 55% of the children who developed cerebral palsy had Apgar scores of 7–10 in the first minute and 73% of 7–10 at 5 minutes. These observations suggest that a significant number of cerebral palsy cases are determined by factors other than intrapartum asphyxia.

Children born before 37 weeks of gestation are considered *premature* and liable to several problems in the neonatal period. Severity is proportional to the degree of prematurity. Newborns at risk are those of very low birth weight (less than 1500 g) and particularly of extremely low birth weight (less than 1000 g). The specific relationship between premature delivery and spastic diplegia was first recognized by Freud in 1897. The risk seems to be directly related to fetal immaturity. Nevertheless, it is not clear whether this is solely due to the effect of prematurity on neuron development at a critical stage or is secondary to other risks such as intraventricular haemorrhage and leucomalacia (Stanley and Alberman, 1984). On the other hand, it is known that, in premature infants, the germinal matrix juxtaposed to the periventricular ependyma (lateral ventricles) has low resistance to hypoxia and that haemorrhages in this area are relatively frequent (Pape and Wigglesworth, 1979). A lesion limited to this region may result in spastic diplegia, which correlates with the anatomy. The cortical tract portion related to the movements of the lower limbs is closer to the lateral ventricles.

Bacterial meningitis is an important cause of neonatal morbidity and mortality. Most cases are caused by Gram-negative bacteria, and the incidence of severe neurological sequelae in this age group is large.

Most *herpes simplex* virus infections in the newborn are acquired during passage through the labour canal. In approximately 50% of infected children, the virus affects the CNS. Caesarean section delivery is indicated for mothers with genital infection. Unfortunately, mothers of infected newborns may not show any clinical evidence at the time of birth.

In *blood incompatibilities* and other newborn haemolytic disorders, unconjugated bilirubin may reach critical levels, e.g. up to 15 mg/dl. Above this level, there is a great risk of deposition in the basal ganglia, and therefore of kernicterus. The more immature the newborn, the greater the susceptibility. Choreoathetosis is directly related with neonatal hyperbilirubinaemia as well as auditory deficit. Anti-D gammaglobulin injection (RhoGam) in the Rh-negative woman shortly after delivery of a Rh-positive child or other circumstances in which placental bleeding may occur, phototherapy and appropriately indicated exchange transfusion have all caused an important decrease in the number of cases of cerebral palsy due to hyperbilirubinaemia (Stanley, 1984).

Severe and prolonged *hypoglyaemia* may be associated with neurological sequelae. Newborns at high risk belong to four main groups: infants of diabetic mothers, low birth weight, prematurity and genetic inborn errors of metabolism, the latter being a very rare condition.

Postnatal cerebral palsy is defined as a disorder of posture and movement secondary to a non-progressive brain lesion occurring between 4 weeks and 2 years of age, realizing that the most important changes in myelination occur before the third postnatal year. Studies carried out in Sweden have also established 2 years of age as a limit (Hagberg *et al.*, 1975; Lagergren, 1981) but Stanley and Blair (1982) have extended the period until 5 years. The main cause of postnatal cerebral palsy is CNS infection (60% with a larger incidence in economically underprivileged populations), followed by head trauma (20%). Studies carried out in North America have not reported cases of cerebral palsy associated with malnutrition but, in Australia, malnutrition was considered as the cause in about 2% of the population studied (Stanley and Blair, 1984).

Finally, it is important to emphasize that the positive association between asphyxia and cerebral palsy is clear, but the conclusion that asphyxia and other perinatal problems are the most frequent causes of cerebral palsy is not supported by long-term follow-up studies (Nelson and Ellenberg, 1986; Blair and Stanley, 1988).

De Sousa (1991) in reviewing the various origins/causes of cerebral palsy concluded that the factors responsible for CP are most often present before birth. However, when birth asphyxia has occurred in an infant who subsequently develop cerebral palsy, prenatal factors have contributed to the asphyxia. No evidence of birth asphyxia was found in 78% of children developing CP, but other prenatal and maternal risk factors were present, e.g. low birth weight, long maternal menstrual cycle, premature placental separation and polyhydraminos.

DIAGNOSIS

The diagnosis of cerebral palsy is essentially clinical and difficult to establish in infants under 12 months until the deformities become evident as the CNS matures. A detailed history of gestation, labour, delivery and of the first 2 years of life must be made. Familial antecedents are also very important, as they can highlight the possibility and the need to investigate a genetic disorder. What usually brings the attention of parents or the paediatrician to the problem is the motor delay; every child with motor delay deserves a neurological evaluation and follow-up. In the older child, where the clinical picture is more defined, diagnosis is clearer. The main objective must be to establish a diagnosis through the evaluation of tonus, deep tendon reflexes, the presence or absence of involuntary movements, co-ordination, balance, active movements and muscle mass. It is important to attempt to define the site of the primary alteration, whether encephalic, spinal or muscular.

In a child with hypotonia, hypo- or areflexia, apparent muscular atrophy, absence of involuntary movements and good cognitive development, the disorder must be due to a lower motor neuron or primary muscular dysfunction. Upper motor neuron lesions may be located in the cerebral cortex, internal capsule, cerebral peduncles, brain stem or spinal cord, and are associated with pyramidal signs (Chusid, 1985). If the motor disorder is secondary to an encephalic lesion, a pyramidal syndrome (spasticity, deep tendon hyper-reflexia, clonus and Babinski), an extrapyramidal syndrome (involuntary choreoathetoid or dystonic movements) or ataxic syndrome (lack of balance, inco-ordination, dysdiadochokinesia, asynergy, hypotonia and pendular reflexes) may be the diagnosis.

In infants, the evaluation of primitive reflexes and postural reactions is essential. If the lesion is anatomically close to the encephalic integration site, some reflexes will remain beyond the age that they should disappear and certain reactions will not arise at the time they normally should.

Although their interpretation is relatively difficult, particularly in infants under 6 months, the evaluation of tonus and deep tendon reflexes is extremely important. Both, hypertonia, usually coupled with hyper-reflexia, and hypotonia may indicate an upper motor neuron disorder. In many children who will develop spasticity, the initial finding is difficulty in free hip abduction due to adductor hypertonia. Clonus and extensor plantar response are normal findings until approximately 7 months of age. Sustained clonus, however, should be considered pathological. In the first months of life, suckling or swallowing difficulties and neck hyperextension are strongly suggestive of a cerebral lesion.

In spite of the fact that in cerebral palsy the lesion is non-progressive, there will be changes in the neurological picture, due to the CNS maturation. The child who is hypotonic in the first few months may later show choreoathetosis, ataxia or even spasticity. In the extrapyramidal forms, the involuntary movements may appear around 12 months. Athetosis in the second semester of life may represent the initial finding of ataxia (Beret, 1974). Nelson and Ellenberg (1982), in a large longitudinal study of 229 children with diagnosis of cerebral palsy at 1 year of age, 118 did not present with any motor deterioration at 7 years.

Depending on the degree of spasticity, articular deformities are frequent and they tend to progress to the extent to interfere with gait performance.

To decrease the possibility of diagnostic error it is very important to determine if the alterations found in following up a child with motor disorder are related to the natural history of a static lesion or to a progressive one.

Computerized tomography (CT) and magnetic resonance imaging (MRI) are now generally used to evaluate the brain structure. These imaging examinations can demonstrate the extension and severity of hydrocephalus, congenital malformations, myelination pattern, atrophy and porencephalic cysts. The skull x-ray may not show calcifications which are easily seen on CT. MRI does not demonstrate calcifications but, is more sensitive than CT in identifying white matter changes and certain congenital malformations of the brain.

DIFFERENTIAL DIAGNOSIS

The conditions that determine neurological alterations or motor development delay are numerous (Table 7.5 and every professional working with cerebral palsy must be able to question and discuss the diagnosis.

Table 7.5 Differential diagnosis

Neuromuscular diseases
Congenital myopathies
Muscular dystrophy
Spinal muscular atrophy
Genetic syndromes
Nervous system metabolic diseases
Amino-acid metabolism disorders
Phenylketonuria
Homocystinuria
Lysosomal diseases
Glycogen storage diseases (glycogenoses)
Mucopolysaccharidoses
Lipid metabolism disorders
Gangliosidoses
Tay–Sachs disease (GM2 gangliosidosis)
Pseudo-Hurler (GM1 gangliosidosis)
Niemann–Pick disease
Gaucher disease
Krabbe disease,
Metachromatic leucodystrophy
Phakomatoses
Sturge–Weber disease
Tuberous sclerosis
Ataxia-telangiectasia
Degenerative diseases
Spinocerebellar ataxia
Familial spastic paraplegia
Hereditary sensory motor neuropathy
Brain tumours
Spinal malformations
Sacral agenesis
Diastematomyelia
Spinal tumours
Spinal cord injury following birth trauma
Congenital AIDS

In *Duchenne muscular dystrophy*, symptoms arise between 2 and 5 years. The diagnosis is rarely made before 3 years of age but there frequently is a history of motor delay. Equinus may be present from the time the child begins to walk. Others show, initially, a gait pattern suggesting lack of balance. All these observations suggest that symptoms actually have begun earlier.

The American Academy of Cerebral Palsy – AACPDM – classification (Minear, 1956) and many authors in this field (Denhoff, 1976; Taft, 1984; Bleck, 1987) consider genetic diseases not as a differential diagnosis but as a cause. Hereditary diseases comprise a large number of pathologies characterized by dysmorphias and errors of metabolism. The first edition of autosomal dominant, autosomal recessive and X-linked phenotypes listed 1487 described diseases; the 1988 edition lists 4344, approximately 10% of which are due to a known metabolic disorder (McKusick, 1988). Chromosomal abnormalities are important causes of mental retardation and congenital structural defects. Approximately one in 150 newborns has a chromosomal abnormality (Hirschhorn, 1987). Down syndrome, followed by the fragile X syndrome, are the two most commonly found chromosomal disorders (Kahkonen *et al.*, 1986). The diagnosis of dysmorphic syndromes due to rarer genic alterations requires a meticulous examination with description of all findings, followed by a search in congenital malformation books, atlases, catalogues or special softwares. In the well described genetic disorders, particularly when the chromosomal alteration or the type of heritage is already determined, it is preferable to increase the level of diagnostic precision rather than label these children with the diagnosis of cerebral palsy.

The initial manifestations of CNS *metabolic* or *degenerative* diseases may be characterized by developmental delay, with or without alterations in the neurological status. Diagnostic confusion is, therefore, perfectly possible until the picture of motor regression becomes evident.

The forms of *hereditary sensory-motor neuropathies* associated with cerebellar signs or spastic paraplegia may also be easily mistaken with cerebral palsy. Both ataxia and paraplegia appear early and, in the initial stages, are not accompanied by the other characteristic findings.

The clinical manifestations of *brain tumours* will depend mainly on their site and the patient age. Motor development delay in infancy progressing to hemiplegia, diplegia or ataxia, with or without seizures, can be confused with cerebral palsy. Due to CNS immaturity, even with a progressive brain lesion, the neurological alterations may not suggest progression until the appearance of motor regression signs or increased severity of the neurological picture. The cranial contrasted CT scan is positive in most tumours but in some cases the lesion may only be identified through MRI scanning.

Intraspinal tumours can cause paraplegia or quadriplegia (when highly located), with pyramidal tract signs, sensory disturbances and loss of sphincter control. Congenital tumours interfere with the growth of the lower limbs with scoliosis or torticollis, depending on its localization. Skin changes on the spine and occult spina bifida are frequent findings. Plain x-ray may be positive but myelography and MRI are the diagnostic methods of choice.

Spinal cord injury following birth trauma, especially in breech presentations, may affect particularly the middle and lower cervical segments. Dislocation and fracture of the spine are uncommon. Flaccidity is observed at birth but spasticity of the lower extremities may gradually arise. Decreased or absent perspiration below the levels innervated by the upper thoracic nerves may interfere with body temperature regulation. Such disturbance may represent a life-threatening condition.

Children with *intrauterine acquired AIDS* usually show developmental delay and neurological changes such as axial hypotonia, deep tendon hyper-reflexia, spastic diplegia or quadriplegia. Acquired microcephaly with cortical atrophy identified on cranial CT scan may also be present (Ultmann *et al.*, 1985).

PROGNOSIS

Motor and cognitive development are affected by the anatomical localization and extent of brain damage. Despite early diagnosis and proper intervention, the disability is permanent and a variety of factors influence the outcome of a child with cerebral palsy. Epilepsy refractory to anticonvulsants, mental retardation, severe visual impairment, poor nutritional status and lack of stimulation are some of the negative factors. According to Molnar (1979), the probability of a child achieving independent ambulation decreases after 4 or 5 years in any type of motor involvement and is unlikely after 8 years of age.

Commonly, all children with spastic hemiplegia achieve independent walking. With respect to diplegia, in a study of 116 children, the majority walked at about 2–4 years (20% needed crutch or walker support), and only 8.5% did not achieve ambulation by 8 years of age (Miranda, 1979). The more severe athetoid or spastic quadriplegic patients have the worst motor prognosis. Usually, these children end up in wheelchairs and a significant number will require total care.

Although there is a strong correlation between clinical type and prognosis, this should be questioned as first predictor due to the difficulty in classifying some children according to motor involvement at an early age (Harris, 1987; Watt *et al.*, 1989).

Bleck (1975), in a study of 73 children with cerebral palsy or delayed motor development, concluded that the presence or absence of certain primitive reflexes and postural reactions after 12 months of age have a predictive value in relation to walking prognosis. Molnar (1979) found significant correlation between sitting at 24 months and ambulation. More recently, a prospective study of 74 neonates – survivors of intensive care units – who were later diagnosed as having cerebral palsy, re-examined factors that might predict the ambulatory potential of children with cerebral palsy at an early age. It was found a positive relationship between sitting at 2 and ambulation at 8 years of age. In addition, the persistence of any of the following primitive reflexes – tonic-labyrinthine, asymmetrical tonic neck (ATNR), symmetrical tonic neck (STNR) and Moro – and absence of postural reactions – foot placement – had a statistically significant correlation with non-ambulatory status (Watt *et al.*, 1989).

Establishing the prognosis for ambulation at an early age is an important step in the general approach to cerebral palsy, and a more comprehensive and rational treatment programme can be better defined.

Campos da Paz and colleagues (1994), from a 22-year retrospective analysis to determine walking prognosis, have clearly demonstrated that the achievement of head balance before 9 months was a good sign for walking and if not developed until after 20 months, this indicated a poor prognosis for walking. Sitting by 24 months and motor control of crawling by the age of 30 months were good predictors of a good prognosis (Figures 7.27, 7.28).

ASSOCIATED DISTURBANCES

Although the defining disability of cerebral palsy is motor dysfunction, additional handicaps are often present. 'Doctors can choose to ignore these complexities simply by referring the child for *therapy*' (Scrutton, 1984). However, the effectiveness, even of the orthopaedic treatment of a cerebral-palsy patient, is also dependent on a comprehensive understanding and proper management of all the possible associated conditions. An Achilles tendon lengthening, for example, may not represent a priority in the presence of some of these disturbances.

Mental retardation

A significant number of children with cerebral palsy have some degree of mental retardation. Hohman (1953) studied 600 cerebral-palsy patients and concluded that 75% had impaired intelligence. A study of 80 children carried out in our Cerebral Palsy Unit demonstrated that children with spastic hemiplegia have the best cognitive level, followed in regressive order by those with choreoathetosis, diplegia and spastic quadriplegia (Braga, 1983). These findings are in agreement with the experimental studies by Hohman (1953) and Young (1989) who also include the ataxic group, which displays similar cognitive level as hemiplegics.

The high incidence of cognitive impairment among cerebral-palsy patients is well established but any judgement based on initial impressions may lead to wrong conclusions. With the advent of the new communication alternative methods, children who

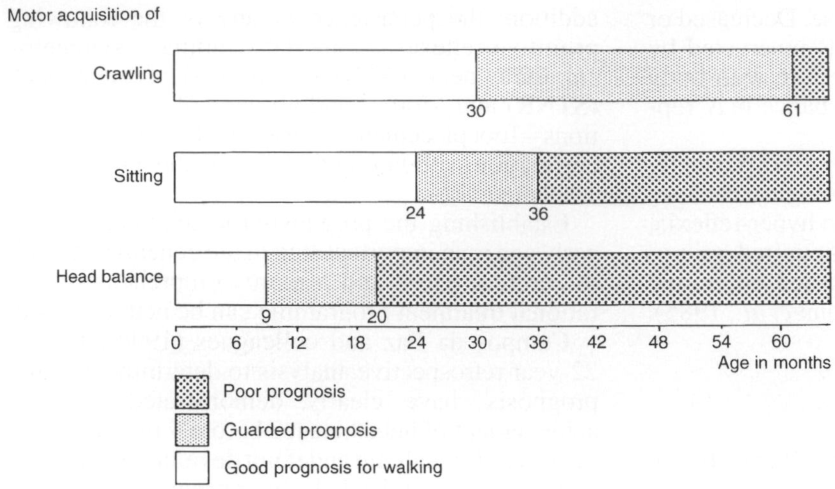

Figure 7.27 The prognosis for walking is based upon the achievement of head balance before the age of 9 months and, if not developed until after 20 months, this indicates a poor prognosis.

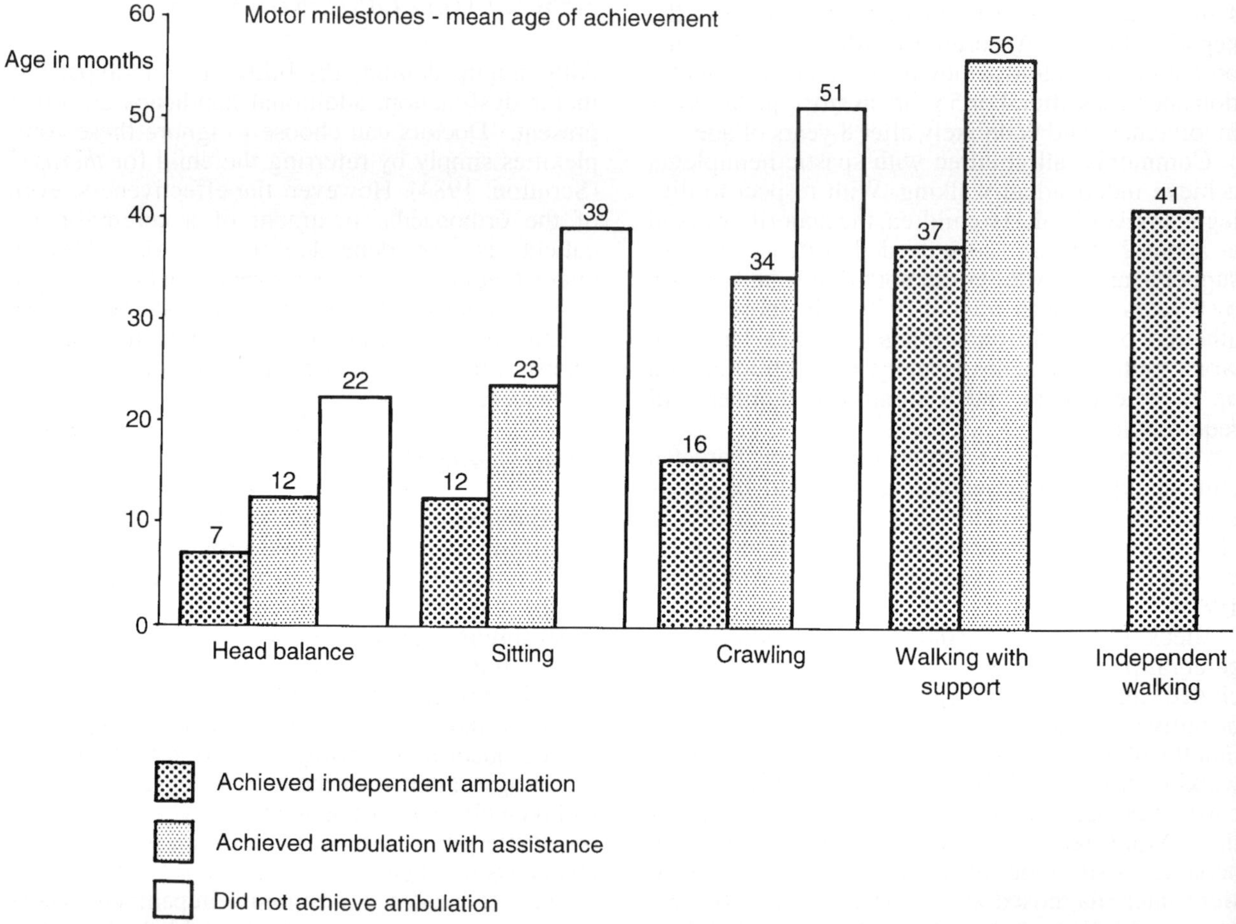

Figure 7.28 A histogram showing the times of achieving head balance, sitting, crawling, walking with or without support, against mean age of achievement in months. (SARAH's chart, Brazil, 1994)

once would have been considered as mentally retarded are now recognized to have better cognitive level than believed.

Epilepsy

Around one-third of children with cerebral palsy have some type of seizure disorder especially in the mentally retarded group. Epilepsy is also more common in spastics than in the extrapyramidal forms. The generalized tonic-clonic convulsions are most common but any type of seizure may be associated with cerebral palsy. In a representative number of children the prognosis is poor, and are resistant to anticonvulsants. Some of the patients with intractable epilepsy may benefit from surgical treatment (Aicardi, 1988). The objective with most procedures is to remove the epileptogenic focus responsible for initiation of the seizure discharge. When resection of a limited area is not possible, sagittal callosotomy may be indicated but the results obtained with this technique are still controversial. Concerning orthopaedic surgery, depending on the type of operation and the goals to be achieved, the intervention should be postponed until reasonable control of the convulsions is reached. Cessation of the attacks is followed by motor and cognitive improvement in some cases.

Auditory impairment

Hearing impairment is more common in children with cerebral palsy than in the general population. Infants at risk should be screened no later than 6 months of age (Cox, 1988). Some of the high-risk factors outlined in 1972, and modified by the Joint Committee on Infant Hearing in 1982 are:

1. parental suspicion that the child does not hear;
2. congenital perinatal infection (e.g. toxoplasmosis, rubella and CMV);
3. malformation of the pinna, face or palate;
4. low birth weight (less than 1500 g);
5. hyperbilirubinaemia at a level indicating need for exchange transfusion;
6. bacterial meningitis;
7. severe neonatal asphyxia; and
8. use of ototoxic drugs (e.g., streptomycin, kanamycin, neomycin and other aminoglycosides).

The screening procedure can consist of behavioural observation and electrophysiological tests such as brain stem auditory evoked response, which does not demand co-operation of the child. This is applicable to young children, or to those who are mentally deficient or multi-handicapped.

The incidence of sensorineural hearing impairment, in infants surviving neonatal intensive care units, may be as high as one in 25 (Stein *et al.*, 1983). Early detection can result in early intervention contributing towards better learning skills with appropriate approach.

Visual impairment

The most common ocular abnormality in cerebral palsy is strabismus. Nystagmus is sometimes seen in ataxia. Myopia is mostly seen in premature babies, and hemianopia is frequently found in hemiplegics who have a cortical sensory deficit. Cataracts, chorioretinitis, and retrolental fibroplasia may also be associated with cerebral palsy, depending on the cause of the movement disorder. In most eye defects, referral for ophthalmological consultation is indicated.

Visual acuity, pupillary responses, confrontal visual fields, and ophthalmoscopy are commonly sufficient for proper diagnosis. In very young infants or retarded children, electrodiagnostic tests such as visual-evoked response (VER) may be mandatory (Scher, 1989).

Perceptual and visual motor disorders

Visual, perceptual, visual motor or spatial inability are names frequently used to define the difficulty in perceiving spatial relationships (Abercrombie, 1964). The tests commonly used to assess perceptual disorders require vision and movement. This condition is fairly common in cerebral palsy with some implication with learning ability (Williams, 1958; Wedell, 1960; Nelson, 1962). Athetoids appear to have fewer perceptual and visual motor disorders than spastics, and it seems that the perceptual ability is not related to the degree of motor involvement. According to Feagans (1983), much of the work concerning treatment programmes for perceptual problems has now been overlooked. Perceptual motor training, in most children with cerebral palsy, does not seem to help reading and writing disabilities.

Feeding disorders

Poor weight gain in cerebral palsy is commonly a consequence of inadequate caloric intake due to refusal of food, vomiting, gastro-oesophageal reflux and impaired swallowing. Malnutrition can result in apathy and increased rate of infection (Fee *et al.*, 1988). Moreover, as in all neurogenic dysphagia syndromes, the child is at risk of aspiration. This condition is very distressing for parents. Some families may spend several hours each day feeding the child, and not rarely the use of non-oral feeding by nasogastric tube (Jones, 1989), or even gastrostomy is required to preserve nutritional status (Shapiro *et al.*, 1986). For the most severe cases, videofluoroscopic investigation is indicated because difficult swallowing, in some children, may be associated with unexpected abnormalities (Griggs *et al.*, 1989).

Contrary to malnutrition, overweight also may present as a problem especially for children in wheelchairs. Once obesity has been established, it may be extremely difficult for the child to lose weight (Bax and MacKeith, 1975).

Dental problems

Enamel hypoplasia occurs frequently in children with cerebral palsy (Kanar, 1976). Furthermore, impaired orofacial motor co-ordination and swallowing may not only interfere with oral hygiene but also contribute to inadequate intake of protein, vitamins, calcium, phosphorus and fluoride, predisposing to dental caries (Fee *et al.*, 1988).

Drooling

Cerebral palsy children with severe motor disability may drool due to dysfunction of oral muscle co-ordination. Some other factors contributing to drooling are head position, sitting posture, tongue size and the ability to breathe through the nose (Koheil *et al.*, 1987). Drooling may predispose to and transmit infection, disturbing child care and education. Feeding programmes and biofeedback training tend to decrease the volume of oral saliva, with more effective swallowing by better oral motor control. A surgical procedure, aiming to alleviate the problem, may be recommended for some of the children who do not get any improvement from those conservative means of treatment. Bilateral submandibular duct relocation seems to be a most acceptable technique (Crysdale, 1982).

Constipation

The accumulation of stools is frequent especially in the total-body-involved children, and in some cases it can progress to severe constipation. Decreased body activity, low fluid intake and increased consumption of constipating foods such as milk and milk products are some of the factors contributing to constipation. Dietary management regarding fibre intake combined with habit training is important if the colon is not dilated. In case of megacolon, the general recommendations are: low-residue diet, mineral oil by mouth, and administration of enemas.

Bladder dysfunction

Cognitive level, communication, mobility and upper limb function are some of the factors implicated in urinary control in patients with cerebral palsy. Although the incidence of incontinence in this population is not well known, studies in symptomatic patients have demonstrated urodynamic abnormalities and upper motor type neurogenic bladder (McNeal *et al.*, 1983; Bauer, 1985; Decter *et al.*, 1987). In a smaller group, the findings suggest both upper and lower motor neuron dysfunction (Bauer, 1985) and in these children, spinal cord damage probably has occurred at the same time as the cerebral insult (Clancy *et al.*, 1989).

It is not known whether detrussor sphincter dyssynergia is as potentially harmful to the kidneys in patients with cerebral palsy as it is in those with spina bifida (Borzyskowski, 1989).

MANAGEMENT

'The aim of treatment for children with cerebral palsy or other conditions involving upper motor neuron is to lead them towards the greatest degree of independence possible' (Bobath and Bobath, 1984). After a complete assessment, the physician should plan recommendations, taking into account the age, motor involvement associated handicaps, and social conditions.

Most therapists consider that early initiation of treatment is preferable but controlled studies

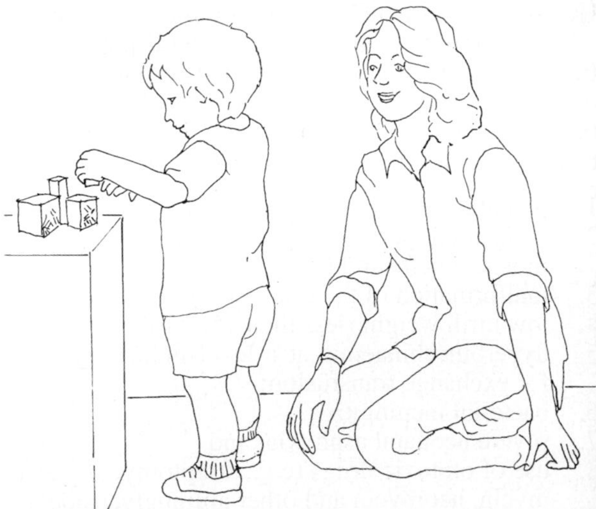

Figure 7.29 The stimulation programme can be developed through integrated activities. The child may be encouraged to stay in standing position, in front of a chair with some selected objects on it, making it possible to be trained in the ability of standing equilibrium. (From SARAH's *Parent Guide to Child Development*, Brazil, 1984)

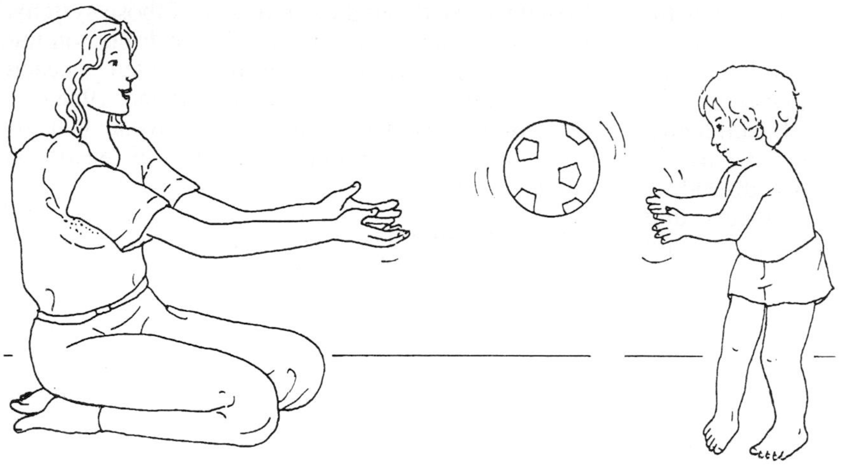

(a)

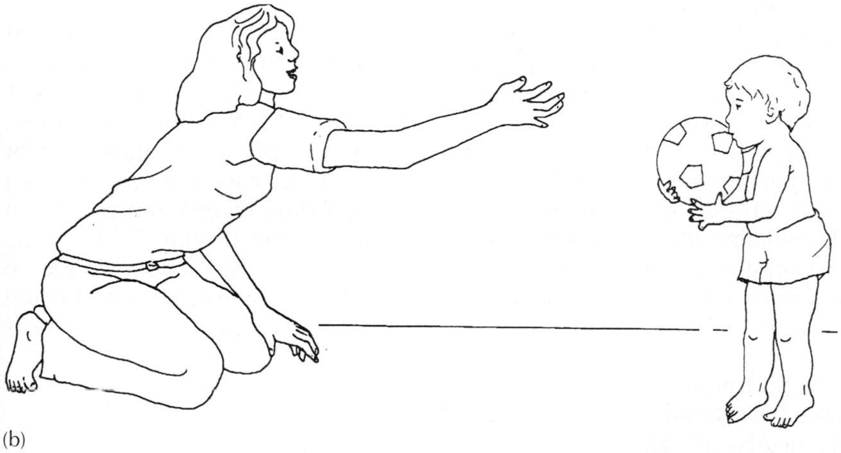

(b)

Figure 7.30 (a) and (b) Motor approach should emphasize active movements through play and games. (From SARAH's *Parent Guild to Child Development*, Brazil, 1984)

(Goodman *et al.*, 1985; Piper *et al.*, 1986) have been unable to demonstrate the efficacy of early intervention. Furthermore, many of the treatment methods are established experimentally with little concern for a conceptual support based on neurophysiology. Clinical experience has shown that early neurological findings can resolve even without therapy, and functional improvement with increasing age can occur without treatment. However, once the diagnosis is established, for the moderately and severely involved children, a comprehensive approach should be started. 'Parents need close contact with someone who understands their problems, gives them something positive to do and can help them to find out and understand the difficulties of their child' (Scrutton, 1984).

Stimulation or enrichment programmes are designed to provide developmental activities to infants who are at risk for conditions (environmentally or biologically caused) that might interfere with their ability to have, in the future, a productive life (Denhoff, 1981). Concerning cerebral damage or maldevelopment, a multidisciplinary approach is required for most cases. Stimulation programmes (usually based on neurodevelopmental therapy – NDT) 'probably work more by avoiding deprivation than by accelerating maturation' (Fox, 1984) (Figures 7.29 and 7.30).

Particularly in children under 5 years of age, the cognitive development in cerebral palsy is negatively influenced by motor disability and consequently sensorial deprivation (Young, 1978). Some aspects of mental retardation in these children can be prevented or even reverted with proper environmental stimulation (Gibbs, 1959). In relation to long-term gains in motor development, further studies are needed to prove the true effectiveness of developmental therapy. Such an approach, however, seems to have a positive effect on social–emotional interaction and integrity of the family of a cerebral-palsy child.

Good results may certainly be achieved if instead of therapists trying to 'normalize' the muscle tone of children with severe cerebral damage or malformation, they should work toward setting realistic functional goals.

Some children will have their equilibrium and co-ordination ameliorated by training. Repetition may improve some movement pattern but all team members working with cerebral palsy must be aware that for children with relevant motor disability, therapists, teachers, rehabilitation engineers and orthotists should work on communication, self-care and mobility.

Ambulatory patients usually need intensive physical therapy or re-establishment of the gait after orthopaedic surgery. In most cases, this intensive programme does not need to continue longer than 3 or 6 months (Bleck, 1987).

Parent training

Several studies support the importance of mother–child attachment for the developmental process of a child (Caldwell, 1967; Spitz, 1979; Rappaport *et al.*, 1981; Braga, 1983) and training of parents to implement stimulation programmes has proved more effective (Browder, 1981). Parents, however, are not always ready to start the programme. Emotional problems, feelings of incompetence to put the programme into practice, or lack of knowledge about the real significance of a chronic, irreversible brain lesion may interfere with their participation in the process. Explanations about the pathology with words that can be easily understood, proper orientation about each activity that should be performed at home, psychological support and home visits aiming to fit the programme to the family needs, are all factors that will influence the final result regardless of the treatment method.

Communication

In the case of brain damage, depending on the type and severity of motor involvement, the child may lack the muscle control for functional speech.

The vocalizing of recognizable sounds by 2 years of age is an indicator of good prognosis for language development. Poor head control is usually associated with poor speech (Bleck, 1982).

Language and cognition have a reciprocal relationship. When speech is not present, depending on the age and cognitive level, augmentative communication systems such as pointing, eye contact, facial expressions, manual sign languages, picture and symbol displays, computers and print-voice synthesizer will be helpful until speech develops or by providing an alternative to speech if it does not develop. A speech pathologist or an experienced teacher should help to select the communication system that can be tested for each child. Parents are often concerned that the use of any of those systems may inhibit the development of speech but, on the contrary, the devices seem to facilitate speech development (McNaughton, 1982; Shane, 1988).

Surveys of persons with severe physical handicaps have pointed out a priority of needs as follows:

- communication;
- independence in daily living activities;
- mobility (Figure 7.31); and
- walking (LeBlanc, 1982).

Thus, providing an alternative in speech for children with severe motor disability must be considered the first objective of any treatment programme.

Seating

A properly seated child has decreased abnormal muscle tone, better control of both hands, improvement of drooling and more ability to concentrate on the various activities rather than be concerned about body orientation in space. Moreover, management and transportation will be easier. Even children with the most severe forms of cerebral palsy can be seated in a special seating (Figure 7.32). Some of them may require surgery such as adductor release to prevent hip dislocation, hamstring lengthening to allow hip flexion, and correction of scoliosis in a small group (Rang *et al.*, 1981).

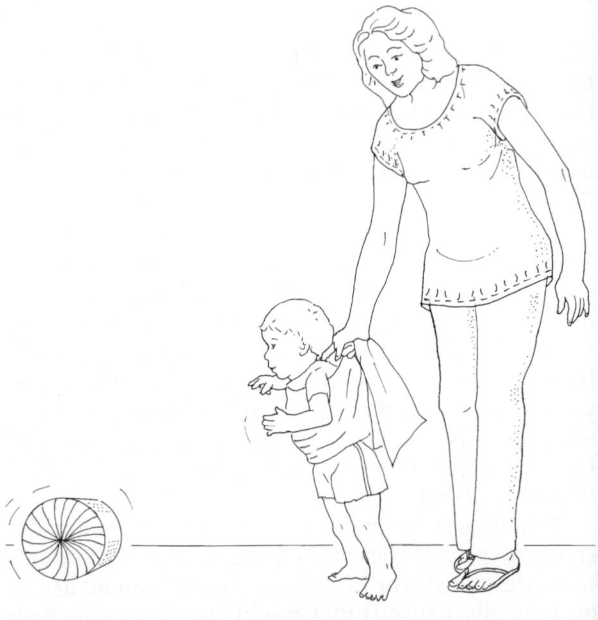

Figure 7.31 Gait training, after achieving standing equilibrium, with support.

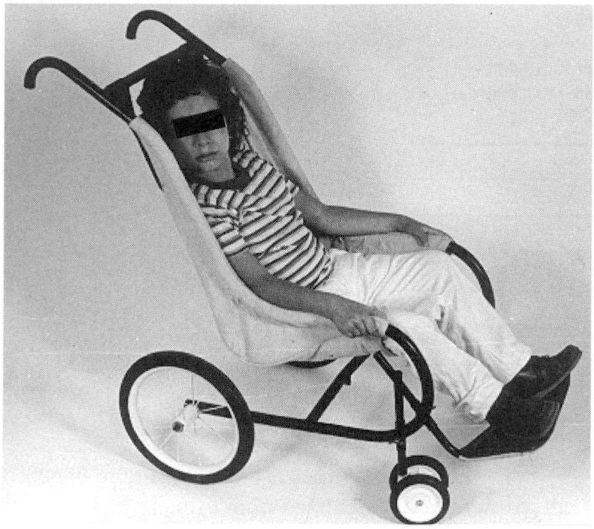

Figure 7.32 Depending on the degree of motor deficiency and cognitive level, strollers can be helpful. Whenever it is possible, the objective should be to give the child independence in locomotion by using hand-driven or power-driven wheelchairs.

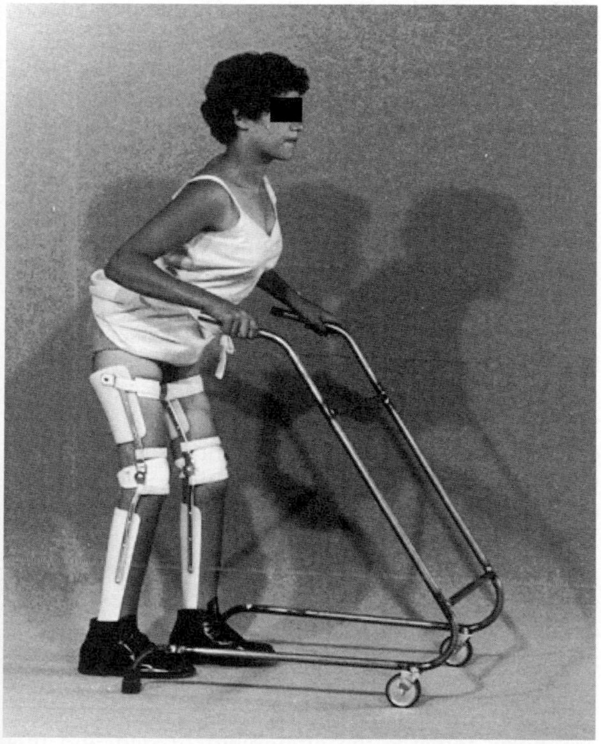

Figure 7.33 The indication of walkers are for children who lack sufficient equilibrium. Some children use this kind of mobility device for a limited time period because as the improvement of balance occurs, they are able to walk independently.

Walking aids and mobility

To promote ambulation, depending on the degree of dysequilibrium, the use of crutches, canes or walkers may be indicated. For children who have not developed functional walking, any means of mobility (e.g. tricycles, bicycles with training wheels, hand or power-driven wheelchairs) should be provided aiming more independence, and community integration (Figure 7.33).

Bracing

In bracing a child with cerebral palsy, the following facts should be understood:

1. Brace design had its origin on the treatment of poliomyelitis in which the aim was to support an unstable joint due to a lower neuron lesion.
2. The natural history of deformities in cerebral palsy, being more complex than in other neurological disorders, must be understood.
3. The mass production of brace components triggered off the need for customizing – fitting – demanding qualified technicians and when it is possible, rehabilitation engineers.

Concerning the prevention of deformities, Sharrard (1976) found that the brace delayed deformities, but no longer than one year, and also concluded that a brace has very little place in the management of cerebral palsy. In a study of 131 patients, the following goals were studied: decrease of progression of deformities; and marked improvement or even achievement of gait. Irrespective of time, long or short leg braces did not produce significant results up to 4 years (Campos da Paz *et al.*, 1983). Upper limb orthoses do not seem to improve function or correct contractures and there are no data to support the efficacy of splinting of the hand aiming to prevent deformities (Bleck, 1987; Koman *et al.*, 1990a). Thus, the use of braces in cerebral palsy might be more related to the demand for some sort of treatment or pressure coming from parents or society. Nevertheless, clinical experience frequently shows that some children can benefit from using a splint, especially if the main objective is to improve stability (Figure 7.34).

The latest development in materials, mainly plastics, injection and moulding techniques, computer design, and robotics have opened the route to a totally different approach to orthoses. However, these advances are still not fully available. From a biomechanical point of view, the difficulty is mainly related to design – the task to match an instant joint centre of movement and the splint centre of rotation.

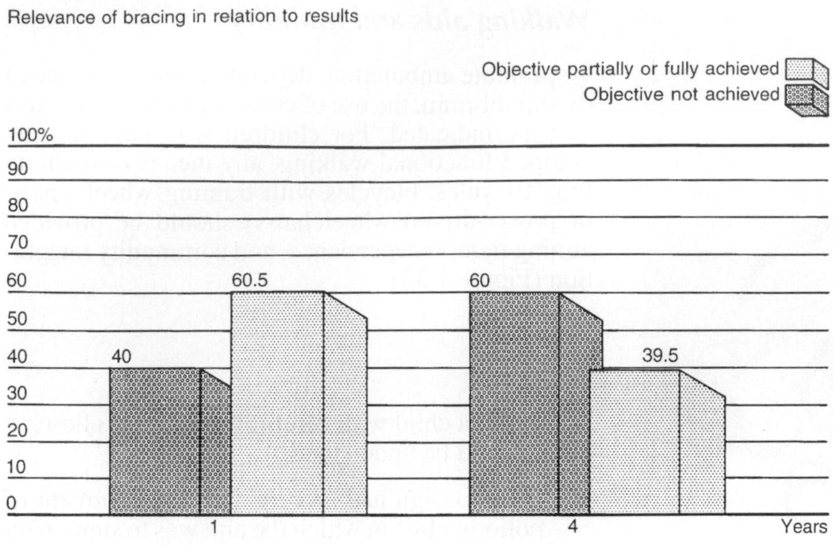

Figure 7.34 Short-term benefit obtained from using braces is reduced with time.

The main indications for bracing in cerebral palsy are:

1. Early postoperative stages to induce early walking.
2. Following cast manipulation and myoneural blocking to postpone tendon lengthening or tendon transfers on the foot.

Drug therapy

Dantrolene, diazepam, and baclofen are the drugs commonly used to control spasticity. However, in children with cerebral palsy these drugs were not found to have any substantial benefits. Dantrolene sodium causes mild to moderate generalized muscle weakness in some patients and is toxic to the liver. Side-effects, such as dizziness, weakness, somnolence, and learning disability, have limited the use of diazepam, which may still be of value in some circumstances (e.g. postoperative care). Baclofen has proved to be effective only in spasticity due to spinal cord lesions (Hudgson and Weightman, 1971; MacDonell *et al.*, 1989; Ochs *et al.* , 1989).

ORTHOPAEDIC AND SURGICAL MANAGEMENT

Eggers in 1963 stated that: 'the ability of a muscle to participate in the movement of more than one joint and to stabilize one joint and move the other signifies a complex mechanism. One must accept the evidence of these complicated dynamics even though he cannot analyze them scientifically and physiologically.' The accumulated experience has now shown that results considered as satisfactory in short-term follow-up tend to deteriorate in time. In our review of 274 patients submitted to surgical treatment from 1966 to 1983, the relapse rate of a deformity, at 4 years postoperation, was found to be around 35% after such procedures as hamstring and Achilles tendon lengthening. The results of hip, knee and foot interventions were dependent on the topography of motor involvement and on the cognitive level. Children with lower motor neuron and cognitive lesions had smaller postoperative gain (Campos da Paz *et al.*, 1983).

The major difficulty in the treatment of a child with cerebral palsy is related to the poor understanding of the changing relationship between growth and muscle imbalance. Furthermore the tendency to misinterpret spasticity as strength contributes to place surgical procedures, in many cases, on the borderlines of experimentation. The orthopaedic surgeon must be aware that when transferring a tendon in cerebral palsy he or she is in fact changing the point of application of a spastic muscle. This may explain the high incidence of unexpected results.

Surgery in cerebral palsy can nevertheless be performed with some degree of success. With complete preoperative analysis, objectives clearly defined according to neurological potential, appropriate surgical techniques and postoperative care, fair results can be achieved.

The spastic quadriplegic patients display a worse prognosis towards the attainment of gait and this justifies a smaller percentage of surgical procedures in this population. For this group, the aims would be basically to gain better sitting and hygiene through improvement of hip abduction.

Spastic diplegia and hemiplegia are the groups in

which surgeries are more frequently carried out aiming at improvement of gait. The most common surgical procedures, which are still of value in the ambulatory child are presented on Table 7.6. Some procedures may be performed under the same anaesthesia. In some circumstances, it is better to proceed gradually, preventing overcorrection and long-term immobilization.

The ambulatory child

The examination of a physically handicapped child on a stretcher may lead to wrong conclusions, which are fundamentally related to the complex interaction of deformities in movement. Frequently, the function observed on an examination table does not occur when the child walks. Only the assessment of the altered movements allows the establishment of a more adequate treatment programme.

Auxiliary assessment techniques

Due to the unexpected results with surgical procedures in cerebral palsy, auxiliary techniques to analyse and simulate situations may be extremely helpful.

Myoneural blocks, under general anaesthesia, may be done by injecting the belly of the muscle with 50% alcohol. Care must be taken to avoid summation of an excessive alcohol dose and anaesthetic effects. The injection points are better determined with the use of an electric stimulator to observe the muscular action. The alcohol reduces the stretch reflex, probably by altering the sensitivity of the muscle spindle receptors. The effects last for 2–6 weeks, sufficient time for proper evaluation and gait analysis. Recent studies using botulinum toxin demonstrate a tendency in improve these techniques (Koman *et al.*, 1990b).

The use of different orthoses to impinge joint movement or to compensate for deformity, frequently needed in equinus, has proved to be helpful mainly to block the interaction of the deformities or even to establish the more appropriate time for surgical intervention.

Motion analysis

The motion analysis represents the difference between a subjective personal evaluation and the quantification of data. This permits a more precise judgement facilitating the decision-making process and follow-up. Non-quantitative gait analysis can be performed with a simple slow motion study recorded with a commercial home TV equipment. Goniometry, dynamic EMG and force-plates are instruments that allow the quantification of data. They complement the study but are not mandatory. Slow motion can bring a great amount of information contributing to more accuracy to the decision-making process. With the development of technology – digital TV and TV photo capture – we are entering a time in which image recording can be an everyday instrument of an out-patient clinic.

The spastic gait is related to the following deformities: hip flexion, hip adduction, knee flexion, pes valgus, pes varus and equinus of the ankle.

Hip flexion

The iliopsoas muscle is the main flexor of the hip. When a flexion deformity is over 20°, physiological lordosis is increased. With an associated fixed knee flexion, a Z-lengthening of the psoas tendon must be combined with lengthening of the medial hamstrings. When this deformity was treated by hamstring transference to the femoral condyle (Eggers, 1952), and lengthening of the Achilles tendon, a crouch gait frequently resulted. Hamstring transfer in cerebral palsy and Achilles tendon lengthening should only be considered after both hip and knee flexion deformities have been reduced by postural measures.

The use of spica plasters after psoas intervention is no longer used because of the need for early and intensive physiotherapy allowing the child to regain early ambulation. The operative correction of any hip flexion deformity must only be performed after a cautious ambulation assessment.

Hip internal rotation

This deformity in gait does not necessarily interfere with performance and represents mainly a cosmetic problem. Therefore derotation osteotomies aimed to correct hip internal rotation are questionable. Depending on the degree of the external tibial fibular compensatory torsion, internal rotational osteotomy of the tibia and fibula have to be carried out if correction of hip internal rotation is undertaken (Figures 7.35 and 7.36).

Hip adductions

Generally, in ambulatory patients, surgery for adduction deformity is indicated when the hip is limited in abduction to 20° or less with flexed knees or when 'scissoring' occurs with gait. When in doubt about the need for surgery, myoneural blocks of the anterior branch of the obturator nerve may be helpful.

Frequently, the final decision must be taken under general anaesthesia. If after a medial hamstring

Table 7.6 The most frequent surgical procedures that are still of value in the ambulatory child*

Procedure	Indication	Expected results	Procedure details	Possible complications	Frequent associated procedures listed with suggested timing (staging)
1. Z-lengthening of the psoas tendon	Flexion deformity of the hip over 20° shifting the centre of gravity forward	Improvement of balance at gait shifting the centre of gravity backwards	Supine position Oblique incision beginning at the anterior superior iliac spine and continuing distally and medially to the level of the lesser trochanter Medial retraction of the femoral nerve vessels Z-lengthening of the tendon Repair stitches at the tendon ends prior to suture Bed rest in prone or supine position for 3 weeks with early bed exercises Immobilization is not necessary	Decrease in hip flexion pull (causing increased difficulty in climbing stairs) Compensatory 'caliper gait' with increased pelvic rotation at swing phase inducing more energy consumption	3, 4, 2, 1, and 6
2. Adductor tenotomy	Scissoring gait causing instability	Improvement of balance	Frog position in supine Longitudinal incision beginning at the origin of adductor longus and continuing along its direction for about 4 cm The adductor longus and the gracilis are isolated and sectioned with electrocoagulator Meticulous haemostasis to avoid haematoma Compressive bandage Plaster only when hamstring lengthening is simultaneously performed	Asymmetrical abduction deformity with pelvic tilt	3, 4, 2, 1, and 6
3. Medial hamstring lengthening	Flexion deformity over 30° during the gait	Increased step length Prevention of patellofemoral pain affecting gait in adolescence	Supine position allowing hip flexion for evaluation of the popliteal angle reduction Incision over the tendon Distal sectioning of the semitendinosus	Patella alta Recurvatum and secondary rotation of the tibia	3, 4, 2, 5, and 6

Table 7.6 Continued

Procedure	Indication	Expected results	Procedure details	Possible complications	Frequent associated procedures listed with suggested timing (staging)
3. Medial hamstring lengthening *(continued)*			Proximal tenotomy of the gracilis The proximal end of the semitendinosus is sutured to the distal end of the gracilis Fractional lengthening of the semimembranosus Long leg plaster for 4 weeks Early walking		
4. Lateral hamstring lengthening (biceps)	Popliteal angle showing insufficient correction after medial release (over 30°)	Increased step length Prevention of patellofemoral pain affecting gait in adolescence	In case of a popliteal angle over 30°, after the medial hamstring lengthening, a fractional lengthening of the biceps must be performed	Patella alta and recurvatum	3, 4 (consecutive if necessary), 2, 5, and 6
5. Distal rectus femoris release	Lack of flexion at swing phase inducing 'caliper gait' EMG studies showing muscle activity throughout the gait cycle	Prevention of patella alta and recurvatum	Supine position Longitudinal incision over the quadriceps tendon above the proximal end of the patella Distal sectioning of the anterior rectus femoris tendon Knee flexion to 90° performing the suture of the tendon to the lateral and medial borders of the vastus medialis and laterallis Long leg plaster for 4 weeks Early walking	Decrease of extension pull inducing relapse of flexion at stance phase	3, 4, 2, 5, and 6
6. Achilles tendon lengthening	Equinus deformity, mainly in boys, difficult to compensate with heel raising Deformities secondary to heel cord shortening (rocker-bottom, valgus and varus feet)	Improvement of gait by increase of step length and decrease of abnormal cadence	Zig-zag incision to minimize scarring Z-lengthening maintaining the foot in neutral position Meticulous closing of the tendon sheath Short leg plaster and/or splintage for 4 weeks Early walking	Insufficient take off with decreased step length (early stages) Progressive crouch gait (late stages)	3, 4, 1, and 6

Prepared by A. M. Nomura MD, paediatric orthopaedic surgeon, SARAH/Instituto Nacional de Medicina do Aparelho Locomotor, Brasília, Brazil.

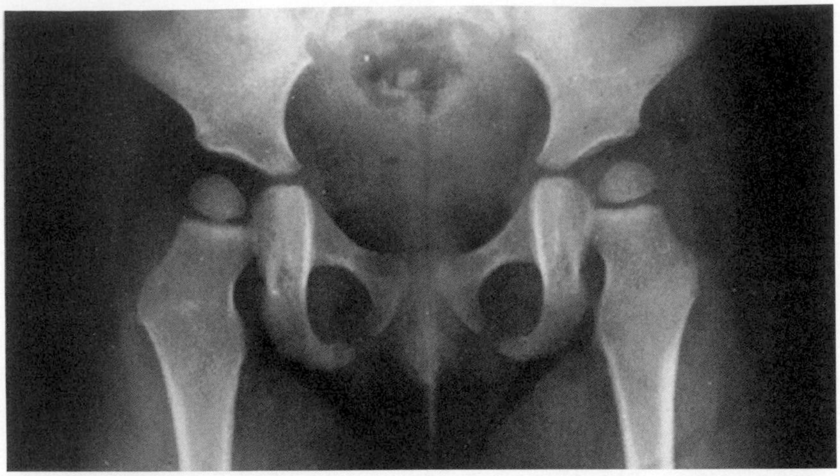

(a)

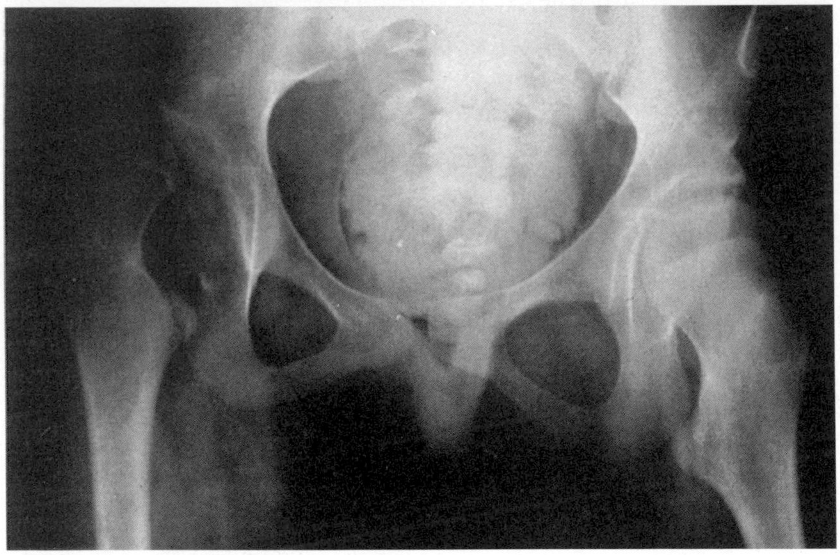

(b)

Figure 7.35 (a) The hip of a spastic diplegic in which there is severe bilateral coxa valga. It was treated at this time by an adductor tenotomy and anterior neurectomy. (b) Dislocation of the right hip has now taken place 8 years following surgery.

lengthening some degree of abduction is obtained, adductor tenotomy should be postponed to avoid an iatrogenic secondary abduction deformity.

A spica plaster cast is now necessary. In the postoperative care, the main objective is to re-establish the gait as soon as possible. The cerebral palsy child loses considerably his performance with any prolonged immobilization.

Outcome studies involves understanding the natural history of the disease, the technical outcome, the functional health assessment and the patients and family satisfaction (Goldberg, 1991).

Subluxation/dislocation of the hip is a frequent complication in children who have total body involvement. Prevention by iliopsoas and adductor tenotomies is most successful when performed before the age of 2–3 years. Recently this complication has been noticed after the procedure of selective posterior rhizotomy and possibly spinal instability may be seen.

When hip dislocation has occurred it is important to ensure success by open operation by achieving complete reduction, good acetabular coverage and restoring some form of muscle balance. Therefore one performs a soft tissue release of adductors/capsule, iliopsoas, open reduction of the hip joint with varus derotation of the femoral neck – often involving a shortening osteotomy – and finally a pelvic osteotomy.

Knee flexion

Excessive energy consumption during walking and standing and the gradual wear and tear of the patellofemoral joint will result from a knee flexion deformity. The indication for medial hamstring lengthening is based upon the popliteal angle. Gait analysis combined with clinical evaluation now

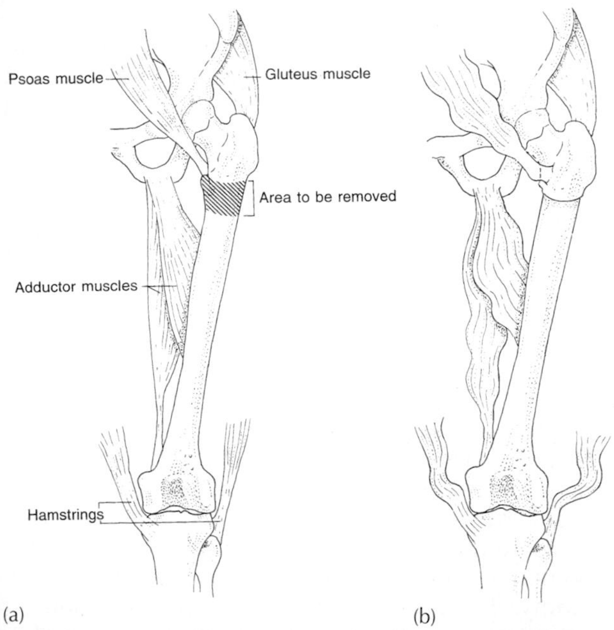

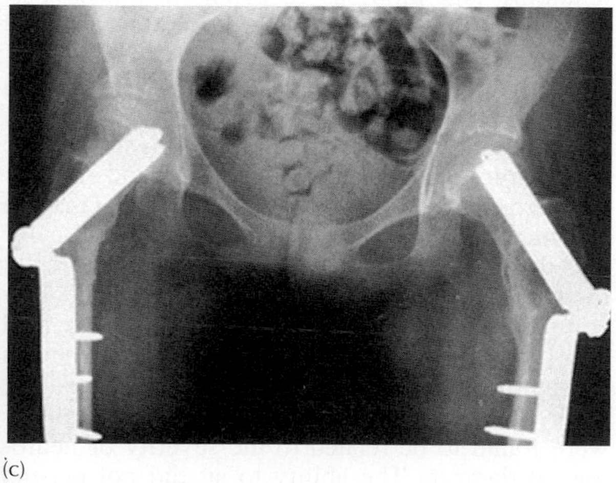

Figure 7.36 (a) It is possible to relieve rotational adduction, hamstring and flexion deformities by femoral shortening with removal of a segment of the femur bilaterally. This is done only in severe involvement. (b) The bone shortening relatively increased the soft tissue functional length. (c) Femoral shortening with removal of the lesser trochanter segment. Both internal fixation and plaster spica immobilization are necessary in the severely affected patients who require this procedure.

show that 30° appears to be the critical point. With an increasing angle, Eggers lengthening must be considered. Knee and hip flexion are common complications due to Achilles tendon overlengthening seen frequently in the crouch gait.

To simplify the surgical procedure, tenotomy of the gracilis is carried out, but maintaining its distal part to which the tenotomized semitendinosus is sutured.

The advantages of medial hamstring release is to decrease the internal rotation pull. If after the lengthening described, the popliteal angle was not decreased, lengthening of the biceps tendon must be considered. The patient is usually lying on his back and the surgeon is carrying out the lengthening procedure through a horizontal plane. Patella alta and recurvatum are not uncommon complications and can be avoided by a distal rectus femoris muscle release procedure. In the postoperative care a long leg plaster for 4 weeks is indicated.

Foot deformities

Farabeuf in studying the movements of the subtalar joint gave a classical description of its unstable condition in the presence of muscle imbalance: 'The calcaneous pitches, turns and rolls under the talus. It pitches and plunges, it rolls on itself like a boat over the waves' (Kapandij, 1974). The recent understanding of the helicoidal movements of the subtalar joint reinforces this important concept. In considering the role of the peroneal, tibialis and triceps muscle in the movements of the hindfoot, correction of fixed varus or valgus depends on achieving a balance of the imbalance (Figure 7.37) by compensating for the

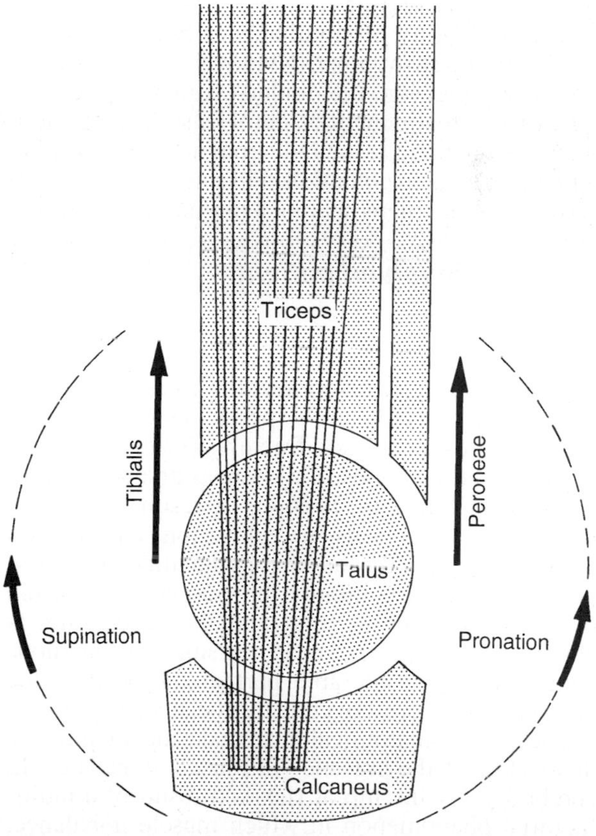

Figure 7.37 The 'calcaneus' joint.

dominance of the spastic muscle groups. Tibialis posterior lengthening, tibialis posterior split techniques with the anchoring of a part of it on the peroneus brevis, peroneal lengthening and Achilles tendon lengthening are all the procedures that are frequently carried out.

When prolonged spasticity produces secondary adaptations, at the appropriate age group, extra-articular or triple arthrodesis may be indicated and often proves to be the definitive procedure.

Equinus is almost always present in early walking. Over a period of time it becomes associated with inversion or eversion of the foot. If possible, the correction of the equinus should be postponed to the last of any surgical programme of a spastic child because overlengthening of the Achilles tendon will increase knee and hip flexion deformities. In the history of cerebral-palsy surgery, equinus was usually the first problem to be tackled. This has proved to be a mistake, producing an embarrassing number of patients with secondary deformities and considerable loss of energy during gait.

The simulation of surgical results with blocking techniques (alcohol) is a most important procedure in the treatment of the spastic foot. The use of plastic splints and intermittent plaster techniques may also be helpful especially to postpone the procedure to a more appropriate time.

The possibility of simultaneous brain and spinal cord lesion due to hypoxia (Clancy *et al.*, 1989), opens a new chapter on the understanding and consequently the treatment of cerebral palsy. The development of magnetic resonance imaging, and sensitive and motor evoked potentials will contribute to a more complete judgement and decision-making process.

The total involved patient

Hip

The unstable hip in cerebral palsy gives rise to pain, to difficult perineal care, to pelvic obliquity, scoliosis, decubitus ulcers, and fractures (Pritchett, 1983). Hip dislocation in these children, as first pointed out by Watson-Jones in 1926, is a result of muscle imbalance, and leads to adduction and flexion contractures, by the adductor and iliopsoas spasticity. In full term infants the normal relationship between the femoral head and the acetabulum is characterized by a large head and small cartilaginous container. A considerable part of the head of the femur is therefore covered by the fibrous capsule. These normal anatomical facts make the hip liable to dislocation in the presence of muscle imbalance. In cerebral palsy the hip at risk is a result of a multifactorial phenomenon in which muscle imbalance, variations in physeal pressure, abnormal growth, all produce gradual incongruence and eventual subluxation interfering with joint stability. Cooke *et al.* (1989) from a large retrospective study of 462 patients have described dislocation as occurring in 10% of all patients with almost all quadriplegias, especially with athetoid features. In patients over the age of 10 years an association with scoliosis was usual especially when the cerebral palsy was severe. The acetabular index was always used as a predictor on radiography.

Sharrard *et al.* (1975) stated that a prophylactic surgical procedure could improve function and control the development of subluxation, and dislocation of the hip, preventing pain. They recommended surgical intervention whenever the range of abduction becomes less than 45°. Kalen and Bleck (1985) reviewed 99 operated patients under the age of five years. Previous surgery was adductor tenotomy with or without neurectomy of the anterior branch of the obturator combined with iliopsoas recession or tenotomy. Better results were found when the adductor tenotomy and iliopsoas recession had been performed on patients who had been ambulatory or had the potential for ambulation, and did not have scoliosis or any pelvic obliquity. The successful cases had been operated upon before the age of 5. Generally, after this age, varus-derotation osteotomy and pelvic osteotomies are required (Figures 7.35 and 7.36).

There are many operative procedures that may be recommended for dislocated hips in cerebral palsy but the question is whether surgery will really facilitate care in the non-walking patient. A study comparing similar groups of treated and untreated total body involved patients with unstable hips showed no significant difference in the frequency of pain or other complications. Pelvic obliquity and scoliosis were found to be related to the severity of neurological damage. The ability to sit did not depend on the status of the hip. Thus, Pritchett (1990) has questioned the usefulness of surgical treatment of an already dislocated hip in patients with severe cerebral palsy.

Long-term studies of patients with untreated congenital dislocation of the hip have shown no real handicap in terms of function for daily living activities up to the fourth or fifth decade. Nevertheless results in treated bilateral congenital dislocation of the hip show that surgical treatment frequently has led to the need for total hip replacement around the fifth or sixth decade. Because hip development and its anatomically liability to dislocate at early stages, early treatment of the hips at risk should be considered. However, the major problem is not related to technical difficulties but to early detection and understanding of the pathomechanics in each case.

The surgeon must be aware that when he or she is able to detect a hip at risk the best moment for the treatment of instability may have been lost. Bony surgery aiming to improve hip containment in the presence of spasticity may increase the joint friction coefficient leading to a painful arthritic hip earlier than one would expect. McHale *et al.* (1990) have described a successful combined operation to decrease pain, increase free movement and to prolong pain free sitting time. It consists of excising the femoral head and supporting the upper femoral segment by a valgus osteotomy.

Spinal deformity

The incidence of scoliosis in cerebral palsy varies from 21% (Balmer and MacEwen, 1970) to 64% (Madigan and Wallace, 1981), depending on the population studied obviously being more frequent in severely involved patients. The curvature in non-ambulatory children is similar to that found in neuromuscular diseases – a long C curve. Although aetiological factors are poorly understood, asymmetrical spinal muscle contractions may play an important role in the mechanism by which this type of scoliosis develops (Bleck) 1987). Despite early diagnosis and conservative treatment the curves tend to progress to a more severe degree than in idiopathic scoliosis and may continue progressing even after skeletal maturity (Sponseller *et al.*, 1986). Severe spinal deformities may be related to disabilities of decreased sitting tolerance, poor sitting balance, back pain and pulmonary impairment (Stanitski *et al.*, 1982).

The use of braces is commonly recommended, aiming to hamper the progression of the curve until the age of 10 years when the arthrodesis can finally be performed but, its effectiveness in cerebral palsy has to be questioned (Bradford, 1987).

Regarding surgical treatment, in spite of the advent of new instruments and techniques, the indications and the methods are still controversial. A careful assessment of each patient is important to evaluate the risks, which are greater in paralytic scoliosis, and to define the rehabilitation potential (Bleck, 1987). Best results are achieved when the curve is less than 60° correction is demonstrated by an x-ray with traction in the lying position. If the pelvic obliquity is not relevant, posterior fusion is sufficient and it is not necessary to include the sacrum. For rigid scoliosis with pronounced pelvic obliquity, surgery in two stages with anterior and posterior fusion including the sacrum, is recommended (Bonnet *et al.*, 1976; Lonstein and Akbarnia, 1983; see Chapter 8).

Upper limb

Concerning the upper extremities, in cerebral-palsy, there are infinite variable patterns of movement, much more complex than the movements observed in the lower limbs during the gait. In the upper limb, the objectives of surgical treatment are frequently related to:

1. improvement of the fingers and wrist extension;
2. improvement of the grasp;
3. increase in active supination;
4. improvement in hygiene; and
5. improvement in the appearance of the hand.

The results are mainly influenced by joint contractures and, to a lesser degree by loss of the sensation of tactile gnosis (Martini, 1986). Severely retarded patients will not achieve good functional results.

The presence of contraction of the multiarticular muscles inhibits voluntary movements of the fingers causing rigidity and profoundly affecting the movement modulation and consequently the total upper limb function. The use of intrinsic muscles can be facilitated by reducing hypertonicity of the multiarticular muscles and by activation of voluntary movements of the fingers. Many patients can then become functionally independent (Matsuo *et al.*, 1990). The classification displayed in Table 7.7 is a good way to assess preoperative and postoperative upper extremity status, aiming to evaluate functional outcome after hand surgery.

In the upper extremity, Samilson and Perry (1975) have emphasized that such conditions as functional dissociation of the limb from body image, lack of cooperation required for re-education, emotional and sensory disorders, cerebellar ataxia or rigidity and athetosis are added difficulties.

The hand is frequently disabled by sensory loss, particularly of spatial relationships. Stereognosis, position sense and two-point discrimination are lost.

It is a matter of interest and speculation as to whether a hand made more functional would in time acquire any sensory usefulness if this sense was deficient to begin with. Green and Banks (1962) showed, in evaluating stereognosis, that there was an

Table 7.7 Hand function classification

Excellent	Good use of hand, effective grasp and release, voluntary control
Good	Helper hand, effective grasp and release, some voluntary control
Fair	Helper hand, no effective use, moderate grasp and release, fair control
Poor	Paperweight, absent grasp and release

From Mowery *et al.* (1985) Upper extremity tendon transfers in cerebral palsy: electromyographic and functional analysis. *Journal of Pediatric Orthopedics* **5**, 69–72.

apparent improvement in this modality of awareness, the only one tested.

Operations on the upper extremity have as their objective the placing of the hand and forearm in a functional position.

Some indications of the paucity of surgery on the cerebral-palsied upper extremity may be gathered from Goldner's experience (1969) of finding surgical indications in 16 out of some 900 cases evaluated. Yet the surgery produced gratifying functional results. It is further evident from examination of the literature and one's own experience that certain fundamentals have slowly evolved.

1. Better results are achieved in the presence of relatively well preserved IQs; this should have been anticipated because those with the better IQs generally have better preservation of motor function, and this type of patient is intellectually aware of the need for rehabilitation.
2. If the wrist can be brought into dorsiflexion and ulnar deviation with the presence of a slight degree of voluntary finger extension, then operative procedures which effectively achieve this attitude will improve hand function with further improvement in finger extension. If forearm supination can be achieved by surgery and training, then improvement of the patient's motor function can be expected; he becomes, at least in part, bimanual.
3. Even a spastic muscle, provided it is partially under voluntary control, will function though its tendon be transferred to achieve another purpose.
4. Better functional results can be expected in hands in which the modalities of sensory awareness are relatively well preserved.

Wrist fusion is now no longer regarded so favourably; indeed, unless the optimum position is accurately determined by preoperative splinting, it may well increase flexor spasm, worsen grip and release, and exaggerate finger and thumb-in-palm deformities (Goldner, 1955). But Eggers and Evans (1963), using a proximal row carpectomy to reduce the tension of the flexors before arthrodesis, believe this to be a most reliable procedure. By placing the wrist in ulnar deviation, either by wrist fusion or tenodesis on the ulnar side, the attitude of the thumb is improved with respect to the remainder of the hand by leaving it away from the main hand mass. This procedure is more often accompanied by cosmetic improvement than are others. The Green adaptation of the Steindler procedure of transfer of the flexor carpi ulnaris into the extensor carpi radialis tendon will achieve dorsiflexion of the wrist and some degree of supination (Green and Banks, 1962). Attempts at transferring the pronators to make them more effective as supinators have not been satisfactory.

Finger deformity

The inability to open the hand and fingers for grasp or release is marked. The spasm in the flexor groups is also seen in the balance between the intrinsics and extensors, which, however, may be weakened. Swan neck deformity is seen not only due to intrinsic plus mechanism but also due to contracture involving the middle bands of the extensor aponeurosis. Therefore interossei releases with tendon grafting and sublimis tenodesis to hold the proximal interphalangeal joints in flexion are indicated (Swanson, 1960).

No procedures have yet been evolved for the effective solution of finger and thumb function. The fingers are difficult enough because of the presence of spasticity of the intrinsics, but some improvement can be achieved by release of the flexor group from the proximal aspect of the ulna and interosseous membrane and permitting the muscle mass to slide distally. This effectively weakens the whole group of flexors and permits the weakened extensors to be brought into play. Transfer of a wrist flexor into the common extensor will also assist in extending the fingers. These procedures will make the hand a holding tool, and, if associated with some degree of active supination, the result is worthwhile functionally, as well as cosmetically.

Thumb deformity

The primary disability results from the adducted, flexed position of 'thumb-in-hand', with a rotational position of the two proximal joints. Inglis *et al.* (1970) described a carefully controlled series of operations for this deformity. They found that the most common procedure was a Z-plasty of the first web space structures with transfer of the flexor carpi radialis tendon through a pulley in abductor pollicis brevis into abductor pollicis longus. This improved grasp in 80%, and pinch in 60%, and 20% had improved pulp-to-pulp pinch. But a prior wrist fusion gave poorer results.

Thompson (1942) advocated fusion of the first two metacarpals in the position of function by bone grafting through the first interosseous space, with the first metacarpal being placed at 90° to the palm. It is also rotated outward from its flexed, adducted and opposed position in the palm. The angle between the first and second metacarpals is made to 45°. This achieves a fixed pincer effect between thumb and index, and although the functional improvement is only slight, any gain is significant.

Lam (1972) has improved this arthrodesis by

using a triangular-shaped cortical graft from the ilium and fixing it in position with a transverse screw. He observed improvement in pinch and opposition in carefully selected spastic patients who had voluntary control of the fingers.

Goldner (1969) described five main patterns of hand and forearm deformities, excluding those with poor sensation, motor power or fixed contractures, which will respond to surgical treatment:

1. The hand with good grasp or release but no contractures except for the thumb in the palm position. Sensation may be poor. Minimal improvement in function as a helper hand can well be achieved by stabilization of the metacarpophalangeal joint of the thumb and plication of the abductor pollicis longus tendon.
2. The hand which cannot actively extend at the wrist or fingers and the thumb pulled into the palm. Spasticity is moderate although the flexor sublimus tendons are overactive. Tactile grasp is good. Arthrodesis of the metacarpophalangeal joint of thumb, transfer of flexor digitorum sublimus tendons through the interosseous membranes into the extensor digitorum longus of fingers or thumb, and transfer of the flexor carpi ulnaris to the extensor carpi radialis brevis to act as a supinator and dorsi flexor will improve function.
3. The hand with greater flexion deformity and inability to extend the digits except when the hand is fully palmar flexed. The thumb is also in the palm. Transfer of flexor carpi ulnaris to the finger extensor with rerouting of the flexor carpi radialis to the extensor pollicis longus and arthrodesis of the metacarpophalangeal of the thumb and even of the wrist may be required for disability.
4. The hand with decreased active wrist flexion and weak finger extensors. The thumb may be hyperextended or lying in the palm. Brachioradialis can be transferred as a wrist flexor and allow extension of the fingers if a motor insertion to them can be provided. An alternative approach is to carry out arthrodesis of the metacarpophalangeal joint of the thumb, plication of abductor pollicis longus, rerouting of extensor pollicis longus and using flexor sublimus longus as a motor.
5. The hand tightly closed with severe flexion deformity of wrist and fingers. Treatment is mainly cosmetic and not functional, with tendon lengthening and arthrodesis of the metacarpophalangeal joint of the thumb and of the wrist joint.

Fortunately, there is little indication for orthopaedic surgical procedures for either the shoulder or elbow. If the hand and forearm can be made functional, and if the patient can be made to employ them, these joints are adequate.

Flexor release

A useful operation to aid the development of hand opening in order to commence grasp is the operation of releasing the flexor origin of the forearm muscles. The long flexor to the thumb may be added where a flexed and adducted thumb remains in the palm. Flexor power overcomes the long extensors of both fingers and thumb, but extensor power must be present as a necessary condition prior to this operation.

The operation was described for the cerebral palsy patient by C.M. Page in 1923 and evaluated by Inglis and Cooper in 1966. Braun *et al.* (1970) extended its use to the hemiplegic stroke patient.

The incision begins on the medial side of the arm well above the medial epicondyle and extends one-half the length of the forearm along the medial border of the ulna. The ulnar nerve is identified. The common origin of the flexors is detached from the medial epicondyle. The flexor carpi ulnaris attachment from the ulna is released. Dissection is continued until the median nerve is exposed. Dissection is sufficient to allow retraction of the common origin 2–5 cm, and it is now recommended that these muscles be sutured to the periosteum of the ulna.

A separate ventral incision identifies the deep flexor of the thumb, with lengthening done in the forearm above the transverse carpal ligament.

A reasonable, but not sensational, improvement can be expected with good follow-through in an active extension programme. The limb is first immobilized with the elbow in flexion for 6 weeks.

Shoulder and elbow deformities

The deformity of adduction, internal rotation and flexion often leads to early contracture but very rarely requires surgery. Indications for surgery are when abduction is less than 45° or external rotation is less than 15° or when there is over 40° fixed flexion deformity at the elbow. Tenotomy of subscapularis, divisions of pectoralis major have all been carried out. Mital (1979) has reported good results from preoperative procaine block – particularly to allow the use of crutches before lengthening the flexors of the elbow joint.

Surgical procedures which are indicated for selected cases are:

1. Transfer of the flexor carpi ulnaris to the extensor carpi radialis longus and/or extensor carpi radialis brevis to obtain some wrist dorsal flexion and grasp (Wenner and Johnson, 1988) as described by Green.

2. Release of the flexor digitorum profundus, flexor digitorum sublimis and extensor digitorum comunis to facilitate the use of the intrinsic muscles by reducing spasticity of the multiarticular muscles (Matsuo *et al.* 1990).
3. Transfer of the flexor carpi ulnaris to the extensor digitoris comunis to correct wrist flexion deformities.
4. Z-Lengthening of the digitorum superficialis in the forearm to cope with finger flexed deformities.
5. Release of the first dorsal interosseous muscle from the first and second metacarpals and division of the proximal or distal insertions of the adductor pollicis, for adduction deformity of the thumb (Koman *et al.*, 1990a).
6. Arthrodesis of the metacarpophalangeal joint of the thumb as adjunctive treatment of thumb-in-palm deformity aiming at thumb radial grasp – associated with intrinsic muscle lengthening and/or extrinsic tendon transfer (Goldner *et al.* 1990).
7. Wrist fusion aiming at improvement in hygiene and cosmetics (Hoffer and Zeitzew, 1988).
8. Pronator teres tenotomy or pronator teres rerouting to increase active supination of the forearm.

The planning for combined surgical procedures on the upper limb requires an understanding of the interaction of the deformities, the compensatory movements and the objectives to be achieved in each patient. It is mandatory for the surgeon to understand not only the complexity of visual-motor co-ordination, allowing some degree of function even in a deformed limb, but also the importance of body orientation in space for enhancing upper extremity function (Nwaobi, 1987). It is sometimes better to accept a twisted hand as an auxiliary element rather than to embark in elaborate procedures that might lead to a disaster.

The presence of involuntary movements demands a precise judgement before any intervention, and the presence of any sensory loss of profrioception and prehension, i.e. tactile gnosis, also requires consideration and they often mitigate against a reasonable outcome.

Selective dorsal rhizotomy

The main objective of this procedure is to reduce spasticity by decreasing incoming sensory information. The posterior roots from L2 to Sl are isolated bilaterally and each rootlet is stimulated electrically to identify those that show abnormal electromyographic response – tonic muscle contractions and spread of the contraction to muscle groups from other segments. Some of these rootlets are selected to be cut and those that show no reaction or only weak response to stimulation are left intact.

This surgery is better indicated for children with good cognitive level and reasonable motor development. They should have some form of forward locomotion or at least sufficient trunk control with only spasticity. After operation the reduced tone appears to help in walking or other functions as side-sitting or weight-bearing in non-walkers (Peacock *et al.*, 1987). Cahan *et al.* (1990) in studying 14 patients for up to one year postoperation found significant improvement gait patterns of walking speed, stride length and motion of hip, knee and ankle. A 7-year follow-up study of 51 spastic children operated upon between 1981 and 1984 found that the reduction of spasticity has persisted in all cases and sensory disturbances were minimal (Arens *et al.*, 1989). However, further studies are required to determine the true effectiveness or long-term risks of selective dorsal rhizotomy (Neville, 1988).

References

Abercrombie, M.L.J. (1964) In: *Perceptual Visuo-motor Disorders in Cerebral Palsy.* Little Club Clinics in Developmental Medicine II. Edited by M.L.J. Abercrombie. Published by Medical Education and Information Unit of The Spastics Society in association with William Heinemann (Medical Books) Ltd: London

Aicardi, J. (1988) Clinical approach to the management of intractable epilepsy. *Developmental Medicine and Child Neurology* **30**, 429–440

Alberman, E. (1984) Describing cerebral palsies: methods of classifying and counting. In: *The Epidemiology of the Cerebral Palsies. Clinics in Developmental Medicine No. 87*, pp. 27–31. Edited by F. Stanley and E. Alberman. S.I.M.P. with Blackwell Scientific Publications: London/ Lippincott: Philadelphia

Arens, L.J., Peacock, W.J. and Peter, J. (1989) Selective posterior rhizotomy: a long-term follow-up study. *Child's Nervous System* **5**, 148–152

Asirvatham, R., Watts, H.G. and Rooney, R.J. (1990) Rotation osteotomy of the tibia after poliomyelitis. *Journal of Bone and Joint Surgery* **72B**, 409–411

Balmer, G.A. and MacEwen, G.D. (1970) The incidence and treatment of scoliosis in cerebral palsy. *The Journal of Bone and Joint Surgery* **52B**, 134–137

Barr, J.S. and Record, E.E. (1947) *Surgical Clinics of North America* **27**, 281

Bauer, S.B. (1985) Urodynamic evaluation and neuromuscular dysfunction. In: *Clinical Pediatric Urology*, 2nd edn. Edited by P.P. Kelalis, L.R. King and A.B. Bellman

Bax, M.C.O. (1964) Terminology and classification of cerebral palsy. *Developmental Medicine and Child Neurology* **6**, 295–297

Bax, M.C.O. and MacKeith, R. (1975) The paediatric role in the care of the child with cerebral palsy. In: *Orthopaedic Aspects of Cerebral Palsy. Clinics in Developmental Medicine Nos. 52/53*, pp. 26–34. Edited by R.L. Samilson. S.I.M.P. with William Heinemann Medical Books Ltd: London

Beret, F.C. (1974) Paralisis cerebral infantil. In: *Exploracion Clinica Y Semilogia en Neuro-Pediatria*, pp. 149–157. Editorial Espax Publicaciones Medicas: Barcelona

Blair, E. and Stanley, F.J. (1988) Intrapartum asphyxia: a rare cause of cerebral palsy. *Journal of Pediatrics* **112**, 515–519

Bleck, E.E. (1987) In: *Orthopaedic Management in Cerebral Palsy. Clinics in Developmental Medicine No. 99/100*. MacKeith Press with Blackwell Scientific Publications Ltd: Oxford/Lippincott: Philadelphia

Bleck, E.E. (1975) Locomotor prognosis in cerebral palsy. *Developmental Medicine and Child Neurology* **17**, 18–25

Bleck, E.E. (1982) Cerebral palsy. In: *Physically Handicapped Children a Medical Atlas for Teachers*, pp. 59–127. Edited by E.E. Bleck and D.A. Nagel. Grune & Stratton: Orlando'

Blodgett, W.H. and Houtz, S.J. (1960) *Journal of Bone and Joint Surgery* **42A**, 59

Bobath, K. and Bobath, B. (1984) The neuro-developmental treatment. In: *Management of the Motor Disorders of Children with Cerebral Palsy. Clinics in Developmental Medicine No. 90*. pp. 6–18. Edited by D. Scrutton. S.I.M.P. Blackwell Scientific Publications Ltd: Oxford/ Lippincott: Philadelphia

Bodian, D. (1949) In: *Proceedings of the International Polio Congress, 1948*, pp. 62, 78. Lippincott: Philadelphia, PA

Bodian, D. (1952) *American Journal of Hygiene* **55**, 414

Bonnet, C., Brown and Grow, T. (1976) Thoracolumbar scoliosis in cerebral palsy. Results of surgical treatment. *Journal of Bone and Joint Surgery* **58A**, 328–336

Borzyskowski, M. (1989) Cerebral palsy and the bladder. *Developmental Medicine and Child Neurology* **31**, 682–689

Bosworth, D.M., Fielding, J.W., Leibler, W.A., Ishizuka, T., Ikeuchi, W. and Cohen, P. (1960) *Journal of Bone and Joint Surgery* **42A**, 1223

Bowker, J.H. and Halpin, P.J. (1978) Factors determining success in reambulation of the child with progressive muscle dystrophy. *Orthopedic Clinics of North America* **9**, 2–10

Bradford, D.S. (1987) Neuromuscular spinal deformity. In: *Scoliosis and Other Spinal Deformities*, 2nd edn. Edited by J.E. Lonstein, D.S. Bradford, R.B. Winter and J.W. Ogilvie. W.B. Saunders Company: Philadelphia

Braga, L.W. (1983) *O Desenvolvimento cognitivo na Paralisia Cerebral. Um estudo exploratorio*. Master Thesis, University of Brasilia, Brazil

Braun, R.M. Mooney, V. and Nickel, V.L. (1970) Flexor origin release for pronation flexion deformity of the forearm and hand in stroke patients. *Journal of Bone and Joint Surgery* **52A**, 902–920

Brody, B.A., Kinney, H.C., Kloman, A.S. and Gilles, F.H. (1987) Sequence of central nervous system myelination in human infancy. I. An autopsy study of myelination. *Journal of Neuropathology and Experimental Neurology* **46**, 283–301

Browder, J.A. (1981) The pediatrician's orientation to infant stimulation programs. *Pediatrics* **67**, 42–44

Bunnell, S. (1938) *Journal of Bone and Joint Surgery* **20**, 275

Cahan, L.D., Adams, J.M., Perry, J. and Beeler, L.M. (1990) Instrumental gait analysis after selective dorsal rhizotomy. *Developmental Medicine and Child Neurology* **32**, 1037–1043

Caldwell, B.M. (1967) What is the optimal learning environment for young children. *American Journal of Orthopsychiatry* **26**, 8–21

Campbell, W.C. (1923) *Journal of Bone and Joint Surgery* **5**, 815

Campos da Paz Jr, A., Nomura, A.M., Braga, L.W., Burnett, S.M. (1983) Cerebral palsy: a retrospective study. Paper, presented at the Autumn Meeting of The British Orthopaedic Association, Nottingham, England

Campos da Paz Jr, A., Burnett, S.M., Braga, L.W. (1994) Walking prognosis in cerebral palsy: a 22-year retrospective analysis. *Developmental Medicine and Child Neurology* **36**, 130–134

Cashman, N.R. (1992) Polio, including postpolio syndrome: facts and myths. *Current Opinion in Orthopedics* **3**, 224–228

Chasnoff, I.J., Burns, W.J., Schnoll, S.H., Burns, K.A. (1985) Cocaine use in pregnancies. *New England Journal of Medicine* **313**, 666–669

Chusid, J.G. (1985) In: *Correlative Neuroanatomy and Functional Neurology*. Lange Medical Publications: Los Altos, CA

Clancy, R.R., Sladky, J.T. and Rorke, L.B. (1989) Hypoxic-ischemic spinal cord injury following perinatal asphyxia. *Annals of Neurology* **25**, 185–189

Clark, J.M.P. (1946) *British Journal of Surgery* **34**, 180

Cooke, P.H., Cole, W.G. and Carey, R.P. (1989) Dislocation of the hip in cerebral palsy: natural history and predictability. *Journal of Bone and Joint Surgery* **71B**, 441–446

Cox, L.C. (1988) Screening the high-risk newborn for hearing loss: the Crib-O-Gram V the auditory brainstem response. *Infants and Young Children* **1**, 71–81

Crysdale, W.S. (1982) Submandibular duct relocation for drooling. *Journal of Otolaryngology* **11**, 286–288

Cwik, V.A. and Brooke, M.H. (1992) Recent advances in diagnosis and treatment of Duchenne muscular dystrophy. *Current Opinion in Orthopedics* **3**, 218–223

Decter, R.M., Bauer, S.B., Khoshbin, S. *et al.* (1987) Urodynamic assessment of children with cerebral palsy. *Journal of Urology* **138**, 1110–1112

Denhoff, E. (1976) In: *Cerebral Palsy a Developmental Disability*. Edited by W.M. Cruickshank. Syracuse University Press: Syracuse

Denhoff, E. (1981) Current status of infant stimulation or enrichment programs for children with developmental disabilities. *Pediatrics* **67**, 32–37

De Silva, S., Drackman, D.B., Mellitis, D. and Kunci, R.W. (1987) Prednisone treatment in Duchenne muscular dystrophy. *Archives of Neurology* **44**, 818–822

De Sousa, C. (1991) Cerebral palsy: new perspectives on its origins, complications and treatment. *Current Opinion in Orthopedics* **2**, 263–268

Dowben, R.M. (1961) *Archives of Internal Medicine* **107**, 430

Dubowitz, V. (1991) Prednisone in Duchenne dystrophy. *Neuromuscular Disorders* **1**, 161–163

Dunn, N. (1922) On stabilising operations in the treatment of paralytic deformities of the foot. *Proceedings of the Royal Society of Medicine* **15**, 14–22

Eggers, G.W.N. (1952) Transplantation of hamstring tendons to femoral condyles in order to improve hip extension and to decrease knee flexion in cerebral spastic paralysis. *Journal of Bone and Joint Surgery* **34A**, 827–830

Eggers. G.W.N. and Evans, E.B. (1963) Surgery in cerebral palsy. *Journal of Bone and Joint Surgery* **45A**, 1275–1305

Elmslie, R.C. (1934) *Modern Operative Surgery*. Cassell: London

L'Episcopo, J.B. (1934) Tendon transplantation in obstetrical paralysis. *American Journal of Surgery* **25**, 122

Feagans, L. (1983) A current view of learning disabilities. *Journal of Pediatrics* **102**, 487–493

Fee, M.A., Charney, E.B. and Robertson, W.W. (1988) Nutritional assessment of the young child with cerebral palsy. *Infants and Young Children* **1**, 33–40

Forgan, L. and Munsat, T.L. (1974) Spinocerebellar degenerative disease. In: *Spinal Deformity in Neurological and Muscular Disorders*. Edited by J.H. Hardy. C.V. Mosby: St Louis, MO

Fox, A.M. (1984) Does infant stimulation work? *Modern Medicine of Canada* **39**, 1045–1053

Gardner, E. (1958) *Journal of Bone and Joint Surgery* **40A**, 831

Geary, N. (1984) Late surgical decompression for compartment syndrome of the forearm. *Journal of Bone and Joint Surgery* **66B**, 745–748

Gibbs, N. (1959) Some learning difficulties of cerebral palsied children. *Spastics Quarterly* **8**, 21–23

Gilbert, A., Brockam, R. and Carlioz, H. (1991) Surgical treatment of brachial plexus birth injury. *Clinical Orthopaedics and Related Research* **264**, 39–47

Goldberg, M.J. (1991) Measuring outcomes in cerebral palsy. *Journal of Pediatric Orthopedics* **11**, 682

Goldner, J.L. (1955) *Journal of Bone and Joint Surgery* **37A**, 1141

Goldner, J.L. (1969) Reconstructive surgery of the upper extremity affected by cerebral palsy or brain or spinal cord trauma. *Current Practice in Orthopaedic Surgery* **3**, 124–138

Goldner, J.L., Koman, L.A., Gelberman R., Levin, S. and Goldner, R.D. (1990) Arthrodesis of the metacarpophalangeal joint of the thumb in children and adults. Adjunctive treatment of thumb-in-palm deformity in cerebral palsy. *Clinical Orthopaedics and Related Research* **253**, 75–89

Goodman, M., Rothberg, A.D. and Houston-McMillan, J.E. (1985) Effects of early neurodevelopmental therapy in normal and at risk survivors of neonatal intensive care. *Lancet* **14**, 1237–1330

Green, W.T. (1949) *Journal of Bone and Joint Surgery* **31A**, 485

Green, W.T. and Banks, H.H. (1962) *Journal of Bone and Joint Surgery* **44A**, 1343

Grice, D.S. (1952) *Journal of Bone and Joint Surgery* **34A**, 927

Griggs, C.A., Jones, P.M. and Lee, R.E. (1989) Videofluorscopic investigation of feeding disorders of children with multiple handicap. *Developmental Medicine and Child Neurology* **31**, 303–308

Hagberg, B., Hagberg, G. and Olow, I. (1975) The changing panorama of cerebral palsy in Sweden 1954–1970 I. Analysis of the general changes. *Acta Paediatrica Scandinavica* **64**, 187–192

Harris, S.R. (1987) Early neuromotor predictors of cerebral palsy in low-birthweight infants. *Developmental Medicine and Child Neurology* **29**, 508–519

Herschkowitz, N. (1988) Brain development in the fetus, neonate and Infant. *Biology of the Neonate* **54**, 1119

Hinman, A.R., Foege, W.H., de Quadros, C.A. *et al.* (1987) The case for global eradication of poliomyelitis. *Bulletin of the World Health Organization* **65**, 835–840

Hirschhorn, K. (1987) Chromosomes and their abnormalities. In: *Nelson Textbook of Pediatrics*. Edited by V.C. Vaughan. W.B. Saunders Company: Philadelphia, PA

Hoffer, M.M. and Zeitzew, S. (1988) Wrist fusion in cerebral palsy. *Journal of Hand Surgery* **13A**, 667–670

Hoffman, E.P., Brown, R.H. and Kunkel, L.M. (1987) Dystrophin: the protein product of the Duchenne muscular dystrophy locus. *Cell* **1**, 919–928

Hohmann, L.B. (1953) Intelligence levels in cerebral palsied children. *American Journal of Physical Medicine* **32**, 284–290

Horstmann, D.M. (1952) *Proceedings of the Society for Experimental Biology and Medicine* **79**, 417

Horstmann, D.M. and McCollum, C. (1953) *Science* **82**, 434

Hudgson, P. and Weightman, D. (1971) Baclofen in the treatment of spasticity. *British Medical Journal* **4**, 15–17

Inglis, A.E. and Cooper, W. (1966) Release of flexor pronator origin of the hand and wrist in spastic paralysis. *Journal of Bone and Joint Surgery* **48A**, 847–857

Inglis, A.E., Cooper, W. and Bruton, R. (1970) Surgical correction of thumb deformities in spastic paralysis. *Journal of Bone and Joint Surgery* **52A**, 253–268

Irwin, C.E. (1947) *Journal of the American Medical Association* **133**, 231

Jahnke, A.H., Bovill, D.F., McCarroll, H.R., James, P. and Ashley, R.K. (1991) Persistent brachial plexus birth palsies. *Journal of Pediatric Orthopedics* **11**, 533–537

Joint Committee on Infant Hearing (1982) Position statement. *Pediatrics* **70**, 496–497

Jones, K.L. (1988) In: *Recognizable Patterns of Human Malformations*, 4th edn. Edited by W. Smith. W.B. Saunders Company/Harcourt Brace Jovanovich, Inc.: London/Philadelphia

Jones, P.M. (1989) Feeding disorders in children with multiple handicaps. *Developmental Medicine and Child Neurology* **31**, 398–406

Kahkonen, M., Leisti, J., Thoden, C-J. and Autis, S. (1986) Frequence of rare fragile sites among mentally subnormal school children. *Clinical Genetics* **30**, 234–238

Kalen, V. and Bleck, E.E. (1985) Prevention of spastic paralytic dislocation of the hip. *Developmental Medicine and Child Neurology* **27**, 17–24

Kanar, H.L. (1976) Dental characteristics. In: *Cerebral Palsy a Developmental Disability*, pp. 343–368. Edited by W.M. Cruickshank. Syracuse University Press: Syracuse

Kapandji, I.A. (1974) In: *The Physiology of the Joints*. Translated by L.H. Honore. Churchill Livingstone: Edinburgh, London and New York

Kaplan, E.B. (1958) *Journal of Bone and Joint Surgery* **40A**, 817

Kinney, H.C., Broddy, B.A., Klonan, A.S. and Gilles, F.H. (1988) Sequence of central nervous system myelination in human infancy. *Journal of Neuropathology and Experimental Neurology* **47**, 217–234

Koenig, M. and Kunkel, L.M. (1990) Detailed analysis of the repeat domain of dystrophin reveals potential hind segments that may confer flexibility. *Journal of Biological Chemistry* **265**, 4560–4566

Koheil, R., Sochaniwiskyj, A.E., Bablich, K., Kenny, D.J. and Milner, M. (1987) Biofeedback techniques and behavior modification in the conservative remediation of drooling by children with cerebral palsy. *Developmental Medicine and Child Neurology* **29**, 19–26

Koman, L.A., Gelberman, R.H., Toby, E.B. and Poehling, G.G. (1990a) Cerebral palsy management of the upper extremity. *Clinical Orthopaedics and Related Research* **253**, 62–74

Koman, L.A., Nicastro, J.F., Smith, B.P., Goodman, A.R. and Mooney, J.F. (1990b) *Cerebral Palsy Management by Neuromuscular Blockade with Botulinum-A Toxin*. Paper, presented at the Combined Meeting of the Paediatric Orthopaedic Society of North America/European Paediatric Orthopaedic Society, Montreal, Canada

Lagergren, J. (1981) Children with motor handicaps. *Acta Paediatrica Scandinavica* **Supplement 289**.

Lam, S.J.S. (1972) A modified technique for stabilising the spastic thumb. *Journal of Bone and Joint Surgery* **54B**, 522–525

Lau, J.H.K., Parker, J.C., Hsu, L.C.S. and Leong, J.C.Y. (1986) Paralytic hip instability in poliomyelitis. *Journal of Bone and Joint Surgery* **68B**, 528–533

LeBlanc, M. (1982) Systems and devices for nonoral communication. In: *Physically Handicapped Children. A Medical Atlas for Teachers*, pp. 159–169. Edited by E.E. Bleck, and D.A. Nagel. Grune & Stratton, Inc.: Orlando, FL

Lonstein, J.E. and Akbarnia, B.A. (1983) Operative treatment of spinal deformities in patients with cerebral palsy or mental retardation. *Journal of Bone Joint Surgery* **65A**, 43–55

MacDonell, R.A.L., Talalla, A., Swash, M. and Grundy, D. (1989) Intrathecal baclofen and the H-reflex. *Journal of Neurology, Neurosurgery and Psychiatry* **52**, 1110-1112

McHale, K.A., Bagg, M. and Nason, S.S. (1990) Treatment of the chronically dislocated hip in adolescents with cerebral palsy with femoral head resection and subtrochanteric valgus osteotomy. *Journal of Pediatric Orthopedics* **10**, 504–509

Mackenzie, I.G. (1959) *Journal of Bone and Joint Surgery* **41B**, 738

McKusick, V.A. (1988) In: *Mendelian Inheritance in Man Catalogs of Autosomal Dominant, Autosomal Recessive, and X-Linked Phenotypes*. The Johns Hopkins University Press: Baltimore and London

McNaughton, S. (1982) Augmentative Communication System: Blissymbolics. In: *Physically Handicapped Children. A Medical Atlas for Teachers*, pp. 146–158. Edited by E.E. Bleck, and D.A. Nagel. Grune & Stratton, Inc.: Orlando, FL

McNeal, D.M., Hawtrey, C.E., Wolraich, M.L. and Mapel, J.R. (1983) Symptomatic neurogenic bladder in a cerebral-palsied population. *Developmental Medicine and Child Neurology* **25**, 612–616

Madigan, R.R. and Wallace, S.L. (1981) Scoliosis in the institutionalized cerebral palsy population. *Spine* **6**, 583–590

Martini, A.K. (1986) Critical evaluation of the results following corrective operations of the spastic hand. *Zeitschrift fur Orthopadie und ihre Grenzgebiete* **124**, 173–178

Matsuo, T. and Tayama, N. (1990) Combined flexor and extensor release for activation of voluntary movement of the fingers in patients with cerebral palsy. *Clinical Orthopaedics and Related Research* **250**, 185–193

Mayer, L. (1931) *Journal of Bone and Joint Surgery* **13**, 1

Mehta, S.N. and Mukerjee, A.K. (1991) Flexion osteotomy of the femur for genu recurvatum after osteomyelitis. *Journal of Bone and Joint Surgery* **73B**, 200–202

Miller, F. and Moseley, C. (1985) Treatment of spinal deformity in Duchenne muscular dystrophy. *Orthopaedic Transactions* **9**, 125–130

Minear, W.L. (1956) A classification of cerebral palsy. *Pediatrics* **18**, 841–852

Miranda, S. (1979) *Outcomes of Spastic Diplegia*. Unpublished study. Children's Hospital at Stanford, Palo Alto

Mital, M.A. (1979) Lengthening of the elbow flexors in cerebral palsy. *Journal of Bone and Joint Surgery* **61A**, 515–522

Mitchell, G.P. (1952) *Lancet* **2**, 451

Molnar, G.E. (1979) Cerebral palsy: prognosis and how to judge it. *Pediatric Annals* **8**, 596–606

Monreal, F.J. (1985) Consideration of genetic factors in cerebral palsy. *Developmental Medicine and Child Neurology* **27**, 325–330

Mowery, C.A., Gelberman, R.H. and Rhoades, C.E. (1985) Upper extremity tendon transfers in cerebral palsy: electromyographic and functional analysis. *Journal of Pediatric Orthopedics* **5**, 69–72

Munsat, T.L. (1991) Poliomyelitis: new problems with an old disease. *New England Journal of Medicine* **324**, 1206–1207

Munsat, T.L., Baloh, R., Pearson, C.M. *et al.* (1974) *Journal of the American Medical Association* **226**, 1536

Mustard, W.T. (1952) *Journal of Bone and Joint Surgery* **34A**, 647

Mustard, W.T. (1959) *Journal of Bone and Joint Surgery* **41B**, 289

Nelson, K.B. and Ellenberg, J.H. (1981) Apgar scores as predictors of chronic neurologic disability. *Pediatrics* **68**, 36–43

Nelson, K.B. and Ellenberg, J.H. (1982) Children who outgrew cerebral palsy. *Pediatrics* **69**, 529–539

Nelson, K.B. and Ellenberg, J.H. (1985) Antecedents of cerebral palsy. I. Univariate analysis of risks. *American Journal of Diseases in Children* **139**, 1031–1038

Nelson, K.B. and Ellenberg, J.H. (1986) Antecedents of cerebral palsy. Multivariate analysis of risk. *New England Journal of Medicine* **315**, 81–86

Nelson, T.M. (1962) A study comparing visual and visual-motor perceptions of unimpaired, defective and spastic cerebral palsied children. Abstract. In: *Perceptual and Visuo-motor Disorders in Cerebral Palsy*. Little Club Clinics in Developmental Medicine II. Edited by M.L.J. Abercrombie. (1964) Published by The Spastics Society Medical Education and Information Unit in association with William Heinemann (Medical Books) Ltd.: London

Neville, B.G.R. (1988) Selective dorsal rhizotomy for spastic cerebral palsy. *Developmental Medicine and Child Neurology* **30**, 395–398

Nwaobi, O.M. (1987) Seating orientations and upper extremity function in children with cerebral palsy. *Physical Therapy* **67**, 1209–1212

Ober, F.R. (1944) AAOS Instructional Course Lectures **1**, 274–276

Ochs, G., Struppler, A., Meyerson, B.A. *et al.* (1989) Intrathecal baclofen for long-term treatment of spasticity a multi-centre study. *Journal of Neurology, Neurosurgery and Psychiatry* **52**, 933–939

Paneth, N. and Kiely, J. (1984) The frequency of cerebral palsy: a review of population studies in industrialized nations since 1950. In: *The Epidemiology of the Cerebral Palsies. Clinics in Developmental Medicine No. 87*, pp. 46–56. Edited by F. Stanley, and E. Alberman. S.I.M.P. with Blackwell Scientific Publications: London/ Lippincott: Philadelphia

Pape, K.E. and Wigglesworth, J.S. (1979) Hemorrhage, ischemia and the perinatal brain. *Clinics in Developmental Medicine. Nos. 69/70.* William Heinemann: London

Partridge, T.A. (1991) Myoblast transfer: a possible therapy for inherited myopathies? *Muscle and Nerve* **14**, 197–212

Paul, W.D. (1955) Medical management of contractures in muscular dystrophy. Proceedings of the Third Medical Conference of the Muscular Dystrophy Association of America, New York, 1954. *American Journal of Physical Medicine* **34**, 172–179

Peacock, W.J., Arens, L.J. and Berman, B. (1987) Cerebral palsy spasticity. Selective posterior rhizotomy. *Pediatric Neuroscience* **13**, 61–66

PHLS Communicable Disease Surveillance Centre (1986) *British Medical Journal (Clinical Research Edition)* **293**, 195–196

Piper, M.C., Kunos, V.I., Willis, D.M., Mazer, B.L., Ramasay, M. and Silver, K.M. (1986) Early physical therapy effects on the high-risk infant: a randomized controlled trial. *Pediatrics* **78**, 216–224

Pritchett, J.W. (1983) The untreated unstable hip in severe cerebral palsy. *Clinical Orthopaedics and Related Research* **173**, 169–172

Pritchett, J.W. (1990) Treated and untreated unstable hips in severe cerebral palsy. *Developmental Medicine and Child Neurology* **32**, 3–6

Rang, M., Douglas, G., Bennet, G.C. and Koreska, J. (1981) Seating for children with cerebral palsy. *Journal of Pediatric Orthopedics* **1**, 279–287

Rappaport, C.R., Fiori, W.R. and Herzberg, E. (1981) In: *A infancia inicial: o bebê sua mãe*. EPU: São Paulo

Ratliff, A.H.C. (1957) *Journal of Bone and Joint Surgery* **39B**, 781

Robins, R.H.C. (1959) *Journal of Bone and Joint Surgery* **41B**, 337

Ross, P.M. and Lyne, E.D. (1980) The Grice procedure: indications and evaluation of long term results. *Clinical Orthopaedics and Related Research* **153**, 194

Russell, R. (1947) *British Medical Journal* **2**, 1023

Russell, R. (1950) *Journal of Bone and Joint Surgery* **32B**, 748

Samilson, R.L. and Perry, J. (1975) Orthopaedic assessment in cerebral palsy. In: *Orthopaedic Aspects of Cerebral Palsy*. Edited by R.L. Samilson. Heinemann Medical: London

Scher, M.S. (1989) Pediatric electroencephalography and evoked potentials. In: *Pediatric Neurology Principles and Practice*, pp. 67–103. Edited by K.F. Swaiman. C.V. Mosby Company, St Louis: Baltimore and Toronto

Schlesinger, E.B. (1951) *Lancet* **2**, 600

Schwartzmann, J.R. and Crego, C.H. Jr (1948) *Journal of Bone and Joint Surgery* **30A**, 541

Scrutton, D. (1984) In: *The Epidemiology of the Cerebral Palsies. Clinics in Developmental Medicine No. 90.* Edited by D. Scrutton. S.I.M.P. with Blackwell Scientific Publications: London/Lippincott: Philadelphia

Seddon, H.J. (1956) *Journal of Bone and Joint Surgery* **38B**, 152

Seddon, H.J. (1965) Volkmann's ischaemia. *British Medical Journal* **1**, 1587–1592

Segal, A., Seddon, H.J. and Brooks, D.M. (1959) *Journal of Bone and Joint Surgery* **41B**, 44

Sever, J.W. (1916) *American Journal of Diseases of Children* **12**, 541

Shane, H. (1988) Communication enhancement: principles and practices. *Exceptional Parent* **May–June** 20–27.

Shapiro, B.K., Green, P., Krick, J., Allen, D. and Capute, A.J. (1986) Growth of severely impaired children: neurological versus nutritional factors. *Developmental Medicine and Child Neurology* **28**, 729–733

Sharrard, W.J.W. (1976) Indication for bracing in cerebral palsy. In: *The Advance in Orthotics*. Edited by G. Murdoch. Edward Arnold: London

Sharrard, W.J.W., Alen, J.M.H. and Heaney, S.H. (1975) Surgical prophylaxis of subluxation and dislocation of the hip in cerebral palsy. *Journal of Bone and Joint Surgery* **57B**, 160–166

Somerville, E.W. (1959) *Journal of Bone and Joint Surgery* **41B**, 279

Spector, S.A. (1987) In: *Pediatrics*. Edited by A.M. Rudolph, and J.I.E. Hoffman. Appleton and Lange: Los Altos, CA

Spencer, G.E. and Vignos, P.J. (1962) Bracing for ambulation in childhood progressive muscular dystrophy. *Journal of Bone and Joint Surgery* **44A**, 234–239

Spires, M.C., Gordon, E.F., Choudhuri, M., Maldonado, E. and Chan, R. (1989) Intracranial hemorrhagy in neonate following prenatal cocaine exposure. *Pediatric Neurology* **5**, 324–326

Spitz, R.A. (1979) *O primeiro ano de vida*. Trad. E.M.B. Rocha. Martins Fontes: São Paulo

Sponseller, P.D., Whiffen, J.R. and Drummond, D.S. (1986) Interspinous process segmental spinal instrumentation for scoliosis in cerebral palsy. *Journal of Pediatric Orthopedics* **6**, 559–563

Stanitski, C.L., Micheli, L.J., Hall, J.E. and Rosenthal, R.K. (1982) Surgical correction of spinal deformity in cerebral palsy. *Spine* **7**, 563–569

Stanley, F. (1984) Perinatal risk factors in the cerebral palsies. In: *The Epidemiology of the Cerebral Palsies. Clinics in Developmental Medicine No. 87*, pp. 98–115. Edited by F. Stanley and E. Alberman. S.I.M.P. with Blackwell Scientific Publications: London/Lippincott: Philadelphia

Stanley, F. and Alberman, E. (1984). Birthweight, gestational age and the cerebral palsies. In: *The Epidemiology of Cerebral Palsies. Clinics in Developmental Medicine No. 87*, pp. 57–68. Edited by F. Stanley and E. Alberman. S.I.M.P. with Blackwell Scientific Publications: London/ Lippincott: Philadelphia

Stanley, F. and Blair, E. (1982) An epidemiology study of cerebral palsy in Western Australia, 1956–1975. III. Postnatal aetiology. *Developmental Medicine and Child Neurology* **24**, 575–585

Stanley, F. and Blair, E. (1984) Postnatal risk factors in the cerebral palsies. In: *The Epidemiology of Cerebral Palsies. Clinics in Developmental Medicine No. 87*, pp. 135–149. Edited by F. Stanley and E. Alberman. S.I.M.P. with Blackwell Scientific Publications: London/ Lippincott: Philadelphia

Stein, L., Ozdaman, O., Kraus, N. and Paton, J. (1983) Follow-up of infants screened by auditory brainstem response in the neonatal intensive care unit. *Journal of Pediatrics* **103**, 447–453

Steindler, A. (1923) *Journal of Bone and Joint Surgery* **5**, 284

Swanson, A.B. (1960) Surgery of the hand in cerebral palsy and the swan neck deformity. *Journal of Bone and Joint Surgery* **42A**, 951–964

Tachdjian, M.O. and Matson, D.D. (1965) Orthopedic aspects of interspinal tumors in infants and children. *Journal of Bone and Joint Surgery* **47A**, 223–248

Taft, L.T. (1984) Cerebral palsy. *Pediatrics in Review* **6**, 35–45

Thompson, C.F. (1942) *Journal of Bone and Joint Surgery* **24**, 907

Thompson, R.A. and Vignos, P.J. Jr (1959) *Archives of Internal Medicine* **103**, 551

Turner, P.R., Westwood, T., Regen, C.M. and Steinhardt, R.A. (1988) Increased protein degradation results from elevated free calcin levels found in muscle from mdx mice. *Nature* **335**, 735–738

Ultmann, M.H., Belman, A.L., Ruff, H.A. *et al.* (1985) Developmental abnormalities in infants and children with acquired immune deficiency syndrome (AIDS) and AIDS-related complex. *Developmental Medicine and Child Neurology* **27**, 563–571

Vignos, P.J., Spencer, G.E. and Archibald, K.C. (1963) *Journal of the American Medical Association* **184**, 89

Walton, J.N. (1964) Muscular dystrophy: some recent advances in knowledge. *British Medical Journal* **1**, 1271–1274

Watson-Jones, R. (1926) Spontaneous dislocation of the hip. *British Journal of Surgery* **14**, 36–57

Watt, J.M., Robertson, C.M.T. and Grace, M.G.A. (1989) Early prognosis for ambulation of neonatal intensive care survivors with cerebral palsy. *Developmental Medicine and Child Neurology* **31**, 766–773

Wedell, K. (1960) The visual perception of cerebral palsied children. Abstract. In: *Perceptual and Visuo-motor Disorders in Cerebral Palsy*. Little Club Clinics in Developmental Medicine II. Edited by M.L.J. Abercrombie (1964) The Spastics Society, Medical Education Information Unit in association with William Heinemann (Medical Books) Ltd: London

Weissman, S.L., Torok, G. and Khermosh, O. (1961) *Journal of Bone and Joint Surgery* **43A**, 1135

Wenner, S.M. and Johnson, K.A. (1988) Transfer of the flexor carpi ulnaris to the radial wrist extensors in cerebral palsy. *Journal of Hand Surgery* **13A**, 231–233

Williams, J.M. (1958) Some special learning difficulties of cerebral palsied children. Abstract. In: *Perceptual and Visuo-motor Disorders in Cerebral Palsy*. Little Club Clinics in Developmental Medicine II. Edited by M.L.J. Abercrombie (1964) The Spastics Society, Medical Education Information Unit in association with William Heinemann (Medical Books) Ltd: London

Wilson, F.C. Jr, Fay, G.F., LeMonte, P. and Williams, J.C. (1965) Triple arthrodesis. *Journal of Bone and Joint Surgery* **47A**, 340–348

Wilson, J.L. (1953) *Pediatric Clinics of North America* **1**, 20

Young, M.H. (1978) Cognitive development in cerebral palsied children. *Dissertation Abstracts International* **38**, 6630–6631

Young, J.H. (1989) Cognitive development in cerebral palsied children. *Journal of Child Cognitive Psychology* **2**, 11–17

Yount, C.C. (1926) *Journal of Bone and Joint Surgery* **8**, 34

CHAPTER 8

Spinal Deformities in Children

ROBERT A. DICKSON

Scoliosis and kyphosis

BASIC PRINCIPLES OF EXAMINATION AND RADIOGRAPHY

When the spine is viewed from the front or back, i.e. in the coronal plane, it is straight and if it is not then the condition of scoliosis, or lateral curvature of the spine, exists. When the spine is viewed from the side, i.e. sagittal plane, it is not straight. At birth there is a gentle kyphosis (spinal curvature convex posteriorly) from crown to rump. Shortly thereafter, increasing awareness of the environment produces neck extension, while the attainment of the upright position sees the development of lumbar extension. The cervical and lumbar regions are therefore naturally lordotic (spinal curvatures convex anteriorly) with the intervening thoracic spine retaining its posterior convex curve.

Scolioses are subdivided into two principal categories: non-structural and structural. *Non-structural scolioses* are lateral spinal curvatures without rotation, rarely progressive and are usually secondary to some other problem, e.g. leg length inequality, producing a tilted pelvis and a compensatory non-structural scoliosis of the lumbar spine to restore balance, or painful lesions of the spine, such as a disc herniation or discitis, which produce a non-structural scoliosis locally due to asymmetric paravertebral muscle spasm. A straight spine is restored by treating these conditions. By contrast, *structural scoliosis* is defined as a lateral curvature with rotation, and is a primary problem of the shape of the spine with significant progression potential during the period of spinal growth.

On radiography, if the scoliosis is non-structural, i.e. there is no vertebral rotation, then it is very adequately represented on a posteroanterior (PA) radiograph. Structural scolioses have concomitant rotation and therefore PA radiographs give relatively poor two-dimensional oblique representations of the deformity. The Scoliosis Research Society (1976) defined a number of parameters to describe and quantify the appearances on plain PA films. If horizontal lines are drawn along the upper surface of the vertebrae above the curve apex and along the bottom of the vertebrae below the curve apex then the amount of vertebral tilt will be seen to vary through the curve (Figure 8.1). The vertebrae that are most tilted from the horizontal at the top and bottom

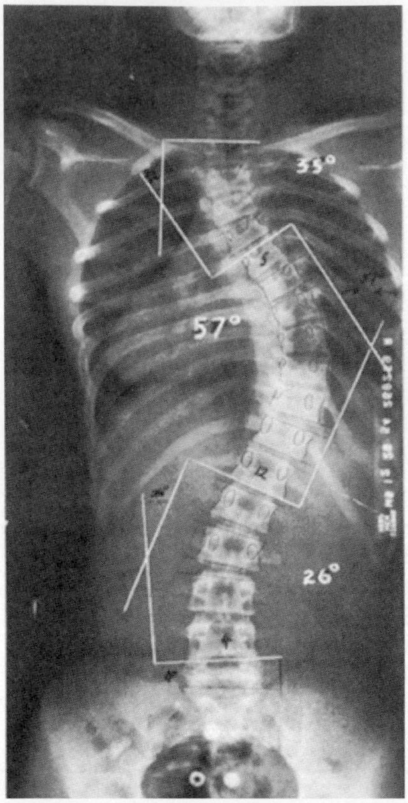

Figure 8.1 PA radiograph of a right thoracic curve. T5 and T12 are the upper and lower end vertebrae respectively being maximally tilted into the concavity of the curve. A line drawn along the upper surface of the upper end vertebra and a line drawn along the lower surface of the lower end vertebra when produced will subtend an angle of 57°. This is referred to as the Cobb angle of the curve. The size of the upper and lower compensatory curves can be similarly measured. Rotation is determined by the relationship of the oval shadows of the pedicles to the side of the vertebral body and can be quantified in degrees using the Perdriolle torsiometer.

of the curve are termed the end vertebrae. If the lines along these vertebrae are extended until they intersect, they subtend an angle which is referred to as the Cobb angle of the deformity (Cobb, 1948). With mild deformities the resultant angle is small so that the two lines do not intersect on the x-ray film and thus perpendiculars are dropped from each so that the angle can be measured on the radiograph. This technique of measuring the Cobb angle is very imprecise. In practice the error can be reduced to less than 2° by using the protractor of Whittle and Evans (1979) from Oxford – a simple template with in-built needle protractor, rather like a compass, obviating the need to draw any lines at all (Figure 8.2).

The vertebra at the curve apex is referred to as the apical vertebra but if there is an even number of vertebrae between the upper and lower end vertebrae there will be two apical vertebrae. The position of the apical vertebra or vertebrae determines empirically the site of the curve. If the apex is at C7 or T1, or at T12 or L1, then these curves are referred to as cervicothoracic and thoracolumbar respectively. Between these two positions curves are referred to as thoracic and below the thoracolumbar region they are referred to as lumbar. Any above the cervicothoracic junction are termed cervical, although these seldom, if ever, exist. Curves are further specified as right or left according to the direction of the convexity of the curve, e.g. right thoracic or left thoracolumbar which are very common curve patterns (Figure 8.3).

Inspection of the PA radiograph demonstrates that the vertebrae in the curve are rotated, with the posterior elements turning into the curve concavity while the anterior vertebral bodies turn into the curve convexity. Rotation is maximal at the curve apex and can be measured by locating the position of the convex pedicle in relation to the side of the relevant vertebral body, by the method of Nash and Moe (1969) or be more precisely estimated using the template of Perdriolle (1979). As the rotational component of the deformity in the transverse plane is usually the chief complaint, measurement of rotation is more clinically relevant than measurement of Cobb angle. Cobb angle is thus a non-linear expression of curve size which progressively underestimates the true size of the deformity (Dickson, 1987). Therefore one should not describe a population of scoliotic patients by way of an average Cobb angle nor express change in Cobb angle as a percentage. Rotation does, however, increase linearly as the deformity increases.

For most curves the upper and lower end vertebrae are still somewhat rotated and are termed 'neutral vertebrae'. A spinal fusion operation must involve the neutral vertebra above to neutral vertebra below or the deformity may subsequently increase with growth.

Above and below the 'structural curve' are nonstructural curves bringing the spinal column straight above and below. These are termed 'compensatory scolioses'. One single structural curve is much less common. Close inspection of the PA radiograph usually indicates that the spine bends in the opposite direction either above or below the seemingly single structural curve and sometimes both (Cruickshank *et al.*, 1989). Double or triple curve patterns are thus common and they are described as a composite of the component parts, e.g. right thoracic and left lumbar, a common double curve pattern.

On studying the spine above what initially appears to be a single right thoracic curve, it is not uncommon to find a truly structural curve above, convex to

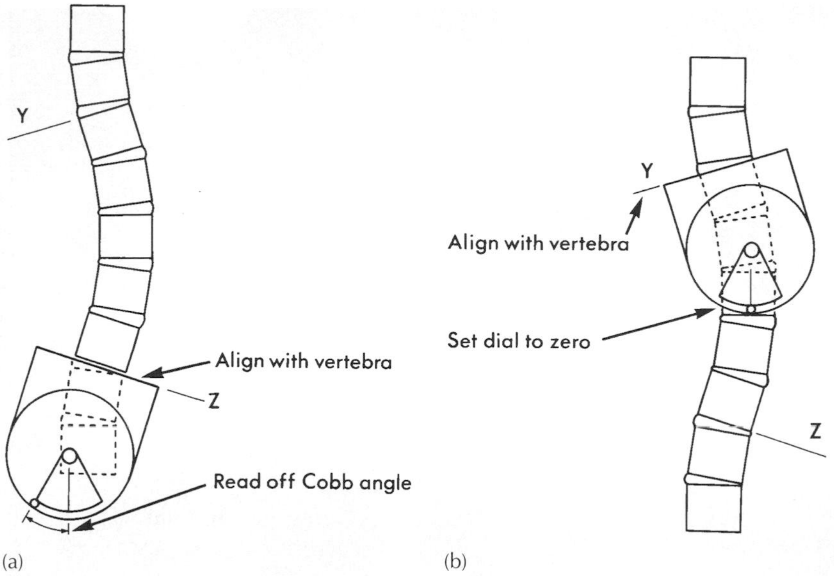

Figure 8.2 (a) and (b) The Oxford Cobbometer. An accurate method of measuring Cobb angle without the need to draw lines or perpendiculars on the radiograph.

the left, and this is called a double thoracic major curve pattern. The height of the shoulders provides a clue to the presence of a double thoracic curve pattern. In the presence of a single thoracic curve the shoulder on the concave side is lower, whereas in a double thoracic curve pattern it is higher. This has been called by the French the *signe d'épaule* (the sign of the shoulder) (Figure 8.4). It is therefore important to image the entire length of the spinal column with full length spinal films to diagnose other spinal problems, as well as for spina bifida occulta or spondylolisthesis.

Although the compensatory scolioses above and below tend to preserve spinal balance this is not always achieved with the result that the trunk may list to one or other side, more commonly to the side of the curve convexity. Such a spine is said to be decompensated and a plumbline dropped from the vertebra prominens either with reference to the patient or an erect full length film will be seen to fall to one side of the midpoint of the lumbosacral junction (Figure 8.5).

Radiographs are also of value for other estimations, e.g. the prognosis of idiopathic thoracic curves in infancy, and for the measurement of the rib/vertebra angle difference (RVAD) at the curve apex (Mehta, 1972). A line is drawn along the neck of the rib attached on each side of the apical vertebra and the angle it subtends with a line drawn down the vertical axis of the vertebra is registered (the rib/vertebra angle) (Figure 8.6). When the one is subtracted from the other the RVAD is calculated and, if greater than 20°, the curve is likely to be of the progressive type.

As the size of the deformity increases so does its rigidity and therefore it is important to assess the flexibility of the curve, especially when surgical treatment is being considered as instrumentation merely takes up the natural flexibility or slack of the curve. Flexibility can be assessed radiographically by obtaining side-bending, supine, or maximum traction films and comparing the size of the deformity with that observed on the erect film (Figure 8.7). Side-bending films are valuable when anterior instrumentation is being considered as the angular appearance of the intervertebral discs dictates the extent of the necessary instrumentation and fusion.

Radiographs are also necessary to estimate bone age and the status of apophyseal maturity. Risser (1958) first described the process of appearance, migration, and maturation of the iliac crest apophysis, ultimate fusion signifying the attainment of maturity (Figure 8.8), In a similar manner the status of ossification of the vertebral ring apophyses can be judged. These ring apophyses take no part in longitudinal spinal growth nor do their maturation have anything to do with vertebral growth (Bick *et al.*, 1950). The vertebral end-plate epiphyses, not the ring apophyses, do not finally fuse until the middle of the third decade, i.e. at the age of about 25 years, a decade beyond growth of the appendicular skeleton (Bernick and Cailliet, 1982). Children grow on average 2 cm in height from spinal growth after general skeletal maturity (Tupman, 1962). This prolonged period of spinal growth is of considerable importance to the individual with a spinal deformity as the forces of three-dimensional spinal buckling can be accommodated in a continuing change of vertebral shape.

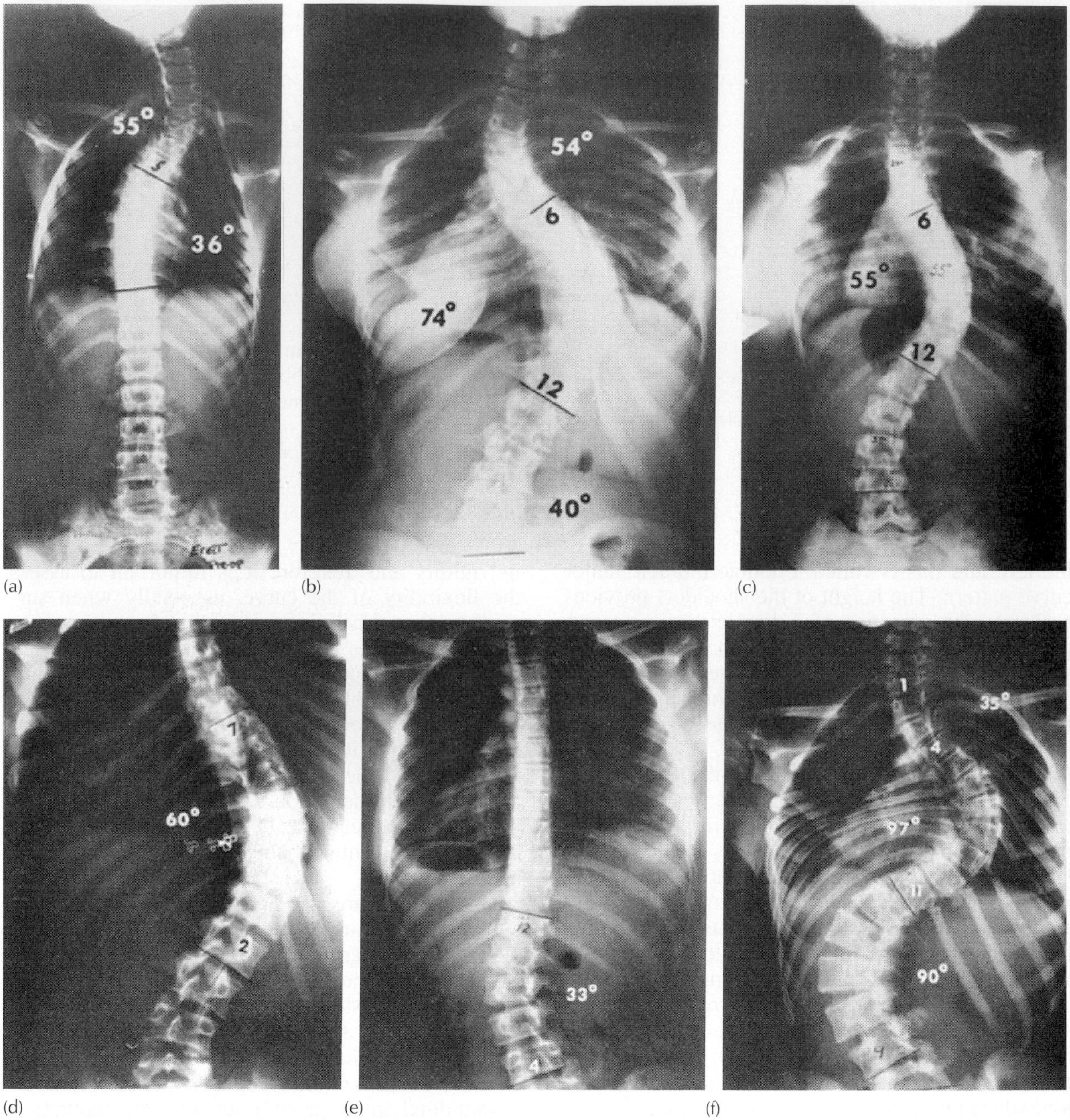

Figure 8.3 Radiographs showing the six basic curve patterns observed in idiopathic scoliosis. (a) Cervico-thoracic, (b) double thoracic, (c) main thoracic, (d) thoraco-lumbar, (e) main lumbar and (f) combined thoracic and lumbar.

The most accurate method of assessing bone age is by comparing a standard film of the left hand and wrist against standards referred to as the Tanner and Whitehouse second (TW2) method (Tanner *et al.*, 1983). Bone age can be assigned accurately to within a tenth of a year and thus a PA radiograph of the left hand and wrist is an integral component of a scoliosis series of x-rays.

Assessing skeletal maturity during adolescence, although identifying the vulnerable period of maximum adolescent growth velocity, has little value in estimating how much the spine will continue to grow beyond general skeletal maturity. Therefore radiographic measures of maturity should be supplemented by direct anthropometric measures of growth plotted sequentially on centile charts (Tanner and Whitehouse, 1975).

In order to rationalize the enormous number of conditions which appear to be causally related to the presence of a spinal deformity, an aetiological

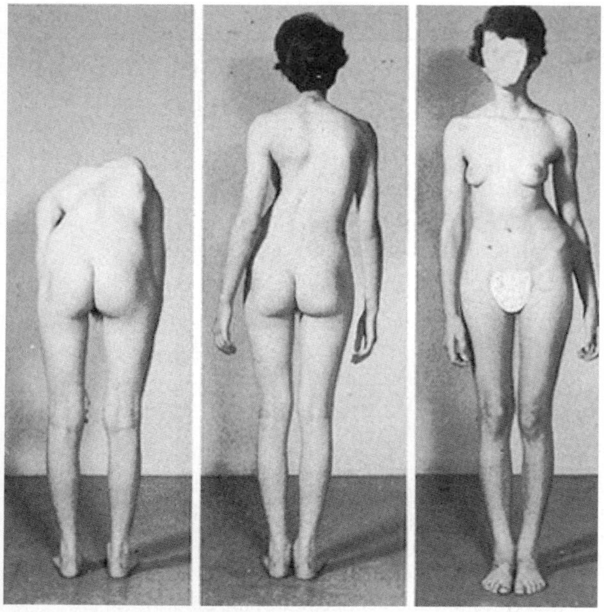

(a) (b) (c)

Figure 8.4 This looks initially like a simple right thoracic scoliosis but note that the left shoulder is appreciably higher than the right. With a single right thoracic curve the left shoulder would be lower than the right. The higher left shoulder is referred to as the '*signe d'épaule*' – the sign of the shoulder, and indicates the presence of an upper left structural curve, making this a double thoracic major configuration.

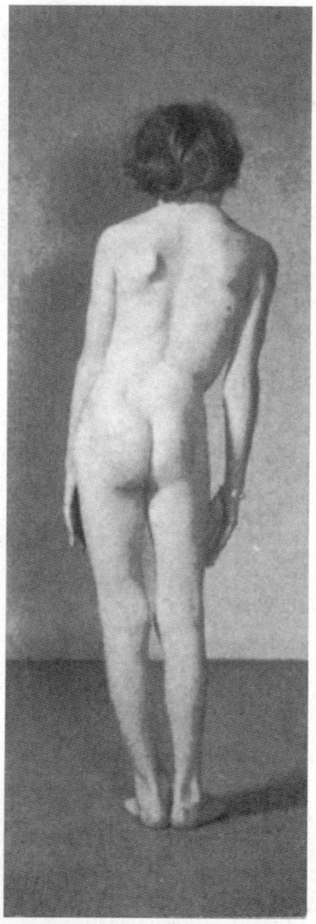

Figure 8.5 Note the list of the torso to the right, i.e. decompensation.

classification (Table 8.1) has been proposed by the Scoliosis Research Society (Goldstein and Waugh, 1973). Idiopathic deformities are the most prevalent and refer to the presence of a spinal deformity in the absence of any associated clinical abnormality or congenital spinal anomaly. Congenital deformities are primarily divisible into two categories – congenital bony deformities, and congenital spinal cord deformities (spina bifida or myelodysplasia). With congenital bony deformities there is always a congenital bony anomaly discernible on radiographs while the congenital cord deformities are always associated with the spina bifida patient who has significant neurological loss. Neuromuscular deformities, e.g. Friedreich's ataxia and the muscular dystrophies, also include related conditions such as cerebral palsy and poliomyelitis with a common clinical denominator of neuromuscular loss or imbalance. Deformities in association with Von Recklinghausen's disease are described, while the term mesenchymal deformities include such conditions as the heritable disorders of connective tissue and the bone dysplasias. Finally, structural spinal deformities can arise as a result of trauma, infection, or tumours.

It is clinically imperative to assess the spinal deformity in association with the underlying condition so that the spine is not isolated from other important aspects of the patient.

THE ANATOMY AND BIOMECHANICS OF SPINAL SHAPE

To appreciate the clinical behaviour of spinal deformities and their response to treatment it is essential to understand how spinal deformities arise from normal spinal shape (Deacon *et al.*, 1984). In order to position adequately the head in space, the cervical spine has a considerable range of movement as does the lumbar region for positioning the trunk. By contrast, the thoracic spine, behind the vital organs, is much less flexible with additional protection and stiffness supplied by the attached thoracic cage, which also provides an adequate chest volume with the spine being kyphotic.

The line of the centre of gravity of the body lies anterior to the entire spinal column, barely coming in contact with the anterior surface of the fourth lumbar vertebra. The spine is thus under a continuous

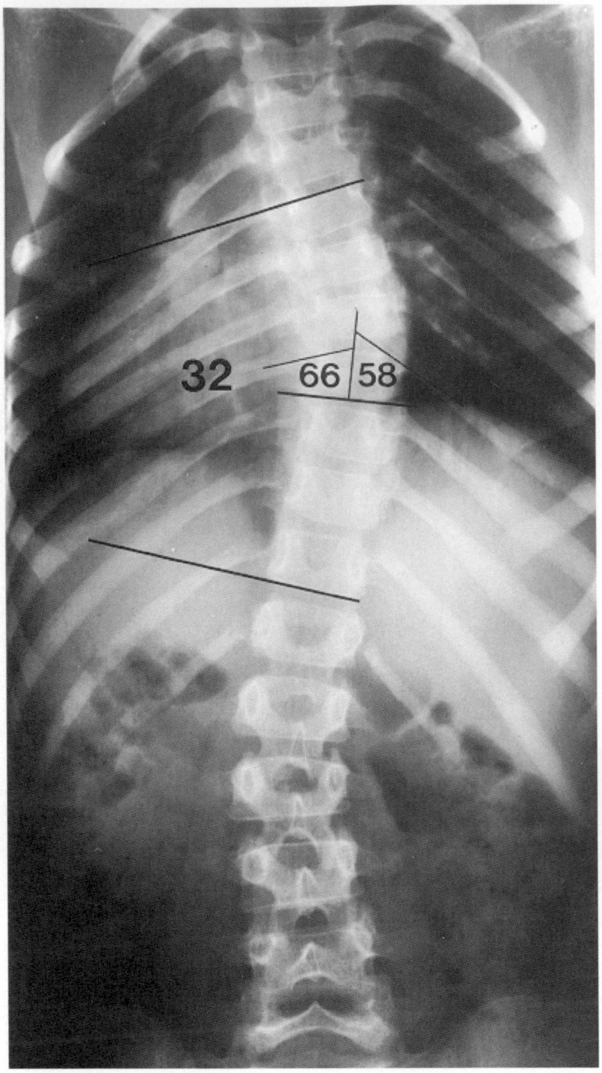

Figure 8.6 Measuring the rib vertebra angle distance (RVAD). Although the Cobb angle is over 30°, the rib/vertebra angle difference (66–58) is only 8°, strongly suggesting a resolving curve.

forwards bending moment and to counteract this there is powerful extending posterior erector spinae musculature, keeping the spine upright. Because it is mechanically illogical to place spinal flexor muscles on the anterior surface of the spine so close to the line of the centre of gravity, there are no spinal flexor muscles attached to the front of the spine from foramen magnum to sacrum. The diaphragm is attached to the thoracolumbar region, while the hip-flexing psoas major muscle is attached to the side of the spine on the upper lumbar transverse processes. The spinal flexors, to give them the best leverage, are as far forward as possible in the anterior abdominal wall.

Because of the differing functional requirements

Table 8.1 Aetiological classification of spinal deformities

Primary, progressive or structural deformities	
Idiopathic deformities	
Idiopathic scoliosis	
Early onset	
Late onset	
Idiopathic kyphosis	
Type I – classical Scheuermann's disease	
Type II – 'apprentice's spine'	
Congenital deformities	
Bone deformities	
Scoliosis	Failure of formation
Kyphosis	Failure of segmentation
Lordosis	Mixed
Cord deformities	
Myelodysplasia scoliosis	
Myelodysplasia kyphosis	
Myelodysplasia lordosis	
Bone and cord deformities	
Syndromes in which congenital spine deformities are prevalent	
Neuromuscular deformities	
Cerebral palsy	
Poliomyelitis	
True 'neuromuscular disorders'	
Familial dysautonomia	
Malignant hyperpyrexia	
Deformities in association with neurofibromatosis	
Dystrophic deformities	
Idiopathic-type deformities	
Mesenchymal deformities	
Heritable disorders of connective tissue	
Mucopolysaccharidoses	
Bone dysplasias	
Metabolic bone disease	
Endocrine disorders	
Traumatic deformites	
Vertebral	
Extravertebral	
Deformity due to infection	
Pyogenic infection	
Tuberculosis	
Deformity due to tumours	
Intradural tumours	
Syringomyelia	
Paravertebral childhood tumours	
Primary extradural tumours	
Metastatic spinal disease	
Secondary, non-progressive or non-structural deformites	
Pelvic tilt scoliosis	
Irritative lesions	
Hysterical scoliosis	

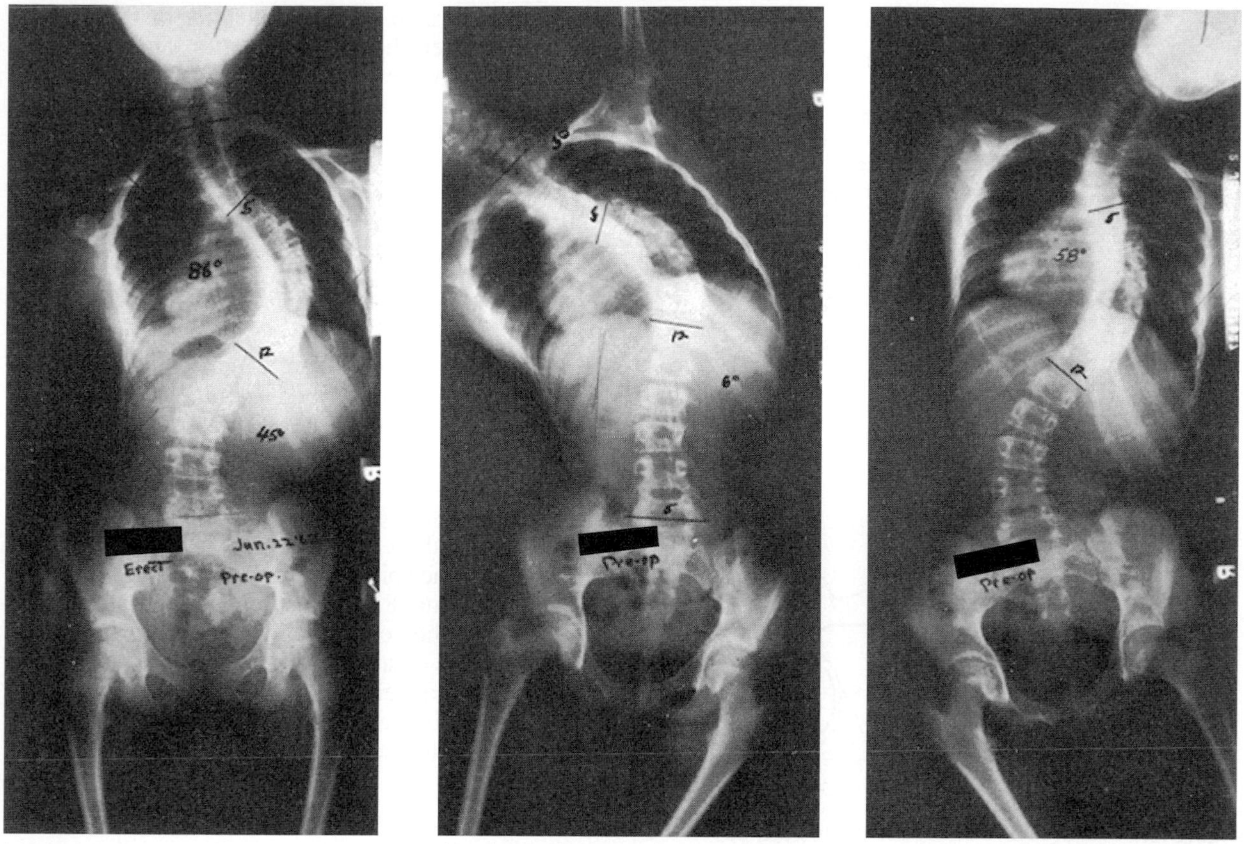

(a) (b) (c)

Figure 8.7 (a) Erect radiograph. (b) Left lateral bending radiograph to assess the flexibility of the compensatory curves. (c) Right lateral bending radiograph to assess the flexibility of the structural curve.

in cervical, thoracic, and lumbar regions, these three areas of the spine have differing geometry and kinematics. The cervical and lumbar regions, being both lordotic, have greater similarity to each other than the intervening thoracic kyphosis, e.g. the greater intervertebral disc height in the cervical and lumbar regions and the posterior facet joint alignment being more in the sagittal than coronal plane,

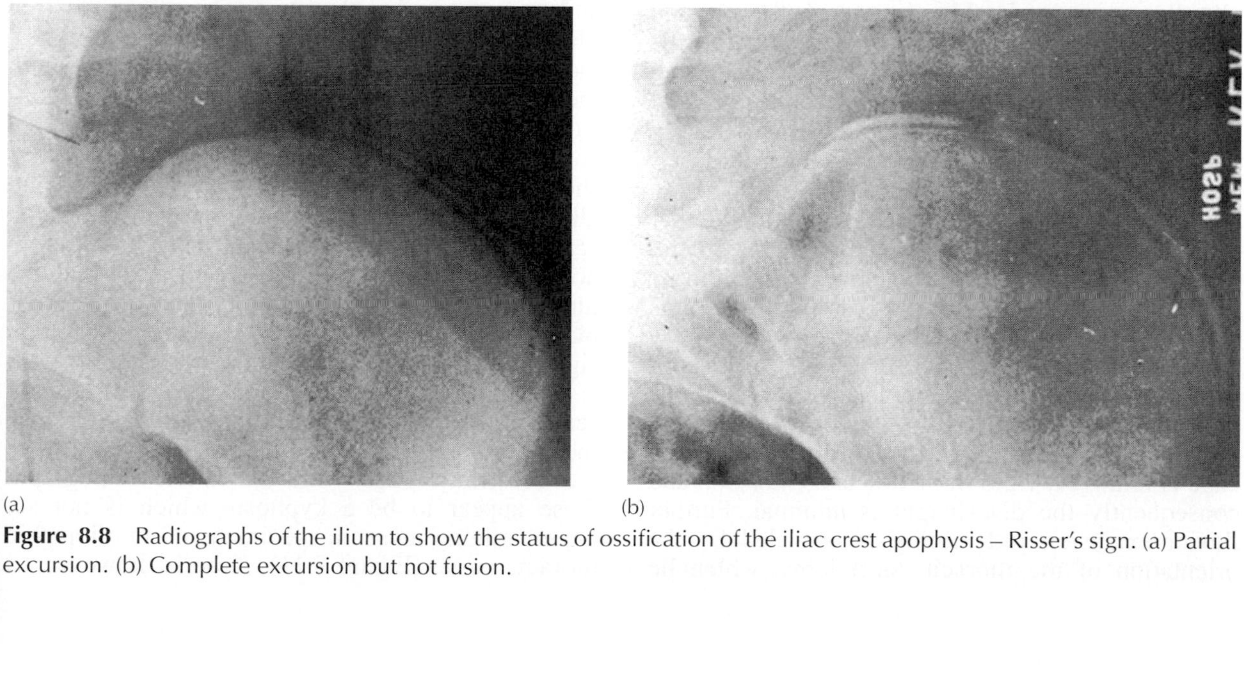

(a) (b)

Figure 8.8 Radiographs of the ilium to show the status of ossification of the iliac crest apophysis – Risser's sign. (a) Partial excursion. (b) Complete excursion but not fusion.

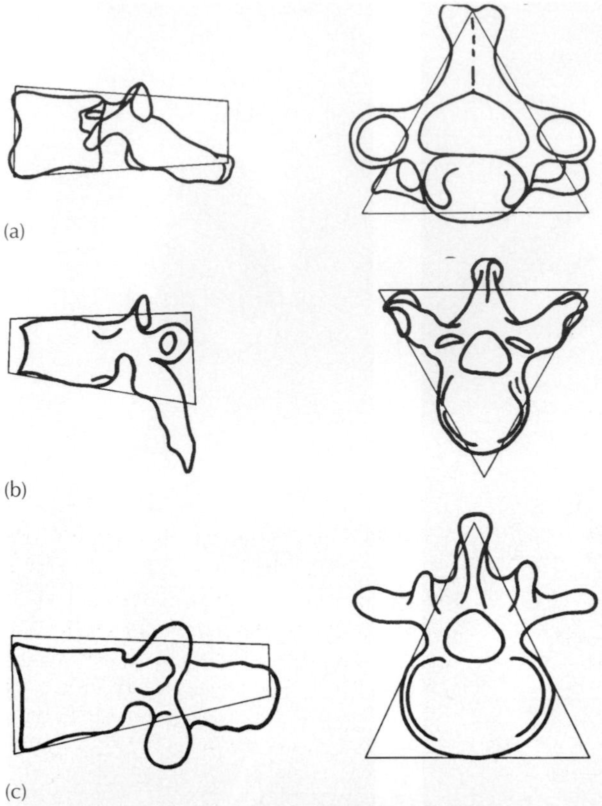

Figure 8.9 Sagittal and transverse plane geometry in the cervical region (a), the thoracic region (b), and the lumbar region (c). In the cervical and lumbar region the vertebrae are lordotic in the sagittal plane and prismatic with the prism base directed anteriorly. The opposite configuration exists in the thoracic region with the vertebrae being kyphotic in the sagittal plane and prismatic in the transverse plane with the apex anteriorly.

all allow a considerable degree of flexion and extension. The chin can readily be placed on the chest and the hands on the ground in full cervical and lumbar flexion. To prevent this happening, except at will, the erector spinae musculature is very strongly developed behind the cervical and lumbar lordoses, as well as additional strong ligamentous support in the form of the ligamentum nuchae and the lumbar fascia. Except for the atlantoaxial motion segment, rotation is inhibited in the cervical and lumbar regions by the alignment of the posterior facet joints and thus rotator muscles in these regions are only represented vestigially, or indeed, as in the case of the sternomastoid, for example, bypass the spine altogether.

By contrast, the thoracic spine with its attached rib cage is relatively rigid in flexion and extension and consequently the disc height is minimal. Further flexion/extension inflexibility is provided by the orientation of the thoracic facet joints which lie obliquely more in the coronal than in the sagittal plane. However, the axes of rotation of the thoracic facet joints in the presence of kyphosis lie well anterior to the spine. Therefore in the thoracic region some rotation occurs at each motion segment which is precisely the opposite configuration to that which occurs in the cervical and lumbar regions.

Transverse plane (cross-sectional) geometry and kinematics are also fundamentally different in the cervical, thoracic and lumbar regions, but again the cervical and lumbar spines show similar properties. The cervical and lumbar vertebral bodies are broader from side to side than front to back, in the lumbar region often being described as kidney-shaped. This 3:2 ratio of side-to-side versus front-to-back body dimensions is reversed in the thoracic region where the vertebral bodies are longer from front to back and are often described as heart-shaped. When the attached neural arches complete the cross-sectional perspective, the spinal column appears triangular or prismatic (Figure 8.9), the bases of the prisms facing anteriorly in the cervical and lumbar regions while the apex of the prism points anteriorly in the thoracic region. These different anatomical and biomechanical features of different spinal regions are important in dictating where and how spinal deformities develop.

THE DEVELOPMENT OF SPINAL DEFORMITIES

Two basic types of spinal deformity are recognized: scoliosis and kyphosis. All structural scolioses involve a lateral spinal curvature with rotation as a three-dimensional deformity. No matter where in the spine the deformity is (i.e. thoracic or lumbar region) and no matter what the underlying diagnosis (i.e. idiopathic, cerebral palsy, Marfan's syndrome), there is a constant direction of spinal rotation with the posterior elements rotating into the curve concavity and the anterior elements into the curve convexity (Figure 8.10). The back of the spine is thus shorter than the front (Deane and Duthie, 1973) and all structural scolioses are therefore lordotic (Deacon *et al.*, 1984; Dickson *et al.*, 1984). There is therefore no such deformity as kyphoscoliosis. While the lumbar spine is naturally lordotic in the sagittal plane, the presence of lordosis in the thoracic region signifies a major change from the norm.

The lordotic nature of structural scoliosis is not seen on ordinary PA and lateral radiographs, because these radiographs are necessarily oblique views of the deformity. Also with the lateral radiograph, these appear to be a kyphosis which is not so. On examining museum specimens of an idiopathic thoracic curve (Figure 8.11), there is, however, so

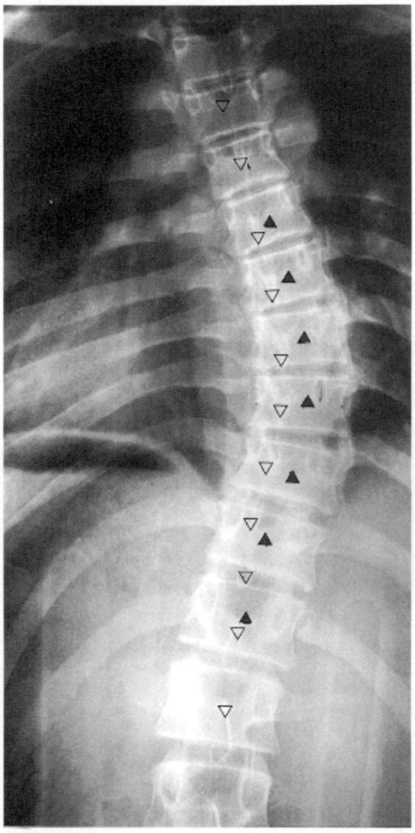

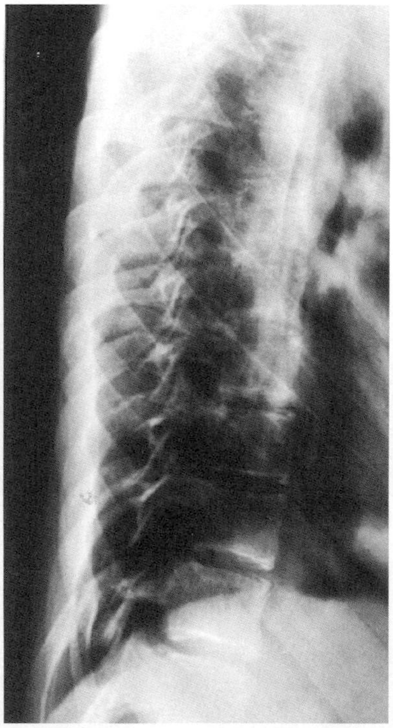

(a) (b)

Figure 8.10 (a) PA radiograph of a right thoracic curve with the centre of the vertebral bodies anteriorly marked with solid triangles and the tips of the spinous processes with hollow triangles. The line down the back of the spine is shorter than the line down the front, indicating the presence of lordosis. (b) True lateral radiograph of the same patient revealing the fundamental lordosis.

much rotation at the curve apex that a PA radiograph of the specimen now looks more like a lateral projection of the curve apex. It is, however, not the back of the spine which points backwards (true kyphosis) but the side of the spine (i.e. the scoliosis). When the x-ray beam is turned truly lateral to the apex the lordosis is unmasked.

Stagnara therefore devised the '*plan d'élection*', or true PA of the deformity (du Peloux *et al.*, 1965). Here the x-ray beam is directed truly posterior–anterior to the apical vertebra to show the true size of the deformity. The nature of this complex three-dimensional deformity can be made to vary merely by varying the radiographic two-dimensional projection (Figure 8.12). The size of the deformity varies in sinusoidal fashion being maximal at the true *plan d'élection* position and minimal when the projection is only lateral to the curve apex.

In a young growing idiopathic thoracic deformity (Figure 8.13) posterior instrumentation and fusion will further tether the back of the young growing spine such that continued spinal buckling occurs with further growth. Progression of the deformity can go beyond the *plan d'élection* position, with increase in the deformity.

The crucial and primary role of the abnormal thoracic lordosis was readily appreciated by Adams, whose classic 1865 text was written well before the discovery of x-rays. He made his critical observations by dissecting cadaver specimens and furthermore described the forward bending test whereby the rotational prominence is much less obvious in the erect than the forward bending position. Forward bending compresses the lordosis and forces it to buckle out to the side and this process would also, but more insidiously, occur with growth. His clear statement that 'lordosis plus rotation equals lateral flexion' indicates succinctly the pathogenesis of structural scoliosis.

This important work has only received very sporadic attention subsequently (Somerville, 1952; Wittebol, 1956; Roaf, 1966). Eleven articulated spines with idiopathic scoliosis were studied by Deane and Duthie (1973) and demonstrated that the shortest distance down the spine was down the back whilst the longest distance was down the front without exception. They also described the important concept of transverse plane geometry being prismatic (see Figure 8.9). These same museum specimens were looked at again and it was shown

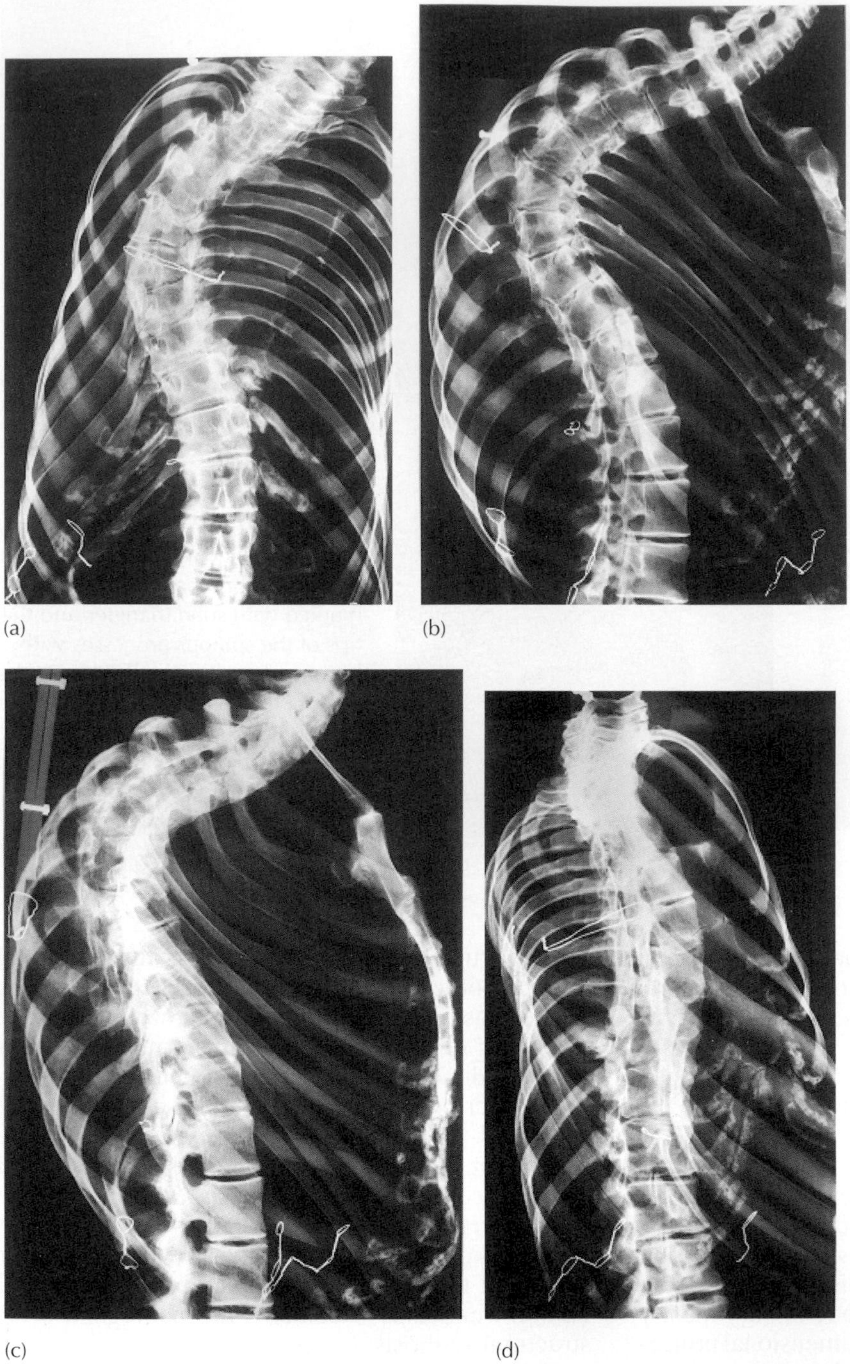

Figure 8.11 Four different radiographic projections of the same museum specimen of a left thoracic scoliosis. (a) PA view. (b) True PA view of curve apex (*plan d'élection* of Stagnara). (c) Lateral view of specimen showing the spurious impression of kyphosis. (d) True lateral projection of the curve apex revealing the constant lordosis.

that the apical vertebral bodies were significantly taller anteriorly than posteriorly and that there were significant correlations between the size of the secondary scoliosis, the amount of axial rotation and the size of the apical lordosis (Deacon *et al.*, 1984).

A similar study was subsequently carried out on 150 patients with single idiopathic thoracic curves and analysis of true lateral radiographs of the curve apex showed lordotic vertebral wedging which could be positively correlated with the degree of apical rotation and the PA Cobb angle (Deacon and Dickson, 1987). The appearance of the apical two or three vertebrae in the true lateral profile, which were lordotically wedged with posterior Schmorl node formation, appeared to be opposite to the appearance of the apical vertebrae in the other idiopathic spinal deformity of childhood and adolescence, i.e. Scheuermann's disease or idiopathic hyperkyphosis

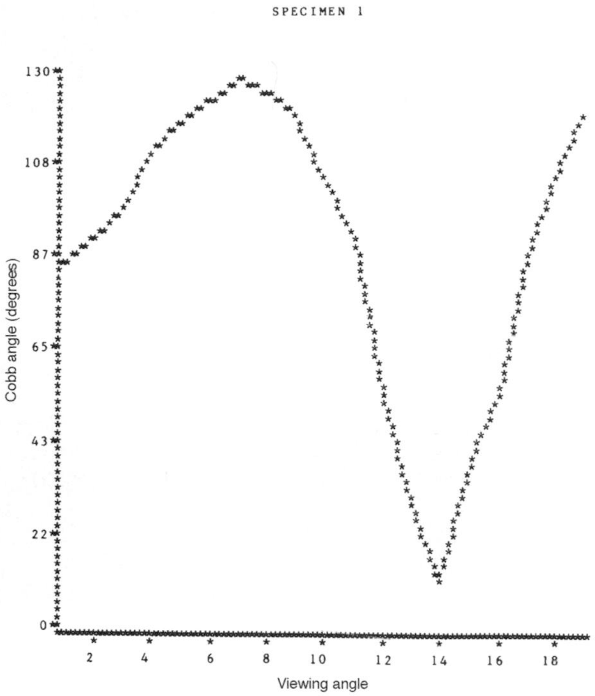

Figure 8.12 The museum specimen has been rotated through 180° with the Cobb angle being measured at 10° intervals. It can be seen that the Cobb angle changes in sinusoidal fashion according to the plane of radiographic projection, being maximal in the position of the *plan d'élection* of Stagnara and being minimal in true lateral profile.

(Figure 8.14). This observation had also been made by Roth (1981). Fifty consecutive patients with thoracic Scheuermann's disease were then investigated with PA and lateral radiographs. True idiopathic scoliosis was commonly found several spinal segments below the apex of the thoracic kyphosis as well as a compensatory hyperlordosis in the lumbar region (Deacon *et al.*, 1985). Willner and Johnsson (1983) have already shown pantographically that the lateral profile of children with thoracic idiopathic scoliosis was flatter than normal children, who in turn were flatter than those with thoracic Scheuermann's disease. Therefore it appears that the two conditions, idiopathic thoracic scoliosis and thoracic Scheuermann's disease, represent the opposite ends of a spectrum with the great majority of normal individuals without a spinal deformity lying in between.

Willner also demonstrated in normal children that lateral spinal profile changed with age, decreasing between the ages of 10 and 12 in both sexes but increasing over the year or two before skeletal maturity. The early phase of flattening of the lateral profile occurs synchronously with the adolescent growth spurt in females. It is the rule that children present with an idiopathic scoliosis following a significant growth spurt (Figure 8.15) (Duthie, 1971; Willner, 1974; Leong *et al.*, 1982) and that progressive scoliosis is much more common in girls. Therefore the natural trend for diminution of the thoracic kyphosis being associated with a significantly increased growth velocity would lead to the development of idiopathic scoliosis with its peak incidence in early adolescence. When the natural thoracic kyphosis increases again, a year or two before maturity, this is the peak incidence time for thoracic Scheuermann's disease in association with the peak adolescent growth velocity. Because Scheuermann's disease develops relatively late in the growth period, the idiopathic scoliosis related to the compensatory area of lumbar hyperlordosis is only of a mild degree, seldom measuring more than 30°, and is not usually a significant clinical problem.

A recent longitudinal cohort study of the lateral spinal profile compared the lateral profiles of those who started with a straight spine and who developed idiopathic scoliosis during the course of the study against those that started straight and remained straight (Mahood *et al.*, 1990). They demonstrated that the abnormally lordotic thoracic spine was present before either of the other two components of the deformity.

There is no single gene for idiopathic scoliosis (Carr *et al.*, 1989), nor would one expect there to be, but familial trends do occur (DeGeorge and Fisher, 1967; Cowell *et al.*, 1972; Riseborough and Wynne-Davies, 1973; Cziezel *et al.*, 1978). Patterns of growth during childhood and adolescence are closely shared by first- and second-degree relatives, i.e. familial as well, the timing of rapid perimenarchal growth spurt and the ultimate height of the spinal column (Tanner, 1962). Some years ago Delmas (1951), a French anatomist, and more recently Stagnara *et al.* (1982) suggested that spinal shape was a familial matter.

There is also clear evidence that lateral profile abnormalities are pathogenetic regardless of curve site. In thoracolumbar and lumbar curves, analysis of lateral profile has shown that the spine is abnormally hyperlordotic (Pelker and Gage, 1982).

In the thoracic spine idiopathic scoliosis and Scheuermann's disease appear to be widely separate but the differences in vertebral morphology are much more subtle than is generally appreciated (Deacon *et al.*, 1985). Typical thoracic vertebrae in a normal-shaped spine are kyphotically wedged by some 3°. Scheuermann's disease is defined as the presence of 5° of kyphotic wedging over three consecutive thoracic vertebrae (Sorenson, 1964), while only just over 3° of kyphotic wedging have to be lost for the idiopathic lordoscoliosis to develop. The spine is growing in three dimensions until the middle of the third decade; it is not perhaps

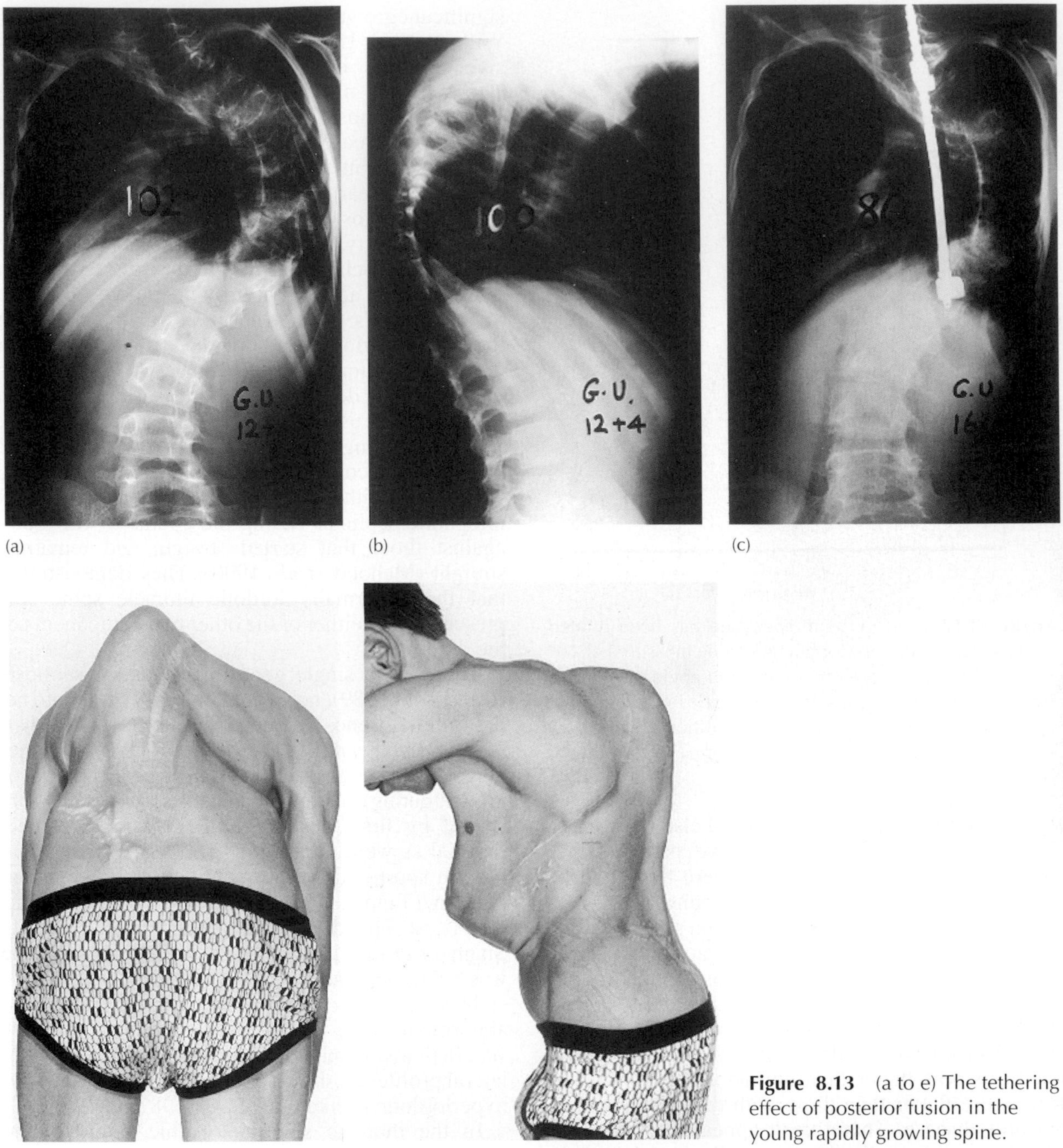

(a) (b) (c)

(d) (e)

Figure 8.13 (a to e) The tethering effect of posterior fusion in the young rapidly growing spine.

surprising to find such a high prevalence rate of minor spinal asymmetries when school children are systematically examined. The apex of Scheuermann's disease varies between the lower thoracic and upper lumbar regions, just as the apex of idiopathic scoliosis does. The lower, thoracolumbar Scheuermann's disease, referred to by Sorenson as 'apprentice's spine', is a well recognized clinical entity.

Careful examination of the patient and inspection of the radiographs demonstrates that double or multiple curve patterns are much more common than single curves (Cruickshank *et al.*, 1989). The King classification of these curve patterns has gained widespread acceptance but is purely descriptive of the coronal plane component of the deformity (King *et al.*, 1983). Analysis of the sagittal plane demonstrates the important balance between kyphosis and

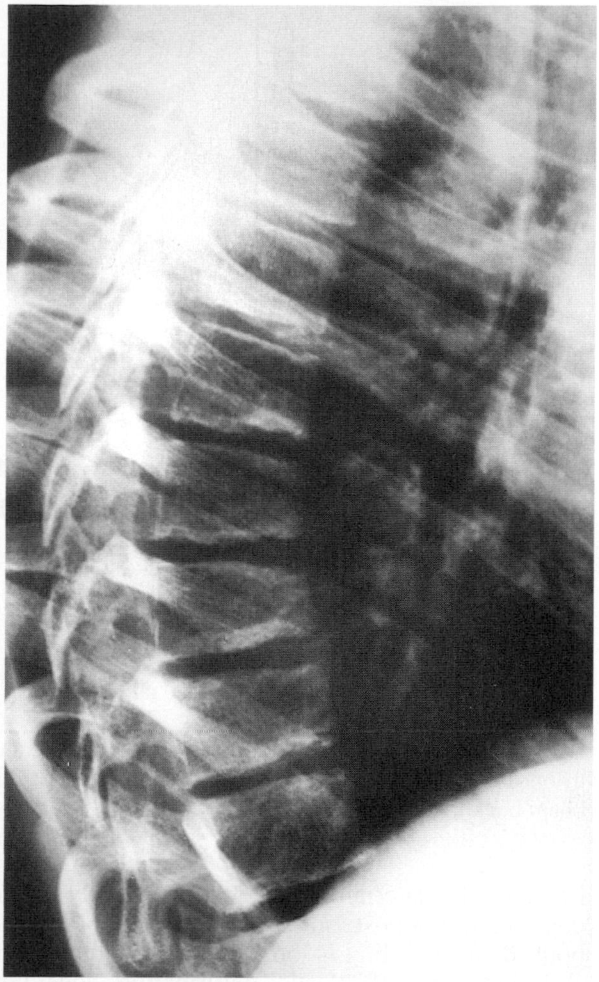

Figure 8.14 Scheuermann's disease. Lateral radiograph of the thoracic spine showing type I Scheuermann's disease – idiopathic thoracic hyperkyphosis.

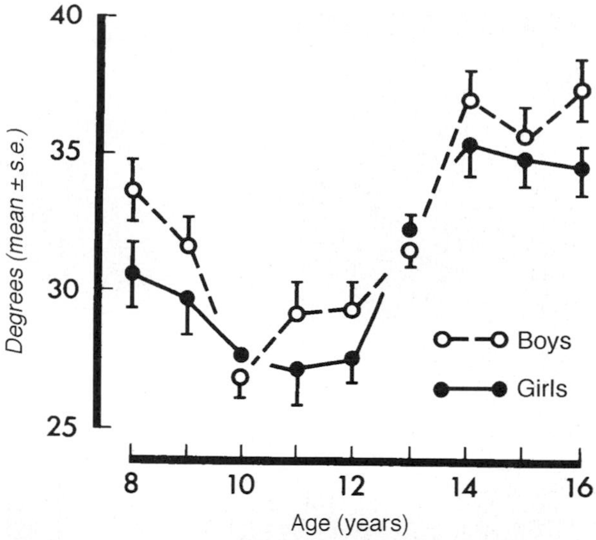

Figure 8.15 A graph of thoracic kyphosis on the vertical axis against age on the horizontal axis. In both boys and girls the thoracic kyphosis naturally reduces during the phase of the adolescent growth spurt.

lordosis in the growing spine. Above and below a single curve are what are termed compensatory scolioses restoring the spine to the vertical. A single curve is characterized by an apical zone of lordosis and if three-dimensional spinal balance is to be preserved there ought to be zones of kyphosis above and below. Therefore the beginnings of the compensatory scolioses are characterized by spinous process rotation to the convexity of the scoliosis, confirming the presence of kyphosis.

Triple curve patterns are also not uncommon (e.g. an uppermost thoracic curve convex to the left, an intervening lower thoracic curve convex to the right, and a lower lumbar curve convex to the left). Inspection of the PA radiograph (Figure 8.16) demonstrates that these three lordoscolioses merge one into the next with no intervening kyphosis, indicating that the spine is lordotic throughout.

Understanding three-dimensional spinal shape in structural scoliosis is important in determining what should be done to the spine operatively and over what length. It is no longer appropriate to throw a long 'blanket' posterior fusion at a spinal deformity. Hitherto there has been far too much reliance placed upon PA and lateral radiographs of the patient and clearly it would be quite inappropriate to obtain multiple radiographic projections of each child so as to determine spinal shape more precisely. A particularly helpful method is by way of computer graphics (Howell and Dickson, 1989). Known landmarks (e.g. vertebral body corners, pedicles) are digitized on PA and lateral radiographs and then a simple PC software program can spin the spinal column round and present it to the observer at any desired position of rotation. Thus, for example, the *plan d'élection* and true lateral appearances can be determined without taking special derotated x-ray views (Figure 8.17).

THE BIOMECHANICS OF SPINAL DEFORMITIES

Engineers have studied flexible columns for centuries and describe only two fundamental ways in which such a column can fail:

- angular collapse (material failure) and
- beam buckling (structural failure) (White and Panjabi, 1980) (Figure 8.18).

Angular collapse is, of course, kyphosis and

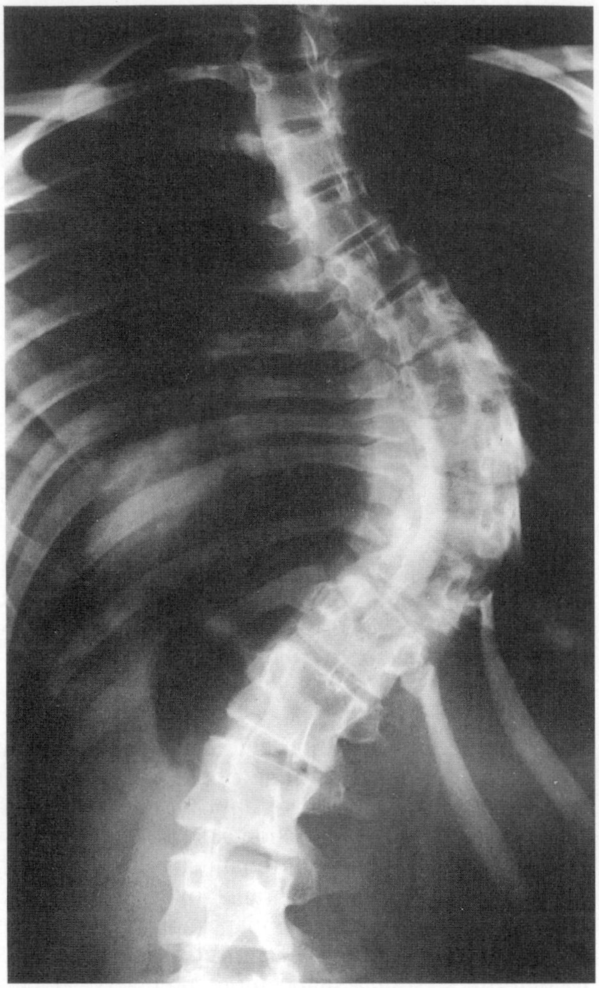

Figure 8.16 PA radiograph of what initially appears to be a single right thoracic curve. The spinous processes in both the upper and lower compensatory curves rotate into the curve concavity, indicating the presence of a triple structural curve pattern.

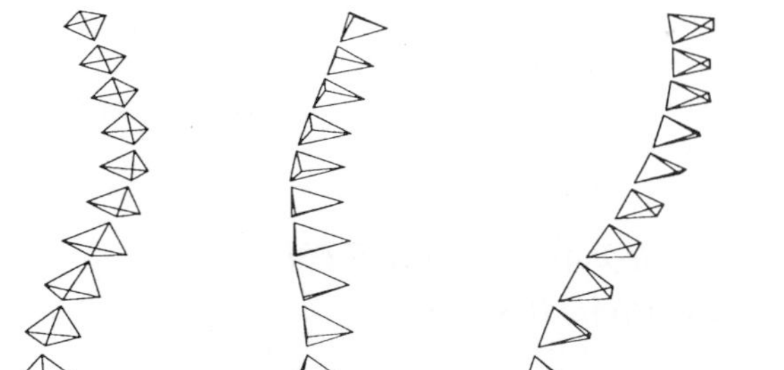

Figure 8.17 Spinal profiles generated by computer modelling with data derived from biplanar AP and lateral x-rays. By this means the spine can be viewed in any plane without the taking of further radiographs.

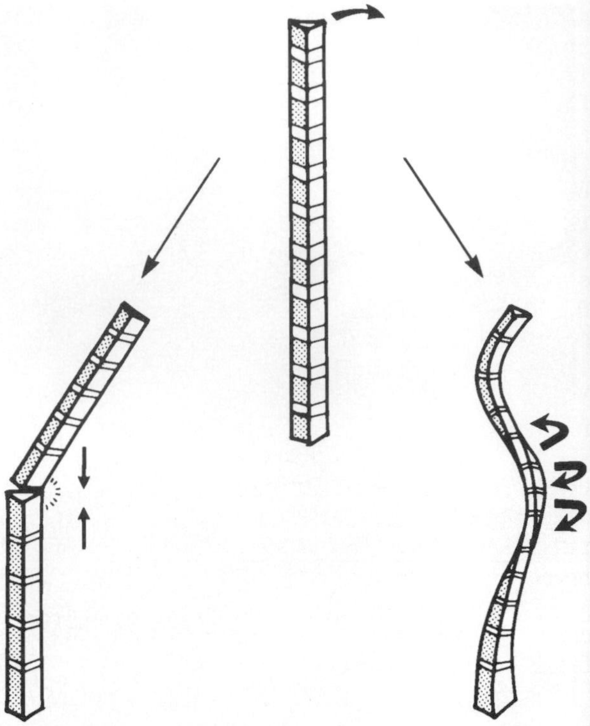

Figure 8.18 A cantilever or beam only fails mechanically in one of two ways: angular collapse (kyphosis, left) or beam buckling (lordoscoliosis, right).

implies true material failure either anteriorly under compression or posteriorly under tension, or indeed both. Beam buckling is lordoscoliosis with rotation and this form of plastic deformation does not necessarily imply true material loss. Moreover, the variables which are important in the mechanical behaviour of flexible columns are well established and are gathered together in the form of Euler's laws (Gordon, 1978). Although these laws in their simplest form pertain to a symmetrical column, such as a cylindrical pole, they are applicable in principle to the asymmetric flexible column of the spine.

Scoliosis

There is a requirement for the head and feet to face the front and therefore the ends of the human flexible column are relatively constrained. Under load the column would therefore fail towards the middle (where idiopathic scoliosis and Scheuermann's disease are particularly prevalent). Slenderness is also an important factor. This refers to the relationship between the length of the column and its cross-section. For columns of the same cross-section a longer column would fail before a shorter one, while for given lengths a thinner column would fail before a thicker one. It would therefore be expected that scoliotic children would be relatively tall and thin and several studies have confirmed this (Willner, 1974; Drummond and Rogalan, 1980; Archer and Dickson, 1985). Stiffness is also an important factor and it is both a material and structural property. Stiffness has important implications as regards bending characteristics and the human anisotropic flexible column is stiffer in females than males (Poussa *et al.*, 1989). A more flexible column moves elastically in response to an applied load, whereas the stiffer female column favours a torsional response to a bending load.

The fourth dimension, time, is also important with Wolff's law. In addition to the static features of material properties and structural geometry there is a super-added biological response of a dynamic nature. Growth and the repetitive cyclical loading of the activities of daily living, particularly flexion, are incrementally taken up by the growth plate. The involved vertebrae progressively adapt their shape and become more and more three-dimensionally asymmetric. Progressive deformation of the column therefore occurs during the phase of growth.

A very important variable in Euler's laws is the critical load to the spine and this is where the aetiological classification of scoliosis comes into play (Dickson, 1988). Idiopathic scoliosis occurs in children who are otherwise entirely normal clinically. Other aetiological categories in the classification are associated with a well recognized clinical condition, e.g. connective tissue disease. They do, however, share precisely the same type of deformity with idiopathic scoliosis, namely a lordoscoliosis with rotation. The incidence and progression potential of the lordoscoliosis in these conditions are very much greater than in idiopathic scoliosis. This is because the underlying condition has disadvantaged the critical load to the spine.

This can occur at bone level, ligament level or neuromuscular level and is all to do with balancing guyropes and reactive forces. Thus brittle bone disease and neurofibromatosis weaken the spinal column at bone level and in neurofibromatosis the more dystrophic the bone change the higher the prevalence rate of scoliosis, the earlier the age of onset, the more angular and sharp and rotated the deformity with greater progression. In mechanical terms there is material (brittle) failure superimposed upon the underlying structural (lordotic) or plastic failure. The heritable disorders of connective tissue such as Marfan's syndrome and Ehlers–Danlos syndrome affect the spine at ligament level with a higher prevalence rate and progression of the idiopathic type of lordoscoliosis. Indeed the deformities of Marfan's syndrome and idiopathic scoliosis are indistinguishable radiographically, although clinically very dissimilar.

With paralytic disorders such as cerebral palsy, poliomyelitis and muscular dystrophy, because of the dysfunction at the neuromuscular level, the spine readily collapses. The most common deformity type is the long C-shaped lordoscoliosis with pelvic obliquity, arising from asymmetric paraspinal muscle weakness in an area of pre-existing natural lordosis. The more severe the neuromuscular problem the higher the prevalence rate and greater progression potential of the deformity. A relatively mild cerebral palsy child with minimal brain dysfunction has a prevalence rate and progression potential of idiopathic-type scoliosis not that much greater than that of a normal child. At the other end of the spectrum with a child with severe spastic quadriplegia there is always a severe collapsing scoliosis by the time of puberty.

Another important biomechanical variable is the size of the deformity in relation to the progression potential. A curve of 40° will have more tendency to progress than a curve of 20° i.e. the further a spinal column has buckled the more likely it is to continue. The cross-sectional geometry of the spine is prismatic and in the thoracic region the prisms are such that their apices point anteriorly (Deacon *et al.*, 1987). This is a vulnerable configuration on forward flexion as a prismatic-shaped column flexed towards one of its apices is very much more rotationally unstable than when it is flexed towards its bases due to the second moment of area. Accordingly, the vulnerable thoracic prisms are protected by the presence of a kyphosis such that they are always behind the axis of spinal column rotation, without any tendency to torsion under bending load. However, when the essential lordosis develops during childhood and adolescence the anterior prismatic apex comes to lie in front of the axis of spinal column rotation and therefore buckles to the side in order to be accommodated.

The mid–lower thoracic vertebral bodies are constantly flattened on the left side by the descending thoracic aorta, a phenomenon well described by anatomists who recognized the existence of physiological thoracic scoliosis of a few degrees convex to the right and attributed it to this aortic effect (Cruveilhier, 1841; Frazier, 1940; Farkas, 1941). These lower thoracic prisms are therefore asymmetric and the anterior apex lies to the right of the midline (Figure 8.19). On flexion, for mechanical, geometric reasons, there will be a strong tendency for the column to be deflected to the right.

No such vertebral asymmetry exists in the lumbar spine to explain the tendency for lumbar curves to be convex to the left but just to the left of the front of the lumbar vertebral body lies the lumbar aorta and the presence of blood at arterial pressure with a significant resistance, therefore favouring a left-sided

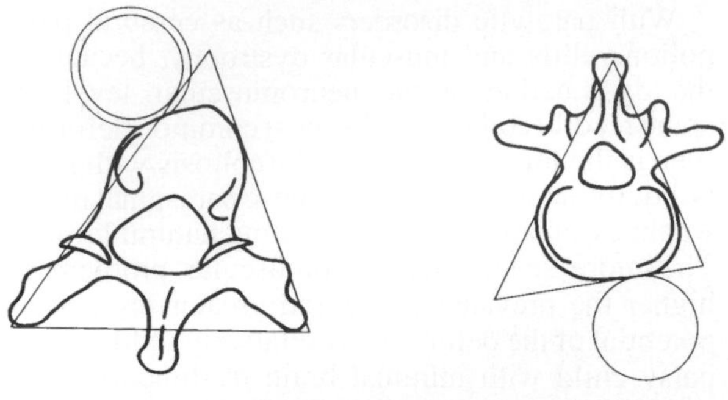

Figure 8.19 The descending thoracic aorta constantly deforms the mid–lower thoracic vertebrae putting the apex of the prism to the right side. There is a similar dynamic effect in the lumbar region favouring left-sided rotation.

rotation. There is no other obvious explanation for the sideness of curves at different sites and handedness has been conclusively disproven (Goldberg and Dowling, 1991).

The cervical and lumbar regions, being naturally lordotic, would appear superficially to be vulnerable to the development of lordoscolioses as the vertebral bodies lie anterior to the axis of spinal column rotation. There are, however, very considerable inbuilt protective mechanisms. The cervical and lumbar regions are towards the end of the flexible spinal column and a column preferentially fails in the middle.

Second, the very considerable amount of flexion available allows these regions to become frankly kyphotic before the limits of flexion are reached, in contrast to the stiff thoracic lordosis in association with thoracic scoliosis. There is little or no anisotropism in the cervical and lumbar regions with similar flexibility in both AP and lateral directions. Also, posterior to the cervical and lumbar lordoses the very powerful paraspinal muscles maintain stability. In the presence of a neuromuscular disorder with weakening of these strong muscles, this natural area of lordosis would increase and readily buckle to the side. Therefore the typical paralytic curve is sited in the lumbar region with hyperlordosis and a collapsing scoliosis with pelvic obliquity.

Kyphosis

The biomechanics of kyphosis is a much more straightforward affair. The relatively mild S-shaped configuration in the sagittal plane of the normal spine does not have to become very much more pronounced before the thoracic kyphosis exponentially and autonomously increases, as seen in progressive Scheuermann's disease. Such a hyperkyphotic spine is, however, naturally protected from buckling although a little right/left asymmetry in the kyphotic process can give rise to a few degrees of non-rotated lateral curvature at the kyphotic apex (Sorenson, 1964; Deacon *et al.*, 1985).

Because the line of the centre of gravity is in front of the entire spine, angular collapse always produces kyphosis, even in an area of natural lordosis such as the lumbar spine. Trauma and the destructive effect of tumours and infection often result in angular kyphosis. Should such insults occur before spinal maturity, and the destabilizing effect of surgical laminectomy on the growing spine is a notable example, then a progressive kyphosis ensues (Figure 8.20).

Experimental production of scoliosis

This has for many years been used to study the pathogenesis of scoliosis. In 1939 Haas damaged surgically the epiphyseal cartilaginous plate of the vertebrae on one side; other authors (Bisgard and Musselman, 1940; Nachlas and Borden, 1950), by unilateral growth arrest of two or three vertebrae, produced rotary lateral curvatures of the spine.

Radiation damage has also been used to produce this lesion in animals. Arkin and Simon (1950) implanted radium seeds next to the intervertebral spaces of the lumbar spine in rabbits and this resulted in suppression of growth of the epiphysis with wedging of the vertebral bodies and a scoliosis, as well as stunting of the iliac crest. Contraction and soft tissue of the concavity of the curve was not rewarded as a major factor in the mechanism of scoliosis. Farkas (1954) believed that in the production of irradiation scoliosis the weakest link lay in the epiphyseal ring which becomes separated from the vertebra. Rubin *et al.* (1962) carried out a longitudinal study of children following radiation for Wilms' tumour and medulloblastoma. Twelve cases developed a measurable scoliosis, but only one deteriorated over 45°. In this series there were marked bony changes in the vertebrae, in the pelvis and ribs, but these curves did not deteriorate even though they had begun in infancy, and should have behaved similarly to that of infantile idiopathic scoliosis.

Schwartzmann and Miles (1945) created muscle imbalance in rats and mice by the selective release of certain muscle groups on the vertebral column which resulted in the development of scoliosis.

Langenskiold and Michelsson (1962) produced progressive scoliosis by removing the posterior end of five or six ribs as well as by hemilaminectomy of five of the thoracic vertebrae. They pointed out the only common factor was the loss of function of the posterior costotransverse ligaments, and by cutting these ligaments in rabbits they produced similar deformities.

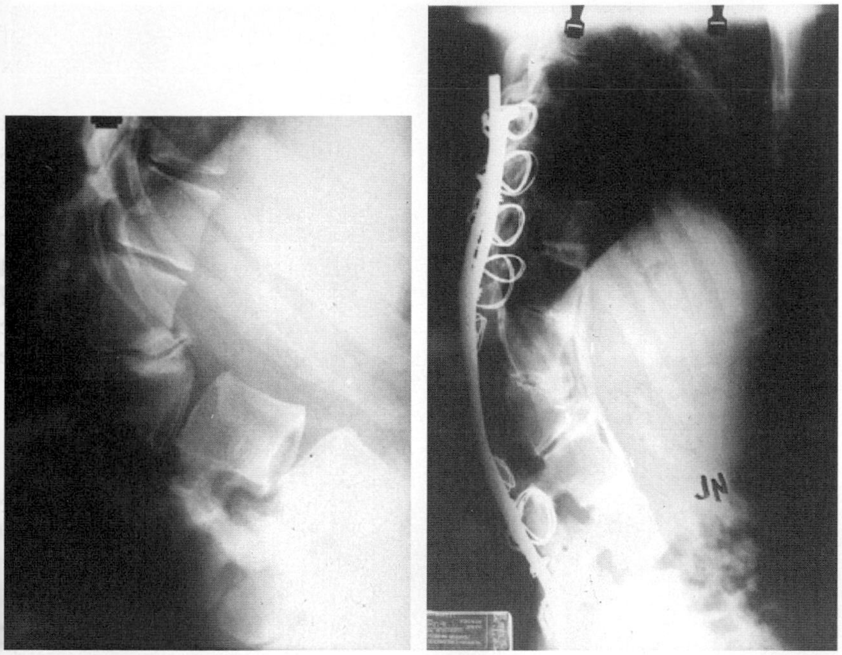

(a) (b)

Figure 8.20 Post-laminectomy kyphosis. (a) This fracture with temporary neurology was dealt with by wide laminectomy. A severe unstable kyphosis has developed. (b) Dealt with by anterior and posterior fusion.

Ponseti and Shephard (1954) produced scoliosis, with other lesions of lathyrism, in rats who had been fed diets containing *Lathyrus odoratus* seeds. These skeletal deformities were due to lesions in the epiphyseal plates, with loosening and detachment of the tendinous and ligamentous insertions.

Experimental work by Liszka (1961) of Poland, repeated by MacEwan (1968) offers a new approach to the further investigation of the aetiology of idiopathic scoliosis. The section of the dorsal and ventral nerve roots on one side of the thoracic spine in 2–3-week-old rabbits produced a scoliosis with rotation and angulation similar to the idiopathic-type curve in the human. Resection of three nerve roots regularly produced a 50° curve. Increasing the number of nerve roots sectioned increased the degree of angulation. Yamada and associates (1969) found eqilibrial dysfunction in 57 out of 70 scoliosis patients during the period of rapid vertebral growth. They suggested a disturbance at spinal cord and brain stem levels as an aetiological factor in scoliosis.

Electromyographic studies have not shown any significant differences between the musculature on the concave and convex sides (Editorial, 1976). Histochemical investigations have shown that there are relatively more slow-twitch muscle fibres on the convex side of the curve (Fidler and Jowett, 1976), but whether these changes are primary or secondary is as yet unknown. Abnormal metachromasia of skin fibroblasts has been detected in idiopathic scoliosis patients (Nordwall and Waldenstrom, 1976), but the significance of these observations remains to be elucidated.

Damage to the posterior sensory nerve roots, degeneration of anterior horn cells in the spinal cord and defects of the basal ganglia are all associated with an increased prevalence of scoliosis (Robin, 1975). Experimental damage to these structures can cause scoliosis in the laboratory animal (MacEwan, 1973).

Equilibrial dysfunction has been incriminated as a factor in the development of idiopathic scoliosis, and indeed has been correlated with curve magnitude and progression (Yamada *et al.*, 1969). Abducent paralysis and nystagmus have been noted in individuals with particularly severe curves. Electronystagmographic studies have revealed vestibular dysfunction in idiopathic scoliosis patients (Sahlstrand *et al.*, 1977). However, equilibrial, postural and vestibular dysfunction are also found in other types of scoliosis and the problem of cause and effect remains unsolved.

By damaging the growth plate by either irradiation or surgery a deformity occurs but such experimental damage has never produced a three-dimensional deformity in the growing animal. The common denominator of these experimental procedures was surgical interference close to the segmental arterial blood supply to the spinal cord. De Salis *et al.* (1980) provided the missing link by demonstrating that in rats and rabbits the spinal cord is supplied by an

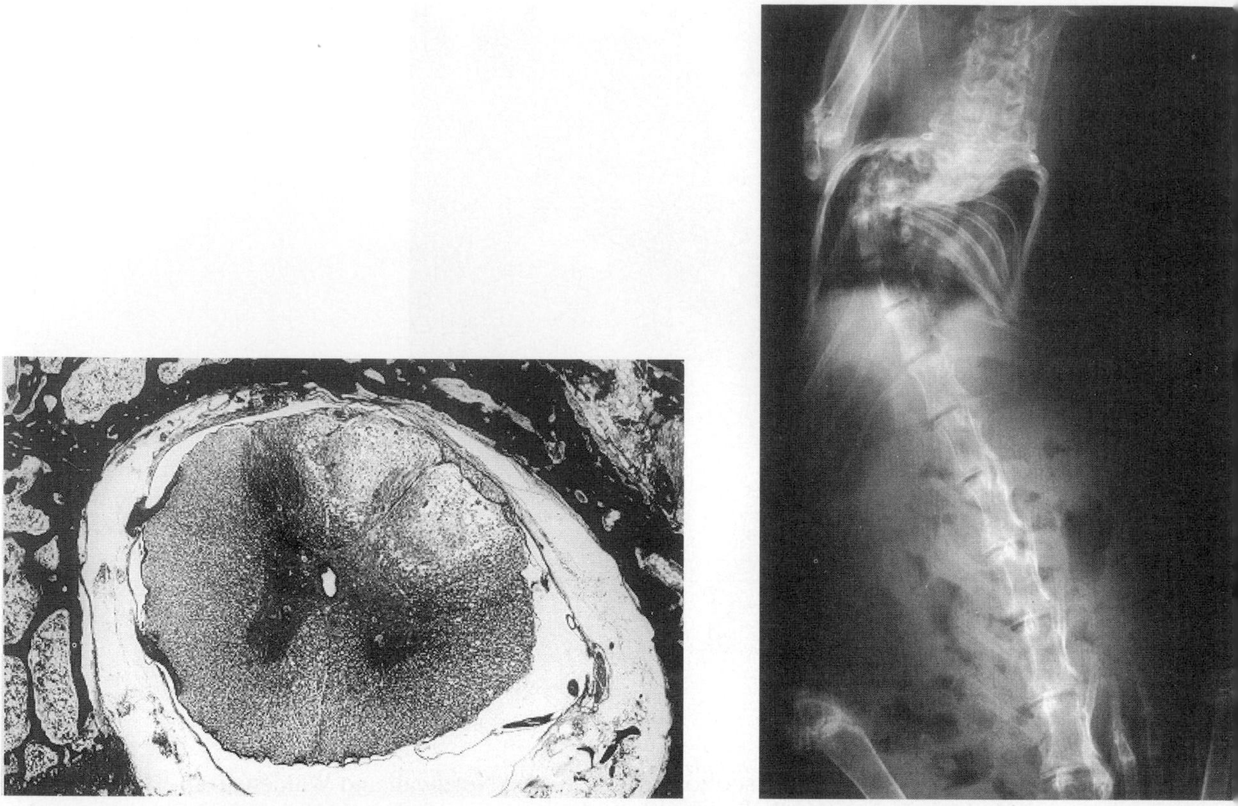

(a) (b)

Figure 8.21 Experimental 'paralytic' scoliosis (a and b). Severe thoracic scoliosis in the rabbit in association with a cord infarct. The Cobb angle was more than 40° by the time the animal woke up from anaesthesia.

important feeder vessel at every segmental level whereas in the human there tends to be one important vessel at one particular level (the artery of Adamkiewicz).

Lawton and Dickson (1986) and Smith and Dickson (1987) have demonstrated that if the segmental blood supply is not interfered with then only a very mild postural scoliosis is produced which resolves quickly. If the segmental arterial supply to the spinal cord is interfered with then a paralytic scoliosis of major proportions is rapidly produced, as well as a large spinal cord infarct at post-mortem examination. These authors had produced an experimental 'paralytic' scoliosis ant not experimental 'idiopathic' scoliosis (Figure 8.21). The only way to produce the deformity in an animal comparable to idiopathic scoliosis is by way of posterior tether to the growing spine. The typical idiopathic lordoscoliosis then develops with all three components that we see in the human – lordosis, lateral curvature and rotation (Figure 8.22).

Idiopathic scoliosis

Although the condition can develop at any time during spinal growth, it has been traditionally subdivided into infantile (under 4 years of age), juvenile (4–9 years of age) and adolescent (10 years of age to maturity) types according to age of onset (James, 1954). These ages of onset were in turn referable to the three phases of increased growth velocity. Thoracic deformities in excess of 60° were regarded as potentially serious, in view of a tendency to produce morbidity and mortality from cardiopulmonary compromise (Nachemson, 1968; Nilsonne and Lundgren, 1968; Collis and Ponseti, 1969). However, cadaver dissection work on children with infantile scoliosis who had perished for other reasons showed that a significant chest deformity could only produce a long-term health problem if it interfered with reduplication of the pulmonary alveolar tree (Reid, 1971). At birth the lungs are not mini-versions of the adult form but consist of only a few million alveoli which reduplicate to about 250 million at the age of 4 before plateauing out at 300 million at the

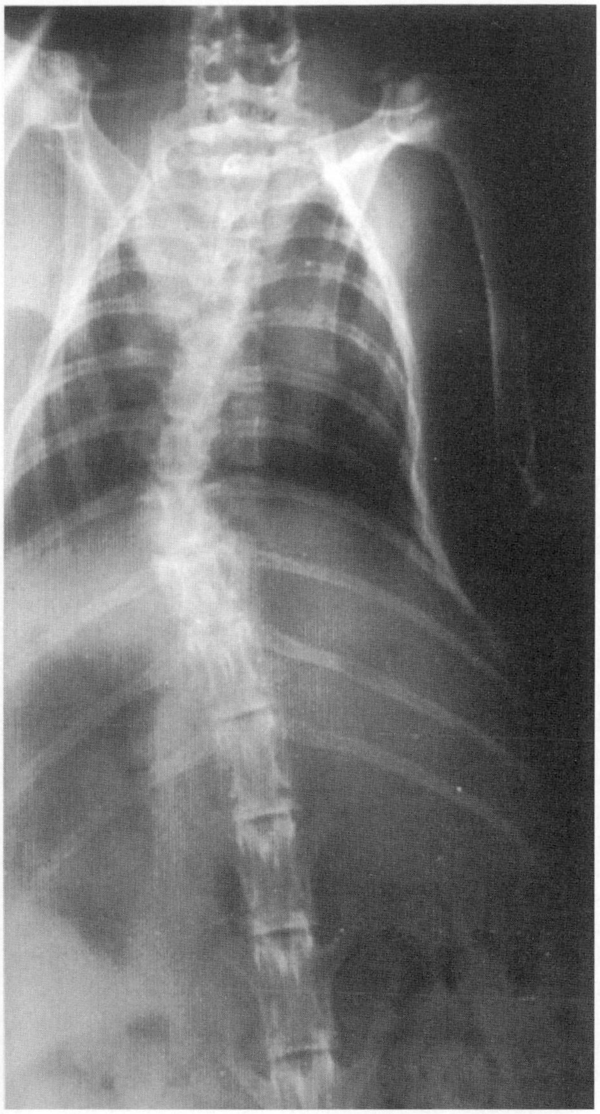

Figure 8.22 Experimental 'idiopathic' scoliosis 4 weeks after posterior cord tether in the growing rabbit.

age of 8. Therefore only infantile progressive scoliosis would significantly interfere with subsequent cardiopulmonary function. Branthwaite (1986) assessed cardiorespiratory function in several hundred untreated scoliosis cases and demonstrated that only if there was a chest deformity of significance before the age of 5 years was the patient subsequently disadvantaged. But when a thoracic scoliosis becomes a severe deformity after the age of 5 years, no significant cardiopulmonary dysfunction occurred.

The older long-term follow-up studies of untreated thoracic scoliosis ignored the age of onset and progression. Indeed, in Nachemson's oft-quoted study there is an identifiable subset of patients with a significant thoracic deformity which was definitely of adolescent onset and this group behaved similarly to other children.

Therefore only two categories of onset of idiopathic scoliosis, early onset and late onset, before and after 5 years of age should be used (Dickson, 1985).

EARLY ONSET IDIOPATHIC SCOLIOSIS

This condition refers to the development of an idiopathic structural scoliosis before the age of 3–5 years. This condition is therefore equivalent to infantile idiopathic scoliosis. There are two basic subgroups – the resolving and the progressive varieties, although there is an intermediate group of children whose deformity having developed then remains static for many years. In the early part of this century the condition was common, almost as common as late onset scoliosis, and the great majority were of the progressive variety, quickly going on to severe deformities with significant cardiopulmonary complications (Harrenstein, 1930; James, 1951; Scott and Morgan, 1955; James *et al.*, 1959).

The condition is now relatively unusual, providing only a small number of cases seen in scoliosis clinics each year (McMaster, 1983). Over 95% are of the benign resolving variety, with the male to female ratio of 3:2. Most curves occur in the thoracic region but lumbar and double curve patterns are not uncommon. Three-quarters of thoracic curves are convex to the left. The pathogenesis of this condition is uncertain and two schools of thought exist:

1. prenatal intratuterine pressure moulding (Browne, 1956; Mehta, 1984); and
2. postnatal moulding from the baby lying in the lateral/oblique position (Mau, 1968; Watson, 1971; McMaster, 1983).

Certainly moulding is an important factor as there is always evidence of skeletal asymmetry elsewhere. Plagiocephaly (on the side of the curve convexity), plagiopelvy, bat ear, wry neck, and hip adduction, all on the same side, are common associated features. In favour of postnatal moulding is the fact that plagiocephaly is not present at birth but develops during the first few days of life, as indeed do the other clinical aspects of the condition (Dempster and Dickson, 1987). Moreover, where infants have been laid prone to stop the harmful effects of the lateral/oblique position, the condition of infantile idiopathic scoliosis has all but disappeared (McMaster, 1983). There is 30 times the expected rate of scoliosis in parents and siblings of affected children but there are not thought to be any genetic differences between early and late onset idiopathic scoliosis (Wynne–Davies, 1975). There is also an increased prevalence rate of congenital heart disease, inguinal hernia, breech delivery, older mothers, congenital hip dislocation, and other congenital malformation such as hiatus hernia (Mehta, 1984).

In an effort to sort out 'progressors' from 'regressors' Mehta (1972) studied the PA radiographs of thoracic curves and measured the rib/vertebra angle on each side of the apical vertebra (see Figure 8.6). Should the difference of angles (rib/vertebra angle difference, RVAD) be greater than 20° the curve was likely to progress and vice versa with lower RVADs. While this is certainly a useful measure, it is only a measure of vertebral rotation. The developmental status of the typical 'progressor' is a low birth weight, floppy baby, with low neurological development scores. Wynne-Davies (1975) recorded a high prevalence rate of mental retardation in the 'progressive group'. This lends support to the notion that neuromuscular factors may be important. By contrast, the normal birth weight, normally developing baby with a mild idiopathic deformity due to pressure moulding is easily able to resist progressive buckling and the deformity resolves with time. It may take several years for resolution to occur and it is typical for the rotational prominence on the curve convexity to be the last deformity to disappear.

Early onset scoliosis, before the age of 5 years, of the progressive variety has a poor prognosis as regards health. A reduction in vital capacity or in forced expiratory volume with larger curves due to increased chest wall stiffness, should not be misinterpreted as having real clinical outcome problems. There is no evidence that the scoliotic back is any more painful than the straight back, at least as regards frequency and severity of episodes of pain. Clinical experience suggests, however, that should a scoliotic spine become painful then it is more resistant to standard measures than the straight back, recalcitrant cases usually coming to spinal fusion (Dawson *et al.*, 1973a; Kostuik *et al.*, 1973; Ponder *et al.*, 1975).

Untreated progressive idiopathic cases have also been associated with social and psychological dysfunction but these Swedish studies included a large number of severe thoracic cases, many of whom were the early onset category (Bengtsson *et al.*, 1974). Patients with the very ugly torso deformity of early onset progressive scoliosis are disadvantaged by lower marriage rates, higher divorce rates, lower numbers of children per marriage, higher psychiatric consultation rates and higher suicide rates. The early onset severely progressive idiopathic case, more uncommon nowadays, should be treated for health, social and psychological reasons. Late onset scoliosis is, however, a matter of deformity only.

LATE ONSET IDIOPATHIC SCOLIOSIS

Epidemiological surveys of school children for torso asymmetry have demonstrated that late onset idiopathic scoliosis is a very common condition (Kane and Moe, 1970; Brooks *et al.*, 1975; Ascani *et al.*, 1977; Bellyei *et al.*, 1977; Lonstein, 1977a; Rogala *et al.*, 1978; Smyrnis *et al.*, 1979). Prevalence studies indicate that 40% of scolioses detected in the community are non-structural curves secondary to a leg length inequality (Dickson *et al.*, 1980). When these are excluded, 10% of normal adolescent school children will have a measurable late onset idiopathic scoliosis. Two per cent will have a curve measuring 10° or more and only 2 per thousand a curve measuring 20° or more (Dickson, 1983). Comparison of prevalence rates 10 years apart indicates that this condition is less prevalent and less progressive than it was. A similar trend is being observed in the United States (Lonstein *et al.*, 1982).

In scoliosis clinics there is a female to male ratio of 10:1, with right thoracic curves being more prevalent and an appreciable progression potential. However, when curves of all magnitudes in school screening programmes are analysed, the female to male sex ratio is equal, there is a preponderance of lumbar curves, with only 1:10 progressing. Ninety per cent of these either remain the same or even improve. With increase in curve size there are more girls, greater number of thoracic curves, and progression more likely.

A recent survey involving the screening of 16 000 Leeds school children derived a cohort of almost 1000 who were then followed for 6 years with annual AP and lateral x-rays of the spine (Mahood *et al.*, 1990).

In particular two subsets were studied: first, those who started with a straight spine and developed idiopathic scoliosis during the course of the study and second, those who started straight and remained straight. Both lateral profile and growth velocity were important discriminant factors in differentiating these two subsets. Those who developed idiopathic scoliosis had a flatter lateral profile to start with in the region of the curve apex and had a significantly higher growth velocity.

AETIOLOGY

Early work described action potential asymmetry by electromyography in the paraspinal muscles (Lefebvre *et al.*, 1961), and histopathological observations of fibre-type disproportion in the same musculature (Zuk, 1962) were subsequently invalidated as being secondary to the presence of the spinal curvature (Alexander and Season 1978; Zetterberg *et al.*, 1983; Saartok *et al.*, 1984). Research involving other musculoskeletal tissues and at one stage or another eye, ear, brain, spinal cord, nerve roots, muscles, more muscles, rib heads, costotransverse ligaments, intervertebral discs, viruses, have all been accused of causing idiopathic scoliosis, but never substantiated.

However, O'Beirne *et al.* (1989) looked at not only idiopathic scoliosis but also congenital deformities and subdivided them into progressive and non-progressive types. The function of the brain stem equilibrium centres was tested and it was found that dysfunctional responses were characteristic of curves that were progressive or had recently progressed irrespective of aetiology. Such phenomena were secondary to the curve itself rather than being of primary aetiological importance in idiopathic scoliosis.

Koch's postulates dictate that if a variable is to be aetiological then all patients must have it. The only abnormality that patients have in structural scoliosis concerns the lateral spinal profile. Some changes that have been identified may have something to do with progression potential of the established condition but are certainly not aetiological, e.g. spinal balance mechanisms when deficient would be less able to resist the buckling potential of a lordosis deformity. Neuromuscular scoliosis is a well accepted phenomenon, with greater incidence of scoliosis in the patients with a more severe degree of paralysis. The small minority of cases of so-called 'idiopathic scoliosis' with an identifiable neuromuscular abnormality (e.g. syringomyelia) are, indeed, true 'neuromuscular scoliosis'. The overwhelming majority do not have any identifiable cause and that is why their condition is termed idiopathic scoliosis.

TREATMENT

Late onset scoliosis

Conservative treatment

As the condition is one of deformity and appearance, and not one of organic ill-health, the decision to treat is based upon whether the deformity is acceptable or not. Acceptability is not necessarily easy to define. A small, e.g. a Cobb angle of 40°, deformity may be totally unacceptable and insist upon treatment whereas other patients and their families find a deformity of a Cobb angle of 60° entirely acceptable. The future of the deformity and the risks and rewards of treatment, must be presented. In immature patients there is considerable time for deterioration to occur whereas if the patient is relatively mature then the deformity remains static.

If the deformity is acceptable and if there is still much growth ahead then the aim of conservative treatment would be to maintain the existing deformity through the rest of growth. If the deformity is unacceptable then the role of treatment, usually surgical correction and fusion, will be to restore the most acceptable state and to maintain it during the remainder of growth, recognizing a number of serious problems, with both conservative and surgical treatments.

A number of contraptions and devices have been used since the time of Hippocrates in an effort to prevent the progression of a structural scoliosis with no great enthusiasm either by patient or protagonist (Jones, 1922–31). The early part of this century saw the use of plaster-of-Paris casts, particularly by the French, but plaster casts were soon superseded by the Milwaukee brace designed by Blount (Blount and Schmidt, 1957) (Figure 8.23). It should be remembered that the Milwaukee brace was designed to support the poliomyelitis scoliosis postoperatively, i.e. after spinal fusion, and was never conceived as an orthosis for the conservative treatment of any form of scoliosis (Blount and Moe, 1973). Mass polio vaccination programmes have markedly reduced the incidence of poliomyelitis scoliosis. The Milwaukee brace was applied to idiopathic scoliosis curves in an effort to prevent their progression, by holding the pelvis below and the head above, and by using a pull strap round the twisted thoracic cage. Blount also observed that if the lower pelvic girdle component of the orthosis was made flat in the sagittal plane (i.e. flattening the lumbar lordosis) then the thoracic deformity above would be seen to improve spontaneously by an important change in lateral profile. With the lumbar lordosis obliterated then the only way the patient could maintain trunk extension was to extend the thoracic spine above and thus make more room for the lordosis which moved back towards the mid-sagittal plane (Dickson, 1985). The Milwaukee brace is an example of a CTLSO (cervico-thoracic-lumbar-sacral orthosis). It became apparent that the Milwaukee superstructure was not necessary and indeed produced mandibular deformities (Watts *et al.*, 1977), and therefore the Boston underarm brace was developed (TLSO) (Figure 8.24). Empirically the brace was prescribed for 23 hours a day with 1 hour out for a wash and some

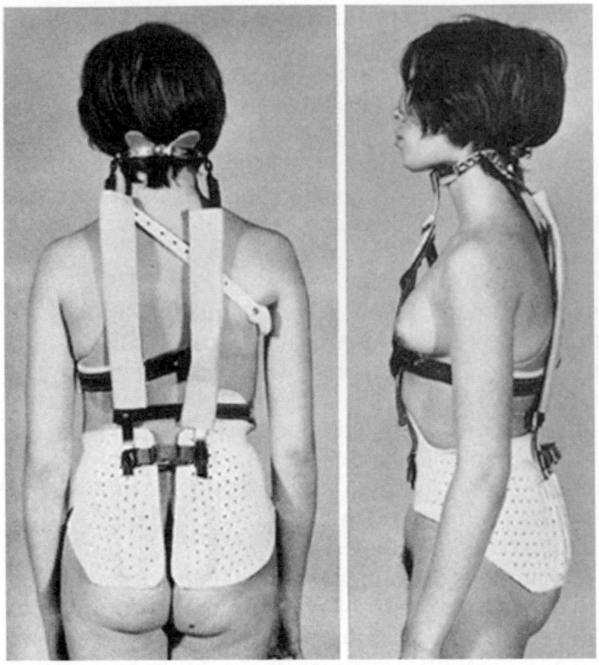

(a) (b)

Figure 8.23 A Milwaukee brace with left thoracic, right lumbar pad. The pelvic girdle is fashioned in Orthoplast, which is washable.

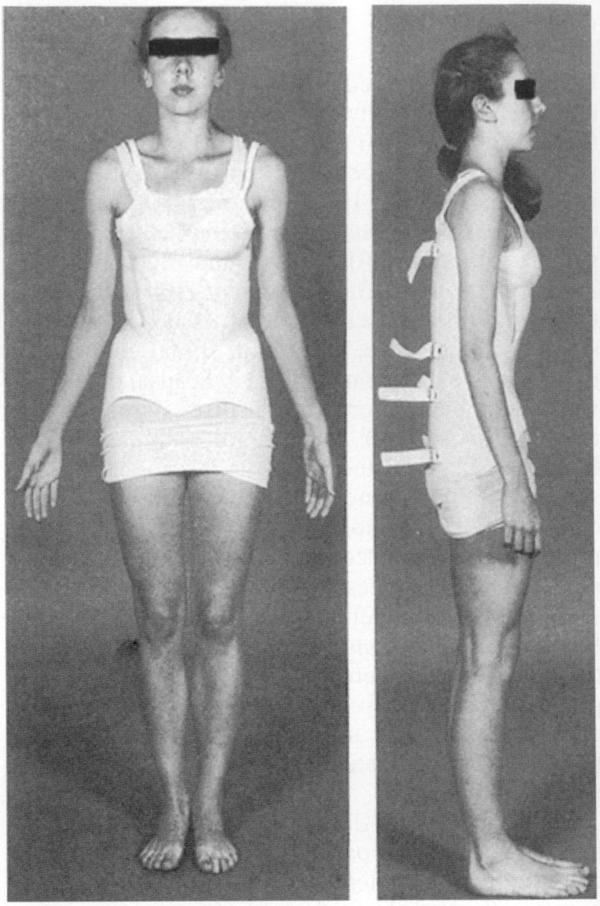

Figure 8.24 The Boston brace system.

exercises. The scientific validity for brace wearing remaining unchallenged by any form of clinical trial or controlled investigation. For curves of 20° or more almost 80% could be prevented from progression, or even improved a little, by brace wearing (Keiser and Shufflebarger, 1976; Mellencamp *et al.*, 1977). With better results seeming to occur with smaller curves, screening for the condition of late onset idiopathic scoliosis produced enormous numbers of relatively small curves. However, it also became apparent from school screening that 80% of curves measuring 20° or more would not progress, or indeed would improve somewhat, even if they were not braced. The Scoliosis Research Society have little confidence in orthotic treatment (Morrissy, 1988). A small controlled study from Sweden showed no benefit on those wearing braces (Miller *et al.*, 1984), while a meticulous controlled study of Boston data demonstrated that braces were ineffective (Goldberg *et al.*, 1992).

Results of the European Brace Trial (Edgar, personal communication, 1994) have shown that if an increase in Cobb angle of 6° is regarded as the threshold for progression then the wearing of a brace exerts a significant preventative effect. Six degrees may be significant statistically but not clinically.

Electrical stimulation of the paraspinal muscles in an effort to correct the curve was shown to be ineffective (Bradford *et al.*, 1983). Investigative work by hidden compliance meters concerning conservative treatment by bracing showed that even in seemingly user-friendly and compliant middle class English families braces were only worn for a fraction of their prescribed time (Houghton *et al.*, 1987). Concern about conservative treatment also raises other important issues. One of the main prerequisites of any screening programme is that there should be 'effective' non-operative treatment for the early curve (Whitby, 1974), but there is none.

As conservative treatment cannot usually prevent the progression of a deformity, let alone improve it, then when the deformity becomes unacceptable only surgical treatment can influence it. Before the days of instrumentation, corrections were achieved by the application of preoperative plaster-of-Paris casts either in the form of localizers or turn-buckle casts (Hibbs *et al.*, 1931). Windows were then made in the back of the cast through which a spinal fusion operation was carried out. This was the correct strategy, i.e. to obtain as good a correction as possible, and then to maintain that correction,

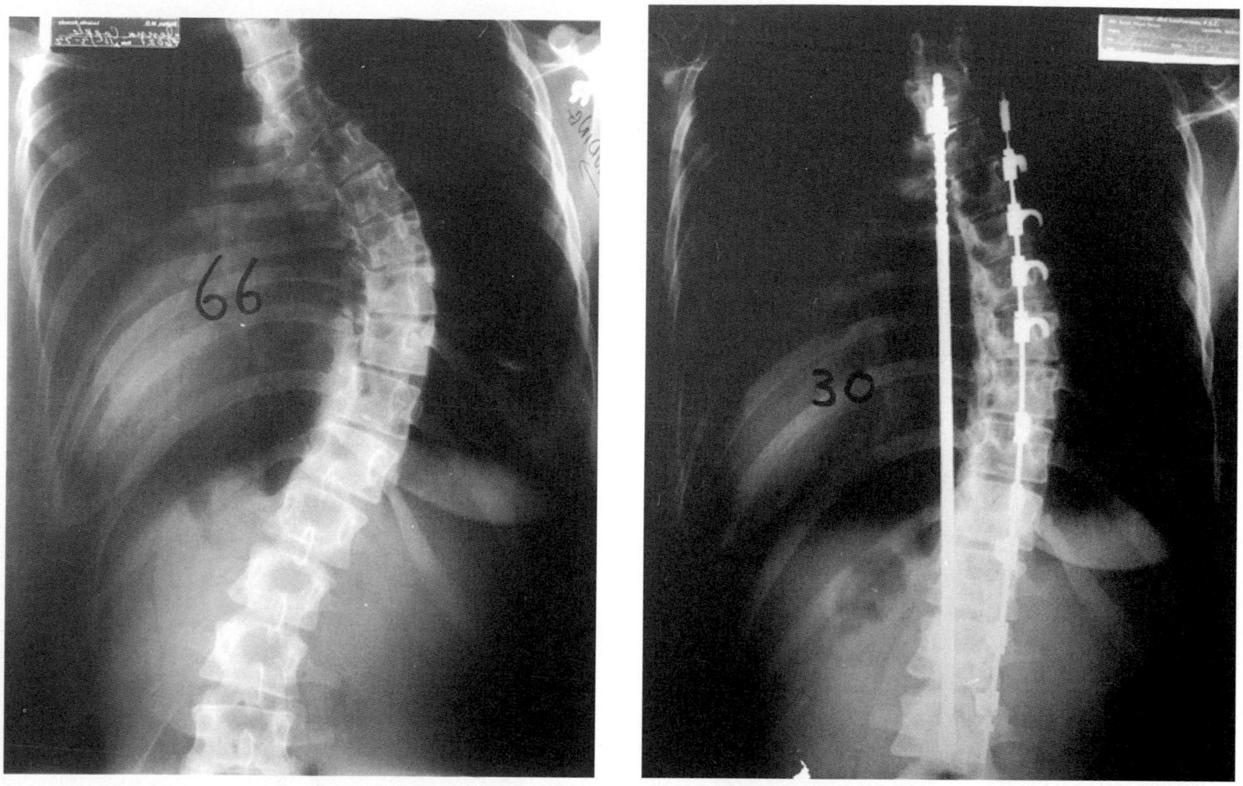

(a) (b)

Figure 8.25 (a) Preoperative and (b) postoperative PA x-rays of a right thoracic idiopathic scoliosis with a good correction in the coronal plane.

through growth by spinal fusion. However, the posterior spinal fusion would tether the spine behind the essential lordosis.

Surgical treatment

In 1962 Harrington described his instrumentation, the essential feature of which was a longitudinal rod fixed by hollow hooks to the spine above and below the deformity, with the ability to extend the rod and elongate the distance of the spine. A compression metalwork system was placed on the convex side of the spine, pulling down on the vertebral elements above the apex and pulling up below, so that the convex side of the spine was shortened (Figure 8.25). Using the two systems it was possible to achieve an appreciable correction of the Cobb angle for flexible curves and this technique gained rapid worldwide acceptance (Goldstein, 1966; Moe, 1972; Harrington, 1973) with meticulous bone grafting.

Moe, comparing Harrington instrumentation with previous plaster corrective treatments, noted that there was no difference in the percentage correction of Cobb angle (Moe, 1958). The pseudarthrosis rate was greatly reduced using instrumentation as well as the need for plaster-of-Paris and the length of hospitalization. Then Schultz and Hirsch (1973), and many others afterwards (Thulbourne and Gillespie, 1976; Benson *et al.*, 1977; Aaro and Dahlborn, 1982), demonstrated that using distraction as a method of correction did not bring about any derotation at the curve apex. The rotational rib prominence with which the patient presented was left unchanged (Figure 8.26). Again, if the patient was immature, then, following a temporary improvement in appearance, this could deteriorate with subsequent growth as the back of the spine was tethered.

Although wiring vertebrae to longitudinal rods was a much earlier design concept (Lange, 1910; Resina and Alves, 1977), it became effective when Luque applied sublaminar wires to longitudinal rods for early flexible poliomyelitis curves (Luque, 1982). The strong strength of the lamina and the multiple segmental fixation provided considerable rigidity and protection to the corrected position. Wires were then added to the idiopathic scoliosis case, either to standard Luque non-hooked-in L-rods or on the concave side to a Harrington distraction rod (a Harrington–Luque procedure). It was possible to improve the Cobb angle over and above standard Harrington instrumentation, but the rotational

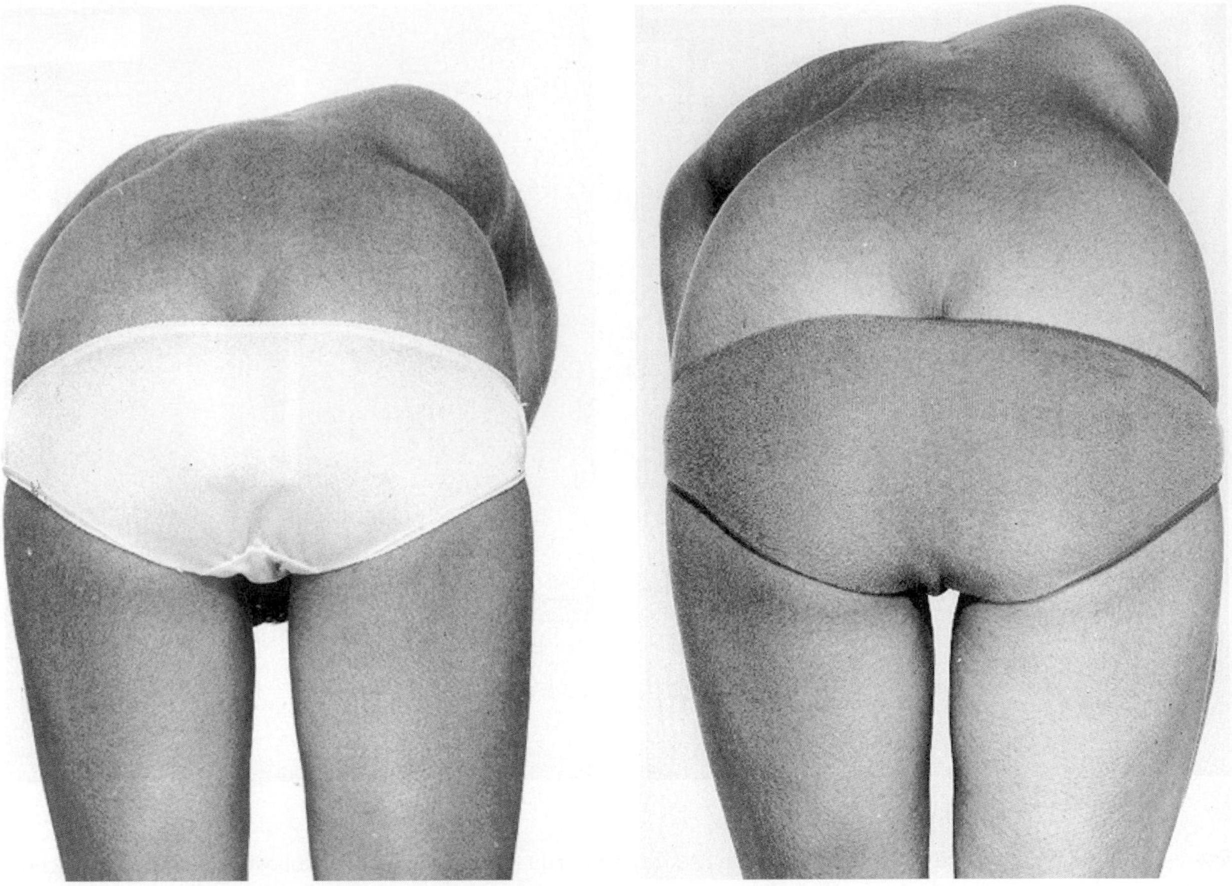

(a) (b)

Figure 8.26 Forward bending view (a) before and (b) 2 years following Harrington instrumentation for a right thoracic curve. There has been no correction of the rib hump which was the patient's chief presenting complaint.

prominence remained unchanged or indeed was made worse. To improve the rotational component the Harrington–Luque procedure has been modified (Dickson and Archer, 1987). The longitudinal rod is prebent into an appropriate amount of kyphosis so that the sublaminar wires on the concave side pull backwards rather than sideways. The Leeds procedure in flexible idiopathic thoracic curves achieves an amount of derotation in excess of 50% (Figure 8.27).

Cotrel and Dubousset (Dubousset *et al.*, 1986), used longitudinal metalwork with hooks not dissimilar to those designed by Harrington. A longitudinal rod is inserted on the concave side and prebent into about half the value of the scoliosis (i.e. if the scoliosis measured 50° then prebending to 20° or so). Then because the rod can be rotated within the hooks before final tightening the scoliosis is turned 90° round into kyphosis before final rod/hook tightening. Then on the compression side a straighter rod is inserted in an attempt to flatten down the convex side of the curve apex. Finally with the aid of two metal clamps the two rods are joined together to make a rectangular stable configuration (Figure 8.28). Their initial results demonstrated a 40° improvement in rotation at the curve apex (Dubousset *et al.*, 1986). Dwyer *et al.* (1969) developed a system of attacking the problem anteriorly and inserting metalwork designed to shorten the too long anteroconvex side of the curve. The intervertebral discs were excised down to the end plates and the posterior longitudinal ligaments. Transverse vertebral body screws were placed, each screw having a hollow head to receive a cable which was then subsequently tightened with the effect that the screw heads were compressed one to another (Figure 8.29). For idiopathic scoliosis this has never achieved great acceptance but the technique has been readily applied for more complex and demanding paralytic curves.

The Dwyer instrumentation was upgraded by Zielke in Germany and the braided cable was exchanged for a threaded rod, rather like a Harrington compression rod, with curve correction being

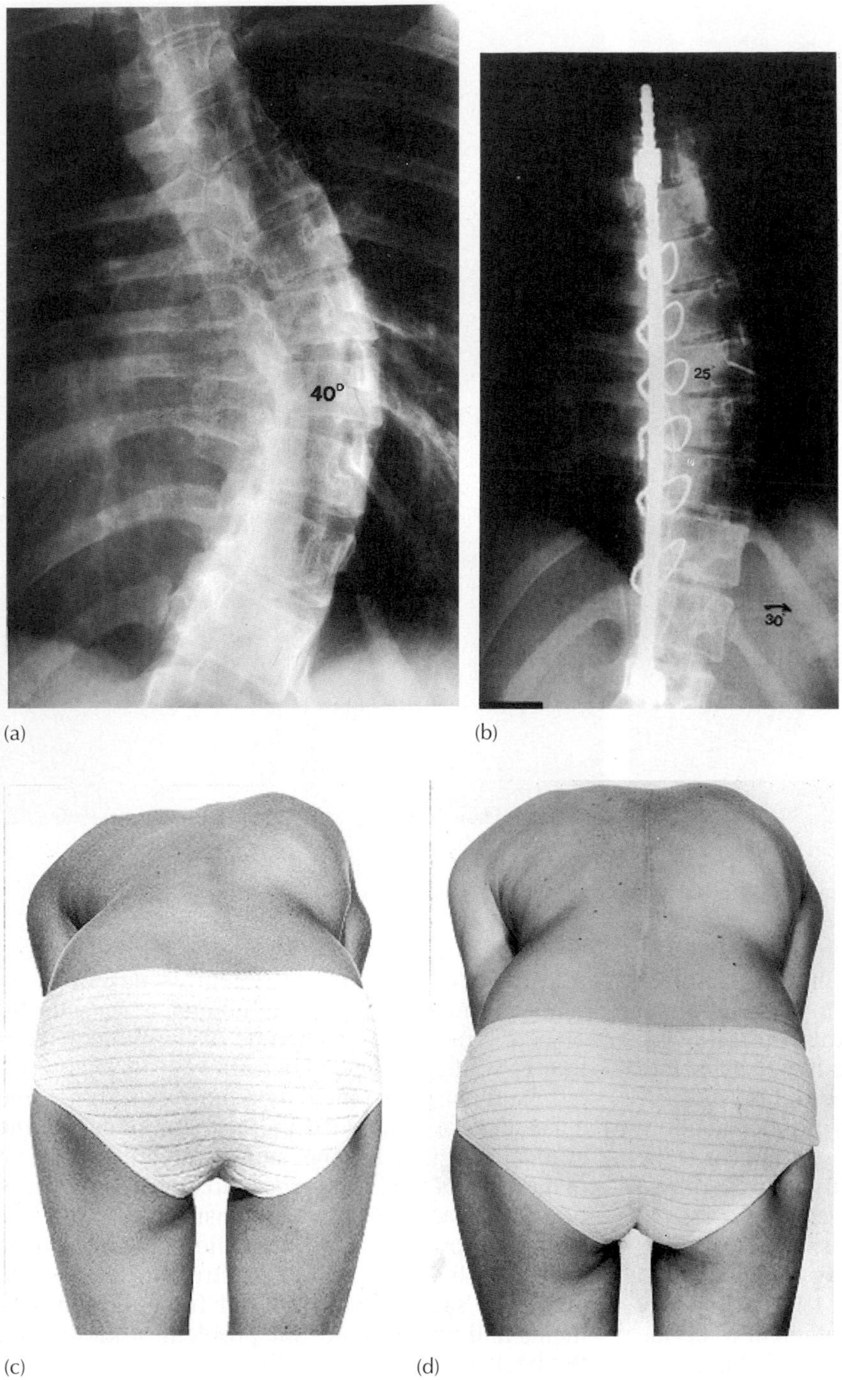

Figure 8.27 One-stage Leeds procedure. (a) PA radiograph of a right thoracic curve before surgery. (b) PA radiograph 2 years after surgery. Little can be said about the degree of correction from frontal plane radiographs. (c) Forward bending view before surgery. (d) Forward bending view 2 years after surgery showing an almost complete and sustained correction of the rib hump.

achieved by tightening nuts on the compression rod (Zielke and Berthet, 1978). There are a number of inherent advantages in using the Zielke VDS system for idiopathic scoliosis. The system is immensely strong as well as segmental. Most importantly, fewer vertebral segments require to be instrumented and fused than by dealing with the problem posteriorly (Figure 8.30). A painful flat back is a significant iatrogenic problem following posterior instrumentation for thoracolumbar or lumbar curves.

The VDS system is equally applicable to the thoracic spine and excellent results have been demonstrated in thoracic idiopathic curves in terms of all three components of the deformity (Figure 8.24) (Griss *et al.*, 1984). The anterior VDS instrumentation also shortens the spine through the

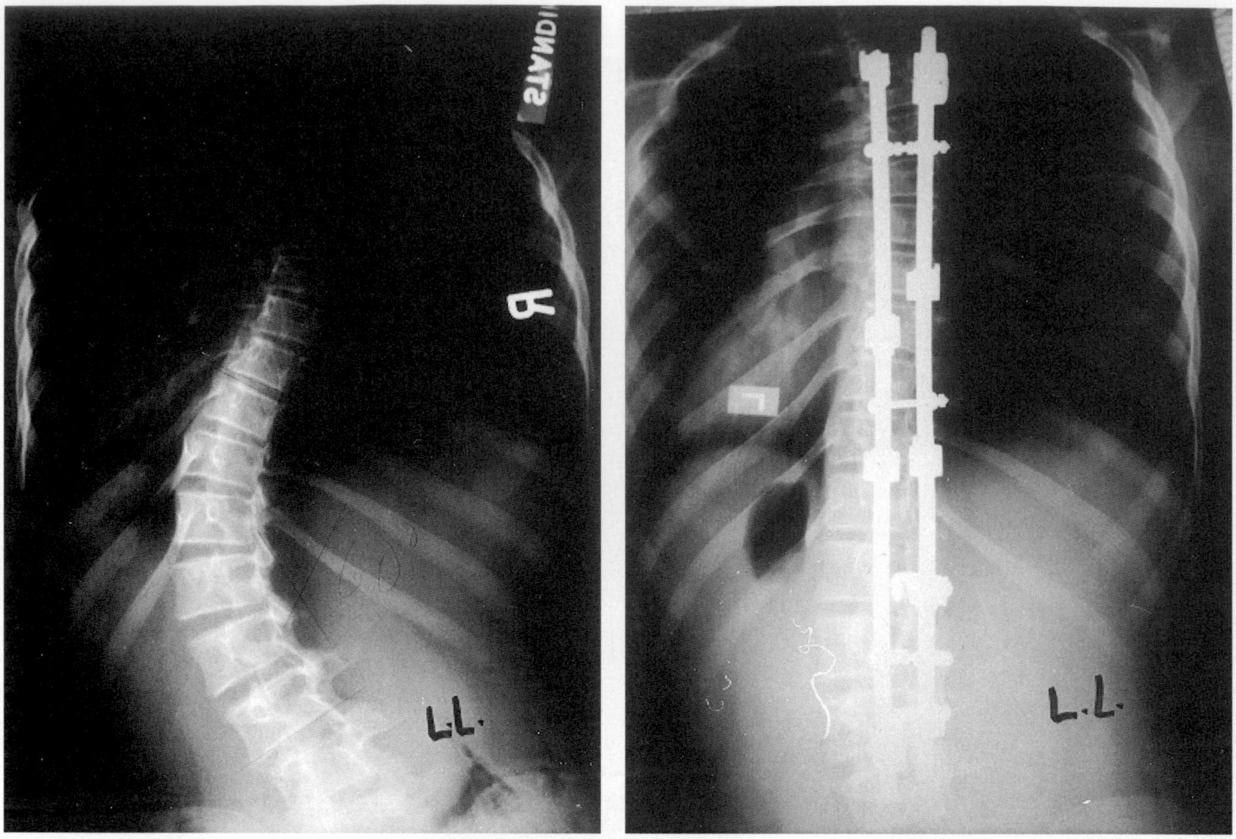

(a) (b)

Figure 8.28 PA radiographs (a) before and (b) 2 years after Cotrel–Dubousset (CD) instrumentation.

deformity by disc excision and then compression of the end plates by the instrumentation whereas other techniques cannot guarantee not to put the spinal cord under tension. The neurological risks following anterior VDS instrumentation are lower than with posterior instrumentation techniques.

For thoracic curves following instrumentation, should the rotational prominence still appear to be unduly deformed this can be readily improved by a costoplasty, by dividing the transverse processes at their bases and flattening of the rib hump or completely excising the ribs forming the hump itself (Schollner, 1966; Manning *et al.*, 1973; Chopin *et al.*, 1979). In practice it is quite sufficient to divide the apical five or six ribs just beyond the costotransverse junction and then to displace the lateral end under the vertebral end (Leatherman and Dickson, 1988). The rib hump is immediately significantly flattened and the ribs rapidly unite. *Costoplasty* for rib prominence deformity in idiopathic scoliosis can be carried out at the time of scoliosis surgery to achieve a greater preportional correction than when carried out as a procedure after fusion has been achieved (Barrett *et al.*, 1993). Indeed, the ribs removed at the time of primary surgery provide enough autogenous bone graft material. The Oxford integrated shape imaging system as described by Turner-Smith and by Houghton is a very useful objective measuring technique of the thoracic contour as well as the spinal deformity.

In summary, for single thoracic curves, or double curve patterns where the thoracic component is the clinically significant one, surgical treatment can be in the form of the Leeds procedure, CD instrumentation, or anterior Zielke VDS instrumentation. Deformities lower than the thoracic spine should be dealt with by anterior Zielke instrumentation which preserves sagittal contours and frees motion segments and thus obviates the problem of the painful flat back.

More severe, and therefore rigid, curves cannot be dealt with by a single posterior surgical procedure. Single posterior instrumentation procedures are thus contraindicated once the Cobb angle exceeds 60°. Multiple anterior discectomies over the apical five or six segments is essential for curves of about 60–90° Cobb angle prior to second stage posterior Leeds or CD instrumentation (Dickson and Archer, 1987). While it is increasingly common to perform the two procedures, i.e. anterior discectomy and posterior

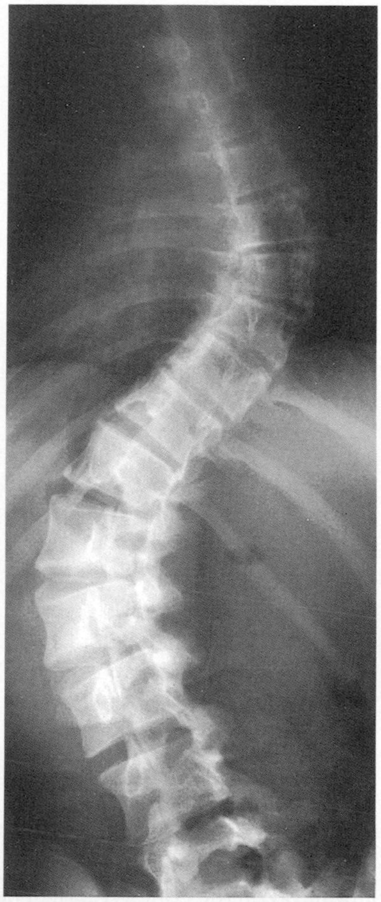

(a)

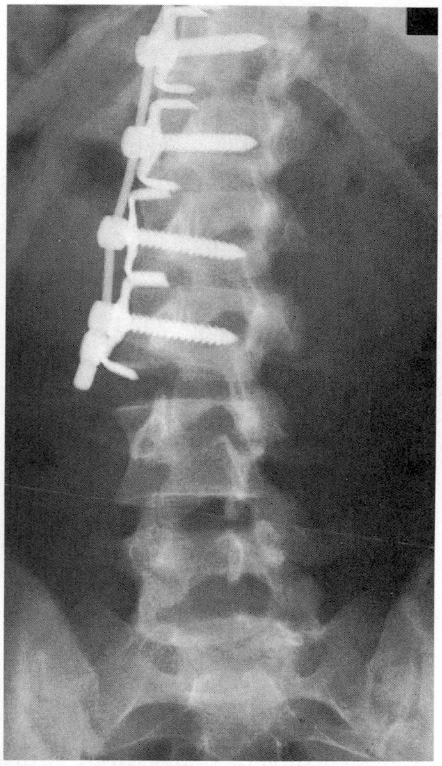

(b)

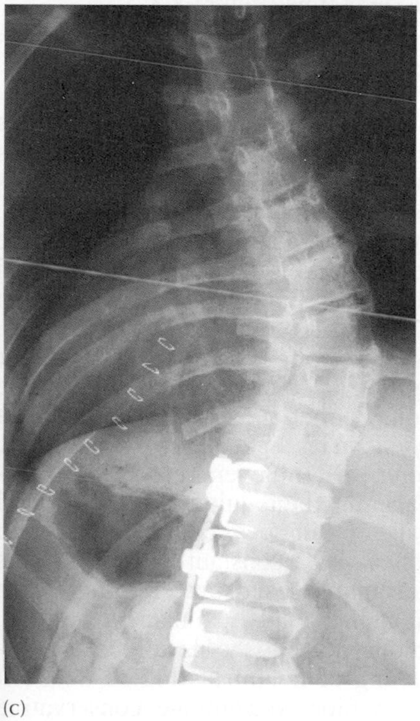

(c)

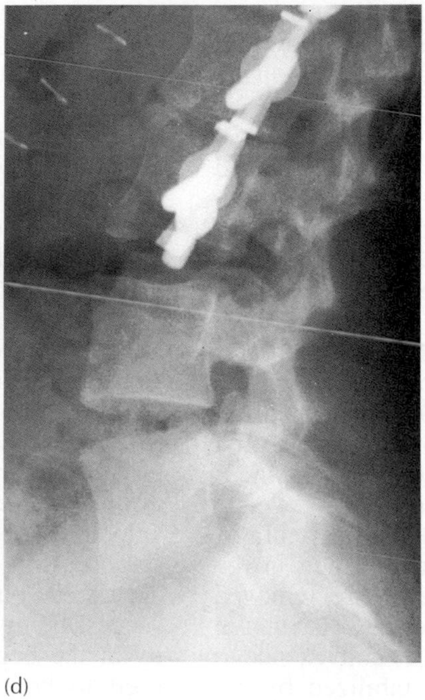

(d)

Figure 8.29 Dwyer instrumentation. (a) Preoperative PA view showing a large left thoracolumbar curve but also a structural right thoracic curve above of lesser magnitude. (b) The lower curve has been very well corrected. (c) There has been a compensatory improvement in the upper right thoracic curve. (d) With anterior instrumentation the fusion is relatively short and motion segments are preserved below the instrumentation along with the lumbar lordosis.

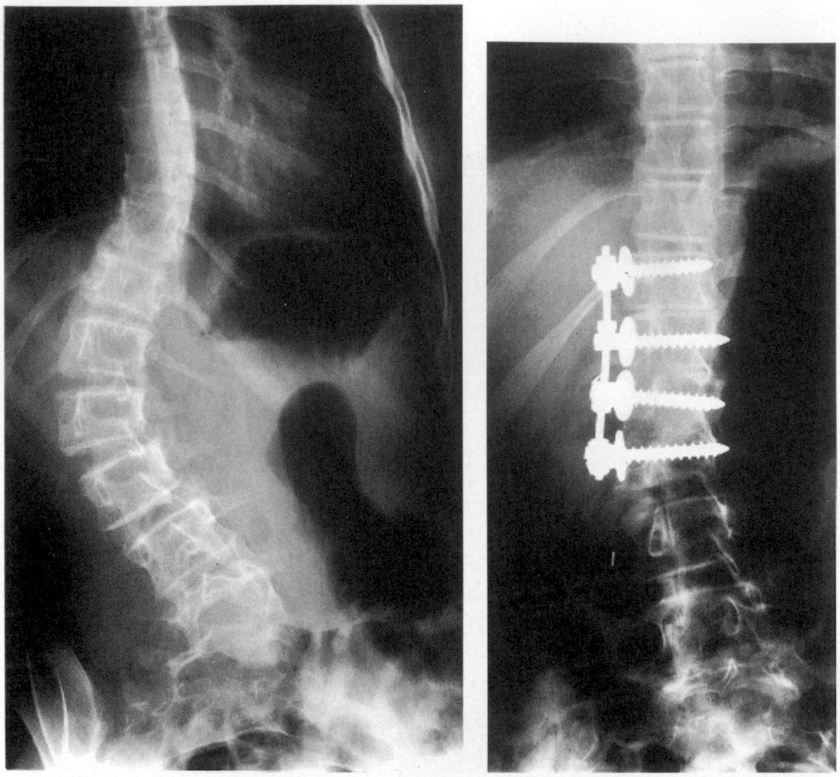

(a) (b)

Figure 8.30 Zielke instrumentation. (a) PA radiograph of a left lumbar curve before surgery. (b) PA radiograph after short segment Zielke instrumentation showing a very good correction.

instrumentation and fusion, in one sitting, it should be noted that, following multiple anterior discectomy, the curve spontaneously collapses into itself with the space thereby made available (Figure 8.31). Therefore there is much to be said for the two stages being separated by a week or two so as to allow this process of spontaneous correction to occur. If, on the other hand, a curve of 60–90° is dealt with by anterior Zielke VDS instrumentation, then of course the instrumentation has to be inserted in the one and only anterior stage.

Once the curve has got beyond about 90° Cobb angle then even multiple anterior discectomy cannot provide sufficient flexibility. For these less common, but important, most severe and rigid cases, it is necessary to provide flexibility at bone level and for this purpose Leatherman's two-stage wedge resection is required (Leatherman, 1973; Leatherman and Dickson, 1979). The apical vertebra is resected first by an anterior and then a posterior stage. The spine is thus shortened and straightened in closing wedge fashion. In the first stage the apical vertebra is resected anteriorly down to dura and then in the second stage the posterior elements are removed in the same closing wedge fashion. A Harrington compression system is applied to the convex side to close the wedge which is then stabilized by the insertion of a distraction rod on the concave side. The spine is therefore straightened but, importantly, shortened at the same time (Figure 8.32).

Early onset scoliosis

No treatment is required for the resolving case although the child should be seen at regular intervals until resolution occurs. For the progressive case it is imperative to start treatment as early as possible. Early treatment is often delayed because of the time interval between the development of the condition and the case being seen by an orthopaedic surgeon experienced in scoliosis problems (Conner, 1984). None the less, as soon as the progressive, or potentially progressive, case presents, a Cotrel-type EDF (elongation, derotation, flexion) plaster cast should be applied under light general anaesthetic (Mehta and Morel, 1979). Several casts, at 3- or 4-monthly intervals, may be required to get the child through to the age of 4 or so when infantile growth velocity curve slows to a constant level. With this serial casting technique, even severely progressive curves can be contained and even made to resolve, success being proportional to the size of the deformity at the beginning of treatment (Figure 8.33). It used to be the fashion to continue conservative

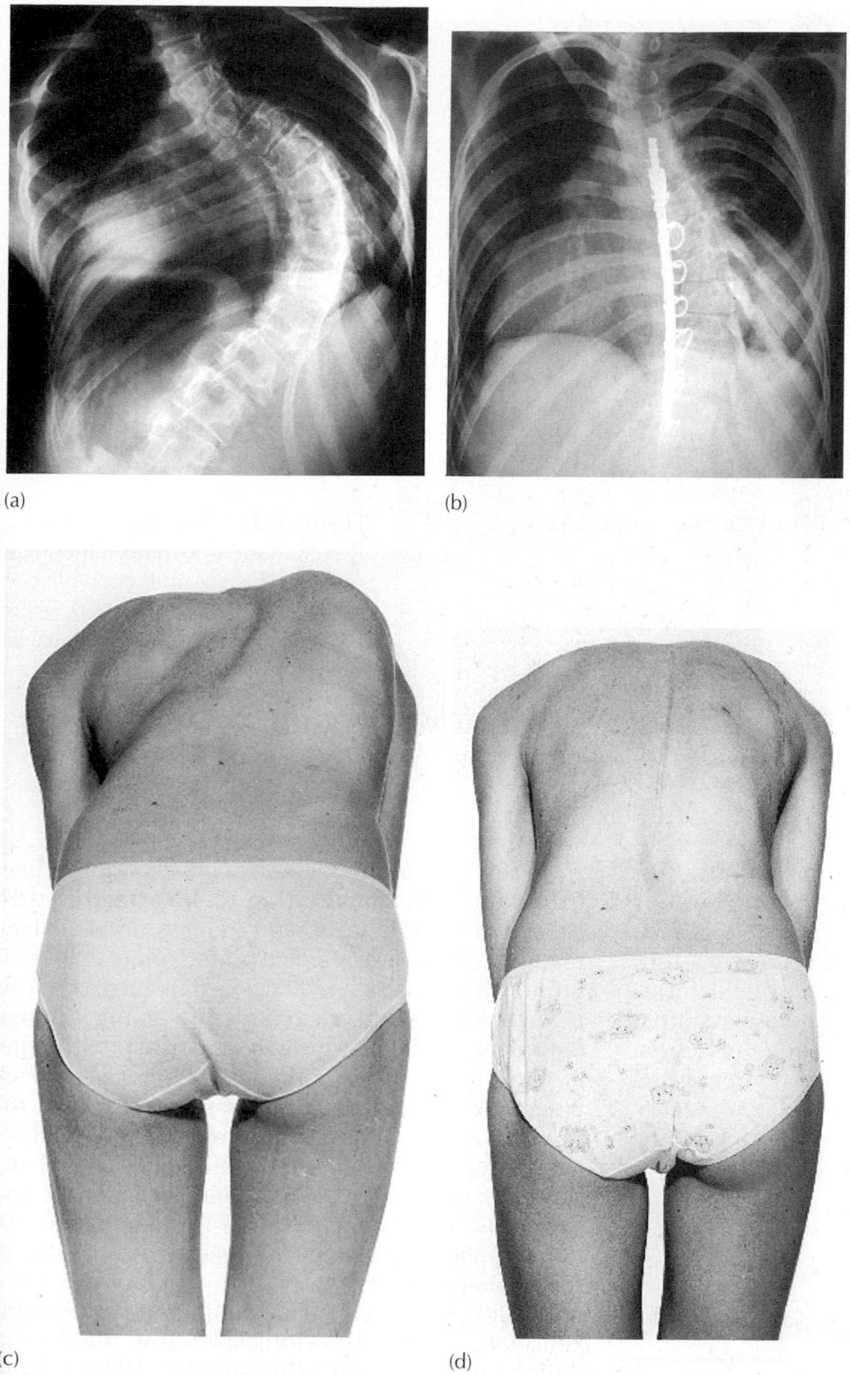

Figure 8.31 Two-stage Leeds procedure. (a) PA radiograph preoperatively showing a severe (100° Cobb angle) thoracic scoliosis. (b) After first-stage multiple anterior transthoracic discectomy and second-stage posterior instrumentation. There appears to have been an excellent correction. (c) Forward bending view before surgery. (d) Forward bending view 1 year after surgery showing an almost complete correction of the severe rotational prominence.

treatment, following serial casting, by bracing but this is unnecessary. Those that go on to resolve do so without bracing while those that remain static do so during this phase of constant growth velocity but require to be followed up through adolescence.

For those progressive cases too late, or too severe, for cast treatment, or for the failures of cast treatment, surgery is indicated. Posterior fusion is contraindicated. It is imperative that anterior spinal growth stops and this can easily be achieved over the apical five or six vertebrae by way of anterior transthoracic multiple discectomy with removal of the growth plates (Leatherman and Dickson, 1988). A Harrington rod can be inserted subcutaneously, and extraperiosteally, so as not to excite the periosteum into producing a spontaneous fusion. Then intermittently as growth dictates the rod can be lengthened or exchanged. It is preferable to try and

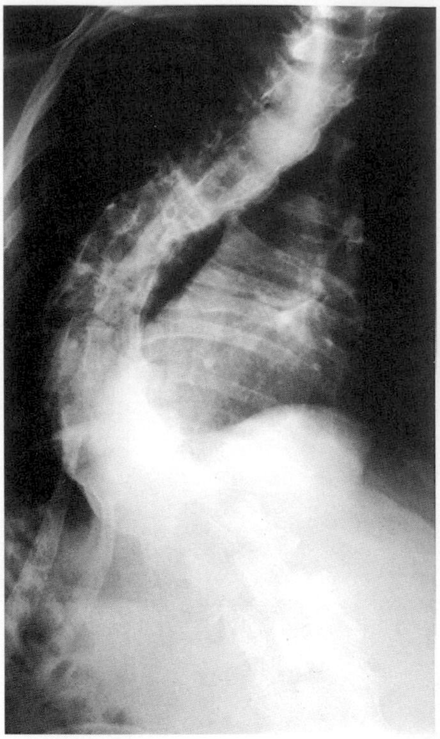

(a)

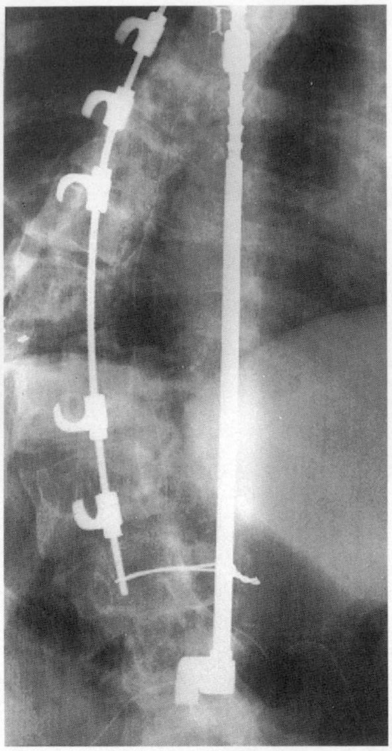

(b)

Figure 8.32 Two-stage wedge resection for a previous tethering posterior fusion. (a) Preoperative radiograph showing a severe left thoracic curve. (b) After two-stage wedge resection there has been a very good correction of these difficult cases.

recreate thoracic kyphosis instrumentally in an effort to prevent further buckling with growth. Posterior fusion is obviously withheld at this stage so that the spine can grow down the metalwork (Figure 8.34). Those that present late with the most severe deformity are not amenable even to anterior multiple discectomy and require two-stage wedge resection. It is most important to assess these children at the severe end of the spectrum for cardiopulmonary function as irreversible damage to the pulmonary alveolar tree may already have occurred.

Idiopathic kyphosis (Scheuermann's disease)

There are two types of Scheuermann's disease: type I, thoracic, and type II, thoracolumbar or lumbar (Figure 8.35). Type I is the commoner.

TYPE I – THORACIC

There is a kyphosis with its apex at the T8–9 level and to satisfy Sorenson's (1964) definition three consecutive apical vertebrae have to be kyphotically wedged by 5° or more. Clinical presentation is later than with idiopathic thoracic scoliosis and is typically during the 2 years preceding general skeletal maturity. Boys are affected more often than girls presumably because it is then, when thoracic kyphosis is increasing again, that boys are going through their peak adolescent growth velocity. Presentation is a result of the hyperkyphotic deformity, back pain, or both. It is extremely rare for the kyphosis to threaten the function of the spinal cord (Bradford and Garcia, 1969). Lateral radiographs reveal the kyphotic wedging with end-plate irregularity and Schmorl node formation (see Figure 8.14). PA radiographs may demonstrate slight asymmetry of the kyphotic process but in 60% of cases there is a mild idiopathic scoliosis in the region of the compensatory lumbar hyperlordosis below the area of thoracic hyperkyphosis (Deacon *et al.*, 1985) (Figure 8.36).

Unlike idiopathic thoracic scoliosis, thoracic Scheuermann's disease is eminently treatable conservatively, as the deformity is restricted to one plane. An extension plaster cast, or an extension underarm brace, will lead to rapid resolution, often within 6 months or a year, provided there is reasonable spinal growth left (Bradford *et al.*, 1974). Anterior vertebral height quickly catches up and leads to a truly physiological correction (Figure

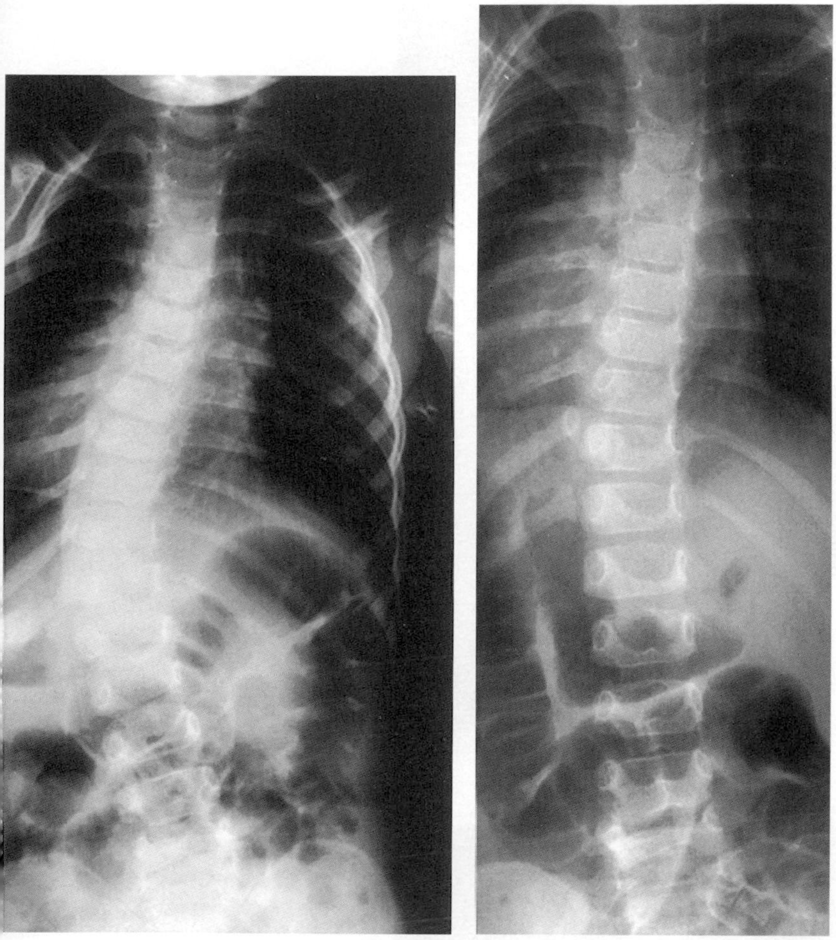

(a) (b)

Figure 8.33 (a) Infantile idiopathic scoliosis before and (b) after several EDF casts.

3.37). Bearing in mind that vertebral end-plate fusion does not occur until the middle of the third decade, even patients in their late teens should be given the opportunity of conservative treatment.

For those that fail conservative treatment, or for those with severe deformities, surgical correction can be contemplated although the results of so doing are neither so predictable nor so good as with idiopathic thoracic scoliosis (Bradford *et al.*, 1975; Taylor *et al.*, 1979). Both one- and two-stage procedures have been advocated. Posterior Harrington compression instrumentation, or posterior CD instrumentation, combined with posterior fusion, forms the basis of the one-stage procedure. However, even with relatively mild cases, the apical three or four segments are rigid and do not correct at all even by firm manual pressure. The cosmetic improvement is therefore more attributable to influencing the flexible part of the kyphosis well above and below the more rigid apical region. More severe cases tend to be dealt with by two-stage surgery with preliminary anterior transthoracic multiple discectomies and bone grafting the interspaces (Streitz *et al.*, 1977; Herndon *et al.*, 1981). Then second stage posterior instrumentation is carried out as before. At best a 40% correction of the kyphosis can be achieved but this is a lot of surgery to go through for this amount of correction. An accurate presentation to the patient and family of the 'risks and rewards' equation is therefore essential.

TYPE II – THORACOLUMBAR

This was referred to by Sorenson as 'apprentice's spine'. This not uncommon condition presents in the late teens and early twenties, i.e. after general skeletal maturity, but not before the attainment of spinal maturity. The presentation is typically of local pain rather than deformity and sometimes the pain can be in the low back region rather than over the kyphosis apex (Hensinger *et al.*, 1982). There is a

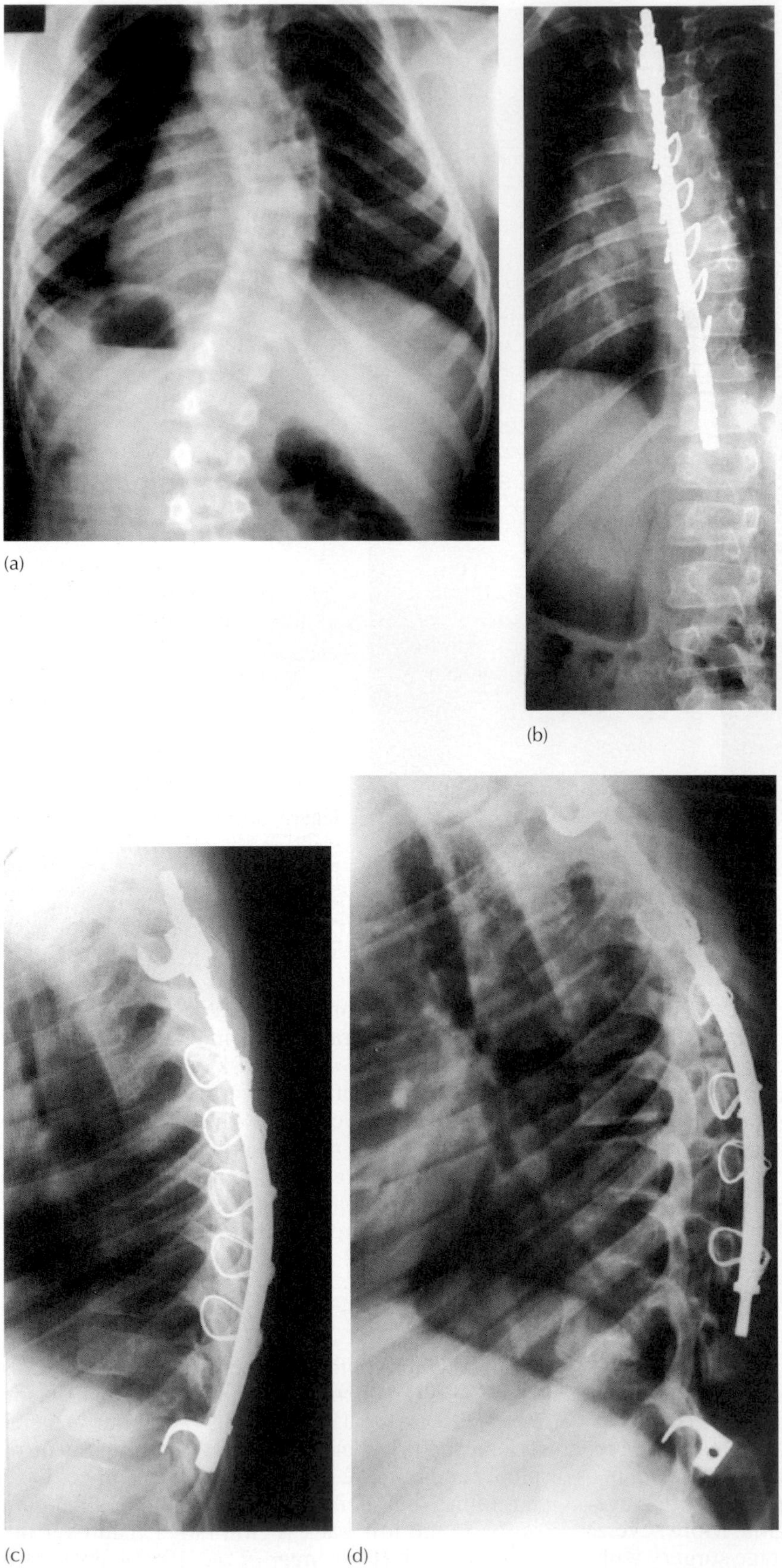

(a) (b) (c) (d)

Figure 8.34 'Growing instrumentation'.

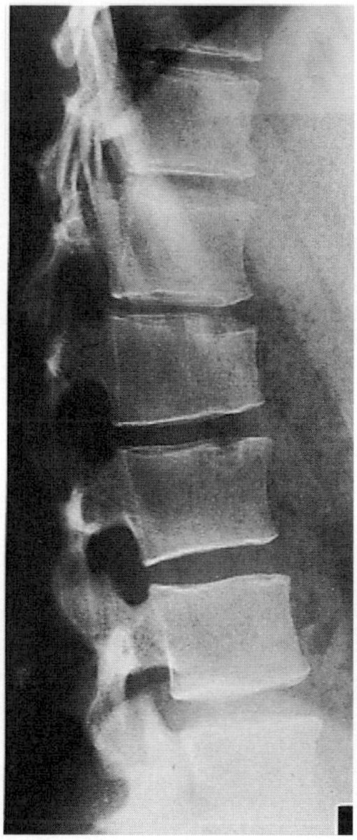

Figure 8.35 Lateral radiograph of the thoracolumbar spine showing type II Scheuermann's disease – 'apprentice's' spine.

much higher prevalence rate of lower lumbar spondylolyses in type II Scheuermann's disease and therefore it is important in the patient with low back pain to perform oblique radiography as well as routine PA and lateral projections. The deformity *per se* does not require surgical treatment and, in the absence of spondylolyses, symptoms respond well to extension exercise treatment.

Congenital spine deformities

There are two basic types of congenital spine deformity, congenital bone deformities and congenital cord deformities. Congenital bone deformities are attributable to a primary congenital bony anomaly, in the form of either failure of formation, or failure of segmentation (Figure 8.38). Bilateral failures, e.g. butterfly vertebra or block vertebra, do not produce a deformity. Anomalies need to be unilateral to produce a progressive problem. If the unilateral problem is in the frontal plane then a progressive scoliosis occurs, whereas if it is in the sagittal plane then a progressive kyphosis occurs.

CONGENITAL BONE ANOMALY

The progression potential of the underlying congenital anomaly depends both upon biological and biomechanical factors. A unilateral failure of segmentation (unilateral bar) does not allow growth on the concave side over how many segments the bar occupies. Therefore convex growth plate activity against no activity on the concave side can lead to a serious progressive scoliosis of early onset (Figure 8.39) (Winter *et al.*, 1968; McMaster and Ohtsuka, 1982). By contrast, a single unilateral failure of formation (hemivertebra) still has growth-plate activity on the concave side, thus only a mild deformity generally ensues, e.g. when the hemivertebra is fully segmented with a disc space and growth plates above and below. Commonly the hemivertebra is semi-segmented with a disc space and growth plates only either above or below, in which case there will be no growth asymmetry and no reason for presentation. The worst anomaly complex is a combination of a unilateral bar on one side and a hemivertebra on the other, one growth asymmetry compounding the other.

Biomechanical factors are important (Deacon *et al.*, 1991). Solitary hemivertebrae produce deformation only in the coronal plane. The sagittal plane is not affected and there is therefore little or no rotation. By contrast, failures of segmentation affect both coronal and sagittal planes and a posterior element rotation. These are progressive lordoscolioses with a super-added buckling potential (Figure 8.40). As these are congenital deformities, present at or before birth, then significantly progressive deformities are of early onset and can considerably jeopardize cardiopulmonary function.

In the sagittal plane failures of formation are more common than failures of segmentation and a particularly dangerous anomaly is the dorsal hemivertebra (Figure 8.41). Here, the anterior half of the vertebra fails to develop whereas the posterior half does, and with progressive growth there is increasing angular kyphosis – the hemivertebra is displaced backwards into the front of the spinal cord. Twenty per cent of cases go on to significant neurological problems as a result of spinal cord tension over the hemivertebra (Winter *et al.*, 1973).

When a patient with a congenital bony anomaly of the spine is encountered it is important to assess other organ systems (MacEwen *et al.*, 1972; Owen, 1976). Routine imaging has demonstrated that 50% of cases have an associated significant anomaly of the urinary tract and 20% have an anomaly of the gut. The embryopathology is thus shared among these organ systems and collectively they are referred to as the 'split notochord syndrome'.

In addition, in 10–20% of cases there is evidence

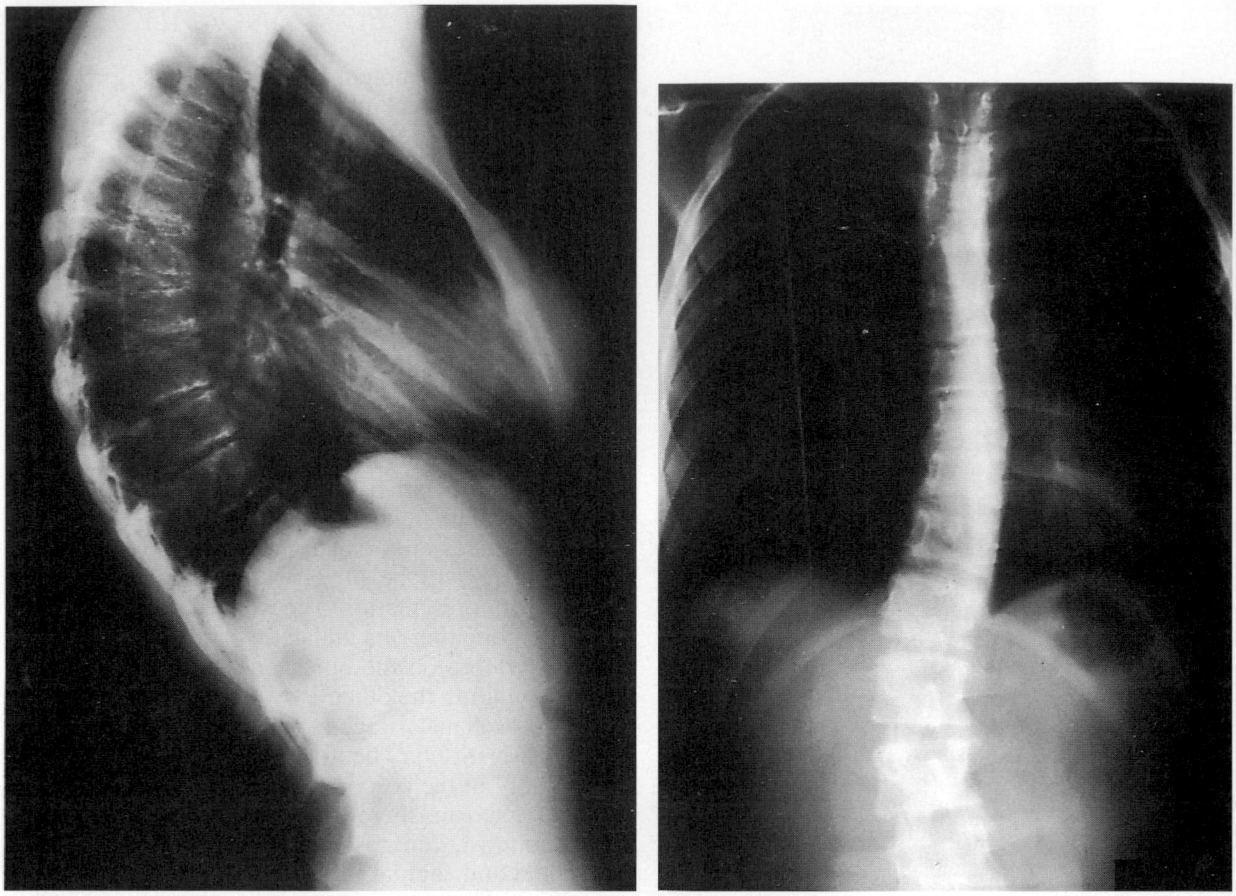

(a) (b)

Figure 8.36 (a) Lateral radiograph of type I thoracic Scheuermann's disease. (b) PA radiograph of the same patient showing an idiopathic lumbar scoliosis below the area of hyperkyphosis.

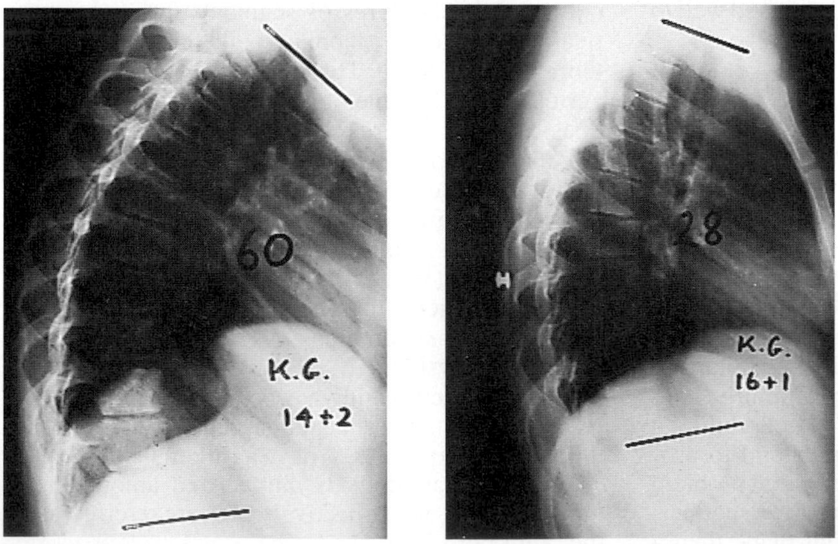

(a) (b)

Figure 8.37 Lateral radiograph of a 14-year-old boy with 60° of thoracic Scheuermann's disease. (b) After 2 years of extension bracing the thoracic kyphosis has been restored to normal.

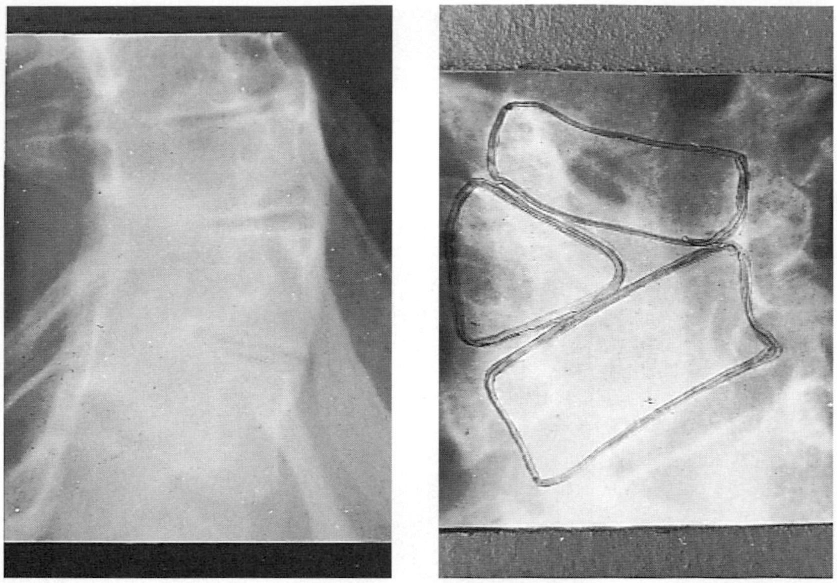

(a) (b)

Figure 8.38 Unilateral failure of segmentation – unilateral bar. Significant progression is the rule. (b) Unilateral failure of formation – hemivertebra.

of associated spinal dysraphism – a tethered conus, dermoid cyst, intradural lipoma, split cord, diastematomyelia, spinocutaneous fistulas, the commonest combination being a tethered conus in association with diastematomyelia (Till, 1969; Gillespie *et al.*, 1973; Winter *et al.*, 1974). Therefore in all cases it is essential to perform a very careful and thorough physical and neurological examination as well as imaging of parts other than the spine. Congenital spine anomalies are also common in certain syndromes such as Apert's syndrome, Crouzon's syndrome, Larsen's syndrome, and Treacher Collins syndrome (Sherk *et al.*, 1982).

Cervicothoracic congenital bony anomalies are commonly associated with a short neck, low hair line, soft tissue neck webbing, and secondary wry neck. This feature complex is referred to as the 'Klippel–Feil syndrome' and may be associated with a high, relatively undescended scapula – 'Sprengel's shoulder' (Hensinger *et al.*, 1974) (see Chapter 3).

It is important in children presenting with what

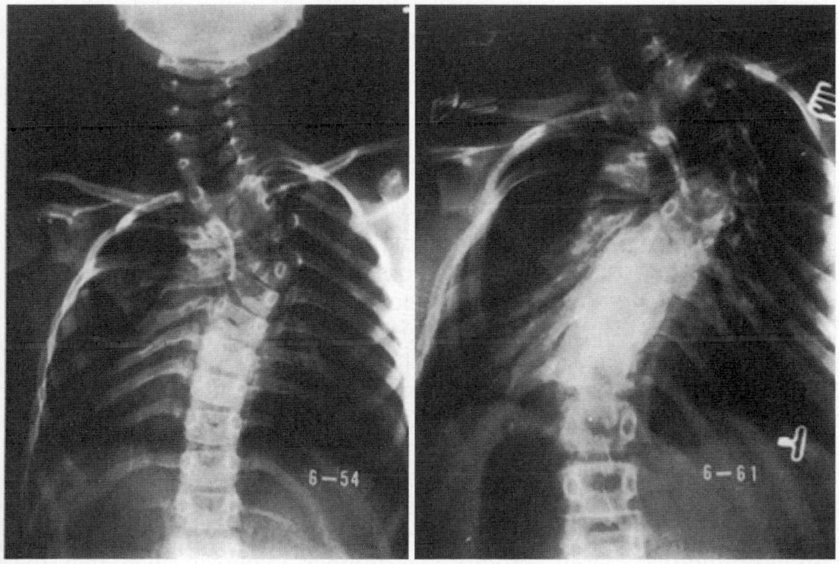

(a) (b)

Figure 8.39 The effects of a unilateral bar. Radiograph (b) is taken 7 years after (a). There has been significant progression.

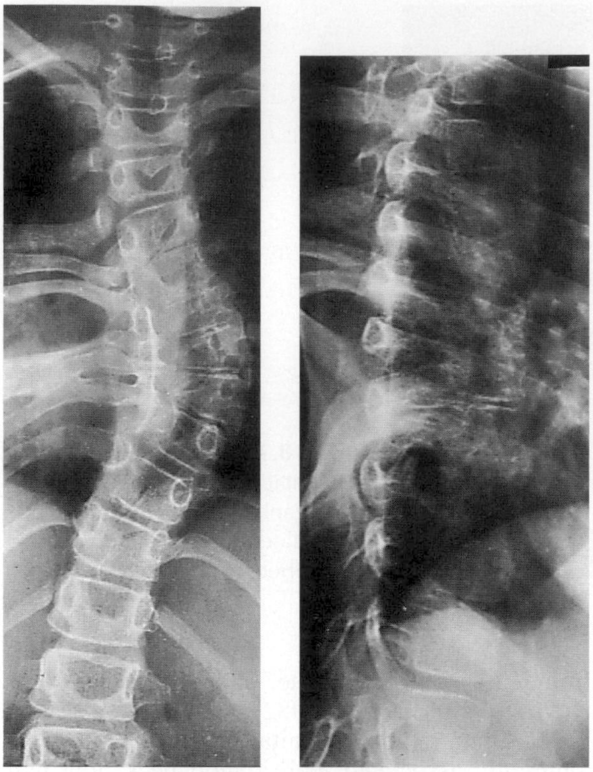

(a) (b)

Figure 8.40 (a) PA radiograph of the unilateral bar. (b) True lateral radiograph of a curve apex showing the lordosis which will add biomechanical buckling to growth asymmetry.

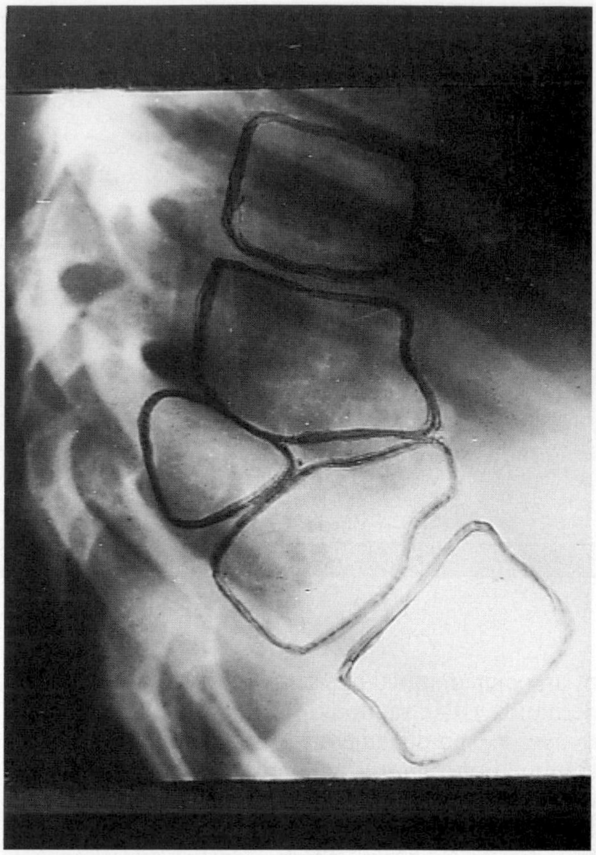

Figure 8.41 Lateral radiograph of the lower thoracic spine showing a dorsal hemivertebra.

appears initially to be a typical idiopathic curve to obtain adequate x-ray views over an adequate length of the spine. In the upper thoracic region it is not uncommon to find two adjacent vertebrae being relatively unsegmented, more on one side than the other. The effect is to throw off a secondary idiopathic-type curve below (Figure 8.42). Such patients are much more at risk than the uncomplicated idiopathic case and the status of the spinal cord must be thoroughly assessed by appropriate CT and MR imaging before surgical treatment is contemplated.

CONGENITAL CORD ANOMALIES

These refer to the spina bifida, or myelodysplasia, syndrome (see Chapter 7). It is important to appreciate that there are two fundamental types of spinal deformity in the spina bifida patient (Raycroft and Curtis, 1972; Leatherman and Dickson, 1977). Sixty per cent of spinal deformities are of the collapsing C-shape neuromuscular variety with pelvic obliquity, but some 40% are attributable to a significant congenital bony anomaly at the thoracolumbar junction. In the sagittal plane there is always a degree of hyperlordosis in association with the collapsing paralytic curve but 10% of spina bifida children are born with the congenital lumbar kyphosis in myelomeningocele always accompanied by a high level neurological paralysis (Hoppenfield, 1967).

Spina bifida children can be disadvantaged functionally as regards their spinal deformity because it either interferes with their walking potential or sitting stability. As with other paralytic conditions, surgical treatment for spinal deformities is better designed and more predictable in the wheelchair sitter. Walkers generally depend upon a mobile lumbar spine and interference with it by spinal fusion can dysfunction them to the point of putting them off their feet. If surgery is to be contemplated then it must be established that the dysfunction is caused by the spinal deformity rather than by any associated feature such as mental deficiency, or expanding hydrosyringomyelia. The congenital kyphosis of myelomeningocele nearly always produces a severely progressive lumbar kyphosis such that the chest comes to lie on the front of the thighs with

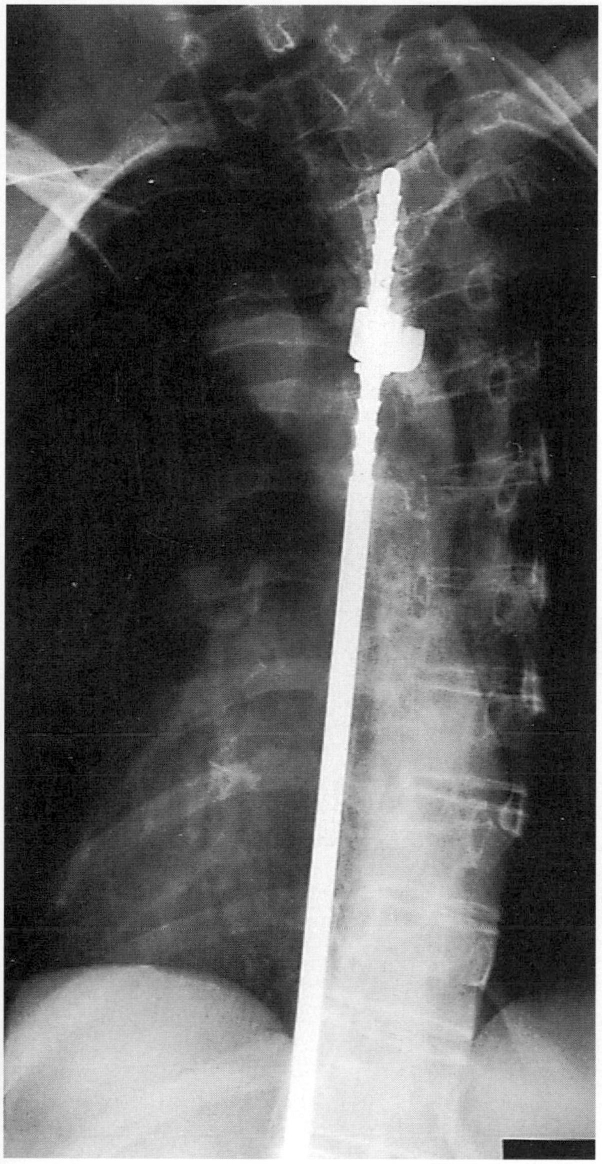

Figure 8.42 'Congenital' idiopathic scoliosis. There appears to be a right idiopathic thoracic curve but inspection of the top of the thoracic spine reveals segmentation failures. The right 'idiopathic' curve below these segmentation failures has been thrown off as a compensatory curve.

patients having great difficulty even sitting, or seeing forward.

TREATMENT

The scoliosis in association with congenital bony anomalies is treated for the same fundamental reasons as its idiopathic counterpart – with early progressive cases jeopardizing organic health and later progressive cases being a question of deformity and appearance only. While the rewards may be similar to idiopathic scoliosis the risks are very much greater, particularly with regard to inducing paralysis (MacEwen *et al.*, 1975). Like other structural scolioses, those attributable to congenital bony anomalies are not amenable to conservative treatment and there is no place for bracing. Unlike the idiopathic case, these curves are quite rigid and there is no flexibility which can be gathered up by instrumentation. Indeed distraction instrumentation is contraindicated because of the high risk of paralysis (Winter, 1983). The problem is one of angular bony rigidity in the region of the curve apex and this requires a spinal osteotomy. In the early pioneering days of anterior spinal surgery there was an unacceptably high incidence of paralysis either by doing too much at one time and thus interfering with the local cord blood supply, or by putting the spinal cord under tension.

Hodgson initially favoured the circumferential opening wedge osteotomy where the concavity was osteotomized and opened out to obtain correction (Hodgson, 1965). Dommisse carried out 68 of these procedures with complete paralysis in four (Dommisse and Enslin, 1970). Leatherman then introduced the concept of closing wedge osteotomy with an apical wedge removed from the convex side (Leatherman, 1969, 1973). When the wedge was closed the spinal canal was shortened rather than being tension lengthened (Figure 8.43). In the early days there was no instrumentation to close the wedge or protect the closed position, but when Harrington instrumentation was introduced the compression system on the convex side was ideal for closing wedge purposes. In the first anterior stage the apical vertebral body is removed and in the second posterior stage the posterior elements are removed to complete the wedge. A compression system is applied to the convex side and when the wedge is closed further stability and correction are obtained by the insertion of a Harrington distraction rod on the concave side. A posterior fusion of the entire structural curve then completes the procedure. Seventy such cases have been reported with no significant neurological complications and with long-term follow-up testifying to the reliability of the procedure (Leatherman and Dickson, 1979). When preoperative spinal cord imaging by CT or MR examination reveals the presence of a diastematomyelia (spur of bone or fibrous tissue cleaving the cord in the sagittal plane), or a tethered conus, this should be dealt with neurosurgically by way of a preliminary laminectomy. When preoperative imaging demonstrates a dystrophic problem over a very considerable spinal extent, the dangers of dealing with it outweigh the rewards and surgical treatment should be withheld. Leatherman's two-stage wedge

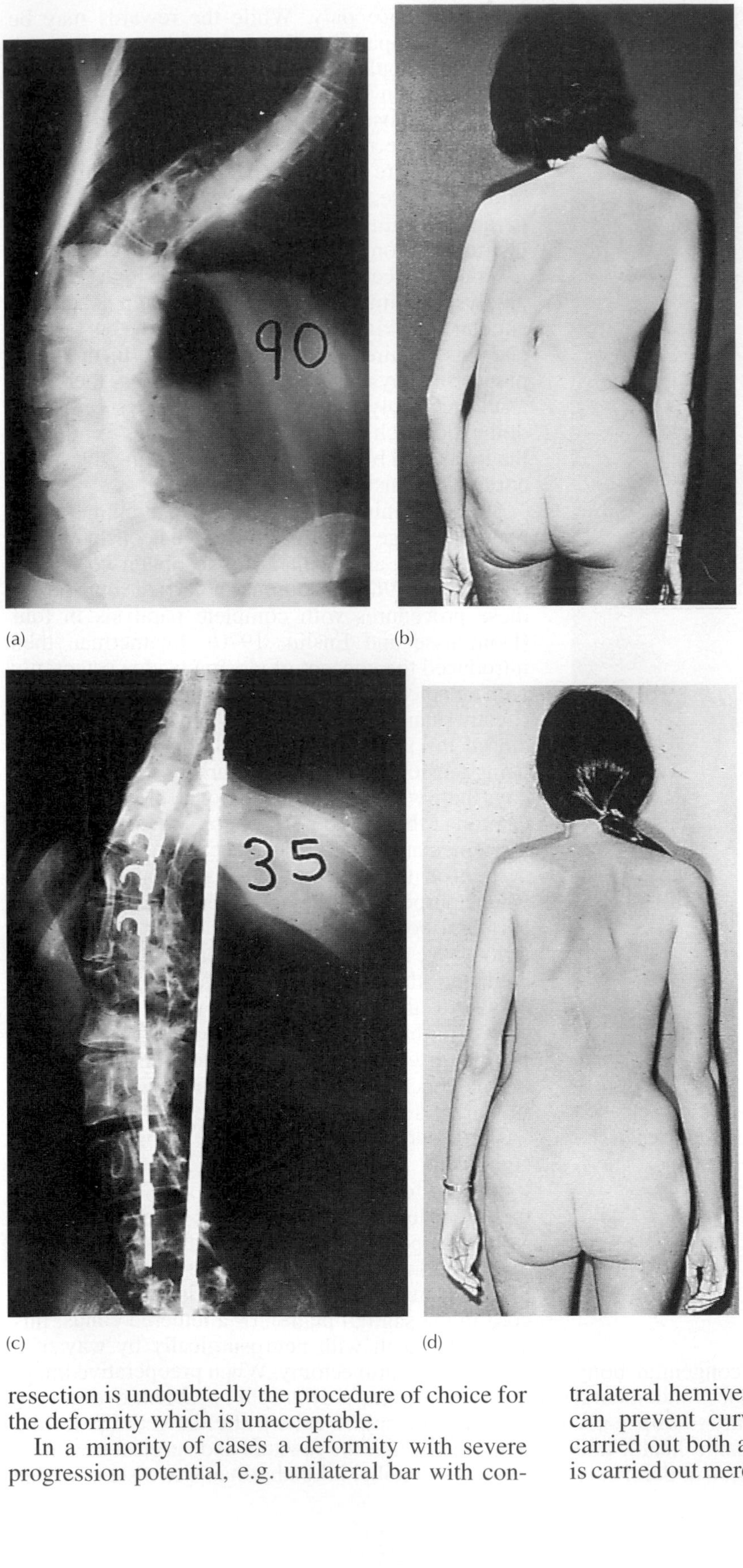

Figure 8.43 Two-stage wedge resection for congenital scoliosis. (a) PA x-ray showing a severe left lumbar scoliosis. (b) Erect view of patient showing the scoliosis and the tell-tale hairy patch. (c) PA x-ray postoperatively showing a good correction. (d) Erect view of the patient 2 years postoperatively showing a complete correction of the deformity.

resection is undoubtedly the procedure of choice for the deformity which is unacceptable.

In a minority of cases a deformity with severe progression potential, e.g. unilateral bar with contralateral hemivertebra, a formidable fusion-*in-situ* can prevent curve progression but this must be carried out both anteriorly and posteriorly. If fusion is carried out merely posteriorly (Moe and Sundberg,

1968; Winter and Moe, 1982) then this has the danger of accelerating further progression by way of posterior tether (see Figure 8.14). Anterior vertebral growth must be stopped by way of disc and growth plate excision over the apical five or six segments. This may be a formidable undertaking in a child of 2 or 3 years of age when the spine is as much cartilage as bone but it is the only way to attenuate progression of the deformity. Posterior metalwork without fusion can be used as a second-stage procedure to splint the deformity but allow it to continue growing (Leatherman and Dickson, 1988).

In an attempt to treat congenital scoliosis physiologically, Roaf (1963) devised the concept of anteroconvex hemiepiphyseodesis. By tethering growth on the convex side of the curve apex anteriorly it was hoped that the spine would subsequently grow straighter. This proved to be effective for the solitary hemivertebra with no buckling potential but such anomalies seldom progress to an unacceptable degree anyway. The exception is the lumbosacral hemivertebra which can produce a progressive list of the torso. Here posterior fusion-*in-situ* can attenuate progression but wedge excision is preferable (Figure 8.44).

For the long C-shaped collapsing 'paralytic' scoliosis in the spina bifida patient with pelvic obliquity the spine must be instrumented and fused both anteriorly and posteriorly as posterior surgery alone has an unacceptably high complication rate (Sriram *et al.*, 1972). After anterior discectomy Zielke instrumentation is extended down to L5, while second-stage posterior segmental instrumentation is carried down into the pelvis (Figure 8.45). The lower ends of the rods can be passed into the iliac blades to better secure them (the Galveston technique) (Allen and Ferguson, 1979). Posterior element absence or deficiency in the spina bifida patient may prevent wire fixation at one or more levels and such levels can be dealt with by pedicular fixation techniques.

The congenital lumbar kyphosis spina bifida patient always has a non-functioning spinal cord to well above the apex of the kyphosis. The spine can be straightened posteriorly by excision of the redundant spinal cord and posterior kyphectomy, followed by posterior instrumentation and fusion (Sriram *et al.*, 1972). However, interference with a seemingly non-functioning spinal cord can provoke reactivation of previously arrested hydrocephalus and can defunction some still active cord-mediated reflex arcs. It is therefore preferable to preserve the spinal cord and

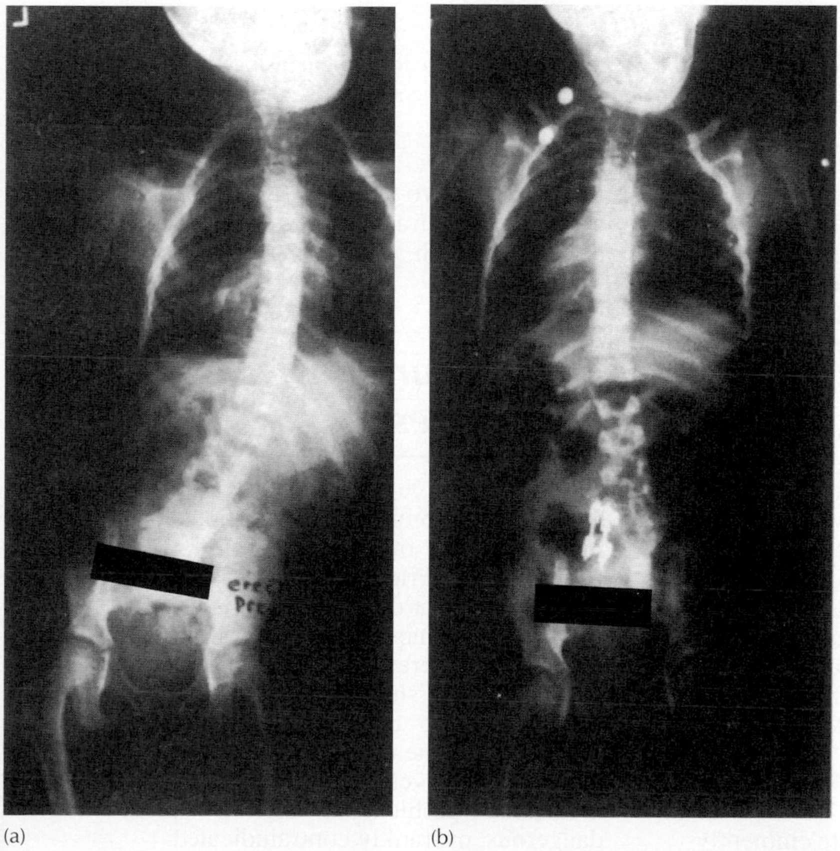

(a) (b)

Figure 8.44 Lumbar scoliosis. Anteroposterior radiographs with the patient (a) erect and (b) 1 week after operation. A wedge resection of a lumbar vertebra segment had been carried out through an anterior approach. Closure of the wedge defect with Harrington's compression instrumentation. (Case of A.R. Hodgson.)

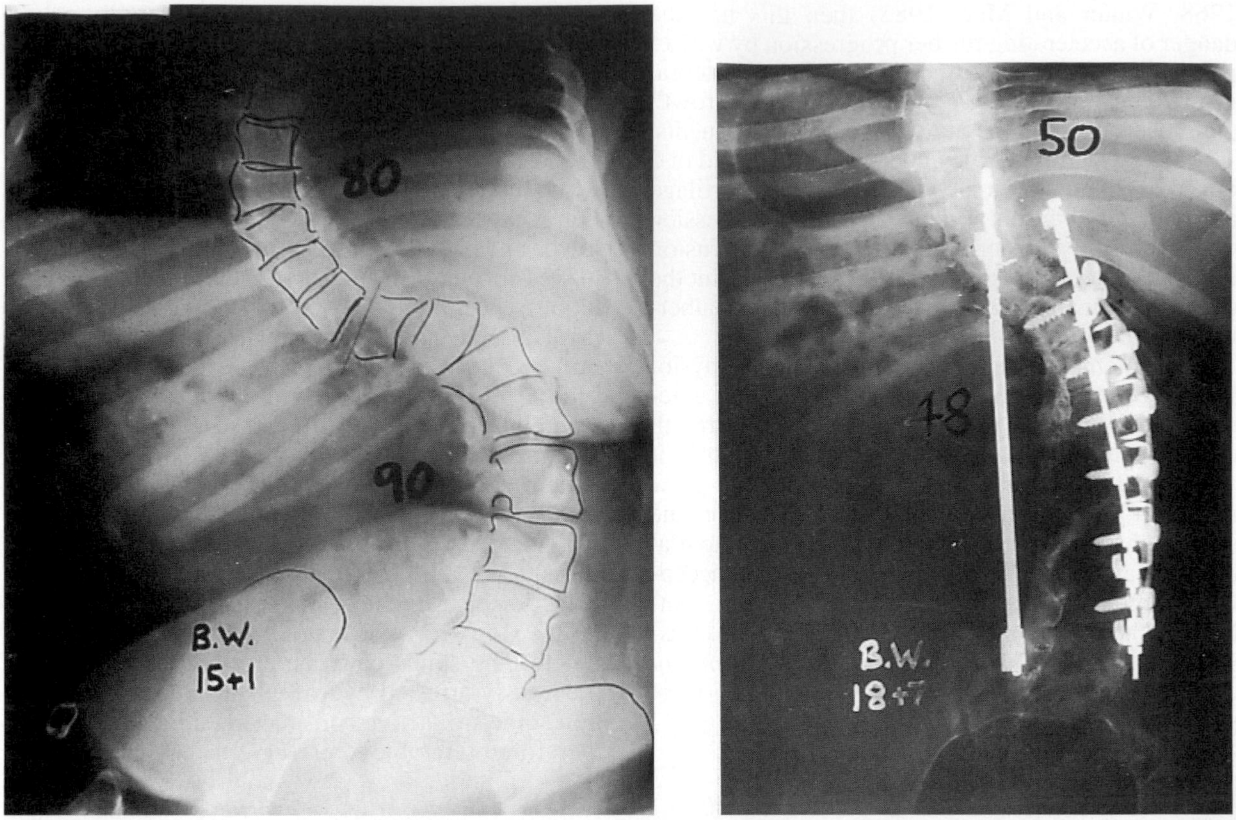

(a) (b)

Figure 8.45 (a) The typical collapsing curve of spina bifida with pelvic obliquity and the hip dislocating on the high side. (b) Four years after anterior and posterior instrumentation and fusion showing a good correction most importantly of the pelvic obliquity.

perform a two-stage anterior release followed by posterior instrumentation and fusion (Leatherman and Dickson, 1978). The anterior longitudinal ligament and annulus fibrosus of the lumbar discs are also tightly contracted. When all these are released anteriorly the kyphosis can become surprisingly flexible such that a good posterior instrumentation correction can be achieved in the second stage (Figure 8.46).

The 'risks and rewards' equation is particularly important in the spina bifida patient with insensitive poor quality scarred skin and potential infection. In addition, lack of quantity and quality of bone leads to a high pseudarthrosis rate with associated instrumentation failure. Further surgical procedures are therefore frequently required. These patients do, however, have a severe disability if they cannot sit unsupported in a wheelchair. They have to use their upper extremities to hold themselves up and are therefore denied prehensile function. This is the prime indication for surgical treatment.

It should be remembered that 40% of spina bifida scolioses are due to a congenital anomaly at the thoracolumbar junction and these are eminently treatable by two-stage wedge resection which is a much more straightforward and predictable procedure than with a collapsing paralytic curve.

Other neuromuscular deformities

The true neuromuscular conditions of childhood include spinal muscular atrophy, the peripheral neuropathies, Friedreich's ataxia, arthrogryposis, and the muscular dystrophies (Shapiro and Bresnan, 1982a) (see Chapter 7). Cerebral palsy and poliomyelitis are therefore not true neuromuscular disorders but do share many common features. It is important to understand the nature of pelvic obliquity and the difference between balanced and unbalanced curves.Many of these conditions have associated problems rendering spinal surgery dangerous, or frankly contraindicated.

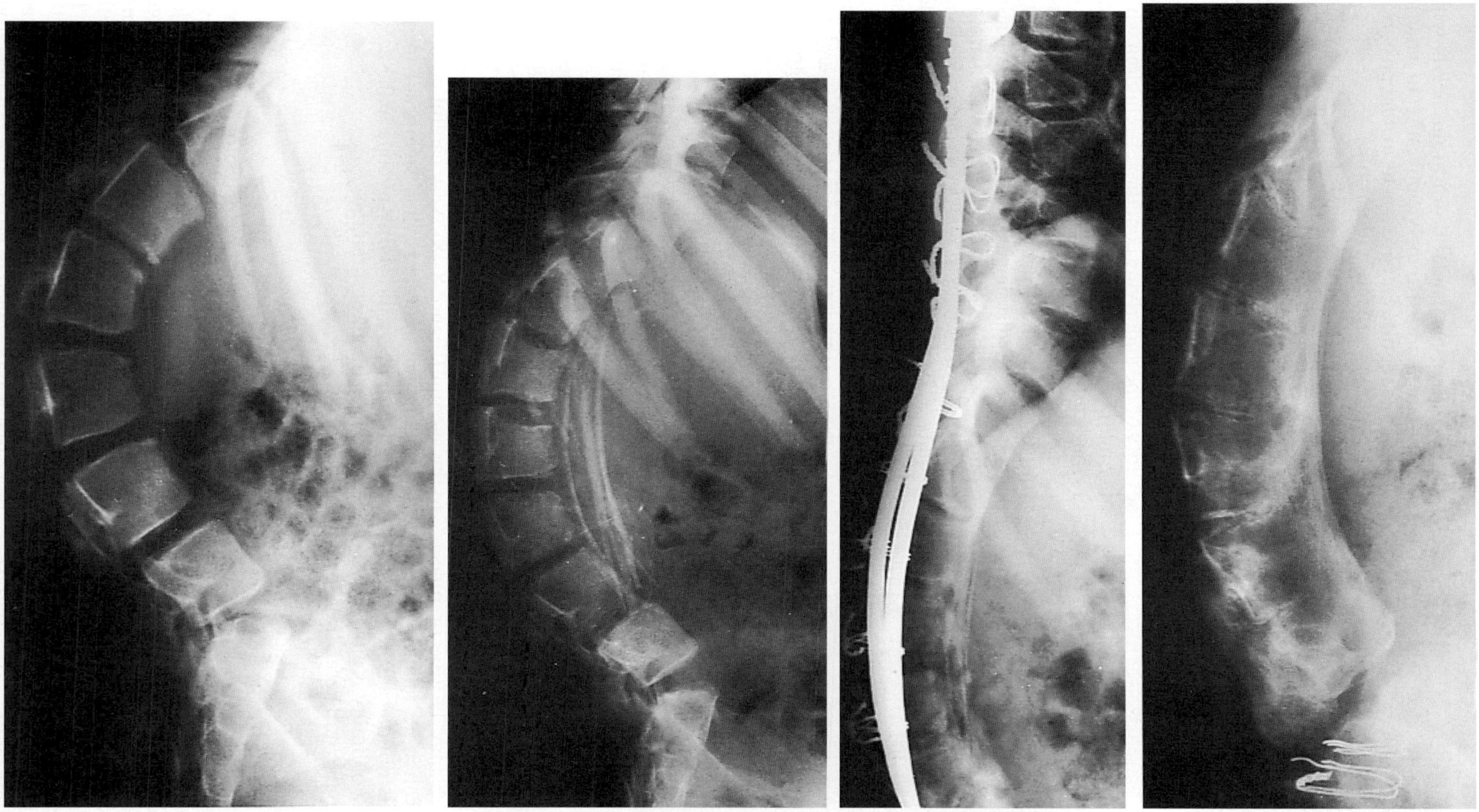

(a) (b) (c) (d)

Figure 8.46 The congenital kyphosis of myelomeningocele. (a) Lateral x-ray of the lumbar spine showing 90° of kyphosis. (b) Lateral x-ray after first-stage anterior strut grafting and interbody fusion. (c) After second-stage posterior segmental instrumentation going well above the kyphosis into the thoracic spine. (d) After removal of metalwork several years later there is a solid fusion and good correction. The lumbosacral segmental level is not fused, as is often the case, but the segment was stable.

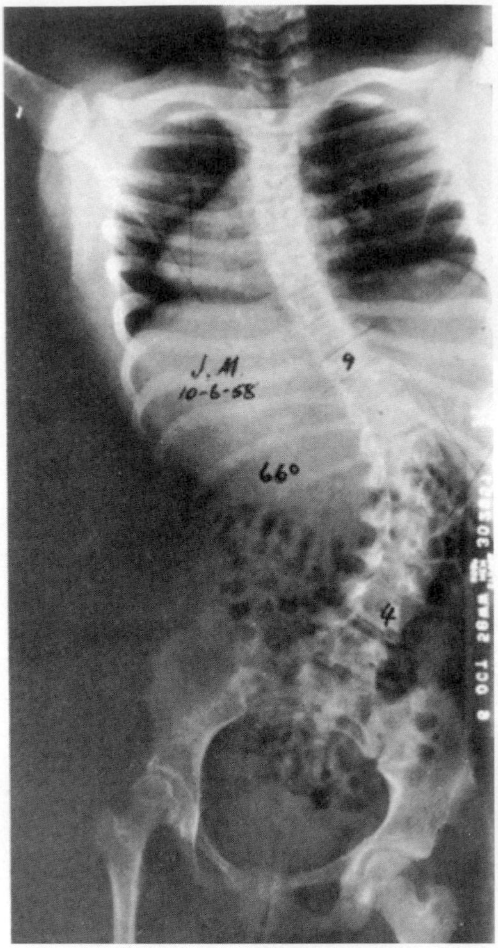

Figure 8.47 Typical paralytic thoracolumbar scoliosis of the long C-shape variety with pelvic obliquity.

There are three types of pelvic obliquity – suprapelvic, transpelvic, and infrapelvic (Raycroft and Curtis, 1972). Infrapelvic pelvic obliquity is due to a leg length inequality which may be true or functional, unilateral hip dislocation, or relative adduction, and renders the pelvis oblique in the upright position. Transpelvic pelvic obliquity is attributable to relative overactivity of the unilateral iliopsoas muscle in cerebral palsy.

Suprapelvic pelvic obliquity is produced by a collapsing paralytic scoliosis above the pelvis with the low side of the pelvis being on the side of the convexity of the scoliosis (Figure 8.47). In assessing these patients, for their functional requirements, it is very important to evaluate the nature of this pelvic obliquity. For example, tendon transfer operations designed to locate and stabilize a dislocated hip always fail if the pelvic obliquity is suprapelvic. Balanced curves do not extend down to the pelvis which is horizontal, and therefore can be dealt with by straightforward procedures. By contrast, unbalanced curves extend down to the pelvis with concomitant suprapelvic pelvic obliquity. In general these curves require extensive anterior and posterior instrumentation support with fusion.

CEREBRAL PALSY

Almost half of all patients with cerebral palsy develop a scoliosis of clinical significance (Rosenthal *et al.*, 1974). The age of onset and progression potential of the scoliosis is directly related to the severity of the underlying condition. In children with only minimal brain dysfunction, balanced scolioses of the idiopathic type are encountered with a prevalence rate close to that of true idiopathic scoliosis. At the other end of the spectrum, patients with spastic quadriplegia will develop clinically significant scolioses by the end of growth, with an unbalanced curve pattern and an associated pelvic obliquity. These children also have appreciable mental impairment, motor dysfunction, as well as significant sensory deficits (Tizzard *et al.*, 1954).

Balanced curves can be dealt with along the same lines as the idiopathic counterpart with an emphasis more on prevention of curve progression than on curve correction, and with the use of traditional techniques rather than aggressive treatment strategies. For children with collapsing unbalanced curves, surgery should not be contemplated for those that are still walking. Lonstein and Akbarnia (1983) showed very poor results, with a very high complication rate, many children losing their walking ability directly as a result of the surgery. Surgery is therefore reserved for the wheelchair sitter who has lost hand function by having to use the upper extremities for support. Anterior segmental instrumentation and fusion is followed by posterior segmental instrumentation and fusion down to the sacrum (Figure 8.48). Very careful preoperative planning is required when significant mental impairment affects the ability to cope with such an extended treatment programme.

POLIOMYELITIS

With poliomyelitis the same pelvic obliquity problems are operative and it is very common to have associated imbalance about the hip (Somerville, 1959). There are two principal curve types – high curves associated with asymmetric paralysis, and low curves with pelvic obliquity associated with symmetric paralysis (James, 1956; Roaf, 1956). It was for the polio scoliosis that Harrington (1960) devised his instrumentation and it was the Milwaukee brace that was designed to provide the postoperative

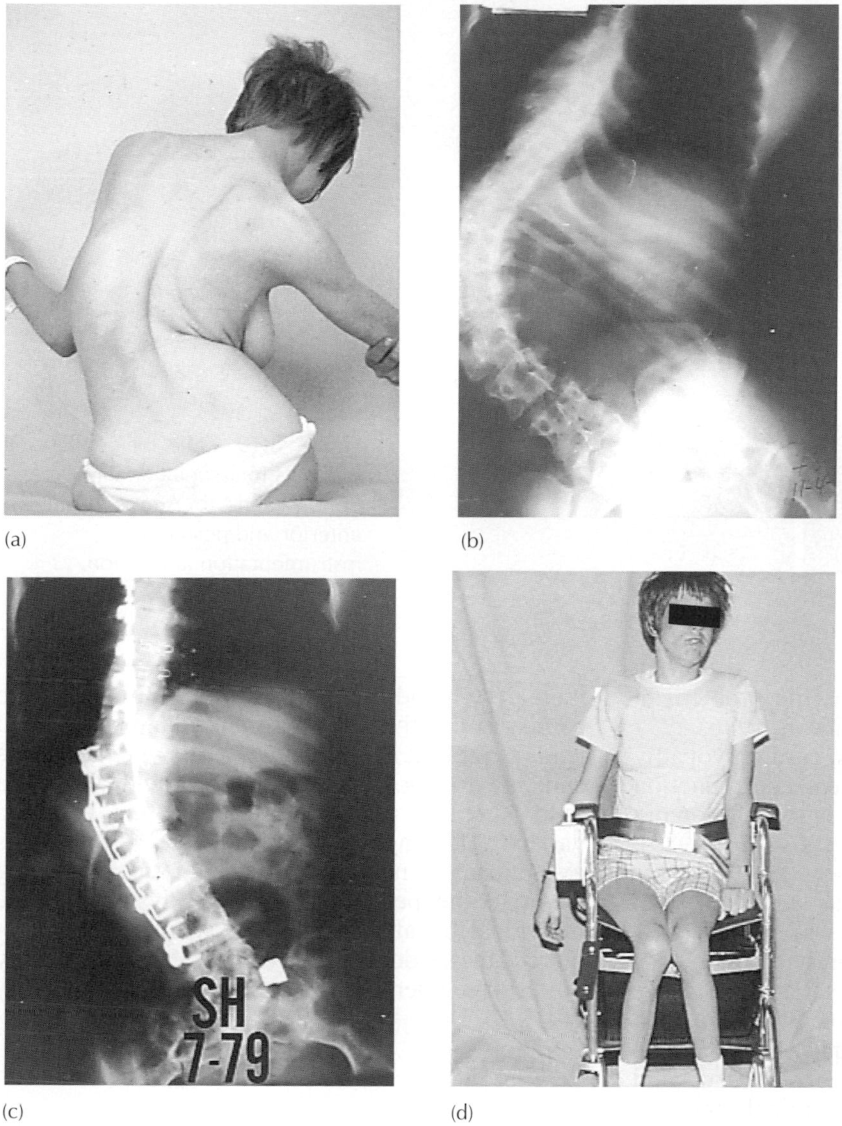

Figure 8.48 (a) The typical paralytic scoliosis in association with cerebral palsy such that there was no sitting stability. (b) The PA radiograph confirms the long C-shape scoliosis with pelvic obliquity. (c) After two-stage anterior and posterior fusion there is good correction of pelvic obliquity as well as the scoliosis. (d) The patient is comfortable in a wheelchair and has sitting stability, the ultimate goal.

support (Blount and Moe, 1973). Initially the instrumentation was inserted without fusion and failed with rapid recurrence of the deformity and the instrumentation cutting out, or displacement. With the addition of a sound bony fusion the results improved dramatically.

The higher curve without pelvic obliquity should be dealt with as for the idiopathic counterpart, while the collapsing C-shaped curve with pelvic obliquity should be dealt with by anterior and posterior instrumentation and fusion (Figure 8.49). The polio patient often gains most and has the lowest complication rate. Luque (1982) demonstrated that progressive curves at the mild end of the spectrum can be dealt with by one posterior segmental instrumentation and fusion procedure.

SPINAL MUSCULAR ATROPHY

Like poliomyelitis, the anterior horn cell is involved in spinal muscular atrophy but as a progressive cell degeneration. There was a subdivision between the early onset Werdnig–Hoffmann and the adolescent onset Kugelberg–Welander varieties but it is now recognized that they all are within a broad spectrum of function and life span (Dubowitz, 1974; Shapiro and Bresnan, 1982a). As with other paralytic conditions the earlier the onset the more severe the underlying condition with the tendency towards an early onset progressive collapsing C-shaped unbalanced curve and pelvic obliquity. Hip instability compounds the pelvic obliquity but scoliosis is the

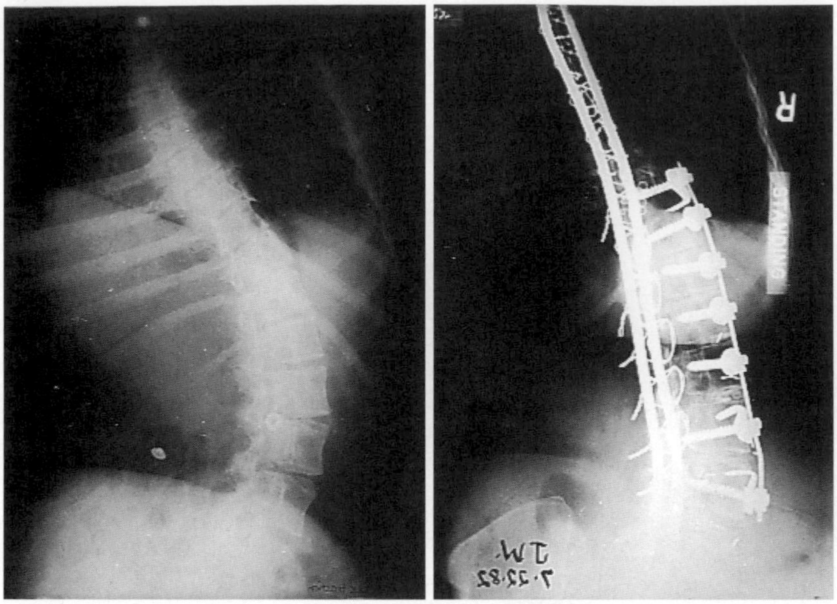

(a) (b)

Figure 8.49 (a) A long collapsing scoliosis in association with poliomyelitis. (b) After two-stage anterior and posterior instrumentation and fusion.

most common and severe orthopaedic problem in these patients (Schwentker and Gibson, 1976).

Although there is no associated cardiomyopathy in the spinal muscular atrophy patient, chest function is at risk and pulmonary complications following spinal surgery are frequent (Riddick *et al.*, 1982). A mobile lumbar hyperlordosis is essential for walking and in such patients spinal surgery is contraindicated. Because of the risks of surgery it is worth trying to reduce curve progression by the use of a 45° reclining wheelchair, a total contact Derby seat, and altering the base of the wheelchair to match the degree of pelvic obliquity. This can be most effective with the early flexible curve and may obviate the requirement for surgical intervention. For those with loss of sitting stability surgical correction and fusion is indicated but it is important to follow these children carefully and regularly. An anterior first stage can be performed with considerable pulmonary risks because of interference to the diaphragm and therefore the ideal case would be the relatively flexible one which can be dealt with by posterior segmental instrumentation and fusion alone. Even so, considerable perioperative pulmonary care is required, including tracheostomy.

THE PERIPHERAL NEUROPATHIES

There are a variety of conditions under this general category of which peroneal muscular atrophy (Charcot–Marie–Tooth disease) is the most common. The condition is neurologically milder in comparison with other neuromuscular disorders and tends to present in the teenage years with pes cavus and claw-toeing. Ten per cent of individuals have a mild idiopathic-type deformity of the balanced variety (Hensinger and MacEwen, 1976). It is exceptional to encounter a true paralytic curve going down to the pelvis sufficient to dysfunction the individual by affecting sitting stability. When required these deformities can be dealt with by posterior segmental instrument and fusion only.

FRIEDREICH'S ATAXIA

This is a condition of progressive cerebellar degeneration and, like peroneal muscular atrophy, presents in the early teens often with pes cavus. In addition, however, there is a progressively more broad-based and unsteady gait. There is continued and often rapid progression to wheelchair sitting in the twenties, and death from cardiomyopathy around the age of 40 years. Three-quarters of all patients do develop a collapsing paralytic deformity in time and again surgical treatment should be addressed to the wheelchair sitter losing stability (Hensinger and MacEwen, 1976). Because of the cardiopulmonary risk, only posterior segmental instrumentation and fusion should be attempted.

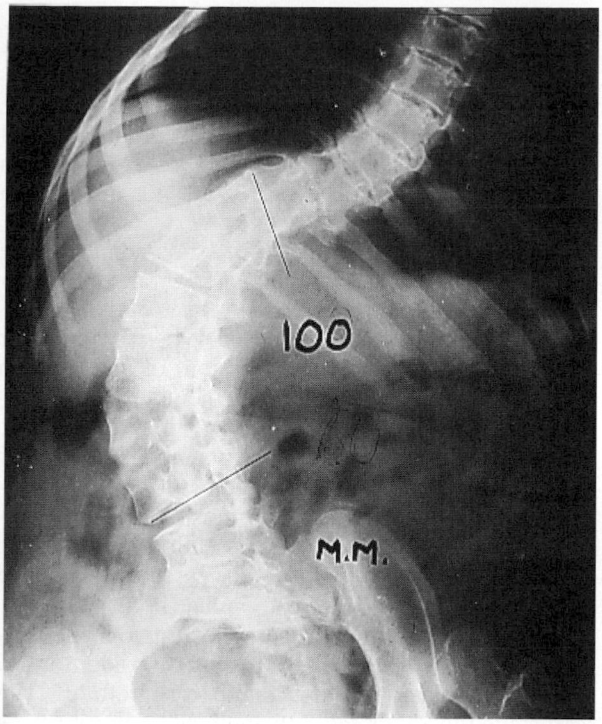

Figure 8.50 Thoracolumbar scoliosis with pelvic obliquity and a dislocating hip on the high side in association with arthrogryposis.

ARTHROGRYPOSIS

This peculiar condition of multiple joint stiffness, deformity and dislocation is now considered to have a neuromuscular pathogenesis (Shapiro and Bresnan, 1982b). A significant structural scoliosis occurs in about a quarter of all patients and while most are of the collapsing paralytic variety, some are due to congenital bony anomalies at the curve apex. Unlike the other neuromuscular conditions, even the collapsing paralytic curve in arthrogryposis is quite rigid from the outset. There is very often hip contracture or dislocation compounding the problem of pelvic obliquity (Figure 8.50). Two-stage anterior and posterior instrumentation and fusion is required for these difficult and rigid deformities which may even require two-stage wedge resection to achieve sufficient correction.

THE MUSCULAR DYSTROPHIES

There is a spectrum of severity in the muscular dystrophies from the severe and universally fatal Duchenne dystrophy at the one end, through the congenital myopathies, to the milder Becker and fascioscapulohumeral dystrophy at the other. The development of segmental instrumentation has seen surgery being increasingly prescribed for these dystrophies and it is common to perform a long thoracolumbar posterior segmental spinal instrumentation and fusion operation as soon as the Duchenne patient begins wheelchair life (Weimann *et al.*, 1983). There is an overall mortality rate of from this procedure and therefore the 'risks and rewards' equation has to be very carefully considered (Swank *et al.*, 1982). These children die from a terminal cardiomyopathic event with the cardiorespiratory reserve being seriously impaired long before death. Surgery should not be performed if the vital capacity is less than 30% and only posterior segmental instrumentation and fusion should be carried out. Any anterior surgical interference with the diaphragm is much too risky. While all Duchenne patients do develop a collapsing spinal deformity, not all are necessarily impaired with it. If curve size is less than 50° it is seldom dysfunctioning (Wilkins and Gibson, 1976) and time can be bought, and thus surgery delayed, or even obviated, by altering the height of the wheelchair base, raising the low buttock, and using a reclining wheelchair.

Although the congenital myopathies are not progressive in the neuromuscular sense (Dubowitz, 1978), surgery is not well tolerated and the question of surgical intervention should be explored along the lines of the Duchenne patient. The other forms of dystrophy at the milder end of the spectrum are not complicated by significant cardiomyopathy and seldom produce an unbalanced spine. These balanced curves should therefore be dealt with as for their idiopathic counterpart by posterior segmental instrumentation and fusion alone.

Neurofibromatosis

As with peroneal muscular atrophy and Friedreich's ataxia, it is often the orthopaedic surgeon who makes the initial diagnosis of this condition because of a musculoskeletal manifestation. Between 30 and 40% of these patients do develop a spinal deformity, while 10% develop a spondylolisthesis (McCarroll, 1950). At the mild end of the spectrum there may be only a few *café au lait* spots (there should be a minimum of six measuring 1.5 cm each before the diagnosis is confirmed) (Crowe *et al.*, 1956). At the other end of the severity spectrum all components of the musculoskeletal system can be involved, including the skin with either nodular or plexiform lesions, limb size discrepancy, multiple neurofibromata along the course of the peripheral nerves, cranial and spinal nerve dumb-bell tumours, and vascular abnormalities such as haemangiomata and thick-walled plexiform veins. Although the condition is genetically expressed as an autosomal dominant, at least 50% are spontaneous mutations.

The more severe the clinical expression of the condition the more obvious is the dystrophic bone change in the axial skeleton; this is characterized by vertebral scalloping, rib spindling, and vertebral pseudo-fusions (Hunt and Pugh, 1961). The more evidence of dystrophic bone change the earlier the onset, the more severely progressive, and the more angular the associated spinal deformity (see Figure 8.46) (Roaf, 1966; Chaglassian *et al.*, 1976; Simmons and Thomas, 1976). However, at the milder end of the spectrum the deformities are indistinguishable from idiopathic scoliosis.

As with other conditions the associated spinal deformities are broadly divisible into two categories – lordoscoliosis, and kyphosis – the latter being much less prevalent than generally appreciated. This is because the angular lordoscoliosis associated with considerable dystrophic bone change is so rotated from the sagittal plane that it gives the impression of kyphosis when the patient is viewed or x-rayed from the side (Deacon *et al.*, 1984). Kyphoses do, however, occur and these tend to be in the thoracic region, although they can be encountered in the neck or cervicothoracic junction, giving rise to a progressive swan-neck deformity of progressive kyphosis and progressive compensatory lordosis in the sagittal plane. Neurological complications caused by tension behind the apex of the kyphosis are not uncommon (Lonstein *et al.*, 1980).

In all but the mildest cases masquerading as true idiopathic scoliosis, both an anterior and posterior fusion are necessary to prevent loss of correction. Thus it should be routine practice to perform anterior multiple discectomy with excision of the growth plates, followed by posterior segmental instrumentation and fusion (Dawson *et al.*, 1973b: Winter *et al.*, 1979). On occasion, even a very soundly performed bone grafting operation often leads to a pseudarthrosis, the graft reabsorbing. The most severe deformities require two-stage wedge resection at the curve apex in addition to multiple discectomy during the first stage (Figure 8.51) (Leatherman, 1973).

Kyphotic deformities again need two-stage surgery with an anterior strut graft in addition to multiple discectomy and interbody grafting. The cervical/cervicothoracic swan-neck deformity is very difficult to manage and is best dealt with by

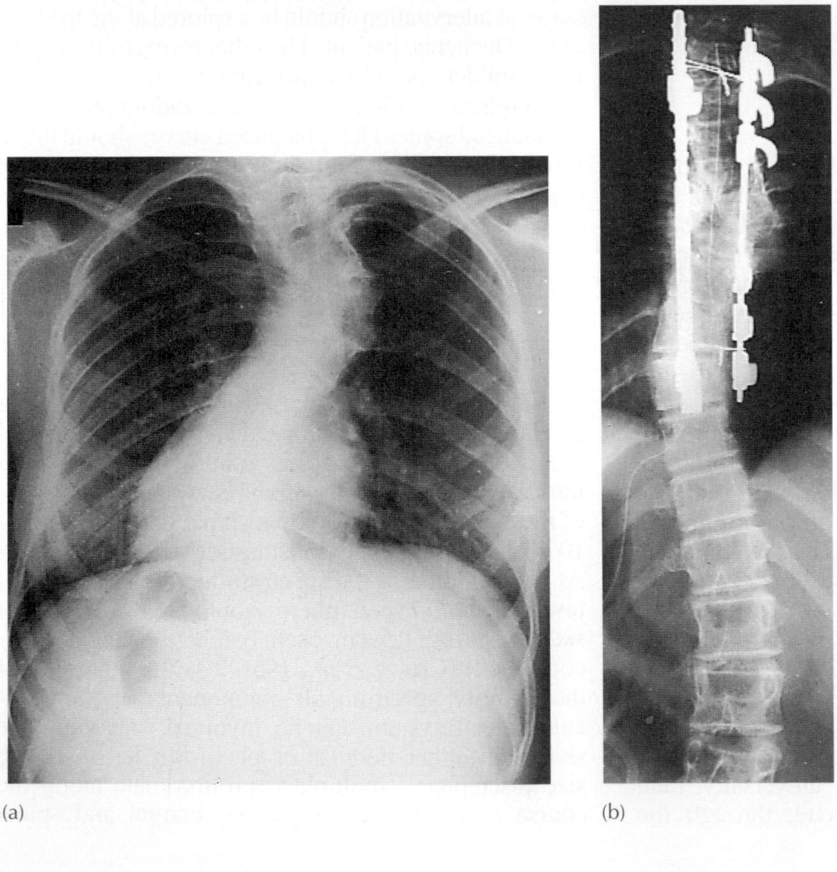

(a) (b)

Figure 8.51 Two-stage wedge resection for a high thoracic curve in von Recklinghausen's disease. (a) Preoperative radiograph. (b) After two-stage wedge resection showing good correction with good spinal balance.

external fixation using a halo vest or cast while the anterior and posterior fusions consolidate.

Mesenchymal disorders

(see Chapter 4)

This group comprises the heritable disorders of connective tissue, the mucopolysaccharidoses, and the skeletal dysplasias. Spinal deformities are common and are due to intrinsic bone or soft tissue weakness, favouring spinal column buckling, or due to deficient anterior vertebral body development, particularly in the thoracolumbar region.

THE HERITABLE DISORDERS OF CONNECTIVE TISSUE

These are problems of collagen formation and affect the musculoskeletal system either by way of bone weakness (osteogenesis imperfecta), or soft tissue weakness (Marfan's syndrome, homocystinuria, Ehlers–Danlos syndrome).

Osteogenesis imperfecta is attributable to defective synthesis of enough type I collagen and this seriously affects the skeleton as bone contains only type I collagen (Smith *et al.*, 1983). The condition is divided into mild and severe types based upon the presence of long bone deformity. At the milder end of the spectrum spinal involvement is indistinguishable from idiopathic juvenile osteoporosis with vertebral osteoporosis, compression fracturing and biconcavity. There is therefore a trend towards thoracic hyperkyphosis with an associated increase in anterior chest deformities such as pectus carinatum or excavatum.

Towards the more severe end of the spectrum the type II congenita form is invariably associated with a spinal deformity (Bauze *et al.*, 1975). Rather like von Recklinghausen's disease, the scoliosis is associated with intrinsic bone weakness. Bracing has been of some benefit in the kyphosis patient but has been ineffective for the scoliosis patient with rib deformities being a common complication (Yong-Hing and MacEwen, 1982). In an attempt to reduce scoliosis progression Harrington distraction instrumentation has been the mainstay of surgical treatment but the results have been disappointing and significant complications occur in over 30%. This is because the metalwork readily cuts out or dislodges from the weakened bone. To overcome this, methylmethacrylate cement has been used to support hook sites (Waugh, 1971) but segmental wiring or a compression system is preferred so as to spread load over as wide an area as possible (Figure 8.52).

Marfan's syndrome is a dominantly inherited disorder of skeletal deformity, arachnodactyly, dislocated lenses, and aortic dilatation (Smith, 1979). Deficient collagen synthesis is expressed clinically in the form of soft tissue laxity and the prevalence rate of structural scoliosis is of the order of 50% (Robins *et al.*, 1975). It is radiographically indistinguishable from idiopathic scoliosis and there tend to be two curve patterns – single right thoracic or double structural. Although life span is reduced by aortic incompetence, dissecting aneurysm or mitral and tricuspid valve disease, these do not constitute contraindications to spinal surgery. Treatment is along the same lines as idiopathic scoliosis but the recurrence rate is high following posterior instrumentation and fusion alone. Preliminary anterior multiple discectomy should therefore be carried out with the objective being to achieve both anterior and posterior spinal fusion.

Marfan's syndrome has many clinical similarities to homocystinuria and Ehlers–Danlos syndrome. In homocystinuria there is additional spinal osteoporosis and platyspondyly with the posterior vertebral borders being particularly concave. As with Marfan's syndrome half the patients have a significant scoliosis (Brenton *et al.*, 1972) but because of the high risk of thrombosis in these patients (Gibson *et al.*, 1964) surgical treatment should not be offered. It is now clear that there are a number of different subgroups of the Ehlers–Danlos syndrome of which type 6 is the ocular-scoliotic form. In addition to loose jointedness there is excessively stretchable and fragile skin. Some degree of scoliosis is present in the majority of cases but tends not to be severe or particularly progressive (Beighton and Horan, 1969). The risk in operating upon patients with Ehlers–Danlos syndrome is haemorrhage due to excessive vascular fragility and the surgery is contraindicated unless the precise subtype of Ehlers–Danlos syndrome is known and safe (Smith, 1979).

MUCOPOLYSACCHARIDOSES

The mucopolysaccharidoses affect the skeleton by way of failure of normal breakdown of complex carbohydrates which thus accumulate in the tissues. Only MPS IV (Morquio's syndrome) is commonly seen by orthopaedic surgeons. In addition to platyspondyly which considerably foreshortens trunk height, there are two major spinal problems in the Morquio patient – thoracolumbar kyphosis and atlantoaxial instability as a result of a dysplastic or an aplastic odontoid peg (Kopits *et al.*, 1972; Bethem *et al.*,

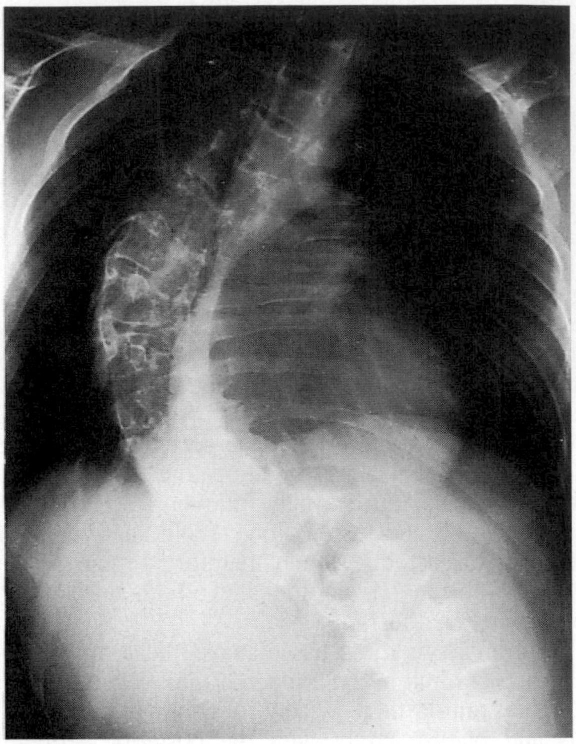

(a)

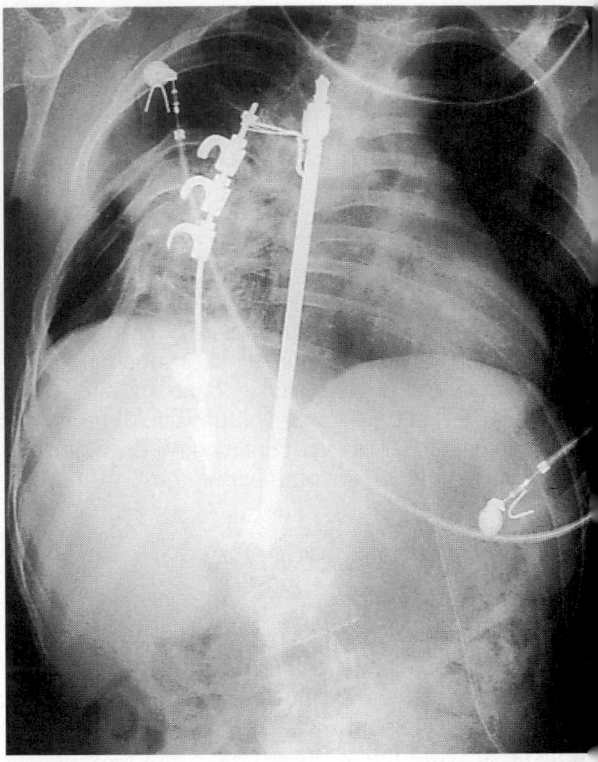

(b)

Figure 8.52 (a) PA radiograph showing a severe thoracic scoliosis in association with type I osteogenesis imperfecta. (b) Following two-stage anterior multiple discectomy and posterior Harrington instrumentation there has been a good correction. It is always advisable to distribute load – hence the compression system on the convex side.

1981) (Figure 8.53). The thoracolumbar kyphosis is due to anterior vertebral beaking with the T12 or L1 vertebra being deficient anteriorly. As with other thoracolumbar kyphoses there is often an associated barrel-shaped chest and prominent sternum. With growth, a progressive thoracolumbar kyphosis occurs and can be severe enough to compromise the function of the spinal cord. Such patients therefore have to be watched neurologically. Any signs of progressive paraparesis must be investigated by spinal cord MR imaging and followed by anterior spinal decompression and strut grafting combined with posterior stabilization. Atlantoaxial subluxation is notorious not only for producing neurological symptoms but also because of its mortality. Presenting neurological symptoms may not be so obvious as with a thoracolumbar kyphosis and may only express itself in terms of tiredness, weakness, vague leg pains, syncope, gait abnormality, or respiratory symptoms. So potentially serious is this problem that prophylactic C1/2 fusion is recommended by the age of 10 years (Kopits, 1976). This is achieved by posterior on-lay bone grafting and external fixation using a halo cast.

SKELETAL DYSPLASIAS

Of the many, and very often rare, skeletal dysplasias significant spinal involvement tends to occur with multiple epiphyseal dysplasia, achondroplasia, spondyloepiphyseal dysplasia, and diastrophic dysplasia (Spranger *et al.*, 1974). Multiple epiphyseal dysplasia is a problem of irregular epiphyseal growth with abnormal endochondral ossification. As a result of this dysplasia multiple joints are involved, usually the hips, knees and elbows. The vertebral epiphyses are also affected with both flattening and irregularity giving rise to a Scheuermann-like thoracic hyperkyphosis. Because of the tendency towards kyphosis, scoliosis is uncommon, but can occur.

The spine is typically, and often severely, involved in achondroplasia. There is, however, a spectrum of severity of spinal involvement (Wynne-Davies *et al.*, 1981). There are two particularly important features with regard to the spine – spinal stenosis and a thoracolumbar kyphosis (Nelson, 1972; Lutter and Langer, 1977). Both can give rise to adverse neurological features and both can be present. There is a tendency to thoracolumbar kyphosis and therefore structural scoliosis is rare. A

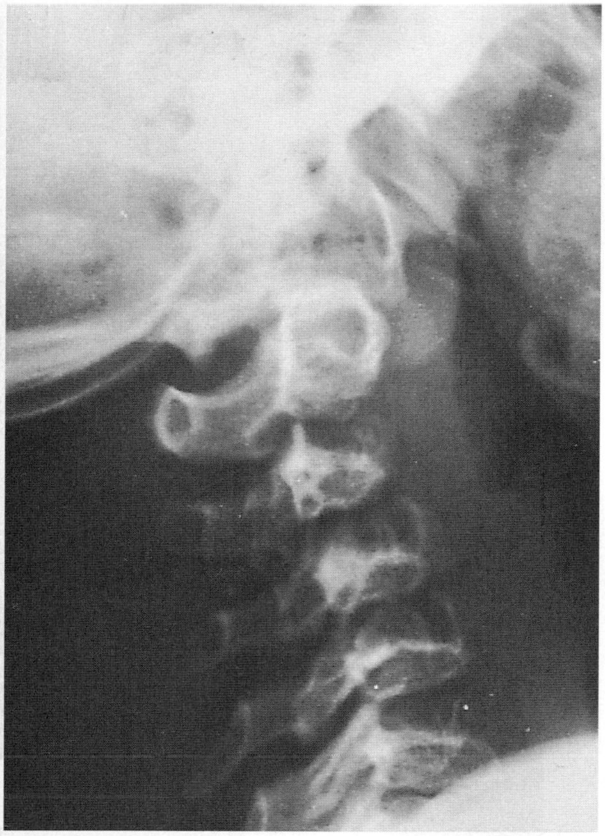

Figure 8.53 Lateral radiograph of the cervical spine in a case of Morquio's disease (MPS IV). There is an absent odontoid and anterior subluxation of the atlas on the axis.

in mucopolysaccharidoses the thoracolumbar vertebra is bullet shaped; being deficient anteriorly results in a local angular kyphosis. In the great majority of cases, however, this thoracolumbar kyphosis resolves with growth and although signs of paraparesis can occur in a few, surgery need not be rushed into unless it be the unusual progressive case for which anterior decompression and strut grafting is the requisite procedure. Spinal stenosis is a much more potent cause of neurological symptoms and signs. This is compounded by lumbar hyperlordosis with impinging facet joints and infolded ligamentum flavum. Measurement of spinal canal dimensions has not been helpful, and of more importance are short pedicles, thickened laminae and articular processes (Lutter *et al.*, 1977). Spinal cord imaging by CT and or MR scanning demonstrates multiple level stenosis often going well up into the thoracic spine. For those with progressive neurological features decompressive laminectomy is necessary and this should be widened by an undercutting facetectomy so as to minimize spinal instability. In the immature patient spinal decompression should be accompanied by spinal stabilization and fusion to prevent a rapidly progressive kyphosis which may in turn adversely affect spinal cord function (Figure 8.54).

There are two types of spondyloepiphyseal dysplasia – the mild tarda variety and the more severe congenita type. In the tarda form there is mild vertebral dysplasia with platyspondyly and a tendency towards kyphosis (Hensinger, 1977). The condition is commonly confused with MPS IV but the vertebrae are not only fat but 'humped' posteriorly (Langer 1964). A thoracolumbar bullet-shaped vertebra producing kyphosis is often aggravated by local flexion/extension instability to produce adverse neurological features. As with other angular kyphoses, anterior vertebral body resection and strut grafting followed by posterior stabilization is required. The congenita form has the same spinal features but more severely expressed.

In diastrophic dysplasia, in addition to the short limbs, club foot deformity, and joint contractures, the spine is commonly involved (Herring, 1978; Bethem *et al.*, 1980). Progressive scoliosis occurs in about 50% of cases and both anterior and posterior spinal fusions are required to stabilize it. Spina bifida occulta, either cervical or lumbar, is a common feature and thus if spinal shape is to be altered by instrumentation the spinal canal must be imaged adequately preoperatively to exclude cord tether. A particularly worrying spinal problem in diastrophic dysplasia is a cervical kyphosis sufficient to produce quadriplegia and, indeed, death. Again both anterior and posterior fusion are required for stabilization.

Spinal deformities due to trauma

Traumatic spinal deformities can occur as a result of trauma to the vertebral column itself (e.g. injury or operation), or from extravertebral trauma as a result of damage to the chest wall or flank by surgery or fibrosis.

DEFORMITIES DUE TO VERTEBRAL TRAUMA

Approximately one-tenth of all spinal injuries occur in children under the age of 15 and about 50% of these have some form of neurological loss (Kewelramani and Tori, 1980). Compared with the adult pattern, in young children the injury tends to occur as a result of a road traffic accident or a fall, while

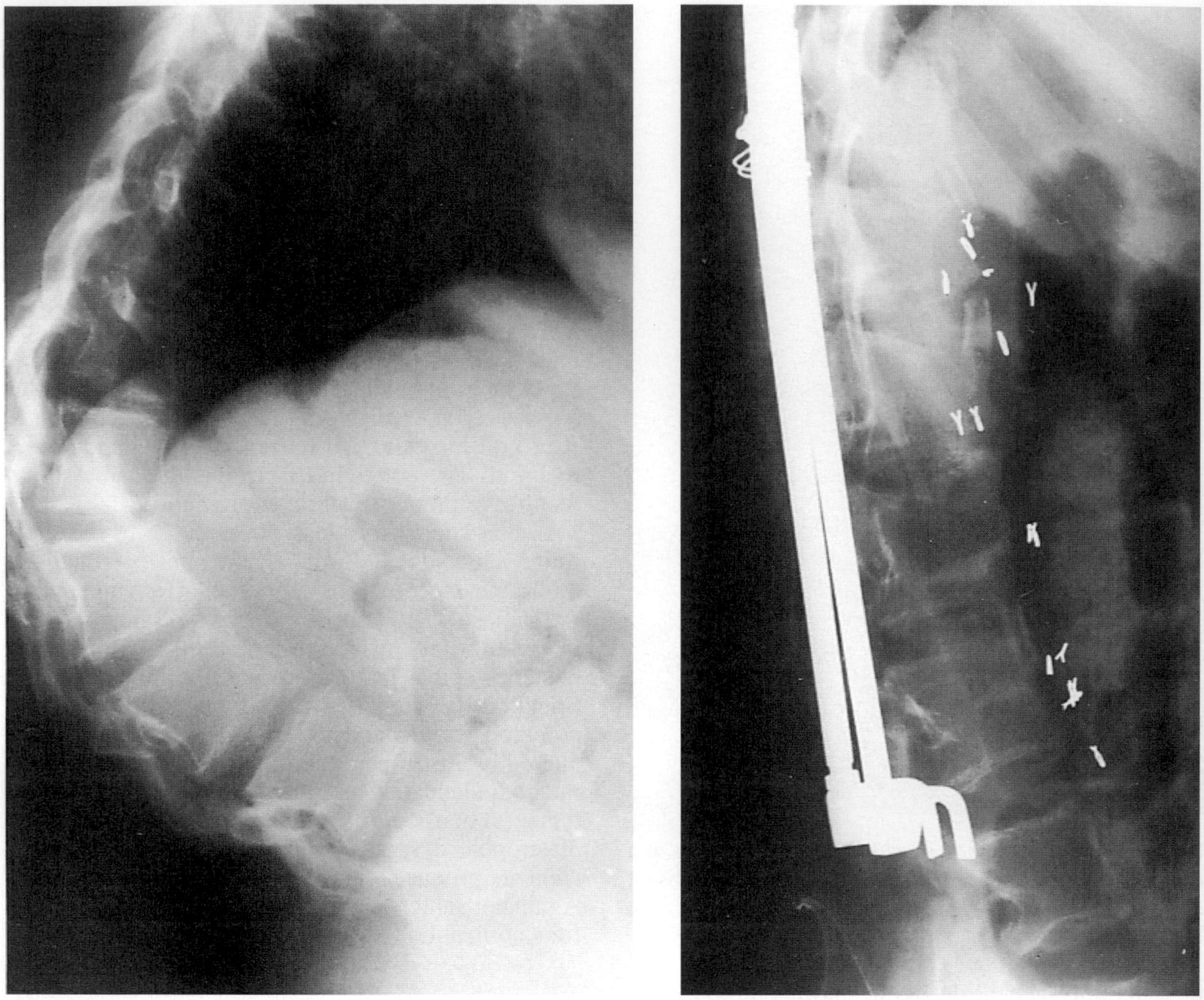

(a) (b)

Figure 8.54 (a) Lateral radiograph in a teenage boy with achondroplasia and significant spinal stenosis after widespread laminectomy showing the development of a severe kyphosis giving rise to its own neurological complications. (b) Lateral radiograph after anterior and posterior fusion. A stable spine resulted in a very much improved position with resolution of the neurological sequelae.

in older children and adolescents a sporting mishap is usually the mechanism of injury. Delay in diagnosis is often common, as a result of being one injury in a multiple injury pattern, e.g. a head injury diverting attention, but the commonest cause of delay is an inadequate lateral spinal radiograph (Davies *et al.*, 1971) or now a CT scan. Non-accidental injury is becoming steadily more prevalent. In children there may be no obvious bony derangement of the spinal column, yet the child has an obvious spinal cord injury. In addition 3 mm of displacement between C1/2, C2/3, and C3/4 is present in 20% of normal children, indicating that physiological displacements or variations are common (Bohlman *et al.*, 1983).

In children upper cervical spine injuries, i.e. 50% of all neck injuries, are greatly over-represented compared with the adult pattern. In addition to plain films, computerized tomography is necessary to assess disc and bone fragments in relation to the spinal cord. In the thoracolumbar region the injury pattern in children is again different from that encountered in adults. Two-thirds are stable compression fractures while one-third are fracture dislocations, with more than a 50% incidence of significant neurological damage (Hubbard, 1974). Autopsy studies have shown that the discs are not damaged but the vascular growth plate preferentially takes the trauma load (Aufdermaur, 1974). One of the important factors determining the presence of a progressive deformity in the injured immature spine is significant growth plate damage, the other being the presence of paralysis, thus favouring the development of the typical paralytic collapsing scoliotic curve, very similar to a neuromuscular scoliosis (see Figure 8.56). A third factor, and one of increasing importance over the past two or three decades, is the injudicious performance of laminectomy in the immature spine. As the line of the centre of gravity of the body passes just in front of the anterior surface of the fourth lumbar vertebra then any material loss in the spine will readily produce kyphosis. In order to prevent late cervical spine instability and kyphosis, Bohlman *et al.* (1983) recommend surgical stabilization, particularly for the child over the age of 8 years with atlanto-occipital instability, or for C3–C7 injuries when the posterior ligament complex is torn.

In the thoracolumbar region, provided the growth plate does not receive irreparable damage, then remodelling is the rule. Indeed, overgrowth readily occurs as the anterior periosteum and longitudinal ligament are relatively lengthened with the anterior parts of the growth plate being stimulated preferentially. While Hubbard (1974) indicated a very benign prognosis in the great majority, a rather different outcome was observed by Pouliquen and Pennecot (1983) with a progressive deformity in almost half their children. Therefore an extension brace, e.g. a Scheuermann's thoracic kyphosis brace, should be fitted, so as to give every opportunity for the traumatic kyphosis to improve with growth. The presence of a type V growth plate injury is seen in an increasing local angular kyphosis and this requires both anterior fusion and posterior instrumental stabilization. For the child with paraplegia, if the level is above T10 a paralytic deformity will inevitably occur. For the older child or adolescent, progression to a dysfunctional sitting stability may occur, but for the more immature, anterior and posterior spinal fusion with segmental instrumentation may be necessary.

DEFORMITIES DUE TO DAMAGE OF CHEST OR ABDOMINAL WALL

In 1934 Bisgard described two types of thoracogenic scoliosis – pleural and thoracoplastic. With chronic pleural thickening there was a long mild curvature with little or no rotation, but a more obvious lateral curvature, sometimes with rotation, was produced by thoracoplasty. The more the ribs resected and the more the transverse processes were interfered with, the more evidence of spinal deformity, rather like the experimental scoliosis produced in animals by Langenskiold and Michelsson (1961). These deformities are almost certainly produced by interference with the spinal reflex arc with 60% of the deformity present within a week of surgery and nearly all of it by the end of the first year (Stauffer and Mankin, 1966; Loynes, 1972).

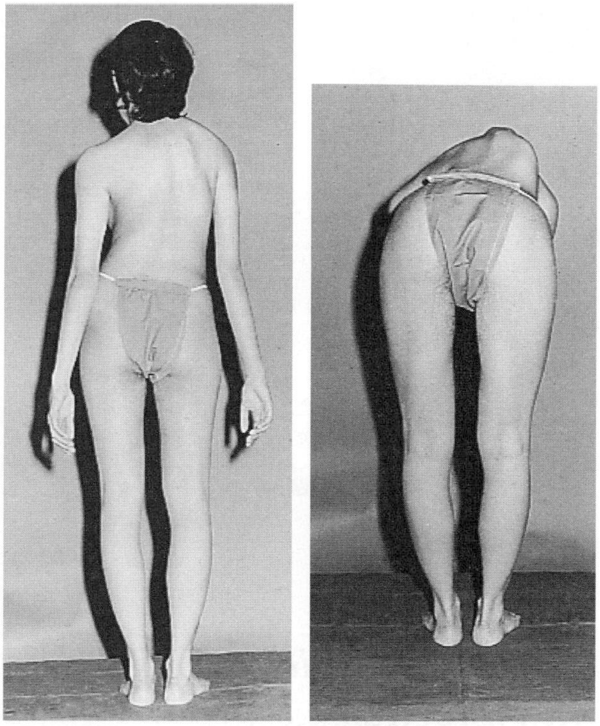

(a) (b)

Figure 8.55 Erect (a) and forward bending view (b) of a thoracic scoliosis due to an extensive thoracoplasty for tuberculosis.

Even the performance of a simple thoracotomy operation, with or without rib resection, can produce a scoliosis, convex away from the side of thoracotomy rather like Bisgard's pleural type of scoliosis. A curvature of real clinical significance is, however, seldom produced (Figure 8.55). These chest-wall-type scolioses are treated as for idiopathic scoliosis at the same site.

Very occasionally burns or retroperitoneal fibrosis can tether the trunk and induce a scoliosis. In the early days when hydrocephalus was dealt with by thecoperitoneal shunting rather than ventriculoatrial shunting, the adhesion and fibrosis formation from multiple operations including several lumbar laminectomies tethered the lumbar spine into hyperlordosis (Steel and Adams, 1972; McMaster and Carey, 1985). In some cases this was severe enough to warrant anterior closing wedge lumbar osteotomy.

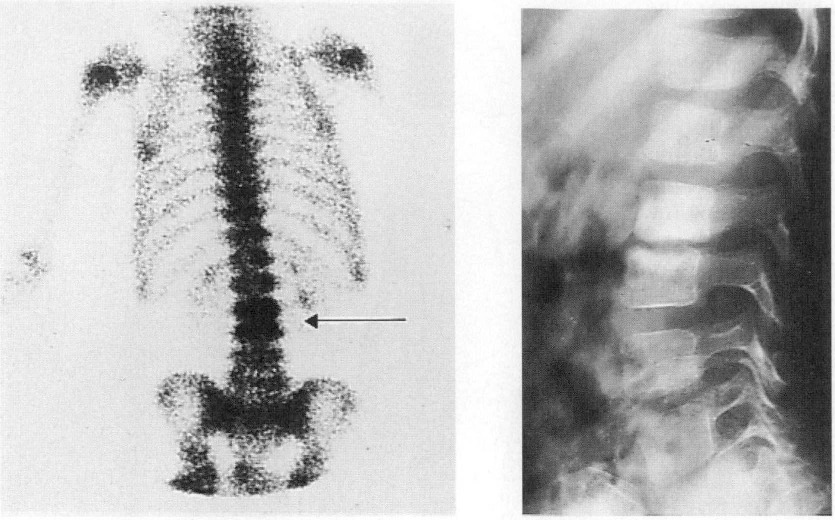

(a) (b)

Figure 8.56 Classical discitis. The lumbar spine is the most commonly affected site and the bone scintography (a) was positive long before plain x-ray changes were visible (b).

Spinal deformities associated with infection (see Chapter 9)

Spinal infection is broadly divisible into two groups, pyogenic or tuberculous, the former accounting for two-thirds of cases. Although certain clinical features are more typical of one type of spinal infection than the other, the modes of presentation can be quite indistinguishable and there is all too frequently a considerable delay in diagnosis (Wedge and Kirkaldy-Willis, 1990). In addition, particularly in children, there is the condition of intervertebral discitis, the cause of which is yet unclear. It is not bacteriological but may well be an immune reaction (Menelaus, 1964). The spine is a favourite site for infection because of the very rich blood supply and the free communication between Batson's pelvic plexus and the vertebral venous plexuses (Batson, 1940). Trueta, however, considered the venous side much less relevant than the very rich arterial supply taking organisms quickly to the metaphyseal regions close to the end plates (Wiley and Trueta, 1959). The septic process with the pressure of local pus and bacterial toxins producing vascular spasm can go on to a septic necrosis with sequestration of bone as well as disc. Unchecked local vertebral collapse occurs with kyphosis formation and abscess accumulation which can spread down tissue planes or compromise the spinal cord.

With pyogenic infections the lumbar spine is most commonly involved (Figure 8.56), followed by the cervical spine, and the posterior elements are only very rarely involved. Fever, back pain, and tenderness constitute the classical triad, along with neurological loss if there is significant kyphosis or abscess formation. Both plasma viscosity and white cell count are raised and bacteriological titres also rise with the infectious process. If a spinal infection is to be biopsied it is important to send material for both pathology and bacteriology with instructions for the latter to be examined for aerobic, anaerobic, tuberculous and fungal infections (Wedge *et al.*, 1977). The condition may arise in the spine *de novo* or spread metastatically from elsewhere as part of a septicaemic process. The non-bacterial discitis tends to present with local pain and severe muscle spasm and, while the sedimentation rate might be mildly raised other blood tests are normal. The typical radiographic features of disc space narrowing may not be obvious for several days and skeletal scintigraphy and now MR imaging are very sensitive investigations in detecting the condition at an early stage. In pyogenic infections abscess formation is limited, spinal cord compromise is unusual, and the process goes on to spontaneous interbody fusion or fibrous ankylosis (Griffiths and Jones, 1971; Wedge *et al.*, 1977).

In tuberculosis of the spine the L1 vertebral body is the most commonly affected (O'Brien, 1977) and the clinical course tends to be more insidious than if pyogenic. An angular kyphosis (gibbus), abscess formation and paralysis as presenting features are also very much more typical of tuberculous spinal disease (Figure 8.57). Again, pathological and bacteriological confirmation by biopsy is important, particularly for appropriate drug therapy of appropriate sensitivity. In tuberculous infection the disc space may survive for a long time but eventual

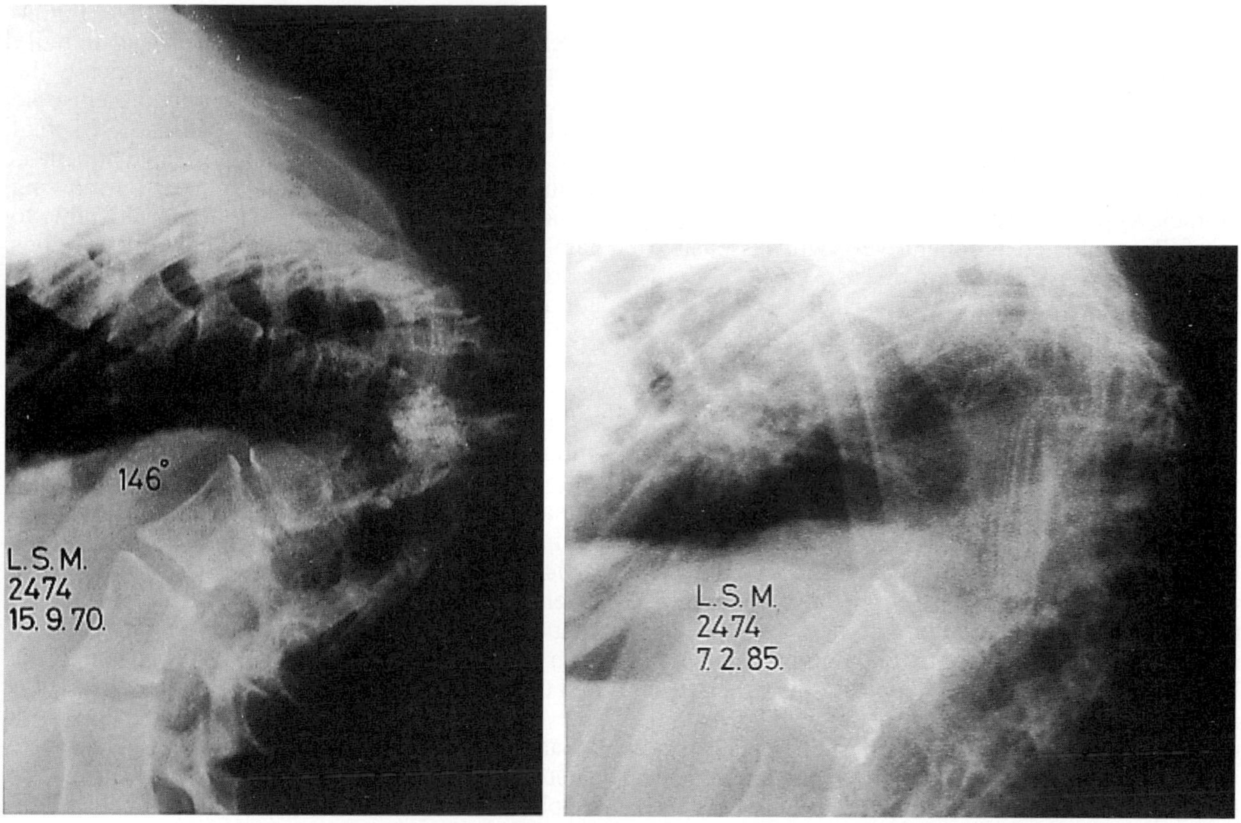

(a) (b)

Figure 8.57 (a) Severe lower thoracic gibbus with impending paralysis in association with long-standing tuberculosis. (b) After anterior decompression and strut grafting the kyphosis has been much improved and the neurological catastrophe averted (case of Professor J.C.Y. Leong).

bone destruction disc sequestration is much more common.

Pyogenic infections are usually attributable to the *Staphylococcus aureus* but in the young child the pneumococcus or *Haemophilus influenzae* organisms are not unusual. Appropriate antibiotic treatment should last for a period of 3 months and spinal discomfort should be mitigated by the application of a spinal support. Only with significant abscess formation or neurological compromise is surgery indicated in the form of anterior decompression and strut grafting with posterior instrumental stabilization.

Over the last two or three decades there has been considerable debate as to how tuberculous spinal infection should be treated and despite the excellent results from Hodgson's radical anterior operation (Hodgson and Stock, 1960) the Medical Research Council still recommend a policy of rest and chemotherapy even for the patient with complete paralysis (Griffiths, 1986). Despite the MRC's views, most modern-day spinal surgeons do recommend anterior excision of the diseased bone with the deficit made good by strut grafting and this is generally followed by posterior instrumentation. This operative procedure is absolutely indicated if there is abscess formation, progressive kyphosis, and neurological compromise (Wedge and Kirkaldy-Willis, 1990). Operative treatment should be supported by antituberculous chemotherapy with rifampicin and isoniazid in daily divided doses orally for a minimum of 9 months.

When radical anterior excision and decompression and fusion are performed in the young spine the growth of the anterior spinal column is tethered and in Fountain *et al.*'s (1975) cases 10% went on to progressive kyphosis. Surgical treatment is still controversial for this type of kyphosis with less than 30% correction (Hodgson, 1973; Yau *et al.*, 1974). There seem to be two situations where surgery should be prescribed – the increasing kyphotic deformity, particularly with evidence of paraparesis, and the established tuberculous kyphosis already with adverse neurological signs. The Hong Kong group have published complex multistage procedures with interval halopelvic traction with a lot of complications and little gain. It is preferable to carry out anterior excision of the apical vertebral body, plus the two discs on each side, and then insert both strut and interbody grafts supported posteriorly by segmental instrumentation. It is awkward surgery at the front of a significant kyphosis and chest function is always reduced in the presence of a significant thoracic kyphosis. Patients should therefore be very carefully evaluated preoperatively with a sensible 'risks and rewards' equation discussion.

Deformities associated with tumours (see Chapter 10)

Spinal or paraspinal tumours can produce a spinal deformity either by their physical presence or by the treatment required to deal with them. Intradural tumours are rare in children and most are gliomas, including astrocytomas and ependymomas, or neuroblastomas. The considerable Boston experience indicates that these lesions affect boys twice as frequently as girls and half of them occur in the first 4 years of life, more being benign than malignant (Tachdjian and Matson, 1965). Limp leg weakness and back pain are the chief presenting symptoms, while pathological reflexes, paralysis, and muscle spasm are the commonest physical signs. There is a true lordoscoliosis in one-third of cases (Figure 8.58). The diagnosis is often delayed and initially incorrect (Fraser *et al.*, 1977). Characteristically the back pain is continuous rather than being episodic and is more pronounced at night. MR and CT spinal cord imaging confirms the diagnosis. Treatment is in the form of microsurgical removal following laminectomy which may have to be considerable to gain access. Radiotherapy is prescribed for lesions that cannot be totally removed but the prognosis is not greatly affected and the 5-year survival for malignant cases is about 60%.

Syringomyelia, a chronic slowly progressive degeneration of the spinal cord and medulla with cavitation and gliosis, can present with a similar initial clinical picture to intradural tumours (Huebert and MacKinnon, 1969; Williams, 1979). While spinal cord tumour or trauma can produce cord cavitation (non-communicating syringomyelia) the typical syrinx is of the communicating variety with patency between the cavity and the posterior fossa (Figure 8.59). There is typically sensory dissociation with pain and temperature involved but not touch, and this is due to the decussating pain and temperature fibres being centrally located in the cord. Meanwhile the sensation of 'touch' is preserved. There is weakness and wasting of the muscles supplied by the involved segments. As with intradural tumours, pain is the most common presenting feature either located to the back but very commonly in the form of severe headache. Both hydrocephalus and

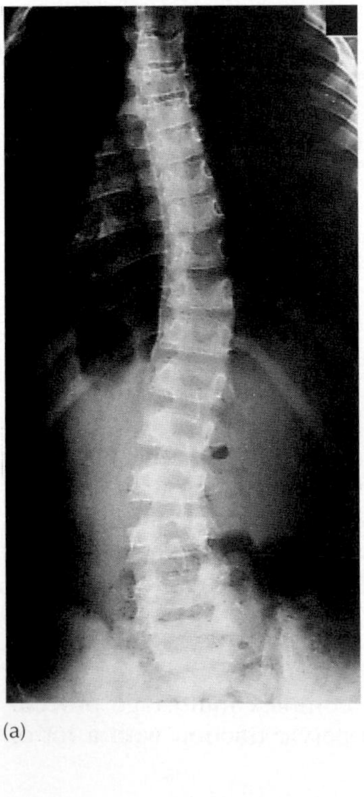

(a)

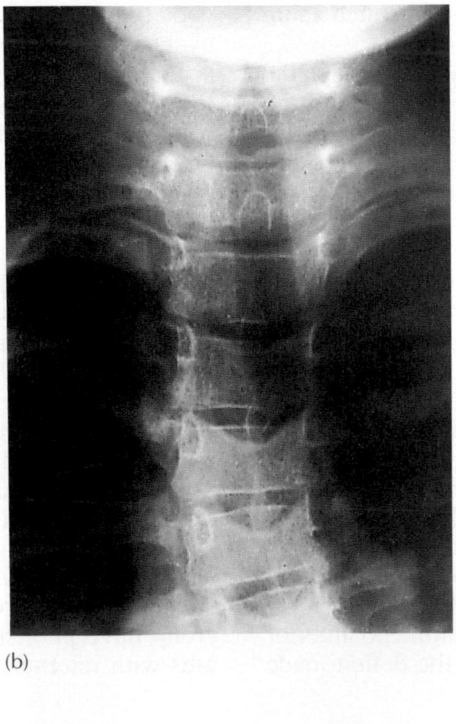

(b)

Figure 8.58 (a) PA radiograph showing a mild idiopathic-type double structural scoliosis in a boy with an intradural astrocytoma. (b) PA radiograph of the cervicothoracic region showing gross pathological widening of the interpedicular distance.

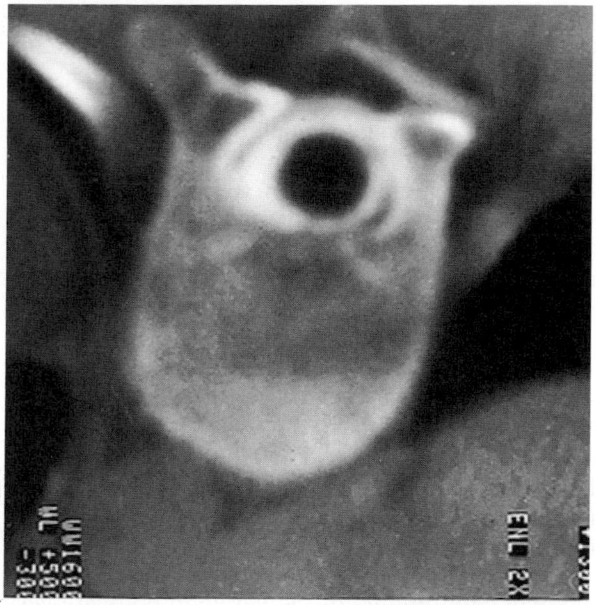

Figure 8.59 CT myelogram showing a large syrinx.

basilar impression are associated but interpedicular widening is the characteristic plain film appearance. Spinal cord imaging confirms the diagnosis.

It would appear from Tachdjian and Matson's series that about 50% of children with intradural neoplasms or syringomyelia present with an idiopathic-type scoliosis but little if any rotation, and without progression. Whether the deformity is produced by asymmetric muscle spasm or true interference of spinal cord or root function is unclear. It is unusual to find a scoliosis clinically severe enough to warrant surgical treatment and, indeed, such spinal deformities that are present tend to resolve or appreciably improve when the underlying spinal cord lesion has been dealt with therapeutically. The important problem posed by the presence of a syrinx is an extremely high rate of paralysis when distraction instrumentation is inserted. Indeed Huebert and MacKinnon's two operated cases became paraplegic and died following posterior Harrington instrumentation. Therefore any scoliosis in association with back pain or headache, or an unusual curve pattern such as a progressive left thoracic curve and, indeed, all significantly progressive scolioses in boys, should undergo preliminary spinal cord imaging prior to any consideration of surgery. Should a cord lesion be found then instrumentation is contraindicated. The best that can be offered is a fusion-*in-situ* although appreciable improvement follows spontaneously upon anterior multiple discectomy.

Loss of posterior spinal column support by way of laminectomy for the treatment of intradural lesions in the immature spine is a potent cause of progressive kyphosis, especially when facet joint stability has been jeopardized (Sim *et al.*, 1974; Lonstein, 1977b). Eighty per cent of such children will develop progressive kyphosis unless the spine is stabilized at the same time (see Figure 8.20). Experienced neurosurgeons have stressed the need for collaborative orthopaedic assistance (Gerlach *et al.*, 1967; Matson, 1969). Posterior fusion is ineffective because the grafts are on the tension side of the spine, resulting in a pseudarthrosis rate of over 50%. As with other kyphoses, anterior fusion is necessary and unless life expectancy is thought to be particularly poor the anterior spinal stabilization should be performed at a second stage following the initial laminectomy (Lonstein, 1977b). Should progressive kyphosis go unchecked, a nasty angular deformity, giving rise to its own neurological compromise, can develop and for this, anterior decompression and strut grafting is required (Leatherman and Dickson, 1979).

The other common type of spinal deformity is the paralytic lordoscoliosis in the thoracolumbar region with pelvic obliquity proportionate to the degree of neurological impairment either as a result of the lesion itself or its treatment. As in other forms of paralytic curve anterior and posterior instrumentation and fusion are necessary.

The paravertebral neoplasms, Wilms' tumour and neuroblastoma, can be associated with a spinal deformity by way of radiation therapy with the spinal column necessarily being in the radiation field. Radiation therapy is not now prescribed for Wilms' tumours limited to the kidney when this been complete resected, wheras a neuroblastoma requires both chemotherapy and radiotherapy, because surgical removal is often incomplete. It has been known since the time of Perthe (1903) that both growing cartilage and bone were particularly susceptible to radiation therapy and that this was in proportion to the radiation dosage received. Thus the activity of the epiphyses is suppressed in both the long and flat bones (Gall *et al.*, 1940). Excessive radiation can produce myelopathy (Burns *et al.*, 1972), while many years after radiation treatment osteochondromas or even osteogenic sarcomas can develop (Murphy and Blount, 1962). The typical vertebral changes following radiation therapy are lines of increased density, giving the appearance of a vertebra within a vertebra, irregularities of the epiphyseal margins, and a bullet-shaped vertebra rather like that seen in some skeletal dysplasias (Rubin *et al.*, 1962; Donaldson and Wissinger, 1967; Riseborough *et al.*, 1976). This bullet-shaped vertebra can be the apex of a local kyphosis, with more than half of these patients having a mild degree of scoliosis, seldom in excess of 20° and without significant rotation.

Treatment of the post-radiation kyphosis has been associated with a catalogue of complications

(Mayfield, 1979; King and Stowe, 1982). Every child who underwent an attempted posterior fusion with Harrington instrumentation developed a pseudarthrosis, with an infection rate of almost one-third, and an unacceptably high rate of neurological complications. Again, anterior fusion is necessary and because of the poor recipient area serious consideration should be given to providing the strut graft with a vascular supply.

Extradural tumours of the spine are uncommon but can produce a spinal deformity. Of particular note are the osteoid osteoma and osteoblastoma, giant cell tumour and aneurysmal cyst, and eosinophilic granuloma. Osteoid osteomas and osteoblastomas share similar histological appearances in that there is a small nidus of vascularized osteoid tissue. Osteoid osteomas are cortical or subcortical and are surrounded by an area of reactive sclerotic bone, whereas osteoblastomas are medullary lesions and are greater than 2 cm in diameter. Continuous pain, worse at night, is typical and is thought to be due to the release of prostaglandins. Accordingly, anti-inflammatory drugs relieve the pain. These lesions tend to be in the pedicle/transverse process junction in the thoracolumbar region and although they are intensely active on skeletal scintigraphy, plain films are seldom, if ever, normal in that an expanded pedicle/transverse process area can be seen (Figure 8.60). The natural history for these lesions is spontaneous resolution; this may take many years (Moberg, 1951). There is commonly a delay in diagnosis and the pain and misery often lead to the child passing through psychiatric departments before the diagnosis of an organic lesion is confirmed. A scoliosis is very common in association, with a lesion at the curve apex. These curves are seldom, if ever, progressive and have little rotation (Sabanas *et al.*, 1956; MacLellan and Wilson, 1967). When the lesion is excised surgically the scoliosis characteristically resolves unless asymmetric posterior tethering and scarring has been caused during the surgery (Ransford *et al.*, 1984).

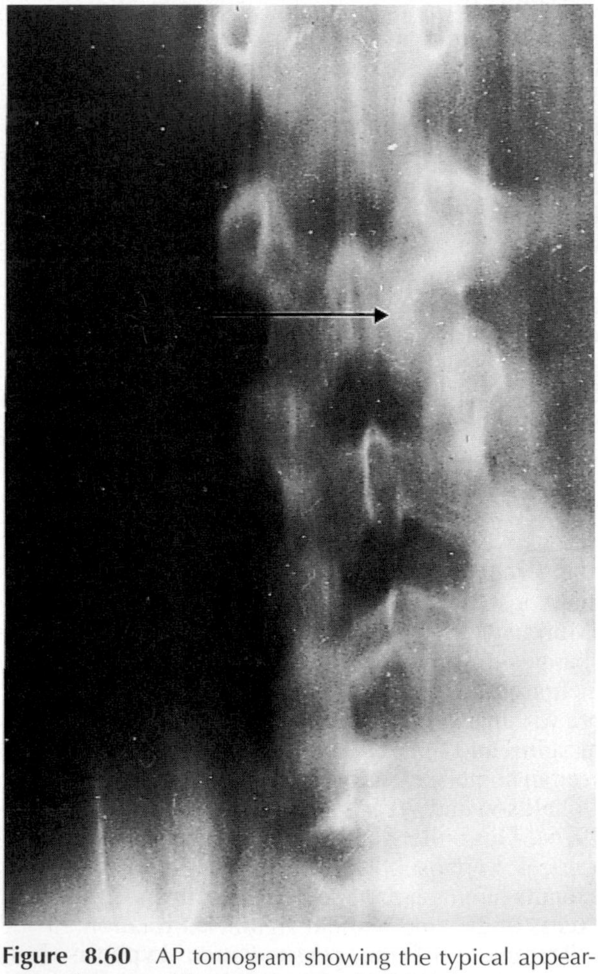

Figure 8.60 AP tomogram showing the typical appearance of an osteoid osteoma at the L1/2 level.

Giant cell tumours of the vertebral body are very rare and what were thought to be giant cell tumours were found on review to be nearly all aneurysmal bone cysts (Jaffe *et al.*, 1940). However, these lesions can produce a local angular kyphosis with signs of impending paralysis. The preferred treatment is complete excision which requires total vertebrectomy with anterior strut grafting and posterior instrumental support. Eosinophilic granuloma is associated with back pain, muscle spasm, tenderness, and a mild kyphos, and shares the same histological pattern as Hand–Schüller–Christian disease. After the long bones of the lower limbs, the vertebral bodies, ribs, and skull are the commonest sites. Unlike in adults where rapid vertebral compression can lead to paralysis, the clinical course is insidious in adolescence with significant flattening of the affected vertebral body, followed by restitution to normal size (Figure 8.61). Treatment is therefore not required but biopsy may be necessary to confirm the diagnosis.

The juvenile or adolescent disc syndrome (see Chapter 13)

This term refers to disc derangements in the immature spine which, as in the adult, have a predilection for the lower lumbar spine. In the adult the term 'disc herniation' is applied but in the adolescent the pathology is quite different with the disc derangement being in the form of a diffuse bulging without annular disruption. The degenerative changes observed in the adult disc, i.e. proteoglycan and

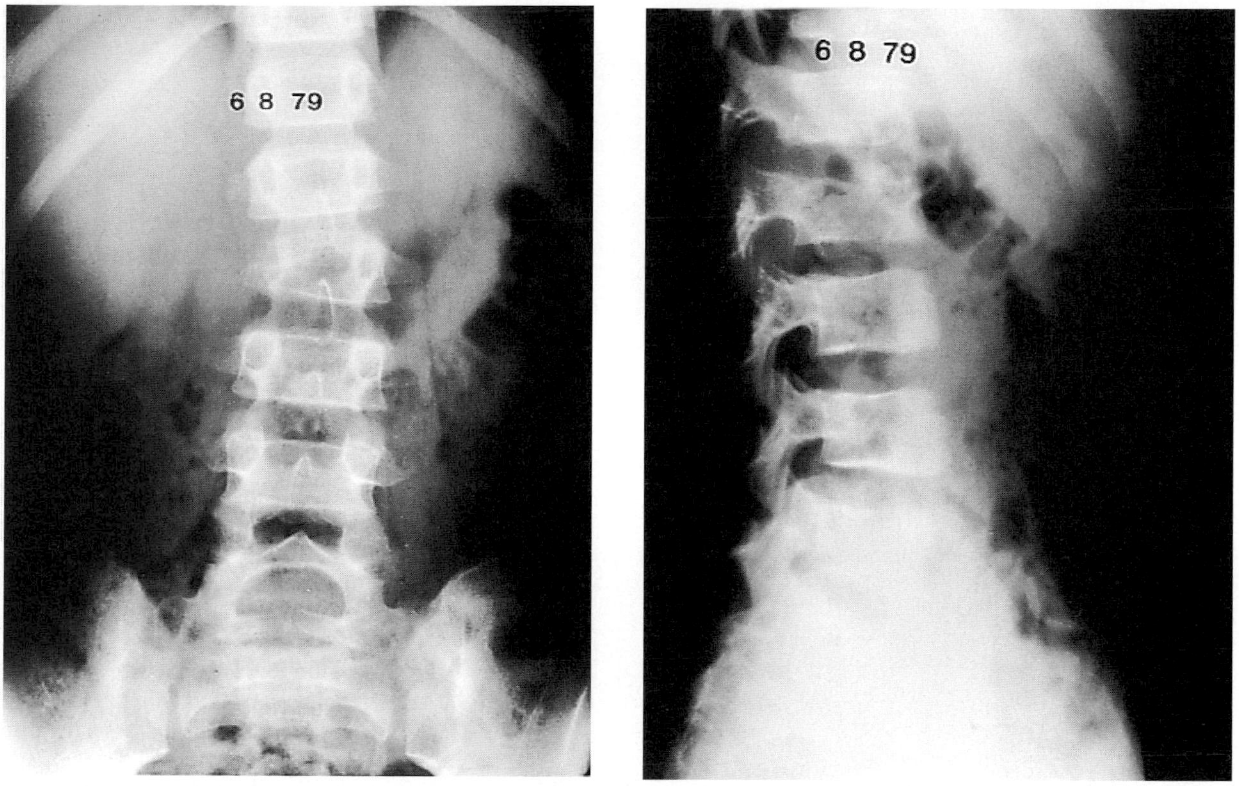

(a) (b)

Figure 8.61 (a and b) Eosinophilic granuloma of the second lumbar vertebra.

collagen degradation, as well as change in water content, are also observed in immature disc derangement but to a very much less degree (Taylor and Akeson, 1971). In addition, the deranged nucleus is not collagenous but rather gelatinous. The incidence is unknown but the condition probably represents the very early end of the spectrum of 'slipped' discs.

Back pain is often present for a long time before clinical presentation and the history of injury is only present in a small minority of patients (Russwurm *et al.*, 1978; Kamel and Rosman, 1984). As with the adult, the back pain is increased by activity and relieved by rest. Evidence of radiculopathy in the form of root pain and neurological symptoms and signs is rare in the adolescent. Muscle spasm with significant flattening or reversal of the lumbar lordosis is, however, a virtually constant finding, as is some degree of 'sciatic scoliosis' (Figure 8.62). There is correspondingly a considerable reduction in lumbar spine movements. An odd protective type of shuffling gait can be produced. Other than showing abnormality of contour with loss of the normal lumbar lordosis consequent upon muscle spasm, plain films of the lumbar spine are unrewarding. Spinal canal imaging reveals a space-occupying lesion, more central in location than lateral, and may be of appreciable size in the absence of any neurological features.

The differential diagnosis includes infection of the spine, as well as that of inflammatory non-bacterial discitis. Spondylolysis and spondylolisthesis can also present with similar back symptoms and should there be any doubt concerning the presence of a serious organic lesion then skeletal scintigraphy and MR imaging should be performed.

It is difficult to define a standard treatment programme for the child or adolescent where both personal experience and too few numbers of reported cases do not allow too definitive recommendations. For the less common patient with all the physical characteristics and a large disc derangement on confirmatory imaging, there is much to be said for early surgical intervention and, as with the adult, this should be in the form of a very limited or microprocedure. Borgesen and Vang (1974) and Touchie and Thompson (1975) reported respectively series of 25 and 26 patients with the adolescent disc syndrome and found results from a standard fenestration discectomy even better than in the adult with excellent results in more than 90% of cases. Although epidural steroids and even chymopapain have been tried, there is a strong tendency for spontaneous

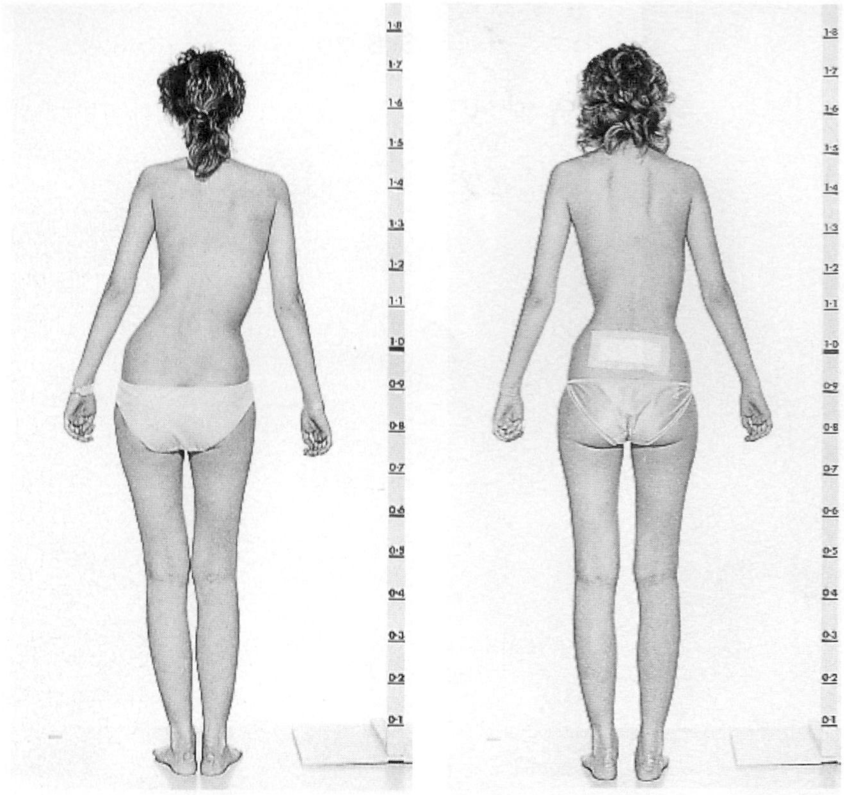

(a) b)

Figure 8.62 (a) Severe sciatic scoliosis in a girl with the adolescent disc syndrome. (b) One day postoperatively the scoliosis has virtually completely resolved.

resolution of clinical features, although this may take some 18 months to 2 years. Curtailing physical activity, the wearing of a daytime spinal orthosis, regular analgesic tablets, and physiotherapy should be tried before surgery is contemplated. This protracted clinical course together with all the uncertainties concerning operating on an immature spine may strain patient/parent/doctor relationships. Patience and time are required by all parties to achieve a satisfactory outcome.

Spondylolisthesis

This condition was first recognized over two centuries ago by obstetricians who encountered significant obstetric difficulties due to reduction in the sagittal diameter of the pelvis because of an anteriorly displaced fifth lumbar vertebra (Herbiniaux, 1782). There then followed much debate as to whether the condition was congenital or acquired but it soon became clear that a defect in the neural arch (spondylolysis) was a crucial factor (Meyer-Burgdorff, 1931). L5/S1 is the commonest level affected; the condition is familial and age related (Frieberg, 1939).

CLASSIFICATION

Newman and Stone (1963) studied more than 300 cases over a 15-year period and put forward a classification which has been slightly modified (Wiltse *et al.*, 1976). There are five principal types – dysplastic, isthmic, degenerative, traumatic and pathological.

Dysplastic spondylolisthesis

Dysplastic spondylolisthesis is the type which was originally termed 'congenital'. It refers to hypoplasia, or indeed aplasia, of the L5/S1 posterior facet joint, which does not allow slippage beyond 25% of the sagittal width of the spine. A complete anterior dislocation (spondyloptosis) occurs when there is a period of attenuation of the pars interarticularis followed by the development of a frank secondary spondylolysis. Because it starts at birth or soon afterwards, there are a number of features which allow clear distinction of this category based upon

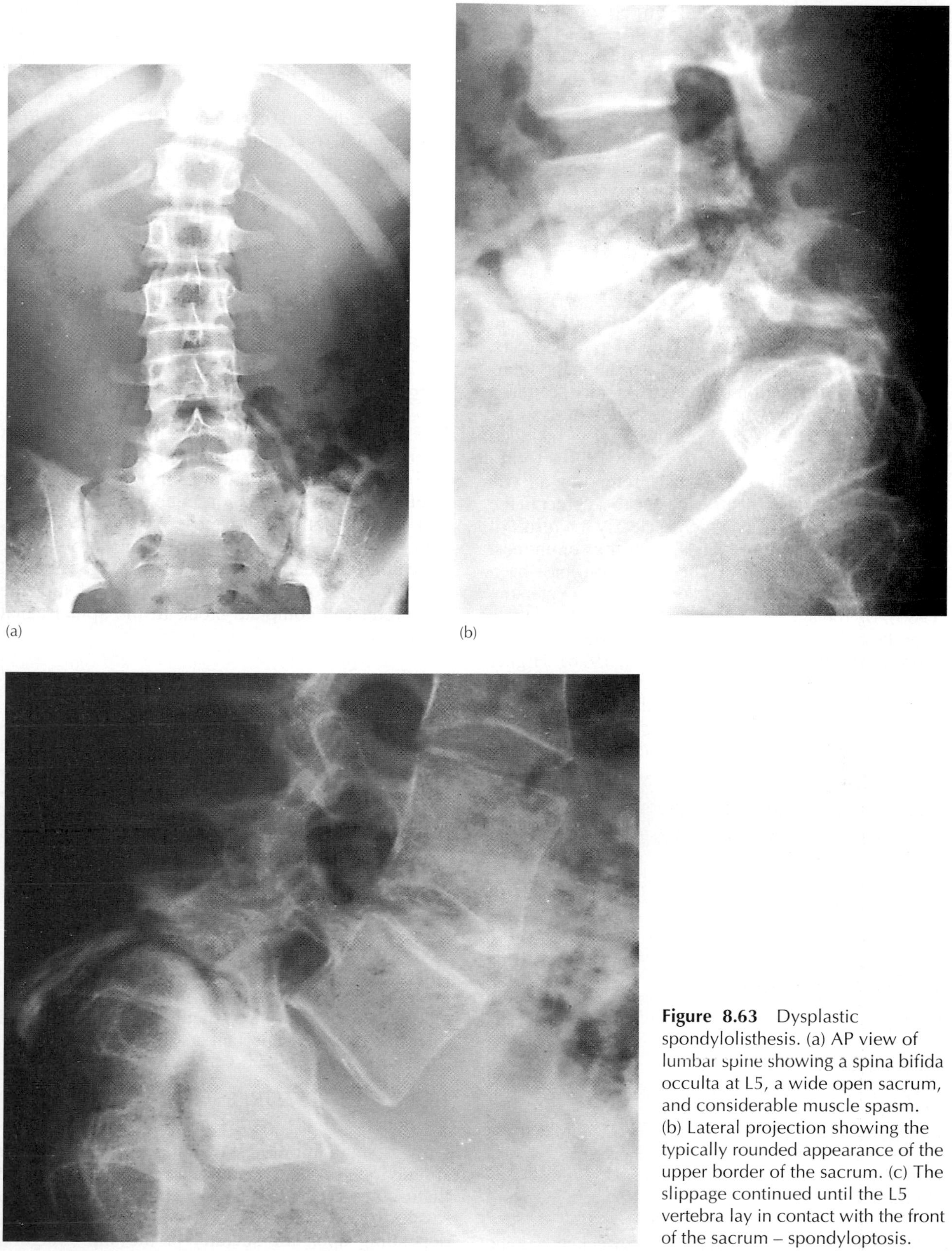

(a) (b) (c)

Figure 8.63 Dysplastic spondylolisthesis. (a) AP view of lumbar spine showing a spina bifida occulta at L5, a wide open sacrum, and considerable muscle spasm. (b) Lateral projection showing the typically rounded appearance of the upper border of the sacrum. (c) The slippage continued until the L5 vertebra lay in contact with the front of the sacrum – spondyloptosis.

plain radiographs (Figure 8.63) or now CT or MR imaging. On the AP projection there is always a spina bifida occulta of L5 and a wide open sacrum. In the lateral projection the upper border of the sacrum is rounded, indicating that the body of L5 has rolled round the top of the sacrum rather than simply having moved forwards. Accordingly, the inferior margin of L5 is reciprocally rounded and the L5 body lordotically wedged. It is the only true developmental type of spondylolisthesis, all others being acquired.

Isthmic spondylolisthesis

This is by far the commonest category and there are two subgroups – associated with a spondylolysis, or associated with attenuation of the pars interarticularis. Attenuation of the pars is only seen as a secondary problem with the progression of dysplastic spondylolisthesis and is incorrectly included under the heading of 'isthmic' (Scott, 1990). Therefore 'isthmic' spondylolisthesis refers to a lytic spondylolisthesis with slippage due to a defect in the posterolateral elements which is clearly the result of stress fracturing (Figure 8.64). L5 is the commonest site for the 'lyses' but the condition has been reported in infancy (Wertzberger and Peterson, 1980). By the age of 5 years or so the prevalence rate is of the order of 3 or 4% and this increases to 10% or more in the late teens (Wiltse *et al.*, 1976). Higher prevalence rates have been noted in gymnasts and trampolinists and this accords with the theory that it is spinal hyperextension stressing the pars which is the weakest part of the neural arch (Jackson *et al.*, 1976). Farfan argues that flexion, shear, and rotation are also required to produce the lesion and further suggests that it is due to one single initial microfracture which never goes on to heal (Farfan *et al.*, 1976). In the immature spine there is a marked tendency towards healing and the defect is filled with a zone of endochondral ossification which generally proceeds to bone formation. However, when skeletal maturity is reached the zone of endochondral ossification can be replaced by a typical hypertrophic non-union which never spontaneously heals. Once the lysis has developed, the repetitive stressing of the gymnast prevents union and accounts for why more than half of the 11% of gymnasts with bilateral L5 lyses also have an obvious spondylolisthesis (Jackson *et al.*, 1976).

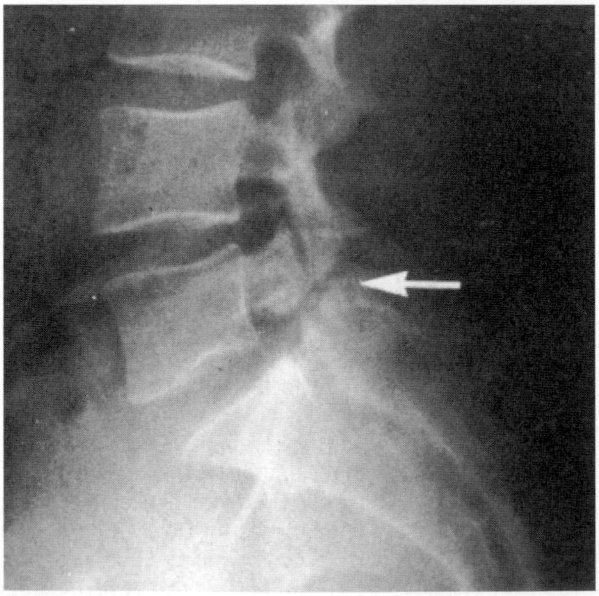

Figure 8.64 Lateral radiograph of the lower lumbar spine showing a mild spondylolisthesis of the lytic variety.

Degenerative spondylolisthesis

This nearly always occurs at the L4/5 level in elderly females with evidence of primary generalized osteoarthritis. It is attributable to L4/5 posterior facet joint incompetence consequent upon degeneration of that motion segment (Newman, 1955). As there is no attenuation or defect posterolaterally these bony elements move forward with the vertebral body and thus only a millimetre or two of slippage can produce a complete block to the spinal canal (Figure 8.65).

Traumatic spondylolisthesis

This refers to a fracture anywhere but in the pars and, as Taillard (1976) rightly points out, should not be regarded as spondylolisthesis at all. A gradual type of slippage can occur below a longstanding fusion of the spine. This is referred to as 'spondylolisthesis acquisita' and belongs to the traumatic category.

Pathological spondylolisthesis

This is where there is pathological spondylolisthesis where bone disease affects the strength of the posterolateral elements and in this respect tuberculosis, Paget's disease, rheumatoid disease, and metastasis are all important aetiological factors.

CLINICAL FEATURES

Only a small minority of individuals with either spondylolyses or spondylolisthesis ever declare themselves clinically. Those who do present as a result of low back pain with other clinical features depending upon the severity of the slip (Magora, 1976). Deformity only occurs with severe slippage

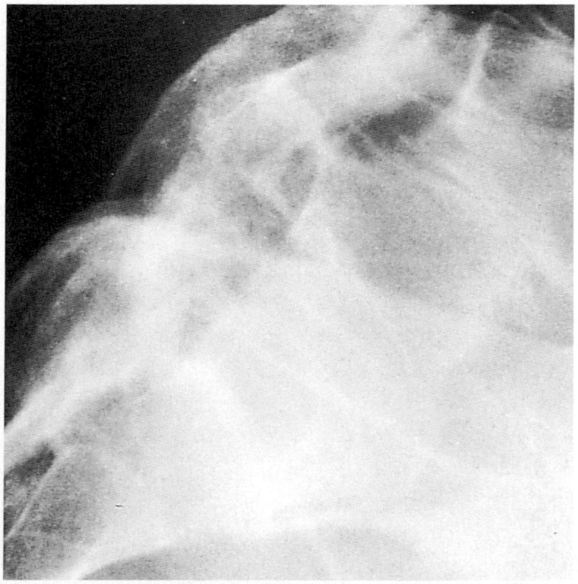

(a)

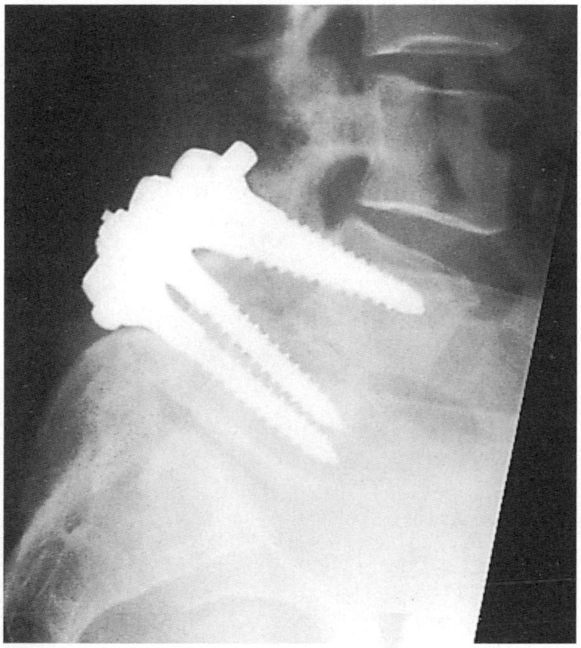

(b)

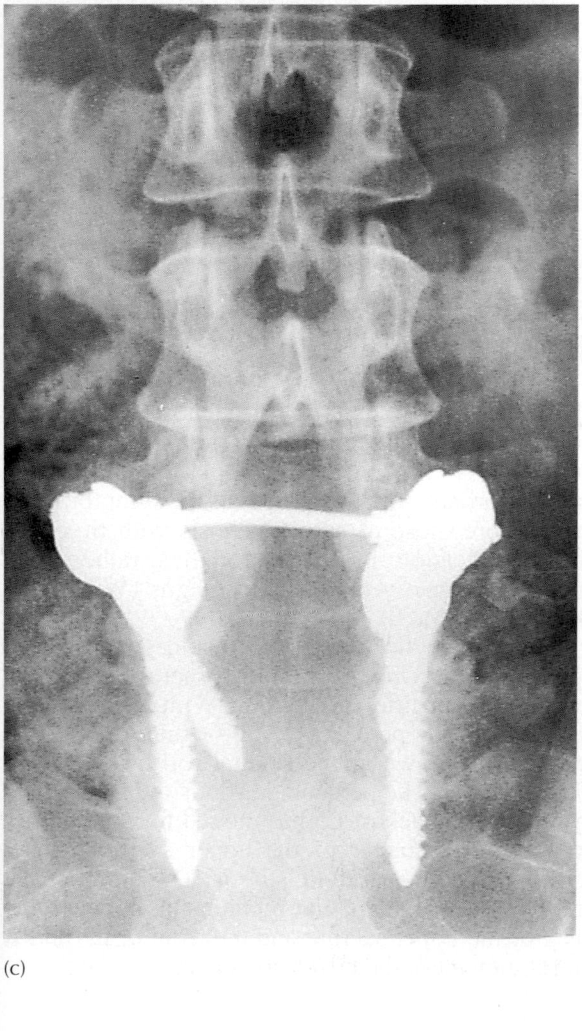

(c)

Figure 8.65 (a) Lateral radiograph of lower lumbar spine showing significant L4/5 degenerative spondylolisthesis. There were symptoms of an impending cauda equina catastrophe. (b) Lateral radiograph after decompression and stabilization using transpedicular CD metalwork. (c) AP view at follow-up showing a solid intertransverse fusion. Symptoms were completely relieved.

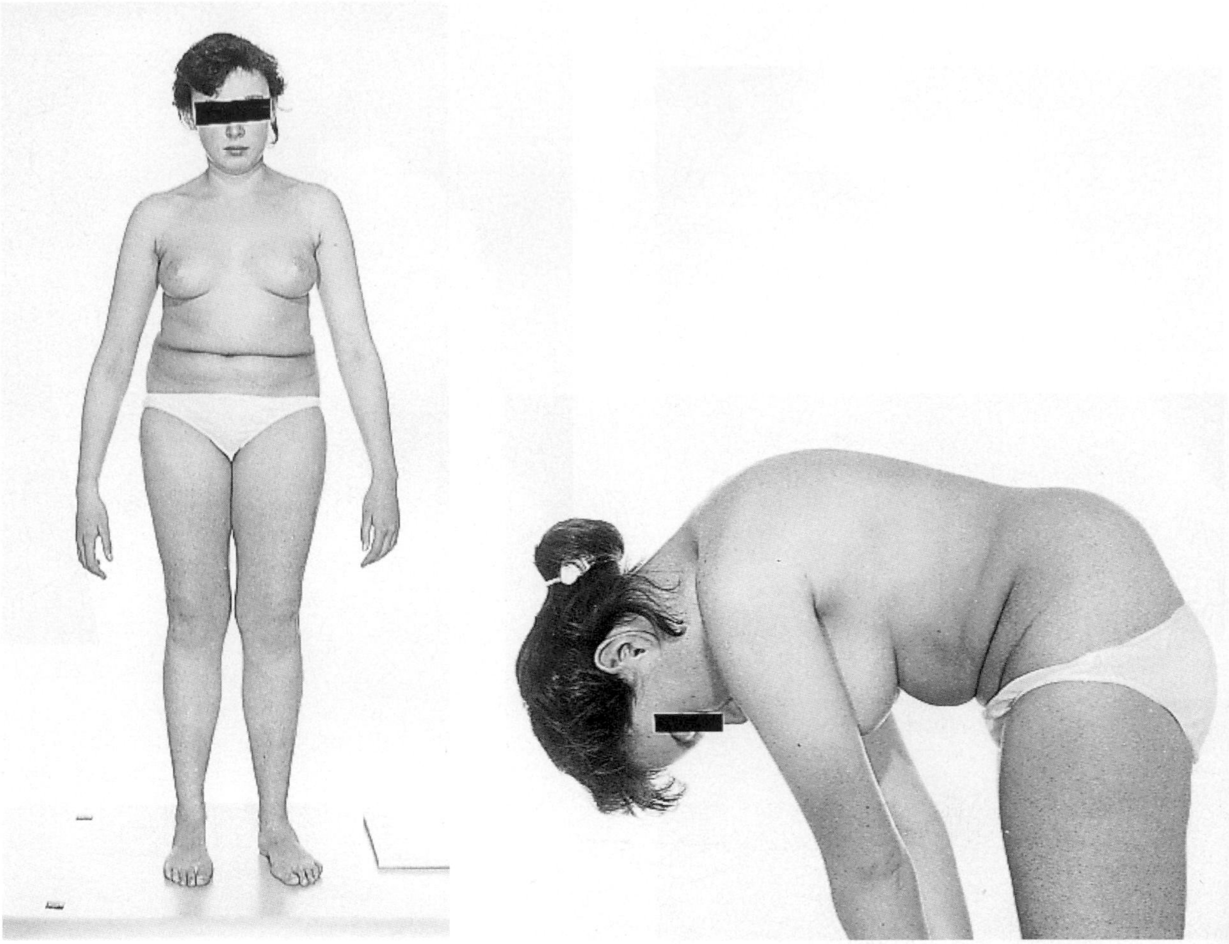

(a) (b)

Figure 8.66 The clinical features of severe spondylolisthesis. (a) Because this is a lumbosacral kyphosis the skin crease necessarily is anterior. (b) Sideways view forward bending to show the very obvious lumbosacral kyphosis.

but some children with severe degrees of slippage can appear normal, particularly so in lytic spondylolisthesis where slippage tends to occur solely in the sagittal plane. With severe degrees of dysplastic spondylolisthesis, however, with L5 rolling round on top of S1, the typical clinical appearance is of lumbosacral kyphosis, significant flattening of the buttocks as the pelvis is tucked under, and horizontal transabdominal skin creases (Figure 8.66). Flexion of the pelvis leads to a flexed position of the hips and a compensatory flexion of the knees to complete the Z-deformity. Accompanying these changes the hamstring muscles secondarily tighten with painful spasms in association with back pain.

Any significant neurological deficit in the lower extremities is rare except in degenerative and pathological spondylolisthesis, even with severe degrees of slippage. Very few have any radicular features of sciatica and even fewer an objective neurological deficit. The process of slippage is slow and, rather like degenerative spinal canal stenosis, the neural tissues can adapt to deformation if it is spread over a long period of time. In severe dysplastic spondylolisthesis approaching spondyloptosis the symptoms are much more those of spinal stenosis with tiredness and claudication in the extremities rather than any frank objective neurological signs (Wiltse and Jackson, 1976).

To measure the degree of displacement based upon a lateral x-ray of the lumbosacral junction in the standing position (Wiltse and Winter, 1983), one can express the percentage slip or the lumbosacral angle, also known as the sagittal roll or slip angle (Figure 8.67). The percentage slip is the percentage by which the back of L5 has moved forward across the sagittal diameter of the upper sacram and is relevant in lytic spondylolisthesis. The lumbosacral angle refers to the angular relationship between the back of the upper sacrum and the front of L5 and is more relevant in the dysplastic form.

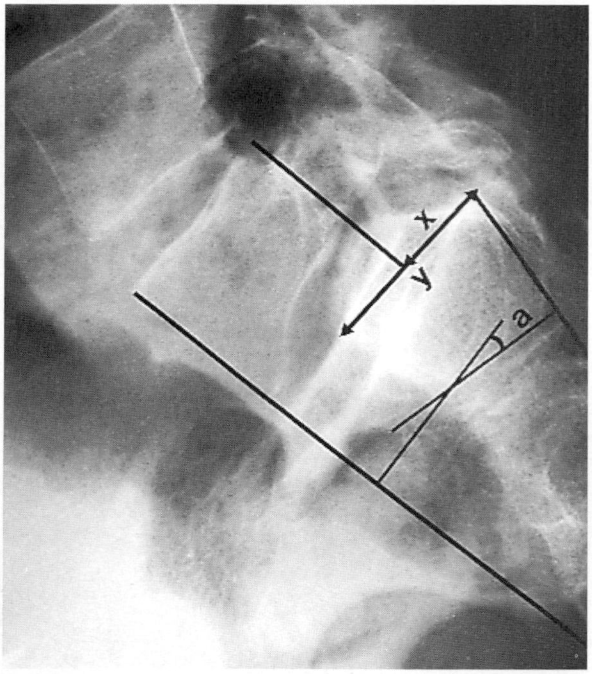

Figure 8.67 The most valuable measurements in spondylolisthesis are the percentage slip (*x* × 100)/*y*, and the slip angle (*a*).

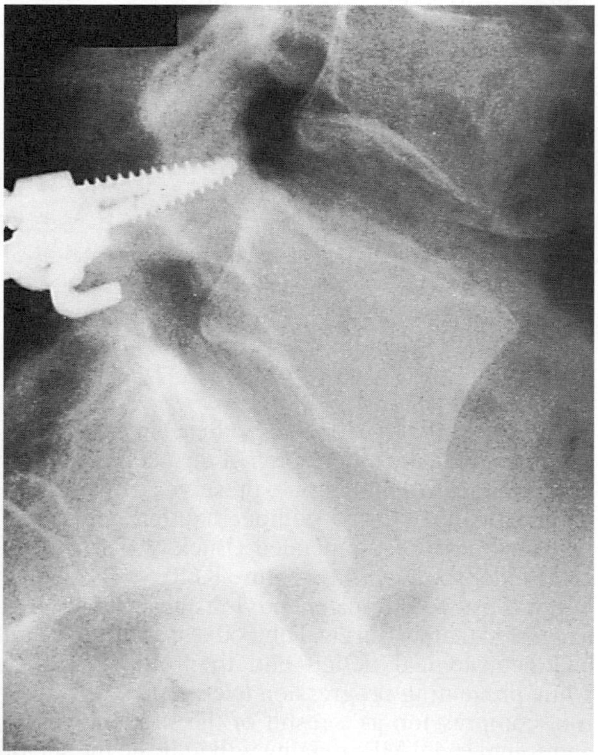

Figure 8.68 For persistently symptomatic lysis. Lateral view of the lumbosacral region of a professional cricketer having undergone lysis repair and fixation using Morscher's hook-screw clamp.

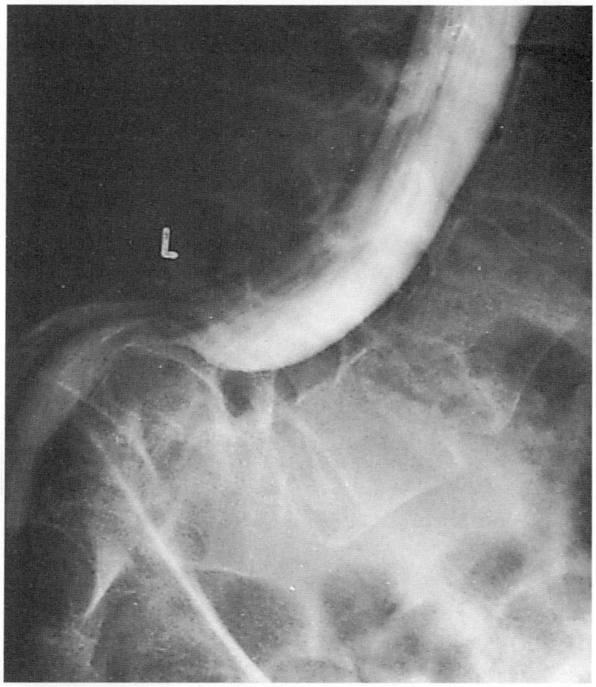

Figure 8.69 Lateral myelogram showing some narrowing of the dye column behind the upper border of the sacrum in a severe case of spondylolisthesis. Objective neurological features are, however, rare even in this degree of spondylolisthesis.

TREATMENT

It is the patient who should be treated rather than the radiographs. Wiltse, with great experience, categorically recommends surgical treatment only if there is a more than 50% slip in a child under the age of 10 years. In this situation prophylactic fusion is recommended (Wiltse and Jackson, 1976). Lesser degrees of slip are dealt with symptomatically by restriction of vigorous sporting activities. Increase in slip only occurs during the first few years, if it ever does (Wiltse and Jackson, 1976). Blackburne and Valikas (1977) only observed a moderate slip in 15% of their patients and noted that if the degree of slip was 30% at presentation then further slipping was extremely rare. Determination of progression in children and young adults still remains a problem. Seitsalo *et al.*, (1991) found in their series of 134 girls and 138 boys that surgical treatment using a posterior or posterolateral technique had no significant effect upon progression; indeed, they did not differ from conservatively treated patients. Ninety per cent of the slip had occurred at the time of the first radiograph and only 10% increased during the first postoperative year or after the first examination.

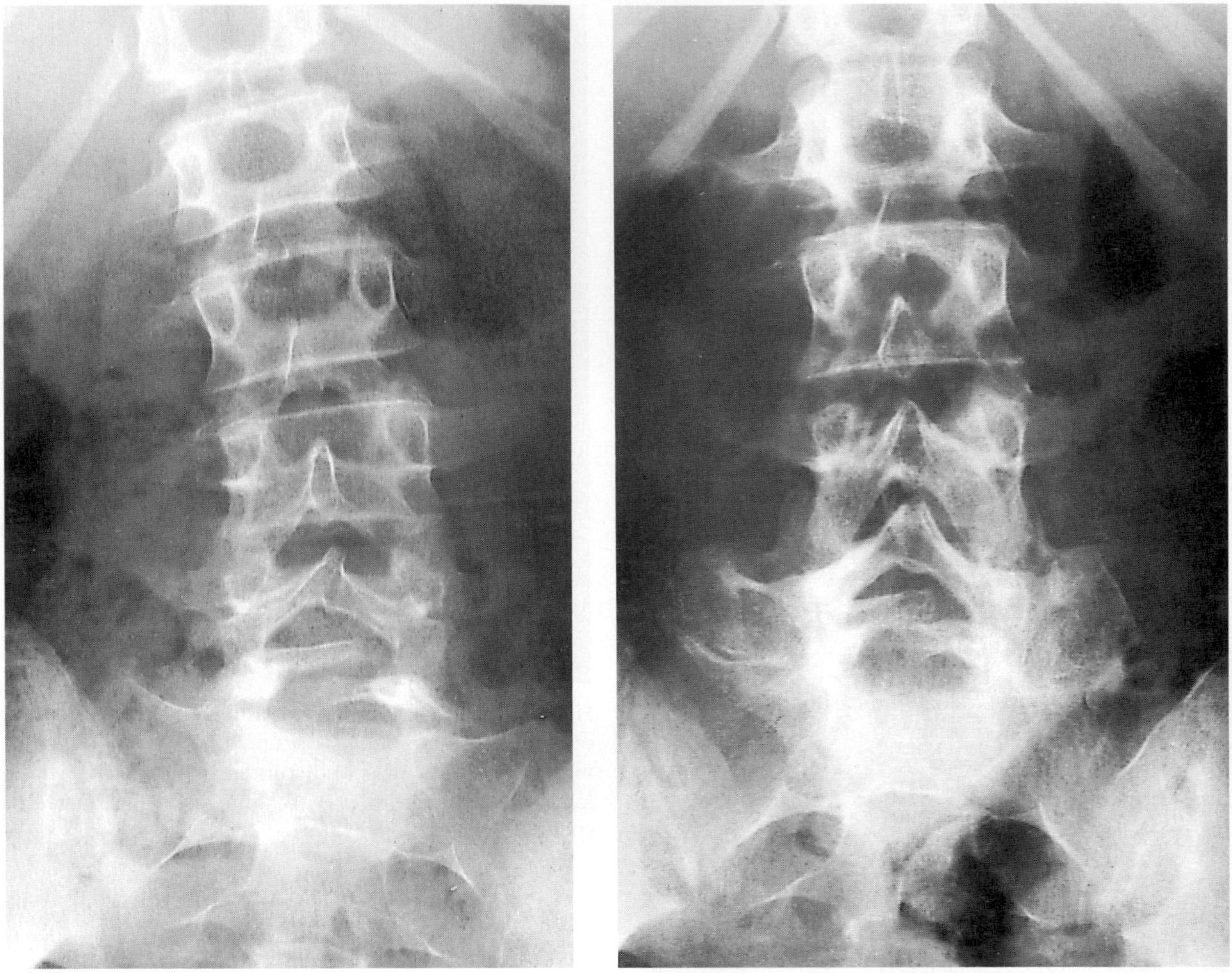

(a) (b)

Figure 8.70 Bilateral intertransverse fusion is the simplest and most effective method of stabilizing the lumbosacral junction in spondylolisthesis. (a) AP radiograph of a dysplastic spondylolisthesis with significant muscle spasm. (b) Following intertransverse fusion which is clearly solid all symptoms resolved.

Other authors also emphasize that spondylolistheses of 20% or less slip have a benign natural history. No clear prognostic factors are known at the present time for predicting progression of larger 'slip' deformities. Lysis in children tends to heal and therefore surgical treatment for spondylolysis without slip is only indicated in the adult with a hypertrophic non-union, and low back pain of a mechanical type, with L5 root irritation. Participants in sports activity in which the back is stressed, e.g. fast bowlers in cricket, are at risk. In mechanical low back pain with radiological evidence of instability, a motion segment fusion is indicated when symptoms fail to respond to a standard conservative treatment regimen. In L5 root irritation due to the hypertrophic callus around the lysis, a sound fusion should lead to resolution of the hypertrophic callus, but excision of the callus with decompression of the nerve root may be indicated. In an attempt to preserve L5/S1 motion simple fusion with or without fixation across the lysis has been recommended (Buck, 1970; Buring and Fredensborg, 1973) (Figure 8.68).

For those with frank spondylolisthesis it has been suggested that the surgical objective is to relieve pain and neurological deficit and to provide stability while preventing progression (Verbiest, 1979). Real root compression as a result of the slippage is rare and spinal canal MR imaging will indicate the site of compression which is usually the upper back corner of S1 (Figure 8.69). A sound intertransverse L5/S1 fusion without surgical attention to this area of root irritation (Wiltse and Jackson, 1976) will improve

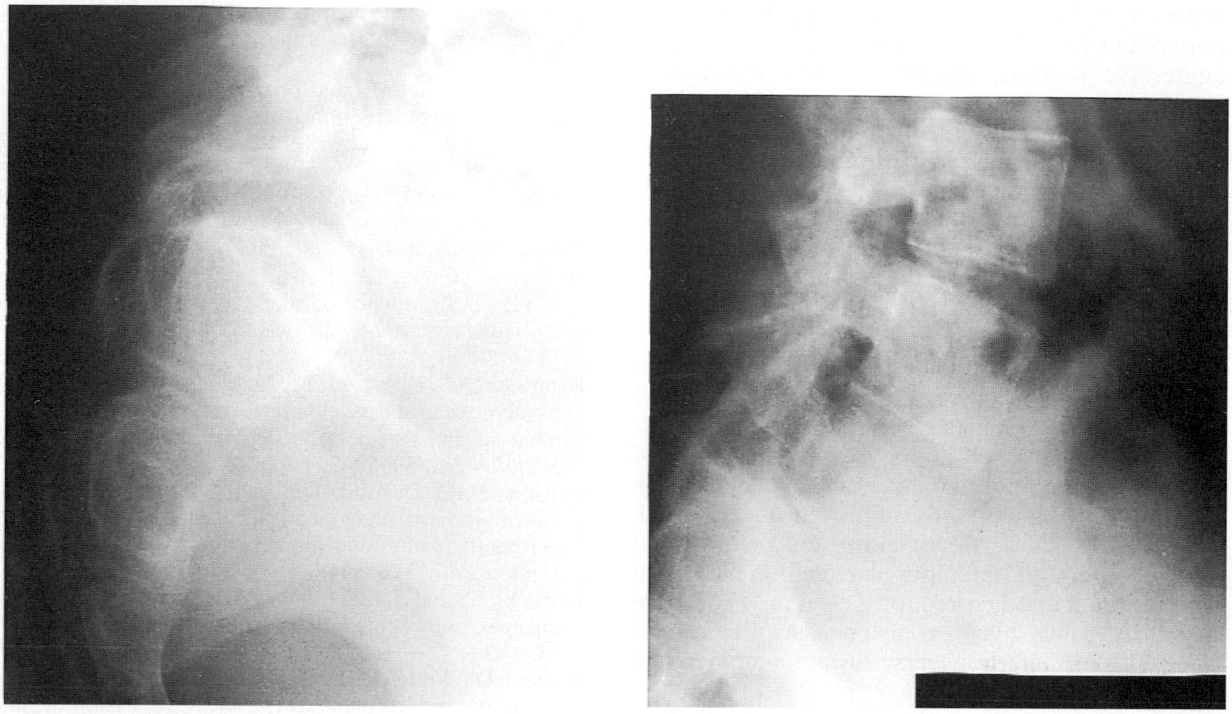

(a) (b)

Figure 8.71 (a) Severe dysplastic spondylolisthesis. (b) After reduction using three successive Scaglietti casts, and sound fusion, there has been an excellent and sustained correction.

the symptoms. The Gill procedure of removal of the 'loose rattle fragment' is of little value (Gill and White, 1965; Crock, 1981) because the root is compressed between the proximal pars and the pedicle, i.e. well proximal to the rattle fragment.

Treatment for mechanical low back pain in association with slippage in the absence of neurological features ranges from the fusion-*in-situ* at one end of the spectrum to radical multistage surgery incorporating an anterior stage plus the insertion of metalwork to the other. Wiltse and Jackson (1976) recommended intertransverse fusion in all but the most severe degrees of slip and demonstrated excellent results in 90% of cases, a figure unmatched by any other reported treatment modality (Figure 8.70). Bilateral posterolateral (intertransverse) fusion was the best as regards stability, and posterior fusion was the worst, not even managing to abolish movement anteriorly (Lee and Langrana, 1984).

Posterior fusion, i.e. fusion medial to the transverse processes, is associated with a significant postoperative progression rate which is not seen following a sound intertransverse fusion (Newman, 1965; Dandy and Shannon, 1971; Turner and Bianco, 1971). Anterior interbody fusion as first described by Mercer in 1934 has had its protagonists over the years, but the clinical results are only fair with a successful result only being achieved in some 50% of cases (Flynn and Hoque, 1979). Concern about injuring the presacral sympathetic outflow with damage to ejaculation is still present. The interbody fusion can, however, only be performed from a posterior approach (posterior lumbar interbody fusion, PLIF) and thus anterior neurovascular complications can be avoided (Cloward, 1963). Interbody fusion should be reserved for the unusual case which did not have a satisfactory result following bilateral intertransverse fusion.

Reduction of the spondylolisthesis prior to a stabilizing fusion has been attempted both by open and closed means. Capener (1932) first attempted open reduction while La Chapelle (1939) attempted closed reduction and Harris, in 1951, recommended preoperative skeletal traction. Verbiest (1979) favoured anterior lumbosacral fusion for severe degrees of spondylolisthesis following posterior decompressive laminectomy with removal of the posterosuperior corner of S1 should a preoperative myelogram indicate this is a compressive structure. In addition to L5/S1 discectomy, tibial cortical struts were inserted between the bodies of L5 and S2. He reported good results with this staged anterior and posterior surgical approach and this has been modified by others (Bradford, 1979; McPhee and

O'Brien, 1979). L5 nerve root damage has been reported and DeWald *et al.* (1981) cautioned against aggressive multiple staged operative procedures. Intertransverse fusions have been reinforced by posterior segmental spinal instrumentation but without improving the degree of slip, or the fusion rate.

Fixation techniques have recently gained considerable popularity in the treatment of spondylolisthesis (Cotrel *et al.*, 1988; Steffee and Sitkowski 1988). During insertion of the pedicular metalwork it is important that the L5 nerve roots are clearly seen from their thecal origin through to their exiting foramen. For spondylolisthesis at the very severe end of the spectrum where L5 sits in front of S1 (spondyloptosis) Gaines recommends anterior excision of the fifth vertebral body with replacement of L4 on top of the sacrum (Gaines and Nichols, 1985). The deformity is certainly improved but the trunk still remains short. Recognizing the neurological risks of operative attempts at reduction Scaglietti demonstrated good corrections, even in very severe cases, by using hyperextension casts for several weeks prior to intertransverse fusion-*in-situ* (Figure 8.71) (Scaglietti *et al.*, 1976).

References

Aaro, S. and Dahlborn, M. (1982) The effect of Harrington instrumentation on the longitudinal axis rotation of the apical vertebra and on the spinal and rib-cage deformity in idiopathic scoliosis studied by computer tomography. *Spine* **7**, 456–462

Adams, W. (1865) *Lectures on the Pathology and Treatment of Lateral and Other Forms of Curvature of the Spine*. Churchill and Sons: London

Alexander, M.A. and Season, E.H. (1978) Idiopathic scoliosis: an electromyographic study. *Archives of Physical Medicine and Rehabilitation* **59**, 314–315

Allen, B.L. and Ferguson, R.L. (1979) The operative treatment of myelomeningocele spinal deformity. *Orthopedic Clinics of North America* **10**, 845–862

Archer, I.A. and Dickson, R.A. (1985) Stature and idiopathic scoliosis. A prospective study. *Journal of Bone and Joint Surgery* **67B**, 185–188

Arkin, A.M. and Simon, N. (1950) Radiation scoliosis: an experimental study. *Journal of Bone and Joint Surgery* **32A**, 396

Ascani, E., Salsano, V. and Giglio, G. (1977) The incidence and early detection of spinal deformities. A study based on the screening of 16,104 schoolchildren. *Italian Journal of Orthopaedic Traumatology* **3**, 111–117

Aufdermaur, M. (1974) Spinal injuries in juveniles. Necropsy findings in twelve cases. *Journal of Bone and Joint Surgery* **56B**, 513–519

Barrett, D.S., MacLean, J.G.B., Bettany, I. *et al.* (1993) Costoplasty in adolescent idiopathic scoliosis. *Journal of Bone and Joint Surgery* **75B**, 881–885

Batson, O.V. (1940) The function of the vertebral veins and their role in the spread of metastases. *Annals of Surgery* **112**, 138–149

Bauze, R.J., Smith, R. and Francis M.J.O. (1975) A new look at osteogenesis imperfecta. A clinical, radiological and biochemical study of forty-two patients. *Journal of Bone and Joint Surgery* **57B**, 2–12

Beighton, P. and Horan, F. (1969). Orthopaedic aspects of the Ehlers–Danlos syndrome. *Journal of Bone and Joint Surgery* **51B**, 444–453

Bellyei, A., Czeizel A., Barta, O., Magda, T. and Molnar L. (1977) Prevalence of adolescent idiopathic scoliosis in Hungary. *Acta Orthopaedica Scandinavica* **48**, 177–180

Bengtsson, G., Fallstrom, K., Jansson, B. *et al.* (1974) A psychological and psychiatric investigation of the adjustment of female scoliosis patients. *Acta Psychiatrica Scandinavica* **50**. 50–59

Benson, D.R., DeWald, R.L. and Schultz, A.B. (1977) Harrington rod distraction instrumentation. Its effect on vertebral rotation and thoracic compensation. *Clinical Orthopaedics* **125**, 40–44

Bernick, S. and Cailliet, R. (1982) Vertebral end-plate changes with aging of the human vertebrae. *Spine* **7**, 97–102

Bethem, D., Winter, R.B. and Lutter, L. (1980) Disorders of the spine in diastrophic dwarfism. A discussion of nine patients and review of the literature. *Journal of Bone and Joint Surgery* **62A**, 529–536

Bethem, D., Winter, R.B., Lutter, L. (1981) Spinal disorders of dwarfism. Review of the literature and report of eighty cases. *Journal of Bone and Joint Surgery* **63A**, 1412–1425

Bick, E.M., Copel, J.W. and Spector, S. (1950) Longitudinal growth of the human vertebra. A contribution to human osteogeny. *Journal of Bone and Joint Surgery* **32A**, 803–814

Bisgard, J.D. (1934) Thoracogenic scoliosis. Influence of thoracic disease and operations on the spine. *Archives of Surgery* **29**, 417–445

Bisgard, J.D. and Musselman, M.M. (1940) Scoliosis: its experimental production and growth correction; growth and fusion of vertebral bodies. *Surgery, Gynecology and Obstetrics* **70**, 1029

Blackburne, J.S. and Valikas, E.P. (1977) Spondylolisthesis in children and adolescents. *Journal of Bone and Joint Surgery* **59B**, 490–494

Blount, W.P. and Moe, J.H. (1973) *The Milwaukee Brace*. Williams & Wilkins: Baltimore

Blount, W.P. and Schmidt, A.C. (1957) The Milwaukee brace in the treatment of scoliosis. *Journal of Bone and Joint Surgery* **39A**, 693

Bohlmann, H.H., Rekate, H.L. and Thompson, G.H. (1983) Problem fractures of the cervical spine in children. In: *Problematic Musculo-Skeletal Injuries in Children*, pp. 101–24. Edited by G.R Houghton and G.H. Thompson. Butterworths: London

Borgesen, S.E. and Vang, P.S. (1974) Herniation of the lumbar intervertebral disc in children and adolescents. *Acta Orthopaedica Scandinavica* **45**, 54–59

Bradford, D.S. (1979). Treatment of severe spondylolisthesis. A combined approach for reduction and stabilisation. *Spine* **4**, 423–429

tion spondylodesis (VDS). In: *Management of Spinal Deformities*, pp. 193–235. Edited by R.A. Dickson and D.S. Bradford. Butterworths International Medical Reviews: London

Hass, S.L. (1939) *Journal of Bone and Joint Surgery* **21**, 963

Harrenstein, R.J. (1930) Die Skoliose bei Saueglingen und ihre Behandlung. *Zeitschrift fur Orthopädie und Chirurgie* **52**, 1–40

Harrington, P.R. (1960) Surgical instrumentation for management scoliosis. *Journal of Bone and Joint Surgery* **42A**, 1448

Harrington, P.R. (1962) Treatment of scoliosis. Correction and internal fixation by spine instrumentation. *Journal of Bone and Joint Surgery* **44A**, 591–610

Harrington, P.R. (1973) The history and development of Harrington instrumentation. *Clinical Orthopaedics* **93**, 110–112

Harris, R.I. (1951) Spondylolisthesis. *Annals of the Royal College of Surgeons* **8**, 259–297

Hensinger, R.N. (1977) Kyphosis secondary to skeletal dysplasias and metabolic disease. *Clinical Orthopaedics* **128**, 113–128

Hensinger, R.N., Greene, T.L. and Hunter, L.Y. (1982) Back pain and vertebral changes simulating Scheuermann's kyphosis. *Orthopaedic Transactions* **6**, 341–342

Hensinger, R.N., Lange, J.E. and MacEwen, G.D. (1974) Klippel–Feil syndrome: a constellation of associated anomalies. *Journal of Bone and Joint Surgery* **56A**, 1246–1253

Hensinger, R.N. and MacEwen, G.D. (1976) Spinal deformity associated with heritable neurological conditions: spinal muscular atrophy, Friedreich's ataxia, familial dysautonomia, and Charcot–Marie–Tooth disease. *Journal of Bone and Joint Surgery* **58A**, 13–24

Herbiniaux, G. (1782) *Traite sur Divers Accouchments Laborieux, et sur les Polypes de la Matrice*. J.L. DeBoubers: Brussels

Herndon, W.A., Emans, J.B., Micheli, L.J. and Hall, J.E. (1981) Combined anterior and posterior fusion for Scheuermann's kyphosis. *Spine* **6**, 125–130

Herring, J.A. (1978) The spinal disorders in diastrophic dwarfism. *Journal of Bone and Joint Surgery* **60A**, 177–182

Hibbs, R.A., Risser, J.C. and Ferguson, A.B. (1931) Scoliosis treated by the fusion operation. An end result study of 360 cases. *Journal of Bone and Joint Surgery* **13**, 91–104

Hodgson, A.R. (1965) Correction of fixed spinal curves. *Journal of Bone and Joint Surgery* **47A**, 1221–1227

Hodgson, A.R. (1973) Correction of kyphotic spinal deformities. *Journal of Bone and Joint Surgery* **55B**, 211–212

Hodgson, A.R. and Stock, F.E. (1960) Anterior spine fusion for the treatment of tuberculosis of the spine. *Journal of Bone and Joint Surgery* **42A**, 295–310

Hoppenfield, S. (1967) Congenital kyphosis in myelomeningocele. *Journal of Bone and Joint Surgery* **49B**, 276–280

Houghton, G.R., McInerney, A. and Tew, A. (1987) Brace compliance in adolescent idiopathic scoliosis. *Journal of Bone and Joint Surgery* **69B**, 852

Howell, F.R. and Dickson, R.A. (1989) The deformity of idiopathic scoliosis made visible by computer graphics. *Journal of Bone and Joint Surgery* **71B**, 399–403

Hubbard, D.D. (1974) Injuries of the spine in children and adolescents. *Clinical Orthopaedics* **100**, 56–65

Huebert, H.T. and MacKinnon, W.B. (1969) Syringomyelia and scoliosis. *Journal of Bone and Joint Surgery* **51B**, 338–343

Hunt, J.C. and Pugh, D.G. (1961) Skeletal lesions in neurofibromatosis. *Radiology* **76**, 1–20

Jackson, D.W., Wiltse, L.L. and Cirincione, R.J. (1976) Spondylolysis in the female gymnast. *Clinical Orthopaedics* **117**, 68–73

Jaffe, H.L., Lichtenstein, L. and Portis, R.B. (1940) Giant cell tumour of bone. Its pathologic appearance, grading, supposed variants and treatment. *Archives of Pathology* **30**, 993–1031

James, J.I.P. (1951) Two curve patterns in idiopathic structural scoliosis. *Journal of Bone and Joint Surgery* **33B**, 399–406

James, J.I.P. (1954) Idiopathic scoliosis: the prognosis, diagnosis and operative indications related to curve patterns and the age of onset. *Journal of Bone and Joint Surgery* **36B**, 36–49

James, J.I.P. (1956) Paralytic scoliosis. *Journal of Bone and Joint Surgery* **38B**, 660–685

James, J.I.P., Lloyd-Roberts, G.C. and Pilcher, M.F. (1959) Infantile structural scoliosis. *Journal of Bone and Joint Surgery* **41B**, 719–735

Jones, W.H.S. (1922–31) *Hippocrates*, 4 vols. Heinemann: London

Kamel, M. and Rosman, M. (1984) Disc protrusion in the growing child. *Clinical Orthopaedics* **185**, 46–52

Kane, W.J., and Moe, J.H. (1970) A scoliosis prevalence survey in Minnesota. *Clinical Orthopaedics* **69**, 216–218

Keiser, R.P. and Shufflebarger, H.L. (1976) The Milwaukee brace in idiopathic scoliosis. Evaluation of 123 completed cases. *Clinical Orthopaedics* **118**, 19–24

Kewalramani, L.S. and Tori, J.A. (1980) Spinal cord trauma in children: neurologic patterns, radiologic features, and pathomechanics of injury. *Spine* **5**, 11–18

King, H.A., Moe, J.H., Bradford, D.S. and Winter, R.B. (1983) The selection of fusion levels in thoracic idiopathic scoliosis. *Journal of Bone and Joint Surgery* **65A**, 1302–1313

King, J. and Stowe, S. (1982) Results of spinal fusion for radiation scoliosis. *Spine* **7**, 574–585

Kopits, S.E. (1976) Orthopaedic complications of dwarfism. *Clinical Orthopaedics* **114**, 153–179

Kopits, S.E., Perovic, M.N., McKusick, V., Robinson, R.A. and Bailey, J.A. (1972) Congenital atlanto-axial dislocations in various forms of dwarfism. *Journal of Bone and Joint Surgery* **54A**, 1349–1350

Kostuik, J.P., Israel, J. and Hall, J.E. (1973) Scoliosis surgery in adults. *Clinical Orthopaedics* **93**, 225–234

La Chapelle, E.H. (1939) Spondylolisthesis. *Nederlands Tijdschrift voor Geneeskunde* **83**, 2005–2010

Lange, F. (1910) Support for the spondylitic spine by means of buried steel bars attached to the vertebrae. *American Journal of Orthopedic Surgery* **8**, 344–361

Langenskiold, A. and Michelsson, J.E. (1961) Experimental progressive scoliosis in the rabbit. *Journal of Bone and Joint Surgery* **43B**, 116–120

Langenskiold, A. and Michelsson, J.E. (1962) The pathogenesis of experimental progressive scoliosis. *Acta Orthopaedica Scandinavica* **Supplement 59**

Langer, L.O. (1964) Spondyloepiphyseal dysplasia tarda. *Radiology* **82**, 833–839

Lawton, J.O. and Dickson, R.A. (1986) The experimental basis of idiopathic scoliosis. *Clinical Orthopaedics* **210**, 9–17

Leatherman, K.D. (1969) Resection of vertebral bodies. *Journal of Bone and Joint Surgery* **51A**, 206

Leatherman, K.D. (1973) The management of rigid spinal curves. *Clinical Orthopaedics* **93**, 215–224

Leatherman, K.D. and Dickson, R.A. (1977) Vertebral body resection for spinal deformity in myelomeningocele. In: *Myelomeningocele*. Edited by B.L. McLaurin. Grune and Stratton: New York

Leatherman, K.D. and Dickson, R.A. (1978) Congenital kyphosis in myelomeningocele. Vertebral body resection and posterior spine fusion. *Spine* **3**, 222–226

Leatherman, K.D. and Dickson, R.A. (1979) Two-stage corrective surgery for congenital deformities of the spine. *Journal of Bone and Joint Surgery* **61B**, 324–328

Leatherman, K.D. and Dickson, R.A. (1988) *The Management of Spinal Deformities*. Wright: London

Lee, C.K. and Langrana, N.A. (1984) Lumbosacral spinal fusion. A biomechanical study. *Spine* **9**, 574–581

Lefebvre, J., Triboulet-Chassevant, A. and Missirliu, M.F. (1961) Electromyographic data in idiopathic scoliosis *Archives of Physical Medicine and Rehabilitation* **42**, 710–711

Leong, J.C.Y., Low, W.D., Mok, C.K., Kung, L.S. and Yau, A.C.M.C. (1982) Linear growth in Southern Chinese female patients with adolescent idiopathic scoliosis. *Spine* **7**; 471–475

Liszka, O. (1961) Spinal cord mechanisms leading to scoliosis in experimental animals. *Acta Medica Poloma* **2**, 45

Lonstein, J.E. (1977a) Screening for spinal deformities in Minnesota schools. *Clinical Orthopaedics* **126**, 33–42

Lonstein, J.E. (1977b) Post-laminectomy kyphosis. *Clinical Orthopaedics* **128**, 93–100

Lonstein, J.E. and Akbarnia, B.A. (1983) Operative treatment of spinal deformities in patients with cerebral palsy or mental retardation. *Journal of Bone and Joint Surgery* **65A**, 43–55

Lonstein, J.E., Winter, R.B., Moe, J.H., Bradford, D.S., Chou, S.N and Pinto, W.C. (1980) Neurologic deficits secondary to spinal deformity: a review of the literature and report of 43 cases. *Spine* **5**, 331–355

Lonstein, J.E., Bjorklund, S., Wanninger, M.H. and Nelson, R.P. (1982) Voluntary school screening for scoliosis in Minnesota. *Journal of Bone and Joint Surgery* **64A**, 481–488

Loynes, R.D. (1972) Scoliosis after thoracoplasty. *Journal of Bone and Joint Surgery* **54B**, 484–498

Luque, E.R. (1982) The anatomic basis and development of segmental spinal instrumentation. *Spine* **7**, 256–259

Lutter, L.D. and Langer, L.O. (1977) Neurological symptoms in achondroplastic dwarfs – surgical treatment. *Journal of Bone and Joint Surgery* **59A**, 87–92

Lutter, L.D., Lonstein, J.E., Winter, R.B. *et al.* (1977) Anatomy of achondroplastic lumbar canal. *Clinical Orthopaedics* **126**, 139–142

McCarroll, H.R. (1950) Clinical manifestations of congenital neurofibromatosis. *Journal of Bone and Joint Surgery* **32A**, 601–617

MacEwen, G.D. (1968) In: *Scoliosis Causation, Proceedings of a Second Symposium*. Edited by P.A. Zorab. Livingstone: Edinburgh

MacEwen, G.D. (1973) Experimental scoliosis. *Israel Journal of Medical Sciences 9*, 714–718

MacEwen, G.D., Winter, R.B. and Hardy, J.H. (1972) Evaluation of kidney anomalies in congenital scoliosis. *Journal of Bone and Joint Surgery* **54A**, 1451–1454

MacEwen, D.G., Bunnell, W.P. and Sriram, K.A. (1975) Acute neurological complications in the treatment of scoliosis. *Journal of Bone and Joint Surgery* **57A**, 404–408

MacLellan, D.I. and Wilson, F.C. (1967) Osteoid osteoma of the spine. A review of the literature and report of six new cases. *Journal of Bone and Joint Surgery* **49A**, 111–121

McMaster, M.J. (1983) Infantile idiopathic scoliosis: can it be prevented? *Journal of Bone and Joint Surgery* **65B**, 612–617

McMaster, M.J. and Carey, R.P.L. (1985) The lumbar theco-peritoneal shunt syndrome and its surgical management. *Journal of Bone and Joint Surgery* **67B**, 198–203

McMaster, M.J. and Ohtsuka, K. (1982) The natural history of congenital scoliosis. A study of 251 patients. *Journal of Bone and Joint Surgery* **64A**, 1128–1147

McPhee, I.B. and O'Brien, J.P. (1979) Reduction of severe spondylolisthesis. *Spine* **4**, 430–434

Magora, A. (1976) Conservative treatment in spondylolisthesis. *Clinical Orthopaedics* **117**, 74–79

Mahood, J.K., Howell, F.R., Howel, D. and Dickson, R.A. (1990) The lateral profile in idiopathic scoliosis – a longitudinal cohort study. *Orthopedic Transactions* **14**, 724–725

Manning, C.W., Prime, F.J. and Zorab, P.A. (1973) Partial costectomy as a cosmetic operation in scoliosis. *Journal of Bone and Joint Surgery* **55B**, 521–527

Matson, D.D. (1969) *Neurosurgery of Infancy and Childhood*, 2nd edn. Charles C Thomas: Springfield, IL

Mayfield, J.K. (1979) Post-radiation spinal deformity. *Orthopedic Clinics of North America* **10**, 829–844

Mau, H. (1968). Does infantile scoliosis require treatment? *Journal of Bone and Joint Surgery* **50B**, 881

Mehta, M.H. (1972) The rib vertebral angle in the early diagnosis between resolving and progressive infantile scoliosis. *Journal of Bone and Joint Surgery* **54B**, 230–243

Mehta, M. (1984) Infantile idiopathic scoliosis. In: *Management of Spinal Deformities*, pp. 102–120. Edited by R.A. Dickson and D.S. Bradford. Butterworths International Medical Reviews: London

Mehta, M.H. and Morel, G. (1979) The non-operative treatment of infantile idiopathic scoliosis. In: *Scoliosis – Proceedings of the Sixth Symposium 1979*, pp. 71–84. Edited by P.A. Zorab and D. Seigler. Academic Press: London

Mellencamp, D.D., Blount, W.P. and Anderson, A.J. (1977) Milwaukee brace treatment of idiopathic scoliosis. *Clinical Orthopaedics* **126**, 47–57

Menelaus, M.B. (1964) Discitis. An inflammation affecting the intervertebral discs in children. *Journal of Bone and Joint Surgery* **46B**, 16–23

Meyer-Burgdorff, H. (1931) *Untersuchungen uber das Wirbelgleiten*. Thieme: Leipzig

Miller, J.A., Nachemson, A.L. and Schultz, A.B. (1984) Effectiveness of braces in mild idiopathic scoliosis. *Spine* **9**, 632–635

Moberg, E. (1951) The natural course of osteoid osteoma. *Journal of Bone and Joint Surgery* **33A**, 166–170

Moe, J.H. (1958) A critical analysis of methods of fusion for scoliosis. *Journal of Bone and Joint Surgery* **4**, 529–554

Moe, J.H. (1972) Methods of correction and surgical techniques in scoliosis. *Orthopedic Clinics of North America* **3**, 17–48

Moe, J.H. and Sundberg, A.B. (1968) Spine fusions in the scoliotic growing child. *Journal of Bone and Joint Surgery* **50A**, 849

Morrissy, R.T. (1988) School screening for scoliosis. A statement of the problem. *Spine* **13**, 1195–1197

Murphy, F.D. and Blount W.P. (1962) Cartilaginous exostoses following irradiation. *Journal of Bone and Joint Surgery* **44A**, 662–668

Nachemson, A. (1968) A long term follow up study of non-treated scoliosis. *Acta Orthopaedica Scandinavica* **39**, 466–476

Nachlas, I.W. and Borden, J.N. (1950) *Surgery, Gynecology and Obstetrics* **90**, 672

Nash, C.L. and Moe, J.H. (1969) A study of vertebral rotation. *Journal of Bone Joint Surgery* **51A**, 223–229

Nelson, M.A. (1972) Spinal stenosis in achondroplasia. *Proceedings of the Royal Society of Medicine* **65**, 1028–1029

Newman, P.H. (1955) Spondylolisthesis: its cause and effect. *Annals of the Royal College of Surgeons* **16**, 305–322

Newman, P.H. (1965) A clinical syndrome associated with severe lumbo-sacral subluxation. *Journal of Bone and Joint Surgery* **47B**, 472–481

Newman, P.H. and Stone, K.H. (1963) The etiology of spondylolisthesis, with a special investigation. *Journal of Bone and Joint Surgery* **45B**, 39–59

Nilsonne, U. and Lundgren, K.D. (1968) Long term prognosis in idiopathic scoliosis. *Acta Orthopaedica Scandinavica* **39**, 456–465

Nordwall, A. and Waldenstrom, J. (1976) Metachromasia of fibroblasts from patients with idiopathic scoliosis. *Spine* **1**, 97–98

O'Beirne, J., Goldberg, C., Dowling, F.E. and Fogarty, E.E. (1989) Equilibrial dysfunction in scoliosis: cause or effect? *Journal of Bone and Joint Surgery* **71B**, 150

O'Brien, J.P. (1977) Kyphosis secondary to infectious disease. *Clinical Orthopaedics* **128**, 56–64

Owen, R. (1976) The association of axial skeleton defects with gastrointestinal and genitourinary abnormalities. In: *Scoliosis*, pp. 209–214. Proceedings of a Fifth Symposium held at the Cardiothoracic Institute, Brompton Hospital, London in September 1976. Edited by P.A. Zorab. Academic Press: London

Pelker, R.R. and Gage, J.R. (1982) The correlation of idiopathic lumbar scoliosis and lumbar lordosis. *Clinical Orthopaedics* **163**, 199–201

Perdriolle, R. (1979) *La Scoliose – Son Etude Tridimensionelle*. Maloine: Paris

Perthe (1903). Cited by Riseborough, E.J. (1977) Irradiation induced kyphosis. *Clinical Orthopaedics* **128**, 101–106

Ponder, R.C., Dickson, J.H., Harrington, P.R. and Erwin, W.D. (1975) Results of Harrington instrumentation and fusion in the adult idiopathic scoliosis patient. *Journal of Bone and Joint Surgery* **57A**, 797–801

Ponseti, I.V. and Shephard, R. (1954) *Journal of Bone and Joint Surgery* **36A**, 1031

Pouliquen, J.C. and Pennecot, G.F. (1983) Progressive spinal deformity after spinal injury in children. In: *Problematic Musculo-Skeletal Injuries in Children*, pp. 32–60. Edited by: G.R. Houghton and G.H. Thompson. Butterworths: London

Poussa, M., Harkonen, H. and Mellin G. (1989) Spinal mobility in adolescent girls with idiopathic scoliosis and in structurally normal controls. *Spine* **14**, 217–219

Ransford, A.O., Pozo, J.L., Hutton, P.A.N. and Kirwan, E.O'G. (1984) The behaviour pattern of the scoliosis associated with osteoid osteoma or osteoblastoma of the spine. *Journal of Bone and Joint Surgery* **66B**, 16–20

Raycroft, J.F. and Curtis, B.H. (1972) Spinal curvature in myelomeningocele: natural history and etiology. *Journal of Bone and Joint Surgery* **54A**, 1335

Reid, L. (1971) Lung growth. In: *Scoliosis and Growth. Proceedings of a Third Symposium*. Edited by P.A. Zorab. Churchill Livingstone: Edinburgh

Resina, J. and Alves, A.F. (1977) A technique of correction and internal fixation for scoliosis. *Journal of Bone and Joint Surgery* **59B**, 159–165

Riddick, M.F., Winter, R.B. and Lutter, L.D. (1982) Spinal deformities in patients with spinal muscular atrophy. *Spine* **7**, 476–483

Riseborough, E.J. and Wynne-Davies, R. (1973) A genetic survey of idiopathic scoliosis in Boston, Massachusetts. *Journal of Bone and Joint Surgery* **55A**, 974–982

Riseborough, E.J., Grabias, S.L., Burton, R.I. and Jaffe, N. (1976) Skeletal alterations following irradiation for Wilms' tumour with particular reference to scoliosis and kyphosis. *Journal of Bone and Joint Surgery* **58A**, 526–536

Risser, J.C. (1958) The iliac apophysis, an invaluable sign in the management of scoliosis. *Clinical Orthopaedics* **11**, 111–119

Roaf, R. (1956) Paralytic scoliosis. *Journal of Bone and Joint Surgery* **38B**, 640–659

Roaf, R. (1963) The treatment of progressive scoliosis by unilateral growth arrest. *Journal of Bone and Joint Surgery* **45B**, 637–651

Roaf, R. (1966) The basic anatomy of scoliosis. *Journal of Bone and Joint Surgery* **48B**, 786–792

Robin, G.C. (1975) *Scoliosis and Neurological Disease*. Wiley: New York

Robins, P.R., Moe, J.H. and Winter, R.B. (1975) Scoliosis in Marfan's syndrome, its characteristics and results of treatment in 35 patients. *Journal of Bone and Joint Surgery* **57A**, 358–368

Rogala, E.G., Drummond, D.S. and Gurr, J. (1978) Scoliosis: incidence and natural history. *Journal of Bone and Joint Surgery* **60A**, 173–176

Rosenthal, R.K., Levine, D.B. and McCarver, C.L. (1974)

The occurrence of scoliosis in cerebral palsy. *Developmental Medicine and Child Neurology* **16**, 664–667

Roth, M. (1981) Idiopathic scoliosis and Scheuermann's disease: essentially identical manifestations of a neurovertebral growth disproportion. *Radiologica Diagnostica (Berlin)* **22**, 380–391

Rubin, P., Duthie, R.B. and Young, L.W. (1962) The significance of scoliosis in postirradiated Wilms' tumour and neuroblastoma. *Radiology* **79**, 539–559

Russwurm, H., Bjerkrein, I. and Ronglan, E. (1978) Lumbar intervertebral disc herniation in the young. *Acta Orthopaedica Scandinavica* **49**, 158–163

Saartok, T., Dahlberg, E., Bylund, P., Eriksson, E. and Gustafsson, J-A. (1984) Steroid hormone receptors, protein and DNA in erector spinae muscle from scoliotic patients. *Clinical Orthopaedics* **183**, 197–207

Sabanas, A.O., Bickel, W.H. and Moe, J.H. (1956) Natural history of osteoid osteoma of the spine. Review of the literature and report of three cases. *American Journal of Surgery* **91**, 880–889

Sahlstrand, T., Petruson, B. and Nachemson, A. (1977) An electronystagmographic study of the vestibular function in patients with idiopathic scoliosis. Proceedings of the Scoliosis Research Society, Ottawa. *Orthopaedic Transactions* **1**, 129

Scaglietti, O., Frontino, C. and Bartolozzi, P. (1976) Technique of anatomical reduction of lumbar spondylolisthesis and its surgical stabilisation. *Clinical Orthopaedics* **117**, 164–175

Schollner, D. (1966) Steigerung der Vitalkapazitat durch Rippenbuckelresktion mit der Brustkorbdehnungstechnik. *Zeitschrift fur Orthopädie und Ihre Grenzgebiete* **101**, 323–333

Schultz, A.B. and Hirsch, C. (1973) Mechanical analysis of Harrington rod correction in idiopathic scoliosis. *Journal of Bone and Joint Surgery* **55A**, 983–992

Schwartzmann, J.R. and Miles, M. (1945) Experimental production of scoliosis in rats and mice. *Journal of Bone and Joint Surgery* **27**, 59–69

Schwentker, E.P. and Gibson, D.A. (1976) The orthopaedic aspects of spinal muscular atrophy. *Journal of Bone and Joint Surgery* **58A**, 32–38

Scoliosis Research Society (1976) A glossary of scoliosis terms. *Spine* **1**, 57–58

Scott, J.C. and Morgan, T.H. (1955) The natural history and prognosis of infantile idiopathic scoliosis. *Journal of Bone and Joint Surgery* **37B**, 400–413

Scott, J.H.S. (1990) Spondylolisthesis. In: *Spinal Surgery – Science and Practice*, pp. 353–367. Edited by R.A. Dickson. Butterworths: London

Seitsalo, S., Osterman, K., Hyvarinen, H., Tallroth, K., Schlenzka, D. and Poussa, M. (1991) Progression of spondylolisthesis in children and adolescents: a long term follow-up study of 272 patients. *Spine* **16**, 417–422

Shapiro, F. and Bresnan, M.J. (1982a) Orthopaedic management of childhood neuromuscular disease. Part I: Spinal muscular atrophy. *Journal of Bone and Joint Surgery* **64A**, 785–789

Shapiro, R. and Bresnan, M.J. (1982b) Orthopaedic management of childhood neuromuscular disease. Part II: Peripheral neuropathies, Friedreich's ataxia, and arthrogryposis multiplex congenita. *Journal of Bone and Joint Surgery* **64A**, 949–953

Sherk, H.H., Whitaker, L.A. and Pasquariello, P.S. (1982) Facial malformations and spinal anomalies: a predictable relationship. *Spine* **7**, 526–531

Sim, F.H., Svien, H.J., Bickel, W.H. and Janes, J.M. (1974) Swan-neck deformity following extensive cervical laminectomy. A review of twenty-one cases. *Journal of Bone and Joint Surgery* **56A**, 564–580

Simmons, E.H. and Thomas, A.F. (1976) Neurofibromatosis associated with scoliosis. *Journal of Bone and Joint Surgery* **58A**, 155

Smith, R. (1979) *Biochemical Disorders of the Skeleton*. Butterworths: London

Smith, R., Francis, M.J.O. and Houghton, G.R. (1983) *The Brittle Bone Syndrome*. Butterworths: London

Smith, R.M., and Dickson R.A. (1987) Experimental structural scoliosis. *Journal of Bone and Joint Surgery* **69B**, 576–581

Smyrnis, P.N., Valavanis, J., Alexopoulos, A., Siderakis, G. and Giannestras, N.J. (1979) School screening for scoliosis in Athens. *Journal of Bone and Joint Surgery* **61B**, 215–217

Somerville, E.W. (1952) Rotational lordosis: the development of the single curve. *Journal of Bone and Joint Surgery* **34B**, 421–427

Somerville, E.W. (1959) Paralytic dislocation of the hip. *Journal of Bone and Joint Surgery* **41B**, 279–288

Sorenson, K.H. (1964) *Scheuermann's Juvenile Kyphosis*. Munksgaard: Copenhagen

Spranger, J.W., Langer, L.O. and Wiedemann, H.R. (1974) *Bone Dysplasias*. W.B. Saunders: Philadelphia

Sriram, K., Bobechko, W.P. and Hall, J.E. (1972) Surgical management of spinal deformities in spina bifida. *Journal of Bone and Joint Surgery* **54B**, 666–676

Stagnara, P., De Mauroy, J.C., Dran, G. *et al.* (1982) Reciprocal angulation of vertebral bodies in a sagittal plane: approach to references for the evaluation of kyphosis and lordosis. *Spine* **7**, 335–342

Stauffer, E.S. and Mankin, H.J. (1966) Scoliosis after thoracoplasty: a study of thirty patients. *Journal of Bone and Joint Surgery* **48A**, 339–348

Steel, H.H. and Adams, D.J. (1972) Hyperlordosis caused by the lumboperitoneal shunt procedure for hydrocephalus. *Journal of Bone and Joint Surgery* **54A**, 1537–1542

Steffee, A.D. and Sitkowski, D.J. (1988) Reduction in stabilisation of grade IV spondylolisthesis. *Clinical Orthopaedics* **227**, 82–89

Streitz, W., Brown, J.C. and Bonnett, C.A. (1977) Anterior fibular strut grafting in the treatment of kyphosis. *Clinical Orthopaedics* **128**, 140–148

Swank, S.M., Brown, J.C. and Perry, R.E. (1982) Spinal fusion in Duchenne's muscular dystrophy. *Spine* **7**, 484–491

Tachdjian, M.O. and Matson, D.D. (1965) Orthopaedic aspects of intraspinal tumours in infants and children. *Journal of Bone and Joint Surgery* **47A**, 223–248

Taillard, W.F. (1976) Etiology of spondylolisthesis. *Clinical Orthopaedics* **117**, 30–39

Tanner, J.M. (1962) *Growth at Adolescence*, 2nd edn. Blackwell: Oxford

Tanner, J.M. and Whitehouse, R.H. (1975) *Height Standard Chart*. Creaseys: Castlemead

Tanner, J.M., Whitehouse, R.H., Cameron, N., Marshall, W.A., Healy, W.J.R. and Goldstein, H. (1983) *Atlas of*

Skeletal Maturity and Prediction of Adult Height (TW2 Method). Academic Press: London

Taylor, T.C., Wenger, D.R., Stephen, J., Gillespie, R. and Bobechko, W.P. (1979) Surgical management of thoracic kyphosis in adolescents. *Journal of Bone and Joint Surgery* **61A**, 496–503

Taylor, T.K.F. and Akeson, W.H. (1971) Intervertebral disc prolapse: a review of morphologic and biochemical knowledge concerning the nature of the prolapse. *Clinical Orthopaedics* **76**, 54–79

Thulbourne, T. and Gillespie, R. (1976) The rib hump in idiopathic scoliosis. Measurement, analysis and response to treatment. *Journal of Bone and Joint Surgery* **58B**, 64–71

Till, K. (1969) Spinal dysraphism, a study of congenital malformations of the lower back. *Journal of Bone and Joint Surgery* **51B**, 415–422

Tizzard, J.P.M., Paine, R.S. and Crothers, B. (1954) Disturbances of sensation in children with hemiplegia. *Journal of the American Medical Association* **155**, 628–632

Touchie, H.W. and Thompson, G.B. (1975) The adolescent disc lesion. *Journal of Bone and Joint Surgery* **57B**, 534

Tupman, G.S. (1962) A study of bone growth in normal children and its relationship to skeletal maturation. *Journal of Bone and Joint Surgery* **44B**, 42–67

Turner, R.H. and Bianco, A.J. (1971) Spondylolysis and spondylolisthesis in children and teenagers. *Journal of Bone and Joint Surgery* **53A**, 1298–1306

Verbiest, H. (1979) The treatment of lumbar spondyloptosis or impending lumbar spondyloptosis accompanied by neurological deficit and/or neurogenic intermittent claudication. *Spine* **4**, 68–77

Watson, G.H. (1971) Relation between side of plagiocephaly, dislocation of the hip, scoliosis, bat ears and sternomastoid tumours. *Archives of Disease in Childhood* **46**, 203–210

Watts, H.G., Hall, J.E. and Stanish, W. (1977) The Boston brace system for the treatment of low thoracic and lumbar scoliosis by the use of a girdle without superstructure. *Clinical Orthopaedics* **126**, 87–92

Waugh, T.R. (1971) The biomechanical basis for the utilization of methylmethacrylate in the treatment of scoliosis. *Journal of Bone and Joint Surgery* **53A**, 194–195

Wedge, J.H. and Kirkaldy-Willis, W.H. (1990) Infections of the spine. In: *Spinal Surgery – Science and Practice*, pp. 483–508. Edited by R.A. Dickson. Butterworths: London

Wedge, J.H., Oryschak, A.F., Robertson, D.E. *et al.* (1977) Atypical manifestations of spinal infections. *Clinical Orthopaedics* **123**, 155–163

Weimann, R.L., Gibson, D.A., Moseley, C.F. and Jones, D.C. (1983) Surgical stabilization of the spine in Duchenne muscular dystrophy. *Spine* **8**, 776–780

Wertzberger, K.L. and Peterson, H.A. (1980) Acquired spondylolysis and spondylolisthesis in the young child. *Spine* **5**, 437–442

Whitby, L.G. (1974) Screening for disease. Definitions and criteria. *Lancet* **2**, 819–821

White, A.A. and Panjabi, M.M. (1980) *Clinical Biomechanics of the Spine*, 2nd edn. J.B. Lippincott: Philadelphia

Whittle, M.W. and Evans, M. (1979) Instrument for measuring the Cobb angle in scoliosis. *Lancet* **1**, 414

Wiley, A.M. and Trueta, J. (1959) The vascular anatomy of the spine and its relationship to pyogenic vertebral osteomyelitis. *Journal of Bone and Joint Surgery* **41B**, 796–809

Wilkins, K.E. and Gibson, D.A. (1976) The patterns of spinal deformity in Duchenne muscular dystrophy. *Journal of Bone and Joint Surgery* **58A**, 24–32

Williams, B. (1979) Orthopaedic features in the presentation of syringomyelia. *Journal of Bone and Joint Surgery* **61B**, 314–323

Willner, S. (1974) A study of growth in girls with adolescent idiopathic structural scoliosis. *Clinical Orthopaedics* **101**, 129–135

Willner, S. and Johnsson, B. (1983) Thoracic kyphosis and lumbar lordosis during the growth period in boys and girls. *Acta Paediatrica Scandinavica* **72**, 873–878

Wiltse, L.L. and Jackson, D.W. (1976) Treatment of spondylolisthesis and spondylolysis in children. *Clinical Orthopaedics* **117**, 92–100

Wiltse, L.L. and Winter, R.B. (1983) Terminology and measurement of spondylolisthesis. *Journal of Bone and Joint Surgery* **65A**, 768–772

Wiltse, L.L., Newman, P.H. and Macnab, I. (1976) Classification of spondylolysis and spondylolisthesis. *Clinical Orthopaedics* **117**, 23–29

Winter, R.B. (1983) *Congenital Deformities of the Spine*. Thieme-Stratton: New York

Winter, R.B. and Moe, J.H. (1982) The results of spinal arthrodesis for congenital spinal deformity in patients younger than five years old. *Journal of Bone and Joint Surgery* **64A**, 419–432

Winter, R.B., Moe, J.H. and Eilers, V.E. (1968) Congenital scoliosis, a study of 234 patients treated and untreated. *Journal of Bone and Joint Surgery* **50A**, 1–47

Winter, R.B., Moe, J.H. and Wang, J.F. (1973) Congenital kyphosis. *Journal of Bone and Joint Surgery* **55A**, 223–256

Winter, R.B., Haven, J.J., Moe, J.H. and Lagaard, S.M. (1974) Diastematomyelia and congenital spine deformities. *Journal of Bone and Joint Surgery* **56A**, 27–39

Winter, R.B., Moe, J.H., Bradford, D.S., Lonstein, J.E., Pedras, C.V. and Weber, A.H. (1979) Spine deformity in neurofibromatosis. A review of 102 patients. *Journal of Bone and Joint Surgery* **61A**, 677–694

Wittebol, P. (1956) Idiopathic scoliosis (experimental investigation). *Archivum Chirurgicum Neerlandicum* **8**, 269–279

Wynne-Davies, R. (1975) Infantile idiopathic scoliosis. *Journal of Bone and Joint Surgery* **57B**, 138–141

Wynne-Davies, R., Walsh, W.K. and Gormley, J. (1981) Achondroplasia and hypochondroplasia. *Journal of Bone and Joint Surgery* **63B**, 508–515

Yamada, K., Ikata, T., Yamamoto, H., Nakagawa, Y. and Tanaka, H. (1969) Equilibrium function in scoliosis and after corrective plaster jacket for the treatment. *Tokushima Journal of Experimental Medicine* **16**, 1–7

Yau, A.C.M.C., Hsu, L.C.S., O'Brien, J.P. and Hodgson, A.R. (1974) Tuberculous kyphosis. Correction with spinal osteotomy, halo-pelvic distraction and anterior and posterior fusion. *Journal of Bone and Joint Surgery* **56A**, 1419–1434

Yong-Hing, K. and MacEwen, G.D. (1982) Scoliosis associated with osteogenesis imperfecta. Results of treatment. *Journal of Bone and Joint Surgery* **64B**, 36–43
Zetterberg, C., Aniansson, A. and Grimby, G. (1983) Morphology of the paravertebral muscles in adolescent idiopathic scoliosis. *Spine* **8**, 457–462
Zielke, K. and Berthet, A. (1978) VDS-Ventrale Derotation Spondylodese – vorlaufiger Bericht uber 58 Falle. *Beiträge zur Orthopädie und Traumatologie* **25**, 85–103
Zuk, T. (1962) The role of spinal and abdominal muscles in the pathogenesis of scoliosis. *Journal of Bone and Joint Surgery* **44B**, 102–105

CHAPTER 9

Infections of the Musculoskeletal System

ROBERT B. DUTHIE AND CARL L. NELSON

INFLAMMATION/INFECTIONS OF THE MUSCULOSKELETAL SYSTEM

Inflammation in bones, joints and muscles is either acute or chronic or granulomatous. Acute inflammation usually resolves without any residual ongoing change except when there has been abscess formation with collagen deposition forming a capsule or wall, or fibrosis. Macrophages, polymorphonuclea leucocytes and lymphocytes are the primary cells involved, acting as scavenger cells, ingesting, degrading inflammatory material as well as organisms or foreign material. Macrophages are derived from the circulating monocytes, and respond to macrophage activating factors. They identify foreign antigens for the T helper (CD4) lymphocyte cells and produce complement products: cytokines (interleukin, interferons, platelet activating and tumour necrosing factors); proteases (elastases and collagenases – for tissue destruction); prostaglandins via the arachidonic acid chain, growth promoting factors on fibroblasts and endothelial cells and free oxygen radicals (Duthie and Francis, 1988). These latter substances are formed from the leucocytes and monocyte/macrophage cellular action which has been called the 'respiratory burst' of white cells by Babior (1978). This superoxide serves to lyse invading bacterial cells.

Chronic inflammation is ongoing and associated

with tissue destruction and its replacement by fibrosis due to persistence of the initiating acute inflammatory stimulus, e.g. micro-organisms, or in particular infections, e.g. tuberculosis, leprosy, syphilis, or certain viral infections where the organisms are intracellular. Tuberculosis gives rise to a granulomatous, lymphocytic response which is characterized by necrosis and the epithelioid cells type of Langhans. In rheumatoid arthritis the chronic inflammation is thought to be a non-organic specific autoimmune disease involving a primary reaction of the autoimmune system against the body's own tissues. The primary cell response is in the lymphocytes and plasma cells with hyperplasia of synovial cells and fibrosis. Other causes are the presence of non-degradable material and radiation toxicity.

The cellular filtrate in chronic inflammation is derived from the mononuclear cells – macrophage, eosinophils, lymphocytes and plasma cells – interacting with the immune system (Sheffield, 1993).

Activated lymphocytes, e.g. T cells, produce lymphokines, e.g. interferon, which interact with macrophages and monocytes to produce cytokines. The B lymphocytes give rise to plasma cells. The cytokines, i.e. growth promoting factors, from the macrophages stimulate the fibroblasts to form collagen and fibrous tissue.

Granulation tissue consists of all the above cells within a stroma of fibroblasts, proliferating capillaries, etc., and has to be clearly differentiated from a granulomatous tissue. The systemic effects of chronic inflammation are marked. There can be lymphadenopathy, splenomegaly chronic pyrexia from increased levels of interleukin-1 and other pyrogenesis, general muscle atrophy from increased tumour necrosis factor – these are all commonly seen in tuberculosis. In chronic osteomyelitis there may be a chronic substantial secretion of serum amyloid A protein to give the systemic disease of amyloidosis. Suppression of the marrow can result in a normochromic normocytic anaemia with a raised ESR.

Granulomatous inflammation is an ongoing response to persistent and irritant antigen and in particular to the cellular response of the lymphocytes and macrophages – the latter assuming an epithelial appearance (Sheffield, 1993).

Granulomas result from foreign body reaction to retained surgical suture material, starch powder, sequestrum in chronic osteomyelitis and urate crystals in gout, etc. The more important form is the hypersensitivity granulomatous formation in which there is a cell-mediated immunological response to an antigen with the formation of the epithelial cell type, e.g. myobacteria of tuberculosis, leprosy and other intracellular infections such as histoplasmosis, brucellosis, syphilis, fungus, e.g. *Aspergillus*, *Cryptococcus*; hypersensitivity reactions to foreign protein, silica, schistosomiosis, in certain tumours, e.g. Hodgkin's disease; and unknown antigens in sarcodosis, Chron's disease, etc.

The epithlioid cell arises from adhesion of large macrophages through cytoplasmic interdigitations and intercellular junction. The cytoplasm is expanded by secretory vacuoles and therefore has a secretory role rather than a phagocytosis, lymphocytes are adjacent and often surrounded by fibroblasts. T lymphocyte cells (CD4) activate the macrophages to form epithelioid cells without involving the Rumeral part of the immune system, e.g. in tuberculosis, serum antibodies to the tuberculosis bacteria are not seen to any extent although a positive Mantoux test is a hypersensitivity, immune response to the antigen in the skin. Deficiency of the T cell CD4 lymphocyte as seen in HIV infection and AIDS disease makes these patients very prone to tuberculosis infection.

Cytokines produced by these cells can be inhibited by giving corticosteroids, thereby reducing the degree of the granulomatous inflammation. When excessive, cytokines produce cell necrosis, i.e. caseation, which is also augmented by the lysosyme secretion from the macrophage. Cytokines also mediate increased fibroblastic activity with resultant fibrosis.

Bacterial infections

GENERAL DESCRIPTION

The presence within, or invasion by, pathogenic bacteria or organisms is an infection, particularly when these organisms are capable of invading and multiplying in the human body to produce adverse effects. Entrance to the body is gained through a defect in the protective tissues, with the survival of the organism depending upon the ability to gain further access into the lymphatic and subepithelial tissues. Table 9.1 lists some bacteria and their portals of entry into the body.

If the bacteria circulate, even without associated clinical manifestations, *bacteraemia* results, and if there is a favourable host response, the reticulo-endothelial system will localize and destroy the organisms. If the infection becomes diffuse, however, a *septicaemia* may result. This implies that organisms as well as their toxins are present within the blood stream. Organisms can become intravascular by three mechanisms:

Table 9.1

Portal of entry	Bacteria
Skin	*Staphylococcus aureus, epidermidis* – coagulase negative
	Diphtheroids
Mouth and throat	Streptococci
	Haemophilus
	Tuberculosis
Stomach	Tuberculosis
Small Intestine	Tuberculosis
	Bacteroides
Nose	Staphylococci
	Streptococci
	Leprosy
Colon	Enterobacteriaceae
	Tuberculosis
	Streptococcus faecalis
	Bacteroides

1. by direct extension into vascular channels;
2. by following lymphatic channels and emptying into the venous system; and
3. by embolic spread from a secondary thrombosis within blood vessels, which has become invaded with bacteria.

Toxaemia is the state in which circulating toxins, rather than any infectious organisms, are present in the blood stream defined by Hopps in 1953. Several factors are involved in bacterial invasion: the anatomy, the portals of entry and the lymphatic flow.

ORGANISMS

Musculoskeletal infections encountered by orthopaedic surgeons include soft tissue infections, open fractures, joint infections, and osteomyelitis. These infections have specific pathophysiologies, particular characteristics, and specific organisms that are associated with each infection. One must be aware of the most likely organism found in particular types of infection so that therapy can be guided. The usual soft tissue infections are cellulitis and wound infection. The most common organisms found in cellulitis are *Staphylococcus aureus*, *Staphylococcus epidermidis*, and *Streptococcus pyogenes* and antibiotics should be chosen which kill these bacteria. Wound infections following surgery can develop from a wide variety of pathogens, although *Staphylococcus aureus* and *Staphylococcus epidermidis* are the most common wound infections. Methicillin-resistant *Staph. aureus* has become more common as well as *Enterobacter* and *Pseudomonas aeruginosa*.

Wound infections also occur in open fractures and the incidence of infection is related to the grade of injury, i.e. the more severe the wound the greater the incidence of infection. Fractures are classified into grades I, II, and III open fractures. Grades I and II open fractures treated appropriately have less than 1% incidence of infection; however, grade III open fractures have infection rates ranging from as low as 10% to 50%. A great variety of bacteria, obviously, can be cultured from open fractures but the most common pathogens are *Staphylococcus aureus*, *Staphylococcus epidermidis*, and non-enterococcal streptococci. In heavily contaminated wounds, Gram-negative organisms may be found and in injuries with soil contamination, *Clostridium perfringens* can be found as well. Knowledge of these bacteria dictate the antibiotic chosen.

The application of preparations to wounds is a long-established custom predating the discovery of bacteria, with the substances acting to eliminate bacteria growth. The terms 'germicide' and 'disinfectant' refer to compounds which have traditionally been regarded as lethal to all types of micro-organisms. 'Antiseptic' comes from the Greek *anti septikos* ('against rotting') and refers to an agent which inhibits the growth, with eventual control of sepsis. Unfortunately, nowadays many disinfectants and antiseptics used to clean hospital wards and used as skin preparations in operating theatres and emergency departments have been found to harbour some extremely harmful bacteria such as the *Pseudomonas* species.

Erhlich in 1906 discovered a synthetic arsenic substance for systemic use called salvarsan, or '606', which, when injected intravenously, destroyed the *Treponema* spirochaete. This was the first antimicrobial chemotherapeutic agent ('antibiotic'); these destroy micro-organisms without destroying the host. Others of the many chemotherapeutic agents now available, if used for longer than a very short period of time (often single doses), would destroy the host. These – for example, actinomycin D and methotrexate – are used as anti-cancer agents.

Domagk in 1930 then discovered the '*in vivo*' antibacterial activity of azo compounds containing a sulphonamide group, and by 1935 sulphonamides and related compounds were being used as chemotherapeutic agents.

The term 'antibiotic', as introduced by Waksman, refers to a substance produced by micro-organisms and which has the property of abolishing growth of, or eliminating, the micro-organisms. Penicillin in 1940 was the first true antibiotic, to be followed by streptomycin, bacitracin, the tetracyclines, erythromycin, neomycin, etc. (Table 9.2).

Table 9.2 Pathogenic bacteria – their infections and chemotherapeutic agents

Organisms	Infections	Chemotherapeutic agents
Gram-positive cocci		
Streptococci	Tonsillitis	Penicillin (erythromycin)
	Cellulitis/erysipelas Endocarditis Pneumococcal pneumonia (*Streptococcus pneumoniae*) Glomerulonephritis	Mostly sensitive to penicillin (erythromycin) but some resistance (e.g. strain 19A) to penicillin. Chloramphenicol, erythromycin, clindamycin, tetracycline. co-trimoxazole.
Staphylococci	Boils Osteomyelitis Pyogenic arthritis Pneumonia (esp. post-influenzal) Wounds	90%+ of hospital infections are benzylpenicillin-resistant. Flucloxacillin initially but actual sensitivities are required before appropriate antibiotics can be given. Resistance to many different antibiotics, including gentamicin, is described. Fusidic acid, lincomycin
Gram-positive bacilli		
Aerobic:		
Mycobacterium	Tuberculosis	Rifampicin, ethambutol
	Leprosy	Isoniazid, streptomycin
Corynebacterium	Diphtheria	Antitoxin. Erythromycin for carriers
Bacillus	Anthrax	Penicillin, chloramphenicol, erythromycin
Anaerobic:		
Clostridia	Tetanus	ATT (ATS penicillin)
	Gas gangrene	Penicillin (benzyl), cephalosporins
Gram-negative cocci		
Neisseria	Gonorrhoea	Increasing incidence of penicillin resistance. Streptomycin
Meningococcus	Meningitis and septicaemia	Penicillin, flucloxacillin, ampicillin. Sulphonamides
Gram-negative bacilli		
Aerobic:		
Escherichia *Klebsiella* *Proteus* *Pseudomonas*	Wound infections Abscesses Pneumonia Upper respiratory tract infection	Ampicillin, carbenicillin, cephalothin. Full sensitivities are required as variable resistance to many antibiotics, including aminoglycosides
Salmonella	Typhoid	Ampicillin
	Paratyphoid	Amoxycillin, chloramphenicol
Haemophilus	Epiglottitis 'Chest infections' Meningitis	Ampicillin or chloramphenicol for type B strains
Campylobacter (microaerophilic)	Gastroenteritis	Erythromycin
Anaerobic:		
Bacteroides	Wound infections Peritonitis ?Other infections	Metronidazole

CHEMOTHERAPEUTIC AGENTS

Antibiotics display certain basic properties:

1. low toxicity to human tissue (if recommended dosages are not strictly kept to, many antibiotics can and will be toxic);
2. high toxicity towards certain pathogenic organisms; and
3. the ability to function in the host.

Table 9.3 Classification of antibiotics based upon chemical structure

Aminoglycosides	Gentamicin
	Kanamycin
	Tobramycin
Cephalosporins	Cephradine
	Cephaloridine
	Cefuroxime
	Cefoxitin (a cephamycin)
Macrolides	Erythromycin
	Rifampicin
Penicillins	Benzylpenicillin
	Ampicillin
	Flucloxacillin
Polyenes	Amphotericin
Polypeptides	Bacitracin
	Colistin
	Polymyxin B
Tetracyclines	Oxytetracycline
	Doxycycline
	Minocycline
Lincomycins	
Chloramphenicol	
Steroid antibiotics	Fusidic acid
Synthetic substances	Sulphonamides
	Metronidazole
	Nalidixic acid
	Ethambutol
	Isoniazid

Table 9.3 lists some of the groups of the antimicrobials available. It has been demonstrated that structural similarity results in similar antimicrobial activity in many instances, and alteration in the chemistry of even a minor nature will result in a change in activity and pharmacological properties.

Mode of action

The essential basic property enabling a compound to serve as a useful chemotherapeutic agent is its selected toxicity towards the pathogenic organism rather than the host (Florey, 1958). Although the basis for the selective toxicity must be based upon biochemical processes, most understanding has been obtained by studying the effect of a new antibiotic substance rather than by studying its biochemical activity.

The success of a chemotherapeutic agent depends upon:

1. limiting the growth or multiplication of bacteria without killing them – bacteriostatic, or
2. killing the organism completely – bactericidal.

The bacteriostatic agents depend upon the natural body defences – humoral and cell-mediated – to complete the destruction. It is evident that the final outcome in either instance is the end result of a combination of factors; i.e. drug concentrations, virulence of organism, natural defences, choice of therapy, route of administration, etc.

Biochemical properties shared by all antibiotics are in their absorption into the susceptible cells (Umbreit, 1955), their ability to react with a substance specific to the sensitive organism, or their ability to inhibit a reaction peculiar to the organism. Occasionally, a certain environment develops antagonistic substances which will lessen the effect of an antibiotic agent.

In recent years the specific mode of action of many antimicrobial agents has been defined. Table 9.4 details the biochemical effect of some of the major antimicrobial groups used in clinical practice.

Table 9.4 Biochemical effects of some antimicrobial agents (after Hoeprich, 1977)

Group	Mode of action
Peptides:	
Cephalosporins	Inhibition of cell wall synthesis
Penicillin	Inhibition of cell wall synthesis. Probably inhibits a transpeptidase which causes cross linking between peptide chains and adjacent glycan strands
Polymyxins	Surface active disruption of cell wall membrane complex
Aminocyclitol:	
Aminoglycosides	30 S ribosomal binding, thus inhibiting protein synthesis
Streptomycin	As for aminoglycosides
Macrolides:	
Erythromycin	Binds 50 S ribosomal subunit Blocks peptide bond formation
Rifampicin	Inhibition of DNA-dependent RNA polymerase
Chloramphenicol	Binds 50 S ribosomal subunit Blocks peptide bond formation Block to RNA formation in the 30 S ribosomal subunit
Lincomycins:	
Clindamycin and lincomycin	Binds 50 S ribosomal subunit Blocks initiation of peptide chain
Tetracyclines	Block to RNA in 30 S ribosomal subunit
Polyenes:	
Amphotericin and nystatin	Interact with sterols of cell membrane
Metronidazole	Causes DNA strand breakage and degradation

Summarizing Table 9.4, antimicrobial agents can be grouped into those which interfere with cell wall metabolism and those which interfere with protein synthesis. Metronidazole is the exception. This group of antimicrobials shows an extremely complex mechanism of action. Originally, metronidazole was used in the treatment of *Trichomonas* infection; it was subsequently shown to be effective against anaerobic organisms. The reason for this seems to be that the active form has a reduced nitro group and it is only the anaerobic organisms which have a redox potential able to reduce that group. It is the reduced form which causes complete disruption of the cell DNA molecules.

The mode of action of some antibiotics still remains unknown (e.g. fusidic acid).

Use of chemotherapeutic agents

In spite of the initial overenthusiastic use and abuse of these agents, it is emphasized that one cannot substitute chemotherapy for asepsis and/or antisepsis. The basic principles of surgical technique are still as important as ever, throughout the total care of the patient. A general principle of chemotherapy was described by Garrod and Scowen (1960) – 'each case must be judged on its own merits, but if these are deliberately assessed, and if treatment has an explicit rational basis, indiscriminate use of agents will thereby be excluded'. In the selection of any particular chemotherapeutic agent, consideration must be given to the following.

1. The establishment of a bacteriologic diagnosis; accurate laboratory identification of the organism and its sensitivity is essential for any chemotherapy.
2. The choice of antibiotic then depends upon matching the known activity of various agents against the identified organisms, using both *in vitro* and *in vivo* studies. (Table 9.2 lists the common pathogens and the drug of choice for their control.)
3. Other factors, such as the emergence of resistant organisms or drug reactions, must be considered, as well as the possibility of superadded infection arising.
4. For effective use, known inhibitory concentrations must be given as quickly as possible and must be sustained until the infection subsides (Garrod *et al.*, 1973). The most effective route of administration must be taken (e.g. intravenously, intramuscularly or orally). In many severe infections, intravenous antibiotics should be used in the initial period, the length of the period depending upon the response to the antibiotic. The antibiotic therapy can thereafter be changed to the oral route. In choosing an antibiotic, it is well to note that some can be given only by a particular route; for example, cefuroxime – a recently developed cephalosporin – can be given only by the parenteral route. Cephradine, another cephalosporin, can be given by both enteral and parenteral routes, thus facilitating an easy transition between intravenous and oral therapy. Such factors as the excretory rates, the site of action, the tissue involved, the pH values and the accessibility of infected areas all influence the outcome of drug therapy. Occasionally, local injection into relatively inaccessible areas is warranted; e.g. penicillin into a joint space infected by *Streptococcus pneumonicle*. Serum levels of antibiotics such as gentamicin can be monitored relatively easily. This has two distinct advantages: first, that the dosage is sufficient and a therapeutic level is being maintained between doses; and second, aminoglycosides are quite toxic antibiotics, so serum concentration measurements reduce the possibility of a toxic dose being given.
5. The duration of treatment depends upon the response. Certain infections are controlled in a short period (e.g. gonococcal), while with others a longer time is required for treatment (e.g. subacute bacterial endocarditis, tuberculosis and osteomyelitis).

Complications of chemotherapy

Reaction can be classified as toxic or allergic.

Toxic effects are those caused by an exaggeration of the drug's principal action These can be produced by overdosage, by intolerance or by an idiosyncrasy and systemically reflect the pharmacological properties of the particular drug being administered. The symptoms develop as the agent accumulates and usually do not respond to antiallergic therapy. An example of toxicity is the drug-induced deafness and renal damage caused by aminoglycosides. Neomycin, thought originally to be non-absorbable, has been detected in serum in sufficient quantity to cause toxic effects.

Allergic reactions are not related to an overdose, nor do they demonstrate an exaggerated pharmacological property, and finally do respond to antiallergic therapy (Wood and Lepper, 1958). The serious allergic complication is that of anaphylactoid reaction, as seen most commonly with penicillin. Some individuals show cross-reactions between various groups of antibiotics. For example, some 10% of individuals showing an allergic response to the penicillins will also be allergic to the cephalosporins. Serum sickness also represents a form of allergic reaction.

The following list, as described by von Oettingen, indicates some of the drug reactions which have been observed: dermatitis, urticaria, angioneurotic oedema, rhinitis, conjunctivitis, bronchial asthma, drug fever, aplastic anaemia, eosinophilia, Herxheimer's reaction, gastrointestinal disturbances, pruritus, renal injury, central nervous system disturbances, visual disturbances, vestibular and auditory disturbances, and cardiac complications. Treatment is that of immediate cessation of the offending drug, and specific therapy directed towards either the toxic or allergic reaction (Dunlop and Murdoch, 1960).

CAUSES OF FAILURE OF CHEMOTHERAPY

Failure of chemotherapy or relapse of an infection after initial improvement, requires the consideration of the following:

1. Bacterial drug resistance.
2. Bacterial 'persistence'.
3. Poor host defences.
4. Poor drug absorption.
5. Drug inactivation by the host's protein or flora.
6. Poor penetration of the drug in tissues or cells.

Drug resistance

McDermott (1970) divides drug resistance into two: primary resistance – resistance of staphylococci to penicillin may be of this type; and emergent resistance – this is clinically more important as it requires the continual updating and development of antimicrobial therapy.

Resistance can arise in the following manner:

1. The specific metabolic process affected by the drug may be absent.
2. A structural peculiarity such as absence of the cell wall renders bacteria resistant to penicillin – this occurs in mycoplasmae and in L-forms which may develop from certain bacterial species.
3. The production of enzymes by the bacteria which destroy the drug – this occurs in the staphlococci which produce β-lactamases which destroy penicillin.

It has been postulated that, because there are several different β-lactamases which are structurally diverse, they evolved prior to the antibiotic era (Richmond, 1973). Five main groups of β-lactamase are described. For simplicity, they can be divided into three:

1. Ia – predominant action against cephalosporins;
2. IVa – action against cephalosporins and penicillins, including cloxacillin;
3. IIIa – action against cephalosporins and penicillins, but not against cloxacillin.

β-Lactamase activity is responsible for much bacterial resistance. Clavulanic acid and mecillinam are both substances which have been shown to inhibit β-lactamase activity and reduce the minimum inhibitory concentrations of penicillin and cephalosporin antibiotics. Mecillinam (a β-amidino derivative of 6-aminopenicillinamic acid) has antibiotic activity of its own, whereas clavulanic acid does not. These substances may be of great clinical value.

An important aspect of drug resistance which is becoming apparent is that of plasmid-mediated resistance which can be transferred between bacteria and, more particularly, between species. Plasmid (R factor) resistance gives resistance to a large number of antibiotics. Datta (1973) has described the history of the discovery of R factors which were first shown in *Shigella flexneri*, and gave resistance to streptomycin, tetracycline, chloramphenicol and sulphonamides. The factors were shown to be transmissible to all the Enterobacteriaceae, to *Vibrio cholerae* and *Yersinia pestis*. Since that time, resistance of the plasmid-mediated type has been shown to occur to many antibiotics, including sulphonamides, aminoglycosides and tetracycline. Several groups (Eisenstein *et al.*, 1977; Roberts and Falkow, 1977; Williams, 1978) have demonstrated the spread of R factor resistance outside the Enterobacteriaceae, specifically to *Neisseria gonorrhoeae*. The importance here is the possibility of further spread to the meningococcus.

Antibiotic therapy must therefore be based upon accurate laboratory analysis of the bacterial species involved. Furthermore, all inappropriate antibiotic use must be stopped. For example, Bridges and Lowbury (1977) recorded a marked fall in the incidence of resistant organisms with the termination of use of topical silver sulphadiazine on burns. They also showed decreased resistance to several other antibiotics, particularly amongst the *Klebsiella* species.

Bacterial persistence

This term is used to describe the survival of fully sensitive (*in vitro*) bacteria in the presence of concentrations of an antibiotic which kills the great majority of the bacterial population (reviewed by McDermott, 1969). These bacteria which persist form only a small proportion of a bacterial population exposed to the drug, but their probable clinical significance is that they are responsible for relapse. They occur especially in old bacterial populations or in the presence of pus, poor drainage and foreign bodies.

These are bacterial cells which happen to be relatively dormant and so only slowly metabolizing at the time of exposure to the drug, hence they are less readily eliminated (Rogers, 1967).

Annear (1976) has described three strains of *Pseudomonas* which showed unstable gentamicin resistance. It was demonstrated that the resistance was directly related to colony size. The large colonies were sensitive, but the small colonies were not. The small colonies developed into further small and large colonies which showed the same sensitivities. The unstable resistance seems to reside in an extrachromosomal plasmid location. This type of variable sensitivity may account for some examples of bacterial persistence.

Host factors

The patient with poor defences is more likely to suffer from diseases due to pathogenic bacteria, less likely to respond to chemotherapy and more likely to sustain a superadded infection with other organisms resistant to the antibiotics being used. There may be a congenital agammaglobulinaemia in which a child suffers from bouts of infection with virulent organisms. The infections are usually treated effectively with antibiotics, but tend to be recurrent and severe. Other children suffer from the congenital Di George's syndrome (absence of T lymphocytes or a combined Swiss type immunodeficiency (B and T lymphocyte absence). In the latter type, the child has to be totally isolated to eliminate the possibility of infection. Marrow transplantation may be of use in treating this syndrome. Other factors include old age, diseases such as diabetes, peripheral vascular disease, the reticuloses, alcoholism, and the use of drugs such as corticosteroids, immunosuppressive agents and cytotoxic drugs. Poor drainage of a body space encourages infection, and the absence of tissue fluid flow across a space may diminish the access-defending cells and antibodies and may decrease the penetration of antibiotics.

Antibiotics are bound to the serum proteins; the majority to albumin, but erythromycin binds to α-globulin. The proportion of antibiotic bound varies greatly from one drug to another.

PROPERTIES OF ANTIBIOTICS

To select the most appropriate antibiotics (Cunka, 1988) it is necessary to know the organism, to understand the properties and action of the appropriate antibiotics and to consider alternative methods of administration and the clinical implications of bacteria resistance to antibiotics.

Description of the spectrum and the effective concentrations of commonly used antibiotics are always available. Concentration can be expressed as minimal inhibitory concentration (MIC) which is the 'lowest concentration of antimicrobial agent that prevents visible growth after an 18–24 hour incubation by serial (two-fold) dilution in ranges of minimal bacterial concentration achievable in man' (Neu, 1987). Bactericidal drugs rather than bacteriostatic, are required when there is a decrease in the general and local defence mechanism, serious infections and poor drug penetration.

Tissue penetration of bone, both cortical and cancellous, is poor for the penicillins, but better for cephalosporins – up to 25%. In cancellous bone the peak bone level can be reached within the first hour. The β-lactam (penicillins, ampicillin, mezlocillin) or aminoglycoside (neomycin, etc.) antibiotics have been shown by Fitzgerald (1984) to have good transcapillary passage in normal and osteomyelitic bone, distributing freely within the plasma and interstitial fluid space. However, in osteomyelitis, debridement of sequestrum and/or involucrum is required. Tissue penetration of flucloxacillin or cephradine into normal intervertebral disc does not occur in noninflamed human material (Gibson *et al.*, 1987).

The use of a tourniquet does not appear to affect the bone and soft tissue penetration if it is inflated 5 minutes or so after the intravenous administration of the antibiotics.

In septic arthritis Neu (1987) has shown that aminoglyosides were still positive in the joint aspirate 72 hours after its being given, although their sensitivity was reduced by the presence of large numbers of polymorphonuclear neutrophils, the local hypoxia and the acidic pH.

The side-effects or adverse effects are important, e.g. aminoglycosides cause real damage, as does vancomycin, cephalosporins, tetracycline, etc. The liver (oxacillin, erythromycin, tetracyclines), blood cells (chloramphenicol), ear (vestibular – streptomycin, gentamicin and auditory – neomycin, vancomycin), bleeding diathesis (carbenicillin), all required to be checked. Combined chemotherapy except for antituberculosis treatment, has to be critically evaluated because of drug interaction at receptor site, elimination route competition, disruption of normal floral and enforced adverse drug reactions (Neu, 1987).

SUMMARY OF THE ACTION OF CERTAIN ANTIBIOTICS

β-Lactam antibiotics

These act on the penicillin binding proteins on the cell wall of the bacteria. These enzymes form the protein peptidoglycan which is necessary for the integrating of the wall as well as producing enlargement of the saccules within Gram-negative bacteria. When blocked there is autolysis of the bacteria. However, autolysis may not occur if the autolytic enzyme system is defective or when a β-lactamase is secreted by the bacteria to inactivate the β-lactam antibiotic. These inhibitors are known as fucidal inhibitors. Substances such as clavulanic acid and sulbactum have been developed to augment the activity of the β-lactam antibiotics against these inhibitors, e.g. ticarcillin (Timentin) or amoxycillin (Augmentin).

Penicillins can now be divided into:

- natural – penicillin G and V whose use is now restricted to β-haemolytic streptococcus.
- semisynthetic – ampicillin and amoxycillin – have a broader spectrum to include *Haemophilus influenzae* and gonococcus.
- anti-staphylococcus group – cloxacillin, flucloxacillin – are restricted for use against *Staph. aureus*.
- anti-pseudomonal group – carbenicillin, mezlocillin – are particularly sensitive to staphylococcal β-lactamase and combine with β-lactamase inhibitors, aminoglycoside antibiotics, but there may be some inactivation of the mixture or in renal failure.

Sensitivity reactions, e.g. anaphylaxis (penicillin C), drug rashes and fever, an increase in the ESR and serum alkaline phosphatase, and/or eosinophilia can occur.

Cephalosporins were developed by Professor Abraham in the same Oxford laboratories used by Professor Florey – the developer of penicillin. The first generation – cephazolin – has a broad Gram-positive spectrum, e.g. for *Clostridium*, and a Gram-negative spectrum, e.g. for *Klebsiella, E. coli, Proteus mirabilis* and *pneumococcus*. Adequate bone levels against *Staphylococcus aureus* and Gram-negative organisms are obtainable. Gut organisms, e.g. *Strept. faecalis*, etc., are highly resistant. The second generation – cefoxitin – is effective against *Haemophilus influenzae*, anaerobics and Gram-negative organism.

The third generation are β-lactamases, stable and active against Gram-negative enteric organisms, gonococcus, *H. influenzae*, but not *Staph. aureus* or *Pseudomonas aeruginosa*. It should be noted that none of the cephalosporins is active against methicillin-resistant *Staph. aureus* (MRSA) or methicillin-resistant *Staph. epidermidis* (MRSE).

Cephalosporins are excreted by combined glomerular filtration and tubular secretion which is inhibited by probenecid and therefore this latter substance can used to prolong their half-life.

Two new drugs which are closely related to the cephalosporins – monolactams and carbapenems – are also β-lactamase stable and are therefore of use against *Ps. aeruginosa* and other aerobic enterobacteriacae and have no hypersensitivity or cross-sensitivity. The cephalosporins have a cross-sensitivity to penicillin.

Aminoglycosides

These pass through the bacterial cell membrane in the presence of oxygen and bind to the ribosomes with inactivation of protein synthesis. Resistance to these antibiotic can occur inside the bacteria.

Aminoglycosides have a wide Gram-positive spectrum except for streptococci and enterococci (aerobus) and against aerobic Gram-negative bacteria. They can be used in combination with penicillin against the pseudomonas.

These are not absorbed by the oral route and therefore require injection, or directly into surgical wound or body cavities. They do not penetrate human cells except the renal tubular cell or the inner ear cell. They can produce a curare-like effect if used in renal failure or muscular dystrophy.

Toxic effects are present when adequate dosage is exceeded, or prolonged, in old age, in dehydrated patients or with the use of other nephrotoxic drugs, e.g. cyclosporrins.

Others

1. Vancomycin is of great use against *Staph. aureus* – especially MRSA and *clostridium difficile*. However, it is both nephrotoxic and ototoxic. A new drug, teicoplanin, has now become available for use against MRSA and MRSE and also fusidic acid compound.
2. Lincomycin and clindamycin.
3. Chloramphenicol because of its excellent cerebrospinal fluid penetration, is of use after infection by *Bacteroides fragilis* which can give rise to meningitis after spinal surgery.
4. Metronidazole is absorbed orally and is active against protozoans, *Bacteroider*, and pseudomembranous colitis.
5. Quinolones, e.g. Ofloxacin, developed from nalidixic acid, are effective against Gram-positive including MRSA and Gram-negative organisms, and anaerobes, especially the *Clost-*

ridium species. They are absorbed orally with a half-life of 3–10 hours and good bone levels are achieved. They are now being used in osteomyelitis, infected sternotomy wounds with MRSA, MRSE, and *Pseudomonas aeruginosa*. Their toxic effects, e.g. gastrointestinal and CNS, are minor, but because of a direct effect upon joint cartilage, their use in children is not recommended.

BACTERIAL RESISTANCE TO ANTIBIOTICS

This is an ever increasing problem. The sensitivity of common pathogens as well as the emerging hospital pathogens to first- or even second-line antibiotics can no longer be guaranteed (Jones and Pallett, 1993). Penicillin G – the naturally occurring and indeed the first antibiotic – is no longer effective against *Streptococcus pneumoniae*; 5% of pneumococci now show resistance in England compared with 44% in Spain. Resistance to erythromycin by the pneumoecoccal infections has increased to 10–25% in Europe, although it is rare in Britain. Since the late 1980s over 50% of *E. coli* isolates are resistant to the penicillins, especially ampicillin, because of developing a plasmoid-derived β-lactamase. Similarly *Haemophilus influenzae* has a plasmid against many antibiotics including ampicillin, choramphenicol and trimethoprim. With the increased use of oral cephalosporins and developing β-lactamases, decreased sensitivity or even resistance is now present.

Significant hospital pathogens have been appearing over the past 20 years, e.g. *Klebsiella*, *Enterobacteria*, *Serratia* and *Pseudomonas*. They contain β-lactamases produced by the administration of certain β-lactam antibiotics. *Staphylococcus epidermidis* – normally a skin commensal – has become resistant to flucloxacillin, aminoglycosides and ciprofloxacin when suboptimal sublethal doses of antibiotics are given for other reasons. The genes of this resistance pattern can be transferred to the *Staphylococcus aureus*, giving rise to the methicillin-resistant *Staph. aureus* – MRSA. Their presence is now endemic in many hospitals in Europe and in the USA, upgrading vancomycin as a first-line empirical antibiotic.

THE USE OF ANTIBIOTICS IN PROPHYLAXIS

The use of antibiotics in patients without any harmful factor who are to undergo operation is based upon the concept of their ability to reduce or destroy organisms which are already present in the host or are introduced by the actual surgery or intervention. Burke (1961) introduced this possibility of prevention by his experimental work on wounds. Charnley (1964) pioneered the use of a clean air operating enclosure to reduce airborne contamination around the operation room. Lidwell *et al.* (1982), from a randomized, controlled milticentre trial in Oxford, showed the efficacy of such a system in which the postoperative infection rate was reduced by over eightfold, up to 2 years postoperatively. Indeed, when combined with prophylactic antibiotics, the rate of infection was as low as 0.6%. They also showed that the greater part of joint implant sepsis is transmitted by the airborne route of the conventional operating room, via carriers.

Elective orthopaedic surgery, excluding fracture work, although clean, by introducing bone cement and metalwork during a prolonged operating time increased the risk of bacterial contamination especially in the presence of dead tissue. Therefore, in total joint procedures, antibiotic prophylaxis is indicated. Appropriate antibiotics are selected, e.g. the cephalosporins, because of their high penetration and their half-life characteristics to maintain minimal inhibitory concentration (MIC) against *Staphylococcus* are well known. A bolus is administered intravenously during the induction of anaestheisa and is now accepted and only needs to be given up to 24 hours postoperatively (Nelson *et al.*, 1983).

Antibiotic cement is now also being inserted since the early work of Bucholz *et al.* (1981) using gentamicin. Antibiotics, e.g. gentamicin, erythromycin, will elute from the cement to give a minimum inhibitory concentration (MIC) up to 80% within the first 24 hours. There has been no report of toxicity nor development of resistance by bacteria nor allergic effect upon the mechanical strength of the cement.

Chemotherapeutic antibiotic agents

Once a bacteriological diagnosis is accurately established and the sensitivity of the organism known, chemotherapy can then be appropriately directed. In selecting the antibiotic for treatment, type of infection, hospital sensitivity resistant patterns, and adverse reactions must be carefully considered. However, initially antibiotics are chosen on the basis of what is known to be the most common organism involving the type of infection (Tables 9.5, 9.6, 9.7).

Table 9.5 Gram-positive organisms: initial choice of antibiotics for therapy of musculoskeletal infections

Organism	Antibiotics of first choice (adult doses)	Alternative Antibiotics
Staphylococcus aureus	Nafcillin 2g q6h *or* Clindamycin 900 mg q8h	Vancomycin, cephalothin
Methicillin-resistant *Staphylococcus aureus*	Vancomycin 500 mg q8h	SXT[a] + rifampin Imipenem
Staphylococcus epidermidis	Vancomycin 500 mg q8h *or* Nafcillin 2 g q6h	Clindamycin, cephalothin
Group A streptococcus	Penicillin G 2×10^6 U q4h	Clindamycin, cephalothin
Group B streptococcus	Penicillin G 2×10^6 U q4h	Clindamycin, cephalothin
Enterococcus	Ampicillin 2 g q6h[b]	Vancomycin[b]

[a]Sulfamethoxazole–trimethoprim.
[b]In a serious enterococcal infection, ampicillin plus an aminoglycoside is used.
From Nelson (1993), p. 4324, with permission of the publishers.

The most often used route of administration for a serious infection is intravenous peripheral or into the right atrium by a Hickman catheter, since it provides optimal, high peak concentrations in the tissue, e.g. osteomyelitis; intramuscular or oral administration reduces the peak serum concentration and thus produces lower tissue levels. The dosing interval of a parenteral antibiotic is based on its half-life and can be calculated by multiplying the half-life of the antibiotic by 4.

The use of Hickman or Broviac catheters is now commonly used in treating osteomyelitis in out-patients for up to 30 days with fewer complications of about 20% due to local infections. Few have required removal before the completion of the antibiotic regimen. The advantages to the patients, especially with osteomyelitis, is reduction in hospital stay, better morale, less phlebitis and pain on changing intravenous sites, etc.

Protein binding and tissue binding are also factors that must be considered in antibiotic choices. The amount of antibiotic binding to albumin will determine the degree of release of the antibiotic. Since only free antibiotic is active against bacteria, highly protein-bound drugs may be a disadvantage because their free antibiotic concentration in the blood and tissue may be low. However, highly protein-bound antibiotics provide high bound serum concentration for extended periods. Although these principles are suggested, the precise effect of protein binding remains elusive.

Factors other than protein and tissue binding may also lead to decreased bioavailability of the drug. Factors that may adversely effect the bioavailability of an antibiotic are pH, purulent material, and decreased blood flow.

CLASSIFICATION

In choosing the appropriate antibiotic, resistance also must be carefully considered as well as the mode of action of the drug. The essential basic property enabling a compound to serve as a useful chemotherapeutic agent is its selected toxicity towards the pathogenic organism rather than the host.

Staphylococcus aureus has several recognized forms of antibiotic resistance which include β-lactamase production. β-Lactamase is an enzyme responsible for resistance in the majority of *Staphylococcus* isolates to penicillin and because of its resistance, the penicillinase-resistant semisynthetic penicillins have become the antimicrobial of choice because of their stability in the presence of *Staph. aureus* β-lactamase

LENGTH OF ANTIBIOTIC THERAPY

The length of antibiotic therapy in orthopaedic patients is dependent upon the clinical response of the patients; soft tissue infections usually are treated for 3–7 days parenterally followed by oral therapy for a 2-week period. Osteomyelitis has traditionally been treated with 6 weeks of intravenous antimicrobials depending upon the age of the patient and based

Table 9.6 Gram-negative organisms: initial choice of antibiotics for therapy of musculoskeletal infections

Organism	Antibiotics of first choice (adult doses)	Alternative antibiotics
Acinetobacter sp.	Tobramycin 5 mg/kg/day q8h[d]	Mezlocillin, imipenem
Enterobacter sp.	Tobramycin 5 mg/kg q8h[d]	Cefotaxime, amikacin,[d] mezlocillin, ticarcillin
Escherichia coli	Ampicillin 2 g q6h	Cephalothin, ticarcillin, tobramycin, amikacin[d]
Haemophilus influenzae	Cefotaxime 2 g q8h	Chloramphenicol, ampicillin,[a] cefuroxime, SXT[b]
Klebsiella sp.	Cefazolin 2 g q8h	Tobramycin, cefotaxime, amikacin[d]
Proteus mirabilis	Ampicillin 2 g q6h	Cefazolin, tobramycin[d]
Proteus vulgaris *Proteus rettgeri* *Morganella morganii*	Cefotazime 2 g q8h, tobramycin 5 mg/kg/ day q8h	Mezlocillin, ticarcillin, amikacin[d]
Providencia sp.	Tobramycin 5 mg/kg/day	Cefotaxime, amikacin,[d] STX, mezlocillin, ticarcillin
Pseudomonas aeruginosa	Ticarcillin 3 g q4h or Mezlocillin 3 g q4h + tobramycin 5 mg/kg q8h[d]	Ceftazidime,[c] amikacin[d]
Serratia marcescens	Cefotaxime 2 g q8h or Gentamicin 5 mg/kg/day q8h[d]	Amikacin,[d] ticarcillin

[a]Non-β-lactamase-producing strain of *H. influenzae*.
[b]Sulfamethoxazole–trimethoprim.
[c]In a serious infection, it should be used with aminoglycoside.
[d]Follows blood levels.
From Nelson (1993), p. 4325, with permission of the publishers.

Table 9.7 Anaerobic organisms; initial choice of antibiotics for therapy of musculoskeletal infections

Organism	Antibiotics of first choice (adult doses)	Alternative Antibiotics
Bacteroides fragilis group	Clindamycin 900 mg q8h	Metronidazole, chloramphenicol, cefoxitin
Bacteroides sp. other than *B. fragilis* group	Penicillin G 2 × 10^6 U q4h	Clindamycin, metronidazole, chloramphenicol, cefoxitin
Peptostreptococcus sp.	Penicillin G 2 × 10^6 U q4h	Clindamycin, metronidazole, cefoxitin
Clostridium sp.	Penicillin G 2 × 10^6 U q4h	Chloramphenicol, metronidazole, clindamycin

From Nelson (1993), p. 4325, with permission of the publishers.

Table 9.8 Osteomyelitis: commonly isolated organisms. Haematogenous osteomyelitis (monomicrobic infection)

Infant (<1 year)	Childhood (1–16 years)	Adults (>16 years)
Group B streptococcus	*Staphylococcus aureus*	*Staphylococcus aureus*
Staphylococcus aureus	*Streptococcus pyogenes*	*Staphylococcus epidermidis*
Escherichia coli	*Haemophilus influenzae*	Gram-negative bacilli
		Pseudomonas aeruginosa
		Serratia marcescens
		Escherichia coli
Contiguous focus osteomyelitis (polymicrobic infection)		
Staphylococcus aureus		
Staphylococcus epidermidis		
Streptococcus pyogenes		
Enterococcus sp.		
Gram-negative bacilli		
Anaerobes		

From Nelson (1993), p. 4326, with permission of the publishers.

on the most common bacteria involved in the different age groups (Table 9.8); however, there is a growing tendency to treat for shorter periods of time.

Osteomyelitis

The term *osteomyelitis* is used to describe an infection of the bone. When the root words *osteon* (bone) and *myelo* (marrow) are combined with *-itis*, they define a poorly understood clinical state in which part of the osseous skeleton is infected by micro-organisms.

The term *osteomyelitis* is usually coupled with additional descriptive terms such as *acute* or *chronic* and *haematogenous* or *exogenous*. Pyogenic or granulomatous, terms which indicate the type of host response to the organism, may also be used with osteomyelitis.

Sequestrum, a term used almost exclusively in association with osteomyelitis, is a microscopic or macroscopic fragment of necrotic, usually cortical, bone found at the nidus of the infection within bone. These fragments usually begin as part of the cortex and are surrounded by pus and infected granulation tissue. The cortex becomes devitalized by bacterial toxins, enzymes, intraosseous pressure, or trauma in the acute phase of the disease. Devitalized bone does not necessarily become a sequestrum, which suggests that osteoclasts revascularize and resorb at least some bone. Occasionally, cure or remission is obtained when the host is able to extrude the sequestrum either spontaneously or surgically. Surgical implants and foreign bodies, i.e. cement may behave similarly. Necrotic-infected bone that is not sequestered is, more often, left behind and the disease process continues. Physiologically, children are more likely to be able to resorb completely a sequestered cortical fragment than adults which may, in part, account for the relatively low incidence of chronic osteomyelitis seen in children. But active osteomyelitis in children should not be considered self-limiting.

Involucrum which is derived from the root *volvere* (to wrap) is also seen in osteomyelitis. This condition takes place when newly formed reactive bone occurs at the interface between diseased bone and healthy tissue. Radiographically, it appears as newly formed radiodense bone and is often inaccurately labeled 'sclerotic' (suggesting scar). Bone injury may stimulate involucra physiologically, which results in the accentuated metabolic coupling of osteoclasts and osteoblasts by bone-inductive cytokines (Dewhirst *et al.*, 1985; Bertolini *et al.*, 1986).

Exogenous and haematogenous (endogenous) are the two basic paths of bacterial transmission that cause the development of bone and joint sepsis. Exogenous infection occurs when micro-organisms are directly inoculated into a bone or joint from trauma, surgery, or a contiguous focus of infection. In contrast, when micro-organisms spread through the vascular system into osseous or synovial tissue, producing a secondary focus of infection, haematogenous osteomyelitis or joint sepsis occurs.

Depending upon the type of infecting micro-organism, one of two patterns of host response will generally occur. A fulminating infection resulting from pyogenic organisms, classically Gram-positive staphylococci, is the most common pattern. The second pattern of host response is an insidious granulomatous reaction resulting from less aggressive non-pyogenic organisms, usually acid-fast bacilli. Micro-organisms are, consequently, associated with specific reactive patterns, and each type of organism will evoke a characteristic pyogenic or granulomatous (non-pyogenic) response (Enneking, 1986).

Septic arthritis, like osteomyelitis, may be classified as acute or chronic, haematogenous or exogenous in origin, and may produce a pyogenic or granulomatous host response, depending upon the infecting organism.

Traumatic or surgical inoculation of bacteria into bone and surrounding soft tissue frequently precedes exogenous osteomyelitis. Trauma to the extremity can range from high-energy open fractures to puncture wounds of the foot with the amount of wound contamination ranging from virtually none to the heavy contamination found in barnyard injuries. The inoculation of bacteria into bone from an adjacent or contiguous focus of soft tissue infection can also cause exogenous osteomyelitis.

Exogenous osteomyelitis and haematogenous osteomyelitis differ in the mechanism of inoculation, the anatomical site of inoculation, and the bacterial species inoculated. The mechanism and anatomical site of inoculation are usually apparent. Although the anatomical sites involved include surgical wounds, the sites most frequently involved are those most commonly injured and which most often contain diaphyseal bone. The tibia is the bone most commonly involved in open fractures thus, it is the most common anatomical site of traumatic osteomyelitis. The contaminating inoculum, which is usually pyogenic and polymicrobial, may be combined with various amounts and types of foreign debris (Gustilo, 1979). With haematogenous osteomyelitis, the mechanism of inoculation is via the blood stream, the site of inoculation is metaphyseal bone, and the inoculum is a single organism, usually *Staphylococcus aureus*. Acute exogenous osteomyelitis, unlike haematogenous osteomyelitis, may go unrecognized as the signs and symptoms that accompany acute infection are often masked by the initial trauma.

Exogenous osteomyelitis is the result of direct inoculation of invading bacteria into a compromised local environment. Disrupted, devascularized, and necrotic soft tissue, periosteum, and bone, which result from the initial trauma and interrupted blood supply, provide an abundant culture medium. An environment that isolates these organisms from any immediate host response is provided by the lack of blood supply. Traumatic osteomyelitis and septic arthritis are different from infections following elective or 'clean' surgery in that they involve increased tissue trauma and devascularization. An adjacent soft tissue infection may also hinder local blood supply and produce local soft tissue and bone necrosis (Fitzgerald and Cowan, 1975; Fitzgerald *et al.*, 1975). If such a compromised, bacterially contaminated, microenvironment is not debrided surgically, the bacteria will proliferate and become established, causing an acute infection.

When trauma and infection occur, bone has a blood supply that favours necrosis. Surgical or traumatic fracture of bone disrupts the endosteal blood supply and strips the periosteal blood supply which results in dead cortical and cancellous bone. As compared with soft tissues, necrotic cortical bone is revascularized, resorbed, and remodelled very slowly, when infection is *not* present (Burchardt and Enneking, 1978; Kahn and Pritzker, 1979). When infection is present, the local defence and repair mechanisms are diverted in an attempt to wall off and eradicate the infection, if possible. The walled-off, dead bone segment then becomes a biological sequestrum, which harbours bacteria, allowing them to proliferate and attack surrounding viable tissue and bone by generating toxins and pressure. Pus, theoretically, is accumulated under pressure and adjacent healthy bone is devascularized via periosteal elevation and spread into the endosteal and intramedullary spaces (Larsen, 1938); thus, healing is obstructed or prevented.

In an attempt to isolate the infection, granulation tissue forms early around the infected area while the inflammatory and immunological defence mechanisms work to eradicate the infection. Formation of new antibodies against microbes is stimulated through this process. Initially, granulation tissue surrounds the infected necrotic area, both in bone and in soft tissue, but is then replaced with a dense, relatively avascular, fibrous tissue membrane which protects the host by more effectively isolating the infectious process. Abscess contents, infected bone, and sequestra lie within this membrane-enclosed cavity. Within the Haversian canals and medullary spaces, and, more frequently, beneath the periosteum, primitive mesenchymal cells are stimulated to form new reactive bone around the abscess cavity (Enneking, 1986). As seen in Brodie's abscess, this reactive bone is the involucrum and is a further attempt to wall off the infection from the host. After fibrous and bony encapsulation has occurred, antibodies, inflammatory cells, and granulation tissue must cross this avascular fibrous membrane and involucrum in order to eradicate the organism (Bergman *et al.*, 1982; Old, 1988). An effective attempt to isolate the host from the infection may also isolate the micro-organisms from the host defences, providing a host-generated bacterial line of defence.

The bacteria respond, with a variety of virulence factors, to the host defences. Numerous exotoxins, enzymes, and endotoxins are produced. Oxygen tension, pH, and tissue nutrition decline, which adversely affect surrounding viable soft tissue and bone as well as the cells of inflammation, repair, and immunity. A wide variety of toxins, many of which are species dependent, are produced by micro-organisms (Sawetz *et al.*, 1977).

An emerging virulence factor that has received much attention is the glycocalyx, a hydrated mucopolysaccharide biofilm synthesized by bacteria. This material, which is slime-like and bacteria-exuded, aids in bacterial adherence and may be produced in such enormous quantities as to provide a mechanical barrier to antibodies (Baltimore and Mitchell, 1980), antibiotics (Govan and Fyfe, 1978) and phagocytosis (Schwarzmann and Boring, 1971), while allowing the bacteria to thrive. Glycocalyx appears to be produced most freely once it has assisted bacterial adhesion to a solid substrate such as necrotic bone, a surgical implant, or a foreign body (Gristina and Costerton, 1984; Savage and Fletcher, 1985; Gristina, 1987; Gristina *et al.*, 1987).

To ensure survival, the bacteria have several offensive and defensive mechanisms. Bacteria use exotoxins, enzymes, and endotoxins offensively, to kill the surrounding tissue and use it as a food source. Additionally, four lines of mechanical defence exist against the host's tissue response. The outermost line of bacterial defence, which limits vascular, inflammatory, humoral, and antibiotic (Kilgore *et al.*, 1982) access and penetration to the bacteria, is the fibrous membrane and involucrum produced by the host. Under decreased oxygen tension, the abscess cavity has a low nutrient concentration, and contains necrotic tissue debris, bacterial toxins, enzymes released by lysis of dead inflammatory cells, and the sequestrum, (e.g. prostaglandins E and F_2 (Dekel and Francis, 1981). The sequestrum, implant, or foreign body harbours the micro-organisms and provides a constant unchanging foundation, allowing bacterial adherence, protection, and proliferation. While not only assisting in initial bacterial adherence, the enveloping glycocalyx provides additional protection by inhibiting phagocytosis and antibody and antibiotic penetration. Once the micro-organisms that are protected by these multiple lines of offence and defence are isolated by the host, surgical ablation is usually necessary to eradicate the diseased tissue and bacterial stronghold.

The host will eradicate the infection and healing will occur, if the anatomical location and host response are adequate to overcome the number and virulence of the micro-organisms. If the local environment is compromised, for example, by vascular insufficiency or massive trauma, or if the host response is compromised by immunological, pharmacological, nutritional, or other pathological processes, extensive infection or even death may result. Usually, however, the host and organism will reach a chronic steady state (chronic osteomyelitis) in which healing will not occur. The abscess and sequestra can exist indefinitely with no healing. The sequestra and bacteria, occasionally, are not eradicated but remain as an inactive chronic osteomyelitis in which no signs of active infection are present. Dormant or inactive osteomyelitis can persist for months or even decades; more often, however, a more dynamic, steady state is reached by the establishment of a draining sinus tract. This prevents toxic products of infection and bacteria from accumulating within the host but does not allow for the eradication of the infection unless the entire infected bone or foreign body is extruded (Orr, 1927). Chronic osteomyelitis is often the end result of both exogenous and haematogenous osteomyelitis and complications include non-union, malunion,epiphyseal growth disturbance, and, less frequently, epithelial carcinoma of a sinus tract or amyloidosis.

Haematogenous osteomyelitis

HISTORY

Preantibiotic era

Surgeons, prior to the twentieth century, appeared to be somewhat apathetic when dealing with the problem of osteomyelitis, and to some degree this attitude persists today. Bone and joint infection has been an insidious and tenacious problem from the start; fossil remains of prehistoric man and animal have revealed paleopathological evidence of traumatic osteomyelitis (Sales, 1930). The first written documentation of osteomyelitis was found in the Sanskrit writings of the Hindu surgeons Charaka and Sushruta, circa 2500 BC (Charaka Samhita, 1888; Sushruta Samhita, 1911).

Invariably associating bone diseases with injury, Hippocrates (500–400 BC) accurately described extrusion of an infected bony sequestrum as well as a surgical procedure for hastening the extrusion (Hippocrates, 1849). In addition, he recognized the connection between a non-healing sinus and the presence of dead bone. Medical wisdom, during the ensuing Roman period, was essentially Greek in origin. The earliest attempts at understanding disease pathology were made during this time. In the first century AD, Celsus (1838) determined that inflammation and fever were caused by stagnation of the four humours, which result in the four cardinal signs *rubor* (redness), *tumor* (swelling), *calor* (heat), and *dolor* (pain). Corruption, ulceration, blackness (negrites), caries, fistula, and gangrene were terms he used to describe bone pathology.

From the collapse of the Roman Empire until the Renaissance, there were virtually no advancements made in the treatment of bone and joint sepsis or in the understanding of its pathophysiology. During the Byzantine Empire, Greco-Roman medicine and science were preserved and, during the Arabic period in Syria and Persia, were combined with the Oriental (Sanskrit) body of medical knowledge. Some of the comprehensive literature of this period, in mediaeval Latin translations, survived and was held within European monasteries and cathedrals until the Renaissance.

A succession of wars and the introduction of firearms, during the fourteenth and fifteenth centuries, did much to change the perspective of medicine in Europe. Missiles from firearms altered the character of wounds, resulting in a higher incidence of infected bone injuries. This led to a class of unqualified practitioners, called 'Wundärzte' in Germany, and 'bonesetters' in England, who wrote many pamphlets proclaiming their current understanding and treatment of bone and joint pathology (Wilensky, 1934).

The development of anatomical knowledge characterized the seventeenth and eighteenth centuries. Howship, Havers, and Scarpa described bony anatomy. Percival Pott, in 1771, described an osteomyelitic lesion from which a bony sequestrum was removed. He speculated that the source of the sequestrum lay in the separation of periosteum from bone which caused the avascularity of the bone.

During the 1800s, after systematic application of the microscope to research, authors, such as Virchow, wrote treatises on pathology. These authors, when dealing with inflammation, invariably mentioned the cardinal signs of Celsus. In 1867, a pupil of Virchow, Cohnheim, observed sequential microscopic changes of inflamed tissue and attributed these to each of the cardinal signs: vasodilation (rubor), acceleration of vascular flow (calor), and increased vascular permeability (tumor). As Cohnheim noted, the pain (dolor) could be assumed. In addition, he described slowing of plasma flow, plasma exudation, margination of leucocytes to the periphery of the red cell stream, and their subsequent attachment to the endothelial wall (pavementing), followed by leucocyte emigration (diapedesis). Phagocytosis and antibodies were also discovered during this period.

'Spontaneous' (haematogenous) osteomyelitis as a separate clinical entity was first described by Cragie, in 1828, and Brodie described nine cases of chronic bone abscess, in 1830. The term 'osteomyelitis' was coined, in 1834, by Nelaton. The study of the treatment of osteomyelitis was intensified by the experiences of the Crimean, Italian, and American Civil wars. Prior to 1874, osteomyelitis had been treated with rest and poultices until discharge of the sequestrum occurred spontaneously. Sequestrectomy and subsequent wound granulation were advocated by Sir W. Howes, in 1874. The principles of sequestrectomy and open wound management were further developed during World War I. Carrel and Dakin developed a relatively effective method of acute clinical sterilization of wounds with Dakin's solution.

The use of maggots in wound sterilization has been attempted since the eighteenth century. Connors, during the American Civil War, used this method, as did Baer and Eastman, during World War I, with Baer reporting excellent results with this treatment as late as 1928. Because it had no advantage over surgical techniques and the maggots introduced other bacteria, not to mention negative aesthetic and psychological effects, the method fell into disfavour.

Antibiotic era

The fundamental principles of wide drainage and rest were restated by Winnett Orr, in 1927. Sulphonamides, in the 1930s, ushered in the antibiotic era and, when combined with the Orr technique, provided a giant leap forward in the treatment of osteomyelitis. Treatment of infection was again stimulated by war, in the 1940s. Penicillin was developed in Oxford and then produced through co-operation between the American and British scientific communities. Multiple antibiotics, refinement of surgical techniques, and increased understanding of the pathogenesis of osteomyelitis have been developed since World War II. Osteomyelitis is still on occasion unresponsive to modern therapy, however; and, although mortality has almost been eliminated, it still often results in morbidity and disability. Effective prevention and treatment of osteomyelitis require a complete understanding of its pathophysiology.

CLASSIFICATION

The duration of disease, aetiological mechanism of infection, and type of host response to the infection are the bases of the classification of osteomyelitis and septic arthritis. Virtually all osteomyelitis and septic arthritis can be classified when described using these three parameters. Consideration of these aspects when classifying is helpful as each identifies the characteristics of that infection, its treatment, and the anticipated response.

Duration of disease is described by characterizing the infection as acute or chronic. Acute infection is distinguished from simple inoculation or colonization when bacteria are present but a host response has not yet occurred. Without colonization or a classic histological response, inoculation occurs very early in the course of disease prior to acute infection, e.g. in a contaminated open fracture immediately after trauma. The differentiation between acute and chronic osteomyelitis often is only in terms of absolute time, although this concept is arbitrary. The term acute always refers to early osteomyelitis; however, acute components may also be found in the chronic condition. Acute osteomyelitis is identified, usually within the first 6 weeks, when signs of acute inflammation, periostitis, and radiolucency are present. Later in the disease course, the term *chronic* is used when involucra, sequestra, radiolucency with surrounding radiodensity, and sinuses or fistulae are formed. Chronic osteomyelitis may also be designated as active or inactive (dormant). The terms *acute* and *chronic* would appear to describe opposite ends of disease progression; however, histological differentiation of the two conditions can be difficult. Additional designations such as *subacute* do not provide any additional information that would change treatment or expected outcome and can even cause more difficulty.

SOURCE OF INFECTION

The onset of haematogenous osteomyelitis may follow slight trauma. In some cases careful enquiry may elicit a history of some general blood infection preceding the injury, since the vast majority are examples of a blood-borne infection. The bacteraemia, however, is of a mild type and often its presence is unnoticed. The organisms may have passed into the blood from the tonsils, the lungs, the middle ear, the intestinal canal, genitourinary tract, or from excoriations, bruises, small wounds or suppurations in the skin.

Certain fevers strongly predispose to the disease by preparing the 'soil' for the growth of pyogenic bacteria. Smallpox, malaria, scarlet fever, measles, diphtheria and influenza, for example, all lessen the vital resistance of bone marrow and favour the development of pyogenic organisms. Typhoid fever is not uncommonly followed by chronic osteomyelitis due solely to the typhoid bacillus, but if pyogenic infection is superadded, acute osteomyelitis results. The resistance of marrow is also lessened by such diseases as leukaemias, lymphomas, diabetes and neutropenia secondary to steroid therapy in rheumatoid arthritis.

When the organisms are introduced directly through a wound, as in a compound fracture, the suppurative process invades the bone at the point where it is in contact with infected tissue, but ultimately the whole length and thickness may be attacked.

BACTERIOLOGY

The most common infecting organism is *Staphylococcus aureus*. Sometimes *Streptomyces albus* may be found, in which case the symptoms are less acute. The streptococcus occurs less frequently and is more apt to produce multiple lesions than the other organisms. When the bone is directly infected – from septic wounds – a greater variety of organisms is likely to be present than in blood-borne infections. In addition to those already mentioned, *Escherichia coli* and *Clostridium welchii* may be found, particularly in cases where the original injury was a compound fracture. The pneumococcus is occasionally isolated and is less virulent than the staphylococcus or the streptococcus. Typhoid osteomyelitis is not uncommon, especially in the bodies of the vertebrae and ribs, but gonococcus is rarely found.

The susceptibility of children with sickle cell disease to salmonella osteomyelitis has been well described. Even so, the clinical features of thrombotic marrow crises have to be differentiated from those of mild pyrexia, bone pain and tenderness which precede the clinical and radiographic signs of bone infections. Stool and blood should be cultured for the organisms, in order to begin the appropriate chemotherapeutic drugs as soon a possible (Engh *et al*., 1971). These workers have described the distinguishing radiographic findings as longitudinal, intracortical diaphyseal fissuring, overabundant involucrum formation, and the involvement of multiple and often symmetrical diaphyseal sites (Figure 9.1). In their 10 patients (7 with SS haemoglobin, 2 with S thalassaemia, and 1 with SC haemoglobin), *Salmonella typhimurium*, *Escherichia coli* and *Haemophilus influenzae* were found. These workers also emphasized the efficacy and complications of chloramphenicol therapy.

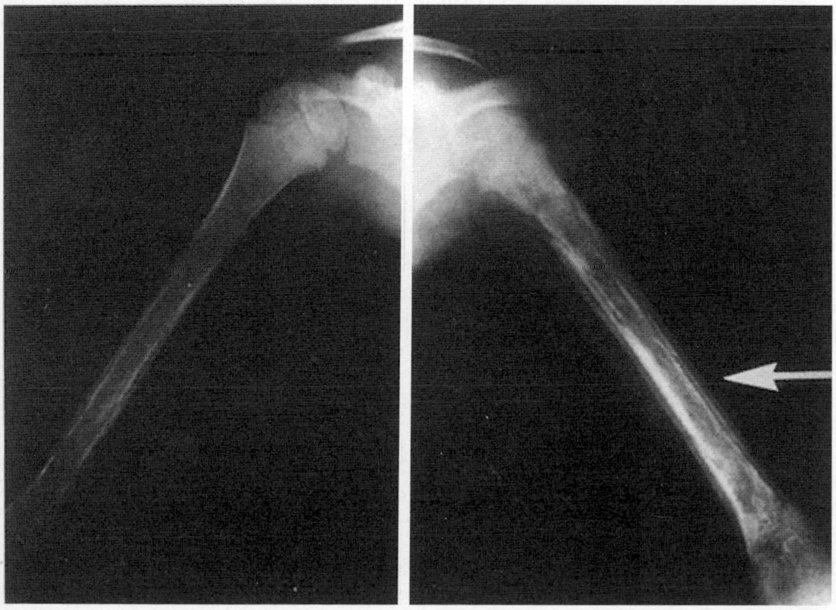

Figure 9.1 Salmonella osteomyelitis with spread from metaphysis to diaphysis.

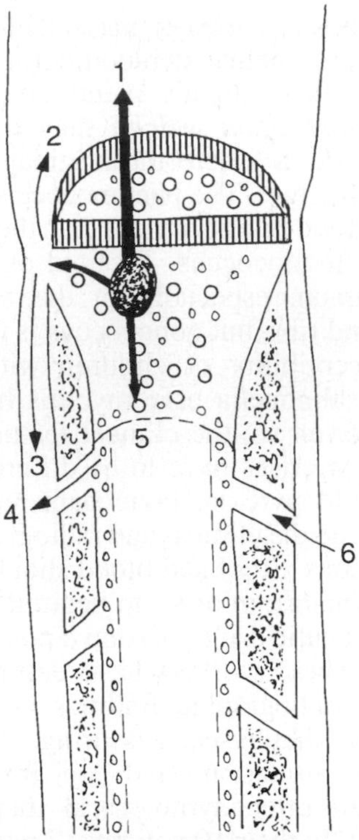

Figure 9.2 Osteomyelitis. The methods of spread (after Platt): 1 and 2, into the joint; 3 and 4, into the subperiosteal space: 5 and 6, into the medulla.

Localizing influences

It is universally agreed that a mild bacteraemia precedes the actual onset of the disease in the metaphysis (Figure 9.2). The vascular arrangements in the metaphysis, and the influence of trauma, are held to be important factors, but the work of Hobo (1921) indicated that lack of active phagocytosis in the metaphysis is of even greater import. It has been pointed out (Duthie and Barker, 1955) that the anatomical arrangement at the epiphyseometaphyseal junction favours localization of bacteria. They described the up-growth of thin-walled primitive blood vessels in between the trabeculae of degenerating cartilage cells and suggested the passage outwards of bacteria during a bacteraemia, into a perfect culture of degenerating cells.

A preceding trauma has an important localizing influence. The usual type of injury is in the nature of an epiphyseal strain. The effect of the trauma is to cause haemorrhage and cell destruction in the region of the epiphyseal cartilage, followed by diminished tissue resistance.

Children are continually receiving slight injuries of this kind, and as they are to some extent painful, there may be definite limitation of the function of the part from protective muscle spasm; in the lower limb, for example, there may be a distinct limp.

Route of infection

The bone may become infected through the blood stream, through the lymph stream, by direct continuity from a neighbouring focus of infection, or by direct inoculation from the body surface. Blood stream infection is by far the commonest, although with the greater frequency of compound fractures and accidental wounds, direct infections are becoming more common.

Incidence of the disease

Careful statistics show that osteomyelitis is a disappearing disease. In spite of this, however, it appears that the condition comes in definite epidemics. It was believed that these epidemics were coincident with a state of staphylococcal infection in the upper respiratory passages. The lessened incidence is explained by the improvement in the general health and in the housing and sanitary arrangements of the people. The disease is commonest during the period of active bone growth; the maximum incidence is therefore between 3 and 15 years of age. The responsible factors are the greater liability to trauma and the frequency of mild bacteraemia at this time of life. Boys are more liable to osteomyelitis than girls, in a proportion of about 4 to 1.

The bones of the lower extremity are more often affected, and, of these, the tibia suffers most frequently. The upper end of the tibia is more commonly involved than the lower end; in the femur, the lower end – the trigone – is the site of election. The greater amount of growing bone at these areas explains their greater liability to infection. The later the epiphysis joins the shaft, the longer the metaphysis persists in a state of activity, and the greater its liability to become infected.

PATHOLOGY

As the bacteria multiply in the metaphyseal locus an inflammatory oedema is set up in the cavity, so that in time the exits and the entrances are completely blocked and what is virtually an abscess results. The focus enlarges, until it appears to the naked eye as a circular patch of oedematous and congested marrow. Microscopically an accumulation of polymorphonuclear leucocytes can be seen around the congested vessels.

Depending to some extent on the type and virulence of the organism, the disease may take one of three courses:

1. When the patient displays a good resistance or the infection is a mild one, the reaction in the

surrounding tissue may be powerful enough to eradicate the organisms before suppuration occurs.

2. When conditions are slightly less favourable – i.e., when the organisms are more virulent, or the phagocytic power less – a chronic, or Brodie's, abscess may form.
3. The usual sequence of a pyogenic inflammation may occur, the congestion being followed by suppuration and sequestration. Prostaglandins E and F_2 are released along with cathepsins and are responsible for the bone destruction (Dekel and Francis, 1981).

When the disease follows either of the first two courses the acute illness gradually abates. Should a Brodie's abscess be formed, the organisms sometimes retain their vitality for a considerable time, and under certain circumstances may undergo a recrudescence of activity. In the centre of the cancellous tissue, a cavity filled with thick pus develops, and, owing to the chronic nature of the disease, the surrounding bone is sclerosed and condensed.

On microscopy, there are areas of necrosis with debris, characteristic cells of the particular organism (e.g. polymorphonuclear leucocytes, lymphocytes, plasma cells and macrophages) in among areas of dead bone with empty lacunae (Figure 9.3). In other cases, new bone formation with osteoblastic activity may be seen.

Usual course of the disease

From the primary focus in the vascular cancellous tissue of the metaphysis, the infection is generally believed to spread with great rapidity to the medullary canal, so that, in a short time, the whole interior of the shaft may be filled with pus. The infection then spreads through the Haversian canals to the periosteum, which is eventually undermined and stripped from the bone by an inflammatory effusion constituting a subperiosteal abscess. The pus is greenish, and may occupy the whole shaft from epiphysis to epiphysis; it may, however, remain limited as a comparatively small focus in the metaphysis, the extent depending upon the intensity of the infection and the patient's resistance.

A large area of cancellous tissue consequently undergoes necrosis, with the formation of sequestra. The compact surface bone is at first more resistant but when the periosteum is raised, its main source of blood supply – the periosteal vessels – is cut off and its vitality impaired. If the pus encircles the shaft, necrosis and sequestration of the entire circumference may ensue, forming the so-called tubular sequestrum. Otherwise the sequestrum consists usually of a portion of the outer layer of the cortex and is more or less flake-like in nature. Should the synovial membrane of a neighbouring joint extend beyond the epiphyseal cartilage to the metaphysis, infection may extend to the joint. In this way an osteomyelitis of the trigone of the tibia may lead to suppuration within the knee joint.

Ultimately the vascularity of the periosteum increases and a deposit of new subperiosteal bone appears, which in time may completely surround the old dead shaft. This envelope of new bone is termed an involucrum, and in the early stages is soft, vascular and easily separated from the underlying bone. It is usually incomplete, owing to the perfora-

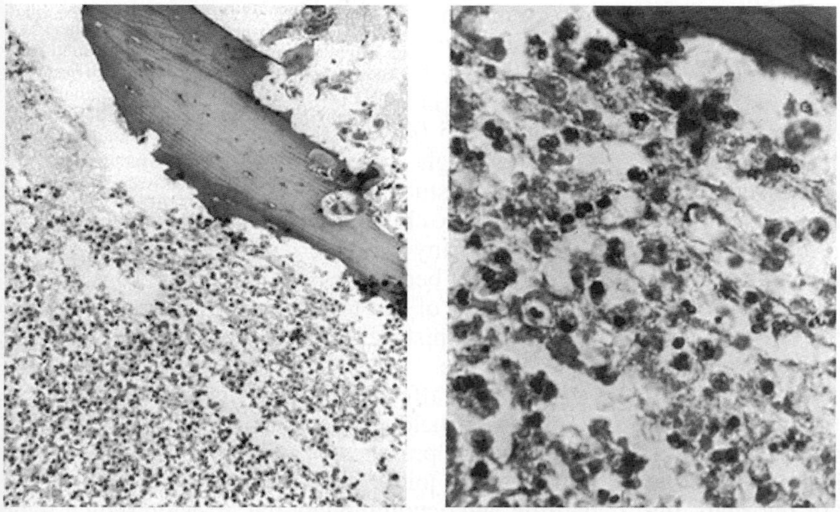

(a) (b)

Figure 9.3 (a) Photomicrograph to show trabecula of dead bone with several empty lacunae and a marked cellular infiltrate (x 70). (b) Photomicrograph showing margins of dead bone with the empty lacunae. Large numbers of mononuclear and some polymorphonuclear cells are present, with much necrotic debris indicating a chronic osteomyelitis (x 325)

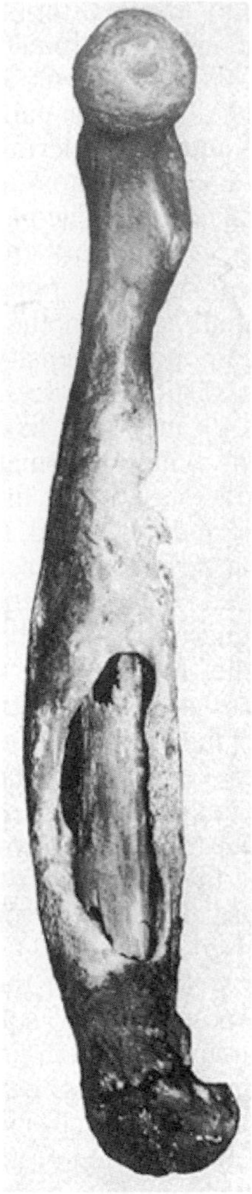

Figure 9.4 Late and untreated osteomyelitis of the femur, the disease beginning in the lower metaphysis. The original shaft has formed an extensive sequestrum.

tions which have taken place through the old periosteum, which remain as holes or 'cloacae' in the enveloping involucrum (Figure 9.4).

In the endosteal areas, a similar reaction occurs and vascular granulation tissue forms on the surface of the still-living bone, between it and the sequestrum. In time it produces separation of the sequestrum, or even absorption should the necrotic bone be small enough. The smaller cortical sequestra may be spontaneously discharged through the cloacae and thence to the surface by way of sinuses through the soft tissues and skin. Large sequestra take a long time to be extruded and the sinuses persist for a very long time. This is one of the reasons for the long duration of convalescence from an attack of osteomyelitis. Another commoner cause of persistent sinus is the presence of a cavity in the interior of the shaft, the walls of which, being rigid, cannot collapse, and which is so deep that the soft tissues cannot fill it up.

Variations with age

The description given is typical for classic osteomyelitis of childhood. However, osteomyelitis may occur at any age. Its clinical and pathological features are different in the infant and the adult.

Trueta (1959) pointed out that the infant under 6 months of age frequently has vascular communication through the epiphyseal growth plate from the metaphysis to the epiphysis. Hence, spread of infection into joints occurs more frequently at this age, and serious involvement and destruction of the epiphysis may ensue. The periosteum is elevated with ease in these babies, to form large involucra. However, because of the growth and bone remodelling potential at this age, little may remain in later life of these gross bony changes.

The adult, like the infant, has re-established vascular connections to the juxta-articular regions and has a higher incidence of secondary septic arthritis. However, the periosteum in the adult is thin and is elevated with greater difficulty from the underlying cortical bone. The adult does not produce large subperiosteal abscesses and instead the pus bursts through the periosteum to produce multiple soft tissue abscesses. Owing to the overall decreased vascularity and much-reduced powers of remodelling, sequestra formation with chronic infection is common.

CLINICAL FEATURES

In the acute stages the child has all the appearances of a severe general illness. He is flushed and restless and complains of headache. The tongue is dry and furred, and vomiting may occur. The pulse rate is high – it may be as much as 120 or 140 – there is marked pyrexia and a leucocytosis which may reach as high as 25 000 cells. The ESR (Westergren) is often very high – e.g. 60 mm in 1 hour – and is of great help in studying the response of the disease to treatment. The child is apprehensive in case the limb should be in any way interfered with. He may object even to the bedclothes being touched. With the development of the toxaemia, however, his apprehension diminishes; he becomes apathetic and finally comatose.

When the affected limb is inspected, it will be found to be held in the position which exerts the minimum of pressure on the inflamed bone. The neighbouring joints are flexed, in order to relax the capsule and accommodate the effusion which they constantly contain. In the early stages no swelling is apparent, but such quickly becomes evident when a subperiosteal effusion has occurred. Reddening of the skin is a late sign; when present, it is localized, like the swelling, to the affected metaphysis. Handling the limb elicits extreme pain, the maximum point of tenderness being situated over the original focus.

In early cases of osteomyelitis, the various bones have specific points of maximum tenderness. When, for instance, the trigone of the femur is affected, it is in the popliteal space; in the case of the head of the tibia it is usually on the anteromedial aspect. When an abscess has formed under the periosteum, it may be possible to detect fluctuation. If the neighbouring joint can be moved without increasing the pain, septic arthritis can be excluded.

On x-ray, Baylin and Glenn (1948) pointed out some soft tissue changes which appear within the first 48 hours. These are a loss of the normal demarcation line between the subcutaneous shadows and muscles, and the appearance of transverse lines of increased densities extending outward from the muscles (Figure 9.5). These changes tend to disappear once there is clinical evidence of breakthrough of one of the cortices (Figure 9.6). White and Dennison (1952) described how periosteal new bone formation is seen within 10–12 days after onset, this change being followed by demineralization in the metaphysis. This is the most reliable of early radiological signs. MRI and CT scanning will help to delineate intramedullary and soft tissue involvement.

CULTURE TECHNIQUES

Perry *et al.* (1991) have compared the efficiency of swabbing of the superficial wound, of needle biopsy and of material obtained during debridement from patients with post-traumatic or postoperative osteomyelitis. Swabbing and needles biopsy were inadequate for determining the presence of aerobic or anaerobic organisms and therefore debridement material should be obtained for culture if all pathogens are to be identified. Additional advantages of such material are that it is suitable for determining fungal infections and for the rare local epidermoid carcinoma. A negative needle biopsy for growth on culture does not rule out sealed pockets of microenvironments of infection and live bacteria. Numerous cultures taken from different sites are essential, stopping the administration of antibiotics for at least 2 weeks before the procedure.

Special testing of white blood cells for leukergy

Leukergy is seen when white blood cells agglomerate in the peripheral venous blood. Fleck first observed this phenomenon in metabolic disorders associated with burns, acute pancreatitis, polycythaemia rubra, some rheumatic disorders and ischaemic heart disease.

Otremski *et al.* (1993) have applied it to diagnosing and monitoring early sepsis of bone. They found

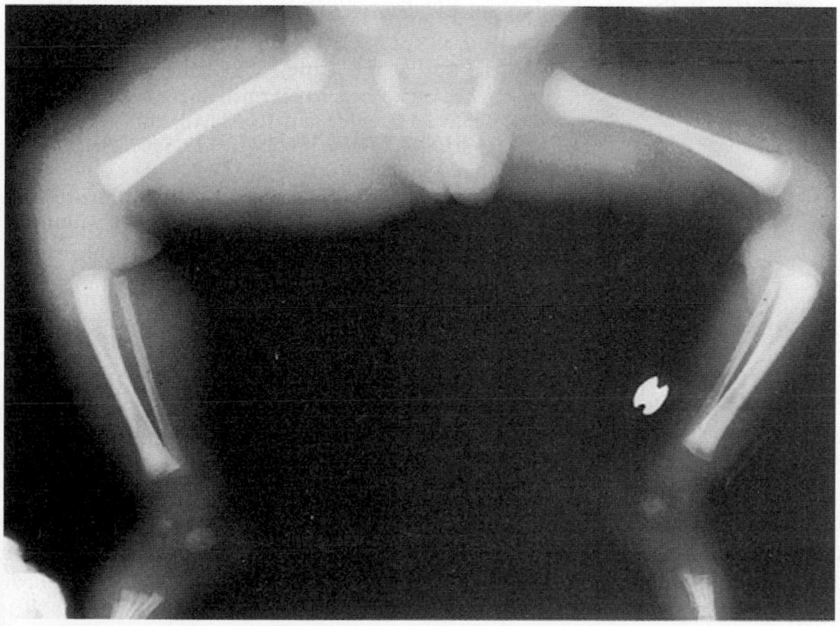

Figure 9.5 Anteroposterior radiograph of the hips and legs of a 2-month-old child with an obvious swelling of the right thigh. The thigh was swollen and tender but the radiograph shows no bony change, and a clinical diagnosis of osteomyelitis was made.

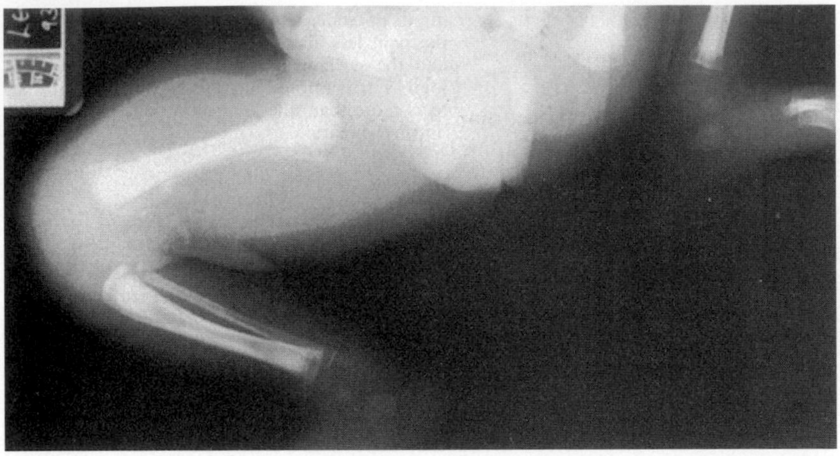

Figure 9.6 Same patient as in Figure 9.5 after 10 days. Extensive subperiosteal new bone formation is seen along the femur.

it to be more accurate than ESR, white blood count or blood culture. The test also detected reactivation of the septic process better than other haematological tests, as well as detecting the eradication of infection. It has been suggested that circulating mediators released during bacteraemia may lead to increased sensitivity of the adhesive properties in white blood cells.

C-reactive protein levels in association with white cell counts and the erythrocyte sedimentation rate have been shown by Unkila-Kallio *et al.* (1994) to be of value in helping to differentiate acute haematogenous osteomyelitis and septic arthritis when associated or not. If a child with clinical features of osteomyelitis has a moderately raised WBC and an elevated CRP level which after admission increases twofold there is a strong possibility that the osteomyelitis is associated with a septic arthritis. If the CRP level does not drop with treatment, septic arthritis should be suspected.

Changes in the ESR gave similar conclusions but much later, e.g. 5–14 days after admission.

DIFFERENTIAL DIAGNOSIS

There are certain conditions which are liable to be confused with acute osteomyelitis.

Acute rheumatism

In acute rheumatism, as in osteomyelitis, there are both pain and swelling, and also sharply localized points of tenderness. However, the onset is more gradual, the pain less acute and more definitely articular, and the swelling confined more definitely to the joint. Furthermore, acute rheumatism usually affects more than one joint at the same time and is 'flitting' in nature.

Erysipelas

Osteomyelitis may be mistaken for erysipelas because of the redness of the skin, but in the latter there is less pain and general toxaemia. In erysipelas the definitely raised margin of the red area is significant.

Haemophilia

A muscle bleed or bleed into a joint will produce marked local pain and tenderness, with general malaise and even fever. A bleeding diathesis should be enquired about and looked for.

Cellulitis

Streptococcal cellulitis in the region of the metaphysis should always suggest osteomyelitis, but in pure cellulitis there is no intense pain and the general malaise is less.

Acute pyogenic arthritis

An acute arthritis sometimes leads to confusion, but the manifestations in the joint are usually sufficient to differentiate the two conditions. In acute arthritis, spasm of the muscles is more marked, movements at the joint are more limited and effusion into the joint space is of earlier onset than in osteomyelitis.

Ewing's tumour or osteosarcoma

These have a much less intense general illness – there is little in the way of local inflammatory reaction. The radiological signs in the metaphysis or diaphysis are obvious much earlier than in osteomyelitis.

PROGNOSIS

Osteomyelitis is a dangerous disease, and before the introduction of modern chemotherapeutic drugs, the prognosis was grave. White and Dennison (1952) reported from their series that there was a 36% mortality rate before the introduction of antibiotics, 12.7% with the use of sulphonamides and 1.2% mortality with penicillin. Chemotherapy has practically eliminated the danger of death from acute osteomyelitis. One is now concerned with the morbidity rather than mortality. Delay in initiating treatment or in the timing of drainage, if indicated, carries the danger of avascular necrosis of bone, chronic abscess formation within the bone (Brodie's abscess) and the possibility of periodic reactivation of the infection throughout life (Figure 9.7). About 90% of cases diagnosed early and treated energetically may be expected to resolve completely without leaving either pathological or surgical complications. The remarkable alteration in the prognosis of acute haematogenous osteomyelitis makes it justifiable to regard penicillin as the greatest advance that has yet been introduced in the treatment of this disease.

Certain factors have a decided influence on the prognosis:

1. *The organism.* Infection by *Staphylococcus aureus* is the most serious and usual type, affecting 70–85% of all patients.
2. *The bone infected.* The nearer to the trunk the affected bone, the more serious is the prognosis.
3. *The age of the patient.* The younger the child, the outlook can be grave not only for life but for destruction of bone and epiphyses.

TREATMENT

Until modern chemotherapy permitted a different approach to treatment, most experienced clinicians advised immediate and thorough drainage with wide opening of the cortex as soon as the diagnosis was made (Figure 9.8).

Osteomyelitis is only part of a general infection and, therefore, immediate intravenous chemotherapy using ampicillin and cloxacillin is started. As the presence of pus within bone or in a subperiosteal abscess is an early and constant feature of osteomyelitis in children, aspiration at the most tender part of the diaphysis is attempted. Aspiration serves several purposes. It confirms the bacteriological diagnosis and sensitivities, allows recognition of the infecting organism and its antibiotic sensitivity prevents the further stripping of periosteum, preserving the blood supply of the bone, and removes a space which penicillin can reach from the blood stream only with difficulty. A blood culture should also be set up to identify the causative organism. This will be especially useful if there is difficulty in tapping a superficial abscess although it is positive in only 70% of cases (Mollan and Piggot, 1977). Indeed, if there is failure – systemically or locally – to the chemotherapy within 24 hours after starting such treatment, it is recommended that an operation

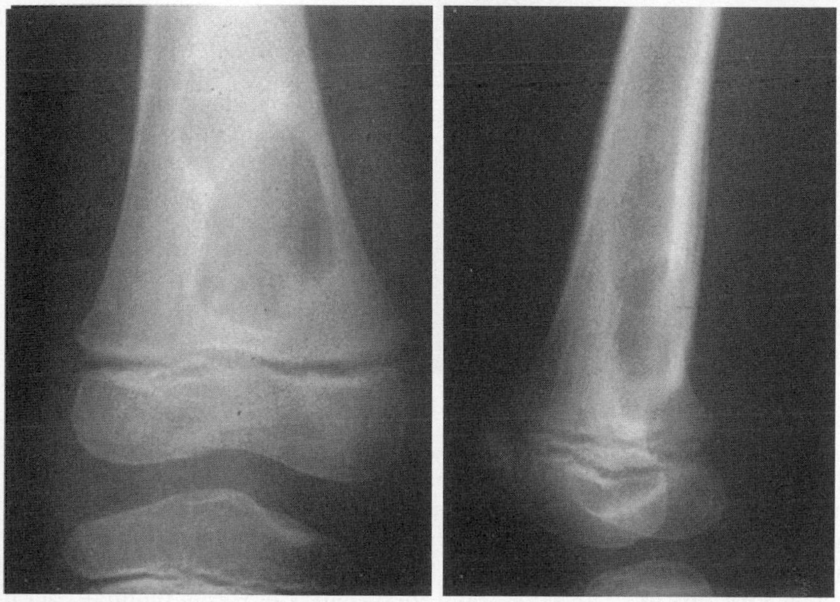

(a) (b)

Figure 9.7 Radiographs of the lower end of the femur of an adolescent girl, showing radiolucent confluent areas of a chronic osteomyelitis with periosteal reaction over the posterior surface.

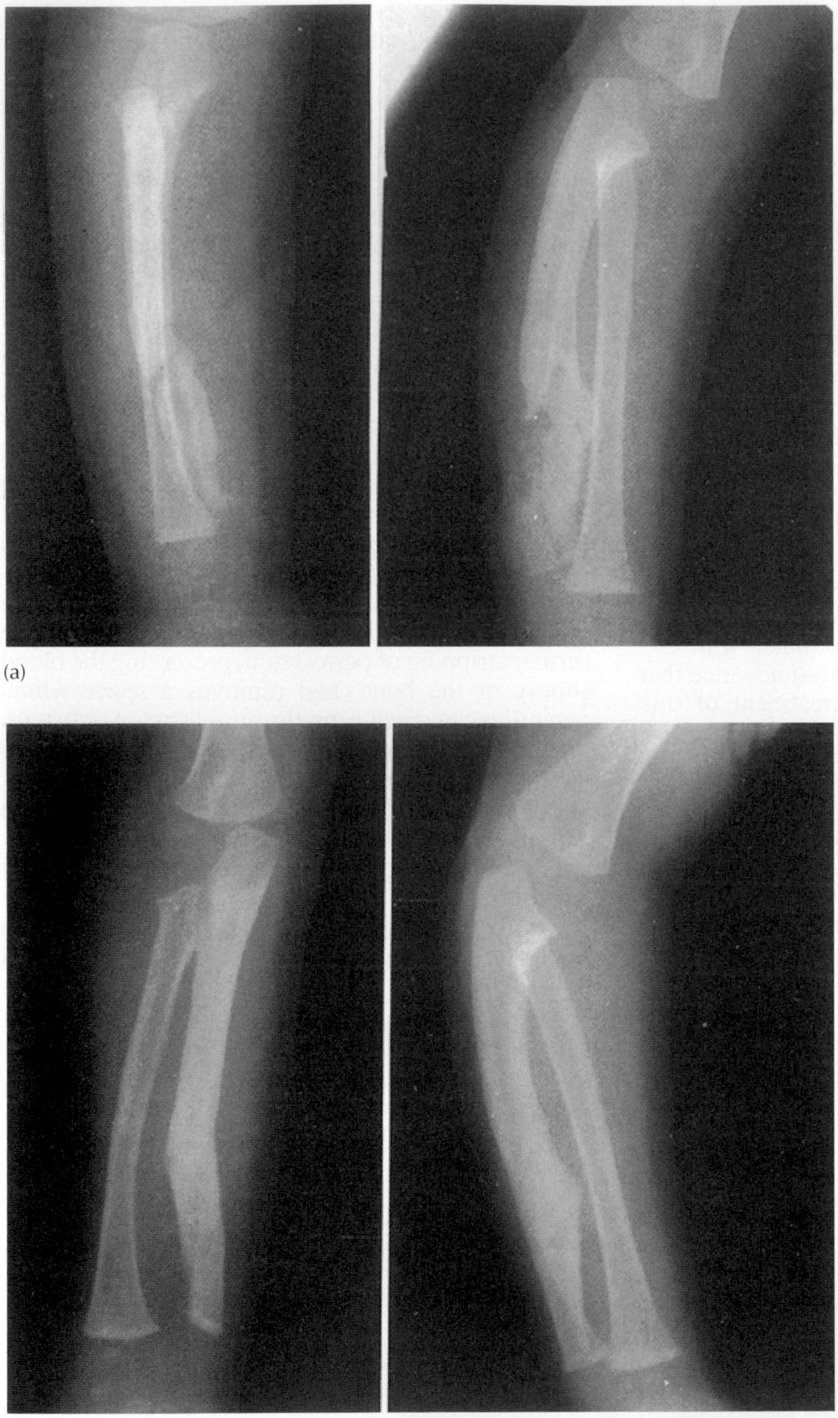

(a)

(b)

Figure 9.8 (a) Radiographs showing a chronic osteomyelitis affecting the distal third of the ulnar bone, with marked periosteal reaction and new bone formation extending up the whole diaphysis as well as destruction of bone. (b) Three months later, after debridement and chemotherapy, showing the healing and remodelling of bone which has taken place.

should be carried out. This consists of multiple drillings away from the epiphyseal line down through the diaphysis until pus-free marrow is obtained. Periosteum should be not stripped off or elevated because this will add to the ischaemia of the cortex as well as opening up further tissue planes for pus to traverse. The wound should be closed primarily to prevent secondary infection and sinus formation.

There has been much discussion about the place of surgery in early, acute osteomyelitis or haematogenous osteitis. Adequate chemotherapy when given early enough has certainly proved to be the method of choice and surgery may never be required, but if there have been localizing signs for over 48 hours and no clinical improvement after 24 hours of antibiotics, drilling must be carried out. The advantages of such treatments are to give an adequate diagnosis of the organism and its sensitivity, and also to reduce vascular damage and bone necrosis (Harris, 1962). Although Blockey and McAllister (1972) believe that most cases can be treated with antibiotics alone, their results were limited to a 1-year follow-up. It is well recognized that flare-up can occur after this length of time.

Immobilization in a cast promotes pain relief and healing and should be carried out for 4 weeks.

Treatment of the general condition

Antibiotics and anti-inflammatory drugs

It is most important to begin antibiotic treatment as soon as the essential investigations have been performed. A combination of flucloxacillin and ampicillin given intravenously will combat most organisms. This combination should continue until blood cultures and sensitivities are available, when a change may be made if necessary. Intravenous antibiotics should continue until the patient responds clinically by the resolution of pyrexia and the disappearance of local swelling, redness and tenderness. Oral antibiotics should be continued for 6 weeks even when clinical progress to recovery is uncomplicated. The ESR, monitored at weekly intervals, indicates overall response. The role of anti-inflammatory drugs in counteracting prostaglandin E and F_2 and thus reducing bone destruction is not established clinically although animal experiments suggest that such treatment may be beneficial in future (Dekel *et al.*, 1980).

Hydration and electrolyte replacement

This must be active with a definite attempt to keep the body in physiological balance.

Protein replacement

Because the patients are extremely ill their protein intake is inadequate. The increased metabolism caused by the disease results in destruction of tissue. The organisms, usually haemolytic, destroy blood cells and a severe anaemia may appear, requiring blood transfusions.

Immobilization

One of the most important of all therapeutic measures is immobilization of an affected extremity to prevent or decrease spread of the infection by reducing the muscle action and blood flow. This is carried out with a compression bandage and a plaster-of-Paris slab, and a window may be cut to observe the local condition. Effective splinting may be continued after the acute stage has passed to prevent deformity arising from contractures and to keep joints in a good functioning position if there is any likelihood of ankylosis occurring – for a period of about 2 weeks.

Treatment of the chronic stage

The chronic stage is marked by the persistence of sinuses and by the repeated breaking down of wounds apparently healed. Three factors are responsible for these:

1. The presence of unabsorbed and retained sequestra.
2. The presence of unobliterated cavities.
3. The change of aerobic cocci infection to Gram-negative (e.g. *E. coli*, *Enterobacter*, *Pseudomonas aeruginosa* and *Proteus* or anaerobes such as *Bacteroides*).

The treatment of the chronic stage is directed to the eradication of these conditions. The operations adopted at this stage of the disease, unlike those appropriate to the early acute stages, are not emergency measures designed to save life. They are methodical and sometimes tedious undertakings, which, if incomplete or lacking in thoroughness, will have to be repeated at a later date.

Removal of sequestra

It is essential that all necrotic cortical bone be removed, otherwise a permanent sequestrum, enclosed by an involucrum, will result. It usually takes from 2 to 3 months before the sequestrum is isolated and separated from its bed, and at this stage it can easily be recognized in a radiograph, since it is more dense than the neighbouring bone and lies free in the cavity.

The limb is rendered bloodless by elevation and the application of a tourniquet. The area in which the sequestrum lies is then exposed by a suitable incision. The involucrum is identified and peeled off the sequestrum by blunt dissection. If the sequestration has extended beyond the limits of the original gutter, the involucrum should be incised longitudinally at either end by a knife or osteotome, and the sequestrum gently extracted. Granulations should not be curetted. If it is still pliable enough, the involucrum should be forced to collapse, so that any cavity left may be made as small as possible.

If the extent of the disease is great, operation may leave an involucrum so weak and fragile that it will be unable to support the limb. In this event the limb should be carefully supported after the operation by plaster-of-Paris or external fixation, and this should be continued until the newly formed bone is sufficiently strong to bear weight or withstand muscular contraction. Radiographs, by demonstrating the amount of new bone formation, are the most efficient indicators of this stage.

Treatment of bone cavities

The history of the case with bone cavities is depressing; there is continuous or intermittent suppuration and sinus formation with acute exacerbations, followed by re-operation and further disappointment.

Before operation on a bone cavity, a clear picture of its location should be obtained by radiography and tomography, both anteroposterior and lateral, after the injection of Lipiodol (Figure 9.9). Methylene blue injected into the sinus tracts aids a block excision.

The obstacles to healing found in chronic bone cavities are the rigid deep walls, the avascular fibrous and infected tissue in the neighbourhood, and the presence of sequestra in the cavity. The operation to deal with these elements is a sculptural procedure designed to ensure the complete removal of devitalized bone and all necrotic soft tissue, so that natural healing may take place.

Preliminary antibiotics

In the chronic stage of osteomyelitis antibiotics have not proved so successful as in the acute stage, mainly because of the difficulty of getting the drug to the part. One of the most important characteristics of the lesion is its poor blood supply. The sequestra and much of the scar tissue are avascular and therefore beyond the reach of any chemotherapeutic agent carried in the blood stream; accordingly it is little use to treat a case of chronic osteomyelitis with any antibiotic unless it is combined with a radical operative attack on the wound. Systemic antibiotics based upon suitable sensitivity, to be given 4-hourly, are begun before operation and continued for 14–28 days. It is probable that the best treatment for chronic osteomyelitis is to space the operation in the middle of a 28-day course so that the wound is saturated with the drug and sterilized so far as possible beforehand; then a radical operation is carried out, with primary closure if possible, followed by another 14 days of systemic antibiotic. If sensitivity of the *Staphylococcus aureus* to penicillin and other chemotherapeutic agents is reduced and they become resistant, other more sensitive agents are given.

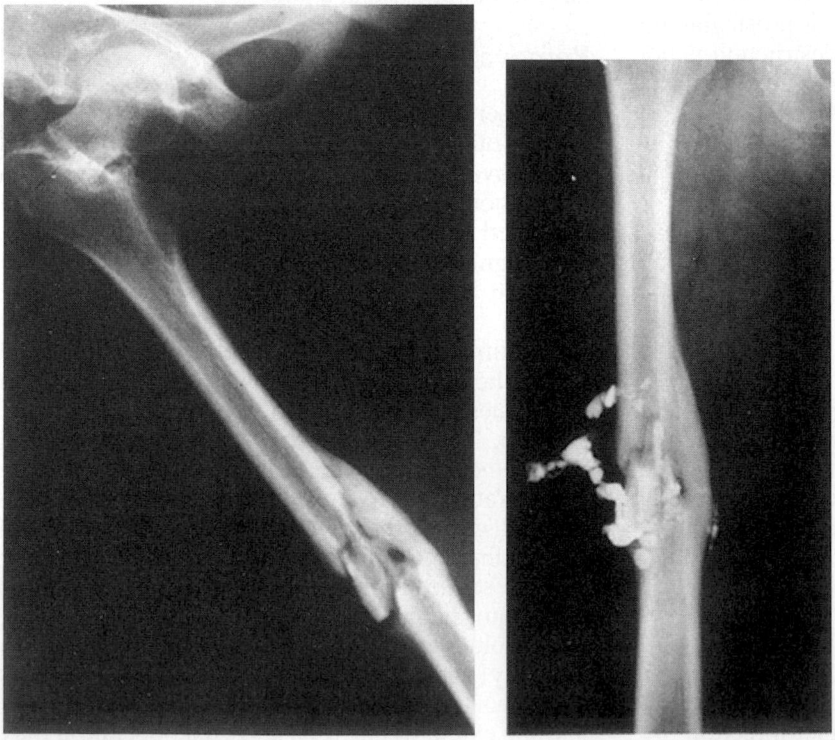

(a) (b)

Figure 9.9 (a) Chronic osteomyelitis following compound fracture of the mid-shaft of the femur. There is also a non-union of the fracture at the base of the neck. (b) Sinogram leading to area of involvement in chronic osteomyelitis.

The operation

An adequate approach is used and extends well into normal tissue, both proximal and distal to the lesion, to allow complete visualization of the diseased tissue, and preservation of important nervous and other structures. All abnormal tissue – sinus tracts and infected granulation tissue, sequestra, eburnated or abnormal bone – is removed radically so that all remaining tissue appears normal and has a good blood supply. Where the cavity is a deep one with high walls, these are gouged or nibbled away to convert the cavity more into the shape of a saucer – hence the name sometimes used of saucerization.

Primary closure of the skin and superficial fascia over the wound should be done. However, if it is under too much tension, the wound may be packed open and dressings continued until there is healthy granulation tissue – when skin grafting can be applied. The limb is placed in a plaster-of-Paris cast and kept in a somewhat elevated position for 3–4 days. In shallow cavities saucerization may be sufficient to produce healing, but in most cases more is required and there are two ways in which the cavity may be filled up, as follows:

1. *Muscle filling.* The bone defect, if shallow, may be obliterated by slight displacement of surrounding muscles; if deep, a muscle pedicle is formed, the gap filled and the flap sutured into the defect.
2. *Bone-fragments filling.* The cavity is filled with cancellous bone fragments from the ilium in those cases where muscle tissue is not available for filling. This method is often done in two stages, the first step being the complete excision of infected and avascular tissue as described. In 10 days' time, when the defect is covered by a thin layer of healthy granulation tissue, the second stage is carried out. Cancellous fragments are removed from the iliac crest and the iliac wound is closed and dressed. The bone defect is now exposed and gently irrigated with normal saline. The grafts are placed in the defect till it is filled. The soft tissue and skin are closed and the part is immobilized in plaster. Closed suction-irrigation drainage with isotonic saline is popular but there is no proven need for detergents or any antibacterial drugs.

COMPLICATIONS

The most important complication of acute osteomyelitis is the development of chronic osteomyelitis, although this occurs in only 5–10% of cases treated promptly and energetically. Septic arthritis of the hip remains an ever-present risk following osteomyelitis of the upper femur even with modern treatment, but metastatic infection is rare.

Chronic osteomyelitis, once established, is liable to the following complications over and above recurrent flares of the infection:

1. Pathological fracture – sometimes resulting in amputation of a major weight-bearing bone. A pathological fracture with infection is still a major hazard to maintaining the limb, especially when there is bone loss. The Papineau treatment is recommended, consisting of:
   - stabilizing the bony fragments by an external fixator device – e.g. the Wagner or Oxford apparatus;
   - extensive debridement;
   - continuous irrigation of the bed with isotonic saline;
   - cancellous bone grafting, with repeat debridement when necessary, onto healthy granulation tissue; and

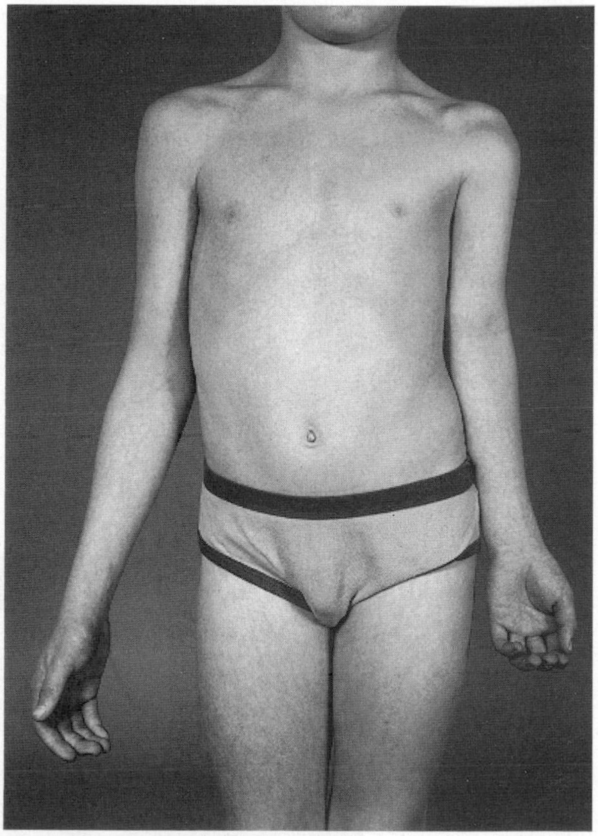

Figure 9.10 Photograph of a 10-year-old boy who had osteomyelitis at the age of 2 years involving the distal humeral epiphysis. This had resulted in marked foreshortening of the left humerus but fortunately the elbow joint had good function.

- secondary skin closure by grafting or transfer. This procedure has reduced the requirement for amputation in un-united infected fractures (Roy-Camille *et al.*, 1976).

2. Epithelioma – to be suspected when a long-standing infection with a quiescent sinus breaks down. Osteomyelitis in infants can spread from the metaphysis to destroy the epiphysis, resulting in a marked longitudinal growth deficiency of a long bone (Figure 9.10). Osteomyelitis can spread and metatasize within the same bone, e.g. the tibia, involving soft tissues, sinus formation

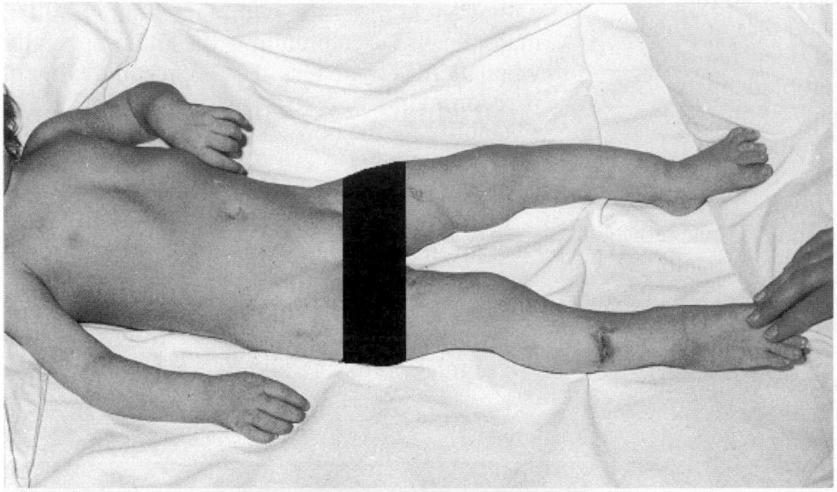

(a)

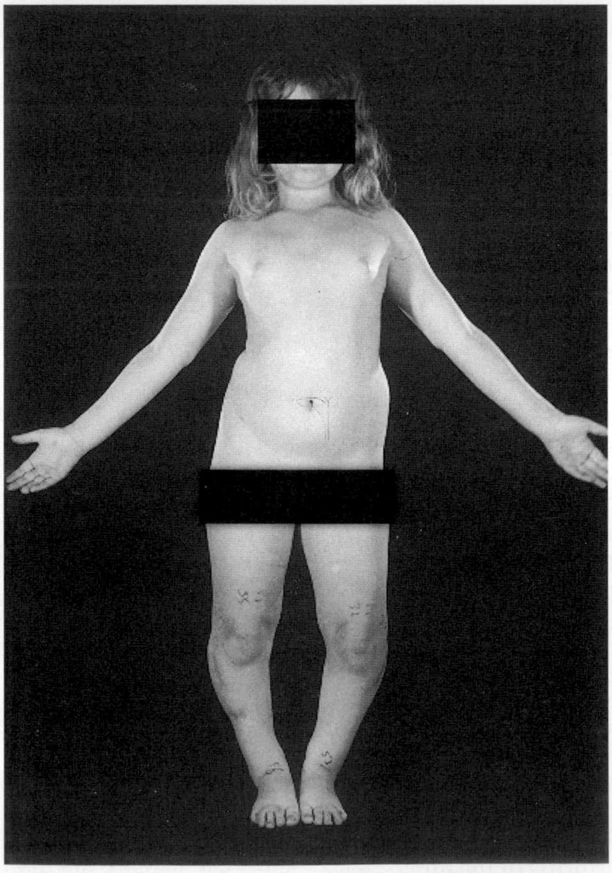

(b)

Figure 9.11 (a) Photograph of an 18-month-old child with a healed right mid-tibial sinus tract overlying a tibial osteomyelitis with healed lesions in both thighs.
(b) Photograph of the same child at the age of 7 years showing the severe tibial varus deformities and loss of leg length.

with marked growth disturbances (Figure 9.11).
3. Growth interference (5% overgrowth, 31% growth arrest, 64% undisturbed) – especially when the upper femur is involved. (Figures 9.10, 9.11).
4. Amyloid disease.

Chronic osteomyelitis requires thorough investigation for the ongoing infection by Tc99 bone scanning, CT scanning for sequestra which may not be visible on radiography by blood examinations for anaemia, raised ESR and CPR and in the presence of a pyrexia blood cultures for a bacteraemia. Accurate bacteriology and sensitivities must be carried out for adequate intravenous chemotherapy before, during and after surgery. In certain circumstances, after removal of segmental involocra, saucerization with deroofing of cavities, removal of sequestrum is carried out, leaving the wound open, but closing muscle. Antibiotic impregnated beads can be left in for up to 3 weeks. Myocutaneous flaps with improvement of the blood supply to the cavities may sometimes be required.

Neonatal osteomyelitis requires early recognition but is obviously difficult in such a young age group. Lethargy, going off feeding, swelling and a pseudoparalysis of the affected limb are the presenting features. Prematurity, skin umbilical sepsis and caesarean delivery are predisposing factors (Jellis, 1992a,b).

Staph. aureus is usually the causative organism but *Streptococcus pneumoniae* and *Haemophilus influenzae* also give rise to a significant number of cases. The upper end of the femur, accompanied by a septic arthritis of thc hip, is the usual site. Characteristic bone changes are seen on radiography with loss of the femoral capital epiphysis and/or subluxation of the hip.

Intravenous antibiotics with an early arthrotomy and drainage is necessary with immobilization on an abduction frame and light traction.

Osteomyelitis in HIV disease

Jellis (1992a) has described how osteomyelitis in adults with HIV infection is now common in Africa. There is comparative lack of new periosteal bone formation with much necrosis even though the usual organism is *Staph. aureus* or *Salmonella* or other Gram-negative organisms. The bones usually affected are upper tibia and lower femur but the disease is often bilateral and septic arthritis common. Treatment consists of antibiotics, drainage and immobilization, but with a poor prognosis for eradication of the bone infection.

UNUSUAL EXPRESSIONS OF OSTEOMYELITIS

Boeck's sarcoidosis

This is an inflammatory disease, granulomatous in nature, which affects primarily the organs of the reticuloendothelial system; i.e. the spleen, lymph nodes, the liver, and also the lungs and bones. Its cause is unknown, but has never been proved to be any form of tuberculosis.

The bones most commonly affected are the short miniature bones (i.e. the metacarpals, metatarsals, etc.), with rare involvement of the long bones. The bone changes are usually found on x-raying a patient who presents with a lymphadenopathy or pulmonary disease. The radiographs show small areas of bone destruction and expansion of the cortex and/or a pulmonary infection. Biochemically there are often changes found in the serum calcium and alkaline phosphatase which are raised because of a vitamin-D-like action by some substance secreted which is possibly by the sarcoid tissues, but may be elevated because of the disease in the liver. Indeed, the hypercalcaemia may lead to urinary calculi formation. There may be a reversal of the albumin/globulin ratio with a raised globulin level. The Nickerson–Kveim skin test is positive.

On microscopy, it is a granulomatous lesion of macrophages, epithelioid cells and giant cells. The caseation of tuberculosis is never seen, although some necrosis of tissue can be produced. The prognosis is relatively good although infection of the lungs or kidneys may, rarely, cause death.

Sclerosing non-suppurative osteomyelitis

This was describcd by Garré in 1891. It may be present acutely with pyrexa, local pain and swelling; more often it is subacute and chronic. The temperature and soft tissue swelling subside, but osseous enlargement persists as a dense fusiform swelling. Tenderness is usually complained of on deep pressure. It has been confused with sarcoma, and it is possible that some sarcomata cured by amputation were in fact examples of this lesion. By many it is attributed to metastases from some undiscovered focus of infection. The long bones, particularly the tibia and femur, are the usual sites. A typical x-ray shows a symmetrical thickening of the cortex with some narrowing of the medulla. The bone production is on the shaft. There is no involvement of the periosteum, no bone destruction and no change in the soft tissues.

Where there is persistent pain, operation of either guttering the bone or the drilling of multiple holes through both cortices may alleviate it.

Syphilitic disease of bone

Syphilitic affections of bone occur in the inherited and acquired forms of the disease, and in the latter they are more serious in the tertiary stage. They differ from tuberculous affections in that the shaft is more frequently involved, while the joints escape. The inflammation is the result of *Treponema pallidum*, which may be demonstrated in the bone marrow 36 hours after infection and prior to the appearance of clinical evidence of disease. The granulation tissue which develops from this inflammation differs from ordinary granulation tissue in that the leucocytes are chiefly of the lymphocytic variety (Figure 9.12). This granulation tissue may develop complete resolution, especially where anti-syphilitic treatment is carried out at an early stage, but if the resolution is delayed long enough, well-formed connective tissue – either fibrous or osseous – may develop. In some cases the granulation tissue may be of such a delicate nature that it dies before any attempt at organization has occurred, and a gumma is formed because many of the vessels are occluded by the proliferation of their endothelial lining, i.e. arteritis.

The tibia, the femur, the humerus and the cranial bones, which are more exposed to extraneous influences, are the most common sites of syphilitic osseous disease.

BONE MANIFESTATIONS

Pain

This may vary from a very slight dull ache up to the most excruciating pains. Often migratory, usually intermittent and not infrequently nocturnal exacerbations interfere with sleep. There are no local abnormalities detectable by clinical or radiological examination and a diagnosis of neuralgia or neuritis is often made. Failure on the part of salicylates to give relief should lead to a suspicion of syphilis, and blood serological tests will invariably confirm this. Anti-syphilitic treatment is rapidly effective.

Periostitis

Periostitis frequently occurs and affects multiple long bones of the extremities. The bone changes may be present at birth or develop later. They are frequently asymptomatic and are often detectable only by routine radiological examination.

The periosteal node

The characteristic lesion is a localized swelling of the shaft, oval or fusiform in shape, which usually involves a portion of the circumference, and may, indeed, even surround the bone. This type of lesion is commoner in inherited syphilis but may occur in the acquired form. The bone most commonly affected is the tibia, which is often thickened for a considerable portion of its length, and usually upon its subcutaneous surface. The sharp anterior crest of the tibia is replaced by a rounded surface, and the

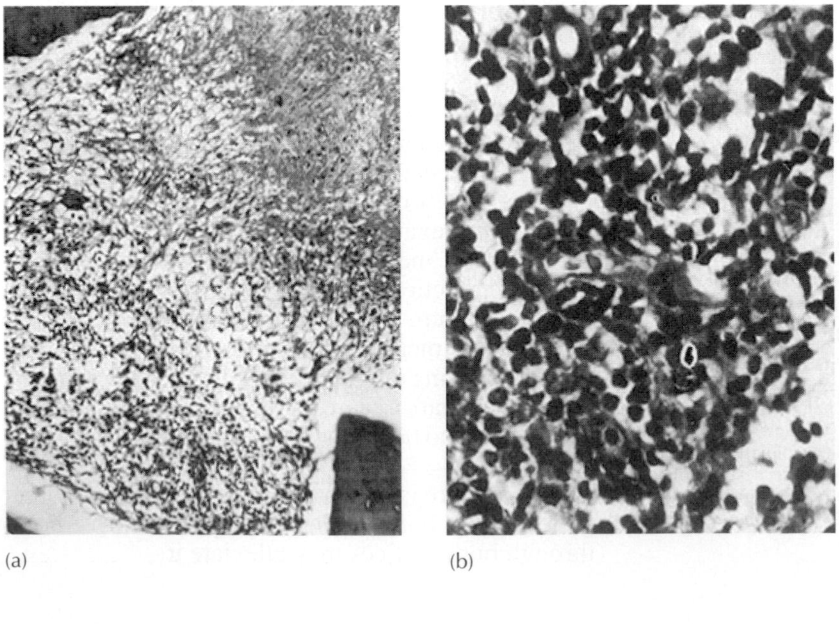

(a) (b)

Figure 9.12 (a) Photomicrograph showing replacement of marrow between two dead bone fragments by fibrous tissue stroma and numerous densely staining round cells of a gumma in bone (x 74). (b) Photomicrograph of some tissue showing the characteristic infiltrate of small round lymphocytic cells without the presence of any polymorphonucleated cells (x 390).

thickening may be so pronounced in front as to give rise to the impression that the bone has become bent. The femur, humerus and ulna may also be attacked.

Important points of differentiation between this rare curvature of the tibia and that seen in rickets are outlined (Table 9.9).

These swellings in the early days are painful, tender and firm, but rarely show any inflammatory redness. As organization of the new tissue occurs, the swelling ossifies and becomes permanent, but it soon begins to attack the bone itself and spread into it. The compact tissue underlying the node is rarefied and then the cancellous tissue adjacent is involved; lastly, the medulla of the central cavity is affected, and in due time the rarefaction gives place to a sclerosing osteitis.

Diffuse osteoperiostitis

This is a chronic inflammation affecting the whole bone, or the greater portion of it, inside its periosteal envelope.

The diffuse character of the affection is due to the permeability of the medullary tissue which fills the spaces in the bone; such a bone is heavier and harder than normal, and shows some periosteal deposit over the whole or greater part of its surface. The interior presents a uniform surface of densely sclerosed bone, involving the cancellous ends, the medullary canal, and the compact bone with its periosteal thickenings. In younger cases the epiphyses may be stimulated and a very marked increase in the length of the bone be produced.

In this osteitis, deep-seated pain in the bone is apt to be specially troublesome, and, when the patient is in bed, it may be of such a distressing and intractable character as to make life almost unbearable.

Occasionally in both of these types, on section or x-ray, a double outline is seen which is very characteristic of syphilis. A second sheath of compact bone overlies or surrounds the original compact layer, but an intervening space exists which may be filled with cancellous bone or granulation tissue. Such an appearance is due to the fact that the periosteum has been lifted from the bone by developing granulation tissue, and a fresh layer of compact bone formed on its undersurface (Figure 9.13). It should be noted that this is, most often, a bilaterally symmetrical polyostotic lesion, affecting tubular bones.

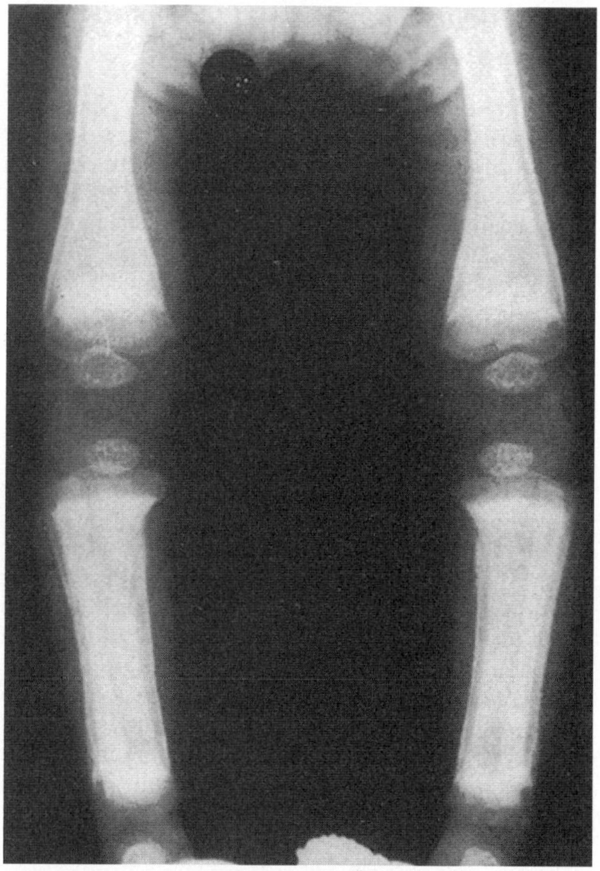

Figure 9.13 Anteposterior radiograph of both legs, showing the extensive subperiosteal new bone formation in a patient with congenital syphilis. (Courtesy of Dr N. Walker)

Table 9.9

	Rachitic curves	Syphilitic curves
Age	Generally under 3	Occurs up to 15
History	Signs of rickets present	Syphilis in parents, and signs of inherited syphilis in child
Direction of curvature	Anterolateral or anteromedial	Generally purely anterior (sabre tibia)
Position of curve	Generally in upper or lower third	Middle of shaft
Crest of tibia	Sharp	Smooth and rounded

Syphilitic inflammation at the epiphyseal line (osteochondritis)

Most children with inherited syphilis show an irregularity of the epiphyseal line. This irregularity is due to abnormal transformation of cartilage into bone, as a result of which not all the cartilage is changed into bone at the same time, but irregular lines of cartilage extend into the diaphysis.

On microscopy, the metaphysis is seen to be replaced by granulation tissue which usually passes upwards between the columns of cartilage, in the epiphysis, which, although they become more mature and calcify, fail to disintegrate and ossify. Indeed, there is an exaggerated subchondral radiolucent zone.

Epiphyseal lesions may be discovered in the early weeks of life by radiological examination, long before the appearance of localizing symptoms or signs. It should be suspected when an infant during the first half-year loses the use of one limb without apparent injury. The upper end of the humerus is the commonest part to be affected.

There is as a rule some thickening about the epiphysis, pain on passive movement, and probably other signs of syphilis. Suppuration may take place and separation of the epiphysis result, but when this occurs it is probably the result of secondary infection.

Gummatous periostitis; gummatous osteomyelitis

Syphilitic inflammation may assume the form of gumma, either on the surface of a bone or in its interior.

The surface gumma resembles an ordinary periosteal node except that it speedily softens at its centre. The skin becomes inflamed and ulcerates, and the well known tough yellow slough is exposed. The slough slowly separates and exposes the bone which is found to be bare and either carious or necrosed. Caries is due to the rarefactive influence of the granulation tissue invading the bone, and necrosis to its caseation or to secondary septic infection.

A gumma in the interior of a long bone is a serious condition because it is apt to be mistaken for a malignant tumour. It may be responsible for spontaneous fracture.

Syphilitic dactylitis

The importance of syphilis of the phalanges lies in the fact that it may be mistaken for tuberculosis. It is met with chiefly in children and affects any of the toes or fingers, but is commonest in the proximal phalanx of the index finger or thumb. More than one finger may be affected, and marked shortening and deformity result. Thickening, increased density, expansion and even absorption of a bone may take place, and open sores may form. The lesion consists of a gummatous osteomyelitis. There is little tendency to break down and ulcerate as in tuberculosis. The finger presents a fusiform swelling and though the movements are impaired the condition is usually painless. The diagnosis may be made from other signs of inherited syphilis. In its early stages the disease is amenable to anti-syphilitic treatment and complete recovery is the rule.

Congenital syphilis

Rasnool and Govender (1989) have reviewed over 190 cases and point out that although rare in the Western world, elsewhere this condition still remains a problem. It can present early up to 4 months with a generalized involvement of the liver and spleen, severe anaemia, a dermatitis or rash, fever and a pseudoparalysis due to joint swelling in the hands or knees, shoulders, elbows and wrists, pathological fractures, actual brachial plexus lesions and osteitis and joint changes after 4 years. The majority of mothers had a positive Wassermann test and most babies gave a positive fluorescent *Treponema* antibody test. The *Treponema* spirochaetes are known to cross the placental barrier after the fourth month of pregnancy.

Differential diagnosis based upon radiology, a multifocal infection of bone, or scurvy, or rickets and/or now the battered baby – child abuse syndrome.

The treatment is by high doses of penicillin over a 10–14 day course, with splintage of the involved limbs, and is usually very successful. Rasnool and Govender reviewed their cases 4 years later and there had been restoration of normal bone and joint anatomy with healing of the pathological fractures.

MISCELLANEOUS DATA REGARDING SYPHILIS OF BONE

1. The fluorescent *Treponema* IgM, IgG serological reactions are positive in all early cases and in approximately 80% of late bone lesions.
2. The ratio of syphilitic arthritis to syphilis of bone is about 1:7.
3. Radiological examination during the first 6 months of life is extremely valuable both in regard to diagnosis and to prognosis.
4. Many case histories do not support the common belief that nocturnal pain is so common as was at one time considered, but it is nevertheless important to bear it in mind.

NON-TUBERCULOUS INFECTIONS OF JOINTS

In this category fall pyogenic arthritis, acute infective arthritis of infants, pneumococcal arthritis, gonococcal arthritis, syphilis of joints and arthritis of brucellosis. They are discussed in the following sections.

Pyogenic arthritis

Purulent infections of a joint cavity are due to the entry of pyogenic organisms. The most common of these is *Staphylococcus aureus*, although streptococci, pneumococci, gonococci, meningococci and *E. coli* infect joints occasionally. It should be noted that, in young children, *Haemophilus influenzae* is quite a common organism, and has been identified in joint aspirates as well as in blood cultures.

The joint reacts by exuding fluid via the inflamed synovial membrane which contains antibodies, leucocytes and plasma proteins which, with dead and dying bacteria, form a purulent effusion. The organisms may be grown from the pus but in some cases there may be very little pus and negative growths from cultures occur in 60% of cases. Infection by *Neisseria gonorrhoeae* may occur, though it is less common nowadays. Pyogenic arthritis of the hip in the neonate is a particularly difficult disease to detect. As a result, it is often diagnosed late and so irreversible damage to the articular cartilage and to the blood supply of the epiphysis of the femoral head follows, with consequent severe shortening and disability (Figures 9.14 and 9.15). Although pyogenic arthritis is less common in children and young adults, it is now more commonly found in the elderly with pre-existing joint disease, in the HIV infected haemophiliac patient and in other immunocompromised patient groups, e.g. rheumatoid arthritis, who have been treated with cytotoxic drugs.

Infective arthritis occurs during a bacteraemia, e.g. Lyme's disease, with the tick-borne spirochaete *Borrelia burgdorferi*, or viraemia, e.g. measles, and the infective organism is rarely found in the knee joint.

Reactive arthritis occurs when there is an infection elsewhere which produces a sterile arthritis or synovitis, e.g. ankylosing spondylitis or gastroenteritis due to salmonella, shigella, etc. The majority of these patients are HLA B27 positive.

Routes of infection

The organisms gain entrance as they do in acute osteomyelitis. Thus the joint may be infected by the direct implantation of bacteria through a puncture wound, by the direct extension of infection from a

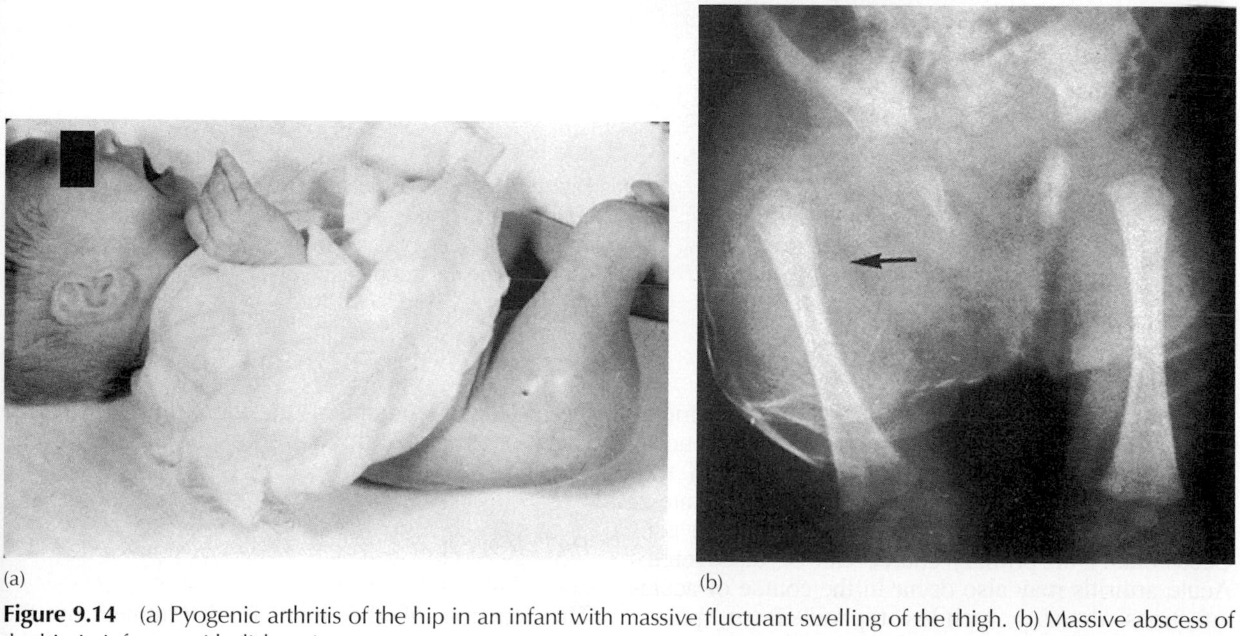

(a) (b)

Figure 9.14 (a) Pyogenic arthritis of the hip in an infant with massive fluctuant swelling of the thigh. (b) Massive abscess of the hip in infancy, with dislocation.

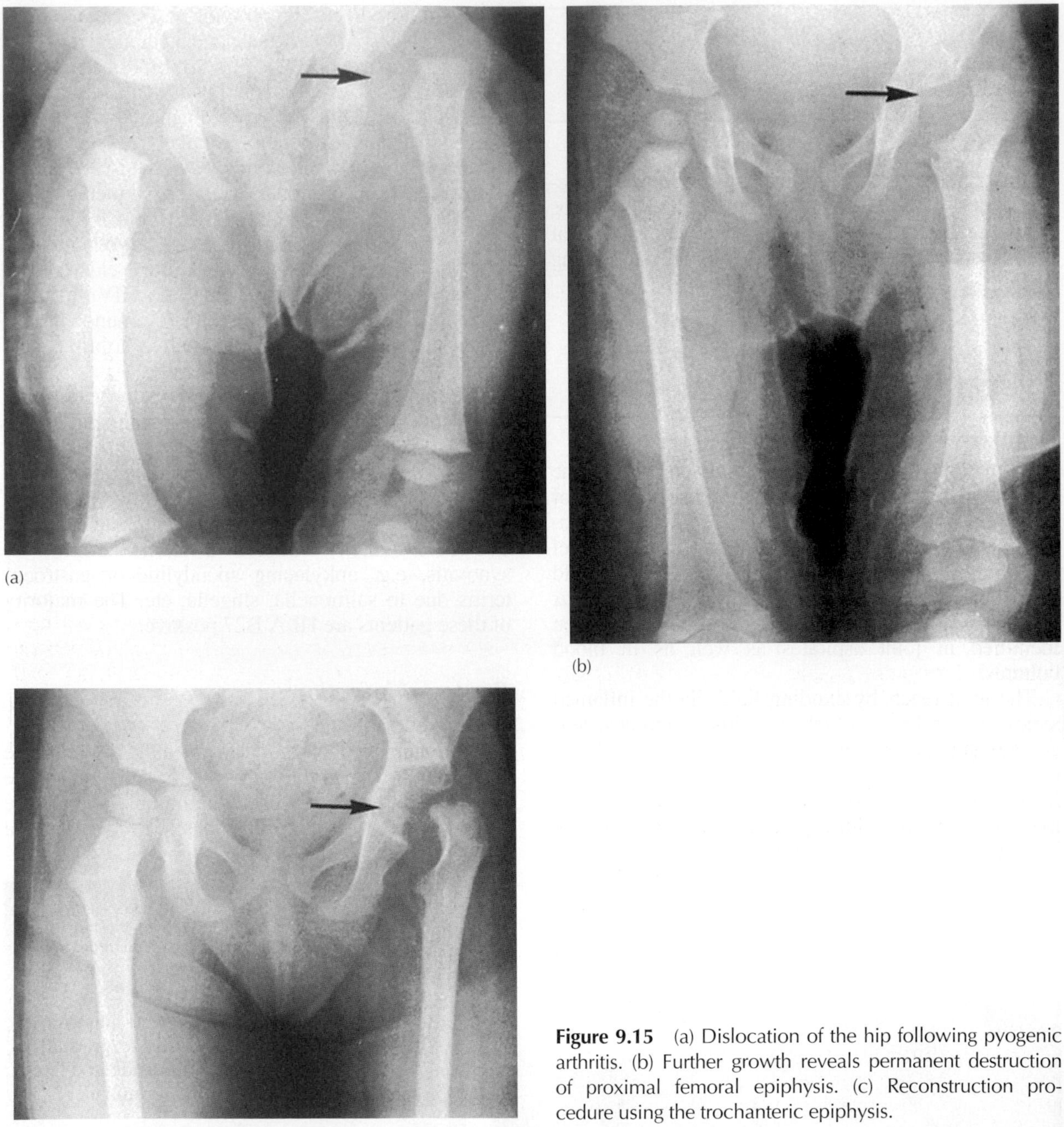

Figure 9.15 (a) Dislocation of the hip following pyogenic arthritis. (b) Further growth reveals permanent destruction of proximal femoral epiphysis. (c) Reconstruction procedure using the trochanteric epiphysis.

compound fracture or an inflamed bone, or, more often, the process may result from a haematogenous infection, the primary focus being situated in the genitourinary tract, the respiratory tract, the intestinal tract, the teeth, the tonsils or the middle ear. Occasionally no primary source can be discovered. Acute arthritis may also occur in the course of acute infectious diseases such as typhoid fever, pneumonia, influenza and scarlet fever, and in such event the responsible organisms are the ordinary pyogenic cocci or the specific bacteria causing the febrile condition.

PATHOLOGY

The reaction of the joint is determined by the virulence of the organisms and the resistance of the individual; in any case there is an exudation of fluid into the synovial cavity, which will be serous, seropurulent or frankly purulent, according to the gravity of the disease.

The serous type

The joint is distended with clear serous fluid and is the site of a mild inflammatory hyperaemia, with dilatation of the vessels of the synovial membrane and capsule. The effusion may subside gradually without further trouble, or it may subside and later recur, or it may eventually become seropurulent, or actually purulent.

Serofibrinous arthritis

Here the synovial membrane is not only hyperaemic but actually inflamed, so that the joint aspect is covered with a serofibrinous exudate and the cavity filled with a cloudy fluid containing a large number of polymorphs and a few large mononuclear cells. Organisms are present in the joint fluid in the early stages. There is usually in addition some periarticular inflammation, and, since adhesions are particularly liable to follow, the ultimate degree of function of the joint depends on the amount of scar tissue and the number of adhesions.

Purulent arthritis

In the most severe type of acute arthritis the whole joint and its surrounding structures are quickly involved. There is a considerable exudate of pus in the joint cavity, containing large numbers of polymorphs, bacteria, red blood corpuscles and fibrin. The capsule and synovial membrane are infiltrated with leucocytes, and engorged, and there may be small areas of focal necrosis or fatty degeneration. The destruction eventually spreads to the articular cartilage. The articular cartilage changes from blue-white to yellow and dies. The articular cartilage is partly destroyed by enzymes – e.g. plasmin, which is produced by inflamed synovial cells from plasminogen breakdown because of the kinases released from staphylococci or streptococci (Lack, 1959) – and by encroaching granulations from the synovia; synovium becomes completely detached, to lie free in the joint cavity in a pool of pus. Other enzymes – i.e. cathepsins B and D – are released from the polymorph as are collagenases, caseinase and proteases from chondrocytes. The role of prostaglandins in particular cartilage destruction is not yet defined, but Robinson and Granda (1975) have described them as being increased. The bone is thus exposed, and if the disease is very acute, osteomyelitis may arise, with its sequelae – suppuration, necrosis and sequestration. The intra-articular ligaments may be destroyed as the tension of the exudate rises, and finally the capsule may be perforated, the pus escaping from the joint to form an extra-articular or periarticular abscess.

The end result depends on the stage at which treatment is instituted; if treatment has been started early, a surprising amount of function may be preserved. In the majority of cases – especially in infants, when the diagnosis may often be delayed – there is gross disorganization of the joint, which is left crippled by adhesions and ankylosis.

CLINICAL FEATURES

In the absence of suppuration – i.e. in the serous and serofibrinous types – the symptoms resemble those of acute rheumatism. Movement, either active or passive, is practically impossible because of the pain, but usually only one joint is involved, in sharp contrast to acute rheumatism. Chronic cases are similar to, and perhaps identical with, rheumatoid forms of arthritis, and many joints may from time to time undergo attacks of pain, swelling and stiffness. The adjacent muscles are also implicated and undergo fibrous changes so that they become weak and stiff. The repeated distension so relaxes the ligaments that the joint becomes more and more unstable and insecure, and the slightest movement then causes extreme pain.

The serous type (acute synovitis)

Acute synovitis is evidenced by a tense painful swelling of the joint. In superficial joints, such as the knee, the bony outline may be completely obliterated. The joint feels hot, and it is usually kept in a position of slight flexion by muscular spasm, and any attempt to move it is attended with severe pain. The temperature is raised, and there is usually a high leucocytosis. If the joint is aspirated at this stage, a clear exudate will be obtained, with a low sugar content.

The serofibrinous type

This is a later stage of the serous type, and is a much more serious condition. The joint is exquisitely tender, fever is high and night pains occur from loss of muscular control.

The suppurative type

In the early stage of the suppurative type, when the disease is limited to the synovial cavity, the symptoms differ little from those of acute synovitis. The patient, however, is more apprehensive; he feels extremely ill and the joint is more painful. The limb wastes rapidly and the temperature is high.

Associated diseases (e.g. infections, boils, otitis media) or a history of injections of corticosteroids or systemic diseases such as rheumatoid arthritis or diabetes mellitus may be found.

DIAGNOSIS

Pyogenic arthritis usually commences rapidly and without previous warning. Malaise and temperature are associated with effusion and pain in the joint. At first a small amount of movement does not produce pain but later spasm of muscles occurs. It is of great importance to aspirate and examine as early as possible some of the synovial fluid in the suspected joint. As well as Gram-staining of a direct smear, which may well provide immediate identification of the organism, culture media for the various types of organisms should be set up: e.g. *blood agar plates* for staphylococci, pneumococci or streptococci; *chocolate agar* for neisseria and haemophilus; *thioglycollate/phenylethyl alcohol blood agar plates* with added kanamycin/vancomycin to destroy aerobic organisms; and *eosin–methylene blue agar plates* for Gram-negative organisms. The blood count is of less importance, as a leucocytosis is often present in the conditions most likely to be confused with pyogenic arthritis. The ESR is usually very high – e.g. over 80 mm in 1 hour (generally of a higher magnitude than in osteomyelitis).

Ward *et al.* (1960) emphasized that the possibility of achieving a positive bacteriological culture is directly proportional to the number of days of chemotherapy before it is taken; i.e. on the first day of therapy they achieved 100% positive culture of the specific organism, whereas during the first week of chemotherapy the incidence was only 50% and after this period the fluid was sterile on culture. Also, accompanying this change there was a reduction of the fluid leucocyte count from over 100 000 before chemotherapy, down to approximately 4000 after some form of chemotherapy had been given for 2 weeks. The characteristic features of the synovial fluid in this condition are a 100 000 white cell count with the polymorphonuclear leucocyte being the predominant cell type. The mucin clot test is poor and there is marked reduction in glucose with elevation in the total proteins. The fluid appears to be very turbid. Penicillin is injected into the joint after the diagnostic aspiration.

The importance of early diagnosis must be emphasized, to prevent vascular complications of ischaemic necrosis, particularly in the hip of young children. The radiographs are of little diagnostic value except for demonstrating the presence of distension by increase in the joint fluid (Figure 9.16). This is followed by demineralization or osteoporosis with cartilage destruction, loss of joint space and, finally, necrosis of bone. Epiphyseal disturbance of slipping or premature closure occurs. Fibrous or bony ankylosis may then result. In the pathological changes, the subchondral plate of calcified cartilage has certain significance in acting as the final barrier to the passage of organisms into adjacent bone where an osteomyelitis can occur. Typical pathology of an infection of a joint and its complications are seen in Table 9.10.

A diagnosis of a septic arthritis or osteomyelitis must be considered in a child who presents with evidence of an acute or generalized infection with:

1. Pain and tenderness in a limb.
2. Swelling of or near a joint.
3. Inability to move a limb because of weakness, pain or spasm.

The differential diagnosis of tuberculosis and pyogenic arthritis still presents a problem. The onset of the former may be quite acute and of the latter insidious. The diseases commonly confused are acute rheumatism, an effusion from a neighbouring suppurative process, such as osteomyelitis, and acute infective (non-suppurative) arthritis.

Disseminated staphylococcal infection

Young children with an osteomyelitis or a septic arthritis may after 2–3 days develop a pyrexia above 38.5°C, become severely ill with heart or lung involvement, e.g. stephylococcal peneumonia, emphysema, myocarditis, pericarditis with or without an effusion. Paterson *et al.* (1990) have reported upon 38 such children in which 79% had the features of toxic shock syndrome. Their mortality rate was 13% and 39% had long-term orthopaedic complications. They emphasize that such patients should be treated in intensive care with a multidisciplinary team. All foci should be identified and drained and aggressive appropriate antibiotic therapy given.

TREATMENT

Joint drainage and antibiotics

It is important to emphasize that, for practical purposes, all joint infections should be regarded as suppurative and, therefore, likely to cause permanent damage to the articular cartilage. It is essential to aspirate on suspicion of infection. Although theoretically it is possible to control septic arthritis by repeated aspirations and systemic antibiotics, the

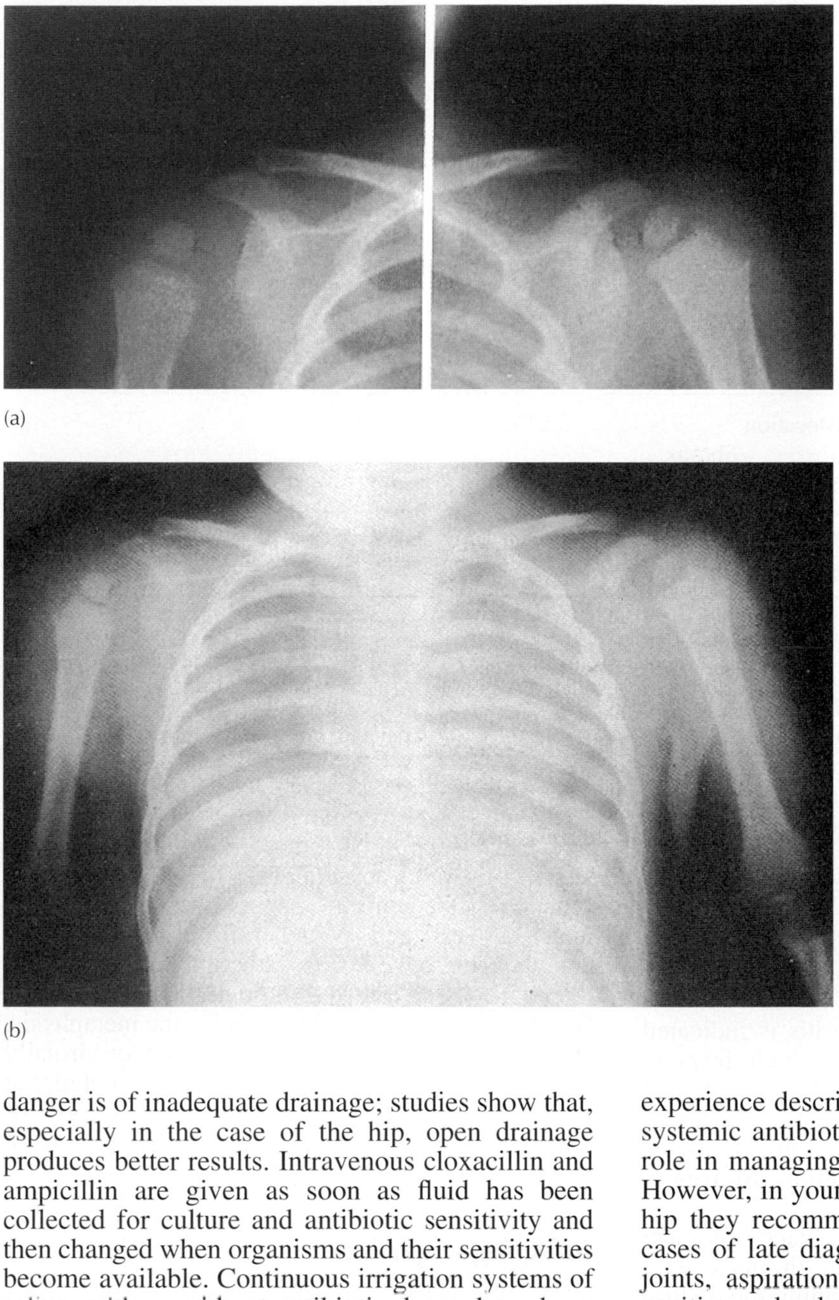

Figure 9.16 An 18-month-old child who presented with inability to move the upper extremity, and these radiographs revealed an outward displacement of the right humeral head. Aspiration of this joint revealed numerous pneumococci on culture.

danger is of inadequate drainage; studies show that, especially in the case of the hip, open drainage produces better results. Intravenous cloxacillin and ampicillin are given as soon as fluid has been collected for culture and antibiotic sensitivity and then changed when organisms and their sensitivities become available. Continuous irrigation systems of saline, with or without antibiotic drugs, have been described but secondary infections have been recorded and there appears to be little gained by such a method. The passage of chemotherapeutic agents across the synovial membrane is affected by the pH and by the viscosity of the synovial fluid but most of all by the amount of debris and dead tissue in the joint. Thus, although antibiotics vary in their degree of penetration of the synovial membrane, all commonly used ones achieve acceptable therapeutic levels if there is adequate drainage and exposure of living tissue in the joint cavity.

Wilson and Di Paolo (1986) from a 10-year experience describe that in addition to bed rest and systemic antibiotics, joint aspiration has a definite role in managing acute septic arthritis in children. However, in young infants with involvement of the hip they recommended hip arthrotomy and in all cases of late diagnosis (i.e. over 4 days), in other joints, aspiration is sufficient. Blood culture was positive and only half as often as joint fluid culture, and *Haemophilus* was the most common organism found from 6 months to 2 years.

Immobilization

Immobilization of the patient and the affected joint is vital to relieve pain and to reduce spread of infection via blood and lymph streams. This may be achieved by light skin traction for the hip or splintage with compression bandages and plaster-of-Paris back slabs for the knee. Immobilization continues until, as with osteomyelitis, the patient is apyrexial, pain-free

Table 9.10 Pathology and complication of joint infection

Synovium → hyperaemia → oedema → cellular { hypertrophy / invasion }
Effusion → pus → abscess
Cartilage lysis + plasminogen + kinase → plasmin + cathepsins + prostaglandins

Joint pathology: subchondral bone reaction < pyogenic / tuberculous

Epiphyseal growth disturbance (Figure 9.15):
Vascular disturbance — bacteraemia, toxaemia, anaemia / thrombosis / embolism

---

Complications

Joint destruction: dislocation
ankylosis — fibrous / cartilaginous / bony
arthritis
amyloidosis

---

and the joint is clinically quiescent. At this stage the joint may be mobilized gradually but antibiotic therapy should continue for at least 6 weeks. Any recurrence of pain, pyrexia or failure or the ESR to fall indicates residual infection, and immobilization should be recommenced whilst a decision is made regarding the necessity for further surgical exploration. Further joint aspiration to detect a change in bacterial behaviour and sensitivity is also indicated. Careful follow-up of the patient is necessary and radiographs at intervals to assess the state of the articular cartilage (Figure 9.17).

Radical treatment of septic arthritis is indicated in all but the very early cases, which respond rapidly within 24 hours to antibiotic therapy and immobilization. In doubtful cases it is better to explore the joint than to risk the destructive effects of an inadequately controlled infection (Morrey *et al.*, 1976).

Delay in obtaining an adequate bacteriological diagnosis and initiating appropriate drainage with antibiotics is the one factor determining the quality of the joint after infection.

Where all the components of the joint are infected and the cartilage has already been destroyed, the best that can be hoped for is ankylosis, and therefore the treatment consists of fixation, free drainage and the prevention of deformity. The joint is immobilized in the position which promises the maximum degree of function. In particular, a careful watch is kept for dislocation which is often spontaneous in the hip and knee, and which should be reduced as soon as the acute inflammatory symptoms have subsided.

Acute infective arthritis of infants

Acute infective arthritis is not a disease of great frequency in children, but carries with it the possibility of serious consequences to life and to future function of the limb. It appears usually in children under 1 year and is generally secondary to a neighbouring bone lesion, although less commonly the joint may be infected through the blood stream. Osteomyelitis has a predilection for the metaphysis, and this in many cases is intra-articular, or virtually so, since the articular capsule of the joint includes at least a portion of the metaphysis. This form of infection is being seen increasingly in neonatal intensive care units.

Infecting organisms

By far the greatest number of cases are caused by infection with *Staphylococcus aureus* or the haemolytic streptococcus. Less commonly, the organism is the influenza bacillus, pneumococcus, *Escherichia coli*, or, in fact, any of the pyogenic organisms. Generally speaking, infections produced by the staphylococcus are the most virulent and most destructive, while those produced by the haemolytic streptococcus are only a little less severe. Of cases of acute coxitis in infants, 70% are due to streptococcal or pneumococcal infection. In later childhood and adolescence, on the other hand, the staphylococcal lesion predominates, while practically all adult cases

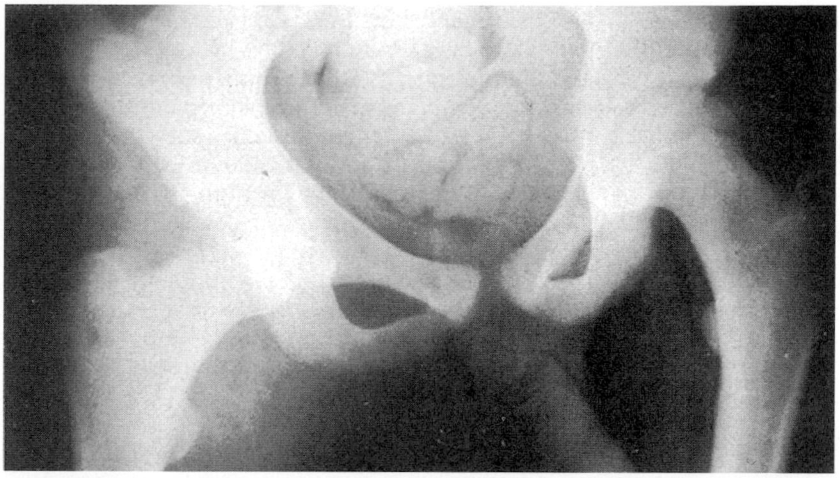

(a)

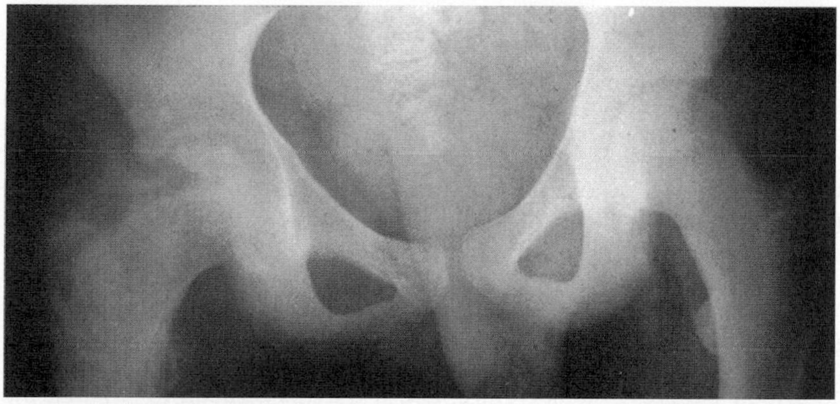

(b)

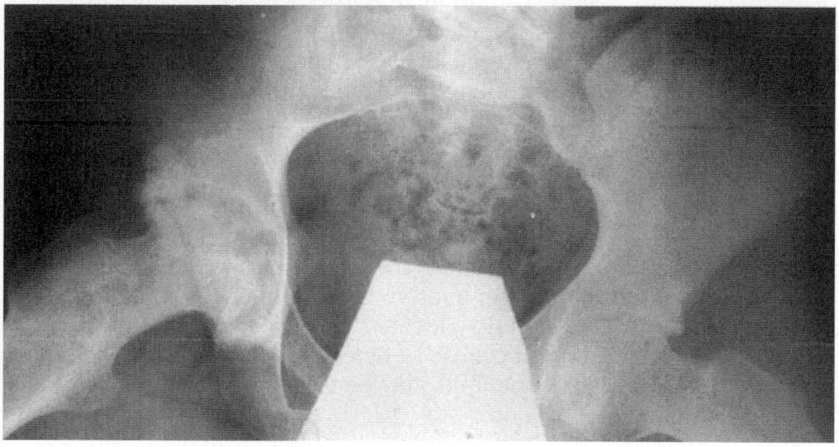

(c)

Figure 9.17 (a) Radiograph of the young adolescent who presented with pneumonia, pain and limitation of movement of the right hip joint. There was some loss of joint space and detail, and on aspiration thick pus was obtained which on culture revealed *Staphylococcus aureus*. (b) Radiograph 2 months later showing the osteomyelitis with loss of bone substance involving both the femur and the acetabulum with further decrease in joint space in spite of chemotherapy and open drainage. (c) Radiograph 1 year later, showing the joint deformation with limitation of adduction and new bone formation at the superior aspect. A fibrous ankylosis had resulted.

are due to streptococcal or pneumococcal infection. Cases of staphylococcal coxitis in adults are recurrences of an earlier infection.

The local source from which the general infection develops may be the oronasal passages, skin, umbilicus or respiratory tract.

PATHOLOGY

The infection starts in the synovial membrane lining the joint. This rapidly becomes inflamed, swollen and oedematous, and from its surface are poured out synovial fluid, plasma and leucocytes, filling the joint cavity with a turbid fluid containing large numbers of polymorphonuclcar leucocytes and much fibrin. The synovial membrane has less power than the peritoneum in combating infection, but as long as it remains comparatively healthy, and especially as long as the joint tension is not excessive, it may deal successfully with a considerable degree of infection. If the infection is severe or prolonged, the mesothelium lining the synovial membrane is destroyed, and its place taken by a mass of granulation tissue. The articular cartilage is less readily involved than the synovial membrane – which is fortunate, since any injury to the cartilage results in greater or less impairment of the function of the joint.

CLINICAL FEATURES

The onset is abrupt and in many cases is preceded by trauma. At an appreciable interval after the trauma, usually 12–24 hours, the joint becomes painful, swollen and hot. Movement and weight-bearing are painful, and quickly become impossible. The patient begins to show signs of toxaemia and fever, and may even at an early stage have one or more rigors. Examination reveals muscle spasm, fluid within the joint capsule and pain on the slightest movement. The joint is fixed, usually in flexion. The temperature is elevated to about 39°C and a polymorphonuclear leucocytosis is present. Blood culture often demonstrates a septicaemia. Finally, the diagnosis is completed by aspiration of purulent fluid from the joint.

In infants the diagnosis may be rendered difficult by the feebleness of their general reaction to the infection, since suppurative arthritis may exist without any elevation of temperature or leucocytosis. In such cases only the local signs of arthritis are present, and aspiration of the joint is the only certain means of diagnosis.

It is to be noted that in early purulent arthritis, when the articular cartilage is still unharmed, there is a small range of movement which is entirely free from pain.

DIFFERENTIAL DIAGNOSIS

Acute rheumatic fever

This is very rarely seen in developed countries.

Suppurative joint infections are most frequently confused with acute rheumatic fever. In acute infective arthritis the slightest attempt at active or passive movement of the affected joint is almost impossible, and induces severe pain. In acute rheumatism there is often a preceding history of tonsillitis, and the multiplicity of the joints involved together with the comparative mildness of the inflammation usually indicate the diagnosis.

In one type of monarticular infection there is occasionally some difficulty. In this group of cases there is a history of a rapidly developing pain in a joint, along with the other signs of arthritis – increased local heat, rigidity, limitation of movement and effusion. Immediately thereafter multiple joint lesions occur in rapid succession, but do not present the definite findings which the original focus demonstrated.

Tuberculous arthritis

Tuberculous arthritis has often to be considered, but in tuberculosis there is no leucocytosis and the progress is usually very insidious. There is also complete limitation of joint movement, except in synovial tuberculosis. In children the tuberculin reaction is an aid to diagnosis and there is usually sufficient x-ray evidence to differentiate the two conditions.

Traumatic synovitis

This must also be seriously considered, for after some trauma there may be pain, limitation of movement, effusion, and occasionally elevation of temperature, and it may be difficult to say that the case is actually not one of infection. There is, however, no increase in local temperature or leucocytosis, and no evidence of the systemic reaction. Pain and muscle spasm are relieved by immobilization, while in purulent arthritis these usually persist.

Haemophilic arthritis

Though rare, haemophilic arthritis must be borne in mind. It may arise without known cause or significant trauma, but there may be associated ecchymoses in the skin overlying the joint. The temperature may be slightly elevated. The history may be of assistance, because of hereditary transmission, and more than one joint may be involved.

TREATMENT

As with the treatment of acute haematogenous osteitis in children or infants, there is a controversy about conservative *vs* operative management for septic arthritis. This revolves around the point of whether a joint and its content can be adequately drained by aspiration. In Baitch's (1962) study, 10 out of the 66 required open incision and drainage, and this he recommended particularly when the condition had failed to respond to more conservative measures over a 72-hour period, and when the material was too thick to aspirate adequately. In children and infants with involvement of the hip and shoulder particularly, he recommended early open drainage. Morrey *et al.* (1976) have recently emphasized the need for open and early drainage to reduce the risk of avascular necrosis of the femoral capital epiphysis.

Pneumococcal arthritis

Pneumococcal infection of a joint, though rare, is occasionally encountered. As a rule a single one of the larger joints is involved, but in 25% of cases the disease is polyarticular. It appears that previous disease of the joint, such as gout or rheumatism, predisposes to the pneumococcal infection.

The condition usually arises in association with some other pneumococcal lesion such as pneumonia or otitis media, and it may begin during the actual septicaemic stage or during convalescence. A common time of onset is about 2 weeks after the commencement of pneumonia. In certain cases the joint manifestation has actually preceded a pneumococcal pulmonary infection, indicating the septicaemic nature of the process. Pneumococci may or may not be obtained by blood culture. Infants and alcoholics are most liable to the infection.

In the so-called 'primary' cases the onset is sudden, the joint becoming distended with fluid, which is at first serous and very soon purulent. The pus is greenish-yellow and contains flakes of fibrin. Pneumococci can usually be demonstrated, and their presence constitutes the main point of distinction between this and other forms of acute arthritis.

In the secondary cases (e.g. those secondary to pneumonia) the clinical features do not differ appreciably.

TREATMENT

The joint should be aspirated and cultured, with ampicillin replacement and the limb immobilized with traction. Frequently then the infection settles down, leaving little permanent damage. Ampicillin is given parenterally in addition to the local injection.

Gonococcal arthritis

The incidence of gonococcal rheumatism or arthritis is now probably less than 1%. It usually develops during the third week of the infection, although occasionally it arises only when the disease is on the decline, even some months after the original urethritis. It is stated to be four or five times more common in men than women, and the usual age period is from 20 to 30 years, largely because gonorrhoea is then more frequent. It may occur in newborn babies from the first week onwards. The joint manifestations have a tendency to relapse and recur.

AETIOLOGY

Among the predisposed causes the most important is the lack of treatment in the earlier stages of gonorrhoea, while activity or heavy exercise during the acute stage also tends to produce an arthritis. Recurrance of infective manifestations in a joint frequently follows reinfection or the lighting up of a chronic focus. The infection of the joint is metastatic, and the organism is carried by the blood stream to the affected joint. The organisms are only likely to be isolated from the joint fluid in the very early stages of the arthritis.

The disease is monarticular in 40% of cases, but frequently a number of joints become infected during some stage of the illness, with recovery in all save one. This residual monarticular affection shows a tendency to resist the routine therapeutic measures and it may be activated by urethral traumatism or prostatic massage. The large joints are involved with greater frequency than the small ones, the knee being most frequently affected. The order of frequency (Lees, 1931) is: knee, ankle, metatarsophalangeal, shoulder, wrist, metacarpophalangeal and elbow joints. Patients who give a history of a previous arthritis, and who subsequently develop a gonococcal urethritis, are very prone to develop gonococcal arthritis.

PATHOLOGY

Acute cases may be divided into four types:

1. Arthralgia, in which one or more joints may be painful but there are no gross physical signs.
2. An acute infection with effusion in one or more of the larger joints.
3. An acute infection with erosion of cartilage in addition to the effusion.

4. An acute infection involving the synovial membrane and the articular surfaces. The intra-articular exudate becomes purulent, and there is marked ulceration and erosion of all the cartilaginous surfaces. This condition is comparatively rare.

Subacute and *chronic cases* may be divided into two main types:

1. A synovial type, involving especially the knee joint. The synovial membrane is thickened, and there is a moderate effusion.
2. A mixed type, involving both the synovial membrane and the articular surfaces, and frequently polyarticular in the smaller joints, in which the serofibrinous exudate is always fibroblastic and leads to adhesions and deformity. Proliferative changes are more evident than destructive ones, and the periarticular tissues are involved in the fibrosis in almost every case.

CLINICAL FEATURES

The acute joint infections other than arthralgia begin suddenly, and are often ushered in by a chill or a rigor. The temperature is raised and the joint is painful. The pain rapidly becomes excruciating, and is attended by muscular rigidity. The skin overlying the joint becomes red and hot, and periarticular oedema soon manifests itself. When the joint effusion becomes purulent, pyrexia is increased and rigors occur.

The acute form may subside into a chronic type, or a subacute or chronic infection may arise *de novo*. The symptoms resemble those of the acute phase, but are milder except during the acute exacerbations which are liable to occur. The associated muscles become atrophied, and there is a persistent joint effusion. When there is gross enlargement of one joint – e.g. the knee – in the absence of febrile and other symptoms, the condition is known as hydrops or hydrarthrosis. Suppuration is rare in this form.

The tendons, the tendon sheaths, the bursae and the periosteum may be inflamed, in association with gonococcal arthritis. This is especially so of the tendons of the wrist and ankle and of the retrocalcanean bursa. In severe cases the adjacent bones are rarefied.

DIAGNOSIS

A painful affection of a joint, whether acute, subacute or chronic, and which is associated with periarticular changes, should prompt tactful inquiries concerning urethral discharge. The latter may be extremely slight (e.g. a 'morning drop') or there may be no discharge but a palpable enlargement of the prostate or of the seminal vesicles. The secretion of these organs may be expressed by finger massage and may show gonococci on examination. When no Gram-negative, intracellular diplococci can be demonstrated in a stained film, it is essential to conduct cultural and sugar fermentation tests and, if necessary, the oxidase reaction, on specimens obtained from the most common foci of residual infection – the prostate and cervix.

Even when there is no obvious focus of gonococcal infection, it is always important to exclude this type of joint lesion by repeated examinations, when an acute, subacute or chronic affection of a joint is painful, persistent and associated with periarticular changes.

It is important in acute cases to be able to differentiate between acute rheumatism and a gonococcal arthritis, as shown in Table 9.11.

Acute gonococcal arthritis must, in addition, be differentiated from arthritis following pneumonia, dysentery, cerebrospinal infection, typhoid or scarlet fevers, acute tonsillitis and tuberculosis.

It is important to bear in mind Reiter's syndrome, which was first described in 1916, because the triad of urethritis, polyarthritis and conjunctivitis is most suggestive of a gonococcal infection. The condition is a form of non-gonococcal urethritis which is probably due to a virus, and certain authorities have demonstrated the presence of inclusion bodies.

PROGNOSIS

The prognosis in the first three groups of gonococcal arthritis – arthralgia, acute and subacute synavitis, and acute and subacute synovitis and arthritis – is invariably good, even when there is involvement of the periarticular structures, if treatment of the original focus of infection, and of the joint, is carried out on correct lines. In the fourth group – acute arthritis with suppuration – surgical intervention may be required, and there may be considerable loss of function. Subacute and chronic cases react well to treatment, but recovery is always slow and the joint condition is apt to recur. In neglected cases the articular cartilage may be destroyed and fibrous ankylosis occur; bony ankylosis is uncommon.

Table 9.11

Acute rheumatism	Gonococcal arthritis
No evidence of genitourinary disease	The genitourinary symptoms and signs may occasionally be well marked but are more frequently of a slight nature
Marked temperature reaction and more prolonged constitutional upset and prostration	Very moderate temperature reaction, and constitutional upsets light, except in purulent cases
Sweating very profuse, with acid odour	Very little sweating except in purulent cases
Pain intense and aggravated by the slightest touch	Pain less intense
Many joints involved, but as pain leaves one it flits to another, and the first affected appears to be free from discomfort	May be limited to one joint, and usually one or two joints only, and pain does not leave a joint rapidly and pass to another
Tendon sheaths and periarticular tissues rarely involved	Tendon sheaths and periarticular tissues very frequently the site of disease
Often some cardiac complication, such as endocarditis or pericarditis, and an active focus of infection in the tonsils	Cardiac complications very rare, and no acute condition in the tonsils
Symptoms and temperature react extremely well to the administration of salicylates	Salicylates have little effect on the pain, the swelling or the temperature
Complement-fixation test of blood negative	The complement-fixation test may be positive but too much reliance should not be placed on this test, which has not attained the same significance or reliance as the Wassermann test in syphilis
Very rarely seen	

TREATMENT

Eradication of the original focus of infection

Local measures

These need not be considered here, but, despite modern systemic remedies, they still play an important part in treatment.

Chemotherapy

Adequate dosage with penicillin compounds is required.

Treatment of the infected joints

Relief of pain is of primary importance and is obtained by rest in a semi-flexed position. While rest is advisable if the pain is severe, it is very important not to continue immobilizing the joint any longer than is necessary to relieve the acute pain. Early mobilization is one of the greatest assets to the recovery of joint function.

Operative treatment has been advocated largely in Europe, but it is doubtful if more than a few acute or subacute cases require operative intervention. Aspiration will undoubtedly relieve the intra-articular pressure. The fluid from the joint may be replaced by 10 000 units of flucloxacillin daily for 3 days.

The response to flucloxacillin is usually excellent, and, provided treatment is begun early and the organism is not resistant, resolution takes place without damage to the joint.

Syphilis of joints

Syphilis as an aetiological factor in arthritis is probably commoner than is generally believed. Anti-syphilitic treatment is clearly indicated in all cases of syphilitic arthritis, but the response – unless in the early stages of the disease, both in the inherited and acquired forms – is in the main not encouraging. Diagnosis is materially assisted by concomitant signs or symptoms of syphilis and blood serological and cerebrospinal fluid tests (Wassermann, *Treponema* immobilization, etc.). The latter are invariably positive in the early stages but are not so reliable in late syphilitic lesions, being positive in only about 50% of these cases. It need hardly be stressed that a negative blood serological test does not exclude syphilis as the cause of the arthritis. Syphilis of the joints may occur at all stages of the disease and in both the inherited and acquired forms.

CLASSIFICATION OF SYPHILITIC ARTHRITIS

Joint lesions in inherited syphilis

1. Parrot's syphilitic osteochondritis
2. Clutton's joint; symmetrical hydrarthrosis (in childhood)

Joint lesions in acquired (early) syphilis

1. Arthralgia
2. Hydrarthrosis
3. Plastic arthritis (very rare)

Joint lesions in acquired (late) syphilis
Gummatous arthritis

1. The synovial form
2. The osseous form
3. Charcot's joints (tabetic arthropathy)

JOINT LESIONS IN INHERITED SYPHILIS

Parrot's syphilitic osteochondritis

This is an epiphysitis, or a juxtaepiphyseal inflammation, which occurs during the first few months of life in children with inherited syphilis. It affects the upper limbs more frequently than the lower, and is often associated with an effusion into the adjacent joint. The gelatinous tissue breaks down to form a greenish-yellow fluid from which a strongly positive *Treponema* immobilization reaction is obtainable. The extremities of the bones at which growth principally takes place – knee, shoulder and wrist – are more frequently involved, the epiphyseal region becoming large and tender. Separation of the epiphysis may occur and give rise to unwillingness to move the joint – syphilitic pseudoparalysis.

The *radiographic changes* are irregularity of the epiphyseal line, cupping of the metaphysis, widening of the articular space, thickening of the periosteum and decalcification of the neighbouring bone.

Anti-syphilitic treatment may produce complete resolution, but the growth cartilage may be so damaged that, later, shortening or deformity arises.

Clutton's joint; symmetrical hydrarthrosis (in childhood)

The joint condition commonly known by this name was first described by Clutton in 1886, and consists of symmetrical hydrarthrosis of the knee in children from 8 to 16 years of age. The onset is insidious and there is no fever. The joints are painless, and in spite of the effusion the patients are able to walk quite well. This condition when associated, as it commonly is, with eye changes and other stigmata of congenital syphilis, constitutes a striking clinical picture.

The condition shows a slow response to treatment and appears to run its own course. Spontaneous recovery may take place. Relapses are unlikely.

JOINT LESIONS IN ACQUIRED SYPHILIS

Arthralgia

Arthralgia forms part of the clinical picture in the secondary stage. It may even appear before the early rashes. The pain is never severe and can often be more correctly described as an ache. As in tertiary syphilis, it is chiefly nocturnal. It usually affects one or more of the larger joints; there is little, if any, muscular spasm; and usually at this stage there is no local swelling, heat or tendency to deformity.

The diagnosis is determined by the history and general phenomena and the positive Wassermann reaction.

Hydrarthrosis

Later in the secondary stage serous synovitis may occur. It usually involves two or more joints, especially the knees, and often in a symmetrical manner. In the earlier cases the synovitis is of a transient nature, but later it is more persistent. Fluid is abundant and the synovial membrane is swollen. Pain is moderate, and gentle passive movement does not hurt, although direct pressure on the joints may do so.

TERTIARY SYPHILITIC ARTHRITIS (GUMMATOUS ARTHRITIS)

Gummatous arthritis may affect a whole joint, or be localized to part of a joint. Its onset is usually insidious, less commonly acute and sudden; usually the joint has been previously normal, though occasionally it is superimposed on a secondary syphilitic joint lesion such as hydrarthrosis.

The synovial form

The commonest joints to be affected are the knee, ankle, elbow and shoulder, but smaller ones, such as the interphalangeal joints, are occasionally affected. There is considerable but painless effusion, but exceptionally, pain may be severe, and the disease simulate tuberculosis. The pathological changes are limited to the outer layers of the capsule, and consist of thickening and perivascular infiltration. The lining endothelium and articular cartilage remain shiny.

The osseous form

The whole of one large joint is affected – as a rule, the knee. The condition resembles osteoarthritis both pathologically and on x-ray examination. Distension of the joint is present, and some increase in the density of the periarticular soft parts can be seen.

The spine is sometimes affected and the disease then closely simulates tuberculosis, the diagnosis being made only when other symptoms or signs of syphilis are present, blood serological tests assist, and/or the response to suitable anti-syphilitic treatment is satisfactory.

Even in well-established gummatous arthritis, timely treatment can produce great improvement, though not so much as in the earlier cases.

A weight-bearing caliper should be worn throughout the active stage of the disease, but it should be taken off daily so that the joint may be put through its full range of movements without weight-bearing. The clinical picture of a painless polyarthritis in a child, without local heat, redness, wasting, pyrexia, night-starting or response to salicylate treatment, makes up a characteristic picture.

Charcot's joints (tabetic arthropathy)

This is considered to be neuroarthropathic in origin. It usually occurs in acquired syphilis but may very occasionally follow inherited syphilis. The large joints – the knee, ankle, hip or shoulder – are commonly affected, but rarely multiple large or smaller joints may be involved. The early stages of rapid exudation into the joint cavity and periarticular structures are rapidly followed by a painless disorganization of the articular and surrounding structures. Radiological examination shows gross disorganization, disappearance of cartilage and articular margins, and bony rarefaction with calcification in the capsule. Fragments of bones are commonly found lying free in the joint.

Diagnosis is arrived at by correlating a history of a rapidly progressive and painless disorganization of a joint, without associated muscular atrophy, with the clinical and serological signs of locomotor ataxia (tabes dorsalis). Other associated neurotrophic features may be present, such as perforating ulcers affecting the sole of the foot, or one of the toes, and pathological fractures may occur. Treatment is most unsatisfactory and very disappointing, but where splinting is impracticable, arthrodesis, preceded by suitable anti-syphilitic treatment consisting chiefly of penicillin, may prove successful.

GENERAL DIAGNOSIS

The family history, that of previous diseases and of the present condition should be most carefully considered. The Wassermann and *Treponema* immobilization tests should be conducted as a routine in every case of chronic arthritis of any degree of severity and, where serological diagnosis presents any doubts or difficulties, it is advisable to examine the CSF and repeat quantitative tests at monthly intervals, over a period of 6 months, in order to observe their variations. The blood serum and, if obtainable, the joint fluid, should be investigated, for in a number of cases a positive result may be obtained from the fluid when the blood serum gives a negative result. It is important to remember that blood serological tests may also be negative in late cases of acquired syphilis although the CSF *Treponema* immobilization tests may be positive. Finally, one must not forget the possibility of a non-syphilitic arthritis occurring in a person with concomitant positive blood serology.

Arthritis of brucellosis

Osteoarticular manifestations in human and animal brucellosis are important and not infrequent. The types of brucellosis are:

1. arthralgias and ostalgias;
2. fibrositis;
3. hydrarthrosis;
4. acute arthritis;
5. chronic arthritis; and
6. osteitis, osteomyelitis and osteoperiostitis.

Spondylitis is the most frequent articular lesion and may simulate Pott's disease or spondylitis ankylopoietica. The microbe may localize in the joints and produce purulent metastatic arthritis in septicaemic cases. In chronic types the articular changes are part of an allergic inflammatory response of mesenchymal tissues. The disease should be suspected when a patient shows musculoarticular changes with psychic asthenia, changes of the eighth cranial nerve and autonomic nervous system disturbances with or without fever. Additional findings of positive intradermal reaction of Bund, anaemia with anisocytosis, leucopenia with neutropenia and lymphocytosis, normal ESR and an agglutination titre to *Brucella* of 1:1280 support the diagnosis of brucellosis.

Treatment is by streptomycin 2 g intramuscularly daily, combined with chlortetracycline 2 g daily for 2 weeks. Methicillin or Chloromycetin may be used in place of chlortetracycline. Others have combined cortisone with the antibiotics.

INFECTIONS IN TOTAL JOINT REPLACEMENT

Infection following total joint replacement is a special but common problem. It is painful, disabling, costly, often requires removal of both components and the cement. It has been shown to have a mortality of from 7% to 62%. Factors predisposing patients to infection following total hip replacement include the large mass of foreign material implanted, the large dead space left in the wound, the mobility of the artificial joint implanted, and the fact that the procedure is usually performed on older and somewhat debilitated patients. The incidence of infection following total hip replacement varies from 0% to 11%.

Specific cohorts of patients have been identified as high-risk group, e.g. patients with obesity, diabetes, alcoholism and rheumatoid arthritis, and those who have been receiving steroids, immunosuppressive drugs or anticoagulants have also been said to have a higher incidence of postoperative infection. The likelihood of infection is said to be increased when the period of hospitalization before surgery is prolonged. Operations lasting more than 2 hours, previous hip surgery with or without infection present, and urinary tract infections have been reported to increase the likelihood of infection. Postoperative haematoma or postoperative necrosis of the skin incision may make infection more likely. Worblewski and del Sel (1980) reported the incidence of deep sepsis in various groups of patients after total hip replacement who did not have routine administration of prophylactic antibiotics: primary osteoarthritis 0.3%, rheumatoid arthritis 1.2%, males with postoperative urethral instrumentation 6.2%, patients with psoriasis 5.5% and patients with diabetes 5.6%.

AETIOLOGY AND EPIDEMIOLOGY

The common bacteria isolated from infected hip replacements are:

- *Staphylococcus aureus*
- *Staphylococcus epidermidis*
- B-streptococci, group G
- *Streptococcus pneumoniae*
- *E. coli*
- *Proteus* sp.
- *Alcaligenes faecalis*
- *Propionibacterium acnes*
- Peptococci
- *Fusobacterium*

Prosthetic replacement infections arise primarily from exogenous or endogenous sources. The patient's skin is the most common source of contamination even though sporadic outbreaks traced to the operating or ancillary personnel have been reported.

It is difficult to assess the role that intraoperative airborne organisms play in total hip replacement infections. Fitzgerald *et al.* (1977) studied 658 consecutive hip replacements in which wound cultures were taken at operation. Many of the organisms isolated corresponded to organisms cultured from the operating room air. Only 4 (2%) of the 195 patients with positive intraoperative cultures later became infected. They concluded that airborne organisms rarely emerged as infecting pathogens following total hip replacement. However, in the same study deep sepsis was twice as frequent (1.7%) when total hip replacements were done in older operating rooms with low rates of air exchange, than when done in rooms with high rates of air exchange.

In a multi-institutional study the lowest rate of infection following hip replacement was noted in centres that use a vertical unidirectional air flow system in association with a personal isolation system or body exhaust suit.

Metastatic sources of infection may be involved as well, e.g. percutaneous sutures, suction drains, intravenous catheters, and indwelling urinary catheters. Fitzgerald *et al.* (1977) found that patients with bacteriuria following total hip replacement had a 3.4% incidence of deep sepsis while those without urinary infection had a 1.5% incidence of deep sepsis. Stinchfield *et al.* (1980) reported 10 patients with late (average 34 months) haematogenous infection following joint replacement surgery. They stated that these infections arose from distal foci of sepsis which included the gastrointestinal tract, cutaneous infections and dental abscesses. There is still controversy about the metastatic spread following dental surgery and indeed whether prophylactic antibiotics are worthwhile (Blackburn and Alarcon, 1991; Thyne and Ferguson, 1991).

Kamme and Lindberg (1981) have stated that the early and the haematogenous infections in total hip replacements are caused by commonly recognized pathogens, while delayed infections are most likely to be caused by aerobic and anaerobic organisms of low virulence inoculated into the wound in small numbers at the time of the operation. In their series, Enterobacteriaceae and *Staph. aureus* accounted for 69% of the isolates in 12 patients with early sepsis. *Staph. aureus* and *Streptococcus pneumoniae* were the only pathogens isolated in 5 patients with haematogenous sepsis. Of the 21 patients with delayed sepsis *Staph. epidermidis*, *Propionibacterium acnes* and *Fusobacterium* account for 88% of the isolates.

CLINICAL STAGING

Many authors, including Fitzgerald, have divided deep sepsis after total joint replacement into three stages in an attempt to standardize the terminology of postoperative prosthetic infections. These stages are based on the time of presentation and the clinical course.

- Stage 1 is an acute, fulminating infection that develops within the first 4 weeks after surgery.
- Stage 2 is delayed sepsis that develops as a low-grade infection from postoperative week 4 to the second postoperative year.
- Stage 3 is defined as a haematogenous infection that develops in a previously asymptomatic patient and usually occurs 2–5 years after surgery.

Stage 1 infections have become relatively infrequent as most patients now receive systemic perioperative prophylactic antibiotics. The infections are easily diagnosed by their clinical presentation, usually after an infected haematoma. Stage 2 and stage 3 infections may be difficult to diagnose as the usual clinical signs of wound infection, fever, drainage, induration and erythema are rarely present. The patient's chief complaint is primarily pain, especially when weight-bearing. The differential diagnosis is that of aseptic loosening at the bone cement interface or loosening secondary to low-grade infection.

Laboratory investigations

The leucocyte count is usually normal in stage 2 and stage 3 infections. The erythrocyte sedimentation rate (ESR) and the C-reactive protein (CRP) are two serological markers of inflammation or infection, although both are quite non-specific. Fitzgerald found the ESR to be frequently elevated: greater than 50 in women; greater than 40 in men. In uncomplicated total hip replacement for osteoarthritis, the CRP levels may be slightly raised before surgery, reach a peak 2 days postoperatively and then returned to normal 3 weeks following surgery. One must realize that a normal ESR or a normal CRP does not exclude infection, particularly in patients who have received antibiotics. Testing for leukergy (Otremski *et al.*, 1993) is proving of interest and value.

Radiographic loosening

Radiographic loosening is defined as a 2 mm radiolucent line circumferentially present around the prosthesis. This is often progressive with time. Radiographic loosening does not differentiate septic loosening from aseptic loosening, nor does endosteal bone resorption or extensive resorption of the medial femoral neck. Evidence of osteomyelitis of the proximal femur is supportive of a diagnosis of deep infection.

Arthrography

Arthrography is indicated in the evaluation of all painful total hip replacements. Plain radiographs alone are quite accurate with respect to loosening of the femoral component, but plain radiographs were poor in the assessment of acetabular component loosening. Arthrography often provided the only preoperative clue that the socket was loose.

Aspiration of contents

Aspiration of the contents from within the periprosthetic pseudocapsule to diagnose subtle sepsis and/or to identify a specific organism is always indicated prior to surgical revision. If a dry aspiration occurs, arthrography is essential to prove correct placement of the needle. Many reports of false-negative aspirations are found in the literature. Important factors for minimizing false-negative results include sterile technique, avoidance of lignocaine and preaspiration antibiotics, and prompt transportation and handling of the laboratory specimen. Conversely, falsepositive hip aspirates have also been reported. False-positive results occurred despite full surgical preparation in the operating theatre. Incidences have been reported as high as 15%. Gould *et al.* (1990) do not believe that routine aspiration prior to prosthetic revision is necessary, but should be reserved for those patients with a suspicion of infection.

Scintigraphic examination

Radionucleotide scanning using bones seeking radionucleotides such as technetium-99m pyrophosphate, gallium and indium may be helpful in defining the aetiology of a painful hip prosthesis. Norris and Watt (1983) studied 110 hips following hip replacement. In the 53 control hips that were scanned from 1 to 24 months postoperatively, 90% exhibited a positive technetium scan (late or fixed phase), due to the preoperative arthritic process. One observes, with increasing time postoperatively, a fall-off in activity on the bone scan. Even so, at more than 24 months postoperatively, a proportion of asymptomatic hips still have a residual bone scan activity around the prosthesis.

In the preoperative perfusion scan, a high proportion of the hips had increased activity. In the postoperative group of asymptomatic hip replacement only a very small portion of hips continued to have high perfusion scans. Even within 3 months of surgery, the perfusion scan was normal in the majority of patients. In comparison, the symptomatic hips were quite different; 95% of the infected hips and 50% of the loose hips had positive perfusion phase technetium scans. In comparison 7% of the asymptomatic hips were positive at 1 year. Using the same group of patients, Norris and Watt (1983) studied the results of gallium scans – 9% of the control group had abnormal gallium scans at 1 year while 90% of the infected hips, and 58% of the aseptically loose hips had positive gallium scans. The sensitivity and specificity of these tests were: the perfusion scan had a 5.9% false-negative rate, and an 18.7% false-positive rate. The perfusion scan in aseptic loosening had a 50% false-negative rate, and a 28% false-positive rate. The bone scan showed no false negatives in infection of loosening, but, a high proportion of false positives in infection (79%) and fewer false positives in septic loosening (19%). The sensitivity and specificity of a gallium scan for infection does not differ markedly from the perfusion scan with 11.8% false-negative incidence and 19.8% incidence of false positives. Likewise, the gallium scan in the aseptically loose hips showed 58.4% false negatives and 29.2% false positives.

Indium granulocyte staining

The use of indium III labelled granulocytes (ILGS) has been suggested as a superior technique for the localization of infection because it reflects quantitatively the presence of granulocytes in the areas under study.

Intraoperative investigations

Kamme and Lindberg (1981) have documented the intraoperative sampling procedure. Antibiotic therapy is discontinued 6 weeks prior to the operation but it is recommenced during the operation as soon as the samples have been taken. The samples consist of five biopsies taken from the tissue immediately adjacent to the cement. Each sample is taken with separate forceps and placed in separate CO_2 filled test tubes and then immediately taken to the bacteriology laboratory for aerobic and anaerobic culture. The most common bacteria found in this study was *Staph. epidermidis* followed by *Propionibacterium magnus*, then *Staph. aureus*, *Streptococcus*, *Neisseria* and *Haemophilus influenzae*.

Much of the confusion experienced in diagnosing infections intraoperatively have been caused by contamination. Intraoperative Gram stain and fresh frozen sections have been advocated by some authors to differentiate septic from aseptic loosening. If either study reveals bacteria to be present, the diagnosis is made. If bacteria are nor present, the diagnosis of infection depends on the number of polymorphonuclear leucocytes present per high power field.

TREATMENT

Diagnosis of the infecting organisms with their sensitivity permits the use of appropriate antibiotic therapy. Debridement is indicated and the removal of the prosthesis with all cement and foreign material if at all possible. Retention of the prosthetic component is rarely successful and usually not indicated (Schoifet and Morrey, 1990). See Chapter 11.

TUBERCULOSIS

Skeletal tuberculosis

There has been a steady decline in the incidence of bone and joint tuberculosis in Britain in recent years, but it is still one of the chief causes of death and crippling in many countries of the world (WHO, 1991). Although it commonly attacks children, its ravages are not confined to the early years. Indeed, in certain areas of the USA it is most commonly found in elderly people who present with some 'chronic' joint disease which has been diagnosed as rheumatoid, gouty or even degenerative arthritis.

Crofton (1960) emphasized that even in economically developed countries 'tuberculosis is very far from being defeated' and pointed out that there might well be over 12 million 'open' or infectious cases throughout the world. He described how it should be possible to eliminate this disease by the use of BCG vaccine, the use of miniature radiography for surveys of communities containing 'high incidence' groups of individuals such as contacts or 'danger groups' such as teachers and doctors, the use of chemotherapy with knowledge of drug resistance, and finally surgery. However, recent studies have shown failure of BCG to prevent infection from already infective cases, so the disease remains a serious health problem and is increasing.

BCG VACCINATION

In the UK this has been carried out on school children aged 10–14 years, reducing the incidence of tuberculosis significantly. Although there has been discussion to discontinue such a programme, reserving vaccination for high-risk groups, e.g. health care workers at risk, tuberculin-negative contacts, immigrants from abroad, etc., this programme will continue. In the USA a significant number of new cases are appearing, not only because of the incidence of HIV infection with their increased susceptibility to tuberulous infection.

It should be noted that BCG vaccine when given to babies and infants has produced a BCG osteomyelitis with lesions in the epiphysis and metaphysis. Some strains of BCG have been isolated from these lesions which have required debridement and chemotherapy for cure.

Infection of a bone or joint with *Mycobacterium tuberculosis* is nearly always secondary to an infection of some other area, usually the lymphatic glands at the root of the lung or in the mesentery. The lymphatic disease is the primary lesion, and, in most cases, more dangerous than the joint lesion, since it is deeply seated, not susceptible to radical treatment and easily overlooked.

AETIOLOGY

Nature of the infecting organism

The tubercle bacillus of bone infections may be of either the human or the bovine type. Bovine infection used to be four or five times more common in skeletal tuberculosis than the human type, but the bovine type is becoming even more uncommon.

Route of infection

Tuberculosis of bone is almost invariably secondary; it is but a local manifestation of a general disease, the original site of which is usually in the bronchial or the mesenteric glands. From the primary focus the bone is usually invaded through the blood stream, but occasionally the bone infection is by contiguity from a neighbouring joint or from infected soft tissues.

Predisposing factors

The factors which favour the development of the disease are general or local. The former may precipitate, or make possible, the infection of the subject with tuberculosis, while the local factors favour its localization in bone. The general conditions include the exanthemata, diseases associated with considerable debility such as influenza, malnutrition and bad hygiene, and now those with immunodeficiency disease of HIV infection.

Influence of injury

A history of trauma is common, and it is possible that injury results in small intraosseous haemorrhages or effusions, in consequence of which some degree of vascular stasis occurs.

PATHOLOGY

A small extravasation of blood within the tubercle bacilli settles and proliferates, and eventually a typical tuberculous follicle is formed, with endothelial cells, lymphocytes and giant cells. As the original follicle enlarges, epithelioid cell granuloma forms and is visible to the naked eye as a small white nodule in the centre of the marrow. Caseation later becomes evident at the centre, while there is an attempt at fibrosis at the periphery (Figure 9.18).

Apart from the actual tuberculous nodule, widespread changes are apparent in the various bony components.

The marrow

During the early days of the disease, immature polymorphonuclear leucocytes proliferate. They are actively phagocytic and contain altered blood pigment. After a few days the polymorphs are replaced by lymphocytes and mononuclear cells, whose presence is characteristic of tuberculosis. If now the disease becomes arrested, fibrotic changes ensue. The lymphocytes disappear, while the fat cells increase in number, and young fibrous tissue appears in their midst. Fibrosed marrow is yellowish-white in colour and firm in consistence.

The lamellae

The lamellar tissue may undergo two types of change. There may be:

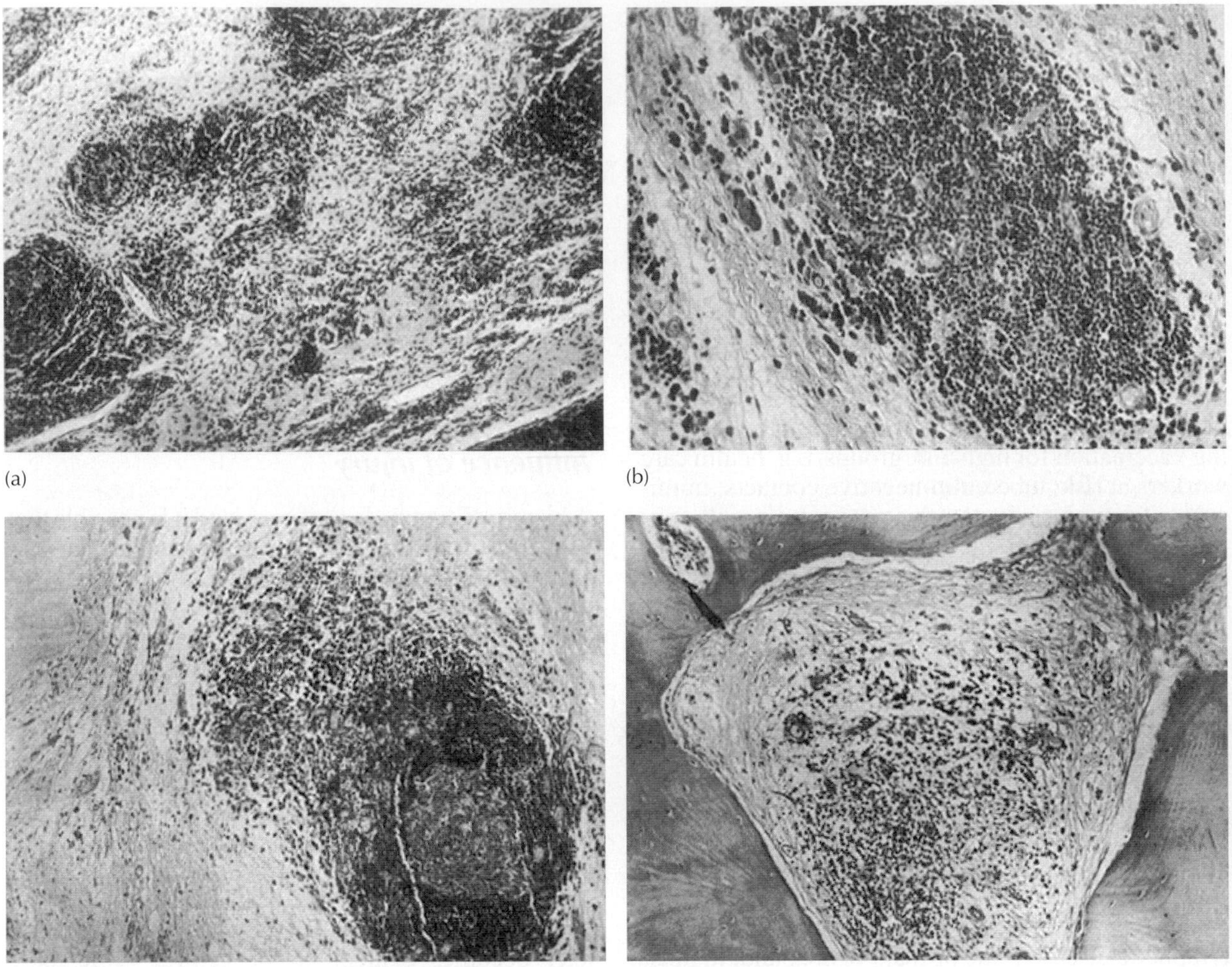

(a) (b) (c) (d)

Figure 9.18 Photomicrographs (x 85) of human synovium, showing (a) the lymphocytic infiltration, giant cell formation and altered vascularity of a tuberculous synovitis; (b) lymphocytic follicle formation with endarteritis of the blood vessels around it; (c) caseation within the centre of a tuberculous follicle; and (d) areas of plasma cell and endothelial cell accumulation, with blood vessel changes in between areas of lamellar bone.

1. *Osteoporosis.* Thinning of the lamellae is brought about by true absorption of bone. In true absorption, the osteoclasts appear beside the lamellae, and produce a series of tiny excavations known as Howship's lacunae. Portions of bone, over a large area, are thus progressively removed and replaced by a fibrocellular marrow, and the individual lamellae in this way acquire a worm-eaten appearance; the fibrous elements at first persist, but ultimately they merge into the fibrous tissue of the adjacent tuberculous nodule.
2. *Osteosclerosis* is the result of osteoblastic activity. The osteoblasts arrange themselves along the surface of the lamellae and, under their influence, successive layers of new bone are deposited. Osteosclerosis is characteristic of the chronic types of disease, and tends to limit their progress.

The periosteum

The increased vascularity of the periosteum is one of the earliest signs of tuberculous infection of bone; it is soon followed by subperiosteal thickening, due to a deposit of new bone, which may be either porous or dense. There is first an activity of the osteoclasts resulting in erosion of the surface of the bone, which therefore becomes rough and irregular. The osteoblasts then proliferate, and a thin layer of new bone is laid down on the uneven surface. The process is repeated until a series of such layers has been deposited, and the circumference of the bone increased.

Course of the disease

The disease progresses slowly, and in the commoner forms caseation occurs in the central portion of the shaft. Ultimately the pus extends peripherally and a subperiosteal abscess forms. If the disease is not healed the periosteum gives way, the tuberculous debris being extruded into the soft parts, where, following the line of least resistance, it tracks along fascial planes to the surface. The skin overlying the abscess reddens but is not warm on palpation (hence the term 'cold abscess'), becomes progressively thinner and ultimately yields, and in this way a tuberculous sinus is formed. If such a sinus becomes infected with pyogenic organisms the prognosis is grave. The child becomes more and more emaciated, the temperature is 'swinging' and, finally, diarrhoea and albuminuria – evidence of amyloid disease – set in.

DIAGNOSIS

Positive evidence of a joint infection is identifying the tuberculous organism on culture from the joint or its neighbourhood, the histological identification of the disease in tissue from the joint, or the reproduction of the disease by the inoculation of a guinea-pig with material from the joint.

Various methods may be used in the attempt to establish the diagnosis of tuberculosis, any one of which may be misleading.

Ziehl–Neelsen stain

Ziehl–Neelsen staining of the acid-fast bacilli may be detected in the aspirate or in excised tissues. Sinnott *et al.* (1990) have described a five-point biopsy, histology and cultural protocol for examining bone biopsy material. This protocol is particularly useful in uncovering tuberculous infections being masked by staphylococcus.

Guinea-pig test

This is the most convenient method when there is fluid available for inoculation. It is better to inject two guinea-pigs in every case. In arriving at a conclusion, distinction has to be made between the case with an actual infection of the joint and a symptomatic synovitis from a periarticular focus; the fluid from the latter is sterile. The guinea-pig test, then, is decisive only when the result is positive, whereas a repeatedly negative result does not preclude tuberculosis.

Tuberculin test

A positive Mantoux test is of significance only in the first 3 or 4 years of life, after which 50% of the population give a positive reaction. On the other hand, a negative Mantoux reaction does not preclude active bone or joint tubercle. The only convincing proofs are, first, the absolutely negative result of all tuberculin tests, including the subcutaneous up to an injection of 10 mg of old tuberculin, and, secondly, a focal reaction which both objectively and subjectively, is undoubtedly positive. The focal reaction is not devoid of danger, however, and it is doubtful, too, whether it is specific.

CLINICAL FEATURES

Pain, swelling, local tenderness with associated muscle spasm around a bone or joint can be seen. Acquired deformities are common. Cold abscess formation, e.g. a psoas iliacus abscess, should be looked for. Involvement of lung, kidney and lymph glands must be excluded by blood counts, ESR, sputum examination by laryngeal swabbing, urine culture, etc. Heaf multiple puncture skin tests are most helpful in testing contacts of known tuberculous patients.

Radiographic appearances

See Figures 9.19 and 9.20.

There is no picture entirely typical of bone or joint tuberculosis in any of its stages. At an early stage, the x-ray examination is usually negative. The earliest sign is decalcification of the bones related to the

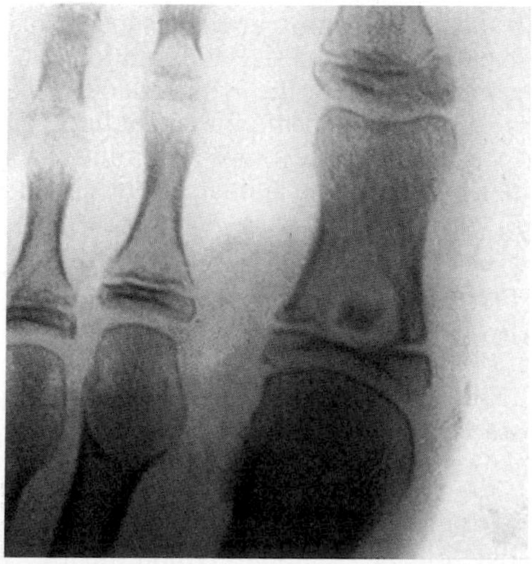

Figure 9.19 Tuberculosis of bone. Disease of the proximal phalanx of the great toe with a small sequestrum.

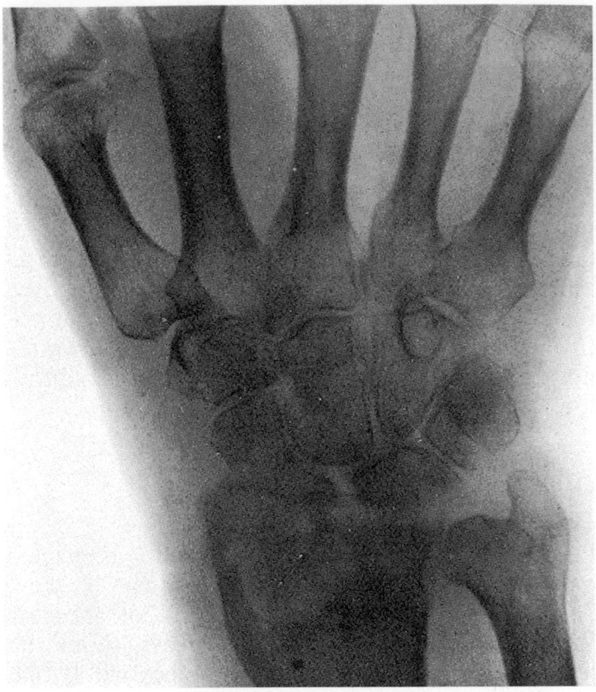

Figure 9.20 Tuberculosis of the lower end of the radius, with involvement of the wrist joint.

affected joint. Later signs are a localized area of diminished density in the bone, an increased joint space, thickening of the synovial membrane and an irregularity of the joint outline. The later films show clearly a gross destructive lesion of the joint with absorption of bone, loss of continuity of the joint and dislocation. With healing there is gradual replacement and condensation of bone, but any gross deformity persists.

Computed tomography (CT) combined with magnetic resonance imaging (MRI) is particularly of value in determining the size and location of the soft tissue component, e.g. the lymphadenitis, the cold abscess formation, and the intramedullary, marrow lesion – as well as the bony and joint changes – particularly of the spine and large joints (Bell *et al.*, 1990).

Wassermann reaction or Treponema *immobilization test*

In all doubtful cases it is the rule to exclude syphilis by one or other of these tests.

Biopsy

A biopsy of the regional lymph nodes, where possible, is often useful. The inguinal gland may show evidence of tubercle in a doubtful knee joint.

Exploratory arthrotomy for debridement and obtaining biopsy material

An exploration of the joint is the most certain way of ascertaining the diagnosis, and should be carried out in any doubtful case. Microscopically, there is marked similarity to syphilis. The tissue may be cultured or a guinea-pig inoculated.

DIFFERENTIAL DIAGNOSIS

Tuberculosis of bone has to be distinguished from the following.

Syphilis of bone

If there is evidence of periostitis and osteitis, there is usually a history of syphilis or other signs of its presence, while syphilis of bone is attended with severe pain. The radiological appearances are dissimilar, and the specific serological tests are positive.

Chronic pyogenic osteomyelitis

In this condition, acute or subacute exacerbations occur at intervals, with fever and local inflammatory signs. On radiological examination, there is more necrosis and sequestration, and more sclerosis.

Sarcoma

Osteogenic sarcoma forms a uniform and more localized swelling at the bone end; its growth is rapid and associated with pain.

PROGNOSIS

The prognosis has become very much better since it is now possible to operate on the infected bone or joint and deal directly, for example, with caries in the infected vertebral bodies. This is possible because of better anaesthesia and the antibiotic cover. Cavities are curetted, sequestra removed and the tuberculous lesion excised. Antibiotics can be applied locally and they become more effective as a result of the hyperaemic reaction following surgery. Excavated areas may be filled with bone grafts. Indeed, with modern methods of treatment it may be considered a curable disease with a good prognosis.

TREATMENT

Treatment must be both local and general. It may be conveniently discussed under five headings – general, chemotherapy, local, operative and the treatment of tuberculous abscesses.

General treatment

Rest, liberal diet and hygienic surroundings are essential. Muscular tone is restored, the bones strengthened and circulation and respiration improved.

Chemotherapy

The traditional triple therapy is still used to discourage the emergence of resistant strains during treatment but streptomycin, para-aminosalicylic acid (PAS) and isoniazid have been replaced by less toxic but equally efficacious drugs. Of the newer drugs, rifampicin has the great advantage of low toxicity although it is bacteriostatic when used alone. Ethambutol has largely replaced PAS in long-term treatment because it is better tolerated and has fewer toxic effects though it may cause visual disturbances. Isoniazid is the most effective anti-tuberculous drug, inhibiting DNA synthesis and intermediary metabolism of the tubercle bacillus, and is retained as a first-line drug despite its hepatorenal or neural toxicity.

The following chemotherapeutic programme is recommended. Rifampicin 600 mg orally daily 1 hour before breakfast combined with isoniazid 300 mg once daily and ethambutol 25 mg/kg once daily for 60 days and then 15 mg/kg. These are continued for 6 months and, if the clinical, serological and radiographic responses are good, rifampicin is stopped and isoniazid and ethambutol are continued for 18–24 months.

In the presence of skeletal tuberculosis with pulmonary involvement, Angel (1992) has recommended a standard drug regimen of isoniazid, rifampicin, pyrazinamide and ethambutol (or streptomycin) for the first 2 months, and then isoniazid and rifampicin for a further 4 months. If bacterial resistance to isoniazid is suspected, e.g. in immigrants from some developing countries (up to 25%) or from India (8–13%), the combined four should be continued.

Pyrazinamide is particularly effective in killing the tubercle bacillis in the acid intracellular environment of the macrophage and therefore is most effective in the first 2–3 months.

The actual duration of giving these drugs will have to be extended if any of them have to be discontinued for any adverse effects. Also compliance has to be constantly checked by tablet counts, regular analysis of urine, particularly in the patient population at risk, e.g. homeless people, alcoholics, drug users, in the elderly and in children.

Adverse effects of nausea, vomiting and jaundice may occur and be investigated before stopping therapy. Liver function tests are essential. Rifampicin reduces the effectiveness of oral contraceptives and can give rise to purpura and acute renal failure. Isoniazid, although cheap and efficient, can cause peripheral neuropathy, insomnia, restlessness and rarely a psychosis. Pyrazinamide can produce a rise in serum uric acid with arthralgia, rashes, etc. Ethambutol, at high dosages, produces ocular disturbances and should not be used in young children or those with visual disturbances. It should not be used in pregnant women for fear of teratological effects.

When sinuses drain persistently there is superinfection with pyogenic organisms which requires treatment with a broad-spectrum antibiotic such as ampicillin.

Chemoprophylaxis

Children under the age of 16 who have not been vaccinated with BCG and have been in contact with tuberculous patients should be given isoniazid 300 mg daily for 6 months. Children. and young adults can also be included in such a regimen particularly in developing and Indian countries, on any form of tuberculosis contact with a positive sputum.

Local treatment

The local treatment includes reduction of any deformity present, traction, fixation of the joint in the desired position, and protection until the healing is complete.

It is of the utmost importance to secure the limb in such a position that, should ankylosis supervene, the greatest possible functional utility will be attained. Attention must therefore be directed to the reduction of any deformity and to the fixation of the joint in the desired position. A flexed knee, for instance, must be extended, and a dropped wrist dorsiflexed. This reduction is commonly effected by gradual traction.

When the deformity is reduced, a decision must be reached on the ultimate aim – a stiff painless joint, or a movable one? The prognosis will be based on the extent of the disease as shown by the radiographs.

When the bone is diseased a stiff joint is probable, though sometimes, after a long period of fixation with ankylosis in view, a surprising degree of movement remains. The joint is encased in plaster-of-Paris, except in very young patients or in those with sinuses, in order to obtain complete immobility; the plaster cast should include the joints on both sides of the affected one. The duration of this treatment depends on many factors – age, site of disease, etc. – but a minimum period of 6 months is indicated.

When the disease is mainly synovial, with little affection of bone, a movable joint should be the aim. The extent of movement will depend on the adhesions between the joint surfaces; hence the object of treatment in these cases is to keep the surfaces as far apart as possible by means of traction, which is more frequently used in the lower limb. The duration of treatment in this phase is until there is no evidence of active disease and healing is far advanced or complete.

Mobilization, using hydrotherapy to restore wasted muscles, is begun, but still under chemotherapy for 6–9 months at least.

Operative treatment

In the majority of cases, conservative treatment is the method of choice, but certain conditions definitely indicate operation. The duration of the disease tends to be shortened thereby.

The operation of joint excision may be advisable in a destructive lesion in an adult, but it is not attended with favourable results in the young child, chiefly because the disease is usually more extensive than is shown in the radiograph and therefore excision of a considerable area of bone is necessary. This would naturally interfere with growing epiphyses and lead to a shortening of the limb in later years. A more direct attack upon the tuberculous area in the joint is now advocated in many cases, along with the administration of anti-tuberculous drugs. Partial capsulectomy and synovectomy removes tissues in which the circulation is defective. These structures re-form easily and quickly and revascularization occurs in the tissue so that the drug obtains access to the subchondral bone on which the integrity of the joint depends. Wilkinson (1965) showed the success of such a method. He operated on 26 children's hips and lost the function of only 4 joints. On the other hand, this method is not successful in adult joints owing to the poor nutrition of the cartilage.

In addition to excision of tuberculous joints, there are important extra-articular forms of operation whereby a joint is fixed by means of an internal bone graft.

Treatment of tuberculous abscesses

A residual abscess is more easily cured than an acute one. The tendency in the treatment of both is to be conservative, and a considerable number of abscesses disappear under this management. A more active therapy is indicated when there is tension of the skin, or where pressure is being exerted on vital parts.

Aspiration

It is sometimes possible to effect a cure by repeated emptying of the abscess. A wide-bore needle is inserted obliquely through healthy skin and pushed on until it enters the abscess cavity, the contents of which are removed by aspiration. Before withdrawing the needle, anti-tuberculous drugs are injected. After withdrawal, the puncture is sealed. The method may be repeated, and if the pus is fluid enough its removal and drug injection may effect a cure. But in many cases the content cannot be aspirated and so a more radical attack is justified.

Chemotherapy

Chemotherapy has its greatest value in reducing the bacteraemia during surgery as well as restoring to tuberculous tissues their powers of healing and thereby allowing tuberculous abscesses to be treated under the ordinary principles of surgery. The abscess is opened and thoroughly evacuated along with any sequestra present. If, as often happens, there is a tract down to bone, the bone may be curetted and soft unhealthy bony debris removed. Bleeding is controlled by packing for a short time. Should there be a large bony defect, it may safely be filled with cancellous bone chips from the iliac crest. Streptomycin and cloxacillin are left in the area and the wound is closed. Systemic cover is continued with the appropriate antibiotic drugs.

Tuberculosis of the hip joint

As a rule, tuberculous disease affects the hip joint before the age of 10. Its incidence is less than that of spinal disease, the ratio being about 7:10. It is slightly commoner in males. The infection, as with all tuberculosis of bone, is invariably secondary to a primary site elsewhere in the body.

PATHOLOGY

The usual initial bone site of the disease is in the upper part of the acetabulum or in the so-called Babcock's triangle (i.e. the lower half of the neck of the femur near the epiphyseal line or in any of the other two sites noted in (Figure 9.21), but it may be synovial in origin. In the neglected case the sequence of the pathology is as follows.

When disease begins near the epiphyseal cartilage of the head of the femur – a place where the circulation is active and the growing bone less

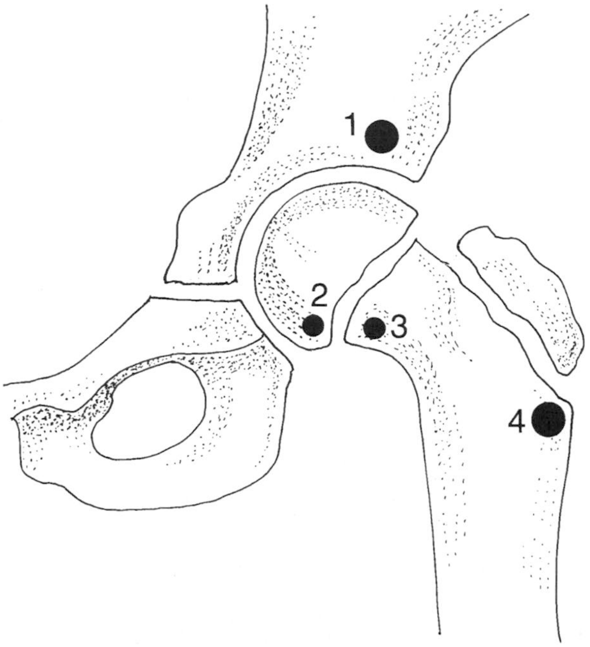

Figure 9.21 The four bone sites of origin of tuberculosis of the hip joint.

resistant – an area of infected granulations forms, which spreads towards the joint. These granulations extend gradually over and under the cartilage, which they ultimately destroy, and finally attack the bones comprising the joint (Figure 9.22). In the early stage there is a simple effusion, but the fluid soon becomes infected with tubercle and the whole joint is invaded by the disease. The synovial membrane becomes thickened, oedematous, grey and ulcerated, and the bones, denuded of their protective cartilage, are eroded, and sequestra may form. Multiple cavitation is typical of tuberculosis of the hip. Cavities in the femoral head and neck are not infrequent but the majority are found in the acetabular roof (Wilkinson, 1965). As the disease progresses, the head of the femur is partly absorbed, the remnants being dislocated from the acetabulum onto the ilium, where a false joint is formed. This is constantly pulled upwards by the muscles acting on the head, giving rise to the so-called 'wandering' or 'migratory' acetabulum.

At a later stage, the pus which has formed bursts through the capsule, and spreads in the lines of least resistance. It may point in the groin, in the neighbourhood of the greater trochanter, or, by perforating the acetabulum, appear as a pelvic abscess.

If left untreated, healing may take place eventually by absorption and connective-tissue encapsulation, but there results much distortion, deformity and ankylosis of the joint.

SYMPTOMS

The disease is insidious in its onset and chronic in its course. Before definite signs appear there is evidence of malaise, the child being pale and apathetic, with a poor appetite and losing weight. One of the first symptoms is stiffness of the limb, which is present on first getting out of bed but passes off during the morning; it returns, however, on a subsequent day and causes the child to limp. Both stiffness and limp tend to persist more and more. Pain may be absent in the early stage or, when present, be referred to the knee. Later the child begins to cry out during sleep, though, on awaking, there may be no complaint of pain. This cry is elicited by the so-called 'starting-pains' caused by the friction of the two diseased surfaces whose movement is permitted by the muscular relaxation that sleep produces. The symptom signifies ulceration of the cartilage surfaces of the joint.

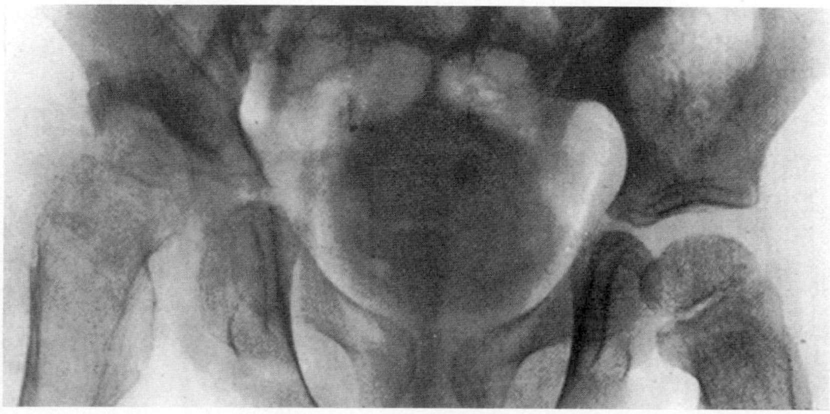

Figure 9.22 Tuberculosis of the hip and sacroiliac joint, after the reduction of the flexion–adduction deformity. Destruction of the articular cartilage is now apparent.

PHYSICAL SIGNS

Lameness is one of the first signs. In the early stages it is caused by stiffness or flexion deformity, the body bending forwards to compensate for inability to extend the hip. Later a further limp is produced by pain. Lastly, there is the limp from real shortening.

Inspection

The examination should be carefully carried out with the patient undressed, and the general effect of the illness may sometimes be seen in the pallor and emaciation. The affected thigh may be visibly wasted, the atrophy extending to the gluteal muscles. The deformity and the resulting limp are now obvious, differing according to the stage of the disease.

Palpation

Palpation corroborates the findings of inspection. The range and freedom of movements are determined by comparison with those on the normal side and are limited in all directions.

Thomas's flexion deformity test is carried out. The good knee and hip are flexed on the abdomen and the child is asked to lay his affected leg on the table. If he cannot do this actively or with slight assistance then there is a flexion deformity present and the test is positive.

Radiographic examination

At an early stage nothing abnormal is noted. The earliest sign is a slight loss of bone density due to synovial oedema. In a few cases, owing to its excessive thickness, it is possible to delineate the synovial membrane, above and below the head. With a large effusion the ends of the bones are farther apart than on the sound side. Bone becomes osteoporotic and, still later, an area of destruction is seen, most commonly in Babcock's triangle on the inferior aspect of the cervical side of the epiphysis (Figure 9.23). It is not uncommon to find on radiography or at operation one or more sequestra. This is usually in the upper and outer quadrant of the femoral head following thrombosis of the lateral epiphyseal vessels supplying this area.

These changes lead to dislocation, with a 'migratory acetabulum'.

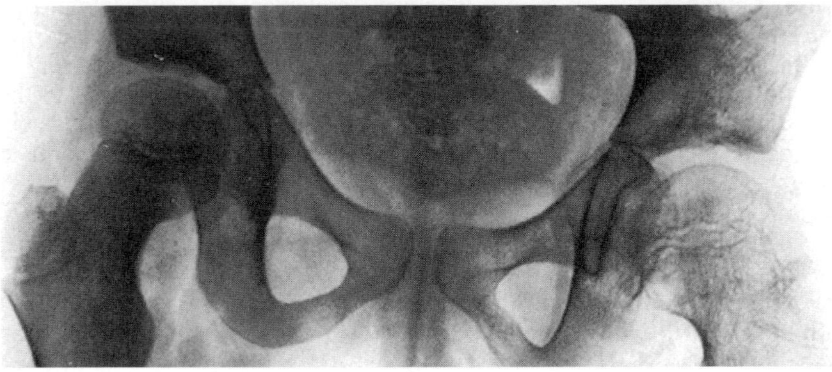

(a)

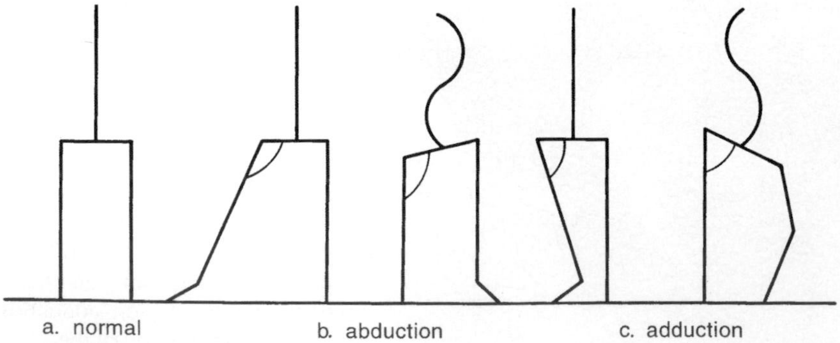

(b)

Figure 9.23 (a) Early case of synovial disease. Note the decalcification especially marked in Babcock's area. (b) Tuberculosis of the hip. Diagrammatic representation of the effects of a fixed joint in abduction and adduction. When abducted, the pelvis is tilted to bring the legs parallel, with an apparent lengthening. When adducted the tilting produces apparent shortening. The spine flexes laterally to allow the head to assume its erect position and scoliosis results.

MRI examination is particularly useful in showing intramedullary spread of the osteomyelitic component as well as for soft tissue abscess formation.

DIAGNOSIS

The diagnosis is made from the history, the symptoms, and from the physical examination, including the radiographs. The results of the tuberculin tests can never be taken as final, and a definite diagnosis can be made only by the discovery of tubercle bacilli, in the fluid or tissue from the joint. In children the Mantoux intradermal test is of some value in that a negative result will count against tuberculosis; but it is only in young children that a positive result can be considered of any particular value. The test should be tried with 1:1000 dilution, and if this is negative repeated with 1:100 dilution. It may be necessary to inoculate a guinea-pig for positive results. Synovial biopsy may show a 'positive' histology as well on involved lymph gland.

DIFFERENTIAL DIAGNOSIS

Various diseases may simulate a tuberculous hip. These may be grouped under the symptoms they produce; viz. limitation of movement, abscess, limp and pain.

Limitation of movement

In tuberculous disease, limitation of movement is caused by spasm of muscles, and is observed in every direction and is often painful.

'Irritable hip' is not uncommon in children. If non-tuberculous, it will disappear after a few weeks' rest and traction with a negative aspiration for organisms.

Upper neurone lesions exhibit spasm which is gradually overcome by pressure. There is no wasting and usually there are signs of the disease in other parts of the limb.

In reflex irritation, as from inflamed glands or injured adductors or phimosis, limitation is not generalized as in hip-joint disease.

Abscesses in the region of the hip

It may be difficult to trace these to their source. If acute, there is little difficulty; if subacute, the possibility of hip disease must be considered. The result of treatment, and the examination of pus from the abscess, should be specially noted. If the abscess is tuberculous, it must be differentiated from a tuberculous infection of the subgluteal or psoas bursa in which the limitation of hip movements is not general. It is in these cases that a complete x-ray examination of the hip, pelvis, and lumbar spine is of diagnostic value (Figure 9.24), as well as an MRI examination.

Limp

Lameness may be due to several conditions.

1. *Congenital dislocation* of the hip is present from birth, the head of the femur is in an abnormal position, and certain movements are increased in range. A radiograph is decisive.
2. *Coxa vara*. Lateral rotation is increased and there is marked deformity. x-Ray examination is of the greatest value.
3. *Pseudocoxalgia (Perthes' disease)*. Many examinations may be required before a diagnosis can be made in this condition. There is less muscular wasting in Perthes' disease, while the radiograph will show more bone changes, which in the early stage of a tuberculous hip are few. In Perthes' disease the movements are not limited in all directions as in tuberculosis.
4. *Irritable hip* in a child with normal radiographs.

Pain

Pain in the region of the hip may be the predominant symptom in the following diseases:

1. *Osteomyelitis and septic arthritis*. The main features in these diseases are local tenderness and toxaemia. A differential white blood count shows a polymorphonuclear leucocytosis; in tuberculosis there is a lymphocytosis.
2. *Slipped upper femoral epiphysis*. The pain, eversion, shortening and absence of wasting are suggestive. x-Ray examination at once reveals the nature of the condition.
3. *Poliomyelitis*. This has a more sudden onset, often arising during an epidemic; the muscles are markedly hyperaesthetic and tender. In a few days the joint can be moved freely in all directions.
4. *Irritable hip*.

PROGNOSIS

In the early case, before irreversible changes have taken place in the cartilage, a good result – freely movable joint – can be expected from conservative treatment; but part of this may well be a biopsy for diagnostic purposes. In later cases, with modern methods of treatment, mortality should be rare.

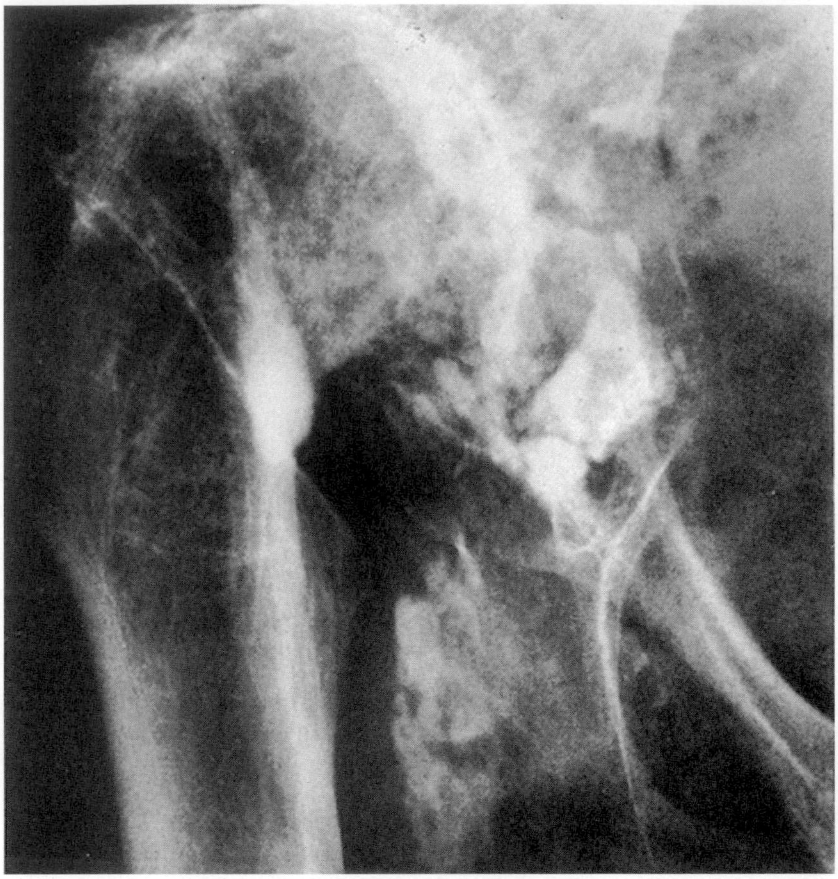

Figure 9.24 Old tuberculosis infection of hip joint with marked calcification of surrounding soft tissues.

When the head is affected, the result is always doubtful, and if there is much bone destruction, ankylosis in a good position is the limit of cure. In this variety there is a marked tendency to adduction, even after treatment has been carried out for a long period.

TREATMENT

General treatment

Liberal diet, fresh air, sunshine, discipline, and education or occupation are still of great importance. Attention, however, must be directed to any local disabilities, and the joint must be placed in the position that will provide the greatest functional position when the cure has been established. The most important part of conservative treatment is, of course, antibiotics.

Local treatment

This will vary according to the extent of the disease. If it is advanced, there is usually some deformity of flexion and adduction, from strong muscular contraction. Before further treatment can be initiated, this deformity must be corrected and any pain that is present alleviated.

Stage of acute symptoms

When the patient is suffering acute pain in the joint, skin traction is applied to the limb by means of strapping. After the application of the traction strapping the limb is placed in a Thomas's knee splint to steady it and ensure traction in the proper direction. The actual pull on the extension may be by a weight led over a pulley at the foot of the bed. If the weight method is used, the amount required is approximately 0.45 kg for every year of age, the foot of the bed being raised so that a counter-extension is formed by the weight of the body.

The actual degree of deformity is estimated, both by obliterating the compensatory pelvic tilt with lumbar lordosis and by abducting the opposite leg, the traction being then arranged to pull in the line of the deformity. This direction can be adjusted. The extension pulls on the opposing joint surfaces, thereby abolishing the spasm of muscle, which causes flexion adduction, providing rest, relieving pain and correcting deformity. Each day this traction is inspected and its direction modified, and in a few weeks the deformity will be corrected sufficiently to ensure a useful position, should ankylosis ensue which is known as the optimum functional position. The greater the real shortening, the more extensive must the abduction be; but, even without bone disease, abduction is advisable, as, with adhesions in the joint, the tendency during convalescence is towards adduction.

Stage of cure

When the acute symptoms, particularly pain and spasm, have subsided, and the deformity has been treated, it is necessary to decide whether or not a movable joint is to be aimed at. This difficult question is decided by radiography. If the head of the bone is much eroded, or there is much disease on the acetabular surface, it is almost certain that ankylosis will ensue. It is true that, occasionally, a much eroded joint, after months in plaster, shows considerable movement. This, however, may be painful, and in any case its functional value is inconsiderable. It is probably wise in all adults, and where destruction of bone is extensive, to aim at ankylosis. When the disease is synovial, or when there is a focus in the neck of the femur, treatment is based on the assumption, or rather the hope, that a mobile joint may result.

Treatment of an average case

Any case likely to retain movement after cure is treated by traction with the object of allowing limited movement and preventing bony ankylosis. An exploratory operation can be carried out for diagnosis, and to permit the antibiotic to get free circulation into the diseased area. The actual operation will be a partial synovectomy which promotes more rapid vascularization of the diseased area. Many of the cases have their period of treatment reduced by this intra-articular operation.

Wilkinson (1965) showed conclusively that all cases are improved by constitutional treatment, antibiotics and intra-articular operation, varying from simple arthrotomies to partial synovectomy with curettage of bone foci.

When the acute symptoms have subsided and the deformity has been reduced, the joint is exposed by a posterior incision and an attempt made to remove most of the tuberculous tissue from the joint and a partial synovectomy is carried out. Cavities in the bone, which are usually posteromedial, are particularly looked for and curetted. The head is not dislocated, for if an attempt is made to do this the neck may fracture, or the blood supply may be compromised.

With this treatment there is quickly an improvement in the patient's general condition; the temperature becomes steady, appetite improves and the patient gains weight. Associated lesions, too, are found to improve, and even more striking is the local improvement in the affected joint. All these changes may follow antibiotic treatment without operation, but they are accelerated by operation and an effective response is usually produced in patients whose response to antibiotics is inadequate.

Following operation, constitutional treatment and traction on the leg on an abduction frame are continued, as, of course, is treatment with antibiotics. Most cases of severe tuberculous infection survive, with return of function.

If complete freedom of movement be allowed within the limits of confinement to bed, and the patient examined daily, it will be found in favourable cases that the joint gains daily in mobility, and that there is an absence of spasm.

Treatment of a case with much bone disease

In such cases ankylosis may be the aim of treatment, and this can best be secured by immobilizing the hip with plaster-of-Paris (Figure 9.25). In applying the plaster cast it has to be borne in mind that the hip will ultimately be fixed in the position chosen. It is important to remember that growth will almost certainly be diminished, and that the only compensation for this, apart from leg-lengthening operations, is an abduction osteotomy. In cases, therefore, where there is much disease in the region of the femoral epiphysis, a moderate amount of abduction is produced. The limb is placed in a neutral position of rotation, or just a few degrees of external rotation. The position of flexion chosen varies with the age, and 1° for each year of life up to 20°, then a little more, is suggested. The patient with an ankylosed hip cannot sit and walk comfortably. He is most comfortable walking with an extended hip, while a flexed hip suits him best for sitting. Something between the two has therefore to be chosen, and his wishes and occupation have to be considered.

Stage of convalescence

At the end of this stage, when there is evidence at the disease is arrested, ambulatory treatment begins. In most cases there is an intervening period of about 3 months when the patient is allowed freedom in bed, unhampered by any apparatus. During this time he is

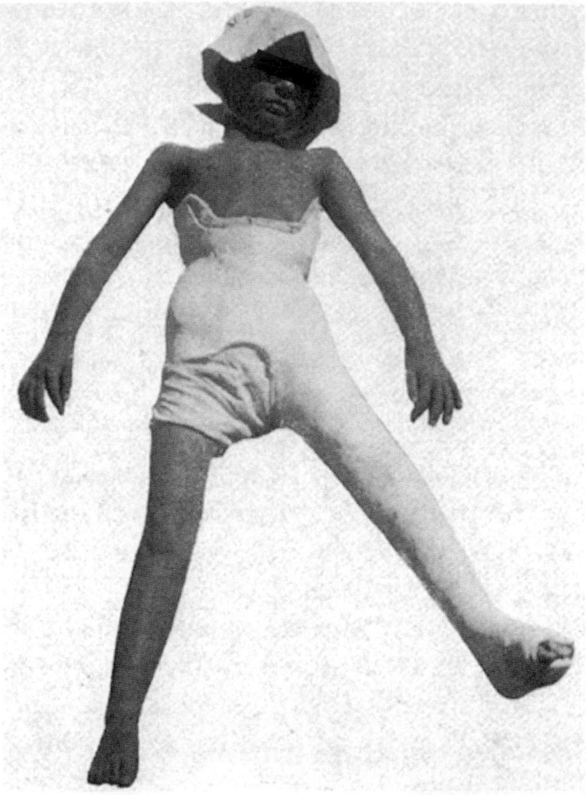

Figure 9.25 Treatment of second stage of tuberculosis by a plaster-of-Paris cast. Note the moulding to secure immobilization.

measured for an orthotic walking caliper, and a raise is fixed to the shoe on the sound side.

Ambulatory treatment is divided into stages so that full function is attained gradually. It is of the utmost importance that the caliper fit the patient correctly. Two things at least are essential for a proper-fitting splint: the tuberosity of the ischium must rest on the ring of the caliper or flange of the orthotic thigh piece, and not slip through it, and there must be a space between the heel of the foot and the heel of the shoe when the patient is standing upright. If these conditions are fulfilled no weight is transmitted through the hip joint, and this avoidance of weight-bearing must be assured during the first stage of ambulatory treatment, when the patient uses his caliper, and crutches, with a raise on the sound side. The patient is usually advised to wear his caliper for at least 6 months, during which time he should be examined at regular intervals.

Anti-tuberculous drugs have allowed a direct attack on the joint; in patients seen early for a mobile joint, and in patients seen late, a shorter period of immobilization, an earlier and quicker fusion, and fewer, if any, complications. There is no doubt that the best results are now obtained by the use of antibiotics and surgery.

It has been pointed out that the hip joint may be affected with tuberculosis in three ways: an extra-articular focus, synovial disease, and an intra-articular lesion with destruction of the cartilage. These lesions may be treated in the following ways.

1. *Extra-articular focus*. Even before the days of streptomycin an extra-articular focus was excised with some measure of success, when it was accessible. It is much safer to do so now, and it should be carried out before the adjacent joint becomes involved. After antibiotics have been administered, the excision is carried out. It is good practice to fill the cavity – after a thorough removal of all diseased bone – with cancellous bone grafts and to use streptomycin and cloxacillin locally. A complete reconstitution of the bone and, of course, a mobile, hip, can be obtained.
2. *Synovial disease*. In synovial disease, with a tense full joint and with the synovial membrane and capsule ballooned out due to an effusion, there is every prospect of obtaining a mobile joint if the antibiotics can reach it in sufficient concentration and if, of course, the joint surfaces are relatively undamaged. The tuberculous exudate does not contain proteolytic enzymes, such as those seen in the exudate of pyogenic infection; the cartilage tends therefore, to persist until a later stage when it is covered by the tuberculous pannus of unhealthy granulation tissue. Early diagnosis and decompression are essential in order to save the joint, and therefore biopsy is justified, apart from diagnosis, to relieve tension and to allow the penetration of the chemotherapeutic agent. Much of the diseased synovial membrane must be removed together with part of the capsule. Synovial membrane regenerates rapidly. After removal of the diseased synovial membrane at operation fresh normal synovial tissues, carrying young blood vessels through which the antibiotics can circulate freely, will form. The only form of immobilization necessary during this treatment is by skin traction.
3. *The intra-articular lesion; intact articular cartilage*. It is unlikely that a joint with good movement will result, but with the use of antibiotics it is surprising how much movement will be maintained and so ankylosis need not necessarily be the aim. Up to a few years ago, even the intra-articular lesion was considered to be cured only when there was bony fusion, but it is recognized that there are still some cases in

which, although the lesion is intra-articular, most of the articular cartilage is still intact. Therefore, there is still the possibility of obtaining a mobile hip, at least for many years. The diseased focus in Babcock's triangle or in the acetabular region is approached and is thoroughly eradicated, the area being packed with cancellous bone chips. It is necessary to immobilize the joint in plaster for a few weeks (in the case of femoral foci) or by fairly heavy traction (in the case of acetabular foci). A certain proportion of hips will still heal by fusion or may require arthrodesis later, but it is remarkable how many will have mobility at the end of treatment. A long period of follow-up, i.e. 2 years, is necessary in order to be able to tell whether the mobility and cure is going to be permanent. If the chemotherapy is continued long enough, reactivation, or flare-up, of the tuberculosis is less likely to occur.

Arthodesis

In every case where ankylosis is to be expected, the question of the operative production of this is to be considered, as in many cases conservative treatment may not produce a sound arthrodesis. It has been stated that there are four main indications for arthrodesis:

1. an adult patient;
2. failure of conservative treatment to arrest the disease after 1 year;
3. relapse, especially the recurrence of pain and deformity after conservative treatment; and
4. certain destructive lesions, e.g. the formation of sequestra in the head or neck of the femur or in the acetabulum.

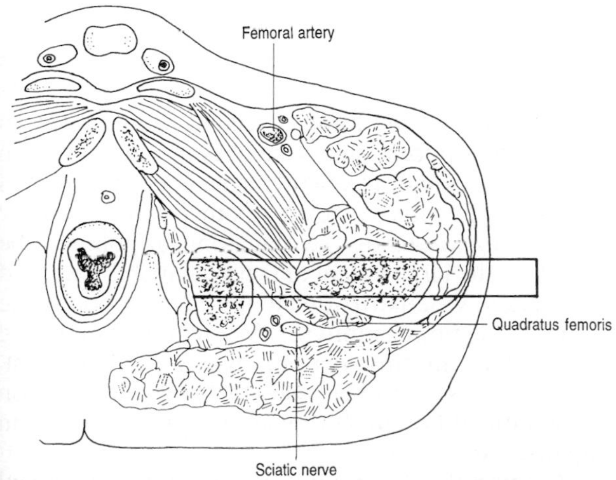

Figure 9.26 The route of Brittain's operation. (After Campbell from *Campbell's Operative Orthopaedics*, edited by A.H. Crenshaw, The C.V. Mosby Company, 1987)

Damaged articular cartilage

If the patient comes under treatment at a late stage when the articular cartilages are irretrievably damaged, then bony fusion must be considered. One need only wait now until the patient's general resistance has been built up in order to overcome the general toxaemia of the bacillary invasion; this is aided greatly by the use of chemotherapy. Arthrodesis is performed on the same lines as an arthrodesis of the spine, and, to the same extent, forms an internal splint. By this means the operation hastens the fusion of the joint and shortens the convalescence of the illness. It is indicated in patients who have frequent painful attacks, with extreme shortening, and a tendency to increasing deformity, especially if there are signs pointing to a relapse.

Various methods of arthrodesis of the hip have been described, some of them opening the joint and removing tuberculous debris before grafting bone into the surfaces as described.

Ischiofemoral method of extra-articular arthrodesis (Brittain)

Brittain pointed out that older methods have a common disadvantage in that, while fusion is taking place, the hip joint is subjected to the predominant force of adduction, and that any graft from the ilium to the greater trochanter may lose contact at each end. There is thus a distracting force on the graft, while in that of Brittain the force is one of compression. This operation 'consists of a subtrochanteric osteotomy through which the ischium immediately below the acetabulum is incised by a wide osteotome and a space made in it to receive a flat massive tibial

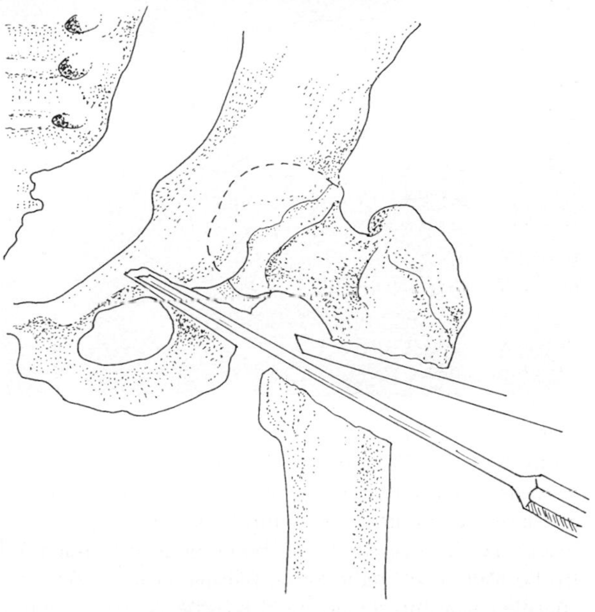

Figure 9.27 Arthrodesis by the ischiofemoral method.

bone graft. This is embedded deeply in the ischium and its outer part remains between the fragments of the osteotomy' (Figures 9.26 and 9.27).

A useful alternative, and a simple one, is the McMurray subtrochanteric osteotomy. Since the disease is now cured by antibiotics, the purpose of this operation is to give a stable weight-bearing surface without tendency to adduction. This operation is useful to correct an old fixed adduction–flexion deformity, as by this means the excess of shortening from the adduction is overcome and the strain on the lumbar spine relieved.

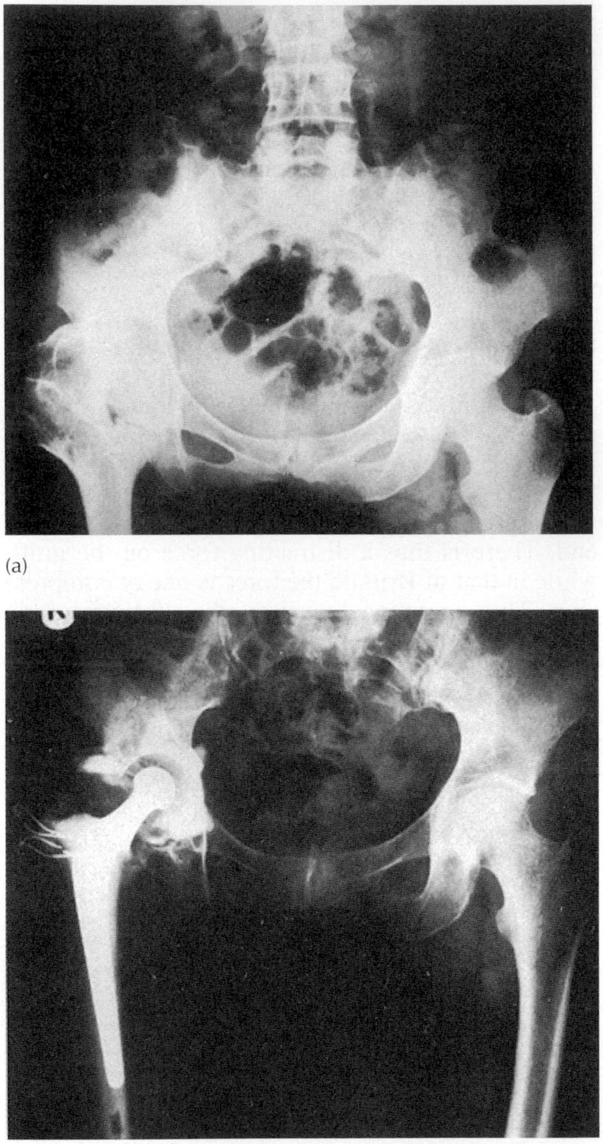

(a)

(b)

Figure 9.28 (a) Anteroposterior radiograph of the pelvis 40 years after tuberculosis of the right hip treated by attempted extra-articular arthrodesis. The hip has an unsound ankylosis and the bone graft has fractured. (b) Postoperative radiograph following insertion of a Charnley total hip replacement prosthesis. The patient is progressing well 1 year after operation.

Secondary operations

To correct an old fixed adduction–flexion deformity some form of osteotomy is usually employed.

In cases of sound bony ankylosis with adduction–flexion deformity, a subtrochanteric or a transtrochanteric osteotomy may be performed and the deformity reduced. By this means the excess of shortening from the adduction is overcome and the strain on the lumbar spine relieved.

Total hip replacement

It should be noted that in a personal series of over 20 such hip replacements no reactivation of the original infection has occurred but chemotherapy was continued for 1 year postoperatively. Shanmugasundaram (1987) has reported another series in which Charnley's low friction total hip replacement has been carried out in tuberculous 'destroyed' hip joints in which over 10% had had reactivation of infection in spite of prolonged chemotherapy but a successful revision was carried out in over half these patients – so this operation is of great benefit in certain societies in which mobile hip joints are required for daily activities.

In old quiescent cases where back pain or contralateral arthritis of the hip has occurred, conversion of the arthrodesed hips to a mobile state by total joint replacement is very worthwhile in selected cases, under chemotherapy (Figure 9.28).

Tuberculosis of the knee joint

Tuberculosis of the knee is second in frequency to that of the hip joint, and, like it, is most common in childhood, though frequently seen later. It is always secondary to active disease in other parts – usually the lymphatic glands. Two anatomical points to be noted are the large extent of synovial membrane, and the marked vascularity due to the late junction of the femoral and tibial epiphyses. Much growth of the leg takes place in this region; disease of the joint, therefore, is serious because of its possible effect on leg length, although shortening is more extensive in hip disease.

Because the knee joint is superficial, synovial swelling is observed earlier and the diagnosis is made frequently before there has been much joint disturbance or necrosis of bone. Even before the anti-tuberculous drug era many knee joints of children recovered with useful function.

PATHOLOGICAL ANATOMY

The disease may begin either in bone, usually in the femoral or tibial epiphysis or, more rarely, in the patella or in the synovial membrane, the latter being the most frequent site. Girdlestone described three groups of cases:

1. Osseous foci without infecting the joint. These foci are extra-articular, but in contiguity. Excision of the focus without entering the joint may save the latter. Patients with this type of disease form only a small proportion.
2. Osseous foci discharging into the joint (Figure 9.29).
3. No visible osseous focus. This group is radiologically synovial. Here the outlook is relatively favourable.

In the later stages these three usually coexist.

The synovial membrane is thickened, grey and translucent, and in places gelatinous or even caseous. Fluid is present in varying amount, and adhesions form so that the outlying synovial pockets become loculated. Granulations spread under and over the cartilage, which, being eroded by pressure and friction, may become detached, leaving the bones exposed. At the same time, softening and stretching of the ligaments tend to produce subluxation of the tibia, which slips backwards and rotates laterally. Inflammation takes place round the joint, leading to thickening, so that the spindle-shaped tumour known as a 'white swelling' is formed.

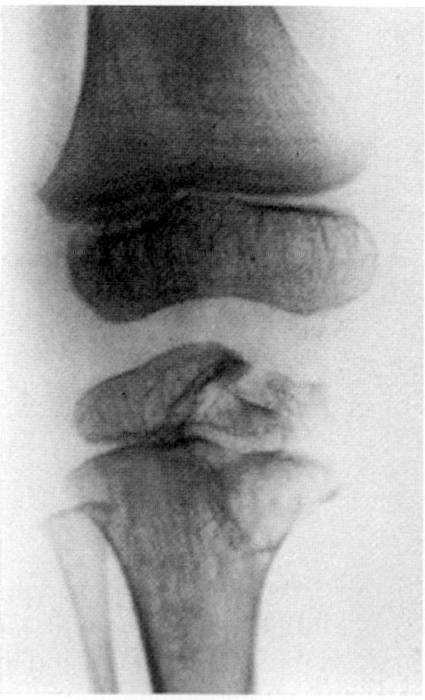

Figure 9.29 Intra-articular disease with spread from epiphyseal focus.

CLINICAL FEATURES

The patient is between the ages of 9 and 20, complaining of some swelling in the knee joint with modest pain and slight heat, and often with a history of injury but with little apparent deterioration of health. In the later cases the combination of muscular atrophy with enlargement of the joint gives an appearance of great swelling. Flexion and subluxation of the tibia are seen in the later stages, followed by periarticular abscesses and sinuses (Figure 9.30).

Swelling

The joint being superficial, swelling is soon apparent, and may be due to synovial thickening or the presence of fluid. Evidence of fluid is obtained by compression of the suprapatellar pouch with the palm of one hand, while the other palpates the patella and the pouches on both sides of it. When due to synovial thickening, the swelling is usually semi-elastic and doughy.

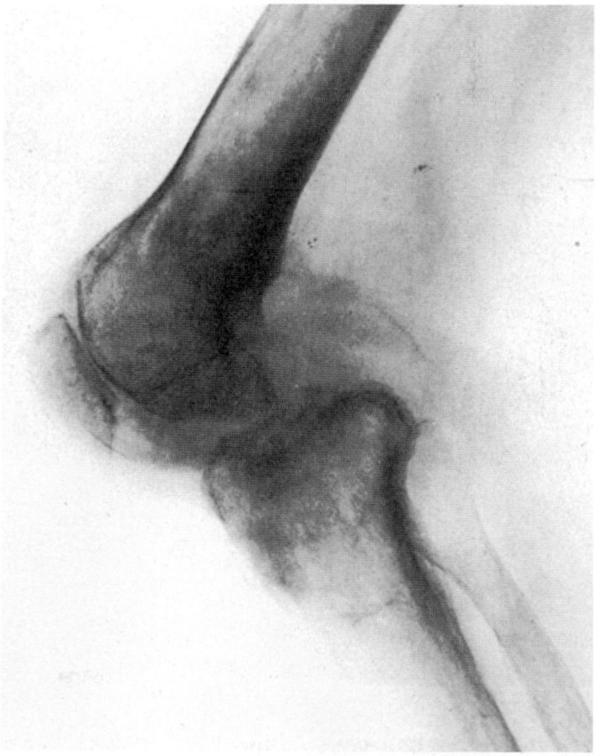

Figure 9.30 Subluxation of the knee from untreated tuberculous disease.

Limp

At first, when walking, the patient holds the knee moderately flexed to lessen the effect of the body weight, but free extension is possible. Later, however, it is limited.

Pain

At first moderate, pain may later become acute. The joint is easily tired and any sudden movement increases the pain. Night cries are common.

Muscular atrophy and spasm

Atrophy is greater than can be accounted for by disuse and probably arises from some trophic disturbance. Spasm affects the hamstrings, and the biceps, acting on the head of the fibula, pulls the leg backwards and rotates it laterally.

Shortening

The disease, by stimulating growth locally, may at an early stage cause lengthening (Figure 9.31); in the more destructive lesions, however, shortening is the rule, from retardation of growth and destruction of bone.

DIAGNOSIS

The history may reveal the likelihood of human infection, some previous manifestation of tuberculosis, or some loss of health and vigour. When a child develops a chronic swelling of the knee joint of an indolent character, with flexion and limitation of movement, diagnosis is, as a rule, easy, but there can be no certainty without histological or bacteriological examination.

Calvé emphasized many years ago the importance of infection of the regional glands in the groin proved by biopsy as an aid in diagnosis. A radiograph shows signs of early disease, especially if comparison be made with the sound knee. Bilateral disease is very rare.

In cases of doubtful synovial disease the authors carry out a biopsy of the synovium and, if this is negative, a diagnostic biopsy.

In considering the diagnosis, chronic traumatic synovitis, subacute infective synovitis, rheumatoid arthritis and acute rheumatism have all to be considered.

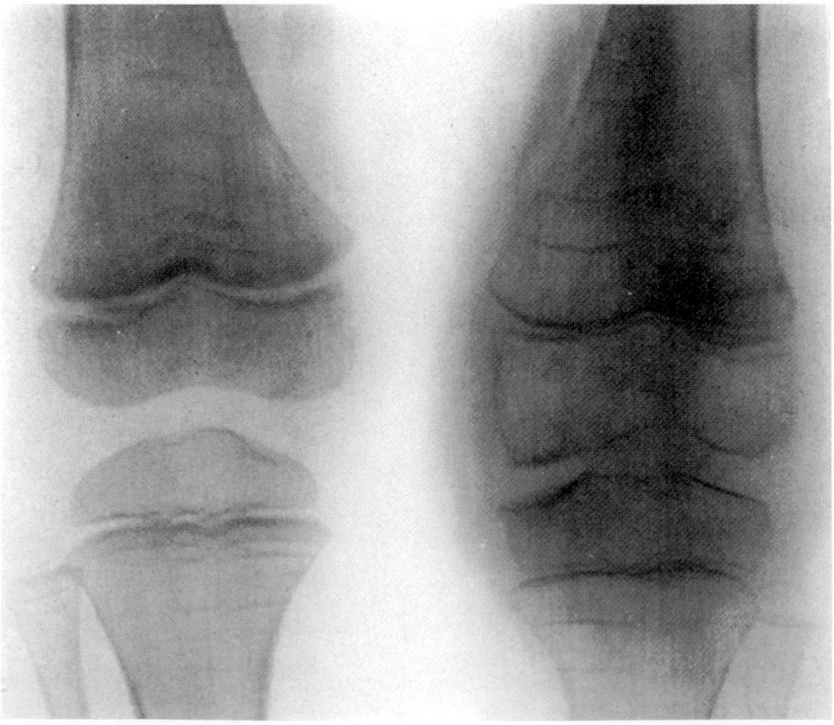

Figure 9.31 Tuberculous disease of the left knee joint. Growth has been accelerated and there is now actual lengthening of the diseased leg. This is unusual though not uncommon.

PROGNOSIS

The functional result improves in proportion to early diagnosis and efficient treatment.

Stevenson, in the 1950s, reported on 33 cases, the majority being of the younger age groups, and found 16 with full mobility, 8 more with over 95° and only 5 ankylosed. All the patients treated with intra-articular chemotherapy retained over 120° of flexion. These results were obtained with the previous average period of conservative treatment more than halved.

TREATMENT

As the patients suffer from tuberculosis of which the arthritis is only one manifestation, all need general treatment – with physical rest, chemotherapy, selected diet, etc.

At an early stage, when the disease is acute and painful, and the joint flexed, rapid relief is obtained by skin traction in the recumbent position and a Thomas's knee splint with a knee-flexion piece applied. The kneepiece allows the pull to be made in the line of the deformity, and, as treatment progresses, it can be adjusted daily until full extension is obtained. Great care must be taken to avoid backward or rotational displacement of the tibia, and this is achieved by reversed dynamic slings (Stein and Dickson, 1975).

When the knee is in a good functional position – that is, just short of complete extension – consideration has to be given, as in hip-joint disease, to the ultimate aim of treatment.

In the child, an attempt may be made to get a movable joint, and, as long as there is a possibility of this, traction may be continued.

In children it is unusual to get much cartilage destruction and it is likely that the majority will recover with antibiotic and constitutional treatment alone, especially if a joint biopsy is performed. Biopsy has a therapeutic value as well as a diagnostic one since local and general improvement usually take place afterwards. It is, of course, necessary where there is any doubt about the diagnosis. Through a small lateral incision over the suprapatellar pouch a piece of the capsule and synovial membrane is excised and sent for histological examination, culture and guinea-pig inoculation.

In most cases, however, a partial synovectomy is more valuable than the minor operation of biopsy. Synovectomy is carried out in those whose knees remain warm and swollen even after antibiotic therapy or whose range of movement does not show improvement. It is reserved for children since adults do not get the same benefit, especially in the way of improving movement.

The operation is undertaken after the preliminary treatment by rest, traction and antibiotics. Wilkinson (1965) said that 'joint clearance' was a more accurate name for the operation. Diseased synovial membrane is removed from the anterior and lateral compartment and from the suprapatellar pouch. The pannus over the articular cartilage is stripped off and the menisci, if fragmented, are removed. The infrapatellar fat pads are also removed because they are likely to become fibrosed. Careful haemostasis is ensured.

Following the operation, rest and traction to the knee should be continued, but in a few weeks voluntary flexion exercises should be instituted. If after a few days without traction the range of movement is less, it is necessary to resume traction. Antibiotics are continued for 6–12 months, by which time the child may be allowed to walk but with some protection – a walking caliper or crutches – for a short time yet. When radiography reveals an extra-articular abscess, this should be evacuated by a small incision over the abscess and removal of overlying bone. The cavity is curetted.

During succeeding years it is recommended that the patient be seen at intervals of from 3 to 6 months for a year or two to prevent, if possible, any deformity or recurrence of the disease.

Arthrodesis

This is usually required where there is marked erosion of bone and most often in adults. It is, in the first instance, an operation to remove pus, necrotic material, sequestra and oedematous synovial membrane. In the second instance it is an operation to obtain bony fusion. A tourniquet is used.

A linear parapatellar incision is made around the knee. The incision is deepened until the ligamentum patellae is exposed this is displaced laterally and the joint is flexed and opened.

Pus and necrotic material are removed from within the joint. The oedematous synovial membrane is removed as thoroughly as possible from all compartments. The cartilage is removed from the patella and from the tibia and femur by saw cuts at right angles to their longitudinal axes. These cuts can be made to correct any genu valgum or varus. A compression arthrodesis is carried out. The compression is continued for about 6 weeks, when the pins are removed and if there is clinical fusion a plaster cylinder from groin to ankle is applied. When the operation is carried out in children care must be taken to avoid damage to the epiphysis by chiselling off the cartilage rather than using saw cuts. Fusion in such a case is slower and may take 3–4 months.

Tuberculosis of the ankle

Tuberculosis of the ankle is relatively uncommon. The joint, although somewhat resistant to treatment – specially in adults – owing to the weight it has to support, its complex character and the free communications of its synovial spaces, usually responds well.

PATHOLOGY

The earlier lesion is usually a focus of erosion in one of the articulating bones, and from this the synovial membrane becomes involved.

In early cases, in children at least, the disease may be seen to be in one of three groups as is common in other joints:

1. The *extra-articular type* may be in the neighbouring soft tissues in the bony structure, as for example the bone abscess seen often in the calcaneum but also in the talus and cuboid.
2. In the *synovial type* there is generalized decalcification of the bones with synovial thickening.
3. The *intra-articular type* forms the largest group, and the ankle joint itself is the usual site though other smaller joints may appear to be the initial site.

Sinus formation occurs in the great majority of cases, though here this does not appear to have the same malign influence that it has in other joints and a sound though fibrous ankylosis usually results in children.

CLINICAL FEATURES

Limp and pain are the earliest symptoms. The pain is more acute in those lesions which spread from the bone, being intensified by pressure on the calcaneus either by increased plantar flexion or by lateral compression of the bone. The first deformity is dorsiflexion, to relieve tension on the talus, but later, with the progress of the disease, plantar flexion and equinovalgus deformities develop, both of which relieve the pressure of the weight of the body on the foot. The patient then walks stiffly, and on his toes. Swelling is evident in front of the joint in bone disease, and round the malleoli in synovial disease. Local heat and redness may be present, and there is the usual limitation of movement from muscular spasm. In the late stages, abscesses and sinuses are common.

DIAGNOSIS

A chronic monarticular arthritis with limitation of

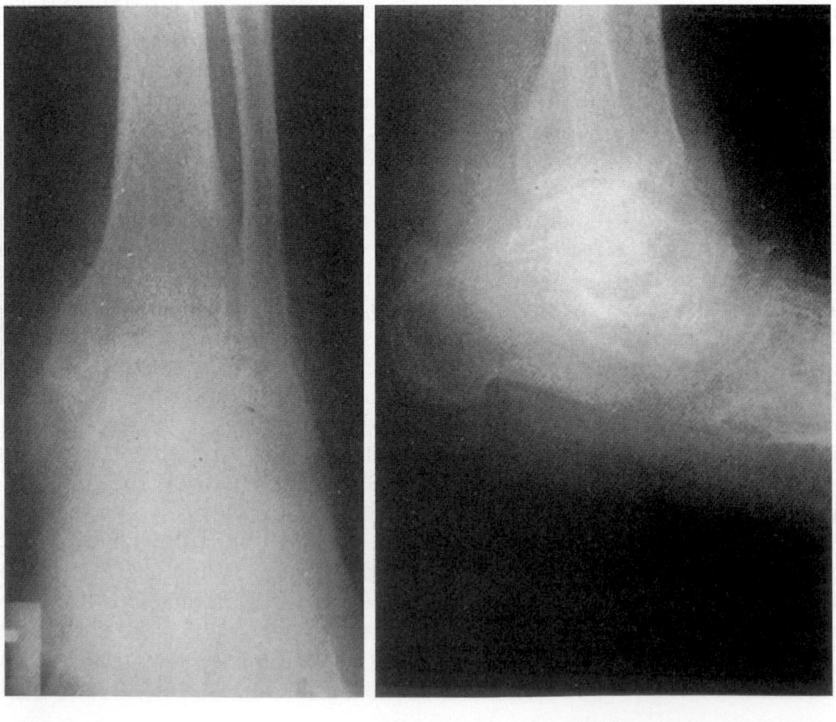

Figure 9.32 Radiographs of the left ankle of an elderly man who presented with a 'gouty' arthritis and with an elevated serum uric acid. Marked loss of bone density and joint space is seen and, on biopsy, a tuberculous synovitis was found.

movement, pain and tenderness and evening pyrexia is probably tuberculous. The osteoporosis seen on x-ray examination (Figure 9.32) is characteristic but may be due to rheumatoid disease. Biopsy may be carried out to verify the diagnosis.

TREATMENT

Most cases of a mild degree are treated conservatively by immobilization in a below-knee plaster and with antibiotics. There should be no weight-bearing but the patient need not be confined to bed. Those of a more severe degree may require an arthrodesis following a joint clearance.

Arthrodesis

The joint is exposed through a curved or lateral J-shaped incision. The peroneal tendons may be retracted or divided and stitched together at the end of the operation. The lateral malleolus is divided at the joint level and this piece of bone is cut up into small chips. Inversion of the foot now exposes the joint from which all cartilage is thoroughly removed. Bone graft material is now inserted into the joint cavity. Internal fixation may be achieved by staples of the Blount type. The ankle is put in a few degrees of plantar flexion and kept in position with a plaster-of-Paris slab. This and the stitches are removed in 10 days and a tighter fitting below-knee plaster of patellar end-bearing type can be applied when the oedema has settled. Firm fusion is obtained in 3–4 months.

This operative method is believed to be the safest treatment in the majority of cases and little or no disability follows if the tarsal joints are mobile.

Tuberculosis of the tarsus

As in the ankle joint, the talus is frequently the seat of the primary disease; it may, however, originate in the calcaneum. The mid-tarsal joint is most frequently involved. Two varieties are described. In one, the disease starts near the surface of the bone and spreads rapidly to the neighbouring joints, while in the other, which is frequently seen in the calcaneus, the disease is deeply seated in the substance of the bone and is difficult to differentiate from a Brodie's abscess. Endarteritis of the nutrient vessel is common.

CLINICAL FEATURES

Pain is an early symptom, but is usually less severe than in disease of the ankle joint. Inversion and eversion are limited when the posterior bones are infected, while in cases of more distal infection, movements at the mid-tarsal joints of the foot are also restricted. Swelling is evident on the dorsum of the foot, over the region of the disease. A limp and an equinovalgus deformity complete the picture.

DIAGNOSIS

A diagnosis is made from the swelling, limp, deformity and x-ray appearances (Figure 9.33). Köhler's epiphysitis of the navicular has to be considered in the differential diagnosis.

TREATMENT

Conservative treatment by immobilization and antibiotics may be effective in cases with little bone affection, but surgical treatment is often necessary. The aims of operation are to remove the necrotic tuberculous material and to fuse the joints. With

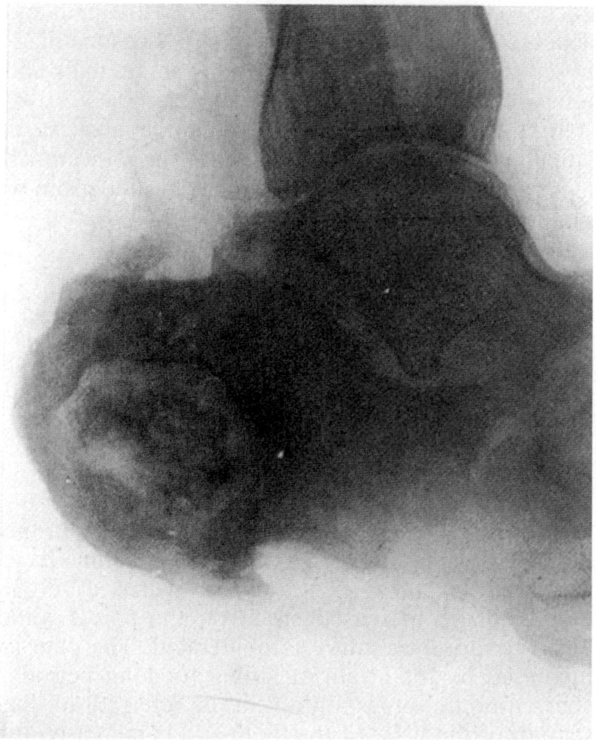

Figure 9.33 Tuberculous disease of the calcaneus with a central sequestrum.

arthrodesis of the subtaloid or the mid-tarsal joint it is necessary to do a standard triple arthrodesis. The only deviation from this is where the bony surfaces do not lie in apposition. This is achieved by inserting bone graft taken from the crest of the ilium.

Sometimes, where the disease is limited to the calcaneum, it may be eradicated by the removal of the area. Similarly, where a phalanx or a metatarsal is infected, the condition is best treated by the removal of the bone.

Tuberculosis of the sacroiliac joint

The sacroiliae articulation is a true arthrodial joint, with all the usual joint structures, and therefore subject to all joint diseases. It is rarely infected with tuberculosis in children, but at the termination of the growth period the disease is more common and is not infrequently bilateral.

The disease may originate in the lateral mass of the sacrum, or may spread thence from the lumbar vertebrae. It is also seen not infrequently in association with a tuberculous hip. The synovial membrane then becomes infected and finally, by extension, the ilium. *Abscess formation* is the rule and usually occurs early in the disease. It is rarely that pain and abscess are coincident, as once an abscess is diagnosed it has broken through its confining walls and relieved the tension that causes the pain.

In the great majority of cases the abscess is situated over the posterior aspect of the joint; much less commonly in other regions such as the groin or gluteal region. It is rare in the pelvis.

CLINICAL FEATURES

The onset is frequently insidious and an abscess is often the earliest indication. Usually, pain and tenderness are the first symptoms.

Pain

Pain is felt most commonly as a sciatica or in the hip or lumbar region, or over the joint. It is increased by movement, and is worse at night owing to the increased strain on the pelvic joint when the lordotic curve is obliterated. The pain is increased by the strain of sitting for long periods, stair-climbing or stooping. It is referred to the sacrum or the back of the thigh and is increased by jars, sudden turns as in bed, and often by coughing or laughing.

Limited motion

Motion is limited in various ways. Forward bending with straight knees is limited; but with the knees flexed and the hamstrings relaxed, as in sitting, the extent of flexion is increased – in this respect differing from what is found in lumbar disease. Extension and lateral flexion are also limited. It will be found that straight leg raising in the recumbent position is limited, and usually pain is produced when the movement is attempted on either side (Goldthwait's sign).

DIAGNOSIS

The following symptom complex is pathognomonic of an affection of the sacroiliac joint.

1. Pain at the joint on turning over while in the recumbent position.
2. Discomfort when lying on the back.
3. Pain on sitting on the affected side, relieved by sitting on the opposite buttock.
4. Pain in the joint on forward bending.
5. Pain on pressure over the joint.
6. Listing of the spine to the opposite side.
7. Positive Goldthwait's sign.

The conditions likely to be confused with sacroiliac disease are arthritis of the hip, disease of the lumbar vertebrae and sciatica. Radiographs are not particularly helpful in the early stages, but in time show erosion of the joint line, foci in the ilium or sacrum, or some alteration in the joint line, but, unlike most tuberculous joints, very rarely decalcification. Tomography may prove specially valuable in revealing early cavitation and joint erosion MR imaging is of great value to show the abscess formation within the pelvis.

The prognosis is reasonably good, especially as an isolated uncomplicated lesion.

TREATMENT

Conservative treatment follows the same lines as that of Pott's disease of the lumbar vertebrae – rest to the joint and chemotherapy. Recumbency with adequate protection and immobilization of the joint are indicated; these can best be carried out with a bed of plaster-of-Paris, extending from below the nipples to below both knees. The pelvic part of the plaster should be firmly moulded to the contour of the pelvis, and retained in place for from 3 to 6 months. Thereafter, prolonged protection of the joint is necessary. This is also useful where sinuses are present. Most cases heal by bony fusion.

Operation

Following a short period of conservative treatment by fusion of the joint, it may be necessary to aspirate an abscess by open operation. Arthrodesis is advisable, as in the absence of operative interference the disease may grumble on for a long time, producing discomfort and ill-health.

An anterior shell is made for the patient some time before, and he gets an opportunity of becoming accustomed to the prone position.

The incision is a semilunar one along the posterior two-thirds of the iliac crest, curving round the posterior iliac spine, then running parallel with the fibres of the gluteus maximus for a distance of 5–8 cm. The fibres of the gluteus maximus are separated and the borders of the great sciatic notch are identified by palpation. The centre of the sacroiliac joint lies 2.5 cm above the anterosuperior angle of the notch. The joint is exposed by cutting through the iliac bone in this area. All tuberculous material is removed with a sharp spoon and gouge, and perhaps enlarging the opening through the ilium with nibbling forceps. The arthrodesis is achieved by filling the cavity with bone graft from the piece of ilium removed from the crest. The patient is then returned to his plaster support for about 3 months.

Tuberculosis of the shoulder joint

Tuberculosis of the shoulder joint is rare, particularly in children. Out of a total of 2922 cases of tuberculous disease of the spine and joints, only 27 affected the shoulder joint – a percentage of less than 1.

PATHOLOGY

The disease originates, as a rule, in the head of the humerus. The commoner form is the so-called caries sicca, an osteoporotic atrophic form with much wasting of muscle, pain and limitation of movement, but no abscess.

The other form is the florid type with much thickening of the synovial membrane. The head becomes eroded, its place being filled by fibromyxomatous and granulation tissue. The muscles contract and pull the head hard against the glenoid which also become eroded. Finally the whole joint becomes destroyed, and filled with pus.

CLINICAL FEATURES

An insidious onset is characteristic, with early limitation of movement – abduction which is to some extent masked by the mobility of the scapula on the chest wall. In the early stage there is dull aching in the front of the joint and at the insertion of the deltoid. This may be referred to the elbow and forearm.

Limitation of abduction and of lateral rotation are marked, the joint swells, the muscles atrophy markedly, and soon it is necessary to support the arm in a sling. An abscess may form at a later stage and rupture through the capsule anteriorly, pointing in front of, or behind, the insertion of the deltoid. Subcoracoid dislocation, from disintegration of the joint and destruction of the ligaments, may follow. A radiograph shows at first an irregular outline of the head of the humerus with erosion of the joint line. Later the destruction of bone is obvious. The initial focus may be in the metaphysis or in the adjacent bone but the joint is soon invaded. The cartilage is destroyed and the adjacent bone eroded and absorbed. Sequestra are common but there is seldom sclerosis or new bone formation. Osteoporosis is extensive.

TREATMENT

General treatment including hospitalization and chemotherapy is just as necessary in this case as in other joints. The patient should be completely rested in bed, at any rate during the early stages.

Local treatment is by immobilization by means of a plaster cast enclosing the arm from the wrist upwards, the chest and body. The shoulder is abducted to an angle of 70° or a little more in a child, the elbow being on the same plane as the anterior chest wall and the humerus rotated laterally so that the forearm is at an angle of 15° with the horizontal. This method provides efficient fixation, is comfortable, lessens pain since it takes the weight of the arm off the joint structures, and, should ankylosis take place, leaves a useful arm.

In the course of such conservative treatment, minor operations such as biopsy or evacuation of an abscess may be required, and in such cases the opportunity should be taken for intra-articular deposition of streptomycin.

After 3 months of this conservative treatment, the top part of the armpiece of the plaster cast is removed and the patient encouraged to lift the arm out of the plaster. When this is possible the plaster spica may be removed and a sling substituted. As long as movement improves, he is allowed more freedom. If it diminishes, or pain, muscle spasm or swelling return, then a further period of more conservative treatment is instituted though, depending on the individual case, an arthrodesis may be considered.

Where the disease is osseous, ankylosis is the aim, and this is more likely to be achieved by some form of operative arthrodesis. Operation will be carried out at an early in adults, and much later in children. In both cases the activity of the disease should have ceased and the resistance of the patient be raised to the optimum degree.

Arthrodesis

Method

The operation, with antibiotics, as in other joints, is a combined debridement–fusion procedure. The joint is exposed by an incision starting behind the acromion and forwards and downwards to some 8 cm below the acromion. A portion of the acromion may be removed and a good exposure of the joint ensured. Tuberculous detritus and the cartilage are removed from the joint. The actual fixation of the joint is produced by a graft from the tibia. A perforation is made through the humerus to the centre of the glenoid and penetrates the scapula for about 4 cm. The graft and nail are hammered home with the joint in the optimum position and chips of bone, from either the acromion or iliac crest, are packed into the cavity of the joint, and also streptomycin. After suture of the wound, the position is further maintained by a shoulder spica of plaster-of-Paris which is best made beforehand and bivalved, and after the operation is joined up by further plaster bandages. After 2 weeks the spica is removed (and also the stitches) and a new well-fitting one applied. At the end of 4 months fusion should be complete.

The low operation of Brittain (Figure 9.34)

This is a good method of maintaining the joint in a functional position though it must be combined with a debridement of the joint, packing with bone graft, and streptomycin.

It is an extra-articular operation carried out by bridging the space between the scapula and the humerus through a posterior incision. It is similar to Brittain's hip arthrodesis in that the force exerted on the grafts is one of compression and much more likely to produce bone fusion than in the high type of operation where the force is a distracting one.

A tibial graft is cut in the shape of an arrow about 13–15 cm in length.

An incision 18 cm long is made from the posterior margin of the deltoid down the axillary border of the scapula to 2.5 cm from its inferior angle. The teres major and minor are identified, and an incision is made through the latter down to the axillary border of the scapula, which is cleared with bone elevators. Five centimetres of the humerus should be cleared

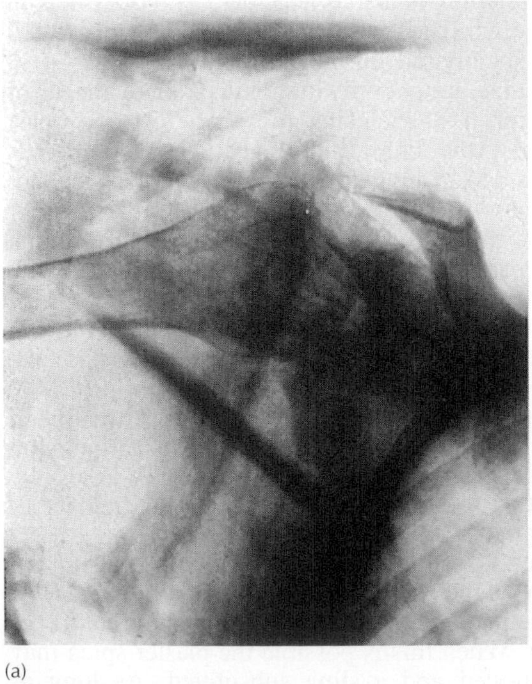

(a)

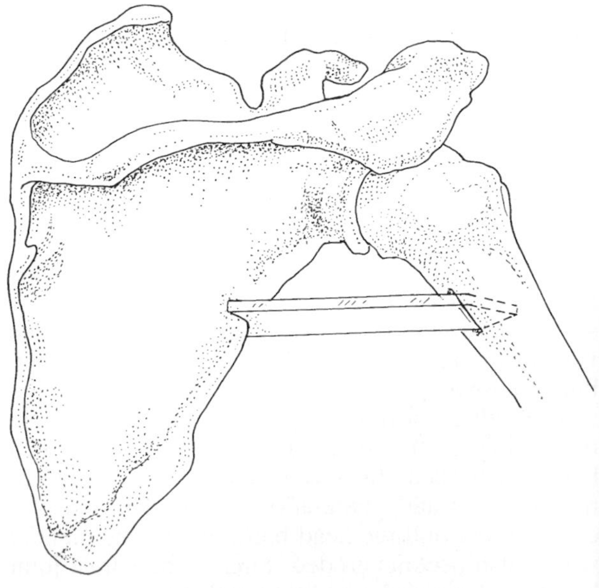

(b)

Figure 9.34 Arthrodesis of the shoulder by the extra-articular method of Brittain. A somewhat modified type of graft is shown. The scapula in contact with the graft should be denuded of periosteum and bare bone exposed.

and bone elevators passed round the bone. Care should be taken not to prolong this incision too proximally, as the circumflex artery may be severed. The circumflex nerve is not so important, as the shoulder is being fused. The point of the arrow graft is inserted into the humerus first, and then by abducting the arm the graft can be carefully inserted into position so that the limbs fall into the notch in the scapula and grasp the bone. The plaster is then completed by long slabs on the arm and across the back and chest, with the patient still lying on his face.

After being worn for 4 months, the plaster cast is removed and an x-ray taken. When fusion is complete, an abduction splint is substituted and the scapular muscles are exercised and re-educated.

Tuberculosis of the elbow

The disease is met with more frequently in this joint than in the shoulder or wrist. It is more common in adults than in children.

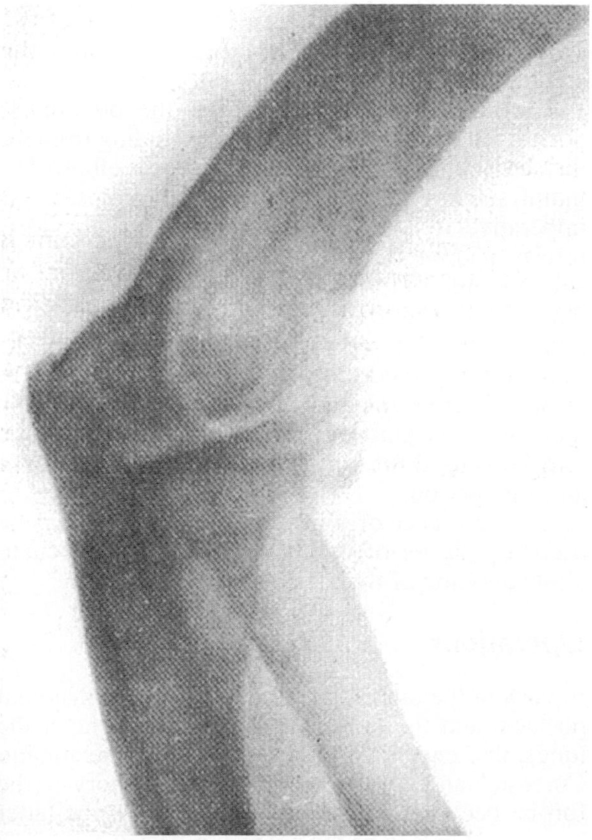

Figure 9.35 Tuberculosis of the elbow joint.

PATHOLOGY

It is commonly synovial, but in some cases there is a bone focus in the olecranon or in the radius, the lateral condyle of the humerus coming next in order of frequency. The disease may be so well established when the patient is seen for the first time that such localization is impossible.

CLINICAL FEATURES

Pain aggravated by movement is at first confined to the joint. At a later stage it may extend to the forearm. Swelling is noted on the back of the elbow on both sides of the olecranon, and the bony prominences are obliterated. Muscular spasm sets in and movement is limited. At first only the extremes of flexion and extension are affected, but later the joint becomes stiff at a mid-position, with the forearm fixed midway between pronation and supination. Muscular wasting is pronounced and, as in the knee joint, this may cause an exaggerated impression of the degree of swelling. Local heat varies with the activity of the disease. When an abscess forms, it points at the lateral side of the olecranon. A radiograph (Figure 9.35) shows a soft tissue swelling, osteoporosis, erosion of the joint surfaces, or possibly disease in the bone.

With early and efficient treatment the outlook is good.

TREATMENT

The aim of conservative treatment is a joint with a useful range of painless movement, and this should be the result in the majority of patients.

Tuberculosis of the elbow joint in children is best treated by conservative measures of rest and chemotherapy. The joint is placed at rest in the position that will be most useful should ankylosis ensue, which in most cases is flexion at a little less than a right angle.

When the position is corrected, a plaster-of-Paris cast or a splint is applied. When the patient feels his arm well and has no pain, he is allowed to use a sling. The sling is lengthened gradually and if, in a few days, the arm can be lifted to the point from which it started, recovery is presumed and the arm may be allowed greater freedom. This is a good test of recovery of the joint. Usually fixation is required for about 6 months.

Operative treatment

In some cases it may be possible to remove small foci

of disease from the olecranon or adjoining bones before the joint is involved.

Where there is gross joint destruction, and in bone disease in adults, operation is usually required after preliminary treatment by chemotherapy and rest. The choice of operation in the elbow lies between a debridement, an excision creating a pseudarthrosis, and an arthrodesis. The patient's work will be considered in coming to a decision, and where it is heavy an arthrodesis will be the operation of choice.

Debridement

A lateral approach is used, and all debris, synovium and loose tissue is removed together with the head of radius. The elbow is rested in a collar-and-cuff sling for 3 weeks, and then gentle active movement is encouraged.

Excision of the joint

The destroyed joint is exposed through a posterior incision and the muscles are stripped from the bones, taking particular care of the ulnar nerve. The humerus is divided transversely 2.5 cm above the articular surface, the ulna just distal to the coronoid process, and the radius just distal to the head. The gap between the divided bones should not be more than 2.5 cm. A right-angled plaster slab from the upper arm to the wrist is applied, particularly to control lateral movements. After 3 weeks the elbow is supported by a sling, and active exercises of the muscles that move the elbow are encouraged.

Arthrodesis

The joint is approached from the medial aspect. The ulnar nerve is dissected free and held forward by a tape. The joint is then opened and cleared of infected material. The lower end of the humerus is squared off and the ulna and olecranon are shaped appropriately to receive it. These bones are transfixed with pins to which compression clamps are afterwards applied. Cancellous iliac bone is packed into the joint and the latter put in an optimum position of 90° and the compression applied. A shoulder spica is now applied, and at the end of 3 months is replaced by an arm plaster for a further 3 months.

Tuberculosis of the wrist

Tuberculosis rarely affects the wrist in childhood, but in adults it is more common.

The disease, though it may be synovial in origin, usually starts in the bone, the commonest site for the primary focus being in the lower end of the radius or the os capitatum. Because of the intricate arrangement of the synovial membrane and the small size of the bones, dissemination is rapid. The disease frequently spreads to the flexor synovial sheaths, causing a fibromyxomatous degeneration. Abscesses and sinuses are common sequelae.

The usual symptoms are swelling, deformity, pain and limitation of movement. Physical signs are soon evident owing to the superficial character of the joint which also makes examination easy. Pain is an early symptom. At first it is felt at the site of the disease but later becomes general throughout the joint. Palmar flexion is the usual deformity. The movement at the wrist joint, and frequently at the inferior radioulnar joint, are limited in all directions. Abscesses are superficial, and they usually break down and form sinuses.

Owing to the superficial nature of the joint, diagnosis is not difficult.

TREATMENT

Conservative treatment

Treatment is usually conservative with antibiotics and immobilization.

The wrist should be fixed in the dorsiflexed position in a plaster-of-Paris cast extending from the metacarpophalangeal joints, to above the elbow. The thumb and fingers should be accurately opposed. It is imperative to maintain dorsiflexion, as ankylosis results and this position gives the optimum of strength and usefulness. Chemotherapy is begun at once. The plaster treatment should continue for 4–6 months, as a shorter period will inevitably be followed by recurrence. The plaster should fit accurately and be skin-tight or over stockinette at the most. After the plaster is removed, a leather or plastic wristlet is used for 6 months to protect the joint for a further period.

In the presence of sinuses a cock-up splint may be used, or a plaster-of-Paris splint with windows cut to allow dressing of the sinuses.

Operations

In view of the multilocular character of the synovial pockets, and the possibility of involvement of the lungs, the tendency is towards operative treatment. Curetting and excision are not satisfactory – the former because it is so often incomplete, the latter because it tends to be too extensive. The one does not eradicate the disease, while the other, although it removes the disease, too often leaves the wrist flail and the limb functionally incapacitated. A superficial abscess may require aspiration and after evacuation streptomycin should be injected. It may be necessary to open the abscess through a small incision over it and even to remove a sequestrum.

Arthrodesis

This is the operation of choice, if it is performed before the formation of sinuses with their inevitable secondary infection. It is carried out after the method of Albee. An ankylosis is produced between the metacarpals and the radius by inserting a bridge of bone. Consequently absolute immobility of the wrist results, and as the bed in the radius is made deeper in its proximal part than its distal, the wrist is ankylosed in the dorsiflexed position.

After a dorsal incision has been made, the carpus is exposed, and periosteum incised and elevated over the distal extremity of the radius and third metacarpal bone. With the power saw a gutter is prepared, measurements of which are taken with a flexible probe, and a bone graft removed from the tibia and inserted in the prepared bed.

An iliac cortical cancellous graft 1 cm longer than the bed and 1 cm wide, is inserted into it, not flatly, but on its edge. Its shape allows it to be firmly slotted into the bed between the radius and the third metacarpal when traction is put on the wrist. The wrist is completely locked in position by the graft.

Tuberculous disease of the vertebral column (Pott's disease)

Tuberculosis of the vertebral column, first described by Percival Pott and since associated with his name, is a slowly developing disease, characterized by pain, spinal deformity and, occasionally, paralysis. It is a disease of early childhood, the majority of cases starting between the ages of 3 and 5, but in recent years the disease has tended to affect an older age group: adults of over 40 years in Madras and in Korea, with women more prone to infection during their reproductive years (Shanmugasundaram, 1987). (See Chapter 8.)

PATHOLOGY

Sites of the disease

Spinal tuberculosis is met with most frequently in the lower thoracic region, T12 to L4 vertebrae, possibly due to the relatively large amount of spongy tissue in the vertebral bodies, the degree of weight-bearing, and the extent of movement demanded of this portion of the column. The infection is a blood-borne one, but the prevertebral lymphatic tissue is also important. Since the tubercle bacillus not infrequently gains entrance to the body through the abdominal glands and lymph vessels, it may well be that the close proximity of such an obvious source of infection as the thoracic duct is responsible for the actual tuberculous infection of these vertebrae.

At an early stage it is not possible to say how many vertebrae are infected even on a radiograph. Double lesions with intervening normal vertebrae are found in 5–10% of cases. Tuberculosis in other parts of the body is seen in about 40% of cases; e.g. renal and pulmonary disease. Over 18% of patients with untreated bone and joint tuberculosis have a tubercular bacilluria, due to an initial papillitis becoming a glomerulonephritis.

Vertebrae develop from sclerotomes which lie on each side of the notocord. The lower half of one vertebra and the upper half of the vertebra below, with the intervertebral joint between them, are formed from each pair of sclerotomes and have the same blood supply. The occurrence of disease involving adjacent halves of vertebrae with early narrowing of the intervening disc is common and is explained on the above vascular basis.

Varieties

The following varieties of vertebral tuberculosis are commonly recognized:

1. *Central*, in which the spongy tissue of the body is affected as diffuse osteomyelitis of the body. It is sometimes apparent at an early stage in an x-ray or MRI examination for abscess formation and CT for bone and joint involvement, as an increase in density of the vertebral body.
2. *Metaphyseal tuberculosis* (intervertebral articular type) where the disease arises near the epiphyses of the body and, therefore, close to the intervertebral disc. The infection in this, the commonest type of disease, is chiefly in the body of the epiphysis. The disc space is rapidly narrowed.
3. *Anterior or periosteal variety*, where the primary focus is deep to the periosteum on the front

of the body, beneath the anterior longitudinal ligament.

4. *Posterior element tuberculosis*. Occasionally the transverse process is affected, and, more rarely, the vertebral arch. CT scanning has proved to be essential in demonstrating bony involvement of these structures where radiography is insufficient (Jellis, 1992b), he has emphasized the importance of these findings in planning operative decompression and stabilizing procedures.
5. *A true tuberculous arthritis* occurs in the occipito-atlanto-axial group of joints.

The sequence of pathology

The disease begins as an infection of a single vertebra. The primary error is a tuberculous endarteritis; the marrow is converted into pale myxomatous tissue. In the devitalized tissue a tuberculous follicle develops until it is visible to the naked eye as a small yellow-grey nodule. As this nodule grows, the lamellae over a wide area are progressively destroyed and eventually disappear. Since the strength of the vertebra depends on the internal structure of its body, it follows that with the disorganization of its lamellar structure its strength is seriously compromised, especially as there is practically never any subperiosteal new bone formation. Indeed, in the vertebral column, tuberculosis seems to exercise an inhibitory effect on new bone formation, in contrast to the long bone in which the deposit of new bone is a striking feature.

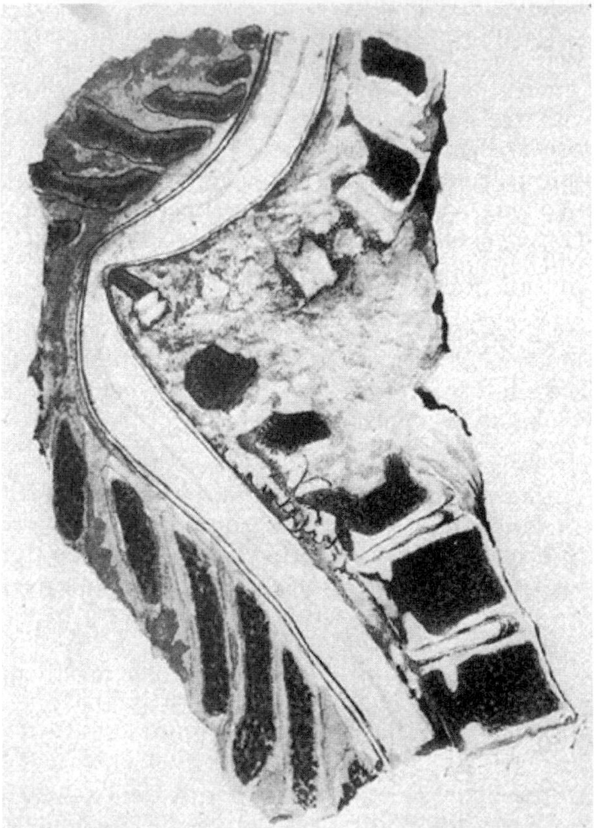

Figure 9.36 Tuberculosis of the spine, producing angulation.

The centre of the body being caseous, the superimposed weight of the vertebral column is now borne by the fragile shell of compact bone, which sooner or later collapses. An angular deformity – kyphus, gibbus or hunchback – now results, for the neural arch is swung upwards on the fulcrum of the articular processes when the short arm lever of the vertebral system, formed by the diseased body, descends (collapses). As a result of the collapse the tips of the adjacent spines are widely separated (Figures 9.36 and 9.37). Such deformity is most marked in thoracic caries, because of the normal anterior curve there. In the cervical region collapse rarely occurs because the weight is transmitted chiefly through the articular processes. The deformity, therefore, is a comparatively slight one. In the lumbar region also the deformity is small, since, owing to the normal lumbar lordosis, the body weight is borne chiefly by the posterior parts of the vertebral body, and collapse is incomplete.

Associated changes – abscess formation

When the body of the vertebra collapses there is expressed from it a collection of tuberculous detritus, consisting of granulation tissue, caseous matter, disintegrated bone lamellae and bone marrow. This is a cold abscess, and is the commonest complication of Pott's disease, occurring in 20% of cases. At first, the debris collects under the anterior longitudinal ligament on the front of the vertebral bodies; then it becomes further disseminated along one or several courses. It may pass backwards and invade the vertebral canal – a serious complication, resulting, as it usually does, in pressure on the spinal cord. It may track forwards and become diverted by various anatomical structures such as blood vessels, nerves or muscles. The abscess may therefore come to be situated at a considerable distance from the site of the original disease, and a knowledge of the possible situations of cold abscesses, and the factors which determine them, is consequently of importance (Figure 9.38). Magnetic resonance imaging is most valuable in delineating paravertebral abscess formation and tracting (Jellis, 1992b).

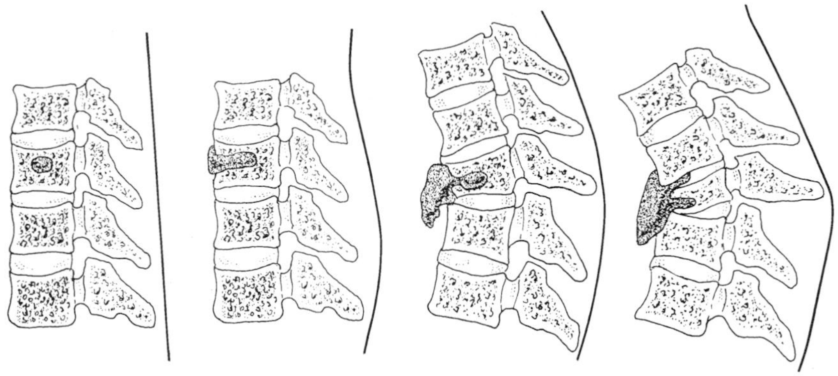

Figure 9.37 Progression of a tuberculous focus in the body of a vertebra, showing the collapse of the body and the production of the gibbus.

CLINICAL FEATURES

Before the actual onset of characteristic local symptoms, there may be lassitude, loss of weight, a poor appetite and often an evening rise of temperature. These symptoms last for a few weeks or months, but eventually the evidence of spinal trouble appears, as follows.

Pain

The occurrence of pain is usually, but not invariably, the first indication of spinal disease. The pain may be either local (i.e. experienced in the back) or referred along one of the spinal nerves. In either case, it is frequently severe, because of the free and complex nature of the movements of the spinal column, and because of the close proximity of the spinal nerves. When felt locally, the pain is acute and stabbing, and situated over the affected vertebrae. It is aggravated by pressure on the spinous process, or by the rotation of the vertebra produced by pressing on the transverse processes.

In caries of the cervical spine the area of referred pain is usually situated over the occiput and in the

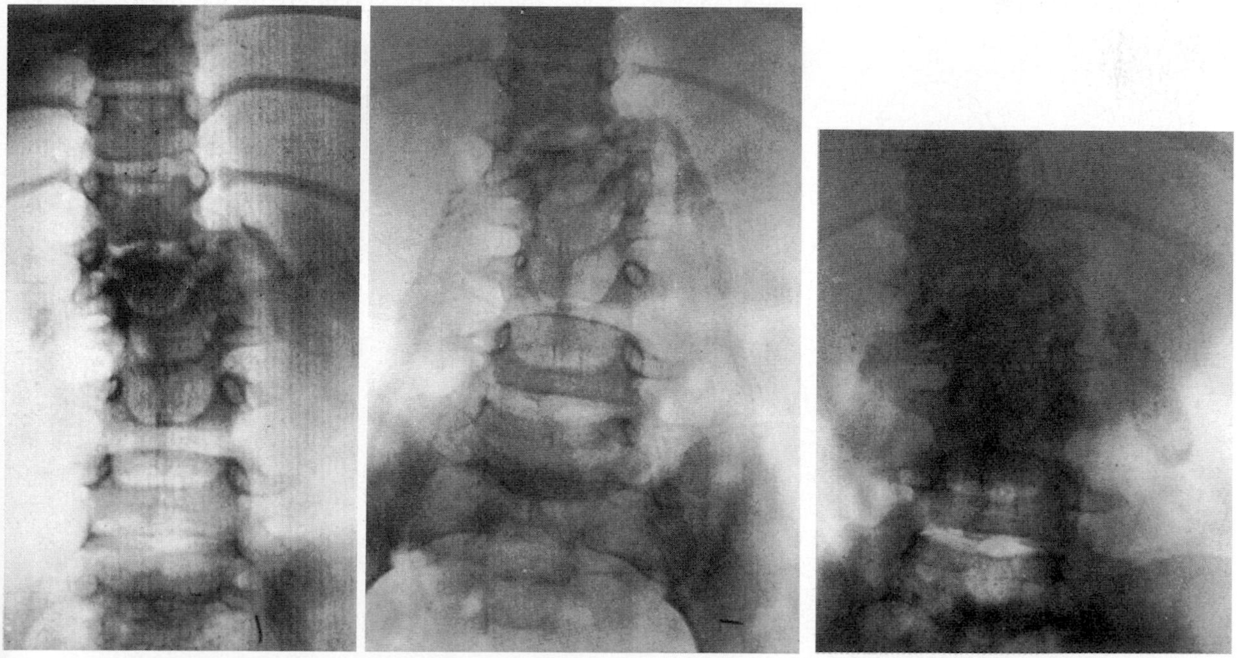

(a) (b) (c)

Figure 9.38 Tuberculosis of the spine. (a) Disease affecting the lumbar region with a typical lateral displacement and the formation of a psoas abscess on the left side. (b) A later stage – 10 months later – of lumbar disease. (c) The appearance after 19 months' treatment: healing is taking place and the bones are better defined; the abscesses are now calcified.

arms; in thoracic disease it takes the form of intercostal neuralgia; in the thoracolumbar disease, of 'girdle pains' or epigastric pain; and in the lumbar spine to the hips and legs.

Night cries

Night cries are less frequent in spinal disease than in tuberculosis of the larger joints, but do occasionally occur in disease of the cervical or thoracic vertebrae. They are reliable evidence of the activity of the tuberculous process.

Abscess formation

The search for abscesses is an essential part of the investigation of any case of spinal caries, but the presence of certain symptoms will attract particular attention to the possibility of abscess formation.

The retropharyngeal abscess of cervical disease is associated with dysphagia and dyspnoea; abscesses in disease of the upper thoracic vertebrae are usually anterior, and may therefore involve the recurrent laryngeal nerves and give rise to dyspnoea and vocal changes.

In the lumbar spine, the debris seeks the surface usually as a psoas abscess, and the presence of infective material is so apt to induce irritation and spasm of the muscle that there is often persistent flexion and lateral rotation of the limb, any attempt to overcome these deformities being attended with great pain.

PHYSICAL EXAMINATION

General appearance

A systematic general examination may demonstrate the presence of other signs of tuberculous infection.

Attitude and gait

There is often a strained and expectant facial expression, for the child (30%) or adult (70%) is in continual dread of any sudden jar or movement. When the disease is active, no matter the situation, the patient walks with the leg joints semi-flexed, to lessen the jar of sudden movements. In addition, disease in each situation is associated with a characteristic gait or attitude – e.g. bending the hips and knees instead of the spine when picking up an object from the floor (Figure 9.39).

In upper cervical disease, the position of the head is similar to that in wry-neck, but the face is not rotated. In lower cervical disease, the head is thrown backwards and to one side, and may be supported by the hand (Figure 9.40).

In upper thoracic disease, the shoulders are raised, and the arms and shoulders drawn backwards. The

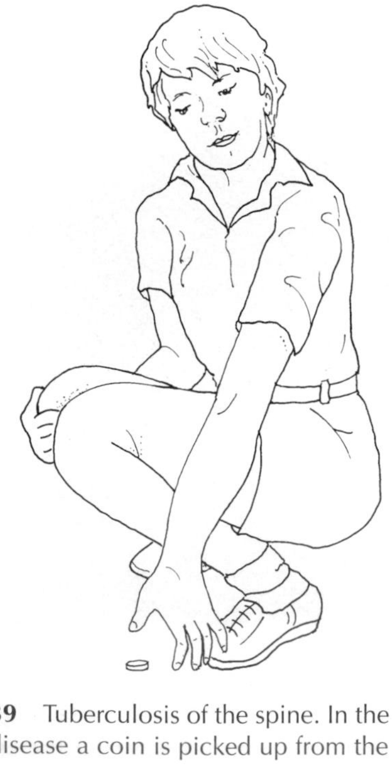

Figure 9.39 Tuberculosis of the spine. In the presence of thoracic disease a coin is picked up from the floor in this way.

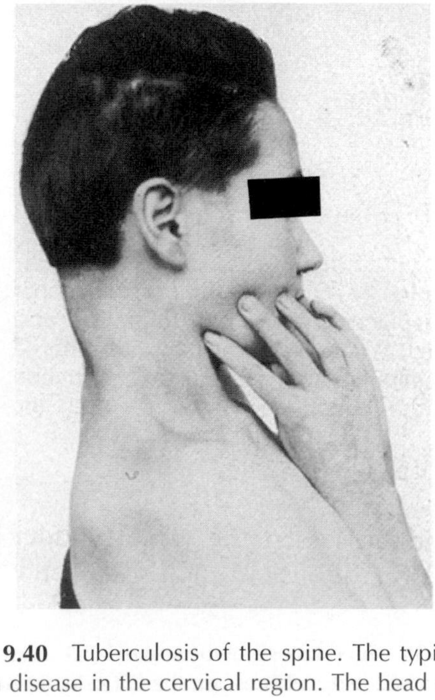

Figure 9.40 Tuberculosis of the spine. The typical attitude in disease in the cervical region. The head requires support.

head appears sunken, owing to the apparent shortening of the neck, and the attitude is aptly referred to as the 'military attitude'. In mid-thoracic disease, the anteroposterior diameter of the chest is considerably increased, and owing to the shortening in stature the patient appears stunted and the arms seem unduly long. In low thoracic and upper lumbar disease, the thorax and head are thrown backwards, the abdomen is prominent, the patient walks with the legs far apart, and waddles – the so-called 'alderman's gait'.

In lower lumbar disease there is pronounced lordosis, and the chest is thrown forwards till the last rib and the iliac crest may be actually in contact.

Deformities of the spine

The patient is stripped to expose the whole spine. Inspection may then reveal the presence of angulation, deformity, lateral deviation, lordosis, flattening or boarding, or paravertebral swelling.

1. *Angulation of the spine* (*kyphosis*) is the result of the collapse of the affected vertebra(e) and varies in degree with the extent of the disease. When a series of vertebrae are affected the projection is slight and gradual, but when only one body is diseased the angulation is localized and prominent. The anterior type of disease, which affects a long segment of the column, is associated with a long gradual curvature similar to that of the ordinary round shoulders.
2. *Scoliosis.* Lateral deviation often complicates kyphosis; indeed, the case may be mistaken for one of simple scoliosis.
3. *Lordosis.* The spines above and below the site of the disease may show exaggerated forward curvature, to compensate for the kyphosis.
4. *Boarding.* The normal anteroposterior curves may be obliterated, even though the vertical axis of the spine is straight. Such 'boarding' or 'flattening' is the result of muscular rigidity, and, as it is one of the earliest clinical signs to appear, its recognition is of great importance.
5. *Paravertebral thickening.* The width of the column at the site of the disease may be increased, or a cold abscess may be seen pointing at one or other side. Such thickening is better distinguished by palpation, the finger being drawn down the back on either side of the spinous processes.

Movements of the spine

The natural efforts to protect the diseased vertebrae result in a spastic condition of muscles which effectively limits the spinal movements. This muscular rigidity is the most characteristic sign of Pott's disease. To elicit it, the anteroposterior, lateral and rotatory movements of the spine are carefully tested.

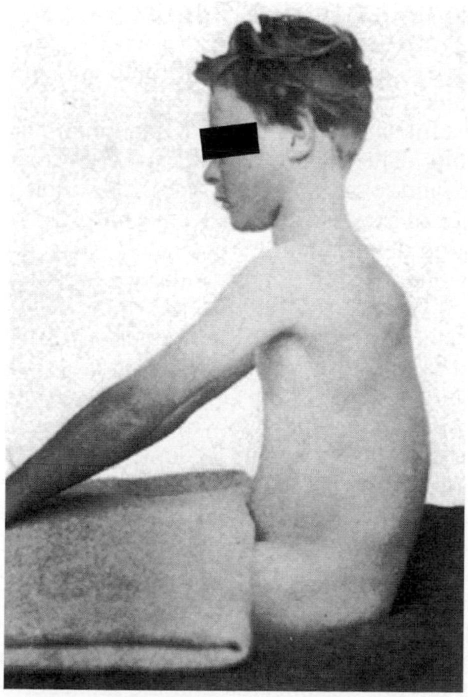

Figure 9.41 Tuberculosis of the spine. The deformity in the region of the upper thoracic vertebrae is indicative of underlying disease.

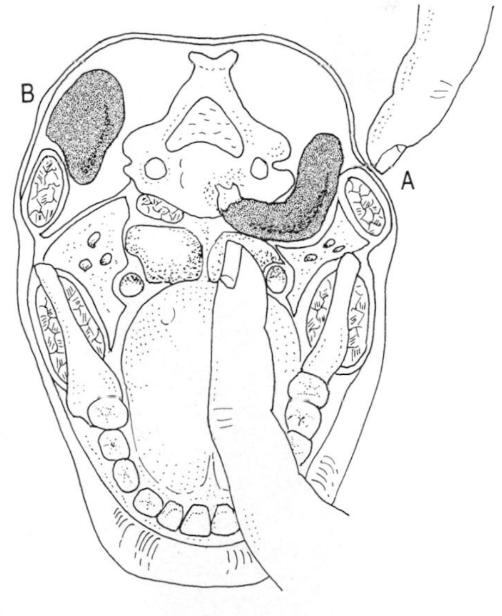

Figure 9.42 Abscess from tuberculosis of the cervical region. It may be palpated bidigitally through the mouth (A) differing in this respect as well as in site from the glandular abscess (B). (After Calot)

Examination for cold abscess

All possible abscess sites should be explored: the pharynx, the triangles of the neck, the loins, the iliac fossae, the groins, the gluteal and the ischiorectal regions (Figures 9.41–9.44). Sometimes the abscess is recognized only on x-ray examination.

Paralysis

The paralysis occurring in about 15% of cases is spastic in the early stages, with occasional involvement of the bladder and rectum; only very rarely are sensory disturbances present. The paralysis may be incomplete, or may at first be complete and become incomplete later. Its extent and nature depend on the level and the amount of cord involvement.

When the infection is in the cervical region, the phrenic, accessory and hypoglossal nerves may be affected. The arms are involved before the legs.

In thoracic disease there is spastic paralysis of the legs, without involvement of the sphincters. In low thoracic and lumbar caries the lower limbs are paraplegic and the sphincters sometimes paralysed as well. There are trophic disturbances. The motor paresis results in awkward jerking movements, an ataxic gait, and stumbling and dragging of the toes; sensory changes are rare, but there may be pain in the body or limbs and derangements of cutaneous sensation. The deep reflexes are exaggerated in the early stages, but disappear progressively as cord degeneration proceeds.

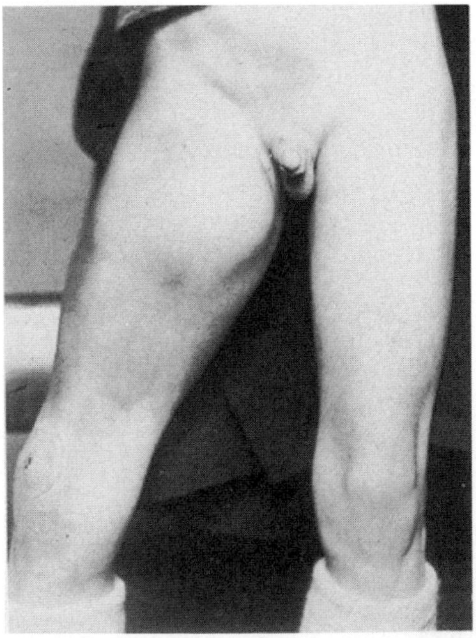

Figure 9.43 Tuberculosis of the spine. A psoas abscess appearing in the thigh, having escaped from the pelvis under the inguinal ligament.

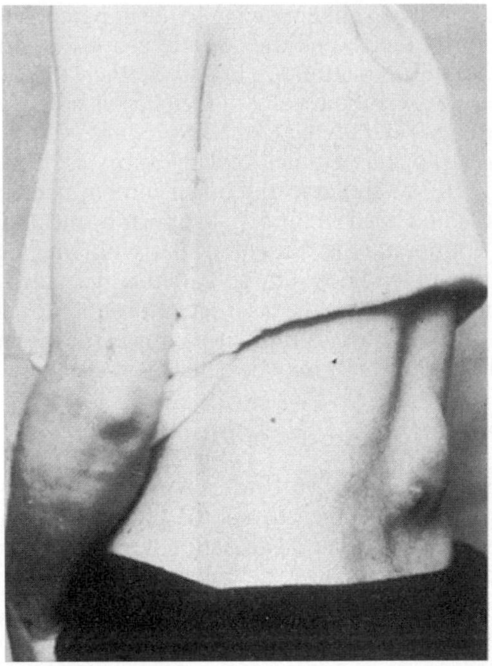

Figure 9.44 Tuberculosis of the spine. Tuberculous abscess coming to the surface through the lumbar triangle.

Radiographic examination

An x-ray investigation includes both an anteroposterior and a lateral view of the spine; tomography is also useful with MRI and CT examinations when available. The diagnosis is thus confirmed, the degree and extent of the disease estimated, the presence of a cold abscess detected and any evidence of healing determined.

The lateral view is particularly valuable, as it shows evidence of the disease long before the other. Narrowing of the intervertebral disc is the earliest and most constant radiographic sign in tuberculosis of the spine (Figure 9.45). Bone scanning with technetium-99 will often show a 'hot spot'. Later, as the spine becomes 'buckled', the vertebral body becomes wedge-shaped (Figure 9.46).

In addition, during the active stage, the affected vertebrae are less dense, decalcification has occurred, and there is want of clarity in the detail of the bones. As healing takes place, the decalcification becomes less marked. Ultimately the diseased vertebrae form a continuous mass, the intervertebral spaces having disappeared and the adjacent bodies fused.

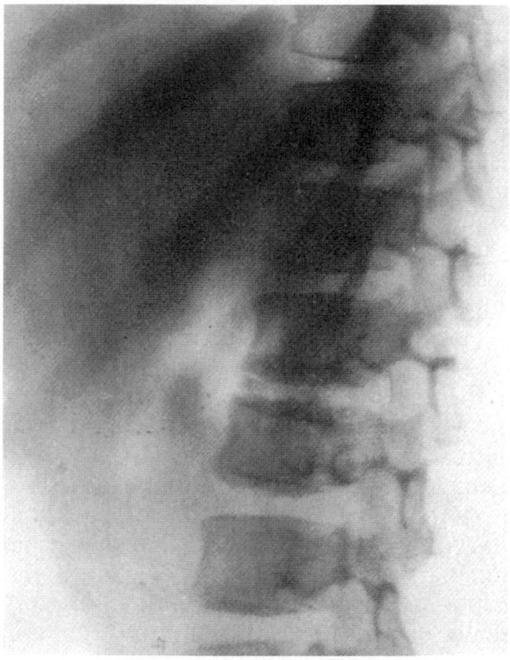

Figure 9.45 Tuberculosis of the spine. Epiphyseal disease of the contiguous epiphyses of the first and second lumbar vertebrae with disc space narrowing.

DIAGNOSIS

The recognition of spinal tuberculosis is not difficult when a well marked kyphosis is present, but if the results of treatment are to be satisfactory, a diagnosis must be made at a substantially earlier stage. Further more, the presence of a gibbus is not invariable; even in late spinal tuberculosis, with paraplegia, the 'hump' may be absent. The important findings which establish the diagnosis are rigidity, pain, slight spasticity, abscess formation (Figure 9.47) and the radiological appearances previously discussed.

The early diagnosis may not be easy, as tuberculosis may be mistaken for a variety of conditions when considered on a regional basis. Cervical Pott's disease may be confused with developmental abnormality or even sarcoma; thoracic Pott's disease must be distinguished from rickets, scoliosis, osteochondritis, Schmorl's disease, aneurysm and Scheuermann's disease. Tuberculosis of the lumbar vertebrae may be mistaken for hip-joint disease, sacroiliac disease, low-back strain, secondary carcinoma, pyogenic disease, spondylitis ankylopoietica and osteoarthritis.

Infection of a spinal segment with paravertebral abscess formation can prove to be a difficult diagnostic problem. Allen *et al.* (1978) have described the various radiological changes resulting from spinal infections. Other organisms (e.g. *Salmonella typhi, S. cholerae*, etc.) have been considered to be tuberculosis clinically until cultures of material obtained locally have shown the correct cause (Schweitzer *et al.*, 1971). Neoplasms also have to be excluded.

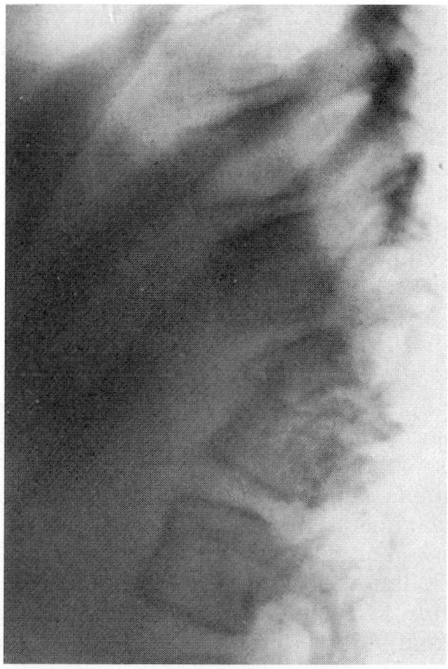

Figure 9.46 Tuberculosis of the spine, affecting the upper lumbar region with collapse of the vertebrae.

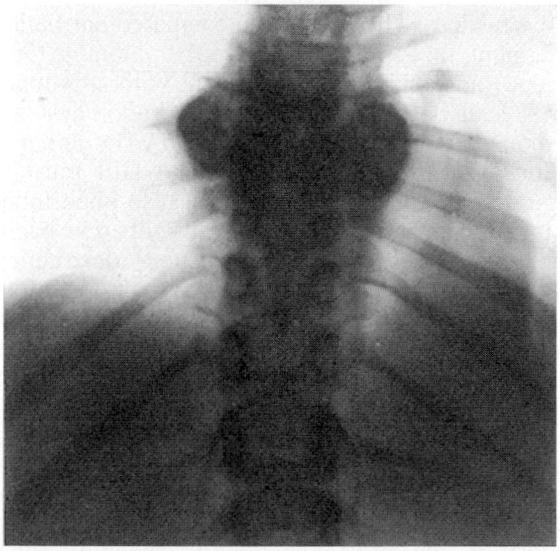

Figure 9.47 Tuberculosis of the spine. A 'dumb-bell' abscess arising from disease of the seventh and eight thoracic vertebrae.

PROGNOSIS

Vertebral tuberculosis before the advent of chemotherapy was a serious condition, especially in children. Sven Johansson in 1926 reported on 91 cases, of whom not quite one-third were treated by surgical fusion and the rest conservatively, the mortality rate was 28%. But results are very different now. Wilkinson (1965), in a series treated between 1948 and 1958 by direct operation and antibiotics, had no operative mortality and, of 128 patients, 120 had sound healing with a stable ankylosis. It is interesting, too, that the lesion in the great majority of cases was in the thoracolumbar region – the area where poor results were formerly frequent. Hodgson and Stock (1960) reported on the first 100 patients treated by direct operation, anterior spine fusion and antibiotics, with sound fusions in 94 patients.

Similar results were reported by Martin (1970), with success in 98% of patients with no relapses, when treated by the same technique.

Direct approach to the spine anteriorly for diagnosis, debridement and stabilization is the method of choice where all facilities are available and drug therapy can be guaranteed. Other methods may be required under less favourable circumstances.

The Medical Research Council Working Party (1974) reported on a comparative study from two centres in South Korea and Hong Kong, and described no statistical differences between two groups (both receiving PAS and isoniazid for 18 months and one receiving a supplement of streptomycin for 3 months); one group had in-patient rest in bed for 6 months followed by out-patient treatment (91% healed), and the other had out-patient treatment from the start (89% healed). The report also compared out-patient treatment in a plaster jacket for 9 months (90% healed) and ambulatory treatment without support (84% healed). Healing was assessed upon systemic response and radiographic change. The latter is notoriously difficult to define, and still must be regarded as a weak end point because bone tuberculosis disease may never lose its tubercle bacilli content – especially with much bone destruction, cavitation and surrounding sclerosis. Therefore, these results confirm that tuberculous spinal disease can be controlled by ambulatory out-patient therapy with some form of spinal support and adequate chemotherapy of isoniazid and rifampicin for 6–9 months, but, for eradication and prevention of deformity, anterior spinal surgery must still be considered. When Potts paraplegia is also present, the Hong Kong procedure of Hodgson and Stock (1960) is the most satisfactory, specially when compared with conservative treatment, or those receiving a costotransversectomy procedure.

The MRC working party on tuberculosis of the spine (1993) from their Korean study emphasize the success of both the 6- and 9-month regimen of isoniazid with rifampicin. They believe that this form of treatment is particularly relevant where the 'Hong Kong' radical operation may not be possible. Sinuses and abscesses resolved – 22% within 2 months, and there was no recurrence. Drug resistance to isoniazid may be found in certain countries and then a third drug, e.g. streptomycin or better pyrazinamide, which can be given orally, should be added for the first 2 months.

Myelopathy with functional impairment, e.g. 'Pott's paraplegia', can be successfully treated with chemotherapy alone, but there is still some debate whether surgical intervention is also required because of limited modern comparative studies.

Leong (1993) in commenting upon the drug trials by the MRC (Great Britain) and their results, points out that the criteria of their patients reaching a favourable status', i.e. no signs or clinical abscess formation, no involvement of the CNS, no surgical treatment or additional drug therapy, etc., did not include as necessary criteria radiological evidence of complete bony fusion, maintenance of vertebral body height and the degree of kyphosis. When these are considered by the end of 3 years only 44% of patients had achieved complete bony fusion, 16% had no radiological evidence of bony fusion at all, and 32–52% of patients had an increase in the kyphotic angle of 11–30°. (18–23% of the patients increased to more than 31°). Since the mean angle of admission to the study was 40%, this observed deterioration was very significant and in the more severe cases could eventually lead to paraplegia of late onset. The MRC trials have shown that this condition can be treated effectively by anti-tuberculous chemotherapy alone but with better definition of the disease process using CT and MR scanning, surgical treatment is still indicated in some patients, especially to obtain a better fusion rate and to prevent the deformity of kyphosis.

GENERAL TREATMENT

Efficient general management is still of the utmost importance in tuberculous disease of the spine. It consists of the usual anti-tuberculous measures, as, for example, improved hygiene, healthy surroundings and a liberal nutritious diet.

Before treatment is begun, other foci in the spine, kidneys and lungs must be treated and a baseline ESR obtained. Skeletal scanning with technetium-99 will often indicate other areas of involvement.

The advent of chemotherapy has fundamentally altered the treatment of tuberculous disease of bone and joint. With antibiotics it is now possible to prevent further spread of the disease, and with surgery to eradicate the primary lesion safely.

The existence of bone or joint tuberculosis always indicates that there has been a haematogenous dissemination of the disease, and one is as concerned in trying to knock out other cryptic foci of tubercle bacilli as to deal with the more obvious lesion. In most orthopaedic lesions it is desirable to continue treatment until the bone lesion is really well healed and in most cases it is wise to continue for 6–12 months. After the first 6 months or so, treatment continues with a combination involving rifampicin, isoniazid and ethambutol.

LOCAL TREATMENT

The local treatment is important; unless it is efficiently carried out, the general treatment is of little avail.

Treatment of an uncomplicated case

The majority of cases of Pott's disease may be placed in this category. The treatment is divided into stages – the first, that of complete recumbency; the second, the stage of ambulation; and the third, the stage of convalescence. The treatment is carefully graduated, the patient passing by degrees from one stage to another, when symptoms pointing to activity or recrudescence of the disease are absent.

Nature, be it noted, in endeavouring to protect the carious vertebrae, immobilizes the vertebral column by keeping the muscles contracted in involuntary spasm. In so doing, however, the spasm increases the tendency of the diseased vertebrae to collapse, and thus inaugurates or aggravates an angular deformity. The ideal method of treatment seeks to ally the spasm, to immobilize the spine, to remove abscess and other dead tissue, to prevent deformity, to arrest the progress of the disease and finally to cure it.

Recumbency

Recumbency, although now very much shortened, should be advocated at the start of treatment in advanced forms of the disease, and both before and after any operation. Fixation of the spine in the recumbent position in full extension affords more complete immobilization than any form of ambulatory fixation, and is therefore attended with greater and more rapid relief of symptoms. Rest alone, however, is not enough to prevent the displacement of the vertebrae. The treatment by plaster is the most efficacious, the most simple and the most practical. Precedence is given to fixation in a properly made plaster shell. Ambulatory forms of immobilization in plaster jackets are preferred on economic, social and compliance terms but there have been no studies to prove they are more efficient as regards the disease process. The plaster shell is made for the individual case and is accordingly much more comfortable and fits more accurately.

Plaster shells may be of two types, posterior and anterior, and in constructing them it is necessary to make the shell with the patient's body hyperextended as far as the activity of the disease allows.

1. *Posterior plaster shell.* As patients who are being treated in a plaster shell should be turned over frequently to have their backs attended to, it is a useful plan to make a lid, or anterior shell, in which they can lie while receiving this attention. The anterior shell is placed in position and the two cases are strapped together, and thus a complete plaster box is formed in which the patient is securely held. The box is now rolled over and the posterior shell lifted off. By this means the skin of the back can be exposed and treated with alcohol and powder without interrupting the immobilization at all. The condition of the skin is of particular importance when methods of correcting the deformity are in use, as the skin is then more subject to pressure necrosis.
2. *Anterior plaster shell.* This is a very comfortable method and the one of choice in treating low thoracic and lumbar disease and is applied with the patient lying on his back. The hyperextension is achieved by allowing his head and neck to drop to a lower level than the area of disease by an appropriate arrangement of small pillows. It is found that defaecation and micturition are performed in an even cleaner manner than with a posterior shell. The anterior shell has the further advantage that when the child tries to look about him the tendency is for the spine to be hyperextended, whereas in the dorsal decubitus the tendency is towards flexion. Contraindications are a large abscess, such as a psoas, sinuses which require dressing anteriorly, paraplegia or spasm. It is quite impossible to have a spastic patient in an anterior shell, since the spasmodic movements quickly initiate sores on his knees.

The recumbent stage of treatment lasts for a varying short period and after the first month the condition will be reviewed with the possibility of operation in view. The operation will be frequently carried out now since it aims at the complete extirpation of the diseased focus and its replacement by bone grafts to stabilize the weakened spine.

On discontinuing recumbent treatment, the patient must be kept under close observation for some time after, since unfavourable symptoms may recur. He is usually kept in bed on a firm mattress. Any return of pain, the appearance of paralysis, deterioration in general condition, the development of abscesses or increase in kyphosis imperatively demand the resumption of recumbent treatment.

RECUMBENT TREATMENT AS APPLIED TO INDIVIDUAL REGIONS

Cervical and upper thoracic regions

As the cervical vertebrae are small, the disease is usually limited in extent. The truly transverse direction of the transverse processes limits the amount of wedging here. The prognosis as regards recovery from the disease is good, and there is usually little or no apparent deformity, since the great mobility of the cervical spine compensates considerably for any local fixation.

Some method of extension should be used during the recumbent stage, carried out for about 1 month. When the tuberculous disease is actually situated in the occipitoatlantoid region, a similar method of treatment is employed, but here the prognosis is not so good because the disease is in close proximity to the vital medullary centres. Sudden death may occur from compression of the spinal cord, and abscess formation is a common and dangerous complication.

Skeletal traction by applying halofemoral traction apparatus is more effective, and greater traction and immobilization can be achieved. There is no skin pressure, particularly under the chin as produced by head halter traction. Although the Hong Kong school have achieved good success with halopelvic traction, other centres have had significant complications from the pelvic transfixation rods and from hyperdistraction of the cervical spinal spaces, with subsequent collapse. The halo component can be subsequently attached to a plaster jacket for ambulation.

Lifeso (1987) has graded tuberculosis lesions involving the atlantoaxial spine from those with minimal ligamentous or bone destruction and no displacement of C1 on C2 to those with marked ligamentous, bone destruction and displacement of C1 forward on C2. Transoral biopsy, decompression, the Fang-Ong procedure, reduction by halo traction and a subsequent occiput to C2 or C3 fusion can be carried out successfully.

Thoracolumbar region

It is difficult either to prevent or to cure deformity resulting from disease of the upper thoracic vertebrae, hence round shoulders and a short neck are frequent sequelae. Paralysis not infrequently occurs, and when it does immobilization must be complete. In thoracic disease the fixation, by means of some form of plaster cast, is the best form of treatment.

In the lumbar region the prognosis is good. Healing takes place quickly and the trunk is left only a little shorter and broader than before, though a peculiar erectness of attitude may persist. Here, too, the preferred method of treatment is by plaster, for it has the additional advantage of preventing the contraction of the psoas muscle which is so common and which may result in grotesque deformity. This contraction is usually evidence of an abscess at the origin or within the substance of the muscle, and during the active stage of the disease is attended by pain. In early cases the psoas contraction yields to sustained traction, but in old neglected contractures the shortened tissues may have to be divided by open incision, and the deformity thereafter corrected by forcible manipulation.

CONVALESCENCE

During the recumbent and ambulatory stages radiographic examinations should be made at frequent intervals. As long as there is any cavitation, unevenness in the bone shadow or evidence of decalcification, it may be concluded that the disease is not yet healed. When the bone density has been restored to normal, when pain and muscular spasm have been entirely abolished and when the general condition is good, the possibility of convalescence may be considered.

The convalescent regimen should extend over a period of about a year. At first the apparatus is removed only for a short period each day, and then reapplied; gradually the intervals of freedom are increased until ultimately the support can be dispensed with altogether. Should there be any return of pain, or any increase in the degree of the deformity, the appliance is replaced.

Ambulatory treatment

When the child is allowed upon his feet, the spine must still be carefully protected, and numerous methods have been devised towards this end. Usually a plaster-of-Paris jacket is used.

When the disease is situated in the higher thoracic vertebrae the jacket should reach well above the affected bones. In cervical caries the support is usually of the Minerva type, the plaster extending upwards as far as the jaw, mastoid, and occiput. Alternatively, a 'halo' support may be employed bonded to a body jacket.

Whichever type of jacket is advocated, it should be worn for at least 6 months; it is then discarded in favour of a removable plastic jacket.

TREATMENT OF THE COMPLICATIONS OF POTT'S DISEASE

The abscess

In most cases of Pott's disease, an abscess is present at one time or another, but unless it is associated with pressure symptoms, is present on radiographs and MRI examination or appears as a palpable tumour, its occurrence can only be presumed. It is more common in connection with disease in the lower parts of the spine, where the size of the vertebrae is relatively large.

The abscess consists of a central mass of caseous debris, with a limiting wall of granulation tissue. The contents are often entirely liquefied; the fluid is then of a creamy colour, with pieces of cheese-like material floating in it. In the absence of secondary infection, the fluid is sterile.

The old dictum of 'where there is pus, let it out' is now just as acceptable for tuberculous collections as pyogenic ones. The risks of preantibiotic days of miliary tuberculosis or of tuberculous meningitis do not now occur. The dominant feature in the treatment of the disease lies in the disposal of the abscess – and there is usually some collection of tuberculous detritus in this affection. So it is good surgical practice to undertake early aseptic evacuation of the abscess.

In some cases where the contents are very fluid it may be possible to aspirate the abscess, but in the majority it is better to evacuate it by open operation. At such an operation the cavity should be cleaned up by removal of its contents, including any loose bony or other debris, using carefully a blunt curette. Streptomycin is inserted into the cavity and the latter closed by suture without open drainage.

Active treatment of abscess debris in various situations

Operative surgery is required for destructive changes with abscess formation. Hodgson and his colleagues (1967) proved the efficacy of the transpleural anterior approach for extensive debridement with anterior rib bone grafting.

Anterolateral decompression (the old costotransversectomy) via a lateral extrapleural approach allows an evacuation of abscess formation, necrotic bone and sequestra, specially when one carries out an excision of one or more pedicles.

Laminectomy via the posterior approach is rarely indicated now except for the unusual 'spinal tumour' case because it removes the stabilizing and strengthening neural arch components.

Cervical region

Abscesses in connection with cervical disease usually become evident in the retropharyngeal space; to avoid their pointing and rupturing into the septic pharynx, they should be evacuated from the neck. Two methods are available:

1. The abscess may be aspirated through a needle inserted behind the posterior border of the sternomastoid. This is the better method, provided the contents are not too thick to be drawn through the aspirator.
2. Should aspiration not be feasible for any reason, the abscess must be evacuated by open operation. A vertical incision is made behind the sternomastoid muscle, care being taken to avoid the accessory nerve. The transverse processes of the vertebrae are exposed between the sternomastoid and the splenius capitis and levator scapulae muscles; the abscess is located by following the anterior surface of the processes. After the cavity has been cleansed with pledgets of gauze, the incision is completely closed. Abscesses from middle cervical disease usually point in the supraclavicular region, and there is no difficulty in their treatment aspiration and incision (Figure 9.48).

Thoracic region

Occasionally abscesses may press on the respiratory tract, and give rise to dyspnoea of a spasmodic nature. If this dyspnoea is frequent and severe, it may be wise to evacuate the abscess contents by costotransversectomy.

Costotransversectomy
A transverse incision 7 cm in length, is made over the vertebral end of the rib corresponding to the apex of the gibbus. The rib is exposed, and the periosteum carefully elevated on the superficial and deep surfaces. Care is required in getting out the rib heads; this may be difficult as they may have developed an ankylosis to the vertebral bodies. The rib is divided with nibbling forceps 4 cm from the tip of the transverse process of the corresponding vertebra. Great care is taken to avoid perforating the pleura.

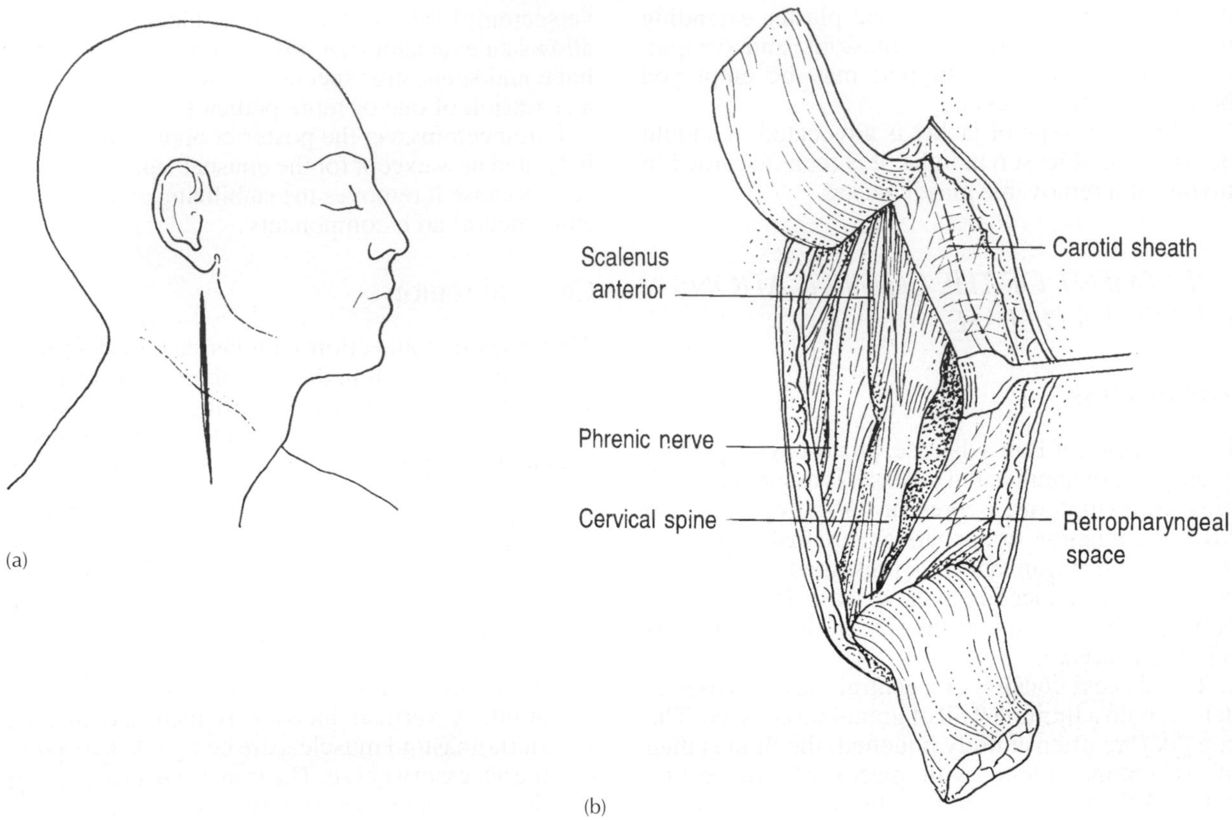

Figure 9.48 (a) The incision for the anterior approach to the cervical spine. (b) The anterior exposure of the cervical spine for drainage of a spinal abscess.

The transverse process is then cut through at its base and removed after its costal attachment has been divided. Occasionally the removal of the rib opens the abscess cavity, but if it does not, the tunnel should be explored gently with the finger, and when the wall of the abscess is located it is opened with a blunt instrument. When more than one rib is resected, the neurovascular bundle between the two is encircled with a double ligature, tied in two places and divided.

Occasionally also when more than one rib is removed, a longitudinal incision in the line of the costotransverse joints may be employed with advantage.

Costotransversectomy has certain advantages: it attacks the main cause of the paraplegia, the abscess cavity, and by emptying the abscess reduces the pressure on the cord and the toxicity of the focus. Drainage of the material after costotransversectomy is away from the cord – not around it as after laminectomy. The operation does not weaken the bony spine. The technique is not difficult, nor is there any great operative risk. A relatively large canal is formed through which it is possible to evacuate not only fluid pus but granulation tissue, necrotic bone and caseous material.

Lumbar region

An abscess should be opened and drained. A vertical incision is made along the lateral border of the sacrospinalis, between the last rib and the crest of the ilium. The tensor fascia is divided, to expose the quadratus lumborum. The muscle is split longitudinally to the lateral side of the transverse process, the lumbar arteries being carefully avoided.

Pun *et al.* (1990) have reported on 37 patients from Hong Kong with lumbosacral tuberculosis and emphasize its rarity with pain as the presenting symptom and often a discharging sinus. Neurological involvement because of the large intraspinal space was uncommon. Anterior debridement with bone grafting can reduce the incidence and degree of kyphosis with its complications.

Radical operation

The approach to the treatment of tuberculosis of

bone and joint has significantly altered in the last two decades and operations of a curative nature, as opposed to stabilization, that would have been highly dangerous before, are now possible with antibiotics. Removal of tuberculous foci was attempted years ago but usually with a high mortality and so was given up. But with the protection from such things as dissemination and sinus formation such operations are now successfully carried out with gratifying and quick results. It is highly improbable that antibiotics can reach the tuberculous area, if the disease is of any duration, as the surrounding fibrosis of attempted healing forms an impenetrable barrier. This is one of the main reasons for opening up the diseased area, and also progressive bone destruction can be stopped by radical intervention.

Cases showing clinical and radiological evidence of activity are subjected to operation. Evidence of activity includes abscess formation, clinically or radiologically confirmed, poor general condition or a rise of sedimentation rate. Operation is considered even though there is no real evidence of an abscess for in any case one is usually present. To ensure a stable spine at the end of treatment the operation should be done before gross vertebral destruction occurs, especially in children in whom destruction of tuberculous bone may be rapid. Where there is gross destruction, stability must be ensured by filling the cavity with bone grafts.

Other tuberculous manifestations are not a contraindication except in extreme cases. Skeletal tuberculosis should be treated before lung or urinary disease. In this way the patient's power of resistance is increased and better conditions are ensured for continued chemotherapy of lungs and kidneys respectively. In cases of slight changes and without noteworthy clinical symptoms the progress is watched before interfering.

The cervical spine is reached by an incision along the anterior border of the sternomastoid, reflecting that muscle backwards and the oesophagus, trachea, larynx and carotid sheath forwards.

The upper thoracic is reached by a periscapular incision, lifting the scapula forwards and outwards by a Tudor Edwards retractor. An anterolateral approach is used as already described. An extrapleural approach is made but the pleura may be opened and, indeed, many operators use a transthoracic approach. In the thoracic region from D4 to D12 the thoracotomy should be performed by rib resection so that the rib is available for the graft. Hodgson and Stock (1960), with considerable experience, suggest for the dorsolumbar spine a Fey's eleventh-rib incision. Through this incision good access is obtained from T11 to L5, but if the lesion is higher the tenth rib may be excised and the diaphragm separated posteriorly so that the peritoneum may be displaced forwards (Figure 9.49).

At the operation the abscess cavity is entered as early as possible. All diseased tissues, pus, sequestra, necrotic bone and devitalized discs are removed. The diseased vertebra is removed as far back as the spinal cord as there is often a posterior intraspinal abscess.

Bone grafts are now inserted. A strut-graft of the requisite length from ribs or iliac crest is introduced to keep the vertebra sprung apart, and the surrounding cavity filled with chip grafts.

Hodgson and Stock (1960), on reviewing their first 100 cases following anterior spinal fusion, found that one-third of the cases showed extension of the paravertebral abscess containing bone sequestra to involve either pleura or lung. They pointed out that by such an approach it is possible to eradicate the disease focus, to provide a raw bleeding bed for adequate access of chemotherapeutic agents and finally to achieve early stabilization of the spine. Their series mortality was less than 4% and fusion was achieved in over 93 patients. In a later report, Kalamchi *et al.* (1976) point out the value of the halopelvic apparatus in correcting and especially holding severe kyphosis.

Rajasekaran and Soundarapandian (1989) have defined accurately the progression of kyphosis. In 41% of cases a stable graft provided structural support, but in the remaining group failure of the anterior graft due to slippage, fracture, resorption was commonly found when the graft spanned more than two disc spaces. They recommended an extended period of non weight-bearing, posterior arthrodesis after 6–12 weeks and prolonged use of a brace until consolidation was achieved. They also confirmed that an anterior spinal arthrodesis was superior to ambulation and chemotherapy alone.

The kyphosis deformity still remains a problem and is little improved by the anterior decompression procedure alone. Louw (1990) has reported on using the Hong Kong technique with vascularized rib grafts, posterior osteotomies with instrumentation. Good correction of the kyphosis was obtained with full neurological recovery and early fusion.

When a psoas abscess is present, it is easily found and usually yields a tract directly to the vertebral lesion. If it does not do so, or when no abscess is present, the lateral parts of the vertebrae are exposed, and, if necessary by the aid of radiographic examination with indicator, the bone lesion can be attacked before it has broken through the cortex.

Irrespective of the site of the lesion the subsequent operative procedure is as follows: The abscesses are thoroughly drained and the tuberculous granulations removed. The sinus tracks are followed, so that no gravitation abscesses are overlooked. No attempt is made, however, to remove the whole wall of the abscess. The outer abscess membrane is left intact.

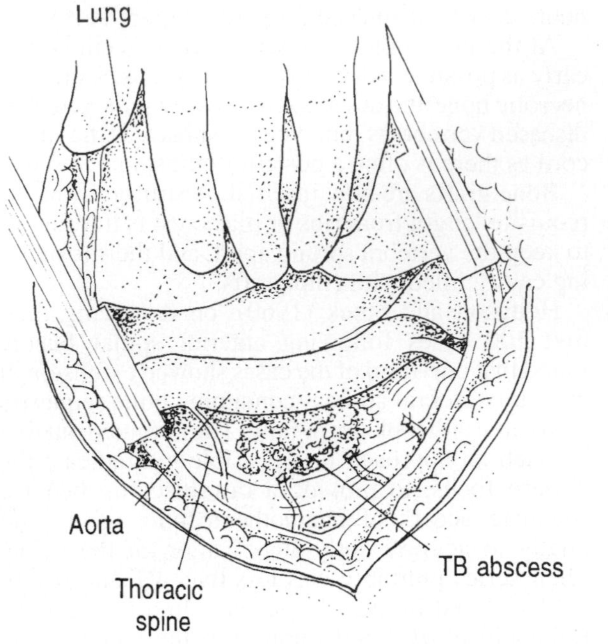

(a)

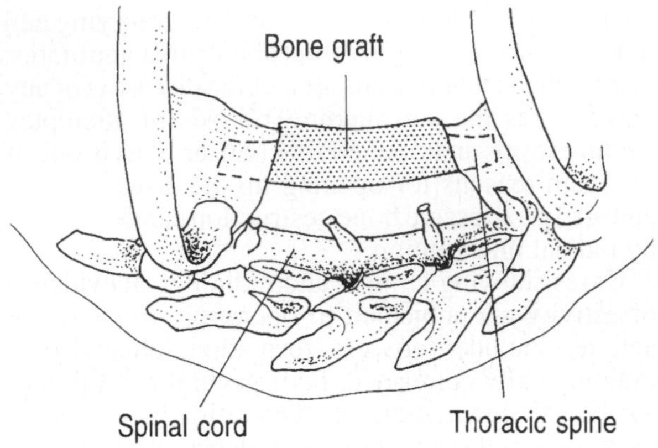

(b)

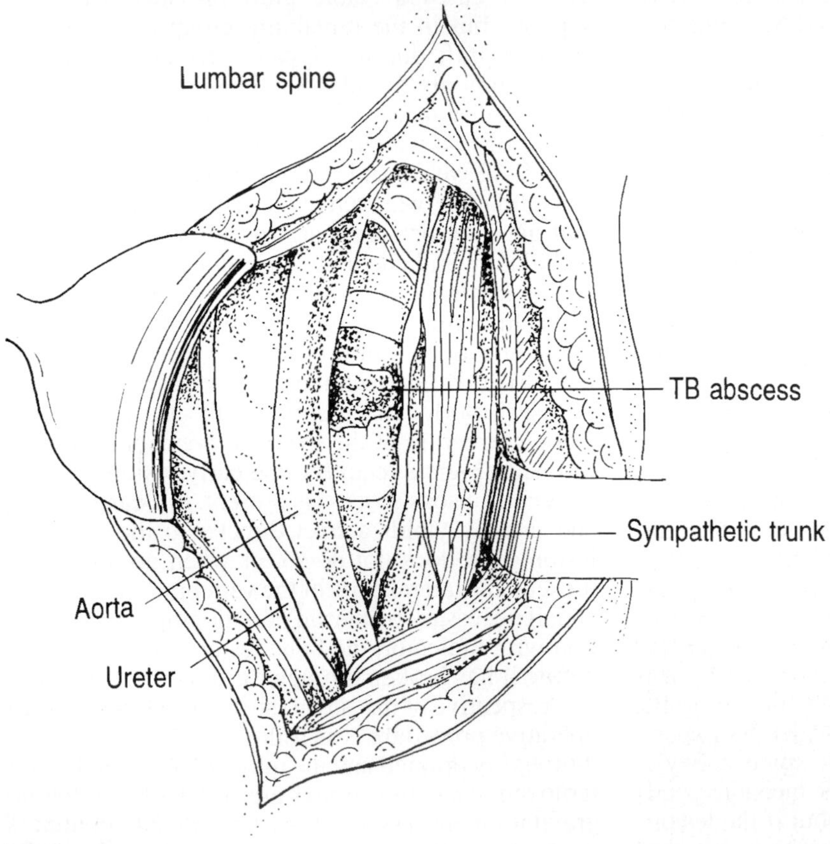

(c)

Figure 9.49 (a) The left transpleural anterior approach to the thoracic spine. The lung and aorta are retracted to the right and the abscess, bone and debris are removed under direct vision to expose and free the spinal cord. (b) The bridging bone graft of rib or iliac crest used to support the spine following the radial drainage procedure. (c) The anterior extraperitoneal approach for drainage of a tuberculous spine abscess in the lumbar region.

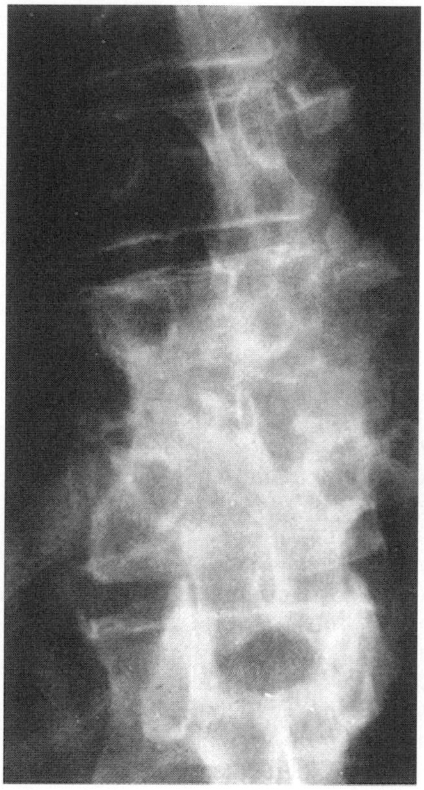

(a)

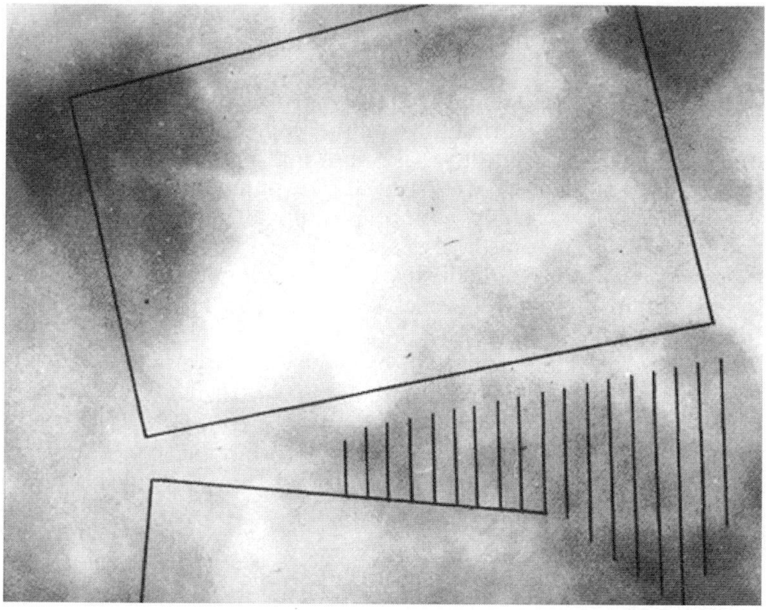

(b)

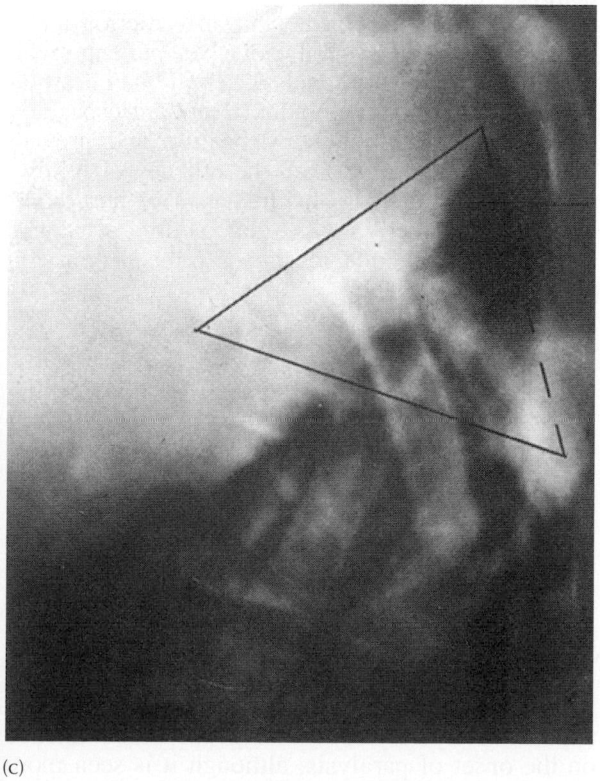

(c)

Figure 9.50 (a) Anteroposterior radiograph of tuberculosis of thoracic vertebrae 11 and 12 with angular collapse but little paravertebral abscess formation. (b) Lateral view of same area, showing bony destruction and minimal abscess formation. (c) Postoperative lateral radiograph showing increased angular kyphosis with fracturing of rib graft. This went on to solid union and healing of disease.

Histologically it may be regarded as the body's defence zone against the tuberculous process and as such it is of value.

Sequestra of bone and of invertebral disc tissue are removed. If it is difficult to see the bone cavity, one has to use a curette to make sure that most of the diseased tissue has been removed. The procedure is completed by washing with physiological saline solution, by which some further sequestra and granulations may appear. Slight diffuse bleeding cannot be avoided, but this usually ceases after washing with hydrogen peroxide. In those cases in which a radical evacuation of the lesion is thought to have been ensured and in which internal fixation is considered to be of value, the cavity is filled with bone chips from the iliac crest. Streptomycin powder is applied both in the bone cavity and in the abscess, and the wound is closed by primary suture.

Pre- and postoperative orthopaedic treatment

Immediately after the diagnosis has been established and the decision to operate has been made, the patient is placed in a plaster bed. When the patient has got accustomed to lying day and night in the plaster bed, the operation is carried out. There is no necessity to wait until the disease has reached a more favourable stage, but the operation should be performed as soon as possible.

After the operation the patient is immobilized in the plaster bed for some months. In uncomplicated cases the patient is then allowed to be ambulant wearing a plaster jacket, which usually after 4–6 months is exchanged for a corset. When the process is considered to have healed, light physiotherapy may strengthen the muscles of the back and eliminate the need for an external support.

In cases of recurrence of sinuses or abscesses the patients are kept in the plaster bed until healing of the sinus is achieved. However, the advantages of such correction must be balanced against its complications.

When the spondylitis is already on the way to healing, as a result of conservative measures, the graft may contribute considerably to the stabilization of the defective spine, and to the maintenance of the result already achieved. Following the necrotic process, subluxations in the intervertebral joints certainly result from the dislocation of the bony fragments. This, no doubt, leads to seriously altered statics in the whole vertebral column and to manifestations of insufficiency of the muscular and ligamentous apparatus, with pain. These are often interpreted as indications of recurrence of the tuberculous inflammation, whereas they are, as a matter of fact, merely signs of static insufficiency. In such cases operation is indicated, towards the relief of symptoms and not against the disease itself (Figure 9.50).

OUT-PATIENT TREATMENT

Out-patient treatment in developing countries remains one of the major orthopaedic problems. Although in this chapter we have described what one might term the standard or classic approach in management, it is obvious that with social and economic restrictions and limited hospital resources this will require much modification. This is particularly seen in lack of in-patient facilities and anti-tuber-culous drugs as well as different attitudes and discipline by involved people. Dickson (1967) reviewed the place of ambulant, non-operative treatment of 32 Nigerian children with the lesion being mainly at the thoracolumbar junction. The majority had pulmonary lesions from hilar adenopathy to bronchopneumonia and 10 children had neurological signs in the lower limbs. The degree of severity depended upon the number of vertebrae involved, the degree of kyphosis and the number achieving intervertebral fusion (14 patients). The outcome was obviously related to the age and severity of the disease at the time of diagnosis and onset of treatment. Only one out of this series came to operation, with four relapsing or failing to respond to this form of conservative treatment. The author believed that these results compared favourably with more radical debridement and anterior spinal fusion. He also pointed out that patients with advanced disease and much vertebral body destruction are less suited for ambulant treatment, especially in hoping to achieve bony healing and prevent increasing deformity. Also, the efficacy of follow-up to ensure adequate maintenance of anti-tuberculous drug therapy is essential, as drug resistance has been described. Dickson described admission to hospital for:

1. very ill children;
2. paraplegics;
3. patients with extensive disease, or those failing to respond to ambulant drug therapy within 3 months clinically and 6 months radiographically; and
4. all patients with a paravertebral abscess.

Pott's paraplegia

Paraplegia occurs as a sequel to Pott's disease in approximately 10% of cases. Age has little influence on the onset of paralysis, although it is seen more commonly in childhood because of the relatively higher incidence of the disease at this age period. Paraplegia is rarely met with in disease below the level of the first lumbar vertebra since the cord has terminated below this point, and as thoracic disease is far more common than cervical disease the majority (85%) of paraplegias accompany thoracic lesions. In addition to the greater frequency of disease in the upper and middle thoracic region, the narrowing of the bony canal here and the difficulty in securing complete fixation during treatment increased the probability of paralysis.

The error responsible for the paralysis may arise in the bones, the membranes or the cord itself.

1. *Bone causes*. Angulation of the anterior wall of the bony canal may, though rarely, give rise to paralysis, a partial dislocation of the vertebra, a sequestrum, the extension of tuberculous granulations into the canal or a cold abscess. A relatively intact disc may be found in the middle of the diseased area pressing on the cord.
2. *Causes in the membranes*. When the meninges are at fault, the cause is usually a pachymeningitis, or more rarely a leptomeningitis; these result in thickening of the membranes and in obliteration of the blood and lymph vessels.
3. *Causes in the cord*. The nervous tissue of the cord is practically never infected with tuberculosis but an early form of paralysis may be due to circulatory change in the cord in the neighbourhood of the lesion without gross compression. This is associated with the early and most active stage of the disease when there is vascular engorgement in the epidural space, infiltration, lymphatic obstruction, and as a rule some mild circumferential compression of the theca. The spinal cord may be flattened from pressure, or oedematous as a result of vascular stasis. In the earlier stages the paresis is transient and as a rule relieved quickly by immobilization.

Hodgson *et al.* (1967) believed that Pott's paraplegia should be classified as due to:

1. Extrinsic cause – e.g. abscess formation, sequestrated bone, discal fibrosis, pathological subluxation or dislocation of vertebrae, transverse ridge of bone anteriorly.
2. Intrinsic causes – e.g. focal meningitis or meningomyelitis, infective thrombosis, spinal cord tumour.

They found in dural biopsies, granulomatous inflammation with epithelial tubercle formation or caseous necrosis.

They also showed that even where there was no myelitis, the inflammatory swelling of the dura and adjacent soft tissues could produce pressure on the spinal cord, which, alone or with other factors, might be a significant factor in the production of paraplegia. This is considered to be further evidence in favour of early surgical decompression of the cord in Pott's paraplegia, since if allowed to progress irreversible changes occur in the spinal cord. Tandon and Pathak (1973) have described how a localized arachnoiditis can cause a common form of paraplegia in India, called primary tuberculous spinal radiculomyelitis.

Girdlestone originally described two main groups of paralysis which are distinguished by their onset in relation to the duration of the disease – early- or late-onset paraplegia.

Paraplegia of early onset

This type is found in early active Pott's disease. Usually the Pott's disease has been recognized before the paresis. Paraplegia may, however, be the presenting symptom. The first symptoms are muscular weakness, inco-ordination and spasticity. Pain in the back or referred to the involved nerve roots is common. The awkwardness of gait and spasticity proceed until walking becomes impossible. There is first a paralysis in extension, with increasingly frequent attacks of general flexor spasm, and it eventually becomes a paralysis in flexion, indicating a complete loss of conductivity of the pyramidal tracts. In exceptional cases the compression is sudden enough to cause an initial flaccid paralysis from spinal shock. Where the paralysis is in extension it is incomplete, the pyramidal or possibly vestibulospinal tracts having partially escaped compression; sphincter involvement is common.

Paraplegia of late onset

In this type the outstanding characteristics are the late and gradual onset, the incompleteness of the paralysis and the high percentage of permanency in comparison to the first group.

The onset is variable from a few months to many years after the apparent quiescence of the disease. Muscular spasticity is usually the first sign. Sensory changes may be lacking throughout but there is usually widespread though incomplete anaesthesia. Pain is rarely felt, but there may be a little backache or irregular pains down the limbs. Even at its height, late onset paresis is typically incomplete and the legs are seldom devoid of slight voluntary power.

PROGNOSIS

In paraplegia of early onset, though often incomplete, if the patient is seen in good time the paralysis is usually curable when the tuberculosis is arrested. None the less, it has to be realized that there are cases where this is not so and the paralysis may be permanent though the tuberculous disease becomes cured. The prognosis is better in the young than the old, while the longer the paralysis has existed the poorer the outlook. Gradual onset is less harmful than a sudden crush. The more complete the sensory loss and the deeper the motor paralysis, the worse the outlook. Loss of sphincteric control indicates a greater pressure and, for that reason, a less favourable prognosis.

TREATMENT

Pott's paralysis is becoming rarer because of earlier diagnosis and more prompt and effective initial treatment. The method of treatment – conservative or operative – will depend on the type of case and whether occurring early or late in the disease. However, adequate chemotherapy must be initiated promptly.

There are three principal indications for operation:

1. A rapidly progressive paresis which is advancing daily. An immediate operation is carried out.
2. The case in which paresis advances over weeks or months in spite of adequate treatment, effective fixation and postural correction.
3. The case in which, in spite of adequate treatment, fixation and postural correction, a slight or moderate paresis develops and persists.

Prompt relief of pressure upon the spinal cord is required if immobilization fails to obtain within a week or two a definite and progressing amelioration in the neurological dysfunctions. If the loss of power has proceeded to a complete paraplegia the situation may become irrecoverable, even if in some cases the paraplegia has become very recently complete. If there is some voluntary control the cord is in little danger of irrepairable damage, but when this is lost decompression should be delayed. Pathological dislocation and displaced sequestra may be seen by tomography, CT and MRI examination and indicate operative relief.

The basis of management in all cases of Pott's paraplegia is general treatment for the tuberculosis, and immobilization in a plaster shell with a turning case. The criteria for traction are not so clear, but in all cervical and upper dorsal cases (as most of them are) better results with less discomfort are achieved by the application of skeletal traction by means of a halofemoral appliance. The shell is tilted down a little at the foot end to provide sufficient counter-traction by body weight and a 2.25–4.50kg weight applied to the traction appliance.

In recent years an aggressive approach has gained popularity with early surgical eradication of the tuberculous forms, decompression of the cord being followed by anterior spinal grafting. Hodgson *et al.* (1964) demonstrated that this approach carried the greatest percentage of cure rate in the shortest time: 74% had complete recovery.

Hodgson also demonstrated that a prolonged paraplegia did not necessarily mean permanent paraplegia, having had recovery in patients paraplegic for as long as 4 and 5 years.

Guirguis (1967) reported his experience of 78 patients treated by an anterolateral decompression extrapleural procedure which left the facets undisturbed maintaining the strength of the spine: 14 patients had complete cure of paraplegia, 22 had satisfactory return of motor power and sphincteric control, 4 patients had no improvement or died. No patient with complete flaccid paralysis was improved. The main indications for this form of surgery were cord compression, sequestra, collapsed vertebrae with gibbus formation, lack of radiographic evidence for compression and spastic paraplegia in flexion.

LEPROSY

This chronic inflammatory disease, although endemic in Asia, Africa and South America, occurs sporadically in other countries, and, with modern travel and migration, cases now require treatment throughout the world. The World Health Organization estimates that there are 11–12 million leprosy patients world wide.

It is caused by the acid-fast bacillus *Mycobacterium leprae*, first described by G. Armauer Hansen in 1874. It can be seen in two major forms although indeterminate cases may be found: *lepromatous*, in which the bacilli are readily found in the widespread inflammatory areas in the skin, peripheral nerves, mucous membranes, lymph nodes, bone marrow, eyes and testis; and *tuberculoid*, in which the bacilli are very frequently seen and skin lesions are rare.

The mode of transmission of the bacillus is thought to arise from the nose of lepromatous leprosy patients by nasal discharge, droplet via coughing and sneezing rather than from ulcerating skin lesions or from intact skin. The portal of entry appears to be skin and nose or mouth. Fluorescent leprosy antibody absorption test (FLA-ABS) and more recently ELISA (enzyme-linked immunoasorbant assay) antigen have been used to determine carriers of leprosy antibodies as well as subclinical states of this disease.

Peripheral nerve involvement with anaesthesia and paralysis occurs early and is widespread. The lepromin test of intradermally injecting a sterilized saline emulsion of the bacilli will aid in differentiating the two types – the lepromatous type having a negative response whereas the tuberculoid type is usually strongly positive.

The characteristic lesion of leprosy is found in the skin, i.e. hypopigmentation and in the nerves which become enlarged and hard. Anaesthesia with the presence of acid-fast bacilli in a skin biopsy is most suggestive. Nerves commonly involved are the corneal, facial, ulnar, median, radial, lateral popliteal and posterior tibial nerves.

There is swelling of the basement membrane of the Schwann cells, with pressure necrosis and a surrounding granulomatous inflammation. This results in a neuritis with pain, paraesthesia or anaesthesia and local tenderness. Deep tendon reflexes remain normal but electromyography shows the denervation lesion. Differential diagnosis is of a peripheral neuritis, syringomyelia and trophic ulceration. Neuropathic joint changes especially in the tarsal joints giving rise to a warm and swollen foot, are commonly seen and plantar ulceration may result from the anaesthesia, from direct injury and from the various classic deformities of the drop and inverted foot with clawing of digits.

The reasons for the predilection of *M. leprae* for peripheral nerves and the sites of involvement are not yet known. Various theories of immunological protection, lower temperature favouring proliferation, repeated trauma with microvascular changes at specific sites which are superficial, around bony prominences, etc. have all been described by Parkes (1988). He has reviewed how the bacteria enter the endoneurium by their direct uptake by Schwann cells of the cutaneous nerves, their uptake by inflammatory cells, e.g. monocytes, and through the blood nerve barrier of the endoneurial blood vessels. Sensory loss precedes motor power involvement, the latter implying that the infection has already spread a long way up the nerve. Segmental demyelination is thought to be due to the direct destruction of Schwann cells by the intracellular proliferation of the mycobacteria as well as ischaemic/pressure effects and a delayed-type hypersensitivity reaction.

The central nervous system is not involved because of its higher temperature and the absolute impermeability of the blood–brain barrier.

The sensory nerve damage results in areas of anaesthesia and no response to harmful stimulus. Therefore trauma from extremes of burns, rat bites, to ill-fitting shoes or no shoes leads quickly to ulceration and secondary infection. Sympathetic/parasympathetic damage leads to loss of vascular or sweating control. Motor impairment with muscle paralysis leads to drop-foot, facial paralysis, development of fixed joint deformities and contracture.

Radiographs of the feet may show gross osteolysis or resorption of the tarsometatarsal bones due to osteomyelitis (Figures 9.51 and 9.52). In the hand subarticular resorption of the phalanges can be seen with soft tissue swelling. Osteoporosis secondary to disuse of a digit or a limb is commonly found. There is a specific leprous osteitis or granuloma which is rare and varies in severity from osteoporosis, to pseudo-cyst formation, to large areas of bone destruction.

TREATMENT

As for tuberculosis, the main object of treatment is to destroy the bacilli in all tissues and produce regression of the inflammation – this taking many months or years to achieve. However, one of the differences is seen in the necessity for a careful dosage pattern in order to prevent the reaction of oedema and cellular infiltration which leads to a worsening of the neuritis with destruction of the eyes, of nerves and of skin.

The drugs commonly used are dapsone, solapsone, thiambutosine (DPT; 4,4-diaminodiphenyl sulphone), thiosemicarbazone, and streptomycin with isoniazid. More recently, rifampicin has been

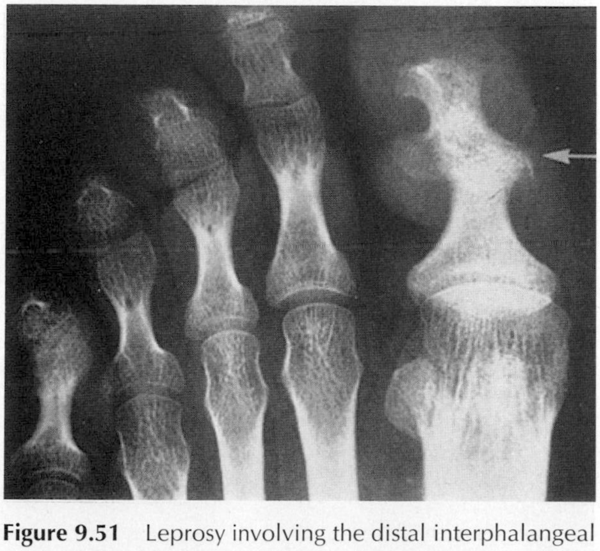

Figure 9.51 Leprosy involving the distal interphalangeal joint of the big toe with marked resorption of all the terminal phalanges surrounded by soft tissue swelling.

used with a successful bactericidal effect (Rees *et al.*, 1970). Local treatment is directed towards preventing complications by splintage, graduated exercises, surgery to decompress any entrapment of peripheral nerves and calipers or braces for the deformities. Chiase and Roger (1985) have described the main indication for neurolysis of the common peroneal nerve in leprosy is for a hyperalgesic neuritis with motor power weakness. In a painless long-standing paralysis with neural fibrosis, the result is poor.

Chronic ulceration, particularly of feet and hands, is commonly found due to loss of cutaneous sensation. Gauze dressings are not effective because of difficulty in keeping in place, their sticking to granulation tissue, etc., and therefore zinc oxide strapping has been used, and more recently semipermeable hydrocolloid occlusive dressings (Duoderm).

The effect of weight-loading spread by orthotic supports, e.g. cork insoles, by plaster casts, even by metatarsal head resection is now most important.

Ulceration and gross osteomyelitis in the feet can be controlled and improved by a carefully performed Syme's amputation, despite anaesthesia of the stump (Srinivasan, 1973).

Horibe *et al.* (1988) have described 146 patients

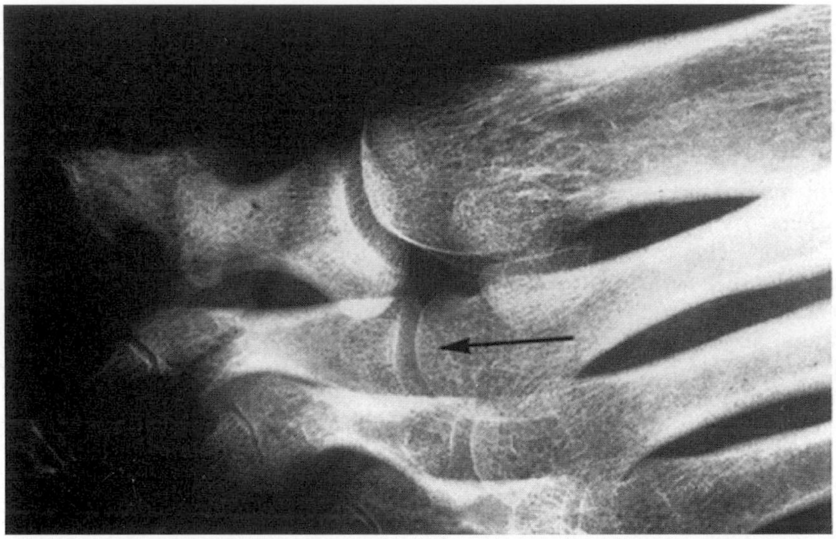

(a)

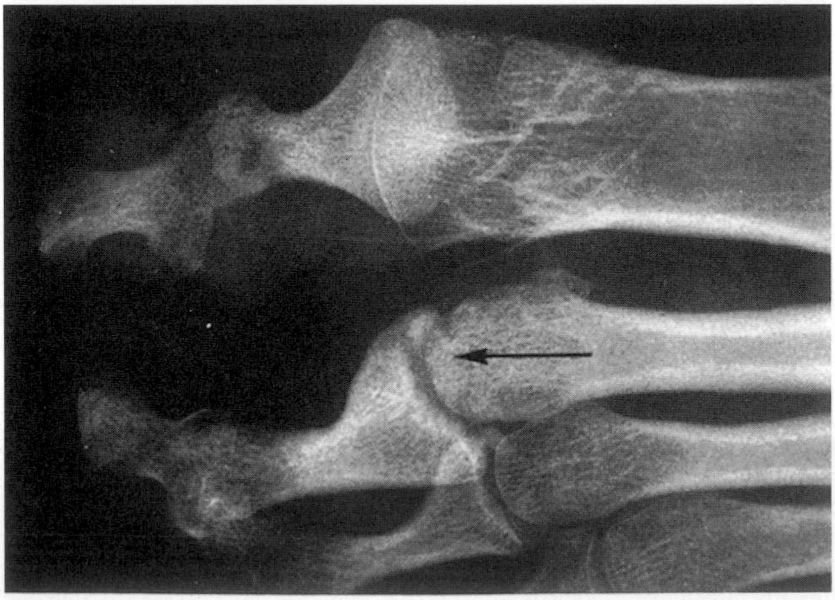

(b)

Figure 9.52 Leprosy involving the terminal aspects of the digits, with rapid destruction of the second metatarsal joint and its diaphysis.

with leprosy develop a neuropathy of the foot and ankle major joints. Lateral popliteal nerve paralysis was common and led to repeated trauma and/or abnormal stresses, with radiographic signs in the ankle and mid-tarsal joints.

Successful arthrodesis of the ankle requires meticulous technique of radical debridement of articular cartilage sclerotic bone, synovial tissue and scarred capsular tissue, with careful fashioning of the excised bone surfaces for apposition and rigid internal fixation. Incisions must heal perprinium (Shibata *et al.*, (1990) to prevent secondary infection.

Stiff fingers are a problem with clawing of the digits and flexion deformities of wrists; these can be treated with wax baths, serial splintage, active assisted and passive exercises. Efficient programmes of this kind give better results than surgery for secondary deformities. Reconstructive surgery is now indicated for deformities but of course complete anaesthesia cannot be corrected. Goodwin (1963) described how the degree of inflammation should be estimated by the Bacteriological Index (BI) test of examining areas of skin for the acid-fast bacilli and the Morphological Index (MI) indicating the percentage of bacilli retaining their morphological normal form. These two indices should be low before considering surgery.

Specific lesions and deformities are considered in Chapters 15 and 17.

HYDATID DISEASE OF BONE (TAENIA ECHINOCOCCUS)

Hydatid disease is endemic in many parts of the world, including Iran, Iraq, Greece, the Balkans, Russia, South Africa, Israel, Cyprus, India, Canada and Alaska, and man gains infection from a variety of mammals such as dogs, sheep, cattle, pigs, horses and camels. Involvement of the liver by the embryos is the commonest sequel producing cysts but bone is involved in only approximately 1% (Alldred and Nisbet, 1964).

The lesions in bone may lie dormant for 10–20 years (Hooper and McLean, 1977) and occur mostly in long bones such as the femur, humerus and tibia but they also arise in the spine where rupture can take place into the spinal canal, producing severe neurological impairment. Flat bones may be affected less frequently. The hydatid cyst begins in the metaphysis, giving rise to a multilocular cyst causing scalloping of the cortex but with little expansion, sclerosis or periosteal reaction. If the cortex is eroded and the soft tissues are involved, calcification occurs in the latter (Figure 9.53), which is typical of the lesion (Booz, 1975). The articular surfaces are never breached. Pathological fracture may occur.

Diagnosis is made on clinical grounds and confirmed by the indirect haemagglutination test or the

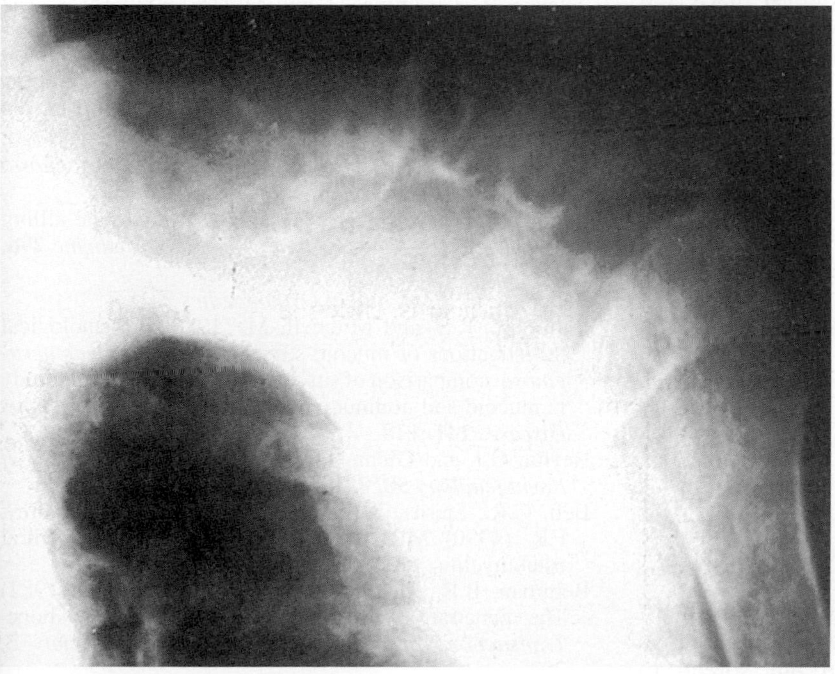

Figure 9.53 Radiograph showing the typical expansile appearance of hydatid disease of the clavicle. (Courtesy of Dr N. Walker)

Casoni or complement-fixation tests. CT and MR imaging are also proving to be helpful.

Treatment is curative only by complete excision of the affected portion of bone or by limb ablation. Curettage is often performed because the nature of the cyst is not recognized preoperatively, in which case the use of hypertonic saline is most effective since it sterilizes the germinal elements of the parasite, the scolices, by osmotic action but recurrence and/or secondary infection is the rule, necessitating radical excision.

FUNGAL INFECTIONS OF BONE

Mycotic osteomyelitis is the general term used to describe a group of rare diseases caused by fungal infection in bone.

Actinomycosis from cattle, occurs in man in the soft tissues such as the mouth, appendix, caecum and lungs, and the skeleton is affected secondarily, the mandible most commonly. The infection may spread from the lung to the thoracic spine and from the caecum to the pelvis. Multiple abscesses result with the typical amorphous yellow granules or 'sulphur granules' formed of fungal colonies. The affected bone has a moth-eaten appearance. In the spine the condition is distinguished from tuberculosis by sparing of the intervertebral discs and absence of vertebral collapse and kyphosis, whilst the transverse processes and heads of ribs are involved.

Treatment is classically with the penicillins, though the addition of streptomycin or one of the tetracyclines may be necessary, and is required for 6 months at least. Surgical excision of the affected bone is required for treatment of multiple abscesses.

Blastomycosis is another rare disease of skin and lungs but secondary extension to bones and joints may occur directly or by haematogenous spread. The disease is endemic in the USA, extending from Wisconsin to Louisiana, across Kentucky and the Carolinas. A chronic granulomatous disease similar to tuberculosis occurs which causes destructive osteomyelitis of the vertebrae, ribs, skull and sometimes of long bones. Diagnosis is established by smear of affected tissues, serology and skin testing. Amphotericin is effective in treatment but is nephrotoxic.

Coccidioidomycosis is endemic to south-west USA. Infection is by inhalation of dust, so that lungs are the primary site of infection but spread to multiple bone sites is recorded; the spine, pelvis, hands, feet, femur and tibia are most common. The infection produces a granulomatous tuberculoid type of tissue reaction with caseation. Transient chest pain and fever are frequent clinical features. The chest lesions are initially circumscribed but later become more diffuse which resolve over several weeks. Diagnosis is by microscopy of the spores. Treatment by amphotericin is employed with bony excision of local lesions.

Candida albicans infection of bone occurs usually secondarily in association with narcotic abuse, hyperalimentation or in immunosuppressed patients. The spine may show vertebral osteomyelitis and narrowing of the intervertebral disc space (Hirschmann and Everett, 1976); involvement of the long bones, knee joints, scapula, pelvis and costochondral sites have been reported (Smilack and Gentry, 1976). Treatment with amphotericin appears to be effective. Other fungal infections have been reported such as *Torulopsis* and *Fusarium*, but these are still very rare. With the increasing effectiveness of antibiotics and the increase in numbers of immunosuppressed or intensively managed patients the incidence of fungal infections will probably steadily increase.

References

Alldred, A.J. and Nisbet, N.W. (1964) Hydatid disease of bone in Australia. *Journal of Bone and Joint Surgery* **46B**, 260–267

Allen, E.H., Cosgrove, D. and Millard, F.J.C. (1978) The radiological changes in infections of the spine and their diagnostic value. *Clinical Radiology* **29**, 21–40

Angel, J.H. (1992) Modern management in pulmonary tuberculosis. *Prescribers Journal* **32**, 144–152

Annear, S. (1975) Unstable gentamicin resistance with linkage to colony size in *Pseudomonas aeruginosa. Pathology* **7**, 281–283

Babior, B.M. (1978) Oxygen dependent microbial killing by phagocytes. *New England Journal of Medicine* **298**, 721–725

Baitch, A. (1962) *Clinical Orthopaedics* **2**, 157

Baltimore, R.S. and Mitchell, M. (1980) Immunological investigations of mucoid strains of *Pseudomonas aeruginosa*: comparison of susceptibility by opsonic antibody in mucoid and nonmucoid strains. *Journal of Infectious Diseases* **141**, 128

Baylin, G.J. and Glenn, J.C. (1948) *American Journal of Roentgenology* **50**, 851

Bell, G.R., Sterns, K.L., Bonutti, P.M. and Boumphrey, F.R. (1990) MRI diagnosis of tuberculous vertebral osteomyelitis. *Spine* **15**, 462–465

Bergman, B.R., Haynes, D.W. and Nelson, C.L. (1982) The penetration of antibiotics into avascular bone. *Transactions of the Orthopedic Research Society* **7**, 202

Bertolini, D.R., Medwin, G., Bringman, T. *et al.* (1986) Stimulation of bone resorption and inhibition of bone formation *in vitro* by human tumour necrosis factor. *Nature* **319**, 516

Blackburn, W.D. and Alarcon, G.S. (1991) Prosthetic joint infections – a role for prophylaxis. *Arthritis and Rheumatism* **34**, 110–117

Blockey, N.J. and McAllister, T.A. (1972) *Journal of Bone and Joint Surgery* **54B**, 299

Booz, M.K. (1975) Radiological diagnosis of hydatid disease of bone. *Journal of Bone and Joint Surgery* **57B**, 111

Bridges, K. and Lowbury, E.J. (1977) Drug resistance in relation to use of silver sulphadiazine cream in a burns unit. *Journal of Clinical Pathology* **30**, 160

Bucholz, H.W., Engelbrecht, E., Lodenkamper, H., Pottiger, H., Siegel, A. and Elson, R.A. (1981) Management of deep infection of total hip replacement. *Journal of Bone and Joint Surgery* **63B**, 342–345

Burchardt, H. and Enneking, W.F. (1978) Transplantation of bone. *Surgical Clinics of North America* **58**, 403

Burke, J.F. (1961) The effective period of preventive antibiotic action in experimental incisions and dermal lesions. *Surgery* **62A**, 161–164

Celsus A. Cornelius (1838) *Of Medicine*. Translated by James Grieve; revised by George Futuoye. 3rd edn. H. Renshaw: London

Chaise, F. and Roger, B. (1985) Neurolysis of the common peroneal nerve in leprosy. *Journal of Bone And Joint Surgery* **67B**, 426–429

Charaka Samhita (1888) *Collected Works*. Translated into English by Arinash Chandia. Kavirotiva: Calcutta

Charnley, J. (1964) A clean air operating enclosure. *British Journal of Surgery* **51**, 195–202, 202–205

Crofton, J. (1960) *British Medical Journal* **1**, 679

Cunka, B.A. (1988) Antibiotics in orthopaedic surgery. In: *Orthopaedic Infections*, pp. 156–174. Edited by D. Schlossberg. Springer-Verlag: New York

Datta, A. (1973) In: *Current Antibiotic Therapy*. Proceedings of a symposium, 1972. Edited by A.M. Geddes and J.D. Williams. Churchill Livingstone: Edinburgh and London

Dekel, S. and Francis, M.J.O. (1981) The treatment of osteomyelitis of the tibia with sodium salicylate. An experimental study in rabbits. *Journal of Bone and Joint Surgery* **63B**, 178–185

Dekel, S, Schmidt, E., Dickson, R.A. and Francis, M.J.O. (1980) *Journal of Bone and Joint Surgery* **62B**, 257

Dewhurst, F.E., Stashenko, P.P., Mole, J.E. and Tsurumachi, T. (1985) Purification and partial sequence of osteoclast activating factor: identity with interleukin-l beta. *Journal of Immunology* **135**, 2562

Dickson, J.A.S. (1967) Spinal tuberculosis in Nigerian children. *Journal of Bone and Joint Surgery* **49A**, 682–694

Dunlop, D.M. and Murdoch, J.McC. (1960) *British Medical Bulletin* **16**, 67

Duthie, R.B. and Barker, A.N. (1955) *Journal of Bone and Joint Surgery***37B**, 304

Duthie, R.B. and Francis, M.J.O. (1988) Annotation. Free radicals and Dupuytren's contracture. *Journal of Bone and Joint Surgery* **70B**, 689–691

Eisenstein, B.I., Sox, T., Biswas, G., Blackman, E. and Sparling, P.F. (1977) Conjugal transfer of the gonococcal penicillinase plasmid. *Science* **195**, 998–1000

Engh, C.A., Hughes, J.L., Abrams, R.C. and Bowerman, J.W. (1971) Osteomyelitis in the patient with sickle cell disease. *Journal of Bone and Joint Surgery* **53A**, 1–15

Enneking, W.F. (1986) *Clinical Musculoskeletal Pathology*. Storter Printing: Gainesville, FL

Evans, R.P., Nelson, C.L., Lange, T.A. and Harrison, B.H. (1988) Acute exogenous osteomyelitis. The role of surgery in a reproducible model. *Transactions of the Orthopedic Research Society* **13**, 437

Fitzgerald, R.H. (1984) Antibiotic distribution in normal and osteomyelitis bone. *Orthopedic Clinics of North America* **15**, 537–546

Fitzgerald, R.H. and Cowan, J.D.E. (1975) Puncture wounds of the foot. *Orthopedic Clinics of North America* **6**, 969

Fitzgerald, R.H. Jr, Landells, D.G. and Cowan, J.D.E. (1975) Osteomyelitis in children: comparison of haematogenous and secondary osteomyelitis. *Canadian Medical Association Journal* **112**, 166

Fitzgerald, R.H., Nolan, R., Ilstrup, D.M. *et al.* (1977) Deep wound sepsis following total hip replacement. *Journal of Bone and Joint Surgery* **59A**, 847–855

Florey, H.W. (1958) *General Pathology*, pp. 871, 895. W.B. Saunders: Philadelphia, PA

Garrod, L.P. and Scowen, E.F. (1960) *British Medical Bulletin* **16**, 22

Garrod, L.P., Lambert, H.P. and O'Grady, F. (1973) *Antibiotics and Chemotherapy*. Churchill Livingstone: Edinburgh and London

Gibson, M.J., Karpinski, M.R.K., Slach, R.C.B., Cowlishaw, W.A. and Webb, J.K. (1987) The penetration of antibiotics into the normal intervertebral disc. *Journal of Bone and Joint Surgery* **69B**, 784–786

Goodwin, C.J. (1963) *Essentials of Leprosy for the Clinician*. Hong Kong Auxiliary of the Mission to Lepers: Hong Kong

Gould, E.S., Polley, H.G. and Boben, S.E. (1990) Role of routine percutaneous aspiration prior to prosthesis revision. *Skeletal Radiology* **19**, 427–450

Govan, J.R.W. and Fyfe, J.A.M. (1978) Mucoid *Pseudomonas aeruginosa* and cystic fibrosis. Resistance of the mucoid form to carbenicillin, flucloxacillin and tobramycin and the isolation of muroid variants *in vitro*. Journal of Antimicrobial Chemotherapy **4**, 233

Gristina, A.G. (1987) Biomaterial-centred infection: microbial adhesions vs. tissue integration. *Science* **237**, 1588

Gristina, A.G. and Costeron, J.W. (1984) Bacterial adhesion and the glycocalyx and their role in the musculo skeletal infection. *Orthopedic Clinics of North America* **15**, 517

Gristina, A.G., Costeron, J.W., Hobgood, C.D. and Webb, L.X. (1987) Bacterial adhesion, biomaterials, the foreign body effect and infection from natural ecosystems to infection in man: a brief overview. *Contemporary Orthopedics* **14**, 27

Guirguis, A.R. (1967) Pott's paraplegia. *Journal of Bone and Joint Surgery* **49B**, 659–667

Gustilo, R.B. (1979) Use of antimicrobials in the management of open fractures. *Archives of Surgery* **114**, 805

Harris, N. H. (1962) Place of surgery in early stages of acute osteomyelitis. *British Medical Journal* **2**, 1440

Hippocrates (1849) *The Genuine Works of Hippocrates*.

Translation with annotations, etc. by Francis Adams. Sydenham Society: London
Hirschmann, J.V. and Everett, E.D. (1976) Candida vertebral osteomyelitis. *Journal of Bone and Joint Surgery* **58A**, 573–575
Hobo, T. (1921) Zur Pathogenese der Acuten haematogenen Osteomyelitis. *Acta Scholae Medicinalis Universitatis Imperialis in Kioto* **4**, 1
Hodgson, A.R. and Stock, F.E. (1960) *Journal of Bone and Joint Surgery* **42A**, 295–310
Hodgson, A.R., Yau, A., Kwon, J.S. and Kim, D. (1964) *Clinical Orthopaedics and Related Research* **36**, 128–150
Hodgson, A.R., Skinsnes, O.K. and Leong, C.Y. (1967) Pathogenesis of Pott's paraplegia. *Journal of Bone and Joint Surgery* **49A**, 1147–1156
Hoeprich, P.D. (1977) *Infectious Diseases: a Modern Treatise of Infectious Processes*, 2nd edn. Harper Medical: New York
Hooper, J. and McLean, I. (1977) Hydatid disease of the femur. *Journal of Bone and Joint Surgery* **59A**, 974–976
Horibe, S., Tada, K. and Nagana, J. (1988) Neuroarthroplasty of the foot in leprosy. *Journal of Bone and Joint Surgery* **70B**, 481–485
Jellis, J.E. (1992a) Haematogenous osteomyelitis. *Surgery* **1**, 145–148
Jellis, J.E. (1992b) Granulomatous and non-bacterial infections. *Current Science/Current Opinion in Orthopaedics* **3**, 65–68
Jones, G.R. and Pallett, A.P. (1993) Clinical implications of bacterial resistance to antibiotics. Editorial. *Hospital Update* **1**, 199–200
Kahn, D.S. and Pritzker, K.P.H. (1979) The pathophysiology of bone infection. *Clinical Orthopaedics* **141**, 143
Kalamchi, A., Yau, A., O'Brien, J.P. and Hodgson, A.R. (1976) Halo-pelvic distraction apparatus. *Journal of Bone and Joint Surgery* **58A**, 1119–1125
Kamme, C. and Lindberg, L. (1981) Aerobic and anaerobic bacterial in deep infections after total hip arthroplasty: differential diagnosis between infectious and non-infectious loosening. *Clinical Orthopaedics and Related Research* **154**, 201–207
Kilgore, R.W., Haynes, D.W. and Nelson, C.L. (1982) The penetration of antibiotics into avascular bone. *Transactions of the Orthopedic Research Society* **7, 202**
Lack, C.H. (1959) *Journal of Bone and Joint Surgery* **41B**, 384
Larsen, R.M. (1938) Intramedullary pressure with particular reference to massive diaphyseal bone necrosis. Experimental observations. *Annals of Surgery* **108**, 127
Lees, D. (1931) *Practice and Methods in the Diagnosis and Treatment of Venereal Diseases*. Livingstone: Edinburgh
Leong, J.C.Y. (1993) Editorial. Tuberculosis of the spine. *Journal of Bone and Joint Surgery* **75B**, 173–175
Lidwell, O.M., Lowbury, E.J.L. and Whyte, W. (1982) Effect of ultra clean air in operating rooms on deep sepsis in the joint after total hip or knee replacement – a randomised trial. *British Medical Journal* **285**, 10–14
Lifeso, R. (1987) Atlanto-axial tuberculosis in adults. *Journal of Bone and Joint Surgery* **69B**, 183–187
Louw, J.A. (1990) Spinal tuberculosis with neurological deficit: treatment with anterior vascularised rib grafts, posterior osteotomies and fusion. *Journal of Bone and Joint Surgery* **72B**, 686–693
McDermott, M. (1969) *Harvey Lectures* **63**, 1
McDermott, M. (1970) *American Review of Respiratory Disease* **102**, 857
Martin, N.S. (1970) *Journal of Bone and Joint Surgery* **52B**, 613–628
Medical Research Council Working Party on Tuberculosis of the Spine (1974) *British Journal of Surgery* **61**, 853–866
Mollan, R.A.B. and Piggot, J. (1977) Acute osteomyelitis in children. *Journal of Bone and Joint Surgery* **59B**, 2–7
Morrey, B.F., Bianco, A.J. and Rhodes, K.H. (1976) Suppurative arthritis of the hip in children. *Journal of Bone and Joint Surgery* **58A**, 388–392
MRC (1993) Controlled trial of short-course regimens of chemotherapy in the ambulatory treatment of spinal tuberculosis. *Journal of Bone and Joint Surgery* **75B**, 240–248
Nelson, C.I., Green, T.G., Porter, R.A. and Warren, R.D. (1983) One day versus seven days of preventative antibiotic therapy in orthopaedic surgery. *Clinical Orthopaedics and Related Research* **176**, 258–261
Nelson, C.L. (1993) In: *Surgery of the Musculo-Skeletal Systems*. Edited by C. MacEvarts. Churchill Livingstone: Edinburgh and London
Neu, H.C. (1987) General concepts of the chemotherapy of infectious diseases. *Medical Clinics of North America* **71**, 1051–1064
Norris, S.H. and Watt, I. (1983) Radioactive isotope scanning in revision arthrography 2. *Proceedings of a Symposium held in Harrogate* 28
Old, L.J. (1988) Tumor necrosis factor. *Scientific American* **May**, 59
Orr, H.W. (1927) The treatment of osteomyelitis and other infected wounds by drainage and rest. *Surgery, Gynecology and Obstetrics* **45**, 446
Otremski, I., Newman, R.J., Kahn, P.J. *et al.* (1993) Leukergy – a new diagnostic test for bone infection. *Journal of Bone and Joint Surgery* **75B**, 734–736
Pales, L. (1930) *Paléopathologie et Pathologie Comparative*. Masson: Paris
Parkes, M. (1988) The mechanism of nerve damage in leprosy. In: *Essays on Leprosy*, pp. 79–100. Edited by T.J. Ryan and A.C. McDougall. Published for St Francis Leprosy Guild
Paterson, M.P., Hoffman, E.B. and Roux, P. (1990) Severe disseminated staphylococcal disease associated with osteitis and septic arthritis. *Journal of Bone and Joint Surgery* **72B**, 94–97
Perry, C.R., Peason, R.L. and Miller, G.A. (1991) Accuracy of culture of material from swabbing of the superficial aspect of the wound and needle biopsy in preoperative assessment of osteomyelitis. *Journal of Bone and Joint Surgery* **73A**, 745–749
Pun, W.K., Chow, S.P. Luk, K.D., Cheng, L.L., Hsu, L.C. and Leary, J.C. (1990) Tuberculosis of the lumbosacral junction. Long-term follow-up of 26 cases. *Journal of Bone and Joint Surgery* **72B**, 675–678
Rajasekaran, S. and Soundarapandian, S. (1989) Progression of kyphosis in tuberculosis of the spine, treated by ante-

rior arthrodesis. *Journal of Bone and Joint Surgery* **71A**, 1314–1323
Rasnool, M.N. and Govender, S. (1989) The skeletal manifestations of congenital syphilis. *Journal of Bone and Joint Surgery* **71B**, 752–755
Rees, R.J.W., Pearson, J.M.H. and Waters, M.F.R. (1970) *British Medical Journal* **1**, 89
Richmond, R. (1973) In: *Current Antibiotic Therapy*. Proceedings of a symposium, 1972. Edited by A.M. Geddes and J.D. Williams. Churchill Livingstone: Edinburgh and London
Roberts, J. and Falkow, W. (1977) Conjugal transfer of R plasmids in *Neisseria gonorrhoeae. Nature* **266**, 630
Robinson, H.J. and Granda, J.L. (1975) Synovial fluid prostaglandin E levels in orthopedic diseases. *Journal of Bone and Joint Surgery* **57A**, 573
Rogers, H. J. (1967) Killing of staphylococci by penicillins. *Nature* **213**, 31–33
Roy-Camille, R., Reignier, B., Saillant, G. and Berteaux, D. (1976) Résultats de l'intervention de Papineau. *Revue de Chirurgie Orthopédique et Reparatrice de l'Appareil Moteur* **62**, 347–362
Savage, D.C. and Fletcher, M.M. (editors) (1985) *Bacterial Adhesion: Mechanisms and Physiological Significance*. Plenum: New York
Sawetz, E., Morwick, S.L. and Adelberg, E.A. (1977) *Review of Medical Microbiology*. Lange Medical Publishers: Los Altos, CA
Schoifet, S.D. and Morrey, B.F. (1990) Treatment of infection after total knee arthroplasty by debridement with retention of components. *Journal of Bone and Joint Surgery* **72A**, 1383–1390
Schwarzmann, S. and Boring, J.R. III (1971) Antiphagocytic effect of slime from a mucoid strain of *Pseudomonas aeruginosa. Infection and Immunity* **3**, 762
Schweitzer, C., Hoosen, C.M. and Dunbar, J.M. (1971) *South African Medical Journal* **45**, 126–128
Shanmugasundaram, T. (1987) Bone and joint tuberculosis. *Surgery* **1**, 1060–1066
Sheffield, E. A. (1993) Granulomatous inflammation. *Surgery* **11**, 451–453
Shibata, T., Tada, K. and Hashizumo, C. (1990) The results of arthrodesis of the ankle for leprotic neuroarthroplasty. *Journal of Bone and Joint Surgery* **72A**, 749–756
Sinnott, J.T., Concio, M.R., Frankle, M.A., Gustbe, K. and Spiegal, P.G. (1990) Tuberculous osteomyelitis masked by concomitant staphylococcal infection. *Archives of Internal Medicine* **150**, 1865–1868
Smilack, J.D. and Gentry, L.O. (1976) Candida costochondral osteomyelitis. *Journal of Bone and Joint Surgery* **58A**, 888–890
Srinivasan, H. (1973) Syme's amputation in insensitive feet. *Journal of Bone and Joint Surgery* **55A**, 558–562
Stein, H. and Dickson, R.A. (1975) Reversed dynamic slings for knee-flexion contractures in the hemophiliac. *Journal of Bone and Joint Surgery* **57A**, 282–283
Stinchfield, F.E., Bigliani, L.U., Neu, H.C., Goss, T.P. and Foster, C.R. (1980) Late haematogenous infection of total hip replacement. *Journal of Bone and Joint Surgery* **62A**, 1345
Sushruta Samhita (1911) Translated by Kaviras Kunsa Lal Bhishagratna, Calcutta
Tandon, P.N. and Pathak, S.N. (1973) In: *Tropical Neurology*, p. 37. Edited by J.D. Spillane. Oxford University Press: London
Thyne, G.M. and Ferguson, J.W. (1991) Antibiotic prophylaxis during dental treatment in patients with prosthetic joints. *Journal of Bone and Joint Surgery* **73**, 191–194
Trueta, J. (1959) The three types of acute haematogenous osteomyelitis. *Journal of Bone and Joint Surgery* **41B**, 671–680
Umbreit, W.W. (1955) *American Journal of Medicine* **18**, 717
Unkila-Kallio, L., Kallio, M.J.T. and Peltola, H. (1994) The usefulness of C-reactive protein levels in the identification of concurrent septic arthritis in children who have acute haematogenous osteomyelitis. *Journal of Bone and Joint Surgery* **76A**, 848–853
Ward, J., Cohen, A.S. and Bauer, W. (1960) *Arthritis and Rheumatism* **3**, 522
White, M. and Dennison, W.M. (1952) *Journal of Bone and Joint Surgery* **34B**, 608
Wilensky, A.O. (1934) *Osteomyelitis, its Pathogenesis, Symptomatology and Treatment*. Macmillan: New York
Wilkinson, M.C. (1965) *Annals of the Royal College of Surgeons of England* **37**, 19–30
Williams, J. (1978) Spread of R-factors outside the Enterobacteriaceae. *Journal of Antimicrobial Chemotherapy* **4**, 6–8
Wilson, N.I.L. and Di Paola, M. (1986) Acute septic arthritis in infancy and childhood. 10 years' experience. *Journal of Bone and Joint Surgery* **68B**, 584–587
Wood, W.S. and Lepper, M.H. (1958) *Year Book of Medicine*, p. 9. Year Book Publications: Chicago
World Health Organization (1991) Guidelines for tuberculosis treatment in adults and children. In: *National Tuberculosis Programme*, vol. 161.
Wroblewski, B.M. and del Sel, H.J. (1980) Urethral instrumentation and deep sepsis in total hip replacement. *Clinical Orthopaedics and Related Research* **146**, 209–212

CHAPTER 10

Tumours of the Musculoskeletal System

KENNETH E. MARKS, GEORGE H. BELHOBEK, THOMAS W. BAUER AND ROBERT B. DUTHIE

MUSCULOSKELETAL ONCOLOGY

Introduction

During the past 20 years, dramatic improvements in the treatment of musculoskeletal neoplasm have enabled more patients than ever to survive with improvement in their functional, psychological and economic outcomes. This has been brought about by 5 factors:

1. improved radiographic techniques for the localization of tumours and metastases;
2. better understanding of the disease process;
3. improved techniques of musculoskeletal reconstruction;
4. expansion of the role of radiation and chemotherapy; and
5. more aggressive treatment of metastatic disease.

History

Gross, in his 1879 paper entitled 'Sarcoma of the long bones', noted that osteoid malignancies had been described by Müller, a European pathologist, as early as 1843. However, Gross's article laid the foundation for the study of sarcomas in the English-speaking world. He described a variety of sarcomas in 83 patients. Amputation of the extremity was clearly the treatment of choice, and 78% of all patients described underwent that operation. Amputation in the nineteenth century was not without risk. Of all those who underwent operation, 22% died of complications. The leading causes of postoperative death were sepsis and haemorrhage. Of those who survived the operation, 27% had local recurrence in the stump. Of the group that Gross classified as having 'periosteal osteoid sarcomas', 23% were described as 'remaining well without local or general return'.

Gross also described local resection of malignant neoplasms. Of the 83 patients with sarcomas, five underwent surgical resection. Everyone in that group died with either local recurrence or residual disease.

Because of the hopelessness of the disease, doctors of that day elected not to treat approximately 16% of sarcoma patients especially those near the trunk.

In the decades that followed the Gross article, surgical techniques improved rapidly with a decrease in postoperative mortality, but there were no significant improvements in survival statistics for osteogenic sarcoma for the next 70 years.

The most important registry in North America was organized by Dr Earnest A. Codman for the American College of Surgeons (Codman, 1926). This registry provided statistical proof of what the treating physician had known for some time, that the prognosis for musculoskeletal tumours was ominous. In fact, it was not until 1913 that Johns Hopkins Hospital could record its first 5-year survival of an osteogenic sarcoma patient (Bloodgood, 1926a, b).

The search to find more effective and less mutilating treatments for patients was helped by the introduction of the roentgen ray to detect bone sarcoma at an early and more treatable stage. Innovative non-ablative techniques were introduced to surgery. Bloodgood advised against curetting metaphyseal and diaphyseal lesions of the long bones and instead suggested resection and bone transplantation. Although Bloodgood did not advocate the abolition of amputation, he did de-emphasize the position of ablative surgery as the sole treatment.

Bloodgood even recommended resection and bone transplantation for metastatic lesions in order to restore function and provide palliation to terminally ill patients (Bloodgood, 1926a, b). Because of his contributions, Bloodgood may be considered the father of limb-sparing surgery for sarcomas.

By the 1920s, radiotherapy was finding its place in the treatment of metastatic and primary musculoskeletal neoplasms. Bloodgood advocated irradiation of 'Ewing's type' tumours.

The use of chemotherapeutic agents for sarcomas did not gain importance until the past two decades. It had been tried from time to time, but some initial reports of success were subsequently disproved. In 1928, Coley mentioned a toxin treatment given to patients with surgically unresectable primary lesions, or known metastatic disease. This 'toxin treatment' was also used 'prophylactically' in hopes of retarding or eradicating pulmonary metastases. This early attempt at chemotherapy was eventually proved useless.

As a group, musculoskeletal neoplasms were viewed as more malignant than most other tumours. In this atmosphere of ultimate hopelessness, most surgeons abandoned resection in favour of amputation and adopted strategies to spare their doomed patients the problem of local recurrence. As Kolodony noted in 1925: 'The average surgeon does not care to take chances. It is much easier to amputate and to forget than to be conservative and worry.'

A paper by McKenna and colleagues (1966) on Memorial Hospital's experience with sarcoma between 1925 and 1955 did much to discredit resection as a mode of treatment for sarcomas arising from bone.

Although there was no significant change during the first 75 years of the twentieth century in the treatment of skeletal tumours, especially osteogenic sarcoma, some institutions observed gradual improvement. Mayo Clinic patients who had undergone amputation for osteogenic sarcoma alone had an increase in 3-year survival rate from about 25% in the early 1960s to 50% between 1972 and mid-1974 (Taylor *et al.*, 1978). This improvement could not be completely explained by the authors of the Mayo Clinic report, but some believe that the improving picture is due to earlier detection and treatment.

The air of despondency was also evident in other disciplines concerned with the treatment of sarcomas. In his paper on treatment of osteogenic sarcoma by radiotherapy alone or radiotherapy followed by delayed amputation, Sir Stanford Cade (1955) noted that his colleagues were very pessimistic concerning the role of radiation treatment. Cade's treatment programme included high-dose (8000–10 000 rad; 80–100 Gy) radiation to the tumour followed by amputation if no metastatic disease had been observed for 2–18 months. If metastatic disease developed amputation would not be performed. This was designed to spare terminally ill patients amputation and to reserve amputation for patients with a chance of survival.

During the 1940s and 1950s, a few surgeons

adopted a more conservative approach to sarcoma treatment, such as resection of a body part without reconstruction of the extremity. The region of greatest use was the shoulder girdle of the upper extremity. Although Linberg first described an interscapulothoracic resection of the shoulder joint in 1928, it was only sporadically employed for over a quarter of a century (Linberg, 1928). It was rediscovered in 1955 by Pack (Pack and Baldwin, 1966) and later used by Francis and Worcester (1962) and Marcove *et al.* (1977).

The greatest use of wide resection without reconstruction has been in the treatment of soft tissue sarcomas. Shiu *et al.* (1975) described 297 soft tissue sarcomas treated from 1949 to 1968 at the Memorial Sloan-Kettering Cancer Center. The overall 5-year survival rate for *en bloc* resections was 63%, whereas the rate for amputation was 45%. The rate of local recurrence after resection was 28% compared with 7% in amputation stumps. It must be noted, however, that larger and more difficult tumours were coming to amputation. Simon and Enneking (1976) employed similar methods of radical local resection in 54 patients with soft tissue sarcomas of the extremities. Their overall survival rate was 62% while their recurrence rate was 16.7%. Both of these large series confirmed the role of *en bloc* resections in the treatment of soft tissue sarcomas.

Concurrent with the development of resection techniques was the development of bone grafting to supply structural integrity to the resected part. In 1926, Bloodgood used bone grafts after resection of long bones; more recent work has been done in the United States by Parrish (1973) and Mankin *et al.* (1982a) and Ottolenghi (1966) and D'Aubigné and Dejouany (1958) in Europe. Parrish (1973), between 1959 and 1970, carried out resections and reconstructions with the use of large allografts for low-grade malignancies such as giant cell tumours, or low-grade chondrosarcomas.

D'Aubigné and Dejouany (1958) of France devised an operation using a massive allograft for reconstruction after resection of tumours around the knee. This procedure was the direct ancestor of the 'turn up–turn down procedure' advocated by Enneking. D'Aubigné advocated massive bone grafts for both malignant and benign conditions. Mankin *et al.* (1982a) reported the Massachusetts General Hospital's experience with massive cadaveric allografts after tumour resection with 61 patients who were followed for 2 or more years, with a 3% local recurrence rate. The overall success rate based on function for those patients who had neither metastatic disease nor local recurrence was 73.8% good or excellent, 10% requiring brace or cane, and 16.5% failures. A high complication rate had its impact on the overall results.

The development of prostheses to replace resected segments of bone and joint was not attempted until 1940. In September of that year, Moore and Bohlman (1943) implanted a Vitallium upper third of the femur endoprosthesis in a patient suffering from a giant cell tumour. After a stormy postoperative course, the prosthesis functioned well until the patient died of cardiac disease 2 years later.

Following Judet's endoprosthesis design, a number of authors in both North America and Europe have reported the use of metal and acrylic endoprostheses after resection of the proximal femur for tumorous conditions (Hudack, 1951; Clark and Bingold, 1952).

Similar acrylic endoprostheses were employed in the early 1950s to replace the distal femur. Kraft and Leventhal (1954) replaced a distal femur after resection for a giant cell tumour. That prosthesis, along with the majority of similar prostheses of acrylic plastic, failed due to the inherent limitations of materials.

Surgeons were reporting limb salvage operations with increasing frequency during the 1960s and early 1970s.

In 1965, Wilson and Lance described 32 patients with low-grade tumours treated with segmental resection and surgical reconstruction of the skeleton. Mostly autografts were used for reconstruction, but Vitallium endoprostheses were employed in 16% of these patients. The local recurrence rate was 16.7%. In the early 1970s, Smith and Simon (1975) and McGrath (1972) reported encouraging results of sarcoma treatment employing resection; and, in most cases, replacement with autografts or allografts. Functioning of salvaged limbs was considered significantly better than that anticipated with amputation (McGrath, 1972; Chuang *et al.* 1981).

Successful limb salvage was being reported with increasing frequency (Goorin *et al.*, 1980; Sim 1981; Mankin *et al.*, 1982a). Sim and Bohlman (1982) reported successful treatment of sarcomas treated with *en bloc* resection and replacement with tumour prosthesis implanted around the hip and knee. Eighty-three per cent of hip prostheses and 80% of knee prostheses were mechanically sound at 5 years. Local recurrence developed in 8 of the 154 patients with primary tumours. With improvements in chemotherapy, radiation therapy and radiographic imaging of sarcomas in concert with advances in musculoskeletal reconstruction, *en bloc* resection is now the treatment of choice for sarcomas. However, this must be done with great care so as not to increase the rates of local recurrence, which would decrease our patients' chances of survival.

Clinical features and evaluation

INITIAL EVALUATION

The patient will present with a mass or musculoskeletal pain.

The goal of the evaluation is to bring every malignant tumour to prompt diagnosis and treatment. A delay in diagnosis can lead to a significantly worse prognosis or the lost chance for a limb-sparing operation. A secondary goal is to spare patients with benign disease the risk, discomfort and expense of an extensive evaluation.

The evaluation should minimize the length of hospitalization and expense to the patient and society. The evaluation should be so structured that at points in the evaluation interim information is provided that will enable the practitioner to refer the patient, if needed, at the appropriate time. To accomplish these goals the evaluation should be carried out in four phases. The first phase is performed in the doctor's office or out-patient clinic. The only tools necessary for the successful completion of the initial evaluation is a high index of suspicion for tumours, routine x-ray facilities, routine laboratory facilities, a meticulous history and a thorough physical examination. The second phase of the evaluation is the prebiopsy regional evaluation. This is to determine the size, location, and types of tissues involved with the tumour. All anatomical structures should be evaluated whether or not they are involved with the neoplastic process. This evaluation may include computerized tomography (CT scan) or magnetic resonance imaging (MRI scan). This phase can be accomplished on an out-patient basis which is preferable for both economic and psychological reasons. The third phase of the evaluation is the actual biopsy which can be an out-patient procedure. If presumptive clinical and pathological evidence suggests that the tumour is malignant the fourth phase of the evaluation is undertaken which is the diligent search for metastatic disease. This includes CT scanning of the lung and a ^{99}Tc bone scan. Other tests may be added when clinically indicated.

PRESENTING SYMPTOMS AND HISTORY

The patient usually presents complaining of either a mass or pain. In addition to these classic complaints, a number of patients are referred because of lesions that are incidentally found on radiograph taken for unrelated reasons. As with any clinical evaluation, the patient's age, sex and race are recorded along with his or her presenting complaint. The sex of the patient is less important than the age in making the diagnosis. Some tumours such as giant cell tumours are found with a great frequency in females while most other primary musculoskeletal tumours are found predominantly in males. Race is almost never helpful in making the diagnosis.

If the presenting complaint is pain, the pain is usually a deep constant pain which is not particularly associated with exercise. The pain may be present for only a few weeks or as long as 3–4 years. Characteristically, the pain has become progressively worse over the preceding weeks, months or years. The discomfort is usually poorly localized and significantly worse at night. Initially, the pain can be controlled by low-grade analgesics but eventually many patients have started to use codeine or other narcotics prescribed by their family doctor. The pain may be associated with an antalgic limp or complaints of muscle wasting or weakness. The patient may also state that the pain currently is related to weight-bearing while initially it was not. When this pattern of pain is volunteered, the orthopaedist must think of a pathological fracture or an impending pathological fracture. Conversely, when the patient states that his pain was severe weeks or months ago and now is progressively getting better, the chances of malignant disease are significantly diminished.

The patient must be questioned concerning both acute and chronic trauma as a cause of his pain. The tumour patient typically cannot remember any episode of initiating trauma; if he does, it is usually trivial and not sufficient to explain the severity of his symptoms. The primary usefulness of a trauma history is to help eliminate such entities as myositis ossificans and stress fractures. The process leading to myositis ossificans is initiated by significant trauma (Figure 10.1). The associated pain from myositis ossificans usually diminishes after the initial episode while tumour pain progressively becomes worse.

Stress fractures can occur without any trauma that the patient can remember. The fracture callus thus produced simulates, in some cases, a radiographic picture that can be mistaken for an osteogenic sarcoma. The pain produced by a stress fracture is increased with weight-bearing and decreased by rest. There is no associated soft tissue mass. Radiographically, a fracture line can sometimes be identified with the aid of tomograms. It is important not to biopsy either a stress fracture or myositis ossificans because pathologically these can be confused with a sarcoma and an inappropriate treatment can then be prescribed.

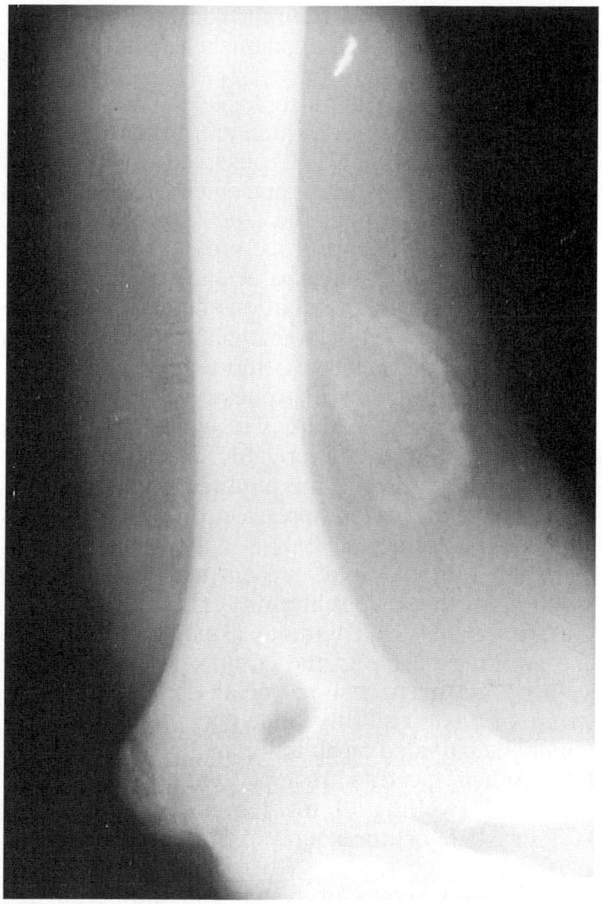

Figure 10.1 Myositis ossificans of the flexor surface of the arm. In myositis ossificans the periphery of the mass has denser more mature bone.

Osteomyelitis may produce pain that is indistinguishable from tumour pain. The patient must be questioned about a history of acute or chronic infection. Fever and chills occur in patients with osteomyelitis and may suggest this diagnosis. Many times patients with osteomyelitis can give a history of relatively recent infections of the respiratory tract, genitourinary tract, skin or soft tissue. A history of penetrating trauma at or near the sight of current pain would strongly suggest infection as the cause of the discomfort.

Chronic infection such as fungal or tuberculosis musculoskeletal disease can mimic musculoskeletal neoplasm. Recently the incidence of musculoskeletal tuberculosis has been increasing due to the spread of the human immunodeficient virus (HIV) in the world population. When a biopsy proven diagnosis of musculoskeletal tuberculosis is made, blood testing for HIV is mandatory. It can be difficult to distinguish neoplasm from chronic infection based on plain radiographs alone. Personal, family and travel histories often help in the diagnosis of chronic bone infection. Various blood antibody titres and skin antigen tests may be useful; however, the definitive test is the biopsy and tissue culture.

Younger children frequently have difficulty in describing the presence of pain. Instead, their discomfort manifests itself in alterations of activity or function. The child's parents may note that the child is not as active as before, is irritable or demonstrates a limp. When any of these symptoms is present, tumour must be included in the differential diagnosis.

Alternatively, the presenting complaint may be a mass which can be either painless or painful. The rate of enlargement is important and should be determined by questioning. It is important to determine whether or not the mass changes in size from day to day because a fluctuating mass is more indicative of a cyst, ganglion or a haemangioma rather than a solid tumour. The patient should be questioned concerning the existence and location of other masses and whether or not there is a family history of masses located near the joints. This point may

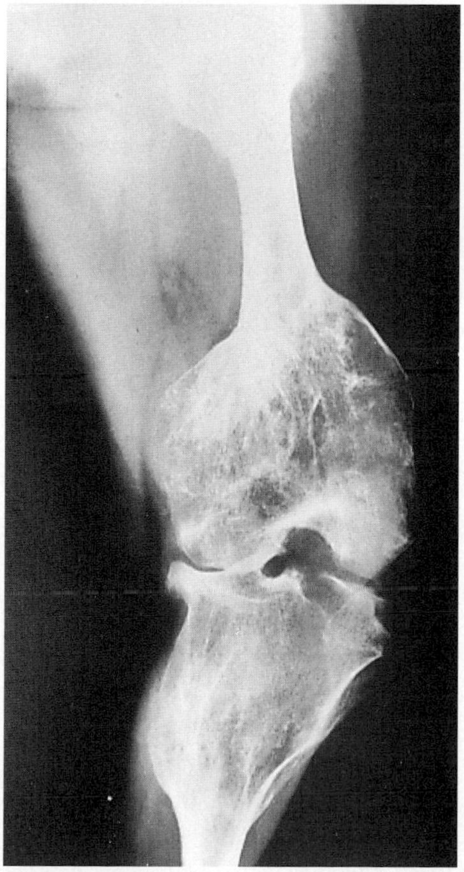

Figure 10.2 Deformity of the femur and tibia due to enchondromatosis (Ollier's disease).

be an indicator of Ollier's disease (Figure 10.2) or Maffucci's syndrome.

Also, a history of von Recklinghausen's disease and its stigmata such as *café au lait* spots or subcutaneous neurofibromas should be sought (Figure 10.3). The patient should be questioned concerning industrial exposure to carcinogens or a previous history of radiation therapy. It has long been known that bone-seeking radionuclides can cause sarcomas. A classic early example of this was the production of osteogenic sarcomas in workers as a result of the ingestion of radium during the painting of luminous dials for watches. A diverse group of chemical carcinogens have also been implicated in sarcoma induction. They include methylcholanthrene, cupric chelated *N*-hydroxy-2'-acetylaminofluorene, zinc beryllium silicate and beryllium oxide (Pritchard *et al.*, 1975b). Currently, the most worrisome and controversial of the possible carcinogens is nickel and nickel compounds (Sunderman, 1973). Nickel is used in many orthopaedic devices. Although a small number of sarcomas have been associated with orthopaedic devices, no definite causative role of the metal implant has been established (Martin *et al.*, 1988).

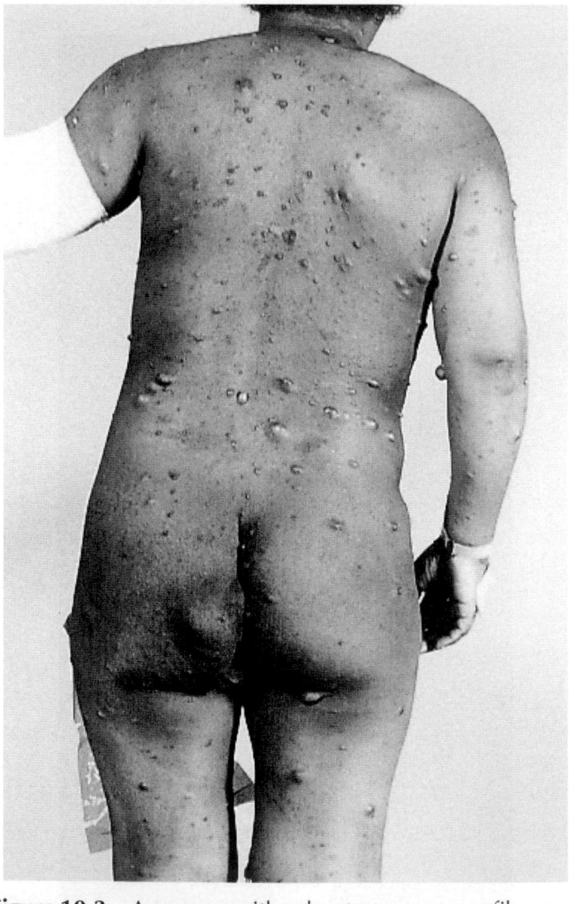

Figure 10.3 A woman with subcutaneous neurofibromas of von Recklinghausen's disease in a sarcomatous degeneration of a buttock neurofibroma.

A few patients with musculoskeletal tumours will present with symptoms which are primarily neurological. Makley *et al.* (1982) observed that in 83% of their series, sacral tumours presented with symptoms that were indistinguishable from a herniated disc. Also, patients with soft tissue tumours arising from a major nerve may have paraesthesia, atrophy and anaesthesia over the distribution of that nerve (Chiao *et al.*1987). At times, tumours located near but not in the nerve will cause nerve compression and a loss of neurological function. Peripheral nerves are compressed by tumours in areas in which the nerve is confined and not freely movable. The sciatic notch, the inguinal canal and the popliteal fossa are locations where nerve compression due to tumour is especially common.

Pelvic tumours may present with unexplained swelling of the lower extremity. The pelvic tumour can be painless and without a palpable mass and the swelling is due to the compression of an iliac vein by the mass. It is especially important to be aware of this possibility since many times the mass cannot be palpated on abdominal or pelvic examination. When faced with a patient complaining of unilateral swelling of the leg, a venogram, scan (CT or MRI) or ultrasound examination should be performed.

A detailed review of systems should be elicited from the patient. This should include a history of recent weight loss or a previously diagnosed neoplasm. Special attention should be paid to the respiratory system, the lower GI system, genitourinary system and the breast and reproductive systems in females. Abnormalities in the system review should be followed up with the appropriate tests to rule out the possibility that metastatic disease is causing the presenting musculoskeletal lesion.

Physical examination

A general physical examination is carried out for metastatic disease or to find a primary carcinoma which has metastasized to the musculoskeletal system. Detailed regional examination is then performed to determine what tissues are involved with the neoplasm and to aid in the logical selection of future tests. The musculoskeletal system is made up of seven types of tissue which are mesenchymal in origin:

1. skin and subcutaneous tissue,
2. lymphatic tissue,
3. vascular structures,
4. musculoaponeurotic tissues,

5. neurological structures,
6. bone and
7. joints.

In every patient with a suspected musculoskeletal tumour, the skin and subcutaneous tissue should be carefully inspected and palpated. Tumours with a soft tissue component can deform the contours of the extremity. This deformation is made more evident when the involved part is compared with the contralateral undraped extremity. In addition, large tumours can produce small dilated superficial veins overlying the mass. The skin of the entire body is inspected for *café au lait* spots and subcutaneous neurofibroma, both of which are signs of von Recklinghausen's disease. Similarly, a venous malformation which is located usually on the same side of the body as a cartilaginous tumour is an indication of Maffucci's syndrome. The detailed examination of the skin may uncover a malignant melanoma that could be responsible for a bone lesion. On palpation, the skin over a tumour may exhibit increased warmth. A warm mass is more indicative of either a malignant tumour or an inflammatory lesion such as an abscess. If the skin is not freely movable, then it must be assumed that it is involved with or closely approximates the neoplastic process. When a mass is felt close to the skin every effort must be made to determine whether or not it penetrates the deep fascia. Skin and fascia involvement become important in staging the tumour and its eventual biopsy and treatment.

The regional lymph nodes in the involved extremity are carefully palpated for signs of metastatic disease. Although musculoskeletal tumours characteristically produce haematogenous pulmonary metastases, all of them can involve regional lymph nodes. Early lymphatic metastases are found frequently in synovial sarcomas, malignant fibrous histiocytomas, and rhabdomyosarcomas.

A thorough vascular examination includes inspection, palpation, auscultation and circumferential measurements. The extremities are inspected for small superficial dilated veins over the tumour mass and larger varicose veins distal to the tumour mass. A tumour located proximally may have obstructed the venous return enough to cause an unilateral increase in the size of the varicose veins or pitting oedema. The peripheral arteries are palpated, graded and compared to the uninvolved side. The mass is also palpated for thrills or pulsations. It is then auscultated to determine the presence or absence of a bruit which may be caused by either a high rate of flow through the tumour or partial compression of an artery. When a haemangioma is suspected, it is useful to measure the circumference of the extremity at the level of the mass and the circumference at the level of the uninvolved extremity. The extremity is then elevated for 2 minutes and remeasured while still elevated. The diagnosis of a haemangioma is favoured when the circumference of the involved extremity decreases after elevation.

The muscles in the vicinity of the tumour and their associated aponeurotic structures are carefully examined. The size of the tumour mass is measured and recorded. It is palpated for hardness (sarcoma and usually hard), contour and tested for mobility. It should be noted whether or not the tumour is adherent to deeper structures such as bone or fascia. When the tumour is adherent to these structures, the excursion of the associated tendons are less than normal, usually producing a decreased range of motion of a nearby joint. The status of the peripheral nerves in the involved extremity is assessed. This examination should include inspection of the extremity for muscle atrophy or fasciculation of the muscle bundle. The muscles near the tumour and distal to the tumour should be tested for strength, but may be difficult to interpret or misleading due to pain in the involved extremity. The sensory examination is less susceptible to the effects of pain and can be quite useful in determining which nerves, if any, are involved with the tumour process. The reflexes are examined and compared to the uninvolved side. Any loss of a reflex is significant and may indicate a neural involvement with the tumour.

The joints at either end of the involved bone or muscular compartment are evaluated for effusion, discontinuity of motion, decreased range of motion or intra-articular masses. The involved bone is then palpated for abnormalities of contour or local tenderness. The metaphyseal areas of other long bones may also be palpated in searching for multiple osteochondromas.

Plain radiography

The time-proven plain x-ray examination remains the basic means of evaluating skeletal neoplasms, and correlating radiographic findings with the biopsy is necessary to obtain the most accurate diagnosis. The use of high-quality x-ray equipment and techniques in the performance of these examinations will assure that the maximum amount of diagnostic information will be available on the films.

Two x-ray projections, usually frontal and lateral, are required for adequate evaluation of a bone neoplasm. Additional views such as oblique and tangential views are occasionally helpful in demonstrating a lesion in profile. The joint nearest the bone tumour should always be included, and adequate coverage of the adjacent areas should be included to demonstrate any skip lesions or the involvement of contiguous bones.

In patients with systemic disorders which may affect multiple bones, a skeletal survey can be obtained and should include at least one projection of the bones of the upper and lower extremities, the pelvis, the spine, the ribs, and a lateral view of the skull. Technetium-99m (^{99m}Tc) radionuclide bone scanning has largely replaced the radiographic skeletal survey as a screening examination for metastatic cancer in bone.

Accurate tissue diagnosis of a bone neoplasm on the basis of its radiographic characteristics is often not possible. However, the radiographic appearance of a lesion does provide reliable information regarding its aggressiveness and rate of growth (Lodwick *et al.*, 1980a, b). Emphasis is placed on such variables as tumour shape and location in the bone, pattern of bone destruction and any associated bony proliferation, the condition of adjacent bony cortex and tumour matrix mineralization.

TUMOUR SHAPE AND LOCATION

Lodwick (1971) has indicated that certain features regarding the shape and location of a lesion in bone can be useful in the differential diagnosis. Most neoplasms grow progressively in all directions and tend to retain a spherical shape. However, certain lesions have a tendency to grow asymmetrically, causing an elongated appearance in bone. Neoplasms which characteristically show this feature include chondromyxoid fibroma, Ewing's sarcoma, primary lymphoma of bone, chondrosarcoma, and angiosarcoma.

The location a primary bone tumour occupies in a particular bone is also of diagnostic importance (Figures 10.1 and 10.4), including whether the lesion has its primary location in the epiphysis, metaphysis, or diaphysis of the bone and whether the lesion occupies an eccentric or central location. The determination of whether a lesion originates from the medullary cavity, the cortex, or from the periosteal layer of bone should also be made. Establishing the position of the centre of a lesion is more difficult when it involves a small tubular bone such as the fibula since an eccentric lesion in a small tubular bone soon appears central in location.

Certain solitary lesions in tubular bones show a remarkable propensity to develop in specific anatomical locations. For example, chondroblastoma in a long bone is never diagnosed without involvement of the epiphysis (Figure 10.5). This tumour, however, can extend through the unfused epiphyseal plate to involve the adjacent metaphysis. Although originating in the metaphysis, giant cell tumours quickly penetrate the closed growth plate, involving the epiphysis with extension to the subchondral bone of the adjacent joint. Other tumours characteristically having a metaphyseal location are chondromyxoid fibroma, non-ossifying fibroma, aneurysmal bone cyst, unicameral bone cyst, osteochondroma, and mesenchymal neoplasms such as chondrosarcoma and osteosarcoma. Lesions that tend to develop in the diaphysis include Ewing's

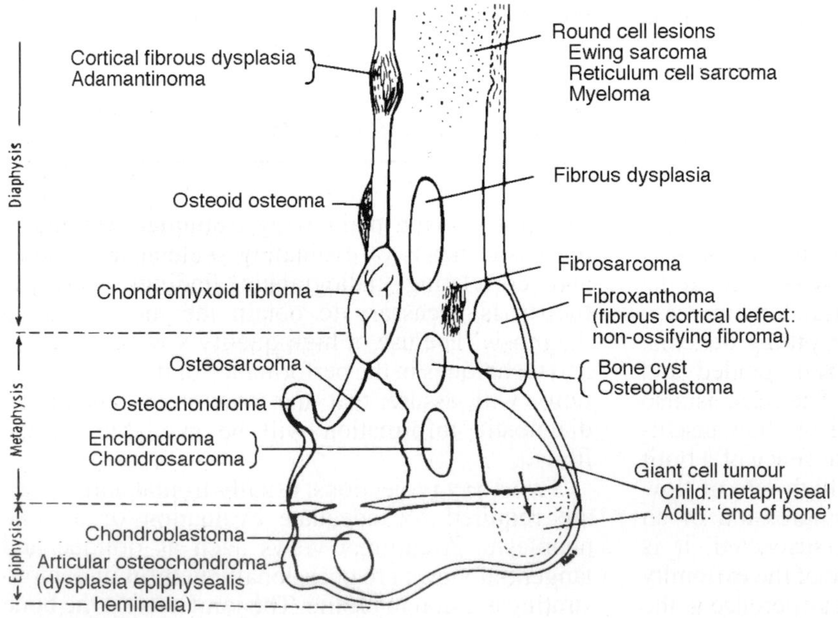

Figure 10.4 The location of a primary tumour within a bone is of diagnostic significance. This illustration demonstrates the characteristic location of several commonly encountered lesions. (From Madewell, J. E., Ragsdale, B. D. and Sweet, D. E. (1981) Radiologic and pathologic analysis of solitary bone lesions, Part 1: Internal margins. *Radiologic Clinics of North America* **19**, 715–748, by permission of the publisher)

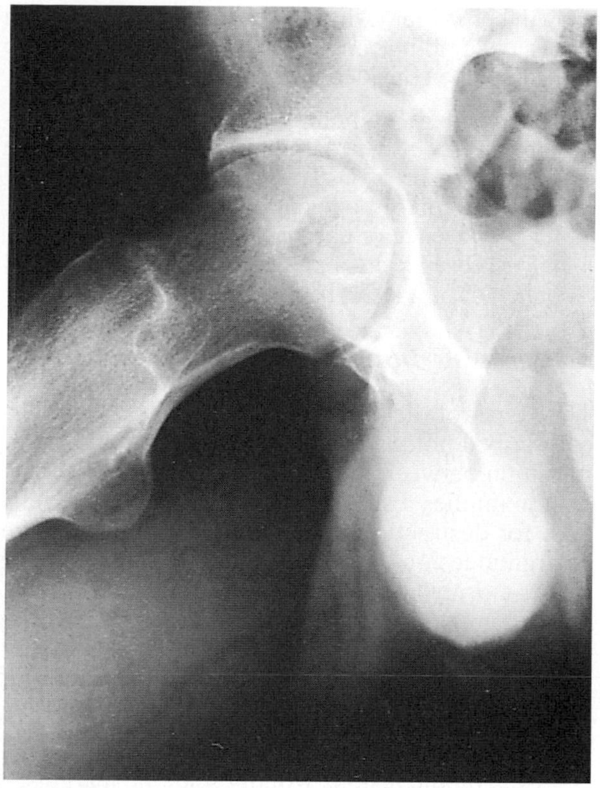

Figure 10.5 This chondroblastoma occupies a typical location in the epiphyseal region of the proximal femur. Stippled calcifications are seen in 50% of chondroblastomas and are demonstrated in this case. In the absence of visible calcifications, the differential diagnosis must be expanded to include avascular necrosis, Brody's abscess, and histiocytosis-X.

sarcoma, primary lymphoma of bone, and myeloma. These neoplasms also occur in the metaphysis. Benign tumours found in diaphyseal locations include non-ossifying fibroma, unicameral bone cyst, aneurysmal bone cyst, enchondroma, osteoblastoma, and fibrous dysplasia. Epiphyseal equivalent areas exist adjacent to articular cartilages in the pelvic and shoulder girdles. Lesions that commonly develop in these areas are those that show a predilection for the epiphyseal regions of the tubular bones. Tumours located in the epiphyses also develop in the small bones of the wrist and mid-foot and in the patella.

Certain lesions develop in the medullary canal on or close to the central axis of the bone. Examples include enchondroma and unicameral bone cyst. Giant cell tumour, chondromyxoid fibroma, and osteosarcoma, chondrosarcoma, and fibrosarcoma can have an eccentric location in the bone. Cortical lesions include osteoid osteoma and non-ossifying fibroma. Tumours arising from the outer surface of the cortex are described as juxtacortical, periosteal or parosteal. Periosteal lesions are often fusiform in shape, erode the underlying cortex ('saucerization'), and elevate the periosteum, causing a Codman's triangle (e.g. periosteal chondroma or periosteal osteosarcoma) (Unni *et al.*, 1976a, b; Bauer *et al.*, 1982). Parosteal tumours appear to have a broader attachment to the cortex and expand into adjacent soft tissue, often wrapping around the bone (e.g. parosteal osteosarcoma) Unni *et al.* 1976a, b). It is particularly important to recognize this group of lesions, because tumours that arise in a periosteal location may have a somewhat better prognosis than the equivalent tumour arising in the medullary canal (Bator *et al.*, 1986).

PATTERNS OF BONE DESTRUCTION AND REPAIR

The radiograph can also demonstrate how aggressively the disease is spreading and how effectively the host bone is repairing the injury. Bone destruction and new bone formation associated with bone neoplasms are mediated by osteoclasts and osteoblasts. Bone destruction is usually not a direct effect of tumour cells but is accomplished by normal host osteoclasts somehow activated by the tumour. A possible exception to this rule is the giant cell tumour, a neoplasm composed of osteoclasts, but even this has been contested (Steiner *et al.*, 1972).

The bone destruction seen on radiographs is a summation of osteoclastic resorptive activity on both the cortical and trabecular bone surfaces. This activity acts in two stages beginning with the removal of mineral content of bone matrix (Handcock and Boothroyd, 1963) and followed by enzymatic digestion (Belanger and Migicovsky, 1963) and possible mechanical abrasion of collagenous fabric (Madewell *et al.*, 1981). Resorption involves the complete removal of a given volume of bone matrix. For this reason, the descriptive terms of destructive change, 'osteolysis', and 'osteopenia', are preferred to the term demineralization. Osteoclasts can destroy bone at a greater rate than osteoblasts can produce it (Johnson, 1964). Both activities always coexist to some degree, and the relative predominance of one process over the other will be perceived as a visible margin to the lesion on the radiograph.

The perception of osteolysis on the plain radiograph depends on the type of bone destroyed (cortical versus cancellous), the amount of bone loss, and the volume of host bone adjacent to the lesion available for contrast (Madewell *et al.*, 1981). Destruction of cortical bone, although slower, is appreciated more easily because of the great contrast in density created by a focal area of lysis in the compact structure of cortical bone. The more loosely organized structure of cancellous bone requires that large amounts of trabecular bone (30–50%) be removed before the loss will be evident on plain radiographs (Ardran, 1951; Lodwick, 1971; Edeiken and Hodes, 1973a). In structures with a predominance of cancellous bone such as the spine, pelvis, ribs, or ends of long bones, large amounts of cancellous bone may be removed with little or no change on the radiograph. For this reason, lesions arising in cancellous bone may go undetected for long periods of time unless accompanied by bone proliferative changes. In the elderly, where there is generalized bone loss due to ageing, early detection of destructive lesions is more difficult.

Bone destruction associated with bone neoplasm manifests itself in patterns that reflect pathological grade in a single frame in time. This concept has been analysed and well summarized by Lodwick *et al.* (Lodwick, 1964, 1965, 1966, 1971; Lodwick *et al.* 1980a, b). Not only is the pattern of bone destruction significant, the interface zone between the lesion and the host bone or periosteum also accurately reflects growth behaviour (Anger, 1952). In order to reach a consistent grading conclusion, the following specific signs must be considered in this order of priority:

1. The pattern of bone destruction and the configuration of the marginal interface zone of the lesion.
2. Penetration of bone cortex by the lesion.
3. The presence or absence of a sclerotic rim.
4. The presence and extent of an expanded cortical shell (Lodwick *et al.*, 1980a, b).

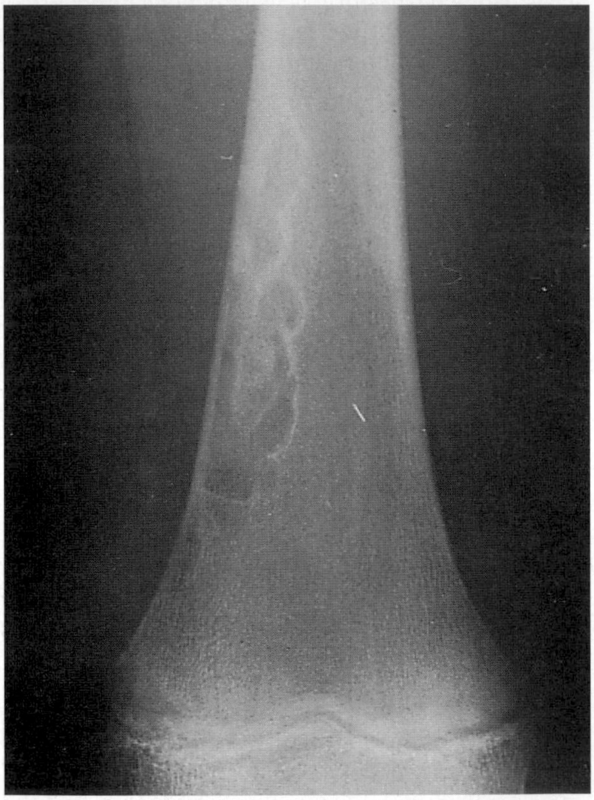

Figure 10.6 This non-ossifying fibroma is an example of a type IA geographic pattern of destruction. The well defined sclerotic margins of the lesion indicate a growth rate which allows time for the host bone to produce reactive bone at the margins of the slowly enlarging neoplasm.

Geographic bone destruction (type I)

This type of destruction is seen as a well circumscribed hole in the bone with a narrow zone of transition between normal and abnormal bone. The pattern implies a slow growth rate, one that permits time for destruction of all bone in the path of the enlarging lesion. The actual edge of the tumour relates closely to the visible edge of the tumour as it is seen on the radiograph. The geographic destruction pattern can be further divided into three subtypes which correlate with the rate and manner of growth:

A – Geographic lesions with sclerotic margin:
B – Geographic lesions without sclerotic margins:
C – Geographic lesions with ill-defined margins.

The relative biological aggressiveness increases from type A to type C.

Geographic lesions with marginal sclerosis (type IA)

This pattern is most commonly associated with benign, slow growing disorders (Figure 10.6). Lesions commonly falling into this category are unicameral bone cyst, non-ossifying fibroma, enchondroma, chondromyxoid fibroma, chondroblastoma, and fibrous dysplasia. Sclerotic rims that gradually fade into the adjacent cancellous bone are commonly seen with chronic osteomyelitis, Brodie's abscess, and histiocytosis X.

Geographic lesions with no sclerosis in the margin (type IB)

Lesions in this category have sharply defined edges (narrow zone of transition) but not sclerotic margins. Normal trabeculae are present up to the edge of the lesion but totally removed along a plane of contact between the tumour and normal bone. This category includes many of the same histological diagnoses included in the group IA category, the difference being a more aggressive behaviour. Giant cell tumours typically have IB margins.

Geographic lesions with ill-defined margins (type IC)

This type of geographic lesion is not only focally destructive but also locally infiltrative with tumour extending into the marrow space in advance of the osteolytic edge. This creates a wider zone of transition at the margin of the lesion which reflects the greater biological activity of these tumours. As the growth rate increases, there is less evidence of circumscription, and the lesion becomes less well defined (Figure 10.7). Vigorous destruction of the cortex will result in complete perforation of the bone. The presence of a soft tissue mass is indicative of complete cortical penetration. Typical lesions with this pattern include giant cell tumour, fibrosarcoma, and chondrosarcoma. Aggressive forms of benign neoplasm such as enchondroma, chondroblastoma, and desmoplastic fibroma can occasionally be classified in this category.

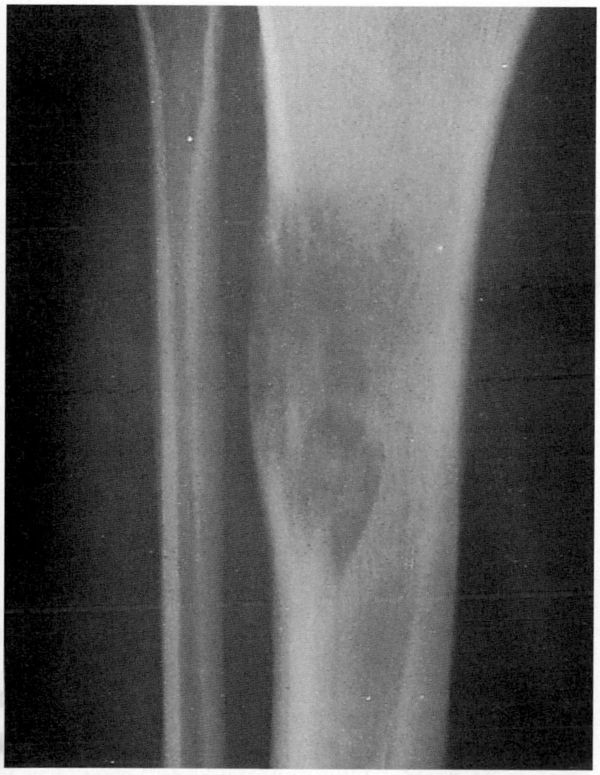

Figure 10.7 This osteolytic osteosarcoma is an example of a type IC geographic pattern of destruction. This type of geographic lesion is not only focally destructive but also locally infiltrative with tumour extending in advance of the osteolytic edge (wide zone of transition).

'Moth-eaten' destruction (type II) (regional invasion)

This is a more aggressive pattern of bone destruction characteristic of a lesion that is growing more rapidly than one with geographic bone destruction. The moth-eaten pattern of destruction consists of multiple scattered holes that vary in size and seem to arise separately. These scattered holes coalesce to form larger areas of bone destruction. Cancellous bone, cortical bone, or both, may be involved. In cancellous bone, normal trabecular markings can be seen between the holes because of the regionally infiltrative nature of this pattern (Figure 10.8). Bone destruction of this type may be difficult to visualize early, especially if there is already a paucity of cancellous bone present as in elderly patients. Total penetration of the cortex is assumed with the moth-eaten pattern (Lodwick *et al.* 1980a). The moth-eaten pattern is frequently seen with malignant

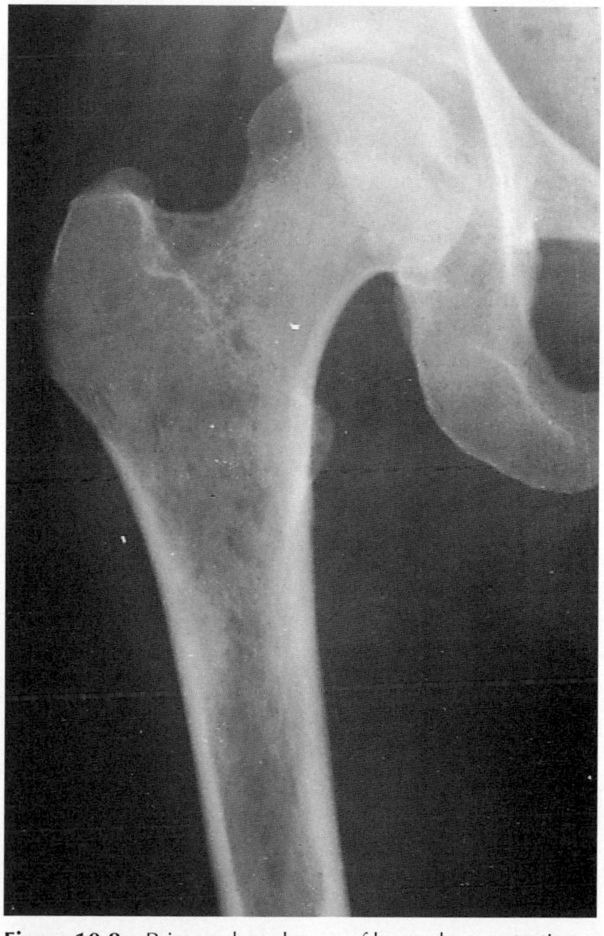

Figure 10.8 Primary lymphoma of bone demonstrating a type II pattern of bone destruction (moth-eaten). This pattern is characteristic of an aggressive bone-destroying process and is frequently seen with malignant neoplasms.

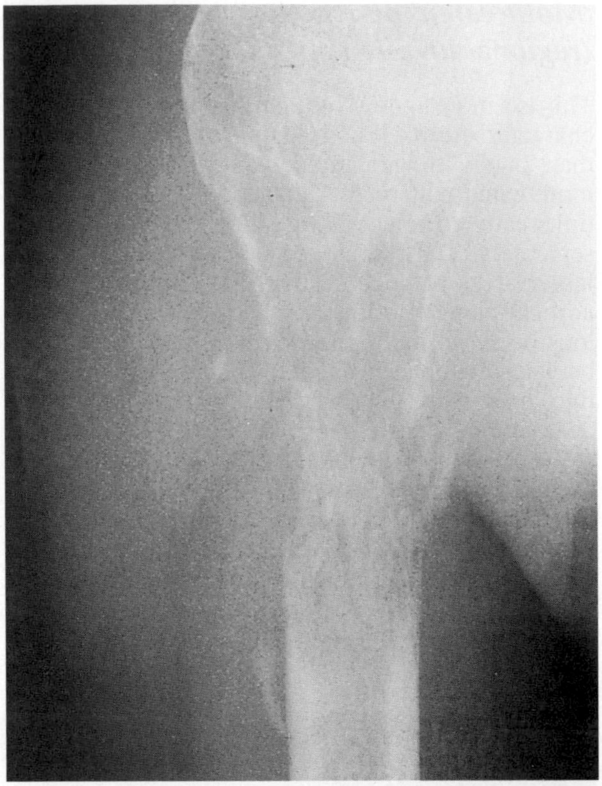

Figure 10.9 Ewing's sarcoma demonstrating aggressive bone destruction including a permeative (type III) bone destruction pattern. It may be difficult to separate moth-eaten and permeative patterns in some cases, a distinction which is probably unnecessary since both patterns indicate an aggressive bone-destroying process.

neoplasms such as Ewing's sarcoma, primary lymphoma of bone, chondrosarcoma, fibrosarcoma, and osteosarcoma. Aggressive forms of osteomyelitis can also destroy bone with a moth-eaten pattern.

Permeative destruction (type III)

The permeative pattern indicates an aggressive bone-destroying process with rapid growth potential. Permeative lesions are poorly demarcated and not easily separated from surrounding normal bone. The permeative pattern is characterized by numerous elongated holes or slots in the cortex that run parallel to the long axis of the bone. They are reasonably uniform in size. The slots are created by osteoclastic cortical tunnelling in an accelerated caricature of the resorption phase of normal Haversian remodelling (Madewell *et al.*, 1981). Total penetration of the cortex is assumed with the permeative pattern (Figure 10.9).

Permeative destruction may be seen in several disease categories including neoplastic, mechanical, inflammatory, and metabolic. Tunnelling may or may not be accompanied by tumour or inflammatory infiltrates. Malignant lesions demonstrating this pattern tend to infiltrate the marrow space diffusely. The list would include primary round cell tumours, fibrosarcoma, high-grade chondrosarcoma, and angiosarcoma. An occasional benign process such as osteomyelitis will also show this pattern.

Lodwick *et al.* have pointed out the difficulty of distinguishing moth-eaten from the permeative pattern of destruction. They question the necessity of making this distinction as both patterns suggest an aggressive bone-destroying process (Lodwick *et al.*, 1980a, b).

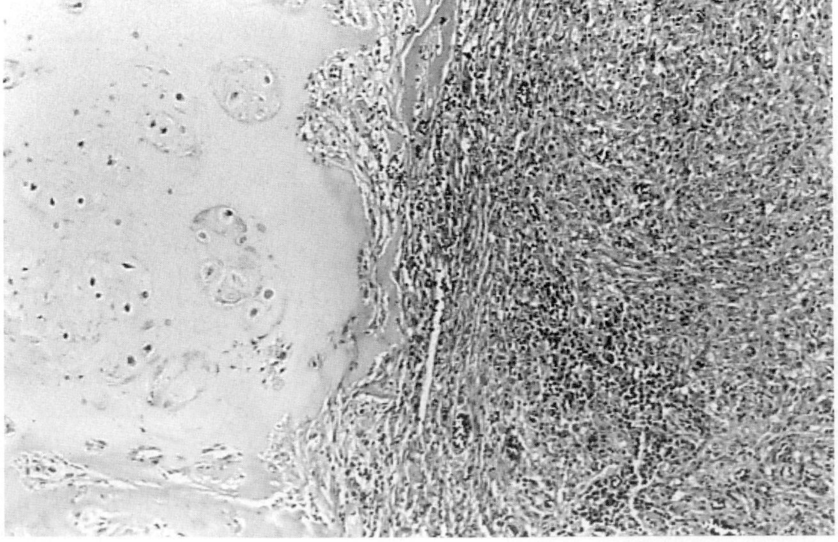

Figure 10.10 Photomicrograph of a dedifferentiated chondrosarcoma. The low-grade cartilage component often corresponds to a geographic radiographic appearance, while the high-grade sarcoma component is responsible for the permeative, 'changed' appearance typical of this tumour.

Combination and changing patterns

Any combination of geographic, 'moth-eaten', and permeative patterns in a single lesion is indicative of a change toward a more aggressive local growth. Combination patterns may be seen when benign lesions become more active, undergo malignant degeneration, or fracture. The development of a combination or a changing pattern can be documented by observing a sequence of radiographs (Madewell *et al.*, 1981).

Madewell *et al.* point out that the fastest rate of tumour growth through a cancellous network is signified by little or no radiographic change in bone density or trabecular pattern. Very rapid filling of the cancellous and diaphyseal marrow space with tumour eliminates elements such as osteoclasts, osteoblasts, and blood vessels, leaving behind an intact bony architecture (Madewell *et al.*, 1981). It is especially important for the musculoskeletal pathologist to recognize radiographic features of a 'changed' lesion in order to determine whether or not the biopsy specimen is representative of the most important process. For example, a dedifferentiated chondrosarcoma (Figure 10.10) and a malignant fibrous histiocytoma arising in association with a pre-existing bone infarct both show radiographic features sug-gesting 'change'. A biopsy specimen showing only a low-grade cartilage tumour or a bone infarct should be considered insufficient, because neither would adequately explain the aggressive component of the radiograph.

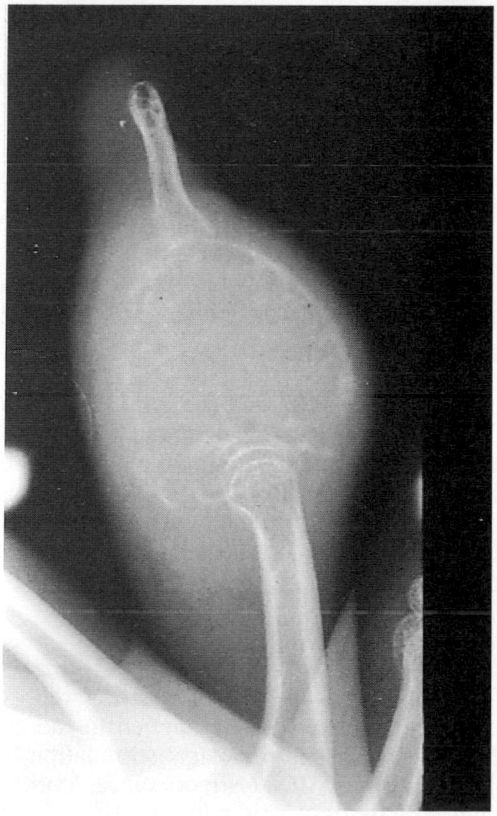

Figure 10.11 The trabeculated appearance of this aneurysmal bone cyst is the result of uneven ridges on the inner surface of the periosteal shell and is due to uneven growth rates in the lesion. The ridges should not be misinterpreted as bony trabeculae traversing the tumour.

PERIOSTEAL REACTIONS

The periosteum of adult bone is minimally cellular and mainly fibrous in its inactive state. The adult periosteum, however, may become thickened and cellular as a reaction to injury. This activated periosteum regains its ability to make new bone. The configuration of a periosteal reaction is an index not only of the nature of the inciting process but also of its intensity, aggressiveness, and duration. Periosteal reactions must mineralize to become visible on a radiograph. The process of mineralization usually requires a period of between 10 days and 3 weeks following the initial stimulus. Basically, periosteal reactions can be classified as solid or interrupted (Edeiken and Hodes, 1973b). Ragsdale *et al.* (1981) have expanded this classification with the addition of several subclasses as follows.

Solid periosteal reactions

Shell formation

Widening of a bone contour represents periosteal activity. The expansion of bone is the result of a relatively slow bone-destroying process that has invoked removal of bone from the endosteal surface of the cortex at a rate balanced by production of new bone on the periosteal surface. The bony margin of the shell is therefore a layer of periosteal new bone and not an expansion of the original bone cortex.

The thickness of a periosteal shell depends on the speed of the destructive process relative to the rate of periosteal new bone formation.

Smooth shells

Shells with smooth outer contours are caused by lesions that apply uniform pressure on the cortex. These shells are usually, but not necessarily, eccentric and are usually associated with benign lesions.

Lobulated shells

A shell with a lobulated margin develops when a lesion has focal variation in growth rate. The

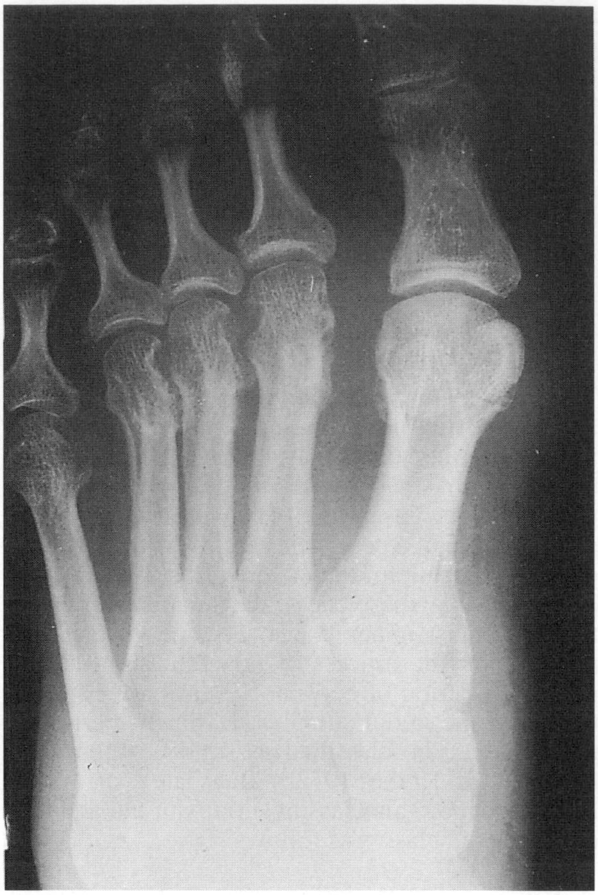

Figure 10.12 The single lamellar periosteal reaction seen with the metatarsal bones of this diabetic patient has been described as the hallmark of a benign process. Such reactions are commonly associated with low-grade inflammation as in this case, histiocytosis X, early stress fractures, and osteoid osteoma.

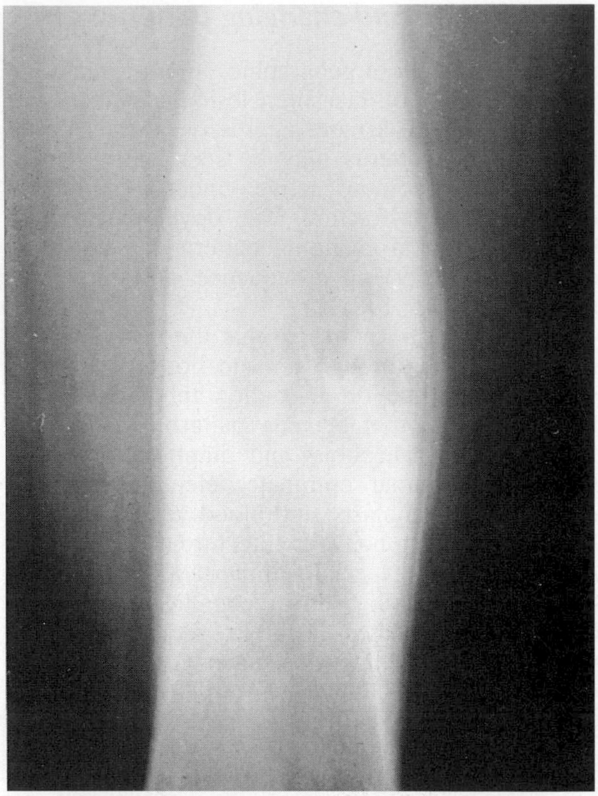

Figure 10.13 The lamellated or 'onion-skin' periosteal reaction associated with this osteosarcoma is seen with aggressive bone-destroying processes such as acute osteomyelitis and cellular bone sarcomas.

more rapidly enlarging areas correlate with cortical bulges.

Ridged shell

A ridged shell, also referred to as trabeculated, septated, or soap-bevel reaction, develops when the growth of a destructive lesion is uneven. Radiographically these ridges may be misinterpreted as bony trabeculae within the lesion (Figure 10.11). The ridged shell is most often seen in benign processes such as non-ossifying fibroma, giant cell tumour, aneurysmal bone cyst, and enchondroma. The ridged shell, however, can also be seen with slowly growing malignant processes such as chondrosarcoma, fibrosarcoma, plasmacytoma, and metastatic neoplasm of renal, thyroid, and melanoma origin.

Continuous periosteal reactions with cortical persistence

Included under this heading are solid, single lamellar, laminated, and parallel spiculated periosteal reactions. With these reactions, the cortex tends to persist, although varying degrees of subperiosteal tumour penetration from the marrow space can and does occur, especially with the laminated and parallel spiculated forms.

Solid periosteal reaction

A solid continuous periosteal reaction represents multiple layers of new bone applied to the cortex resulting from chronic periosteal stimulation by an indolent lesion in the marrow space, cortex, or adjacent soft tissues. This pattern, also referred to as cortical thickening or hyperostosis, connotes a very slow rate of progression. Intracortical osteoid osteoma, chronic low-grade infection, and large enchondromas are examples of lesions often accompanied by solid periosteal reaction.

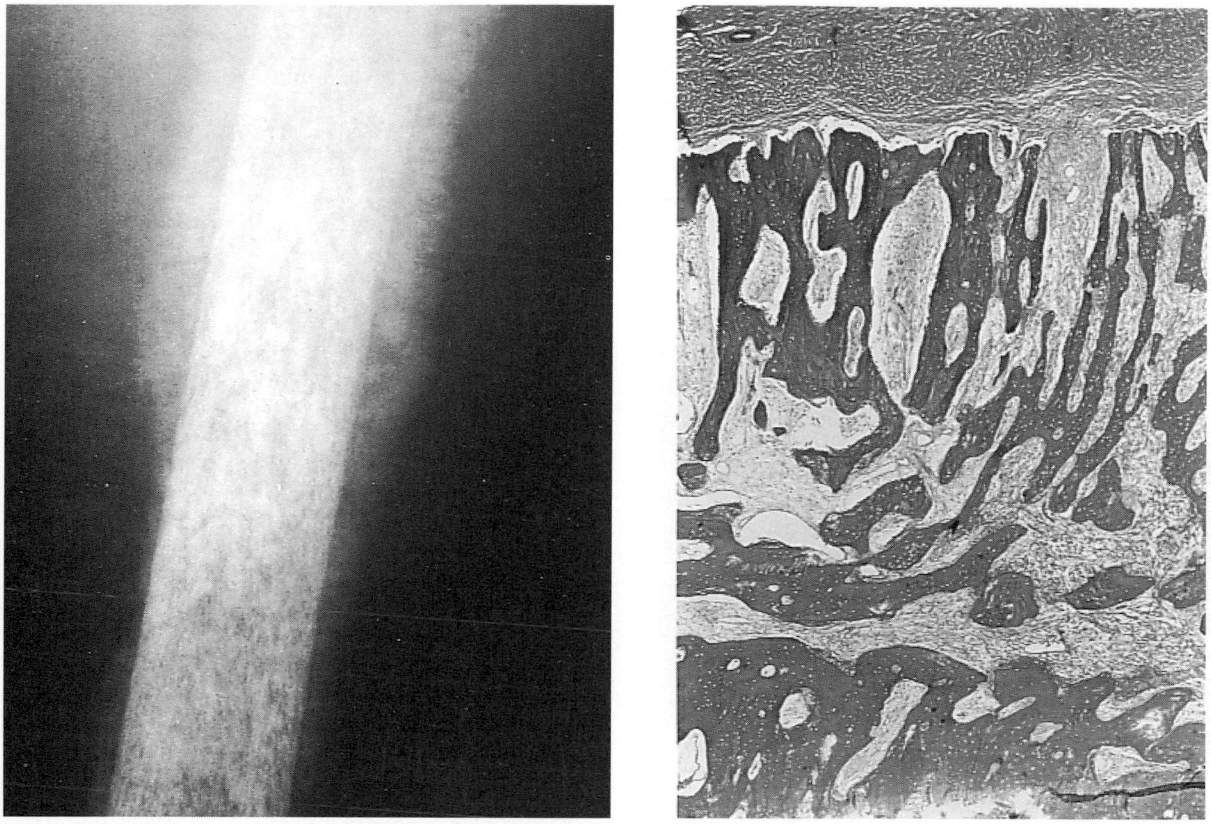

(a) (b)

Figure 10.14 (a) The parallel spiculated periosteal reaction demonstrated here implies a more rapidly progressing process than the solid or lamellar reactions. It is usually seen with malignant processes, in this case metastatic prostate carcinoma. (b) Histologically, the parallel, spiculated periosteal reaction shows trabeculae of bone oriented perpendicular to the cortex. This pattern, here associated with an osteosarcoma, usually indicates a highly aggressive lesion.

Single lamellar reaction

The lamellar reaction consists of a single layer of new bone that appears as a uniform radiodense line 1–2 mm from the cortical surface which may or may not join the cortex at its proximal and distal extremes, and persists relatively unchanged for weeks (Figure 10.12). This form of periosteal reaction has been described as the hallmark of a benign process and is commonly seen with such lesions as histiocytosis X, osteomyelitis, osteoid osteoma, and fractures (Edeiken and Hodes, 1973b). Dense undulating periosteal reactions are a variant of single lamellar reactions and are commonly seen with low-grade osteomyelitis, hypertrophic osteoarthropathy, long-standing varices, and chronic osteitis.

Lamellated reactions

The lamellated continuous periosteal reaction is created by multiple concentric planes of ossification. This form has also been referred to as 'onion-skin' (Figure 10.13). Lamellated periosteal reaction occurs with active bone-destroying lesions such as acute osteomyelitis and cellular bone sarcomas, especially Ewing's sarcoma and osteosarcoma.

Parallel spiculated reaction

The parallel spiculated reaction (hair-on-end) implies a more rapidly progressing process than the solid or lamellar reaction. The spicules are the result of new bone formation along the radially oriented periosteal vessels that extend from the periosteum to the cortex. The spicules range from uniform, fine, velvet-like structures to long, drawn-out linear shadows (Figure 10.14). This pattern is usually seen with malignant processes.

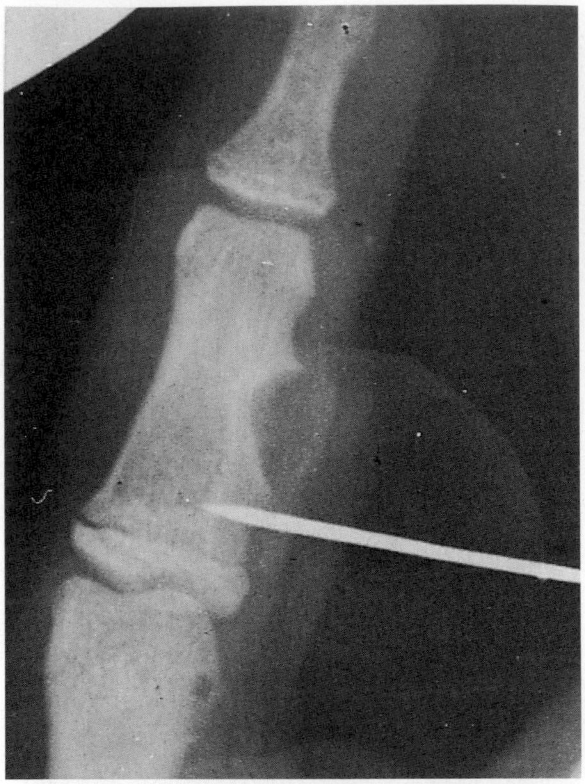

Figure 10.15 Periosteal buttress formation, as seen with this periosteal chondroma, is usually a feature of a slowly growing, benign lesion. (Reproduced, with permission, from Bauer, T. W., Dorfman, H. D. and Latham, J. T. (1982) *American Journal of Surgical Pathology* **6**, 631–637)

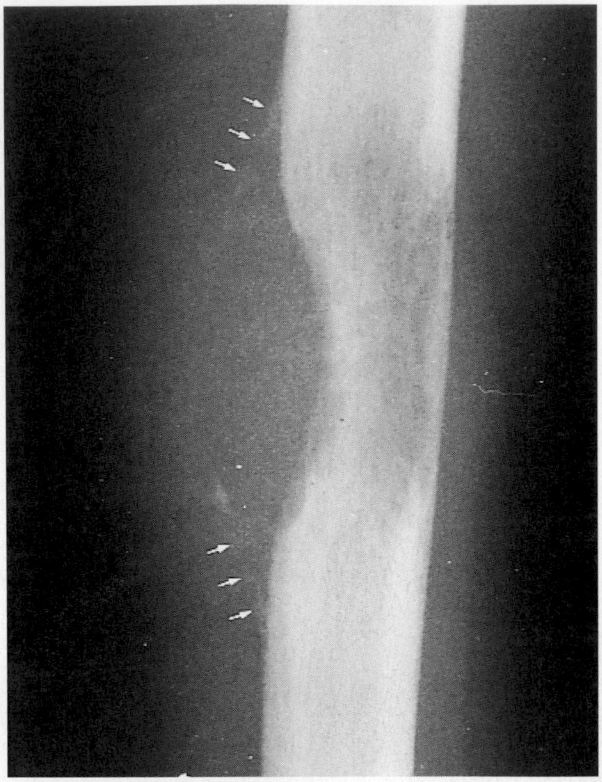

Figure 10.16 Codman angles (arrows) may result from any process, benign or malignant, which lifts the periosteum so aggressively that the periosteal reactions associated with the most aggressive portions of the process are rapidly destroyed, leaving only wispy tufts of periosteal reaction at the margins of the lesion. The Codman angles shown here are associated with an aggressive aneurysmal bone cyst. Note also the permeative pattern of bone destruction.

Interrupted periosteal reactions

Interrupted periosteal reactions occur when aggressive bone tumours reach a subperiosteal position. These reactions develop when either the aggressive nature of the lesion denies space for elaboration of new bone in the areas of most active tumour growth or when pressure by the tumour stimulates osteoclasts to remove reactive bone before it becomes radiographically visible (Ragsdale *et al*., 1981).

Buttress

Buttressing refers to the formation of a solid wedge of new bone at the cortical margins of a slowly expanding lesion. The cortex beneath the buttress is frequently intact, but the cortex just beyond it is usually absent with or without the creation of a shell. Buttress formation is generally associated with benign bone neoplasms (Figure 10.15).

Codman angle

The Codman angle essentially represents the analogue of the buttress in the aggressive bone-destroying lesion. Originally described by Ribbert in 1914 and later elaborated upon by Codman (1926), the Codman angle was long believed to be a manifestation of malignant bone disease only. It is now appreciated that the Codman angle may result from any process that aggressively lifts the periosteum (Figure 10.16). Included among these processes are a few cases of acute osteomyelitis and some very aggressive aneurysmal bone cysts as well as osteomas. Codman angles are usually tumour free since they result from periosteal elevations secondary to bleeding and oedema in advance of an aggressive bone-destroying process.

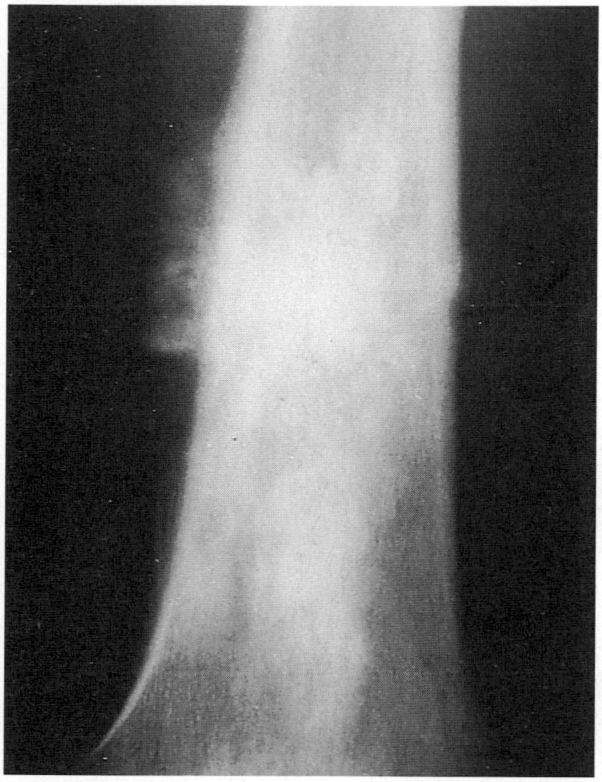

Figure 10.17 The divergent spiculated or 'sunburst' periosteal reaction pictured above is most commonly seen in osteosarcoma. Occasionally, however, this reaction will occur with osteoblastic metastases and haemangiomas.

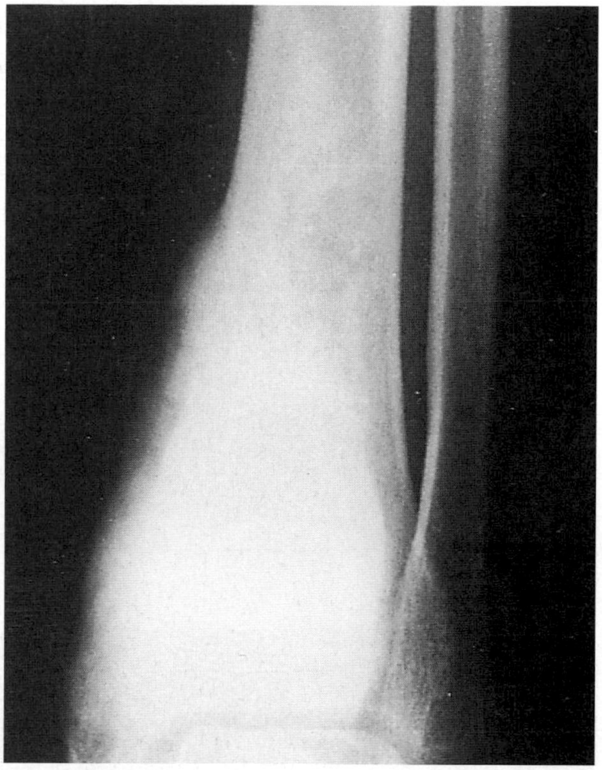

Figure 10.18 This osteosarcoma demonstrates the confluent, dense cloud-like mineralization characteristic of tumour osteoid. The mineralization of neoplastic bone is initially observed in the centre of the lesion where cellular activity is the greatest.

Complex periosteal patterns

Divergent spiculated pattern

The divergent spiculated pattern, also known as the sunburst pattern, is a combination of reactive bone formation and malignant osteoid production. 'Histologically, the individual rays consist of various combinations of reactive and sarcoma bone with spaces between the individual rays occupied by cellular tumor and tumor products' (Madewell *et al.*, 1981; Figure 10.17). The sunburst reaction is highly suggestive but not diagnostic of osteosarcoma. Occasionally this reaction can also be seen with osteoblastic metastases and haemangioma.

Periosteal reactions may be helpful for tumours that arise in the diaphysis or metaphysis, but it should be noted that periosteum is replaced at the end of the bone by the joint capsule. Tumours that arise within the zone of insertion of the joint capsule may be associated with a joint effusion and hyperplasia of synovium, without the radiographic features of a periosteal reaction. For example, an osteoid osteoma arising at the end of a long bone may require a bone scan followed by tomograms or CT for localization, as the 'usual' periosteal reaction will not occur (Bauer *et al.*, 1991)

TUMOUR MINERALIZATION PATTERNS

Deposition of additional mineral in and around focal lesions of bone is seen as:

- mineralization of tumour matrix;
- reactive bone proliferation in response to injury;
- mineral deposition in areas of degenerated or necrotic tissue.

The identification of characteristic mineralization patterns has diagnostic significance.

Bone tumours and tumour-like conditions can be divided into categories of matrix-producing lesions, non-matrix-producing lesions, or as a combination. The term matrix refers to the acellular/intracellular substance produced by mesenchymal cells and includes osteoid produced by osteoblasts, chondroid produced by chondroblasts, and myxoid and col-

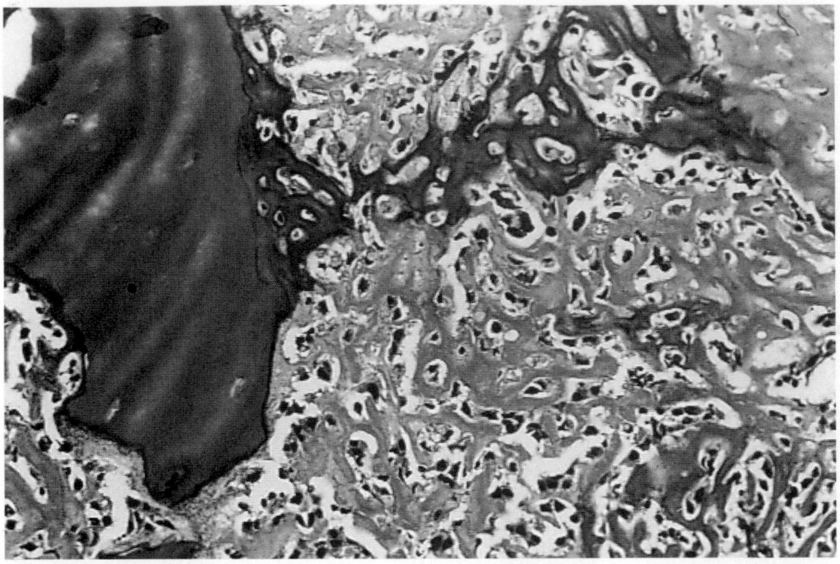

(a)

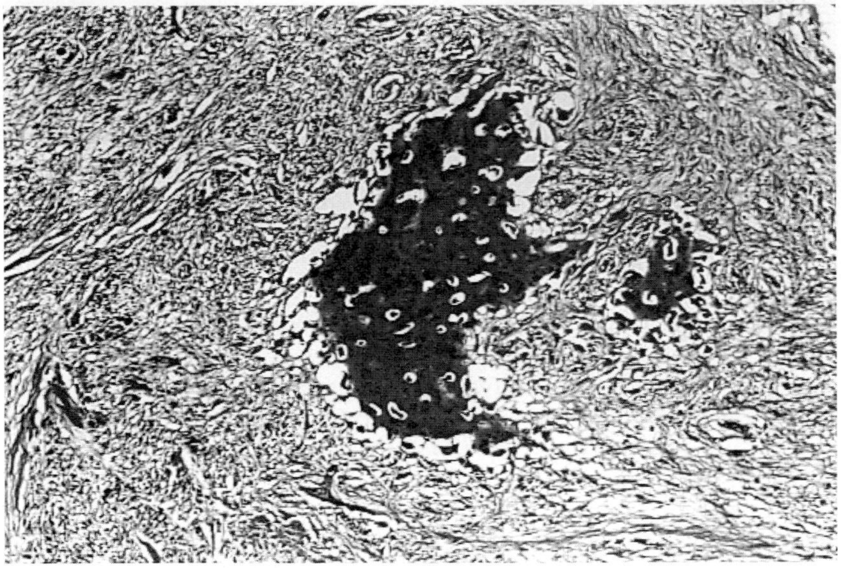

(b)

Figure 10.19 (a) The osteoid of high-grade osteosarcomas may be incompletely mineralized, producing a permeative, radiolucent appearance on plain radiographs. (b) Osteoid produced by parosteal osteosarcomas, on the other hand, is usually more uniformly mineralized, imparting a more uniform density to radiographs.

lagen fibres produced by fibroblasts (Sweet *et al.*, 1981). Two of these matrices, chondroid and osteoid, calcify and ossify in characteristic patterns.

Osteoid matrix

Mineralization of osteoid elaborated by neoplastic osteoblasts is the final step in the creation of tumour bone. Osteoid tissue mineralizes in a confluent manner that results in a radiographic density ranging from a hazy ground-glass appearance to a dense ivory-like pattern (Figure 10.18). Rapidly growing neoplasms such as osteosarcoma usually produce immature woven tumour bone which is seen as ill-defined poorly structured clouds of density (Figure 10.19). On the other hand, slowly growing, osteoid-producing tumours such as parosteal osteosarcomas produce solid mature tumour bone which is seen as well defined, heavily mineralized masses radiographically (Lodwick, 1971) (Figure 10.19). The mineralization of neoplastic bone is initially observed in the centre of the lesion where cellular maturity is the greatest.

Tumour bone is occasionally produced by fibroblastic cells that have been converted to functional osteoblasts through the mechanism of metaplasia. When this occurs in fibrous lesions such as fibrous dysplasia, the pattern of bone formed is woven

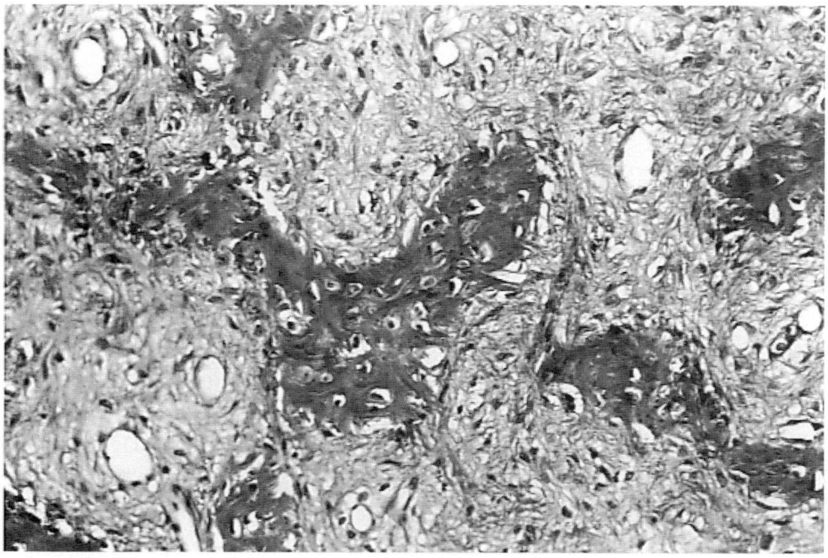

Figure 10.20 Fibrous dysplasia is characterized by 'C' or 'S' shaped trabeculae of woven bone, usually without osteoblastic rimming, associated with a fibrous stroma. This lesion is usually less uniformly mineralized than normal trabecular bone, resulting in a hazy, 'ground-glass' radiographic appearance.

or fibrous in appearance (Figure 10.20). Woven bone of this type is usually less densely mineralized than tumour bone formed directly from neoplastic osteoblasts. The result is a hazy ground-glass appearance.

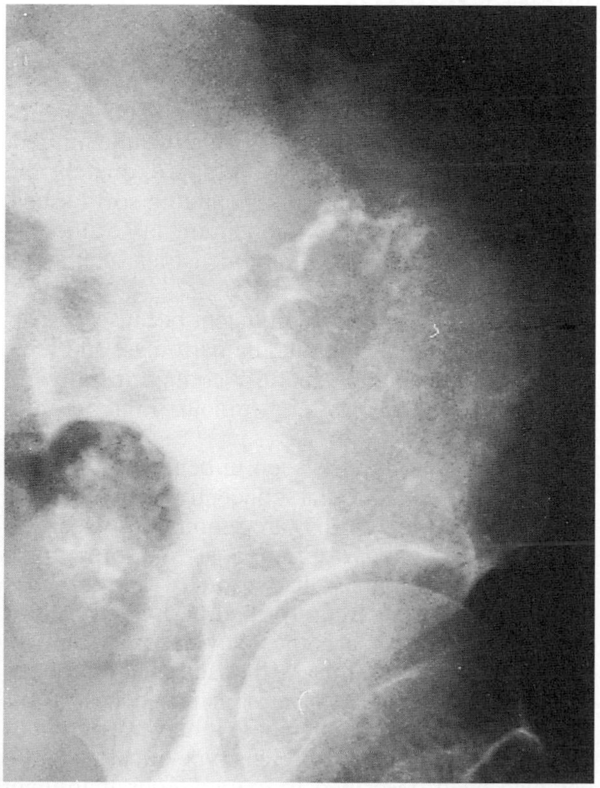

Figure 10.21 In neoplastic cartilage, mineralization is typically seen as stipples, floccules, arcs, and rings. The calcification within this chondrosarcoma is an example.

Chondroid matrix

In neoplastic cartilage, calcification in the form of stipples, floccules, arcs, and ring-like shapes conforms to the lobulated configuration of the cartilaginous matrix (Figure 10.21). Since this calcification usually occurs in the most mature cartilage, it is characteristically found in the centre of a lesion. An admixture of stipples and floccules is seen with considerable frequency in both benign and malignant cartilaginous tumours (Phemister, 1930).

Reactive bone mineralization

Reactive bone is formed either through modulation of normal marrow or soft tissue elements to osteoblastic activity or from periosteal reaction (Sweet *et al.*, 1981) at tumour margins. Slowly progressive neoplasms including certain malignant lesions such as primary lymphoma of bone and Ewing's tumour can stimulate reactive bone activity along with osteolytic activity. This results in a coarsened and mottled trabecular pattern of combined radiolucency and increased radiodensity. Endosteal and trabecular sclerosis can also be stimulated by inflammatory disorders such as chronic low-grade osteitis and osteomyelitis. Only when mineralized osteoid matrix is demonstrated outside of the bone proper can an absolute radiographic diagnosis of tumour bone be made (deSantos, 1980).

Dystrophic mineralization pattern

Dystrophic calcification results from the deposition of mineral salts in degenerating or necrotic tissue, primarily necrotic fat and densely hyalinized con-

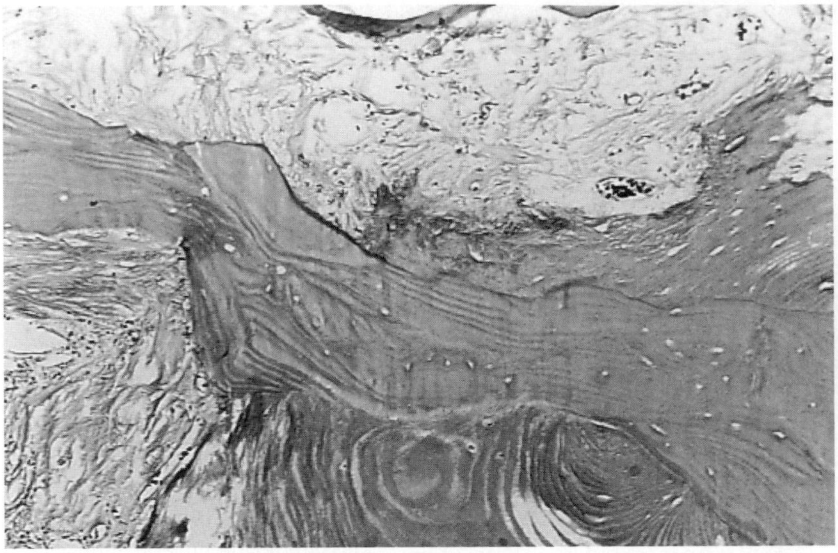

Figure 10.22 Bone infarcts show different radiographic and histological appearances based on the age of the lesion. Remote infarcts tend to show necrotic bone with fibrous marrow. Dystrophic calcification of the marrow appears radiographically as punctate calcification.

nective tissue. This process can result in stippled, flocculent, solid, patchy, and linear density patterns in bone (Sweet *et al.*, 1981). This type of mineralization can be seen in such lesions as ossifying lipomas, bone infarcts, and in areas of bone radiation necrosis (Figure 10.22). The mineralization in bone infarction occurs in the periphery of a lesion. Uncommonly, necrotic portions of non-matrix-producing tumours, e.g. Ewing's tumour and primary lymphoma of bone, will mineralize which can be misleading.

INFLUENCE OF AGE ON DIAGNOSIS

Since tumours of different histological types can present with similar radiographic appearances, it is fortunate that many neoplasms demonstrate peak incidence at different ages, allowing the age of the patient to be a factor in making the diagnosis. Because malignant neoplasms are more likely to be discovered early after onset than benign neoplasms, age is a more useful criterion when dealing with malignant tumours (Nelson, 1966). For instance, the peak incidence of bone lesions of leukaemia and neuroblastoma is in the first decade of life. Osteosarcoma and Ewing's tumour are more common in the second decade, and giant cell tumours are uncommonly seen before the third decade. Tumours such as fibrosarcoma, chondrosarcoma, and primary lymphoma of bone are more likely to occur after the third decade, whereas myeloma and metastatic neoplasms are the predominant forms of malignant tumour after the fifth decade (Ginaldi and deSantos, 1980). It must be understood, however, that age alone cannot be an absolute indication of a particular diagnosis since there are wide variations in the overall incidence of most lesions.

PLAIN X-RAY EVALUATION OF SOFT TISSUE TUMOURS

The diagnostic information available on plain radiographs of soft tissue tumours is usually quite limited. Most soft tissue neoplasms are approximately the same radiodensity as their surrounding soft tissues. The exceptions are lesions containing large amounts of tissue with contrasting radiodensities such as fat or calcium.

Tumours that appear radiolucent because of their fat content include lipomas, hamartomas, and teratomas. Liposarcomas generally contain insufficient fat to be recognized as fatty tumours radiographically.

Calcifications may be seen in benign and malignant neoplasms. Circular concentric calcifications representing phleboliths are commonly seen in haemangiomas and arteriovenous malformations. Myxomas, xanthomas, hamartomas, and lipomas may have sharply circumscribed peripheral calcifications. Soft tissue sarcomas may undergo haemorrhage and necrosis that will result in amorphous calcification. Such calcification is particularly common in synovial sarcoma where it may be seen in as many as 20–30% of cases. This type of calcification has also been described in extraosseous malignant fibrous histiocytomas and in rhabdomyosarcomas (Alazraki *et al.*, 1980). Extraskeletal osteosarcoma and extraskeletal chondrosarcoma characteristically show irregular, poorly marginated calcifications and ossifications. These calcifications must be differentiated from the more sharply circumscribed peripheral calcifications seen in the mature stage of myositis ossificans.

Neoplastic masses characteristically displace soft tissue fat planes while soft tissue planes are characteristically obliterated by oedema with inflammatory conditions. Distortion and blurring of part of the interface between malignant neoplasms and their surrounding soft tissues can be seen (Martel and Abell, 1973).

Smooth resorption of cortical bone adjacent to a soft tissue mass reflects a reaction to local hyperaemia or a pressure effect from the adjacent mass (Martel and Abell, 1973). Sclerosis of the margin of this erosion would indicate a slowly progressing lesion while the absence of such a border would suggest a more aggressive process (Chew and Hudson, 1982). Irregular cortical and cancellous bone destruction is indicative of malignancy or infection (Chew *et al.*, 1981). Metastasis of soft tissue sarcomas to distant bones is not uncommon (Wong *et al.*, 1982; Kirchner and Simon, 1984).

Imaging of musculoskeletal neoplasms

The plain radiographic examination today as in the past is the first step in the evaluation of musculoskeletal neoplasms. Valuable information concerning the location of a skeletal lesion and indication of its aggressiveness can be obtained from the plain radiographic examination. Plain radiographs usually do not provide the contrast resolution and spatial information necessary to allow a decision of limb salvage or local excision to be made. In past years, preoperative angiography had played an important role in demonstrating the local extent of tumour masses and their relationships to neurovascular bundles and fascial planes. The development of CT scanning soon replaced angiography as the primary method of localizing disease processes. More recently, magnetic resonance imaging has become an important method of providing information for accurate staging of musculoskeletal neoplasms.

CT SCANNING

Computed tomography has the ability to determine intramedullary and extramedullary extension of disease, to localize the lesion in a cross-sectional display and to define the relationships between tumour and vital structures. Numerous authors have reported that CT gives a better indication of the extent of disease than conventional radiographic techniques (Wilson *et al.*, 1978; deSantos *et al.*, 1979a; Levine *et al.*, 1979; Ginaldi and deSantos, 1980).

The entire length of the tumour must be visualized so that at least one normal scan above and one below the lesion are obtained. If the lesion involves the end of the bone, scans through the adjacent joints should be obtained. The contralateral extremity is included in the field whenever possible.

Information will be maximized by scanning after the injection of intravenous contrast material (deSantos *et al.*, 1978; Heelan *et al.*, 1979; Levine *et al.*, 1979; Levine, 1981; Hudson *et al.*, 1983). Enhancement of soft tissue tumours or soft tissue extensions of bone tumours occurs with intravenous contrast, and there is generally improved visualization of neurovascular bundles on post-contrast studies (Levine, 1981).

Conventional axial images are in most instances adequate for diagnosis and treatment planning. Several authors have shown good correlation between CT estimates of tumour size and measurements obtained from resected specimens (deSantos *et al.*, 1979a; Heelan *et al.*, 1979; Levine *et al.*, 1979). These estimates can be obtained in the transverse direction by assessing the cross-sectional diameter of the tumour on the CT image itself. The longitudinal measurement is determined from the number of axial scans on which the tumour is demonstrated. Multiplanar reconstruction of CT scans, when available and when feasible, and direct longitudinal scanning of a lesion can also assist in the determination of tumour size (Levine, 1981).

Overestimation of tumour size will occur when oedema surrounding a tumour mass is mistaken for the neoplasm itself (Egund *et al.*, 1981). Imaging following biopsy can result in overestimation of tumour size and location because of the inability to differentiate between tumour and post-biopsy haematoma (Jones and Kuhns, 1981). For this reason, imaging studies should be completed prior to a biopsy of the lesion (Mankin *et al.*, 1982b).

Underestimation of tumour size can occur in patients with a paucity of adipose tissue between muscle bellies and fascial planes. Fat provides the contrast necessary for demonstration of a mass. Images of tumours arising in anatomy of small cross-section such as the calf and forearm and in emaciated patients and children may be compromised by a lack of fatty tissue.

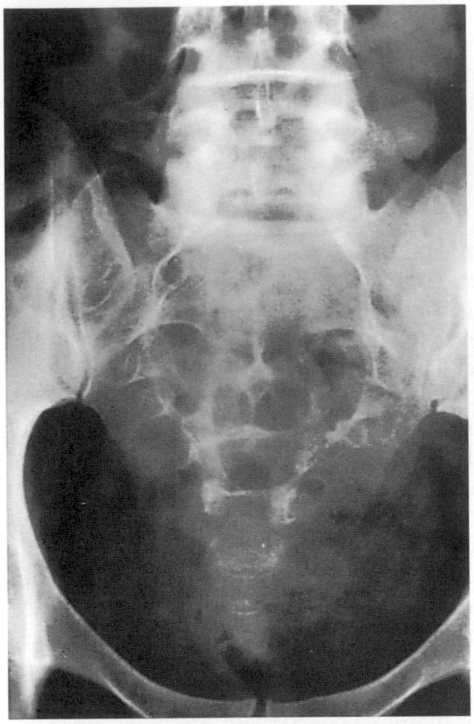

(a)

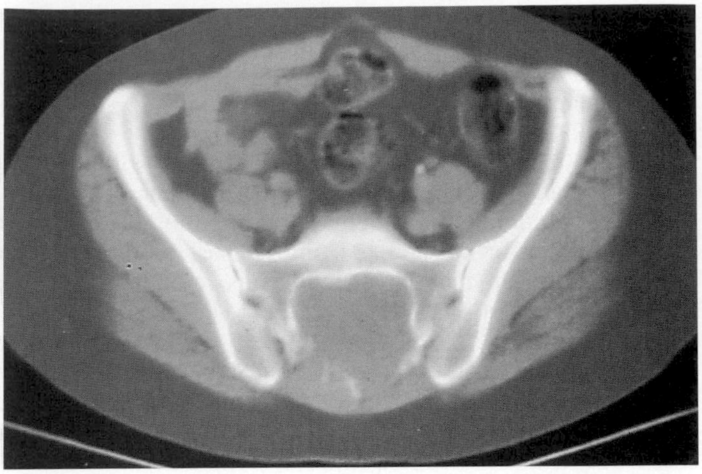

(b)

Figure 10.23 This plain radiograph (a) of the sacrum demonstrates subtle distortion of the bony architecture suggesting the presence of a mass. The CT image (b) greatly enhances the demonstration of the lesion.

Role of CT in the diagnosis of musculoskeletal tumours

Levine *et al.* (1979) found CT useful in establishing a primary diagnosis in only 26% of 50 patients. Wilson *et al.* (1978), however, found that CT provided unique information leading to a correct diagnosis in 45% of 55 patients studied. CT is particularly helpful in providing diagnostic information about bony lesions located in the axial skeleton such as the pelvis, sacrum, chest wall, and vertebral appendages (Figure 10.23). CT may be of value in differentiating solid from cystic bone lesions, and occasionally CT will demonstrate subtle tumour matrix mineralization not apparent on routine radiographs. Computed tomography may also be more accurate in demonstrating the integrity of the cortex in an area containing tumour (Figure 10.24). CT can be useful in excluding soft tissue tumours in patients with palpable masses relating to exaggerated normal anatomy. Although soft tissue neoplasms generally exhibit tissue densities less than normal muscle, demonstration of masses by CT still depends on surrounding fat for optimum contrast resolution. Benign lesions are often sharply marginated on CT scans while malignant neoplasms will often have

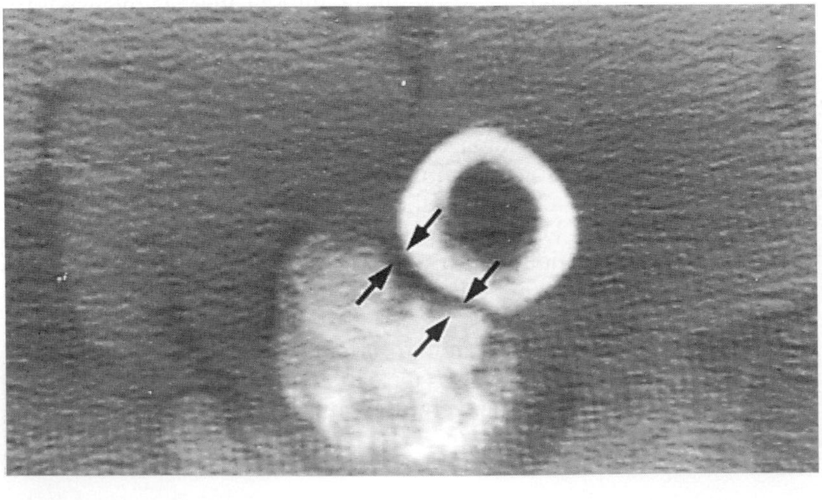

Figure 10.24 A CT scan through the proximal thigh demonstrates an ossified mass in the soft tissue adjacent to the femur. The clear separation of the mass from the femur helps support the diagnosis of parosteal osteosarcoma. The centrally concentrated matrix ossification is also characteristic of this lesion.

infiltrative growth patterns. Benign masses tend to demonstrate a more homogeneous density than malignant neoplasms (Rosenthal, 1982). But absolute differentiation between benign and malignant lesions, however, is not possible with CT scanning.

CT evaluation of pulmonary metastases

It is generally accepted that computed tomography is the procedure of choice for detecting pulmonary metastases in patients with musculoskeletal neoplasms. Multiple studies comparing CT with chest radiography and chest linear tomography (Muhm *et al*., 1978; Schaner *et al*., 1978; Pass *et al*., 1985) have demonstrated that CT is the most sensitive test. Screening CT of the thorax should be considered in patients with high-grade tumours. CT is valuable for determining the exact location of pulmonary lesions before invasive procedures such as biopsy or surgical resection are undertaken (Davis, 1991).

CT scanning for possible pulmonary metastasis is usually performed with 10 mm contiguous CT images without intravenously administered contrast material. Thin-section (less than 5 mm) scans can occasionally be helpful in providing additional information about an individual nodule.

Haematogenous dissemination of metastases generally results in pulmonary nodules which are multiple, spherical, and variable in size. They are usually bilateral and peripheral in location. Pulmonary metastases from osteosarcoma, chondrosarcoma, and synovial sarcoma may be calcified (Davis, 1991).

Differentiation between metastatic and benign lesions can be problematic. With a solitary nodule, primary lung carcinoma must be considered. Where there is a question, percutaneous needle aspiration biopsy is often helpful (Westcott, 1985). Biopsy can generally be accomplished with fluoroscopic guidance if lesions are of sufficient size. CT-guided biopsy may also be performed but is generally more time-consuming (Weisbrod, 1990).

MAGNETIC RESONANCE IMAGING

This technology produces high-resolution tomographic images similar to those of x-ray computed tomography but without involvement of ionizing radiation. Images can be primarily obtained in multiple planes if desired without the need for computer image reconstruction.

The intensity of the MR signal is determined by

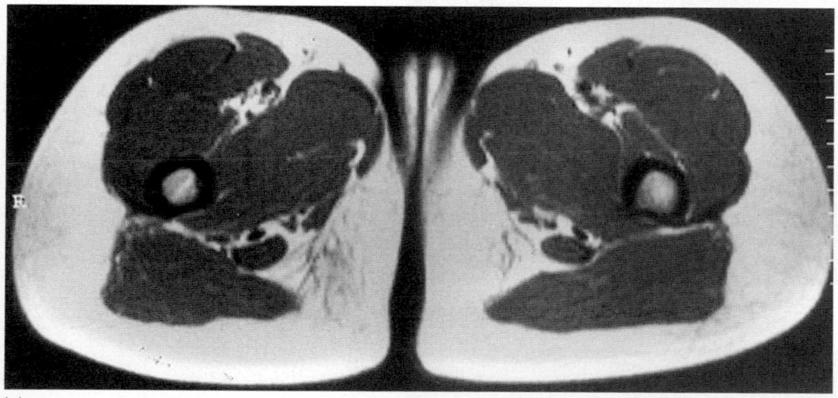

(a)

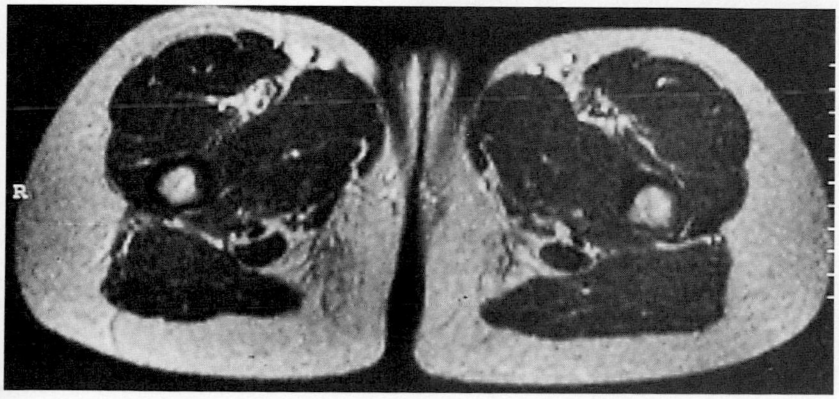

(b)

Figure 10.25 These axial magnetic resonance images through the proximal thigh demonstrate normal T1 (a) and T2 (b) tissue signal characteristics with spin-echo image acquisition techniques. The bright signal in subcutaneous regions and the bone marrow is characteristic of fat. Normal muscle has less signal intensity than fat (grey), and cortical bone shows very low signal intensity (black).

the density of the resonating nuclei, by flow, and by two chemical parameters called relaxation times, T1 and T2. Both normal and abnormal tissues can be characterized by their T1 and T2 values (Figure 10.25). When tissues are altered by disease, their T1 and T2 values may change, allowing pathological structures to be distinguished from normal anatomy on MR images. In general, pathological tissues, including neoplasms, will show lengthening of the T1 and T2 values so that, compared to normal muscle, abnormal tissue will have slightly decreased or increased MR signal on T1-weighted images and significantly increased MR signal on T2-weighted images. Neoplastic masses are therefore demonstrated on the basis of intrinsic signal differences between abnormal and normal tissue.

MR imaging of musculoskeletal neoplasms should be performed before biopsy. In the immediate period after biopsy, the difficulty in distinguishing tumour from oedema, haemorrhage, and reactive fibrosis may result in overestimation of tumour extent (Sundaram and McLeod, 1990).

The standard MR examination for staging must include both T1- and T2-weighted pulse sequenced images. T1-weighted sequences differentiate tumour masses from fat while the T2-weighted sequence generally separates tumour masses from surrounding muscle. T1- and T2-weighted pulse sequences are always made in the axial plane. These images are often complemented by a T1-weighted set of images in the coronal or sagittal plane to include the entire length of the extremity and adjacent joint. Coronal or sagittal images are useful in demonstrating intramedullary extent of tumour and skip metastases. Axial images should include the entire dimension of the tumour mass as well as any skip metastases (Alazraki *et al.*, 1980).

Additional pulse sequences may be employed in a

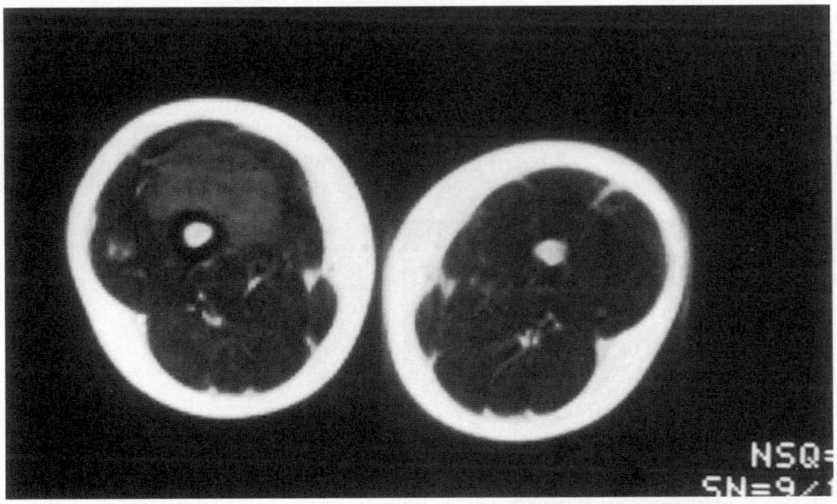

(a)

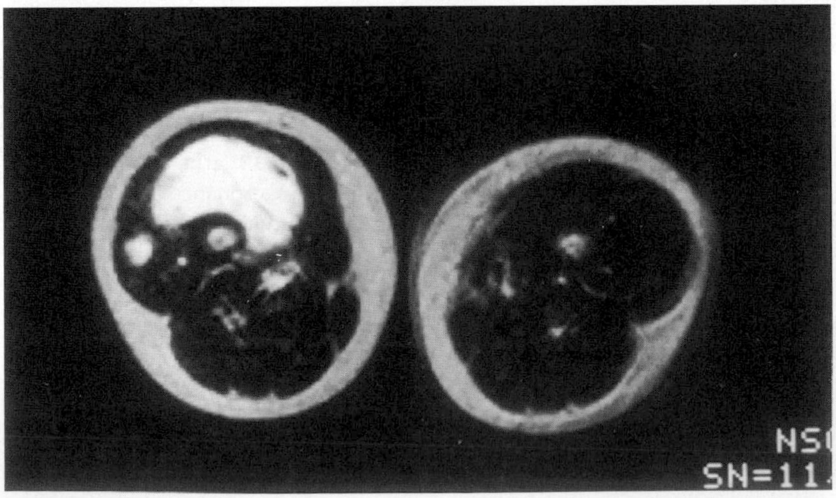

(b)

Figure 10.26 T1-weighted (a) and T2-weighted (b) spin-echo images demonstrate a large mass in the anterior aspect of the right thigh and a smaller lesion laterally (soft tissue haemangioma). The T1 image demonstrates a slight increase in magnetic resonance signal in the masses compared to muscle, while the T2-weighted image demonstrates bright magnetic resonance signal in the masses, greatly enhancing their conspicuity.

given case to increase or clarify diagnostic information, e.g. gradient recalled pulse sequences for the evaluation of vessels adjacent to tumour or the short IT inversion recovery (STIR) pulse sequence for separating neoplastic from normal tissue (Dwyer *et al.*, 1988).

MR characterization of tumours

In most cases, MR signals are not specific in characterizing musculoskeletal tumours. In general, musculoskeletal neoplasms demonstrate MR signal slightly greater or slightly less than normal muscle signal on T1-weighted spin-echo images. Differences are often slight, making a separation of masses from normal surrounding muscle difficult. Because of the long T2 values generally seen in neoplasms, the lesions are much more easily seen on T2-weighted images (Pettersson *et al.*, 1987) (Figure 10.26). Lipomas demonstrate high MR signal on both T1- and T2-weighted sequences (short T1 and T2 characteristics) and are the same intensity as normal subcutaneous fat. Subacute haematomas, lipoblastic liposarcomas, some haemangiomas, and haemorrhage into a pre-existing mass compose a spectrum of conditions demonstrating high signal intensity on T1-weighted MR images (Sundaram and McLeod, 1990; Davis, 1991). A few soft tissue masses have little or no signal on T2-weighted pulse sequences, e.g. clear cell sarcoma, aggressive fibromatosis, malignant fibrous histiocytosis, and malignant schwannoma. Pigmented villonodular synovitis will have foci of low signal on T1- and T2-weighted sequences due to the deposition of haemosiderin into the tissues (Sundaram and McLeod, 1990; Wetzel and Levine, 1990). Aneurysms and vascular malformations may have regions of low signal because of flow void (Sundaram and McLeod, 1990; Wetzel and Levine, 1990). Mature fibrotic scarring produces low signal intensity on all pulse sequences (Pettersson *et al.*, 1987). Ossification or gas within soft tissue masses will also show decreased MR signal on T1- and T2-weighted images (Zimmer *et al.*, 1985).

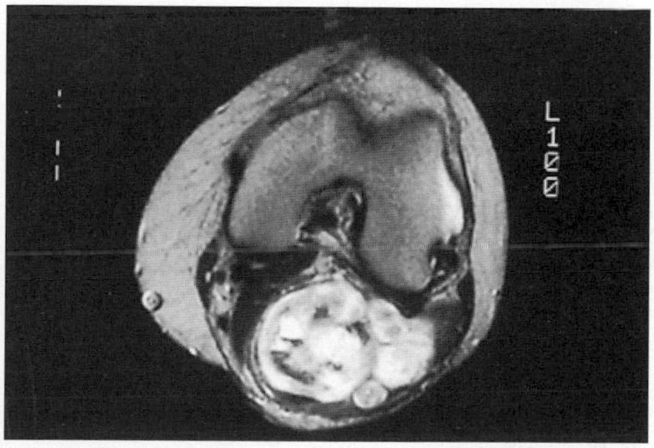

Figure 10.27 This T2-weighted spin-echo image in the axial projection demonstrates a mass in the popliteal fossa. Characteristics of the mass, including irregular borders, inhomogeneous signal intensity, and peritumoral oedema, suggest malignancy, in this case synovial sarcoma.

Magnetic resonance imaging does not provide an absolute prediction of malignancy or benignancy based on signal intensities or relaxation times. Criteria used to help differentiate benign from malignant soft tissue tumours include signal intensity, signal homogeneity, signal changes in adjacent soft tissue, tumour margins, extracompartmental extension, and evidence of bone destruction and neurovascular invasion. No single criterion has been found to be reliable (Kransdorf *et al.*, 1989). A mass with well defined margins, homogeneous signal, and no associated reaction in peritumour tissues is more likely to be benign. A mass with irregular borders, inhomogeneous signal intensity, and a peritumoral oedematous reaction makes the diagnosis of a malignant lesion more probable (Figure 10.27).

Berquist *et al.* (1990) found benign desmoid tumours and necrotic benign neoplasms most often confused with malignant lesions. The malignant lesion most commonly misclassified as benign was synovial sarcoma. MR imaging has become the procedure of choice for local staging of bone and soft tissue neoplasms. The tissue contrast between mass and normal tissue is far better with MR compared to CT based on the intrinsic tissue contrast provided by the signal changes in pathological tissues. MR imaging therefore more clearly defines the extent of soft tissue masses and soft tissue extension of bony masses than computerized tomography (Figure 10.28). As with CT scanning, however, MR is unable to accurately separate neoplasm from peritumoral oedema since both inflammatory tissue and neoplastic tissue display similar signal intensity changes (Beltran *et al.*, 1987). MR imaging has the ability to visualize directly bone marrow content and is a more effective means of demonstrating intramedullary extension of neoplasm and skip metastases than CT.

MR imaging evaluation of recurrent neoplasm

An important use of MR imaging is for post-therapy follow-up of patients. In the early postoperative period, there may be difficulty in distinguishing residual or recurrent neoplasm from postoperative signal change based on tissue inflammation and

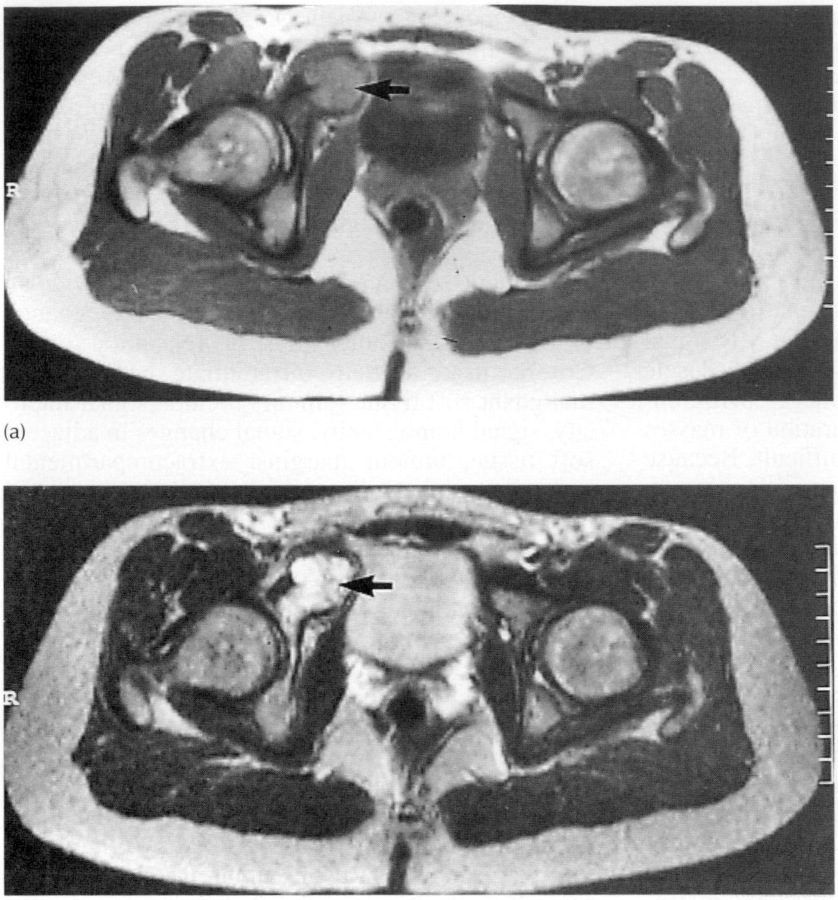

(a)

(b)

Figure 10.28 Axial T1-weighted (a) and T2-weighted (b) spin-echo images of the pelvis demonstrate a bone lesion in the anterior aspect of the right acetabulum and superior pubic ramus with obvious soft tissue extension of tumour mass (arrow). The tissue contrast available with magnetic resonance imaging makes it the preferred method of documenting soft tissue and intramedullary extension of bone neoplasms.

oedema. With time, surgical beds will demonstrate low signal intensity on both T1- and T2-weighted pulse sequences which is characteristic of surgical fibrotic scarring. Vanel *et al.* (1987) found that low signal intensity indicated the absence of active neoplasm in the therapy or surgical bed with 100% accuracy in those patients who had not received radiation therapy. For patients who had undergone radiation therapy, they found it impossible to differentiate between radiation-induced inflammatory changes and active tumour. Post-radiation inflammatory changes were seen up to 4 years post-radiation therapy. Recurrent neoplasm also generally has a mass-like configuration compared to the more longitudinal configuration seen with acute and subacute scarring.

Artefacts resulting from metallic implants which degrade CT images are less of a problem with MR images since artefacts on MRI are usually localized. They may not impair the diagnostic quality of the image.

MR Imaging after chemotherapy or radiotherapy

MR imaging has been used to evaluate the response of bone and soft tissue sarcomas to chemotherapy and radiation therapy (Holscher *et al.*, 1987; Vanel *et al.*, 1987). Tumour volume decrease and the development of pseudocapsules can be estimated accurately (Holscher *et al.*, 1987; Vanel *et al.*, 1987). The extent of tumour necrosis and the presence of viable tumour are more difficult to determine. However, decreasing tumour volume and signal intensity or the development of a short T2 after treatment appears to reflect a good treatment response (Holscher *et al.*, 1987; Vanel *et al.*, 1987).

Magnetic resonance imaging versus computerized tomography scanning

Magnetic resonance imaging is now considered the examination of choice for local staging of tumours of bone and soft tissue masses (Sundaram and McLeod,

1990). MR and CT scanning should not routinely be considered complementary studies, and it is uncommon for both studies to be justified in the staging process. CT scans are justified as adjuncts to plain radiographs to clarify the morphology of skeletal lesions, particularly those located in the flat bones such as the pelvis, ribs, scapulae, and vertebrae. Bony lesions in the axial skeleton are often poorly characterized with plain radiographs alone. CT is preferred to MRI in the peripheral skeletal when osteoid osteoma is strongly suspected (Sundaram and McLeod, 1990). CT is also better for the demonstration of tumour mineralization.

Gadolinium-enhanced MR imaging

Laredo (1993) has emphasized the value of this technique in differentiating intrathecal tumours from arachnoiditis, tumours from normal soft tissues during spread or extension and recurrent tumour from scar tissue.

TECHNETIUM RADIONUCLIDE IMAGING

The development of the automatic scanner (Cassen *et al.*, 1951) along with improvements in gamma camera technology (Anger, 1952) have resulted in a more efficient radionuclide imaging system.

Technetium-99m-labelled phosphate compounds were found to have excellent physical characteristics for gamma camera imaging and allowed bone scanning to become a simple, fast, and highly sensitive technique capable of detecting a wide variety of bone diseases. The technetium-99m phosphate compound utilized in the evaluation of musculoskeletal neoplasms is technetium-99m methylene diphosphate.

Scintography

Modern whole-body bone imaging scans are obtained after the intravenous administration of 15–25 mCi ([5.5–9.2] $\times 10^{11}$ Bq) of technetium-99m-labelled methylene diphosphate. Standard delayed images are obtained beginning 3–4 hours following injection to allow optimal skeletal uptake of radionuclide and clearance of tracer from the soft tissue. Thirty to 50% of the radiopharmaceutical localizes in the skeleton. A small percentage remains in the soft tissues, and the remainder is excreted by the kidneys (Thrace and Ellis, 1987). In special circumstances where the relative blood flow to a lesion is considered important diagnostic information, for instance osteoid osteoma, the three-phase scan technique should be employed.

Whole-body imaging demonstrates multiple sites of neoplasm while spot images at the site of a primary lesion provide high resolution for better demonstration of tracer characteristics of a primary musculoskeletal neoplasm. A commonly employed approach is to combine a whole-body scan technique with high-resolution supplementary images localized to the site of primary tumour.

Physiology of radionuclide localization

Radionuclide bone scintigrams are sensitive for demonstrating altered local metabolism in areas of active bone remodelling. The factors that affect increased tracer localization in bone neoplasms are primarily related to increased vascularity, increased rate of bone mineralization, and increased extraction efficiency (uptake) of the radiopharmaceutical by osteoid tissue involved in the process (Subramanian *et al.*, 1975; Davis and Jones, 1976; Alazraki *et al.*, 1980). The increased localization of radiopharmaceutical in a bone neoplasm is due to newly formed osteoid tissue. The tracer does not localize in the neoplastic tissue *per se*, but in the remodelling, metabolically active bone surrounding the lesion. The exception would be osteosarcoma or osteoid osteoma where radionuclide is attracted to neoplastic osteoid formed by these lesions. When reactive bone formation does not accompany a bone-destroying process, the bone scan image will appear normal if the size of the lesion is too small to be resolved by the gamma camera system. If the lesion can be resolved by the system, the lesion will be recognized as a photon-deficient area on the scan (Bataille *et al.*, 1982).

Localization of technetium-99m phosphate complexes occurs in primary malignant soft tissue tumours even when local bony structures are uninvolved. This most likely relates to hyperaemia in the tumour and/or to the influx of calcium ion with the formation of hydroxyapatite crystals. In many of these lesions, however, tracer localization is not associated with any demonstrable formation of hydroxyapatite crystals (Chew *et al.*, 1981).

Clinical application of radionuclide scanning in metastatic neoplasm in bone

The most frequent indication for technetium-99m bone imaging is for the detection of skeletal metastases from primary neoplasms. It is a sensitive method of localizing skeletal metastases with a very low incidence of false negative scans. Skeletal scintigraphy with a technetium-labelled compound

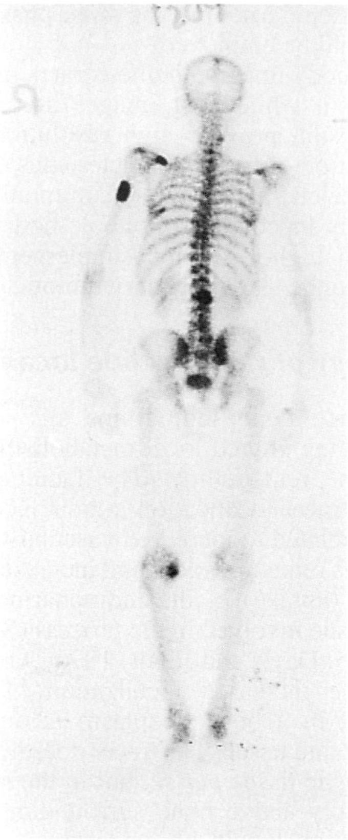

Figure 10.29 This whole-body delayed image of a technetium-99m phosphate scan demonstrates skeletal metastases from prostate carcinoma in the proximal right humerus, the right scapula, and in the left L2 pedicle. The increased radionuclide uptake in the medial aspect of the right knee reflects degenerative joint disease.

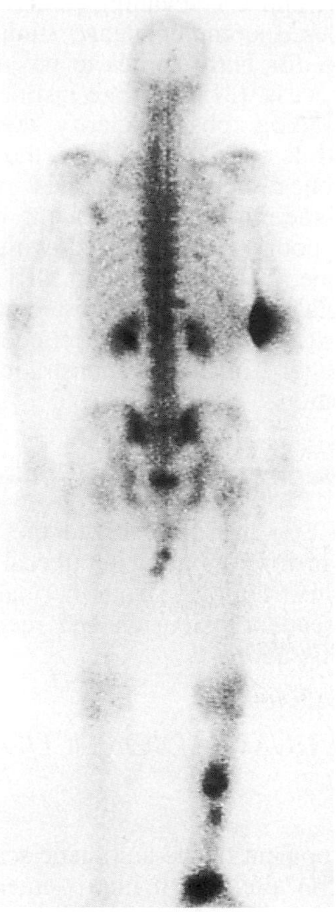

Figure 10.30 A delayed whole-body image of a technetium-99m phosphate scan demonstrates a primary bone neoplasm in the left talus (aggressive chondroblastoma) and distant metastases in the left tibia and several left ribs.

is a more reliable and simple screening examination for skeletal metastases than the radiographic skeletal survey (Brady and Croll, 1979) (Figure 10.29). The whole-body radiation dose from a standard bone scanning procedure is similar to that of a radiographic skeletal survey. False negative scans can result from symmetrical or diffuse disease patterns and with metastatic deposits from an extremely aggressive primary tumour, e.g. multiple myeloma. The overall sensitivity of the radionuclide bone scan in demonstrating myeloma lesions is 80% which is significantly lower than with the radiographic skeletal survey (Wahner *et al.*, 1980; Woolfenden *et al.*, 1980; Bataille *et al.*, 1982).

In primary bone neoplasms

The most important indication is for technetium radionuclide bone imaging to differentiate monostotic from polyostotic involvement (Figure 10.30). Baseline radionuclide bone scans have been reported to show skeletal metastases in 2% and 12% of osteosarcoma and Ewing's sarcoma respectively (McNeil, 1978). About 15% of patients who have received adjuvant chemotherapy after surgical resection of osteosarcoma have been shown to develop bone metastases in the absence of prior pulmonary metastases. The technetium-99m bone scintigram should therefore be included with the chest radiograph and the chest CT scan to rule out metastatic sites in these patients (Larson, 1978).

The radionuclide bone scan has been utilized as one of several preoperative imaging studies to assess the intraosseous extent of tumour and to attempt localization of skip metastases. Radionuclide uptake beyond the margins of neoplasm tissue is common so that it is difficult to document the exact extent of tumour on skeletal scintigrams. This so-called 'extended pattern of uptake' is based on the presence of peritumoral oedema and hyperaemia and disuse osteoporosis (Thrall *et al.*, 1975; Simon and Kirchner, 1980). The technetium-phosphate bone scan has not been shown to be a reliable method of detecting skip metastases (Chew and Hudson, 1982).

MRI based on its ability to image primarily the marrow space and its contents has become the standard method of estimating intraosseous extent of tumour and demonstrating skip metastases. However, MR scans are also unable to differentiate accurately between peritumoral oedema and neoplasm.

In primary soft tissue neoplasm

The technetium-99m-labelled phosphate compounds will also localize in a variety of soft tissue sarcomas, more commonly on blood pool images than on delayed images (Kirchner and Simon, 1984). Chew and his group found that nearly all malignant soft tissue tumours and about 50% of benign lesions take up bone-seeking radiopharmaceuticals (Chew *et al.*, 1981).

Enneking *et al.* (1981) have demonstrated that an increased radionuclide uptake in bone adjacent to a soft tissue sarcoma indicates bone involvement with neoplasm. Since bone is the second most common metastatic site for soft tissue sarcomas (after lung), a preoperative scintigram provides additional information for clinical staging and follow-up.

ARTERIOGRAPHY

It is of interest that some of the earliest efforts in the field of angiography were directed toward the study of bone neoplasms (Caldas, 1934; Farinas, 1937; Dos Santos, 1950).

Authors have described characteristic abnormal patterns of abnormal vascularity which they felt would allow differentiation between benign and malignant tumours. The demonstration of tumour vessels (irregular calibre, distorted, coarse, abrupt angulations), amputation of vessels, vascular laking, and arteriovenous shunting were considered characteristic of malignant lesions. Hypervascularity, parenchymal staining, and early venous drainage were considered non-specific findings seen in both malignant and benign processes.

However, even high-quality modern angiographic techniques are not always capable of providing information which consistently separates benign from malignant bone and soft tissue neoplasms or allowing an accurate differentiation between inflammatory and neoplastic disease processes (Halpern and Freiberger, 1970; Levin *et al.*, 1972; Viamonte *et al.*, 1973; Hudson *et al.*, 1975, 1981).

The main contribution of angiography over the

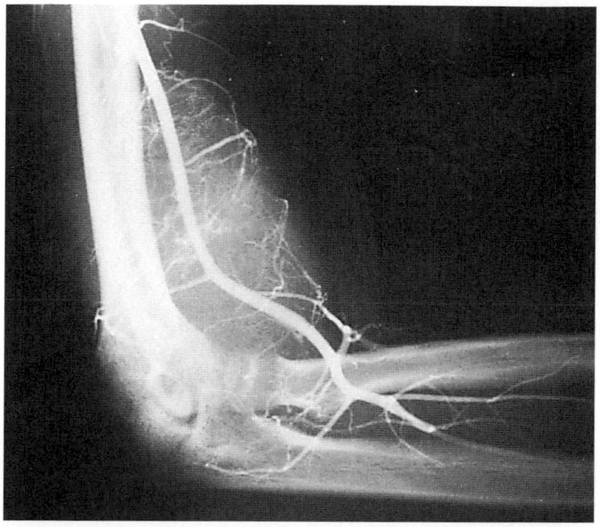

Figure 10.31 This brachial arteriogram demonstrates a large soft tissue mass anterior to the distal humerus. Assessment of the extent of tumour based on the intrinsic increase in vascularity in the neoplasm as well as displacement of normal vessels adjacent to the mass.

years has been in the assessment of the total extent of the neoplastic process. The improved contrast compared to plain radiographs is based on tissue enhancement due to a tumour's intrinsic increased vascularity and on displacement of normal vessels adjacent to the tumour mass (Figure 10.31). Preoperative angiography is no longer the standard practice for demonstrating the extent of tumour masses, however, being replaced by preoperative CT or MRI examinations. Preoperative angiography, however, may still be indicated when questions concerning tumour-vessel relationships remain unanswered on CT or MR scans. Angiography can also help demonstrate variations in normal vascular anatomy.

Preoperative angiography will demonstrate tumour vascularity and help predict surgical blood losses. Based on this knowledge, the radiologist may be asked to suppress selectively the blood supply of a highly vascular tumour by means of iatrogenic arterial embolization. The use of this technique in the therapy of musculoskeletal neoplasms was first described by Feldman *et al.* in 1975. A number of materials have been suggested as therapeutic emboli including absorbable gelatin sponge (Gelfoam, Upjohn, Inc.), steel coils, plastic or glass beads, detachable balloons, ethyl alcohol, and rapidly setting polymers (Figure 10.32).

There are indications for transcatheter embolization to be employed as a definitive treatment in some benign vascular tumours. Chuang *et al.* (1981) reported ten cases of giant cell tumours and aneurysmal bone cysts treated with transcatheter arterial

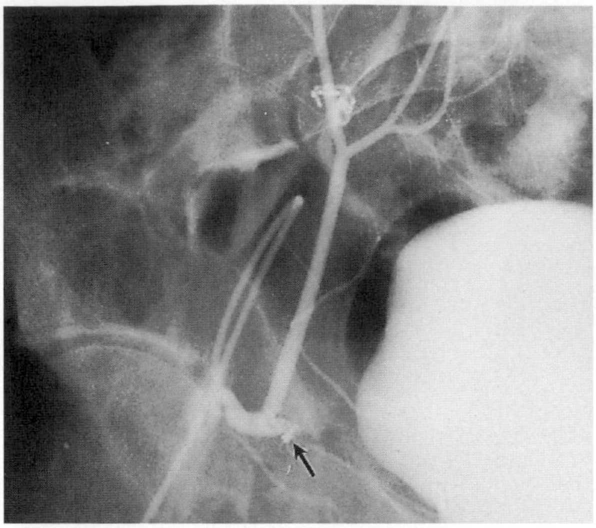

Figure 10.32 Transcatheter tumour embolization with a variety of materials (steel coils in this case) can be helpful in controlling intraoperative blood losses during resection of hypervascular benign and malignant neoplasms.

embolization. His results show complete or marked pain relief in 70% of these patients. Embolization can also be an effective definitive treatment for such vascular deformities as arteriovenous fistulae, aneurysms, and haemangioma. Arterial blockade can be used to reduce the vascularity of hypervascular benign and malignant tumours preoperatively, thereby reducing intraoperative blood losses. Transcatheter embolization can also be used for control of intractable pain or recurrent bleeding in unresectable primary and secondary neoplasms (Chuang *et al.*, 1979).

Laboratory studies

Blood tests are particularly helpful in the evaluation of metastatic disease to the musculoskeletal system. When evaluating a bony lesion in a male over the age of 50, prostatic acid phosphatase and prostatic specific antigen levels can be important in making the diagnosis of metastatic prostatic carcinoma. It is important not to draw the blood for testing immediately after a rectal examination since the massaging of a prostate will markedly elevate the acid phosphatase level. A high acid phosphatase level along with a blastic lesion on plain radiographs is enough to make a presumptive diagnosis of metastatic prostatic carcinoma. Blood tests can also be useful in the diagnosis of multiple myeloma. Multiple myeloma produces lytic lesions that are usually widespread throughout the skeleton. Serum electrophoresis abnormalities coupled with lytic lesions on radiography can lead to the diagnosis of multiple myeloma. At the same time as the blood tests, urine should be obtained for protein electrophoresis and for Bence Jones protein. Tests of a patient with suspected metastatic carcinoma and primary sarcomas should include a complete blood count, C-reactive protein (CRP) and a sedimentation rate. Anaemia may be present due to the replacement of the bone marrow by a neoplastic process. Infection is associated with a high white blood cell count and elevations in the sedimentation rate and CRP. An elevated sedimentation rate can also be seen in primary neoplastic conditions which affect marrow elements such as multiple myeloma and Ewing's sarcoma. Laboratory tests are less helpful in diagnosing primary tumours of the musculoskeletal system. An increase in the alkaline phosphatase level is frequently, but not always, observed with patients with osteogenic sarcoma when there is a destructive bone-forming lesion of the skeleton. In patients with chondrosarcomas, the glucose tolerance test is sometimes abnormal. With the exception of the abovementioned tumours, the typical musculoskeletal tumour presents with normal blood chemistries and counts.

Biopsy

The biopsy is the single most important step in the staging of a musculoskeletal neoplasm, to determine the histological diagnosis of the tumour and the type and extent of the treatment. Errors in the technique of biopsy can cause significant changes in the plan of treatment, thus adversely affecting the prognosis. Mankin (Mankin *et al.*, 1982b) studied 329 patients with musculoskeletal neoplasms to determine the effect of a biopsy on the ultimate outcome of treatment. Two hundred and twenty-two lesions were primary in bone and 107 in soft tissue. Of those tumours biopsied, 18.2% had major errors in diagnosis and 10.3% had non-representative tissue or technically poor biopsies with a complication rate of 17.3%. In 4.5% of the patients an unnecessary amputation was performed as a result of biopsy-related complications. More importantly, the prognosis and outcome were adversely affected in 8.5% of the patients. These biopsy-related problems occurred from three to more than five times more frequently when the biopsy was performed at a referring institution rather than in a treating centre.

The biopsy skin incision should be placed in such a manner so as not to compromise subsequent surgery, with sufficient amount of the lesion so that the pathologist can provide a definitive diagnosis.

There are two types of biopsy, open incisional and closed biopsy techniques, requiring careful planning, skin handling, asepsis, haemostasis and wound closure. To leave unexcised a biopsy site is to invite a local recurrence. In the open technique an incisional biopsy is preferred over an excisional biopsy. Excisional biopsies usually have a limited margin and are inadequate for definitive tumour control. Except for the small tumours that can be excised with wide margins, it is best to do an incisional biopsy and leave the tumour mass intact. The part of the tumour to be biopsied is chosen with the aid of the scans to ensure that viable tumour is obtained. Frequently, the soft tissue mass of a bone tumour is the best place to obtain a biopsy. If the tumour is located within a bone, a cortical window is carefully made and the tumour sample removed. For tumours containing a component of non-calcified tissue a frozen section is obtained to ascertain that viable and representative tissue has been obtained. At the time of biopsy, especially frozen section, it is imperative to share with the pathologist all appropriate clinical information as well as radiographic studies. It is also helpful for the surgeon to view the frozen section and discuss the case with the pathologist. This communication helps both physicians to determine the adequacy of the sample. For a large, painful geographic lytic lesion with endosteal scalloping of the femur in an adult, for example, the simple recognition of cartilage on the frozen section may be sufficient to guide further treatment. In other cases, it may be sufficient for the pathologist to simply classify the tumour as benign or malignant, without attempting to determine the specific histological classification at frozen section. It is particularly important to bring to the attention of the pathologist radiographic or clinical features of a 'changed' lesion (e.g. dedifferentiated chondrosarcoma, or malignant fibrous histiocytoma arising in association with a bone infarct), to help ensure adequate sampling of the most important tissue component.

Frozen sections are also helpful in determining whether or not tissue should be saved frozen or placed into different fixatives for special studies. For example, some immunohistochemical stains necessary for thorough classification of malignant lymphomas require either frozen sections, flow cytometry, or special fixatives. Similarly, if Ewing's sarcoma or rhabdomyosarcoma is suspected, then fixing a small portion of the tissue in glutaraldehyde will permit subsequent electron microscopy. Specific chromosomal abnormalities are being recognized in an increasing number of tumours, including Ewing's sarcoma, neuroectodermal tumours, and synovial sarcoma. If facilities exist, submitting sterile tissue for cytogenetics can be extremely helpful in making a precise diagnosis for some lesions. The final diagnosis for many musculoskeletal tumours requires correlation of the clinical and radiographic findings with the histological appearance and the results of special stains. These variables can be most efficiently handled by promoting close communication between the surgeon, radiologist, and pathologist. After biopsy the cortical window is filled with acrylic bone cement to prevent bone bleeding. A post-biopsy haematoma can spread tumour cells, increasing the risk of recurrence or forcing a change in the plan for surgery.

Because of the many inherent risks, haematoma, infection and skin problems of the open biopsy technique, a number of centres have increasingly relied upon closed percutaneous needle biopsy techniques. Needle biopsy obtains a core of tissue a few millimetres in diameter. This technique should be differentiated from fine-needle aspiration that obtains cells for cytological examination. It can be done under CT or ultrasound control, for deep tumours. Its main disadvantage is the small amount of tumour tissue obtained for pathological interpretation. With experience a pathologist can gain efficiency and confidence in making the diagnosis on small tumour samples. DeSantos *et al.* (1979b) reported on 34 suspected primary bone neoplasms evaluated by needle biopsy, with adequate material from 31 tumours. The accuracy rate of the procedure was 93% for bone tumours. The use of closed biopsy techniques has been established to an even greater extent in soft tissue neoplasms. Ball *et al.* (1990) reported on 52 consecutive patients with soft tissue tumours biopsied with a percutaneous needle, and these provided 96% adequate material for diagnosis with an accuracy of 98% for the diagnosis of malignancy and 94% for the diagnosis of sarcoma. It was recommended that closed needle biopsy should replace open biopsy as the primary means of diagnosis of soft tissue tumours unless a satisfactory tissue sample cannot be obtained.

Surgical staging

Many factors are involved in choosing the proper therapy for the patient. They include the stage of the disease, the expected functional result after surgery, the age of the patient, the type of adjuvant therapy preoperative and postoperative, whether or not there is a pathological fracture and the patient's wishes and his tolerance for risk-taking. A surgical staging system developed by Enneking has gained acceptance throughout the world (Enneking *et al.*, 1980). It has been clinically tested and found to be relevant to both surgical planning and result studies. The surgical staging system is simple, clear cut and easy to use, thus making the staging of sarcomas possible in the community hospital, as well as the cancer centres. The surgical staging system for musculoskeletal sarcomas is based on three factors which are the surgical grade (G), the local extent (T) and the presence or absence of regional or distant metastases (M).

Enneking points out that from the standpoint of surgical planning, tumours may be divided into two surgical grades: low-grade (G1) and high-grade (G2). The histological grade is important since high-grade lesions are treated more aggressively than low-grade lesions, e.g. with radical margins or procedures that produce wide margins, while low-grade lesions may be managed with wide margins or in some cases marginal margins. Generally, low-grade lesions have a low risk of metastases (less than 25%), are slow growing and late to metastasize. High-grade lesions have a significantly higher incidence of metastasis. Most histological grading schemes for sarcomas are based on either three or four grades. If the Enneking grading and staging system is to be consistently used, then the pathologist should also provide a tumour grade of either 'high' or 'low'. This is difficult, as specific criteria for a two-level grading scheme are not available for most musculoskeletal tumours. Although some tumours are high-grade by definition (e.g. round cell liposarcoma or rhabdomyosarcoma), others show a broad range of histological grades (e.g. fibrosarcoma or chondrosarcoma). While specific histological features may carry more or less importance in certain histological tumour types, as a general rule high-grade sarcomas show more nuclear anaplasia, a higher mitotic rate, less differentiation, and more necrosis than low-grade tumours. Although not true in every case, as a general rule we find that most tumours considered grade 'one' by conventional grading are 'high-grade' by the Enneking classification. This concept is based on the relatively arbitrary presumption that most grade one tumours have a propensity for local recurrence, while most grade two and grade three tumours bear a significant risk of distant metastasis. In the absence of metastases the histological grade determines the stage: Stage I = G1; stage II = G2.

The surgical staging system of Enneking divides the anatomical extent of the tumour into intracompartmental (A) or extracompartmental (B) subdivisions. This division is not necessarily related to the size of the tumour; however, larger tumours have a tendency to invade more than one anatomical compartment. Anatomical compartments have natural barriers, e.g. fascial septae, muscles origins, etc., to prevent the extension of the tumour into adjacent compartments. A bone forms a compartment in itself. This compartment extends to the articular cartilage, cortical bone and its investing periosteum. Joints are also compartments with their surgical boundaries being the articular cartilage and the joint capsule. Throughout the patient's body, there are many soft tissue compartments, e.g. quadriceps, hamstrings, biceps and triceps. It is important to note that the adequacy of the surgical margin is determined by whether or not there is a barrier between the plane of resection and the tumour. If there is a barrier, then a few millimetres of tissue is an adequate surgical margin.

The last major determinant in the surgical staging system is whether or not the patient has metastases to a distant site or the regional lymph nodes: Stage III = metastatic disease. The presence of metastatic disease denotes a poor prognosis.

Surgical resection

The importance of a preoperative staging system to the treatment design is that the stage of the disease is linked to the type of surgical margin dictated by the histological grade which is required for definitive local control. Generally speaking, extracompartmental lesions are more likely to require amputation or adjuvant radiation therapy than intracompartmental lesions. There are a number of modifying circumstances to be considered before the decision for surgery is made, e.g. the patient's age, wishes and expectations, lifestyle and expected function after reconstruction.

Enneking (1983) has described four types of surgical margins based on the relationship of the margins to the tumour, as follows.

INTRALESIONAL MARGIN

An intralesional surgical removal of a tumour can be accomplished by either a planned excision or inadvertently by amputation through the tumour. In this procedure, the tumour is actually entered and then removed piecemeal, leaving behind microscopic and macroscopic foci of tumour in both the tumour bed and the tissues bordering the surgical approach. It is most commonly employed in benign tumours and metastatic malignant tumours such as enchondromas, chondromyxofibromas and benign osteoblastomas. Its usefulness has been extended to more aggressive tumours by also using cryotherapy in conjunction with the intralesional excision. Marcove *et al.* (1973) have achieved excellent results in giant cell tumours using curettage of the lesion and cryotherapy employing liquid nitrogen. The repeated freezing of the curetted cavity devitalizes a margin of tissue surrounding the cavity. This kills microscopic and macroscopic foci of tumour left behind by the curettage. Intralesional excision with cryotherapy has been used in an increasing number of bone tumours such as ameloblastomas and aneurysmal bone cysts and now in low- and medium-grade chondrosarcoma and more recently central osteogenic sarcomas (Marcove, 1982). The treatment by intralesional excision with cryotherapy of high-grade sarcomas remains controversial.

In a similar manner, giant cell tumours have been treated by cauterizing the tumour bed with phenol and filling the cavity with methylmethacrylate bone cement (Persson *et al.*, 1987). This method was originally developed in Europe and has now gained acceptance in North America. The treatment with phenol extends the surgical margins and the filling of the defect with methylmethacrylate bone cement provides immediate support for the load-bearing bone. In addition, since bone cement is homogeneous and radiopaque, small recurrences, if they should occur, can be easily visualized at the margins of the cement. Recently the phenol has been omitted because it is frequently hard to control and often causes chemical burns to nearby soft tissues. It has been found that the monomer of methylmethacrylate and the heat of polymerization of the cement kill residual tumour cells and reduce the chance of local recurrence.

The greatest use of intralesional excision for malignant disease is found in the treatment of pathological fractures caused by metastatic carcinomas. When combined with rigid internal fixation, and methylmethacrylate bone cement, it provides an excellent means for palliation and preservation of limb function.

MARGINAL MARGIN

This is a more extensive type of surgery which removes a lesion in one piece by dissecting along the pseudo-capsule or through the reactive tissue around the lesion. Enneking believes that this type of surgery, when used for malignant tumours, leaves microscopic disease at the margin of the wound in a high percentage of the cases. Marginal excision is adequate for most benign tumours and a very few low-grade malignant tumours. Lindberg *et al.* (1981), however, have proposed combining marginal excision with high doses of radiation. With this combination, they were able to preserve the function of the limb in 80% of the patients and tumour control was achieved in 78% with only 22% experiencing local recurrence.

WIDE MARGIN

A wide excision or amputation is accomplished when the plane of the resection is entirely through normal tissue and away from the pseudo-capsule and the reactive zone around the tumour. There is no effort made to remove the entire compartment that contains the tumour. Wide amputation has been the procedure of choice in many institutions. The Istituto Ortopedico Rizzoli reports a 5% incidence of recurrence after a wide (through the bone) amputation for osteogenic sarcoma (Campanacci *et al.*, 1981). Wide excision is usually adequate for both low-grade and high-grade soft tissue sarcomas. The width of the margins, however, is controversial. Some surgeons recommend a margin of 5–8 cm when resecting soft tissue sarcomas. Other surgeons, however, are able to achieve local control of low-grade sarcomas with considerably narrower margins.

RADICAL MARGIN

Radical amputations and excisions are procedures in which the lesion, pseudo-capsule, reactive zone and the entire compartment involved are removed in one block. Most centres have now stopped using radical margins for all but a few extensive high-grade sarcomas. Local control can usually be achieved by a wide resection with or without adjuvant radiation therapy.

Surgical decision-making

Factors other than the histological grade of the sarcoma and the anatomical location and extent of the tumour also play an important part in the treatment planning.

EXPECTED FUNCTIONAL RESULT

After the tumour has been staged, the patient will either be a candidate for an amputation or an excision with the appropriate margins. If an excision is contemplated, the postoperative functional result for the involved extremity must be projected and be compared to the expected functional result of an amputation at an appropriate level. If the result of the excision is significantly worse than the expected result of the amputation, then the amputation would be preferred.

AGE

Excision of the growth plate or radiation in a growing child condemns the extremity to be shorter than the opposite side. It has been observed that young children adapt to amputation more easily than adults. Because of these factors amputation has been the treatment of choice for these growing children. The situation has been slowly changing due to the advancement of technology and surgical technique. Expandable endoprostheses have been developed to mimic the growth of the extremity (Lewis, 1986). Although successful, this technique requires multiple operations and eventually replacement of the expandable device with a more permanent endoprosthesis.

In the older growing child non-expandable endoprostheses and allograft can be use for reconstruction.

ADJUVANT CHEMOTHERAPY AND SURGERY

The majority of orthopaedic oncologists believe that adjuvant chemotherapy decreases the rate of local recurrence and allows the surgery to be less radical. It would seem likely that by killing tumour satellites in the malignancy's reactive zone the chance of recurrence would be less even if the reactive zone was entered during a wide resection. This hypothesis is supported by the observation that it is not unusual to find a rim of thick nearly acellular fibrous tissue surrounding a sarcoma that has been successively treated by preoperative chemotherapy. Presumably this rim has less viable tumour cells and therefore the chance of recurrence would be less.

LIFESTYLE

Occupational and recreational activities both affect the final choice of treatment. A procedure that leaves the patient with a limb that excludes him from the possibility of employment or prevents him from undertaking recreational activities is of little benefit to the patient. In addition, *en bloc* excisions frequently require longer hospitalization and convalescence than amputation. A patient's occupation may be lost if he is away from his job for an extended length of time.

GOALS OF TREATMENT

Whether the treatment is designed to be curative or palliative bears heavily on the decision on what type of treatment should be carried out. If the treatment is palliative, then it should be so designed as to achieve palliation while keeping hospitalization and convalescence down to a minimum, e.g. a tumour located in the extremity that would be a candidate for a radical or wide local excision with reconstruction may be better treated by palliation with either amputation or a modified wide excision with radiation.

PATHOLOGICAL FRACTURES

Pathological fractures markedly decrease the possibility of successfully resecting the tumour while maintaining the limb. When pathological fractures occur, the surrounding tissues are infiltrated with haematoma and neoplastic material. Since the pathological fracture can change a lesion from intracompartmental to extracompartmental, it may necessitate an amputation where otherwise an excision would have been indicated.

SURGICAL EXPERTISE

Certainly, the expertise of the surgeon is an important factor in choosing surgery. If the surgeon is not familiar with *en bloc* techniques, then it would serve the patient best to either refer the patient or to perform an amputation.

Surgical reconstruction

Skeletal reconstruction is frequently necessary after tumour resection to achieve the best functional results. In recent years there have been great improvements in the equipment and techniques used in skeletal reconstruction, thus decreasing the need for amputation. The preoperative planning should include an estimate of soft tissue loss with a plan for soft tissue reconstruction. Depending on the circumstances, soft tissue reconstruction can include split thickness skin grafts, local flaps or vascularized musculocutaneous flaps from remote locations.

Resection of certain bones or anatomical sites requires *no reconstruction* because the functional loss is slight, no adequate reconstruction is available or other body structures are able to compensate for the loss. No reconstruction is necessary for tumours involving the clavicle, scapula distal to the scapular spine, pubis, ischium, parts of the ilium excluding the acetabulum, and the proximal two-thirds of the fibula. The functional results after the resection of these bones are usually good to excellent.

Resection of the shoulder including the proximal humerus, clavicle and the scapula is followed by the loss of shoulder function. However, if the elbow and hand function remain normal, or nearly so, then the upper extremity function remains adequate and no reconstruction is warranted. Reconstruction is necessary after resection of all other skeletal parts.

Many muscle groups and compartments may be resected with surprisingly little functional loss. No soft tissue reconstruction is necessary after resection of the triceps, gluteus maximus, hip abductors, hamstrings or the adductors of the thigh. If only one of the quadriceps muscles is spared then the extremity's function is adequate for daily use. Muscle transfers similar to those described for poliomyelitis can be used in those patients who have suffered significant functional loss from their tumour resection, waiting until after the critical period for local recurrence because of the risk of locally spreading tumour cells from a potentially contaminated field to an uninvolved compartment or muscle group.

BONE CEMENT

To fill the cavity created by the intralesional excision of a benign bone tumour, e.g. giant cell tumour, with methylmethacrylate bone cement, has four advantages:

1. It requires very little additional operating time,
2. The material has adequate compressive strength for anticipated loads,
3. The chemical monomer and the heat of polymerization kill tumour cells, thus making recurrences less likely,
4. Bone cement is homogeneous on x-ray examination and small recurrences usually located at the cement/bone interface can be detected and treated at an earlier stage (Figure 10.33).

For these reasons, bone cement has been widely used to augment the internal fixation of bone metastatic carcinoma that has gone on to pathological fracture. While it may also be helpful in benign or low-grade bone tumours, it should be recognized that methymethacrylate is not remodelled by bone, and does not have the same mechanical properties as bone. If placed immediately beneath the subchondral plate, secondary osteoarthritis is a likely consequence. Nevertheless, the advantages of methacrylate in some clinical settings outweigh the disadvantages.

BONE GRAFTS

The oldest form of skeletal reconstruction is bone

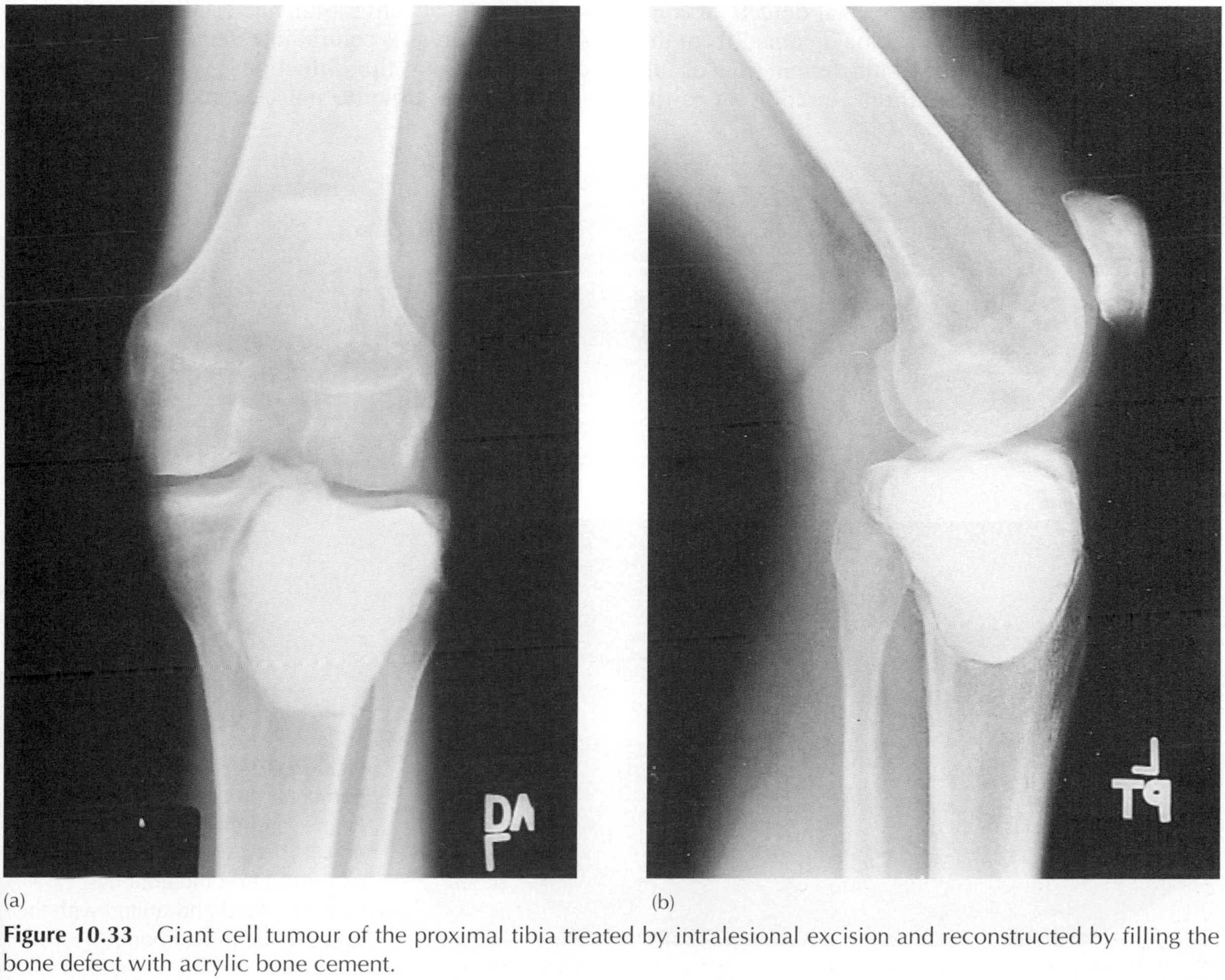

(a) (b)

Figure 10.33 Giant cell tumour of the proximal tibia treated by intralesional excision and reconstructed by filling the bone defect with acrylic bone cement.

grafting. The bone can come from the individual (autograft), or another individual of the same species (allograft).

Autografts

Cancellous autograft material is commonly obtained from the iliac crest, the trochanteric area of the femur or the proximal tibia. It is used to graft small to medium size post-resection defects in bones that have not lost their structural continuity. It is most commonly used in a patient with a benign tumour of bone who has undergone an intralesional resection. Autografts are easily available, immunologically compatible and are high quality grafts with superior osteogenic capacity that do not subject the patient to the risk of transmitted disease and are the most quickly incorporated into the skeleton. The disadvantages of cancellous autografts are they require a second incision, graft site morbidity and limited quantity. This last limitation becomes especially important in children.

Non-vascularized cortical autografts are useful for the reconstruction of some skeletal defects of long bones. Cortical autografts can be obtained from the proximal two-thirds of the fibula, femur, tibia or full thickness grafts from the ilium. In addition to the general advantages of autografts, cortical grafts restore the structural integrity and strength of long bones that have undergone segmental resection for tumour. They are used in both benign and malignant tumour cases. Because of the size of the cortical autografts they find their greatest use in the reconstruction of the upper extremity, e.g. distal radial defects. Long fibular segmental autografts, either singularly or paired, can be used to reconstruct defects in the humerus (Figure 10.34). Fibular autografts are less desirable for the reconstruction of lower extremity defects because they are usually too weak to withstand the stress of weight-bearing. Although non-vascularized fibular autografts do hypertrophy, they are subject to frequent stress fractures throughout their postoperative course. To overcome the limitations of fibular cortical autografts in weight-bearing long bones Enneking and Shirley (1977) popularized methods of excision/arthrodesis for tumours located in the distal femur or proximal tibia (Figure 10.35). Bicortical iliac autografts are frequently employed to reconstruct the spine after vertebral body resection. The use of any type of cortical autograft in bacterially contaminated or infected areas is contraindicated due to the chance of potentiating the infection. While donor site morbidity is usually not severe, a decrease in

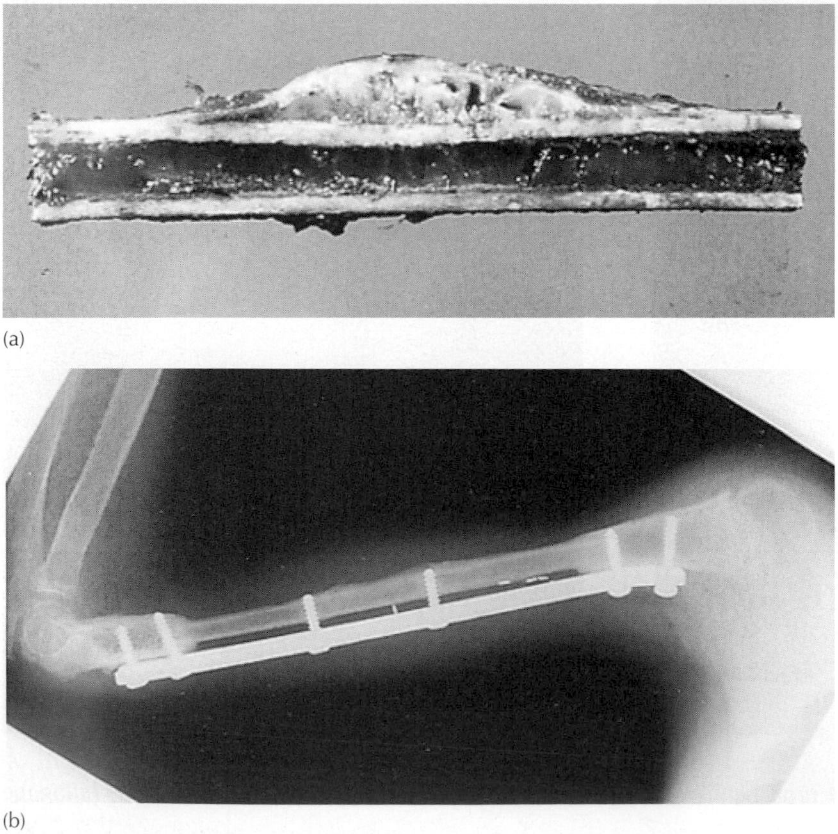

(a)

(b)

Figure 10.34 (a) Diaphysis of the humerus resected for a periosteal Ewing sarcoma in a 12-year-old boy. (b) Two years after reconstruction the graft has hypertrophied and united with the host's metaphyseal bone.

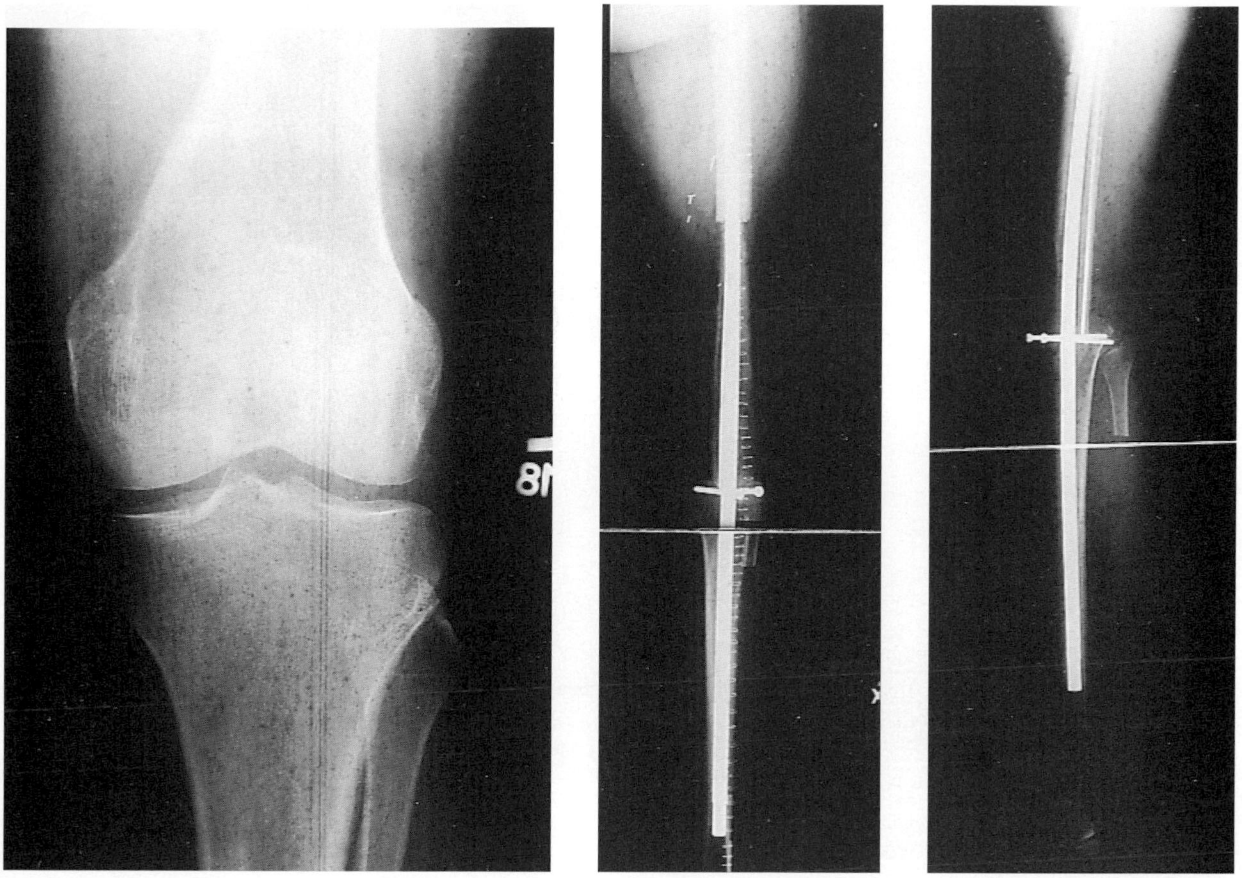

(a) (b) (c)

Figure 10.35 (a) Giant cell tumour of the distal femur. (b) and (c) Enneking's technique for excision/arthrodesis.

strength due to detachment of muscle origins can be observed. With the increased use of allografts the use of non-vascularized cortical autografts has decreased.

Vascularized autografts have found a small but useful part in reconstruction procedures. The donor sites are most commonly the proximal fibula and the anterior iliac crest. These grafts are ideal for diaphyseal defects greater than 10 cm long, a poorly vascularized bed, or when bone healing is delayed by radiation therapy or chemotherapeutic agents (Figure 10.36). The disadvantages to vascularized autografts are donor site morbidity and the prolonged operative time.

Allografts

There are many types of allografts currently in use and most major musculoskeletal oncology centres have tissue banks to supply this vital biological material. Allograft can be deep frozen for years before use; thus, large inventories of bone and joints can be accumulated. It is necessary to have a large inventory so that an allograft of proper size and shape can be chosen for implantation. Bone allografts can be used as intercalary grafts or to reconstruct a part of a resected joint. Articular cartilage is partially freeze protected by pretreatment with DMSO or glycerol before freezing. The freeze protection is to increase the number of viable cells transplanted, thus reducing in theory the risk of early osteoarthritis seen in patients with osteoarticular allografts. Since ligament and tendon attachments are left on the allograft, remaining soft tissue structures of the recipient can be reattached; this is the major advantage that osteochondral allografts enjoy over endoprostheses. The disadvantages of osteochondral allografts include early osteoarthritis and joint instability or stiffness. Both intercalary and osteochondral allografts share other drawbacks that include size incompatibility, graft reabsorption, stress fractures, high rate of infection and the possibility of transmitting disease, e.g. HIV disease. Many of these drawbacks can be obviated by using a total joint endoprosthesis/allograft composite (Figure 10.37). Allograft replacement is the treat-

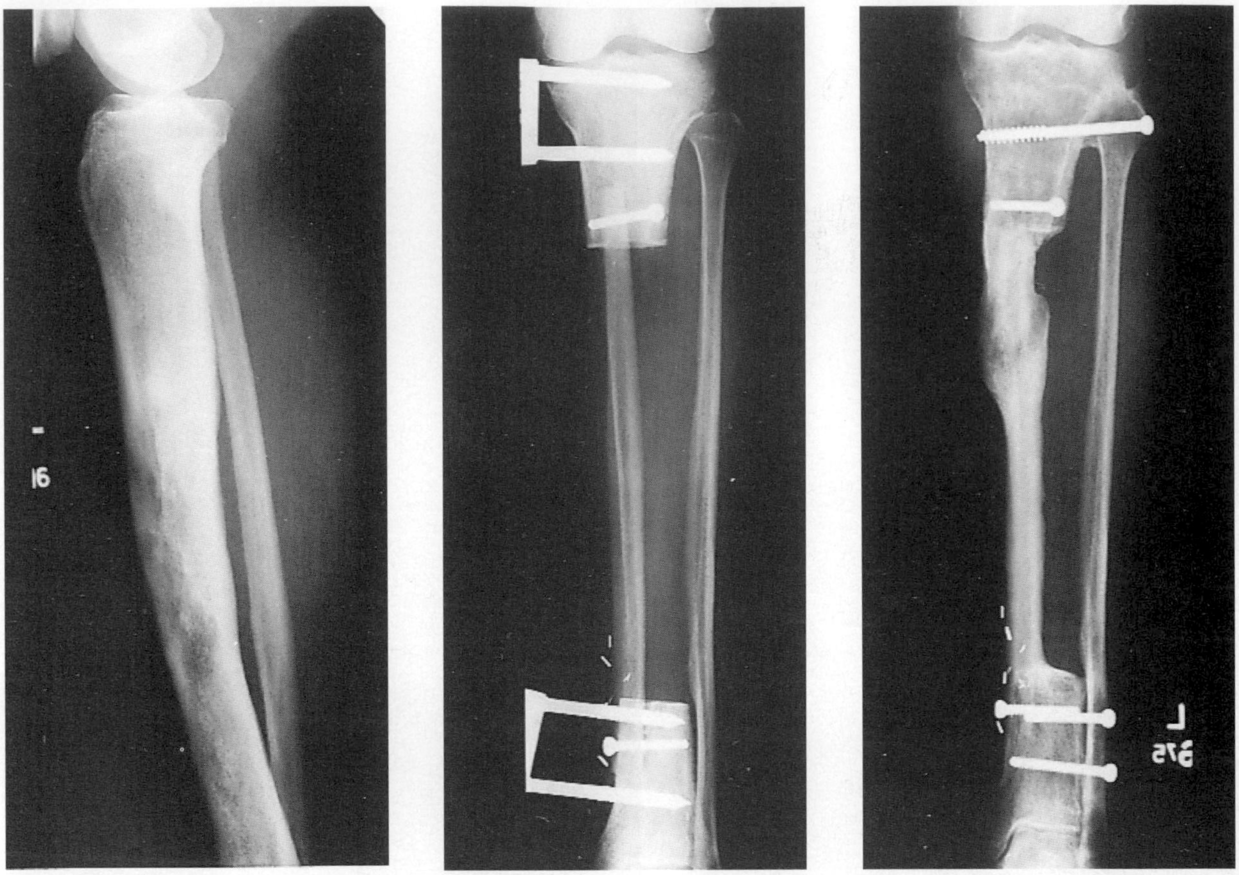

(a) (b) (c)

Figure 10.36 (a) Squamous cell carcinoma occurring in the site of chronic osteomyelitis. (b) Vascularized fibula autograft reconstruction of the surgical defect in the tibia. (c) The vascularized fibula autograft 5 years later free of infection and tumour.

ment of choice for reconstruction of the hemipelvis (Figure 10.38) and replacement of the diaphysis of weight-bearing long bones (Figure 10.39). Although intercalary endoprostheses have been tried with limited success, they are currently inferior to allografts. A modification of the intercalary allograft technique is joint fusion using an allograft to bridge the resected part of the joint (Figure 10.40). Improvements in biomaterials and endoprosthesis design are gradually eroding the remaining relative advantages of allograft over endoprostheses for massive joint reconstruction.

Bone graft substitutes

While autograft and allograft remain the most commonly used osteoinductive materials in reconstructive surgery, the limited availability and high cost of bone graft, as well as concerns of transmitting infectious diseases have led to the development of several synthetic bone graft substitutes. Granules of hydroxyapatite and tricalcium composite are available, and appear to be most effective when mixed with host bone or bone marrow. Similarly, blocks of porous, highly crystalline hydroxyapatite are somewhat brittle, but may also be useful in filling bone defects. At the present time, however, neither of these compounds by itself is likely to be satisfactory in weight-bearing applications. In the near future, however, synthetic growth factors coupled with calcium phosphate carriers are likely to provide osteoinductive as well as osteoconductive materials useful for skeletal reconstruction.

ENDOPROSTHETIC REPLACEMENT

Endoprostheses are improving rapidly and will be the dominate technology in the near future for major skeletal reconstruction. Endoprostheses enjoy many advantages over allografts. First, they can be made in any size or shape. Because of modularity of the

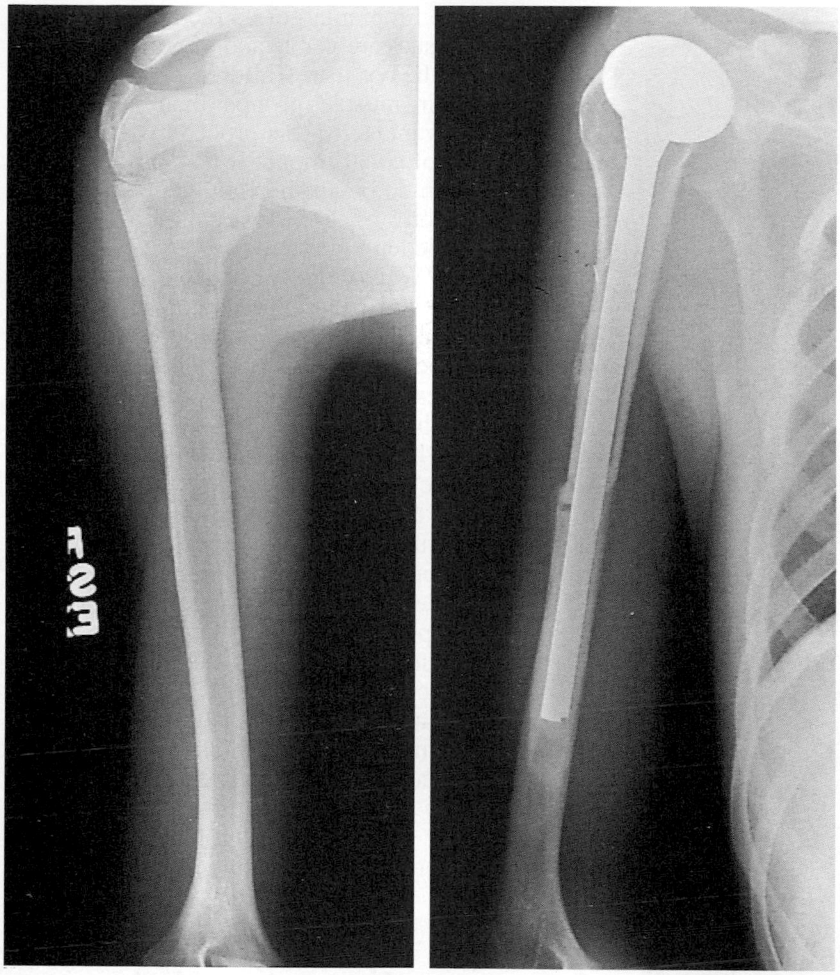

(a) (b)

Figure 10.37 (a) Osteosarcoma of the proximal humerus in a 16-year-old boy. (b) Neer endoprosthesis and proximal humeral allograft and allograft/host rotator cuff repair.

components an endoprosthesis can be fabricated or modified at the time of surgery to reflect any changes in the operative plan. Skeletal reconstruction using an endoprosthesis requires less operative time than an allograft and the surgical infection rate is less. Unlike allografts, endoprostheses can be sterilized, thus, have no chance of spreading transmittable diseases, e.g. HIV disease. Postoperative rehabilitation is shorter which is important for patients that may have a shorter life expectancy. They are far stronger than bone graft, and mechanical breakage is not a current problem. The endoprosthesis attachment to the host bone has also improved due to the advances in bone ingrowth technology and hydroxyapatite coatings. When endoprostheses eventually loosen or wear out their revision is less technologically demanding than revising an allograft to a total joint replacement. The main disadvantage of endoprosthetic design relates to the inability of soft tissue structures, such as tendons, ligaments, and muscle origins, to attach to the device's biomaterial. Endoprostheses are used mainly around the knee and hip (Figures 10.41 and 10.42), or in combination with allografts to reconstruct the shoulder and proximal tibia.

ROTATIONPLASTY

In Europe the Van Nes rotationplasty has gained acceptance as a method of reconstruction after an intercalary amputation for malignant disease (Kotz and Salzer, 1982). While not as popular in North America, it is useful for the post-resection reconstruction of the lower extremity in the growing child. Most commonly, the tumour is located in the distal femur adjacent or involving the knee but must not involve the sciatic nerve. If the sciatic nerve is involved then amputation is imperative. The resection includes the knee and as much of the femur as

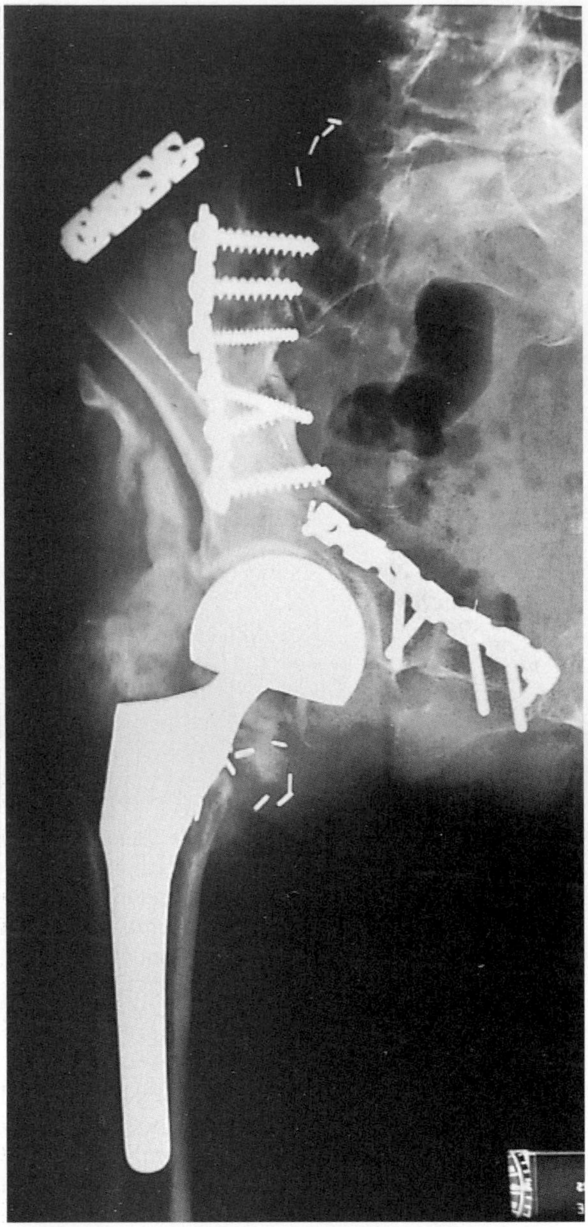

Figure 10.38 Proximal femoral endoprosthesis and pelvic allograft (acetabulum and part of the ilium) 4 years after pelvic reconstruction for a chondrosarcoma.

necessary. The lower leg is externally rotated 180° and the tibia is internally fixed to the proximal femur. In effect the ankle joint functions as a knee joint and the calf muscles act as the flexors and extenders of the new knee. The foot simulates a below the knee amputation stump. A prosthetic orthosis is fitted. The child functions like a person with a below-knee amputation instead of the poorly functioning patient with a high above-knee amputation. Because the proximal femoral and distal tibial epiphyseal plates are spared, the limb enlarges as the child grows. In addition, all tissues are viable and of normal strength, thus allowing heavy use. Children do better at re-educating their muscle groups than adults. The primary disadvantage to this procedure is cosmetic and the psychological impact it has on the patient. Again, children do better than adults in adjusting to their altered body image. Most children are happy that they avoided amputation.

Gottsauner-Wolf (Gottsauner-Wolf *et al.* 1991) reported on the Austrian experience with 70 young patients that had undergone rotationplasty for sarcoma. The procedure was found to be excellent for eradicating local disease with only one local recurrence out of the 70 treated, but there were many complications, both early and late, the most severe of which were occlusion of the re-anastomosed vessels in 10% of the cases, that led to three amputations. The patients' function was found to be comparable with that of below-knee amputees. Many of the patients returned to sports activities. None of the patients had phantom pain or symptoms of an amputation neuroma. In North America, Cammisa *et al.* (1990) functionally tested 12 patients that had undergone rotationplasty and concluded that these patients performed as well as those who had endoprosthetic replacement and better than those who had above the knee amputation. From these studies it is reasonable to conclude that rotationplasty is a favourable alternative to amputation.

Intraoperative adjuncts to surgery

The role of an intraoperative adjunct is to extend the surgical margins to reduce the chance of recurrence. Phenol is commonly used to sterilize the tumour bed after giant cell tumour resection. It is an example of a chemical adjunct to surgery. The main disadvantage to phenol is that it is hard to control and injury to surrounding soft tissues can occur. In addition, phenol does not penetrate deeply into the bone, thus it is possible to leave viable tumour behind.

Cryosurgery has a number of advantages over phenol as a surgical adjunct. Marcove *et al.* (1973) performed the first bone cryosurgery in 1964. The first patient to be treated with cryosurgery had metastatic lung carcinoma. The indications for this mode of therapy expanded to include many benign but aggressive neoplasms including giant cell tumours, chondroblastomas and aneurysmal bone cysts. The treatment of giant cell tumour of bone had

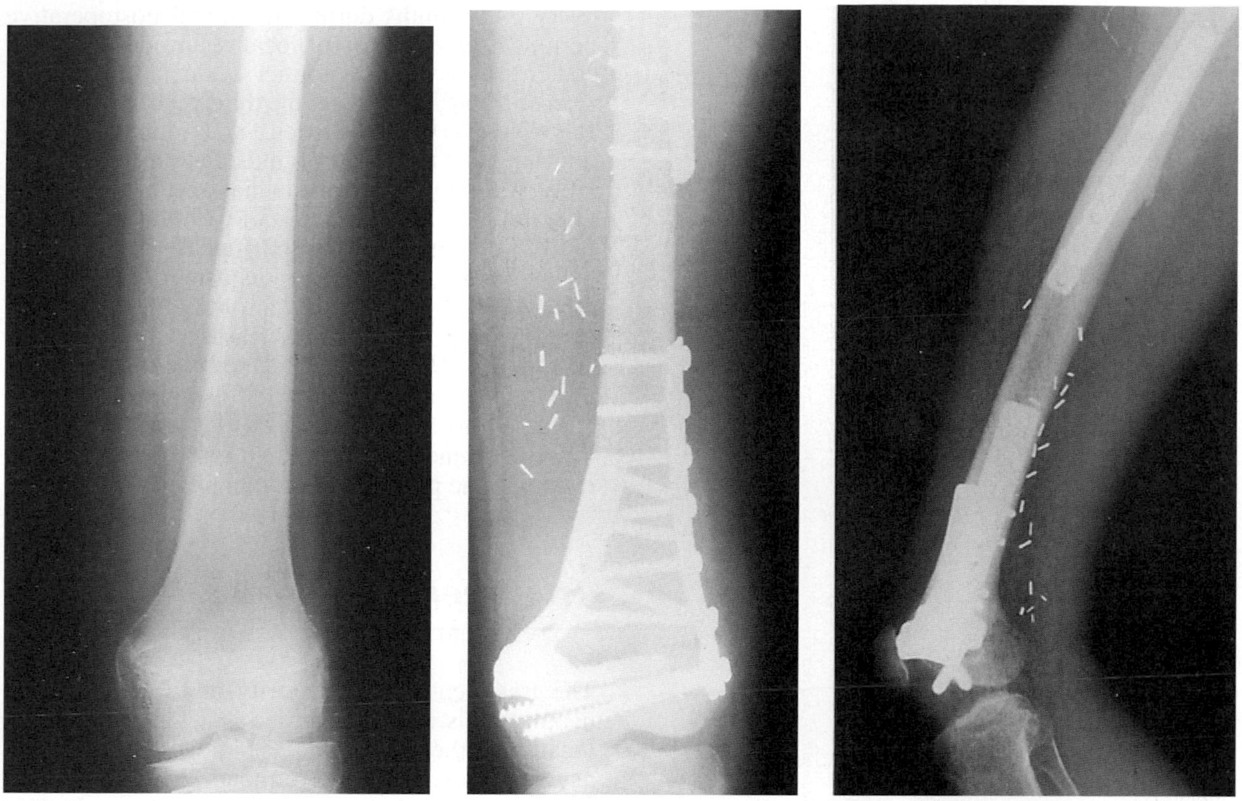

(a) (b) (c)

Figure 10.39 (a) Osteosarcoma of the distal femur in a 12-year-old girl. (b) and (c) Intercalary femoral allograft 4 years after excision and reconstruction.

always been marked by a high local recurrence rate. Marcove *et al.* (1973) reported on 25 giant cell tumours treated by cryosurgery and found lower rate of recurrence than had been reported before. Only 8% had obvious clinical recurrence at the time of a second-look biopsy with an additional 24% with microscopic disease. In a subsequent paper Marcove (1982) reported on the extension of the indications for cryosurgery to include unicameral bone cysts, fibromyxoma of bone, fibrous dysplasia, eosinophilic granuloma, haemangioma of bone and large chondromas. The limiting factor of cryosurgery is size with the largest tumour not exceeding 12 cm in diameter. Marcove reported a 2% recurrent rate in the last 50 patients treated. With this method the margins of the resection can be extended for over 1 cm. The factors involved in the extent of freezing and subsequent necrosis are density and vascularity of bone, presence or absence of tourniquet, size of lesion, duration of the freeze, the rate of freezing and thawing. For malignant disease the author uses cryotherapy for the treatment of symptomatic metastatic lesions that are either radioresistant or recurrent after the maximum dose of radiation has been given. The main drawback to this technique is the high rate of complications, include local flap necrosis, secondary fractures, nerve injuries and bone infection. While useful, this technique has been supplanted in part by cementation for benign bone tumours.

Persson *et al.* (1987) reported a study done in Sweden on giant cell tumours treated with intralesional excision and reconstruction with acrylic bone cement. This method of treatment achieves tumour control similar to cryosurgery while subjecting the patient to a lower rate of complications. It is our preferred method for the treatment of giant cell tumour and similar aggressive benign lesions of bone.

While intraoperative radiation therapy has been found useful in other disciplines, it is rarely used in the treatment of musculoskeletal tumours. It is also very expensive and poses considerable logistic problems to the surgeon and operating room personnel. Most importantly, external beam radiation and brachial therapy are better suited for the extremities.

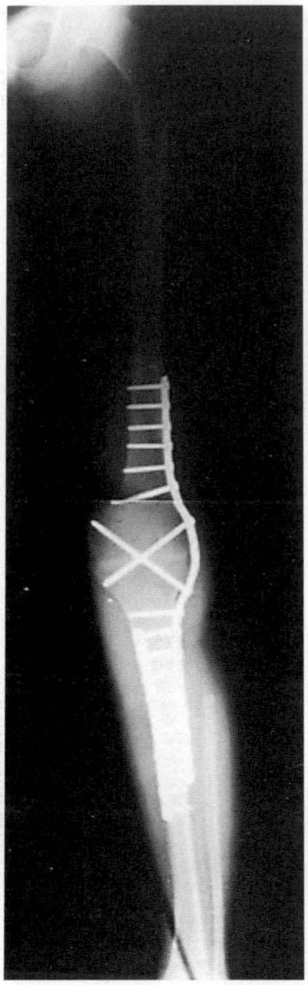

Figure 10.40 One year after wide resection of proximal tibia for osteosarcoma. Knee was fused with an intercalary tibial allograft.

Postoperative follow-up

The initial treatment marks only the beginning of the total treatment plan. In selected patients postoperative radiation and/or chemotherapy play essential roles in the local and general control of the disease. Even after treatment with these modalities have been completed the patient requires careful follow-up in order to discover local recurrence and metastatic disease at the earliest possible and most treatable stage. Recurrent tumour and metastatic deposits can also metastasize and add to the mortality rate, but with early treatment further spread can be prevented. Local recurrence becomes clinically apparent usually in the first 2 years after the initial treatment, varying with the histological grade of the neoplasm. During this 2-year period patients with high-grade tumours are seen every 2 months for clinical examination of the tumour site and a biplanar chest x-ray. Patients with low-grade tumours are seen every 3–4 months during this initial postoperative period. Any suspicion of local recurrence or metastatic disease requires further evaluated with a CT scan or a MRI scan. After the third year the patient is followed every 6 months for 2 additional years. The total length of follow-up for most sarcomas is 5 years. However, chondrosarcomas may recur many years after initial treatment and should be seen once a year for the rest of their lives. Clinical evaluation by palpation and inspection is adequate for some but in others, e.g. thighs, pelvis and back, are best evaluated by either MRI or CT scans. During the critical early period the scans are obtained two to three times a year depending on the type of the tumours and the adequacy of the initial treatment. The discovery of local recurrence or metastatic disease is followed by restaging the patient and prompt treatment.

Treatment of unusual tumours

The treatment of the majority of musculoskeletal neoplasms is very similar and is determined by the location of the tumour and its biological aggressiveness. However, certain tumours deserve special mention due to the controversy that surrounds their treatment or the uniqueness of their behaviour.

DESMOID TUMOURS OF SOFT TISSUE

The treatment of desmoid tumours has been marked by frequent recurrence of this benign but locally aggressive soft tissue tumour. Rock *et al.* (1984) report a recurrence rate of 68% at an average of 1.4 years after the first treatment. This recurrence rate is much higher than what could be expected in a sarcoma of equal size and location. They recommend wide local excision when feasible or marginal excision and postoperative radiation therapy. Zelefsky *et al.* (1991) agreed that conservative surgical resection and postoperative interstitial iridium-192 is effective therapy for desmoid tumours.

McDougall (McDougall and McGarrity, 1979) reported three cases of extra-abdominal desmoid tumours in which two tumours disappeared after the patients went through the menopause and the desmoid in the third patient varied in size during the patient's menstrual cycle. The authors tested this third tumour and found oestrogen receptor sites. Tamoxifen was prescribed, but the results were inconclusive.

Other forms of non-surgical therapy have been tried with varying success. Klein *et al.* (1987) found only one patient in the seven studied showed a

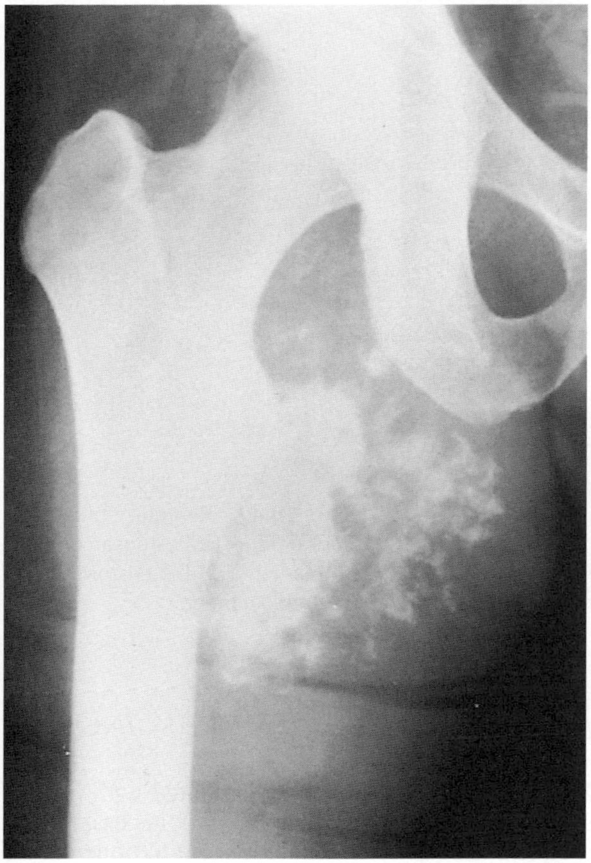

(a)

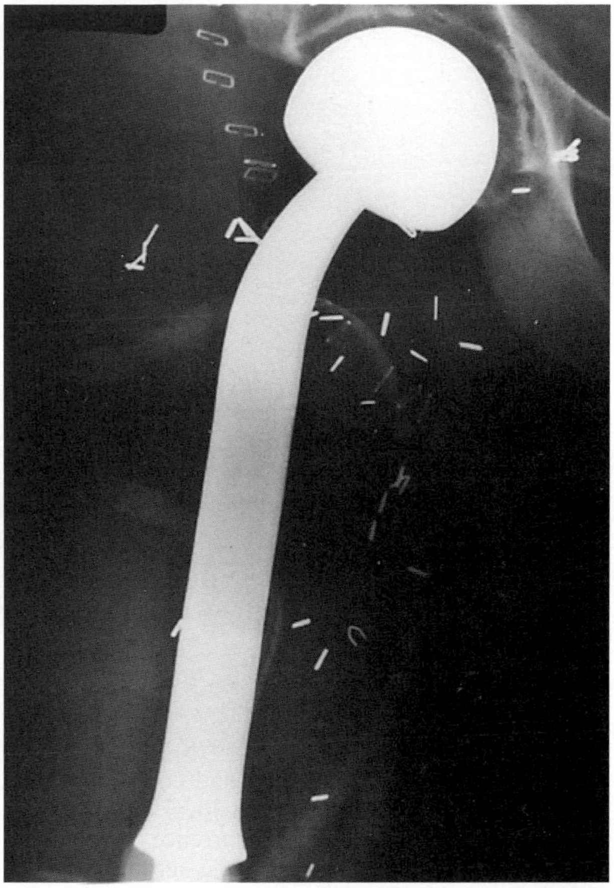

(b)

Figure 10.41 (a) Chondrosarcoma of the proximal femur. (b) After resection and reconstruction with a proximal femoral endoprosthesis.

response to indomethacin, sulindac or tamoxifen used as a single agent or in combination. Low-dose vinblastine and methotrexate has been used with success by Weiss and Lackman (1989) to treat eight patients with desmoid tumours. They concluded that chemotherapy was an acceptable alternative to radical surgery in selected patients.

The Cleveland Clinic describes a less surgically aggressive protocol for the treatment of desmoid tumours. After the desmoid is diagnosed by open or needle biopsy the patient is either followed by close observation and measurement if there is no history of rapid progression of the tumour mass or by tamoxifen therapy if there is a history of rapid progression. For those desmoids that do increase in size during observation tamoxifen is prescribed. The patients that fail tamoxifen treatment undergo wide surgical resection. Only those patients with involved margins or gross tumour left behind are treated with radiation therapy. The conservative use of radiation therapy is because of the real chance of producing a post-radiation sarcoma in these usually young patients. Chemotherapy is reserved for patients with desmoid tumours located in a surgically inaccessible location.

EWING'S SARCOMA

In 1921 James Ewing described a malignant small cell sarcoma of bone with a dismal prognosis that bears his name. The treatment of choice was radiation therapy to achieve local control. Most centres experienced a very high local recurrence rate and a 5-year survival rate of less than 10%. Macintosh *et al.* in 1975 reported the experience of the Bristol Royal Infirmary with Ewing's sarcoma, in which he reported 2-year disease-free survival rates of 24% for tumours of long bones and 5% for other bones mostly located in the axial skeleton. All the sarcomas were initially radiosensitive; however, one-third of the tumours recurred locally. In that series neither whole bone radiation nor higher doses ensured local control. Therefore surgery for local control should be considered.

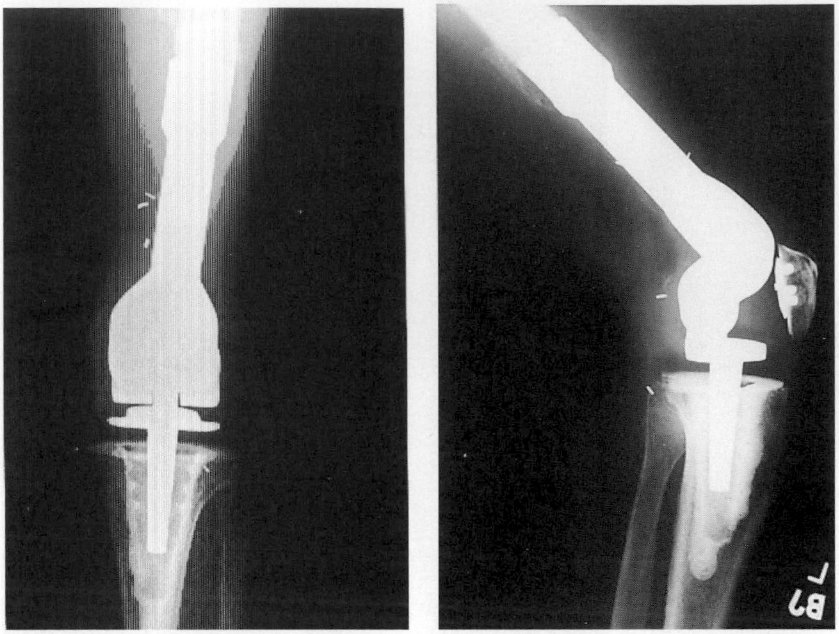

(a) (b)

Figure 10.42 Resection of a distal femoral periosteal osteosarcoma reconstructed with a custom total knee replacement.

In 1975, Pritchard *et al.* (1975) studied 229 patients with Ewing's sarcoma and concluded that patients treated with surgery for local control, e.g. amputation, had fewer local recurrences and better survival than patients treated by non-surgical means. Other authors in Europe and North America confirmed Pritchard's findings. Bacci *et al.* (1989) reported the experience of the Istituto Ortopedico Rizzoli with 144 localized Ewing's sarcomas. All the patients were treated with chemotherapy. Patients treated with amputation or resection plus radiotherapy had a significantly better prognosis (60% versus 28%) than those patients treated with radiation alone. Bacci found that Ewing's sarcomas located in the pelvis had a poor prognosis. Since 1980 all authors report significant improvement in prognosis in all groups receiving chemotherapy.

It is recommended that all patients with Ewing's sarcoma receive preoperative chemotherapy followed by surgical resection or amputation. If the margins of the resection are compromised, then radiation therapy should be added to the protocol. Only the most surgically inaccessible lesions should be treated locally by radiation alone. The need for surgery is most apparent in pelvic Ewing's sarcoma. After surgery a prolonged course of chemotherapy is given.

METASTATIC RENAL CELL CARCINOMA

Most metastatic disease can be treated with intralesional excision, internal fixation if necessary and radiation therapy. Metastatic disease to bone can be considered a late and incurable stage of many cancers with the goal being palliation and restoration of function because solitary metastatic deposit is usually followed by widespread musculoskeletal disease. However, renal cell carcinoma can follow a different clinical course with a solitary deposit being the only and potentially curable manifestation of metastatic disease. Long-term, disease-free survival can be achieved after wide resection for cure. In all but the most accessible solitary lesions it is our protocol to radiate the lesion first and wait 6–12 months, and if there is no additional metastatic disease, perform a wide resection of the solitary focus. If there is an impending pathological fracture a wide resection should be considered as the initial treatment.

Treatment of metastatic sarcoma

In the past patients who had metastatic sarcoma to the lung eventually died. In 1971, Martini *et al.* reported long-term survival of patients with solitary pulmonary metastases who had pulmonary resections. The success of this treatment was made possible by the biological behaviour of sarcomas. Haematogenous spread of sarcoma to the lung is the most common metastatic route, and may be the only site of spread until late in the course of the disease. The aggressive surgical removal of metastatic pulmonary nodules was incorporated into most treatment protocols for osteogenic sarcomas and soft tissue sarcomas. Roth *et al.* (1985) of the American National Cancer Institute studied this form of treatment and found that for soft tissue sarcomas the number of metastatic nodules, disease-free interval and tumour doubling time significantly correlated with postoperative survival. Patients with four or fewer nodules survived longer than patients with more than four. Patients with a disease-free interval longer than 12 months had a longer survival than patients with a disease-free interval less than 12 months. In addition, Roth observed that patients with a tumour doubling time of more than 20 days did better. In this study the only significant predictor of survival for osteogenic sarcoma was the number of nodules. Generally, between 20 and 40% of patients with metastatic sarcoma to the lung can be salvaged by careful postoperative follow-up and aggressive surgical treatment of metastatic disease. All sarcoma patients with metastatic disease confined to the lung should be considered for pulmonary resection.

Treatment of locally recurrent sarcoma

Local recurrence of a sarcoma after surgical treatment is a serious problem that is frequently associated with widespread disease and death. However, some of the patients may have their life and limb salvaged by further treatment. When local recurrence is detected then careful and complete restaging is mandatory. The presence of metastatic disease is a major determinant of future local treatment. If the metastatic disease is extensive then the goal of treatment is palliation to improve the quality of the patient's remaining life. Limited local resection of the recurrence with radiation therapy can be considered. If the sarcoma is locally confined and there are only a few metastatic lung nodules in addition to the local recurrence then long-term survival can still be achieved. In that case the local disease should be surgically treated for permanent control and the pulmonary nodules resected. The type of treatment for local recurrence depends on the extent of the local disease and the likelihood of previous surgical spread into neighbouring compartments. When limb-sparing operation is undertaken then the margin must be either radical or wide. If there is any doubt concerning involvement of the surgical margin with tumour then radiation therapy is prescribed. When the possibility exists that the neighbouring anatomical compartments are involved with recurrent tumour, then amputation should be considered the best treatment.

Radiation therapy

Although surgical removal provides the greatest opportunity for cure of patients with malignant primary bone and soft tissue neoplasms, a large number of patients having primary surgery cannot be cured by surgery alone. Multiple disciplines should be involved in developing and carrying out the appropriate plan of patient management, in order to achieve the best result. Chemotherapy and radiation therapy have greatly improved survival rates and local recurrence rates. Chemotherapy finds its greatest use in the treatment of systemic disease while radiation therapy is primarily concerned with the local control of the disease either in combination with surgery or less frequently as the sole modality. The treatment of metastatic carcinomas of the skeleton depends to a great extent on radiation therapy.

Amputation provides better local control for extremity sarcoma than limb-sparing surgery. The higher local recurrence rates in patients treated with limb-sparing surgery have been attributed to inadequate excisions that leave viable tumour cells at the surgical margins. The goal of providing a patient with a functional limb after excision of an osseous or soft tissue sarcoma often is challenged by anatomical constraints, such as tumour impingement on a critical neurovascular structure. In such cases, the surgeon is faced with the dilemma of deciding whether to leave intact a functional limb potentially compromised by microscopically positive surgical margins or to amputate the extremity. The incidence of microscopically positive margins is 13–36% in patients undergoing limb-sparing surgery (Collin *et al.* 1986, 1987; Potter *et al.*, 1986; Brennan *et al.*, 1991). Microscopically positive margins lead to local recurrences. It is important to avoid local recurrence because it places the patient at further risk of developing metastatic disease that may lead to death.

Lindberg *et al.* in the 1960s pioneered the concept of postoperative adjuvant high-dose radiation therapy (Lindberg *et al.*, 1981). The initial reports of high-dose radiation therapy (5000–6500 cGy) after complete local excision of these tumours described a very impressive local control rate of 80% with a decrease in the need for amputation to approximately 10%. The effectiveness of radiation therapy decreases proportionally to the amount of residual disease left behind by the surgery. The surgeon should make every attempt to achieve a wide surgical margin when dealing with a high-grade sarcoma.

There are two types of radiation therapy in musculoskeletal oncology. The first type is external beam megavoltage photons of electron beam radiation. The radiation may be given to the tumour preoperatively or to the tumour field postoperatively. The total dose can be split between the pre- and postoperative periods. A strip of normal tissue is spared along the length of the irradiated limb and the joints are shielded where possible. The usual dose of radiation in the extremity is between 5000 and 6500 cGy. Twenty-five to thirty fractions over 5–6 weeks are usually necessary.

Brachytherapy is another method of adjuvant radiation therapy. It is a postoperative technique where the soft tissue sarcoma is first excised with marginal or wide margins and immediately thin plastic catheters are inserted into the tumour bed at 1 or 2 cm intervals. These catheters are brought out lateral to the wound closure (Figure 10.43). Two to eight days later the catheters are after-loaded with iridium-192 seeds. The time and number of seeds are determined by a nomogram based on the wound and tumour bed size and seed strength. The average dose of radiation delivered by this technique is 4500 cGy and the sarcomas of the extremity and superficial trunk (Harrison *et al.*, 1993). All patients underwent a grossly complete resection with a limb sparing operation. On histological examination 20% had

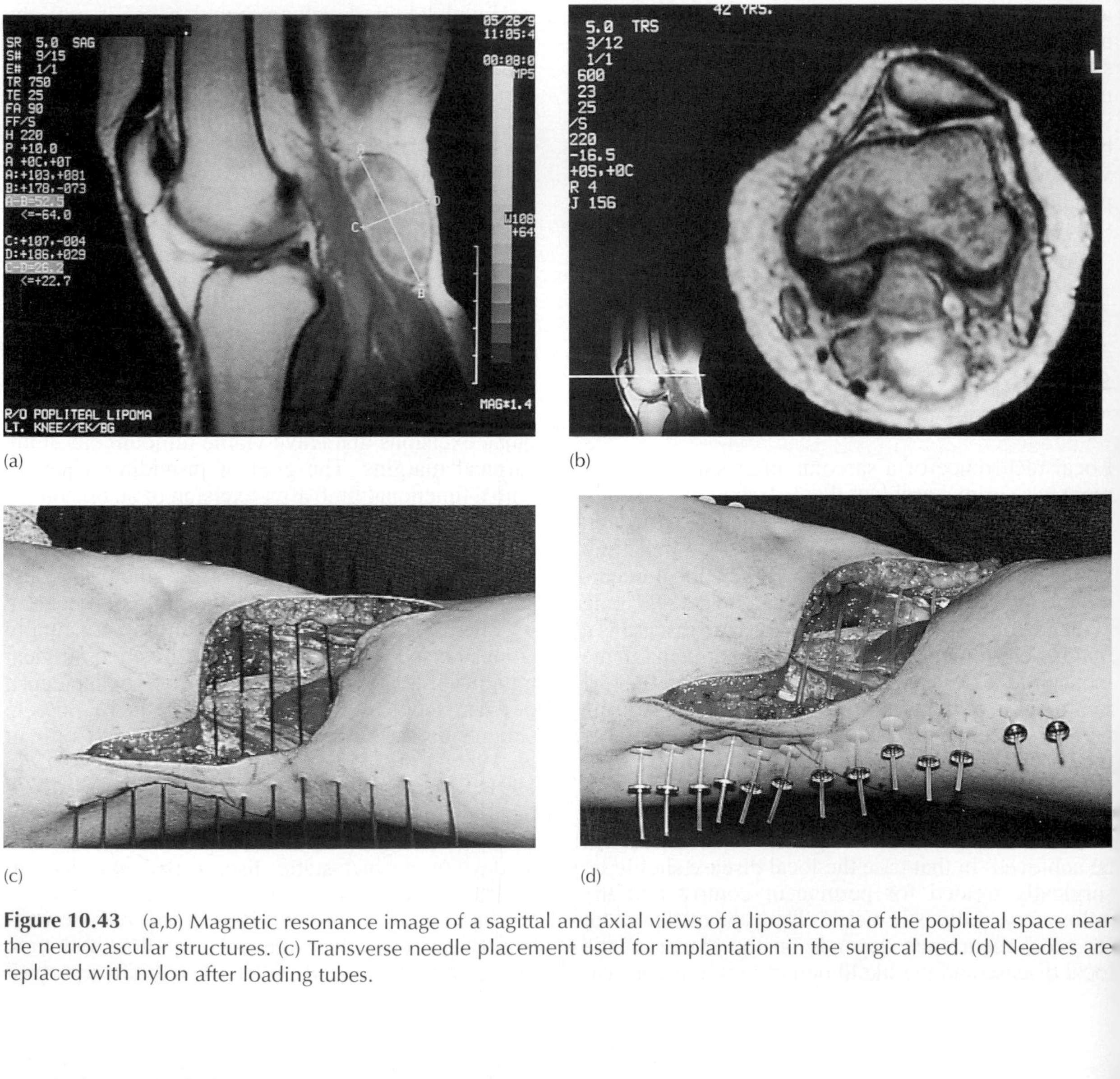

Figure 10.43 (a,b) Magnetic resonance image of a sagittal and axial views of a liposarcoma of the popliteal space near the neurovascular structures. (c) Transverse needle placement used for implantation in the surgical bed. (d) Needles are replaced with nylon after loading tubes.

positive margins. At 5 years, local control was 82% in the brachytherapy treated group compared with 67% in the control group that did not receive radiation therapy. Brachytherapy provides excellent local control and significantly shortens the treatment time when compared to adjuvant external beam radiation.

Either type of radiation can cause early or late local complications. Wound healing is often a problem in irradiated tissues and wound infections are more common. Bones that have been irradiated are slow to heal any osteotomies or fractures. Bones included in the radiation port may develop pathological fractures. Muscles may become more fibrotic and lose their strength and excursion. If joints are included in the radiation port the ensuing joint fibrosis often decreases its range of motion. Extremity swelling can be a great problem to the patient. A small number of extremities that have undergone radiation therapy will need to be amputated to improve function and to alleviate the local problems caused by the radiation.

The complication of most concern is post-radiation sarcoma. The latent period between radiotherapy and diagnosis of sarcoma averaged 14.3 years in a series from the Mayo Clinic reported by Weatherby *et al.* (1981). In that series only about 30% of the patients survived 5 years without recurrence. The low risk of sarcoma following radiotherapy for treatment of malignant disease in adult patients should not be a contraindication for its use in these patients. Childhood tumours should be treated by radiation therapy with great caution due to the many years that the young patient is at risk following treatment. Radiation therapy for benign bone or soft tissue tumours should be reserved for lesions that are not amenable to surgical treatment.

Chemotherapy

The introduction of systemic chemotherapy has dramatically improved survival rates for patients with osteosarcoma and Ewing's sarcoma. The current role of chemotherapy in the management of patients with soft tissue sarcoma, however, is unclear.

Up until recently osteosarcoma was treated by through-the-bone amputation or disarticulation of the involved extremity. Even with amputation more than 80% of the patients went on to develop metastatic disease. Those patients must have had microscopic, subclinical pulmonary metastases at the time of ablative surgery. Reasoning that chemotherapy should be most effective against microscopic disease, adjuvant clinical trials were initiated in the early 1970s using high-dose methotrexate with leucovorin rescue. The adjuvant use of doxorubicin or cisplatin as single agents was similarly employed. These clinical trials demonstrated the efficacy of each agent as an adjuvant in the treatment of osteosarcoma when compared to historical controls. In trials using these adjuvants approximately 60% of patients remain continuously free of disease at 5 years.

Similar success was achieved by adjuvant chemotherapy in the treatment of Ewing's sarcoma. Surgery and radiotherapy were the mainstays of therapy for Ewing's sarcoma prior to the 1960s. The prognosis was dismal and because of that local control by radiotherapy was adequate. After several agents were noted to be active in metastatic Ewing's sarcoma, adjuvant trials were begun (Hustu *et al.*, 1972; Jaffe *et al.*, 1976; Rosan *et al.*, 1981). In all these studies, the failure rate declined when compared to the failure rate among historical controls.

Chemotherapy can be given preoperatively, postoperatively or in combination. Preoperative chemotherapy was first given to osteosarcoma patients while they waited for their endoprosthesis to be fabricated. Casper *et al.* (1994) has pointed out that preoperative chemotherapy is desirable for several reasons. First, occult micrometastases would be subjected to chemotherapy before acquiring resistance. Second, preoperative chemotherapy may be expected to limit tumour spread before the operation. Third, the experimentally observed postoperative growth spurt of micrometastases is ablated by preoperative treatment. Fourth, the effect of chemotherapy on the size of the tumour may permit a less radical operation. Finally, response to preoperative chemotherapy may have prognostic significance and could be used to guide postoperative treatment.

There are general and local risks associated with preoperative chemotherapy. Primary among these risks is that non-responding patients to chemotherapy delay their surgery while the tumour grows and possibly spreads. Complications of chemotherapy may further delay the needed surgery. All chemotherapy to varying degrees debilitates and immunosuppresses the patient, thus adding to the risk of surgery. Postoperatively, infections and wound complications are more frequently observed in patients who have undergone preoperative chemotherapy and can, when encountered, delay the postoperative chemotherapy or radiation therapy. However, most surgical oncologists believe that the benefits of neoadjuvant chemotherapy outweigh the risks.

McDonald *et al.* (1990) studied the influence of chemotherapy on perioperative complications in limb salvage surgery for bone tumour. He found that patients who did not receive any chemotherapy had a

25.2% incidence of complications. This compares with a 55.4% incidence in patients that received chemotherapy prior to surgery. The most common complication was infection in 11.8% of the patients. After neoadjuvant chemotherapy, reconstruction with an uncemented prosthesis led to the fewest complications.

The value of adjuvant chemotherapy for the treatment of patients with high-grade soft tissue sarcomas remains unknown. Some trials have indicated an improved disease-free survival advantage with a trend toward improved survival in patients with extremity sarcomas (Edmonson *et al.*, 1984; Chang *et al.*, 1988) but others have not reported significant improvement in disease-free or overall survival times with adjuvant chemotherapy (Wilson *et al.*, 1986; Eilber *et al.*, 1988). Until the role of chemotherapy in soft tissue sarcoma is better defined we have reserved chemotherapy for those patients with poor prognostic factors. Generally, younger patients in good health, with large (greater than 5 cm) high-grade sarcomas are treated by chemotherapy. In addition, those patients with metastatic sarcoma are also treated.

PATHOLOGY OF MUSCULOSKELETAL TUMOURS

The subject of 'bone tumours' is confused because there has been failure between pathologists, radiologists and clinicians to agree upon a generally acceptable terminology.

1. In response to injury, infection, or in consequence of maldevelopment or hormonal disturbance, localized overgrowth of bone, cartilage or fibrous tissue may occur. These lesions present as bony swellings and the clinician has by custom (and, for many reasons, convenience) described these as 'tumours' although they are not, in a pathological sense, neoplasms. Such 'tumours' are self-limiting, yet structurally they have a similar appearance to true neoplasms (e.g. 'osteoma' or 'chondroma').
2. In bone there are not only cells concerned with the formation and the maintenance of the osseous structure – the truly 'osteogenic' tissues – but many other elements are present: marrow (haemopoietic) tissue, fat, nerves, blood vessels, and, forming a sheath over the surface of the bone, there is a condensation of fascia (fibrous outer layer of the periosteum). Further, certain tissues are included within bony spaces and canals – teeth, epithelial linings of air sinuses, the notochord. From each of these structures tumours may arise and, again by custom, they are often described as 'bone tumours'.
3. The presence of bone in a tumour is not of diagnostic significance and the term 'osteogenic' has, in consequence, been frequently misused.
   (a) In certain tumours ossification may be a function of the tumour cells, and in such instances these cells can be regarded as neoplastic osteoblasts. It is correct, therefore, to employ the terms osteoma, osteosarcoma or osteoblastic sarcoma. It is often difficult to differentiate between *malignant* ossification (i.e. bone formed by malignant osteoblasts) and *benign* ossification (i.e. bone formed by normal osteoblastic activity in malignancy in cartilage, osteoid or collagenous tissues) or from other normal bone formed in response to malignant tissue.
   (b) Ossification within the stroma of a neoplasm may arise from local changes in the calcium metabolism and circulation, but in such cases it is usually possible to differentiate between the true tumour cells and those which are in juxtaposition to the new bone spicules and by which the bone is obviously formed.
   (c) A further difficulty arises from the reaction of the normal tissue adjacent to the tumour – especially a malignant one. As a result of increased vascularity, or by pressure of the tumour in a direction perpendicular to the normal lines of stress on the trabeculae, there may be marked absorption. There may be mechanical compression of the blood vessels with consequent ischaemic necrosis and sequestrum formation. Thus around any tumour there may be seen decalcified osteoid tissue, necrosed bone and multinucleated giant cells (osteoclasts) removing the debris.
   (d) There is frequently beneath the periosteum new bone formation which is reactionary in type. The degree of this reaction varies, and is observed in tumours which arise primarily in bone as well as in metastatic lesions – e.g. in secondary tumours of the prostate and in relation to the meningiomata. In part at least the 'sunray' spicules observed in the osteosarcoma and the new bone laid down parallel to the shaft and called 'Codman's triangle' by the radiologist is a non-neoplastic reaction.

A very striking example is the 'onion layers' seen in Ewing's tumour.

4. Bone develops from primitive mesenchyme. From this by differentiation there develops a common immediate precursor of those cellular elements which are identified in growing and adult bone as the osteoblast, the chondroblast, the osteoclast and the fibroblast, to produce bone, cartilage, the absorption of bone or collagen.

   In tumours derived from these cells the same power of metaplasia is commonly manifest, and accordingly within the same tumour widely different histological pictures are observed. Thus while the predominant feature may be cartilage formation, in other areas there may be well marked ossification or only fibroblasts with collagen fibres. In anaplastic tumours the dedifferentiation may have been so marked that it is impossible to adduce the cell type from which it came – the pathological diagnosis being an undifferentiated sarcoma.

Biological properties of musculoskeletal tumours

In order to classify and to characterize particular tumour types it is important:

1. *To define the cell of origin.* Often in tumours of bone, whether benign or malignant, it is difficult to determine from what cells they arise; e.g. an osteogenic sarcoma may arise from 'malignant' osteoblasts or from primary mesenchymal cells. However, other tumours such as chordoma arising from notochordal remnants, adamantinoma (particularly of the jaw, which is thought to arise from dental epithelium) and the various haemopoietic and lymphoid tumours all arise from more recognizable origins.
2. *To identify the cytology of the tumour cell and its stroma as well as their degree of differentiation.* Cells which show lack of differentiation or fail to represent any recognizable cellular type, or vary in size or shape, or demonstrate increased nuclear staining (e.g. hyperchromatism), or possess nuclei exhibiting mitotic figures or reduplication, are considered more malignant. Malignancy is confirmed by the biological properties of infiltration, metastasizing and the wide field of origin of the cells.
3. *To observe the behaviour and growth of the tumour.* The multipotency of skeletal tissues, and therefore the neoplasia which can result, makes it unlikely that the histological appearances will be the same in all cases. Therefore, on microscopy of small areas or biopsies, there may be difficulty in diagnosis. The presence of giant cells can indicate a response of the host to the tumour or a response of the tumour stroma to the host cells or may be an actual part of the tumour differentiation such as seen in a giant cell tumour or an osteoclastoma. Their presence can confuse a diagnosis, and skilled interpretation of adequate specimens is essential. Johnson (1953), in relating the site of origin of musculoskeletal tumours to the usual cellular activity in that area (Figure 10.44), demonstrated that the giant cell tumour commonly arises in the juxtametaphyseal area because of the usual presence there of osteoclastic activity, which is required for remodelling. An aneurysmal bone cyst is also found here. The osteogenic-osteolytic sarcoma is usually seen just below this area, whereas the fibrosarcoma is in relation to the endosteum and the round cell sarcoma occurs within the medullary cavity as well as a Ewing's sarcoma myeloma. From the parosteal site sarcoma, chondromyxoma fibroma, osteoid osteoma, adamantinoma can all arise. Under the periosteum and within the cortex a fibrous cortical defect can be seen.

In determining the behaviour of tumours, the expressions 'benign' and 'malignant' are often used, but these are relative terms and, indeed, Foulds (1954) considered they have little meaning in evaluating the clinical or experimental behaviour of tumours. He emphasized that it is the tumour's response to its environment, or any change in this environment, which should be used as a guide to the subsequent behaviour of the tumour and, hence, prognosis.

The frequency of *distribution* of the various types of bone tumours has been reviewed by Dahlin (1986) (Table 10.1) and is still the most comprehensive review. The *incidence* of bone tumours as regards the community or population in which it appears, is often difficult to obtain because it is usually based upon analysis of mortality rates. Stout (1961) described the distribution of malignant tumours of soft tissues and peripheral nerves (Table 10.2).

The relative age incidence is shown in Figure 10.45. The first curve of greatest mortality appears between the ages of 15 and 20 years of age (being greater in males), and after this there is a steady secondary peak from the age of 30 years onwards to about 75 years of age. The initial curve is due to primary malignancies of bone, such as osteogenic sarcoma, whereas the latter age grouping is due to

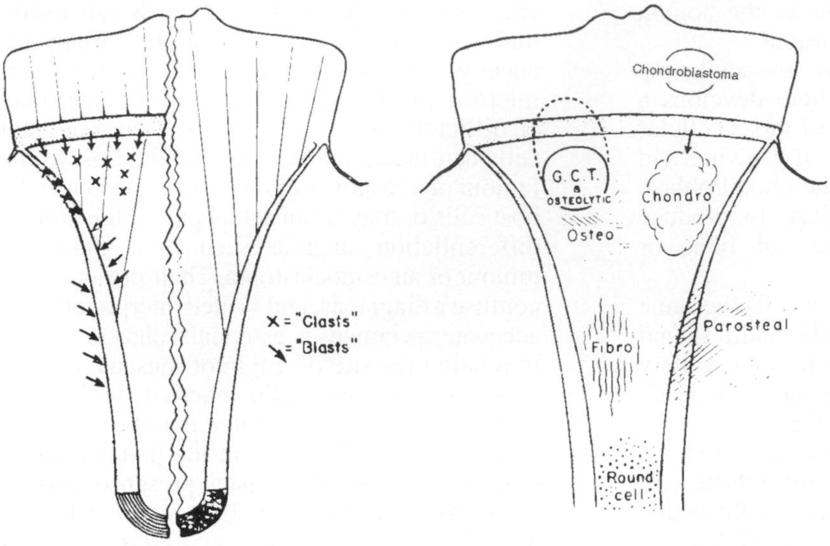

(a) (b)

Figure 10.44 Showing the sites of origin of bone tumours in relation to their cells of origin and their activity. (Reproduced with permission, from Johnson, L. C. (1953) *Bulletin of the New York Academy of Medicine* **27**, 164)

malignant neoplasia in such pre-existing conditions as Paget's disease.

In considering the nature of neoplasia or the development of malignancy in cells (Table 10.3), Burnet (1957) defined it 'as a primary change in the character of cells, which undergo a series of somatic mutations with an increased growth potential rendering them insusceptible to normal growth control'. Goodpasture (1957) defined a malignant tumour as being 'an autonomous new growth which arises from

Table 10.1 Classification of 6221 primary tumours of bone by Dahlin (1986)

Histological type	Benign	Cases	Malignant	Cases
Haematopoietic (41.3%)	–	–	Myeloma	2245
			Reticulum cell sarcoma	327
Chondrogenic (20.9%)	Osteochondroma	579	Primary chondrosarcoma	367
	Chondroma	162	Secondary chondrosarcoma	52
	Chondroblastoma	44	Dedifferentiated chondrosarcoma	51
	Chondromyxoid fibroma	30	Mesenchymal chondrosarcoma	15
Osteogenic (19 3%)	Osteoid osteoma	158	Osteosarcoma	962
	Benign osteoblastoma	43	Parosteal osteogenic sarcoma	36
Unknown origin (9.8%)	Giant cell tumour	264	Ewing's tumour	299
	(Fibrous) histiocytoma	7	Malignant giant cell tumour	20
			Adamantinoma	17
Fibrogenic (3.8%)	Fibroma	72	Fibrosarcoma	158
	Desmoplastic fibroma	4		
Notochordal (3.1%)	–	–	Chordoma	195
Vascular (1.6%)	Haemangioma	69	Haemangioendothelioma	25
			Haemangiopericytoma	5
Lipogenic	Lipoma	5		
Neurogenic	Neurilemmoma	10		
Totals		1447		4774

Reproduced with the permission of the author and of the publishers, Charles C Thomas, Springfield, Illinois, USA.

Table 10.2 Location of malignant tumours of the soft tissues and peripheral nerves

	Upper extremity	Lower extremity
Differentiated fibrosarcoma	62	47
Malignant fibrosarcoma	26	94
Liposarcoma	49	216
Rhabdomyosarcoma	17	64
Synovial sarcoma	25	45
Osteogenic sarcoma	3	11
Chondrosarcoma	6	14
Reticulum cell sarcoma	30	27
Malignant schwannoma	10	15
Neuroepithelioma	7	5

Reproduced with permission, from A. P. Stout, 1961, *Cancer Journal for Clinicians* **11**, 210.

found a high incidence of antibody produced by a irreversible change in a new direction so that the cells fail to respond to normal cellular control'.

VIRUSES

Fujinaga *et al*. (1970) used the Harvey and Moloney sarcoma viruses to induce osteosarcomata in rats and hamsters. In humans, Eilber and Morton (1970)

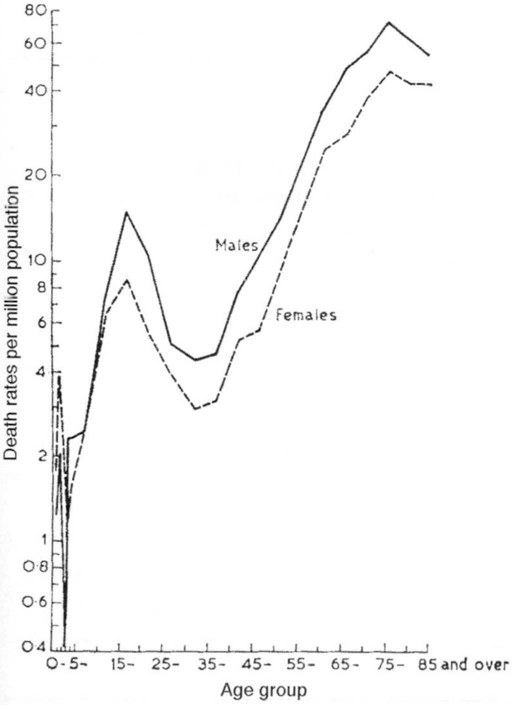

Figure 10.45 The incidence of bony tumours as determined by mortality as regards age and sex. (By courtesy of HM Stationery Office)

sarcoma-specific antigen in patients with different types of sarcomata, and they also isolated the antibody in close relatives. Cell-free extracts from the sarcoma induced the formation of the sarcoma-specific antigens in normal human cells. Because of these findings it was suggested that this virus may be related to the aetiology of sarcoma in man.

IRRADIATION

Irradiation by radioactivity is now well documented as a cause of bone sarcomata; e.g. the dial painters as described by Martland in 1931. Finkel and Biskis (1968) used a variety of isotopes and viruses to induce osteosarcoma in experimental animals.

In the development of a malignancy, the factors must be either (1) chromosomal or genetic, or (2) extrachromosomal in origin. These were reviewed by Sissons and Duthie (1959). At the present time, no single aetiological agent has yet been determined and, indeed, the varying patterns of age incidence, as well as the numerous types, suggest that there are a number of aetiological factors taking part. One of the

Table 10.3 Development of malignancy – an outline of various aetiological factors producing neoplasia

Chromosomal or genetic	Extrachromosomal factors
In animals	Hormones
In tissue culture *in vitro*	Extraneous carcinogens
In humans	Viral
	Irradiation
	Chronic irritation or infection
	Metabolic diseases
	Immunological

difficulties in studying skeletal neoplasia has been the rarity of being able to observe premalignant change of the tissues. There are only four known examples of such lesions:

1. Diaphyseal aclasis (10–15) – chondrosarcoma.
2. Fibrous dysplasia (few) – fibrosarcoma.
3. Irradiated tissues – osteogenic sarcoma.
4. Paget's disease (10–20) – multiple sarcomata (both osteogenic and chondrosarcomata).

In diaphyseal aclasis, which is a strongly inherited condition from an autosomal dominant gene, 10% have been recorded as undergoing chondrosarcomatous changes. In Paget's disease, which is present in about 3–4% of the European population over the age of 40 years (Collins, 1956), 10–20% of these patients have been observed on post-mortem to have developed sarcomatous changes. Indeed, Thomson and Turner-Warwick (1955) reported that 30% of patients over the age of 30 years, with malignant bone change, have Paget's disease. In humans, viruses as carcinogenic agents cannot be implicated as yet although Stewart and Eddy (1956) developed an SE polyoma virus which can produce osteo- and fibrosarcomata experimentally in rodent animals. Duthie (1972), using this virus, has demonstrated some of the properties of lung metastases, after successive excision of the primary osteosarcoma.

Growth patterns and their hormonal background may have some significance in the development of osteogenic sarcoma in males and females. Price (1958) showed that the greatest incidence in females occurs between the ages of 5 and 14 years, whereas in males it is between the ages of 15 and 24 years (Table 10.4). He believed that the higher incidence at this later age in males occurs because they grow longer and larger and, therefore, there are more cells available to undergo malignant mutations. Extraneous carcinogenic agents are now well recognized (e.g. hydrocarbons, aromatic and azo dyes which can produce fibrosarcoma); and radiation from both internal (e.g. plutonium, radium, yttrium, strontium) and external sources of x-irradiation are also well known in producing osteosarcoma both experimentally and accidentally.

Classification of bone tumours

1. *True bone tumours*. Arising from cells of mesenchymal origin, derived from a common ancestry and whose function is primarily skeletal bone formation, these neoplasms fall into four main groups (Table 10.5) according to the predominant cell type present. By reason of the mutability of the cells metaplasia is common and intermediate stages are found.
2. *Tumours arising from tissues normally in bone but not participating in bone formation*. These are outlined in Table 10.6.
3. *Tumours arising from included tissue*. These include chordoma and adamantinoma.
4. *Metastatic tumours of bone*.

Diagnosis

(see 'Musculoskeletal oncology' section)

In diagnosis one has three primary aims:

1. To assess the extent of the primary tumour.
2. To assess the extent or presence of metastases.
3. To delineate the histological type.

Table 10.4 The relative incidence of osteogenic sarcoma in males and females, corrected for population at risk

	0–4 years		5–14 years		15–24 years		25+ years	
	Male	Female	Male	Female	Male	Female	Male	Female
Number of osteogenic sarcoma in series	–	–	25	24	42	22	5	2
Percentage of tumours in series	–	–	34.6	50	57	45.7	8.4	4.3
Percentage of population	13.8	12.9	29.1	28.2	30.3	30.7	26.8	28.2
Relative percentage incidence, tumours/population	–	–	1.2	1.88	1.88	1.5	0.3	0.2

Note that the highest incidence in males is between the ages of 15 and 24, whereas in females it is between the ages of 5 and 14 years.
Modified, with permission from C. H. G. Price, 1958, *Journal of Bone and Joint Surgery* **40B**, 574.

Table 10.5 True bone tumours

Cell type predominating	Simple tumour types	Malignant
Osteoblast Tumour cells show active ossification	Osteoma: Osteoid osteoma Benign osteoblastoma	Osteosarcoma: Primary Parosteal
Chondroblast Tumour cells show active cartilage formation	Chondroma: Benign chondroblastoma Chondromyxoid fibroma	Chondrosarcoma: Primary Secondary
Fibroblast Tumour cells show active collagen formation	Fibroma: ?Solitary bone cyst Non-osteogenic fibroma Fibrous dysplasia	Desmoid sarcoma: Malignant fibrous histiocytoma
Osteoclast Osteoclast probably arises from coalescence of stromal cells which in turn arise from the non-bone forming supportive connective tissue	Osteoclastoma Aneurysmal bone cyst Adamantinoma Chordoma (notochordal remnants)	Malignant osteoclastoma

Table 10.6 Tumours arising from tissues normally found in bone, but not participating in bone formation

Tumours arising from fibrous tissue forming the non-osteogenic outer layer (fascial) of the periosteum:
- Periosteal fibroma
- Periosteal fibrosarcoma
- Malignant fibrous histiocytoma

Tumours arising from the elements of bone marrow:
- Myeloma
- Reticulum cell sarcoma
- Hodgkin's disease of bone
- Lymphosarcoma
- Ewing's sarcoma

Tumours from blood vessels:
- Haemangioma
- Haemangioblastoma
- Aneurysmal bone cyst
- Angiosarcoma

Tumours arising from adipose tissue:
- Lipoma
- Liposarcoma

Tumours arising from nerves:
- Neurilemmoma
- Neurofibroma

Tumours of synovium

Tumours of striated muscle:
- Rhabdomyosarcoma

True bone tumours

True bone tumours comprise osteoma, osteosarcoma, chondroma, multiple enchondromata, chondrosarcoma, fibrosarcoma and osteoclastoma, and are discussed in the sections which follow.

*OSTEOMA**

A true osteoma, though rare, is found in the orbit, nasal sinuses, external auditory meatus and the oral side of the mandible. This tumour is usually composed of tissue as dense and hard as ivory, and is frequently termed 'ivory exostosis'. It is usually small, sessile, single and grows slowly; its surface is smooth, but may be slightly nodular. As it grows it tends to become more conical. When these tumours grow from the inner table of the cranial bones, they may cause pressure on the brain.

In the differential diagnosis from a biotrophic osteoma the clinical course is decisive but is of little importance as the indications for surgical interference are identical.

* Descriptive terms commonly include the following: (1) osteophyte – when localized and tendritic; (2) hyperostosis – when growth is diffuse; (3) enostosis – when growth occurs into the medullary cavity; (4) compact osteoma – osteoma durum or eburneum – when it is smooth and hard; (5) cancellous osteoma (osteoma spongiosum or osteoma medullare) – when it consists of soft, spongy bone; (6) parosteal osteoma – when it occurs outside the periosteum; (7) movable periosteal osteoma, or disconnected osteomas – when growing in tendon, muscle, or fascial planes; (8) heterologous osteoma – occurring in meninges, lung, diaphragm, parotid or skin.

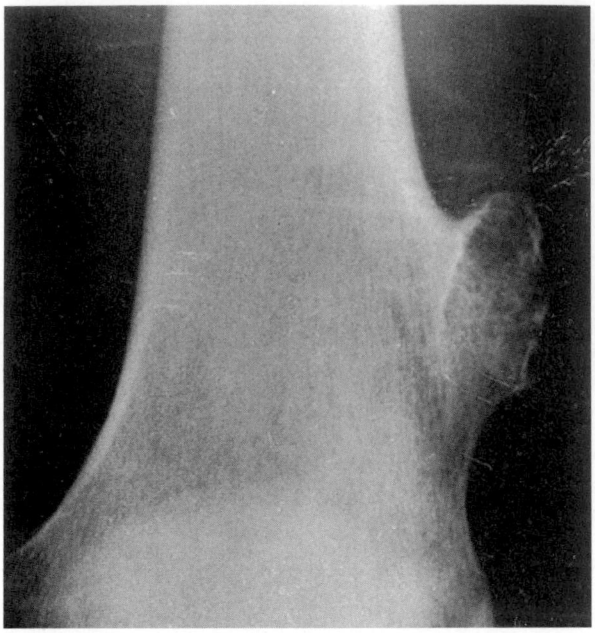

Figure 10.46 Exostosis of the distal femur.

Exostosis

Bone may form due to abnormal growth or imperfect remodelling to an excessive degree in varying parts of the skeleton and to these a variety of names have been given depending on the site and aetiology. These are not true tumours, as their growth will cease with the removal of the underlying cause or with cessation of general skeletal growth. The term 'exostosis' is used to differentiate such lesions from true neoplasms (Figure 10.46).

Traumatic osteoma

Traumatic osteomata are most frequently observed in relation to the femur, beneath the quadriceps, in relation to the adductor magnus (the so-called 'rider's bone') or in relation to the medial collateral ligament of the knee joint (Pellegrini–Stieda's disease). The condition is also not infrequent at the elbow, the exostosis forming in the intermuscular planes of the brachialis following dislocation.

Injury leads to the formation of a subperiosteal haemorrhage, the periosteum being detached by muscular traction. If the periosteum remains intact, the haematoma may become absorbed; but if the periosteal reapposition and the absorption of the blood clot are prevented by ill-advised movements or massage, the clot is invaded by mesoblastic elements and bone is laid down. The resulting exostosis in this case is smooth and firmly adherent to the bone.

If the periosteum ruptures, the blood escapes into and along the fibrous tissue planes and septa, and the subsequent deposit of new bone is therefore rough, or irregular in shape, and elongated, in the long axis of the muscle amongst whose fibres it is being deposited.

Occasionally a similar effect may follow tears of tendon and muscle fibres, without actual damage to the periosteum. In such cases, the new bone laid down has, apparently, no continuity with the adjacent bone.

Biotrophic osteoma (osteochondroma)

In structure and aetiology such osteomata are identical with those occurring in metaphyseal aclasis. A process of bone develops, projecting towards the diaphysis, and is capped by a detached fragment of epiphyseal cartilage. As the shaft of bone grows in length, the 'osteoma' assumes an acute angle with the shaft and is directed away from the epiphyseal plate. The 'osteoma' continues to grow, new bone being formed by the cartilaginous cap, but this growth ceases simultaneously with the fusion of the adjacent epiphysis or if the cartilaginous cap is removed. When fully developed, the marrow of the shaft is continuous with that of the cancellous tissue of the osteoma. When fully formed, the osteoma consists of a shell of compact bone enclosing cancellous tissue, with a cap or tip of cartilage. It is

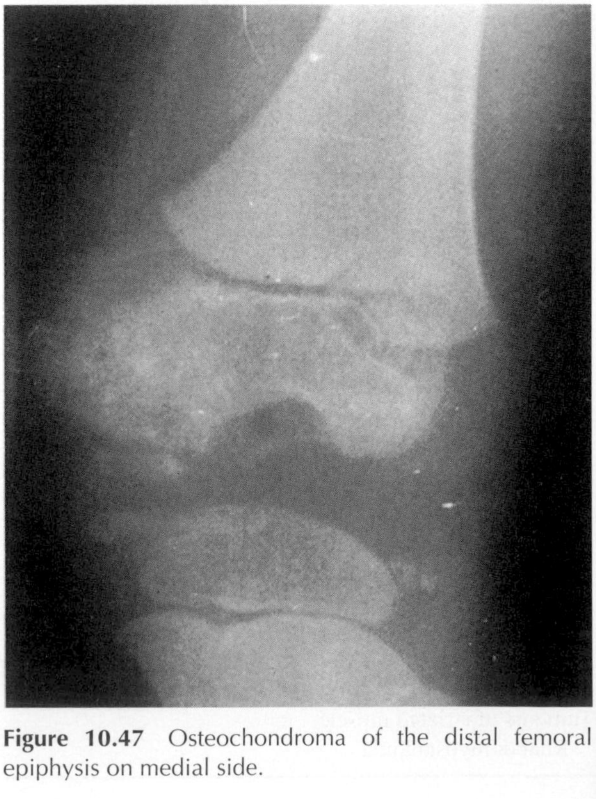

Figure 10.47 Osteochondroma of the distal femoral epiphysis on medial side.

usually pedunculated, with a bulbous extremity. It occurs during adolescence, never after the epiphysis has united, equally in boys and girls. The condition may be familial.

These exostoses are commonest at the extremities of the bones, especially at the ends where the epiphyses are the last to join the shaft. The lower end of the femur (Figures 10.47 and 10.48), the upper end of the tibia and the upper end of the humerus are consequently the commonest sites.

The summit of these growths is often covered by an adventitious bursa, and not uncommonly they interfere with the free action of muscles or tendons, or with the movement of joints. Exostoses are frequently found growing from the epiphyses of flat bones such as the scapula and the innominate.

Osteoid osteoma

This tumour is commonly diagnosed in young males and females between the ages of 10 and 30 years, with the bones of the lower extremities being predominantly involved (e.g. tibia and femur) although it is found in the vertebrae.

Jaffe (1935) believed it to be a very slow-growing neoplasm, but, because of its self-limiting nature its shell of bony sclerosis and its characteristic location, some believe that it is infective in origin or in some cases a staphylococcus has been cultured. A vascular lesion or embryonic rest has also been suggested.

This lesion presents with pain, frequently in the night, which is not aggravated by exercise or position, but is often relieved specifically, although empirically, by salicylates. There may be a tender swelling in a superficial site (e.g. in the tibia) but no increase in local tenderness, oedema or heat. The pain is believed to result from the lesion being very vascular with numerous nerve fibres. Oedema and increased tension result in stimulation of these nerve endings.

On x-ray examination, the usual findings are a zone of bony sclerosis surrounding a radiolucent nidus of variable size, although these classic features may take some months to develop or several projections in different planes to visualize the central nidus (Figure 10.49). The bone reaction of sclerosis or increased bone density can arise from either endosteal or periosteal surfaces, as it may lie within the cortex.

This condition has to be distinguished from:

1. The sclerosing non-suppurative osteomyelitis of Garré.
2. Brodie's abscess.
3. Osteogenic sarcoma.
4. Ewing's sarcoma.
5. Non-ossifying fibroma (in its early stages) (Figure 10.50).

On *complete* removal of the lesion, there are seen on histology three characteristic regions as described by Jaffe: an inner region of vascular granulation tissue containing osteoblasts and, outside this, calcification and osteoid formation surrounded by trabecular formation of bone in various stages of reorganization (Figure 10.51).

Complete resection, if possible, will provide cure,

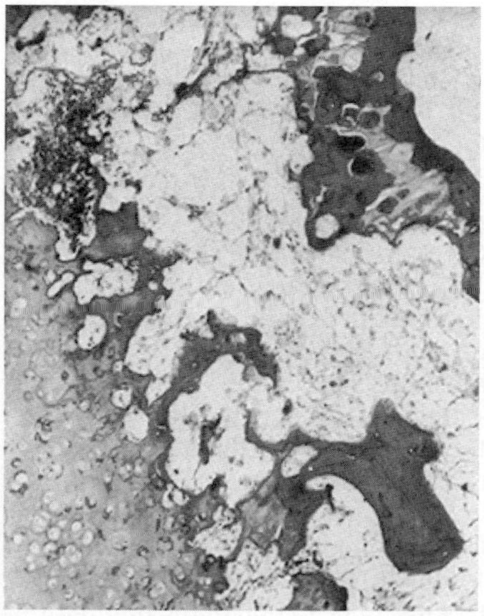

(a)

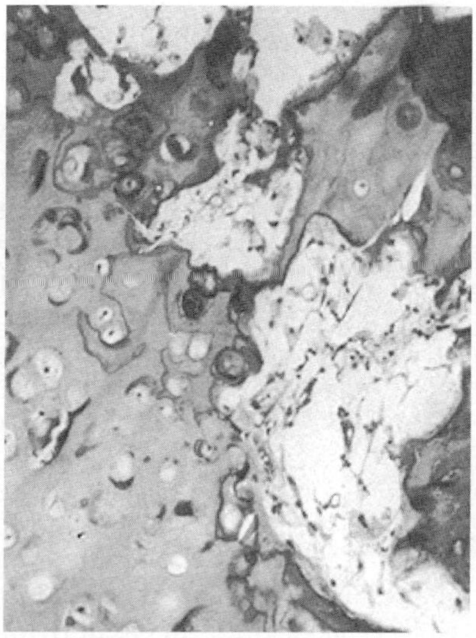

(b)

Figure 10.48 (a) Photomicrograph showing the definite but irregular activity of a cartilaginous cap overlying cancellous bone. (× 58). (b) Photomicrograph of the same exostosis showing the irregular multiplication of epiphyseal cartilage cells and early ossification at the growth plate. (× 144).

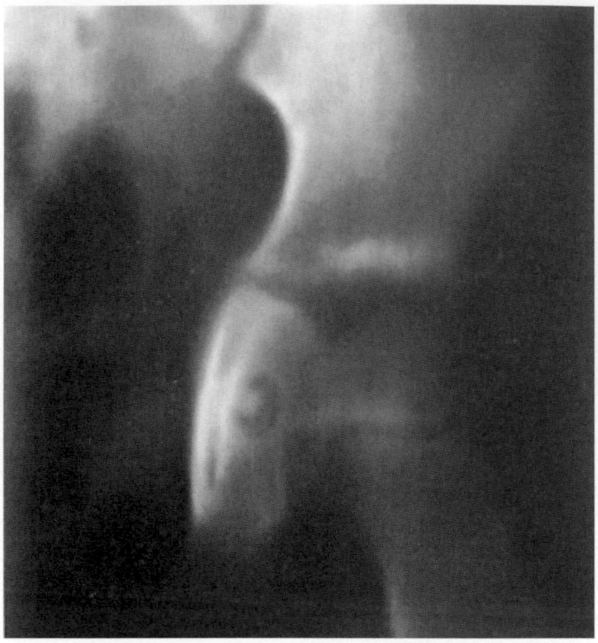

Figure 10.49 Scanogram showing osteoid osteoma in the depths of the acetabulum with central calcific density in the radiolucent nucleus.

but partial removal of the sclerotic bone and the nidus is often sufficient for symptomatic improvement. Malignancy has not been reported after surgical treatment.

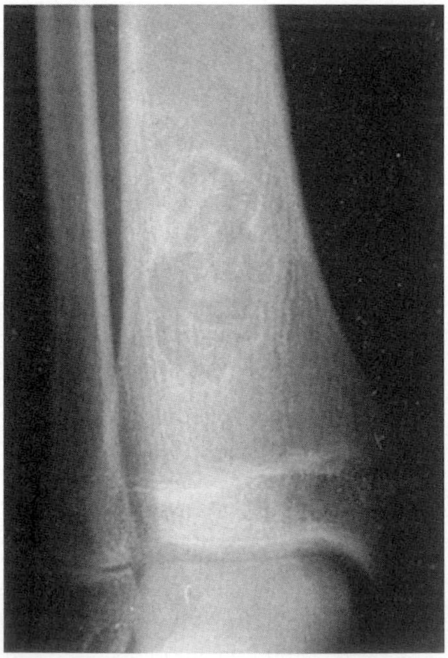

Figure 10.50 Radiograph showing a non-ossifying fibroma of the distal tibia, in which the typical 'bubbled' appearance of the sclerotic margin can be seen.

Benign osteoblastoma (osteogenic fibroma)

This is a relatively rare tumour, most commonly seen in the vertebrae as well as in limb bones such as the femur (Jaffe, 1935). It may be a coincidental finding, although it can present with pain and tenderness in any age group. On x-ray examination it is seen as a circumscribed expanding osteolytic lesion with some radiopaque mottling of osteoid or bone content.

On biopsy, the lesion is commonly 'gritty' and vascular and its histology shows a fairly regular orientation of new bone formation with trabeculation. The osteogenic cells have the appearances of malignancy, although the presence of giant cells sometimes confuses the diagnosis.

An ossifying fibroma is almost exclusively limited to the jawbones, it is most commonly seen in adolescents, with a slight predilection for females. It is often asymptomatic, being discovered as an ancillary finding in dental examinations. Radiographically it is seen as an area of 'ground-glass' radiolucency progressing to more or less marked sclerosis.

Microscopically (Figure 10.52) it appears as an area of rather dense fibroblastic proliferation within which are many 'puddles' of dense bone, whose margins are sharp and more basophilic than the areas within. It is thought now by many to be a local manifestation of fibrous dysplasia, with cytology peculiar to the area, and progressing in increasing ossification as it matures, as does its skeletal counterpart. Lesions in the vertebrae may present with pain as well as evidence of cord pressure including motor and sensory disturbances (Lichtenstein, 1977). Pathological fractures are unusual.

Treatment is a resection if possible, otherwise curettage with bone grafting. Radiotherapy may be indicated in inaccessible areas such as vertebrae.

OSTEOSARCOMA

The term 'osteosarcoma' is employed to designate those tumours which arise from cells principally concerned with bone formation and in which this characteristic is maintained as a predominant feature of the neoplasm.

Where the bone absorption is predominant, due either to the degree of vascularity or to the malignancy of the tumour, the terms 'telangiectatic' or 'osteolytic sarcoma' have been applied. In very vascular tumours with pulsation the name malignant bone aneurysm has been given.

The osteosarcoma is relatively rare, the incidence in Great Britain being 1 per 75 000 of the population. It may occur at any age period, but has a decided

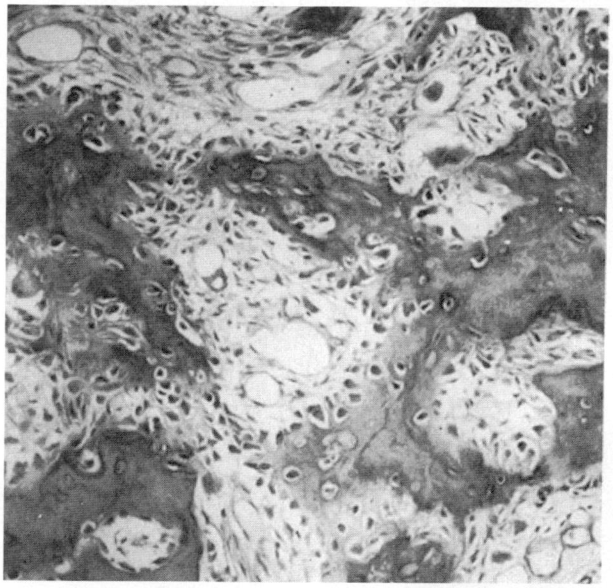

(a)

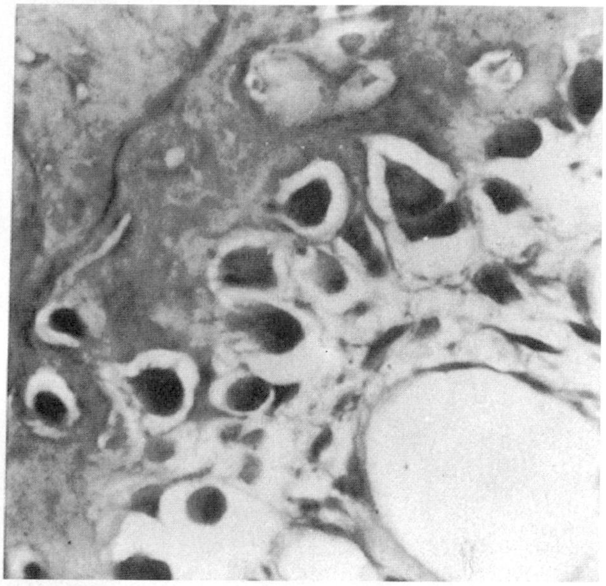

(b)

Figure 10.51 (a) Photomicrograph of tissue taken from an osteoid osteoma, showing the very active and malignant-appearing osteoblast activity and new bone formation commonly seen in the centre of this lesion. (× 166). (b) Photomicrograph showing the appearance of very active osteoblasts in the central position. (× 500).

predilection for the second decade. Price (1958) described a significant similarity between osteochondroma and osteogenic sarcoma of male predominance, peak incidence between the ages of 15 and 20 years, and anatomical distribution. This is of interest because of the hereditary background exhibited by the osteochondroma. In older individuals it is an occasional sequel to Paget's disease, and, rarely, to other osteodystrophies.

The tumour arises in the metaphysis where nor-

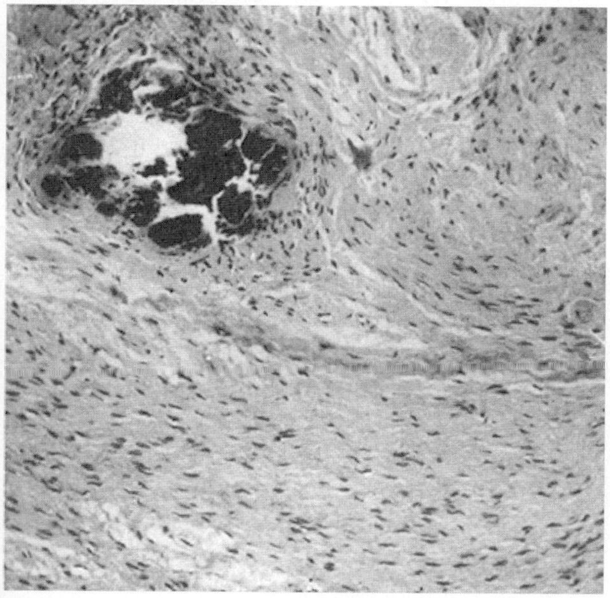

(a)

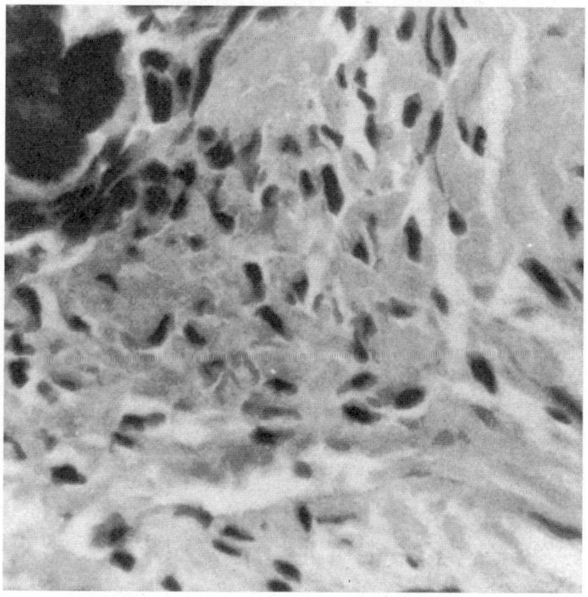

(b)

Figure 10.52 (a) Photomicrograph showing a normal-appearing dense fibrous tissue and one area of calcification. (× 167). (b) Photomicrograph showing in detail the fibroblastic activity at the margin of the calcified area. (× 536).

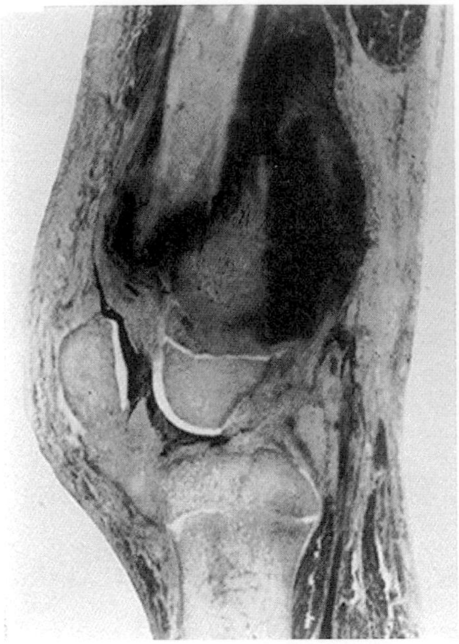
(a)

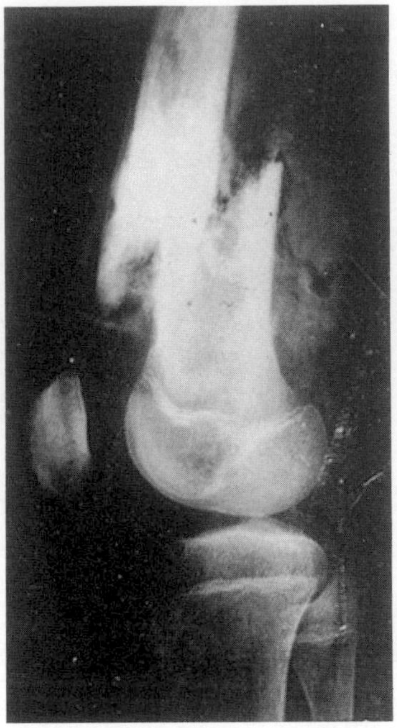
(b)

Figure 10.53 (a) Osteosarcoma of femur. Male aged 17 years. (b) Showing pathological fracture.

mally the growth is more active. The large majority are found in the lower limb, especially the lower metaphysis of the femur and the upper end of the tibia (Figure 10.53), 52% occur in the femur, 20% in the tibia and 9% in the humerus. In the femur, 82% occur at the lower end and 9% in the greater trochanter; they are very rare in the head and neck. In the tibia, 90% affect the upper medial aspect (Figures

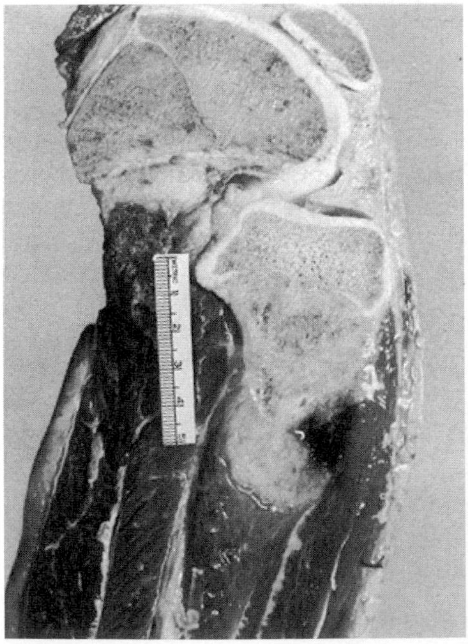
(a)

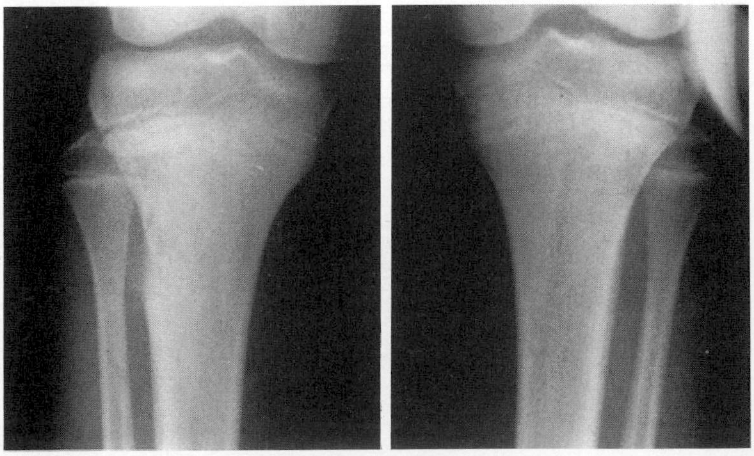
(b)

Figure 10.54 (a) An osteosarcoma of proximal tibia in an adolescent boy. Note the persistence and continuity of the epiphyseal line with the erosion and destruction of cortex anteriorly. Compare this site with the diagram in Figure 10.44. (b) Radiograph of the same tumour, showing the lesion in the outer upper aspect of the right tibia (left tibia included for comparison).

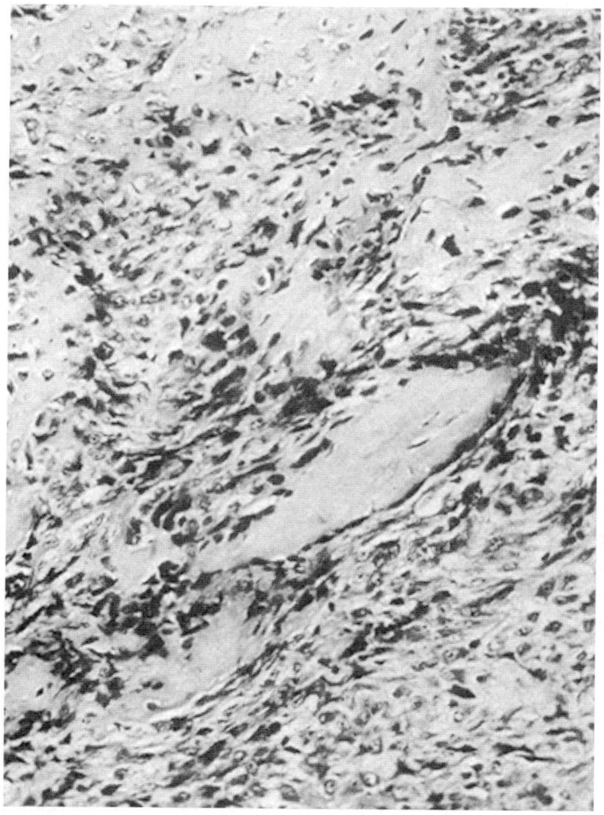

Figure 10.55 Photomicrograph of osteosarcoma with marked variation in cell size, shape and staining properties of the nuclei, as well as the irregular structure of the bone formed. (× 269).

10.54 and 10.55). In the humerus the upper end is the most commonly involved, and it is very rare to find osteogenic sarcoma below the deltoid tubercle. Less usual sites are the radius, where it is extremely rare to find osteogenic sarcoma at the lower end – a common site for osteoclastoma; the ulna, where there is also an immunity of the lower end; the ilium and the scapula. For some reason, the short long bones appear to be rarely affected (Figure 10.56).

The tumour initially may appear to originate beneath the periosteum or more centrally in the shaft of the bone, but there would appear to be no reason to assume that these constitute different types of tumour.

From its initial situation the tumour extends in two directions – (1) towards the medulla and (2) to the subperiosteal area (Figure 10.57). In the medulla, the bone trabeculae are destroyed, and the tumour appears as an irregular mass permeating and frequently extending for a considerable distance along the medullary canal. At first the periosteum offers an impenetrable barrier and is only raised off the bone. Beneath the membrane the tumour may extend widely, ensheathing the bone and producing a fusiform swelling. The periosteal separation stops short at the attachment of the periosteum to the epiphyseal cartilage. Similarly, the intramedullary part of the tumour does not transgress the cartilage of the epiphysis – a useful point in distinguishing it from an osteoclastoma. Canadell *et al.* (1994) had reported on an innovative method to preserve the epiphysis when resecting metaphyseal malignant bone tumours. They point out that frequently it has been necessary to sacrifice the adjacent epiphysis. However, this has been avoided by carrying out a preliminary procedure of physeal distraction – during the course of adjunct chemotherapy and then following this by an *en bloc* resection without exposing the metaphyseal surface of the epiphysis. The final phase is to reconstruct the bone defect when the pathologist has reported absence of any tumour from the margin of the resected segment. At a mean follow-up of 54 months there were no local recurrences, although three patients had died of pulmonary metastases out of 28 patients with various sarcomata. Also 'skip' lesions were rare.

The tumour varies greatly in appearance. It may be soft, fleshy and vascular, with areas of haemorrhage

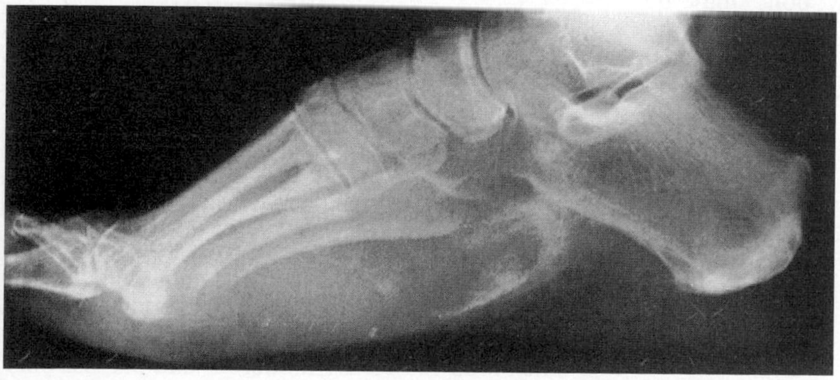

Figure 10.56 Radiograph showing an ossifying expanding tumour in a middle-aged woman, involving soft tissues under foot arch. Histology was that of an osteogenic sarcoma.

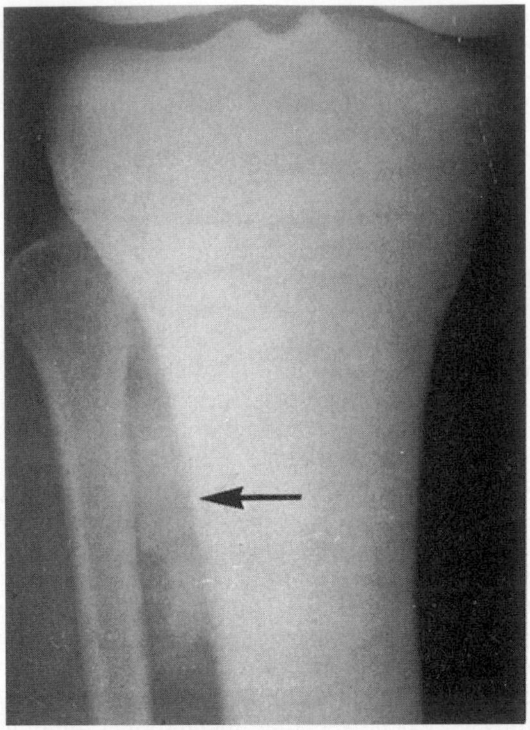

Figure 10.57 Radiograph showing an osteosarcoma of the proximal tibial metaphysis with much subperiosteal new bone formation on the lateral aspect.

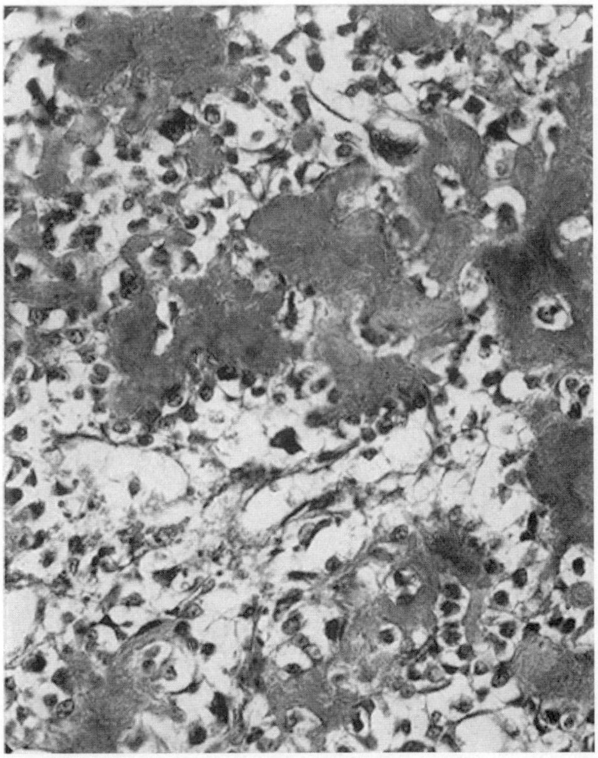

Figure 10.58 Photomicrograph from tumour in Figure 10.57, showing the formation of osteoid tissue by malignant 'bone cells'. (× 196).

and necrosis, or it may be greyish-white and solid when it contains cartilage or bone. In the first type, there is little or no new bone formation; the tumour is largely a destructive one. The new bone may be arranged as scattered islands throughout the tumour which impart a gritty sensation on cutting, and that found beneath the periosteum is sometimes arranged at right angles to the cortex as a series of radiating spicules. To this arrangement is attributable in part the 'sunray' appearance in the radiographs. This peculiar arrangement is due to the vessels which pass perpendicularly from the periosteum to the cortex and along which the bone is laid down, and, as already noted, some of this new bone may be reactionary. On the diaphyseal side of the tumour the periosteum is often stripped for a short distance, and here there may be deposited layers of new bone arranged parallel to the shaft. This area is triangular in shape and is usually referred to as Codman's reactive triangle.

If the sarcoma grows rapidly and the periosteal reaction is weak, pathological fracture may occur. This at once provides an outlet for the expanded tumour and leads to its ultimate phase of infiltration of the soft tissues.

Histology

While the most frequently observed cell is small and spindle shaped and with a hyperchromatic nucleus, great variation in cell form is invariable (Figure 10.58). In shape the cells may be polyhedral or round, or, less commonly, cuboidal or even columnar; they vary considerably in size, and the arrangement, too, varies; in some the spindle cells are arranged in bands as in a cellular fibroma, in others they assume palisade, alveolar or columnar formation and simulate epithelium. The degree of pleomorphism is most marked in the extreme anaplastic tumours in which there are often giant multinucleated cells of bizarre shapes. Mitosis is usually well marked and these cells are often surrounded by a delicate eosinophilic matrix.

The intercellular matrix may be scanty or considerable, and in character may be myxomatous, cartilaginous, osteoid or osseous, according to the degree of differentiation and metaplasia which are occurring (Figure 10.59) When there is rapid destruction of bone, cells of the osteoclast type are found (Figure 10.60). Cartilage cells may be found when it is termed 'chondroblastic' osteosarcoma, but the malignant osteoid matrix gives the diagnosis.

The blood vessels are numerous and possess only

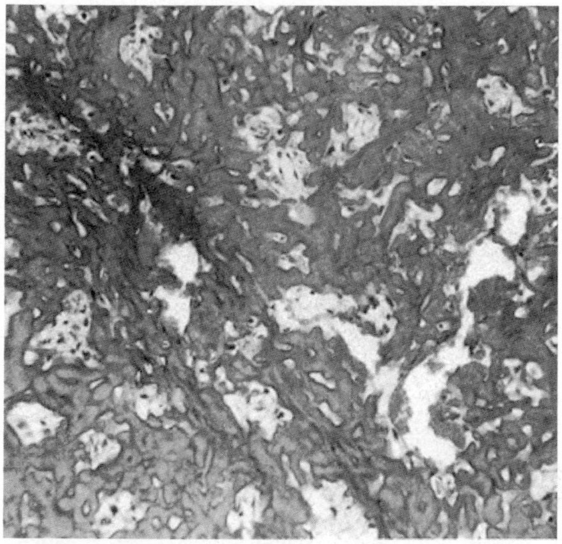

(a)

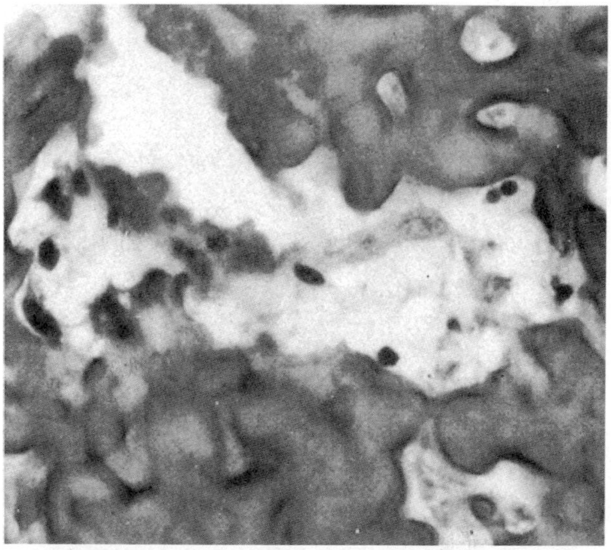

(b)

Figure 10.59 (a) Photomicrograph of a sclerosing osteosarcoma showing dense but irregular bone formation with widely scattered osteoblasts and only an occasional osteocyte. (× 160). (b) Photomicrograph of the same tissue to show the variation in size and shape of the malignant osteoblasts. (× 509).

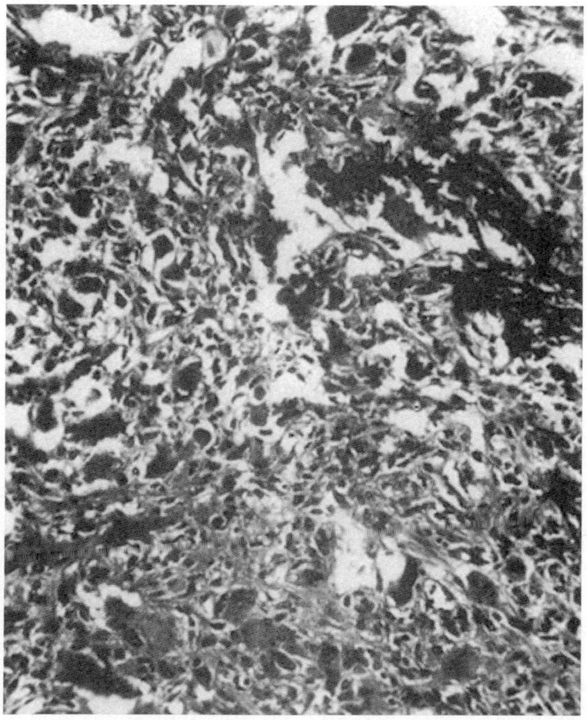

(a)

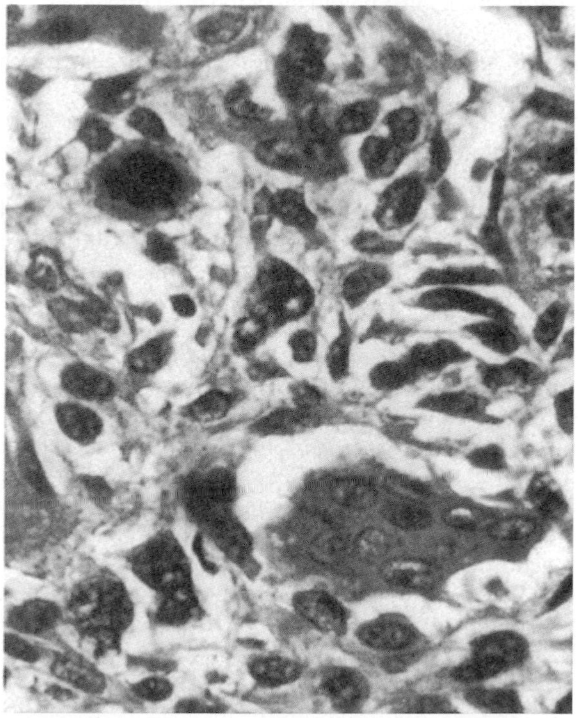

(b)

Figure 10.60 (a) Photomicrograph of an osteolytic osteosarcoma, showing marked cellular activity with minimal bone formation. (× 189). (b) Same tissue to show variation in size and staining reaction of the cell, with marked pyknosis and active mitosis in progress with the presence of giant cells. (× 600).

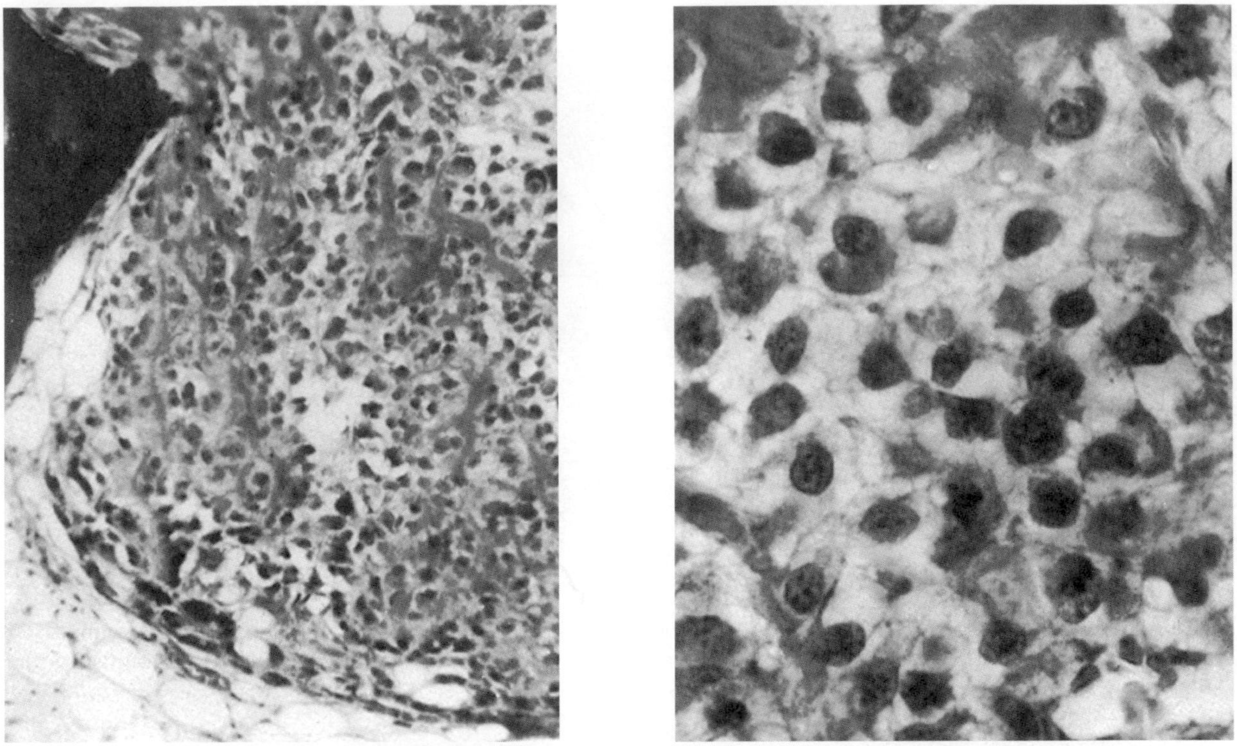

(a) (b)

Figure 10.61 (a) Photomicrograph of an osteoid osteosarcoma with less dense cellular matrix of an osteoid nature rather than malignant bone formation, but marked cellular activity and irregularity. (× 188). (b) Same tissue showing the intercellular osteoid material with mitosis of cells which have a slightly more uniform cell pattern. (× 579).

thin walls. The degree of vascularity varies within wide limits – in some instances being so extreme that the tumour may pulsate and simulate an aneurysm.

The formation of bone in these tumours would appear to proceed from the primitive malignant cell to ossified tissue directly (Figure 10.61) without any intervening stage of chondrification, but where cartilage is present in these tumours this, too, may become ossified.

The histological picture varies not only between different tumours but also between different sections taken from the same tumour. It is said that different areas of the same tumour may show, when integrated, the complete range of structural variation exhibited by osteosarcomatous lesions.

These variations have in the past led to much confusion and a variety of names purporting to distinguish distinctive tumours have been employed.

Clinical course

Pain, especially at night, is usually the first symptom and precedes the tumour by days, weeks or months. The pain is intermittent. It is due to the severe sensitiveness of the periosteum, and such pain in the long bone of a young adult should arouse suspicion of sarcoma. Less commonly there is only a tired feeling, and a slight limp. A second common feature in the clinical history is trauma, which, however, is often unreliable.

The general condition is good until a late stage in the disease, although night pains may keep the patient in misery and cause rapid deterioration. Occasionally there is pyrexia accompanied by leucocytosis. The clinical picture in the terminal stages is unlike that seen in carcinoma. The patients tend to become anaemic rather than cachectic; their haggard, pallid appearance is characteristic. The skin, too, reacts differently; it preserves its mobility and natural colour for a long time and becomes stretched instead of infiltrated as in carcinoma. Dilated veins may be evident at an early stage (Figure 10.62).

The size, shape, outline and consistency of the tumour are well perceived on palpation (Figure 10.63). In very vascular tumours a pulsation and bruit can be felt. The rapidity of growth and the increase of size depend on the malignancy, but after the periosteal capsule has been perforated the rate of growth increases rapidly. Pathological fracture is not typical of osteogenic sarcoma, since the swelling and pain usually keep the patient off his feet. There may be some initial pain and

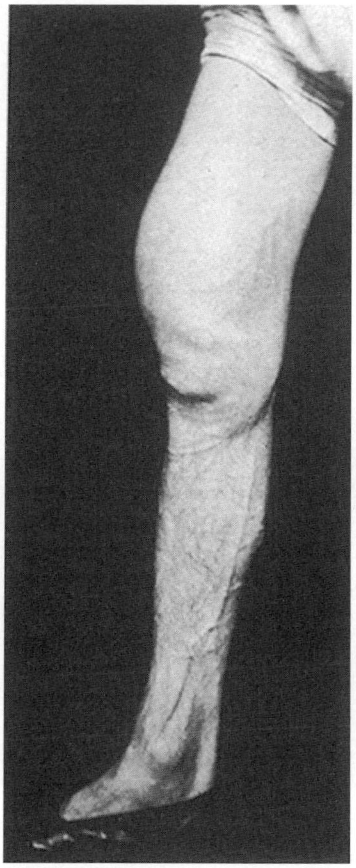

Figure 10.62 Osteogenic sarcoma involving the distal end of femur, with overlying dilated veins.

effusion into the nearest joint, but movement is free and painless.

Later, general dissemination of the tumour takes place. While the lymphatic stream occasionally plays a definite role with regional lymph-node involvement in 30% of patients at post-mortem examination, spread by the blood vessels is predominant. Pulmonary metastases are the most frequent. The first clinical signs of these are usually those of a diffuse bronchitis, but occasionally the cough, dullness, fever and leucocytosis suggest a diagnosis of pneumonia.

Diagnosis, prognosis and treatment

See section on 'Musculoskeletal oncology'.

Osteosarcoma in Paget's disease

It has been estimated that in approximately 5–10% of cases of Paget's disease sarcomatous changes occur on post-mortem examination. While histologically the disease is similar to that arising *de novo* in younger patients, the neoplastic change takes place at a much later age – usually over 50 years. The tumour is more diffuse in character and appears to arise simultaneously at multiple sites.

Parosteal sarcoma; juxtacortical osteosarcoma

Aakhus *et al.* (1960) reported on five patients with this condition which appears to occur in older age groups and presents as a painful tumour mass, particularly in the vicinity of the knee joint. It is juxtacortical in position, and is always densely ossified, but within it there may be areas of less ossified or calcified cartilage. There are usually no periosteal reactions or 'sunrays'. The rate of development is slow, but eventual destruction of the cortex with invasion of the medullary cavity occurs. This lesion makes up 4% of all osteosarcomas, but occurs at a later age and most commonly in females. The distal femur, the proximal tibia and the humerus are the most common sites. It is a slow and late metastasizing tumour with a better prognosis, slowly growing in size locally with minimal and late-in-onset symptoms. Because it is parosteal in site, it usually appears on the surface, rather than intracortically, producing large homogeneous lobulated new bone outside the bone shell and into soft tissue – often palpable.

Histologically, it consists of trabeculae of malignant bone and osteoid tissue with a definite malignant connective-tissue stroma, encapsulated by fibrous tissue. Its general prognosis is better than that of osteogenic sarcoma, particularly when treated with a primary amputation – i.e. 50–70% 5-year survival (Johnson, 1968). Simple excision leads to a recurrence, but for small tumours, early wide resection will give a cure of 80–90% long-term survival (Unni *et al.*, 1976b).

Okado *et al.* (1994), reporting from a large series of parosteal sarcoma, characterized the lesion as having arisen from the surface of the bone and that the tumour is well differentiated, i.e. a well formed osteoid matrix within a spindle-cell stroma, with less than 25% of the medullary cavity being affected. They found that dedifferentiation was more common, i.e. 16% of their patients, and by CAT cross-sectional imaging they demonstrated medullary involvement in 22%, and adjacent soft tissue invasion in 45%. At an average follow-up of 13 years, just under 17% had died of the tumour, almost all with a dedifferentiated histology. There is an increased risk of local recurrence which was associated with incomplete resection.

For diagnosis and treatment see section on 'Musculoskeletal oncology'.

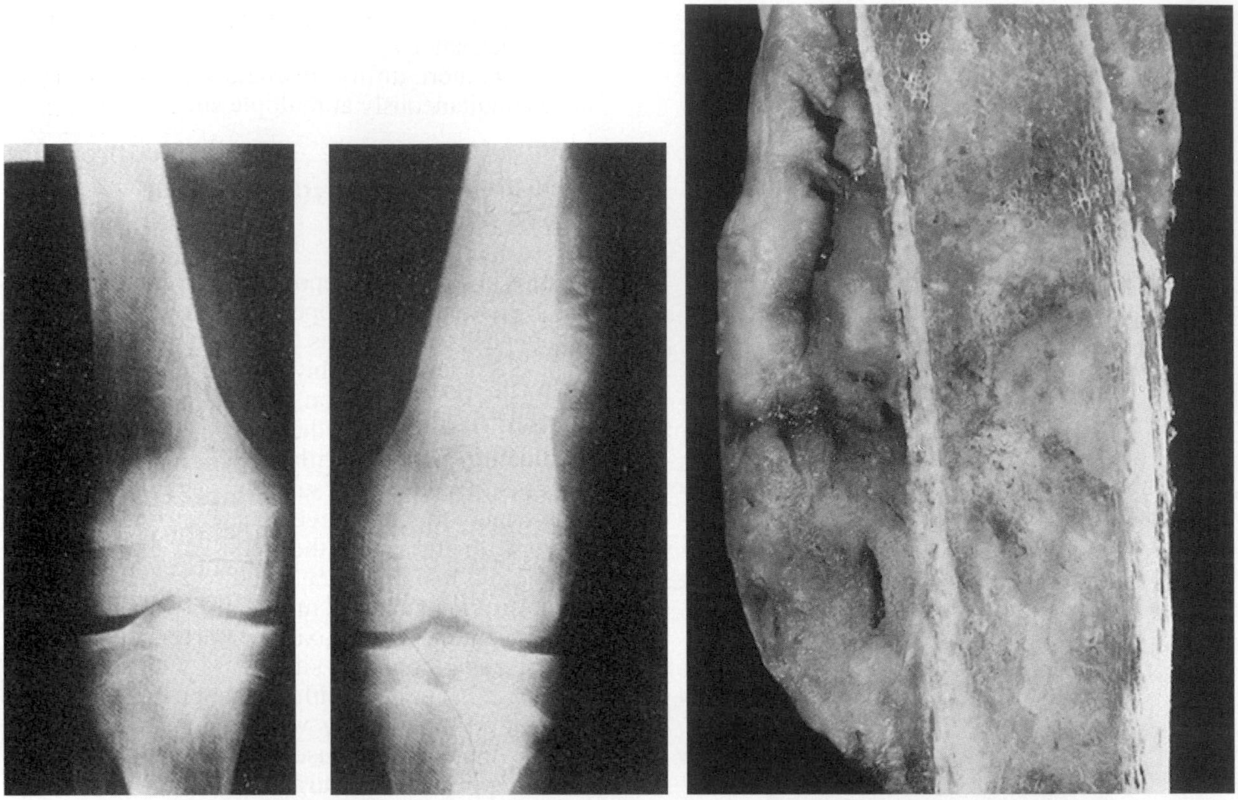

(a) (b) (c)

Figure 10.63 Osteosarcoma of femur showing in (a) a marked lytic response with destruction of bone and in (b) an osteoblastic response with rapidly growing subperiosteal new bone formation to give the 'sunray' appearance. (c) Pathological specimen, showing intra- and extramedullary lesions.

CHONDROMA

A chondroma is a benign tumour arising from the cartilaginous elements of the developing bone. It grows slowly, and is generally lobulated and encapsulated by fibrous tissue. Calcification frequently occurs in the fibrous septa dividing the lobules, while the intercellular matrix may undergo mucoid degeneration, particularly in the large chondromata which grow from the innominate bone.

Malignancy has been reported occurring after the trauma of operation in incomplete removal. The usual sites of growth are the fingers, toes, sternum and ribs; more rarely, the vertebrae and metaphyses of long bones, especially of the lower limbs. It usually appears in the third decade, and when malignancy supervenes it frequently does so after the age of 35 and occurs most commonly in tumours of the large long bones. Indeed, if this type of tumour presents as a centrally placed mass of such a bone or of a flat bone (e.g. the ilium or scapulae), one must seriously consider a low-grade chondrosarcoma.

Microscopically there is a chondroid matrix containing cartilage cells, encapsulation and lobulation are present, and calcification and mucoid degeneration are common.

The capsule is formed by vascular connective tissue which sends septa into the tumour substance, thus dividing it into lobules.

The arrangement of the cells is irregular and the fibrous content varies so that there is a mixture of hyaline and fibrocartilage, and frequently elastic tissue. The tumour may be lobulated by septa from the vascular connective tissue capsule. The tumour grows by apposition of cartilage cells derived from the connective tissue perichondrium. When ossification does occur, the tumour is known as osteochondroma.

Clinical features

The tumour may attain a very large size and destroy the adjacent bone undermining its structure without showing the histological criteria of malignancy. Occasionally pathological fracture may be the first evidence of its presence or by its position and size it may give rise to deformity, pressure on nerves, or interfere with movement of adjacent joints.

When a chondroma occurs in the small bones of the hand or foot it is known as a solitary cystic chondroma, and when it occurs elsewhere within a bone as a single enchondroma. This latter term may give rise to confusion as it includes both chondromas and cartilaginous hypertrophy.

The differential diagnosis is mainly by that of its clinical course – true tumours will not stop growing at the cessation of general skeletal growth.

Radiological appearances

The x-ray picture is generally held to be characteristic – a dense shadow, with a feathery outline composed of calcified spicules. In the absence of calcified or ossified areas in the tumour, the tumour is virtually invisible, though it may be suspected from the greater density of the soft tissues in relation to the bone.

The solitary cystic enchondroma

In the short long bones of the hand and foot there is occasionally found a solitary enchondroma. They usually occur in the metaphyseal region of a proximal phalanx or metacarpal, and seem to be especially common in the little finger. The tumour arises insidiously, and remains symptomless for a long time; attention is often directed to it through trauma, or the occurrence of a pathological fracture.

The tumour is at first composed of cartilage cells, but has a decided tendency to undergo myxomatous degeneration. In the process of growth it may greatly expand the cortex of the affected bone. Usually benign, malignant change has supervened on numerous occasions.

Treatment

During the stage of active cortical expansion, or after the occurrence of pathological fracture, the cyst should be curetted and its cavity cauterized, bone grafts being inserted where the integrity of the parent bone has been threatened. In this way, rapid and permanent healing results. When the cyst wall is thick, and is not giving rise to symptoms, it should be left alone.

MULTIPLE ENCHONDROMATA (ENCHONDROMATOSIS, OLLIER'S DYSCHONDROPLASIA)

Multiple enchondromata occur in childhood and affect the short long bones of the hand and foot, so that the part may be distorted and appear to be of excessive size (Figure 10.64). They arise in the centre of the shaft as a collection of cartilage cells

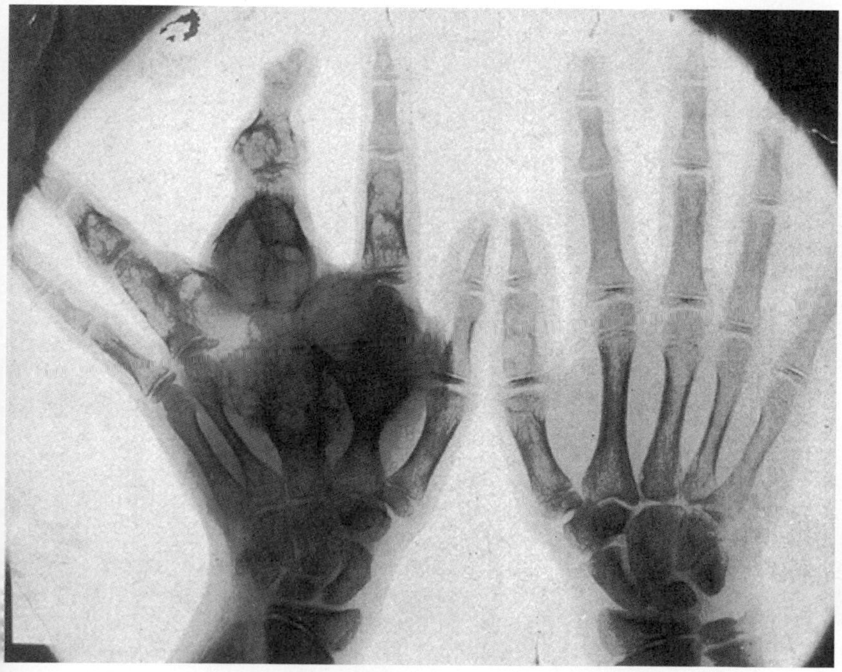

Figure 10.64 Multiple enchondromata of the hands. An x-ray showing the extensive and disabling deformity which this disease can produce.

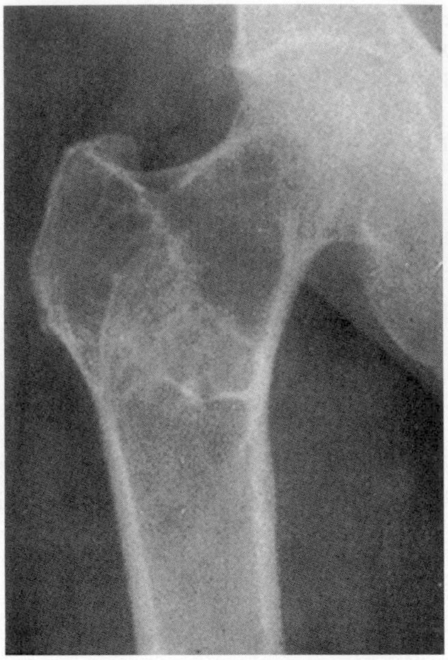

Figure 10.65 Radiograph of an elderly woman, showing a central enchondroma of bone occupying the upper half of the femur. The cortex is maintained, which aids in differentiating it from a bone cyst or a giant-cell tumour.

which, in the process of growth, gradually expand the surrounding cortex (Figures 10.65, 10.66, 10.67). It has been suggested that these tumours arise as a result of deficiency in the nutrient vessel, and an imperfection in the early vascularization of the cartilaginous framework has left within the centre of the shaft isolated islands of cartilage which have later assumed proliferative activity.

The tumours are simple, they are deforming and ugly, but otherwise harmless; if left alone they may disappear when growth in length ceases. See Chapter 4.

Treatment

Operative treatment is indicated when the tumours are rapidly growing and have become unsightly or a source of inconvenience. Complete excision, with curettage and cauterization of the tumour bed, is essential. Should this procedure lead to the collapse of the fragile bony shell of the affected bone, the shell should be packed with autogenous bone graft. The tumours should be dealt with at successive operations.

Other cysts of the short bones of the hands and feet

Reference may here be made to cysts of the hand and foot of other than chondromatous origin. Cysts can be subdivided into:

1. A group corresponding histologically to osteitis fibrosa.
2. A group in which amongst the fibrous stroma of the tumour, there are a few scattered giant cells smaller than those of the typical giant cell tumour – the giant cell variant of the bone cyst.

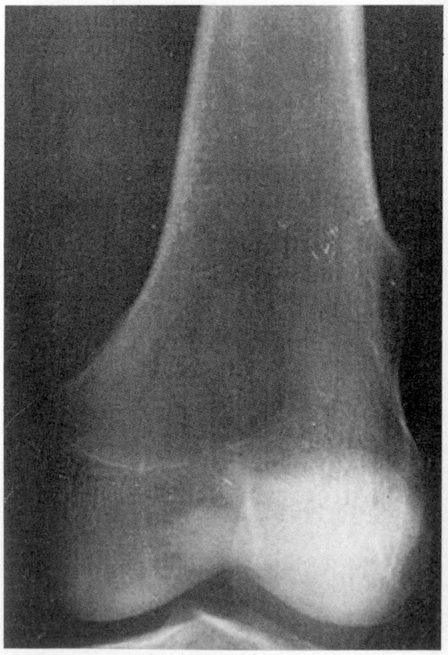

(a)

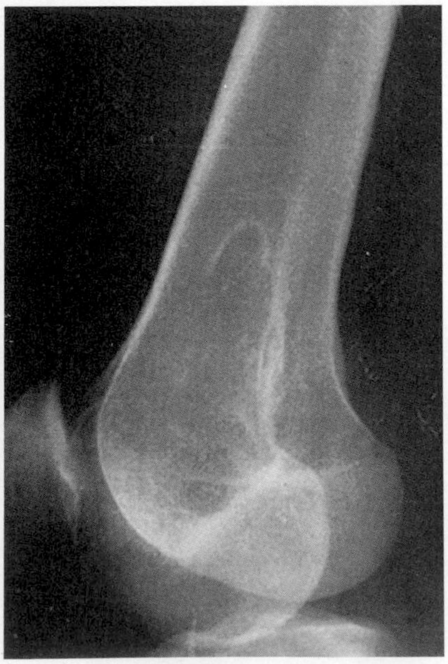

(b)

Figure 10.66
(a) Osteochondroma of the distal femur, showing the rather sessile outgrowth from the diaphysis, orientated in a retrograde direction. (b) Lateral view of the same lesion.

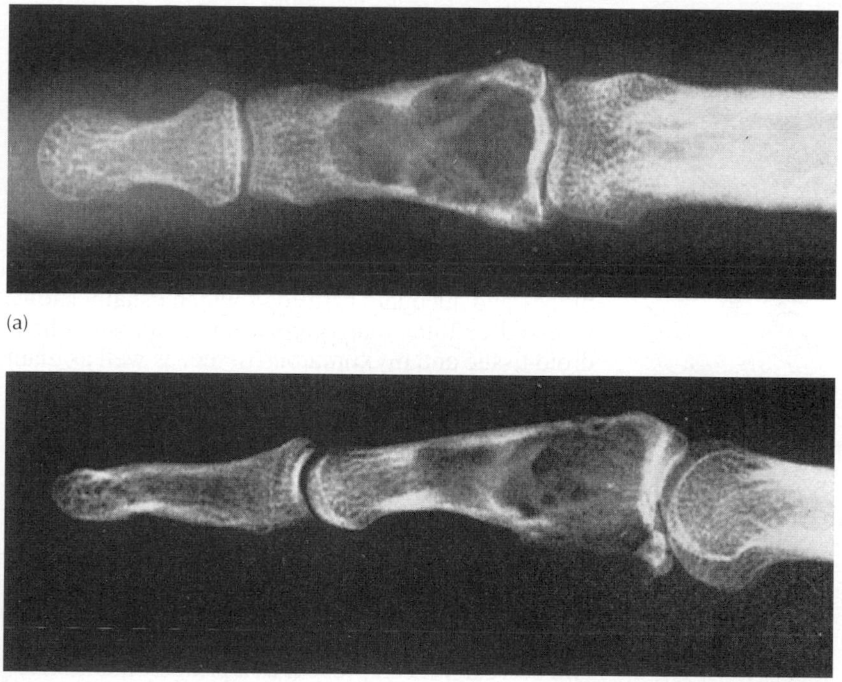

Figure 10.67 Enchondroma of middle phalanx: (a) anteroposterior and (b) lateral view.

3. A group in which large numbers of typical giant cells are scattered throughout the stroma of spindle-celled connective tissue which, however, predominates – the spindle-celled variant of the giant cell cyst.

In this way one can note the frequent relationship between osteitis fibrosa and giant cell tumour, though the latter, in its classic form, is not found in the short bones of the hand and foot.

Symptoms arise when trauma results in a fracture, or when the enlarging cyst produces pain, and this directs attention to a gradually increasing swelling. The hand is affected more often than the foot.

Radiological appearances

At first the cyst is located at the metaphyseal area of the affected bone but gradually becomes displaced down the shaft as the bone grows. The cortex is usually expanded, and the trabeculae are largely destroyed though traces of them may be seen as fine streaks running through the otherwise structureless area. There is no subperiosteal new bone reaction.

The radiological signs are similar to those of the cystic enchondroma; the two lesions cannot therefore be distinguished on x-ray examination, but only at operation – the chondroma is filled with bluish-white radiolucent material, the cyst with crumbly brown tissue – and on histological examination.

Benign chondroblastoma

This tumour was first identified by Codman (1925) and named a 'chondromatous giant-cell tumour'. However, it occurs in an earlier age group – i.e. the first and second decades, in which the epiphyseal

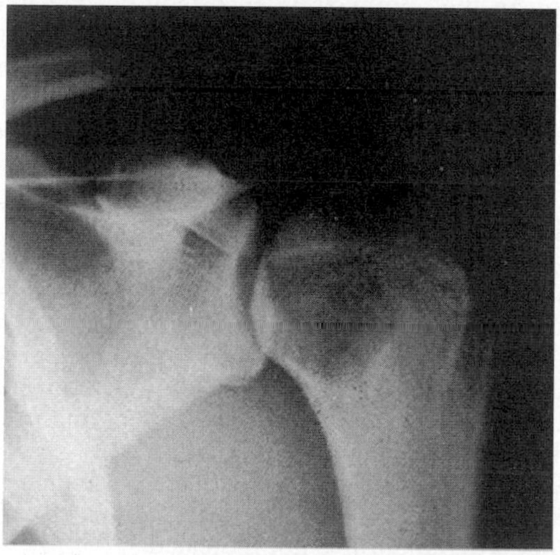

Figure 10.68 Radiograph of a benign chondroblastoma of the upper end of the humerus whose epiphysis has closed. The tumour has invaded the metaphysis. The epiphysis is the usual site for this tumour, which does not expand bone. Within the radiolucent lesion there are dense areas of calcification.

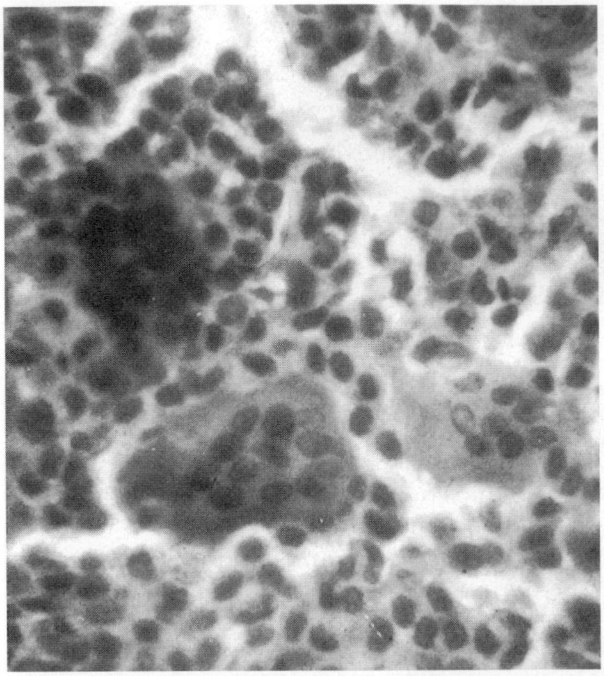

Figure 10.69 Photomicrograph showing the large cells which appear as primitive chondroblasts – vacuolated cytoplasm and large round nuclei. (× 281).

line has not yet closed; indeed, Jaffe believed the origin to be from a primitive cartilage cell type.

There is often a long history of a painful swelling with loss of joint function. On x-rays, the typical lesion in the epiphysis is an osteolytic one which contains flecks of calcium phosphate deposits. Extension into the metaphysis and articular cartilage may occur, but the margin is always discrete and demarcated by a zone of sclerotic or condensed bone (Figure 10.68). This tumour is most commonly confused with a sarcoma or an inflammatory process such as tuberculosis.

On biopsy, the lesion is found to be very vascular and gritty. Histology shows much chondroid material with 'chondroblastic' appearing cells, which exhibit strong metachromasia and a positive periodic acid–Schiff reaction (Figure 10.69). Osteoid tissue and calcified areas are seen as well as giant cells (Schajowicz and Gallardo, 1970).

Treatment consists of adequate curettage and cancellous bone grafting, and this gives excellent results. x-Irradiation is not indicated.

Chondromyxoid fibroma

This lesion was first described in 1958 by Jaffe (1978) and in 1959 by Lichtenstein (1977); although their cases were localized to the bones of the lower extremity, it can be found in both small and large bones elsewhere.

It presents as a painful swelling which on x-ray is a non-specific-appearing osteolytic lesion expanding the cortex in an eccentric position. It appears as an eccentric lesion in the tibia and in the femur but is central in the fibula and foot bones. It is usually well defined with periosteal new bone on the outer surface and sclerosis on the inner.

Diagnosis in young adults or adolescents requires biopsy and adequate histology which usually shows a mixed cellular matrix containing fibrosis, chondroid tissue and myxomatous tissue, as well as giant cells and attempts at osteoid formation. There may be partitions of fibrous tissue between myxoid pseudolobules which do not stain for mucin.

Treatment is an *en bloc* resection or curettage.

CHONDROSARCOMA

This tumour occurs mainly between the ages of 20 and 60 years. It can present as a primary malignancy in the earlier age groups and as secondary malignant change in previous conditions such as an osteochondroma, or in Paget's disease or diaphyseal aclasis.

Their clinical presentation is often vague, although when a change in size and symptoms of a known osteochondromatous mass occurs, or recurrence of an excised 'benign' cartilage tumour takes place, this is suggestive of sarcoma.

The bones most commonly involved are the pelvis, the ribs and sternum, and the femur. Dahlin and Henderson (1956) stated that the nearer the cartilaginous tumour is to the axial skeleton and the larger it is, the more likely it is to be malignant. Commonly these tumours are divided into central or peripheral types depending upon their location, with the peripheral lesion having a better prognosis in being secondary, circumscribed and operable (Lichtenstein, 1977). About 60% occur in the pelvic bones or upper femora. Intrahepatic lesions present late with neurological symptoms and signs, e.g. referred pain, sciatica, bladder and venous obstruction signs.

Clinically there are described five types of chondrosarcoma:

1. Central which is usually intramedullary and primary. It varies in its grade of malignancy and rarely extends into soft tissues. Calcification within it is minimal.
2. Mesenchymal – also intramedullary, primary and containing small compact round cells in sheets of cartilage matrix. High-grade malignancy is usual.

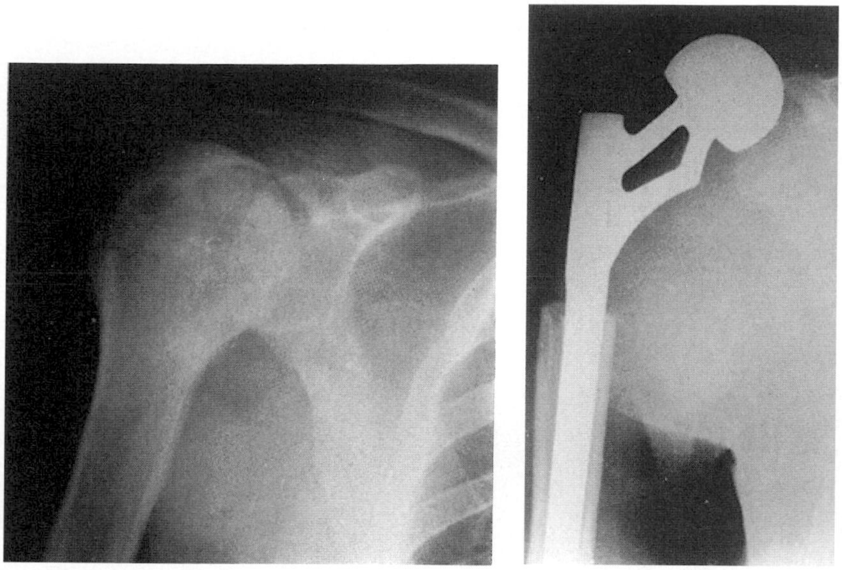

(a) (b)

Figure 10.70 (a) Radiograph of a chondrosarcoma, involving the upper end of a humerus in a middle-aged man, which was considered secondary to a previous enchondroma. (b) The upper end of the humerus with its surrounding musculature was radically excised and replaced with a metal prosthesis.

3. Peripheral – cortical in site but spreading out into soft tissues; usually low grade in malignancy, heavily calcified and secondary to osteochondroma, and diaphyseal aclasis.
4. Clear cell sarcoma – may be mistaken as a chondroblastoma but is low grade and locally recurrent with round clear cells and few mitoses.
5. Dedifferentiated-anaplastic – high grade of malignancy with osteoid of an osteosarcoma or malignant fibrous histioma changes predominate. It erodes through the cortex with adjacent soft tissue involvement.

On x-rays there is often frank destruction of

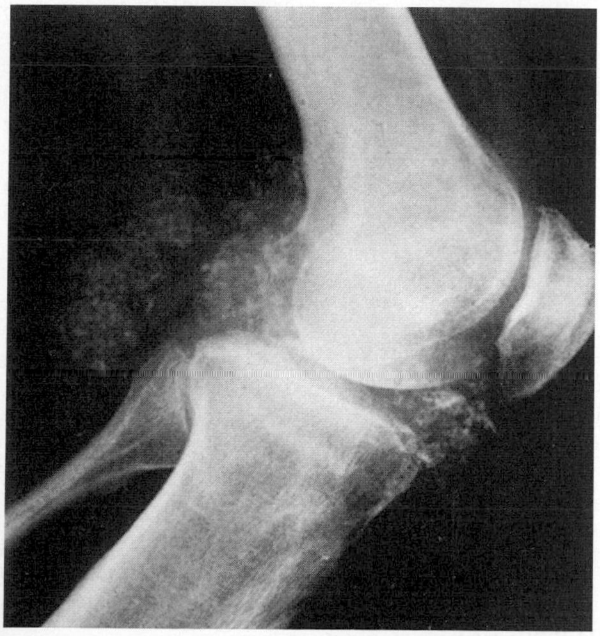

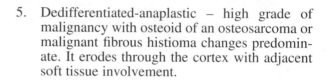

Figure 10.71 Chondrosarcoma involving the knee joint (lateral radiograph). The irregular calcification is typical and more discrete than that associated with synovial sarcoma.

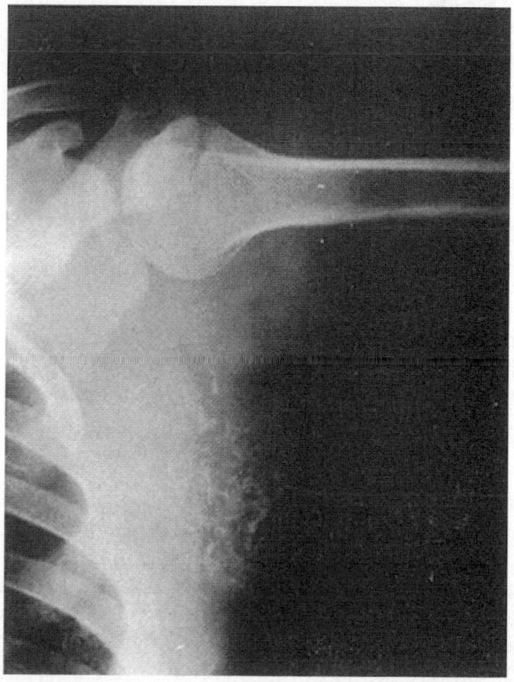

Figure 10.72 Recurrence of chondrosarcoma after partial resection of the scapula.

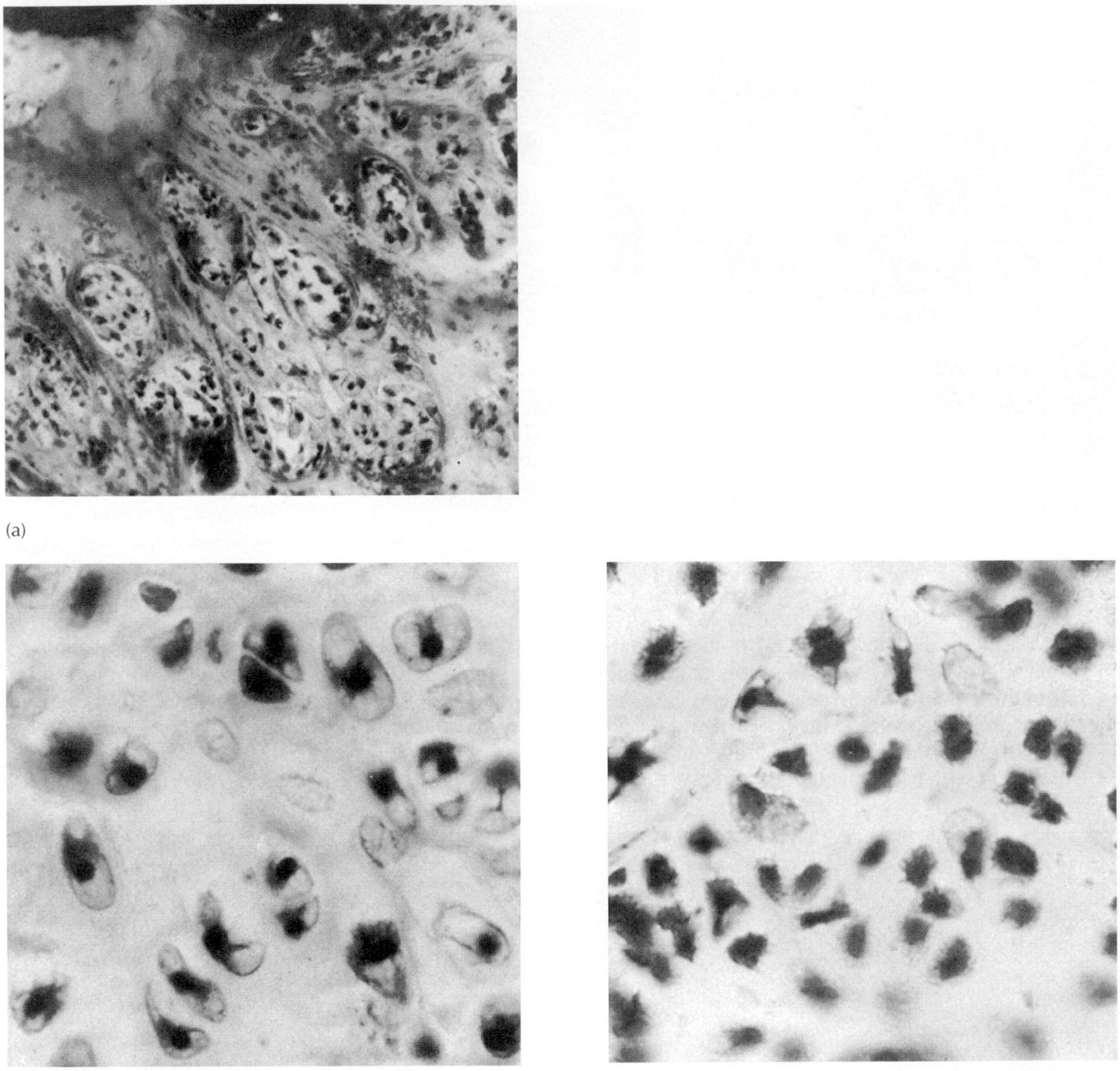

(a)

(b)

(c)

Figure 10.73 (a) Photomicrograph of a chondrosarcoma, showing the general appearance of tissue suggestive of malignancy. (× 165). (b) Photomicrograph of (a), showing marked variation in size of the cells and the presence of several double nuclei, those being major criteria for diagnosing malignancy in chondromatous tumours. (× 528). (c) Further detail to show evidence of pleomorphism and the presence of double nuclei within the large malignant cartilage cells. (× 520).

trabecular bone and cortex with an expanding lesion which contains irregular flecking or mottling of calcified tissue (Figure 10.70). There may or may not be periosteal new bone formation to this tumour which often can be seen invading soft tissues (Figures 10.71 and 10.72).

On biopsy the sarcomatous mass appears as greyish, translucent, fairly vascular tissue which may be lobulated or containing areas undergoing cystic degeneration and liquefaction. Histologically, varying degrees of pleomorphism, hyperchromatism, mitotic figures, enlarged nuclei, chondroid formation with calcification and ossification are seen (Figure 10.73).

Discrete sarcomatous masses may be separated from the main tumour mass in the medullary cavity – hence the local recurrence after inadequate excision or amputation.

Attempts have been made to grade the degree of malignancy and, hence, prognosis, but since the total mass of the specimen is rarely examined, the total pathology can rarely be appreciated. However, Thomson and Turner-Warwick (1955) divided this tumour simply into three types:

1. *Low grade* – well differentiated, in which the cells are cartilaginous in type although increased in number, with the matrix being well formed. Local infiltration of host's tissues at the periphery is seen. Nearly three-quarters of these patients were alive 10 years after treatment.
2. *Average grade* – in which there is a reduction in the amount of matrix and an increase in the cellularity, the cells varying in size and shape with nuclear irregularities. Less than half of these patients were alive at 5 years and only one-third were alive at 10 years.
3. *High grade* – poorly differentiated cartilaginous pattern with anaplastic cells being common, frequent mitoses and only occasional islands of cartilage being seen. Areas of myxoid matrix are commonly seen. This type behaves similarly to the osteogenic cell (i.e. only 1 in 10 survived 3 years). In their series, out of the 38 patients who died, at least 17 had metastasis to the lungs and to other sites. There is rarely, if ever, osteoid formation.

Mankin (1978), from an extensive and exhaustive study of 49 separate cartilage tumours and of articular cartilage samples, found that the tumours had:

1. Increased water and ash content (probably in the form of calcium salts).
2. No differences in the amounts of proteoglycans or DNA.
3. 'Excess' protein (probably from collagen and proteoglycans) was markedly increased and varied directly with the malignancy of the tumour.
4. An alteration in the distribution of glycosaminoglycans with a marked increase in chondroitin-4-sulphate and a reduction in keratan sulphate and chondroitin-6-sulphate.
5. Marked qualitative similarity to the values obtained from articular cartilage and therefore a similar metabolic pattern in both malignant and normal chondrocytes.

However, there were wide ranges in the amounts of the various biochemical components. Statistically it was possible to show significant differences between the benign, low-grade and high-grade malignant tumours. This, he believed, may result from the malignant cells reverting to a more immature or embryonic type of cell and metabolism. To distinguish a high grade of malignant tumour from a low grade, Mankin described the six most important factors as: water content greater than 85%; DNA content greater than 5.5 μg/mg; 'excess' protein greater than 350 μg/mg; chondroitin-4/chondroitin-6 ratio greater than 1; a galactosamine/xylose ratio of less than 10; and a hexosamine concentration of less than 75 μg/mg. Such work is obviously very important for the future biochemical indexing of malignancy.

Basic biological investigations in biochemistry, DNA ploidy analysis, cytogenetics and molecular biology are being applied to the aetiology of sarcomas (Gebhardt, 1991). These will in time improve our knowledge about the heterogeneity of response to both adjuvant chemotherapy and to the actual surgery by similar histological types of tumours, as well as to develop biological markers for diagnosis and for treatment.

Kreichberg *et al.* (1982) have defined the prognostic value of cellular DNA, different clinicopathological factors and ploidy. They found a significantly higher 10-year survival rate in the diploid (with normal DNA content) chondrosarcomas than in the hyperdiploid (abnormally increased DNA content) chondrosarcoma. Ploidy and treatment were significantly related to the 10-year recurrence rate.

Treatment

See section on 'Musculoskeletal oncology'.

Secondary chondrosarcomata

Secondary chondrosarcomata arise in a pre-existing chondroma, osteochondroma, multiple exostoses and Ollier's disease, and occur mainly in the pelvis, the vertebrae, the femora and the humeri. Malignant change has been reported after x-ray therapy for other malignancies. When an enchondroma of the long bone in the adult becomes painful, it is probably malignant, especially if it is penetrated through the cortex of the bone on radiography (Figure 10.74). Treatment should be excision, using a wide margin, or by amputation, especially if recurrence takes place after resection. After local resection recurrence is higher than after an amputation carried out through the proximal joint. Marcove (1977) has described a recurrence rate at 5 years of 63% for grades 1 and 2, and 85% for grade 3. At 10 years, Dahlin and Henderson (1956) described a recurrence rate of 41%.

Prognosis in chondrosarcoma is dependent upon early diagnosis and upon the feasibility of adequate, though usually radical, surgery. When amputation is carried out, it should involve the biopsy site and therefore avoid the likelihood of implantation growth.

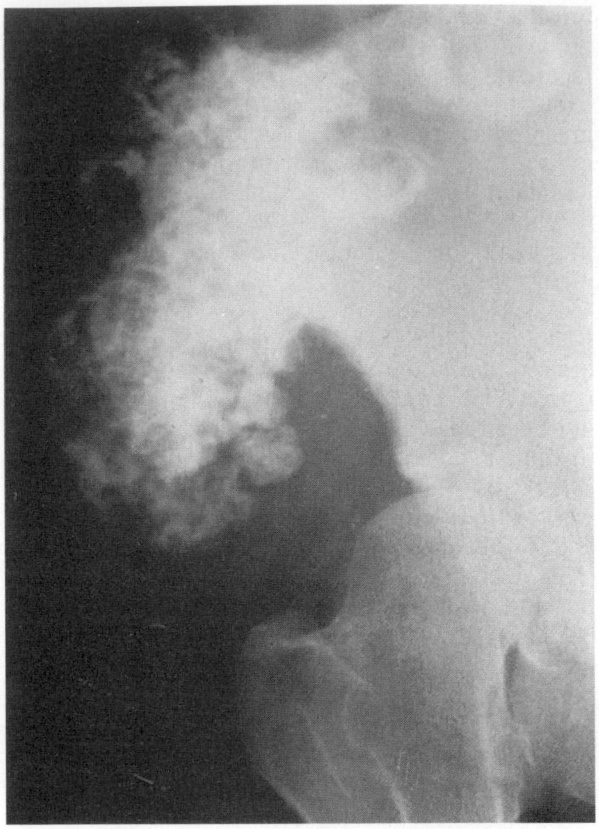

Figure 10.74 Chondrosarcoma of the ilium arising in an osteochondroma.

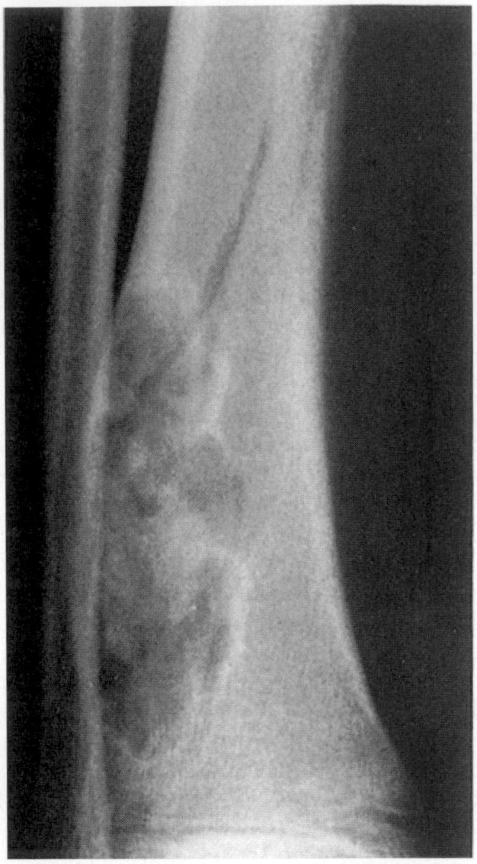

Figure 10.75 Fracture involving non-osteogenic fibroma of the distal tibia: when involving the cortex, they tend to be linear and are always metaphyseal.

Fibrous lesions

Benign fibrous tumours of bone are rare lesions and are closely allied to the fibrous dysplasias. Accordingly they may be regarded as derived from cellular elements of the bone-forming series, but the exact histogenesis is still obscure and indefinite; they are described as arising chiefly in the second decade and characteristically situated in the metaphysis.

The cellular and collagenous fibrous content of the tumour varies; the fibres are usually arranged in whorls. Growth is slow and unlimited, and mucoid or necrotic degeneration frequently occurs. Ossification is also common but differs from the normal in that the bone is laid down in an irregular manner because of the original irregular pattern of the fibroblasts. Very rarely does organized compact bone make its appearance. When the bony structure is organized and growth, although slow, is unlimited, this is known as a true osteoma.

When situated periosteally, it is known as a periosteal fibroma or exostosis if calcification has occurred; when in the medullary cavity, central fibroma; when in the bone substance, it has the clinical picture of a bone cyst. The condition is closely allied to fibrous dysplasia of bone but the presence in the latter of bone trabeculae undergoing resorption is regarded as of differential significance.

Included in this group there is the non-osteogenic fibroma (non-ossifying fibroma).

Non-osteogenic fibroma

This lesion is usually discovered incidentally on x-rays for other conditions in children as small cortical areas of radiolucency, although, rarely it presents as a pathological fracture in the first and second decades (Figure 10.75).

It usually begins in a metaphyseal location and during growth some will disappear (Figure 10.76). However, a few are displaced towards the centre of the bone, where they may grow large with thinning of the cortex but usually with a sclerotic margin.

On biopsy, the tissue is fibrous and nodular and contains variable amount of cells (Figure 10.77) – both fibroblasts and 'small' giant cells in a relatively large amount of collagenous fibrous tissue in which there is, rarely, delicate trabeculae of

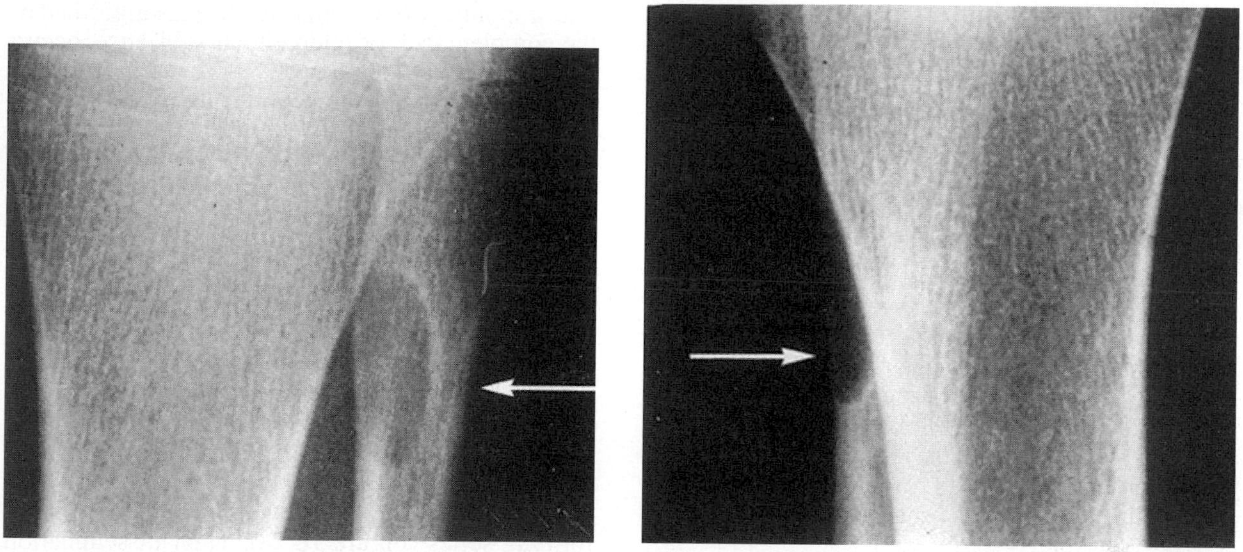

(a) (b)

Figure 10.76 (a) Anteroposterior and (b) oblique radiographs showing a non-ossifying fibroma as a benign cortical defect on the medial border of the proximal fibula bone.

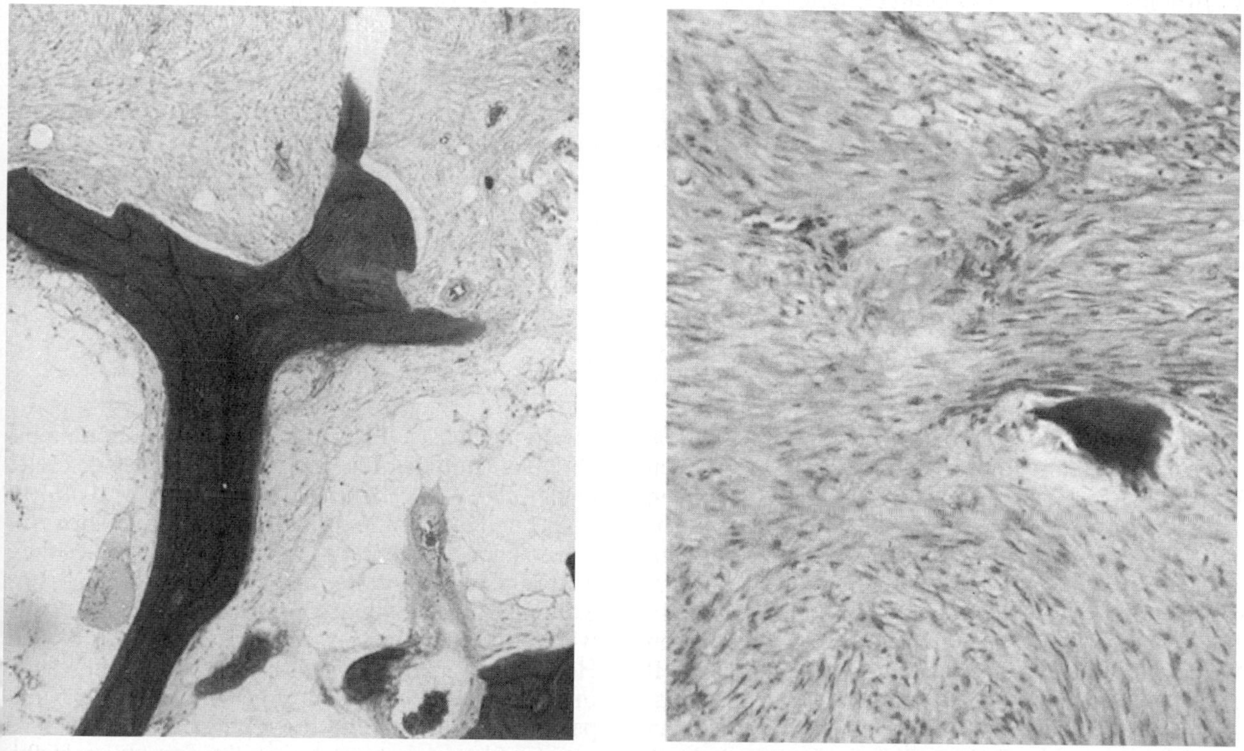

(a) (b)

Figure 10.77 (a) Photomicrograph of a non-ossifying fibroma, showing the invasion of normal marrow and trabeculae of bone by this dense but evenly formed cellular fibrous tissue. (× 58). (b) Photomicrograph showing the combination of dense but regular fibrous tissue and loose 'xanthoma' cells with their large foamy cytoplasm on the right. (× 179) bone, which aids in differentiating it from fibrous dysplasia.

Curettage or local resection is indicated, and adequate in amount to prevent recurrence.

Many now consider that the non-ossifying fibroma arises from a fibrous cortical defect which continues to proliferate and enlarge within the subcortical medullary surface.

Fibrous cortical defect

This is very common in children – up to 40% of all children aged between 4 and 8 years – and arising from the fibrous tissue of the periosteum. It is a peripheral lesion, located in the femur or tibia, healing by sclerosis. The histology consists of whorls of fibrous tissue in continuity with the periosteum. Treatment is usually one of observation.

Malignant fibrous histiocytoma

Malignant fibrous histiocytoma is a high-grade malignancy of bone, involving the metaphysis of long bones, especially around the knee in adults.

It is markedly osteolytic with destruction of cortex, periosteal reaction but no intracalcification. Histologically there are spindle-shaped fibroblasts, histiocyte-like cells, forming sheets of radiating cells which contain mitotic figures and some are multinucleated. Occasional osteoclasts are seen through the stroma. Metastatic renal carcinoma is one of the differential diagnoses. For treatment see section on 'Musculoskeletal oncology'.

FIBROSARCOMA

Examples of osteosarcoma with a predominantly fibroblast element are recognized but are regarded as variants of the osteosarcomata rather than a separate type of tumour.

Medullary fibrosarcomata, which comprise 10% of primary malignant bone tumours, have been distinguished by Thomson and colleagues (Thomson and Turner-Warwick 1955); in these tumours definite collagen formation has been the predominant feature. They occasionally arise in fibrous dysplasia, bone infarctions, post-radiation bone and very rarely after osteomyelitis. There has been early destruction of bone, but in some ossification has been present. It is of possible significance that these tumours appear to have a much more favourable prognosis than osteosarcoma, there being a 25% 5-year survival rate following radical surgery or x-irradiation and local excision. Over 50% of their patients who died had pulmonary metastases and a few had malignant deposits in lymph nodes. The same authors differentiate a spindle cell sarcoma which is distinguished by the complete lack of intercellular substance, occurs in a younger age group and is more radiosensitive.

These tumours were reported by Thomson and Turner-Warwick (1955) at all ages and as a secondary malignant degeneration in Paget's disease of the skull. They usually occur in middle age, affecting the long bones, either central – intramedullary – or cortical – periosteal (which have the best prognosis). They usually occur in long bones around the knee joint, as a central lesion which expands and partially destroys the cortex.

It is difficult to classify these tumours which are not yet clearly distinguished or generally recognized. It may be that they have a similar histogenesis to the simple tumours noted above, and from their location within the bone there is *prima facie* evidence that they arise from tissues of the bone-forming series (Figure 10.78). Their dissemination is usually via the blood stream to the lungs, but occasionally regional lymph nodes are involved. These tumours have been grouped, from their histological appearances, into two main types – one being well differentiated and the other poorly differentiated and anaplastic with a very poor prognosis.

Wide radical excision can be considered for low-grade, well differentiated and circumscribed intramedullary tumours of small size. Amputation, however, may be required. Radiotherapy is not indicated. Pritchard *et al.* (1977), from an excellent series but including soft tissue involvement, reported that 60% of all their patients treated since 1950 were alive without metastases. But over all for all types of this bone tumour alone, the 5-year survival is only 29%. See section on 'Musculoskeletal oncology'.

OSTEOCLASTOMA OR GIANT CELL TUMOUR

The typical osteoclast is a large cell containing a variable number of centrally placed, but discrete, nuclei. They are identical in appearance, ovoid in shape, and basophilic on staining with haematoxylin and eosin. Their cell of origin is unknown, since they are found in many states and conditions of bone. For example, these cells are commonly found in areas where bone is being remodelled, in recesses named Howship's lacunae. They also follow haemorrhage into the marrow or during cyst formation and are particularly prominent in hyperparathyroidism or osteitis fibrosa cystica during the formation of the 'brown node' which consists of granulation tissue infiltrated with new and old extravasated blood. They are also found in such bone lesions as non-osteogenic fibroma, unicameral bone cysts, aneurys-

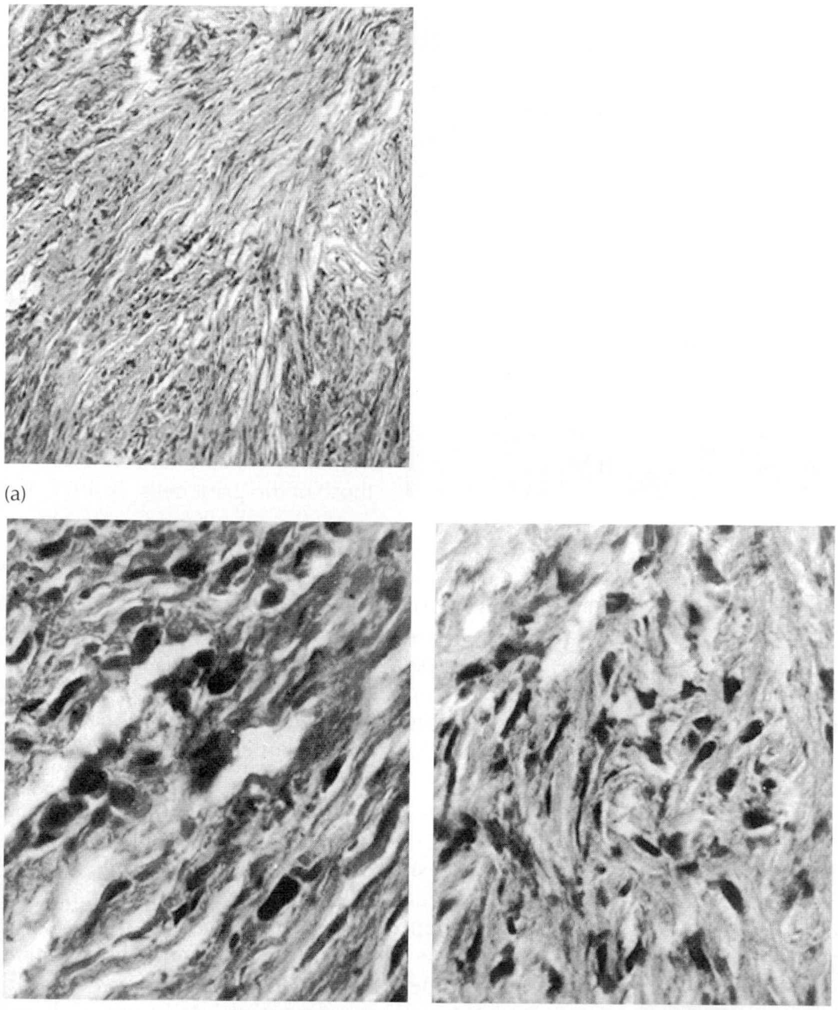

(a) (b) (c)

Figure 10.78 (a) Photomicrograph of a fibrosarcoma, showing the flowing dense but irregular fibrous tissue containing less organized and arranged pleomorphic cell shapes. (× 130). (b) and (c) Further detail, showing the irregularity of these spindle cells, with marked pleomorphism and the densely staining nuclear pattern characteristic of malignant cells. (× 408).

mal bone cyst, fibrous dysplasia, chondroblastoma, osteogenic sarcoma and histiocytic granulomatosis, but these must be clearly differentiated from a giant cell tumour.

The critical feature of this tumour is the vascular and cellular stroma which is made up of oval-shaped cells containing a small elongated, darkly stained nucleus with little eosinophilic cytoplasm on staining with haematoxylin and eosin. The giant cell is a large cell with pink-staining cytoplasm and is filled with numerous and centrally placed nuclei which are vesicular in character and appear very similar to the stromal cells, so much so it is considered that they arise from fusion of the stroma cells. The stroma cells show a varying degree of malignancy with the typical features of mitotic activity, pleomorphism and hyperchromatism (Figure 10.79). In the more frankly malignant giant cell tumours, the giant cells become anaplastic with areas of necrotic material and haemorrhage. These true neoplasms occur mainly in the second and third decades, with an equal sex distribution. They are seen mainly in the ends of long bones, particularly in the vicinity of the knee and at the lower end of the radius. Osteoclastoma commonly arises in the metaphyseal-epiphyseal area and is related to the usual osteoclastic activity of remodelling in this area. On x-rays, the epiphyseal-metaphyseal areas are seen to be enlarged and occupied by clear cystic tumour (Figure 10.80). The cortex is thin and may sharply limit the tumour from the surrounding soft tissues, with a sharp line of demarcation between the tumour and the unaffected shaft, in contradistinction to sarcomata and bone cysts. The expanding osteolytic lesion can continue to destroy the cortex, although usually it leaves some external rim. The tumour grows eccentrically to destroy the epiphyseal cartilage and it may penetrate the articular cartilage, but rarely does it extend into a joint. Pathological fractures do occur (Figure 10.81).

Clinically these patients present because of pain

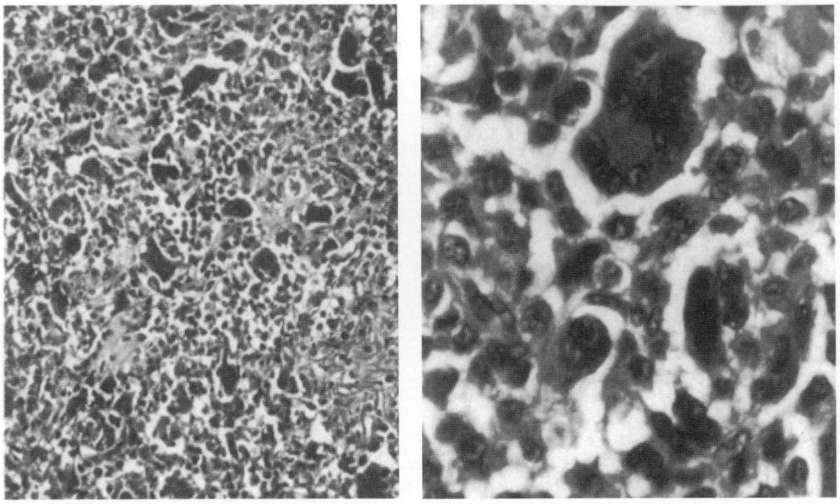

(a) (b)

Figure 10.79 (a) Photomicrograph of a giant cell tumour, showing the centrally placed and oval-shaped nuclei of the stromal cells and the many giant cells whose nuclei appear to be similar to those of the stromal cells. (× 130).
(b) Photomicrograph showing in greater detail the marked similarity between the nuclei of the mononuclear stromal cells and those of the giant cells. (× 407).

and loss of function around the joint, which may even suggest a possible inflammatory lesion and a swelling of an asymmetrical nature. Radiologically it is an eccentric lytic lesion, with poorly defined borders usually metaphyseal or juxtaepiphyseal in site, expanding the cortex which may be destroyed,

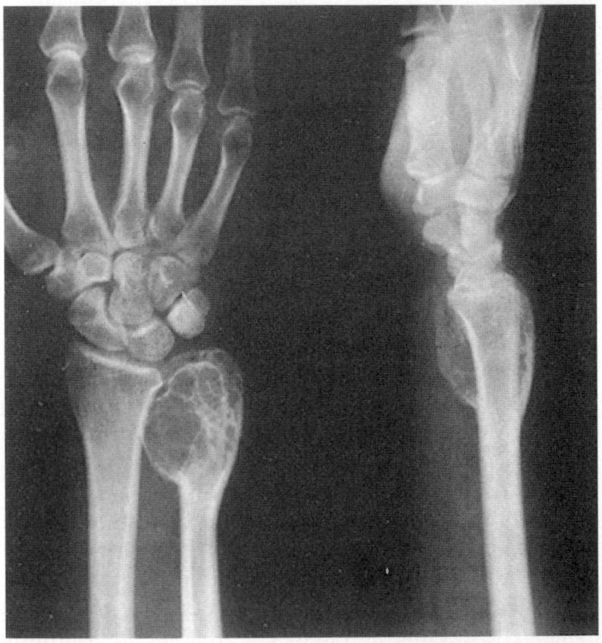

Figure 10.80 Radiograph showing a giant cell tumour of the distal ulna. The junction of the lesion with the normal bone is typical. The old cortex has been destroyed, new bone has been laid down around the lesion and this bone abuts the old cortex on its lateral side rather than being in direct continuation with it.

resulting in soft tissue extension. Upon biopsy, the tumour mass is seen to be contained by a thin-shelled cortex and appears to be red, greyish and haemorrhagic, often under some pressure. There may be cystic areas containing fatty areas and bone debris. It can spread along the intramedullary space.

Although in the past these tumours have been regarded as relatively benign, Thomson and Turner-Warwick (1955) showed that there is approximately a 60% 5-year survival rate. However, they emphasize that there are varying degrees of malignancy of this tumour, depending upon the sarcomatous nature of the stroma. Therefore, treatment is directed towards complete and total local resection if at all possible; otherwise, amputation. Amputation is required in about 30% of giant cell tumours. This is because of the rapid expansion of the primary tumour into adjacent tissues (which may undergo destruction) and because, after radical excision, infection may occur. Radiotherapy has not been shown by Dahlin's group to decrease the recurrence rate, and indeed 10% of their tumours with such treatment underwent sarcomatous degeneration. There is still some controversy about such a possibility and, therefore, x-irradiation is not recommended except in inaccessible lesions. However, it should be mentioned that out of all malignancies of bone, the giant cell tumour has the best prognosis. 'Complications' of this tumour are recurrence of about 35% (Goldenberg *et al.*, 1970); malignant degeneration with metastases in about 30% (Hutter *et al.*, 1962); irradiation sarcomata, with or without pathological fracturing (Figures 10.82 and 10.83); and bone grafting problems.

Treatment is often restricted by these tumours being adjacent to a weight-bearing joint. Where possible (e.g. lower end of ulna, upper end of fibula),

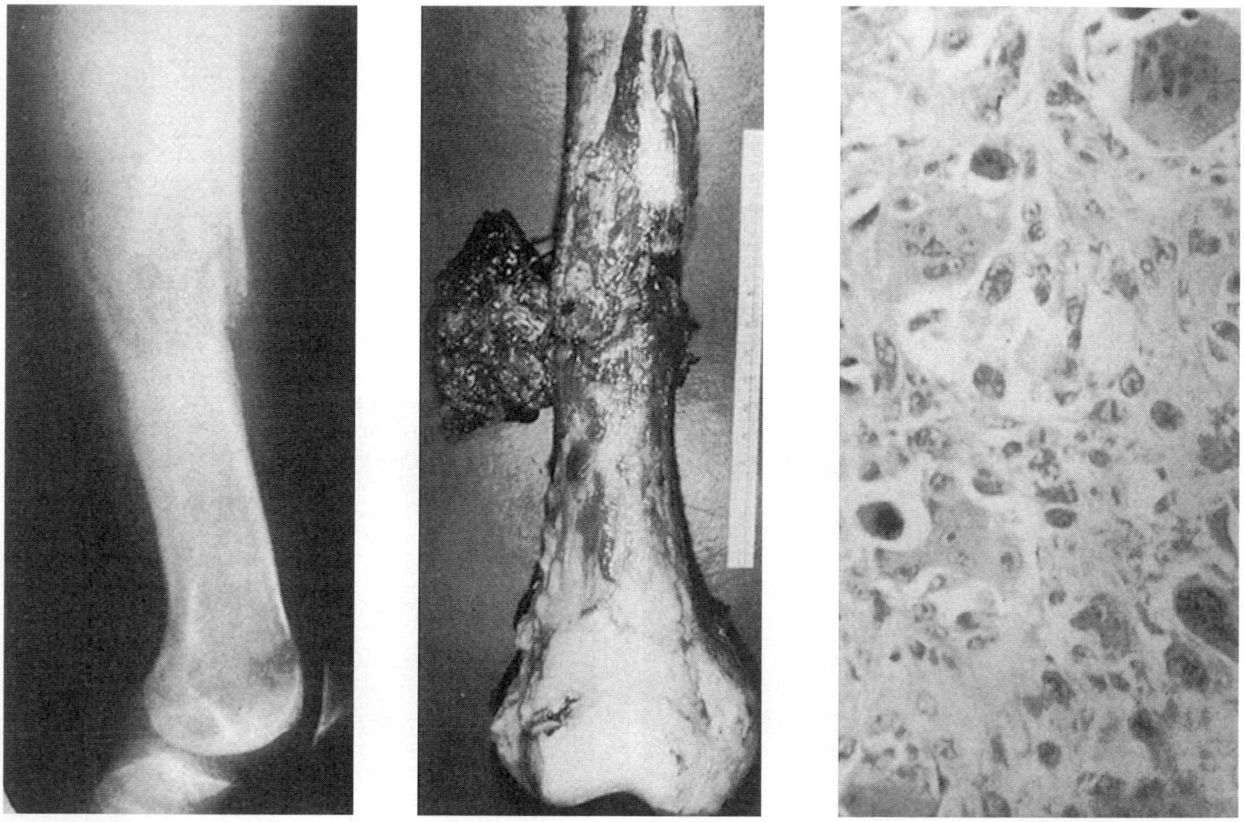

(a) (b) (c)

Figure 10.81 (a) Lateral radiograph of a young man's femur showing a pathological fracture through an osteolytic area involving the shaft. (b) Photograph of the specimen from (a), showing the extension out of the soft tissues of the tumour. (c) Photomicrograph showing giant cells with varying numbers of nuclei, some of which look similar to the large vesicular nuclei of the stroma cells. (× 500). This tumour, in spite of the unusual situation in the diaphysis, was diagnosed as a giant cell tumour, and its metastases to the lungs also appeared to be those of a giant cell tumour. However, other more rare malignancies of bone such as a liposarcoma have to be considered, with the giant cells being a reaction to the malignancy rather than part of the neoplasia.

complete resection of the tumour and adjacent bone should be carried out. Resection of a giant cell tumour in the vicinity of the knee joint, with arthrodesis of the knee, is also recommended by Campanacci and Costa (1979).

Extensive resection and prosthetic replacement can now be carried out, but, being in the younger adult groups, it is likely that this procedure will have to be repeated.

Thorough curettage with extensive cancellous bone grafting is still the operation of choice – even though a recurrence rate of 50% is found – because it can be repeated. Radical excision with cryosurgery offers the best cure and this tumour rarely metastasizes. However, after multiple local procedures for local recurrence, between 8 and 22% become malignant, although local radiotherapy is thought to play a significant role in this transformation (see section on 'Musculoskeletal oncology').

Giant cell tumour, in making up about 5% of all primary bone tumours, occurs most commonly in the lower end of the femur, the upper tibia, the lower end of the radius, rarely in the sacrum and even more unusually in the pelvic bones. Sanjay *et al.* (1993) have reviewed 19 patients with giant cell tumours involving a pelvic bone – predominantly of the ilium. The patients were 30–40 years of age. Treatment of the 'active' lesion was curettage with only one local recurrence which developed at 12 months. Eight patients who had an 'aggressive' lesion received a resection of most of the lesion accompanied by a local curettage of the margin. Four had in addition post-resection irradiation. None had local recurrence, six had no evidence of any disease, but one died of post-radiation sarcoma 13 years later and one died of pulmonary metastases 3 years after operation. Four patients who had recurrent tumours when first seen were managed by hemipelvectomy, wide re-

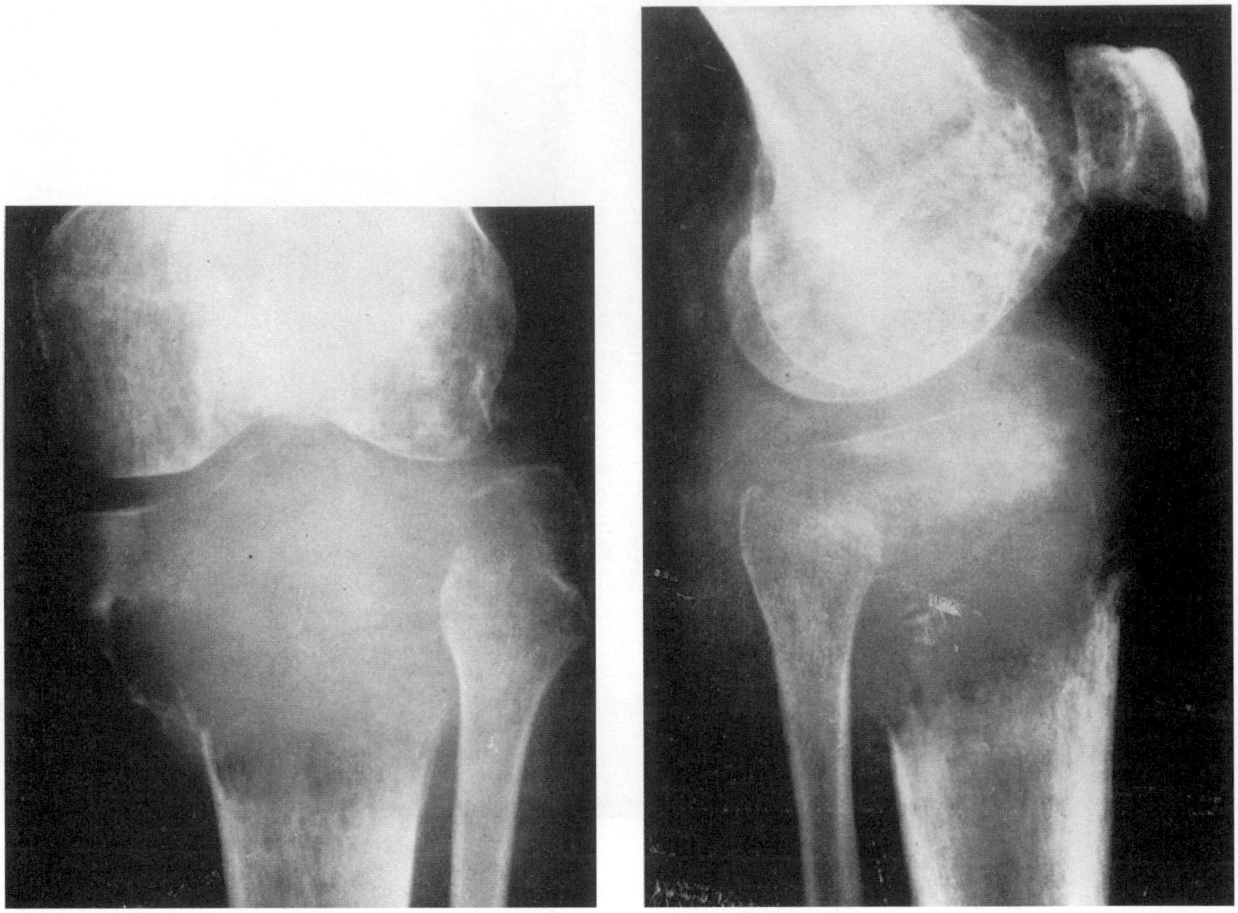

(a) (b)

Figure 10.82 (a) Anteroposterior and (b) lateral radiographs, showing expansile giant cell tumour involving upper end of tibia. A pathological fracture has taken place at the distal pole.

section, etc. Three had no evidence of disease up to 20 years after operation, and one died with post-radiation metatastic osteosarcoma 8 years after operation.

Vander Griend and Funderburk (1993) have reported on their results of treating giant cell tumours involving the distal radius in 23 patients. Where possible extensive curettage using a high speed burr or pulsating lavage and electrocautery with packing of the cavity by methylmethacrylate should be used to preserve function. This can be carried out when the lesion is intraosseous or when there is minimal cortical penetration.

When there has been cortical penetration and extraosseous extension of the tumour, resection of the distal part of the radius and a radiocarpal arthrodesis using an intercalary bone graft and stabilizing with a long plate is recommended. In only one case was a below-elbow amputation required.

Non-osteogenic tumours of bone

These are discussed under the headings of periosteal fibrosarcoma, Ewing's tumour, reticulum cell sarcoma, blood vessel tumours and fatty tumours.

PERIOSTEAL FIBROSARCOMA

This tumour originates in the outer non-osteogenic fibrous layer of the periosteum. It is in character a fascial sarcoma and similar in character to those arising in other sites in the soft tissues. It is extracortical and neither invades nor infiltrates the bone. The tumour remains encapsulated for a long time, and as it grows it pushes aside the soft tissues, but rarely infiltrates them.

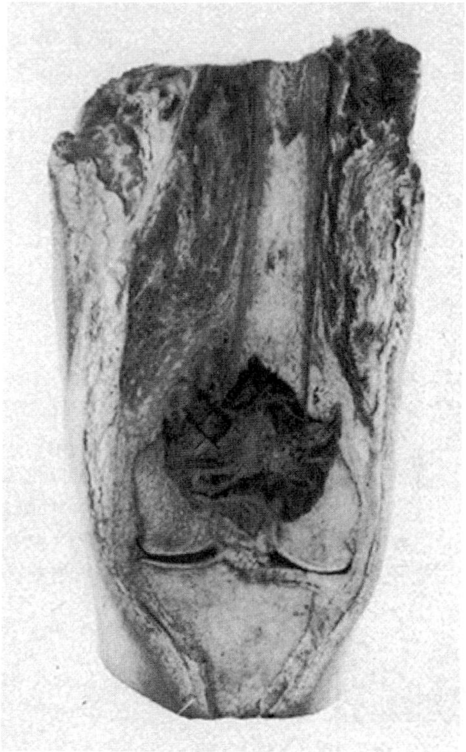

Figure 10.83 Amputation specimen of an osteoclastoma of distal femur, showing a pathological fracture and the biopsy site.

Secondary changes eventually appear in the underlying bone, but they result from the pressure and the contact of the tumour. Saucer-shaped erosions may occur where the cortex is in contact with the tumour, and areas of new periosteal bone formation at the periphery.

The tumour is firm, fibrous, white and glistening, with easily distinguishable fasciculi. Occasionally it is cellular, soft and crumbly, containing cysts. The degree of vascularity varies with the cellularity of the tumour. The tumour may appear to be encapsulated, but the capsule merely consists of the condensed sur-rounding tissues. It remains localized for a considerable time, but ultimately, as the vascularity and cellularity increase, it becomes more malignant. At this stage, secondary metastases usually occur in the lungs.

Histologically the tumour is a spindle cell fibrosarcoma with a variable degree of collagen formation. There is no true ossification but calcification can occur.

Clinical features

While these tumours may arise at any age, and one has been observed in a newborn child, the majority are seen in patients about 30 years of age. Localized swelling, steadily increasing in size and initially with little pain or disability, are the main features. While the tumours have a broad attachment to the periosteum they appear to have considerable mobility on examination.

A very well recognized site for these tumours is at the lower end of the femur (Figure 10.84).

Diagnosis

The radiograph shows a faintly outlined soft tissue shadow, the cortex opposite which often shows a shallow saucer-shaped depression. Beyond this, bone changes are conspicuous by their absence.

Treatment

Radical removal of the tumour is the operation of choice. The prognosis is especially favourable when the tumour is encapsulated. (See section on musculoskeletal oncology.)

EWING'S TUMOUR

In 1928 Ewing described a rare lesion of bone characterized by the development of a tumour in the diaphysis of the long bones, occurring in childhood and associated with febrile attacks, anorexia, weight loss and anaemia. The tumour rapidly involved other parts of the skeleton and was radiosensitive. Histologically the identification of the origin of the tumour was difficult and Ewing believed that it arose from endothelial elements in the marrow. Largely by the work of Willis it was demonstrated that in many of the cases, diagnosed clinically and radiologically as Ewing's tumour, the histological pattern demonstrated a rosette formation which was suggestive if not characteristic of neuroblastomata, and further that in these cases which were submitted to full post-mortem examination a primary tumour, usually in the adrenal, could be found. In other instances the lesion could be identified as a reticulum cell sarcoma (Figure 10.85). In a number of other cases the lesion on fuller examination proved to be metastatic, the primary tumour being located in different sites.

While it is accepted that a majority of the cases presenting these clinical and histological features are in fact examples of metastasizing neuroblastomata or reticulum cell sarcomata, there yet remain a small group of reports in which the fullest examination gives no evidence of any primary neoplasm outside the skeleton. In these the microscopical examination differs from both reticulum cell sarcoma and secondary disease originating in the neural tissues or

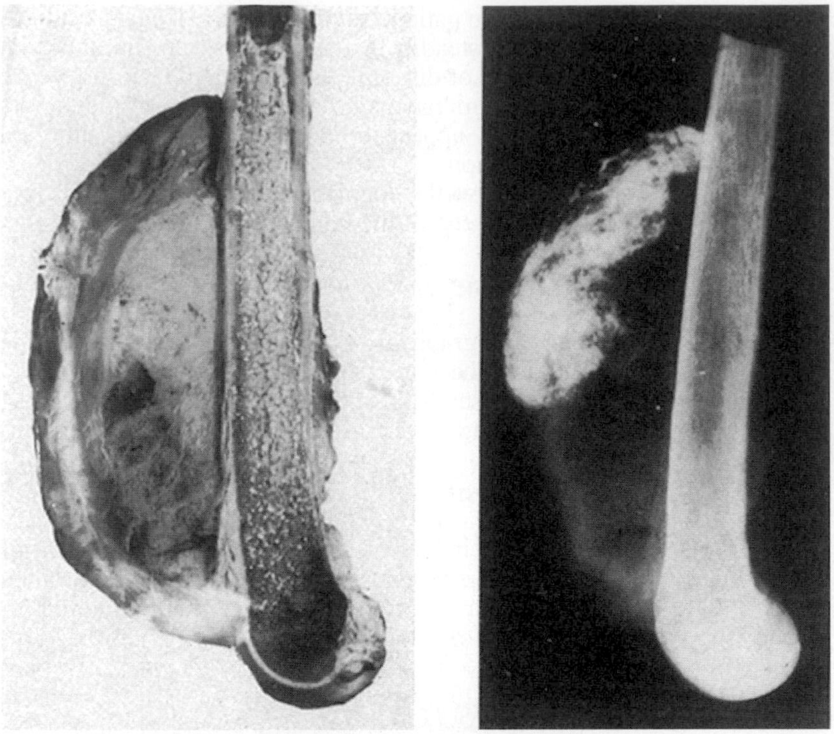

(a) (b)

Figure 10.84 Periosteal fibrosarcoma of femur. Female aged 25 years. (a) History of injury 12 years previously, followed by development of a slowly growing tumour. One year prior to admission the tumour began to grow rapidly. (b) Radiological examination shows extensive calcification.

elsewhere. In differentiating 'round cell' tumours, histochemical techniques are proving much more helpful for identifying intracellular glycogen in Ewing's tumour, intracellular reticulin in reticulum cell sarcoma and catecholamines in metastatic neuroblastoma.

The typical Ewing's tumour usually occurs between the ages of 5 and 15, and is somewhat more common in males. The bones most commonly affected are the flat and axial bones, the long bones, and of them it is most frequently found in the tibia. Next in frequency, the fibula, the humerus and the femur are involved. The tumour has a decided tendency to the involvement of other bones after the primary focus has been established; indeed it may be diffused throughout the whole skeleton, and the skull and small bones may be affected. Regional lymph glands may be involved.

Pathology

The tumour almost invariably begins in the marrow about the middle of the shaft, a feature which serves to distinguish it from the osteogenic and benign giant cell tumours. In colour it is greyish-white. Areas of necrosis and haemorrhage with cyst formation are often present. The lamellae in relation to the tumour mass are destroyed, and necrotic lamellae suggests osteomyelitis.

From the medulla the tumour extends in the Haversian canals to the surface. Under the periosteum compensatory layers of new bone are deposited, only to be destroyed. Such shells of new bone are deposited parallel to the shaft of the bone and have been aptly described as 'onion layers'.

Histology

The microscopical features in these lesions are not specific. The tumour is intensely cellular and usually the cells conform to one type – small, round or polyhedral, arranged in solid cords or sheets. Intercellular substance is minimal. Necrosis is common, and the remaining cells arranged round the central blood vessel have sometimes given the appearance which has justified the term 'perithelioma'. The nuclei are always prominent and mitosis frequent.

Many tumours show a rosette arrangement and within the centre of the rosette, by special staining methods, fibrils can sometimes be demonstrated. Such a structure is characteristic of a neuroblastoma. Pseudorosette formation is, however, more common, but this does not exclude the possibility that these cells are in fact neuroblasts but lacking in fibril formation by reason of the dedifferentiation which has occurred in a rapidly growing tumour.

Despite the bone destruction, giant cells or osteoclasts are never found; nor is new bone to be dis-

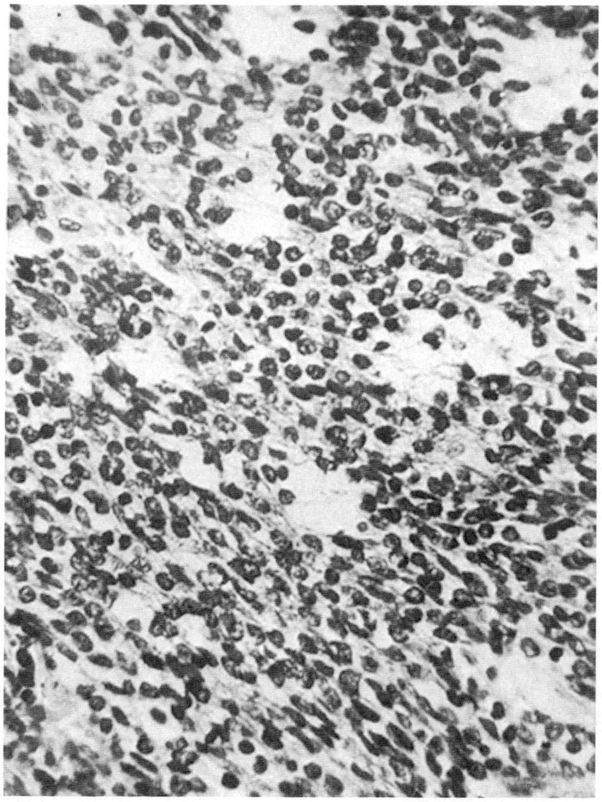

Figure 10.85 Photomicrograph showing cells which are regular in appearance and round, but around this area there are others having a more oval configuration with a moderate amount of reticular intercellular matrix, suggesting the possibility of a reticulum cell carcinoma. (× 263).

covered, apart from the subperiosteal deposits. The vessels of the tumour and the lymphatics may both contain obvious emboli, for the tumour spreads by the blood and lymphatic systems. Liver, spleen and bone marrow scans are required as well as MR and CT scanning for lungs and the primary site.

Clinical features

There is usually a history of preceding trauma, often associated with pain. There occur intermittent attacks of pain followed by the appearance of a slow-growing tumour in relation to the shaft of one of the long bones. During the attacks of pain the tumour may enlarge visibly, and there may be febrile attacks and a leucocytosis. The overlying skin is never affected unless surgical exploration is carried out during one of the acute phases; then the tumour may fungate through the skin. Pathological fracture seldom occurs.

In the late stages multiple deposits appear in the skull, ribs, sternum, pelvis and other, long, bones. There is then marked cachexia and secondary anaemia. When the vertebrae are involved there is severe root pain or paralysis, and death usually results from metastatic involvement of the lungs.

Radiological appearances

There is a diffuse rarefaction (Figure 10.86) towards the centre of the shaft, and extending for a considerable area. In the early stages there is condensation without other change. Later, from reactive irritation the periosteum throws off 'onion-skin layers' parallel to the shaft and rather like osteomyelitis, or, more commonly, small spicules appear (Figure 10.87). The last stage is that of gross tumour formation with destruction of the original bone structure and pathological fracture. In the flat bone, the appearance is of bone destruction and a large adjacent soft tissue mass.

Diagnosis

Classically the differential diagnosis of Ewing's tumour is from chronic osteomyelitis, metastatic neuroblastoma, histiocytosis and, rarely, an osteolytic osteosarcoma. The chief difficulty lies in an

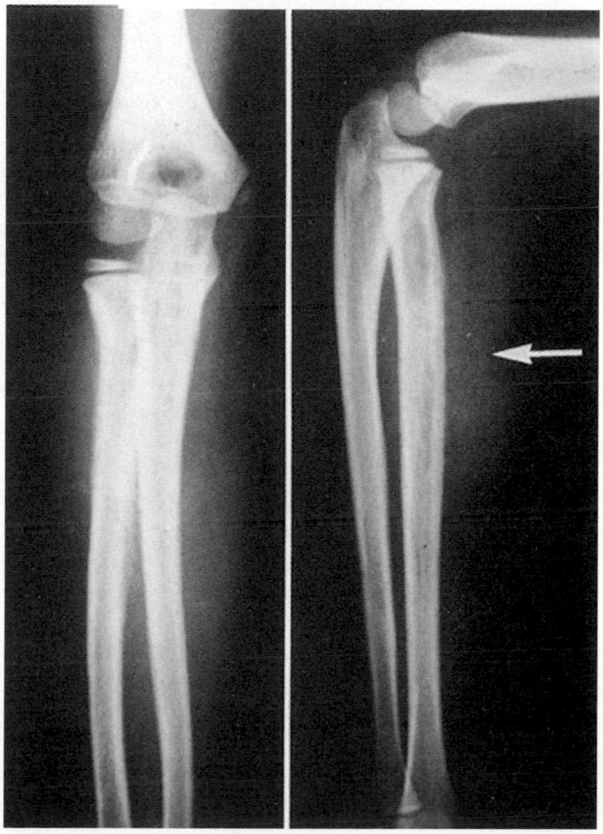

Figure 10.86 Ewing's sarcoma of the radius with linear destruction of an infiltrative type.

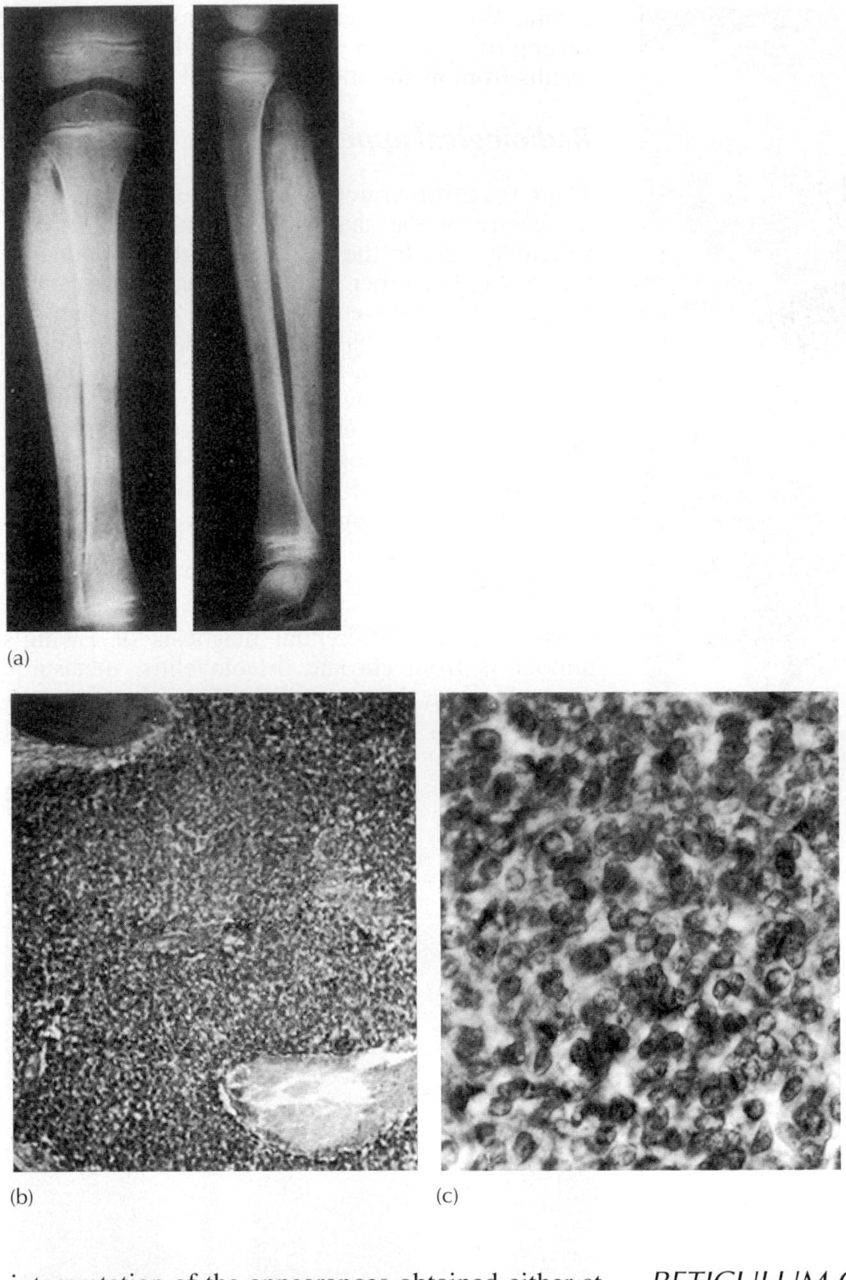

Figure 10.87 (a) Radiograph showing an advanced Ewing's sarcoma of the fibula with marked periosteal new bone formation and loss of the medulla.
(b) Photomicrograph showing the striking homogeneity of this massively cellular lesion. The cells are large, rounded and have regular shaped nuclei and scanty cytoplasm with an almost total absence of any intercellular matrix. (× 115).
(c) Photomicrograph emphasizing the marked similarity between the nuclei and reduced amount of intercellular substance. (× 370).

interpretation of the appearances obtained either at biopsy (Figure 10.88) or at operation, and in those cases where the lesion is metastatic it may be difficult to demonstrate the primary source of the tumour.

The rapid response of many cases labelled Ewing's tumour to radiotherapy was considered to be of diagnostic significance, but this is no longer regarded as correct.

Treatment

See section on 'Musculoskeletal oncology'.

RETICULUM CELL SARCOMA

This is a non-bone-producing tumour which occurs in the second to the fourth decades of life and affects particularly the femur, tibia and humerus. Pain is often the first complaint, preceding the formation of a tumour. This may invade a large part of the shaft of the long bone but without affecting the health of the patient materially.

The x-ray picture is not characteristic. There is an osteolytic lesion in the end of a long bone, which later extends throughout the length. There is fragmentation of the cortex and pathological fracture may occur.

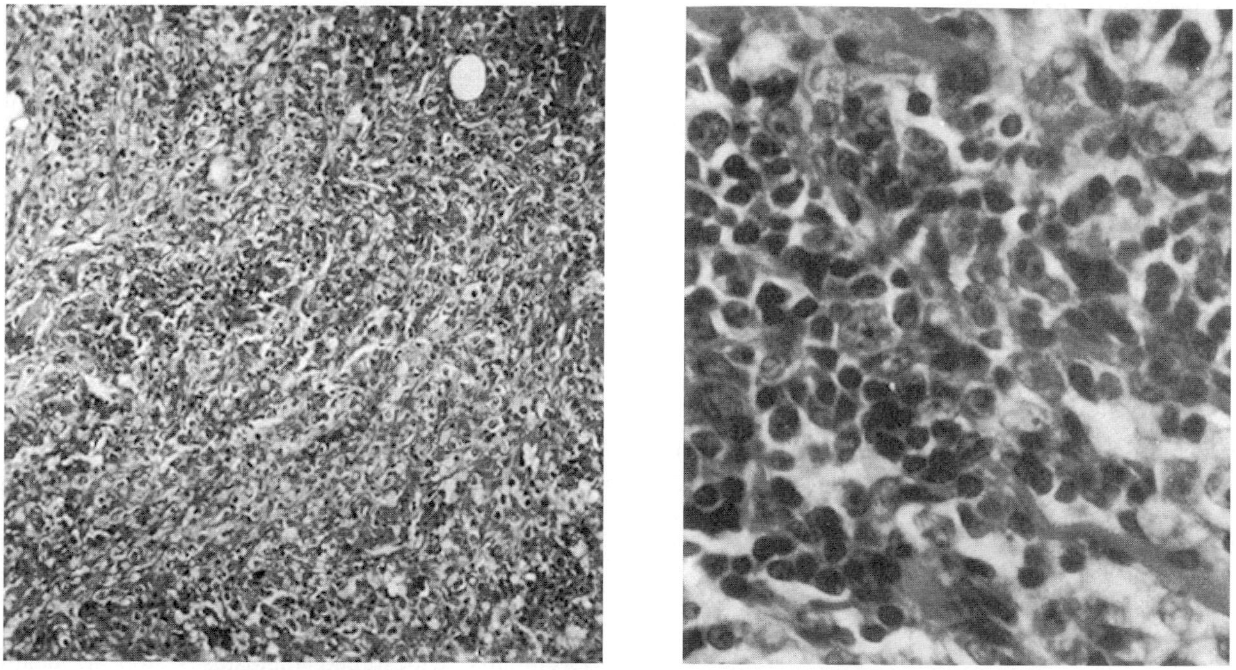

(a) (b)

Figure 10.88 (a) Photomicrograph of a reticulum cell sarcoma. This lesion is less cellular than a Ewing's sarcoma and has a considerable amount of intercellular matrix. (× 177). (b) Photomicrograph showing the cells to be more oval appearing and frequently indented or 'reniform' in outline. (× 532).

Pathology

The shaft is occupied by a pinkish-grey granulation tissue and this in time invades the soft tissue. The cells, which are identical with those of reticulum cell sarcoma of a lymph gland, are larger than a lymphocyte, and have round, oval, indented or lobulated nuclei with considerable cytoplasm. Delicate reticulum fibres pass between the cells, which often show a large number of mitotic figures (Figure 10.89).

The tumour is relatively benign. Although the initial response to irradiation is good, there is usually local recurrence. A primary course of irradiation followed by amputation or radical resection is the most promising method of treatment.

Differential diagnosis

See Table 10.7.

BLOOD VESSEL TUMOURS

Blood vessel tumours in tissue – whether benign or malignant – manifest themselves as lesions of rarefaction with compensatory distal bone formation. These tumours are rare but present an interesting problem of diagnosis.

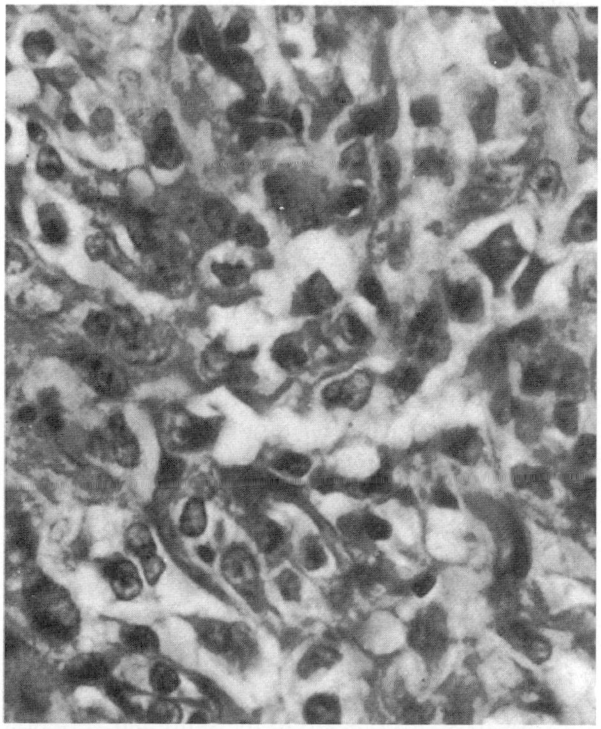

Figure 10.89 Photomicrograph showing the reticular and cellular material with greater variation in both shape and size of all nuclei as well as staining reaction of a reticulum cell sarcoma. (× 468).

Aneurysmal bone cyst

This lesion also occurs in the region of the metaphysis in young people. It can occur in the ends of long bones or in the vertebrae. x-Rays show a characteristic lesion of an eccentrically placed osteolytic expansion of the cortex, with some extension into the surrounding soft tissues (Figure 10.90). However, there are attempts at periosteal new bone formation.

Table 10.7

Ewing's sarcoma	Reticulum cell sarcoma
Aged under 20 years	Aged 35–40 years
Much periosteal reaction with bone destruction	Little periosteal reaction, but destructive and expanding lesion
Small cells with compact chromatin and less defined cytoplasm, which contains glycogen	Larger, round or oval cells with indented nucleus or kidney-shaped, but poorly defined and stained cytoplasm. Delicate framework of interlacing fibres with pattern
Radiosensitive	Radiosensitive
Few 5-year survivors	50% 5-year survivors

Trabeculation may be present at the periphery, but is not so clearly delineated towards the centre. It may be a coincidental finding or present because of pain. On biopsy, it is seen to be a mass of blood spaces filled with frank blood. On histology, the characteristic feature is of cavernous spaces, the walls of which are made up of fibrous tissue containing some thin strands of osteoid tissue, but rarely an endothelial lining. Giant cells may be present, particularly in the more cellular areas of the tumour. Stroma cells are usually fibroblastic and have to be differentiated from that of a giant cell tumour. Local curettage, with or without bone grafting, appears to give adequate results. It is almost diagnostic when the tumour is cut into and there is marked, brisk haemorrhage.

Haemangioma

Vascular tumours of bone are rare, but a number of case reports have established that the most common sites for these lesions are in the skull and vertebral column. Very characteristically in the flat bones bony spicules radiate from the surface, giving what is known as the 'sunburst' appearance. In the vertebrae the characteristic appearance in an x-ray is the presence of vertical parallel lines and increased density. In the vertebral column, when the body is affected the appearance may suggest tuberculosis, secondary neoplasm or Paget's disease. Collapse of the vertebral body occurs and there may be pressure on the cord.

These tumours are benign in character in a majority of instances. Treatment is difficult on account of the location of the tumour, but should the lesion be present in the more peripheral bones radical excision is advised.

Angiosarcoma

Angiosarcoma (angioendothelioma) is *extremely* rare and must be differentiated from the reticulosarcoma which may mimic it closely because of the potential endothelial function of reticular cells. It occurs in patients of any age and apparently any bone in the skeleton may be affected. The clinical course of the tumour is similar to that of osteogenic sarcoma, save that the pain is later in appearance. Eventually widespread metastases appear, death usually resulting from pulmonary involvement.

FATTY TUMOURS

Lipoma

Simple lipomata have been described both as arising within the medullary cavity and in relation to the periosteum. These tumours are innocent, but by their pressure some absorption of adjacent bone may occur (Figure 10.91). Liposarcoma is an exceedingly rare lesion and the pathological diagnosis is the subject of considerable controversy.

Tumours arising from included tissues

Under this heading are discussed adamantinoma, neurilemmoma, chordoma, malignant tumours of the soft tissues and tumoral calcinosis.

ADAMANTINOMA

Adamantinoma, or adamantine epithelioma, has long been known as an entity and ordinarily occurs in the jaw but also affects the tibia; rarely other long bones. Baker *et al.* (1954) reviewed 27 cases occurring in the long bones. The name indicates a

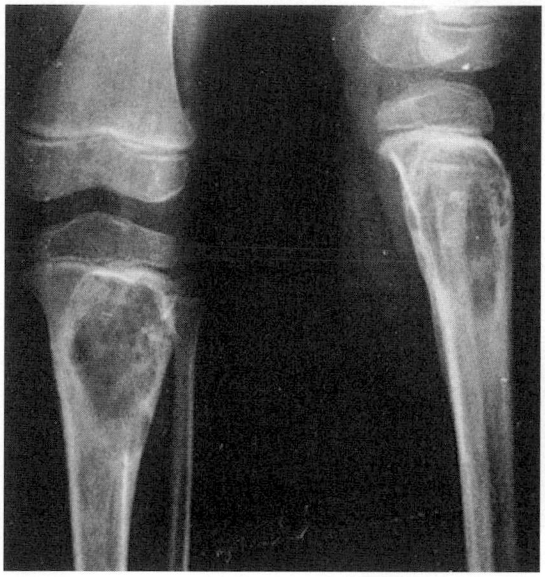
(a)

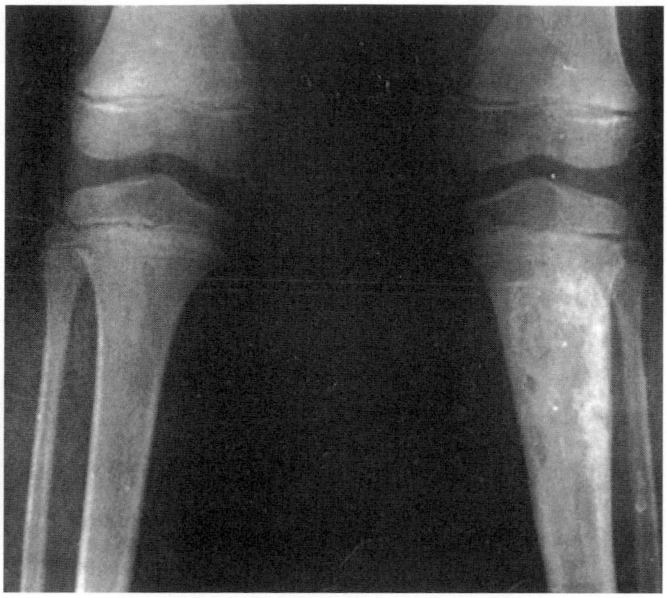
(b)

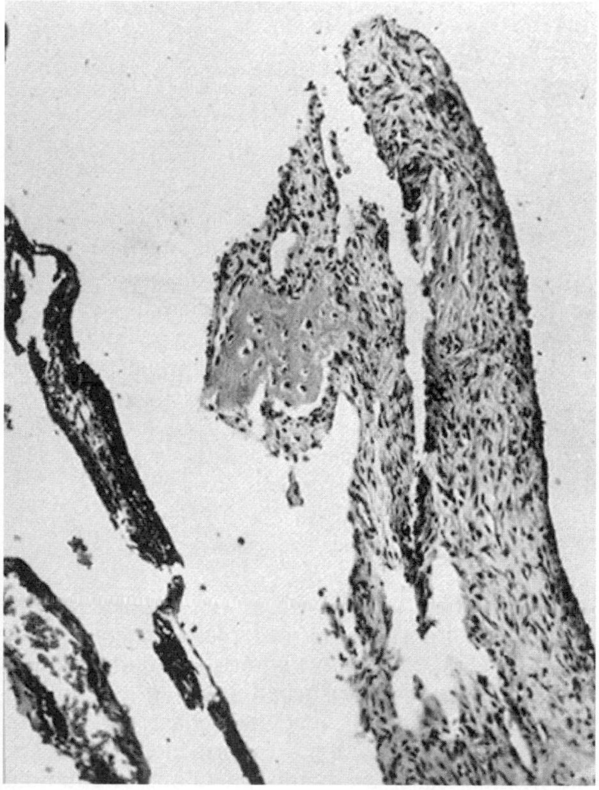
(c)

Figure 10.90 (a) Aneurysmal bone cyst, eccentric in location and destroying the lateral cortex of the proximal tibia. (b) Repair of lesion by a bone grafting procedure but with continuing growth discrepancy of the epiphyseal line laterally. (c) Photomicrograph showing the thin septa of aneurysmal bone cyst with some giant cell formation. (× 108).

tumour consisting of enamel and is misleading, so that until more is known of their pathogenesis it would seem wise to refer to them as 'adamantinoma (so-called)' of the long bones or, after Lichtenstein, 'dermal inclusion tumours'. There is some doubt as to whether these long-bone tumours are in any way related to such named tumours of the jaw, especially as no enamel has been found in them. In the above-

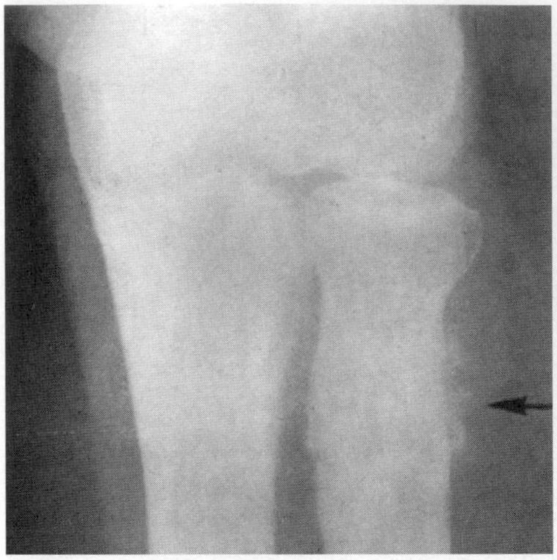
(a)

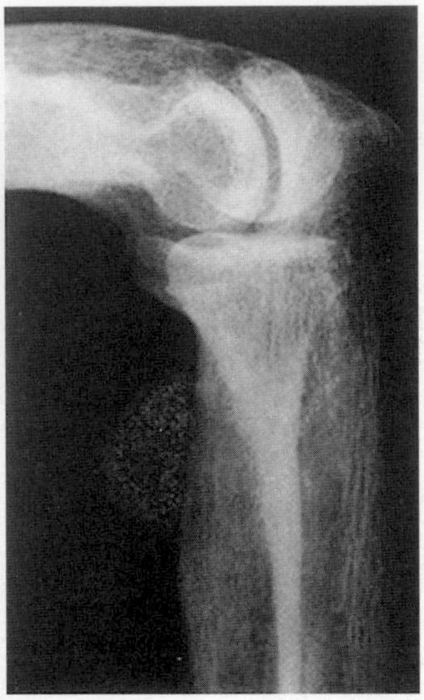
(b)

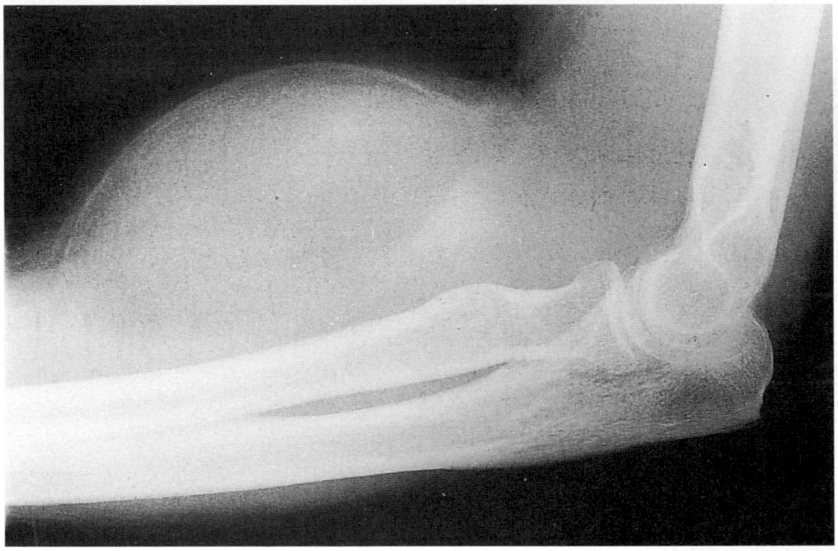
(c)

Figure 10.91 (a) Anteroposterior and (b) lateral radiographs showing the bone reaction in the vicinity of the radial neck of a periosteal lipoma. (c) A 'soft tissue' radiograph to show the large fatty tissue mass – homogeneous in content and contrast. There was a posterior interosseous nerve palsy.

mentioned review, pain was commonly the first symptom and had been present for from 6 weeks to 17 years. Tenderness was the initial symptom in one case. Sometimes the presence of a tumour or mass first attracted attention.

It is a slow-growing tumour whose origin is unknown. There is no agreement as to whether the epithelial tumour is a basal cell or squamous cell carcinoma. There are several theories of origin: e.g. derived from deep-seated, aberrant embryonal nests of epidermoid epithelium; or implanted epidermoid cell nests following trauma; or a variant of a malignant angioblastoma.

x-Rays show a finely trabeculated, expanded, osteolytic shaft lesion with a well defined margin and an intact cortex. Microscopically it consists of solid strands, sheets or whorls of dark-staining polygonal or spindle-shaped cells, often with a tendency towards a syncytial character (Figure 10.92). It shows a tendency to form clefts and cysts, and in most cases there are collections of cuboidal cells arranged in irregular acini. The treatment of choice is amputation, preferably through the more proximal bone. The tumour is said to be highly radioresistant. It is almost certain to recur. In 17 of their 27 cases recurrence took place, followed by death in 8 cases. Metastasis was proved by biopsy in 4 cases, further emphasizing the need for radical

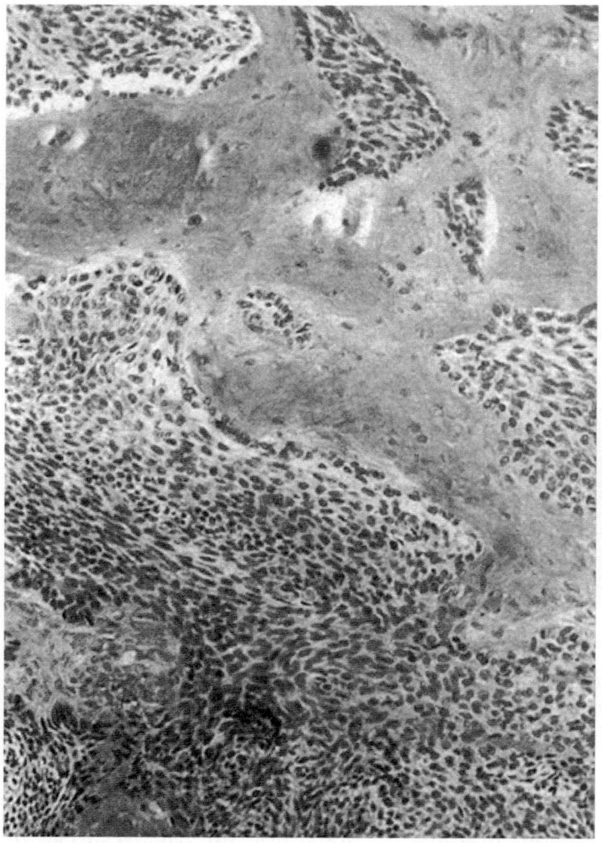

Figure 10.92 Photomicrograph of an adamantinoma of the tibia, showing large oval 'epithelial-like' cells loosely grouped around areas of dense, homogeneous-appearing fibrous tissue in which are a few cells similar to those at the periphery. (× 179).

surgery. Metastases to the inguinal glands have been described.

NEURILEMMOMA

This is a type of nerve sheath tumour which has had a variety of names in the past, but, as it is generally agreed that it is a tumour of the neurilemma, the term neurilemmoma is in general use.

The tumour has been described as growing in long bone and in the sacrum. Clinically the tumour may show as a cystic swelling. The x-rays show destruction of the bone. The common and often only symptom is the physical presence of a tumour. This is always single and circumscribed (Figure 10.93). The clinical course appears to be benign and local removal appears to be adequate. Diagnosis is not made clinically or by radiology, but only by the histology.

CHORDOMA

Chordoma is a rare malignant neoplasm found at either extreme of the spinal axis (i.e. basioccipital or sacrococcygeal) and occasionally elsewhere in the spinal column. It is generally accepted as originating from embryonic remnants of the notochord. In the adult, remnants of the notochord persist in the intervertebral disc nucleus pulposus. The physical presence of a tumour is usually the first symptom, though there is often pain in the back in sacral tumours. The tumours are locally invasive and tend to recur after removal, but some have been reported as producing widespread soft tissue metastases.

The radiograph usually shows destruction of bone with a shadow of a tumour in the soft tissues (Figure 10.94). There is nothing characteristic in the bony erosion, and the diagnosis, though it may be guessed at from the site, is usually made by biopsy. The tumour is slow-growing but malignant, and kills by invasion of vital structures. At least 27% of the growths metastasize. This is most common in sacrococcygeal tumours.

Microscopically chordomas are distinguished with difficulty from atypical chondromas and mucoid or signet-ring carcinomas arising in the gastro-intestinal tract. Myeloblastomas originating in the sacrococcygeal region are usually interpreted as chordomas. The chordoma cells are more epithelial in appearance than cartilage and more variable in size. There is a great tendency for vacuolization and variability in the size of the nuclei.

An attempt at complete surgical extirpation must be made, since these growths are radio-resistant. Paavolainen and Teppo (1976) described a 5-year survival rate of 35% after surgery and high-dosage radiotherapy, but only 18% after 10 years.

MALIGNANT TUMOURS OF THE SOFT TISSUE

These can arise in any connective tissue of the limb.

Fibrosarcoma of plain muscle

These can either be differentiated fibrosarcoma with malignant fibroblasts or malignant fibrosarcoma with anaplastic cells. They usually infiltrate widely, interfering with function, and the patient presents with painful but large tumour mass, particularly in the thigh or the lower extremity.

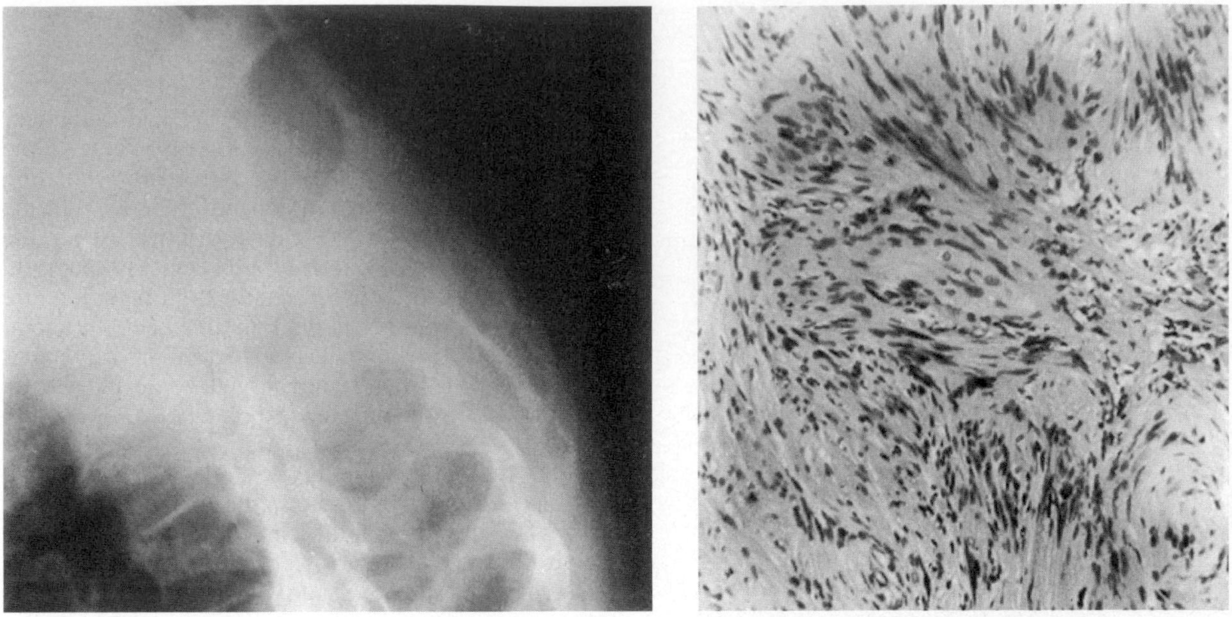

(a) (b)

Figure 10.93 (a) Radiograph showing the cystic and destructive lesion of a neurilemmoma at the root of the scapular spine with elevation of the superficial cortex. (b) Photomicrograph of tissue from a neurilemmoma, showing the whorled and streaking appearance of cells with elongated nuclei and indistinct cytoplasm. (× 212).

Liposarcoma

Liposarcoma of soft tissues of the extremities forms one of the more common malignant tumours. It occurs in the middle age groups, with little difference between the sexes. It occurs commonly in the thigh, in the popliteal area as well as in the inguinal and gluteal regions. It does not appear to arise in previously occurring lipomas. Like the fibrosarcoma, they can be differentiated into two types: one group are well differentiated but atypical lipoblasts, and the other are anaplastic. Curative treatment is directed towards wide surgical excision because their radiosensitivity varies.

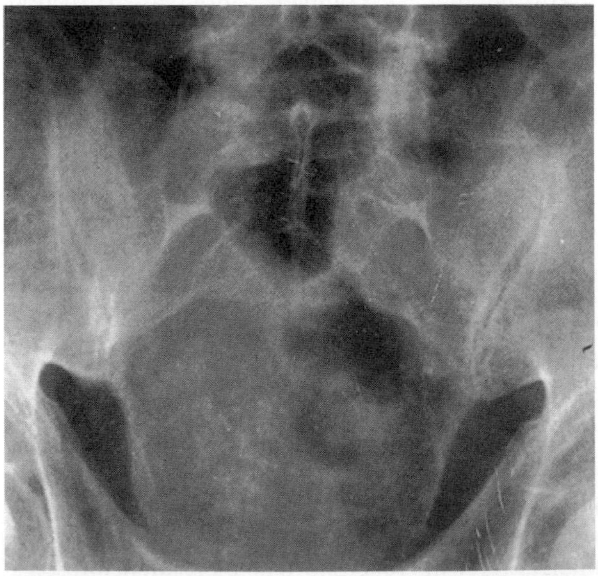

Figure 10.94 Radiograph showing an enlarged and diffuse lytic lesion of a chordoma involving almost all of the sacral body.

Rhabdomyosarcoma

Rhabdomyosarcoma is a malignancy involving the striated muscle cells. It occurs commonly around the head and neck in infants and young adults but in the limbs of adults, making up 10–20% of all soft tissue sarcomas and presenting as a fleshy tumour within muscle where it may be mistaken for haematoma or abscess. About 20% have enlarged regional lymph nodes, and bone metastases do occur. It has a high incidence of blood metastasis with rapid growth and fungation. Histologically it is characterized by giant rhabdomyoblasts with multiple nuclei which attempt to form myofibrils (Figure 10.95). It is rarely radiosensitive.

Synovial sarcoma

Synovial sarcomas occur in subcutaneous tissue as well as in deeply placed muscle layers and have no obvious continuity with joint tissue, although it is

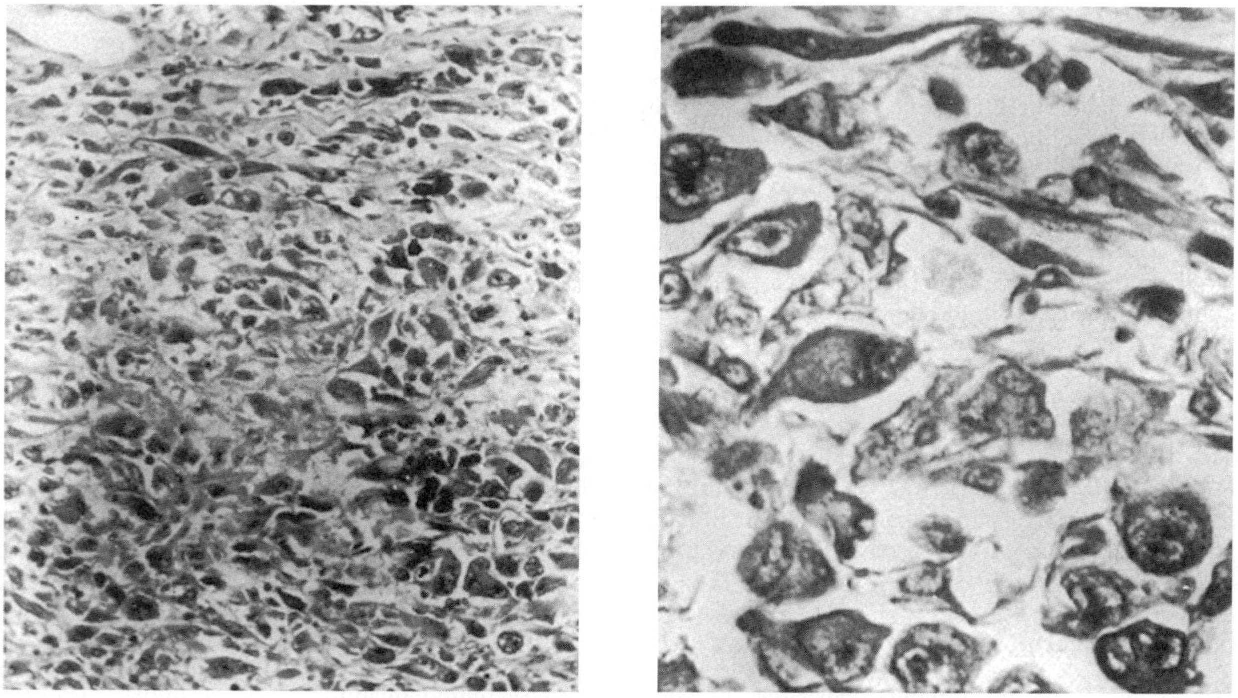

(a) (b)

Figure 10.95 (a) Photomicrograph of tissue from a rhabdomyosarcoma, showing large, irregularly nucleated cells with little cytoplasm arranged in sheets of little stroma. (× 183). (b) Photomicrograph of (a), showing the very characteristic 'strap' cell on the right and the 'racket' cell in the middle with minimal cytoplasm and surrounding stroma. (× 587).

supposed that they arise from embryologically secreted 'synovioblastic cells' (Figure 10.96). They infiltrate and spread locally although metastasis by blood stream has not been reported. Total radical local excision should be carried out to include the main muscle mass involved.

This tumour can arise from synovium or a bursal wall in the third and fourth decade of life, and involves the upper limb more frequently than the lower limb, with a painless swelling. x-Rays may show an extra-articular shadow with or without calcification. The tumour is soft with a false capsule

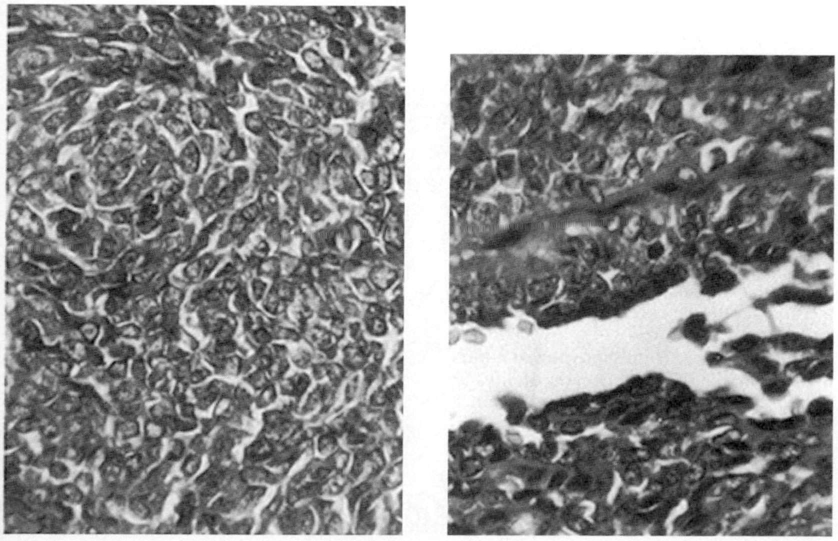

(a) (b)

Figure 10.96 (a) Photomicrograph of a synovial sarcoma, showing sheets of polygonal and plump-appearing nucleated cells with an irregular outline. (× 185).
(b) Photomicrograph of (a), showing further detail of the cells which are organized in a manner suggesting a synovial villus. (× 380).

and may show areas of haemorrhages, mucin and foci of calcification. The histology shows a very cellular stroma made up of spindle cells. There may be areas containing gland-like structures lined with cuboidal or columnar pseudoepithelial cells.

Spread is to lungs and/or bones, with a 20% incidence to regional lymph nodes. There is a 5-year survival rate of about 35%.

Treatment should be radical local excision with block dissection or radiotherapy for regional lymph nodes. Amputation should be carried out for recurrence.

Reticulum cell sarcoma

This also arises in subcutaneous as well as in muscle layers, and develops at any age, growing rapidly and infiltrating widely with metastasis via the blood stream to the lungs. It has to be differentiated from Ewing's sarcoma.

Malignant giant cell tumour

Malignant giant cell tumours can arise in subcutaneous tissues as well as joint structures, tendons and tendon sheaths. Their malignancy is variable and can be evaluated by their histological pattern.

Desmoid tumour

This appears to be a very low-grade fibrosarcoma which is locally invasive, but does not tend to metastasize by blood. It occurs in the deep muscle masses as a painful tumour or swelling. It has a much better prognosis than a fibrosarcoma even though it occurs in young people, but it can recur on inadequate resection and, therefore, it is advisable to remove entirely the involved muscle mass (Figure 10.97) (Musgrove and McDonald, 1948).

General principles of treatment of soft tissue malignancies

These have been reviewed by Simon and Enneking (1976). Usually no capsule surrounds the malignant cells though by rapid growth the surrounding soft tissues may be compressed to form a pseudocapsule; more often, however, this capsule is made up of the peripherally situated neoplastic cells. Therefore, if the malignant tumour is only enucleated, a shell of neoplastic cell will be left behind. The entire muscle bundle surrounding the sarcoma must be removed from its point of origin and insertion, by sharp dissection, as well as ligation of all major tributaries. However, amputation is indicated when the anatomical location warrants it. Extensive resection of soft tissues will offer salvage equal to that obtained by amputation.

Although during the past 30 years heroic attempts have been made to reduce the morbidity and mortality of malignant tumours in the upper aspect of both extremities, by such operations as the forequarter and hindquarter amputations, for such tumours as osteogenic sarcoma, Ewing's sarcoma, etc. these procedures have proven of little value in prolonging life. Their main indication appears to be to prevent fungation or ulceration and to relieve local symptoms, except in such malignancies of soft tissues arising high in the buttock or thigh, such as liposarcoma, fibrosarcoma, secondary chondrosarcoma, etc. Indeed, modification of the classic hemipelvectomy was described (Sherman and Duthie, 1960) in which there is less deformity and dysfunction, but still an adequate tumour excision. With

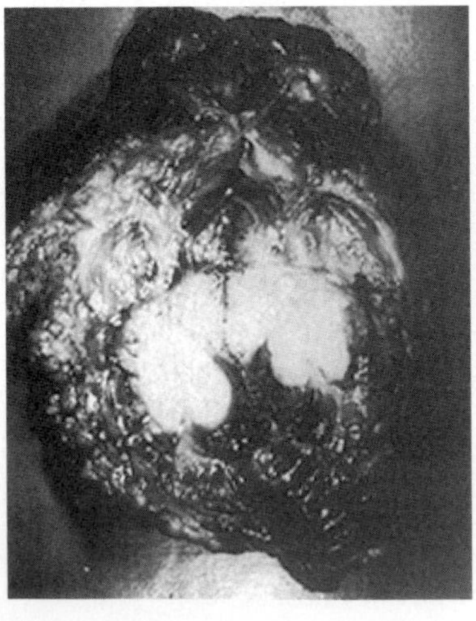

(a)

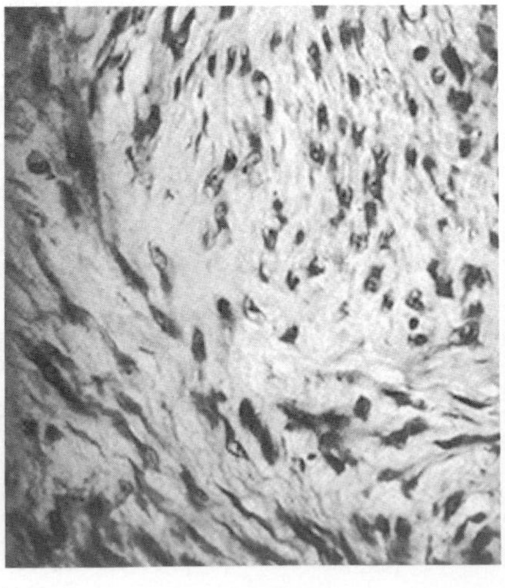

(b)

Figure 10.97 (a) A resected gluteus maximus muscle from a young boy, showing the desmoid tumour enclosed within it. (b) Photomicrograph of tissue from this desmoid tumour, showing the fibroblastic-appearing cells with little cytoplasm and large dark-staining nuclei in some areas and some mitotic figures which, although irregular in shape, have few characteristics of malignancy to suggest a fibrosarcoma. (× 152).

operation it is possible to obtain a 30–40% 5-year survival rate. Saddegh *et al.* (1992) have compared predicting outcome by the Enneking, Spanier and Goodman staging of IA, IB, IIA and IIB with theirs of histological grade and tumour size in soft tissue sarcomas. They found that the 'Enneking' staging was inferior in such prognosticating and that there was very little difference in prognosis techniques between stage IA and IB and stage IIA and IIB lesions, indicating that the significance of those staging distinctions is limited. In their series they also describe with surgical resection alone, local resection alone and amputation with a mean follow-up of 10 years, an overall projected 7-year survival rate of 65% with 31% dying because of metastases and 30% who had a local recurrence rate.

See section on 'Musculoskeletal oncology'.

TUMORAL CALCINOSIS

This is a rare condition, with perhaps a genetic background being inherited as an autosomal recessive and occurring in families. It occurs in children, who present with firm non-tender tumour-like masses in the soft tissues around joints. Occurring around the shoulder, hips, elbows and ankles, they grow in size and deformity and sometimes ulcerate. Hyperphosphataemia has been reported in one family (Baldurasson *et al.*, 1969).

Tumoral calcinosis is an uncommon inherited metabolic disease which is now characterized by para- and periarticular calcified tumours and an evaluated serum phosphorus and 1,25(OH_2)D vitamin levels. It has been suggested that this disease is caused by a defect in the renal tubular phosphate transport mechanism which may be modulated in part by parathormone activity.

These cystic masses, which are gritty on palpation and extend throughout the soft tissue plane without a true capsule, are difficult to excise completely. Inside there is a fluid or putty-like material made up of calcium phosphate embedded within a fibrous proliferation, giant cells and lymphocytes.

These discrete lesions should be differentiated from calcinosis universalis involving the skin and muscles, calcinosis circumscripta, Raynaud's disease and scleroderma.

Recurrence is frequent, with multiple scarring and deformities of the adjacent joints.

Metastatic tumours of bone

There are two stages of malignant disease, irrespective of the primary site of the tumour, to differentiate before embarking upon therapy. A lesion is 'early' if it is localized and therefore is potentially curable by radical surgery. However, once the disease has disseminated it is advanced and the prognosis cannot be improved by ablative surgery.

The skeleton is one of the commonest sites for metastases. This incidence is probably higher than that recorded since the skeleton is usually inadequately examined at necropsy (Lichtenstein, 1977; Jaffe, 1978). The carcinomas which commonly metastasize to bone arise in the breast (about 30%), prostate, thyroid, kidney and lung, as well as from adrenal neuroblastoma. However, skeletal metastases have been found in virtually all types of malignant tumours including melanomata, carcinoid, testicular, ovarian and intestinal tumours.

Carcinoma of the stomach shows bone involvement in only 5% of cases (Figures 10.98 and 10.99).

In the male, carcinoma of the prostate and lung account for 70–80% of skeletal metastases.

METHOD OF SPREAD

Bone may be involved as a result of direct spread from an overlying tumour such as from squamous carcinoma of the skin in the facial bones and in the calvarium; the maxilla, ethmoid and nasal bones

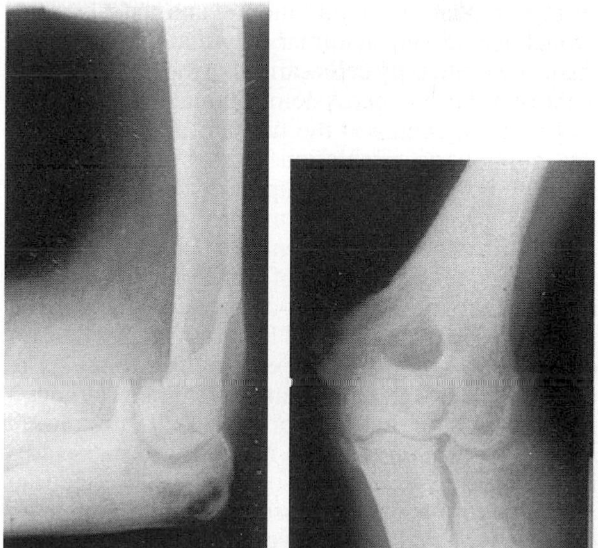

Figure 10.98 Radiographs of the elbow joint of a young man who had presented with symptoms from a 'tennis elbow' of 4 months' duration. Destruction of the upper aspect of the radius by a metastasis from an adenocarcinoma of the stomach, with an obvious soft tissue mass, is seen.

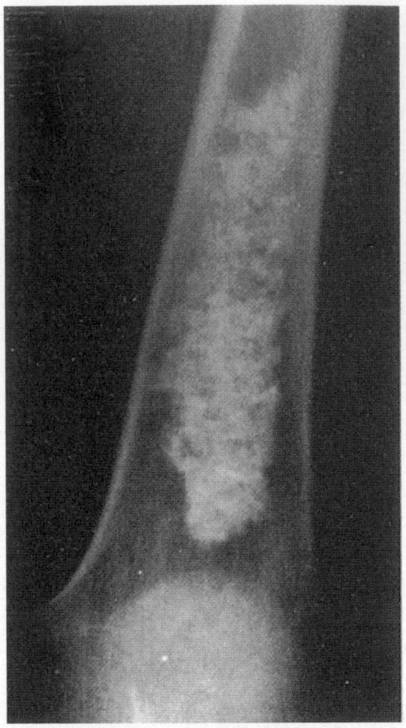

Figure 10.99 Radiograph of the lower aspect of the opposite femur of the patient in Figure 10.65, showing a large, irregular, radiodense area filling the medullary cavity, but the surrounding cortex is normal (i.e. a bone infarct).

from nasopharyngeal carcinoma, and the ribs from bronchogenic and mammary carcinoma. However, the usual route is by cells carried in the blood stream. This may be by the systemic circulation with the cells entering veins in the tumour, passing through the pulmonary circulation to the arterial blood stream and then to the capillary beds. Since the cells pass through the pulmonary circulation, this accounts for the high incidence of pulmonary metastases found in the majority of carcinomata. This does not explain the selective distribution of skeletal metastases in the dorsal and lumbar spine, pelvis, rib cage, skull and proximal end of the femur. The appendicular skeleton is relatively immune although metastases have been described at all sites. In an attempt to explain the high incidence of metastases in the axial skeleton, Batson (1940) described an alternative route for the dissemination of malignant cells. He showed that the vertebral venous system, which contains no valves, communicates freely with venous channels of the chest wall and the intrathoracic and abdominal viscera. When the intrathoracic or intra-abdominal pressure rises, as in coughing or sneezing, a reversed flow of blood in the venous vertebral system can occur. By this method malignant cells may be carried into the bodies of the vertebrae or reach the central nervous system.

There is also no doubt that many more cells are shed into the circulation than eventually develop into metastases. The local factors which stimulate metastatic growth from some cells, whilst destroying others, are ill understood.

It is unusual to find skeletal metastases below the elbows and knees, but, if there is one, one should strongly consider the possibility of myeloma. In general, most carcinomata tend to be *irregularly osteolytic*; they are invasive and tend to penetrate the cortex, in contrast to benign bone lesions which have smooth walls and cause expansion of the cortex without penetration. The lesions are usually destructive (osteolytic), some provoke significant osteosclerosis (osteoblastic) and some give rise to a mixed type of reaction. Milch and Changus (1956) pointed out that osteoblastic metastases were seen in carcinoma of prostate, metastatic carcinoid, carcinoma of the breast and, sometimes, carcinoma of the urinary bladder. Breast carcinoma is notorious for giving rise to osteoblastic lesions in some bones and osteolytic in others at the same time.

These authors described possible mechanisms for metastatic bone destruction by:

1. The direct action of the tumour cell.
2. The action of osteoclasts, although these were not seen.
3. The elaboration of specific bone resorption substances.
4. The mechanical compression effect of the tumour cells.

They also found that there was no real histological dlfferentiation between the so-called 'osteolytic' and 'osteoblastic' metastases. The radiological appearance of osteolysis was indicative of further bone destruction, whereas the appearance of increased bone density or 'blastic' response was due to an increased rate of bone repair rather than any true tumour bone formation.

CLINICAL FEATURES

Skeletal metastases may be present because of pain, localized tenderness, pathological fracture, the majority of which are induced by metastases from mammary carcinomas (Parrish and Murray, 1970), or the development of hypercalcaemia. They may also be found on routine screening of the skeleton of a patient known to have malignant disease.

Hypercalcaemia is found particularly in association with bronchogenic and mammary carcinoma. It is usually produced as a result of the destruction of the skeleton by metastases. As the bone is destroyed, the calcium is released into the circulation. If the kidneys are functioning the calcium is excreted in the urine, as a hypercalciuria. However, if the kidneys are unable to excrete the increased load serum calcium rises to give a hypercalcaemia. This appears to be related more to the rapidity of skeletal destruction rather than the extent of skeletal involvement (Galasko, 1972). Hypercalcaemia may also be caused by the secretion of parathyroid-hormone-like principle by the tumour which is sometimes found in a bronchogenic carcinoma; or the excretion of a vitamin-D-like principle (Grimes *et al.*, 1967); or the excretion of specific osteolytic steroids which have been isolated from mammary carcinoma (Gordan, 1967).

There are two types of hypercalcaemia – first, an 'incidental' variety of about 12 mg/dl which is symptomless and is only found on routine examination of the serum, and second, an 'acute' type of over 13 mg/dl which is potentially fatal if untreated. It is often associated with gastrointestinal disturbances (i.e. anorexia, nausea, vomiting and dehydration) as well as neurological disturbances, including lassitude, confusion and coma.

Other systemic manifestations associated with cancer of the lung, breast, ovary, uterus, etc., have been summarized by Johnston (1970).

1. *In the skin* are: herpes zoster, ichthyosis, hypertrichosis, dermatomyositis (15% of all skin, lesions being associated carcinoma of the stomach, breast or ovary).
2. *In the nervous system* are: corticocerebellar degeneration, acute mental changes, vertigo, ataxia, myelopathy, muscle atrophy, weakness, paraesthesia, cerebellar dysfunction and peripheral neuropathy (sensory or mixed).
3. *In the muscle* are: polymyositis, proximal muscle syndrome, myasthenic syndrome which resembles myasthenia gravis but differs in that 85% of these patients have oat cell carcinoma of the lung.
4. *In the cardiovascular system*: thrombophlebitis in unusual sites, recurrent migratory phlebitis, bleeding diathesis, fibrinogen deficiency which is usually caused by circulating fibrinolysin, occasionally by lytic agents for fibrinogen, prothrombin or factor V. Anaemia which is moderate (the haemoglobin rarely being less than 8 g/dl), normochromic, normocytic due to poor utilization of iron and impaired erythropoiesis.
5. *In the digestive system*: serum proteins lowered (e.g. albumin) and an elevated α-globulin in 'wasting' diseases. Lactic dehydrogenase whose serum level is elevated in a variety of conditions, including malignancy. Acid phosphatase serum levels are increased in patients with carcinoma of the prostate, but may also be elevated in a wide variety of other conditions – e.g. Gaucher's disease, visceral or breast cancer with metastases to bone and liver. Alkaline phosphatase serum levels are elevated in obstructive or hepatocellular hepatic disease and in skeletal disease with increased osteoblastic activity, including metastases.
6. *In the endocrine system*: pituitary effects:
   (a) ACTH-like substances are produced by tumours with Cushing's syndrome of few physical changes but severe biochemical derangements by undifferentiated oat cell tumours of lung and pancreatic carcinoma;
   (b) antidiuretic hormone (ADH)-like substances produce water retention, hyponatraemia, hypotonic plasma and hypertonic urine;
   (c) Thyrotrophic substances are secreted by carcinomas, chiefly originating in the gastrointestinal tract, lung and prostate, and chlorionepithelioma.

   Parathyroid-hormone-like secretion gives rise to hypercalcaemia which is potentially fatal. Apparently, this effect is independent of metastases to bone and is reversible by removal of the primary tumour. It occurs principally in association with carcinoma of the breast, lung and kidney, and osteoclastic resorption of bone has been described.

   Pancreas: 21% of liver carcinomas have hypoglycaemia.

   Hyperglyeaemia: the onset of unstable diabetes in the seventh decade, without family history, should arouse suspicion of pancreatic carcinoma.

   Zollinger–Ellison and related (pluriglandular) syndromes: non-beta islet cell tumours of the pancreas (about one-half of these being malignant); one-third had metastasized when first discovered. Hypersecretion by tumour of a gastrin-like substance is believed to be responsible for extreme gastric hyperacidity and intractable atypical peptic ulceration

   Carcinoid syndrome: originally associated with carcinoid tumour of small intestine, carcinomas of stomach and pancreas, and oat cell carcinomas. These result in abnormal amounts of 5-hydroxytryptamine (serotonin) or 5-hydroxytryptophan secretions.
7. *In the reticuloendothelial system*: tissue immunological suppression relevant to cell-mediated (lymphocytic) immune responses may result (e.g. homograft rejection).
8. *In the skeleton*: pulmonary osteoarthropathy with clubbing of fingers (soft tissue 'hypertrophy'), periosteal new bone in long bones

and pain – all develop rapidly in pulmonary malignancy and tend to regress rapidly with removal of the tumour. These are most frequently encountered in lung cancer but may occur with mesothelioma.

DIFFERENTIAL DIAGNOSIS

A 'solitary' metastasis with the appearance of osteosclerosis has to be differentiated from the simple lesion of a *bone infarct* (Figure 10.100). This occurs in the medulla near the metaphysis, but may extend up the shaft. There is never involvement of the cortex. It appears as an area of irregular bone density due to calcified cartilage and new bone formation although the surrounding bone is always normal. Other lesions to be differentiated are:

1. Chronic sclerosing osteomyelitis.
2. Sclerosing osteogenic sarcoma.
3. Calcifying enchondroma.
4. Multiple myeloma.
5. Hyperparathyroidism.

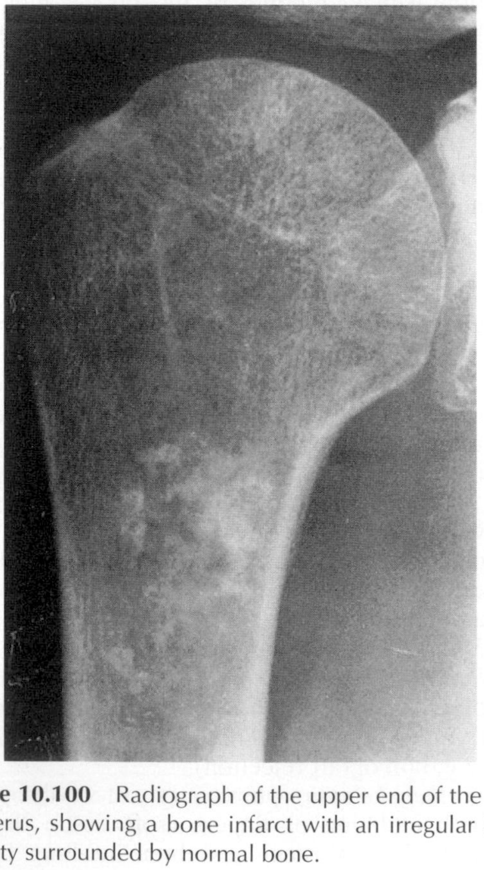

Figure 10.100 Radiograph of the upper end of the right humerus, showing a bone infarct with an irregular bone density surrounded by normal bone.

DIAGNOSIS

Conventional methods of diagnosing skeletal metastases are inaccurate. Of 86 patients with advanced mammary carcinoma, all of whom had skeletal metastases evident on x-ray, pain was complained of by only 65.1% at any stage in their disease, tenderness was elicited in only 16% and the alkaline phosphatase was raised in only 66%. There was no relationship between the presence or absence of pain and the degree of skeletal involvement by the metastases. Occasionally, small lesions which appear as a 'solitary' one may cause extremely severe pain whereas patients with metastases involving almost the entire skeleton may not complain of pain at any stage in their disease. Pain may be localized to a few sites and is not associated with every metastasis.

The serum phosphate is only raised when there is associated renal failure with phosphate retention. The serum acid phosphatase is usually elevated in patients with skeletal metastases from prostatic carcinoma. Elevation of the urinary 24-hour hydroxyproline excretion or abnormality in the urinary hydroxyproline/creatinine ratio may precede clinical and radiological evidence of skeletal metastases by several months (Guzzo *et al.*, 1969).

x-Rays are also unreliable. Metastases start growing in the medulla and from there involve the cortex. It has been shown that at least 50% of the medulla must be destroyed before a lesion will be seen radiologically (Edelstyn *et al.*, 1967). Tomograms are more sensitive but can be used only if the patient has symptoms referable to a specific site. They can not be used for routine screening of the skeleton before deciding the stage of the disease for a particular patient.

The use of technetium-99m phosphate in skeletal scintigraphy is now routine for outlining skeletal metastases. Galasko (1975), from studies of postmortem specimens of bones containing metastatic cancer and implanted rabbit bones, described the pathological basis of scintigraphy. Both bone destruction and new bone formation (from intramembraneous ossification of the fibrous stroma around the tumour) occur with a marked affinity for this bone-seeking isotope. The advantages of this form of bone scanning are that metastases are detected earlier and are thus smaller in size than on routine radiography. Also, Galasko and Doyle (1972) showed that it is a more sensitive index to the response of these lesions to radiotherapy or even chemotherapy, and is most helpful in planning treatment along with pulmonary tomography and a liver scan.

Computed axial tomography (CAT) is now used widely, particularly for suspected spinal, pelvic and around the hip area metastases. Not only does it show accurately small areas of destruction but also soft tissue deposition, i.e. in the lung fields. CAT directed needle biopsy is valuable for exact localization.

Magnetic resonance scanning is particularly valuable for the spine, for the involvement of soft tissue extension within the spinal canal and lung fields and for 'skip' lesions within the medullary space of long bones.

The histomicroscopy varies considerably within the primary lesion which may have been 'silent', only being diagnosed at the time of biopsy. Needle biopsy is of value particularly as the material may well show epithelial features with acinar or papillary formation, mucine production with the tumour cell vacuoles – suggesting gastrointestinal cancer, lung or pancreas. Immunochemical stains are being developed and used specifically for prostatic or thyroid cancers.

In a survey of 2400 consecutive autopsies reported by Johnston (1970), which included 653 malignant neoplasms, he found the following:

1. Total malignant lesions: 653.
2. Cases with skeletal metastases: 212 (32.5% of total malignancies).
3. Solitary skeletal metastasis: 19 (9% of skeletal metastases).
4. Patients with pathological fractures: 13 (6% of skeletal metastases; 2% of total malignancies).

The data are broken down in Table 10.8.

The separation of skeletal metastases into lytic or sclerotic, depending on their radiological appearance, is reinforced by their histological examination. In all metastases there is a combination of destruction due to the tumour and new bone formation caused by the reaction of the bone to the lesion.

TREATMENT

Treatment of skeletal metastases is essentially palliative although there have been cases described where a solitary metastasis from a hypernephroma has been removed, after the primary was treated, with apparent cure. Many patients may live for months or years with skeletal metastases and it is important to relieve their symptoms and improve the quality of their life.

See section on 'Musculoskeletal oncology'.

Table 10.8 Analysis of 653 malignant tumours

Primary source	Proportion of total cancer patients	Metastatic rate to skeleton
Lung	19%	44%
Breast	11.5%	57%
Prostate	5%	55%
Pancreas	6%	12.5%
Stomach	6%	10%

Pain

Pain may only occur in association with hypercalcaemia; once the hypercalcaemia has been treated, the pain will settle. It may be associated with a pathological fracture and again the pathological fracture must be treated. Large lytic metastases with impending fracture may also produce pain and require treatment. The origin of the pain from bone invasion, destruction, fracture or from any adjacent soft tissue or nerve compression, or even visceral extension from pelvis, chest wall or spine, must be carefully looked for and assessed.

In administering the selected medication with its appropriate dosage, careful timing is essential to maintain the desired effect rather than a fixed regimen of, say, three times a day. Sleep should be disturbed in order to be given the appropriate drug rather than the patient awakening with the pain.

When non-narcotic analgesia is inadequate, oral preparations of morphine in dosages varying between 5 and 30 mg should be used without the concern about addiction, depressing respiration, decreased tolerance to it, sleepiness, etc. (Twycross, 1974). Other intermediate-strength narcotics such as dextromoramide (Palfium) which has proved to be most useful in haemophiliac bone cysts, dipipanone (Diconal) or papaveretum (Omnopon) may be better for an active functioning patient, and where the nausea induced by morphine is not controlled by an antiemetic such as prochlorperazine. Morphine can be augmented by prednisolone (15–30 mg daily) for soft tissue or nerve root involvement, or even aspirin for bone destruction. Corticosteroids are important for hypercalcaemia, as are the benzodiazepines or tricyclic antidepressants for anxiety or depression (*Drug and Therapeutics Bulletin*, 1980)

If the patient has a hormonally dependent tumour, such as carcinoma of the breast or prostate, the pain is often relieved by hormonal therapy. In carcinoma of the prostate, stilboestrol therapy, orchidectomy or a combination of both frequently relieves pain. In mammary carcinoma approximately 27% of patients respond objectively to hormonal therapy. In the premenopausal woman this usually consists of an oöphorectomy. In the post-menopausal woman stilboestrol is usually given. In both groups, when the primary treatment fails to produce a remission androgens, progestogens or corticosteroids have been tried; if this, too, fails, endocrine ablative surgery is usually indicated. This includes procedures such as adrenalectomy, hypophysectomy or pituitary ablation using rods of yttrium-90.

Where hormonal therapy is not indicated or not effective, radiotherapy to a localized area of pain will frequently produce relief. Interruption of the nerve supply to the painful area is sometimes indicated. This may take the form of phenol blocks, rhizotomies and even a spinothalamic tract division.

In the incidental type of hypercalcaemia, where the serum calcium is found to be elevated on a routine estimation but where no symptoms have been produced, the exclusion of milk and milk products from the diet usually suffices. In the acute symptomatic form of hypercalcaemia the patient is placed on a low-calcium diet. If necessary, intravenous fluids are given – usually in the form of saline. There is a constant sodium/calcium ratio in the urine so that a greater calcium diuresis is produced by saline than any other form of diuresis. If this fails to control the hypercalcaemia, neutral phosphate should be given (either orally or intravenously) in doses up to 1 g every 6 hours. Many other forms of treatment have been suggested. Cortisone is useful in some patients, and good results have been obtained with mithramycin and with sodium sulphate.

Pathological fractures

More than 50% of patients who develop a pathological fracture die of their disease within 3 months although there have been survivals of 6 years or more after a pathological fracture. Without treatment, the fracture will not heal. Harrington (1977) reported a series of 399 pathological fractures. The types of primary cancers are listed in Table 10.9 and the distribution of pathological fractures is given in Table 10.10.

Treatment of patients with pathological fractures in metastatic bone disease consists of:

Table 10.9 Types of primary cancers involving in 399 pathological fractures

Carcinoma:		
of breast	162	41%
of kidney	38	43%
of lung	36	
of prostate	24	
of bowel	21	
of thyroid	6	
undifferentiated (original unknown)	26	
of other primary origins	24	
Myeloma	36	16%
Lymphoma	26	

Table 10.10 Distribution of 399 pathological fractures

Femoral neck	69	258 in the femur
Trochanteric	50	
Subtrochanteric	84	
Femoral shaft	38	
Supracondylar	17	
Acetabulum	34	
Tibia	36	
Humerus	68	
Ulna	3	

1. Improvement in the health of the patient.
2. Specific treatment for specific cancers (e.g. hormonal therapy for carcinoma of the breast or prostate; radioactive iodine for carcinoma of the thyroid).
3. Chemotherapy.
4. Surgical management.
5. Radiotherapy.
6. Amputation.

Surgical management

See section on 'Musculoskeletal oncology'.

Since the early 1950s, there have been many series reporting on the internal fixation of pathological fractures on long bones in metastatic bone disease.

Parrish and Murray (1970) reported on 104 fractures in 96 patients: 60% of patients were mobilized with at least partial weight-bearing; 26% survived more than 12 months. In 5 patients, large cavities were packed with cancellous bone graft in addition to internal fixation. Parrish and Murray suggested that breast secondaries respond better to fixation and radiotherapy than do other secondaries. Galasko (1974) reviewed 96 long bone fractures treated in Oxford: 19% of patients survived for more than 1 year. He advocated prosthetic replacement of transcervical femoral fractures which will not unite if treated by reduction and fixation. Radiotherapy is an essential adjunct for fracture healing but lytic areas should be stabilized prior to radiotherapy, which weakens the bone and may itself cause fracture.

Methylmethacrylate

In the early 1970s the first reports of the use of methylmethacrylate to supplement fixation of pathological fractures in metastatic bone disease appeared in the English language literature (Harrington *et al.*, 1972).

Histological studies of human bone (Charnley, 1970) and canine femurs (Harrington, 1975) showed that the trabeculae in contact with methylmethacrylate cement undergo necrosis. A layer of fibre cartilage derived from compressed fibrous tissues forms at the interface between cement and bone. The endosteal bone undergoes eventual revascularization, but, in the dog, there is vigorous periosteal new bone formation. An early study of fracture healing in the presence of cement was performed by Wiltse *et al.* (1957). They demonstrated that the fracture united and periosteal new bone invested the cement. Similar experiments were performed in rabbits and sheep by Syzskowitz and Cockin (1974). There was extensive necrosis of the bone ends, thought to be caused by the exothermic reaction upon polymerization of the cement. However, the fractures united by bridging callus, external to the cement and the dead bone ends were revascularized. These authors also reported on the use of cement to fix pathological fractures (metastatic or osteoporotic) in 200 patients. Other studies have suggested that cement may be harmful to fracture healing.

Harrington *et al.* (1976) reported on the operative stabilization of 375 pathological fractures in 323 patients in which the tumour and diseased bone were resected and the resultant defect was packed with cement. The purpose of this technique was to provide early 'rigid' fixation so as to allow early weight-bearing and to overcome the problem of providing any form of fixation where there was marked bone destruction. The mean survival was 15.4 months; 36 patients survived for more than 2 years; 94% of lower limb fractures were allowed early weight-bearing. Failure of fixation occurred in 4 patients. The incidence of complications (e.g. infection) was also very low. There is no clinical evidence that radiotherapy adversely affected the cement. Their indications for prophylactic internal fixation were lesions more than 3 cm in diameter or persistent pain. The surgical techniques used were essentially intramedullary rods for diaphyseal lesions, nail plates for pretrochanteric fractures and prosthetic replacement for proximal femoral fractures. Lesions of the acetabulum were treated by total hip replacement.

Zickel and Mouradian (1976) reported on the internal fixation of 46 pathological subtrochanteric fractures with a stout intramedullary rod, thickened proximally, through which could be passed a nail into the femoral neck and thus provide rotational stability. This form of fixation allowed early mobilization and ambulation, and bone union occurred in 14 patients in 4–5 months.

Many authors have advocated prophylactic internal fixation for long bones containing lytic lesions. The indications are lytic areas which cause pain, with radiological evidence of cortical destruction. Pain usually occurs some weeks prior to fracture and is probably due to minor infractions associated with normal stresses on the weakened bone.

Internal fixation carries the theoretical risk that tumour cells will be disseminated, and tumour cells have been found in blood taken from the inferior vena cava during intramedullary nailing (Hoare, 1968). Many other investigators have isolated cancer cells in the blood of patients with solid lesions during surgical procedures, but there is no clinical evidence that this alters the long-term prognosis (Brostrom *et al.*, 1979).

Amputation or radical excision

Amputation is rarely required in the treatment of pathological fractures but the indications are fungation, intractable pain and vascular insufficiency.

In a series of 1676 malignant melanomas (Stewart *et al.*, 1978), 116 had osseous metastases, the mean time from diagnosis to appearance of the bone secondary being 21 months. The mean survival after the appearance of bony secondary was only 6 months. There were only six fractures of long bones and these were treated by internal fixation and radiotherapy. Prophylactic fixation of lytic areas in the bone was not recommended because of the extremely poor prognosis, but complete excision and total joint replacement is indicated (Figure 10.101).

The management of spinal metastases

Painful spinal metastases are treated by radiotherapy. Surgical treatment may be required if there is associated spinal cord damage or if there is spinal instability due to vertebral body destruction.

In a retrospective review of 154 cases of spinal cord lesions due to extradural metastases, Hall and McKay (1973) found that decompressive laminectomy produced worthwhile results in 38 patients with incomplete paraplegia. These patients regained ambulation, and bladder function which lasted for more than 6 months. There was no neurological recovery if the paraplegia was complete preoperatively, but only 19% survived for 1 year or more.

Radiotherapy

See section on 'Musculoskeletal oncology'.

THE ASSESSMENT OF RESPONSE

The relief of pain does not necessarily mean that the metastases have remitted, since pain may be relieved although the lesions continue to enlarge, as seen on serial x-rays. When a metastasis is brought under

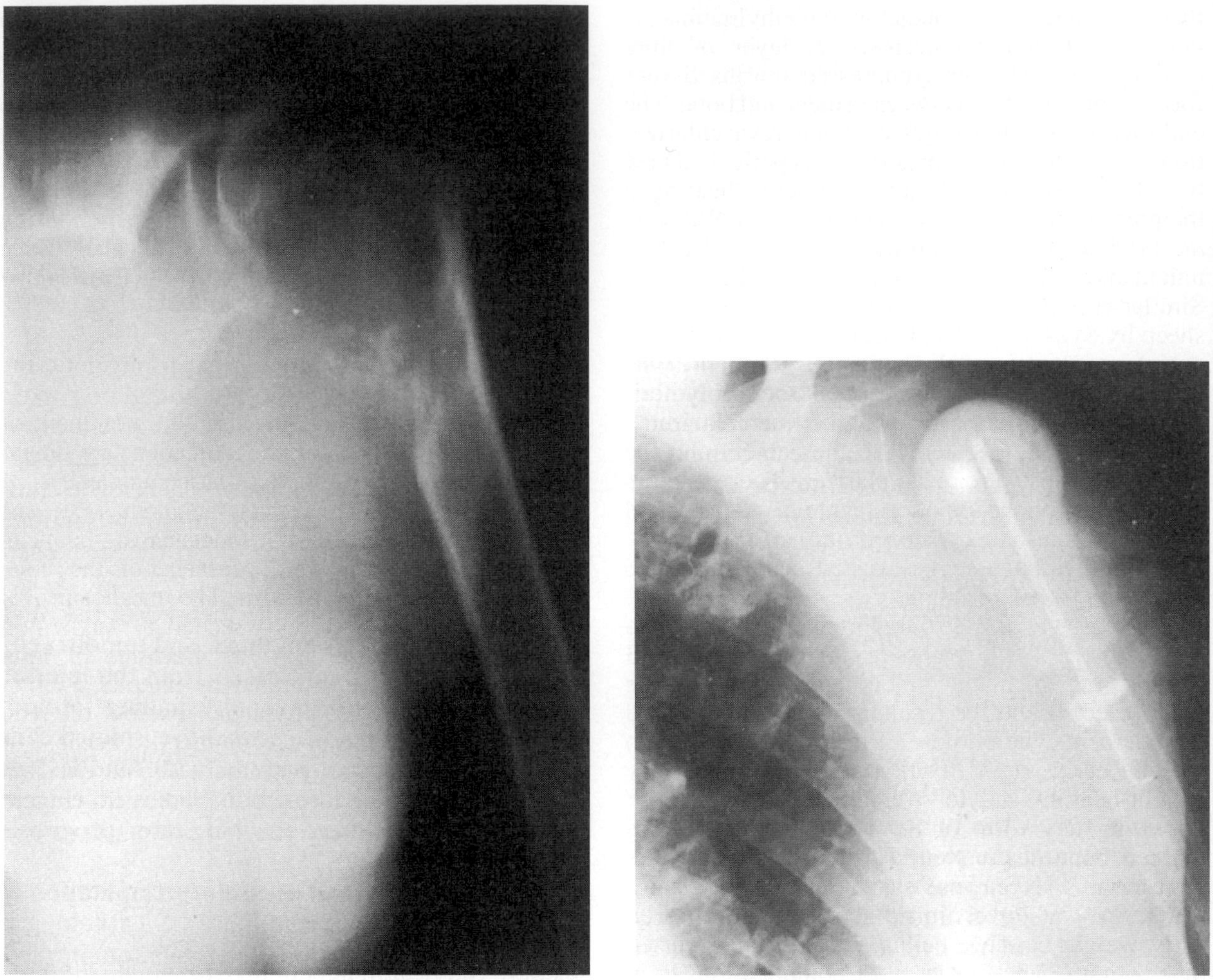

(a) (b)

Figure 10.101 Secondary melanoma, primary removed 20 years ago, occurring as a solitary metastasis and with replacement by isoelastic shoulder prosthesis.

control the radiological appearance alters: the bone either returns to normal or a lytic lesion may regain bone density. However, it is impossible to differentiate new sclerotic lesions due to healing of previously unrecognized metastases from those due to progression of the disease. This may be particularly important in prostatic or mammary carcinoma in order to decide if the patient is responding to therapy or not.

A 'healed' lesion tends to lose its uptake of the bone-seeking isotopes, and what was previously an area of increased uptake may return to normal if the metastasis is brought under control as a result of radiotherapy, hormonal therapy or chemotherapy.

A raised alkaline phosphatase which returns to normal and remains normal usually indicates remission, although occasionally this pattern has been seen in advancing disease. Continuing or increasing elevation indicates progression of the skeletal metastases.

References

Aakhus, T. Eide, O. and Stokke, J. (1960) *Acta Radiologica* **54**, 29

Alazraki, N. P., Davis, M. A., Jones, A. G. *et al.* (1980) Skeletal system: malignant tumours. In: *Nuclear Medicine Review Syllabus*, pp. 284–297. Edited by P. T. Kirchner. Society of Nuclear Medicine: New York

Anger, H. O. (1952) Use of a gamma-ray pinhole camera for in-vivo studies. *Nature* **170**, 200

Ardran, G. M. (1951) Bone destruction not demonstrable by radiography. *British Journal of Radiology* **244**, 107–109

Bacci, G., Toni, A., Avella, M. *et al.* (1989) Long-term results in 144 localised Ewing's sarcoma patients treated with combined therapy. *Cancer* **6**, 1477–1486

Baker, P. L., Dockerty, M. B. and Coventry, M. B. (1954) *Journal of Bone and Joint Surgery* **36A**, 704

Baldurasson, H., Evans, E. B., Dodge, W. F. and Jackson, W. T. (1969) Tumoral calcinoses with hyperphosphatemia – a report of a family with incidence in four siblings. *Journal of Bone and Joint Surgery* **51A**, 913–925

Ball, A. B. S., Fisher, C., Pittam, M., Watkins, R. M. and Westbury, G. (1990) Diagnosis of soft tissue tumours by Tru-Cut biopsy. *British Journal of Surgery* **77**, 756–758

Bataille, R., Chevalier, J., Rossi, M. *et al.* (1982) Bone scintigraphy in plasma cell myeloma. A prospective study of 70 patients. *Radiology* **145**, 801–804

Bator, S. M., Bauer, T. W. and Marks, K. E. (1986) Periosteal Ewing's sarcoma. *Cancer* **58**, 1781–1784

Batson, O. V. (1940) *Annals of Surgery* **112**, 138

Bauer, T. W., Dorfman, H. D. and Latham, J. T. (1982) Periosteal chondroma. *American Journal of Surgical Pathology* **6**, 631–637

Bauer, T. W., Zehr, R. J. and Belhobek, G. H. (1991) Juxta-articular osteoid osteoma. *American Journal of Surgical Pathology* **15**, 381–387

Belanger, L. F. and Migicovsky, B. B. (1963) Histochemical evidence of proteolysis in bone: the influence of parathormone. *Journal of Histochemistry and Cytochemistry* **11**, 734–737

Beltran, J., Simon, D. Katz, W. *et al.* (1987) Increased MR signal intensity in skeletal muscle adjacent to malignant tumours: pathological correlation and clinical relevance. *Radiology* **162**, 251–255

Berquist, T. H., Ehman, R. L., King, B. F. *et al.* (1990) Value of MR imaging in differentiating benign from malignant soft-tissue masses: study of 95 lesions. *American Journal of Roentgenology* **155**, 1251–1255

Bloodgood, J. C. (1926a) Bone sarcoma–periosteal and diffuse type, and their diagnosis from benign lesion. *Journal of Bone and Joint Surgery* **8**, 727–749

Bloodgood, J. C. (1926b) How to diagnose and treat a bone lesion: I. Central lesions. *Journal of Bone and Joint Surgery* **8**, 471–478

Brady, L. W. and Croll, M. N. (1979) The rule of bone scanning in the cancer patient. *Skeletal Radiology* **3**, 217–222

Brennan, M. F., Casper, E. S., Harrison, L. B., Shiu, M. H., Gaynor, J. and Hajdu, S. (1991) The role of multi-modality therapy in soft-tissue sarcoma. *Annals of Surgery* **214**, 328–338

Brostrom, L. A., Harris, M. A., Simon, M. A., Cooperman, D. R. and Nilsonne, U. (1979) The effect of biopsy on survival of patients with osteosarcoma. *Journal of Bone and Joint Surgery* **61B**, 209–212

Burnet, F. M. (1957) *British Medical Journal* 1:779 and 841

Cade, S. (1955) Osteogenic sarcoma: a study based on 133 patients. *Journal of the Royal College of Surgeons of Edinburgh* **1**, 79–111

Caldas, J. P. (1934) Radiodiagnosis of bone tumors by arteriography. Presented at the Fourth International Congress of Radiology, Zurich.

Cammisa, F. P., Glaser, D. B., Otis, J. C., Kroll, M. A., Lane, J. M. and Healey, J. H. (1990) The Van Nes tibial rotationplasty: a functionally viable reconstructive procedure in children who have a tumor of the distal end of the femur. *Journal of Bone and Joint Surgery* **72A**, 1541–1547.

Campanacci, M. and Costa, P. (1979) Total resection of distal femur or proximal tibia for bone tumours. Autogenous bone grafts and arthrodesis in twenty-six cases. *Journal of Bone and Joint Surgery* **61B**, 455

Campanacci, M., Bacci, G., Bertoni, F., Picci, P., Minutillo, A. and Franceschi, C. (1981) The treatment of osteosarcoma of the extremities: twenty years' experience at the Istituto Ortopedico Rizzoli. *Cancer* **48**, 1569–1581

Canadell, J., Forriok, F. and Cara, J. A. (1994) Removal of metaphyseal bone tumours with preservation of the epiphysis. *Journal of Bone and Joint Surgery* **76B**, 127–132

Casper, E. S., Gaynor, J. J., Harrison, L. B., Panicek, D. M., Hajdu, S. I. and Brennan, M. F. (1994) Preoperative and postoperative adjuvant combination chemotherapy for adults with high grade soft tissue sarcoma. *Cancer* **73**, 1644-1651

Cassen, B., Curtis, W., Reed, C. *et al.* (1951) Instrumentation for use in medical studies. *Nucleonics* **2**, 46

Chang, A. E., Kinsella, T., Glatstein, E., Baker, A. R., Sindelar, W. F. and Lotze, M. T. (1988) Adjuvant chemotherapy for patients with high-grade soft-tissue sarcomas of the extremities. *Journal of Clinical Oncology* **6**, 1491–1500

Charnley, J. V. (1970) *Journal of Bone and Joint Surgery* **52B**, 340–353

Chew, F. S. and Hudson, T. M. (1982) Radionuclide bone scanning of osteosarcoma: falsely extended uptake patterns. *American Journal of Roentgenology* **139**, 49–54

Chew, F. S., Hudson, T. M. and Enneking, W. F. (1981) Radionuclide imaging of soft tissue neoplasms. *Seminars in Nuclear Medicine* **11**, 266–276

Chiao, H. C., Marks, K. E., Bauer, T. W. *et al.* (1987) Intraneural lipoma of the sciatic nerve. *Clinical Orthopaedics and Related Research* **221**, 267–271

Chuang, V. P., Wallace, S., Swanson, D. *et al.* (1979) Arterial occlusion in the management of pain from metastatic renal carcinoma. *Radiology* **133**, 611–614

Chuang, V. P., Soo, C. S., Wallace, S. *et al.* (1981) Arterial occlusion: management of giant-cell tumor and aneurysmal bone cyst. *American Journal of Roentgenology* **136**, 1127–1130

Clark, J. M. P. and Bingold, A. C. (1952) Acrylic replacement after segmental resection of bone. *British Medical Journal* **1**, 903–905

Codman, E. A. (1926) The registry of bone sarcoma. *Surgery, Gynecology and Obstetrics* **42**, 381–393

Codman, E. A. (1925) *American Journal of Roentgenology* **13**, 105

Coley, W. B. (1928) The differential diagnosis of sarcoma of the long bones. *Journal of Bone and Joint Surgery* **10**, 420–473

Collin, C., Hadju, S. I., Godbold, J., Shiu, M. H., Hilaris, B. S. and Brennan, M. F. (1986) Localized, operable soft tissue sarcoma of the lower extremity. *Annals of Surgery* **121**, 1425–1433

Collin, C., Hajdu, S. I., Godbold, J., Friedrich, C. and Brennan, M. F. (1987) Localised operable soft tissue sarcoma of the upper extremity: presentation, management, and factors affecting local recurrence in 108 patients. *Annals of Surgery* **205**, 331–339

Collins, D. H. (1956) *Lancet* **2**, 51

Dahlin, D. C. (1986) *Bone Tumours*. Charles C Thomas: Springfield, IL

Dahlin, D. C. and Henderson, E. D. (1956) Chondrosarcoma: a surgical and pathological problem. *Journal of Bone and Joint Surgery* **38A**, 1025–1038

D'Aubigné, R. M. and Dejouany, J. P. (1958) Diaphyso-epiphysial resection of long bones. *Journal of Bone and Joint Surgery* **40B**, 385–395

Davis, M. A. and Jones, A. G. (1975) Comparison of ^{99m}Tc-labelled phosphate and phosphonate agents for skeletal imaging. *Seminars in Nuclear Medicine* **6**, 19–31

Davis, S. D. (1991) CT evaluation for pulmonary metastases in patients with extrathoracic malignancy. *Radiology* **180**, 1–12

deSantos, L. A. (1980) The radiology of bone tumors: old and new modalities. *Cancer* **30**, 66–91

deSantos, L. A., Goldstein, H. M., Murray, J. A. and Wallace, S. (1978) Computed tomography in the evaluation of musculoskeletal neoplasms. *Radiology* **128**, 89–94.

deSantos, L. A., Bernardino, M. E. and Murray, J. A. (1979a) Computed tomography in the evaluation of osteosarcoma: experience with 25 cases. *American Journal of Roentgenology* **132**, 535–540

deSantos, L. A., Murray, J. A. and Ayala, A. G. (1979b) The value of percutaneous needle biopsy in the management of primary bone tumors. *Cancer* **43**, 735–744

Dos Santos, R. (1950) Arteriography in bone tumors. *Journal of Bone and Surgery* **32B**, 17–29

Drugs and Therapeutics Bulletin (1980) **18**, 69–72

Duthie, R. B. (1972) In: *Bone – Certain Aspects of Neoplasia*, pp. 367–377. (Colston Papers, no. 24). Edited by C. H. G. Price and F. G. M. Ross. Butterworths: London

Dwyer, A. J., Frank, J. A., Sank, V. J. *et al.* (1988) Short-TI inversion-recovery pulse sequence analysis and initial experience in cancer imaging. *Radiology* **168**, 827–836

Edeiken, J. and Hodes, P. J. (1973) General radiological approach to bone lesions. In: *Roentgen Diagnosis of Diseases of Bone*, 2nd edn, pp. 36–37. Williams & Wilkins: Baltimore

Edeiken, J. and Hodes, P. J. (1973) New bone production in periosteal reaction. In: *Roentgen Diagnosis of Diseases of Bone*, 2nd edn, Chapter 4. Williams & Wilkins: Baltimore

Edelstyn, G. A., Gillespie, P. J. and Grebbell, F. S. (1967) *Clinical Radiology* **18**, 158

Edmonson, J. H., Fleming, T. R., Ivins, J. C., Burgert, O., Soule, E. F. and O'Connell, M. J. (1984) Randomized study of systemic chemotherapy following complete excision of nonosseous sarcoma. *Journal of Clinical Oncology* **2**, 1390–1396

Egund, N., Ekelund, L., Sako, M. *et al.* (1981) CT of soft tissue tumors. *American Journal of Roentgenology* **137**, 725–729

Eilber, F. R. and Morton, D. L. (1970) *Cancer* **26**, 588

Eilber, F. R., Giuliano, A. E., Huth, J. F. and Morton, D. L. (1988) A randomized prospective trial using postoperative adjuvant chemotherapy (adriamycin) in high-grade extremity soft-tissue sarcoma. *American Journal of Clinical Oncology* **11**, 39–45

Enneking, W. F. (1983) *Musculoskeletal Tumor Surgery*, vol. 1, pp. 643–648 and 91–95. Churchill Livingstone: New York

Enneking, W. F. and Shirley, P. D. (1977) Resection-arthrodesis for malignant and potentially malignant lesions about the knee using an intramedullary rod and local bone grafts. *Journal of Bone and Joint Surgery* **59A**, 223–236

Enneking, W. F., Spanier, S. S. and Goodman, M. A. (1980) A system for the surgical staging of musculoskeletal sarcoma. *Clinical Orthopaedics and Related Research* **153**, 106–120

Enneking, W. F., Chew, F. S., Hudson, T. M. *et al.* (1981) The role of radionuclide bone scanning in determining the resectability of soft tissue sarcoma. *Journal of Bone and Joint Surgery* **63A**, 249–257

Ewing, C. J. (1928) *Neoplastic Disease*. Saunders: Philadelphia

Ewing, J. (1921) Diffuse endothelioma of bone. *Proceedings of the New York Pathology Society* **21**, 17–24

Farinas, P. L. (1937) Differential diagnosis of bone tumors of the extremities by arteriography. *Radiology* **29**, 29–32

Feldman, F., Casarelle, W. J., Dick, H. M. *et al.* (1975) Selective intra-arterial embolization of bone tumors. *American Journal of Roentgenology* **123**, 130–139

Finkel, M. P. and Biskis, B. O. (1968) *Progress in Experimental Tumor Research* **10**, 72

Foulds, L. (1954) *Cancer Review* **14**, 327

Francis, K. C. and Worcester, J. N. (1962) Radical resection for tumors of the shoulder with preservation of a functional extremity. *Journal of Bone and Joint Surgery* **44A**, 1423–1430.

Fujinaga, S., Poel W. E. and Dmochowski, L. (1970) *Cancer Research* **30**, 1698

Galasko, C. S. B. (1972) Skeletal metastases and mammary cancer. *Annals of the Royal College of Surgeons of England* **50**, 3–28

Galasko, C. S. B. (1974) Pathological fractures secondary to metastatic cancer. *Journal of the Royal College of Surgeons of Edinburgh* **19**, 351–362

Galasko, C. S. B. (1975) Pathological basis of skeletal scintigraphy. *Journal of Bone and Joint Surgery* **57B**, 353–359

Galesko, C. S. B. and Doyle, F. H. (1972) The response to therapy of skeletal metastases from mammary cancer. *British Journal of Surgery* **59**, 85–88

Gebhardt, M. C. (1991) Recent basic science investigations of sarcomas. *Clinical Science* **2**, 775–780

Ginaldi, S. and deSantos, L. A. (1980) Computed tomography in the evaluation of small round cell tumors of bone. *Radiology* **134**, 441–446

Goldenberg, R. R., Campbell, C. J. and Bonfiglio, M. (1970) *Journal of Bone and Joint Surgery* **52A**, 619

Goodpasture, E. W. (1957) *Texas Reports on Biology and Medicine* **15**, 451

Goorin, A., Link, M., Jaffe, N., Risenborough, T., Watts, H. and Abelson, H. T. (1980) Adjuvant chemotherapy and limb salvage procedures for osteosarcoma – a seven year experience (abstract). *Cancer Research* **21**, 472

Gordan, G. S. (1967) *California Medicine* **107**, 54

Gottsauner-Wolf, F., Kotz, R., Knahr, K., Kristen, H., Ritschl, P. and Salzer, M. (1991) Rotationplasty for limb salvage in the treatment of malignant tumors at the knee: a follow-up study of seventy patients. *Journal of Bone and Joint Surgery* **73A**, 1365–1375

Grimes, B. J., Fisher, B., Finn, F. and Danowski, T. S. (1967) *Acta Endocrinologica* **56**, 510

Gross, S. W. (1879) Sarcoma of the long bones, based on a study of one-hundred and sixty-five cases. *American Journal of Medical Science* **78**, 338

Guzzo, C. E., Pachas, W. N., Pinals, R. S. and Kraut, M. J. (1969) *Cancer* **24**, 382

Hall, A. J. and McKay, N. M. S. (1973) *Journal of Bone and Joint Surgery* **55B,** 497–505

Halpern, M. and Freiberger, R. H. (1970) Ateriography as a diagnostic procedure in bone disease. *Radiologic Clinics of North America* **8**, 277–288

Handcock, N. M. and Boothroyd, B. (1963) Structure–junction relationships in the osteoblast. In: *Mechanism of Hard Tissue Destruction*, Chapter 18, pp. 497–514. American Association for Advancement of Sciences: Washington DC

Harrington, K. D. (1975) *Journal of Bone and Joint Surgery* **57A**, 744–750

Harrington, K. D. (1977) The role of surgery in the management of pathological fractures. *Orthopedic Clinics of North America* **8**, 841–859

Harrington, K. D., Johnson, J. O., Turner, R. H. and Green, D. L. (1972) The use of methylmethacrylate as an adjunct in the internal fixation of malignant neoplastic fractures. *Journal of Bone and Joint Surgery* **58A**, 1665–1676

Harrington, K. D., Sim, F. H., Enis, J. E., Johnston, J. O., Dick, H. M. and Gristina, A. G. (1976) Methylmethacrylate as an adjunct in the internal fixation of pathological fractures. *Journal of Bone and Joint Surgery* **58A**, 1047–1055

Harrison, L. B., Franzese, F., Gaynor, J. J. and Brennan, M. F. (1993) Long-term results of a prospective randomized trial of adjuvant brachytherapy in the management of completely resected soft tissue sarcomas of the extremity and superficial trunk. *International Journal of Radiation, Oncology, Biology, Physics* **27**, 259–265

Heelan, R. T., Watson, R. C. and Smith, J. (1979) Computed tomography of lower extremity tumors. *American Journal of Roentgenology* **132**, 933-937

Hoare, J. R. (1968) Pathological fractures. *Journal of Bone and Joint Surgery* **50B**, 232

Holscher, H. C., Bloem, J. L., Wooz, M. A. *et al.* (1987) The value of MR imaging in monitoring the effect of chemotherapy on bone sarcomas. *American Journal of Roentgenology* **154**, 763–769

Hudack, S. S. (1951) Restitutive approach to lesions of bone. *Cancer* **4**, 823–834

Hudson, T. M., Haas, G., Enneking, W. J. *et al.* (1975) Angiography in the management of musculoskeletal tumors. *Surgery, Gynecology and Obstetrics* **14**, 11–21

Hudson, T. M., Enneking, W. F. and Hawkins, I. F. Jr (1981) The value of angiography in planning surgical treatment of bone tumors. *Radiology* **138**, 283–292

Hudson, T. M., Schiebler, M. and Springfield, D. S. (1983) Radiologic imaging of osteosarcoma: role in planning surgical treatment. *Skeletal Radiology* **10**, 137–146

Hustu, H. O., Pinkel, D. and Pratt, C. B. (1972) Treatment of clinically localised Ewing's sarcoma with radiotherapy and combination chemotherapy. *Cancer* **30**, 1522–1527

Hutter, R. V. P., Worcester, J. N. Jr, Francis, K. C., Foote, F. W. Jr and Stewart, F. W. (1962) *Cancer* **15**, 653

Jaffe, H. L. (1935) *Archives of Surgery* **31**, 709

Jaffe, H. L. (1978) *Tumours and Tumorous Conditions of the Bones and Joints*, 3rd edn. Kimpton: London

Jaffe, N., Traggis, D., Sallan, S. and Cassady, J. R. (1976) Improved outlook for Ewing's sarcoma with combination chemotherapy (vincristine, actinomycin D, and cyclophosphamide) and radiation therapy. *Cancer* **38**, 1925–1930

Johnson, L. C. (1953) *Bulletin of the New York Academy of Medicine* **27**, 164

Johnson, L. C. (1964) Morphologic analysis in pathology. The kinetics of disease and general biology of bone. In: *Bone Biodynamics*, Chapter 29, pp. 543–654. Edited by H. M. Grost. Little Brown: Boston

Johnson, R. S. (1968) *Clinical Orthopaedics and Related Research* **68**, 78

Johnston, A. D. (1970) Pathology of metastatic tumours in bone. *Clinical Orthopeadics and Related Research* **73**, 8–33

Jones, E. T. and Kuhns, L. R. (1981) Pitfalls in the use of computed tomography for musculoskeletal tumors in children. *Journal of Bone and Joint Surgery* **63A**, 1297–1304

Kirchner, P. T. and Simon, M. A. (1984) The clinical value of bone and gallium scintigraphy for soft-tissue sarcomas of the extremities. *Journal of Bone and Joint Surgery* **66**, 319–327

Klein, W. A., Miller, H. H., Anderson, M. and DeCosse, J. J. (1987) The use of indomethacin, sulindac and tamoxifen for the treatment of desmoid tumors associated with familial polypsosis. *Cancer* **60**, 2863–2868

Kolodony, A. (1925) Diagnosis and prognosis of bone sarcoma. *Journal of Bone and Joint Surgery* **7**, 911–948

Kotz, R. and Salzer, M. (1982) Rotation-plasty for childhood osteosarcoma of the distal part of the femur. *Journal of Bone and Joint Surgery* **64A**, 959–969

Kraft, G. L. and Leventhal, D. H. (1954) Acrylic prosthesis replacing lower end of the femur for benign giant-cell tumor. *Journal of Bone and Joint Surgery* **36A**, 368–374

Kransdorf, M. J., Jelinck, T. S., Moser, R. P. *et al.* (1989) Soft, tissue masses: diagnosis using MR imaging. *American Journal of Roentgenology* **153**, 541–547

Kreichberg, A., Boquist, L., Borssen, B. and Larsson, D. E. (1982) Prognostic factors in chondrosarcoma, a comparative study of cellular DNA content and clinical pathological features. *Cancer* **50**, 577–583

Laredo, J. D. (1993) Gadolinium enhanced MRI in orthopaedic surgery. *Journal of Bone and Joint Surgery* **75B**, 521–523

Larson, S. M. (1978) Mechanisms of localization of gallium-67 in tumors. *Seminars in Nuclear Medicine* **8**, 193–203

Levin, D. C., Watson, R. C. and Baltaxe, H. A. (1972)

Arteriography in the diagnosis and management of acquired peripheral soft-tissue masses. *Radiology* **104**, 53–58

Levine, E. (1981) Computed tomography of musculoskeletal tumors. *CRC Critical Reviews on Diagnostic Imaging* **16**, 279–309

Levine, E., Lee, K. R., Neff, J. R. *et al.* (1979) Comparison computed tomography and other imaging modalities in the evaluation of musculoskeletal tumors. *Radiology* **131**, 431–437

Lewis, M. M. (1986) The use of an expandable and adjustable prosthesis in the treatment of childhood malignant bone tumors of the extremity. *Cancer* **57**, 499–502

Lichtenstein, L. (1977) *Bone Tumours*, 5th edn. C. V. Mosby: St Louis, MO

Linberg, B. E. (1928) Interscapulo-thoracic resection for malignant tumors of the shoulder joint region. *Journal of Bone and Joint Surgery* **10**, 344–449

Lindberg, R. D., Martin, R. G., Romsdahl, M. M. and Barkley, H. T. (1981) Conservative surgery and post-operative radiotherapy in 300 adults with soft tissue sarcomas. *Cancer* **47**, 2391–2397

Lodwick, G. S. (1964) Reactive response to local injury in bone. *Radiologic Clinics of North America* **2**, 209–219

Lodwick, G. S. (1965) A systematic approach to the roentgen diagnosis of bone tumors. In: *M. D. Anterson Hospital and Tumor Institute: Tumors of Bone and Soft Tissue*, pp. 49–68. Year Book Medical Publishers: Chicago

Lodwick, G. S. (1966) Solitary malignant tumors of bone: the application of predictor variables in diagnosis. *Seminars in Roentgenology* **1**, 293–313

Lodwick, G. S. (1971) The bone and joints. In: *Atlas of Tumor Radiology*. Edited by P. J. Hodes. Year Book Medical Publishers: Chicago

Lodwick, G. S., Wilson, A. J., Farrell, C. *et al.* (1980a) Determining growth rates of focal lesions of bone from radiographs. *Radiology* **134**, 577–583

Lodwick, G. S., Wilson, A. J., Farrell, C. *et al.* (1980b) Estimating rate of growth in bone lesions: observer performance and error. *Radiology* **134**, 585–590

McDonald, D. J., Capanna, R., Gherlinzoni, F. *et al.* (1990) Influence of chemotherapy on perioperative complications in limb salvage surgery for bone tumors. *Cancer* **65**, 1509–1516

McDougall, A. and McGarrity, G. (1979) Extra-abdominal desmoid tumors. *Journal of Bone and Joint Surgery* **61B**, 373–377

McGrath, P. J. (1972) Giant-cell tumour of bone. An analysis of fifty-two cases. *Journal of Bone and Joint Surgery* **54B**, 216–229

Macintosh, D. J., Price, C. H. G. and Jeffree, G. M. (1975) Ewing's tumour. *Journal of Bone and Joint Surgery* **57B**, 331–340

McKenna, R. J., Schwinn, C. P., Soong, K. Y. and Higinbotham, N. L. (1966) Sarcomata of the osteogenic series (osteosarcoma, fibrosarcoma, chondrosarcoma, parosteal osteogenic sarcoma, and sarcomata arising in abnormal bone): an analysis of 552 cases. *Journal of Bone and Joint Surgery* **48A**, 1–26

McNeil, B. J. (1978) Rationale for the use of bone scan in selected metastatic primary bone tumors. *Seminars in Nuclear Medicine* **8**, 336–345

Madewell, J. E., Ragsdale, B. D. and Sweet, D. E. (1981) Radiologic and pathologic analysis of solitary bone lesions. Part I: internal margins. *Radiologic Clinics of North America* **19**, 715–748

Makley, J. T., Cohen, A. M. and Boada, E. (1982) Sacral tumors: a hidden problem. *Orthopedics* **5**, 996

Mankin, H. J. (1978) The fourth Shands Annual Lecture. *American Orthopedic Association News* **X**, 8–10

Mankin, H. J., Doppelt, S. H., Sullivan, T. R. and Tomford, W. W. (1982a) Osteoarticular and intercalary allograft transplantation in the management of malignant tumors of bone. *Cancer* **50**, 613–630

Mankin, H. J., Lange, T. A. and Spanier, S. S. (1982b) The hazards of biopsy in patients with malignant primary bone and soft tissue tumours. *Journal of Bone and Joint Surgery* **64A**, 1121–1127

Marcove, R. C. (1977) Chondrosarcoma – diagnosis and treatment. *Orthopedic Clinics of North America* **8**, 811

Marcove, R. C. (1982) A 17-year review of cryosurgery in the treatment of bone tumors. *Clinical Orthopaedics and Related Research* **163**, 231–234

Marcove, R. C., Lyden, J. P., Huvos, A. G. and Bullough, P. B. (1973) Giant-cell tumors treated by cryrosurgery: a report of twenty-five cases. *Journal of Bone and Joint Surgery* **55A**, 1633–1644

Marcove, R. C., Lewis, M. M. and Huvos, A. G. (1977) En bloc upper humeral interscapulo-thoracic resection: the Tikhoff–Linberg Procedure. *Clinical Orthopaedics and Related Research* **124**, 219–228

Martel, W. and Abell, M. R. (1973) Radiologic evaluation of soft tissue tumors: a retrospective study. *Cancer* **324**, 352–365

Martin, A., Bauer, T. W. and Manly, M. T. (1988) Osteosarcoma at the site of total hip replacement. *Journal of Bone and Joint Surgery* **70A**, 1561–1567

Martini, N., Huvos, A. G., Mike, V., Marcove, R. C. and Beattie, E. J. (1971) Multiple pulmonary metastases in the treatment of osteogenic sarcoma. *Annals of Thoracic Surgery* **12**, 271–297

Martland, H. S. (1931) *American Journal of Cancer* **15**, 2435

Milch, R. A. and Changus, G. W. (1956) *Cancer* **9**, 340

Moore, A. T. and Bohlman, H. R. (1943) Metal hip joint. A case report. *Journal of Bone and Joint Surgery* **25A**, 688–692

Muhm, J. R., Brown, L. R., Crowe, J. R. *et al.* (1978) Comparison of whole lung tomography for detecting pulmonary nodules. *American Journal of Roentgenology* **131**, 981–984

Musgrove, J. E. and McDonald, J. R. (1948) *Archives of Pathology* **45**, 513

Nelson, S. W. (1966) Some fundamentals in the radiologic differential diagnosis of solitary bone lesions. *Seminars in Roentgenology* **1**, 244–267

Okada, K., Frassica, F. J., Sim, F. H. *et al.* (1994) Parosteal osteosarcoma. *Journal of Bone and Joint Surgery* **76A**, 366–378

Ottolenghi, C. E. (1966) Massive osteoarticular bone grafts. Transplant of the whole femur. *Journal of Bone and Joint Surgery* **48B**, 646–659

Paavolainen, P. and Teppo, L. (1976) Chordoma in Finland. *Acta Orthopaedica Scandinavica* **47**, 46–51

Pack, G. T. and Baldwin, J. C. (1966) The Tikhor–Linberg resection of shoulder girdle. Case report. *Journal of Bone and Joint Surgery* **48B**, 646–659

Parrish, F. F. (1973) Allograft replacement of all or part of the end of a long bone following excision of a tumor: report of twenty-one cases. *Journal of Bone and Joint Surgery* **55A**, 1–22

Parrish, E. F. and Murray, J. A. (1970) Surgical treatment for secondary neoplastic fractures. *Journal of Bone and Joint Surgery* **52A**, 665–680

Pass, H. I., Dinger, A., Maknch, R. and Roth, J. A. (1985) Detection of pulmonary metastases in patients with osteogenic and soft-tissue sarcomas: the superiority of CT scans compared with conventional linear tomography using .dynamic analysis. *Journal of Clinical Oncology* **3**, 1261–1265

Persson, B. M., Rydholm, A., Berlin, O. and Gunterberg, B. (1987) Curettage and acrylic cementation in surgical treatment of giant cell tumors. In: *Limb-sparing Surgery in Musculoskeletal Oncology*, pp. 476. Edited by W. F. Ennekinge. Churchill Livingstone: New York

Pettersson, H., Gillespy, T., Hamlin, D. J. *et al.* (1987) Primary musculoskeletal tumors: examination with MR imaging compared with conventional modalities. *Radiology* **164**, 237–241

Phemister, D. B. (1930) Chondrosarcoma of bone. *Surgery, Gynecology and Obstetrics* **50**, 216–233

Potter, D. A., Kinsella, T., Glatstein, E., Wesley, R., White, D. E. and Seipp, C. A. (1986) High-grade soft tissue sarcomas of the extremities. *Cancer* **58**, 190–205

Price, C. G. H. (1958) *Journal of Bone and Joint Surgery* **40B**, 574

Pritchard, D. J., Dahlin, D. C., Dauphine, R. T., Taylor, W. F. and Beabout, J. W. (1975a) Ewing's sarcoma: a clinicopathological and statistical analysis of patients surviving five years or longer. *Journal of Bone and Joint Surgery* **57A**, 10–16

Pritchard, D. J., Finkel, M. P. and Reilly, C. A. (1975b) The etiology of osteosarcoma. A review of current considerations. *Clinical Orthopaedics and Related Research* **111**, 14

Pritchard, D. J., Sim, F. H., Ivins, J. C., Soule, E. H. and Dahlin, D. C. (1977) Fibrosarcoma of bone and soft tissues of the trunk and extremities. *Orthopedic Clinics of North America* **8**, 869–881

Ragsdale, B. D., Madewell, J. E. and Sweet, D. E. (1981) Radiologic and pathologic analysis of solitary bone lesions, Part II: periosteal reactions. *Radiologic Clinics of North America* **19**, 749–783

Rock, M. G., Pritchard, D. J., Reiman, H. M., Soule, E. H. and Brewster, R. C. (1984) Extra-abdominal desmoid tumors. *Journal of Bone and Joint Surgery* **66A**, 1369–1374

Rosen, G., Caparros, B., Nirenbery, A. *et al.* (1981) Ewing's sarcoma ten-year experience with adjuvant chemotherapy. *Cancer* **47**, 2204–2213

Rosenthal, D. I. (1982) Computed tomography in bone and soft tissue neoplasm: applications and pathologic correlations. *CRC Critical Reviews in Diagnostic Imaging* **18**, 243–278

Roth, J. A., Putnam, J. B., Wesley, M. N. and Rosenberg, S. A. (1985) Differing determinants of prognosis following resection of pulmonary metastases from osteogenic and soft tissue sarcoma patients. *Cancer* **55**, 1361–1366

Saddegh, M. K., Lindholm, J., Lundberg, J. *et al.* (1992) Staging of soft tissue sarcomas. Prognostic analysis of clinical and pathological features. *Journal of Bone and Joint Surgery* **74B**, 495–500

Sanjay, B., Frassica, F. J., Frassica, D. A. *et al.* (1993) Treatment of giant cell tumour of the pelvis. *Journal of Bone and Joint Surgery* **75A**, 1466–1475

Schajowicz, F. and Gallardo, H. (1970) *Journal of Bone and Joint Surgery* **52B**, 205

Schaner, E. G., Chang, A. E., Doppman, J. L. *et al.* (1978) Comparison of computed and conventional whole lung tomography in detecting pulmonary nodules: a prospective radiologic-pathologic study. *American Journal of Roentgenology* **131**, 51–54

Sherman, C. and Duthie, R. B. (1960) *Cancer* **13**, 51

Shiu, M. H., Castro, E. B., Hadju, S. I. and Fortner, J. G. (1975) Surgical treatment of 297 soft tissue sarcomas of the lower extremity. *Annals of Surgery* **182**, 597–602

Sim, F. H. (1981) Total hip arthroplasty in the management of tumors. *Orthopedic Transactions* **5**, 361

Sim, F. H. and Bohlman, W. E. (1982) Custom prosthetic replacement following skeletal reconstruction in primary and metastatic bone tumors. *Orthopedic Transactions* **6**, 133

Simon, M. A. and Enneking, W. F. (1976) The management of soft-tissue sarcomas of the extremities. *Journal of Bone and Joint Surgery* **58A**, 317–328

Simon, M. A. and Kirchner, P. T. (1980) Scintigraphic evaluation of primary bone tumors: comparison of technetium-99m phosphonate and gallium citrate imaging. *Journal of Bone and Joint Surgery* **62A**, 758–764

Sissons, H. A. and Duthie, R. B. (1959) In: *British Surgical Practice: Surgical Progress*, p. 157. Butterworths: London

Smith, W. S. and Simon, M. A. (1975) Segmental resection for chondrosarcoma. *Journal of Bone and Joint Surgery* **57A**, 1097–1103

Steiner, G. C., Ghosh, L. and Dorfman, H. D. (1972) Ultrastructure of giant cell tumors of bone. *Human Pathology* **3**, 569–596

Stewart, S. E. and Eddy, B. E. (1956) In: *Perspectives in Virology*, p. 242. Edited by M. Pollard. Wiley: New York

Stewart, W. R., Gleberman, R. H., Harrelman, J. N. and Siegler, H. F. (1978) Skeletal metastases of melanoma. *Journal of Bone and Joint Surgery* **60A**, 645–649

Stout, A. P. (1961) *Cancer Journal for Clinicians* **11**, 210

Subramanian, G., McAfee, J. F., Blair, R. J. *et al.* (1975) An evaluation of technetium-99m labelled phosphate compounds as bone imaging agents in radiopharma-ceuticals. In: *New York Society of Nuclear Medicine*. Edited by G. Subramanian, R. A. Rhodes, J. F. Cooper and V. J. Sodd

Sundaram, M. and McLeod, R. A. (1990) MR imaging of tumor and tumor-like lesions of bone. *American Journal of Roentgenology* **155**, 817–824

Sunderman, F. W. (1973) The current status of nickel carcinogenesis. *Annals of Clinical and Laboratory Science* **3**, 156

Sweet, D. E., Madewell, J. E. and Ragsdale, B. D. (1981) Radiologic and pathologic analysis of solitary bone lesions, part III: matrix patterns. *Radiologic Clinics of North America* **19**, 785–814

Syzskowitz, R. and Cockin, J. (1974) Internal fixation of bone defects using bone cement and plates, an experimental study. *Journal of Bone and Joint Surgery* **56B**, 198–199

Taylor, W. F., Ivins, J. C., Dahlin, D. E., Edmonson, J. H. and Pritchard, D. J. (1978) Trends and variability in survival from osteosarcoma. *Mayo Clinic Proceedings* **53**, 695–700

Thomson, A. D. and Turner-Warwick, R. T. (1955) *Journal of Bone and Joint Surgery* **37B**, 266

Thrace, J. H. and Ellis, B. I. (1987) Skeletal metastases. *Radiologic Clinics of North America* **25**, 1155–1170

Thrall, J. H., Geslein, G. E., Corcoron, R. J. *et al.* (1975) Abnormal radionuclide deposition patterns adjacent to focal skeletal lesions. *Radiology* **115**, 659–663

Twycross, R. G. (1974) *International Journal of Clinical Pharmacology, Therapeutics and Toxicology* **9**, 184–198

Unni, K., Dahlin, D. C. and Beabout, J. W. (1976a) Periosteal osteogenic sarcoma. *Cancer* **37**, 2476–2485

Unni, K. K., Dahlin, D. C., Beabout, J. W. *et al.* (1976b) Parosteal osteogenic sarcoma. *Cancer* **37**, 2466–2475

Vander Griend, R. A. and Funderburk, C. H. (1993) The treatment of giant cell tumours of the distal part of the radius. *Journal of Bone and Joint Surgery* **75A**, 899–908

Vanel, D., Lacombe, M., Couanet, D. *et al.* (1987) Musculoskeletal tumors: follow-up with MR imaging after treatment with surgery and radiation therapy. *Radiology* **164**, 243–245

Viamonte, M. Jr, Roen, S. and Lepage, J. (1973) Non-specificity of abnormal vascularity in the angiographic diagnosis of malignant neoplasms. *Radiology* **106**, 59–63

Wahner, H. W., Kyle, R. A. and Beabout, J. W. (1980) Scintigraphic evaluation of the skeleton in multiple myeloma. *Mayo Clinic Proceedings* **55**, 739–746

Weatherby, R. P., Dahlin, D. C. and Ivins, J. C. (1981) Postradiation sarcoma of bone. Review of 78 Mayo Clinic cases. *Mayo Clinic Proceedings* **56**, 294–306

Weisbrod, G. L. (1990) Transthoracic percutaneous lung biopsy. *Radiologic Clinics of North America* **28** (3), 647–655

Weiss, A. J. and Lackman, R. D. (1989) Low-dose chemotherapy of desmoid tumors. *Cancer* **64**, 1192–1194

Westcott, J. L. (1985) Percutaneous biopsy of intrathoracic lesions. *Seminars in Interventional Radiology* **2**, 232–244

Wetzel, L. H. and Levine, E. (1990) Soft-tissue tumors of the foot: value of MR imaging for specific diagnosis. *American Journal of Roentgenology* **155**, 1025–1030

Wilson, J. S., Korobkin, M., Genant, H. K. *et al.* (1978) Computed tomography of musculoskeletal disorders. *American Journal of Roentgenology* **131**, 55–61

Wilson, P. D. and Lance, E. M. (1965) Surgical reconstruction of the skeleton following segmental resection for bone tumors. *Journal of Bone and Joint Surgery* **47A**, 1629–1656

Wilson, R. E., Wood, W. C., Lerner, H. L., Antman, K., Amato, D. and Corson, J. M. (1986) Doxorubicin chemotherapy in the treatment of soft-tissue sarcoma. *Archives of Surgery* **121**, 1354–1359

Wiltse, I. L., Hall, R. H. and Stenheim, J. C. (1957) Experimental studies regarding the possible use of self-curing acrylic in orthopedic surgery. *Journal of Bone and Joint Surgery* **39A**, 961–972

Wong, W. S., Kaiser, L. R., Gold, R. H. *et al.* (1982) Radiographic features of osseous metastases of soft tissue sarcomas. *Radiology* **143**, 71–74

Woolfenden, J. M., Pitt, M. J., Durie, D. G. M. *et al.* (1980) Comparison of bone scintigraphy and radiography in multiple myeloma. *Radiology* **134**, 723-728

Zelefsky, M. J., Harrison, L. B., Shiu, M. H., Armstrong, J. G., Hajdu, S. I. and Brennan, M. F. (1991) Combined surgical resection and iridium-192 implantation for locally advanced and recurrent desmoid tumors. *Cancer* **67**, 380–384

Zickel, R. E. and Mouradian, W. H. (1976) Intramedullary fixation of pathological fractures and lesions of the subtrochanteric region of the femur. *Journal of Bone and Joint Surgery* **58A**, 1061–1066

Zimmer, W. D., Berquist, T. H., McLeod, R. A. *et al.* (1985) Bone tumors: magnetic resonance imaging versus computed tomography. *Radiology* **155**, 709–718

CHAPTER 11

Arthritis and Rheumatic Diseases

ROBERT B. DUTHIE

Chronic arthritis

Chronic arthritis can develop in a large group of diseases, often called the rheumatic diseases, which, because of their prevalence, the deformity and disability produced and the associated economic and social consequences, are among the most serious of all joint affections. The economic importance is reflected by the 37 million working days lost each year in Great Britain due to the rheumatic diseases, representing 11.6% of the total time lost due to sickness (Figure 11.1); 13 million days lost are due to low back pain problems.

Studies suggest that approximately 10% of the population of Great Britain and the United States of America are disabled to some degree by chronic arthritis. Degenerative joint disease (7%) and rheumatoid arthritis (3%) account for most of this total.

Lawrence (1967) showed, in a population study in north-west England, that 2.8% of adult males and 6.3% of adult females have an inflammatory polyarthritis. In a similar survey it was found that 50% of adult males and 52% of adult females had osteoarthrosis affecting one or more joints. This incidence

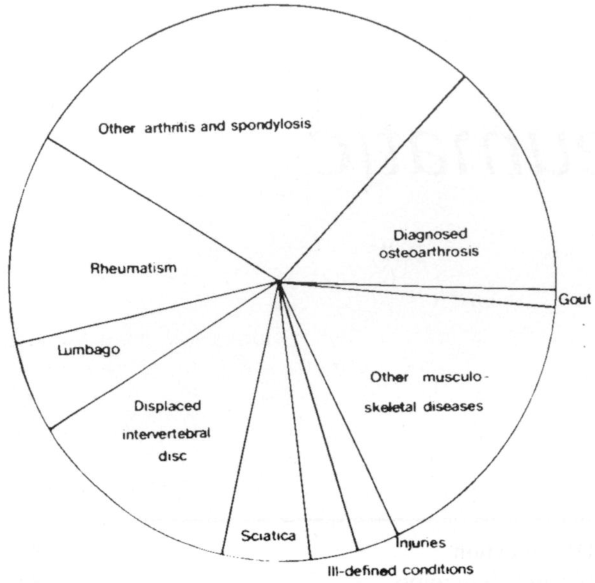

Figure 11.1 Absence from work due to sickness and industrial injuries attributable to rheumatic diseases. (Reproduced, with permission, from DHSS, 1972)

for osteoarthrosis rose to 98% for the age group of 65–74 years (Figures 11.1 and 11.2).

Classification of the causes of chronic arthritis remains difficult because many of them remain unknown. However, a modified version of the classification of the American Rheumatism Association is:

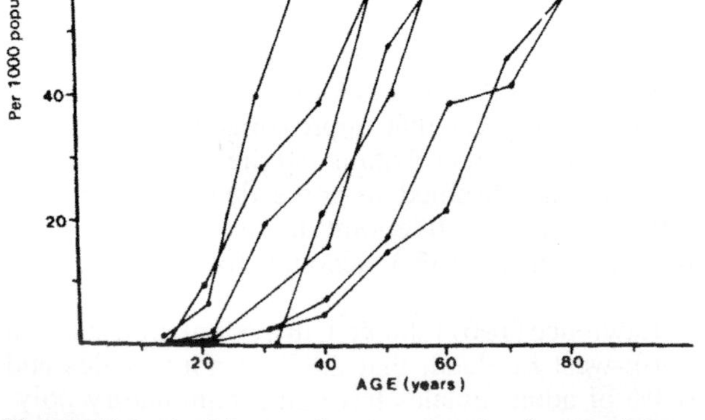

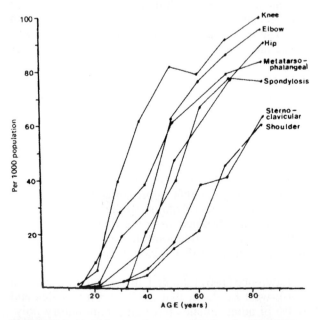

Figure 11.2 Incidence of osteoarthrosis of major joints. (After Danielsson, L.G. (1964) *Acta Orthopaedica Scandinavica*, Suppl. 66)

1. Polyarthritis of unknown cause:
   (a) rheumatoid arthritis;
   (b) juvenile rheumatoid arthritis;
   (c) ankylosing spondylitis;
   (d) psoriatic arthropathy;
   (e) Reiter's disease.
2. Arthritis associated with the connective tissue diseases.
3. Arthritis associated with rheumatic fever.
4. Degenerative joint disease – osteoarthritis, -osis.
5. Arthritis due to infections.
6. Arthritis due to traumatic and/or neurogenic disorders.
7. Arthritis associated with biochemical or endocrine abnormalities. This group includes gout, pseudogout, haemophilia, the haemoglobinopathies, ochronosis, etc.
8. Arthritis due to tumours. This group includes tumours of bone, cartilage and the soft periarticular structures, villonodular synovitis, metastatic deposits, multiple myeloma and the leukaemias.
9. Arthritis due to congenital and inherited disorders. This group includes Marfan's, Ehlers–Danlos and Hurler's syndromes, Morquio's disease, etc. It is likely that the disorders of mucopolysaccharide and collagen metabolism are the causes of most of these conditions.
10. Arthritis due to a miscellaneous group of diseases, including sarcoid ulcerative bowel disease, hypertrophic pulmonary osteoarthropathy, etc.

Chronic arthritis is as old as man himself, it has affected both man and the lower animals from the remote periods in the earliest history, and there are ancient Egyptian bones which exhibit all the typical changes of the disease.

GENERAL CLINICAL FEATURES OF ARTHRITIS

Pain resulting from arthritis of a joint – even though still not fully understood – has been described (Duthie and Harris, 1969) as arising from:

1. Disease involving the *soft tissues* of muscle with spasm or contracture; of capsule which is the most sensitive of all joint tissue (Kellgren and Samuel, 1950); of synovium or periosteum; and of ligaments especially when the joint is unstable.
2. Disease involving the *subchondral bone*, which contains blood vessels and their nerve plexuses in the adventitial coat. Kellgren (1939) showed

that bone is sensitive to pressure and percussion stimuli whereas cartilage is insensitive.

The other clinical features of arthritis of a joint have been reviewed (Kenwright and Duthie, 1971) as:

1. *Loss of mobility* – due to:
   (a) Loss of bone and articular cartilage symmetry leading to incongruity.
   (b) Atrophy, spasm or contracture of muscles with the appearance of intrafibrillary fibrosis within the muscle, in overlying fascia and at the musculotendinous junctions.
   (c) Capsular contractures.
   (d) Mechanical blockage by loose bodies, osteophytes, and cartilaginous or bony debris (Figure 11.3).
2. *Instability* – due to:
   (a) Muscle atrophy and inco-ordination especially in response to effusion and pain. DeAndrande *et al.* (1965), by experimental injection of saline solution, showed that marked atrophy of the quadriceps muscle mass follows distension of the knee joint.
   (b) Joint surface incongruity and roughness, with pain accompanying movement.
   (c) Loose bodies.
   (d) Meniscal degeneration and/or looseness with or without frank tear, as well as abnormality of glenoid cartilages when involved with deforming osteophyte formation/degeneration, etc.
   (e) Trapping of intra-articular synovial folds (e.g. the intrapatellar fold).

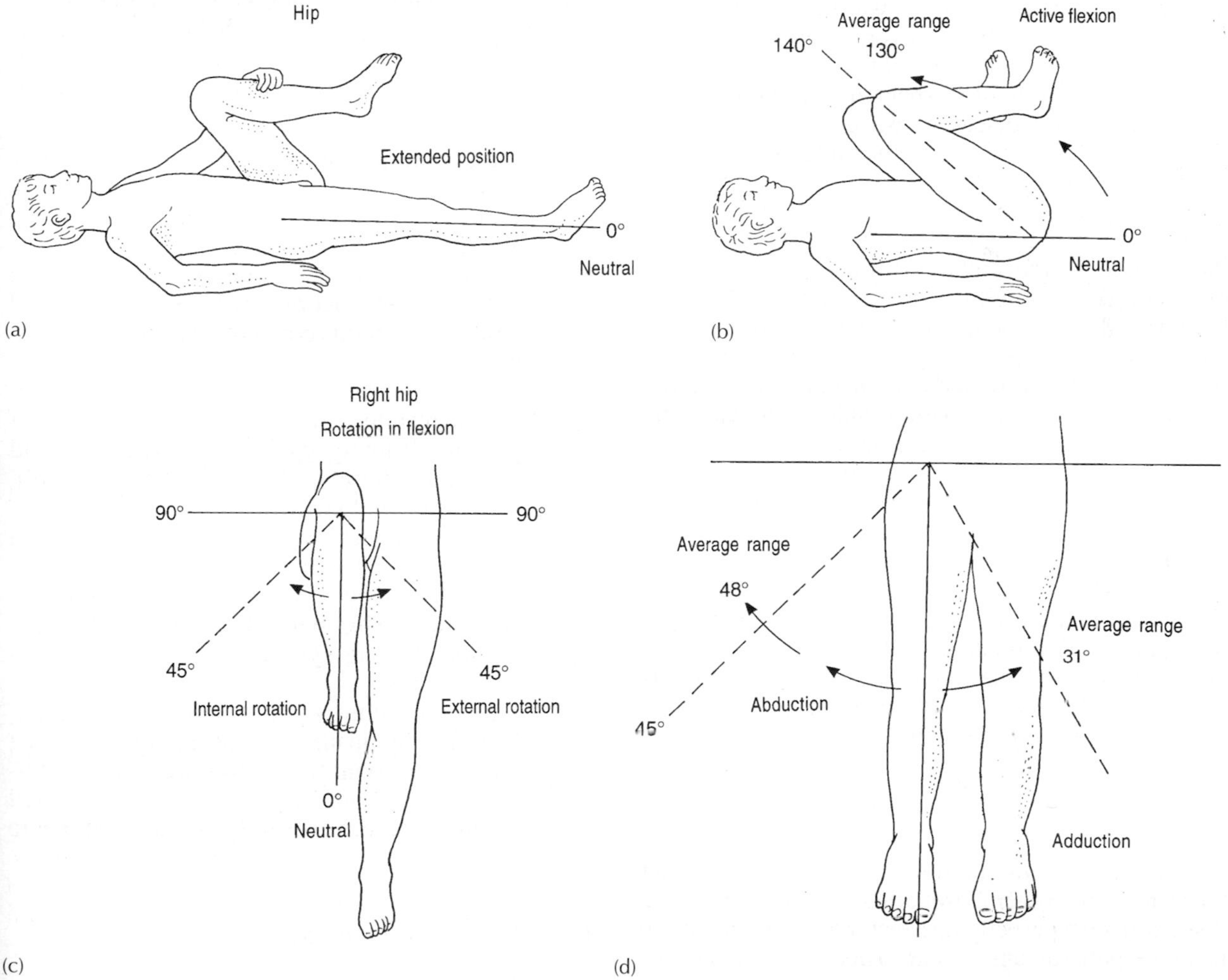

Figure 11.3 (a) Full extension, and (b) full flexion of the hip. (c) Internal and external rotation of the flexed hip joint. (d) Abduction and adduction ranges of motion of the hip joint.

3. *Deformity* – resulting from a swelling of either the joint due to distension by a synovial effusion or the mass of synovial tissue itself; or from soft tissue contractures into flexion, adduction, etc; or from frank angular deformities in valgus or varus positions.

Rheumatoid arthritis

Rheumatoid arthritis is considered to affect approximately 3% of the population in Great Britain and the United States of America, of whom 80% are women. Although it was once thought only to affect populations living in temperate climates, it is now clear from population studies that the incidence of the disease is much the same throughout the world. However, it seems that the disease causes less disability in those living in warmer climates and that the incidence and severity of the disease appear to be altered in many of the developing countries by the shorter life expectancy, the prevalence of infective joint diseases, especially tuberculosis, and the high incidence of other infective diseases such as malaria.

The mean age of onset of rheumatoid arthritis is 40 years but no age group is exempt. An acute onset of the disease in the eighth or ninth decade is well documented although the disease tends to be more benign and spontaneous remissions are more common. The onset in older patients should raise the possibility of an underlying neoplasm or other serious disease exacerbating mild, long-standing rheumatoid arthritis. The disease affects females and males in the ratio 3:1, but the sex incidence of severe disease is almost equal since males appear more liable to the systemic manifestations of the disease. The serious systemic manifestations of the disease, most of which can be ascribed to a widespread vasculitis of small arterioles, have been increasingly recognized. Rheumatoid arthritis is not only a polyarthritis, and the name rheumatoid disease is preferable since it directs attention to the whole patient and not just the joints.

AETIOLOGY

The cause remains unknown. It seems likely that there may be several initiating factors which are distinct from a perpetuating factor about which there is more general agreement. There is evidence of immune overactivity:

1. The presence in the serum of abnormal immunoglobulin–rheumatoid factors – IgG and IgM.
2. The infiltration of the synovial tissue by immunologically competent cells, lymphocytes, and plasma cells, which are responsible for the local production of immunoglobulins including rheumatoid factor.
3. The presence of immune antigen–antibody complexes within leucocytes in synovial fluid and peripheral blood.
4. The finding of lowered complement levels in synovial fluid.

It has been suggested that the basic mechanism in the production of the inflammation is the combination of rheumatoid factor and an altered immunoglobulin with the utilization of complement; the ingestion of the resulting immune complexes by neutrophils causes the release of lysosomal enzymes which act as mediators of the synovitis (Weissmann, 1972). The alteration or production of the immunoglobulin with which rheumatoid factor combines is a vital step. If the alteration appears *de novo*, rheumatoid arthritis can be called an autoimmune disease. However, other aetiological factors may be involved, including:

1. A genetic influence (DR4): there is a tendency for the disease to be aggregated in families.
2. Trauma: many patients have mentioned traumatic incidents as a precipitating cause.
3. Psychological stress: the study of identical twins in one of whom rheumatoid arthritis developed tends to support this concept (Meyerowitz *et al.*, 1968).
4. Infectious agents: renewed interest in this subject has resulted in isolation of a variety of organisms from synovial tissue, synovial fluid and blood. These include diphtheroid bacilli, mycoplasma and viruses.
5. Vascular changes: alteration of the normal peripheral vascular bed, perhaps by autonomic influence, has been suggested as the primary abnormality. This has been implicated to explain the striking symmetry of the arthritis in many patients.
6. Neurogenic: neuropeptides can cause inflammation. Reflex sympathetic areas through the spinal cord could account for the contralateral distribution. Rheumatoid affects the non-paralysed side much more severely in a hemiplegic patient.

CLINICAL FEATURES

The disease is characteristically polyarticular, and although the onset may be monarticular the spread to involve other joints, frequently producing symmetrical disease, is often rapid. The small joints of the hands and feet are first affected in about 70% of patients. In older patients the shoulder joint is commonly involved first and this may present diagnostic difficulty. The onset is acute, with fever and serious constitutional symptoms, in about 20% of cases.

The patients complain of pain and stiffness, most characteristically in the morning. The joints and the surrounding periarticular structures, tendons, ligaments and joint capsules are tender and swollen. Synovial proliferation and joint effusions may be marked. Limitation of joint movement, with the development of correctable flexion deformities at many joints, follows. The flexion deformities accommodate the swollen and proliferating tissues with a reduction in pain. If the inflammatory process is unchecked, further deformities and disabilities will result due to the progressive damage to joint cartilage, subchondral bone and periarticular structures and the muscle spasm. Flexion contractures are the common deformities of the large joints although these may be modified by local mechanical factors. In the hands more characteristic deformities such as ulnar deviation, swan neck and boutonnière deformities of the fingers and in the feet broadening of the forefoot, clawing of the toes and plantar callosities may develop, due to alterations in the intricate mechanical arrangements of the tendons, ligaments and joints. Any diarthrodial joint may be affected but involvement of the sacroiliac joints and the spinal joints except those in the cervical spine is uncommon. Progressive disease causes further loss of cartilage and subchondral bone with subluxation of joints. The end result is fibrous or even bony ankyloses (Table 11.1).

EXTRA-ARTICULAR FEATURES

Rheumatoid arthritis is a systemic disease. Anorexia, weight loss, general malaise, lassitude and depression are common. A low-grade fever may be present. Generalized osteoporosis with more marked juxta-articular osteoporosis occurs. There is lymph node enlargement, with the glands, particularly those draining active joints, being discrete and non-tender. Splenic enlargement is common and the organ is palpable in about 5% of patients.

Subcutaneous nodules

These characteristic features, which are present in 20% of patients, develop over any pressure areas. The extensor surfaces of the forearms are the commonest site but they may develop over unusual sites, such as the occiput, if these become pressure areas. The nodules are usually subcutaneous but they

Table 11.1 Rheumatoid arthritis (peri- as well as polyarticular in site)

Pathological process	Tissues involved	Results in	Deformities
Vasculitis Necrosis Fibrosis	Joint structures	Synovitis – effusion Articular cartilage destruction Pericapsulitis Ligamentous instability Arthritis	Swelling Stiffness Instability-subluxation – dislocation Intrinsic-plus deformity
Plasma cell proliferation	Tendon	Tenosynovitis Rupture	Ulnar deviation of fingers Concertina collapse of fingers
Granulation tissue and pannus formation	Muscle	Wasting Atrophy Fibrosis	Contracture Ankylosis
Synovial hypertrophy: in joint in tendon	Bone	Osteoporosis-thinning of cortex and loss of trabecular structure Cyst formation – subchondral erosions (adjacent to metaphysis) Destruction	
	Subcutaneous	Nodules	

may become fixed in deeper tissues or attached to the periosteum. They may occur in tendons and cause triggering. They have been found and implicated in disease in many internal organs such as the heart, the meninges, retina and bone, but it is in the lung that they cause diagnostic difficulty. They develop in the lower, peripheral lung fields and may undergo cavitation. Their finding on chest radiographs will require the exclusion of tumour, tuberculosis, etc. Subcutaneous nodules occur only in patients with a positive serological test for rheumatoid factor. Their removal, unless they become infected or for mechanical reasons, is probably unwise since they frequently recur and the underlying vasculitis may impair wound healing. Generally their presence is associated with a poor prognosis.

Tendons and bursae

Tendons, in synovial sheaths, and bursae become involved in the same pathological process as affects the joint synovium (Figure 11.4). Involvement may impair their function, and stretching or rupture of tendons, particularly the extensors of the fingers, may occur. The exact mechanism responsible for tendon damage remains undetermined. Simple mechanical damage due to the movement of the tendon over the eroded bone surfaces may be a contributory factor but is probably too simple an explanation. Direct invasion of the tendon by the inflammatory process, the presence of nodules and ischaemic changes due to compression and vasculitis are factors involved in most cases.

The skin

Thinning of the skin due to loss of the subcutaneous fat and connective tissues is common. Shearing stresses on the skin tend to cause an ecchymosis since the small blood vessels are poorly supported. The additional presence of vasculitis may produce difficulties in skin healing after minor trauma or surgical procedures.

Arteries

Many of the complications of rheumatoid disease can be attributed to vascular involvement. Medium or large artery involvement in a process indistinguishable from polyarteritis nodosa is rare. However, inflammatory change in the smaller arteries and arterioles is common. This will cause small necrotic lesions at the periphery, particularly around the nailfolds, and may even lead to small areas of gangrene. Such vascular changes are the basis of the neurological, cardiac and pleural lesions to be described and are the cause of the rheumatoid nodule. They occur only in those with a positive serological test for rheumatoid factor.

There have been suggestions that these vascular lesions and the abnormalities dependent on them are exacerbated or even produced by corticosteroid therapy. This is difficult to prove since those with more severe disease tend to have vasculitis *and* to receive corticosteroids. The increasing incidence of these problems probably reflects increasing awareness of their existence.

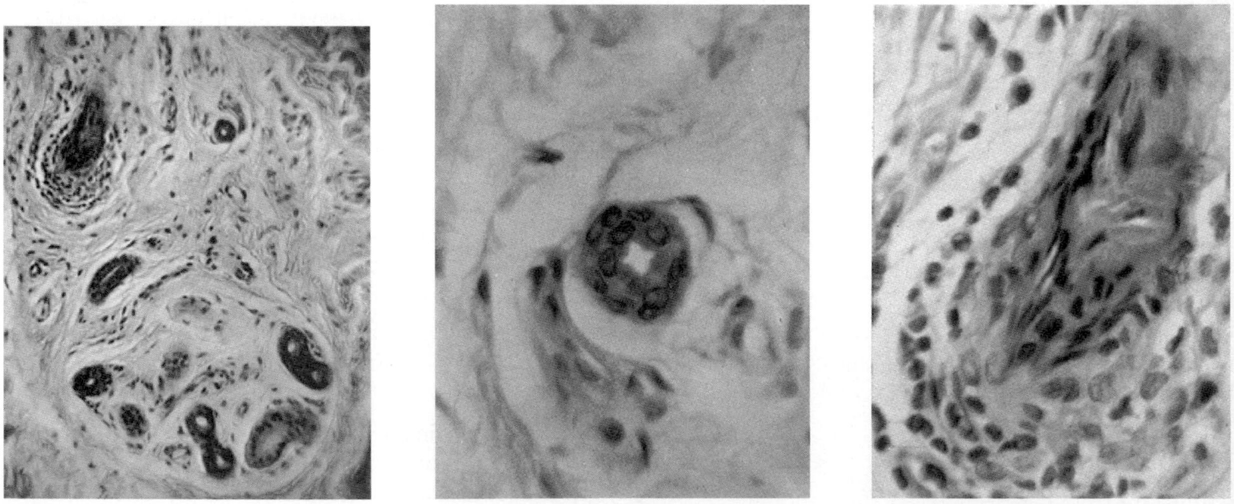

(a) (b) (c)

Figure 11.4 (a) Photomicrograph of synovium from rheumatoid arthritis, showing collection of blood vessels surrounded by plasma cells and connective tissue. (× 25). (b) Photomicrograph showing the endarteritis with narrowing of the lumen because of hyperplasia and hypertrophy of the wall structures. (× 328). (c) Photomicrograph showing vasculitis of a vessel which is surrounded by small round cells. (× 332).

Nerves

Localized digital neuropathy, mononeuritis multiplex with involvement of one or more major nerves producing such signs as foot-drop, and the very serious symmetrical peripheral neuropathy are all due to vasculitis of the vasa nervorum.

Entrapment neuropathies are a common feature of rheumatoid disease and may be the presenting complaint. Carpal and tarsal tunnel compression and entrapment of the ulnar nerve at the elbow and the lateral popliteal nerve at the head of the fibula are well documented. Proliferation of tendon sheath or joint synovial tissue in an area of limited space is responsible. Carpal tunnel compression occurs in 60% of patients at some time. Surgical decompression may be required.

Spinal cord compression may occur. Instability of the atlantoaxial joint with subluxation of the atlas on neck flexion is a radiological finding in 25% of patients. The patients complain of pain, particularly with jolting movement, C1–2 root compression symptoms and occasionally demonstrate long tract signs due to spinal cord compression. Symptoms and signs are less common than the radiological findings would suggest. Sudden death due to cord compression is recorded and might be more common if the possibility were considered in all patients with rheumatoid arthritis who die unexpectedly. Management of pain and root compression is by the use of soft cervical collars, but the presence of persistent symptoms with evidence of cord compression requires surgical fixation. A variety of different methods have been described. Symptomless radiological abnormalities do not require treatment but the anaesthetist should be warned if surgery is planned so that appropriate protective measures can be taken.

Lungs and pleura

Rheumatoid nodules in the lower peripheral lung fields and their association with pneumoconiosis to produce larger nodules often with cavitation (Caplan's syndrome) have been mentioned. Pleuritic lesions also occur and the pathological findings can be considered as a nodule which has been opened out and spread over the pleura. Diffuse interstitial fibrosis occurs in 1.6% of patients. The disease is progressive, resulting in dyspnoea, and there is no useful treatment. Pleural effusions may occur with any of these lung lesions or independently. The characteristics of the fluid are diagnostic. The effusion is rarely large enough to cause symptoms, but aspiration and the instillation of hydrocortisone into the pleural cavity may be beneficial.

Other tissues

The commonest cardiac lesion in rheumatoid disease is pericarditis. This may occur in 10% of cases and occasionally progresses to constrictive pericarditis.

Various inflammatory changes in the eye may impair vision and further disable the patient.

Muscle wasting due to simple atrophy is very common but recent work has confirmed the presence of true myopathy in rheumatoid disease.

Anaemia

Although mild megaloblastic anaemia, usually due to folate deficiency, occurs in 20% of patients, almost all have some degree of anaemia due to abnormalities in iron metabolism. A haemoglobin concentration of 11 g/dl or less is very common and adds to the patient's disability. Oral iron therapy is of no value. The anaemia can be improved by controlling the disease or by parenteral iron therapy.

DIAGNOSIS

The American Rheumatism Association have revised their diagnostic criteria (Arnett, 1989):

1. Morning stiffness, lasting at least 1 hour.
2. Arthritis of three or more joint areas with soft tissue swelling or fluid – observed by a physician – in upper and lower limbs.
3. Arthritis of hand joints (including wrist and/or metacarpals).
4. Symmetrical arthritis – simultaneous involvement of the same joint areas on both sides of the body.
5. A positive serum rheumatoid factor.
6. Radiological changes – especially of hands and wrist, ankle and foot, showing subchondral erosions, bony decalcification, symmetrical articular cartilage loss.
7. Subcutaneous nodules (Figure 11.5).

Criteria 1–4 should be present for at least 6 weeks to make a diagnosis of rheumatoid arthritis.

The American Rheumatism Association no longer believe that the term 'classic', 'definitive' or 'probable' should be used.

PROGNOSIS

It is difficult to give a prognosis in individual cases. Follow-up studies on large numbers of patients treated by simple methods show that after 10 years 50% will have improved and 50% deteriorated. This

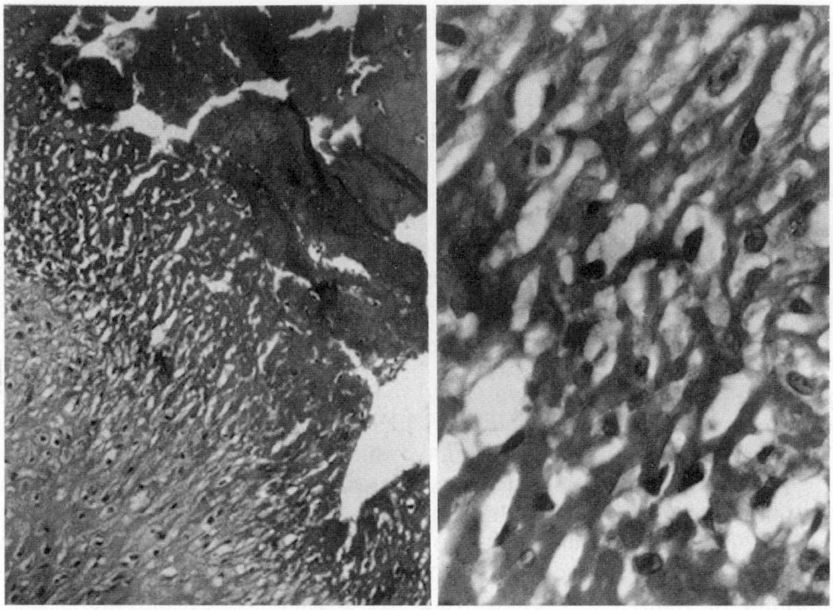

(a) (b)

Figure 11.5 (a) Photomicrograph from a rheumatoid nodule, showing the palisading but relatively acellular connective tissue surrounding the central area of necrosis and granulomatous tissue. (× 36). (b) Photomicrograph of the same section, showing the character of the connective tissue cells making up the wall of subcutaneous nodule, with large cyst-like spaces. (× 310).

important fact, which underlines the known tendency of remissions and relapses in the disease, must be remembered when any form of therapy is being evaluated. Grading of these patients according to their disabilities shows that 21% have no disability; 41% have moderate disability; 27% have more severe disability but remain independent in the home and usefully employed; and 11% are dependent upon others. In these patients the disease was inactive in 24%. The concepts that large numbers of patients become crippled and that the disease becomes burnt out are erroneous. Factors which suggest a poor prognosis include insidious onset, unremitting disease, the presence of nodules and other vasculitic phenomena, severe systemic involvement with a high ESR and anaemia, and the presence in the serum of rheumatoid factor in high titre and HLA DR4. Although few patients die from rheumatoid arthritis *per se*, the disease reduces life expectancy by 5–8 years. Death from bacterial infection and renal disease is commoner than in the general population.

COMPLICATIONS

Amyloidosis is found at post-mortem examination in about 20% of cases. However, few patients show signs of amyloidosis, and proteinuria leading to nephrosis is the usual presentation.

Septic arthritis superimposed upon rheumatoid arthritis is a recognized complication and will occur in 3% of patients. Although the septic process – which is usually due to *Staphylococcus aureus* – may be silent, the apparent flare-up of rheumatoid arthritis in only one joint should be considered as septic arthritis until proved otherwise.

A radiographic diagnosis of rheumatoid disease of the hip was described by Duthie and Harris (1969) as being based upon one or both of two major changes:

1. Subchondral sclerosis over an osteoporotic femoral head which was deformed with joint space narrowing. This loss of cartilage with narrowing of joint space and an increase in the subchondral bony layer may result from a venous or arterial vasculitis and/or from altered attrition and replacement of articular cartilage because of some unspecified enzymatic changes. There may well be an increased shearing effect on the articular cartilage because of altered biomechanics from pathological changes in the muscle, capsule and ligamentous structures as well as from the weight-bearing forces. The increase in bone density may have been produced by the collapse and compaction of surface bony trabeculae if not new bone formation.
2. A radiographic progression of sclerosis, of joint space narrowing, of protrusio or of osseous resorption with actual loss of bone substance, but the last need not necessarily be that of an avascular necrosis (Figure 11.6). The bony changes in avascular necrosis are: first, an apparent increase in bone density because of surrounding osteoporosis; second, a true loss of

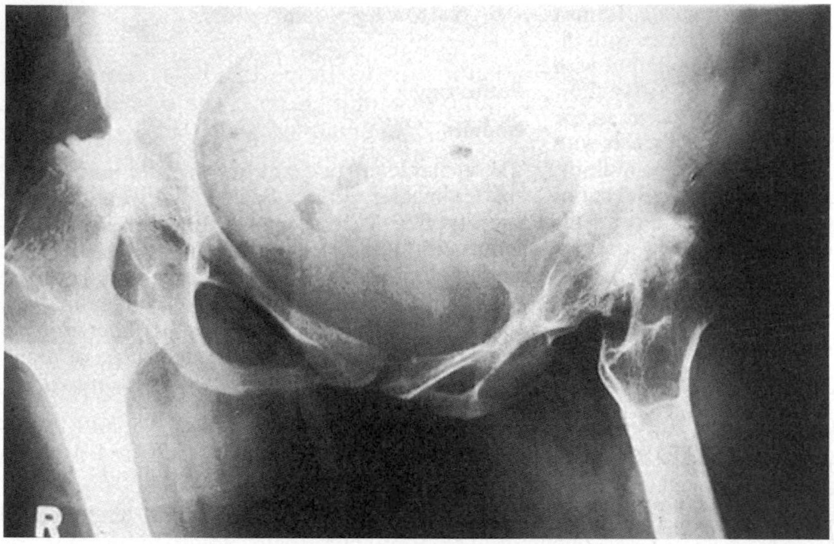

Figure 11.6 Radiographic appearances of severe rheumatoid disease of both hips.

bone density as seen in bone destruction or subchondral cyst formation; and finally, a true increase in bone density due to fracture and/or collapse leading to compaction of bone, or from new bone formation around trabeculae giving rise to subchondral sclerosis. Several of these pathological changes have been described in rheumatoid hip disease, but the incidence of frank avascular necrosis as specifically resulting from rheumatoid changes rather than from degenerative is difficult to record when based solely upon radiographic interpretation (Table 11.2).

Table 11.2 Radiographic appearances

Changes	Patients with	
	Rheumatoid hip disease	'Non-rheumatoid' hips
Bone density:		
Diffuse osteoporosis	27	18
Subchondral sclerosis	25	6
Resorption with collapse	13	0
Joint space		
Narrowing	33	14
Changes in bony outline:		
Acetabulum	30	30
Femur	28	19
Osteophyte formation	16	30
Acetabular deformity:		
Protrusio	14	0
Protrusio with femoral head changes	11	0
Static deformity of hips:		
Adduction	28	19
Abduction	0	0

LABORATORY FINDINGS

The haemoglobin concentration is reduced and values of 11 g/dl are common. The anaemia is usually of a normocytic, hypochromic type. The white cell count is normal or reduced and the proportion of lymphocytes is increased. A neutrophil response with a rise in the white cell count to 10–15 × 10^9/l (10 000–15 000/mm^3) occurs with corticosteroid therapy as well as with bacterial infection. The ESR may be markedly elevated, and in those with long-standing disease may never return to normal values. The tests for rheumatoid factor are positive in 70% of cases. Positive tests are less common in those with disease onset late in life. It must be remembered that positive results occur with increasing frequency in the normal population with age, and that by the age of 70 years 10% may show positive results. Positive results also occur in the other connective tissue diseases and in diseases with marked changes in the γ-globulins such as multiple myeloma, macroglobulinaemia, chronic infections and liver disease. Unaffected relatives of patients have a higher than expected incidence of positive tests.

RADIOLOGICAL APPEARANCES

The sequence of early radiological signs of rheumatoid arthritis in general are:

1. Soft tissue changes around a joint due to an effusion.
2. Perarticular osteoporosis, especially symmetrical, with reduction in the width of the shaft cortices and loss of the normal trabecular pattern.
3. Periosteal reaction with new bone formation along the shaft adjacent to where the capsule is attached.
4. Subchondral cyst formation.
5. Subchondral erosions due to actual loss of bone substance by erosion along the marginal areas of the joint.
6. Narrowing of joint spaces.
7. The place and usefulness of CT scanning and MR imaging is still being evaluated although their value in cervical spinal complications is now well established.

PATHOLOGY

Nodules

These characteristic features consist of non-encapsulated masses, often lobulated and with a central necrotic area. Microscopically the nodule is a granuloma with a central area of fibrinoid necrosis, a surrounding area of epithelioid cells arranged in a palisade and an outer zone of chronic inflammatory cells. Other nodules can usually be differentiated from rheumatoid nodules although those of granuloma annulare may have a very similar appearance (see Figure 11.5).

Synovium

Inflammation of this tissue in joints, tendons and bursae is the essential change. The tissue becomes thickened and oedematous, and granulation tissue (pannus) spreads onto the articular cartilage (Figures 11.7 and 11.8). This synovial pannus produces erosions of the cartilage surface and, by breaching the cartilage–synovium junction, erodes into the subchondral bone. These erosions may become large and cystic with synovial cells which release proteolytic enzymes, disrupting the glycosaminoglycans of the matrix. Such changes, together with the loss of cartilage, lead to joint destruction. The size of these erosions is partly dependent on joint use and this is consistent with a pumping of synovial fluid through the breached cortex. Reparative changes are rarely found and the disease progresses to fibrous and occasionally bony ankylosis. Microscopically the synovium is vascular and infiltrated with lymphocytes and plasma cells which are clumped together in follicles. It must be emphasized that at present pathological techniques alone do not allow a firm diagnosis of rheumatoid arthritis when biopsy material is examined. Very similar changes are present in many types of inflammatory joint disease.

TREATMENT

General principles of management

Team work is essential throughout the course of treatment of this disease, the team being composed

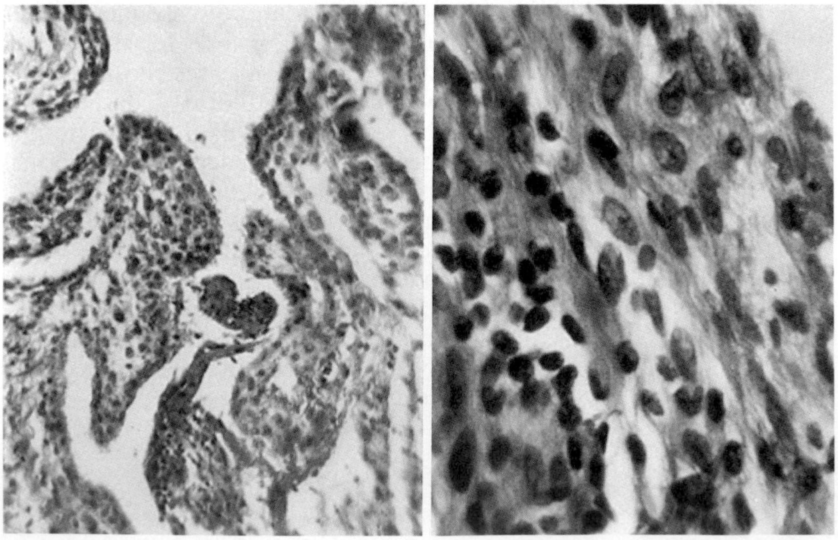

(a) (b)

Figure 11.7 Photomicrographs (a) × 150 and (b) × 357 of tissue from rheumatoid synovitis, showing the cellular infiltration and marked hypertrophy of the synovial villi.

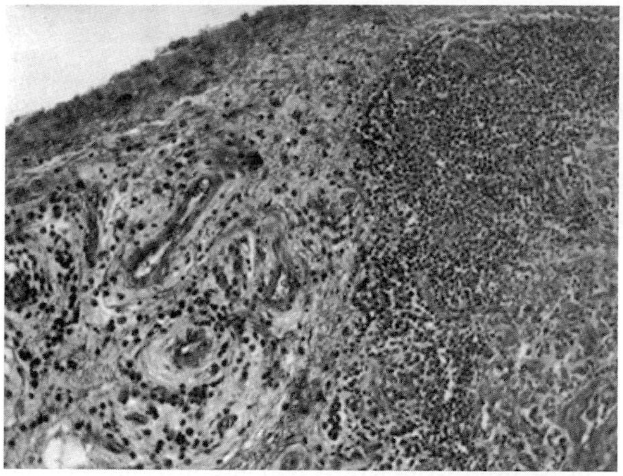

Figure 11.8 Photomicrograph of rheumatoid granulation tissue, showing a pannus with synovial cells on the left. In the central area there is vascular granulation tissue with small round cell infiltration. (× 43).

of physician, orthopaedic surgeon, social worker, occupational and physiotherapists. Effective treatment should combine the best remedial measures of all groups. The better results achieved in patients admitted to hospital early in the course of their disease probably reflect how important it is that the nature of the disease and the aims of treatment be fully understood by the patient, his family and his medical advisers from the onset. Once the diagnosis is reasonably certain, the same basic principles of management can be applied with varying emphasis to all cases. Treatment has five main aims:

1. Relief of inflammation and pain.
2. Correction and control of systemic manifestations.
3. Prevention of deformity (Figure 11.9).
4. Correction of existing deformity.
5. Improvement of functional capacity.

It is a great advantage in planning rational treatment to stage the local disease changes seen radiologically according to severity (Barron, 1969) Table 11.3).

Table 11.3

Stage	Extent of disease	Radiological appearance
1	Synovium	Soft tissue shadowing Marginal erosions
2	Synovium and articular cartilage	Joint space narrowing
3	Synovium, articular cartilage and subchondral bone – skeletal collapse	Bony destruction and joint deformities

Rest

There is much evidence that the continued use of joints during a phase of active disease increases pain, muscle spasm and wasting, exaggerates the constitutional symptoms, and tends to cause flexion deformities in the weight-bearing joints. It is generally accepted that a period of rest in bed relieves these symptoms and improves the general well-being of the patient. There are dangers, however, in uncontrolled bed rest in the form of general physical deterioration, muscle weakness and joint contractures. Accordingly, splints for arms and legs are provided. The use of a firm mattress and a back rest to ensure adequate support, proper posture and comfort are necessary. A fixed bed cage with padded foot rest to keep the weight of the bedclothes off inflamed joints, to prevent foot-drop during periods when leg splints are not worn, and to prevent the patient from slipping down the bed, is also necessary.

Splints – orthotic devices

These have three main functions: (1) rest and relief of pain; (2) prevention and correction of deformity; and (3) fixation of damaged joint in a good functional position.

Rest splints

Splints which hold the limb in a good functional position without muscle spasm are bandaged on at night and for periods of rest during the day for as long as active disease persists. Contrary to what might be expected, morning stiffness is decreased by the use of night splints as inflammation is controlled. The fear of permanent joint stiffness leading to ankylosis has led many physicians to combine splinting with active exercises, and in many centres a daily programme of exercises continues even during the most active phases of the disease. However, it has been shown that there is no substance in these fears and that, as long as cartilage remains, joints do not become ankylosed. Continuous immobilization, perhaps for 3 weeks, has a place in the early stage of the disease. It is probably best avoided in those with severe joint damage and in elderly patients who more readily develop complications such as venous thrombosis, fluid retention, hypostatic pneumonia, constipation and osteoporosis.

Corrective splints

Correction of deformity before contractures have occurred can be achieved at any joint, but especially the knee, with the use of serial splints. New splints

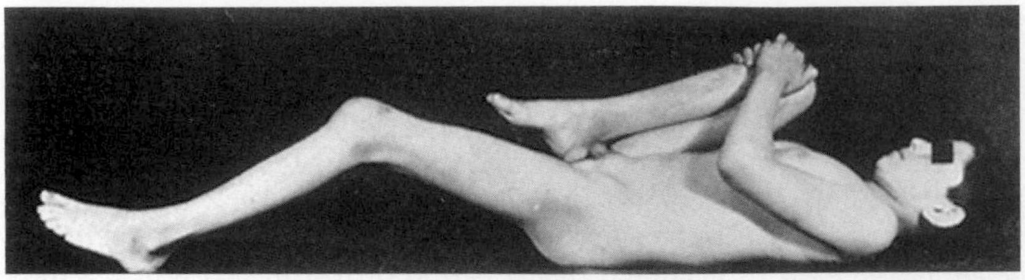

Figure 11.9 Thomas' test showing a hip flexion contracture resulting from a synovitis of the hip.

can be made at weekly intervals. Flexion deformities of the knees are common in the early phases of the disease and must be corrected to prevent serious disability in the later stages. Correction of the deformity is followed by graduated quadriceps exercises to ensure that adequate muscle power is provided to support the joints.

Fixation splints

Static support for persistently painful, unstable or permanently deformed joints is provided by removable splints. The splint is used to hold the joint in a position of function and to improve the performance of everyday activities (Figure 11.10). A variety of suitable materials exist such as polythene, leather and fibreglass, all of which combine lightness, strength and durability with ease of construction and use. 'Velcro' or similar simple fastenings should be used, and care taken to ensure that they are placed so that the patient can use them. Splints of this type allow the activity in a single joint or limb to settle without the need for complete rest. In addition, they can be used to reassure patients that any planned surgical fixation of a joint will not produce the disability that they fear. They are particularly useful long-term aids to function in patients who, for various reasons, may not be considered suitable for surgical fixation.

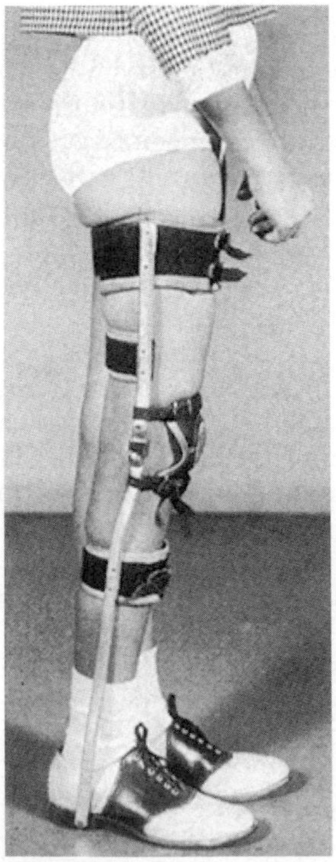

Figure 11.10 Bracing of the lower extremity of a case of juvenile rheumatoid arthritis.

Physical therapy

There is little benefit in instituting physical therapy until joint inflammation has settled as it is difficult and painful to increase muscle bulk or strength around an inflamed joint. However, once the joints are quiescent, the carefully planned programme of graduated exercises is essential because considerable muscle wasting occurs in association with the joint disease. Passive movements tend to produce protective muscle spasm and are discouraged. Active isotonic exercises against increasing resistance are the most satisfactory; where pain is still present on joint movement, however, the exercises are performed isometrically. Care is taken not to allow the patient or physiotherapist to increase the workload too quickly, or fatigue, increased pain and muscle spasm will result. Weight-bearing is permitted only when adequate muscle support has been developed. Various forms of walking aid or splint may be necessary to allow older or more severely affected patients to achieve maximal functional capacity. Patients may need to be shown how to walk with a normal gait, climb stairs, rise from a chair, bath and dress. During periods of bed rest, active exercises can be used on non-involved joints, especially the trunk. A period of 45 minutes prone and supine lying each day encourages good spinal posture and corrects and prevents flexion deformity at the hip joint. Various forms of local heating and cooling may be used to reduce muscle spasm before a period of active exercises, and wax bath therapy for the hands is particularly useful.

Domestic and occupational factors

A consideration of the domestic and occupational problems caused by rheumatoid arthritis involves chiefly an assessment of the part played by the occupational therapist and the social worker. However, the achievement of a satisfactory adaptation to the disease depends not only upon the occupational therapist and social worker but also upon the combined efforts of the whole medical team. In addition, all these efforts are wasted unless the full co-operation and understanding of the patient and his family is obtained. Rheumatoid arthritis imposes more severe problems than many chronic illnesses, as the average age of onset is 40 years and patients are thus likely to have serious economic and family responsibilities.

Drug therapy

Analgesic–anti-inflammatory agents

Drugs in this group constitute the main initial and continuing form of drug therapy. Analgesic agents with no anti-inflammatory effect are of little value until the active disease has been superseded by degenerative arthritis. Such agents are paracetamol, the codeine group and pentazocine. Phenacetin, which is a weaker analgesic, should be avoided because of its relationship to renal papillary necrosis.

Salicylates

These remain the drugs of first choice. None of the newer agents is either more effective or less toxic. A dose of 3–4 g of aspirin per day is required and a blood salicylate level of 20–25 mg/dl should be achieved. Dyspepsia is a troublesome side effect which may be avoided by the use of soluble or enteric-coated preparations or aloxiprin. The tendency for these drugs to cause a small, regular blood loss into the gut is probably not important but the occasional large, idiosyncratic gastrointestinal blood loss requires the avoidance of these drugs in future management.

Indomethacin

This is a useful drug for those tolerant of other preparations. The dosage should be increased gradually from 50 to 150 mg/day. This reduces the side-effects of headache, confusion, gastrointestinal disturbances and loss of libido. Suppositories containing 100 mg of the drug are useful in treating morning stiffness. Dyspepsia is not usually avoided by using suppositories because of a systemic effect of the drug on the gastric mucosa.

Other drugs

Fenamic acid derivatives (mefenamic acid 2000 mg/day or flufenamic acid 600 mg/day) and other drugs (e.g. naproxen 400–500 mg/day or ibuprofen 60–120 mg/day) may also be effective. The frequent need to change drugs in the absence of side-effects suggests not that the drugs are ineffective but either insufficient dosage is being utilized or that other problems, often psychological, posed by the disease have not been fully treated.

Gold and chloroquine compounds

These drugs are considered to suppress the disease and improve the outcome. The choice of these drugs as an addition to the basic programme of analgesic therapy depends to a large extent on personal preference and both compounds carry the risks of serious side-effects.

Gold salts

The chief action of these drugs appears to be the inactivation of enzymes released from neutrophil lysosomal granules. A course of a compound containing 1000 mg of metallic gold given in 20 weekly intramuscular injections, each of 50 mg of gold, after suitable test doses, remains the standard regimen. Improvement in the disease is rarely seen until 500 mg of gold has been given. A beneficial response should be followed by the indefinite continuation of the gold injections at 3- or 4-week intervals. Such a beneficial response is considered to be related to tissue concentration of the gold, and newer methods of measurement should allow a more individual dosage regimen to be employed. The side-effects of the drug, which occur in 20–30% of cases, result from genuine allergic responses or overdosage. These include albuminuria occasionally leading to nephrosis, skin rashes, bone marrow suppression, stomatitis and gastrointestinal tract disturbances. Regular urine and blood examination is therefore necessary.

Chloroquine compounds

The exact mode of action of these drugs is unknown. As with gold, no response is seen for several weeks after starting treatment. Both chloroquine and hydroxychloroquine are used in doses of 200–400 mg/day. The disrepute suffered by these drugs results chiefly from overdosage. Corneal deposition of the drug with blurring of vision and the irreversible retinopathy are the chief side-effects. Protection from these side-effects can be achieved in almost every case if the drug is stopped for a month in each year and regular ophthalmological examinations are undertaken.

Corticosteroid preparations

Undoubted suppression of the symptoms of the disease can be achieved with these drugs but they have no real effect on the progress of the disease. Furthermore, dosage in excess of the equivalent of 10 mg of prednisolone per day will be accompanied by the usual side-effects of these drugs. Used in small dosage, no preparation holds any advantage over any other in terms of fluid retention, muscle wasting and other side-effects. The indications for the use of prednisolone in doses of less than 10 mg/day are:

1. In older patients in whom relief of symptoms offsets the risks.
2. In patients whose employment of domestic needs require that they be kept active for short periods of time.
3. To control severe morning stiffness by taking the drug at night.
4. In patients with severe unremitting disease.

Anabolic steroids

These do not prevent osteoporosis in these patients and indeed no drug therapy has been shown to affect this aspect of the disease or its exacerbation by corticosteroid therapy.

Immunosuppresive drugs

A variety of drugs such as azathioprine, 6-mercaptopurine, cyclophosphamide and penicillamine have been employed in small series of patients with severe disease. The rationale behind their use is based upon their effect on immunological reactions and the hope that they might affect the basic pathological mechanisms in rheumatoid arthritis. Although these drugs appear to impart varying degrees of benefit to patients, the exact mode of action of most of them in this disease is unknown and may not be immunosuppressive. Their use is associated with a variety of side-effects, including leucopenia, opportunist infections and renal tract damage; they should be used with caution, and only in patients in whom other modes of therapy have failed

Dick (1977) has proposed the following as a rational approach to drug prescribing as the disease increases in severity, emphasizing a minimum number of drugs and a low toxicity drug as first choice:

First-line drugs

Alclofenac	Azapropazone
Aspirin	Fenoprofen
Feprazone	Ketoprofen
Flufenamic acid	Mefenamic acid
Flurbiprofen	Naproxen
Ibuprofen	Sulindac
Indomethacin	Tolmetin

These drugs are prescribed singly on a 3-week trial, assessed by patient opinion on the lowest dose to relieve symptoms with minimum side-effects.

Second-line drugs

Chloroquine	Penicillamine
Gold	

These drugs may take 6–8 weeks to achieve a response but all are highly effective in responding patients. Toxic effects on skin, blood, kidneys and eyes require careful monitoring.

Third-line drugs

Corticosteroids	Cytotoxic drugs

These are to be considered only in patients with life-threatening disease when all general methods and other drugs have failed.

A scheme of drug therapy in relation to severity and time, suggested by Dick, is shown in Figure 11.11.

This drug programme has been updated in recent years (*Drugs and Therapeutic Bulletin*, 1993). The slow acting anti-rheumatic drugs (SAARD) – gold, penicillamine, chloroquine derivatives etc. – are now being administered early in some patients in order to limit joint damage, bone demineralization and other catabolic effects. It is hoped to improve the long-term outcome by limiting progressive joint disease or dangerous extra-articular manifestations.

Local corticosteroid therapy

Local injections of a corticosteroid preparation into joints or surrounding soft tissues can be helpful in controlling inflammation. Such injections are not without risk and, in particular, the dangers of superinfection, a crystal reaction and serious bone necrosis have been well documented. However, these risks are minimized if an aseptic injection technique is used and clear indications for the use of these preparations are recognized. Injections given to a site should not be repeated too frequently: perhaps weekly in an acute process and 3-monthly in a continuing process. If two injections to the same site are ineffective, it is pointless to continue. Indications for the use of local corticosteroid injections in rheumatoid arthritis include:

1. Intra-articular injections for the patient with one or two active joints.
2. Tendinitis and tendon nodules; although the benefit in the latter is likely to be transitory and

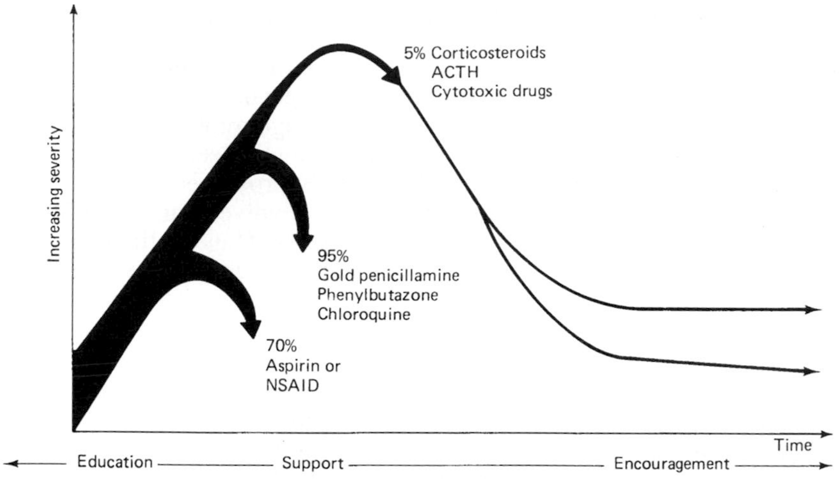

Figure 11.11 Use of drugs in rheumatoid arthritis. (NSAID, non-steroidal anti-inflammatory drugs). (Reproduced, with permission, from Carson Dick, W. (1977) in *Copeman's Textbook of the Rheumatic Diseases*, edited by J.T. Scott, Churchill Livingstone: Edinburgh and London)

surgical clearance may be required (e.g. trigger finger).

3. Capsular or ligamentous involvement (e.g. shoulder).
4. As a temporary measure in the treatment of carpal tunnel and other compression syndromes.

Contraindications to the use of local corticosteroids include:

1. Uncertain diagnosis.
2. Proven or possible infection.
3. Severe joint damage.
4. Severe local osteoporosis.
5. A neurological deficit – because of the risk of producing a Charcot-type arthropathy (Steinberg *et al.*, 1962).

Other drugs of value

These include:

1. Antidepressants.
2. Muscle relaxants.
3. Iron given parenterally.
4. Vitamin supplements.

These drugs may be added in patients who demonstrate a clear indication for such therapy. The addition of unnecessary medication must be avoided in these patients who frequently need to take many tablets each day.

OPERATIVE TREATMENT

Surgical procedures are being increasingly used at all stages of the disease but it is essential that such treatment form a part of the continuing management of the patient by the whole medical team. Active disease is not a contraindication to surgery and there is no evidence that surgery causes a flare-up in general disease. Likewise, corticosteroid therapy is not a contraindication to surgery, although an increase in dosage for 48 hours over the period of the operation may be required. Special problems posed by surgery in this group of patients include: poor skin and vasculitis; osteoporosis; anaemia; problems of incubation for anaesthesia because of reduced neck movement, atlantoaxial subluxation and cricoarytenoid arthritis; and an increased susceptibility to infection. Postoperative mobilization should begin early because of the risk of losing movement in the operated and other joints by prolonged immobilization. Finally, the involvement of multiple joints may impose difficulties in the selection of suitable crutches and other walking aids. This involvement of many joints means that patients with rheumatoid arthritis make fewer demands on their joints than do patients with other forms of chronic arthritis, and the life of various procedures and prostheses may be longer than expected. The indications for surgery are the same as those listed under general principles of management and fall into two groups: prophylactic, which means synovectomy, and radical tendon and reconstructive joint procedures.

Selection of operative procedures

It must be emphasized that procedures should be selected according to a clear understanding of the results to be expected and an overall plan for the patient. Long-term results of most procedures are now available and can act as a guide. Patterns of joint involvement are also important; e.g. in the upper limb there is a significant trend towards affection of proximal joints early in the disease and a high incidence of wrist involvement (Stein *et al.*, 1975). In the lower limb greater benefit accrues from joint replacement at the hip than the knee. With this knowledge it is possible to plan surgery to achieve the maximum benefit for the patient.

The multiple operations are very demanding of the patient's mental and physical stamina, and it is a great boost to morale to perform a procedure (e.g. excision of the lower end of the ulna and dorsal synovectomy of the wrist) as a first step to demonstrate to the patient the potential benefits of surgical treatment.

Synovectomy

Removal of the synovial membrane is employed in those joints in which this tissue is readily accessible, and includes the knee, elbow and the small joints of the fingers. In addition, synovectomy of tendon sheaths, particularly the flexors and extensors of the fingers, should be undertaken as a prophylactic measure.

Tendon synovectomy relieves pain and improves tendon function, and in some cases may be required urgently to protect the extensor tendons of the fingers from stretching or rupture.

Joint synovectomy is carried out in patients with no or minimal radiological evidence of erosions in grade 1 disease in the presence of persistent pain and swelling of about 6 months' duration. It is rarely possible to remove all synovial tissue from a joint. In the knee it is unusual to attempt to remove more than two-thirds of the tissue, which is all that can be achieved by the usual anterior, parapatellar incision and the operation is better performed arthroscopically with a powered shaver. The mechanism by which pain and swelling are relieved in over 90% of cases is not clear since regeneration of the synovial tissue occurs within a few months. In many cases the new synovial tissue looks little different from the original tissue but the presence of a thick connective tissue base may be important in the relief of symptoms. Whether the operation is also prophylactic is still debatable.

The controlled trial of synovectomy of metacarpophalangeal joints and knee joints reported by the Arthritis and Rheumatism Council and British Orthopaedic Association (1976) showed that synovectomy relieved pain in grade 1 disease and slowed down progression in the knee. In the metacarpophalangeal joints of the hand the effects were not so obvious but all the patients who had undergone synovectomy were pleased with the result. Certainly this trial showed some beneficial effects of synovectomy and there is further evidence of improved joint function and radiological appearances – presumably due to reduction of pain and osteoporosis – in grade 2 disease at the elbow (Stein *et al.*, 1975).

Radical surgery

Operations in this group are undertaken to relieve pain, restore function, correct deformity and provide stability. Any surgical programme must include a full assessment of the patient's needs and a detailed assessment of the likely improvement in function in the light of other joint involvement. A series of operations may be necessary. Thus the full benefit of knee surgery may not be achieved without the addition of an operation on the hip. The patient may not be the best judge of his surgical requirements. These considerations and the increasing availability of satisfactory arthroplasties have reduced the number of joints that are arthrodesed. However, arthrodesis remains a useful procedure in selected cases. Individual joints will now be discussed in general and in greater detail under the various anatomical areas in subsequent chapters.

Hand and wrist (see Chapter 15)

In the fingers, periarticular, tendon and muscle involvement as well as joint disease contribute to the symptoms and the characteristic deformities of ulnar deviation, swan neck and boutonnière deformities. In addition to synovectomy of the metacarpophalangeal and proximal interphalangeal joints, soft tissue release, repair of the extensor apparatus and realignment of the tendons may be required. Although such procedures produce cosmetically satisfactory results there is usually some loss of joint movement and finger function is not always improved. Some surgeons prefer to wait until more extensive changes have taken place, often with subluxation of the metacarpophalangeal joints, before operating since an improvement in function is then achieved. Silastic prostheses of several types offer equally satisfactory results (Figure 11.12). Flexion of the fingers is usually limited by tendon involvement but adequate grip and pinch movements result.

From a large series of 144 silicone rubber Swanson arthroplasties of the MCP joints in 27 patients (36 hands), after an average duration of follow-up of 8.5 years, Kirschenbaum *et al.* (1993) have concluded that there was excellent correction of ulnar drift, increased motion of the MCP joints with a more functional arc of motion and an enhanced hand function can be expected. They found that there was a major deterioration in the function of the proximal interphalangeal joints. The overall results – long-term – makes this procedure acceptable when properly indicated, with good technique and postoperative regimen, particularly for relief of pain. Arthrodesis of the metacarpophalangeal joint of the thumb may substantially improve pinch movements, but complex deformities are often present.

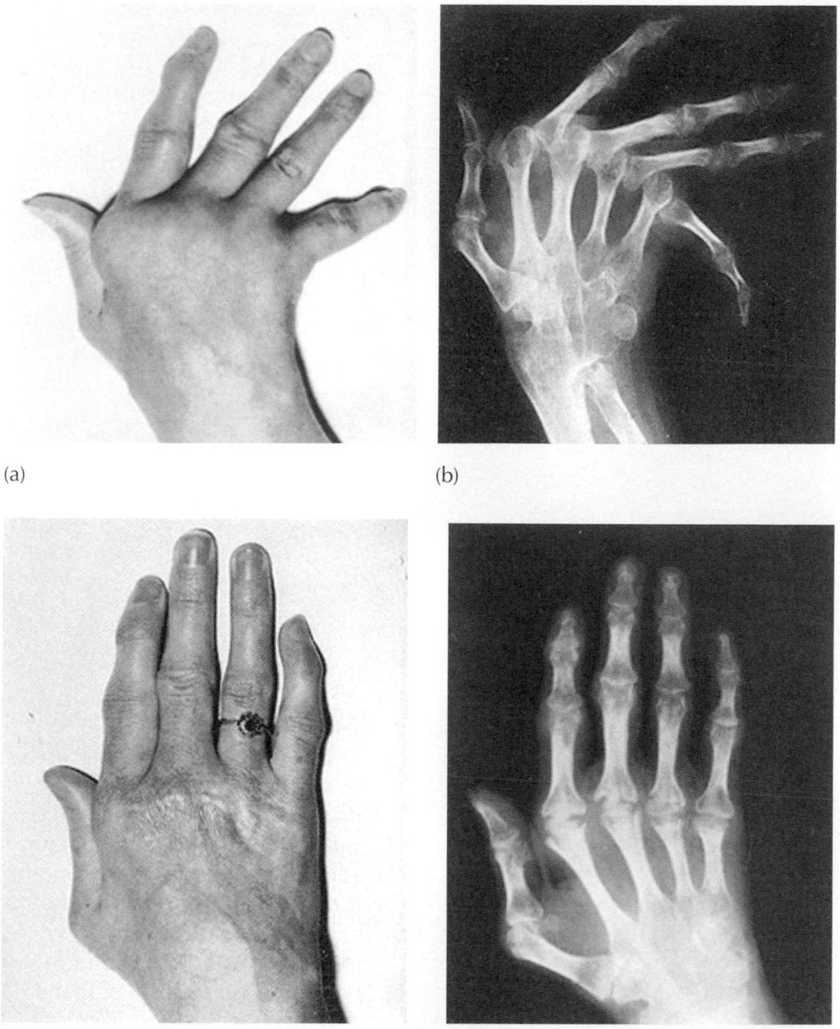

(a) (b) (c) (d)

Figure 11.12 (a) and (b) Photograph and radiograph showing the ulnar deviation deformity of the MCP joints with an ankylosed wrist joint. (c) and (d) Postoperative photograph and radiograph showing the appearance of the same hand after Silastic prosthetic replacements of the MCP joints.

Synovial proliferation and capsule stretching results in anterior subluxation of the wrist with disruption of the inferior radioulnar joint, and consequent prominence, tenderness and springing of the lower end of the ulna. Excision of the distal 1.3 cm of the ulna with synovectomy of the distal radioulnar joint and extensor tendons relieves pain and increases strength without reducing wrist or forearm movement. In those with severe wrist damage, arthrodesis, either radiocarpal or carpal, is a useful procedure. The loss of movement is more than offset by the gain in hand function.

Carpal tunnel decompression may be required in those with evidence of median nerve compression, which must be looked for carefully.

Elbow (see Chapter 14)

Synovectomy may be useful in grade 1 and grade 2 disease. Excision of the radial head increases the range of pain-free motion, especially pronation and supination, and although joint stability may be reduced, this is rarely important in patients with rheumatoid arthritis due to their reduced requirements (Figure 11.13). Various types of arthroplasty have been used in the elbow joint with excision of the ends of the humerus and/or ulna and radial bones. In some instances the insertion of a strip of fascia lata will achieve a reasonable range of pain-free movement but lacks collateral stability (Figure 11.14). Experience with metal or plastic hinge arthroplasties is still not totally satisfactory, but results are improving (Kudo and Awano, 1990; Souter, 1992). Arthrodesis may occasionally be required; the optimum position is 90° of elbow flexion with the forearm in the neutral position. Such a procedure demands good shoulder function and a mobile contralateral elbow.

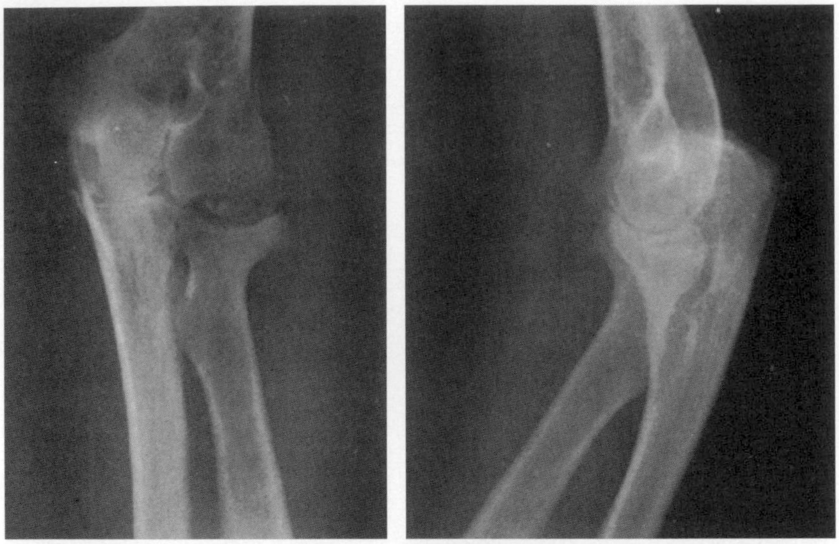

(a)

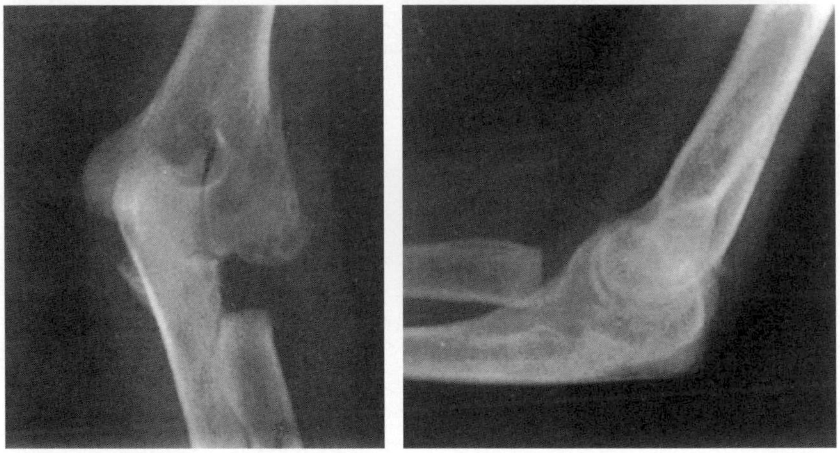

(b)

Figure 11.13 (a) Radiographs showing rheumatoid arthritis of the left elbow joint with loss of joint space, subchondral cyst formation and sclerosis particularly in the radiohumeral joint, and osteoporosis of bones (i.e. grade 2 disease). (b) Radiographs taken after excision of the head of the radius to give marked improvement in the movements of flexion and of rotation.

Shoulder (see Chapter 14)

MR imaging is used to assess the integrity of the soft tissues, particularly the rotator cuff. Excision of the acromion and the underlying bursa relieves pain and improves movement. However, joint stability may be impaired and abduction is often severely restricted. Arthrodesis of the shoulder is technically difficult to achieve but may improve upper limb function if care is taken in selecting the optimum position for fusion. The replacement for the humeral head (Neer's prosthesis) is rarely used alone and probably relieves pain rather than increasing movement. Glenoidectomy produced good function in 8 or 9 patients followed for 6 years (Wainwright, 1974) and should therefore be considered for the persistently painful shoulder. Total joint replacement by prosthetic components is, as in the elbow, indicated for severe disease and the results have improved greatly in the last decade (Jonsson *et al.*, 1990; Kudo and Awano, 1990).

Comparison between a Neer hemiarthroplasty and a total joint replacement for rheumatoid patients has been made by Boyd *et al.* (1990). They found that the total joint replacement gave a much better result with less pain and fewer radiographic changes around the cup. They recommend this operation particularly where there has been little bone response around the glenoid to the rheumatoid process.

Foot and toes

Synovitis of the metatarsophalangeal joints and the associated structures results progressively in broadening and rigidity of the forefoot, loss of the transverse arch, hallux valgus and lateral deviation of the other toes, clawing of the toes, subluxation of the joint and the development of callosities over prominent areas,

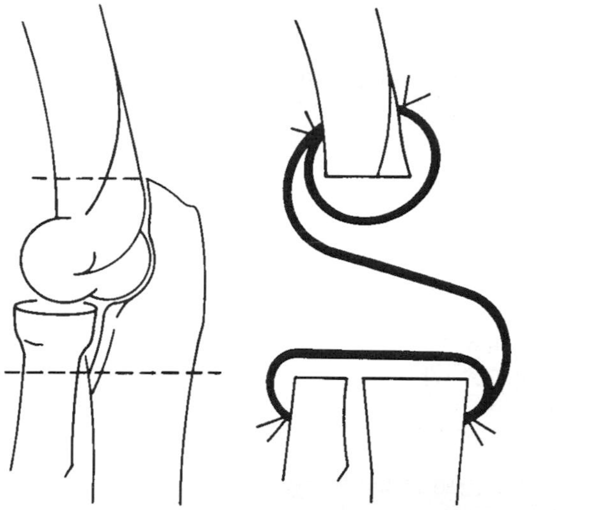

Figure 11.14 The method of covering the excised ends of the humerus, ulna and radius with fascia lata to form an arthroplasty.

particularly the metatarsal heads in the soles. Synovitis of the other toe joints, unlike the hands, is minimal. In the early stages the provision of suitable shoes, to accommodate the foot and prevent the development of pressure areas, and of suitable domed insoles to redistribute the weight are all that are required. Synovectomy of the metatarsophalangeal joints is rarely performed. Excision arthroplasty with removal of the metatarsal heads and/or the bases of the proximal phalanges produces satisfactory results in 90% of cases (Figure 11.15). Poor results are due to insufficient or irregular excision of bone. Grossly deformed toes may be amputated without loss of function of the foot.

Mid-tarsal, subtalar and ankle joints

Involvement of these joints is best treated by the provision of suitable shoes or boots with valgus insoles. Various forms of anklet, plastic heel caps and even a leg iron and T-strap may adequately support these joints. Arthrodesis is the most satisfactory operation. The ankle should be fused in 5° of plantar flexion in men and 10° in women. The foot and heel should be fixed in the neutral position. Ankle replacement is now being practised in patients with severe pain and limited mobility goals.

Knee (see Chapter 16)

Synovectomy is an excellent and well-tried operation for early disease in the knee. Schuller, in 1887, described the first complete synovectomy in four cases of rheumatoid arthritis, but it was Swett (1923) who popularized the operation for rheumatoid arthritis and who put forward a rational explanation as to why synovectomy should be effective. He recorded good recovery of painless function, and suggested that removal of the organized inflammatory exudate would prevent further joint damage. It was also felt at that time that there were added advantages of synovectomy in that the operation would remove 'metastatic foci of infection' and correct the 'metabolic abnormality of suboxidation'.

Synovectomy is performed in order to relieve the patient's symptoms from the painful synovitis and

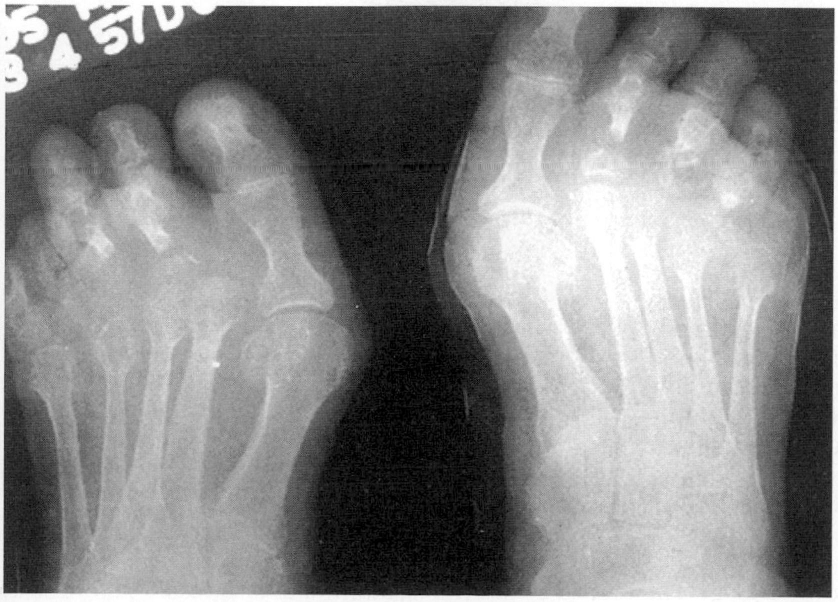

Figure 11.15 Radiograph of rheumatoid arthritis involving the feet in a middle-aged person who had spontaneous resorption of the proximal phalanges of the middle three toes on both feet.

also to prevent further damage to the joint cartilage and adjacent bone by removing the lymphoid tissue with its antigenic IgG protein and rheumatoid factor. These can destroy cartilage by releasing lysozymal enzymes. This is still regarded as being controversial. Even so, favourable results of synovectomy have been described. Garièpy *et al.* (1966), in reviewing 56 unselected synovectomies, showed that 79% of patients experienced good symptomatic relief of pain, with a 6% recurrence rate. It seems that synovectomy is a useful operation for the relief of pain and swelling in the knee joint in patients with symptoms arising from a proliferative synovitis (Arthritis and Rheumatism Council and British Orthopaedic Association, 1976).

It has been described that regenerated synovium was more fibrous with less subsynovial areolar tissue. Mitchell and Cruess (1967) showed experimentally, by using labelled tritiated thymidine, that new synovium forms by metaplasia of existing mesenchymal elements. Patients have come to further surgery following synovectomy in rheumatoid arthritis, and Bränemark and Goldie (1969) found that although these patients did not have clinical synovitis the new synovium was not usually normal, having a microscopic appearance similar to that removed at the initial synovectomy.

Selection of patients for synovectomy

1. Those with persistent, painful synovitis with proliferative synovium not responding to medical management over a period of 3 months.
2. There should be a useful range of movement – i.e. at least (45° of flexion) without any persistent flexion contracture.
3. The radiological changes should not show severe destruction of the joint space or subchondral bone (grade 1 disease).
4. The knee should have reasonable ligamentous stability.

Generalized disease activity is not a contraindication.

The open operation

The open operation is usually carried out through a single lateral parapatellar incision, which usually gives adequate exposure with careful dissection of the synovium from the suprapatellar pouch, carefully preserving the suprapatellar fat pad. This is an important structure for maintaining quadriceps muscle function and preventing fibrosis.

Synovium is removed from the intercondylar notch, the edges of the condyles and the medial and lateral gutters alongside the femoral condyles. The average weight of tissue removed is 200 g. The menisci should not be removed unless very degenerate.

The posterior compartment is not explored through a separate incision unless there is marked tenderness and swelling or a semimembranous cyst in the popliteal fossa (Figure 11.16).

The patella is inspected, but rarely requires removal. The knee is placed on continuous passive motion immediately after operation and progressively increased motion is achieved.

A routine manipulation is not performed, but if the flexion range is not progressing beyond 60° after 7 days' mobilization a gentle manipulation is indicated.

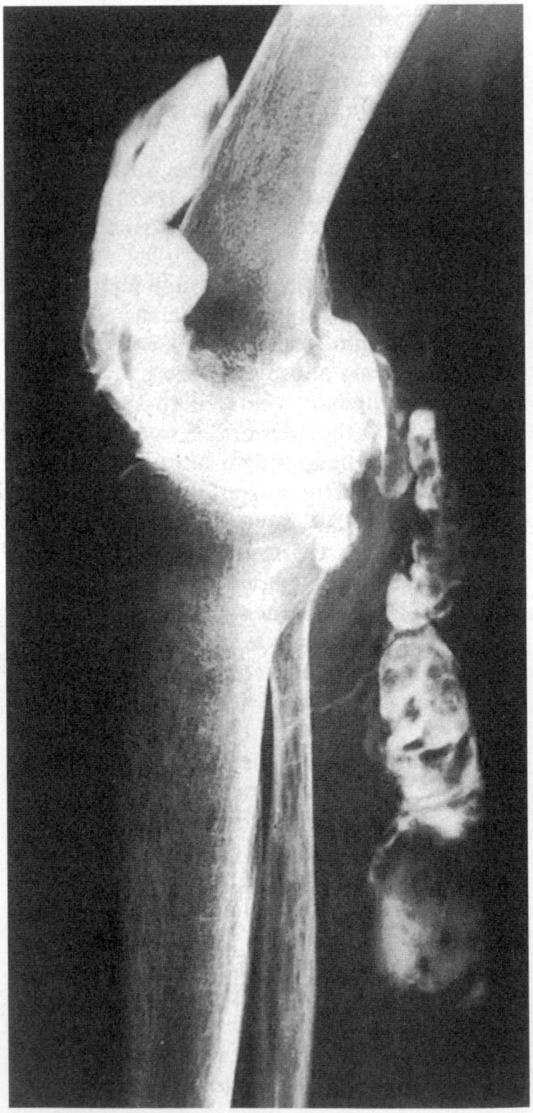

Figure 11.16 Lateral radiograph of knee joint showing radiopaque arthrogram with a semimembranous rheumatoid cyst extending downwards to the calf.

Posterior synovectomy may be required in those with persistent symptoms and particularly in those with an enlarged posterior cyst. Such cysts, which are usually extensions of the normal semimembranous gastrocnemius bursae, may become grossly enlarged, prevent full knee extension and cause venous obstruction (Figure 11.16). In addition, since they are connected to the knee joint by a one-way valvular mechanism, they are subjected to markedly increased fluid pressures. This may result in the enlargement of the cyst into the calf or the sudden rupture of the cyst with the release of irritant synovial fluid. Symptoms and signs of joint rupture, which have also been recorded at the wrist and elbow, mimic those of a deep venous thrombosis. Arthrography should be used to establish the diagnosis. Rupture of the cyst should be treated by cystectomy when the acute symptoms have settled, and the enlarged calf cyst, which is unlikely to rupture, by excision when symptoms demand.

Replacement arthroplasty

Many forms have been utilized for the problem of the stiff, painful, unstable and severely affected knee.

Several types of prosthetic replacements are available.

Metallic tibial plateau hemiarthroplasty

MacIntosh (1967) described the relief of pain and deformity in 70% of 103 knees with rheumatoid arthritis as the underlying pathology between 6 months and 6 years after the operation.

One of the authors (RBD) has employed the MacIntosh prosthetic replacement for over 20 years in grade 2 and grade 3 disease, and feels that this method has a definite role in the treatment of rheumatoid arthritis (Figure 11.17).

This view is supported by the literature (Schorn *et al.*, 1978) but the prosthesis is no longer available. Unicompartment bipolar replacement offers similar results (Marmor, 1988; Scott *et al.*, 1991) but revision to total joint replacement is less straightforward than following a MacIntosh prosthesis (see section on osteoarthritis of the knee, Chapter 16).

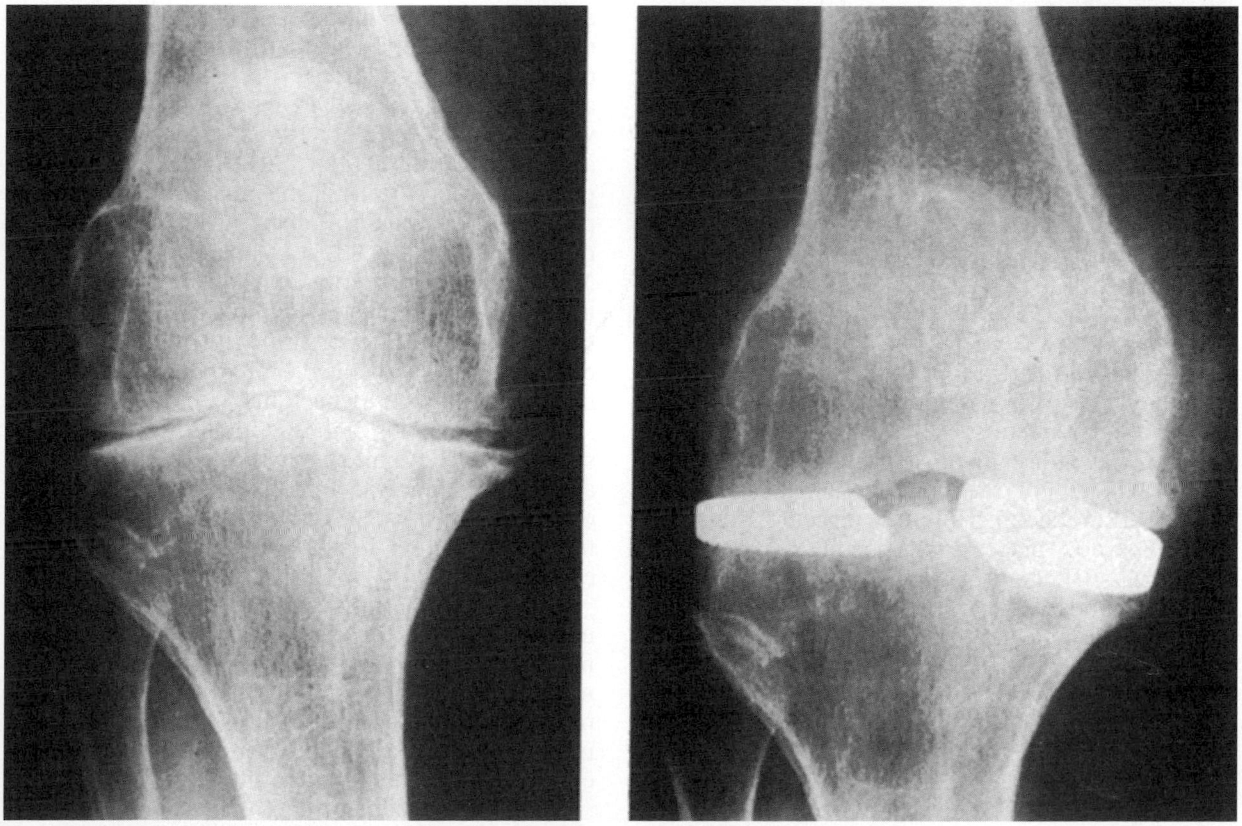

(a) (b)

Figure 11.17 (a) Anteroposterior radiograph showing preoperative rheumatoid arthritic changes. (b) Postoperative radiograph with two MacIntosh plateaux prostheses in position.

Total knee prosthetic replacement

There are numerous models of total prosthesis available but none has proved entirely satisfactory as yet, because of the difficulty of allowing flexion and extension with rotation while reducing the excessive stresses of the cement/bone interface, particularly on the tibial side, although the results of 10–15 year follow-up studies are impressive (Vince *et al.*, 1987; Ranawat *et al.*, 1993). The earliest models were constrained, allowing only flexion and extension in the sagittal plane. Although initially stable and aligned, loosening and fracture occurred rapidly. This led to the development of unconstrained prostheses with some correction of development but stability depending upon the ligamentous integrity of the joint. Semi-constrained types are now used with flexion and some degree of rotation and lateral medial deviation possible. Almost all employ a metal convex femoral surface and a high-density polyethylene concave tibial surface to give the lowest friction and maximum wear properties. Good results – i.e. freedom from pain, a stable knee and a range of movement of 0–90° or more – have been achieved in 90% of patients with rheumatoid arthritis in several series (Laskin, 1990). See Chapter 16.

Stanley *et al.* (1990) have answered the question of whether it is preferable to carry out simultaneous or staged bilateral knee replacements. In a randomized consecutive prospective study of 100 patients, there was no increased perioperative complication rate in those receiving a simultaneous bilateral knee replacement procedure. Certainly rehabilitation is greatly facilitated.

Arthrodesis

Arthrodesis of the knee will give stability for painless weight-bearing. Green *et al.* (1967) described the long-term results following arthrodesis and showed that although most patients adapted very well to a fixed knee, there were certain disabilities in sitting and in reaching into low places. Arthrodesis of the knee does place a load upon the ipsilateral hip, the ankle and the lumbar spine, but surprisingly little upon the opposite knee.

The operation is therefore especially indicated in the young patient with such a severely disorganized knee joint that any other surgical procedure would not give a functional range of movement. The pathological process should involve the one knee joint only, and the hips, ankles, opposite knee and lumbar spine should be normal. When both knees are involved, arthrodesis of one with arthroplasty of the other frequently can give good results.

In rheumatoid arthritis the pathology frequently affects both knees and perhaps the hips and lumbar spine also. These factors tend to influence the surgeon against the use of arthrodesis. There are also difficulties with immobilization which apply in rheumatoid arthritis. However, there is still a place for this operation for the severely disorganized joint.

Many operative procedures have been devised to arthrodese the knee but the authors favour a compression arthrodesis (Charnley, 1953) but using four pins with an external fixator.

Hip

New materials and revision arthroplasty

After 25 years of experience the problems of total hip replacement using high density polyethylene (HDP) against chrome-cobalt steel cemented with PMMA cement are clearer. Some prostheses have lasted for 20 years but wear of HDP does occur and produces particles which cause osteolysis of bone around the prosthesis. This is less with cemented components and in any event is most marked with femoral components. Osteolysis leads to loosening and is aggravated by weight-bearing on a loose prosthesis once it has occurred so that revision is sometimes difficult. The use of ceramic for femoral heads articulating against HDP appears to produce less wear but data beyond 10–12 years are still not available (Sedel *et al.*, 1993). Infection has not proved to be a serious problem and if the surgery is performed in 'clean-air' operating theatres the sepsis rate is less than 1% (Bentley and Simmonds, 1976; MRC, 1982). Late infection can occur and it is advisable to administer prophylactic antibiotics if the patient should have a serious infection elsewhere, especially in the operated limb to prevent colonization of the implant by bacteria.

Synovectomy is rarely employed. Arthrodesis should never be employed in this joint in rheumatoid arthritis. Displacement osteotomy has not proved of value and indeed is often accompanied by non-union. Some form of arthroplasty should be employed.

The excision arthroplasty of Girdlestone is now used rarely but is a useful operation if total replacement arthroplasty fails since the scar tissue formed is more extensive than with a primary procedure giving more stability. Hip movement is good but the joint unstable, particularly in heavier patients, and up to 6 cm of leg shortening may result.

The use of uncemented porous-coated prostheses has been disappointing for the hip since, even when osteointegration occurs there is a 20–50% reported incidence of thigh pain. At present cemented hip replacements remain the best treatment for osteoarthritis and rheumatoid arthritis particularly where the bone is soft.

The investigation of a patient with a painful prosthesis involves a careful history and physical examination. A history of a fall may rarely be given but usually there has been gradual onset of pain. 'Start-up' pain when the patient rises from a chair to walk, which imposes rotational stress on the prosthesis–cement bone interface, is very suggestive of loosening.

Radiographs may show radiolucent lines exceeding 3 mm around the cement but may not be very helpful. Aspiration/arthrography of the hip is rarely useful either to obtain an organism or show definite tracking of dye around the prosthesis.

ESR and CRP may be raised but these are not diagnostic.

Where the prosthesis can be shown to be definitely loose and infected we remove the prosthesis, take biopsies and perform debridement. A custom-designed prosthesis (CAD-CAM) is made for the femur with hydroxyapatite coating on the proximal shaft. The limb is placed on traction for 3 weeks whilst appropriate antibiotics are given. The CAD-CAM prosthesis is then inserted together with an uncemented porous-coated metal acetabular component and an HDP liner. Antibiotics and weight-bearing with crutches continue for 3 months postoperatively (Figure 11.18).

See also Chapter 16.

Rheumatoid arthritis of the cervical spine

This region is commonly involved; of recent years the clinical consequences have been better recognized but are of a special nature. As early as 1890, Garrod noted that 36% of his rheumatoid arthritis patients had involvement of the cervical spine. It is only recently, however, that further reviews and clinical surveys have indicated that, after the metacarpophalangeal joints, the most common region to be involved is the neck.

Pathology of this condition in the neck is unusual but there are rheumatoid granulomata involving all the diarthrodial joints, particularly in the upper four or five segments. Attenuation and laxity of the transverse ligament and of the anterior atlanto-occipital ligaments are marked. Cavitation and invasion by granulation tissue of the intervertebral discs are commonly seen, with adjacent destruction of subchondral bone, eburnation, etc. Blood vessels are involved but not the tissues of the nervous system.

Radiology gives better definition of multiple disc space narrowing with little osteophyte formation, and erosion of adjacent and osteoporotic vertebrae with multiple subluxations at all levels. Within neck supportive collars, both CT and MR scanning have given greater definition of the bony changes, the soft tissue enlargement and the indentation of the cervical cord. Einig *et al.* (1990) have described in detail the indications for the use of MR imaging in this

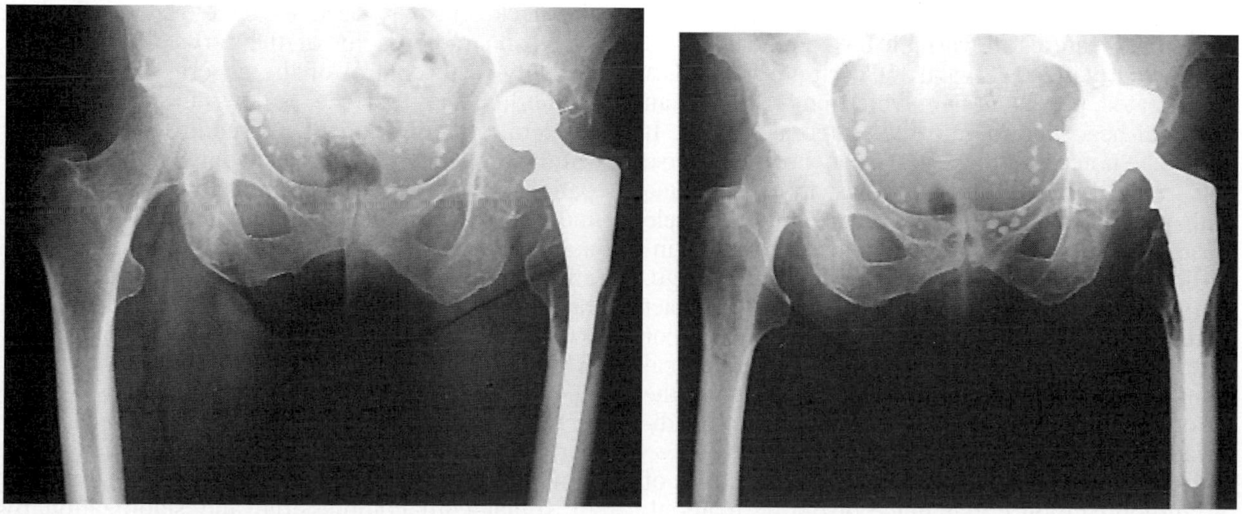

(a) (b)

Figure 11.18 (a) Anteroposterior radiograph of both hips showing a loose Ring total hip prosthesis with osteolysis around the acetabular and femoral components. (b) The same patient after revision of the left hip to a CAD-CAM hydroxyapatite-coated femoral component and porous-coated acetabular component.

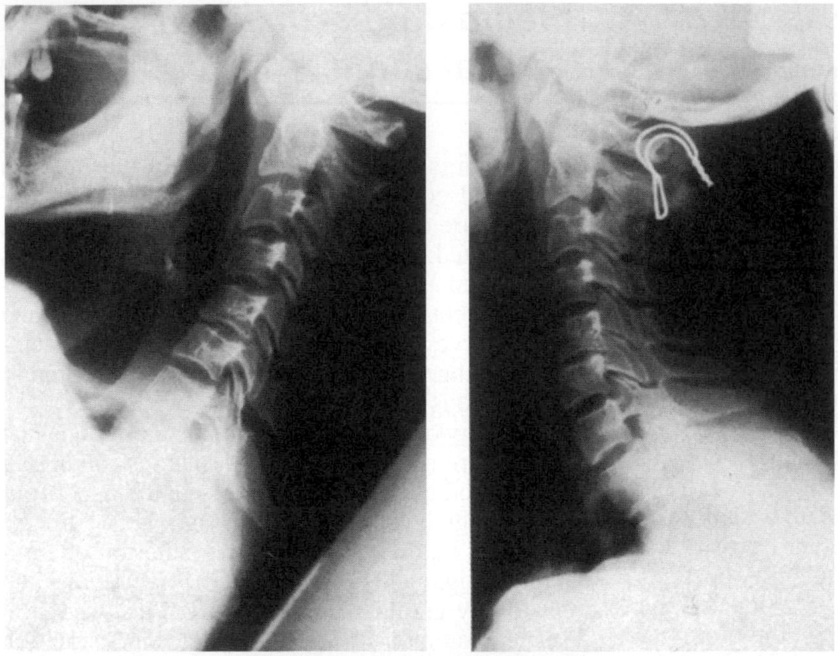

(a) (b)

Figure 11.19 (a) Preoperative flexion radiograph of the cervical spine in rheumatoid arthritis, showing atlantoaxial subluxation. (b) Radiograph 16 months after fusion, showing the stability of the joint with the posterior wires and bone grafts.

condition. There may be atlantoaxial subluxation of 2.5–3 mm or more (Figure 11.19) in 25% of patients with obvious erosion or absorption of the odontoid process. Wedging posteriorly between the posterior arches of the atlas and the axis, and narrowing between the posterior arches of the atlas and the occiput ('platybasia', similar to acetabular protrusion) are commonly found. Subaxial subluxation of C4–5 occurs less frequently but is most likely to be associated with neurological complications.

Clinical features are variable but commonly noted – particularly in the cervical and occipital areas – is a deep-seated, persistent pain which may radiate as an occipital headache or into the temporal regions. It should be noted that these pains may be made worse by cervical traction. Rarely is there a true brachialgia with paraesthesia, weakness of the limbs, muscle wasting, loss of deep tendon reflexes, arterial insufficiency syndromes of the cerebrum (vertigo, eye changes) or spinal cord (pyramidal tract changes) or with involvement of the vertebral or anterior spinal arteries. Severity of neurological symptoms and signs cannot be correlated to the severity of pathological changes as seen on radiography.

Treatment is usually conservative in the form of an immobilization collar made of plastic material. Physiotherapy in the form of traction, heat and exercises usually aggravate the symptoms.

Aside from wedge fractures of the spine occurring from osteoporosis, especially in patients treated by steroids, there may be special complications of rheumatoid arthritis which are life-threatening and which must be excluded before manipulation of the neck for induction of general anaesthesia.

The atlantoaxial joint may be involved by rheumatoid synovitis with stretching of the transverse ligament of the dens and the alar ligaments. This gives rise to subluxation of the joint so that the atlas vertebra rides forwards on the axis during flexion of the neck and may be detected by lateral flexion/extension radiography of the cervical spine. Fortunately, with control of the general disorder, this instability may not be serious in the older or moderately active patient and requires no treatment (Smith *et al.*, 1972). In the younger more active patient or if there is any sign of long tract involvement, fusion of the joint is required. This can be achieved by a posterior approach combining wiring and onlay corticocancellous bone grafting. A much rarer complication of involvement of the atlantoaxial joint is an upward subluxation of the axis tebrae, which is very likely to produce spinal cord pressure and always requires fusion.

Surprisingly, the subluxation of the mid or lower cervical spinal vertebrae is a much more dangerous condition. Such displacement carries a high incidence of spinal cord compression, and stabilization by posterior fusion is an urgent necessity (Figure 11.20). The use of the 'halo' incorporated into a brace which is applied before the operation greatly facilitates the procedure and the patient is able to

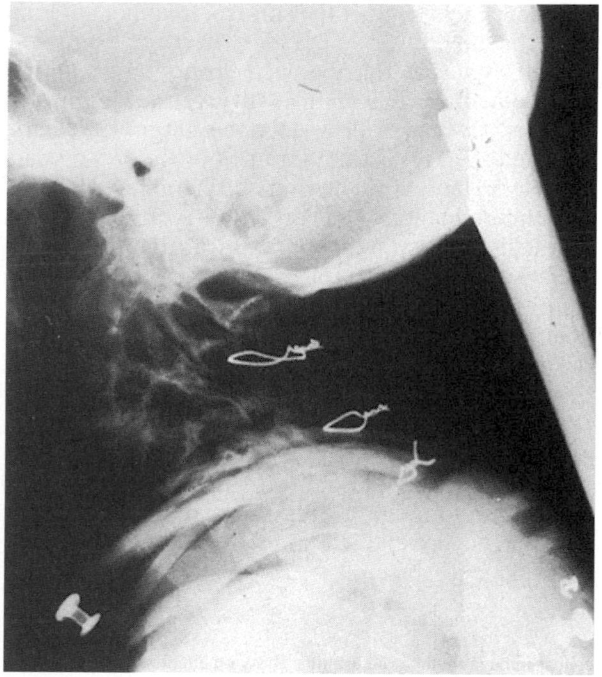

Figure 11.20 Lateral radiograph 6 months after extensive posterior spinal fusion for rheumatoid cervical spine subluxation at C3/4 and C5/6. Incorporation of the posterior bone graft is seen, and the patient has lost all long bone tract compression signs. The halo-body jacket was then removed.

begin walking as soon as the operative wounds are healed.

Boden *et al.* (1993) from a long-term follow-up of 73 patients for 7 years found in over 50% of the cases that paralysis occurred. In these, 35 required operative stabilization, the remainder were treated conservatively and their paralysis increased in severity.

The severity of paralysis and recovery could be correlated to the posterior atlanto-odontoid interval and the diameter of the subaxial sagittal spinal canal measurement, e.g. less than 14 mm. The anterior atlanto-odontoid interval did not correlate with paralysis. Neurological recovery after operation was related to the severity of the paralysis and not to its duration. If basilar invagination was superimposed (5 mm +) clinically important neurological recovery only occurred where the posterior atlanto-odontoid interval was at least 14 mm. They recommended operation of stabilization in all patients with less than those measurements in the presence or absence of any neurological deficit.

Juvenile chronic arthritis

This disease differs in a number of important respects from rheumatoid arthritis in adults and is probably a different disease. Ansell and Bywaters (1959) defined juvenile chronic polyarthritis as 'arthritis starting before the age of 16 years manifest by two of the following: pain, swelling and limitation of movement in four or more joints reliably observed over a period of at least 3 months, or in one joint for a similar period with biopsy confirmation, other diseases being excluded as far as possible, up to 1 year from the onset of symptoms'.

The annual incidence of new cases is 0.12 to 0.19 per 1000 children.

The peak age of onset is between 2 and 4 years with a second peak around puberty. The disease may be entirely confined to the joints or there may be a systemic illness. Monarticular arthritis, commonly involving the knee, is the usual presentation. The disease may remain monarticular but in the majority becomes polyarticular with involvement of the knees, hands, wrists and feet in most cases. Early involvement of the hips, sacroiliac joints and cervical spine is common. Although the increased thickness of articular cartilage seems to retard the appearance of erosions, unremitting disease leads to joint damage often with bony ankyloses. Increases in periarticular vascularity, the presence of systemic disease and the use of corticosteroid drugs may cause a variety of skeletal growth abnormalities due to premature closure of the limb epiphyses. The small chin is a striking abnormality.

Although general malaise, anorexia and weight loss may occur in any case, more characteristic systemic signs are found in some children with polyarthritis. These include fever, lymphadenopathy, splenomegaly, rash (a dusky pink maculopapular eruption) the distribution of which may vary from hour to hour, anaemia, leucocytosis (often up to $20 \times 10^9/l$; 20 000/mm^3) and pericarditis. Iridocylitis – which occurs in 8% of cases – is most common in the monarticular group. Amyloidosis occurs in 3.5% of cases. The ESR is elevated but tests for rheumatoid factor are negative except in a small group of children with late onset of disease, particularly adolescent girls. ANA is found in about 30% of children as antinuclear antibodies.

About 5% of children carry the disease into adult life, when it follows the chronic unpredictable course of adult rheumatoid arthritis. However, involvement of the neck, sacroiliac and hip joints is commoner, the serological tests for rheumatoid factor remain negative and the systemic symptoms disappear. Of those in whom the disease remits, 50% will have no residua, 45% will have moderate deformity and disability, and 5% will be severely incapacitated. A better prognosis is enjoyed by those whose disease starts in early childhood, whose disease is treated within a year of onset and whose involvement is monarticular.

Juvenile rheumatoid arthritis must be differentiated from rheumatic fever, viral and septic arthritis, the connective tissue diseases, the leukaemias and Lyme disease, caused by the spirochaete *Borrelia burgdorferi*, with its arthritis and rash now requires a positive serology for its differentiation.

Treatment involves chiefly the proper management of the patient as a child, with the provision of the necessary hospital, home and educational facilities to achieve this end, and good parental support (Ansell and Bywaters, 1977). Prevention of deformity in a disease with a high remission rate is crucial. All the methods described for adult rheumatoid arthritis are of value except that sustained immobilization in splints is inadvisable because of the tendency of joints to ankylose. Drug therapy in appropriate dosage follows similar lines to that in adult rheumatoid arthritis. However, gold, chloroquine and the immunosuppressive drugs are rarely used. Corticosteroid therapy must be used with care because of the effect on growth. There are reports of the beneficial effect of both ACTH and alternate-day oral steroids on the disease and the absence of growth effects.

Surgical therapy is largely confined to reconstructive procedures, often in early adult life when the disease has remitted. Swann (1990) has written an overview of the place of surgery for these children and emphasized the importance of soft tissue release, particularly of the hip and knee, with closely supervised physiotherapy after all procedures. The prognosis for these children is good in that about 60% will be in remission 10 years after onset, 45% will have a mild degree of disability after the age of 18 years. The remaining group will be more severely affected. There is a mortality of 14% after 15 years of disease in systemic onset juvenile arthritis because of infection, myocarditis and renal failure secondarily to any lordosis (Leak, 1991). Harris and Baum (1988) have carried out a longitudinal study in 35 children with rheumatoid arthritis over 22 years. In group 1, 13 children had mild disease and slight radiographic changes; in group 2, two children had episode activity and disability; in group 3, 14 patients had progressive disability, radiographic changes and required the majority of operations, and in group 4, six patients had dramatic clinical and radiographic findings with little functional disability. All the children had psychosocial problems but responded well to counselling and multiprofessional group management. These problems did influence the timing of the surgical treatment of joint replacements.

Witt *et al.* (1991) reviewed 96 primary total hip replacements in 54 patients with juvenile rheumatoid arthritis, over a follow-up averaging 11.5 years; 25% required revision after an average of 9.5 years with a further 20% having radiographic signs of loosening. Factors such as body weight, reduced physical activity, osteoporosis of the bone with increased vascularity (60% of the patients were on steroids at the time); the accompanying soft tissue contractures and bony deformity; the greater stress on the new hip by disease involving the adjacent joints of the lumbar spine, knees, etc.; deep infection (74%); were all operating against a good result. However, in spite of the figures, the operation and outcome as regards quality of life was remarkable and the authors hope to improve the figures by customized prosthetics and better cementing techniques.

Psoriatic arthropathy

Psoriasis and rheumatoid arthritis are fairly common conditions and will occur coincidentally in the same patient.

The presence of skin changes is essential for the diagnosis. However, only small patches on the extensor surfaces of the elbows or knees or in the scalp may be found. Nail involvement with pitting, ridging and subungual hyperkeratosis is regarded as necessary for the diagnosis by most authors. The arthropathy typically includes involvement of the terminal interphalangeal joints of the hands and feet and often the sacroiliac joints.

The prognosis is better than rheumatoid arthritis, although a few develop a very destructive arthropathy (arthritis mutilans) and in this group a patchy sacroiliitis and spondylitis are common. Multisystem involvement does not occur. Elevation of the serum uric acid is found in a proportion of cases due to the increased cell turnover in the skin and joints, and secondary gout may occur.

Skin lesions should be treated initially with a descaling ointment, and various tar-based preparations are suitable. Subsequently local steroid therapy should be employed. Treatment of the joints should follow the line suggested for rheumatoid arthritis. However, chloroquine should not be used since it may exacerbate the skin lesions. Methotrexate, of value in those with severe skin lesions, is much less beneficial to the arthritis.

As for rheumatoid arthritis, the surgery of replacement of diseased joints is indicated and can be safely carried out with careful operative and perioperative antisepsis, and systemic prophylactic antibiotics since these patients are particularly susceptible to infection of wounds and prostheses.

From family studies of patients with psoriatic arthritis, ankylosing spondylitis, inflammatory bowel disease (e.g. ulcerative colitis, Crohn's disease), because of their similar clinical features, anodular, asymmetrical small joint arthritis, pustular rashes, iridocylitis of the eye although serum negative, have given rise to the concept of 'seronegative spondyloarthritides'. This group of diseases also has an increased frequency of HLA B27.

Reiter's disease

The association of urethritis and arthritis is sufficient for the diagnosis of Reiter's disease. Some authors demand conjunctivitis to make the diagnosis but this occurs in only 40% of cases. Mouth and genital ulceration and characteristic skin lesions – keratoderma blennorrhagica – each occur in 10% of cases.

The cause of the disease is unknown although a variety of organisms have been implicated. The disease develops from the urethritis, which in Great Britain and the USA appears identical to non-specific urethritis, is transmitted sexually and responds to antibiotic therapy. About 1% of males with non-specific urethritis develop Reiter's disease; the usual group affected is those aged 20–50 years. The venereal type of the disease is rare in women and the disease in children is always of the dysenteric type. In many tropical and developing countries and in time of war an identical disease, including urethritis, follows various specific and non-specific types of dysentery. The annual recurrence rate is about 15% and can be precipitated by trauma or intercurrent infection as well as by urethritis or dysentery.

The acute arthritis with marked effusions involves the ankles and knees most commonly although no joint is immune. With persistent or recurrent disease sacroiliac joint involvement occurs in 40% of cases, and the differentiation from ankylosing spondylitis and other causes of sacroiliitis may be difficult. The disease may lead to an erosive arthritis similar to rheumatoid arthritis, and foot changes of a similar type develop in some cases. The disease is self-limiting in almost every case. However, the time to remission varies from 3 weeks to 2 years. There is no specific therapy and the aims of treatment are to induce an early remission and so prevent serious joint disease with deformity. There appears to be a relationship between the promptness of the initiation of treatment and the time to remission of the disease. Simple rest, splintage of involved joints and the prescription of analgesic anti-inflammatory drugs are all that are required in most cases. The ESR is often markedly elevated and its return to normal values may be delayed and thus not provide a good index of disease activity. The decision to mobilize the patient should be taken on clinical grounds. Considerable muscle wasting occurs and adequate physical therapy must be employed before and after weight-bearing. In a few cases corticosteroids may be required to suppress signs of the disease but there is no evidence that they alter the course of the disease. Antibiotic therapy, effective in treating the urethritis, does not usually alter the remainder of the disease. Experience with the immunosuppressive agents is limited but methotrexate and cyclophosphamide may occasionally be beneficial in severe cases.

Synovectomy may be required for persistent synovitis, and reconstructive arthroplasties for seriously damaged joints, particularly the feet, may be undertaken.

Connective tissue diseases

In this group of diseases, there is little evidence of collagen damage and the older name of 'collagen diseases' should be discarded. The group includes systemic lupus erythematosus, polyarteritis nodosa, dermatomyositis, polymyositis and scleroderma (Figure 11.21). A widespread vasculitis is responsible for a variety of pathological changes in many different tissues. Small arterioles are chiefly involved but medium-sized arteries may also be affected, especially in polyarteritis nodosa, with the production of more obvious vascular abnormalities. Symptoms referable to the skin, muscles and joints are common, and renal involvement, often leading to death, occurs frequently. It is important that the musculoskeletal symptoms be distinguished from those of rheumatoid arthritis since the prognosis and management are very different. Arthralgia with mild synovitis, usually of the joints of the hands and feet, is a common presenting symptom. The diseases rarely progress to an erosive arthritis, and any deformities that occur are usually secondary to muscle or skin disease. Myositis is more obvious than in rheumatoid arthritis and is diagnosed by the finding of raised muscle enzyme values in the serum. Avascular necrosis of bone, particularly of the head of the femur, is a recognized complication of these diseases. The cause may be due to underlying

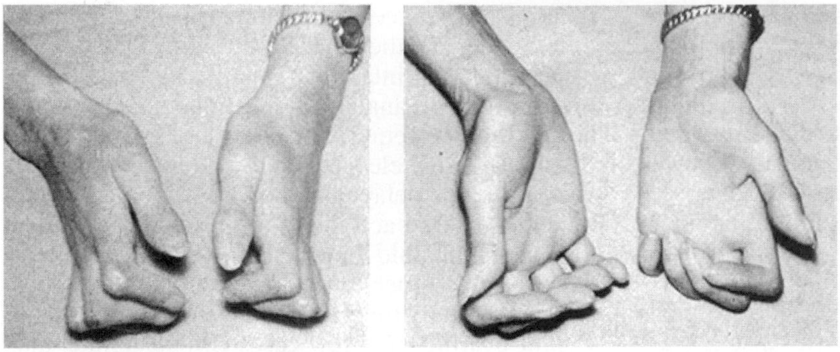

Figure 11.21 The hands of a young woman with scleroderma, showing the marked flexion deformities involving the proximal interphalangeal joints with some degree of hyperextension of the metacarpophalangeal joints. There is marked loss of subcutaneous tissues and ulceration over the proximal interphalangeal joints.

vasculitis or perhaps to the corticosteroid drugs commonly used in the treatment of these diseases.

SYSTEMIC LUPUS ERYTHEMATOSUS

Characterized by multiple arthralgias without a deforming or erosive arthritis, SLE is accompanied by both dermal as well as epidermal involvement; e.g. facial swelling and erythema, and vasculitis in the nail beds. Renal disease with haematuria, proteinuria and urine casts, and an elevated serum creatinine are commonly found. Pleurisy, pericarditis, neurological disturbances of the central nervous system and of the peripheral nerves are reported. Diagnosis is based upon a positive LE cell test, or upon demonstrating a fluorescent antinuclear antibody (ANA test), anaemia, leucopenia, as well as carrying out a skin and kidney biopsy. Non-steroidal anti-inflammatory drugs are preferred to salicylates, and corticosteroids should be reserved for haemolytic anaemia, neutropenia, thrombocytopenia, myocarditis, etc., as well as severe involvement of the kidneys.

SCLERODERMA

The basic pathology of this chronic disease is cellular infiltration of mononuclear cells around small arterioles with abnormal amounts of collagen in the dermis, and thinning of the overlying epidermis. When progressive, there is inflammation, fibrosis, atrophy involving the lung, the heart and pericardium, the kidney, the oesophagus and lower bowel, and Raynaud's phenomenon. The arterioles show necrosis with fibrinoid degeneration and intimal sclerosis. Arthritis of the hands is very common, with marked contractures of the tendons and wasting of adjacent muscles (Figure 11.21). Calcinosis may be associated with sclerodactyly, Raynaud's phenomenon and telangiectasis as a specific syndrome. Ulceration of the skin with absorption of the terminal phalanges can be seen in the late stages.

Ointments, physiotherapy, vasodilator drugs to try to improve the capillary blood flow, anti-inflammatory drugs and antifibrotic drugs (e.g. penicillamine or colchicine) have all been used in skin care.

MIXED CONNECTIVE TISSUE DISEASE

This has many of the features of SLE, scleroderma and polymyositis but only mild renal disease. It can be distinguished by the lack of anti-DNA antibodies found in SLE and the demonstration of high titres of antibodies to ribonucleoproteins (RNP).

Polymyalgia rheumatica

Polymyalgia rheumatica is a clinical syndrome of unknown cause in which severe pain and stiffness of the muscles of the neck, shoulder and pelvic girdles are accompanied by a variety of systemic symptoms and signs. There is often marked morning stiffness without joint swelling. The onset of symptoms is frequently sudden, producing severe disability. Joint involvement is minimal. The ESR is often markedly elevated but there are no specific laboratory findings. There is no evidence of muscle disease.

An underlying vasculitis can be found by temporal or other artery biopsy in 25% of cases and is probably the basis of the disease in all cases. Corticosteroid therapy in a dose of 20 mg of prednisolone per day rapidly controls the symptoms and prevents the development of serious vascular symptoms and signs, particularly blindness. The disease, which occurs most often in patients over 60 years of age, is self-limiting and treatment can be reduced and ultimately discontinued after 2 years or so.

Gout

Much knowledge has accumulated over the past two decades about the nature of purine metabolism and many of the older concepts of hyperuricaemia and gout have been discarded. The end point in purine metabolism is the production of uric acid which is excreted by the kidney. The three major factors in purine metabolism are:

1. The breakdown of body purines (endogenous production).
2. The breakdown of ingested purines (exogenous production).
3. The renal excretion of uric acid.

The distribution curve of plasma uric acid levels in the population depends upon the interaction of these factors. The upper limits of normal – 0.357 mmol/l (6.0 mg/100 ml) in men and 0.325 mmol/l (5.5 mg/100 ml) in women – are merely arbitrary points on the curve. Approximately 5% of the population is hyperuricaemic on these criteria but only a small proportion will develop gout.

The breakdown of body purines

The major pathways in purine metabolism are shown in Figure 11.22. The first stage in purine synthesis is controlled by the enzyme phosphoribosyl-pyrophosphate aminotransferase (PRPP-ATase) and this is the site of action of a feedback control based upon the production of adenine and guanine nucleotides. A second enzyme, hypoxanthine-guanine phosphori-

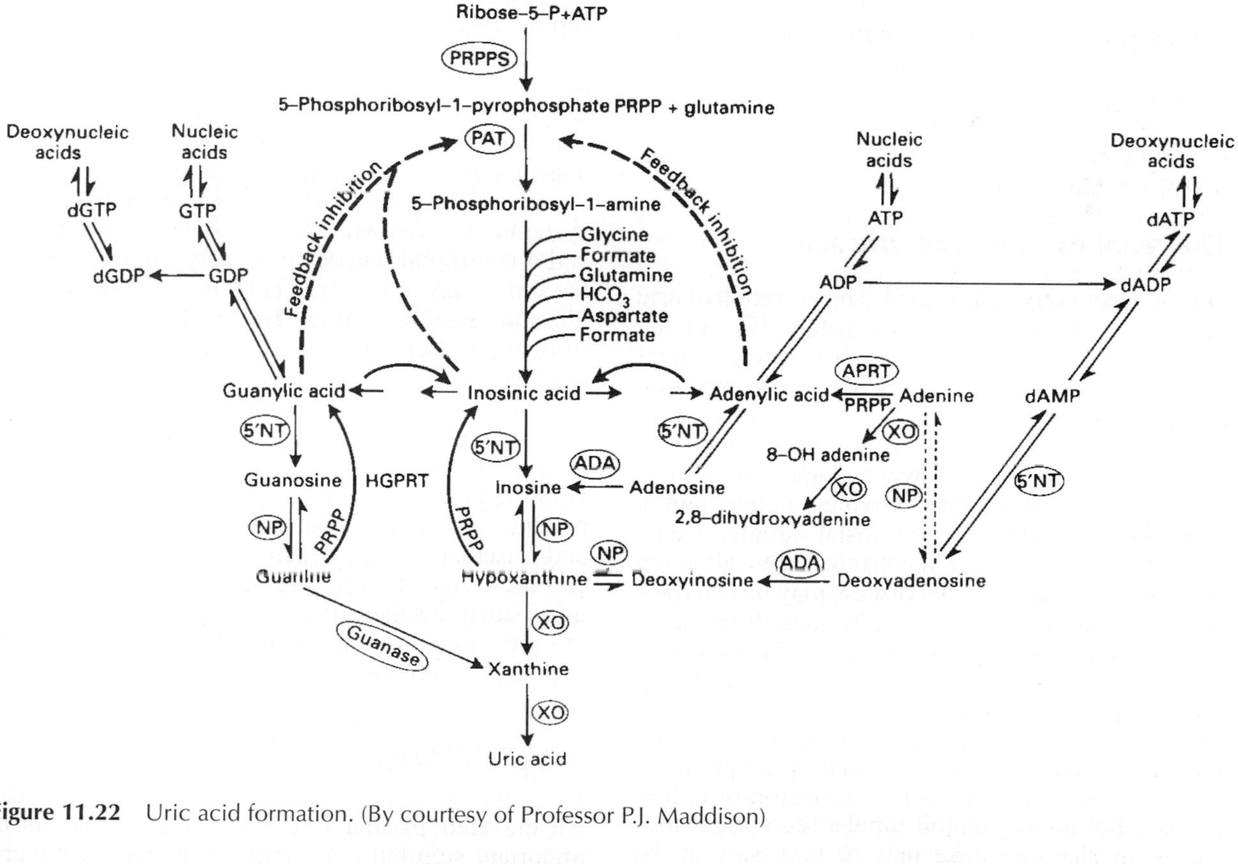

Figure 11.22 Uric acid formation. (By courtesy of Professor P.J. Maddison)

bosyl transferase (HG-PRTase), catalyses a number of stages, all of which are designed to salvage purines for reutilization and hence, by way of the feedback mechanism, to reduce purine synthesis. HG-PRTase occurs in many body cells and can be assayed in erythrocytes. Congenital absence of the enzyme occurs in the Lesch–Nyhan syndrome and reduced levels have been found in a number of patients with gout, and represents part of the genetic basis of the disease. A third enzyme, xanthine oxidase, catalyses the conversion of hypoxanthine to xanthine to uric acid. This fact is utilized in the management of gout with the xanthine oxidase inhibitor, allopurinol. An increase in endogenous purine metabolism occurs in certain diseases, particularly the myeloproliferative diseases, leukaemias, psoriasis, etc., and in a variety of stress situations such as infections and surgery. These increases may overload the metabolic pathways and cause hyperuricaemia and gout.

The breakdown of ingested purines

This represents a relatively unimportant cause and it is exceptional for patients to produce hyperuricaemia with even severe dietary excess unless there is already some metabolic abnormality of the type indicated above. Dietary restriction is rarely necessary with current drug therapy.

The renal excretion of uric acid

This is genetically determined. The excretion of uric acid, which represents approximately 10% of the load filtered by the renal glomerulus, is proportional to the plasma uric acid level. However, the excretion rate in some patients is set at a slightly lower level and hyperuricaemia results. Uric acid is completely removed from the plasma by the glomerulus; almost all is reabsorbed in the proximal tubule and a proportion secreted in the distal tubule. Renal disease may alter these mechanisms but although subjects with chronic renal disease may have hyperuricaemia, gout rarely occurs. Various drugs interfere with the renal handling of urate. The uricosuric drugs, such as probenecid, reduce tubular reabsorption. Salicylates in large doses have a similar effect but in low dosage impair tubular secretion. Many diuretics impair tubular secretion. Conditions of ketosis, produced by diabetes, starvation or excessive alcohol intake, inhibit tubular secretion. Moderation of alcohol intake may be necessary in the management of gout.

PATHOLOGY

The acute attack of gout is caused by the ingestion of microcrystals of urate by neutrophils with the subsequent release of lysosomal enzymes. Such acute attacks occur either when the solubility of urate in body fluids has been exceeded and deposits are accumulating, particularly in articular and periarticular tissues, or when the plasma uric acid level is lowered and such deposits are going into solution. The second mechanism is responsible for the acute attacks of gout which occur during the first weeks of therapy.

CLINICAL FEATURES

Gout is commoner in males, usually after the age of 20, and is rare in women until the menopause. The disease presents as an acute attack of crystal synovitis which clears completely in a week or so, to be followed at intervals of weeks, months or years by further attacks. After a time tophaceous deposits appear on the ears, in tendons and in joints. The joint disease becomes more chronic and leads to severe secondary degenerative joint disease. The acute attack, which frequently involves the metatarsophalangeal joint of the great toe, causes severe pain, swelling and skin erythema. There is usually a systemic reaction with malaise, fever, a raised ESR and a neutrophil leucocytosis. Any joint, including the spine, may be involved but it is uncommon in the hip and shoulder. About 2% of cases are chronic from the outset. The incidence of tophi increases with the length of the history of gout and will reach 90% in untreated cases. Tophi are occasionally radiopaque. They may involve many organs, causing interference with function, and although they involve approximately 10% of the kidneys in these patients, the major renal abnormalities of fibrosis and vascular change leading to hypertension and chronic renal failure are caused by other ill-understood mechanisms. Renal stones occur in 10% of cases. Renal disease is the major cause of death in patients with gout.

INVESTIGATIONS

An elevated plasma uric acid value is the most important sign but only indicates a state of hyperuricaemia. Gout is diagnosed on the clinical symptoms and signs and of the finding of urate crystals in joint effusions. These can be identified using a polarizing microscope, and are usually found as needle-shaped crystals inside neutrophils. These can

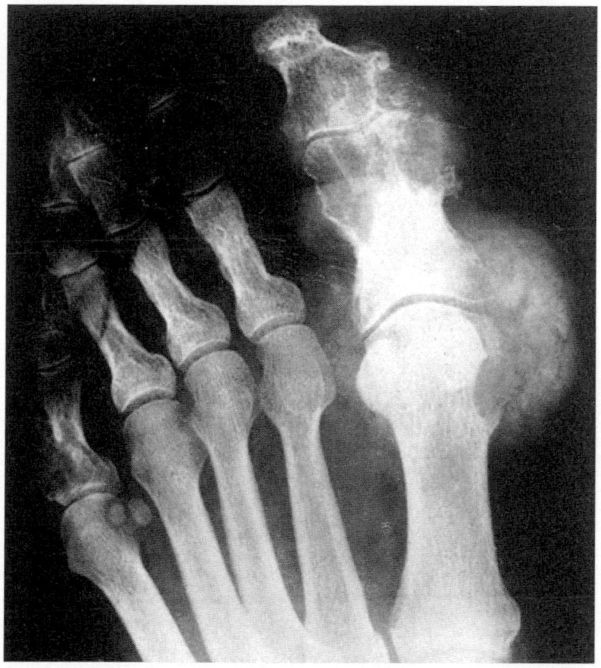

Figure 11.23 Radiograph of the forefoot of a 49-year-old man suffering from gout, showing the marked subchondral bone erosions of big and little toes with radiopaque tophaceous deposits.

be distinguished from the calcium pyrophosphate crystals of pseudogout because the latter are pleomorphic and show weak positive birefringence. Radiographs do not show any diagnostic features except in those cases with radiopaque tophaceous deposits or in marked subchondral erosions of distal interphalangeal joints (Figure 11.23).

TREATMENT

Indomethacin (200 mg per day) is effective. It is occasionally necessary to use corticosteroids intra-articularly. Ideally a patient should have only one attack of gout. To achieve this limitation the plasma uric acid levels must be reduced and it is essential that the patient understands the purpose of the drug therapy, as it must be maintained for life. This can be achieved with a xanthine oxidase inhibitor (allopurinol 300 mg/day). The dose must be adjusted in the light of the serial plasma uric acid values. During the first 3 months it is usual to add a small dose of indomethacin to prevent acute attacks. In patients with severe gout and/or renal disease allopurinol has an advantage, since the purine metabolite xanthine is completely cleared by the kidney compared with the clearance of urate of 10% without and 30% with uricosuric drugs. Dietary restrictions are not necessary. In those liable to renal stone formation it is necessary to ensure that they pass large volumes of dilute, alkaline urine.

Chondrocalcinosis (pyrophosphate arthropathy)

Chondrocalcinosis, or pseudogout, is due to synovitis caused by crystals of calcium pyrophosphate dihydrate. The pathological mechanism and the symptoms are similar to those of gout. The crystals have a characteristic appearance under the polarizing microscope with weak birefringence. The large joints, particularly the knee, are usually involved and present with severe pain, swelling and a low-grade pyrexia over 24–48 hours. Radiographs show calcification in both fibro- and hyaline cartilage (Figure 11.24) but this is a matter of degree, since many elderly patients show such features. The term 'chondrocalcinosis' is thus best used to describe the radiological feature and not a disease. The disease is occasionally associated with hyperparathyroidism, haemochromatosis and gout. The most effective therapy is joint aspiration and the instillation of local steroid. Indomethacin and phenylbutazone help to control acute attacks and prevent recurrences.

As well as calcium pyrophosphate crystals, hydroxyapatite crystals which can be stained by alizarin red 5 are found in ageing joints, synovial fluid or peritendonitis tissue regardless of clinical diagnosis of osteoarthritis. Whether they cause disease or result from the joint disease is not known. However, Halverson *et al.* (1990) have described them in joints rapidly being destroyed. When occurring in the shoulder it is now called 'Milwaukee shoulder' and is believed to result from the discharge of the apatite crystals into the joints from the periarticular tissues.

Tietze's syndrome

This condition usually presents in a middle-aged person, who complains of a painful tender enlargement of at least one of the costosternal junctions, usually opposite the fifth, sixth or seventh ribs. It has been called costochondritis. The pain is aggravated by deep breathing, coughing or any pressure on the thoracic cage.

On examination there is usually a tender mass at the costochondral junction, with an increased local

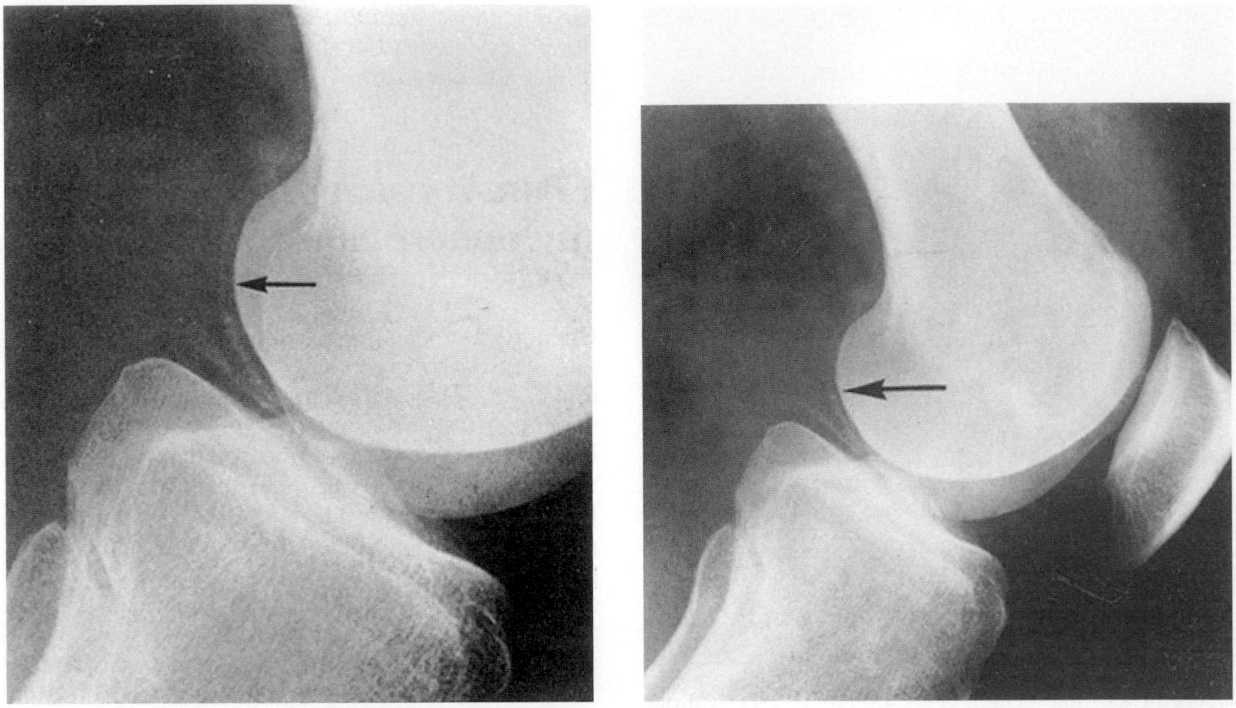

(a) (b)

Figure 11.24 Radiographs showing an example of chondrocalcinosis with calcification in both meniscus and hyaline cartilage of the knee.

temperature, but no definite redness of overlying skin. Biopsy has been carried out on a few cases, and oedema of the perichondrium as well as the soft tissues was found, but nothing more specific than this. The aetiology of this condition is vague, but some form of trauma, mechanical stresses or perhaps the onset of calcification into the chondral aspect of the rib may be a precipitating factor. This is a slow but self-limiting disease. Treatment is usually supportive, with analgesics and local heat, and some have recommended the injection of hydrocortisone solution directly into the most tender area.

Dialysis amyloidosis joint and periarticular disease

Patients undergoing haemodialysis for up to 20 years or continuous ambulatory peritoneal dialysis, develop in joint tissues (hip, knee, shoulder, wrist, cervical and lumbar spine, sacroiliac joints) the β_2 microglobulin amyloid as demonstrated by Congo red and by antibody techniques (Athanasou *et al.*, 1991) in the presence of radiographic changes or not. This material was deposited over the superficial and deep zones of articular cartilage, in hip capsule, in reactive fibrosis tissue and fibrocartilage covering erosions, in subchondral pseudocysts, in disc material and in the carpal tunnel ligamentous tissue. Systemic amyloid deposition was very rare, and in tiny amounts in the wall of small and large blood vessels and in the limbs, liver, myocardium, tongue, etc. These authors emphasize that the degenerative changes in articular cartilage and erosive change occur where the β_2 microglobulin is heavily deposited secondarily to the presence of highly sulphated glycosaminoglycans, e.g. heparin sulphate.

Osteoarthritis (osteoarthrosis)

This disease is characterized by degenerative changes in the articular cartilage of diarthrodial joints and subsequent new bone formation at the articular margins. It results from the rate of degeneration being greater than the rate of repair and/or regeneration of articular cartilage. Basically it is excessive ageing although very little is known about the biochemistry of ageing. By the age of 40 years, about 40% of the population have radiographic signs of osteoarthrosis of major weight-bearing joints (e.g.

knee or hip) and 50% of these will have symptoms (Danielsson, 1964).

Kellgren (1961) preferred the title 'osteoarthrosis' since there is no evidence of synovial thickening or inflammatory infiltration in the uncomplicated condition. He emphasized that there is a different expression of this disease by the male and the female, and this may result from inherited metabolic abnormalities as well as dietary and other environmental factors. In males, the hip joint tends to be more affected, whereas in women the hands are more affected in a polyarticular manner in association with Heberden's nodes. Kellgren described a familial form of osteoarthritis, affecting multiple joints in association with Heberden's nodes, and called it 'primary generalized osteoarthritis'. Primary osteoarthrosis occurs in joints without any previous pathology or any predisposing cause.

AETIOLOGICAL FACTORS IN OSTEOARTHRITIS

Geography

In a review of osteoarthritis in six populations living in different climates, as determined by latitude, the highest prevalence was in Leigh, Lancashire (53°N) and the lowest in Heinola, Finland (61°N) (Lawrence, 1967). Since that time more results have become available and are shown in Table 11.4.

Racial groups

Prevalence surveys have been carried out in non-caucasian populations which show that the prevalence of OA of the hip in the latter is significantly lower than in Europeans.

A survey of 500 Hong Kong Chinese found only 1% of adults over 55 years old had OA of the hip, although the prevalence of OA of the hand was similar to that in Europeans (Hoaglund, 1967). The lower prevalence of hip OA was thought to be due to the low rate of hip developmental abnormalities in Chinese people, possibly secondary to the posture assumed by infants when carried on the mother's back.

The prevalence of OA in American Indians lies intermediate between high European rates and low rates from other parts of the world. Of those aged 55 and above in a Blackfeet Indian population, 8% of men and 11% of women had hip OA. In the same study, comparable European population rates varied from 12% to 22% in men. In black populations, however, the rates varied from 1% to 3%.

OA of the hip is clearly less common in African blacks as a group, save for one area in Africa, Mseleni, where females have an unusually high prevalence of hip arthritis. An investigation showed hip OA in 23% of women over 60 secondary to either protrusio acetabuli, which increased in prevalence with age, in epiphyseal dysplasia, which was part of a polyostotic dysplasia. However, a histomorphometric analysis by Schnitler of the osteopenia associated with Mseleni joint disease concluded that calcium deficiency was the most potent factor in aggravating and speeding up the destructive arthritic changes.

Age

This is probably the most consistently associated factor with generalized and nodular specific OA. The peak incidence of OA is 45 years in the interphalangeal joints and the first carpometacarpal; and that OA occurs later in the knee and latest in the hip (Peyron, 1986). The increase in the prevalence of OA with age is apparently independent of socioeconomic status in the United Status and in the UK. One of the reasons for age-related increases in prevalence of OA is the loss of mechanical resistance of ageing cartilage, due to a defect in stabilizing components of the matrix.

Table 11.4 Prevalence of OA in population samples aged 35–64 years based on x-rays of hands, feet and neck (Lawrence *et al.*, 1963)

Population	Latitude (degrees)	Total x-rayed	% OA No. joints affected		
			1+	3+	5+
Leigh (Caucasian)	53	923	58	1	1.9
Oberhorlen (Caucasian)	50	210	43	5	0.6
Montana (Blackfeet Indian)	48	759	42	8	0.8
Arizona (Pima)	33	632	50	13	2.2
Jamaica (Negro)	18	528	48	8	1.0
Nigeria (Negro)	6	392	31	2	0.2

Some biomechanical factors associated with OA have been identified, but little is known about how these factors change with age and their precise role in the development of OA. The cervical spine is probably the most commonly affected area in the over 75 age group with the lumbar spine next.

Gender

The crude prevalence of OA is the same in both sexes, but in females more joints are affected. Five or more joint groups were affected in 9% of males and 12% of females in population samples in Leigh and Wensleydale (Kellgren and Lawrence, 1957). These figures were based on x-rays of the hands, feet, cervical spine, lumbar spine, knees and pelvis. These studies, in general, have indicated that men have higher prevalence and severity of OA of the body trunk, spine and hips. At ages above 45 years OA appears slightly more frequently in men and involves one or more joints. At ages greater than 55 years OA is more frequent in women and involves multiple joints. It has been shown that OA in post-menopausal women was associated with higher body weight, higher subcutaneous fat and stronger muscles linked to hormonal deficiencies.

Socioeconomic groups

In males in the monarticular form associated with trauma there is a gradient between social class and osteoarthritis. The prevalence of this form of OA is significantly more in social class V than in social classes I and II. There is no relationship between social class and generalized OA. In females there appears to be no association between social class and OA of any kind. Heberden's nodes are unrelated to social class in either sex.

Occupation

Occupations with physical activity involve repetitive use of particular joints over long periods of time. Sports enthusiasts and professional athletes may be conditioned so that their muscles protect their joints, but the manual labourer, factory worker or docker may continue to use the joints even after muscular exhaustion.

Obesity

Obesity has been associated with increased bone mass. Bone mass may be calculated by measuring cortical width in metacarpal bones by radiogrammetry, with mass being expressed as:

$$\text{cross-sectional cortical area} = \pi/4\,(\text{overall width } D)^2 - (\text{medullary width } D)^2.$$

$\pi/4$ is omitted by convention. Radin and Paul (1972) have suggested that a major cause of OA is the failure of subchondral bone to deform with an impact load, leading to increased cartilage damage. If this is true then disorders where bone is stiffer than normal would be associated with higher prevalence of OA and patients with OA would have higher bone masses than normal – a situation seen in Paget's disease.

Metabolic factors

There has been some evidence for a link between diabetes and OA, possibly through elevated growth hormone levels that alter cartilage metabolism and increase bone density. Hyperuricaemia has been found more frequently in people with generalized OA.

Mechanical factors

It has been long considered that mechanical stress, such as single impact stress, gross anatomical damage, subtle mechanical derangement (e.g. long-standing internal derangement of the knee), joint hypermobility and repeated impacts, has been associated with OA but other factors are also operating. Indeed, direct articular cartilage damage is not the sole source of change.

In a study of surgically treated patients 6 months to 21 years Jacobson (1977) showed that after cruciate ligament rupture (usually anterior only) cartilage changes of OA were frequent even in patients in their twenties. It was unclear from this study, however, whether cartilage damage occurred at the time of cruciate rupture or was a consequence of it, or both.

Developmental factors

A substantial proportion of OA of the hip may be accounted for by developmental diseases of the hip. The three major developmental abnormalities are:

1. Congenital dislocation of the hip.
2. Perthes' disease.
3. Slipped capital femoral epiphysis.

Long-term follow-up reports have suggested that patients aged 30–50 have mild functional impairment, but radiographs often show joint space narrowing and other evidence of OA.

Genetic influences

In certain subsets of OA there is a hereditary factor present. This is particularly the case with Heberden's nodes which are twice as frequent in first-degree relatives to females with the nodes. A familial trait has also been noted in generalized OA associated with Heberden's nodes. This trend has been confirmed by studies of twin pairs. As yet, however, no significant link between osteoarthritis and a histocompatibility group has been found.

The extent to which genetic control of enzyme production is involved is at present uncertain, although genetic factors may intervene at any of the levels of chemical or structural organization of collagen. Disruption of collagen is an integral part of the OA lesion, but the collagen concentration is virtually unchanged. Various degradable enzymes with access to cartilage matrix are involved and possibly their inhibitors. Joint laxity may also be a feature in familial predisposition to OA (e.g. OA of the knees in Marfan's syndrome and OA of the hips in CDH).

Rheumatoid arthritis and osteoarthritis may coexist in the same joints. Possible causes include cartilage abnormalities, neuromuscular disorders (altering the biomechanics of the joint), mild inflammatory arthritis and crystals.

Rare disorders such as haemochromatosis, ochronosis and acromegaly can cause cartilage changes and secondary osteoarthritis. Gout can, through repeated episodes of inflammation, lead to chronic joint damage and secondary OA. Most studies have not confirmed the link between generalized OA and raised serum urate levels. Gout is clinically obvious and usually acute, whereas the natural history of OA is insidious without the local inflammatory episodes that typify gout. Rarely, urate crystals are found in osteoarthritis joint effusions.

Doherty *et al.* (1990) have attempted to categorize arthritis by:

1. Distribution of joint disease – generalized, pauciarticular or monarticular.
2. Radiographic features of atrophy or hypertrophy.
3. Associated crystal deposition – pyrophosphates, apatites.
4. Obvious dysplasia or abnormal shape or form.

They also showed that there was an association between obesity and osteoarthritis but it was not consistent for all joints or for the two sexes, e.g. obesity was associated with OA of the knee in women, but not the hip.

Obesity is thought to be a primary and not a secondary factor on the outcome of OA by increasing the impulse loading. Radin *et al.* (1978) believes that the impulse load results in microfractures of the trabeculae which become stiffer and less protective to the overlying articular cartilage. Endogenous oestrogens are other potential factors (Coppens and Dequeker, 1991). Generalized arthritis in women showed a marked peak at the age of 50 years. Spector *et al.* (1988) have shown that these women have had twice the number of hysterectomies compared with age-matched controls. Oestradiol has been shown to suppress the proteoglycan synthesis in both normal and osteoarthritic cartilage (Rosner *et al.*, 1982). Oestrogens have complex interactions with other hormones, e.g. testosterones, growth hormones, insulin-like peptides, interleukin 1 and 2, thus affecting both cartilage and bone.

PATHOLOGY

The primary lesion consists of degeneration of the hyaline cartilage (Figures 11.25 and 11.26). As a result, the cartilage is easily and rapidly eroded until ultimately the bone matrix is exposed. The erosion of the cartilage is not uniform, so relatively at first areas of bone are exposed in a patchy fashion and there are intervening islands of relatively normal cartilage. The perichondrium and the cartilage round the periphery of the joint are stimulated into activity, and, as a result, the non-articular areas of the bones are elevated above the remainder of the surface, and project circumferentially to give the appearance known as 'lipping'. In addition, irregular outgrowths appear in this area, at first cartilaginous but eventually becoming ossified to form osteophytes.

There is a synovitis with fibrosis involving the capsule and subsynovial connective tissues. There is also a reaction to the presence of cartilage debris shed from the joint surface and absorbed between the surface layers of the synovial membrane.

Harrison *et al.* (1953) showed that in osteoarthritis there is proliferation of blood vessels and probably an increase in blood supply to the subchondral bone with thinning of cartilage over the pressure areas, but proliferation of cartilage where there is no pressure. This degenerates and is invaded by larger blood vessels and finally replaced by bone. Venous engorgement with increased pressure in segments of osteoarthritic femoral heads has been reported.

Johnson (1959) described that in the formation of subchondral cysts in osteoarthritis there is initially an oedema in the subchondral marrow, which is followed by the formation of a mucinous fatty marrow and dilatation of surrounding sinusoids. There is mucoid secretion within the centre of this area and the expansion of the cyst cavities by osteoclastic resorption of bony trabeculae. Surrounding this there is some osteoblastic response and a sclerotic wall is formed. Other theories are that these cysts arise from herniation of synovial fluid through cracks within the denuded subchondral bone plate.

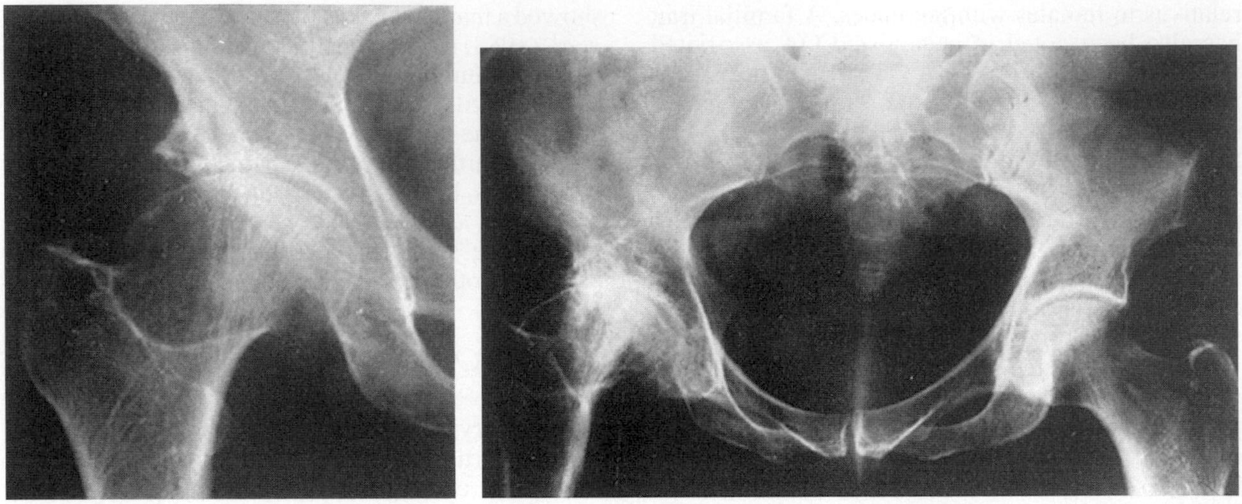

(a) (b)

Figure 11.25 Progression of osteoarthritis of the hip over an 8-year period. (a) Narrowing of joint space, early cyst formation and early thickening of the bone of both femoral head and acetabulum. (b) Further joint space narrowing with increased radiodensity and cyst formation.

Johnson believed that the osteophytic lipping may be due to outward cartilage growth followed by ossification, and local periosteal new bone formation, particularly around the capsular attachments.

The synovial membrane and capsule are involved in the later stages, and are the site of inflammation and adhesions. The synovial tags or polypi are insinuated into the joint, and when very exuberant the process is referred to as 'lipoma arborescens'. Occasionally, cartilage formation occurs in these tags and they are then liable to be broken off into the joint, when they form loose bodies. The exposed bone ends of the articular surface are subjected to considerable friction; in consequence the bone trabeculae in the immediate neighbourhood fracture and repair and the marrow spaces are obliterated. The change involves only a thin layer abutting on the joint, and when the surface of this layer gradually becomes more and more smooth and polished as a result of the continual rubbing, the process is known as eburnation.

An osteoarthritic joint rarely, if ever, becomes completely ankylosed, in contrast to the rheumatoid form in which ankylosis is frequent. Nevertheless,

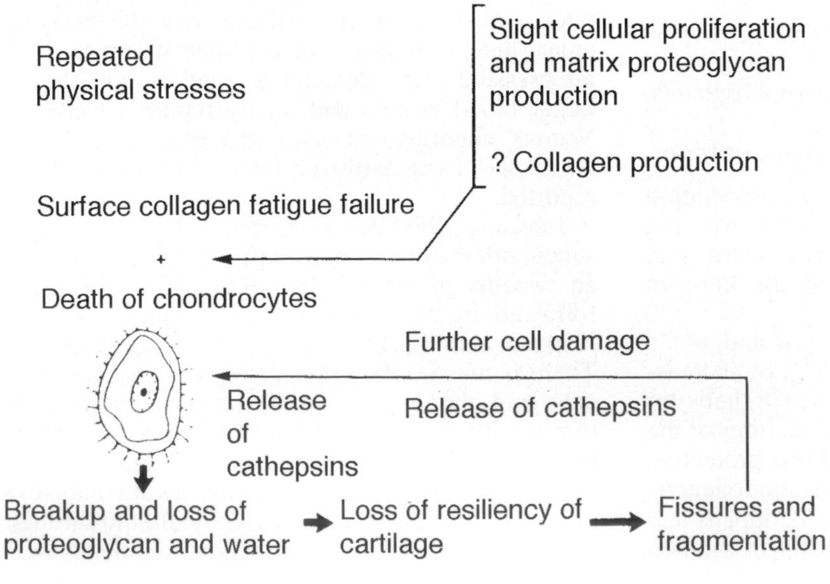

Figure 11.26 The steps in articular cartilage breakdown in osteoarthosis.

the gross peripheral proliferation and the presence of osteophytic outgrowths and dense capsular fibrosis may impede the free movement of the joint, and even simulate a degree of fusion which does not, in fact, exist.

Changes in the individual joint constituents

The articular cartilage

The earliest change in osteoarthritis begins in the hyaline cartilage. Harrison *et al.* (1953) believed that this is not at the summit of the head of the femur (i.e. at the main pressure area) but at the non-pressure area of the lower part of the head which is opposite to the part of the acetabulum without an articular lining. These changes in 71% of femoral heads were in the non-pressure areas, in 26% in both pressure and non-pressure areas, whereas in only 3% were the changes restricted to the pressure areas. Harrison *et al.* argued that use and compression are necessary to maintain the nutrition of the articular cartilage. The intermittent pumping action of alternate pressure and rest forces the synovial fluid into the cartilage. Hence where pressure is absent, nutrition is likely to be absent and degeneration occurs more readily (Figure 11.27).

The immediate reaction of the cartilage is proliferation of the subchondral blood vessels, which is interpreted as an attempt to bring about repair. Calcification and ossification take place in the deeper layers of the cartilage; then the blood vessels enter this calcified cartilage and further calcification takes place ahead of them. In the non-pressure areas this process continues indefinitely, the vessels spread outwards preceded by a vanguard of calcification capped with a layer of fibrocartilage, this gradually increasing the size of the bone, to form osteophytes. In the vascular zone beneath the pressure area cysts are formed, and these cysts always communicate with the joint through small openings. The cysts increase in size from the intermittent pressure of the synovial fluid. At a later stage the hyperaemic bone, no longer protected by its covering of articular cartilage, decreases in height as a result of successive trabecular fractures. Areas of hyperaemia, as well as venous stasis, are seen and cause the severe, constant night pain in later disease.

In response to the progressive breakdown of articular cartilage with loss of matrix proteoglycan and collagen and death of chondrocytes, there is a response in the residual tissue of cellular division (Rothwell and Bentley, 1973) and increased glycosaminoglycan synthesis (Mankin, 1974). Production of new type II collagen, characteristic of hyaline cartilage, has not been convincingly demonstrated although Repo and Mitchell (1971) have demonstrated increased uptake of tritiated proline after lacerative injury of articular cartilage in animals. In any event the repair response of the cartilage is never sufficient to effect repair (Bentley, 1972). Thus inevitable gradual progression of the disease occurs.

The synovial membrane and capsule

As matrix proteoglycan begins to leak out of the damaged articular cartilage, it produces direct irritation and inflammation of the synovial membrane, which undergoes hyperplasia of the lining layer and

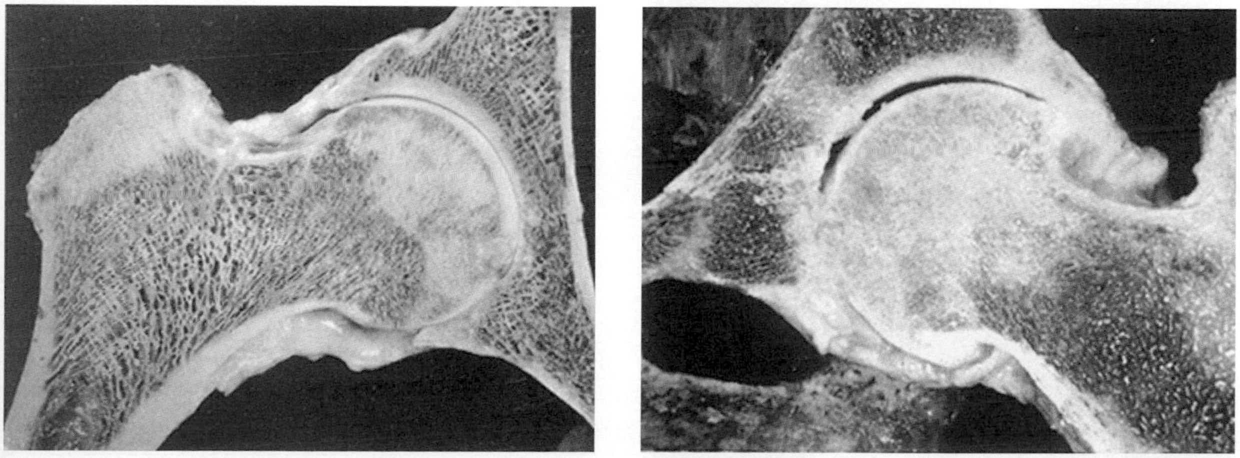

(a) (b)

Figure 11.27 (a) A normal hip in sagittal section. The healthy cartilage is thickest in the weight-bearing area. The capsule is smooth and redundant. (b) The osteoarthritic hip with incongruous seating of the femoral head in the acetabulum. The capsule is thickened and the cartilage over the femoral head is thinned.

hyperaemia. With the progressive accumulation of more cartilage and later bone debris the inflammation persists and inflammatory cells are seen in the subsynovial tissue. With the hyperplasia, the synovium is thrown into folds and villi though these are never so profuse as in rheumatoid arthritis. Fragments of cartilage and bone are engulfed by the synovial membrane and are seen in the subintima. Metaplasia of the synovium may occur with the formation of cartilage or even bone, especially at the point of attachment to the articular margins. These pedunculated masses may break off into the joint to form loose bodies or 'joint mice'. Loose fragments of cartilage and bone from the degenerating articular surface or from osteophytes may also remain free in the joint, giving rise to symptoms of 'locking'. The underlying capsule also becomes involved by the inflammatory process. As fibrosis commences in the synovium and capsule, the latter becomes thickened and shortened with resultant reduction in joint movement (Figure 11.28).

CLINICAL FEATURES

The primary generalized form of osteoarthrosis is manifested by involvement of the distal interphalangeal joints of the hands with Heberden's nodes (osteophytes) and more or less symmetrical involvement of other joints, especially the knees, metatarsophalangeal joints of the toes, the posterior spinal joints and, sometimes, the carpometacarpal joints of the hands and the elbows. Rarely, the hips may be involved also. Such patients are often first seen in a rheumatology clinic because of the hand involvement. It is important to remember that Heberden's nodes occur frequently in isolation without generalized osteoarthrosis.

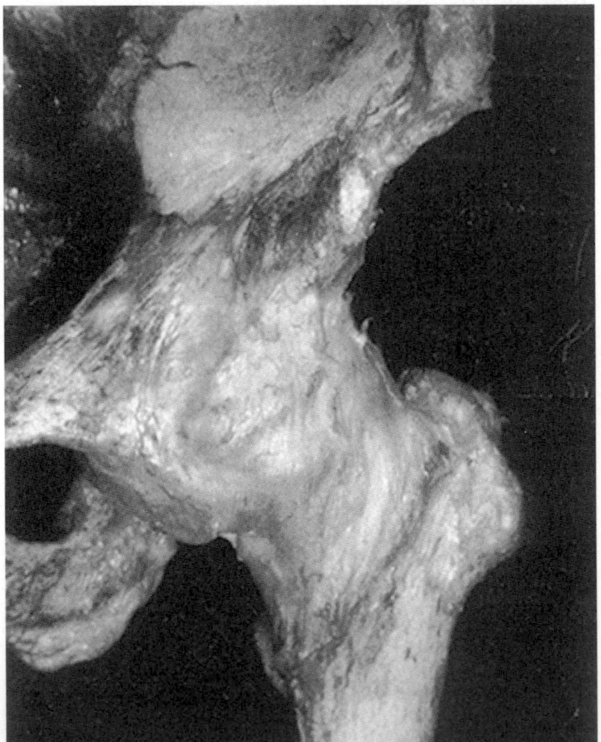

Figure 11.28 The capsule enclosing an osteoarthritic femoral head.

Primary osteoarthrosis affects most commonly the knee and hip, and is usually seen after the age of 40 years. The carpometacarpal joint of the thumb, the metatarsophalangeal joint of the great toe, the posterior spinal joints and the elbows are affected less commonly. Interestingly, primary osteoarthrosis of the ankle never occurs. The earliest symptom is low-grade aching and some stiffness experienced after rest, which is probably due to inflammation of the synovial membrane and resulting joint effusion, and disappears after some movement. As the disease progresses and the subchondral bone is exposed, pain ensues from bone collapse and friction of the surfaces. Reflex muscle spasm occurs to protect the joint from unnecessary movement which would stretch the already contracted inflamed synovium and capsule, and this also is painful. As further bone collapse and new bone formation occur there are areas of hyperaemia and venous stasis in the bony surfaces, producing severe constant pain which is unrelieved by exercise and rest. The presence of osteophytes may rarely be felt on the margins of the joint (Figure 11.29), and the crepitus, due to grating of the bony articulating surfaces on each other, is easily palpable and audible. With the muscle spasm

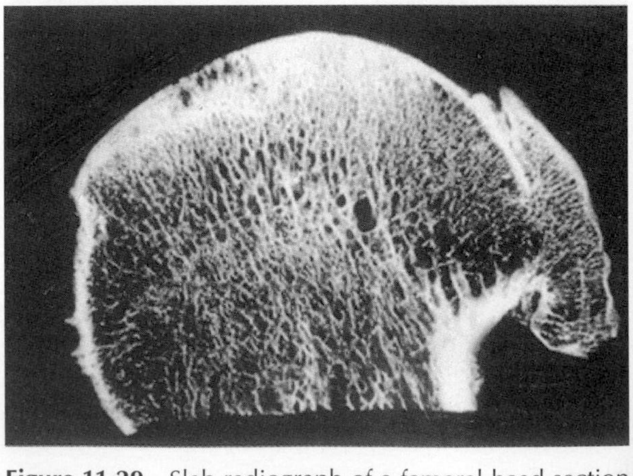

Figure 11.29 Slab radiograph of a femoral head section showing the thickening of trabeculae to meet weight-bearing stress, and cysts. New bone formation results in osteophytes outside the old subchondral bone.

and capsular contracture deformities become established; e.g. flexion, adduction and external rotation at the hip. Where extensive bone loss occurs, angular deformities result (e.g. varus at the knee).

Osteoarthritis can be more adequately controlled, and is more amenable to treatment, in its early phases, than rheumatoid arthritis. The influence of trauma is very important and not sufficiently appreciated. Injury will serve to determine the onset of arthritis in a joint in individuals who already suffer slightly from generalized arthritis. For example, an injury to the knee or the hip is likely to precipitate a troublesome form of arthritis in the injured joint. For this reason, joint injuries in arthritic persons assume an unusual importance and should be prevented or efficiently cared for.

DIFFERENTIAL DIAGNOSIS

The diagnosis of chronic arthritis is seldom difficult unless pain and swelling are limited to one joint. When the onset is acute, gout, pseudogout, rheumatic fever and infective arthritis have first to be considered. The diagnosis soon resolves itself by the course of the disease. In those aged over 50, osteoarthritis is the probable cause. In younger people it may be necessary to distinguish between rheumatoid arthritis, gouty diathesis, gonococcal arthritis and tuberculosis.

PROGNOSIS

The prognosis in osteoarthritis is governed by three factors:

1. The cause of the condition.
2. The joint affected.
3. The state of the cartilage.

TREATMENT

Weight reduction is a valuable way of reducing load through osteoarthritic joints and is an integral part of all non-operative treatment. Dietary modifications otherwise have no proven value.

Local treatment

The affected joint should be protected from injury, and extremes of movement should be prevented since they may tear the capsule or break off peripheral osteophytes into the joint. The joint, however, should not immobilized. It is also essential to prevent deformity, as the altered mechanics resulting from deformity throw added strain on related structures, and may even precipitate the development of degenerative change in other joints. This is particularly important in the hip joint, where a flexion–adduction deformity is likely to be followed by lumbar or sacroiliac joint pain. The use of a walking stick is extremely valuable in lower limb osteoarthrosis and temporary splints are useful in the upper limb joints. Active, non-weight-bearing exercises such as swimming and cycling are helpful.

Drugs which combine an analgesic with an anti-inflammatory effect are valuable in the early stages. Some of these drugs, such as aspirin, indomethacin, and flurbiprofen, reduce synovial inflammation and may slow down the progress of the disease by their 'lysosomal-stabilizing' and 'anti-prostaglandin' effects on the articular cartilage.

Operative treatment

Surgical treatment is necessary in the presence of persistent pain and progressive deformity. The decision to operate is influenced by the severity of rest pain and the number of joints involved. In cases where only one joint is seriously affected, and there is no general affection, then operation is advisable and likely to be successful. The procedures which may be adopted in osteoarthrosis are:

1. Arthrodesis – giving pain relief and stability but no mobility.
2. Juxta-articular osteotomy – giving pain relief, stability and maintaining mobility in a mobile painful joint.
3. Arthroplasty – total joint replacement, giving pain relief, stability and mobility.
4. Joint debridement and drilling – rarely.
5. Joint surface allografting.

Osteoarthritis of the hip

Primary osteoarthritis of the hip is a common disease occurring in up to 40% of the population over the age of 60. It occurs in otherwise healthy though 'ageing' individuals. It is commonest in females but is not limited solely to the older age groups and affects many individuals in the second and third decades. This is particularly so where there are obvious predisposing causes leading to secondary osteoarthrosis.

Cockin and Duthie (1971) explained why hip joints 'wear out' with ageing as follows.

They are required to undergo repetitive movements which are slow in velocity with longitudinal

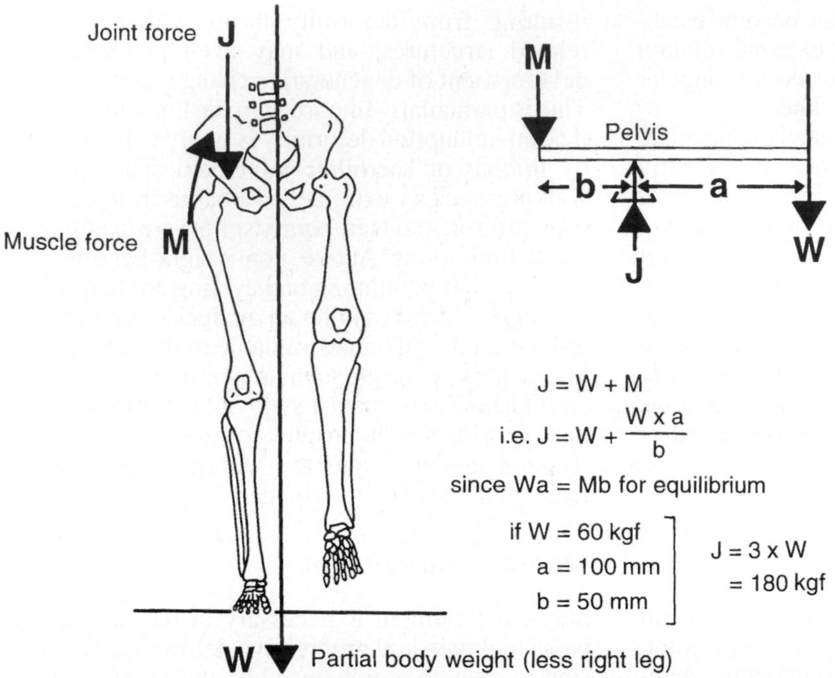

Figure 11.30 The equilibrium of the pelvis about the hip joint in one-legged stance, simplified to consider only the vertical components of force. If the partial body weight has a great lever arm about the hip joint than the abductor muscles, then the muscle force must exceed the partial body weight to achieve equilibrium. (After Denham. R.A. (1959) *Journal of Bone and Joint Surgery* **41B**, 550)

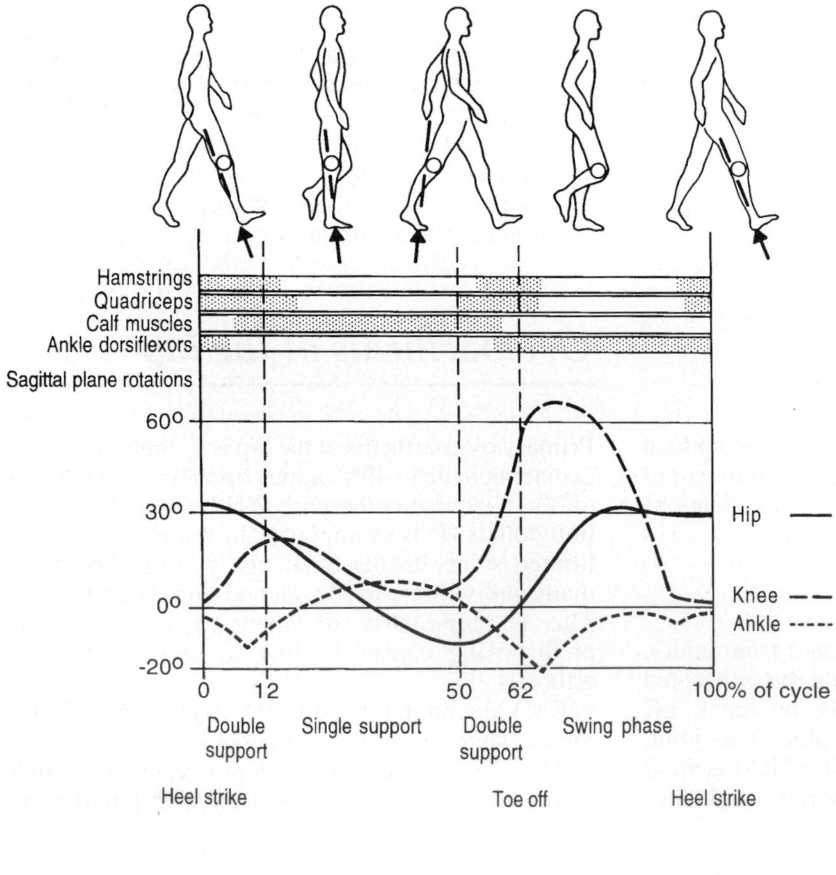

Figure 11.31 Summary of the function of the lower limb when walking. Sagittal plane movements of the joints, the direction of forces on the limb and the periods of activity of the major muscle groups are shown. The normal duration of foot contact and the 'double support' time are indicated. The force acting on the foot is normally directed just posterior to the knee joint, so it tends to flex the knee. Just as the heel leaves the ground it may be directed anterior to the joint, and thus would tend to extend it. (Courtesy of I.A.F. Stokes)

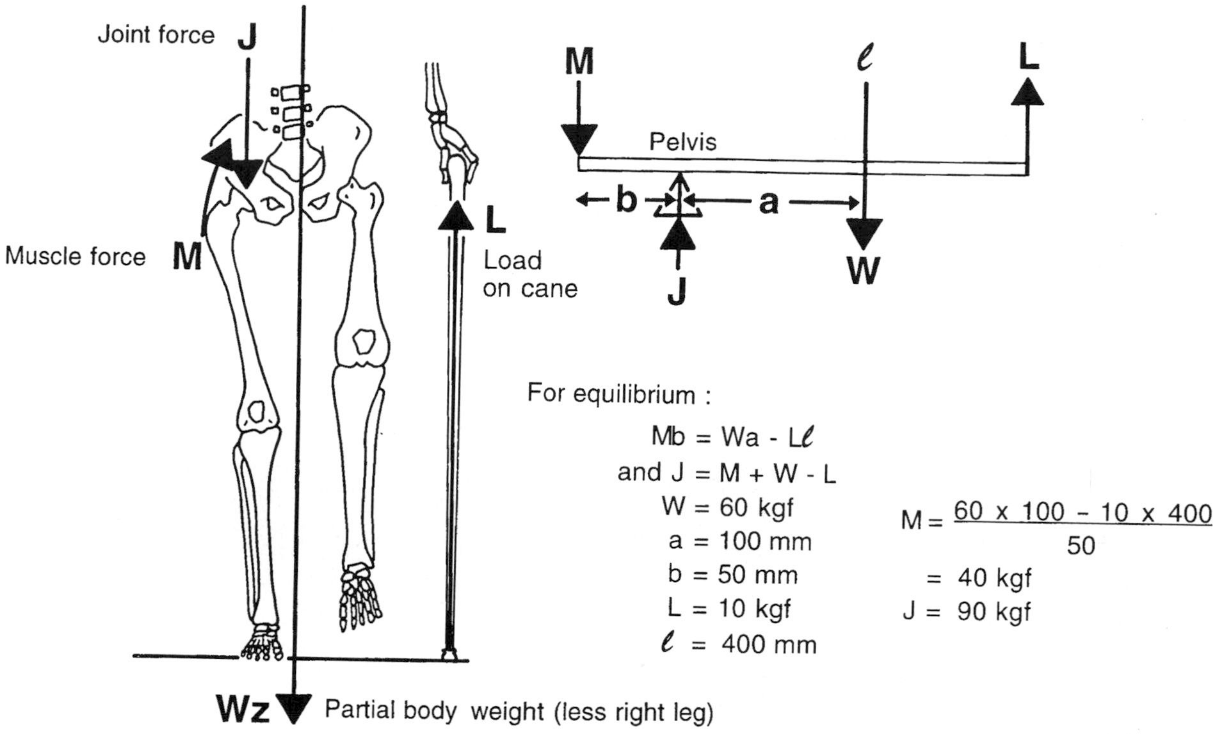

Figure 11.32 The alteration in the forces estimated in Figure 11.30 when a cane is used on the opposite side to the weight-bearing limb. A mere 10 kgf carried by the cane has reduced the hip joint force by about one-half, to 90 kgf. (Courtesy I.A.F. Stokes)

and compressive forces produced by muscle activity of a static or dynamic type and by gravitational loads of body weight.

High loadings are sustained by the hip joint because of the powerful muscles which cross it. When standing on one leg or walking, the weight of the body (excepting the supporting limb) is imposed on the hip, though not directly above it. There is a moment of this weight about the hip which must be counteracted by the abductor muscles (Figure 11.30). Other muscles, especially the gluteus medius and minimus and tensor fascia lata, are active in walking to provide propulsion (Figure 11.31). The result is a hip joint force of about three times body weight in patients after surgery (Rydell, 1966), and somewhat more in the healthy hip (Paul, 1966). Because this force is mainly due to muscle forces rather than body weight, it is not vertical, but inclined anteriorly and laterally into the femoral neck, the actual line of weight-bearing being 5 cm behind the line joining the two femoral heads (Williams and Lissner, 1962). Since the hip joint is dependent upon the distribution of the body weight above it, the type of gait can affect its magnitude. Walking with a side-to-side rocking action to swing the body weight more closely above the hip – a Trendelenburg limp – is one way of achieving this. An 'antalgic' limp which reduces the duration of loading on the affected limb is another common way of favouring a hip joint, although at the expense of the other limb. The walking stick used on the side opposite to a painful hip is an effective way of reducing the joint loading by giving an alternative support to the partial body weight otherwise balanced over the hip by the abductor muscles and reduces joint loading by 50% (Figure 11.32).

Johnston and Smidt (1969) used mechanical analyses to investigate the effects of moving the acetabulum centre, reducing the angle between the prosthesis neck and femoral shaft and transferring the greater trochanter. Significant reduction of loading on the prosthetic joint could be achieved by the surgeon by moving the acetabulum medially, inferiorly and anteriorly, by minimizing the angle of the prosthesis neck, and by lateral transfer of the greater trochanter. The disadvantages of such measures are that they tend to reduce the range of joint movement, and complicate the surgical procedures required for implantation.

In walking and climbing there is vertical movement of the body utilizing gravity through potential energies. This use of gravity as a positive force is a more efficient reservoir for energy than that of muscles with a limited energy storage. Gait depends

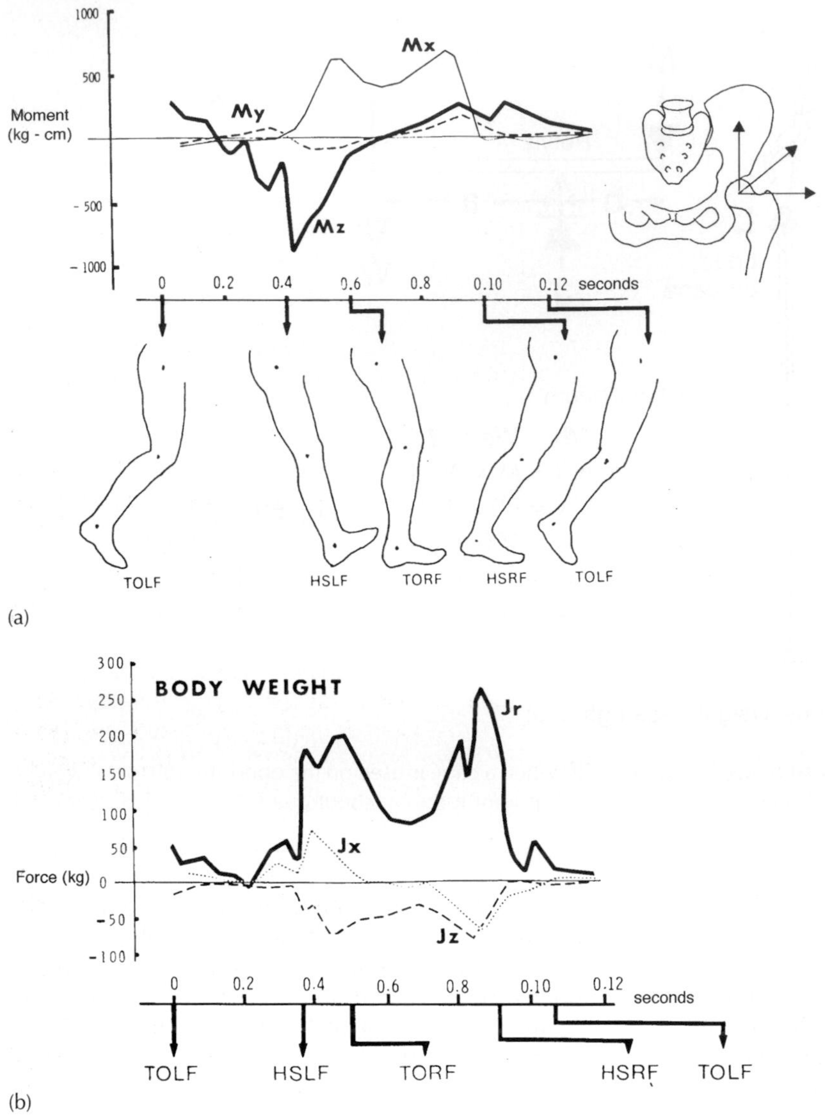

Figure 11.33 Moment relationships (a) during gait and (b) with body weight. (After Paul, J.P. (1966) *Proceedings of the Royal Society of Medicine* **59**, 943)

upon using gravity as much as possible and muscles as little as possible. Muscles are required to hold gravity by adjusting the trajectory of the body in a smooth oscillatory fashion. This smoothness is obviously disturbed with energy loss on heel impact (Figure 11.33).

Changes occur in articular geometry by reduction in surface area, symmetry and stability of joint surfaces. Damage to the supporting capsule, tendon and ligaments also alters the articular geometry. This alteration in surface size influences the force being exerted across the joint. Also, crucially, it interferes with normal lubrication of the joint which depends on the maintenance of incongruent joint surfaces for the circulation of synovial fluid.

There is decrease in the resilience of cartilage from loss of matrix proteoglycans and water caused by the release of cathepsins (especially B and D) into the matrix of the cartilage.

There are also described marked changes in the collagen fibres. Fibre width, cross-linkage and thermal contraction property are altered and there is a decrease in the susceptibility of the collagen meshwork to the collagenase. Avascularity of subchondral bone with posterosuperior collapse of the femoral head, formation of subchondral cysts, fractures of bony trabeculae with healing and compaction all lead to further incongruities of the joint.

The lubrication of the joint is severely disturbed by the alteration in joint congruity and alteration of viscosity of the fluid due to the joint effusion.

The disease appears to represent a balance between localized abnormal stresses and the ability of the joint tissues to repair. It is important to emphasize that repair of joints never occurs in osteoarthrosis but there is a feeble proliferation of cells and an increase

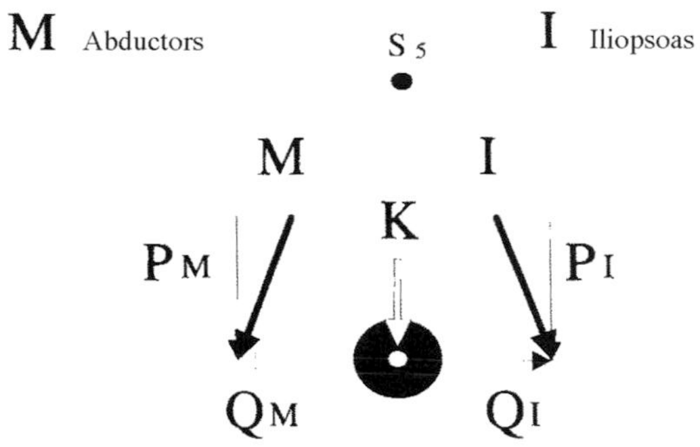

Figure 11.34 The resultant forces of the abductor muscles M, and of the iliopsoas I, are vectors caudolaterally and caudomedially. The normal weight-bearing surface (WBS) is horizontal and therefore those vectors are resolved into vertical components P_M and P_I. Q_M, expulsion force on the head; Q_I, centring force; K, body weight less the weight of the supporting limb, which is centred above the centre of rotation. The quadratus lumborum of the opposite side acts synchronously with the iliopsoas. (Reproduced, with permission from, Bombelli, B. (1993) *Structure and Function in Normal and Abnormal Hips*, 3rd Edition, Springer Verlag: Berlin, London)

in matrix proteoglycan production in response to cartilage breakdown and this may explain periods of lessened symptoms during the progression of the disease. In their study of 400 cases of degenerative arthritis of the hip, Pearson and Riddell (1962) found that only 7 hips became painless spontaneously and none improved radiologically.

Bombelli (1993) has described additional biomechanical features. To balance the body through one foot on the ground on the ipsilateral side the abductors and the ibiacus balance the pelvis, but on the contralateral side the psoas and quadratus lumborum shift the centre of gravity to above the centre of rotation in the femoral head (Figure 11.34).

There are four hip parameters:

1. The orientation of the pelvis when horizontal, the muscle equilibrium is within the weight-bearing surface (WBAS).
2. The inclination of the abductors 'M'.
3. The inclination of the iliacus and psoas 'I'.
4. The anatomical sphericity of the head of the femur.

The weight-bearing surface can be inclined abnormally craniolaterally or craniomedially. When the hip becomes painful this is seen as:

1. An antalgic gait – trunk muscles help iliopsoas to shift centre of gravity; or
2. A Duchenne gait – (short leg) gliding function; or
3. A Trendelenburg gait – (the trunk muscles contribute to shift the body weight but the pelvic tilt reverses the direction).

PATHOLOGY

The normal hip is dislocated only with difficulty. Atmospheric pressure provides a seal, as suggested by Ferguson and Semlak (1970). The ligamentum teres is not an obstacle to dislocation; it is an elongated structure lying loosely coiled in the inferior recesses of the joint with no pressure from the articular surfaces. The capsule is also relatively loose, allowing retraction of the femoral head from the acetabulum once the cohesive tension of the concentric hip joint is broken. When the hip is hyperextended or internally rotated, the capsule tightens and it is easy to see how rigidity of the capsule limits hip motion. Load-bearing occurs below the zenith of the femoral head in a circular band, the 'round' head fitting incongruously in the arch-shaped acetabulum.

The articular cartilage is thickest over the area of maximum weight-bearing on both the acetabulum and the femoral head. It is very resistant to compression and shearing stresses by virtue of the criss-cross pattern of collagen fibres which are bound deeply into the subchondral bone and blend with a thin layer of finer fibres near the surface of the cartilage. This thin layer forms the 'lamina splendens' seen on polarized light microscopy. The collagen meshwork is supported by the osmotic pressure of the proteoglycan molecules intertwined within the cartilage which draw in water by their negative charge. Thus, 70% of articular cartilage is water. It follows that loss of the matrix and water leads to loss of resilience of the cartilage and to splitting of the superficial collagen fibres. Whether this occurs primarily due to release of cathepsins from the lysosomes of the chondrocytes which digest and break up the proteoglycans is not clear. Primary fatigue failure of the superficial collagen has been proposed by Freeman (1980) as an alternative mechanism for cartilage breakdown. The surface of the cartilage has many microscopic grooves which are important for the complex lubrication mechanisms involving the binding of hyaluronic acid to the surface. Lubrication depends on the maintenance of incongruity of the joint surfaces and if the surfaces become more congruent there is a danger of lubrication failure and cartilage surface damage. A sharply defined basophilic line seen on histological sections separates the deep layer of the cartilage (zone III) from the calcified zone IV and the subchondral bone. This is a calcification front and in early osteoarthrosis it may be breached by blood vessels which initiate calcification in the zone III cartilage (Figure 11.35).

EARLY CHANGES

The first observed change in the cartilage is a loss of the white, glistening appearance of the surface, which becomes duller and yellowish. Histologically the upper layers of the cartilage show loss of matrix staining, with metachromatic stains and superficial cell death, with slight fibrillation of the surface collagen fibres. The electron microscopic appearances are of disorganized and fractured collagen fibrils and many dead cells (Figure 11.36). This process begins in the areas which do not habitually take full load and then spreads later to the weight-bearing areas, especially superiorly (Harrison *et al.*, 1953). Hence, the first radiological change observed is narrowing of the joint space, followed closely by osteophyte formation and subchondral bone sclerosis as the disease progresses.

As articular cartilage damage develops and spreads, there is a feeble response of the cartilage to produce new cells (Rothwell and Bentley, 1973) and new matrix (Mankin and Lippiello, 1970) but this is never sufficient to effect repair. Fragments of cartilage break off into the joint and produce a synovitis due to a direct irritant effect of chondroitin sulphate on the synovial membrane. Also, the primitive mesenchymal cells at the margins of the joint in the synovial reflections are stimulated by the synovitis and collagen fragments to produce new cartilage and bone as outgrowths of the femoral head and acetabulum. Thus extracapital osteophytes are produced. Indeed, the amount of cartilage debris is greater in the inferior part of the joint than in the superior and thus the inferior osteophyte is usually larger than the superior on a radiograph.

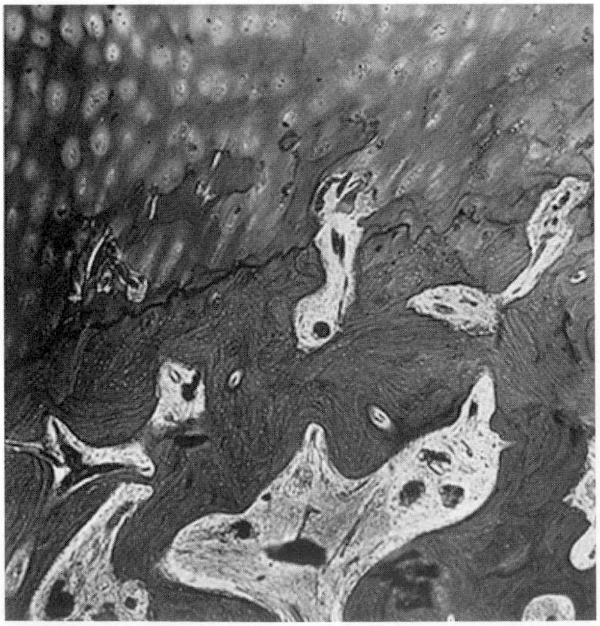

Figure 11.35 Blood vessels progressing through the 'tidemark' to enter the articular cartilage.

The lubrication of the joint is severely impaired by loss of cartilage substance, by fragments of cartilage in the joint and by the effusion of fluid into the joint from the inflamed synovial membrane.

The subchondral bone in the weight-bearing zones is thus exposed and cannot withstand the stresses imposed directly upon it. Fractures of the bony trabeculae occur and these may result in areas of bone necrosis and cysts. As a response there is new bone formation, and the appearances of bone collapse and new bone formation are seen on radiographs as increased density or 'sclerosis'. The thickened bony surface becomes polished, or eburnated, by movement. The 'tidemark' becomes less distinct, particularly at the periphery of the head, and ossification progresses in the base of the cartilage, producing so-called 'intracapital' osteophytes (Figure 11.37). Harrison *et al.* (1953) suggested that this ossification was a response to poor nourishment of the overlying cartilage due to habitual underuse. Cysts may occur or become enlarged also as a result of increased intra-articular pressure and the driving of joint fluid through small cracks in the damaged subchondral bone (Landells, 1953). Fracture callus and cartilage tissue are seen in the femoral head below the eburnated surface in the weight-bearing zones. Cysts appear to develop as a result of degeneration within the repair callus and communicate with the surface as it is worn down. Small cysts may coalesce to form larger cysts within the line of load-bearing of the femoral head and the acetabulum (Figure 11.38).

Where the marrow cavity is exposed to the surface, highly cellular granulation tissue emerges and, under the combined influence of movement and load-bearing, undergoes metaplasia to fibrocartilage. Tufts of fibrocartilage are seen scattered over the surface of the joint, but a complete confluent covering layer cannot be produced because of the constant destructive action of load-bearing. This tissue may form a useful continuous layer over the original cartilage defect if load-bearing is reduced by altering the mechanics of the joint by, for example, femoral intertrochanteric osteotomy. This tissue may resemble hyaline cartilage but does not contain type II collagen and usually degenerates slowly over a period of time.

With progression of the disease, the osteophytes on the medial and posterior aspects of the femoral head and acetabulum continue to enlarge and extend downwards towards the femoral neck. In some cases, additional osteophytes stud the femoral neck, formed

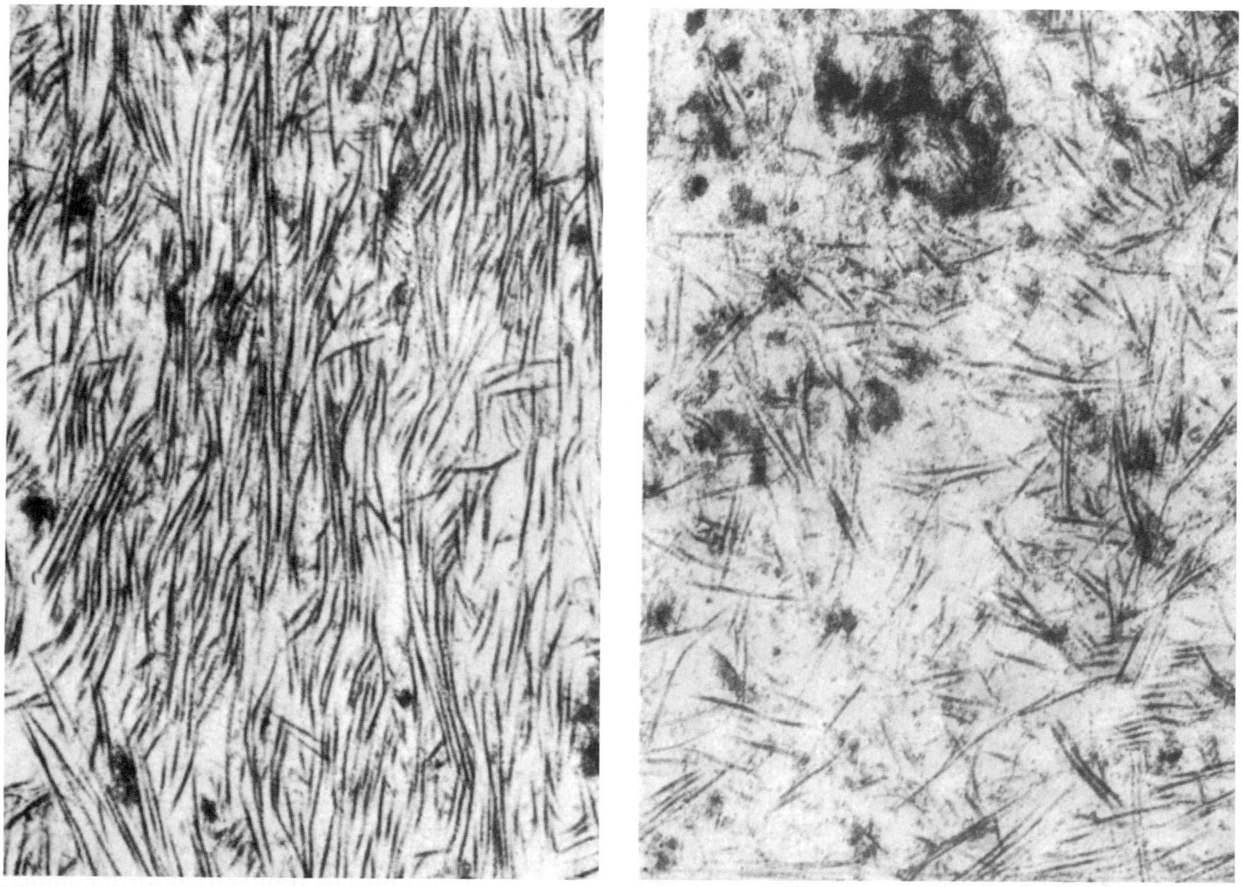

(a) (b)

Figure 11.36 Transmission electron micrographs of: (a) a section cut tangential to the synovial surface in intact cartilage, showing the orderly arrangement of surface collagen fibres; and (b) a section cut tangential to the synovial surface in early cartilage degeneration, showing abnormally wide separation of the surface collagen fibres suggestive of increased water content. (Reproduced, with permission, from Meachim, G. (1980) in *The Aetiopathogenesis of Osteoarthrosis*, edited by G. Nuki. Pitman Medical: Tunbridge Wells)

by the extracapital process (Figure 11.39). Thus the shape of the femoral head and of the acetabulum are changed and the large inferior osteophyte tends to push the head superolaterally into a more subluxed position.

The capsule of the joint becomes increasingly inflamed and thickened by the underlying fibrosis. This leads to the restricted motion characteristic of the late stages of osteoarthrosis and the characteristic deformity of adduction, external rotation and flexion, this being the position of the hip where the joint cavity pressure is least. Stretching of the capsule by exercise and movement will cause pain and tearing with consequently greater fibrosis. Although small fragments of articular cartilage are taken up and phagocytosed by the synovial membrane in established disease, the fragments of cartilage and bone can be seen engulfed in the membrane and maintaining inflammation.

The four characteristic radiographic changes of osteoarthrosis – joint space narrowing, osteophyte formation, sclerosis and cysts in the subchondral bone – thus occur in sequence in response to loss of articular cartilage. The repair response in the joint is inadequate to cope with the breakdown and spontaneous healing does not occur.

SYMPTOMATOLOGY

The usual first complaint is of an ache in the hip (probably due to synovitis) felt particularly in the early morning, and at the same time there is some limitation of movement. These gradually wear off in the course of the day but as the disease progresses they become more and more frequent. Later, a prominent feature is the deformity, initially the result of muscular spasm. The thigh is flexed, adducted and

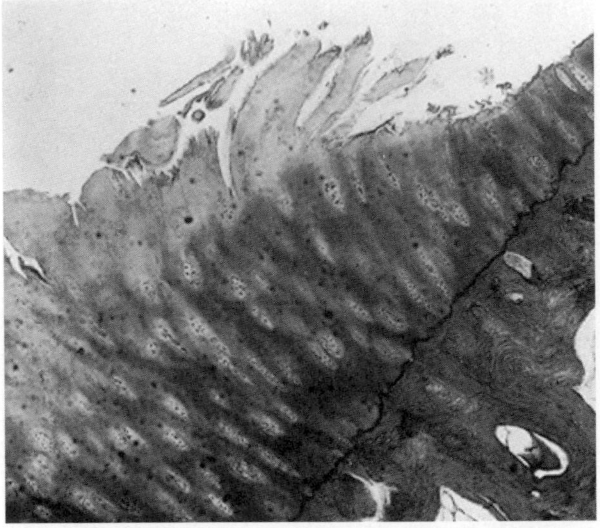

Figure 11.37 Fibrillated cartilage at the edge of the initial lesion. The dark line separating the cartilage from the subchondral bone is known as 'the tidemark'.

externally rotated, and the resulting shortening causes the patient to limp. The deformity has another effect – of placing the lumbar spine and the sacroiliac joints at a mechanical disadvantage and producing pain. As the hip becomes more and more stiff, flexion is progressively limited and sitting is difficult and uncomfortable. Dressing and undressing become difficult, and bathing and pedicure become impossible. With the continued progress of the disease, deformity increases and stiffness in a bad position results. The pain increases in severity, restricting walking to a short distance and becomes present at rest, disturbing sleep.

The pain of osteoarthrosis arises from the inflamed and thickened synovial membrane and capsule, and is aggravated by tears in the capsule produced by movement. Reflex muscle spasm is also painful. Despite the inability to demonstrate nerve fibres by histological staining in subchondral bone, there is little doubt that pain emanates from the irregular and eburnated joint surfaces which can be felt and heard to be grating.

The deformities of the hip are seen in three main patterns:

1. In 80% there is an adduction, external rotation and flexion deformity with joint space narrowing, cysts and sclerosis in the superior segment of the femoral head and acetabulum. There is a somewhat valgus position of the femoral neck and a bony buttress develops on the inferior aspect of the neck (Wiberg, 1939).
2. In 10% there is external rotation of the femur but the leg is in neutral or slightly abducted. The radiological changes are seen mostly in the medial segment of the joint and there is a varus deformity of the femoral neck. Pearson and Riddell (1962) thought that the deformities were due to muscle spasm and secondary capsular contracture.
3. In a further 10% there is concentric loss of cartilage space on the radiographs, and the deformity is of flexion and slight abduction. The appearances may be similar to those of rheumatoid arthritis except that there is hypertrophy of bone rather than atrophy with subchondral sclerosis.

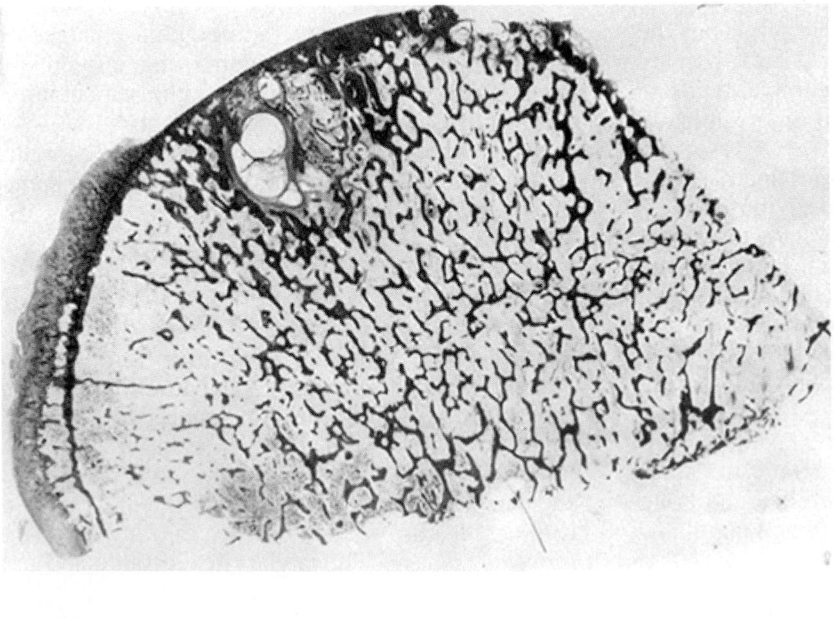

Figure 11.38 Section of femoral head showing eburnated subchondral bone with the overlying cartilage removed. Beneath this area cyst formation begins in the femoral head. The cartilage is fibrillated at the edge of the denuded bone and osteophyte formation begins away from this area.

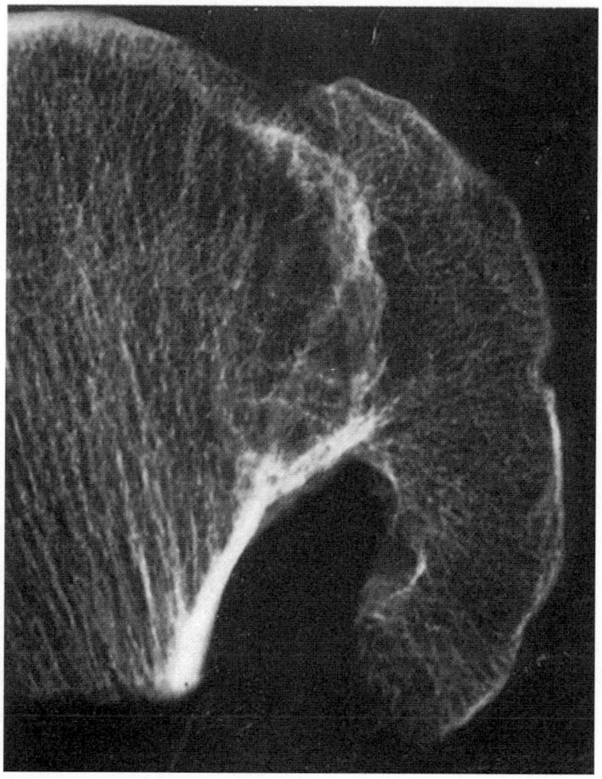

Figure 11.39 Osteophyte formation exterior to the femoral head.

PROGNOSIS

The disease is a progressive one. However, careful attention to mechanical factors, including the use of a walking stick in the opposite hand, analgesic and anti-inflammatory drugs and active exercises, will reduce the symptoms in approximately 30% of cases.

LOCAL TREATMENT

If the patient is seen in the early stages and pain is the pronounced feature, rest is the first requirement, not only to alleviate the pain but also to prevent progressive flexion and adduction of the limb. Therefore, while the symptoms are severe and pain and muscular spasm are present, reduction of activities and the use of a stick are indicated. Use within limits, short of irritating the joint, is desirable in maintaining function. If such exercise produces pain which is persistent and lasts for a period after the activity ceases or comes on at night sufficiently to interrupt sleep, then it is apparent that the joint has been used too freely. Muscle training by non-weight-bearing exercises should be encouraged and a heel-raise may relieve pain by reducing limp. If joint destruction is not severe, gentle manipulation of the hip under general anaesthetic may reduce pain.

OPERATIVE TREATMENT

General indications

Pain unrelieved by conservative treatment is the predominant indication for operation in osteoarthrosis of the hip. *Limitation of movement* is much less disturbing to the patient if only one joint is affected, though it is important when both are involved in the process and in such a case some form of surgery is usually indicated to prevent complete crippledom. *Flexion – adduction deformity* is a third indication in the monarticular case where there is a pelvic tilt and distortion of the lumbar spine producing pain and, eventually, degenerative spondylosis.

Contraindications

These are mainly due to the general condition and age of the patient. Surgery is major but with modern anaesthesia it is rare for a patient who requires operative treatment to be unable to withstand the operation. A full assessment of the patient from the cardiorespiratory point of view, together with the exclusion of any potential sources of infection such as the renal tract, are necessary before operation is undertaken.

The choice of operation will depend upon the age, sex, general condition, build and occupation of the patient. Clinically, three types of individuals present for treatment:

1. The youthful patient in the third and fourth decade with a unilateral affection of the hip. Often there is a history of early pain in the hip and the radiological appearances suggest old trauma to the epiphysis, a dysplastic hip or possibly old Perthes' disease. The femoral head may be large and misshapen and the acetabulum may be deficient. Such patients represent a considerable challenge and the correct treatment for this particular type of patient is not yet clear.
2. A group of patients in which there is bilateral hip disease, which may or may not be part of a generalized primary osteoarthrosis (Stecher, 1965).
3. The patient is older and often the disease is monarticular.

Arthrodesis of the hip

Arthrodesis is now largely of historical interest in the

management of primary osteoarthrosis though it may be indicated rarely in cases of secondary osteoarthrosis due to trauma in the young male patient. Although claims were made that the procedure did not cause disability in later life, it is now apparent that a considerable proportion of patients have complaints of low back pain and develop spondylosis, and the efficiency of walking with a fused hip is much less than that of a hip treated by arthroplasty.

The operation is probably best carried out by an intra-articular type of arthrodesis of the Watson-Jones type in which the articular surfaces are excised and shaped to match one another and the hip is secured by a transarticular nail. In addition, a pelvic graft is screwed superiorly across the arthrodesis to give additional stability and to increase the rate of fusion. Bony fusion may be expected in 94% of cases, and painless knee movement to 90° or more of flexion occurs in 91%. With the obvious disability that arises over many years following an arthrodesis of the hip it is best to restrict this procedure to a young male who carries out a heavy occupation and requires stability of the hip and freedom of pain as priorities. The advances in reconstructive procedures of the hip will probably make this operation obsolete in due course.

Juxta-articular osteotomy

For many years the intertrochanteric displacement osteotomy of the McMurray type (1939) was the mainstay of treatment of the arthritic hip in which there was 90° of flexion and a few degrees of rotation together with the radiological appearance of good bone structure in the hip. Many reviews indicated that the good results of this procedure could be as high as 80% (Osborne and Fahrini, 1949; Ferguson, 1964) but the predictability of this operation was always a problem. Although internal fixation was improved by the use of compression devices, it was found that the best results were generally achieved when the femoral head displaced into some degree of varus, thus removing the heavily loaded superior segment of the femoral head from major weight-bearing. There was undoubted formation of fibrocartilage on the denuded area as described by Bentley (1972) and Byers (1974) but the development of effective replacement arthroplasty has made this operation less favoured.

A major indication for juxta-articular osteotomy is in the vigorous younger patient under age 50 with radiologically early osteoarthrosis who maintains 90° of flexion of the hip and a few degrees of rotation and who, because of the nature of his occupation, requires high stability and strength in the hip (Figure 11.40).

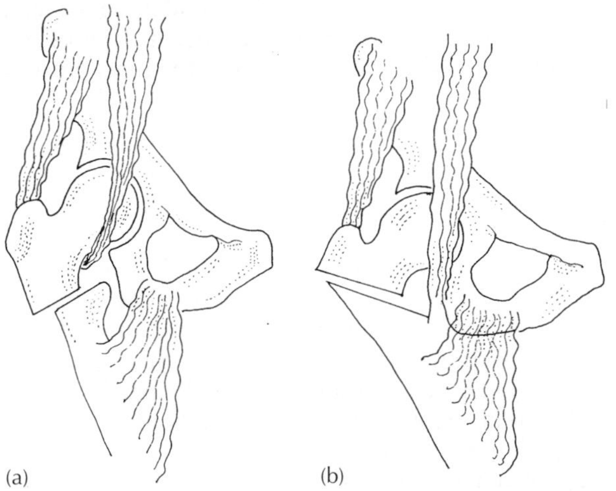

(a) (b)

Figure 11.40 (a) The effect of a displacement osteotomy by relaxing the iliopsoas and adductor muscles, and the upward movement of the greater trochanter to accompany the inward rotation of the neck and head with foreshortening of gluteus medius muscle. (b) Pauwels' varus osteotomy with resection of a small wedge of bone in the upper aspect of a femur and the resultant muscle relations and alteration in articulating surfaces.

Ferguson's rotational osteotomy

The McMurray displacement has the disadvantages of occasional non-union and production of hip mechanics leading to a lurching gait. Both these disadvantages can be overcome by simple internal rotation of the distal fragment by an osteotomy done in the same area. Internal fixation is used to avoid unnecessary immobilization of the patient. Ferguson (1964) described the use of this operation in early osteoarthritis while there is still sufficient anatomy of the femoral head left to save the joint with reasonable expectation of good function and a good result – i.e. patients having 70–90° of flexion under anaesthesia. Rotation may not be present. Twenty degrees of abduction is helpful.

Pauwels' varus adduction osteotomy

Pauwels (1951) reviewed in detail this procedure (Figure 11.40b) and explained the excellent results it achieved by causing:

1. A reduction in the muscle forces by relaxing the adductors, the abductors and iliopsoas (which is divided).
2. A reduction in the static forces by moving the greater trochanter away from the head – the length of the lever arm has been increased.
3. Increase in the articular surface for weight-bearing.

Bombelli (1993) with his three-dimensional, engineering analysis of the osteoarthritic hip has claimed that pelvic and intertrochanteric osteotomies are still reliable operations, not only for relieving the symptoms of pain, often the deformity, but also for the young patient to utilize his/her own bone structures before being replaced by artificial material in 10–15 years' time.

Pelvic osteotomy

This is indicated for pain in the young patient, when the weight-bearing surface WBS is sloping, and the femoral head is spherical. It is also of value to give further acetabular cover for the femoral head, to make the WBS line horizontal, or to increase the contact area. Acetabuloplasty by a shelf operation – the 'tennis racket type' – or pelvic and innominate osteotomies, all have a place.

Intertrochanteric osteotomy

Bombelli describes this operation as indicated for abnormal geometry (congenital or acquired) for the overuse type (high dynamic force or overweight) for the mechanical type of OA in unilateral cases and in relatively young patients (below 50 years of age). The biological reaction is usually normotrophic or hypertrophic. In general the 'spherical head' morphology requires a varus osteotomy and the 'elliptical head' morphology a valgus extension osteotomy.

The valgus-extension osteotomy

This operation is indicated with an elliptical shaped femoral head in contact with a craniolateral inclined pelvic weight-bearing surface level. Osteophyte formation requires analysis so that it does not reduce the efficacy of the osteotomy. Bombelli believes that relief of pain and deformity results from:

1. Stretching of the ligaments and its synovial sheath as well as the superior joint capsule.
2. Shifting the CR (centre of rotation) medially.
3. Roof 'osteophyte' forms or hypertrophies to reduce the extruding force.

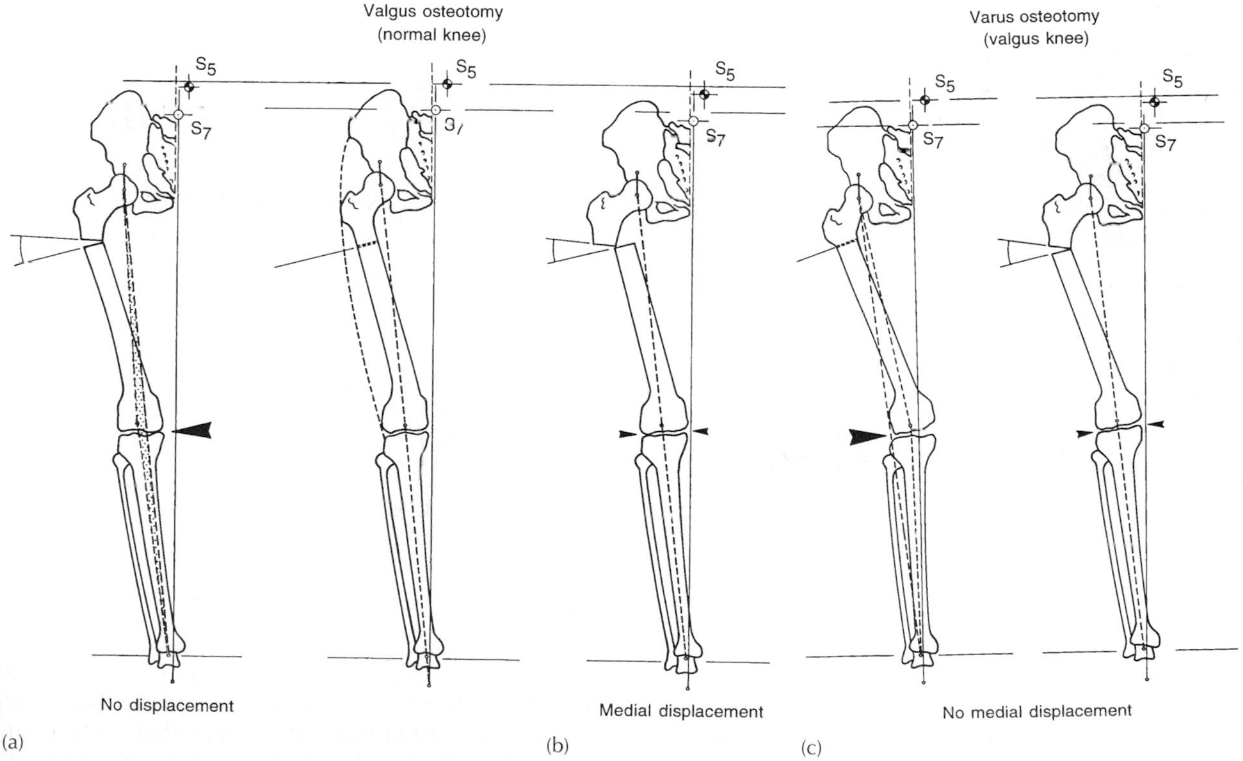

Figure. 11.41 (a) A valgus osteotomy: when carried out in the presence of a normal knee, the shaft should be displaced laterally to avoid excessive strain/stress in the lateral compartment. (b) The medial displacement with elevation and rotation of the femoral head into varus will balance the knee joint stress. (c) If carried out with a valgus deformity of the knee and lateral displacement is not also carried out, it may well be necessary to carry out a supracondylar osteotomy to prevent deterioration of the lateral compartment of the knee. (Bombelli, 1993)

4. The extension part reducing the risk of anterior subluxation of the head.
5. All of these reducing the unit load, producing a more horizontal weight-bearing surface, reducing the compressive forces and improving the hydraulic mechanism.

Consideration of the effect of this operation on leg length and on the likelihood of producing valgus or varus of the knee is essential (Figures 11.41, 11.42).

The varus osteotomy

This is indicated in OA when the head is spherical with a valgus neck, when the weight-bearing surface level is horizontal or craniolateral inclined. It is the most successful of all osteotomies carried out and works by shifting the greater and lesser trochanters upwardly, reducing the tension of the abductors and iliopsoas and therefore vertical compression forces. It improves the Trendelenburg gait pattern. However, it can shorten the leg. The medial displacement of the femoral shaft, by moving the mechanical axis of the lower limb through the centre of the normal knee, helps to prevent the development of arthritis in the medial joint compartment (Figure 11.43).

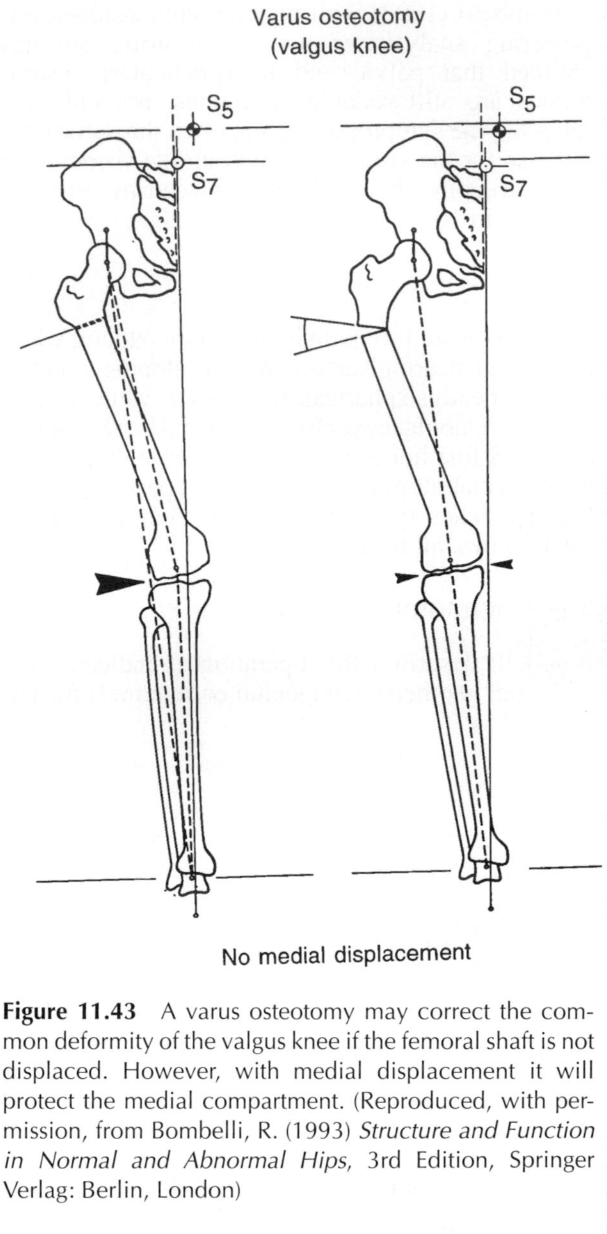

Figure 11.43 A varus osteotomy may correct the common deformity of the valgus knee if the femoral shaft is not displaced. However, with medial displacement it will protect the medial compartment. (Reproduced, with permission, from Bombelli, R. (1993) *Structure and Function in Normal and Abnormal Hips*, 3rd Edition, Springer Verlag: Berlin, London)

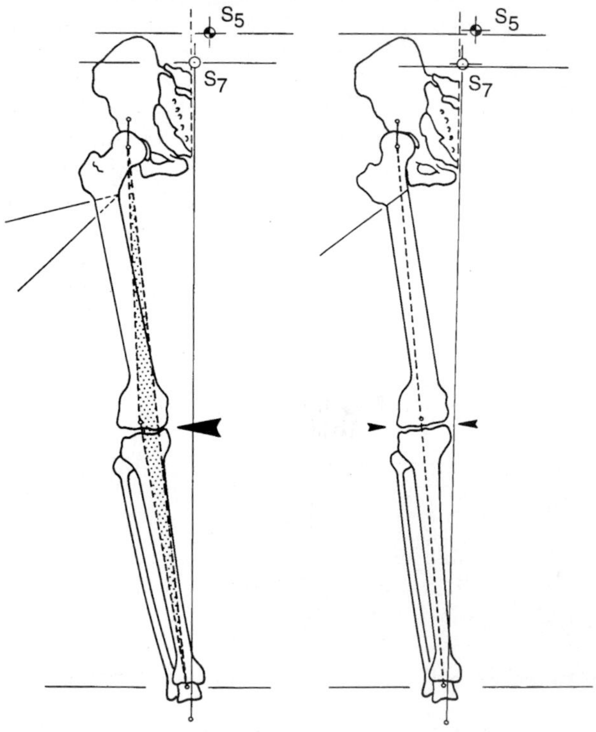

Figure 11.42 When a valgus osteotomy is carried out with the knee in varus, which is quite common, no displacement is necessary to correct the varus and reduce stress through the knee. (Bombelli, 1993)

Trochanteric osteotomy

As seen in a Voss osteotomy, this operation reduces the load on the femoral head by increasing the lever arm of the abductors and makes them more horizontal in action. Bombelli emphasizes that the lateral and distal shift should only reach as far as the level of the femoral head centre of rotation point, for greatest effect.

Nishina *et al.* (1990) described their results after Chiari pelvic osteotomy for early osteoarthritis in a dysplastic hip. Satisfactory results were obtained in nearly all cases with a normal or torn acetabular labrum, but when there was a detached labrum only 50% were satisfactory because of clinical failure. They therefore recommend other operations should be considered.

Werners *et al.* (1990) in a survivorship analysis of patients having had an osteotomy for osteoarthritis of the hip from our centre, found that, 10 years after the osteotomy, 47% had required no further surgery, and after 20 years 23% still had not required a hip replacement. The best results were found in hips with moderate arthritis. Varus angular osteotomies with medial displacement showed the longer survival.

Maistrelli *et al.* (1990) in reviewing 277 valgus extension osteotomies over a 10–15 year follow-up found that 67% were good or excellent. The better results were obtained in patients under 40 years with a unilateral, mechanical type of osteoarthritis, an elliptical femoral head, minimal subluxation and a good range of preoperative motion. There was radiographic evidence of improvement of the arthritis in 39% of the hips.

Total hip replacement after McMurray's intertrochanteric osteotomy, when carried out as a secondary procedure, requires extensive soft tissue dissection to obtain near normal hip mechanics as well as a trochanteric osteotomy (Nagi and Dhillon, 1991). These authors achieved marked improvement in pain and function with no cases receiving a femoral shaft fracture intraoperatively.

Arthroplasty

Arthroplasty of the hip may be achieved by:

1. Interposition (cup) arthroplasty
2. Excisional arthroplasty
3. Total replacement arthroplasty.

Mould arthroplasty

The original Smith-Petersen Vitallium cup arthroplasty was modified by Aufranc (1967), who reported relief of disabling pain in 85% of patients – including 25% with complete relief of pain, 25% with unlimited walking and a need for supplementary revision surgery of only 10% of cases.

Whilst there is no doubt that the good results of this operation were very satisfactory and had the great advantage of longevity, sometimes lasting for 30 years, the period of postoperative mobilization and exercises was very prolonged – as was the period of non-weight-bearing, which would be for up to 3 months. Furthermore, the operation was unpredictable and in most series the revision rate for development of painful 'high spots' was in the order of 20%. This operation has been largely superseded by replacement arthroplasty.

Girdlestone pseudarthrosis

This operation (Girdlestone, 1924) is no longer carried out as a primary procedure for osteoarthrosis of the hip. It is still a valuable procedure following failure of a replacement arthroplasty, and the results after failure for loosening or infection of a total hip replacement arthroplasty are good since there is considerable fibrosis around the hip and, therefore, more stability than seen in a primary case.

Girdlestone described a complete resection of the femoral head and neck down to the base of the trochanters, as well as the superior acetabular margin, so that there is a symmetrical surface between the pelvic surface and the sloping trochanteric line. It has been found that stability is often lost with this form of pseudarthrosis, which then necessitates the wearing of an ischial-bearing brace, particularly in an obese patient. Stability can be improved sometimes by performing a Batchelor or a Milch angulation osteotomy at the same time, with tilting of the femoral fragment in a more horizontal plane up against the side of the ilium.

Total hip replacement arthroplasty

In 1966 McKee and Watson-Farrar described a Vitallium metal-to-metal hip replacement prosthesis. This prosthesis was inserted in many thousands of patients, but as time passed it became apparent that the relatively high friction led to loosening in many cases (Bentley and Duthie, 1973). Total hip arthroplasties are composed of a high-density polyethylene cup and a stainless steel, Vitallium or titanium femoral component. The friction in this prosthesis is much less than in a metal-to-metal one but, interestingly, is still approximately six times higher than that of a normal hip joint. The Charnley prosthesis has led the field and the results have been reviewed on several occasions. In 1972, in a review of 379 primary Charnley prostheses performed between November 1962 and 1965 and followed for between 4 and 7 years, Charnley reported relief of pain and excellent ability to walk in 90% of patients (infection rate was 3.8%: 1.6% early and 2.2% late). Loosening occurred in only 1.34% when the acetabular sockets were cemented in position and average wear of the polyethylene socket was 0.13 mm per year. Non-union of the trochanter occurred in 4.2% and extopic ossification in 5%.

In a review of a further series of 547 patients operated on between 1967 and 1968 and followed up for a period of 8.3 years, the results were maintained at the same high level (Griffith *et al.*, 1978a). In this study, stringent radiological criteria were applied to the results in an attempt to identify features on the radiographs which might indicate incipient mechanical failure at the cement/bone interface. On clinical assessment, 86% were free of pain and 11% had slight discomfort. In patients with unilateral disease, 85% had normal function, and in bilateral disease 78%. Deep infection occurred in 2.2%. Cavitation of the calcar occurred in 4.5%, demarcation of the cement in the femur in 7.9% and subsidence of the femoral component in 8.9%. However, only 0.91% showed loosening and only 5 femoral prostheses fractured during the study. Socket demarcation – i.e. a radiolucent zone between the radiopaque cement and the condensed layer of the cancellous bone of the acetabulum – was seen to some degree in 53.7% but socket loosening ensued only when demarcation was in excess of 2 mm wide and actually occurred in only 0.55%. Over all, 2.18% of mechanical failures could be attributed to failure of the cement/bone interface. Signs of incipient failure were present in 12% of cases. The average rate of wear in this series of polyethelene sockets was 0.07 mm per year (Griffith *et al.*,1978b). Death from pulmonary embolism was 0.9% but no anticoagulant prophylaxis was employed.

Thus, the results indicate that the Charnley type of total hip replacement prosthesis gives a very high level of success – in the region of 95% for unilateral hip disease and 85% for bilateral hip disease where the technique and operating conditions are optimal. Numerous later studies have confirmed this (Bentley, 1994).

With the passage of time it is becoming apparent that the major complication of hip replacement arthroplasty is not wear or toxicity of the wear products but loosening of the prosthesis at the junction between the methylmethacrylate bone cement and the bone itself. In particular, loosening of the femoral component may occur and sinking of the prosthesis in the femoral shaft (Figure 11.44). Controversy exists as to the requirement for loading the calcar of the femur with the prosthesis but the consensus is that it is better to use a prosthesis which loads the calcar rather than one which relies on transmission of stress entirely through the cement to the bone of the calcar femorale. Where loosening of the proximal end of the femoral prosthesis occurs, breakage follows due to fatigue-failure of the metal. This may very well be reduced by avoiding removal of the greater trochanter and thus obtaining better fixation of the prosthesis in the upper part of the femoral shaft (Figure 11.45). Similarly, the radiological appearances of resorption of the calcar of the femoral neck are seen as predisposing to loosening, although in Charnley's series the incidence of calcar resorption was low and such patients did not all develop loosening. Only further long-term follow-up will determine which factors are important in the prevention of loosening of the total hip replacement prosthesis.

A notable failure of total hip replacement has been in its use for too-young patients who have hip dysplasia. In this group of patients the combination of poor bone stock in the acetabulum and poor muscle development appears to predispose the patient to poor functional results and loosening of the prosthesis.

Newer types of total hip replacement arthroplasty

At this time there is no prosthesis which gives

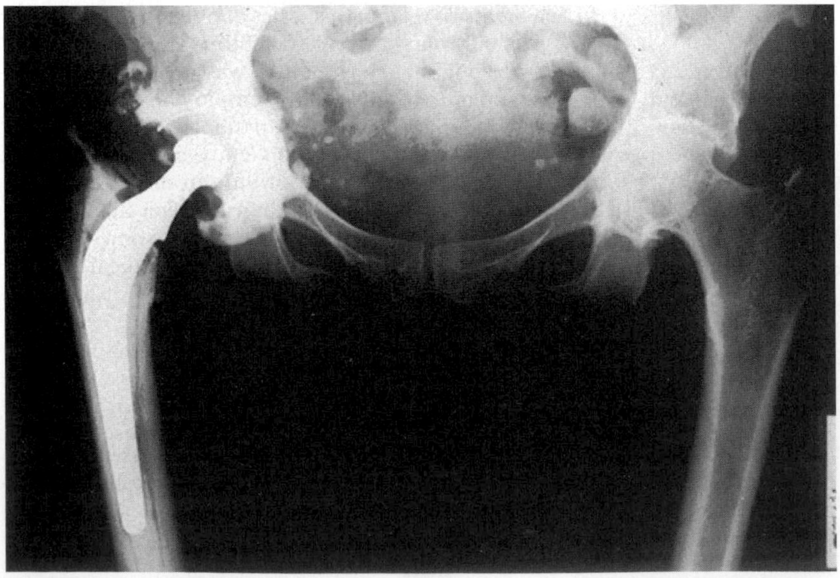

Figure 11.44 Radiograph 2 years after insertion of a Charnley total hip replacement prosthesis. Resorption of the calcar femorale and sinking of the prosthesis are seen. The prosthesis is obviously loose, and the patient experiences pain on walking.

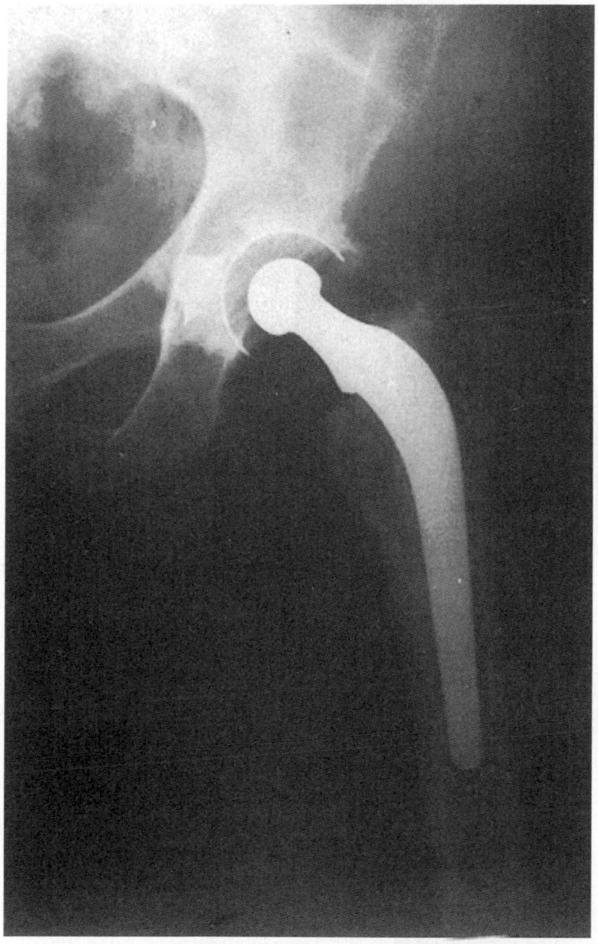

Figure 11.45 Radiograph of a Charnley total hip replacement inserted without removal of the greater trochanter.

superior results to the Charnley type of replacement. Interest has centred around uncemented prostheses (Lord *et al.*, 1979) and the use of a ceramic femoral head articulating against a high-density polyethylene acetabulum. The results achieved with uncemented prostheses with specially scintered surfaces are still provisional and the reports of the ceramic-on-polyethylene prostheses are conflicting. In this latter type of prosthesis the low-friction matrix of the articulation requires to be balanced against the disadvantages of the brittle nature of the ceramic and the high cost.

Uncemented total hip replacement

The early reports of cemented prostheses in the young, i.e. less than 50 years, suggested that they were not satisfactory. Dorr *et al.* (1983) studying a series ranging in age from 14 to 45 years found that, after 2–5 years, 78% were satisfactory, dropping to 72% after 5 years with the poorest results in those under the age of 30 years. The patients with such a poor prognosis had either osteonecrosis or osteoarthritis as the primary pathology, were alcoholics, had had a previous hip infection or operation.

However, although the complication of aseptic loosening was one of the main reasons behind the development of the uncemented prosthesis, other reasons such as dropping the age group below 65 years, leaving better bone stock for the revisions were as important. It should be noted that with improved femoral components and their design, as well as the actual techniques of cementing, all have reduced the femoral loosening rates; for example Milroy and Harris (1990) have had a loosening rate of 3% for cemented femoral components after 10 years.

Callaghan (1993) in a review article pointed out the difficulty of comparing one series to another because several generations of techniques and designs have occurred with the experience of surgeons improving. He illustrated this point by describing how the first generation of total hip prostheses involved hard packing of cement, the next included plugging of the meduallary space distally by using a gun injection system, next porosity interphase, and now nodular components. A similar picture can be found in the rapid evolution and change in non-cemented prostheses, press fit, proximal porous-coated, enhanced coating with hydroxyapatite crystals, etc.

Schulte *et al.* (1993) have reported on a 20-year follow-up of the outcome following a Charnley hip replacement procedure. Out of 330 patients, 83 patients were still alive, 85% of whom had no pain; 53% required no walking aid. At the follow-up time 10% had required revision (2% loosening with infection, 7% aseptic loosening and 1% dislocation). Acetabular loosening was greater than femoral. It was noted that 90% of those still alive had retained their original implant.

This long-term analysis reveals once again the success of this operation and provides the challenge to those propagating the use of non-cemented prostheses.

Recently interest has developed in the use of a more limited type of total hip replacement (Freeman *et al.*, 1978), using a resurfacing technique for the femur and the acetabulum (Figure 11.46). The concept of minimal bone removal is attractive but the problem of loosening of the components appears to be significant, probably due to the higher friction generated within a larger size of prosthesis than the Charnley type (Figure 11.47). Therefore, much longer-term experience is required than presently available to justify the use of such prostheses.

The special problem of osteonecrosis of the

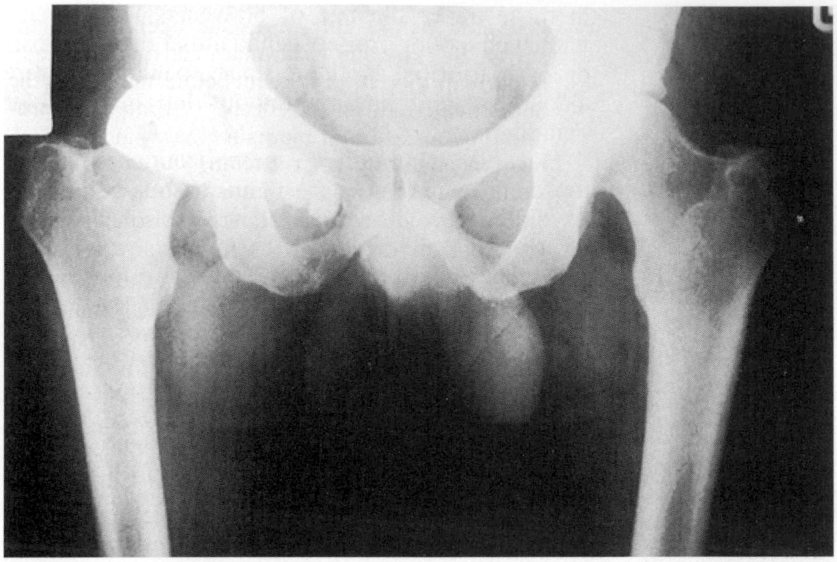

(a)

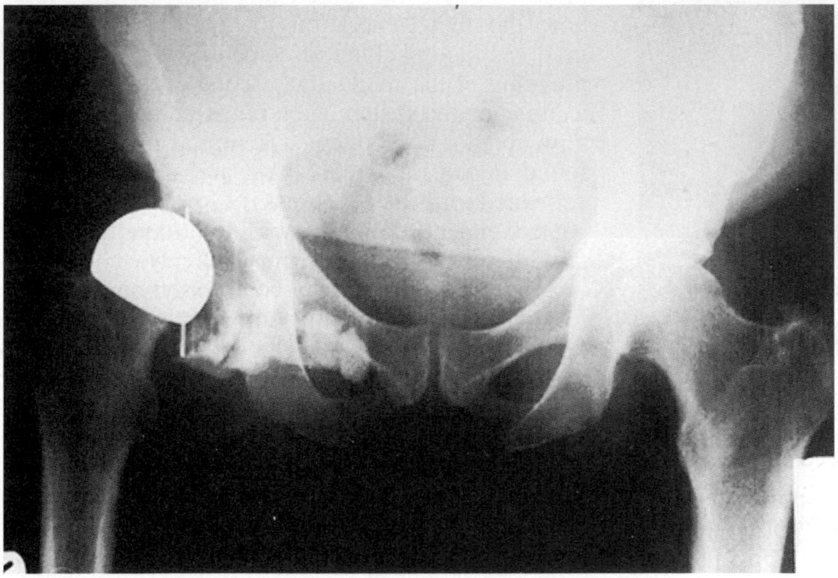

(b)

Figure 11.46 (a) ICLH double-cup arthroplasty for osteoarthrosis of the hip in a 50-year-old man.
(b) Radiograph 1 year after operation. The acetabular cup is obviously loose, and the patient complained of severe pain.

femoral head is the young patient – averaging 35 years of age on following up surface replacements after 8 years – 12% had failed and only 70% were considered to be good or better (de Meulemeester and Rozing, 1989).

At present we consider that it is inadvisable to employ a Charnley total hip replacement in a patient under the age of 40 years, particularly if that patient is energetic and requires to be very active in his work or recreation. The outstanding problem which is emerging for all types of hip replacement is that of loosening and we, therefore, avoid replacement prostheses in the younger patient with osteoarthrosis and attempt to manage such patients by use of femoral osteotomy if the hip is mobile.

Operative technique

Prior to operation it is essential to ensure that the patient is generally fit from the cardiovascular point of view and has no obvious foci of infection. As a result, throat swab, perineal swabs and urinanalysis are carried out. In addition, routine blood count and

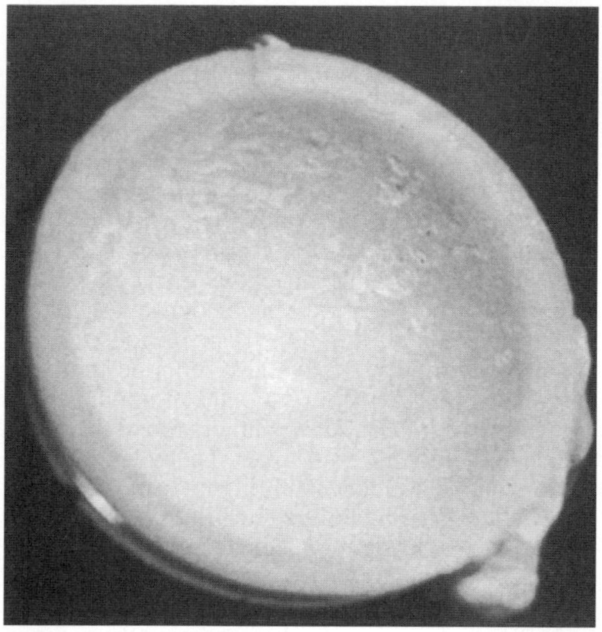

Figure 11.47 High-density polyethylene acetabular cup removed from the patient in Figure 11.46, 1 year after the ICLH prosthesis which had loosened. The obvious pitting and wear of the cup can be seen.

ESR are assessed, together with a chest radiograph. The patient's skin is carefully examined for any signs of low-grade infection, varicose ulceration or psoriasis, all of which predispose the prosthesis site to infection. The patient is given a loading dose of 1 g of ampicillin (Magnapen) with the premedication 2 hours before the operation, or cephalosporin where there is a history of allergy to pencillin. The antibiotic is continued for 48 hours after the operative procedure in a dose of 500 mg four times a day. Where possible, the patient should be operated on in the ultra-clean environment provided by a vertical or horizontal laminar flow enclosure. The Charnley type of Ventile gowns and body exhaust systems do not confer any advantage over the use of a 3-dose regimen of antibiotics in prevention of infection and are, therefore, optional.

The authors prefer a straight lateral approach to the hip in which the incision is deepened through the deep fascia posterior to tensor fasciae latae, to expose the gluteus medius and minimus, the greater trochanter and the upper shaft of the femur. Rather than remove the trochanter from the femur, the anterior 2.5 cm or more of the insertion of the gluteus medius and minimus is divided by a sharp knife from its attachment to the trochanter. The interval between the short abductors and the vastus lateralis is developed and opened to expose the anterior capsule of the hip joint.

The capsule is opened by a T incision and a minimal capsulectomy is carried out in order to give sufficient access to dislocate the hip. The hip is then dislocated by adduction and external rotation. Ordinarily, when the hip joint is dislocated, the state of the femoral head and the acetabulum is recorded with care and the femoral head is excised using a hand saw, to avoid any necrosis of femoral neck bone, at the level of the inferior osteophyte. The line of this excision of the head is decided by placing a trial prosthesis alongside the femur at this point. The acetabulum is then prepared, using expanding reamers. The largest size of polyethylene cup is placed in the acetabulum but this must be a slack fit before cementing is carried out. Radiating drill holes are made into the ilium, ischium and pubis, and the long posterior wall-type of acetabular cup is then inserted in position at an angle of approximately 40° with the horizontal and cemented in place with methylmethacrylate bone cement. The cup is neutralized with regard to anteversion. The femoral shaft is then prepared with flexible reamers, a large curette and rasps, and a trial positioning of the femoral component is carried out. It is important to avoid varus of the prosthesis.

A trial reduction is then attempted, the femoral component being brought onto the flat outer surface of the cup but not fully reduced.

Postoperatively the patient is nursed with the hip in a slightly abducted position on a foam gutter, and active movements of hip, knee and ankle are commenced as soon as consciousness is recovered.

On the second postoperative evening, therapy is begun at a level to maintain the warfarin INR between 1.5 and 2.0. After 48 hours the patient begins to walk around the room using two crutches and with the aid of the physiotherapist. Gradual mobilization commences and by 7–10 days the patient should be able to walk independently with two or one stick. At this point the anticoagulant therapy is stopped. Discharge from hospital is permitted when this stage is reached, and the patient is followed up periodically in the out-patient clinic with serial x-rays at 1 month, 3 months, 6 months and then at yearly intervals to check the clinical and radiological state of the artificial joint.

Uncemented prostheses

Metal backing of polyethylene implants which was introduced to reduce the stress in the polyethylene cup or disc has not been shown to offer any advantages. Indeed Cates *et al.* (1993) have found a 37% increase in wear of the polyethylene at about 6 years after insertion.

An uncemented THR is basically one of two types: press fit or screw fit, with or without a porous-coated surface for bone ingrowth and remodelling.

Reasonable series are now becoming available for study with sufficient follow-up time for a clinical evaluation, especially for persistent thigh or groin pain. This common symptom results from either a poor initial fit or instability after reaming out the femoral medullary space, as well as altered stress transfer directly to the bone compartment or stress shielding. Haddard *et al.* (1990) compared three commonly used non-cemented porous-coated prostheses which had been on average 3 years *in situ*. They found that the Dupuy AML prostheses had average postoperative scores of 80.7 and thigh pain present in 30%, the Howmedica PCA was 83.8 with thigh pain in 30% and the Implant Tech LSF had a score of 91.5 with thigh pain in only 8%. The latter also had a better clinical and radiographic review at this early stage of follow-up.

Other series with uncemented prostheses are now appearing with varying success rates up to 85%, including the younger age groups. However, one of the reasons presented for using uncemented total hip replacement is that they are easier to revise, leaving behind a better bone stock.

In a laboratory cadaveric testing of non-cemented Depuy's Microlock, Howmedica porous-coated and a cemented Harris Precoat prostheses, Phillips *et al.* (1990) found that all cemented stems were more resistant to loosening than uncemented and therefore provided the greatest immediate fixation. They concluded that cementless stems should be protected from rotational loading until porous ingrowth or bone remodelling had occurred. Initially after their insertion a period of non-weight-bearing of at least 6 weeks to 3 months is imperative.

At the present time it is very difficult because of insufficient evidence to demonstrate that one type of successful modern cemented or uncemented prosthesis is better than another. There is now available hydroxyapatite coating of prostheses. Overall, although hydroxyapatite coating of prostheses appears very promising, no uncemented hip replacement has proved superior to the cemented Charnley over a 15-year period.

Hydroxyapatite coating of prostheses

A ceramic coating of hydroxyapatite crystals is sprayed on to the surface of the femoral component in order to stimulate osteoinduction at the bony interface with improved 'locking' of the prosthesis. All cementless prostheses require osseous integration for its fixation without any interposed connective tissue. Morscher (1991) has pointed out that the long-term binding strength of the hydroxyapatite ceramic to the metal is still unknown and that the chemical and physical disintegration of the hydroxyapatite crystals is yet to be studied, particularly as it is a brittle substance with a high modulus of elasticity. He believes that the problem has now been shifted from the bone coating junction to the coating metal interface.

Furlong and Osborn (1991) have reported on four post-mortem specimens of implanted hydroxyapatite coated Furlong prostheses. The implantation periods were from 10 days to 7 weeks. They found woven bone on the hydroxyapatite ceramic, similar to that deposited on surviving cancellous trabeculae of the femoral shaft. There was no evidence of inflammatory reaction or of fibrous tissue response.

Hardy *et al.* (1991) have also reported upon the early response, i.e. within 9 months of implantation, from four specimens. These authors found that there was newly formed bone over the hydroxyapatite coating with new trabecular bridging to the endosteal bone layer. They believed their findings indicated that biological integration had taken place. No loose particles of titanium or hydroxyapatite were found within the joint space. No bone ossification of the endochondral type was seen and therefore direct ossification via differentiation of loose connective tissue had taken place.

Complications of total hip replacement

Infection

Patients selected for such a procedure should be free from clinically obvious infection of the upper respiratory tract, urinary tract, skin, interdigital and any other apparent infection. Obesity, advanced age, metabolic diseases, steroid therapy and alteration of the immune defence mechanism might contribute to the development of deep wound infection.

Rheumatoid arthritis, liver disease, diabetes mellitus and malignant tumours are usually related to deep wound sepsis. Patients with rheumatoid arthritis have more than 0.05 higher incidence of postoperative sepsis. Rheumatoid patients with elevated levels of IgM, peripheral manifestation of the disease and those with low leucocytic chemotaxis are unusually susceptible to sepsis. Patients with previous hip surgery are at greater risk of having deep sepsis. In these patients, ESR determination and x-rays should be studied for evidence of infection. Aspiration of the hip and examination of the aspirate for aerobic and anaerobic cultures should be carried out if there is any reason to suspect infection.

The final decision on whether or not to perform a total hip replacement is delayed until the results of histological examination of frozen sections of tissue specimens obtained at surgery are known. Dense scar tissue has limited ability to heal after incision, retraction and suture. Patients who have had multiple previous surgical procedures may need a preliminary soft tissue plastic procedure to provide healthy tissue at the proposed operation site.

Prophylactic antibiotics (e.g. cloxacillin) can be given systemically but the widespread abuse of the drugs has resulted in the prevalence of an increasing number of resistant strains of pathogenic bacteria.

Pollard *et al.* (1979) found that three doses of cephaloridine is as effective as a 2-week regimen of flucloxacillin. Cephaloridine 1 g i.v. was given at induction of anaesthesia, and the mean concentrations were measured in the excised femoral head, serum and tissues of the operation field. A time/concentration curve of cephaloridine was constructed which gave a mean level of 74 μg/ml immediately after injection, and a decline to 4.5 μg/ml 6 hours later. At this time i.m. injection of cephaloridine was given and repeated after a further 6 hours.

Alternatively, prophylactic antibiotics can be given locally. Local irrigation of the wound during the operation, using antibiotic compounds or anti-septic compound – e.g. noxythiolin (Noxyflex) – has been recommended. Operative drainage should reduce haematoma formation and, so, deep wound infection.

During the operation, behaviour in theatre and control of traffic of the staff in theatre are important factors. In addition, the time of day, the type of operating theatre and the position on operating schedule could also be important factors.

Charnley and Eftekhar (1969) paid special attention to the air in the theatre. With 85 infections in 5800 total hip replacements between 1960 and 1970, the incidence rate fell purely as a result of measures taken to prevent exogenous infection in the operating room. Prophylactic antibiotics were not used in this study.

Andrews *et al.* (1981) claim that a dislocation after operation is particularly liable to lead to infection; it occurred in 16% of 68 infected patients in their series (out of a total of 1746 patients with hip replacements). Deep haematoma occurring in 7 of these series could be a predisposing factor to sepsis. Heparin (subcutaneously) increases the incidence of haematoma formation and, hence, deep sepsis. Aspirin 1 g daily has no effect on the incidence of deep sepsis.

Early infection can be either superficial or deep. Superficial infection is manifested by a pyrexia, high ESR (high ESR is found normally postoperatively and returns to normal after 6 months) and a leucocytosis as well as local redness, swelling or haematoma. Treatment consists of supportive therapy in the form of blood transfusion, and i.v. fluids must be given as necessary. Antibiotics are given intravenously for 4–6 weeks, followed by oral administration for 4–6 months.

Deep wound sepsis after total hip replacement is not usually manifested by fever, erythema of the wound or drainage, except for infected haematoma deep to the fascia which may drain spontaneously. Usually the hip is painful and there is moderate elevation of the sedimentation rate with no fever and a normal leucocyte count.

An arthrogram may be helpful, but it will not always detect a loose or infected prosthesis. It may show permeation of contrast medium into the bone–cement interface about a loose prosthesis in infected hips. There may be lateral pocketing of the medium in the soft tissue structures, enlarged capsular space or sinus formation.

Aspiration of the material for culture and sensitivity during arthrography frequently differentiates between a loose and an infected prosthesis.

A scan with radioactive isotopes can be of value in detecting deep sepsis.

A postoperative haematoma which drains spontaneously should be treated by aggressive surgical intervention together with parenteral antibiotics.

A patient with a painful hip following total hip replacement should have ESR determined, and aspiration of the hip and culture of the aspirate. Histological examination of frozen sections can be helpful in deciding whether low-grade sepsis is present. Treatment ranges from removal of the prosthesis and cement with radical debridement to insertion of a second implant or a pseudarthrosis procedure.

Hunter (1979), in his series, reinserted 65 total hip arthroplasties after sepsis around the hip, and positive cultures were obtained from 56 cases. Although 65% of patients still have their implant in position, only 16 of the 65 (25%) show an excellent or good result. Twenty-three of the 65 (35%) subsequently required an excision arthroplasty. A second implant after sepsis is contraindicated when reasonable function can be obtained from pseudarthrosis or when there is a persistently high ESR in the absence of any other systemic disease.

The patient who is undergoing this salvage should be psychologically prepared and encouraged to accept a Girdlestone pseudarthrosis which will give him a good, functional hip after an infected one has been removed.

Decision about a two-stage reimplantation is based upon the sensitivity of the organism, the spreading extent of the tissue infection and its severity. Gram-negative or streptococcal organisms have a poor prognosis for a successful reimplantation. Reimplantation can be delayed as long as 1 year in order to treat the infection.

Dall *et al.* (1976) tested the mechanical strength of the cement after mixing the methylmethacrylate with various antibiotics. Most of the mixtures retained their antibacterial activity after prolonged storage, despite the heat of polymerization. The mechanical strength of the cement was not much altered provided the antibiotics had been in powder form and added to the dry monomer in the proportion of 1:40.

Buccholz (1979) claim that certain antibiotics will slowly diffuse from methylmethacrylate and cause a local inhibition of bacterial growth. However, the very antibiotics they favour – gentamicin and erythromycin – have been found to be rather ineffective when used with Surgical Simplex P. The long-term release from the cement in amounts sufficient to inhibit bacterial growth were seen only with clindamycin and, to a lesser extent, with cephalothin. Elson *et al.* (1977) confirmed that fucidin and gentamicin mixed with the cement were liberated from the surface. One gram of antibiotics to 40 g of powder Palacos R was five times as effective in releasing the antibiotics as other cements (Simplex, CMW), and the surface concentration of eluting antibiotics was sufficient to cause diffusion across the whole thickness of cortical bone from cadaveric human femoral shafts.

It should be noted, however, that antibiotic loaded cement is described as being mechanically less strong than plain cement.

Levin (1975) has pointed out that there is no clinical evidence that local diffusion of antibiotics from cement is more effective than the use of the same antibiotic systemically. Nevertheless, it is possible that such local action could have a bactericidal effect on bacteria trapped in the minute cracks in the cement and out of reach of systemic circulation.

Salvati *et al* (1986) have shown that gentamicin impregnated cement delivers seven times higher local concentrations than obtained by using the intravenous route. The serum and urine levels are very low and transient and therefore there is little risk of systemic toxicity.

However, antibiotic-loaded cement is highly indicated in revision hip surgery. The drawback of this is allergic reaction and the possible emergence of resistant bacteria. See Chapter 9.

Aseptic loosening

Loosening is the most frequent long-term complication after joint replacement because of bone resorption. Particulate matter or debris is commonly found at the time of revision arising from polyethylene or Teflon (the original cup material) or polymethylmethacrylate cement or metal. These give rise to a foreign body reaction through the giant cells or macrophages which are commonly found in the membrane of the bone implant interphase. Murray and Rushton (1990) have shown experimentally that particles of bone cement and of polyethylene activate macrophages which then are mediators of resorption through the release of prostaglandins.

Anthony *et al.* (1990) have described that localized bone endosteal lysis may occur in the femur without radiographic evidence of loosening. They found that these areas were directly related to a local defect in the cement material around the stem which allowed the joint space contents to reach the femoral endosteal surface.

Santavirta *et al.* (1990) have described 'aggressive granulomatous' lesions in cemented hips, and now have described this as occurring in cementless hip replacement which had required revision on average 4.8 years after its insertion. Histopathologically the granulomas contained large numbers of histiocytes and were thought to have been caused by the plastic debris from the acetabular socket. Pain on weight-bearing was the first symptom with subsequent migration of the acetabular component and fracture of the femoral stem.

Prosthetic loosening which usually requires revision may be due to mechanical loosening with particulate debris activation of bone resorbing agents or low-grade sepsis. Haematological tests (ERS, WBC count, CRP reaction), plain radiography, isotope scanning and labelled white cell scanning are all frequently non-specific. Biopsy with culture is often required. Open biopsy with frozen section is specific and sensitive but obviously a major undertaking and commits the surgeon to follow on. Needle aspiration has proved to be disappointing with many false-positive results. However, Roberts *et al.* (1992) have described their technique of using a liquid enrichment primary culture medium inoculation in the theatre, and then a radiometric culture method – 94% of the aspiration results were correct with sensitivity of 87% and specificity 95%.

Lieberman *et al.* (1991) have reviewed the increasing recognition of the role of metallic wear debris on loosening both from the prosthetic components but also from the screw heads of mechanically fixed acetabular components. They conclude that it is the formation of particulate debris which is the key factor leading to bone resorption and that there may well be a synergistic role of all particulate debris arising from the polyethylenes, the methacrylates and the metal.

Hodge and Chandler (1992) have compared unconstrained and constrained designs over an average period of 55 months and found that with unconstrained replacement 98% had a good or excellent result with constrained only 70% having an equally good result. Of the unconstrained replacements 8% eventually required a revision total joint replacement because of loosening and failure compared with 27% of the constrained design. Only one of their patients developed substantial degenerative changes in the opposite compartment. Cemented replacement gives better results than the porous-coated types for ingrowth fixation, which is often delayed and weaker (Vince and Brien, 1991). In a follow-up of 10–16 years they found that the probability of femoral component failure after 20 years was 86%; acetabular surgery after 20 years was 84%; the probability of both was 75%.

Migration of all femoral components is expected to a varying amount particularly during the first 3 months after isolation. However, Soballe *et al.* (1993) have compared titanium (Ti) alloy coated biometric femoral prostheses with hydroxyapatite (HA) coated biometric femoral prostheses using roentgen stereophotogrammetric markers. All types migrated during the first 3 months after insertion but the HA coated components then appeared to stabilize and the Ti coated components continued to migrate for the next 9 months, although the maximum subsidence in both groups was only 0.2 mm. The HA coated group appeared to have a better Harris hip score.

Causes of bone resorption in loosening

Jirancek *et al.* (1993) in studying the membranous layer between bone and cement in aseptic loosening of the acetabular component found particular debris of polyethylene, methylmethacrylate and metal throughout the membrane, but intracellularly only in the macrophages and in the multinucleated giant cells. By using nucleic-acid probes, hybridization and immunohistochemical techniques they demonstrated interleukin 1 predominantly in macrophages but not in fibroblasts or in T lymphocytes. In contrast the interleukin 1B protein was seen on both macrophages as well as the fibroblasts and therefore had been released by the macrophages. Platelet-derived growth factor was also found in both macrophages and fibroblasts. They postulate that these cytokines are involved in bone resorption, fibroblastic proliferation and loosening.

Fractures

Femoral stem fractures

With improved cementing techniques and materials, fewer fractures of the cemented femoral stems are now presenting (Mollan *et al.*, 1984), but still can be caused by fixation around the distal third of the prosthesis with loosening around the proximal third and gradual distal migration, an increase in body weight and a retroverted, valgus or varus positioning of the prosthesis. Wilson *et al.* (1992) have reported on a 4.1% incidence of fracturing the stem of a Ring Ti Mesh cementless hip prosthesis and the difficulty of retrieving the distal fragment. In their cases there was deliberate damage distal to the tip of the femoral stem in order to remove them.

Fractures of the femoral shaft

Intraoperative fractures of the femoral shaft may occur during a revision procedure during attempts to remove cement or the fractured distal portion of the stem; during the reduction of the two components or of a dislocation; during reaming of the shaft for the femoral component or its insertion (Fitzgerald *et al.*, 1988). Circlage wiring is often adequate to control the fractures which, with careful weight-bearing postoperatively, do not give great problems.

Only 17 fractures of the stainless steel femoral stem components occurred in 10 000 Charnley hip replacements between $1^1/_2$ and 5 years after insertion (Charnley, 1976).

Fractures result from inadequate valgus insertion of the prosthesis, inequality of spread and filling of the intramedullary cavity by the cement, and from inadequate design of the thickness, contour and shape of some femoral stems, especially in relation to the weight and age of the recipient patient. Impurity and poor quality of the steel composition, even when falling below the now established national standards, are rare causes.

Heterotopic ossification

Heterotopic ossification can commonly be seen after total hip replacement of either the cemented or more frequently the non-cemented types, around the neck of the femoral prosthesis. It must be differentiated from the myositis ossificans lesion which develops in the incisional operative scar area. Kjaersgaard-Andersen and Ritter (1991) have suggested a simple clinical classification:

- Grade 1 – no ossification or ossification occupying less than two-thirds of the space between the femur and the pelvis. It is usually without symptoms and not requiring treatment.
- Grade 2 – ossification occupying more than two-thirds of the distance between the femur and the pelvis, including apparent osseous ankylosis. This grade forms about 10–15% of all cases, usually symptomatic with pain and loss of mobility and some will require surgical excision with prophylaxis.

These authors have described the risk factors to be in the male sex over the age of 60 years, with previous history of heterotopic ossification; probably in patients who have hypertrophic osteoarthritis (Goel and Sharp, 1991), ankylosing spondylitis, Forestier disease or Paget's disease – although such conditions have not been documented accurately as likely factors.

There are no known biochemical tests which are of use to determine this disease process.

Effective postoperative prophylaxis can be achieved by lower dosage irradiation with selective shielding of 1000 cGy (Ayers *et al.*, 1986) or by giving anti-inflammatory drugs such as ibuprofen, aspirin or indomethacin (Schmidt and Kjaersgaard-Andersen, 1988). However, it should be noted that there is concern that these drugs could adversely effect the ingrowth of bone into non-cemented porous-coated implants (Keller *et al.*, 1989; Trancik *et al.*, 1989).

Thromboembolism

About 5% of patients, without prophylaxis, having elective total hip replacement, develop symptomatic pulmonary embolism of whom 0.2–5% die of this condition. Risk factors for venous thromboembolism can be divided into:

- *Patient factors* – over the age of 40 years, obesity, presence of varicose veins, bed immobilization, pregnancy, high dose oestrogen therapy (e.g. the pill), previous history of thrombosis, embolism and thrombophilia.
- *Diseases* – malignancy (especially pelvic), heart failure, myocardial infarction, paralysis of lower limbs, infection, paraproteinanaemia, Behçet's disease.
- *Surgical procedures* – trauma or surgery to the pelvis, hip, lower limb, with duration of surgery over 30 minutes.

Lowe (1992) has summarized the work of a consensus group describing the risk, and the incidence, of prophylaxis of venous thromboembolism:

- *In low-risk groups* – in minor surgery lasting more than 30 minutes, minor trauma or illness, age of 40 years, major surgery less than 30 minutes; deep vein thrombosis is less than 10%, proximal vein thrombosis less than 1% and a fatal pulmonary embolism is 0.01%.
- *In moderate-risk groups* – in major general, urological gynaecological operations, age 40 or more with other risk factors, e.g. major illness of heart or lung, cancer, major trauma or burns, minor surgery with previous history of thrombosis; deep vein thrombosis 10–40%; proximal vein thrombosis 1–10% and fatal embolism 0.1–1%.
- *In high-risk groups* – in fracture or major orthopaedic surgery of pelvis, hip or lower limb, major pelvic surgery for cancer; previous deep vein thrombosis, pulmonary embolism, stroke or paraplegic patients, major lower limb amputation; deep vein thrombosis 18–40%; proximal vein thrombosis 10–30%; fatal pulmonary embolism 1–10%.

Proximal vein thrombosis is responsible for the majority of fatal pulmonary embolisms, and is most probably due to damage to the femoral vein intraoperatively. The calf deep vein thrombosis is probably caused by stasis and a hypercoagulability state.

Diagnosis is by ascending venography which is the most expensive and has some complications, e.g. extravasation of material, allergy, phlebitis. Even so it outlines the severity as well as location of the thrombi. Planes *et al.* (1990) studied by venography heparin-treated patients having received a total hip replacement; 10% had a positive venography with 23 distal, 44 proximal, 5 mixed and a further 9 were from calf to thigh. From a post-mortem study they demonstrated clearly the folding over of the femoral vein as the hip was manipulated for dislocation and inspection of the femoral head.

Ultrasound scanning using the B-mode has now become more widely used because of its ease, quickness and non-invasive nature. However, it cannot detect iliac or calf vein thrombosis.

Treatment should be directed at adequate prophylaxis. Warfarin has been used extensively and effectively but it does require daily monitoring to prevent the complication of bleeding in about 4% of cases. Amstutz *et al.* (1989) have reported a less then 0.5% incidence of pulmonary embolism. Unfractionated heparin which inactivates factors IX and X and fibrin conversion, although effective at adjusted high dosages, has now been superseded by low molecular weight heparin given in low dosage, subcutaneously. It prevents over 60% of deep vein thromboses, over 60–70% of fatal pulmonary embolisms and it also reduces total hospital mortality by 25%. It is easier to administer and has far fewer bleeding complications. Turpie (1990) has found from a double blind prospective study after total hip replacement that when low molecular weight heparin was given 30 mg subcutaneously twice daily compared with a control placebo group, this drug reduced the deep vein thrombosis to 12% (versus 45% in controls) and proximal thrombosis to 4% (versus 20% in the control).

Pneumatic intermittent compression leg and boot appliances are now being used prophylactically with effect. Woolson and Watt (1991) have demonstrated that their use can reduce the proximal thrombosis rate to 10%, and there was no significant difference in thrombosis between patients treated with boots alone, boots with warfarin or boots with aspirin.

Epidural spinal anaesthesia, in total hip replacement patients, does reduce the deep venous thrombosis rate because of a decreased need for blood transfusion, earlier mobility, etc.

Surgery of the hips in ankylosing spondylitis

The hip joints are involved in about one-half of patients with ankylosing spondylitis, and 25% suffer pain and stiffness which can usually be controlled. The main indications for surgery are ankylosis combined with poor posture, or disabling pain combined with poor posture (Bisla *et al.*, 1976). It would appear that when the prime indication for hip surgery in patients with ankylosing spondylitis is restricted motion alone, the operation may not be beneficial (Resnick *et al.*, 1976). Operations which should be considered are primary pseudarthrosis, cup arthroplasty and total hip replacement.

PRIMARY PSEUDARTHROSIS

Williams *et al.* (1977) followed up five primary pseudarthroses performed in three patients. Four hips, operated upon for fixed flexion deformity, were graded as fair, and one hip which was operated on primarily for pain was graded as a good result. However, all three patients, two of whom had been bed-bound prior to surgery, were delighted with the results of their operations.

CUP ARTHROPLASTY

Williams *et al.* (1977) have described six patients on whom eight cup arthroplasties were performed but, in spite of improved movement in all cases, the cup had either been removed or was awaiting removal because of pain. One was converted to a pseudarthrosis with a fair result, and six were converted to a Charnley replacement with a good or excellent result in three cases and deep infection occurring in the other three. Better results in cup arthroplasties are probably obtained in patients with ankylosing spondylitis and in those with classic rheumatoid arthritis.

TOTAL HIP REPLACEMENT

Welch and Charnley (1970) and Bisla *et al.* (1976) have described special features of this operation for ankylosing spondylitis. In patients with this condition, the osteotomy of the neck of the femur is done *in situ*, and the femoral head may have to be removed in sections. It is sometimes difficult to identify the margin of the acetabulum before reaming is begun, and three cases are reported in Bisla's series where malpositioning of the cup occurred in a high position with shortening of the leg ranging from 2 to 6 cm.

Results

The results from total hip replacements were:

1. *Range of motion*. Bisla *et al.* (1976) described 23 patients who underwent 34 total hip arthroplasties, with an average follow-up of almost 4 years. In the patients who had had bony ankylosis the average arc of flexion achieved was 37.5°, and in those who had fibrous ankylosis it was 81°. In patients operated on because of pain, the arc of flexion was improved from an average of 50° preoperatively to an average of 96° on follow-up.

   Welch and Charnley (1970), in a series of 20 ankylosing spondylitides followed up for 2–4 years, found that each of their patients gained a total of over 100° of movements in the hips. These patients experienced muscle cramp and some weakness in their immediate postoperative period. They regained excellent muscular control of motion, despite functional inactivity of the muscles in the preoperative state. There were no cases in which the hip re-ankylosed in this series.
2. *Pain relief*. From the Bisla *et al.* series, preoperatively 7 patients with bony ankylosis had no pain whilst 6 patients with fibrous ankylosis and the 10 remaining patients had moderate to severe pain. Williams *et al.* (1977) studied 86 hips in patients with ankylosing spondylitis who received a total hip replacement, and they found that 73% were graded as good or excellent with regard to pain and movement up to 10 years later.

COMPLICATIONS

Infection

Williams *et al.* had 4 cases of deep infection in 86 hips (5%). Three had a secondary pseudarthrosis operation performed within 6 months of replacement and the others remained well on continuous antibiotic therapy.

Fibrous ankylosis

This occurred bilaterally in 3 patients. All had exhibited a progressive pattern of disease before operation and 2 of them had an ESR of over 100 mm. Immediately after operation a good range of movement returned, but within a week pain and stiffness became troublesome.

Bony ankylosis

The first case of re-ankylosis of the hip joint in ankylosing spondylitis after total hip replacement was reported in 1972 (Wilde *et al.*) The occurrence of the postoperative complication coupled with the appearance of bony outgrowths at the site of ligament attachment throughout the axial and extra-axial skeleton in patients with ankylosing spondylitis suggests the presence of an underlying ossifying diathesis and/or diffuse idiopathic skeletal hyperostosis (DISH) (Resnick *et al.*, 1976). A significant number of these patients possess antigen HLA B27, a feature they share with individuals with other arthropathies, characterized by abundant ossification. This gene may be closely related to one which influences bone formation with a possible association of post-operative heterotopic ossification. x-Ray examination of the vertebral column for ankylosing hyperostosis of the spine in patients undergoing hip surgery may be a useful screening procedure. This ossification may be classified as follows:

- I Islands of bone within the tissues about the hip.
- II Bone spurs in the pelvis or proximal end of the femur, leaving at least 1 cm between opposing bone surfaces.
- III Bone spurs from the pelvis or proximal end of the femur, reducing the space between opposing bone surfaces to less than 1 cm.
- IV Apparent bony ankylosis of the hip (Brooker *et al.*, 1973).

Brooker and associates reported an incidence of myositis ossificans in 21% of total hip replacement patients with non-ankylosing spondylitis.

In a 6-year follow-up study of replacement in ankylosing spondylitis, Kilgus *et al.* (1990) have described the excellent durability of the cemented conventional hip prosthesis in the young population (average age of 43 years). Indeed only one – after 17 years – required revision for aseptic loosening. In patients who had had a previous operation on the hip or had bony ankylosis preoperatively, only 11% developed significant heterotopic bone formation. Their conclusions were that prophylactic therapy should be reserved for patients who are at greatest risk for heterotopic ossification. Improved motion (averaging 176° of combined motion) was found and was most gratifying to the patients, although it has to be compared with 214° of motion achieved in patients who had received a similar operation for osteoarthrosis.

Loosening

No patient in the Williams *et al.* series developed loosening of the acetabulum, but in the Bisla *et al.* series there was one case of loosening of the femoral component and two developed acetabular loosening. These and other late mechanical failures may appear in long-term follow-up of these young subjects because patients with ankylosing spondylitis are more active than patients with rheumatoid or osteoarthritis. In addition, an ankylosed spine may impose excessive strain upon the artificial joint, causing late failure of the prosthesis.

Total hip replacement is the procedure of choice for patients with ankylosing spondylitis in whom hip surgery is indicated although primary pseudarthrosis is sometimes a good operation in very disabled patients.

Intrapelvic protrusion of the acetabulum (*protrusio acetabuli*)

Intrapelvic protrusion of the acetabulum was originally described by Otto in 1824, and is often known as the 'Otto pelvis'. Its main characteristic is a bulging of the acetabular floor towards the pelvic basin, so that the socket becomes extremely deep and the head of the femur embedded in it. Otto originally attributed the condition to gout; however, it is now generally assumed that the deformity is not a specific one but may occur in a variety of lesions of the hip joint. Gilmour (1938) suggested there are two main types: primary and secondary, resulting from disease of or injury to the acetabular floor.

Primary protrusio

Gilmour pointed out that the changes are due to the increased plasticity of the acetabular floor so that it yields to the pressure of the femoral head, and that this is due to an acceleration in the rate and an advancement in timing of primary epiphyseal ossification which he termed 'premature acceleration'. Its manifestation in the Y-shaped epiphyses of the innominate bones would convert the normally resistant cartilage of the acetabular socket into young vascular bone – a tissue ill-adapted to resist the stress of the increasing weight of adolescence.

Secondary protrusio

Medial displacement of the acetabular floor may follow gross lesions at the hip. Thus, old fractures, rheumatoid arthritis, osteomalacia and Paget's disease may be causative factors. While these must be borne in mind in investigating a hip which shows protrusio acetabuli, it is certain that such gross and usually obvious lesions play no part in the development of what is generally known as an 'Otto pelvis'.

CLINICAL FEATURES

Primary protrusio

The deformity is common in females in the proportion of 30:7. Bilateral and unilateral protrusio are almost equal in number. For practical purposes, three clinical types of deformity can be recognized:

1. *Deformities without arthritic changes*. This is the uncomplicated type of deformity. Its recognition is usually accidental and due to a radiographic examination for other reasons. In the early stages there is gradual development of a flexion deformity without pain, but as the condition progresses there may be limitation of movement, pelvic tilt from the fixed hip flexion and hyperlordosis of the lumbar spine. The gait may be affected and there may be inability to cross the legs or internally rotate the hips. This type of deformity may persist for years without producing serious arthritic changes.
2. *Deformities associated with unilateral arthritis*. This group is characterized by the development of progressive stiffness and pain in the joint with the deep protrusion, the other remaining sound. These symptoms may develop gradually or date from a specific injury.
3. *Deformities associated with bilateral arthritis*. Both hips have well marked arthritis such as rheumatoid arthritis or osteoarthrosis. The hips tend to stiffen in both conditions, and may do so completely in rheumatoid but never in osteoarthrosis. Later, the lumbar spine and even the knees may show signs of osteoarthrosis. On examination, there is restriction of motion in the hip and particularly restriction of adduction so that the patient may not be able to place the knees together.

RADIOLOGICAL APPEARANCES

The acetabular deformity is readily recognizable on radiographic examination. In early cases the floor of the acetabulum appears thin and may protrude from a few millimetres up to 1 cm into the pelvis. The first sign of protrusio acetabuli on a radiograph is loss of the 'teardrop' shadow which is the inferomedial wall of the acetabulum seen end on. The head of the femur is sunk into the socket and the margins of the acetabulum appear to overhang the femoral neck. The articular surfaces are intact though there may be some symmetrical loss of joint space. With the onset of osteoarthritic change the subchondral bone of the femoral head and acetabulum becomes sclerotic and osteophytes form at the margins of the joint. Often there is formation of new bone on the pelvic surface of the acetabular floor which acts as a reinforcement to prevent complete breakdown of the floor.

Protrusion is often seen in association with varus deformity of the femoral neck. The medial migration of the femoral head can be measured against the 'tear drop' inner wall of the acetabulum, the pelvic wall being either compressed together or indeed obliterated. Wiberg (1939) described the C/E angle – an angle between the perpendicular through the femoral head and the upper and outer acetabulum – in normal as 20–40°. Hooper and Jones (1971) reviewed clinically, radiographically and biochemically 11 patients with primary protrusion. In the younger age groups there was an equal sex incidence with an increasing clinical severity from mild to ankylosis. Pain and stiffness, particularly loss of abduction, were common. They divided the cases into juvenile, middle age (which contained evidence of osteoarthrosis), and elderly, always with symptomatic osteoarthritis. No associated skeletal abnormalitics were found and no metabolic or endocrine disturbance. The authors reviewing the surgical treatment even in those early days found that total hip replacement offered the best result and the worst result was found following osteotomies. The measurement of the C/E angle did not help in either diagnosing or planning treatment.

Acetabular protrusion with its deeply lying thinned medial wall creates a problem for accepting a cemented or an uncemented cup. Reconstructions of the medial wall by bone grafting, metal grid or mesh have all been tried with varying success or failure (Nunn, 1987).

TREATMENT

In the early stages, non-operative treatment in the form of active exercises, swimming or cycling may relieve symptoms. Gentle stretching under anaesthesia may help to overcome the contractures.

In osteoarthrosis, similar treatment may be successful at an earlier stage with the addition of local heat therapy. Operation is indicated for pain. Where the symptoms are severe and the patient is very disabled with bilateral stiff painful joints, the only effective treatment is total hip replacement. In the

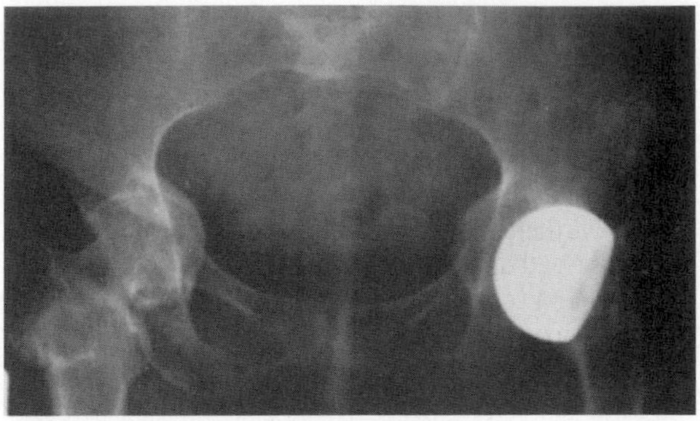

Figure 11.48 Treatment of Otto's pelvis by osteotomy on the right and a large cup arthroplasty on the left hip.

rare unilateral case in a younger patient, cup arthroplasty (Figure 11.48) may be considered.

Gates *et al.* (1990) have reported on their experience of treating 39 hip acetabular protrusion deformities in 32 patients with a follow-up of 12.8 years, by hip replacement and autologous bone grafting (from the femoral head) in 31 hips, three with graft material from the ilium and homologous bone bank material in five. Twenty-four patients had survived for the final assessment, although there was some functional deterioration, 20% showing definite loosening, 10% probable and 60% possible with 10% requiring revision. Interestingly, hips which showed progressive migration demonstrated superior migration rather than medial. These results were better than using cement and wire mesh alone.

The neuropathic joint (Charcot's disease of joints)

This condition, which arises frequently in cases of tabes dorsalis and syringomyelia, was long regarded as being exclusively syphilitic in origin, but is now known to occur following non-specific conditions such as prolonged steroid therapy, rheumatoid arthritis, chronic liver disease and administration of drugs such as indomethacin. A neuropathic ankle has been described following division of the sciatic nerve at the mid-thigh. This case substantiates the theory that the changes are the result of excessive trauma to a joint when there is impairment of the sensory nerve supply.

The affection occurs in 4–10% of cases of tabes and in 25% of cases of syringomyelia. It is rare before the age of 40. In order of decreasing frequency of involvement, the joints most commonly affected are the knee, foot and ankle, hip, intervertebral joints, elbow, shoulder and wrist.

AETIOLOGY

The importance of trauma in the production of this condition was shown by the experimental work of Eloesser (1917). After anaesthetizing a limb by section of the posterior nerve roots, typical Charcot's joints were produced only after trauma to the anaesthetic joints. This resulted in a remarkable proliferation of the surrounding tissues, with thickening of the synovial membrane, formation of polypoidal processes and osteocartilaginous formation in the neighbouring tissues.

The mechanism of the process is evidently a reversion of the cells of the capsule – and of the bone – to a primitive mesenchymal state, a rapid proliferation of them, and subsequent redifferentiation as cartilage, bone and osteoid tissue.

In the neuropathy the pathology is, of course, more grotesque, but there is destruction of articular surfaces and marginal exfoliation.

PATHOLOGY

The outstanding feature is the pronounced and rapid destruction of the articular surfaces. The compact bone underlying the cartilage is also destroyed, until

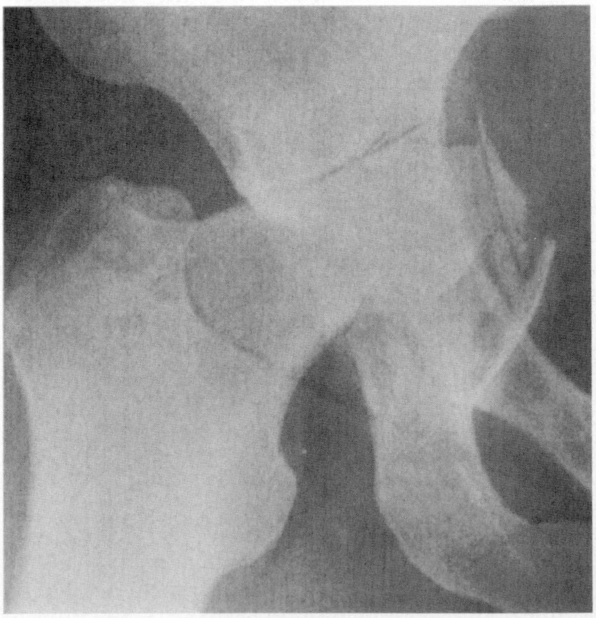

Figure 11.49 Charcot joint disease of syphilis in which there is massive destruction without repair and the accumulation of amorphous debris.

eventually the cancellous tissue is laid bare. The bone ends are therefore extremely irregular and, owing to the great instability of the joint, liable to become displaced (Figure 11.49).

The capsule is thickened, and the intra-articular ligaments are destroyed. The joint cavity is enlarged, due partly to the destruction of bone and partly to the recession of the capsule, which gradually acquires more and more peripheral attachments as the articular margins are worn away. Neighbouring joints or bursae may also become involved and lead to still further deformity. Eventually bones, such as the talus, may come to lie loose in the joint cavity.

The joint cavity is lined by a ragged-looking synovial membrane, bearing numerous villous processes and polypoid masses. This membrane may be continued over the bone ends. Its structure is fibrocartilaginous, and the polypoid bodies are also formed of cartilage.

In certain cases there is a remarkable tendency for new bone to be deposited in the form of osteophytes, or of plaques, in the capsule. Occasionally a layer of new bone is deposited around the diaphysis for some distance beyond the articulating ends – a condition never met with in osteoarthritis. Not infrequently bone is also formed in the interfascial planes outside the capsule. To this form of the disease the term 'hypertrophic' is applied; when the excessive destruction of bone takes place without any attempt at new bone formation, the condition is described as 'atrophic'. The atrophic type is said to affect particularly the joints of the upper extremity, especially the shoulder and the wrist (Figure 11.50).

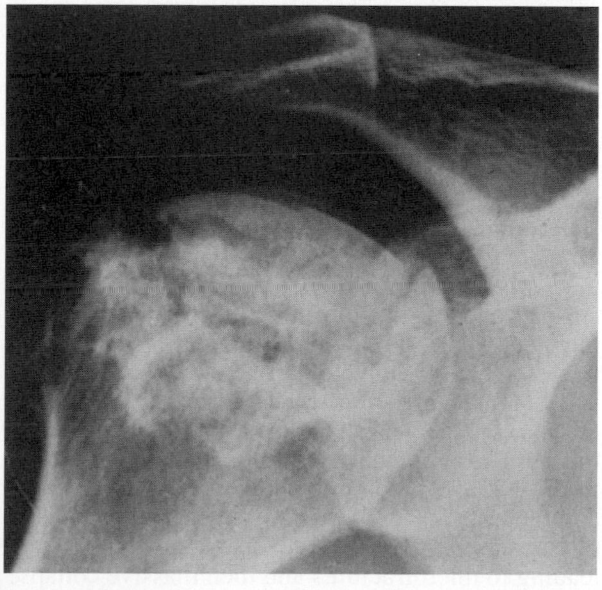

Figure 11.50 Charcot disease involving the upper humerus with very little new bone formation but segmental collapse is obvious.

Brailsford (1950) produced some suggestive evidence to show that the hypertrophic and atrophic types of the disease are really stages in the same process. He followed a case by serial radiography, and his findings apparently show that in neuropathy there are three distinct stages:

1. A stage of *hydrarthrosis*, with distension of the joint by serous effusion – ligamentous laxity.
2. A stage of *atrophy* – or, better, destruction.
3. A *hypertrophic stage*, associated with new osseous deposits about the joint.

These are of some interest in view of the observations on the pathology of the neuropathic joint.

Charcot (1892) distinguished also between 'benign' and 'malignant' forms of tabetic arthropathy. In his benign cases the disease completely disappeared, or did not proceed to complete disorganization of the joint. The malignant group included those in which the bone destruction was advanced, and where absolute disorganization and dislocation of the joint were invariable sequelae.

Pathologists have not yet been able to assign, with any degree of definiteness, the responsibility for maintaining the trophic nutrition of the joints to any one area of the spinal cord.

King (1931) gave a complete account of the microscopic anatomy in a typical case. He found that, while the histological picture varied in different parts of the joint, the following features could be typically observed:

1. In some areas small fragments of dead bone were present, some still attached to the articular surface, others situated in the neighbouring connective tissue. The bone around the Haversian canals was necrotic in places; the fibrous tissue was granular and the vessels degenerated (Figure 11.51).
2. There was marked cellular activity in many parts, consisting of fibroblastic proliferation, and excessive development of bone and cartilaginous tissue, particularly in relation to pieces of necrotic bone. The bone and cartilage showed a great variety of appearances. In the areas of proliferation, the vessels were well developed, and the completely formed vessel walls suggested neoplastic rather than inflammatory vascular proliferation.
3. There was no microscopic evidence of syphilis. Old trauma was suggested by the irregular distribution of large numbers of cells containing blood pigment, indicative of haemorrhage.
4. That the new growth of bone was associated

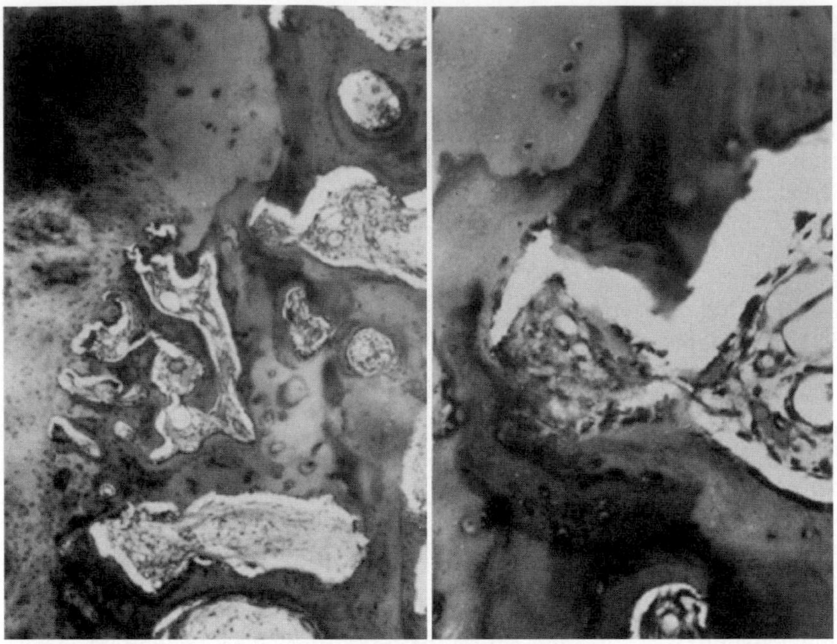

(a) (b)

Figure 11.51 (a) Photomicrograph of the articular and subchondral areas of a Charcot joint, with disruption of the normal articular cartilage on the top left, and the invasion of the subchondral area by vascular granulation tissue. (× 40). (b) Photomicrograph showing the invasion of the subchondral area by a villus-like granulation tissue mass. (× 303).

with architectural remodelling was shown by the decalcification of certain areas. In some of these, osteoclastic activity was evident, but in others osteoclasts were completely absent, and the mechanism of bone removal in them is apparently by halisteresis.

Collins (1950) described the process as being 'a progressive disorganization of an insensitive joint'.

Soto-Hall and Haldeman (1940) described the instability due to the presence of an effusion and ligamentous laxity as being the basis of the disorganization in allowing shearing stress.

Steinberg *et al.* (1962) reviewed the lesion of a Charcot-like arthropathy following the use of intra-articular hydrocortisone.

CLINICAL COURSE

The onset is often sudden and unexpected; premonitory signs are rare. The patient may find on going to bed that one of his joints, usually the knee, has become greatly swollen. The swelling gradually increases, and is eventually associated with a firm diffuse oedema of the leg and foot. The swelling gradually subsides, and the joint is then found to be unduly lax; the bones can be freely moved one upon the other in abnormal directions, and to an unusual extent.

Later, deformity arises as a result of the destruction of the bone ends, of subluxation, of a copious effusion into the enlarged cavity, or of the formation of osteophytes. Throughout the whole course there is a striking absence of pain. The process may occupy only a few weeks, or months; and by the end of that time the joint is often flail, and the patient completely crippled (Figure 11.52a). The disease then gradually diminishes in seriousness, and may even be completely arrested, so that the subject may live for years without any material change in the disabled joint. Other joints may in the meantime pass through a similar series of changes.

Not infrequently a diffuse erythema may be found over a neuropathic joint, particularly at the onset of the disease, when the joint is swollen and oedematous.

Charcot's joints are more common in females. Though the absence of joint pain is noteworthy, the subject suffers the other evidences of tabes in the shape of lightning pains and sensory phenomena; the *Treponema* reaction is usually positive.

Charcot's arthropathy of the spine is rare and consists of a localized form with pathology in one or more segments, or a more diffuse form – more than two segments with loss of disc spaces, bone sclerosis, and large paravertebral ossification masses (Holland, 1953). Even rarer is the development of this condition in the spine after a spinal cord lesion. Sobel *et al.* (1985) described five such patients with a complete spinal cord lesion. With the resultant distal neuropathy, instability between segments occurs, leading to microfractures and then massive collapse and pseudarthrosis. There is marked hypertrophic bone formation around several vertebrae below the spinal cord level. Laminectomy had been performed

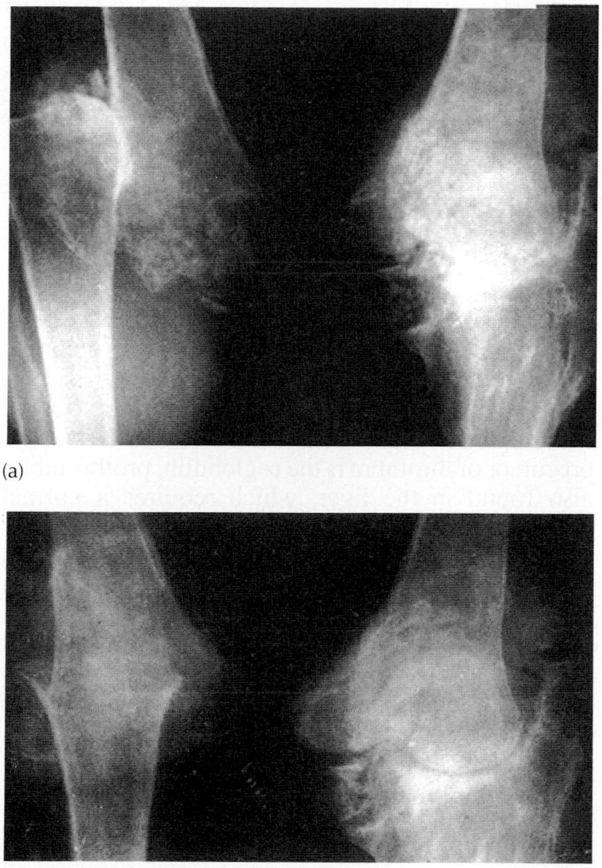

(a)

(b)

Figure 11.52 (a) Radiograph of bilateral Charcot knees with dislocation, marked disorganization and loss of joint structures, with abnormal new bone formation. (b) Radiograph showing the result following a compression arthrodesis of the right knee joint in which stability was achieved through fibrous ankylosis, without evidence of bony union. This was sufficient for this old man to walk using crutches, whereas before he had been limited to a wheelchair.

in four of their patients and was thought to have initiated the breakdown of any stability. These authors describe the success of stabilizing the neuropathic segments with Harrington rods, bone grafting for arthrodesis, turning frames and orthotic support. By such means the deformity was corrected, sitting balance restored and helped to prevent the complication of obstructive uropathy, progressive gibbus formation and decubitus ulcer.

TREATMENT

The knee joint often requires treatment. An arthrodesis should be attempted using Charnley's compression arthrodesis, although the likelihood of obtaining bony ankylosis is poor in comparison with using this procedure for other forms of joint disease. However, the degree of stability which one achieves by fibrous ankylosis is often sufficient for the patient to have, once again, sufficient mobility and freedom (Figure 11.52b). Efficient bracing still has a major part to play in the treatment of this disease.

Successful arthrodesis of a painful, deformed neuropathic ankle joint in leprosy is difficult to achieve because of poor circulation to the skin, secondary to the nerve involvement. Also the shin is vulnerable during the exposure and operation but it is imperative to excise all joint debris, synovial tissue and necrotic bone down to bleeding bone. The talus is largely avascular and necrotic and when complete a tibiocalcaneal fusion should be attempted. Shibata *et al.* (1990) have described their technique and their 73% fusion rate with relief of preoperative pain, swelling, deformity and instability. They used an intramedullary nail with staples or wiring to control rotation. Chronic osteomyelitis and/or sinuses and ulcers of the forefoot indicate a poor prognostic outcome.

The haemophilias

Bleeding diseases of the skeletal tissues can be considered under three main headings based upon their anatomical origin:

1. *Vascular* as seen in direct trauma, in inherited telangiectasis and in allergic purpuras such as Henoch–Schönlein syndrome.
2. *Extravascular* in such conditions as Cushing's syndrome with fragility.
3. *Intravascular* which, in turn, consists of two main types:
   (a) *platelet deficiencies* as seen in thrombocytopenic purpura;
   (b) *coagulation defects* due to:
   (i) varying degrees of deficiency of haemostatic factors – i.e. factor VIII (about 60% of all cases), factor IX (about 12%), von Willebrand's disease (about 15%); the other factors V, VII, X, XI, etc., are very rare;
   (ii) hypoprothrombinaemia which can be either congenital or acquired in the newborn, in vitamin K deficiency and produced by use of anticoagulant drugs;
   (iii) hypofibrinogenaemia either congenital or acquired;
   (iv) circulating anticoagulants, i.e. drugs (e.g. coumarin series or heparin); in dis-

seminated lupus erythematosus, or inhibitors due to circulating antibodies.

John Otto wrote the first important description of this disease in 1803, and in it he postulated Nasse's law that the disease is transmitted as a sex-linked character by females and manifests itself only in males. Sporadic cases are reported, however, so it is not safe to rule out the condition because of an absence of a family history of the disease. Haemophilic arthritis, also known as 'bleeder's joint', was first described by Volkmann in 1868. König in 1892 divided the condition into three stages:

1. haemarthrosis;
2. pan-arthritis; and
3. the regressive stage.

He warned against operation under a mistaken diagnosis.

Factor VIII is a glycoprotein with a molecular weight in the region of 280 000 or more. It is found in normal plasma in a concentration of about 0.2 μg/ml but not in serum, is labile on storage and, following transfusion into a haemophiliac, has a half-life in his circulation of approximately 12 hours.

The site of synthesis of the factor is not known. The little evidence available concerning its site of synthesis suggests that it is made throughout the body in the reticuloendothelial system, chiefly in the liver, in the hepatocytes, kidney, spleen and lymph nodes.

Until recently, it was thought the haemophiliac failed to synthesize the factor VIII protein and this was why his plasma lacked factor VIII activity. During the past 2–3 years, however, it has been shown by means of immunological techniques that in fact haemophiliacs, the proportion varying in different studies, make the protein substance but the protein for some reason or other lacks factor VIII clotting activity.

Fibrin, when formed, is stabilized by the action of activated factor XIII (fibrin stabilizing factor) to give strength to the fibrin clot. If this process does not take place fibrin clot breaks down easily and becomes sensitive to the action of the fibrinolytic enzymes in the blood. This stabilizing factor's action is reinforced by the caproic acid derivatives.

Factor VIII acts as a cofactor in the reaction of factor IX and activates factor X in the presence of calcium ions and phospholipids.

Factor IX is a plasma serine protease which becomes activated when it undergoes proteolytic cleavage. It is a glycoprotein with a molecular weight of 55 000, present in normal plasma in a concentration about 4 μg/ml. In the chain, activated factor IX in the presence of calcium ions, factor VIII and phospholipid assists in cleaving prothrombin to thrombin. It is synthesized in the liver and requires the presence of vitamin K to become active. Its half-life is about 18 hours.

CLOTTING MECHANISM

The clotting mechanism was summarized by Macfarlane (1958). Fibrin formation, which is required for final clotting, arises by action of the proteolytic enzyme, thrombin, on fibrinogen in the presence of ionized calcium and a 'fibrin-stabilizing factor'. Fibrinogen is a globulin formed in the liver. The precursor of thrombin is the α-globulin, prothrombin, also found in the liver, which requires a normal content of vitamin K and bile salts for its production. In the conversion of prothrombin to thrombin, a substance called 'thromboplastin' is required, which is produced from damaged tissues as well as from damaged blood cells such as platelets. The essential factor in platelets to produce thromboplastin appears to be associated with the substance ethanolene phosphatide. In addition to these, factors V and VII, ionized calcium and tissue extracts, particularly of the phospholipid type of protein, are necessary (Figure 11.53).

In the haemophilic patient, blood clot will form in the normal fashion if blood is mixed with haemophilic tissue fluids *in vitro*, but the usual failure to clot following injury *in vivo* is the basic disturbance and, therefore, there are still uncertain mechanisms present (Figure 11.54). Haemophilia is thought to result from a deficiency of an anti-haemophilic globulin, factor VIII, which results in failure of sufficient amount and of the right type of thromboplastin. This condition is caused by an X-linked recessive gene which is handed down to the male of each family by the female – the primary defect being insufficient coagulation. Other entities are recognized, such as Christmas disease, in which there is also a deficiency of the plasma thromboplastic component and, in particular, factor IX. Other syndromes are being separated out, such as pseudohaemophilia, in which there is abnormality of the blood vessels, as well as the lack of various antihaemophilic factors.

Tests to be carried out for the diagnosis of bleeding dyscrasias are:

1. *Bleeding time*. Following a small prick through the skin a macroscopic clot will form within 2–5 minutes. It should be noted that the bleeding time of haemophilics is normal for thrombocytopenia, platelet deficiency, von Willebrand's disease.

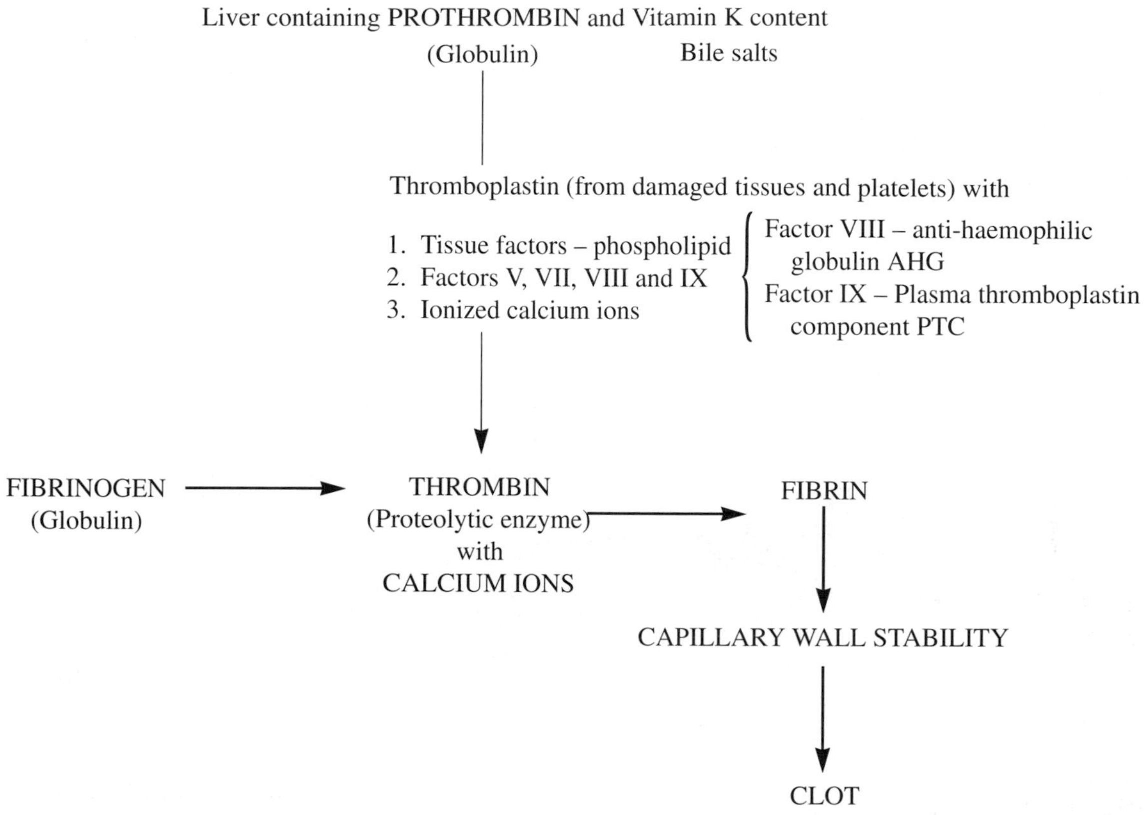

Figure 11.53

2. *Clotting time*. This is an indication for all stages of coagulation and is not sensitive enough to determine those stages which usually occur very rapidly The normal time is 4–10 minutes, and in haemophilics this time may be increased up to 60 minutes.
3. *Prothrombin time*. This indicates the amount of time required for plasma, with adequate ionized calcium ions added and certain tissue extracts, to clot. This is normal in both haemophilics and people with Christmas disease. However, it is abnormal in deficiencies of prothrombin as seen in liver disease, vitamin K deficiencies, dicoumarin toxicity, etc.
4. *Thromboplastin generation test of Biggs and Douglas*. This measures the rate and amount of thromboplastin generated both in the plasma and in the serum components. These are inactive in both haemophilia and Christmas disease patients.
5. *Platelet count*. This will show obvious platelet deficiency, either primary or secondary in nature. Platelet aggregation test for qualitative defects.
6. *Capillary fragility test of Hess*. A sphygmomanometer cuff is inflated to a point halfway between the systolic and diastolic pressures. The skin distal to this is examined for petechiae formation. This indicates the strength of the capillary endothelium and is particularly disturbed in vitamin C deficiencies or scurvy. It is normal in haemophilics.
7. *von Willebrand's factor and antigen*.

Abnormal bleeding into the musculoskeletal system can be differentiated into its two main defects, depending upon certain clinical features (Tables 11.5 and 11.6).

CLINICAL HISTORY

Careful questioning of the patient's personal and family history of bleeding is imperative – for easy bruising, epistaxis, excessive bleeding from cuts, scratches, dental extraction, tonsillectomy (requiring blood transfusion), haematuria, bleeding into joints and muscles.

INCIDENCE

The prevalence of haemophilia in the UK is 90 per million of population and that of Christmas disease 19 per million. The number of patients with bleeding disorders in the Haemophilia Centres of the UK is

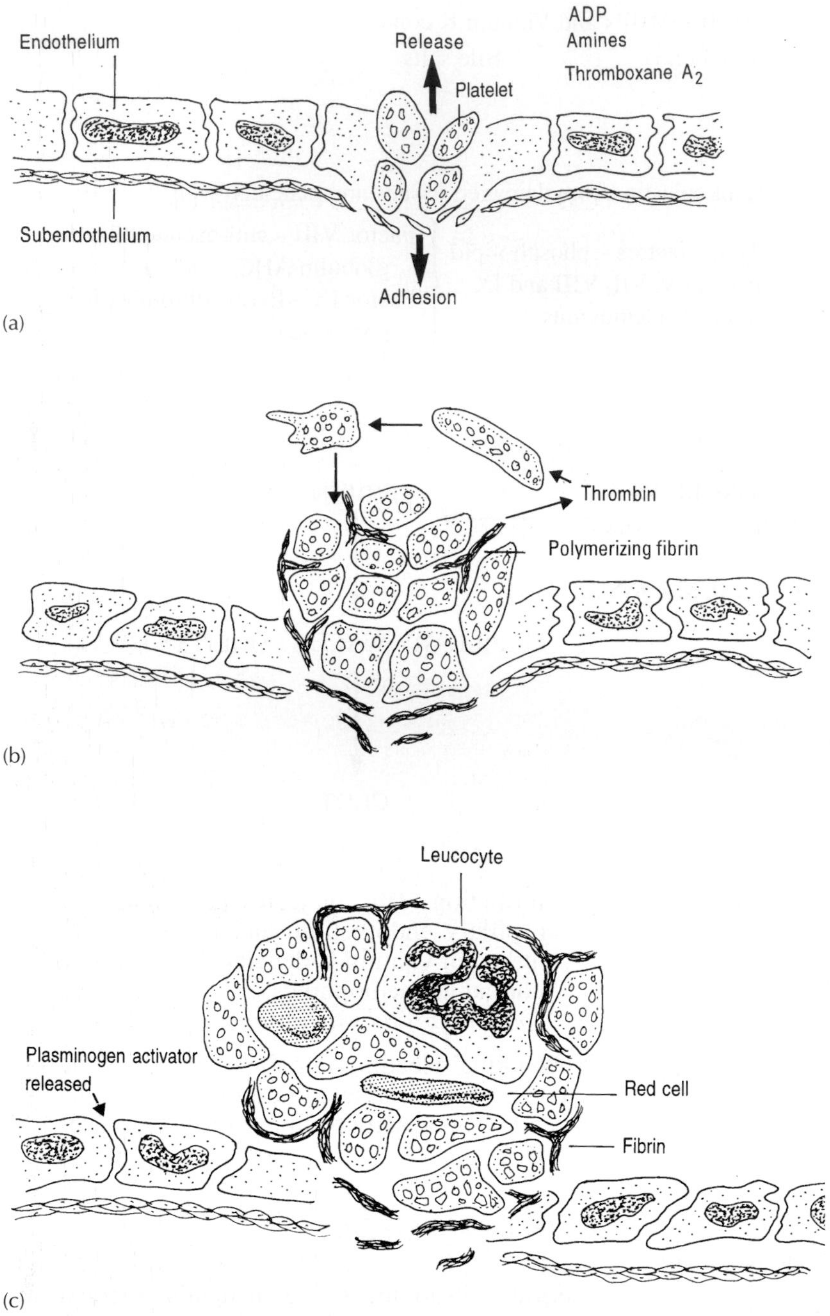

Figure 11.54 (a) Breakdown in the endothelial wall, with platelet plugging and the release of ADP, amines and thromboxane A_2. (b) The development of thrombin and polymerizing fibrin. (c) The release of the plasminogen activator and fibrin formation to give the clot plug. (Redrawn, with permission, from Mason, R.G. (1981) in *Haemophilia*, edited by U. Seligsohn, A. Rimon and H. Horozowski. Castle House Publications: Tunbridge Wells)

seen in Table 11.7. It is of interest that von Willebrand disease, which is inherited as an autosomal dominant disability, is associated with a prolonged bleeding time as well as factor VIII deficiency. This occurs with the same frequency as that of Christmas disease.

The inheritance pattern of haemophilia is well known as an *X-linked recessive*. One-third of all cases are sporadic, and the others occur after several generations from female carriers. The degree of the defect, as well as the clinical severity, is usually uniform throughout the same family.

An X-linked recessive inheritance occurs when the recessive gene is on the X chromosome. Since the male receives an X chromosome from his mother and a Y from his father, the son of a heterozygous female has an equal chance of inheriting the X chromosome which carries the recessive allele and

Table 11.5 Distinction between clotting and capillary defects

Special features	Clotting defect	Capillary defect
Bleeding from small superficial cuts (e.g. shaving cuts)	Often no excessive bleeding	Bleeding often profuse
The time of onset of bleeding	Often delayed 1–3 hours	Usually immediate
The effect of pressure on the lesion	Bleeding restarts after the pressure is released	Bleeding often stopped permanently
The most common sites in severely affected cases	Joints and muscles and massive subcutaneous bruises Any form of internal haemorrhage common	Gastrointestinal bleeding, epistaxis and menorrhagia Large bruises less common Joints and muscles rarely affected
The symptoms of the mildly affected case	Large haematomata following injury Persistent and often dangerous bleeding after trauma	Epistaxis, menorrhagia, traumatic bleeding much less dangerous than in patients with clotting defects
Inheritance	Most are X-linked and recessive	Mainly dominant
Laboratory tests by which abnormalities are most commonly found	Clotting time Prothrombin consumption index Assay of individual factors	Bleeding time Tourniquet Platelet count

therefore has a 1 in 2 (50%) possibility of being affected (Figure 11.55).

This form of inheritance shows the following characteristics:

1. The clinical entity appears almost always in males with unaffected mothers who are carriers.
2. Each son of a carrier has a 1 in 2 (50%) chance of being affected.
3. Affected males never transmit the gene to their sons but do transmit it to their daughters who will in time be carriers. It has been reported that an affected male has married a female carrier and produced several females suffering from haemophila.
4. Unaffected males never transmit the gene to their descendants.

As regards prognosis, only 2 out of the 520 of the Oxford series under the age of 18 years have died. Between 1939 and 1962, Registrar General statistics showed 56 cases dying of haemophilic complications, at an average age of 36.

Macfarlane (1958) described an important relationship – how the circulating amount of factor VIII present in blood relates to the frequency and severity of the bleed. Those who had less than 1% factor VIII were associated with marked deep tissue bleeding and serious haemarthrosic episodes. Up to 5% there was usually gross bleeding episodes but only after a minor trauma to give either haemarthrosis and/or spontaneous bleeding. With 5–25%, severe bleeding occurred only after trauma or surgery. With 25–50% factor present, bleeding occurred only after excessive trauma or injury.

Table 11.6 Tests of clotting function

Whole blood clotting time
Prothrombin consumption index
Activated partial thromboplastin time (APTT)
One-stage prothrombin time
Screening test for factor XIII
Fibrinogen titre
Thrombin time
Assays of factor II
V
VII
VIII
IX
X
XI
XIII
Assays of antithrombin

Table 11.7 Patients with bleeding disorders in UK

Diagnosis	Number of patients
Haemophilia (factor VIII)	5387
Christmas disease (factor IX)	1092
von Willebrand's	2956
Others (factor IX 292, factor XII 160, etc.)	717

Haemophilia Centres Directors (1991).

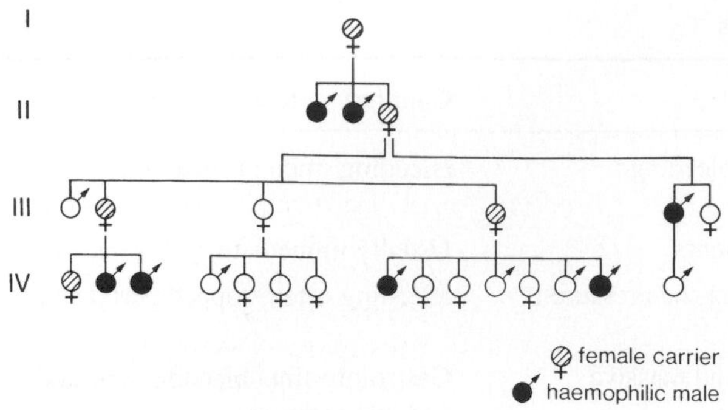

Figure 11.55 A pedigree chart to show the characteristic pattern of X-linked recessive inheritance of haemophilia.

TREATMENT

Treatment is always directed towards correcting the factor deficiency and then attacking the local manifestation. Biggs (1967), of the Oxford Haemophilia Centre, described the sources and strengths of therapy material which are presently available. For the concentrations of factor VIII required for various lesions, and dosage levels to be aimed at, see Table 11.8. The amount of factor administered is calculated approximately using the following formula:

$$\frac{\text{Patient's weight (in kg)} \times \text{Desired rise in factor}}{\text{Total units of factor in dose}} = K$$

In the above formula the patient's weight is known, the desired factor level has been decided upon and K is a constant for a given type of therapeutic material, being 2 for fresh plasma, 1.5 for human AHG concentrates, 1 for animal AHG and 0.7 for Christmas factor concentrates.

For example, if it is desired to raise the factor VIII level of a 70 kg patient from 0% to 50% using human AHG concentrate, the dosage is calculated as follows:

$$\frac{\text{Weight (in kg)} \times \text{Desired rise in factor VIII}}{\text{Total units of factor VIII in dose}} = 1.5$$

i.e.

$$\frac{70 \times 50}{X} = 1.5$$

Therefore $X = 2333$ units of factor VIII.

Agents employed for replacement therapy

Whole blood

The level of factor VIII which may be achieved by the use of whole blood is small. This is particularly so in blood which has been stored, because factor VIII level falls progressively. Transfusions of whole blood should not be given to replace factor VIII in the patient's blood but only to replace blood loss.

Fresh-frozen plasma

Plasma separated from cells within 3–4 hours of donation and then rapidly frozen and stored at –20°C to –40°C may maintain 60–80% of its original factor VIII activity for 2–3 months.

Plasma is effective in the management of some spontaneous haemorrhages into muscles and joints, but has little place in the management of many post-traumatic haemorrhages. When levels of factor VIII higher than 20% of normal are required, one of the concentrated AHG preparations should be employed. The advantages of fresh-frozen plasma are that it is easy to prepare and easily available. The disadvantages are that it takes 30–45 minutes to thaw a bottle of plasma and a further hour to transfuse the dose into the patient. Furthermore, because of the volume transfused, it is not possible to give repeated doses for long without overloading the circulation.

Cryoprecipitate

When frozen plasma is allowed to thaw slowly over several hours at +4°C, some plasma proteins remain in an insoluble state. This cold insoluble fraction or cryoprecipitate is rich in fibrinogen and also factor VIII, and can be separated from the rest of the plasma by centrifugation in the cold to yield a useful concentrate of factor VIII (Pool *et al.*, 1964; Pool and Shannon, 1965). Cryoprecipitate contains 50% of factor VIII activity and 2–3% of the total protein content of the original plasma, giving a 16-fold purification of factor VIII on a protein basis. The chief advantage of cryoprecipitate is that its preparation is relatively simple. It may also be prepared from blood collected for transfusion purposes. The number of donors is few, thus reducing the risk of transfusion hepatitis. The chief disadvantage of cryoprecipitate is that the factor VIII content of the dose is not known before administration because it is not assayed until it has been reconstituted for transfusion and antigenic reactions are frequent.

Freeze-dried human AHC concentrates

These are prepared from plasma by precipitation with alcohol. They are reconstituted for intravenous injection by using distilled water or saline. The concentration of factor VIII in the infusion is approximately four to six times that of plasma.

These freeze-dried concentrates are of great value

Table 11.8

Material	Reasonable dosage (units/kg)	Levels in % normal post-infusion	Lesion
Whole blood	4–5	4–6	Replacement of blood loss only
Fresh-frozen plasma	8–12	15–25	Spontaneous bleeding
	(15–20 ml/kg)		
	(4 litres to give adequate levels for surgery)		Haemarthrosis
Cryoprecipitate	40	60–80	Bleeding, surgery
Human AHG	10–40	40–60	Serious haematoma and surgery
Animal AHG	80–100	100–150	Major trauma and surgery

1 unit is the activity in 1 ml of average normal plasma.

in replacement therapy, for major surgery, for serious bleeding episodes and for the treatment of bleeding episodes in children. The potency of this material may make prophylactic treatment of haemophilia feasible by means of daily injections of a small volume of AHG (Table 11.8).

Blood factors and HIV infection

Up until the early 1980s great strides had been made in blood transfusion techniques, the extraction and concentration of the various factors from plasma had been achieved and had been made available world wide. Suddenly the discovery of the human immunodeficiency virus (HIV) and its transmission by these biological products has decimated the haemophilic population. From 1985 onwards virucidal methods were introduced into the manufacturing process of coagulation factor concentrates, and the preparation of factor VIII by genetic engineering was begun.

Haemophiliacs are known to have been infected with the HIV between 1979 and 1985 – most before the end of 1982 – and there has been no further conversion in the UK after the introduction of heat-treated concentrates (Giangrande *et al.*, 1994).

Factor VIII concentrates have varied greatly in terms of purity and contamination by protein immunoglobulins, fibrinogin, etc., depending upon the manufacturer. With improved techniques of immunoaffinity chromatography with monoclonal antibodies, ion exchange, purity and concentration have improved but also with the removal of the virus of hepatitis B and C and HIV. In addition, these materials are treated by solvent or detergent material or heating. All of these processes have almost doubled the cost.

Factor IX concentrates contain prothrombin concentrates, as well as vitamin K dependent coagulation factors such as factors II and IX. There is a definite risk of thromboembolism, myocardial infarction or disseminated intravascular coagulation. Therefore, heparin has been added to these concentrates. Purer factor IX concentrates are now available with higher specific activities.

There is an increasing incidence of septic arthritis in the haemophilic joint, particularly in those patients with HIV infections (Duthie *et al.*, 1994). Diagnosis by aspiration and fresh culture (plating for both aerobic and anaerobic growth) is essential to discover the invading organism which can be varied, e.g. *Streptococcus pneumoniae*, *Salmonella choleraesuis,* resistant *Staphylococcus aureus*. This aspiration requires full factor replacement. The C-reactive protein can be significantly raised (Gregg-Smith *et al.*, 1993).

Animal AHG concentrates

Porcine and bovine AHG are commercially available as freeze-dried powders, each ampoule of which is reconstituted in 50 ml of saline or distilled water and contains approximately 800 units of factor VIII. With the advent of cryoprecipitate and human AHG concentrates, the use of animal AHG should be used for the treatment of:

1. Patients requiring life-saving surgery when no human AHG or cryoprecipitate is available.
2. Life-endangering haemorrhages in a patient with factor VIII antibodies.

With the administration of these materials, daily estimation of the factor level in the blood is usually carried out to ensure that an adequate haemostatic dosage has been given; i.e. levels of 25–50% for factor VIII or 15–25% for factor IX. Also, assays are carried out for the presence of antibodies to factor VIII, because their presence is a serious feature and indicates difficulty in building up adequate blood levels for controlling bleeding or the effects of bleeding (Duthie *et al.*, 1994).

Factor VIII antibodies

About 5–10% of patients with haemophilia develop antibodies which rapidly inactivate infused factor VIII. These antibodies have been identified as immunoglobulins (IgG) and are thought to arise as a response to infusion of factor VIII. Haemophiliacs who develop factor VIII antibodies do not usually have more frequent spontaneous haemorrhages, although when bleeding does take place it is more difficult to control. If a patient with antibodles to factor VIII bleeds dangerously, he should be treated vigorously with large doses of cryoprecipitate, human AHG or animal AHG. Animal AHG has the advantage that it is available in large quantities commercially and is very potent. In addition, most antibodies to factor VIII are less active against animal factor VIII than against human factor VIII.

Special prothrombin complex concentrates are also of value in treating patients with high levels of inhibitory antibodies. The technique of immune tolerance by giving high doses of factor VIII concentrates over prolonged periods of time will eventually lower the inhibitory levels.

Side-effects are less common with materials of greater purity but transient mild thrombocytopenia is frequent and allergic reactions are seen.

Home therapy

Over the past few years, a home care programme has been developed in which patients or their family members transfuse replacement factors in their own homes. This allows early treatment with instant relief of pain and resolution of joint and muscle bleeds, permitting them to continue at school or at work with little interruption. Not all patients are fitted for this type of programme and certain criteria must be met:

1. The patient and his family must be carefully screened for their psychological balance which might interfere with judgement or alter the manner in which therapy should be given.
2. The patient and his family should be carefully instructed about haemophilia, the type of bleeding episodes, replacement therapy and exactly when they are required to come to the hospital.
3. They should be educated in the technique and hazards of home transfusion.
4. Patients under 4 years of age and without laboratory-proven haemophilia should not be admitted to the programme. Those with inhibitors should be excluded.
5. Every single transfusion, detailing the site of bleeding and the therapy given, should be recorded.
6. A routine follow-up examination must be made – in the severe cases every 3 months and for the others every 6–12 months.

At present, one-third of all infusions given to patients who attend the Oxford Haemophilia Centre are given at home.

If the patient undergoes one of the following conditions, he should be taken to hospital:

1. Severe pain and swelling in any muscle or joint, causing limitation of movement or loss of sleep.
2. Some headache, related or not to any previous injury or swelling in the region of the neck or the floor of the mouth.
3. Severe abdominal pain, haematemesis, melaena or haematuria.
4. Skin wounding requires inspection.

HIV infection

The appearance and identification of the human immunodeficiency virus, HIV, occurred in 1983. Monkey or ape immunodeficiency viruses have become adapted to man. Simian trappers and handlers, through scratches and bites, have been infected by blood from these animals. With change of sexual behaviour, e.g. multiple sex partners and homosexuals, grouping into the larger urban type of life with disruption of the African stable village community, HIV from the middle of Africa has spread throughout the world (Smith, 1993). This has been aggravated by intravenous drug misuse and needle sharing and feeding in the manufacture of blood products material, particularly in the USA, has resulted in its spread into the haemophilic and the rest of the world's population.

PROPERTIES, PREVALENCE AND INFECTIVITY

After the first description of this immunodeficiency viraemia and disease in 1981, much information has been produced about this retrovirus which is 90–120 mm in diameter with a nucleoprotein core. It is an RNA virus which, by possessing a reverse transcriptase enzyme, enters through the CD4 receptor cell wall of the membranes of lymphocytes/monocytes, macrophages, myeloid and microglial cells. It catalyses a new DNA in the chromosomes of the cells. The viral DNA is transcripted back into RNA which makes further virus. The human T4 lymphocyte macrophages are killed to produce a thombocytonia, a lack of response to skin test antigens and reduction in all cells including erythrocytes to produce a severe anaemia.

It is now world wide. It is estimated that there could now be 20 million people infected with the HIV virus and 400 000 with AIDS. The prevalence rates are 2 cases/100 000 in the UK; 30 cases/100 000 in the USA and 60 cases/100 000 in Zaire. In 1990 15 000 HIV people were positive in the UK with 3500 having AIDS, half of whom have already died. A plasma viraemia occurs in the early stages after initial infection and the viral load in the blood mononuclear cells progressively increases (Wooley, 1993). The phenotypic changes in the virus are important in the rate of development of AIDS disease, e.g. patients with syncytia inducing (SI) strain have increased rate of reduction in CD4 cell counts and are therefore more likely to progress to AIDS than those with non-syncytia inducing (NSI) strains. The switch from NSI to SI occurs in early disease when the median CD4 count is about 400 cells/mm^3. It has been shown that after heating and drying cell-free cultures, the virus survives for up to 15 days at room temperature (23–27°C) (Resnick *et al.* 1986) but is very heat labile at 56°C. This property has been used to treat the blood products, factors VIII and IX in order to eradicate the virus, but has doubled the cost of production and therefore placed these factors out of reach of poorer countries. The virus is also sensitive to α-radiation at 2.5×10^5 rads (2.5×10^3 Gy) of γ-radiation (Spire *et al.*, 1985).

Patients who have been infected by the HIV are infectious before the antibody response, at times prior to development of full-blown AIDS and obviously even more so after the development of AIDS. The risk of transmission depends upon the virus titre in the patient, his/her lymphocyte count, the susceptibility of the exposed individual and the treatment after exposure. During actual transmission the important facts are the volume of the inoculum, the site and depth of the inoculation. Under certain conditions there is a 0.3% seroconversion rate with a risk of occupational exposure, one episode in every 20 000 operations.

Since this virus is carried in most body fluids (e.g. blood, semen, CSF), it is transferred both heterosexually and homosexually, from mother to fetus and infant and during intervention such as operations, injections and aspiration procedures. An analysis based upon the surveillance figures from the Centers for Disease Control and Prevention (CDC) of over 6000 registered health care workers has shown that the numbers of health care workers with AIDS were similar in number to the proportion of AIDS amongst the general population. It was seen that relatively few surgeons appear to have AIDS, especially being occupationally derived. However, there are many more nurses and there are now over 32 health care workers who have acquired the infection during their occupation, i.e. a 0.4% infection rate based upon exposure knowledge. The CDC estimated from 4.5 million health care workers in the USA that there are over 360 surgeons, 50000 physicians and 35 000 other workers HIV infected but unrecognized. Mandatory testing for all surgeons, physicians, etc. and other health care workers is not required at the present, although it is arousing fierce debate.

SURGICAL CONSIDERATIONS

An increased risk is a percutaneous inoculation of a large volume of blood such as from a hollow needle, or deep intramusculature exposure to the virus. There is also an increased risk during any operation when the blood loss is more than 300 ml with the operation lasting more than 3 hours, particularly in vascular, intra-abdominal and gynaecological procedures, and of course orthopaedic procedures, e.g. total joint replacement, osteotomies and operations on fractures. In the largest reported series of total hip replacement of 39 cases for haemophilic arthropathy the peroperative blood loss ranged between 300 and 1000 ml (Nelson *et al.*, 1992). Another specific pathological entity – the haemophilic cyst – also during surgery of excision or amputation can lose up to 4 litres of blood during the procedure with gross spillage and soaking of fomites (Duthie *et al.*, 1994).

It is important to appreciate that there is no vaccine, there is progression to AIDS in 50% of the patients and there is no proven treatment. In addition, rates of infection are not based upon one percutaneous exposure but over successive years of potential exposure by the surgeon or health care worker after entering this field at a young age. Screening for antibodies has become a controversial subject and indeed there is no actual figure for seropositivity in the general population. These methods of determining high- or low-risk patients by history or by screening can no longer be regarded as reliable because of the heterosexual spread. Therefore the majority of patients in certain areas must be regarded as positive until proven otherwise. Improvement in all working practices is absolutely essential to reduce the risk, rather than depending upon the results of screening.

A very infectious phase and contraindication to elective surgery is the onset of clinical AIDS with its presentation of opportunistic infections, e.g. *Pneumonocystis carinii* pneumonia, Kaposi's sarcoma, non-Hodgkin's lymphoma, cytomegalovirus and *Mycobacterium tuberculosis* (the lung is affected in more than 70% of AIDS patients at some time during the illness) (Wooley, 1993). In the central nervous system toxoplasmosis, progressive multifocal leucoencephalic tuberculoma, meningoencephalitis and progressive spinal cord myelopathy are all described. There are gastrointestinal syndromes of ulceration and such infections as herpes. In the skin and musosal surfaces ulcerations, malignant changes and lymph node adenopathy can be found. Fever of known aetiology is also a contraindication to surgery. However, it should also be noted that there are other infections not commonly occurring in patients with full-blown AIDS who, because they are susceptible to other infections, develop *Salmonella typhimurium* with septicaemia and enteritis, pneumococcal bacteraemia and tuberculosis. These too are contraindications to elective surgery.

A very important biological consideration was triggered from an observation that surgery may promote clinical AIDS in seropositive patients (Konotey-Ahulu, 1987). Indeed, there have been anecdotal reports on HIV patients who had received total joint replacements and who developed clinical AIDS within a few years of surgery with increasing mortality. On first diagnosing this condition in 1983 it was observed that HIV positive patients had a decreased natural killer cell activity with a reduced number of T4 helper cells (Gottlieb *et al.*, 1983). A similar immunological response of reduction in helper and lymphocytic populations was recorded in the postoperative period after major surgery in other patients than those with HIV (Lennard *et al.*, 1985). However, this depression of the immune system after surgery in 'normal' patients is regarded as being transient. Obviously these interesting observations must be carefully considered before operating electively upon a haemophilic patient or any other HIV positive patient.

In 30 haemophilic patients who were seropositive for HIV, pre- and postoperatively there was subsequent progression of the infection in most, as determined by the CD4 lymphocyte count and the Walter Reed classification. Indeed AIDS was diagnosed in 6 patients who had a low CD4 lymphocyte count preoperatively. Patients with a CD4 lymphocyte count of less than 200/mm^3 should not have an operation if it can be avoided, and the measurement of intradermal skin test antigens was of help. The normal value for CD4 cells is over 700/mm^3.

According to the CDC occupationally transmitted hepatitis B virus (HBV) occurs in an estimated 18 000 health care workers annually, and about 250 of them die each year as a result of the acute and chronic sequelae of HBV, e.g. hepatitis, cirrhosis and cancer. However, infection with the immunodeficiency virus (HIV)-1, has occurred in a smaller number of health care workers who have no non-occupational risk factors for the disease. Therefore the risk of acquiring HIV from patient care activities is very low. The documented episodes of seroconversion have usually followed percutaneous exposure (80% were accidental needlesticks, 89% cuts with sharp objects, 7% open wound contamination and 5% mucous membrane exposures) to infected blood. The risk of seroconversion after an accidental needlestick exposure to blood from a patient carrying HIV-1 is about 0.5%. This has to be compared to the 30% infection rate after similar exposure to HBV infected blood. In the USA fewer than 75 health care workers have developed HIV infection in the workplace whereas an estimated 12 000–18 000 workers became infected with hepatitis B virus.

Universal precautions are easy to implement and, for the most part, this happens in hospitals (Raginer, 1991). However, a study in an American university hospital showed that universal precautions were not adhered to in 30% of procedures that took place in the intensive care unit, and were not followed in 75% of procedures carried out on a surgical ward. Rigorous precautions are essential with isolation of the operating team and patients within a vertical laminar flow operating room to allow control of contaminated materials, decontamination at the end of the procedure, with restriction of staff and movement during procedures. A manual of general principles and guidelines must be available for immediate reference by all staff, with details of the preparation of operating and anaesthetic rooms, equipment, handling of sponges and their disposal, of spillages, instrument cleansing, all spillages, donning and removal of disposable protective clothing, etc.

Protective impervious clothing and waterproof aprons, face masking to including visors, are all required. The full Charnley positive pressure vertical laminar flow 'tents' with closed extraction systems is recommended (Duthie *et al.*, 1994).

In orthopaedic surgery such as total hip replacements, osteotomies, etc., glove perforation or puncture can be as high as 20% per operation, therefore double and protective gloving are essential. Inspection of hands for blood staining after removing gloves is sensible and thorough washing of the hands with an antiseptic soap is carried out. Wound dressing of the operation site at the end of the procedure should be by a water repellent, impervious dressing to contain any exudate. Redressing of wounds should be carried out in designated areas which can be decontaminated, dressings and discharged material 'bagged' for incineration; and the health care team should be properly dressed and protected with impervious aprons, gloves, eye and mouth protection, etc.

If exposure of inoculation is thought to have taken place, careful inspection for needle marks, wounding or penetration is carried out and recorded. Thorough washing with soap and water is as efficacious as an hypochlorite solution. Mucous membranes should be irrigated with sterile saline. The surgeon or nurse should be tested for HIV and HBV and if the patient is known to be hepatitis B surface antigen positive, should then receive hepatitis B immunoglobulin and hepatitis B vaccine. Follow-up testing for HIV after the initial, immediate one should be carried out at 6 weeks, 3 months and 6 months. During this time atypical skin lesions and any unexplained lymphadenopathy are looked for. Counselling and advice are imperative during this period.

A positive HIV seroconversion means no further operating room duties and no giving of injections. All of this results in a complete change in professional activities and, indeed, everyday activities.

An anti-HIV viral drug, zidovudine, was developed in 1985 and the first randomized clinical trial was completed in 1987. It has a similar structure to thymidine with the properties of inhibiting the phosphates important in HIV function as well as blocking the synthesis of viral RNA by inhibiting the HIV reverse transcriptase enzyme.

It is licensed to be used in patients with asymptomatic HIV infection and early symptoms where the CD4 counts are reduced, and in the treatment of patients with AIDS (acquired immunodeficiency syndrome) or ARC (AIDS related complex, e.g. fever, diarrhoea, weight loss and oral candidiasis).

The value of zidovudine prophylaxis after HIV exposure is yet to be established. However, it has been suggested that strong indications for its use are massive parenteral exposure or a deep penetrating injury and weak indications are mucous membrane or subcutaneous exposure, larger bore needle perforations or exposure to anonymous blood in a high-risk setting, i.e. in an emergency department. Zidovudine is considered to prolong survival and to reduce the frequency and severity of opportunistic infections in AIDS patients but it does not necessarily prevent seroconversion. The drug does have a variety of significant side-effects. It is contraindicated in pregnancy, or if there has been cutaneous exposure with intact skin or exposure to other body fluids other than blood, e.g. cerebrospinal fluid, semen, etc.

In haemophilia there is an increasing prevalence of septic arthritis; Gregg-Smith *et al.*, (1993) have shown that this relatively rare complication in haemophilia has now, with HIV infection, become more widespread. The routine aspiration of the joints for bacterial diagnosis as well as blood cultures must be carefully carried out with full precautions. Infection with HIV may predispose to any bacteria involving the haemarthrosis and with the common practice of the haemophilic patient injecting himself with coagulation factor concentrates at home with varying aseptic techniques, infection is now more likely.

Another field now requiring special attention is the harvesting and use of tissues for research or of bone graft material taken either at the time of operation or in the post-mortem room for the control of transmission of HIV and other blood-borne pathogens in biomechanical cadaveric testing. The required precautions against blood and body fluids are described as for infectious control outlined by the Centers for Disease Control. HIV and hepatitis B are screened for, using the enzyme-linked immunosorbent assay as well as HIV P24 core antigen testing but it is emphasized that false negatives can be found during the first 4–12 weeks after infection with HIV. Bone graft material for clinical use now requires negative screening results on taking the bone and then waiting 120 days for another negative result from the same patient before its use. Tissues themselves can be tested for the presence of the virus or not and γ-radiation can be used to kill the virus. All instruments require cleansing, disinfection of the virus with formalin or hypochlorite solutions, but the biochemistry of these tissues may well be affected by such measures.

Bleeding into joints

Bleeding into joints, or haemarthrosis, is the most common manifestation of the haemophilias (about 55% of all 'haemophiliac' hospital admissions are due to this complication). It occurs when the child with less than 1% of factor VIII begins to walk or run at about the age of 1 year or so. The joints most commonly involved are knees, elbows, ankles (all hinge articulations with angulatory and rotational strains), with the wrist, hip, shoulder, hand and foot being quite infrequently involved.

ACUTE HAEMARTHROSIS

After minor injury, or even spontaneously, bleeding is thought to arise from numerous vessels of the stratum synoviale (Figure 11.56). This produces a polymorphonuclear leucocytosis as well as a lymphocytic and histiocytic cellular invasion leading to a synovitis with hyperplasia. Large amounts of the pigment haemosiderin accumulate throughout the synovial tissues. As the swelling rapidly increases, pain becomes a prominent feature with a stiffness of the joint usually in a flexed position as well as inhibition of muscle function. DeAndrade *et al.*

(1965) demonstrated that a rapid filling of a volunteer's knee joint with saline produced severe pain and inhibition of quadriceps function due to capsular distension. A feeling of abnormal sensation – pricking, increased warmth, slight weakness – may precede the actual bleeding with its distension pain.

Distension of the knee joint is easily seen but less so in the elbow or in the ankle joint. Radiography for soft tissue detail will often show a soft tissue outline. Palpation will reveal tenderness and an increased local temperature of the skin is usually present. Differential diagnosis from an infective arthritis, especially as both may produce a pyrexia with acute local tenderness, will be made by a white cell count and a blood culture. Acute joint swelling resulting from rheumatic fever, rheumatoid arthritis or tuberculosis can usually be distinguished.

Treatment is directed towards stopping the bleeding by factor replacement, relieving the pain and swelling by immobilization in compression bandaging with a POP back splint, aspiration to relieve the absorption of blood content and physiotherapy to restore muscle function under factor cover (Figure 11.57). Often early and small acute haemarthroses can be treated on an out-patient basis with the prompt infusion of appropriate factor concentrates, but about 25% will require hospital admission for 2–3 weeks' duration. Protection of the limb by a plastic splint (Figure 11.58) or by the use of a long leg caliper for several months may be necessary, particularly of the knee when there is persistent quadriceps muscle atrophy and/or weakness and joint thickening. This support should be removed frequently for physiotherapy – if necessary, under factor control.

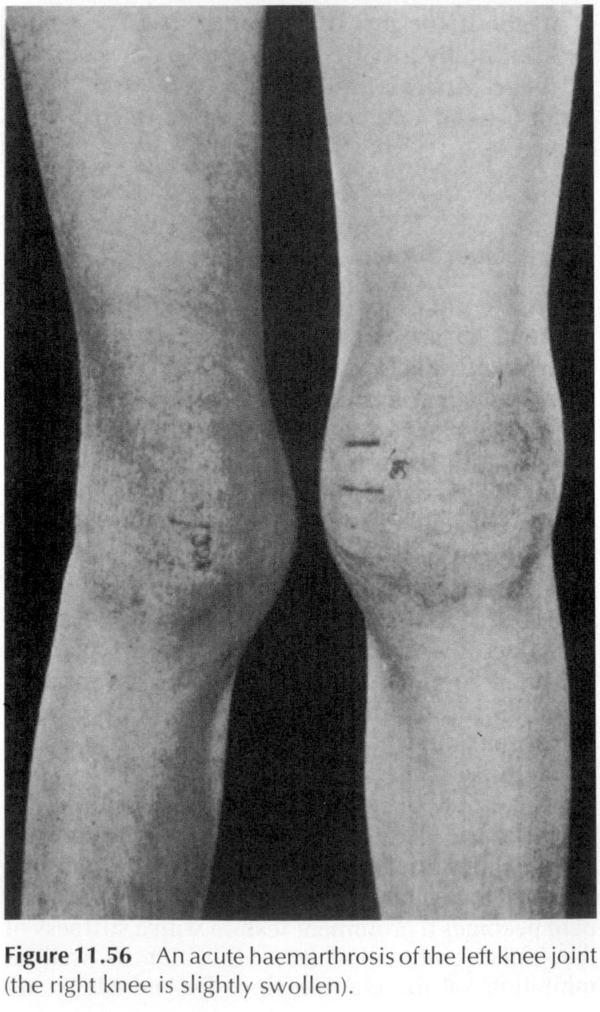

Figure 11.56 An acute haemarthrosis of the left knee joint (the right knee is slightly swollen).

Aspiration of joints

With earlier treatment of haemarthroses, aspiration of joints is required less often. The decision to aspirate is based on the following factors:

1. The size of the haemarthrosis and resulting pain and tension. If severe, aspiration will relieve pain.
2. The interval between onset of bleeding and admission to hospital. If this is more than 24 hours, aspiration is difficult and complete emptying of the joint seldom possible due to clotting of the haemarthrosis.
3. The type of joint involved. Haemarthroses in the elbow or ankle joint usually resolve rapidly and therefore aspiration is rarely required. By contrast, the knee joint may contain large volumes of blood which take many weeks to be reabsorbed.
4. The presence or absence of factor VIII antibodies in the patient's blood. Aspiration in the presence of antibodies is dangerous and may lead to serious extensive bleeding within and without the joint.

Aspiration is carried out with strict aseptic technique.

Chronic haemophilic arthropathy

With prompt and effective replacement therapy and correct treatment of the joint bleeds, such deformities should be fewer. However, haemophilic patients are now living longer and the total number is increasing so that chronic arthropathy remains a problem.

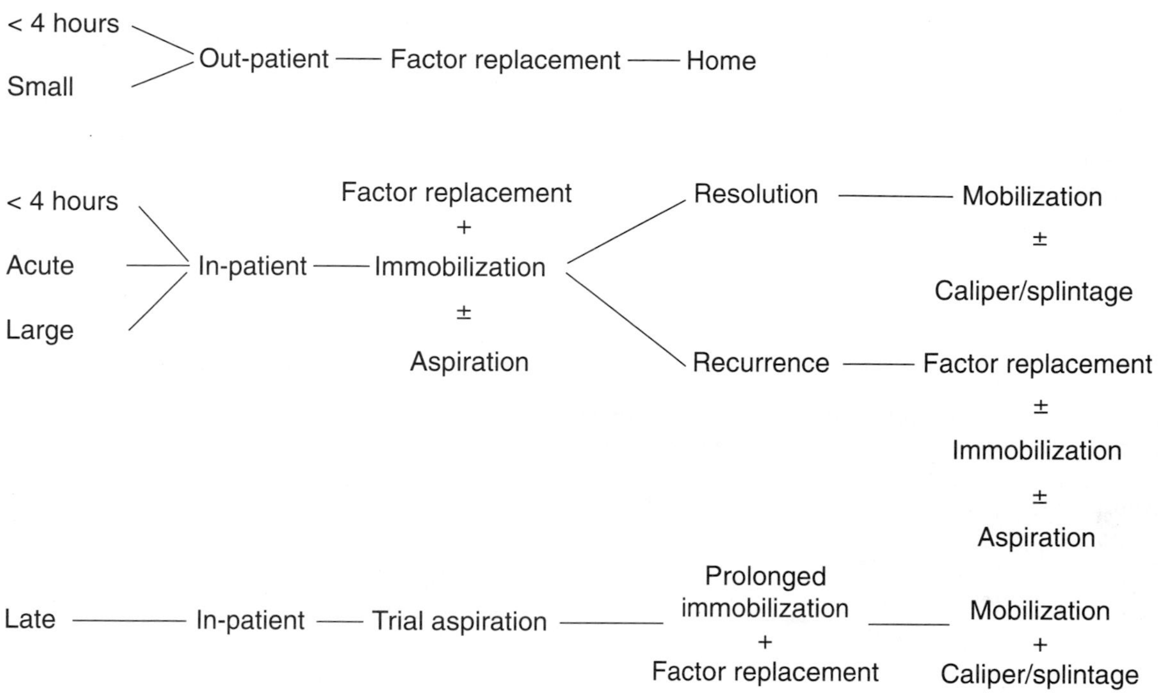

Figure 11.57 Summary of treatment of acute haemarthrosis.

AETIOLOGY

Combined pathological and experimental investigations demonstrated that repeated haemorrhages into joints produce synovial hyperplasia, haemosiderin deposition and fibrous scarring (Hoaglund, 1967; Mankin, 1974).

Azarin *et al.* (1985) have produced experimentally an ongoing haemarthrosis into the knee of dogs by creating a popliteal arteriovenous aneurysm bleeding into the joint. They studied not only the effect of blood on the tissues, but an increased intra-articular pressure of 120–140 mmHg which is also very important in the pathogenesis. Intra-articular ad-

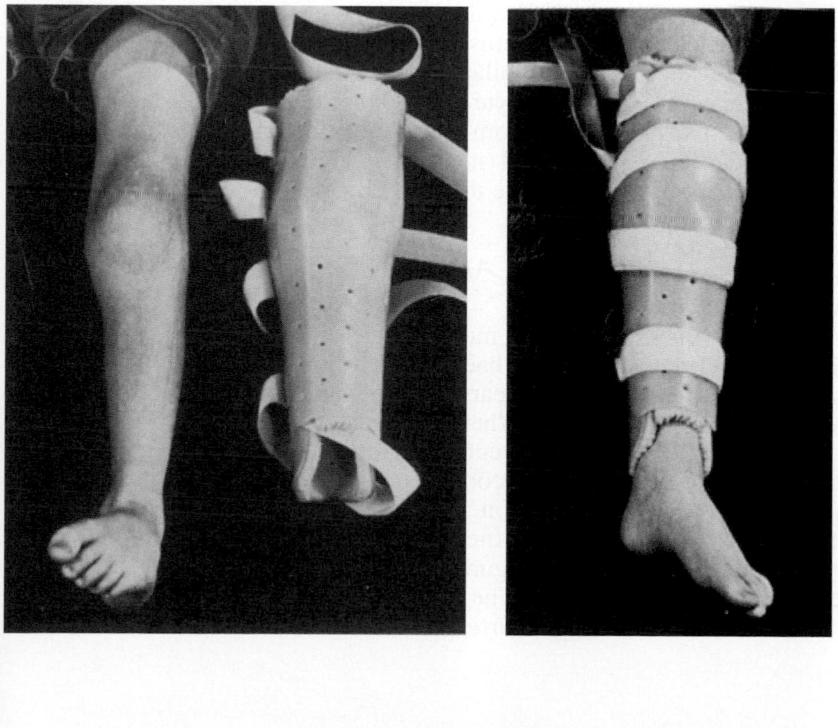

Figure 11.58 Protection of a haemarthrotic knee by plastic splint.

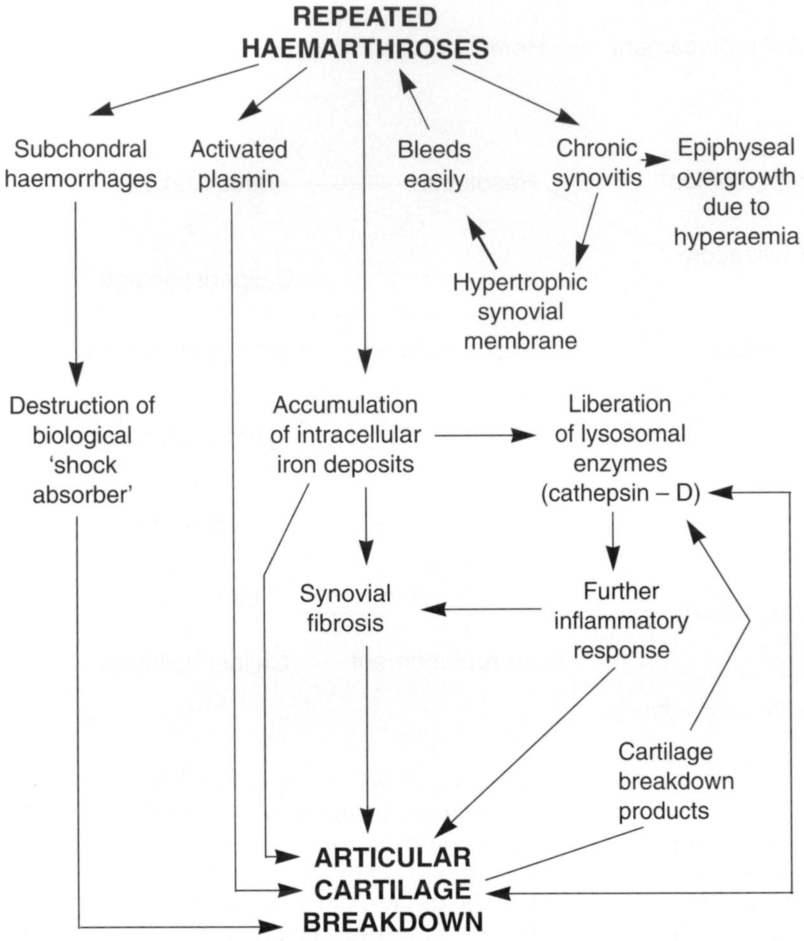

Figure 11.59 Diagnosis of articular cartilage breakdown mechanism (Stein and Duthie, 1981).

hesions will result in reduction of the joint cavity and limitation of movement. The restriction of motion will reduce the circulation of nutrients in the articular cartilage and lead to progressive articular cartilage breakdown (Figure 11.59). The bone changes are attributed partly to disuse osteoporosis and partly to secondary osteoarthrosis following cartilage breakdown. It appears that the initiation of cartilage breakdown is due to the combined effect of immobilization with poor nutrition and the release of enzymes from both the blood within the joint and the inflamed synovial membrane which causes breakdown of the glycosaminoglycans of the matrix (Stein and Duthie, 1981). McLardy-Smith *et al.* (1984) have shown that haemophilic synovium in culture produces more prostaglandin E at much higher levels than normal but less than found in rheumatoid synovitis, with significant loss of chondroitin sulphate from human cartilage.

The late radiographic appearances of the involved joints result from the effects of haemarthrosis, local immobilization osteoporosis and mechanical changes in alignment. The most common features seen in the knee joint are epiphyseal overgrowth, patellar squaring and widening of the intercondylar notch, followed by diminished joint cartilage space, subchondral bone collapse and cyst formation with marginal osteophyte formation (Figure 11.60). Pathologically, apart from the deposition of haemosiderin in the synovial membrane, the late appearances in the joints are those of advanced osteoarthrosis.

CLINICAL FEATURES

Loss of movement is the most frequent finding in chronic haemophilic arthropathy. This often occurs many years before pain and gross deformity are noted. Where moderate or severe radiological changes are present, 80% of involved knees have a fixed flexion contracture. As the changes progress, the correction of flexion deformity becomes increasingly difficult due to posterior subluxation of the tibia (Figure 11.61) and lateral shift of the tibia on the femur. The elbow shows a loss of extension following recurrent bleeding but limitation of flexion is

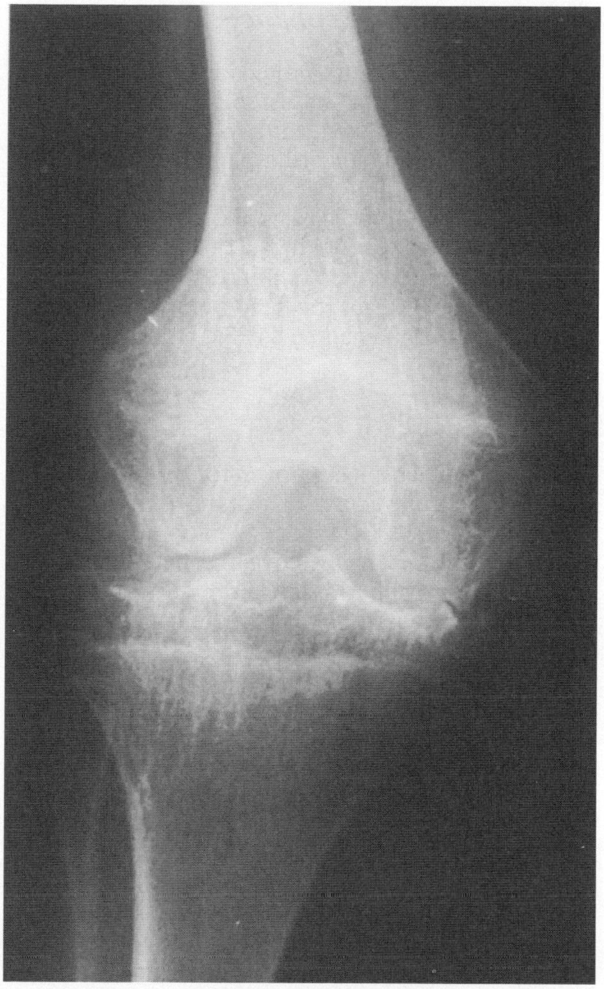

Figure 11.60 Radiograph of chronic haemophilic arthropathy of the knee joint.

slight. Ankle motion appears to be less restricted than that of the knee or elbow.

Joint deformities may be apparent before gross radiological changes are seen. In the knee, valgus and external rotation deformities are frequently observed in joints subject to recurrent bleeding. These follow flexion of the knee and overaction of the lateral hamstrings with the tensor fascia lata opposing the severely wasted quadriceps muscle.

A reduction in the capacity of the joint cavity follows the fibrosis and scarring of repeated haemarthroses. Intra-articular adhesions lead to a small, stiff contracted joint. Bleeding into the joint in these circumstances may result in a small but nevertheless tense and painful haemarthrosis.

Pettersson *et al.* (1980) have described a radiological classification with a points system (Table 11.9).

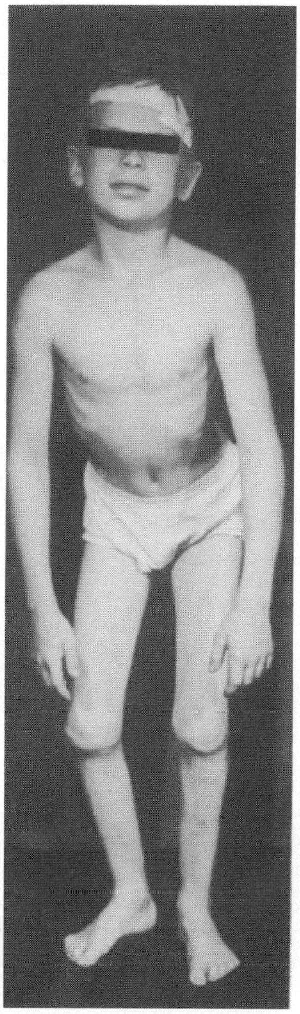

Figure 11.61 Knee contracture affecting stance in a haemophiliac.

CONSERVATIVE TREATMENT

A summary of treatment is given in Figure 11.62.

Physiotherapy

The maintenance of good muscle power, especially of the quadriceps in the case of the knee, is one of the most important aspects of physical therapy in chronic haemophilic arthropathy. This is handicapped by severe wasting which follows each haemarthrosis, and the presence of a flexion contracture makes build-up of the extensors more difficult.

Table 11.9 Radiological classification of haemophilic arthropathy

Type of change	Finding	Score (points)
Osteoporosis	Absent	0
	Present	1
Enlarged epiphysis	Absent	0
	Present	1
Irregular subchondral surface	Absent	0
	The surface partly involved	1
	The surface totally involved	2
Narrowing of joint space	Absent	0
	Present; joint space > 1 mm	1
	Present; joint space < 1 mm	2
Subchondral cyst formation	Absent	0
	1 cyst	1
	> 1 cyst	2
Erosions at joint margins	Absent	0
	Present	1
Gross incongruence of articulating bone ends	Absent	0
	Slight	1
	Pronounced	2
Joint deformity (angulation and/or displacement between articulating bones)	Absent	0
	Slight	1
	Pronounced	2
Possible joint score: 0–13 points		

Adapted from Pettersson *et al.* (1980).

Bracing/orthotic appliances

Employing calipers to protect knees and ankles which are subject to recurrent haemarthroses is useful. They are also useful in supporting lower limbs in which severe arthropathy of the knee or ankle is present. A balance must be achieved between external bracing and the development and maintenance of adequate muscle power.

Pneumatic intermittent compression bags (Allen, 1994) have been used for fixed flexion deformities of less than 40° and can be used at home.

Dynamic splintage

This method has been employed for the correction of knee flexion contracture. The limb is placed on a Thomas' splint with a knee flexion piece, and a reverse sling is placed above the patella exerting pressure on the femur in a posterior direction against the counterpressure of slings on the undersurface of the upper calf. Longitudinal skin traction is applied to the lower leg (Figure 11.63). In this apparatus the patient can carry out active quadriceps exercises and also flex the knee slightly. Emphasis is placed on quadriceps exercises. This technique requires very careful supervision to prevent damage to the skin by the longitudinal traction on the lower leg and bruising from the reverse sling. Good correction of marked deformities has been achieved. This method is particularly useful where posterior subluxation of the tibia has occurred. Dynamic splintage has the great advantage that muscle power and tone are

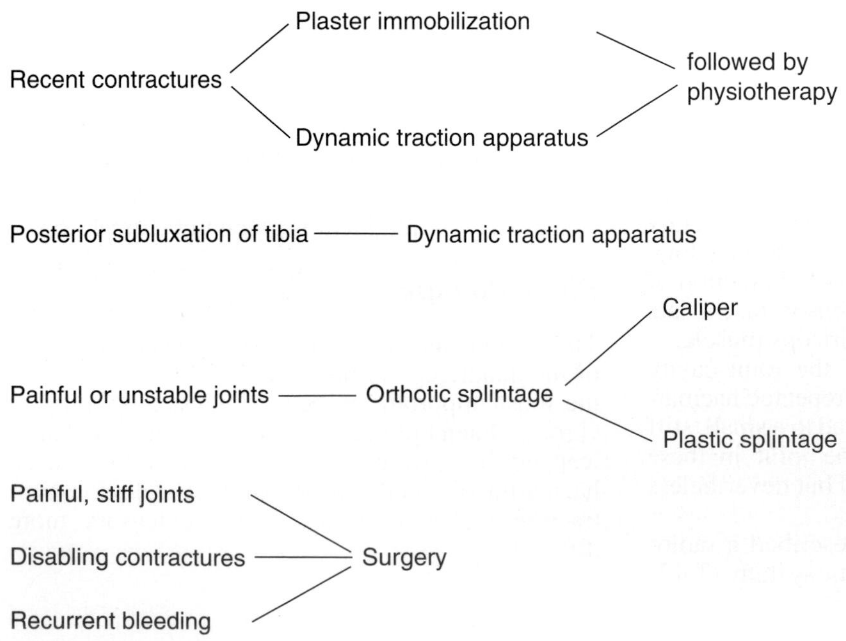

Figure 11.62 Summary of treatment of chronic haemophilic arthropathy.

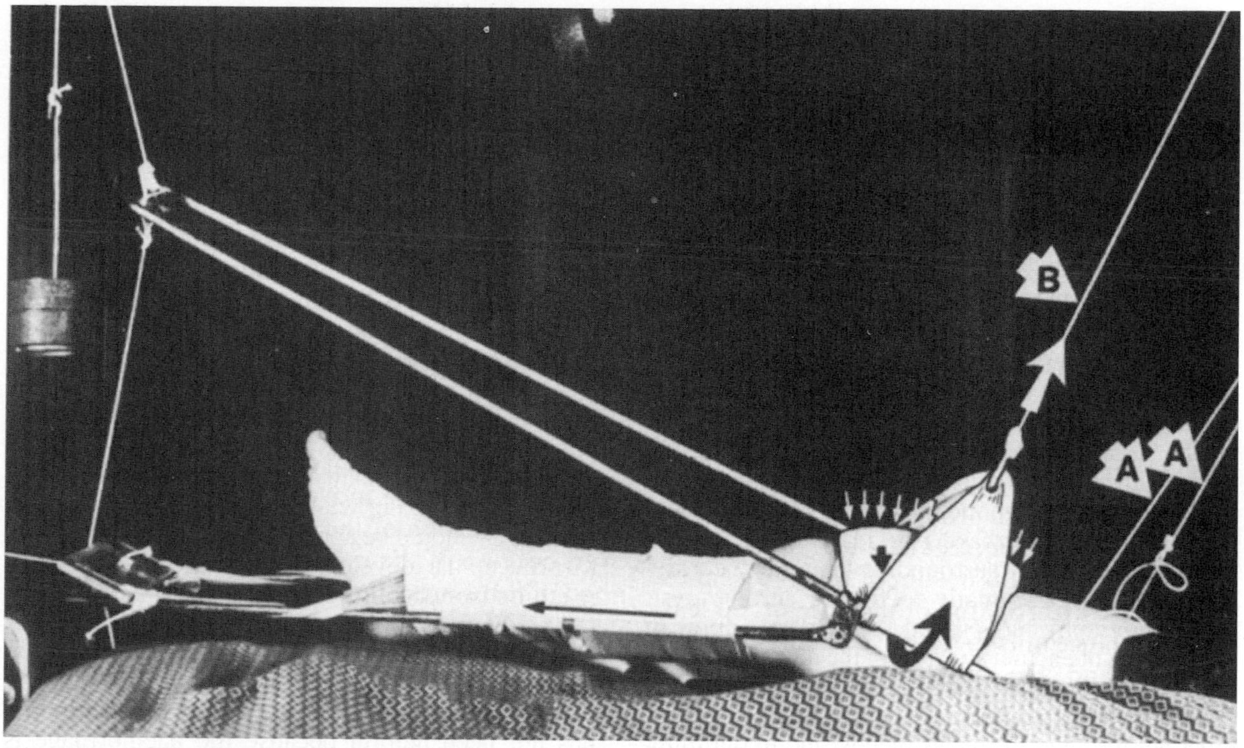

Figure 11.63 Dynamic splintage apparatus. The cords A control the Thomas' splint whilst the pull in cord B is reversed around the splint on to the front of the thigh.

improved, resulting in clearance of fluid from the joint and repair of synovial membrane, and the movement of the joint maintains the nutrition of the articular cartilage. Moreover, because of the movement, there is less likelihood of intra-articular adhesion formation.

Pain relief is improved and factor replacement is rarely required (Stein and Dickson, 1975).

Synovectomy

Synovectomy for the treatment of joints in which repeated bleeds have occurred and in which there is chronic thickening of the synovial membrane has been proposed by some authors (Pietrogrande *et al.*, 1972). It is postulated that the hyperplastic synovium is more likely to bleed than is normal synovium membrane, and also that the synovium is producing proteolytic enzymes which break down the cartilage. Removal of this membrane appears to be a logical method of preventing recurrent haemarthroses and also diminishing the likelihood of further articular cartilage damage. However, it has not proved to be very helpful except in a few cases which have failed to respond to in-patient rigid immobilization and compression with adequate factor replacement.

Synoviorthesis

The destruction of the synovitis membrane and its bleeding hazard can be achieved by synovectomy or by the injection of various radioisotopic materials. This latter approach has been pioneered using radioactive gold, and yttrium (Fernandez-Palazzi *et al.*, 1979). Concern has always been expressed about leakage of the radioactive material, resulting chromosomal breakage with mitoses. Therefore its use in children has to be restricted. However, it is a relatively simple procedure, requiring much less factor replacement. Indeed it can be given in the presence of inhibitors, much less hospitalization and rehabilitation, and now for patients who have the HIV virus. Rivard *et al.* (1994) have recently reported on their 15-year experiences using colloidal P22 chromic phosphate in 48 patients. They found that in half the joints they remained stable or improved as regards range of motion, but the radiographic scores deteriorated. The frequency of bleeding decreased in most of the patients.

Surgery

See pages 838–842.

Bleeding into muscle

This occurs very much less frequently than haemarthrosis; e.g. 14% as against 60% of all 457 bleeding episodes admitted to hospital. Even so, it is the second most frequent cause of spontaneous bleeding.

The most common sites are in the forearm and upper arm and in the calf, iliacus, thigh and buttock. Unlike joint bleeds which predispose to recurrent bleeds, recurrence into the same muscle mass rarely takes place except in the iliac fossa.

Trauma such as by a blow or by unfortunate injection may be the predisposing cause.

The pathology is that of clot formation, muscle fibre death and cellular exudation with polymorphonuclear leucocytes, mononuclear cells or phagocytic cells. If the haemorrhage is extensive, haematoma may persist with surrounding muscle necrosis (Figure 11.64) eventually to form a chronic cyst. Ultrasonography has proved to be most helpful in delineating the actual site within the muscle but also its volume, its adjacency to nerves and vessels and the response to treatment. MR imaging is now also most helpful, e.g. in iliacus bleeds, and in outlining adjacent vital structures, e.g. nerves (Figure 11.64). In the face of severe arthropathy with pain, fixed deformities and disability interfering with the patient's everyday activities, joint stabilization, osteotomies, and arthroplasty all have to be considered and performed.

Clinically, pain becomes progressively more severe, with development of a palpable tumour. Protective muscle spasm may give rise to flexion–adduction deformity of the hip, equinus of the ankle, etc. A neurapraxia lesion of neighbouring peripheral nerves occurs quite frequently (e.g. a femoral nerve paralysis in an iliacus bleed, posterior tibial nerve paralysis in a calf bleed). Volkmann contracture after forearm bleeds has also been seen (Figure 11.65).

TREATMENT

Treatment is directed towards complete rest with splintage. Careful and frequent evaluation for any nerve or vascular complication is necessary by measurement for motor power or sensation; pulses are palpated and tape readings taken of limb circumferences.

Adequate factor replacement is essential for the arrest of bleeding and for relief of pain. Usually more potent sources of factors VIII or IX (AHG material) are required, especially for the more extensive bleeds. Splintage in well padded plasters – but not encasing – should be applied in a functional position to prevent the development of fixed contractures resulting from healing by fibrosis. A greater time is required for immobilization than for a haemarthrosis – until softening of the tumour mass, no pain on isometric contraction of the muscle mass and a decrease in tape measurement are found. Aspiration has not been helpful because the haemorrhage is usually not anatomically circumscribed and the risk of infection is very great. Bleeding into the iliacus muscle with its secondary effect upon the psoas major muscle requires immobilization in a comfortable position of flexion and external rotation of the hip. If large and severe, a hip spica may be required temporarily to relieve pain. Residual contractures require gradual correction in traction, with static and isometric exercises.

Fixed flexion contractures, if allowed to occur, may well require surgery, especially when conservative measures of dynamic splintage fail.

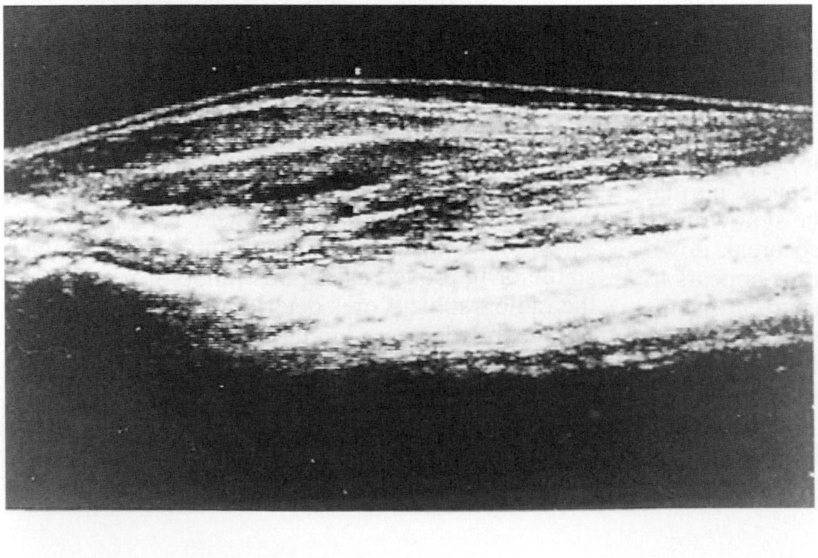

Figure 11.64 Ultrasonic photography to show the infiltrating blood between muscle fibres to produce swelling.

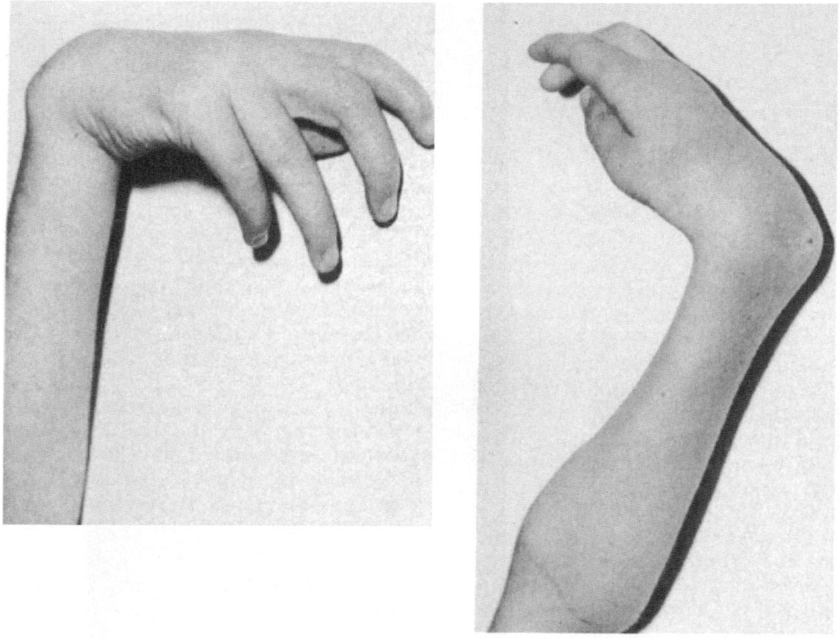

Figure 11.65 Volkmann's contracture of forearm after a bleed in a haemophiliac.

Peripheral nerve bleeds

Peripheral nerve involvement is uncommon and is usually the result of an intramuscular bleed in adults, although extraneural compression by bleeds around the ulnar nerve or by pseudotumours has been described. There has been no proof of an intraneural bleeding lesion. The most common nerve involved is the femoral, followed by the median, ulnar, posterior tibial and sciatic nerves.

CLINICAL FEATURES

In a femoral nerve bleed the patient complains of acute pain in the groin, and this may be present for some hours before femoral palsy becomes evident. Difficulty may be experienced in distinguishing a right-sided iliacus haematoma from an acute appendicitis. The presence of neurapraxia confirms the diagnosis. A mass can be palpated in the iliac fossa in most cases, which is tender at first but then becomes a firm painless swelling. The first manifestation is the localized impairment of sensation over the front of the thigh, which quickly spreads (Figure 11.66). In complete lesions, where total anaesthesia has occurred rapidly, quadriceps paralysis accompanies the sensory changes and the patellar reflex is lost. The recovery of neurological function is prolonged in complete lesions. Full return of motor and sensory function is not usually observed until at least 6 months after haemorrhage.

Anterior and posterior tibial nerves can also be involved, as well as median and ulnar lesions in association with pseudotumour of the lower end of the radius, a large bleed into the forearm flexor muscle leading to a classic Volkmann's contracture. The incomplete recovery of the sciatic and median nerve lesions may be due to intraneural haemorrhage from the relatively large artery which runs beneath the epineurium.

By administering the factor treatment, the pain eases and the flexion contracture gradually lessens. However, a complete neurapraxia will take at least 6 months to recover. Splintage may be required for ambulation or to prevent contracture formation.

The median and ulnar nerve paresis, usually secondary to bleeding into the forearm, may well result in an axonotmesis, with recovery taking up to 9 months. Full passive mobilizing of the wrist and fingers should be carried out to prevent flexor contractures, and plaster splints are required for maintaining a functional position.

Patients who have factor VIII antibodies are significantly less likely to recover full motor and sensory function, and the time for full recovery is much longer (Katz *et al.*, 1991).

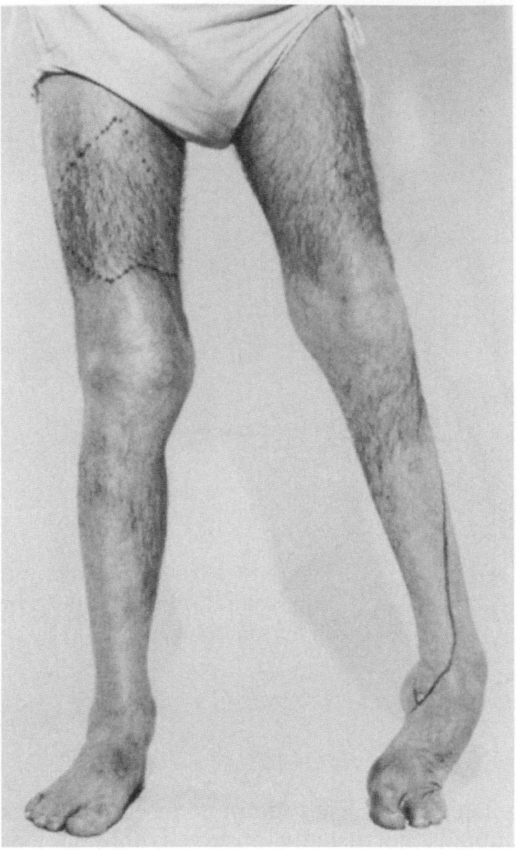

Figure 11.66 Femoral nerve anaesthesia over the right thigh following a bleed. Also present is talipes equinus varus deformity of the left foot with outlined anaesthesia resulting from a lateral popliteal nerve lesion.

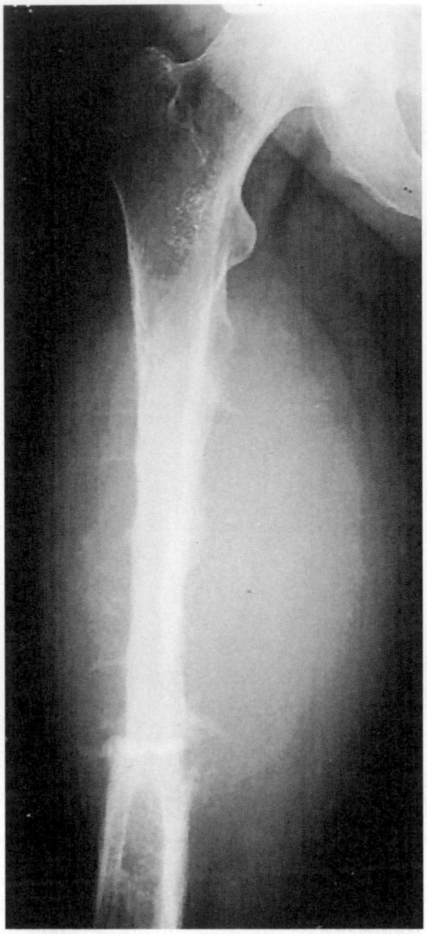

Figure 11.67 Pseudotumour of a femur with a soft tissue swelling and marked periosteal reaction and attenuation of the shaft leading to pathological fracture.

Haemophilic cyst (pseudotumour)

This is a very rare lesion in the haemophilias; in a review by Steel *et al.* (1969) only 47 published cases were found. Fernandez de Valderrama and Matthews (1965) classified these lesions into:

1. Simple cysts within muscle without involvement of bone.
2. Cysts in muscles with extensive periosteal attachment, resulting in bony involvement.
3. True pseudotumours of bone arising from subperiosteal haemorrhages (Figure 11.67).

Steel *et al.* from their experience suggested a fourth category of a true pseudotumour arising from an intraosseous haemorrhage.

Muscle cysts are even more uncommon in spite of the frequency of intramuscular bleeding episodes. This is probably related to the size of the haematoma, the amount of necrosis of muscle and the ability to resorb the clot. Another cause may be an inadequate surgical drainage with insufficient factor replacement which may well lead to a muscle cyst (Figure 11.68).

The cysts involving bone may show massive bone destruction and expansion with periosteal reaction and new bone formation (Figures 11.69–11.71), hence the confusion with neoplastic lesions both in children and in adults. The epiphyseal plate does not act as any barrier to this expanding lesion.

Clinically, an increasing mass in the limbs or pelvis which fails to respond to factor replacement therapy without the presence of antibody formation to factor VIII or IX suggests a pseudotumour. Great care must be taken not to carry out a biopsy procedure without adequate factor control or defining exactly what is to be done. The radiographs are very helpful. In the intraosseous lesion, osteolysis predominates without any real defined margin or new bone response and often there is an overlying

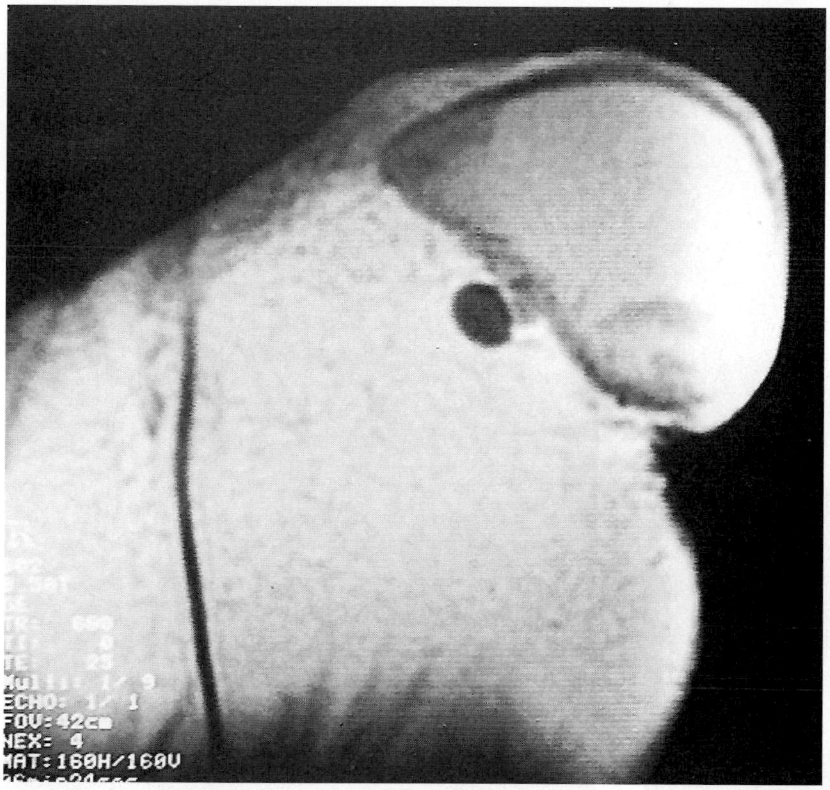

Figure 11.68 Haemophilic cyst within the gluteus maximus of the buttock with the sciatic nerve being outside its wall.

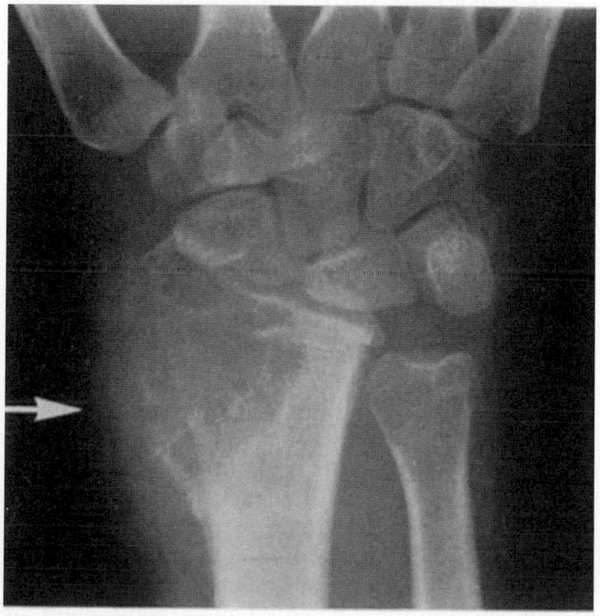

Figure 11.69 Haemophilic bone cyst of lower end of radius with massive bone destruction.

soft tissue shadow. A CT scan is proving to be a most important investigation to delineate both the soft tissue lesion and the bone destruction (Figure 11.72). In the subperiosteal lesion the stripping of the periosteum is characterized by new bone formation but this is, of course, a non-specific bone reaction.

Before 1961 the mortality rate from pseudotumours was over 50% due not only to errors in diagnosis but also to inadequate coagulation control leading to fatal haemorrhages and/or infections due to skin ulcerations, etc.

However, with expert replacement, surgery (i.e. amputation) is less hazardous especially in those cases which fail to respond to conservative treatment, i.e. firm immobilization of the part with AHG or factor IX preparations in sufficient dosages over extended periods of time until all evidence of bleeding has ceased. Resolutions of these pseudotumours is now well documented, but if there is evidence of progressive nerve or vascular complications, spontaneous rupture with haemorrhages and/or infection, excision with obliteration of the cavity by muscle or even bone and, if this is not possible, amputation must still be considered especially if a pathological fracture has developed. Fernandez-Palazzi and Rivas (1985) have reported on their early experience of injecting a 'fibrin seal' into the cavity, after aspiration.

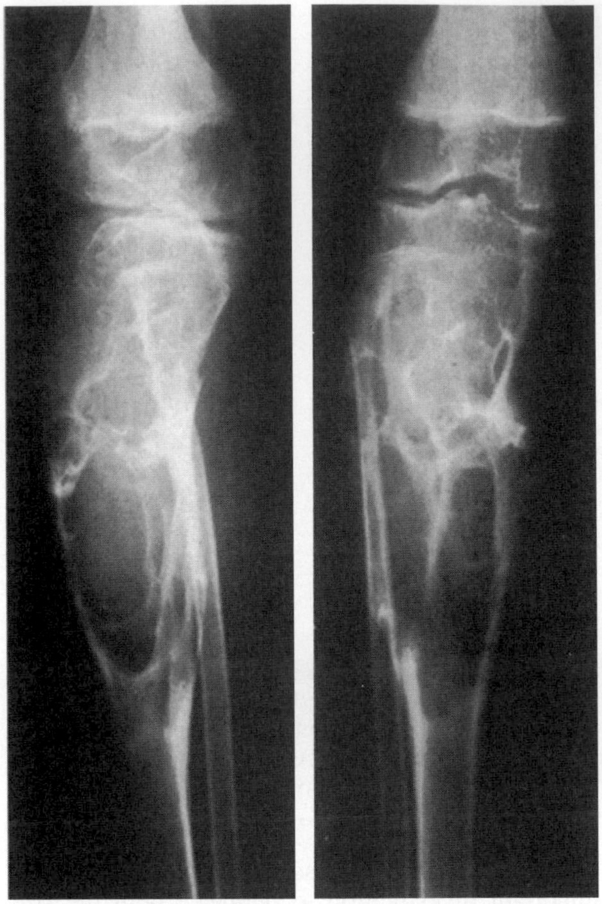

Figure 11.70 Anteroposterior and lateral views of a haemophilic cyst involving the upper end of the tibia.

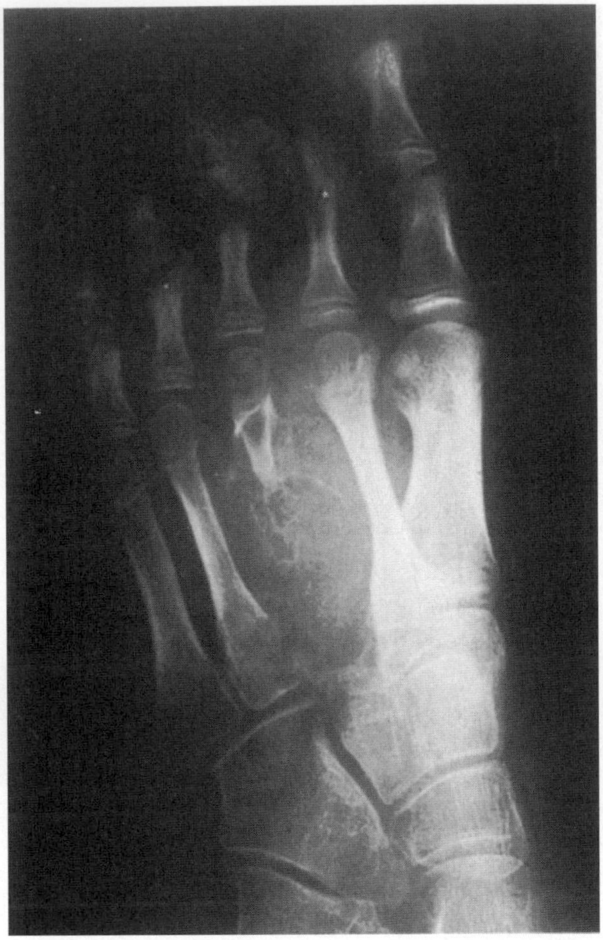

Figure 11.71 Radiograph showing the complete destruction of the third metatarsal by a haemophilic cyst.

Fractures in the haemophilias

These are a rare event but are described here to emphasize that, except for the coagulation factor deficiency state, these fractures do unite well with no untoward bleeding or large haematoma formation. Rigid immobilization (e.g. a POP hip spica) for a fractured femur in a boy with AHG concentration for 4 days gave no concern. Clinical union was achieved in 10 weeks and then the limb was supported by a caliper for an additional 6 weeks.

A conservative approach with rigid immobilization but accepting some degree of deformity usually gives a good result. Open reduction with internal fixation under adequate factor replacement (for at least 14 days' duration) can be carried out where indicated; e.g. in cases of delayed or non-union, in unstable fractures or involving joint surfaces.

Any antibody against factor Vlll is an absolute contraindication.

Surgery in the haemophiliac

The complications of the haemophilias are now better understood and treated more effectively, and it is this experience, especially with the availability of more potent sources of factors VIII and IX, which makes elective surgery reasonable in special centres. Patients with haemostatic deficiency states are living longer and do require surgical correction of their deformities, especially those which lessen function and increase the risk of further haemorrhage.

Operations for stabilization by arthrodesing deformed joints such as the knee or ankle (Figure 11.73); correcting by total hip replacement the pain and limitation of motion due to arthritis of the hip (Figure 11.74), soft tissue debridement or a bony rotation osteotomy for Volkmann's contracture of the forearm; patellectomy, meniscectomy and synovectomy are all well documented (Houghton and

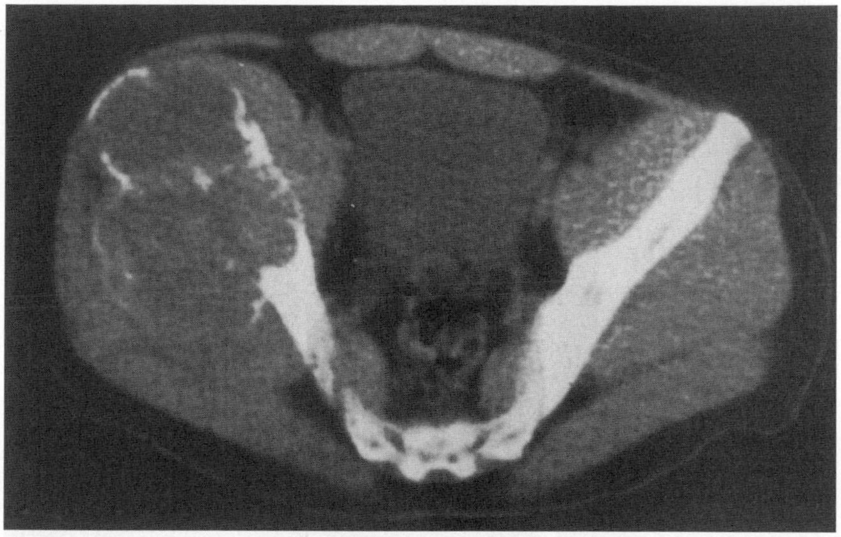

Figure 11.72 A CT scan through the pelvis at the level of the second sacral segment, showing the destruction of the left illium and the haemophilic cyst outlined by an expanding cortical shell of bone.

Duthie, 1979). The surgical technique is meticulous but standard, with use of internal fixation, with or without external immobilization and compression by plaster-of-Paris casting. The key to success is, of course, adequate and skilled haemostatic control. It is essential to raise the concentration of the missing clotting factor VIII or IX in the patient's blood (e.g. 25–50% for factor VIII and 15–25% for factor IX) for not only the period of wound healing but also for that of rehabilitation (Figure 11.75). The details of such management are described elsewhere (Duthie *et al.*, 1994) but emphasis must be given here to the necessity of having available not only the factor material in adequate dosage and for the required duration but also skilled physicians and laboratory workers. In addition to factor replacement, one of two drugs – ε-aminocaproic acid or tranexamic acid – which are fibrin/clot stabilizers and prevent lysis of the newly formed clot – is given orally. It should be emphasized that with such support there is no untoward secondary haemorrhage or anaemia, delay in wound or bone healing or the setting up of a

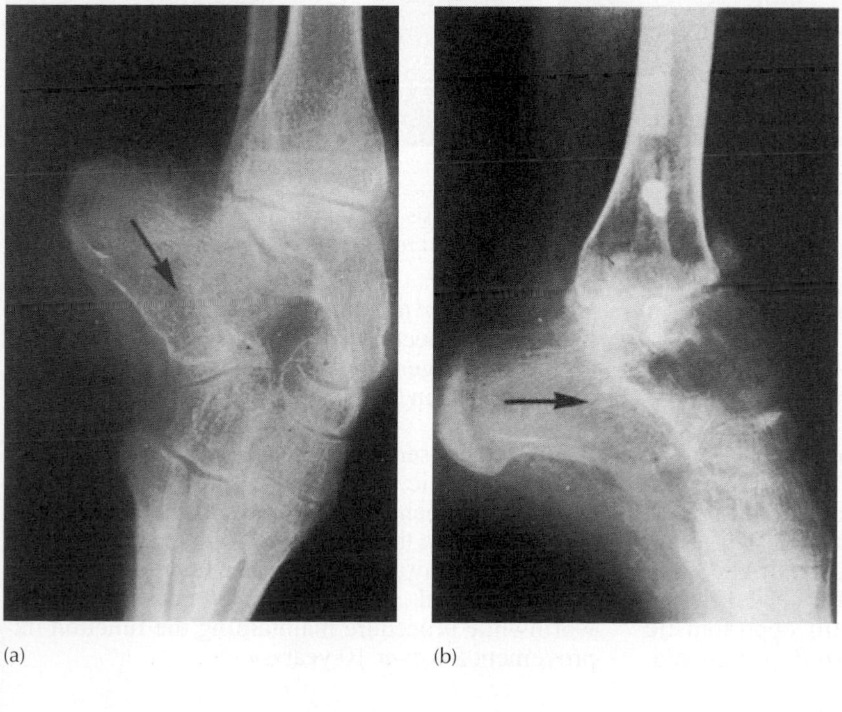

(a) (b)

Figure 11.73 Radiographs of the ankle, showing (a) the fixed equinus deformity resulting from haemophilia, and (b) fusion of the ankle with the hindfoot now plantigrade to the tibial shaft.

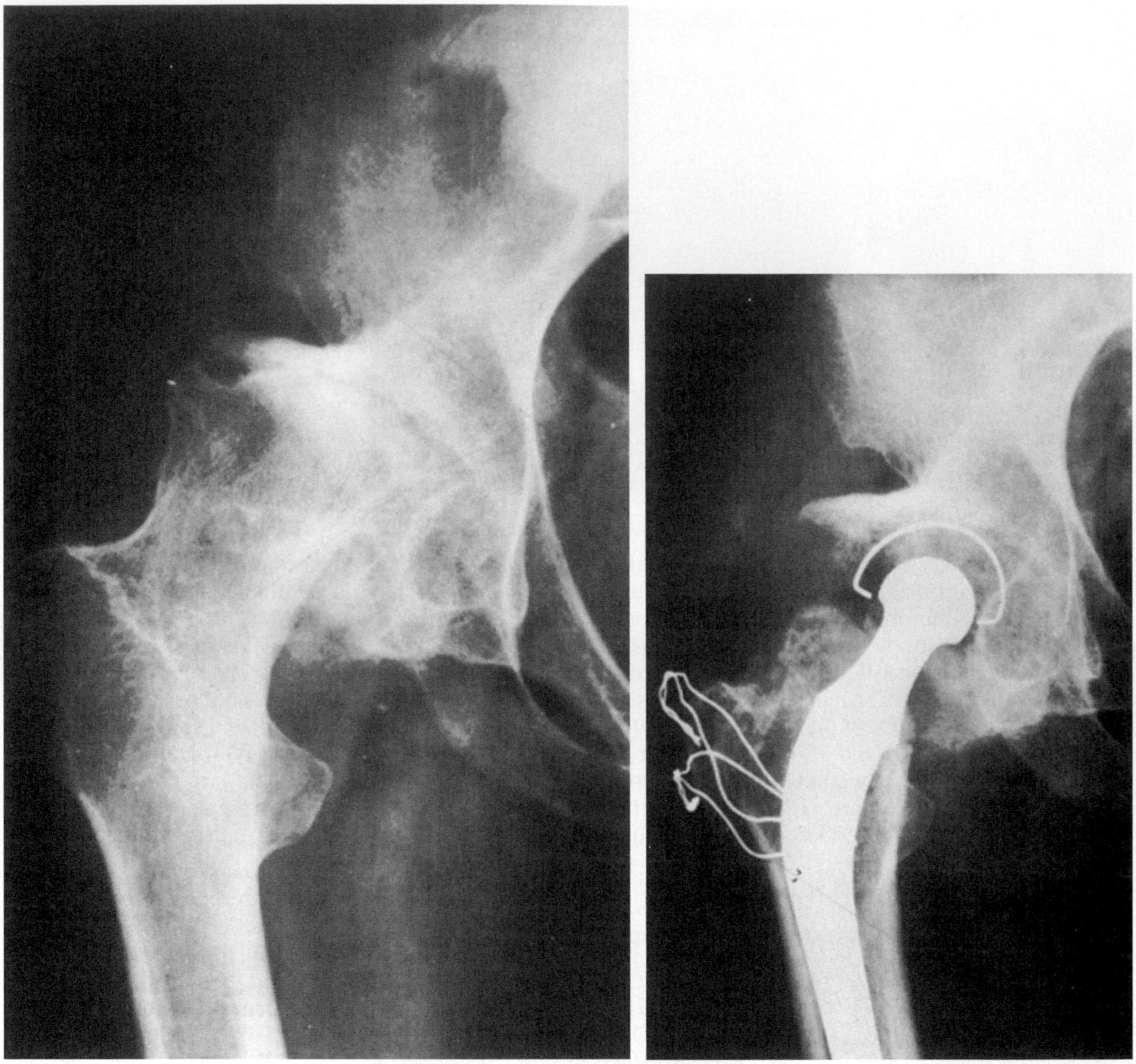

Figure 11.74 Radiographs of a haemophilic patient (a) with avascular necrosis and a painful arthritis of the right hip, and (b) after total hip replacement procedure – with excellent relief of pain and restoration of movement.

bleeding cycle in the operated area or elsewhere in the body.

All patients require screening for factor VIII antibodies, for hepatitis B and C and now for HIV virus indicators by TA/CD helper cell counts. The presence of factor inhibitors is a contraindication for all elective surgery. Phillips (1989) by studying the C44 lymphocyte counts up to 8 years after seroconversion found that at a mean time of 5.5 years after seroconversion 20% had developed AIDS and by 15 years after seroconversion 73% had developed AIDS. The presence of AIDS with opportunistic infections, e.g. *Pneumocystis carinii* pneumonia, *Mycobacterium tuberculosis*, etc., is also a contraindication for elective surgery. There is also debate that major surgery may promote the appearance of clinical AIDS in seropositive patients (Duthie *et al.*, 1994).

Surgery in seropositive patients, about 43% of all haemophilic patients, requires rigorous precautions and techniques for the surgical and nursing team, similar to those required for hepatitis B and C.

Synovectomy and radial head excision for patients with a painful stiff elbow has proved to be a worthwhile procedure maintaining the function improvement for over 10 years.

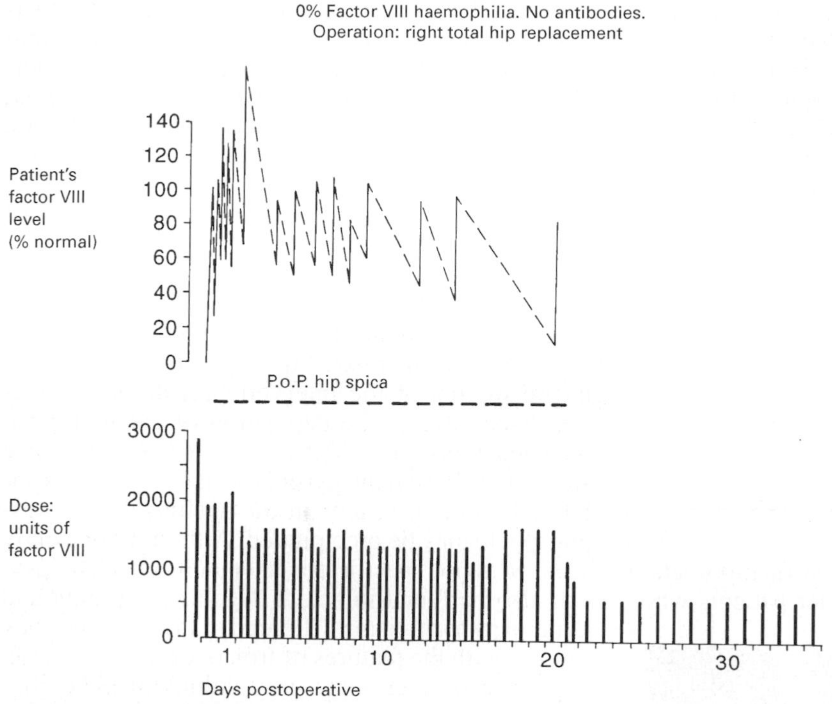

Figure 11.75 The dose schedule and the patient's factor VIII level as a percentage of normal after a total hip replacement.

Total hip replacement (Nelson *et al.*, 1992) has been successfully carried out in 39 patients. A mean follow-up period of 7.5 years has shown a survivorship of less duration than for osteoarthrosis with five requiring revision – two for sepsis and three for aseptic loosening, i.e. 27% loosening rate. Even so, the functional improvement with pain relief is outstanding.

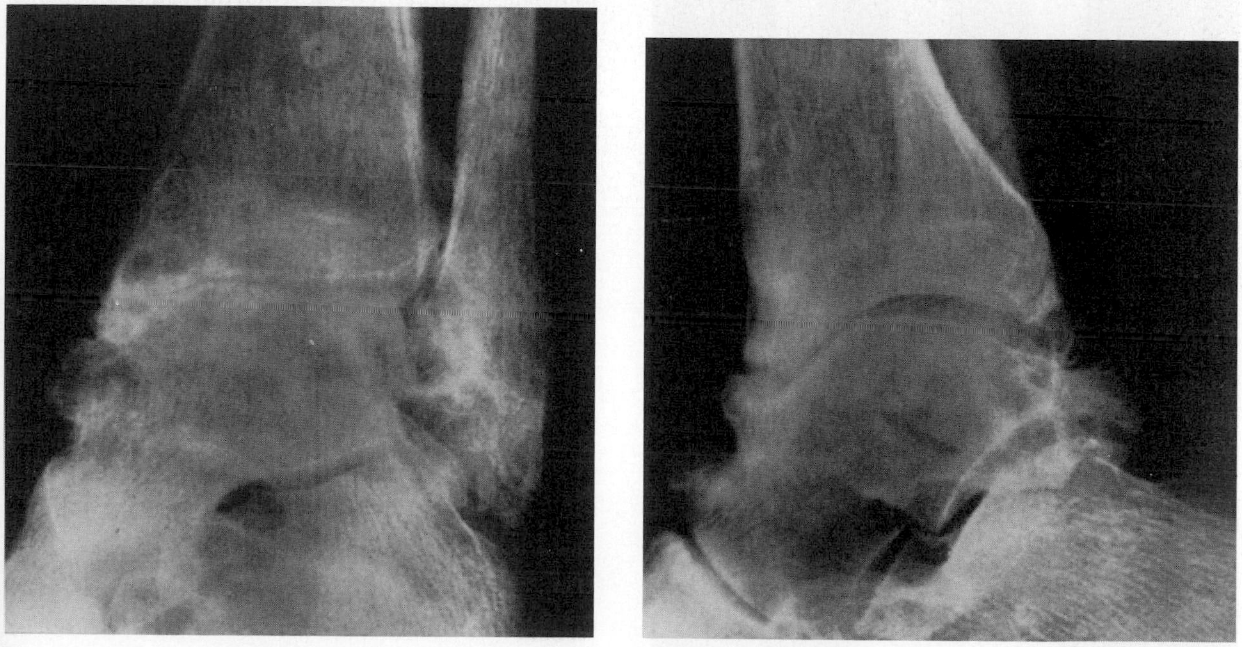

(a) (b)

Figure 11.76 (a) Anteroposterior and (b) lateral radiograph showing the marked disruption of the ankle joint and tibiofibular joint with sclerosis in a patient with haemochromatosis.

Total knee replacement as yet has not become such a standard procedure as that of the hip. Technically it is a more difficult operation with severe contractures, lateral and posterior subluxation of the tibia, poor quality of the tibial bone, with necrosis and defects or cysts. Weidel *et al.* (1989), reviewing their experience of 76 haemophilic patients undergoing total knee replacement, although achieving good results found in this series a recent increase in the occurrence of acute infections. The patients were clearly predisposed to this complication, because of their high incidence of HIV positivity.

Haemochromatosis

Arthritis is a common manifestation of this metabolic disease of iron, usually in older patients who have had the disease for a long time. The arthritis is more like that of osteoarthritis than that of rheumatoid although the metacarpophalangeal and interphalangeal joints are most often affected. However, involvement of larger joints such as wrists, elbows, shoulders, hips, knees and ankles (Figure 11.76) may cause severe disability.

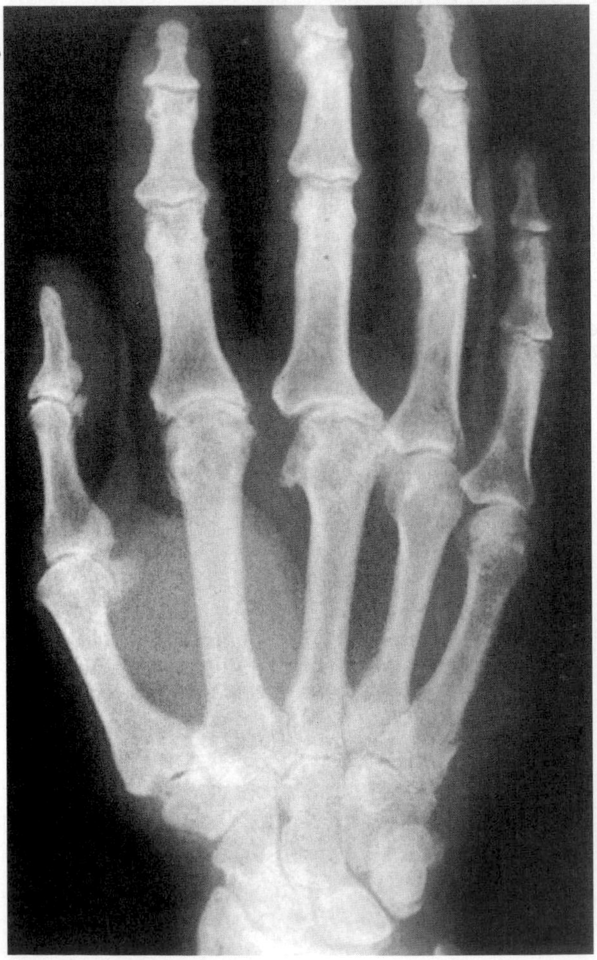

Figure 11.77 Radiograph of a hand showing the early changes of haemochromatosis.

On radiographic examination there is loss of joint space, juxta-articular sclerosis rather than osteoporosis, subchondral cyst formation, but not marginal erosions which are more typical of rheumatoid disease (Figure 11.77). Chondrocalcinosis in the knee joint menisci, hips, symphysis pubis and lateral margin of the intervertebral discs is sometimes seen due to the deposition of calcium pyrophosphate crystals. McCarty *et al.* (1970) have suggested that when pyrophosphate activity is inhibited by the iron ions in the haemosiderin, pyrophosphate may be precipitated. Although frequently seen, it is not specific for haemochromatosis, as it can also be found in senile degeneration, gout and hyperparathyroidism. Clinically the patient may present with the features of iron overload – malaise, very pale or even slate grey colour of skin. Biochemically an elevated serum ferritin and saturation iron-binding tests may be found. Biopsies from liver and synovium are most significant. Mortality is higher when the condition is associated with diabetes mellitus and cirrhosis of the liver (De Jonge-Bok and MacFarlane, 1989).

Stabilization of badly disorganized and painful joints has been carried out. Total hip replacement has proved to be an excellent procedure for relief of pain (Figure 11.78).

The main therapy is directed towards reducing the high circulating iron in order to prevent or reduce the marked haemosiderin deposits in the reticuloendothelial system, in the synovium and in other joint components. Acute inflammatory reactions of joints can be alleviated with such drugs as phenylbutazone or indomethacin.

Avascular necrosis – osteonecrosis of the femoral head in adults

Partial or total interruption of the blood supply of the femoral head results in partial or complete death of the femoral head and can arise from many causes:

1. *Local* – trauma, dysplasia, post-radiation (intrapelvic), arterial disease.

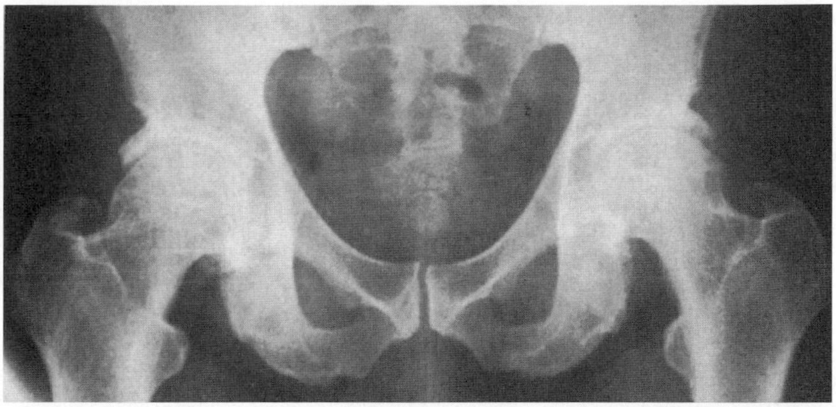

(a)

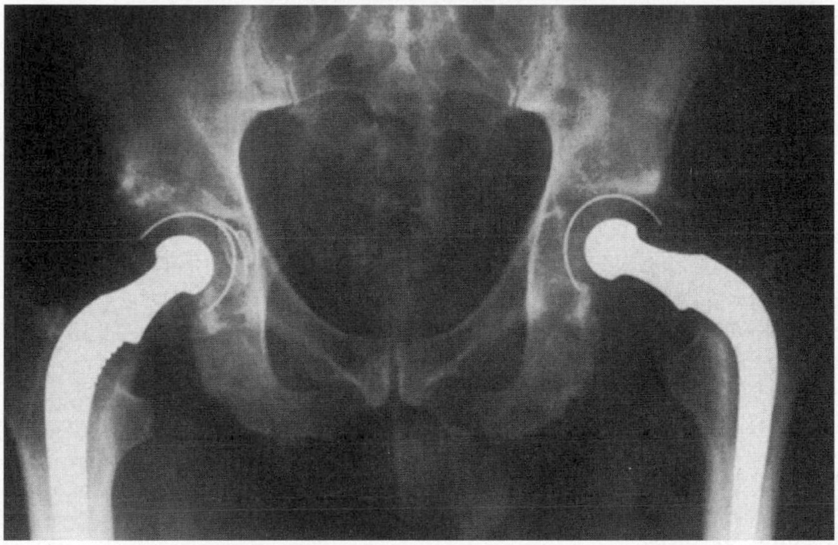

(b)

Figure 11.78 Radiographs showing (a) the typical appearance of hip joints in haemochromatosis, and (b) their replacement by total hip prosthesis.

2. *Systemic disease* – Gaucher's disease, sickle-cell disease, cirrhosis of liver, pancreatitis, gout, connective tissue disease (e.g. systemic lupus erythematosus).
3. *Acquired* – alcoholism, hyperbaric disease, renal transplantation with steroids, renal dialysis (Athanasou *et al.*, 1991) with amyloidosis, indomethacin drug induced, in osteoarthrosis.

Ficat (1985) believed this condition resulted from a blockage of the osseous microcirculation with intramedullary stasis and increased pressure. Extraosseous vessels may be involved by thrombosis, embolism, rupture, stenosis or compression; intraosseous vessels by gas, lipids, thrombosis or vasospasm. He described five successive stages of bone necrosis:

- *Stage 0* – the contralateral hip is involved and symptoms appear, but no clinical or radiographic signs are present.
- *Stage 1* – sudden onset of groin pain, often progressive and radiating. Clinically there is limitation of movement. x-Ray changes are minimal and subtle; loss of trabecular outline and blurring, with mineral patchy osteoporosis.
- *Stage 2* – progression of pain and loss of movement. x-Rays show definite trabeculae pattern loss, with diffuse sclerosis or in an arc form. Decalcification is either general or localized as cysts. This can be confirmed by an increased bone marrow pressure (30 mmHg and above), an intramedullary outflow venography showing obstruction and a core biopsy of marrow changes, some necrosis of medullary content and trabeculae.
- *Stage 3* – on x-rays a sequestrum appears preceded by a crescentic line due to a subchondral fracture, with subsequent flattening of the femoral head. This leads to collapse of the head with a broken contour. The joint space can still appear

normal. There is increased pain and restricted movement, usually with a limp. On core biopsy there is dense medullary fibrosis, new bone formation around dead trabeculae.

- *Stage 4* – x-rays show loss of articular cartilage over a deformed head, with osteoarthrosis supervening, and there are typical signs and symptoms including night pain.

Bilateral hip involvement is seen in 50% of idiopathic osteonecrosis and in over 70% of steroid-induced necrosis.

Ficat recommended core decompression or forage for stages 0, 1 and 2 – although in stage 2 the results were not so good, i.e. 93% for stages 0 and 1 and 82% for stage 2. Results of this procedure still have to be confirmed, especially in stage 2.

Further *in vivo* pathological definition of osteonecrosis has been described from MR imaging. Lang *et al.* (1992) have analysed the 'double line' sign of osteonecrosis. This consists of a peripheral low signal intensity rim representing the thickened trabecular bone, fibrous tissue, cellular debris and an inner border of high signal intensity on the T2 weighted images – which indicates granulation tissue and necrotic bone not yet vascularized.

Very early changes of ischaemia may not be picked up on MR imaging and therefore its value as a scanning technique for early detection, without clinical signs in populations at risk, e.g. renal transplanatation or, indeed, renal dialysis patients, may be low. In such populations, Kopecky *et al.* (1991) found that 14 patients out of 104 renal transplant recipients who were asymptomatic had small segmental changes. Indeed, some of these reduced in size or regressed to normal. They also found that there was no relationship between the

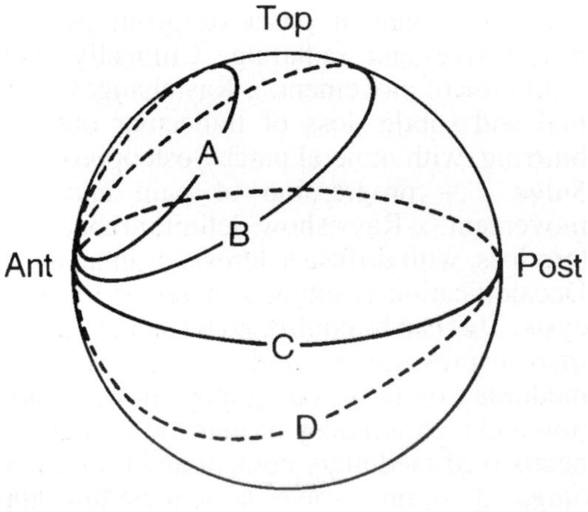

Figure 11.79 Diagram to show the zones demonstrated by MRI scanning of four types of avascular necrosis. (Reproduced, with permission, from Takatori, Y. *et al.* (1993) *Journal of Bone and Joint Surgery* **75B**, 219)

onset of osteonecrosis and the mean cumulative dose of steroids given for the transplantation.

Avascular necrosis of the femoral head is now being extensively studied by MRI (Figure 11.79), especially in those patients at risk because of alcoholism, steroid administration, marrow substitution diseases (e.g. Gaucher's, sickle-cell disease, etc.), who may well be radiographically normal. Takatori *et al.* (1993) from such a series have defined two groups: group 1 or type A in which the fat intensity area was confined to the medial antero-superior portion of the femoral head but did not extend across the zenith of the femoral head on the mid-sagittal MR scan. These did not go on to a subsequent segmental collapse. They also may resolve. Group 2 included three types: type B, the fat intensity area lay beyond the zenith into the posterior part of the femoral head; type C, the intensity occupied the proximal half of the femoral head; and type D, the intensity area was even larger. Collapse ocurred in all within 43 months (a mean time between MRI and collapse being 15 months, range 2–43 months).

SPECIFIC CAUSES OF OSTEONECROSIS

Steroids

There is a definite relationship between steroid use and the incidence of avascular necrosis (AVN) of bone, especially associated with the use of steroids in systemic lupus erthyematosus (SLE) and in renal transplantation. Peak doses of steroids appear to be of more importance than the overall length of treatment, but a further relationship was that between Raynaud's phenomenon, SLE and AVN. It was found that patients with Raynaud's more frequently developed AVN, perhaps suggesting that AVN is in some way caused by a generalized vascular insufficiency.

Dysbaric osteonecrosis

Air workers and divers are at particular risk from this type of AVN (Hungerford and Lennox, 1985).

The period between exposure and radiological changes in the bone are thought to be about 4–12 months, 15% of the lesions are in the femoral head adjacent to the joint surface.

Gaucher's disease

In this disease the enzyme β-glucosidase which helps to metabolize glucose is absent, resulting in accumulation of the precursor of glucose (glucosidase) in the reticuloendothelial system. This appears to be one disease in which the femoral head in particular is affected (Hungerford and Lennox, 1985). Liver disease is also common in children with Gaucher's disease, and this may cause fat embolism, which in turn may cause AVN.

Haemoglobinopathies

Sickle-cell disease and thalassaemia are associated with AVN. The cause of the problem is almost certainly coagulation of blood within the sinusoids of the femoral head (or other part of the skeleton) causing interruption of the blood supply to the bone. The commonest site for AVN is the femur, and the femoral head is the most frequent juxta-articular site. Thirty per cent of patients have radiological evidence of bone infarcts. Sickle-cell disease in osteonecrosis of the femoral head is a common complication with severe pain and marked disability. Total hip replacement is now an accepted form of treatment in spite of its limited and guarded prognosis. Infection and loosening are likely postoperatively and preparation for this major operation by exchange transfusion, antibiotic therapy, intravenous fluid, and oxygen are all necessary. Acurio and Friedman (1992) have described their complication rate of 49% with high revision rates for early technical loosening and infection. Because of this Harrington *et al.*(1993) have described a technique of injecting methylmethacrylate under the elevated articular cartilage shell and necrotic bone. Not only does this give immediate relief of pain and improved mobility but it also restores congruity of the femoral head with its cartilage covering, for several years, before total hip replacement is required.

Irradiation

The relationship between irradiation and osteonecrosis of bone is well established. An incidence of 1.6% and 0.12% has been found in patients with Hodgkin's and non-Hodgkin's lymphoma respectively, and the highest risk appears to be in those who have intermittent steroid and radiotherapy with multiple agent chemotherapy. Trabecular bone may be replaced by fibrous tissue or calcification of the bone marrow may occur. The damage may either be caused by direct cell damage within the bone or possibly due to damage to the cells within the walls of blood vessels with obliteration of the vessels.

Trauma

Dislocation of the hip or fracture of the femoral neck is often followed by avascular necrosis of the head of the femur. It is also well known that the incidence of avascular necrosis after fracture is related to the grade of fracture, with grade 1 having the lowest rate and grade 4 the highest rate of AVN. It is probably direct interruption of the blood supply to the head of the femur due to direct damage to the blood vessels, due to kinking or clotting within the vessels, but it is also possible that a high pressure from blood within the capsule of the joint may interfere with the vascularity of the bone.

Alcoholism

Fat embolism is almost certainly one cause of AVN. Difficulties arise in the definition of alcoholism, and in the screening of large numbers of alcoholics, and therefore the actual incidence of AVN in alcoholics is not known for sure, but most authors consider that there is a causal relationship between the two. Most recent estimates suggest that about 40% of patients with AVN affecting the femoral head are alcoholics (Hungerford and Lennox, 1985). The most commonly affected site is the head of the femur (as in Gaucher's disease), suggesting that the cause of the problem may be the same in the two diseases (fat necrosis). It has also been shown that pancreatitis can directly cause fatty necrosis of the bone marrow and necrosis of the bone trabeculae, so there may be a multifactoral cause.

Hyperuricaemia

Gout and other causes of high blood uric acid may cause AVN of bone. There is, however, doubt about this because many patients with gout have other illnesses such as steroid ingestion, alcoholism or lymphoma (Hungerford and Lennox, 1985).

Idiopathic osteonecrosis

This is a diagnosis of exclusion. There must be some pathological entities causing the necrosis, but to date these have not been discovered, and about 25% of cases remain in this group.

This condition was originally thought to be due to thrombosis of the vessels supplying the femoral head, but Martel and Sitterley (1969) reviewed 33 patients with osteonecrosis who, without any history of trauma, gradually developed pain and restriction of movement in one or both hips. Six of these patients had systemic lupus erythematosus treated with steroids, 5 were alcoholics, 2 had liver cirrhosis and 2 had ankylosing spondylitis. They described a diffuse osteoporosis with loss of trabecular structure which was surrounded by a zone of bone sclerosis. There was also separation of a subchondral fragment from the rest of the bone with deformation of the main femoral head outline.

In a report from renal dialysis and transplant

centres in Europe, the main radiological diagnosis of avascular necrosis of the femoral head was found in over 70% of patients (91% in transplant patients and 22% in those on dialysis). Renal osteodystrophy was present in 17% of dialysis patients but in only 3% of the transplant group. Total hip replacement was carried out in 146 patients with an overall success rate – i.e. pain relief and return to full physical activity or restricted but adequate mobility – in 94% of the transplant patients and in 82% of the dialysis patients.

Radiology

Glimcher and Kenzora (1979) have carefully analysed the radiographic changes which accompany AVN. The density of the bone is dependent on the volume of the bone and the amount of phosphate and calcium in it. The death of bone does not actually change the radiographic appearance of the bone, but the changes seen are the result of revascularization or other changes taking place.

The earliest radiological sign of AVN is the crescent sign seen most clearly in the lateral or frog lateral projections. Although the sign is sometimes not visible until later in the disease, gross examination of the bone always shows this sign and it represents a fracture through the subchondral bone trabeculae. At the periphery of the crescent the fracture becomes more superficial into the subchondral bone and through into the articular cartilage. Much of the remainder of the dead bone ultimately becomes more radiodense than normal, and this is due to new bone being laid down on dead trabeculae.

The next stage of radiographic change reveals flattening of the dome of the head of the femur or a step at the junction between the living and dead bone at the edge of the crescent sign. The bone collapses, there may be cyst formation and ultimately degenerative changes start to occur, initially on the side of the femoral head, but ultimately on the acetabular side as well.

Glimcher and Kenzora (1979) have correlated the pathological and radiological changes as follows:

- *Stage 1* – no radiological change; death of bone cells, cells in the marrow and osteocytes (occurs after as little as 6 hours' ischaemia).
- *Stage 2* – crescent sign, but no collapse; structural failure of subchondral trabeculae, initial resorption adjacent to the fracture (lucency) followed by increasing radiodensity (due to new bone formation on the dead trabeculae).
- *Stage 3* – collapse of the femoral head; attempt at repair of the defect with fibrocartilage with spread ing of a pannus across the articular cartilage lead ing to cartilage degeneration.
- *Stage 4* – degenerative change; occurs secondary to the cartilage degeneration.

TREATMENT

Sugioka and Ogata (1991) have described their results from a transtrochanteric rotational osteotomy as being excellent both clinically and radiographically. They found that in 93% of the cases progression of collapse could be prevented by relieving the mechanical stress of weight-bearing. These authors point out that necrosis does not progress, it is the collapse and deformity which can progress.

There is no place for electrical stimulation. Trancik *et al.* (1990) in a small series of patients with Ficat stage 2 osteonecrosis who had received core decompression and an electrical input, 50% required revision within an average of 13 months and the remainder deteriorated in function.

Maistrelli *et al.* (1988) have reviewed the results of the valgus intertrochanteric osteotomy of Bombelli, performed for osteonecrosis of the femoral head. At 2 years from the date of operation 71% had a clinical satisfactory result and at the final review, i.e. 8.2 years after operation, 58% continued to be excellent or good. Twenty-four hips came to total hip replacement or arthrodesis because of pain. They found that for patients under 55 years of age, hips which were ideopathic or post-traumatic in origin did very much better than alcohol or steroid-induced cases.

Cornell *et al.* (1985) noted that total hip replacement for osteonecrosis had an overall failure rate four times greater than patients with osteoarthrosis.

Bone marrow oedema syndrome

This clinical syndrome consisting of severe pain, reduced mobility with a radiographic transient osteoporosis of one or both hips, affecting women in the first trimester of pregnancy was first described by Curtis and Kincaird in 1959. It usually resolved over the following 6–12 months with normal function and bone density without treatment. Because of the increased uptake with radioisotope bone scanning the differential diagnosis included infective arthritis and osteomyelitis, rheumatoid disease, pigmented villonodular synovitis. Wilson *et al.* (1988) studied ten such patients by MR scanning and found low signal intensity on T1 weighted images with high signal corresponding T2 weighted images, extending from the femoral head out to the trochanteric area.

Such changes were described as being due to bone marrow oedema and resolved. However, some patients have been reported as going on to develop osteonecrosis, i.e. an ischaemic disorder for which core decompression may be considered if the lesion is in the appropriate anterosuperior area. If head collapse occurs total hip replacement may be required.

Hypertrophic pulmonary arthropathy

A syndrome affecting the osseous and other tissues of the extremities may arise in association mainly with chronic intrathoracic disease. The most characteristic features of the syndrome are:

1. clubbing of the fingers;
2. changes in the bones; and
3. changes in the joints.

When all these are present they are spoken of as Marie's sign group, after the observer who first drew attention to the disease in 1890. It is found in a variety of conditions:

1. *Pulmonary suppuration* – bronchiectasis, empyema, pulmonary tuberculosis and abscess (especially the first-mentioned).
2. In some cases of *chronic valvular disease of the heart*, especially when there is chronic venous congestion.
3. In *syphilis of the lung*.
4. In *malignant disease of the lung*.
5. In some cases of *aneurysm of the thoracic aorta* or its branches. When one of the branches is affected, the condition may be unilateral.
6. In some cases of *gastrointestinal or hepatic disease* – e.g. chronic diarrhoea and hypertrophic biliary stenosis.
7. Occasionally in *spinal caries* and *psoas abscess*.

AETIOLOGY

Many theories have been advanced to explain the occurrence of the curious changes associated with this condition.

Compere and Adams (1961) showed that the diseases which are associated with Marie's syndrome are all productive of dyspnoea, cyanosis and a disturbance of the acid–base equilibrium of the peripheral blood. These views are supported by two facts:

1. Similar bone changes are occasionally encountered in those who for a long time live at high altitudes.
2. In certain cases they studied, the carbon dioxide content of the blood serum was increased and the oxygen content diminished.

Campbell and Phillips (1960) described oedema as the primary pathological basis in this disease. They believed that the diseased area through which the blood flowed prevented proper ventilation and accordingly the oxygen tension of the whole arterial blood was lowered. The transference of oxygen from the blood to the tissues depends on the difference in tension of the oxygen in the blood and in the tissues. It will be clear that if from any cause the arterial oxygen tension be lowered, the tissue respiration will be defective. A small defect in tissue respiration may not produce any demonstrable effect on the individual, but, if it does, this will be seen in parts of the body where the defect is increased by a slow circulation. These parts, for mechanical reasons, are the tips of the fingers and toes, and the nose. This imperfect oxygenation, or anoxaemia of the parts, produces oedema and later, if long-continued, it may be hypertrophy of the connective tissue.

PATHOLOGY

The terminal part of the finger is swollen and enlarged. The nail is enlarged so that it overlaps its bed, while it is curved over the end of the fingers, producing the so-called parrot's beak effect. It is markedly striated and breaks easily. Under the nail there is a vascular turgescence and a hyperplasia of the connective tissue.

The joint lesions are the result of swelling and turgescence of the synovial membrane, which shows an infiltration with granulation tissue and with small round cells. Later there may be erosion of the articular cartilage, with exposure of the underlying bone.

The thickening of the bone is due to the deposit of successive layers of new subperiosteal bone. The subperiosteal sheath is loose and friable, and especially marked at the muscular or tendinous insertions.

CLINICAL FEATURES

Clubbing of the fingers

The terminal phalangeal portion of the fingers is swollen, the nail wide, curved, striated and brittle. The finger ends are often congested or cyanosed.

Bone lesions

The osseous lesions consist of symmetrical increase in size of the bones of the extremities, beginning with the distal bones – metacarpals and metatarsals, radius and ulna, tibia and fibula.

Arthritic lesions

There are intermittent attacks of swelling, pain and tenderness, and movements are painful. The swelling can be appreciated as due to increased thickening of the synovial membrane, which persists to some extent when the acute phase is past. In some cases true arthritis may supervene, and lead to fibrous ankylosis and deformity.

Radiation necrosis of bone and joint

It is clearly recognized that growing bone and cartilage are radiosensitive, whereas mature bone and cartilage are considered to be radioresistant. In growing bone, the most sensitive region is in the area of endochondral ossification, where there is derangement in the cartilage column formation, matrix formation, failure of capillaries to appear, with retardation and arrest of growth. However, adult bone, although more resistant, does respond to radiation by becoming devitalized, friable and sclerotic with areas of resorption. The trabeculae become thickened and are heavily mineralized. There is also vascular ischaemia which produces a secondary death of bone with abnormal resorption and proliferation of connective tissues. Sequestration may take place and is secondary to the vascular disturbances or to osteomyelitis which is rare, except in the mandible. These changes are usually without symptoms, until pathological fractures or a secondary osteomyelitis occurs. Sarcomatous changes have been recorded, particularly of the chondrosarcomatous type. Pathological fractures will heal usually without true evidence of bony union.

Radiation necrosis occurs most commonly in the femoral neck and hip joint area because of the frequency of pelvic irradiation for carcinoma of the cervix or other pelvic malignancies. In this condition the patient usually presents with referred pain in the groin or the knee area, and the history of therapy for carcinoma of the cervix may be several years before. Radiographs show fine sclerosis and increased trabecular pattern extending out into the ilium and towards the vicinity of the sacroiliac joint. Changes may be seen in the pubic bones with sclerosis involving the femoral neck and loss of joint space (Figure 11.80). In this lesion the inner cortex and iliopectineal lines are well preserved, with sclerosis being a prominent feature rather than osteolysis. It has to be differentiated from metastatic disease, as well as from a direct extension of the intrapelvic neoplasm (Rubin and Prabhasawat, 1962). Treatment is directed to restricting weight-bearing by an ischial-bearing caliper and rest, although once a fracture has occurred it may be necessary to use internal fixation. Bickel *et al.* (1961) described in detail the management and relatively successful outcome of treatment by internal fixation of post-irradiation fractures of the femoral neck.

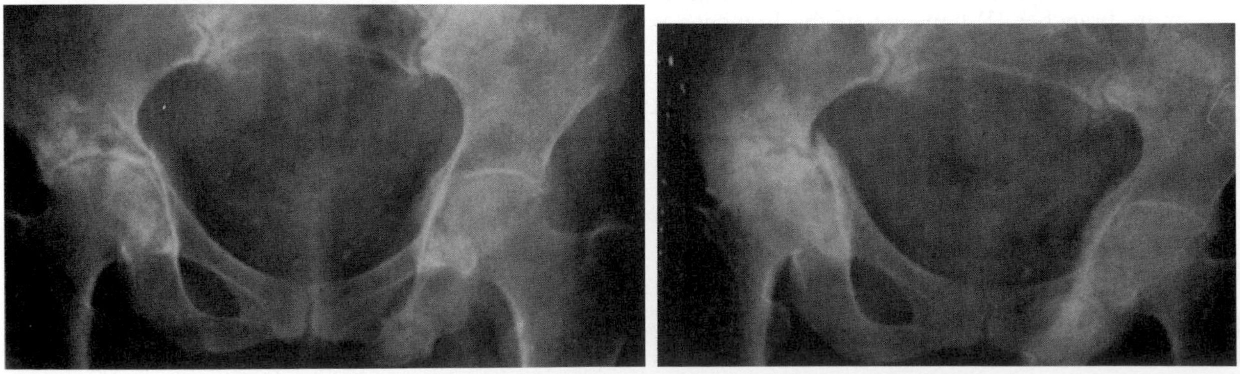

(a) (b)

Figure 11.80 (a) Radiograph of the pelvis and upper femora of an elderly woman who had received treatment with radium implants for cervical carcinoma 4 years before, showing the narrowing of the right hip joint space with sclerosis. There is a pathological fracture involving the left pubic ramus. (b) Radiograph taken 3 years later to show the further disruption of the right hip joint with pathological fracturing and intrapelvic protrusion of the deformed femoral head. Sclerosis is still a marked feature. The iliopectineal line does not show any evidence of osteolytic destruction.

Alkaptonuric arthritis (ochronosis)

An inherited defect in a single enzyme system causes a metabolic disorder in alkaptonuria. Large quantities of homogentisic acid are excreted in the patient's urine. Homogentisic acid is an intermediate compound in a sequence of enzyme-catalysed reactions normally involved in the metabolism of phenylalanine and tyrosine in mammals (Figure 11.81). There is apparently a complete absence of homogentisic acid oxidase in the liver of an alkaptonuric patient.

Although generally described as a recessive Mendelian type of inheritance, the defective gene may be a dominant with incomplete penetrance.

Homogentisic acid is present in the urine, and on standing or on adding an oxidation agent it turns dark brown. This is one of the few conditions which shows ossification of the lamellar structure of the intervertebral disc material; i.e. ossification is taking place within mucopolysaccharide complexes of soft tissues (Figure 11.82). Homogentisic acid pigment is also deposited in the pericardium and other heart structures, bronchial cartilages, kidneys and adrenal glands. After the fifth decade of life, this condition has to be differentiated from other forms of arthritis and metabolic deposition of pigments. The arthralgia is often crippling, and may require an arthroplasty procedure, especially in bilateral hip involvement.

Almost all alkaptonurics by the time they reach middle life develop ochronosis, a pigmentation of the cartilage and fibrous tissues of the body. Secondary degenerative changes in articular cartilages and intervertebral discs cause a widespread arthritis.

CLINICAL FEATURES

It is rare for joint symptoms to be noticed before the age of 40. Most cases develop a stiff spine, although only half of them have serious pain. Deformity is usually a kyphosis caused by the narrowing of the discs. The joints of the shoulder girdle are frequently involved, usually the shoulder but also the sternoclavicular joint. Knees and hips are affected but the smaller joints rarely so. There is evidence of ochronosis in the small pigmented patches in the

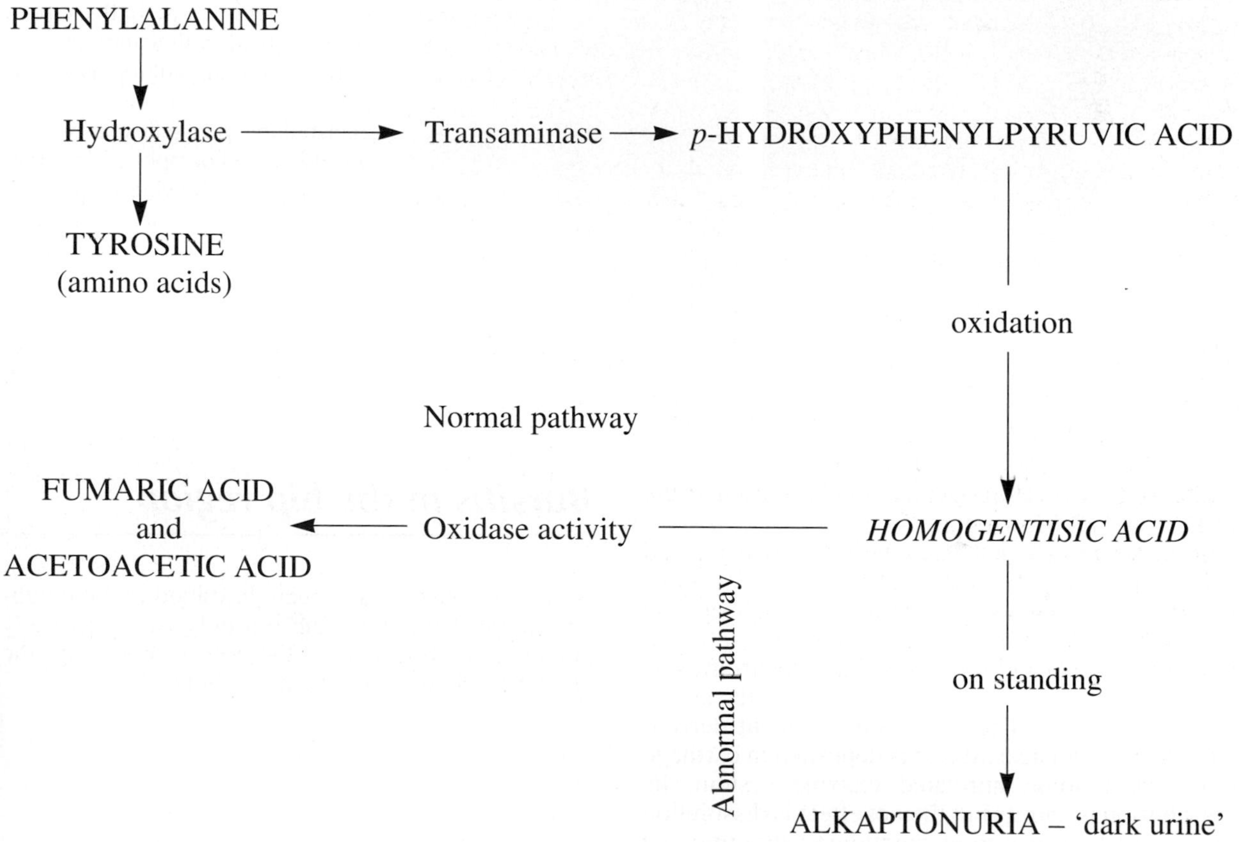

Figure 11.81 Metabolic pathway in the production of homogentisic acid and its breakdown.

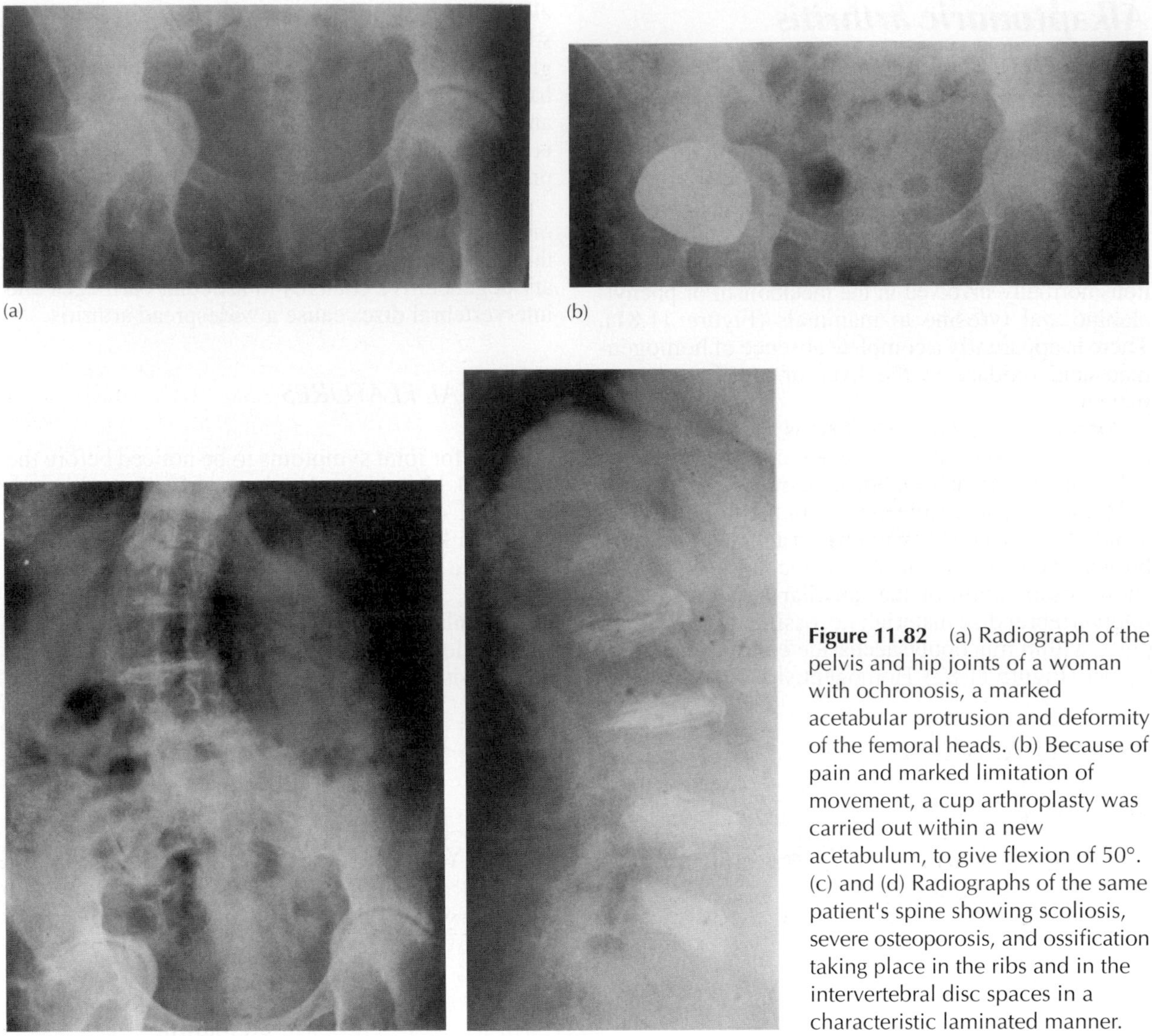

(a) (b) (c) (d)

Figure 11.82 (a) Radiograph of the pelvis and hip joints of a woman with ochronosis, a marked acetabular protrusion and deformity of the femoral heads. (b) Because of pain and marked limitation of movement, a cup arthroplasty was carried out within a new acetabulum, to give flexion of 50°. (c) and (d) Radiographs of the same patient's spine showing scoliosis, severe osteoporosis, and ossification taking place in the ribs and in the intervertebral disc spaces in a characteristic laminated manner.

whites of the eye. Homogentisic acid is present in the urine as a dark brown pigment.

Radiographs show a characteristic narrowing and calcification of the intervertebral discs. The symphysis pubis may be affected, being blurred and sclerosed. In the larger joints the main feature which may distinguish ochronosis from osteoarthritis is periarticular calcification. The severity of the arthritis varies greatly. The ochronotic pigment derived from homogentisic acid that is deposited in cartilage may affect some unrelated enzyme system. Its distribution is spotty, but the net effect is dissolution of the cartilage as a joint functioning structure and subsequent arthritis.

Bursitis in the hip region

Numerous bursae have been described in the neighbourhood of the hip joint, but only two are of any practical significance – the bursa overlying the greater trochanter and the psoas bursa.

Trochanteric bursitis (subgluteal bursa)

The trochanteric bursa is one of some size which lies between the tendons of the gluteus maximus and the lateral surface of the greater trochanter. In inflammatory conditions, pain and tenderness, usually not very severe, are situated just behind the greater trochanter; the tenderness can be elicited by direct palpation over the area or by rotating the limb. When the bursa is distended, the hollow behind the greater trochanter is obliterated, and the limb usually rotated laterally to relax the gluteus maximus. Passive movement of the hip joint is not painful, and there is no flexion contracture. Bursitis has to be distinguished from an acute epiphysitis, from osteomyelitis of the greater trochanter and from the inflammatory diseases of the hip joint. The bursa is not infrequently the seat of a tuberculous infection. Radiographs may show calcification in the area of the trochanteric bursa.

TREATMENT

In the presence of pus the bursa should be incised and drainage established. The incision is made immediately behind the greater trochanter, and care must be taken not to go too far from the trochanter. The sciatic nerve, which lies close to it when the hip is laterally rotated, can be jeopardized.

In non-suppurative lesions, rest, physiotherapy and the injection of lignocaine/steroid compounds are usually sufficient.

Psoas bursitis

The large psoas bursa lies between the iliopsoas muscle and the pelvis. Posteriorly and above, it is in relation to the iliopectineal eminence, and below to the capsule of the hip joint. It accompanies the femoral nerve and frequently communicates with the hip joint. When inflamed, pain and tenderness are present in the medial part of Scarpa's triangle. In the late stage it may suppurate, and fluctuation may then be demonstrated in the same region. The swelling in the triangle may be sufficient, indeed, to obliterate the normal inguinal groove. The bursa is liable to compress the femoral nerve, and pain referred down the limb and to the knee is common, as in hip joint disease. Flexion of the thigh is painful, and the pain increases when the leg is extended. The diagnosis of this condition from hip joint disease, and from psoas abscess, may be extremely difficult. Before any question of aspiration is entertained, it must be remembered that an obturator hernia produces a swelling in this region.

TREATMENT

The treatment, in acute suppurative conditions, consists of incision and drainage, and in chronic infections of complete excision. The bursa is best reached by a vertical incision lateral to the line of the femoral artery; the fibres of the iliopsoas muscle are retracted medially to expose the distended sac. It should be borne in mind that the bursa often communicates with the joint cavity, and it may be necessary, therefore, to drain the hip joint also in purulent infections of the bursal sac.

Snapping hip

An audible sound or click may be heard or felt during certain movements of the hip joint. It may have a variety of explanations, some of which are intra-articular, while others are due to factors outside the joint.

The rare intra-articular type occurs in children, and is due to slight voluntary displacement of the head of the femur over the upper and posterior border of the acetabulum so that the thighs are sharply flexed and adducted. The displacement eventually becomes a habit, and is best prevented by firm bandaging to prevent hip flexion.

The more common extra-articular type is analogous to luxation of the peroneal tendon at the ankle. The snap is heard, and felt, when the knee is flexed and the hip rotated medially. At times a tight band may be seen to slip backwards and forwards over the greater trochanter. This form occurs both in adults and in children, and is apparently due to friction between the anterior border of the gluteus maximus and the trochanter, or between the iliotibial band and the bony prominence. A radiograph should be taken to exclude the presence of osteomata or of osteochondritis. The snapping may become habitual and a source of considerable discomfort to highly strung nervous people On examination of a snapping hip, local tenderness and thickening may, on occasions, be found over the posterior margin of the iliotibial tract, distal to the tensor fascia lata muscle and along the posterior margin of the greater trochanter.

Brignall and Stainsby (1991) have reviewed sev-

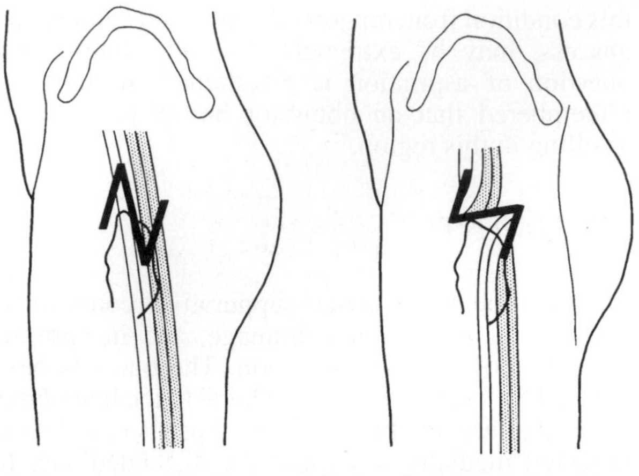

Figure 11.83 The Z-plasty of Brignall and Stainsby (1991) for lengthening the iliotibial band and transposing the proximal part.

eral release techniques, e.g. V-Y plasty, Z-plasty, ellipsoidal excision, a cruciate incision, all with varying success in relieving the snap and the pain. Because of this they carry out a Z-plasty which lengthens the tight iliotibial band and transposes the proximal part of the tract anterior to the greater trochanter (Figure 11.83).

If operative treatment becomes necessary, division of the offending band or tendon or surgical resection of the prominence of the trochanter and a fibrous mass arising from the tensor opposite the trochanter may give a good result. If an osteoma or exostosis is present, it is, of course, removed.

References

Acurio, M.T. and Friedman, R.J. (1992) Hip arthroplasty in patients with sickle cell haemoglobinopathy. *Journal of Bone and Joint Surgery* **74B**, 367–371

Allen, A.L. (1994) Physiotherapy and orthotics in Duthie *et al.* (1994) *The Management of Musculo-Skeletal Problems in the Haemophilias*, pp. 218–251. OUP: Oxford

Amstutz, H.C., Friscia, D.A., Dorey, F. and Carney, B.T. (1989) Warfarin prophylaxis to prevent mortality from pulmonary embolism after total hip replacement. *Journal of Bone and Joint Surgery* **71A**, 321

Andrews, H.J., Arden, G.P., Hart, G.M. and Owen, J.W. (1981) Deep infection after total hip replacement. *Journal of Bone and Joint Surgery* **63B**, 53–57

Ansell, B.M. and Bywaters, E.G.L. (1959) Prognosis in Still's disease. *Bulletin on the Rheumatic Diseases* **9**, 189

Ansell, B.M. and Bywaters E.G.L. (1977) Juvenile chronic polyarthritis. In: *Copeman's Textbook of the Rheumatic Diseases*. Edited by J.T. Scott. Churchill Livingstone: Edinburgh and London

Anthony, P.P., Gie, G.A., Howie, C.R. and Ling, R.S.M. (1990) Localised endosteal bone lysis in relation to the femoral components of cemented total hip arthroplasties. *Journal of Bone and Joint Surgery* **72B**, 971–980

Arnett, F.C. (1989) Revised criteria for the classification of rheumatoid arthritis. *Bulletin on the Rheumatic Diseases* **38**, 1–6

Arthritis and Rheumatism Council and British Orthopaedic Association (1976) *Annals of the Rheumatic Diseases* **35**, 437

Athanasou, N.A., Ayers, D., Rainey, A.J., Olivier, D.O. and Duthie, R.B. (1991) Joint and systemic distribution of dialysis amyloid. *Quarterly Journal of Medicine* **78**, 205–214

Aufranc, O.E. (1967) In: *Modern Trends in Orthopaedics* 5. Edited by W.D. Graham. Butterworths: London

Ayers, D.C., Evarts, C.McC. and Parkinson, J.R. (1986) The prevention of heterotopic ossification in high risk patients by low dosage radiation therapy after total hip arthroplasty. *Journal of Bone and Joint Surgery* **68A**, 1423–1430

Azarin, L., Marques, F. and Gomar, F. (1985) Morphology of haemophilic joints. In: *Orthopaedic Problems in Haemophilia*, pp. 12–13. Edited by S. Dohring and K.P. Schultz. W. Zuchschwendt Verlag: Munchen, Berne, Wien

Barron, J.N. (1969) *Annals of the Rheumatic Diseases* **28**, Supplement 74

Bentley, G. (1972) *Degradation Repair and Replacement of Articular Cartilage*. ChM Thesis, University of Sheffield

Bentley, G. (1994) The current state of total hip replacement. Paper presented at the Second G.C.C. Orthopaedic Meeting, Dubai, October 23rd–27th, 1994

Bentley, G. and Duthie, R.B. (1973) A comparative review of the McKee-Farrar and Charnley total hip prostheses. *Clinical Orthopaedics and Related Research* **95**, 127–142

Bentley, G. and Simmonds, A.B. (1976) Workshop on Control of Operating Room Airborne Bacteria. National Academy of Science: Washington DC

Bickel, W.H., Childs, D.S. and Pirretta, C.M. (1961) *Journal of the American Medical Association* **175**, 204

Biggs, R. (1967) *British Journal of Haematology* **13**, 452

Bisla, R.S., Ranawat, C.S. and Inglis, A.E. (1976) Total hip replacements in patients with ankylosing spondylitis with involvement of the hip. *Journal of Bone and Joint Surgery* **58A**, 233–238

Boden, S.D., Dodge, L.D., Bohlman, H.H. and Rechtine, G.R. (1993) Rheumatoid arthritis of the cervical spine. *Journal of Bone and Joint Surgery* **75A**, 1282–1297

Bombelli, R. (1993) *Structure and Function in Normal and Abnormal Hips*. 3rd edition. Springer Verlag: Berlin, Heidelberg, New York, London, Tokyo, Paris, Hong Kong, Barcelona, Budapest

Boyd, A.D., Thomas, W.H., Scott, R.D., Sledge, C.B. and Thornhill, T.S. (1990) Total shoulder arthroplasty versus hemiarthroplasty indications for glenoid resurfacing. *Journal of Arthroplasty* **15**, 329–336

Brailsford, J.F. (1950) *The Radiology of Bones and Joints*. W. Wood: Baltimore, Maryland

Bränemark, P.I. and Goldie, I. (1969) Physiologic aspects on the timing of synovectomy in rheumatoid arthritis. *Early Synovectomy in Rheumatoid Arthritis*. Excerpta Medica: Amsterdam

Brignall, C.G. and Stainsby, G.D. (1991) The snapping hip. Treatment by Z-plasty. *Journal of Bone and Joint Surgery* **73B**, 253–254

Brooker, A.F., Bowerman, J.W., Robinson, R.A. and Riley, L.H. (1973) *Journal of Bone and Joint Surgery* **55A**, 55–58

Buccholz, K. (1979) Late infections after artificial joint replacement with a septic course. *Chirurg* **50**, 573–575

Byers, P.D. (1974) *Joumal of Bone and Joint Surgery* **56B**, 279

Callaghan, J.L. (1993) Results of primary total hip replacement in young patients. *Journal of Bone and Joint Surgery* **75A**, 1728–1734

Campbell, A.M.L.G. and Phillips, D.G. (1960) *British Medical Journal* **1**, 481

Cates, H.E., Faris, P.M., Keating, E.M. and Ritter, M.A. (1993) Polyethylene wear in cemented metal backed acetabular cups. *Journal of Bone and Joint Surgery* **75B**, 249

Charcot, J.M. (1892) *Nouvelle Iconographie de la Salpêtrière* 121

Charnley, J. (1953) *Compression Arthrodesis.* E & S Livingstone: Edinburgh

Charnley, J. (1972) The long-term results of low-friction arthroplasty of the hips performed as a primary intervention. *Journal of Bone and Joint Surgery* **54B**, 61–76

Charnley, J. (1976) *Journal of Bone and Joint Surgery* **58B**, 390

Charnley, J. (1979) *Low Friction Arthroplasty of the Hip*, p. 65. Springer Verlag: Berlin

Charnley, J. and Eftekhar, N. (1969) Postoperative infection in total prosthetic replacement arthroplasty of the hip. With special reference to the bacterial content of the air in the operating room. *British Journal of Surgery* **56**, 641–649

Cockin, J. and Duthie, R.B. (1971) In: *Modern Trends in Rheumatology – 2*, pp. 267–291. Edited by A.G.S. Hill. Butterworths: London

Collins, D.H. (1950) *The Pathology of Articular and Spinal Diseases.* Williams & Wilkins: Baltimore, Maryland

Compere, E.L. and Adams, W.E. (1961) *Surgery, Gynecology and Obstetrics* **61**, 312

Coppens, M. and Dequeker, J. (1991) Osteoarthritis, obesity and hormones. *Clinical Sciences: Current Opinions in Orthopaedics* **2**, 482–487

Cornell, C.N., Salvati, E.A. and Pellicci, P.M. (1985) Long-term follow up of total hip replacement in patients with osteonecrosis. *Orthopedic Clinics of North America* **16**, 757–769

Curtis, P.H.J. and Kincaird, W.E. (1959) Transitory demineralization of the hip in pregnancy: a report of 3 cases. *Journal of Bone and Joint Surgery* **41A**, 1327–1333

Dall, D., Ger, E., Miles, T. and Forder, A. (1976) A preliminary report on material strength and antibacterial activity of methylmethacrylate antibiotic mixtures. *Journal of Bone and Joint Surgery* **58B**, 390

Danielsson, L.G. (1964) Incidence and prognosis of coxarthrosis. *Acta Orthopaedica Scandinavica Supplement* **66**

DeAndrade, J.R., Grant, C. and Dixon, A. St J. (1965) Joint distension and reflex muscle inhibition in the knee. *Journal of Bone and Joint Surgery* **47A**, 313–322

De Jonge-Bok, J.M. and MacFarlane, J.D. (1989) The articular diversity of early haemochromatosis. *Journal of Bone and Joint Surgery* **69B**, 41–44

Dick, W.C. (1977) In: *Copeman's Textbook of the Rheumatic Diseases.* Edited by J.T. Scott. Churchill Livingstone: Edinburgh and London

Doherty, M., Patrick, M. and Powell, R. (1990) Nodal generalised osteoarthritis in an autoimmune disease. *Annals of the Rheumatic Diseases* **49**, 1017–1020

Dorr, L.D., Takei, G.K. and Conaty, J.P. (1983) Total hip arthroplasties in patients less than 45 years old. *Journal of Bone and Joint Surgery* **65A**, 474–479

Drugs and Therapeutic Bulletin (1993) Slow acting antirheumatic drugs. **31**, 17–20

Duthie, R.B. and Harris, C.M. (1969) A radiographic and clinical survey of the hip joint in sero-positive rheumatoid arthritis. *Acta Orthopaedica Scandinavica* **40**, 346–364

Duthie, R.B., Rizza, C., Giangrande, P.F. and Dodd, C.A.F. (1994) *The Management of Musculo-skeletal Problems in the Haemophiliacs.* Oxford Medical Publications, Oxford University Press: Oxford

Einig, R.B., Higer, H.P., Meairs, S., Faust-Tinnefeldt, G. and Kapp, H. (1990) Magnetic resonance imaging of the cervico-cranial junction in rheumatoid arthritis: value, limitations and indications. *Skeletal Radiology* **19**, 341–346

Eloesser, L.H. (1917) *Annals of Surgery* **66**, 201

Elson, R.A., Jephcott, A.E., McGechie, D.B. and Verettas, D. (1977) Antibiotic-loaded acrylic cement. *Journal of Bone and Joint Surgery* **59B**, 200–205

Ferguson, A.B. Jr (1964) High intertrochanteric osteotomy for osteoarthritis of the hip. *Journal of Bone and Joint Surgery* **46A**, 1159–1175

Ferguson, A.B. Jr and Semlak, K. (1970) Joint stability maintained by atmospheric pressure: an experimental study. *Clinical Orthopaedics and Related Research* **68**, 294–300

Fernandez de Valderrama, J.A. and Matthews, J.M. (1965) *Journal of Bone and Joint Surgery* **47B**, 256

Fernandez-Palazzi, F. and Rivas, S. (1985) The use of fibrin seal. Surgery of coagulation diseases. In: *Orthopaedic Problems in Haemophilia Patients.* Edited by S. Dohring and K.P. Schultz. W. Zuckschwedt, Verlag: Dusseldorf, Munchen, Berne, Wien

Fernandez-Palazzi, F., Bosch, N.B. and Varga, A.F. (1979) Chromosomal study after radioactive synoviorthesis for haemophilic haemarthrosis. *International Orthopedics* **3**, 159–164

Ficat, R.P. (1985) Idiopathic bone necrosis of the femoral head. *Journal of Bone and Joint Surgery* **67B**, 3–9

Fitzgerald, B.H. Jr, Brindley, G.W. and Kavanagh, B.F. (1988) The uncemented total hip arthroplasty; intra-operative femoral fractures. *Clinical Orthopaedics and Related Research* **235**, 61–66

Freeman, M.A.R. (Ed.) (1980) In: *Adult Cartilage*, 2nd edition. Pitman Medical: Tunbridge Wells

Freeman, M.A.R., Swanson, S.A.V., Camron, H. and Brown, G. (1978) ICLH cemented double-cup total replacement of the hip. *Journal of Bone and Joint Surgery* **60B**, 137

Furlong, R.J. and Osborn, J.F. (1991) Fixation of hip prostheses by hydroxyapatite ceramic coatings. *Journal of Bone and Joint Surgery* **73B**, 741–745

Garièpy, R., Demers, R. and Laurin, C.A. (1966) The prophylactic effect of synovectomy of the knee in rheumatoid arthritis. *Canadian Medical Association Journal* **94**, 1349

Gates, H.S., McCollum, D.E., Poletti, S.C. and Nunley, J.A. (1990) Bone grafting in total hip arthroplasty for protrusio acetabuli. *Journal of Bone and Joint Surgery* **72A**, 248–251

Giangrande, P.L.F., Dodd, C.A.F. and Gregg-Smith, S.J. (1994) Knee replacement in haempophilia. Correspondence. *Journal of Bone and Joint Surgery* **76B**, 166

Gilmour, J. (1938) *British Journal of Surgery* **26**, 700

Girdlestone, G.R. (1924) *Journal of Bone and Joint Surgery* **6**, 519

Glimcher, M.J. and Kenzora, J.E. (1979) The biology of osteonecrosis of the human femoral head and its clinical implications. II The pathological changes in the femoral head as an organ and in the hip joint. *Clinical Orthopaedics and Related Research* **139**, 273–312

Goel, A. and Sharp, D.J. (1991) Heterotopic ossification after hip replacement. *Journal of Bone and Joint Surgery* **73B**, 255–257

Gottlieb, M.S., Groopman, J.E., Weinstein, W.Y. *et al.* (1983) The acquired immunodeficiency syndrome. *Annals of Internal Medicine* **99**, 208–220

Green, D.P., Parkes, J.C. and Stinchfield, F.E. (1967) Arthrodesis of the knee. *Journal of Bone and Joint Surgery* **49A**, 1065–1075

Gregg-Smith, S.J., Pattison, R.M. and Dodd, C.A.F. (1993) Septic arthritis in haemophilia. *Journal of Bone and Joint Surgery* **76B**, 368–370

Griffith, M.J., Seidenstein, M.K., Williams, D. and Charnley, J. (1978a) Eight year results of Charnley arthroplasties of the hip with special reference to the behavior of cement. *Clinical Orthopaedics and Related Research* **137**, 24–36

Griffith, M.J., Seidenstein, M.K., Williams, D. and Charnley, J. (1978b) Socket wear in Charnley low friction arthroplasty of the hip. *Clinical Orthopaedics and Related Research* **137**, 37–47

Haddard, R.J., Cook, S.D. and Brinker, M.R. (1990) A comparison of three varieties of non-cemented porous-coated hip replacements. *Journal of Bone and Joint Surgery* **72B**, 2–8

Halawa, M., Lee, A.J.C., Ling, R.S.M. and Vanagala, S.S. (1978) The shear strength of trabecular bone from the femur, and some factors affecting the shear strength of the cement in bone interface. *Archives of Orthopaedic and Trauma Surgery* **92**, 19–30

Halverson, P.B., Carrera, G.F. and McCarty, D.J. (1990) Milwaukee shoulder syndrome: report of fifteen additional cases and description of contributing factors. *Archives of Internal Medicine* **150**, 677–682

Hardy, D.C.R., Frayssinet, P., Guilhem, A. *et al.* (1991) Bonding of hydroxyapatite-coated femoral prostheses. *Journal of Bone and Joint Surgery* **73B**, 732–740

Harrington, P., Bachir, D. and Galacteros, F. (1993) Avascular necrosis of the femoral head in sickle cell disease. *Journal of Bone and Joint Surgery* **75B**, 847–848

Harris, C.M. and Baum, J. (1988) Involvement of the hips in juvenile rheumatoid arthritis. A longitudinal study. *Journal of Bone and Joint Surgery* **70A**, 821–833

Harrison, M.H.M., Schajowicz, F. and Trueta, J. (1953) *Journal of Bone and Joint Surgery* **35B**, 598

Hoaglund, F.T. (1967) *Journal of Bone and Joint Surgery* **49A**, 285

Hodge, W.A. and Chandler, H.P. (1992) Unicompartmental knee replacement: a comparison of constrained and unconstrained designs. *Journal of Bone and Joint Surgery* **74A**, 877–883

Holland, H.W. (1953) Tabetic spinal arthropathy. *Proceedings of the Royal Society of Medicine* **46**, 747–753

Hooper, J.C. and Jones, E.W. (1971) Primary protrusion of the acetabulum. *Journal of Bone and Joint Surgery* **53B**, 23–29

Houghton, G.R. and Duthie, R.B. (1979) Orthopedic problems in hemophilia. *Clinical Orthopaedics and Related Research* **138**, 197–216

Hungerford, D.S. and Lennox, D.W. (1985) The importance of increased intraosseous pressure in the development of osteonecrosis of the femoral head. *Orthopedic Clinics of North America* **16**, 635–684

Hunter, G.A. (1979) The results of reinsertion of a total hip prosthesis after sepsis. *Journal of Bone and Joint Surgery* **61B**, 422–423

Jacobson, K. (1977) OA following insufficiency of the cruciate ligaments in man. *Acta Orthopaedica Scandinavica* **48**, 520–526

Jiranek, W.A., Machado, M., Jasty, M. *et al.* (1993) Production of cytokines around loosened cemented acetabular components. *Journal of Bone and Joint Surgery* **75A**, 863–879

Johnson, L.C. (1959) *Laboratory Investigation* **8**, 1123

Johnston, R.C. and Smidt, G.L. (1969) *Journal of Bone and Joint Surgery* **51A**, 1082–1094

Jonsson, E., Lidgren, L., Mjoberg, B., Rydholn, V. and Selvick, G. (1990) Humeral cup fixators in rheumatoid shoulders. *Acta Orthopaedica Scandinavica* **61**, 116–117

Katz, S.G., Nelson, T.W., Atkins, R.M. and Duthie, R.B. (1991) Peripheral nerve lesions in hemophilia. *Journal of Bone and Joint Surgery* **73A**, 1016–1019

Keller, J.C., Trancik, T.M., Young, F.A. and St Mary, E. (1989) Effects of indomethacin on bone in growth. *Journal of Orthopaedic Research* **7**, 28–34

Kellgren, J.H. (1939) Some painful joint conditions and their relation to osteoarthritis. *Clinical Science* **4**, 193

Kellgren, J.H. (1961) Osteoarthritis in patients and populations. *British Medical Journal* **2**, 1–6

Kellgren, J.H. and Lawrence, J.S. (1957) *Annals of the Rheumatic Diseases* **16**, 494

Kellgren, J.H. and Samuel, E.P. (1950) The sensitivity and innervation of the articular capsule. *Journal of Bone and Joint Surgery* **32B**, 84–92

Kenwright, J. and Duthie, R.B. (1971) Surgical management of the knee. *Arthritis and Rheumatism* **1**, 58–87

Kilgus, D.J., Namba, R.S., Gorek, J.E., Cracchiolo, A. and Amstutz, H.C. (1990) Total hip replacement for patients who have ankylosing spondylitis. *Journal of Bone and Joint Surgery* **72A**, 834–839

King, E.J.S. (1931) *British Journal of Surgery* **18**, 133

King, E.J.S. (1940) *Surgery, Gynecology and Obstetrics* **70**, 150

Kirschenbaum, D., Schneider, L.H., Adams D.C. *et al.*

(1993) Arthroplasty of the metacarpo-phalangeal joints with use of silicone rubber implants in patients who have rheumatoid arthritis. *Journal of Bone and Joint Surgery* **75A**, 3–12

Kjaersgaard-Andersen, P. and Ritter, M.A. (1991) Prevention of formation of heterotopic bone after total hip arthroplasty. *Journal of Bone and Joint Surgery* **73A**, 942–947

Konotey-Ahulu, F.I.S. (1987) Survey and risk of AIDS in HIV positive patients. *Lancet* **2**, 1146–1148

Kopecky, K.K., Braunstein, E.M., Brandt, K.D. *et al.* (1991) Apparent avascular necrosis of the hip. Appearance and spontaneous resolution of MR findings in renal allograft recipients. *Radiology* **179**, 523–527

Kudo, H. and Iwano, K. (1990) Total elbow arthroplasty with a non-constrained surface replacement prosthesis in patients who have rheumatoid arthritis: a long term follow-up study. *Journal of Bone and Joint Surgery* **72A**, 355–362

Landells, J.W. (1953) The bone cysts of osteoarthritis. *Journal of Bone and Joint Surgery* **35B**, 643–649

Lang, P., Genant, H.K., Jergesen, H.E. and Murray, W.R. (1992) Imaging of the hip joint: computed tomography versus magnetic resonance imaging. *Clinical Orthopaedics and Related Research* **274**, 135–153

Laskin, R.S. (1990) Total condylar replacement in patients who have rheumatoid arthritis: a ten year follow-up study. *Journal of Bone and Joint Surgery* **72A**, 529–535

Lawrence, J. (1967) *Occupation and Disease*. A report to the World Health Organization

Leak, A.M. (1991) Juvenille chronic arthritis. Topical reviews. *Reports on Rheumatic Diseases*, series 2, **19**, 1–5. Arthritis and Rheumatism Council

Lennard, T.W.J., Shenton, B.K. and Barzotta, A. (1985) The influence of surgical operations on components of the human immune system. *British Journal of Surgery* **72**, 771–776

Levin, P.D. (1975) The effectiveness of various antibiotics in methylmethacrylate. *Journal of Bone and Joint Surgery* **57B**, 234–237

Liebermann, J.R., Patterson, B.M. and Salvati, E.A. (1991) Complications in total hip arthroplasty. *Current Opinion in Orthopaedics. Current Science* **2**, 455–462

Lord, G.A., Hardy, J.R. and Kummer, F.J. (1979) An uncemented total hip replacement: experimental study and review of 300 Madreporique arthroplasties. *Clinical Orthopaedics and Related Research* **141**, 2–16

Lowe, G. (1992) Thrombeombolic risk factors (THRIFT) consensus group: risk of and prophylaxis for venous thromboembolism in hospital patients. *British Medical Journal* **305**, 567–574

McCarty, D.J., Pepe, P.F., Solomon, S.D. and Cobb, J. (1970) *Arthritis and Rheumatism* **13**, 336

Macfarlane, R.G. (1958) In: *General Pathology*, p. 162. Edited by H. Florey. W.B. Saunders: Philadelphia and London

MacIntosh, D.L. (1967) Arthroplasty of the knee in rheumatoid arthritis using the hemi-arthroplasty prosthesis: synovectomy and arthroplasty in rheumatoid arthritis. In: *2nd International Symposium on Rheumatoid Arthritis*, Basle

McKee, G.K. and Watson-Farrar, J. (1966) *Journal of Bone and Joint Surgery* **48B**, 245

McLardy-Smith, P.D., Ashton, I.K. and Duthie, R.B. (1984) A tissue culture model of cartilage breakdown in haemophilic arthroplasty. *Scandinavian Journal of Haematology* **33**, Supplement 40, 215–220

McMurray, T.P. (1939) *Journal of Bone and Joint Surgery* **21NS**, 1

Maistrelli, G., Fusco, V., Aval, A. and Bombelli, R. (1988) Osteonecrosis of the hip treated by intertrochanteric osteotomy. *Journal of Bone and Joint Surgery* **70B**, 761–766

Maistrelli, C.L., Gerudini, M., Fusco, U., Bombelli, R., Bombelli, H. and Avai, A. (1990) Valgus extension osteotomy for osteoarthritis of the hip. *Journal of Bone and Joint Surgery* **72B**, 653–657

Mankin, H.J. (1974) The reaction of articular cartilage to injury and osteoarthritis. *New England Journal of Medicine* **291**, 1285, 1292, 1335–1340

Mankin, H.J. and Lippiello, L. (1970) *Journal of Bone and Joint Surgery* **52A**, 424

Marmor, L. (1988) Unicompartmental knee arthroplasty: 10 to 13 year follow-up study. *Clinical Orthopaedics and Related Research* **226**, 14

Martel, W. and Sitterley, B.H. (1969) Roentgenologic manifestations of osteonecrosis. *American Journal of Roentgenology* **106**, 509–522

Meachim, G. (1980) In: *The Aetiopathogenesis of Osteoarthrosis*, pp. 16–28. Edited by G. Nuki. Pitman Medical: Tunbridge Wells

de Meulemeester, F.R. and Rozing, P.M. (1989) Uncemented surface replacement for osteonecrosis of the femoral head. *Acta Orthopaedica Scandinavica* **60**, 425–429

Meyerowitz, S., Jacox, R.F. and Hess, D.W. (1968) Monozygotic twins discordant for rheumatoid arthritis: a genetic, clinical and psychological study of 8 sets. *Arthritis and Rheumatism* **11**, 1–21

Milroy, R.D. and Harris, W.H. (1990) The effect of improved cementing techniques on component loosening in total hip replacement. *Journal of Bone and Joint Surgery* **72B**, 757–760

Mitchell, N.S. and Cruess, R.L. (1967) Synovial regeneration after synovectomy. *Canadian Journal of Surgery* **10**, 234

Mollan, R.B., Watters, P.H., Steele, R. and McClellad, C.J. (1984) Failure of the femoral component in Hoye total hip arthroplasty. *Clinical Orthopaedics and Related Research* **190**, 142–147

Morscher, F.W. (1991) Hydroxyapatite coating of prostheses. *Journal of Bone and Joint Surgery* **73B**, 705–706

MRC (1982) MRC trial on ultra-clean air. *British Medical Journal* **285**, 10–14

Murray, D.W. and Rushton, N. (1990) Macrophages stimulate bone resorption when they phagocytose particles. *Journal of Bone and Joint Surgery* **72B**, 988–992

Nagi, O.N. and Dhillon, M.S. (1991) Total hip arthroplasty after McMurray's osteotomy. *Journal of Arthroplasty* **6**, 517–522

Nelson, I.W., Sivamurugan, S., Latham, P.D., Bulstrode, C.J.K. and Matthews, J. (1992) Total hip arthroplasty for haemophilic arthropathies. *Clinical Orthopaedics and Related Research* **276**, 210–213

Nishini, T., Saito, S., Ohzoma, K., Shimizu, N., Hosoya, T. and Ono, K. (1990) Chiari pelvic osteotomy for osteoarthritis. *Journal of Bone and Joint Surgery* **72B**, 756–769

Nunn, D. (1987) The ring uncemented polyethylene cup in the abnormal acetabulum. *Journal of Bone and Joint Surgery* **69B**, 756–760

Osborne, G.V. and Fahrini, W.H. (1949) *Journal of Bone and Joint Surgery* **31B**, 148

Paul, J.P. (1966) *Proceedings of the Royal Society of Medicine* **59**, 943

Pauwels, F. (1951) Des affections de la hanche d'origine mécanique et de leur traitement par l'ostéotomie d'adduction. [Mechanical disabilities of the hip and their treatment by adduction osteotomy] *Revue de Chirurgie Ortopédique* **37**, 22–30

Pearson, J.R. and Riddell, D.M. (1962) Idiopathic osteoarthritis of the hip. *Annals of the Rheumatic Diseases* **21**, 31–39

Petterson, H., Ahlberg, A. and Nilsson, I.M. (1980) A radiographic classification of haemophilic arthroplasty. *Clinical Orthopaedics and Related Research* **149**, 153–159

Peyron, J.G. (1986) Osteoarthritis. The epidemiologic viwpoint. *Clinical Orthopaedics and Related Research* **213**, 13–19

Phillips, A. (1989) Prediction of progression to AIDS by analysis of CD4 lymphocyte counts in haemophilia. *AIDS* **3**, 737–741

Phillips, T.W., Messieh, S.S. and McDonald, P.D. (1990) Femoral stem fixation in hip replacements: a biochemical comparison of cementless and cemented prostheses. *Journal of Bone and Joint Surgery* **72B**, 431–434

Pietogrande, V., Dioguardi, N. and Mannucci, P.M. (1972) *British Medical Journal* **2**, 378–381

Planes, A., Vochella, N. and Pagola, M. (1990) Total hip replacement and deep vein thrombosis. *Journal of Bone and Joint Surgery* **72B**, 9–13

Pollard, J.P., Hughes, S.P.F., Scott, J.E., Evans, M.J. and Benson, M.K.D. (1979) Antibiotic prophylaxis in total hip replacement. *British Medical Journal* **1**, 707–709

Pool, J.G. and Shannon, A.E. (1965) *New England Journal of Medicine* **273**, 1443

Pool, J.G., Hershgold, E.J. and Pappenhagen, A.R. (1964) *Nature* **203**, 312

Radin, E.L. and Paul, I.L. (1972) A consolidated concept of joint lubrication. *Journal of Bone and Joint Surgery* **54A**, 607–613

Radin, E.L., Ettinger, M., Chemack, R., Abermathy, P., Paul, I.L. and Rose, R.M. (1978) Effect of repetitive impulse loading on the knee joint of rabbits. *Clinical Orthopaedics and Related Research* **131**, 288–293

Raginer, S.J. (1991) Symposium-probes risks and future concerns of operating staff. *Bulletin of the American College of Surgeons* **76**, 8–110

Ranawat, C.S., Flynn, W.F., Saddler, S., Hansraj, K.K. and Magreed, M.J. (1993) Long-term results of the total condylar knee arthroplasty: a 15 year study. *Clinical Orthopaedics and Related Research* **286**, 94–102

Repo, R.U. and Mitchell, N. (1971) Collagen synthesis in mature articular cartilage of the rabbit. *Journal of Bone and Joint Surgery* **53B**, 541–548

Resnick, D., Dwosh, I.L., Goergen, T.G. *et al.* (1976) Clinical and radiographic re-ankylosis following hip surgery in ankylosing spondylitis. *American Journal of Roentology* **126**, 1181–1186

Resnick, L., Verank, C., Salahuddin, S.J. *et al.* (1986) Stability in inactivation of HTLV-III/LAV under clinical and laboratory environment. *Journal of the American Medical Association* **255**, 1887–1891

Rivard, G.E., Girard, M., Belanger, R., Jutras, M., Guay, J.P. and Marton, D. (1994) Synoviorthesis with colloidal ^{32}P chromic phosphate for the treatment of hemophilic arthropathy. *Journal of Bone and Joint Surgery* **76A**, 482–488

Roberts, P., Walters, A.J. amd McMinn, D.J.W. (1992) Diagnosing infection in hip replacements. *Journal of Bone and Joint Surgery* **74B**, 265–269

Rosner, I.A., Malemud, C.J., Goldberg, V.M., Papary, R.S., Geitz, L. and Moskowitz, R.W. (1982) Pathologic and metabolic responses of experimental osteoarthritis to estradiol and estadiol antagonist. *Clinical Orthopaedics and Related Research* **171**, 286

Rothwell, A.G. and Bentley, G. (1973) Chondrocyte multiplication in osteoarthritic articular cartilage. *Journal of Bone and Joint Surgery* **55B**, 588–594

Rubin, P. and Prabhasawat, D. (1962) *Radiology* **76**, 703

Rydell, N.W. (1966) *Forces Acting on the Femoral Head Prosthesis*. Tryckeri, AB Litotyp: Göteborg

Salvati, E.A., Callaghan, J.J., Brause, B.D., Klein, R.F. and Small, R.D. (1986) Reimplantation in infection. Elution of gentamicin from cement and beads. *Clinical Orthopaedics and Related Research* **207**, 83–93

Santavirta, S., Hoikka, V., Eskola, A., Konttingen, Y.T., Paavilainen, T. and Tollroth, K. (1990) Aggressive granulomatous lesion in cementless total hip arthroplasty. *Journal of Bone and Joint Surgery* **72B**, 980–984

Schmidt, S.A. and Kjaersgaard-Andersen, P. (1988) Indomethacin inhibits the recurrence of excised ectopic ossification after hip arthroplasty. *Acta Orthopaedica Scandinavica* **59**, 593

Schorn, D., Bentley, G., Deane, G. and Mowat, A.G. (1978) Knee arthroplasty in rheumatoid disease. *Annals of the Rheumatic Diseases* **47**, 295

Schuller, M. (1887) *Die Pathologie und Therapie der Gelenkentzundurgen*. Urban and Schwarzenberg: Vienna

Schulte, K.R., Callaghan, J.J., Kelley, S.S. and Johnson, R.C. (1993) The outcome of Charnley total hip arthroplasty with cement after a minimum of twenty year follow-up. Results of one surgeon. *Journal of Bone and Joint Surgery* **75A**, 961–975

Scott, R.D., Cobb, A.G., McQueeny, F.G. and Thornhill, T.S. (1991) Unicompartmental knee arthroplasty: eight to 12 year follow-up evaluation with analysis. *Clinical Orthopaedics and Related Research* **271**, 96–101

Sedel, L., Nizard, R., Meurier, A., Dorlot, J.M. and Witvoet, J. (1993) In: *Long Term Behaviour of Alumina/Alumina Coupling for T.H.R. Bioceramics*, Vol 6. Edited by P. Ducheyne and D. Christensen. Butterworth/Heinemann: Philadelphia, USA

Shibata, T., Tada, K. and Hashizume, C. (1990) The results of arthrodesis of the ankle for leprotic neuroarthropathy. *Journal of Bone and Joint Surgery* **72A**, 749–756

Smith, J. (1993) The threat of new infectious diseases. *Journal of the Royal Society of Medicine* **86**, 373–378

Smith, P.H., Benn, R.T. and Sharp, J. (1972) Natural history of rheumatoid cervical luxations. *Annals of the Rheumatic Diseases* **32**, 431

Soballe, L., Tohsurg-Larsen, S., Gelineck, J. *et al.* (1993) Migration of hydroxyapatite coated femoral prostheses. *Journal of Bone and Joint Surgery* **75B**, 681–687

Sobel, J.W., Bohlman, H.H. and Freehafer, A.A. (1985) Charcot's arthroplasty of the spine following spinal cord injury. *Journal of Bone and Joint Surgery* **67A**, 771–776

Soto-Hall, R. and Haldeman, K.O. (1940) *Journal of the American Medical Association* **114**, 2076

Souter, W.A. (1992) Souter-Strathclyde arthroplasty in the management of the adult rheumatoid elbow. Results at 5 and 10 year follow-up. *Journal of Bone and Joint Surgery* **74B**, supplement, 268

Spector, T.D., Brown, G.C. and Silman, A.J. (1988) Increased rates of prior hysterectomy and gynaecological operations in women with osteoarthritis. *British Medical Journal* **297**, 899–900

Spire, B., Dormont, D., Barre-Sinousse, F. *et al.* (1995) Inactivation of lymphadenopathy associated virus by heat, gamma rays and ultraviolet light. *Lancet* **1**, 188–189

Stanley, D., Stockley, I. and Getty, C.J.M. (1990) Simultaneous or staged bilateral total knee replacements in rheumatoid arthritis: a prospective study. *Journal of Bone and Joint Surgery* **72B**, 772–774

Stecher, R.M. (1965) Heredity of osteoarthritis. *Archives of Physical Medicine and Rehabilitation* **46**, 178

Steel, W.M., Duthie, R.B. and O'Connor, B.T. (1969) *Journal of Bone and Joint Surgery* **51B**, 614

Stein, H. and Dickson, R.A. (1975) Reversed dynamic slings for knee-flexion contractures in the haemophiliac. *Journal of Bone and Joint Surgery* **57A**, 282–283

Stein, H. and Duthie, R.B. (1981) The pathogenesis of chronic haemophilic arthroplasty. *Journal of Bone and Joint Surgery* **63B**, 601–609

Stein, H., Dickson, R.A. and Bentley, G. (1975) Rheumatoid arthritis of the elbow. Pattern of joint involvement, and results of synovectomy with excision of the radial head. *Annals of the Rheumatic Diseases* **34**, 403

Steinberg, C., Duthie, R.B. and Piva, A.E. (1962) *Journal of the American Medical Association* **181**, 851

Sugioka, Y. and Ogata, K. (1991) Avascular necrosis of the femoral head. *Current Science, Current Opinion in Orthopaedics* **2**, 437–441

Swann, M. (1990) The surgery of juvenile chronic arthritis. An overview. *Clinical Orthopaedics and Related Research* **259**, 70–75

Swett, P. P. (1923) Synovectomy in chronic infectious arthritis. *Journal of Bone and Joint Surgery* **5**, 110

Takatori, Y., Kokubo, T., Ninomiya, S. *et al.* (1993) Avascular necrosis of the femoral head. *Journal of Bone and Joint Surgery* **75B**, 217–221

Trancik, T.M., Mills, W. and Vinson, N. (1989) The effect of ibruprofen, aspirin and indomethacin on bone growth into a porous coated implant. *Clinical Orthopaedics and Related Research* **249**, 113– 121

Trancik, T., Luncefore, E. and Strum, D. (1990) The effect of electrical stimulation on osteonecrosis of the femoral head. *Clinical Orthopaedics and Related Research* **256**, 120–124

Turpie, A.G.G. (1990) Enoxaparin prophylaxis in elective hip surgery. *Acta Chirurgica Scandinavica Supplementum* **556**, 103–107

Vince, K.G. and Brien, W.W. (1991) Arthritis surgery of the knee. *Current Opinion in Orthopaedics* **2**, 22–30

Vince, K.G., Trusall, J.N., Kelly, M.A. and Silva, M. (1987) Total condylar knee prosthesis: 10 to 12 year follow-up and survival analysis. *Orthopaedic Trauma* **11**, 443

Wainwright, D. (1974) *Annals of the Rheumatic Diseases* **33**, 110

Weidel, J.D., Luck, J.V. and Gilbert, M.S. (1989) Total knee arthroplasty in the patient with hemophilia. Evaluation of long term results. In: *Musculo-skeletal Problems in Hemophilia*, pp. 152–157. Edited by M.S. Gilbert and W.B. Greene. New York National Hemophilia Foundation: New York

Weissmann, G. (1972) Lysosomal mechanisms of tissue injury in arthritis. *New England Journal of Medicine* **286**, 141–147

Welch, R.B. and Charnley, J. (1970) Low friction arthroplasty of the hip in rheumatoid arthritis and ankylosing spondylitis. *Clinical Orthopaedics and Related Research* **72**, 22–32

Werners, R., Vincent, B. and Bulstrode, C. (1990) Osteotomy for osteoarthritis of the hip. *Journal of Bone and Joint Surgery* **72B**, 1010–1013

Wiberg, G. (1939) *Acta Chirurgica Scandinavica* **83**, Supplement 58

Wilde, A.J., Collins, H.R. and MacKenzie, A.H. (1972) Ankylosis of the hip joint in ankylosing spondylitis of the total hip replacement. *Arthritis and Rheumatism* **15**, 493–496

Williams, E., Taylor, A.R., Arden, G.P. and Edwards, D.H. (1977) Arthroplasty of the hip in ankylosing spondylitis. *Journal of Bone and Joint Surgery* **59B**, 393–397

Williams, M. and Lissner, H.R. (1962) *Biomechanics of Human Motion*. W.B. Saunders: Philadelphia and London

Wilson, A.J., Murphy, W.A., Hardy, D.C. and Totty, W.G. (1988) Transient osteoporosis: transient bone marrow edema. *Radiology* **167**, 757–760

Wilson, L.F., Nolan, J.F. and Heywood-Waddington, H.B. (1992) Fracture of the femoral stem of the ring TCH prosthesis. *Journal of Bone and Joint Surgery* **74B**, 725–728

Witt, J.D., Swan, M. and Ansell, B.M. (1991) Total hip replacement for juvenille chronic arthritis. *Journal of Bone and Joint Surgery* **73B**, 770–773

Wooley, P. (1993) HIV management in the 1990s. *Hospital Update* 261

Woolson, S.T. and Watt, M. (1991) Intermittent pneumatic compression to prevent proximal deep vein thrombosis during and after total hip replacement. *Journal of Bone and Joint Surgery* **73A**, 507–512

CHAPTER 12

Neurocirculatory Disturbances of the Extremities

I.M.R. LOWDON

LESIONS OF THE PERIPHERAL NERVES

The great frequency of peripheral nerve lesions during and after the World Wars afforded an invaluable opportunity and provided a strong stimulus for the study of such injuries in all their phases and complexities (Tinel, 1917; Woodhall and Beebe, 1956; Sunderland, 1968; Seddon, 1972). Nerve injuries remain of great economic and industrial importance because of their frequency in civilian life, both as a consequence of acute trauma and due to chronic compression syndromes and diseases.

ANATOMY OF A PERIPHERAL NERVE

The separate nerve fibres, or fibrils, are loosely bound together by a fine meshwork of collagen, known as the endoneurium (Figure 12.1); the anatomical distinction between this layer and the neurolemma or fine outer sheath of the individual myelin tubes is a fine one, and has no direct surgical relevance. Collections of nerve fibres, both myelinated and unmyelinated, bound together by endoneurium, are enclosed by the perineurium to form a fascicle (or funiculus). The perineurium is continuous proximally with the arachnoid matter, and distally with the sarcolemmal sheath of muscle fibres, or the capsule of sensory end organs. The perineurium acts both as a structural support to the nerve fibres, protecting particularly against stretch injury (Sunderland and Bradley, 1949) and also as an epithelial membrane which maintains the pressure and chemical composition of the extracellular fluid bathing the nerve fibre (Figure 12.2) (Soderfelt *et al.*, 1973; Low *et al.*, 1977; Myers *et al.*, 1978). An individual nerve is composed of a variable number of fasciculi bound together by connective tissue. This connective tissue is called epineurium, which condenses on the surface of the nerve to form a distinct fibrous sheath to provide mechanical support to the nerve fibres (Figure 12.2). Sunderland has described the great complexity of the fascicular arrangement in the major peripheral nerves. Proximally in the limbs the fasciculi form a plexus with multiple interconnections; more distally, fasciculi are arranged in identifiable groups which may ultimately leave the nerve as branches (Sunderland, 1968) (Figure 12.3).

Sunderland also demonstrated that between 25% and 70% of the cross-sectional area of a nerve could be occupied by the fibrous tissue and blood vessels running within the epineurium (Sunderland and Bradley, 1949). This, and the great complexity of the fascicular arrangement may, in part, explain the poor results of nerve repair following proximal nerve injuries.

PATHOLOGY OF NERVE INJURY

Waller, in 1850, described the process of degeneration and subsequent regeneration of a nerve following injury (Boyes, 1976). Nerve injuries were subsequently classified by Seddon (1949, 1954) into three types (Table 12.1).

Whilst individual nerve fibres will suffer an injury that can be classified according to Seddon's description, it should be noted that the injury sustained to a nerve trunk, particularly in cases of compression or traction injury, is often of a mixed nature involving more than one of the injury modalities described.

Neurotmesis

When a nerve is completely divided, or the injury is so severe as to be equivalent to a division, the injury

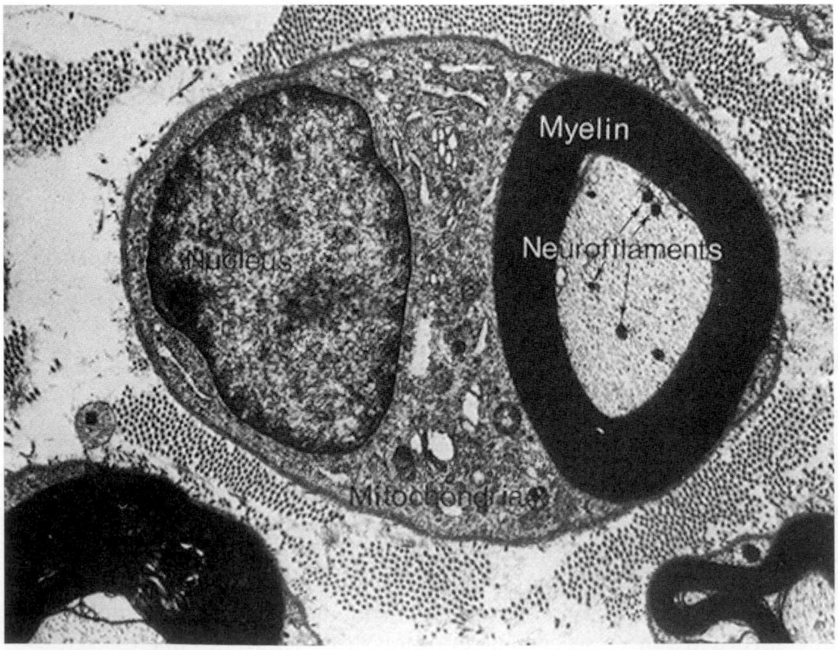

Figure 12.1 Electron micrograph showing a myelinated nerve fibre containing neurofilaments, surrounded by a Schwann cell containing a large nucleus and mitochondria.

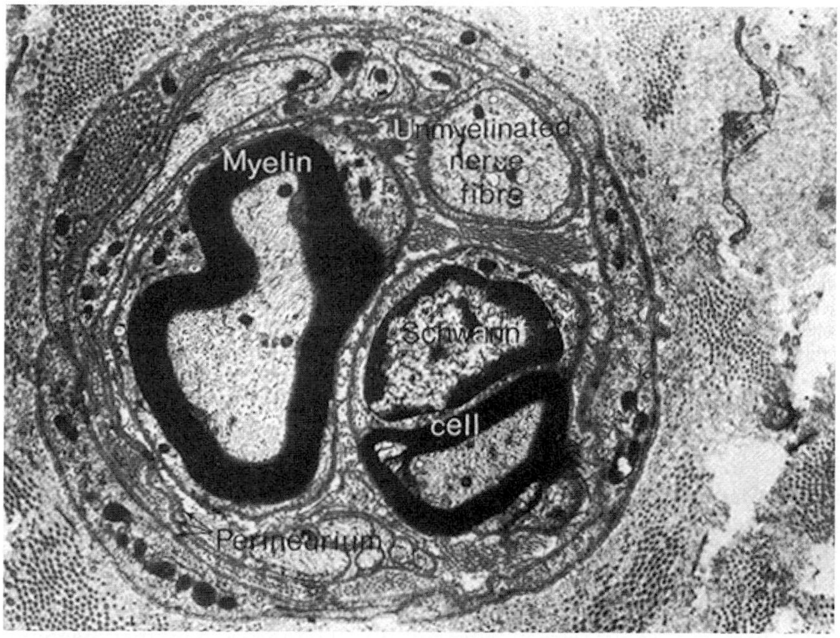

Figure 12.2 The electron microscope anatomy of a peripheral nerve: the axon cylinder is surrounded by a myelin sheath, along the length of which are nodes of Ranvier. The individual nerve fibres are bound together by the endoneurium and groups of nerve fibres are surrounded by the perineurium. A nerve is composed of multiple fascicles bound together and surrounded by a condensation of connective tissue called epineurium.

is called neurotmesis. There is an immediate complete paralysis of the muscles, with rapid diminution of tone and progressive muscular atrophy. Anaesthesia follows immediately after the nerve is divided. Wallerian degeneration follows this injury, in which the distal segment of the interrupted nerve fibre undergoes degeneration due to separation from its trophic centre, which, for the motor fibres, are the anterior horn cells and for the sensory fibres, the posterior root ganglia.

In the first two or three days following nerve division, the myelin sheaths break down and Schwann cells become filled with myelin breakdown products. (Figure 12.4). Many of these Schwann cells assume the appearance and function of macrophages and phagocytose the myelin debris – usually within 2 weeks – but foamy macrophages containing myelin breakdown products may still be seen at 3 months. The macrophages discharge their contents into nearby blood vessels and then either form Schwann cells around new regenerating axon sprouts or differentiate into fibroblasts.

Proximal to the injury, degeneration takes place in a retrograde fashion for one or two nodes only. By the fifth day, regenerating axons reach the proximal cut surface. These axon sprouts are multiple within the same basement membrane, which may be an old Schwann cell membrane. Structural and ultrastruc-

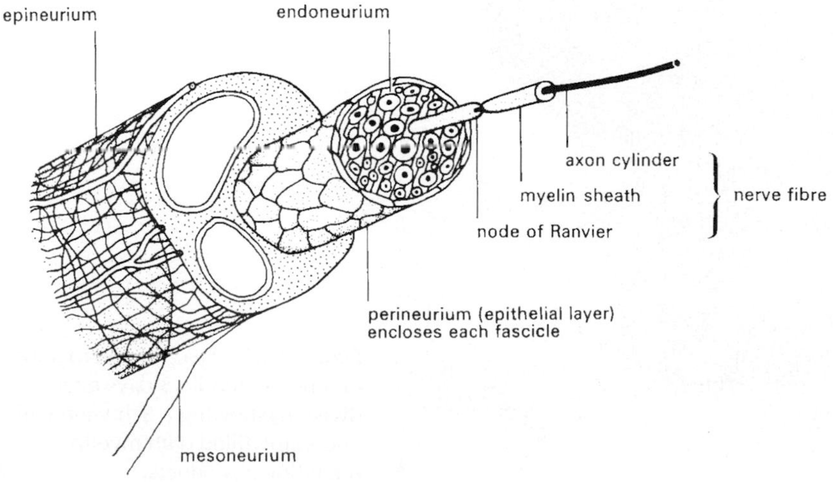

Figure 12.3 Anatomy of a peripheral nerve. Within the epineurium fasciculi form a plexus with multiple interconnections.

Table 12.1 The pathology of peripheral nerve injury

Type	Mechanism	Pathology	Result
Neurotmesis	Transection Stretching (rupture)	Wallerian degeneration Destruction of nerve	Terminal neuroma
Axonotmesis	Stretching Compression	Wallerian degeneration Preservation of structure	Regeneration 1 mm/day
Neurapraxia	Compression	None or local demyelination	Recovery

tural studies demonstrate that regenerating axons progress forward in a haphazard manner through a mass of macrophages and collagenous connective tissue.

Wallerian degeneration provides a chemotactic mechanism in the re-establishment of physiological function as a final result of nerve regeneration (Attardi and Sperry, 1963). Proximal changes occur in the nerve and metabolic studies have shown that the cells of origin of a transected nerve are in maximal metabolic activity after a period of 1 month (Ducker *et al.*, 1969). The chromatolysis seen in the central cell after peripheral nerve division has been shown to represent RNA transformation into a more active form, associated with increased enzymatic activity and the incorporation of amino acids (Gersh and Bodian, 1943). These changes are maximal at 2–3 weeks, thereafter neural tube diameters shrink by as much as 50% and this trend is irreversible (Cragg and Thomas, 1961).

Following division of a nerve, if primary repair is not undertaken, a neuroma forms on the end of the proximal stump, as a consequence of the attempted regrowth of the neurons in association with the local Schwann cells and fibroblasts, into a bulbous amorphous mass of neural and fibrous tissue.

Neuromas in continuity may occur following partial division of a nerve trunk. The structure is the same as a terminal neuroma unless the nerve ends retract substantially, leaving a gap that becomes filled with fibrous tissue alone.

By using the scanning electron microscope Matsuda *et al.*(1988) have demonstrated the morthological changes at the neuromuscular junction or subneural apparatus (Figure 12.5) during denervation and re-innervation in the hamster penoneus longus muscle. After resecting 5 mm of the nerve in the thigh at 4 weeks the whole of the subneural apparatus was elevated above the sarcolemma as a flat plate (Figure 12.5b) which persisted as a bulge for 8 weeks with

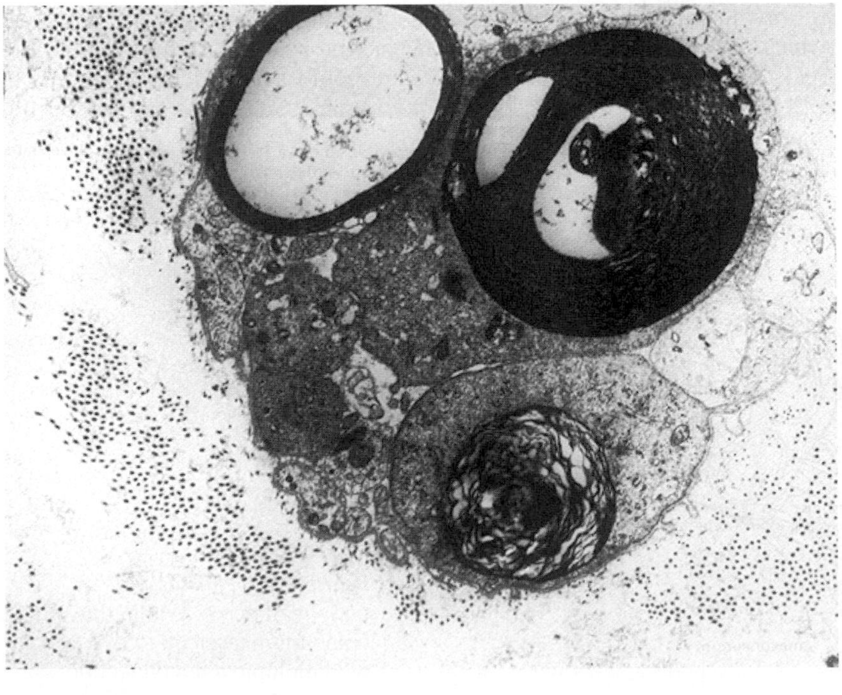

Figure 12.4 Electron micrograph of a nerve bundle 3 days after division, showing a Schwann cell becoming filled with myelin breakdown products.

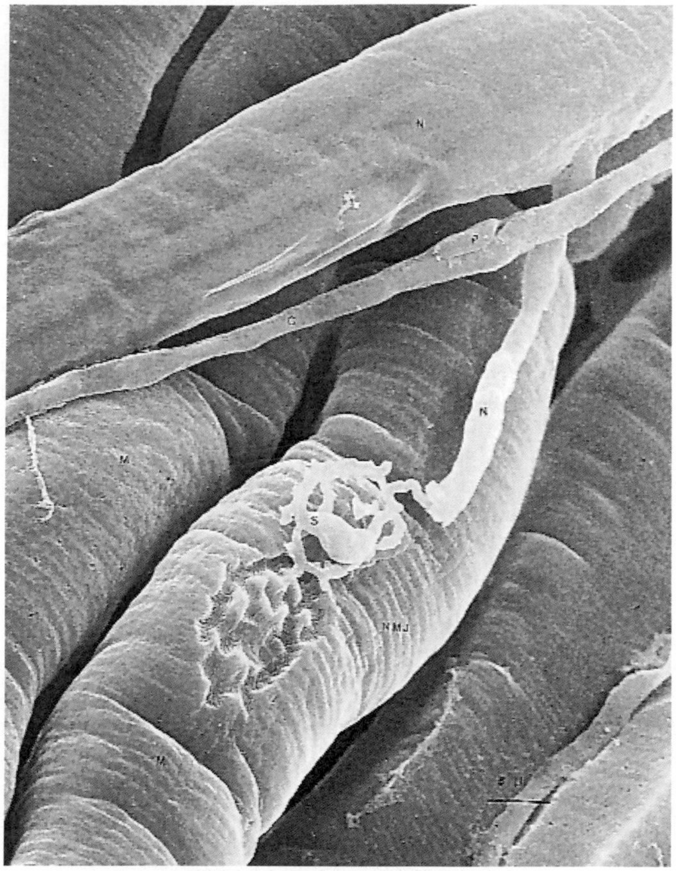

(a)

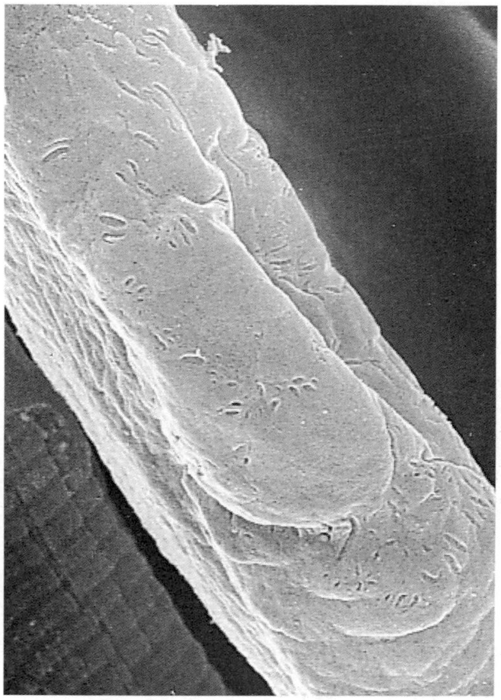

(b)

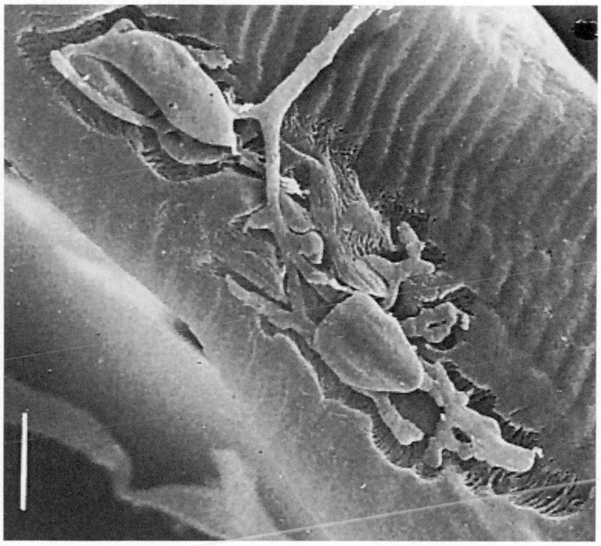

(c)

Figure 12.5 (a) A neurovascular junction with the nerve fibre leaving the main trunk proximally and running down into the middle of muscles fibres (NMJ). One Schwann cell can be seen (S). Just below the main nerve (N) there is a capillary (C) with a pericyte (P) on its wall. (b) After 4 weeks of denervation the neuromuscular junction has lost its junctional fold and the abnormal subneural apparatus is elevated. (c) After 20 weeks there is restoration of the synaptic grooves and junctional folds. (Reproduced, with permission of the senior authors and publishers, from Matsuda *et al.*, 1988)

decrease in the number of the junctional folds. After epineural nerve suture the synaptic grooves and junctional folds so that by 20 weeks the subneural apparatus has recovered its normal structural organization. The persisting junctional folds are thought to be used for the formation of new end plates although it is well established that reinnervation preferentially takes place in the old end plates of the individual muscle fibres.

Axonotmesis

When the nerve is less severely injured, a 'lesion in continuity' or axonotmesis occurs. In this lesion the nerve trunk structure is basically preserved, although the individual nerve fibres do undergo Wallerian degeneration. Regeneration then occurs within the same basement membrane to the original end organ reinnervation occurring in orderly sequence from proximal to distal. Fibrils reach the cut surface by 5 days, and subsequent regrowth down the distal nerve occurs at an estimated rate of 1 mm/day or 2.5 cm/month.

Neurapraxia

A 'transient block', or neurapraxia, is the least severe lesion of peripheral nerves and often follows compression. A conduction block occurs and there may be local demyelination at the site of injury but Wallerian degeneration does not occur and recovery is complete. Large myelinated fibres, serving particularly motor function are most susceptible to compression, and the recovery occurs in an unpredictable manner.

CHANGES IN DEPENDENT STRUCTURES

Many other structures and functions besides motor paralysis and sensory anaesthesia are liable to suffer following peripheral nerve division (Table 12.2). The loss of proprioceptive and autonomic control leads to smooth atrophic skin, with loss of hair, and skin papillae, poor temperature response and loss of subcutaneous fat. The skeletal tissue of a denervated limb undergoes bony osteoporosis, with fibrotic and degenerative changes occurring in joints unless careful measures are taken to keep the limb moving passively. Most of the structures and organs in a limb, including muscles and sensory end organs, are apparently capable of surviving for about a year without innervation, but after this time they become increasingly less likely to regain function, even if successful axonal regeneration occurs. As a consequence of the slow rate of regrowth of nerve fibres (1 mm/day) it is apparent that, in an adult with a brachial plexus injury, even after primary suture and regeneration, some 2 years may elapse before axons reach the hand, by which time many motor end plates will have disappeared and few sensory organs will be capable of reinnervation and function.

Mechanisms of injury

A peripheral nerve may be injured by direct or indirect means.

DIRECT INJURIES

A nerve may be wounded by a stab from a knife, by a bullet or by the ragged ends of a fractured bone. In these cases it may be either completely severed or partially divided. In addition, however, it may be directly compressed by haemorrhage or oedema following nearby injury. Nerves may also be involved by direct vascular ischaemia as seen in Volkmann's contracture of the forearm. The brachial plexus is often injured as a consequence of violent traction

Table 12.2 Consequences of peripheral nerve injury

Type of fibre		Function	Loss seen as:
	Motor	Voluntary muscle	Paralysis; atrophy; electrical changes
Heavy myelinated			
		1. Vasomotor	Vasodilation and vasoconstriction
	Autonomic	2. Sudomotor	Loss of sweating
		3. Pilomotor	Loss of follicular pimples
Less myelinated			
		1. Touch	Altered cutaneous sensibility
		2. Temperature	
	Sensation	3. Deep structures	Altered muscle and bone sensation, reflexes
Unmyelinated		4. Proprioceptive	Altered joint position sense

applied to the limb, resulting in stretching or rupture of the nerve trunks, as in obstetrical paralysis or in motor cycle injuries. Chemical or burn injuries may also be produced by the injection of drugs into a nerve, or the adjacency of methylmethacrylate material to the sciatic nerve during total hip replacement.

Chronic injury is often caused by compression as a consequence of local pressure on a nerve such as occurs in carpal tunnel syndrome or ulnar nerve entrapment at the elbow. Compression of a nerve may cause partial or complete interruption of conduction. Consequently the examination may demonstrate partial motor and sensory loss. Pain is often a feature of a chronic partial compression syndrome (e.g. carpal tunnel syndrome).

Entrapment neuropathies have been described affecting many of the nerves in the body. These may be classified as:

1. *Acute* – when the recumbent body allows the nerve to become compressed by a hard object such as at the elbow (ulnar), hip (sciatic), knee (lateral popliteal), but the paraesthesia and numbness or even muscular weakness last only for a short time after relieving the physical force.
2. *Subacute* – When the compression force is applied over hours; e.g. during the application of a tourniquet (radial nerve) or of a plaster cast (lateral popliteal nerve) or during an anaesthetic, coma or sleep. In haemophilia, bleeds into the iliopsoas muscle are often accompanied by femoral nerve neurapraxia. Ochoa *et al.* (1972) have demonstrated in primates that at the margin of a pneumatic tourniquet there is displacement of the nodes of Ranvier with their myelin sheaths away from the site of compression, causing invagination of the internodes and demyelination, the large myelinated fibres being particularly vulnerable.
3. *Chronic* – Anatomical structures can be rigid and comparatively too small or reduced in volume for their contents, especially in the vicinity of a joint or against a fascial edge covering a muscle. The carpal tunnel is smaller in people with median nerve compression than in asymptomatic controls as demonstrated by computerized axial tomography (Dekel *et al.*, 1980) and the cross-sectional area is reduced further by flexion or extension of the wrist as shown by magnetic resonance imaging (Skie *et al.*, 1990). Congenital or acquired malformations of bones (e.g. cervical rib or cubitus valgus) or of muscles (scalenus anterior) can produce chronic compression syndromes. Systemic diseases may also increase pressure within confined compartments as a consequence of increased volume of the contents (e.g. rheumatoid synovitis, myxoedema, renal dialysis, pregnancy, acromegaly, etc.).

INDIRECT INJURIES

Although a nerve may escape injury at the time of accident, it may be surrounded by callus or enclosed by cicatricial fibrous tissue some considerable time after an injury to a bone or to the soft tissues in its neighbourhood.

Clinical examination

The efficient investigation of the condition of the nerve demands a knowledge of its anatomy and physiology; i.e. its course, it branches, the muscles it supplies and the cutaneous territory to which it is distributed. The examination of the nerve should be repeated at intervals in order to monitor the progress of this recovery and the signs of regeneration as they appear.

The examination of the patient should be undertaken under proper physical conditions since sensory tests and, in particular, electrophysiological examination are unreliable when a limb is cold.

The history is important in identifying the mechanism, type and severity of injury that has been sustained. If delay has occurred from the time of injury, a history of sepsis should be sought and in missile injuries the site of the track, the direction of travel and whether the injury was of high or low energy is of relevance.

Clinical examination should then be undertaken.

POSITION

Lesions of the various nerves often result in a characteristic attitude. Ulnar nerve injuries lead to clawing of the little and ring fingers, characterized by extension of the metacarpophalangeal joints with flexion of the interphalangeal joints; median nerve injuries produce the characteristic flat hand with wasting of the thenar eminence muscle and the thumb lying in the plane of the palm; radial nerve injuries cause a dropped wrist; and lateral popliteal nerve injuries result in a dropped foot.

MUSCLE ASSESSMENT

Zachary (1954) developed a method that was adopted by the Medical Research Council nerve injury centre. In this, the motor power of a particular muscle is calibrated from 0 to 5, i.e. from no contraction to full contraction against resistance (Table 12.3). In cases where the muscle is very weak, it may be necessary to eliminate gravity by lying the patient on his back or by testing the function of certain muscles on a polished surface, which is used to support the part to eliminate gravity and to reduce friction to a minimum.

At 2–4 weeks after denervation, muscles exhibit spontaneous fibrillations and then progressively atrophy to approximately 50% of the normal bulk at the end of 2 months.

Muscular tone is abolished completely. Tone is the state of latent and permanent contraction that persists, even when the normal muscle is at rest; its total disappearance is recognized by the complete flaccidity of the muscular belly on palpation.

A paralysed muscle is painless when compressed. The complete insusceptibility to pressure is one of the clearest signs of complete nerve interruption. Conversely, if the muscle belly is sensitive, although paralysed, the injury is likely to be a neurapraxia with preservation of some conducting fibres (Table 12.4).

Following nerve injury and consequent muscle paralysis, deep tendon reflexes are lost, i.e. a lower motor neuron syndrome.

SENSORY ASSESSMENT

This is also performed according to Medical Research Council principles (Figure 12.6). The area of anaesthesia (loss of light touch sensibility) has particularly sharp boundaries, and can be mapped out to within a few millimetres, particularly if the hand is the affected area. Within this area of anaesthesia, which is marked out on the patient with a continuous line, there is a smaller and usually completely enclosed area of analgesia (loss of pin prick sensibility – which should be marked out with a dotted line. The total area of anaesthesia and analgesia is referred to as the 'autonomous zone'. Moberg (1958) has detailed more sensitive methods of sensory testing following injury, including two-point discrimination. This latter test can be performed on the finger tips with nothing more sophisticated than a modified paper clip and is a useful semi-quantitative method of assessment of a partial nerve injury or of monitoring recovery following injury. In addition, functional impairment in the manipulation of fine objects and identification of shapes can be used to assess the severity of nerve function and recovery. Nerve regeneration can also be monitored using the sensory threshold testing as described by Smith and Mott (1986) (Table 12.5).

The autonomous zone diminishes in size soon after a peripheral nerve injury as branches from adjacent nerves begin to take over the function of the injured nerve. This does not imply nerve recovery, as the sequence of events is too early to be accounted for by regeneration following degeneration.

Table 12.3 MRC method of grading muscle power

0	Complete paralysis
1	Flicker of contraction
2	Contraction with movement of joint when gravity eliminated
3	Contraction against gravity only
4	Contraction against gravity and some resistance
5	Contraction against powerful resistance. Normal power

Table 12.4 MRC method of grading sensory recovery

S 0	Absence of any sensory recovery
S 1	Recovery of deep cutaneous pain sensibility
S 2	Return of some superficial pain and tactile sensibility
S 2+	Recovery of touch and pain sensibility throughout the autonomous zone but with persistent over-reaction
S 3	Return of superficial pain and tactile sensibility throughout the autonomous zone with disappearance of over-reaction
S 3+	As S 3 but with good localization and some return of two-point discrimination
S 4	Return of sensibility as in S 3, with recovery of two-point discrimination

AUTONOMIC ASSESSMENT (Table 12.6)

The autonomic modalities of a peripheral nerve are vasomotor, pilomotor and sudomotor. Sympathetic nerve fibres travel with the nerve trunk in the extremities near to the point of their termination (Flatt, 1980) Thus, in the autonomous zone there is loss of sweat, loss of pilomotor response, and vasomotor paralysis. In the first 2 weeks the affected part is warmer and pinker but thereafter becomes pale, cold and cyanotic. The skin becomes glazed, cutaneous folds disappear, and the capillary crests of the pulp are smoothed out, leaving a flat and polished appearance. The skin is dry and desquamated, which may lead to trophic changes or frank ulceration. There is wasting of the subcutaneous tissue and denervated digits have a tapered conical appearance.

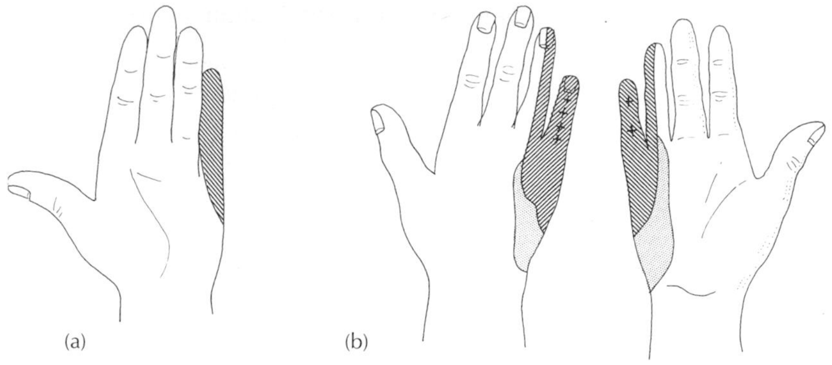

Figure 12.6 Method of recording sensory loss following ulnar nerve injury according to MRC principles. In (a) is shown the typical extent of absolute sensory loss. In (b) the dotted area is insensitive to light touch (anaesthesia) and the shaded area encloses the area of loss of sensation to pin prick (analgesia).

In addition, as a result of disuse, osteoporosis occurs in the bones of the denervated part. Sweat tests are probably most reliable in the earlier stages, immediately following trauma, when the denervated areas may be easily and clearly demarcated with tests, such as the ninhydrin method of Moberg.

EXAMINATION OF THE NERVE

The nerve itself should also be examined for local tenderness. If present, this indicates an incomplete lesion. An attempt should be made to elicit formication, or what is usually known as Tinel's sign. This is evidence of the presence of young axon sprouts and, therefore, of an attempt at regeneration. It is particularly seen after the nerve has been repaired. If the nerve is gently compressed or percussed below the level of the injury a sensation of 'pins and needles' can be elicited in the area supplied by the nerve. This formication can gradually be elicited by more and more distal stimulation as the regeneration proceeds. The distal extent of regeneration can therefore be determined and the rate of progress monitored. The test is unreliable in partial divisions and inapplicable in deeply placed nerves.

The nerve should also be examined for the presence of a neuroma, although this is frequently difficult to determine because of the presence of surrounding encasing fibrous tissue.

Table 12.5 Signs of motor denervation

Paralysis
Loss of tone
Insensitivity to compression
Atrophy
Areflexia

ELECTROPHYSIOLOGICAL ASSESSMENT

Electromyography and nerve conduction studies are important objective estimates of peripheral nerve function. Wallerian degeneration may occur within 72 hours of injury and consequently early electrophysiological examination of distal conduction may indicate the presence of axonotmesis or neurotmesis. Unfortunately, electrophysiological testing is not capable of distinguishing between these two severities of injury, thereby being of little value in identifying injuries that should undergo early surgical exploration. In this technique a nerve is stimulated along its course by skin electrodes and the resultant potentials are recorded along the nerve for sensory nerve conduction studies or from the belly of the target muscle for motor nerve conduction studies.

After 2 weeks, not only will the distal nerve fail to conduct but spontaneous fibrillation potentials may be detected which subsequently decrease in time with reinnervation or fibrosis. Highly polyphasic potentials, becoming more frequent and more normal in configuration, spreading distally, are the electromyographic features of regeneration.

Nerve conduction studies are particularly useful in determining the anatomical site of compression of a nerve. Delay in conduction velocity across the carpal canal is helpful in diagnosing carpal tunnel syndrome. Nerve action potential recordings are more sensitive than conduction velocity studies but require

Table 12.6 Signs of autonomic denervation

Loss of sweating	
Vasomotor paralysis:	early – warm/pink
	late – cold/cyanotic
Loss of cutaneous ridges and folds	
Atrophy of subcutaneous tissue	
Trophic ulceration	

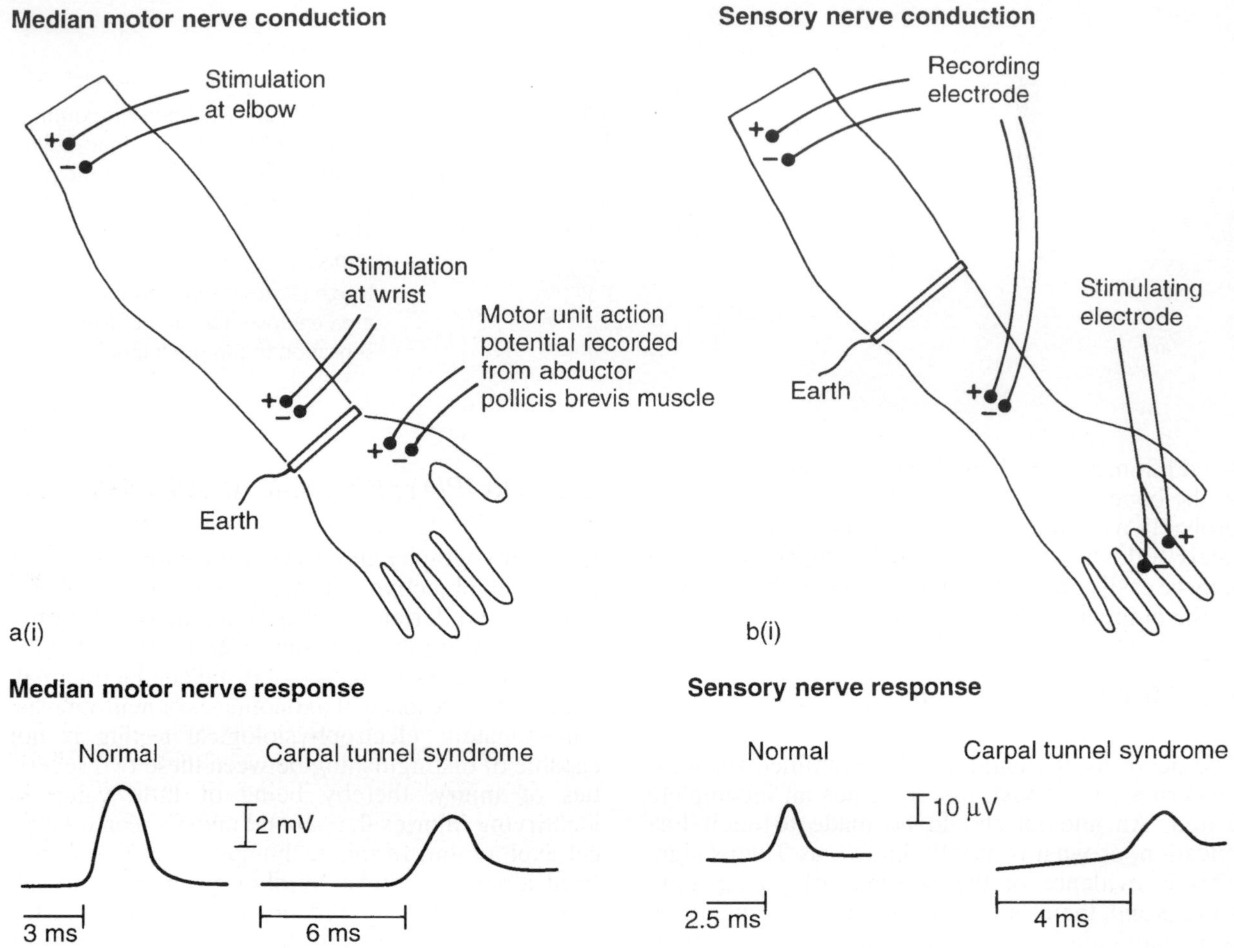

Figure 12.7 (a) Median nerve motor conduction with measuring of the response in the abductor pollicis brevis muscle – normal and in a carpal tunnel syndrome. (b) Median nerve sensory conduction by stimulating the median nerve digital branches and measuring the response above the wrist and the median nerve in the cubital fossa – normal and in a carpal tunnel syndrome. (Redrawn from Cole J. Clinical neurophysiological testing. *Surgery* 1993; 11:12:564 by kind permission of the Medicine Group (Journals) Ltd

a highly refined technique because nerve action potentials are 20 μV whereas muscle action potentials are several mV (Figure 12.7).

IMAGING TECHNIQUES

Plain radiographs are of value in excluding the presence of fracture or foreign body. Assessment of brachial plexus lesions is aided by the performance of computerized axial tomography with myelography (Marshall and De Silva, 1986) which may demonstrate root avulsion from the spinal canal. The value of magnetic resonance imaging in the assessment of these lesions has not yet been fully established.

DIFFERENTIAL DIAGNOSIS

The diagnosis of the nerve injury should not be difficult, and by careful examination, certain confusing conditions can be excluded. These are:

1. Central paralyses, such as monoplegias and cord lesions (e.g. amyotrophic lateral sclerosis, multiple sclerosis).
2. Peripheral polyneuritis due to some form of toxic poisoning or metabolic disturbances (e.g. uraemia, diabetes, carcinomatoas when the motor loss is proximal, vitamin B deficiency and alcoholism, drugs, lead poisoning, organic solvents).
3. Functional paralyses. Some of these are hysterical or mimetic paralyses and correspond to no

definite anatomical distribution. They do not affect so much the movement, as the function, or use of the part. Atrophy and loss of tone such as occur in peripheral nerve lesions are absent, and the area of anaesthesia corresponds to no anatomical nerve distribution; it is more often of the glove or stocking type.
4. Pseudoparalyses from muscular contractures or tendon adhesions.
5. Ischaemic paralyses, which arise from venous or arterial obstruction and result in infarction, fibrous contracture, tendon adhesion and postural deformity.
6. 'Medical' neuropathies usually affect more than one peripheral nerve, especially distally with symmmetrical involvement. The motor, sensory or mixed form can be found, especially of the lower motor neuron type with muscle weakness and atrophy, fasciculation, decreased or loss of reflexes, decreased loss of sensation to pain, light touch, vibration, proprioception, two-point discrimination and Moberg's test.

Treatment of peripheral nerve lesions

The decision to treat a peripheral nerve lesion, either conservatively or by surgical exploration is dependent upon the findings on clinical examination, often supplemented by specific tests such as electrophysiological studies or diagnostic imaging techniques. Over the last few years there has been a swing towards more aggressive surgical management with earlier exploration, in particular of brachial plexus injuries, to define the lesion and allow primary operative repair following neurotmesis.

Conservative treatment is indicated where there is a high probability that the injury is an axonotmesis or neurapraxia, and must in any case be considered part of the postoperative management following surgical intervention.

CONSERVATIVE TREATMENT

The main objective is to preserve the mobility of the whole limb and every part of it, protecting the anaesthetic areas from injury, whilst nerve recovery is awaited. Dynamic and static splintage are carefully used and of great value in maintaining function with isolated peripheral nerve lesions (e.g. cock-up splint for radial nerve paralysis) but it is essential that every joint must be put through its full range of movement at least once every day.

Physiotherapy is of value in maintaining this mobility. During World War II attempts were made to preserve the tone and function of denervated muscles by the use of electrical stimulation of the muscle bellies, with disappointing results. The emphasis should therefore be on passive exercising of the extremity to avoid joint stiffness and the full development of unaffected, or partially affected, muscles to substitute for missing movements where possible, together with the aid of suitably designed splints and braces. The patient is taught to use individual muscles and so gradually restore them to normal. In children this type of treatment may be camouflaged by the use of toys and musical instruments which bring into action the desired muscles.

As recovery occurs, following axonotmesis or neurotmesis, the level at which formication can be elicited (Tinel's sign) indicates the level of regrowth of the nerve. Motor and sensory reinnervation occurs in an orderly manner as the nerve regrows. Following neurapraxia, reinnervation occurs in a random manner due to the differential severity of the injury to individual nerve fibres. As the muscles are reinnervated the patient may complain of some tenderness prior to the commencement of twitching, which is followed by the return of voluntary power. As sensory reinnervation occurs an area initially becomes hyperaesthetic, and often painful, prior to the return of more normal sensibility.

OPERATIVE TREATMENT

Operative treatment is indicated for a neurotmesis. Direct repair or grafting of the nerve to restore continuity may be undertaken, or reconstructive procedures to compensate for the nerve injury, such as arthrodesis or tendon transfer, may be done when operations on the nerve itself are not appropriate.

Evolution of present-day methods of repair

William of Saliceto, Professor of Surgery at Bologna in the thirteenth century, is attributed with being the first surgeon to attempt to resuture divided nerves. Early attempts at restoring the continuity of the divided peripheral nerve depended solely on as accurate as possible a coaptation of the epineurium. Local fibrosis and neuroma formation were frequently encountered, particularly when the nerve was repaired under tension.

Various materials were introduced as barriers against fibrous tissue formation in the form of tubes around the anastomosis. Tantalum shields stopped the ingrowth of fibrous tissue and gave improved structure and initial function but later fragmentation produced secondary scar tissue and functional reduction (Weiss, 1944). Millipore membrane was then used but was later shown to calcify *in vivo*, leading to further secondary scarring (Bassett and Campbell, 1960). In the experimental animal, the use of a silicone rubber cuff around the anastomosis appeared to provide a restraining influence on fibrosis (Campbell and Luzio, 1960), but Sanders and Young (1942) found no benefit in the human by using tubes of plastic, vein or artery.

Various attempts were made to gain length by extensive nerve mobilization or by relaxing the positions of local joints; thereby, lengthening of over 7 cm could be achieved. However, when the joints were subsequently extended, tension was produced on the nerve causing secondary Wallerian degeneration (Highet and Holmes, 1943).

Phillipeaux and Vulpian in 1870 demonstrated that nerve fibres grow through nerve grafts and shortly thereafter the first nerve homograft was used to bridge a deficit in a human median nerve (Albert, 1885). These nerve homografts were, however, subject to immunological rejection. Marmor (1967) attempted unsuccessfully to overcome this by irradiating grafts prior to transplantation and immunological agents were also used (Pollard *et al.*, 1966), although cortisone had previously been shown to inhibit the deposition of myelin by Schwann cells (Lytton and Murray, 1954). In addition, Ochs *et al.* (1970) showed that the transport of proteins down the axoplasmic pathway was strongly inhibited by immunosuppression treatment in patients with irradiated homografts. Ballance and Duel (1932) introduced the use of nerve autografts to overcome these immunological problems and these soon became firmly established as a surgical procedure (Seddon, 1963). The classic technique of cable grafting bridged the gap between the two nerve ends by using several lengths of cutaneous nerve to make up the same diameter as the nerve under repair.

Although in the seventeenth and eighteenth centuries the Dutch microscopy school and the Italian naturalist school demonstrated the detailed structure of the mammalian peripheral nerve, this information could be not utilized by surgeons interested in peripheral nerve repair until the advent of the operating microscope some 30 years ago. The application of microsurgical principles has been responsible for the increased interest in improving methods of reconstituting the divided peripheral nerve. Since then, although the controversy of macroneurorrhaphy versus microneurorrhaphy has not yet been resolved adequately, there is little doubt that improved surgical technique has caused an improvement in the results of nerve repair.

The principles of neurorrhaphy, however, remain the same: tension must be eliminated, an atraumatic technique should be used, the fasciculi should be properly mapped out and aligned, gaps should be prevented, mobilization of a long segment of nerve with its devascularizing effect should be avoided, there must be meticulous haemostasis and minimization of foreign body reactions (Van Beek and Kleinert, 1977). These are all facilitated by the use of the operating microscope.

Epineurial repair

The divided nerve is exposed in a bloodless field and dissected free from local soft tissues. The nerve must be held only gently with non-toothed dissecting forceps at the outer epineurium. Haemostasis in the region of the nerve itself is achieved using bipolar electrocautery. If the nerve is divided obliquely then it can be repaired obliquely. It is not necessary to have cut surfaces at right angles to the longitudinal axis of the nerve.

Rotational alignment of the proximal and distal ends is ensured by inspection of the pattern of longitudinally running blood vessels in the epineurium and by inspection of the fascicular pattern of each cut surface. Using a monofilament non-absorbable suture material, the epineurium is coapted, maintaining the appropriate alignment (Figure 12.8). In the median nerve a 9/0 suture has the appropriate strength, but failing approximately 50% of the time by snapping and 50% of the time by pulling out from the epineurium (Giddins *et al.*, 1989).

Interfascicular repair

In a cleanly severed nerve, individual fascicles, or groups of fascicles, may be aligned and held with fine suture material passed through the perineurial membrane achieving accurate fascicular coaptation in over 90% of cases (Millesi, 1977) (Figure 12.8). If repair is undertaken within 72 hours of injury electrostimulation may be used peroperatively to identify a motor fascicle distally and neuroleptic anaesthesia may be employed to allow identification of the motor fascicle proximally by exclusion as a consequence of stimulation of sensory fascicles. Tension should not be a problem in a clean, fresh incised laceration, particularly as the initial portion of the force displacement characteristic of the mammalian peripheral nerve is almost horizontal, significant displacement being achieved with minimal force.

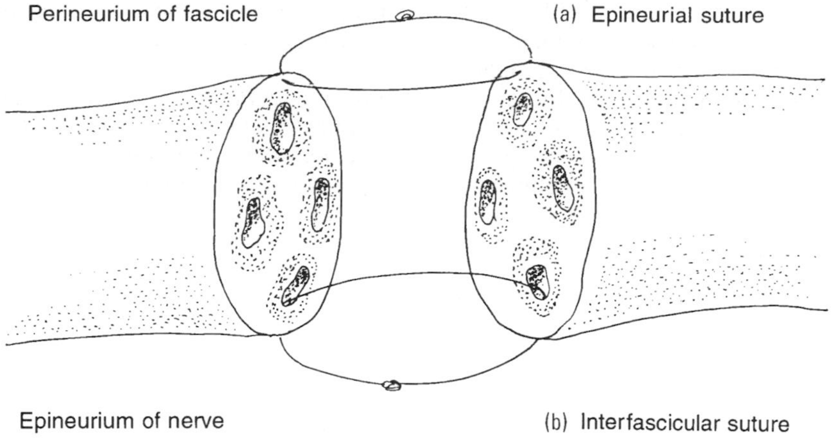

Figure 12.8 Techniques of nerve repair. (a) Epineurial suture – the outer condensation of the epineurium of the nerve only is picked up by the suture material. (b) Interfascicular suture – the perineurium of individual fascicles is sutured, sometimes in addition to passing the suture through the epineurium.

Nerve grafting

Interfascicular

Grafting is indicated when primary nerve repair cannot be performed without excessive tension, when there is significant loss of nerve substance, or when there has been considerable delay between injury and repair. There are no definitive criteria for the selection of a primary repair or graft, and experience and skill are necessary for judgement (Millesi, 1977). Grafting is, however, definitely indicated when primary nerve repair has failed with a resultant neuroma in continuity. The excision of the proximal and distal neuromata and the intervening fibrous connective tissue provides a gap too large to be closed by direct repair.

The nerve is exposed as for primary nerve repair, the fasciculi are identified proximally and distally and are dissected clear of the surrounding epineurium or scar tissue. If a neuroma in continuity is present, each fascicular group should be transected until there is absence of interfascicular scar tissue; it is preferable for fascicular groups to be transected at different levels so that any scar tissue associated with an anastomoses does not occur all at one level (Figure 12.9). The fascicular patterns of proximal and distal cut surfaces are then identified. The length of autograft necessary is determined by measuring the distance between the proximal and distal fasciculi and adding to that half again the length required to allow for retraction and to reroute the graft through a more favourable bed should local scarring be extensive.

The most useful donor site is the sural nerve, which has a length of almost 40 cm, a distinct fascicular pattern and no branches in the calf. Furthermore, the only residual disability from removal of this nerve is a mild hypoaesthesia behind the lateral malleolus. The nerve should be removed through separate incisions rather than using a nerve stripper which damages the outer layers of the nerve substance. One sural nerve autograft is all that is normally required in a great majority of cases of peripheral nerve injury; only in brachial plexus injuries may it be necessary to obtain additional graft material. Other nerves that may be used as graft material include the medial cutaneous nerve of the forearm, the lateral cutaneous nerve of the thigh or the posterior cutaneous nerve of the forearm. The graft is cut into appropriate length segments and the epineurium is removed from each end of each piece

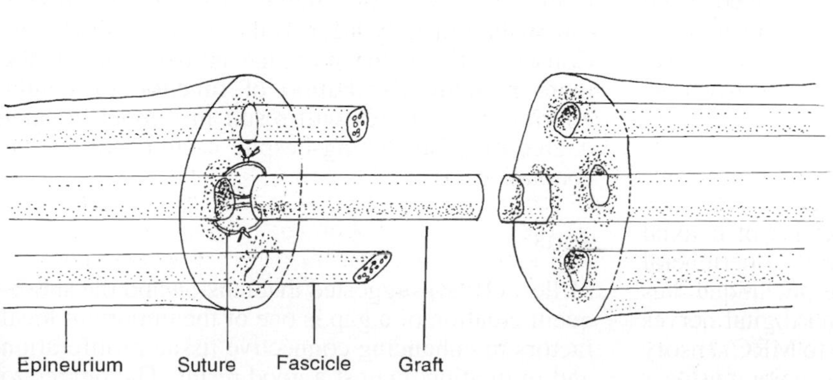

Figure 12.9 Interfascicular nerve grafting: individual fascicles are identified at either end of the divided nerve and are cut at different lengths in order to spread the suture material and anastomoses along the length of the nerve. The gap is bridged by a graft, usually taken from the sural nerve, using an interfascicular suture technique.

of graft material in order to reveal the intrinsic fasciculi. The two anastomoses, proximal-fasciculus-to-graft and graft-to-distal-fasciculus, are fashioned in precisely the same way as for an interfascicular nerve repair.

Cable graft

Epineurial suture may also be employed in nerve grafting. The process is the same as for interfascicular grafting, except that the nerve itself is resected to the extent of the lesion and cable grafts are attached with epineurial sutures or, alternatively, using histoacryl glue.

Epineurial versus interfascicular repair

The advent of microsurgical technique permitted introduction of microdissection of the nerve and interfascicular repair and grafting. Comparative results of this technique as opposed to epineurial suture are, however, not readily available, though Young *et al.* (1981) in a randomized prospective trial of epineurial and interfascicular suture of digital nerves showed no difference between the two techniques. Whilst interfascicular suture is likely to be more accurate in aligning individual fascicles, the necessary intraneural dissection and application of suture material is likely to result in increased fibrosis. It would appear likely, however, that where a large nerve has few fascicles, interfascicular repair may be the method of choice and where the nerve contains multiple fascicles, the likelihood of internal fibrosis being excessive is greater and consequently epineurial repair should be performed.

Vascularized nerve grafts

The use of the ulnar nerve on a pedicle in brachial plexus reconstruction has been described by Bonney *et al.* (1984). Free vascularized grafts, using the dorsal radial nerve supplied by the radial artery, have been utilized by Taylor and Ham (1976). The clinical results have not, however, been proved to be superior to those of conventional grafting techniques and experimental studies have provided contradictory results (McCullough *et al.*, 1984; Koshima and Harii, 1985; Pho *et al.*, 1985).

Degenerated muscle graft

Glasby *et al.* (1986) described the use of coaxial degenerated skeletal muscle autograft in peripheral nerve repair in primates and the technique has subsequently been applied to human digital nerves (Norris *et al.*, 1988) with a recovery to MRC sensory category 3+. A segment of pectoralis major muscle is used, denatured in liquid nitrogen then returned to room temperature in distilled water prior to insertion as a single block.

Initial results appear encouraging, although the results of further studies, including the use of the technique in more demanding situations such as brachial plexus repair, are still awaited. There may be a length limit for the muscle graft of about 4–5 cm. Glasby *et al.* (1990) have reported the use of this technique to repair sheep femoral nerve and the results compare favourably with cable grafts.

Neurolysis

When a nerve is caught up in fibrous scar tissue or callus formation, neurolysis is indicated. It is particularly useful following partial recovery of a complete lesion or failure of improvement following partial injury to a nerve. In such a case, exploration of the site of the nerve may reveal extensive fibrous contracture. The operating microscope is utilized to identify and dissect out the nerve and to remove as much epineurial fibrosis as possible by sharp dissection, in addition to local scar tissue or callus. In some cases, the local scarring is so extensive and nerve function so poor, that excision of the fibrotic neuroma and nerve grafting may be a preferable procedure to undertake.

Factors influencing the outcome of nerve repair

Many factors have bearing on the final outcome.

Age

Children and young adults invariably achieve superior results following nerve injury.

Site of nerve injury

Proximal injuries have a poorer prognosis. This is probably because the degree of organization of the fasciculi into groups of nerves of similar function is established distally, near to the origin of branches. Consequently in the proximal part of a nerve the more random distribution of function of neighbouring nerve fibres will result in a much greater degree of mismatching despite accurate fascicular coaptation.

Tension

Millesi (1968) suggested that tension and the subsequent creation of a gap is one of the important local factors in enhancing connective tissue proliferation and mitigating against a good result. The degree to which a nerve can be stretched without causing direct injury is uncertain. Liu *et al.* (1948) suggested that the perineurium was destroyed by an elongation of as little as 6%. In contradistinction, Hoen and Brackett (1956) found little evidence of structural damage when permanent elongations of the order of 100% were created and Tricker *et al.* (1979) indicated that an elongation of up to 20% had no significant effect on the structure, ultrastructure or electrophysiological function of a nerve.

Timing

The optimal interval between injury and repair has not been clearly determined. Ducker *et al.* (1969) have suggested that nerve repair should be delayed until the nerve cell body is entering the anabolic stage and nerve sprouting is commencing. Dickson *et al.* (1977) suggested this optimal period is at approximately 2–3 weeks following injury. Bolesta *et al.* (1988), however, in studies on rabbit sciatic nerves, have demonstrated that immediate neurorrhaphy produces a superior result as assessed by function, electrophysiological and quantitative techniques and Birch and Raji (1991), in reviewing a personal series of 108 median and ulnar nerve repairs, has demonstrated that the clinical results of primary repair are superior to those of delayed repair or grafting.

Following a closed injury and initial conservative management, the timing of subsequent exploration has to be chosen in order to allow for evidence of potential spontaneous recovery due to axonotmesis or neurapraxia to appear, without jeopardizing the potential for recovery following delayed neurorrhaphy or nerve graft if the injury proves to be a neurotmesis.

Muscle fibres and nerve muscle end plates degenerate after a period of 18 months to 2 years from injury. Consequently, exploration of proximal injuries should not be delayed much beyond 6 months in order to allow adequate time for axonal regrowth and reinnervation prior to irreversible endplate degeneration.

Fibrosis

Mackenzie and Woods (1961), in their study of causes of failure after repair of the median nerve, emphasized the necessity for adequate resection of the nerve ends prior to suture. On serial sections of tissue, removed at the time of median nerve suture, they found that only 50% had had a sufficient amount of fibrotic material removed. Gschmeissner *et al.* (1991) have described an interesting technique to assess rapidly nerve stump excision for use in the operating room to obtain improved visualization of the nerve stump resected material. Each individual slide is frozen, cut to 7 mm and stained with osmium tetroxide, and under the microscope both quantitative and qualitative assessment of myelinated fibres both proximally and distally are readily available with good detail.

General factors

The condition of the patient, the degree of local contamination and contusion of a wound and the possible presence of sepsis must also be taken into consideration in determining the time of repair. The availability of a surgeon with appropriate microsurgical skill is necessary, although Marsh and Barton (1987) demonstrated no clinical difference in the final clinical outcome following primary neurorrhaphy performed by a single trained microsurgeon when epineurial suture was performed with or without an operating microscope.

The median nerve

AETIOLOGY

The median nerve is most frequently injured in wounds of the forearm, especially penetrating injuries, such as those caused by broken glass. It may also be injured in fractures of the lower end of the humerus, and occasionally in fractures of the radius and ulna. Volkmann's ischaemic contracture often causes injury to the median nerve, as do missile wounds of the forearm.

CLINICAL FEATURES

A complete division of the median nerve above the elbow involves the flexors of the wrist, fingers and thumb, the pronator teres and the pronator quadratus as well as the opponens pollicis, abductor pollicis and the superficial head of the flexor pollicis brevis.

Atrophy of the whole thenar eminence is usually a conspicuous sign, but the flexor pollicis brevis may occasionally remain intact owing to its deriving an anomalous supply from the ulnar nerve.

The sensory loss involves the thumb, index and middle fingers, and half the ring finger (Figure 12.10). Injuries of the median nerve are notable for the frequency with which irritative syndromes of all grades develop. Trophic disturbances are best seen in the wasting of the terminal phalanx of the index finger, which is usually thin, pointed and conical.

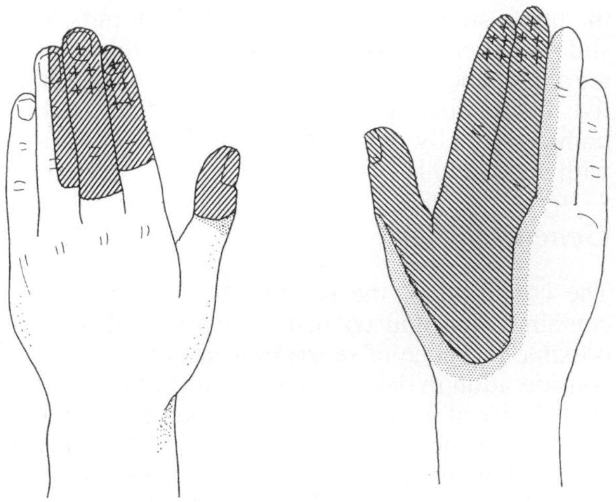

Figure 12.10 Sensory loss in division of the median nerve, shaded area encloses the area of anaesthesia, dotted area encloses the area of analgesia.

DIAGNOSIS

The characteristic attitude of a hand deprived of its median nerve supply is one of flattening, the thenar eminence being entirely wasted and the thumb rolled laterally from paralysis of the opponens pollicis.

In high median nerve injuries the index finger almost entirely loses its power of flexion, and when an attempt is made to close the fist, the thumb and index finger remain extended. Also, when the palm of the hand is laid on a table, the patient is unable to flex the index finger with the other fingers remaining flat on the table.

A good clinical test for the loss of median nerve sensation is to ask the patient to button his coat: this manoeuvre cannot be carried out unless the movements are directed by vision.

In injuries at the level of the wrist joint the limited muscular paralysis may pass unnoticed. The anaesthesia, however, is usually just as complete as in lesions at a higher level.

In complete median nerve lesions, the functional incapacity of the hand is quite out of proportion to the actual motor paralysis, as the median nerve is the 'eye' of the hand, and without sensibility in the thumb and index finger, the hand is almost useless.

PROGNOSIS

After suture of the median nerve at the wrist in an adult, recovery of protective sensation is usual but that to light touch and the development of two-point discrimination is unpredictable, as is recovery of the thenar muscle function.

TREATMENT

Primary repair

Fresh, cleanly incised wounds at the wrist involving median nerve injury should be explored: primary end-to-end repair of the median nerve without tension can invariably be achieved.

More extensive injury at the wrist or more proximally in the arm with damage of a segment of the nerve may result in excessive tension for primary repair and may thus require nerve grafting.

Delayed repair

Median nerve injury, particularly partial divisions of the nerve at the wrist, are occasionally missed on initial examination and present later with a painful neuroma in continuity. Microsurgical intraneural dissection to resect the neuroma whilst leaving intact fascicles undamaged is required, followed by primary end-to-end suture, or grafting. Because of the intraneural scarring the differentiation between neuroma and intact nerve is difficult and great care must be taken lest normal nerve tissue is resected and intact function thereby lost.

Reconstruction following median nerve injury

Following median nerve injury and repair, sensibility may recover without adequate motor function of the small muscles. Reconstructive procedures are then appropriate, in particular to achieve opposition of the thumb and thereby improve function.

In cases of low median nerve injury, where the innervation of the forearm flexor muscles is normal, an opponens-plasty, using the flexor superficialis tendon to the ring finger, provides a satisfactory functional result. This may be performed using the classical Bunnell (1938) technique in which the tendon is passed superficially from proximal to the wrist, through a pulley fashioned from a slip made of 50% of the flexor carpi ulnaris tendon attached distally, to its insertion point into the base of the proximal phalanx of the thumb. An alternative method, as described by Royle (1938) and subsequently modified by Thompson (1942), uses a pulley which is created by passing the tendon subcutaneously from a point distal to the intercarpal ligament and radial to the palmar fascia, the distal insertion being twofold – into the neck of the metacarpal and into the extensor hood over the proximal phalanx. Littler (1949) recommended insertion distally by weaving the tendon into that of the abductor pollicis brevis and Riordan (1964) supplemented this insertion with an extension into the extensor hood.

In more proximal median nerve injuries the function of the superficialis muscle is affected and alternative methods of opponens-plasty should be considered. Muscles that have been used are the extensor carpi ulnaris, elongated with the tendon of the extensor pollicis brevis (Phalen and Millar, 1947), the extensor indicis proprius (Burkhalter, 1974) and the extensor digiti minimi (Steindler, 1918; Schneider, 1969).

Huber (1921) described the use of the abductor digiti minimi, though the functional loss to the ulnar border of the hand as a consequence of this transfer may mitigate against its use.

In low median nerve injury the Camitz transfer, using the palmaris longus, extended by a strip of palmar fascia, is attractive, particularly because the donor muscle has no functional use and there is consequently no risk of deficit (Camitz, 1929). The procedure can usefully be combined with carpal tunnel decompression when motor loss is severe.

Carpal tunnel syndrome

The carpal tunnel syndrome (see also Chapter 15) was first described by Sir James Paget in 1865 as the compression irritation syndrome of the median nerve as it transverses the carpal canal. The condition occurs most commonly in females with no obvious underlying cause, although computerized tomographic studies have demonstrated significantly smaller carpal canals in such individuals (Dekel *et al.*, 1980). The condition may also be caused by fluid retention during pregnancy and the menstrual period, and in systemic conditions characterized by fluid overload including cardiac failure, renal failure, myxoedema, and in the amyloidosis seen in renal dialysis patients.

Eckman-Ordeberg *et al.* (1987), from a large series of over 2000 pregnant women tested by both sensory and motor examinations found that 2% of all pregnant women complained of this syndrome. Eighty-two per cent obtained relief by splinting at night, 16% had no benefit and 2% required a carpal tunnel release. The majority of the women recovered within 6 weeks after delivery, but persistence of symptoms should receive release of the transverse carpal ligament.

The patient characteristically complains of painful paraesthesia and numbness affecting the median nerve-innervated territory of the hand, particularly at night. The patient is awakened after 2–3 hours of sleep and seeks symptomatic relief by vigorously shaking the affected hand. This discomfort precedes motor symptoms or constant sensory loss and is often the presenting feature to the physician.

Sometimes a history of previous trauma, such as a Colles' fracture, can be elicited, and this implies that malunion has led to a reduction in the volume of the carpal canal. Finally, the other contents of the carpal canal may be enlarged, thus encroaching upon the median nerve. This includes local synovitis of a mechanical or rheumatoid variety, and ganglion formation on the volar aspect of the wrist joint.

Carpal tunnel syndrome also occurs with increased frequency in diabetes, in patients on haemodialysis, due to amyloid deposition, and in paraplegia.

Examination of the median nerve function is often entirely normal, though wasting of the thenar eminence, usually localized to the abductor pollicis brevis muscle, with weakness of thumb abduction, occurs in severe cases. There may be hypoaesthesia to light touch and pinprick over the palmar aspect of the radial three and half digits. The skin overlying the palm and the thenar eminence is, however, unaffected, being supplied by the palmar cutaneous branch of the median nerve which arises proximal to the carpal ligament. Phalen (1966) described a provocative test in which passive flexion of the affected wrist reproduces the sensory symptoms within 1 minute. Prolonged digital pressure over the carpal ligament may reproduce the symptoms (Nicolle and Woodhouse, 1965) and Tinel's sign of percussion over the carpal ligament is often positive. A blood pressure cuff applied to the upper arm and used as a venous tourniquet may also precipitate symptoms within 1 minute.

In a recent study of the value of the provocative diagnostic tests, Gellman *et al.* (1986) showed that the Tinel's test was the most specific, Phalen's wrist flexion test the most sensitive, and the tourniquet test was the least sensitive and specific in confirming carpal tunnel compression.

The differential diagnosis in some cases can be difficult, particularly in the elderly individual with associated degenerative osteoarthrosis of the cervical spine. More than one compression syndrome may coexist (Upton and McComas, 1973), and other conditions that may confuse the picture include a coexistent thoracic inlet syndrome or a peripheral neuropathy such as may occur in diabetes or rheumatoid arthritis. Where doubt exists about the diagnosis, electrophysiological studies may be of value, although negative results do not preclude resolution of the clinical symptoms following surgical decompression (Grundberg, 1983). Nerve conduction abnormalities, particularly of the sensory nerve conduction type with a delayed response and diminished amplitude, may be found on comparing one side to the other.

Where a specific cause for the condition can be identified, non-surgical treatment may be of value; thus during pregnancy or in symptoms related to the menstrual period, a wrist splint may be all that is required. An injection of steroid into the carpal canal often produces relief, although this is seldom permanent (Green, 1988). For the majority, whose carpal tunnel syndrome is of idiopathic aetiology, relief of the symptoms can be obtained by surgical division of the carpal ligament, as first described by Learmonth (1933). It is most important to approach the carpal ligament through an incision longitudinally in line with the ring finger (Figure 12.11), thus avoiding the palmar cutaneous branch of the median nerve or one of its larger branches which lie in the axis of the middle finger (Taleisnik, 1973). Lack of attention to this important surgical detail gives rise to a painful neuroma in the region of the scar with hypoaesthesia over the palm and the thenar eminence.

Intraneural neurolysis has not been demonstrated to be of additional value in the treatment of severe cases (Gelberman *et al.*, 1987).

A long-term review of over 200 cases of carpal tunnel syndrome treated surgically indicates that one-third of patients may be expected to recover symptomatically very promptly, a further third may take up to 6 months, while the final third may take up to 2 years to recover fully. Furthermore, those who have had symptoms and physical signs for longer than 6 months achieve a proportionately less satisfactory result (Semple and Cargill, 1969). Failure may be due to incomplete division of the transverse ligament, damage to the motor division of the nerve with neuroma formation or secondary scarring.

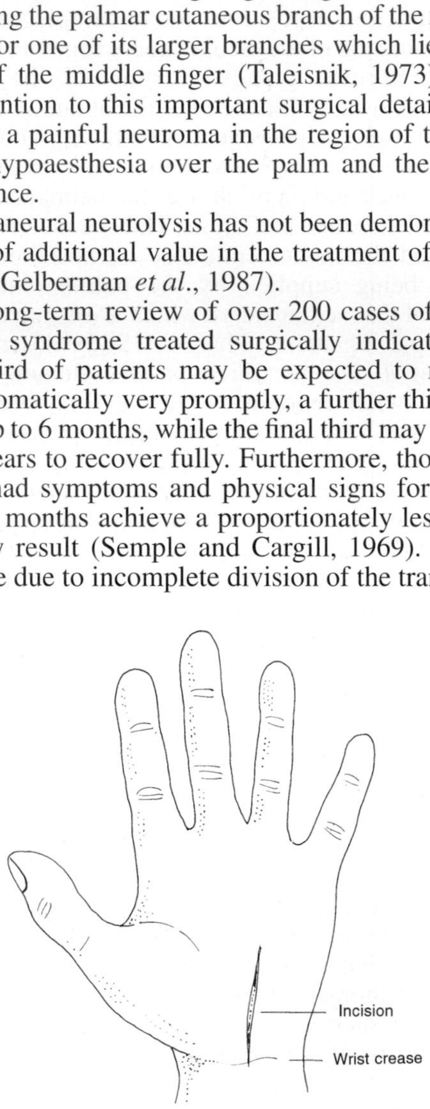

Figure 12.11 Carpal tunnel decompression: the incision must be in line with the ring finger in order to ensure that the median nerve, and in particular the palmar cutaneous branch, is not injured during the exposure.

Complications following carpal tunnel release are common and are incomplete release of the transverse ligament, either its distal or proximal margin, division of the palmar cutaneous branch or the thenar motor branch to the thenar muscle (this can be extraligamentous in 46%, subligamentous in 31% and transligamentous in 23%), excessive neurolysis, adhesions and hypersensitivity of a keloid, haematoma formation and reflex sympathetic dystrophy or algodystrophy.

The ulnar nerve

The ulnar nerve is most commonly injured in incised wounds of the forearm, or in fractures of the lower end of the humerus, particularly those affecting the medial epicondyle. Occasionally it is contused by crutch pressure in the axilla or in the palm of the hand, and it is frequently implicated in osteoarthritic outgrowths about the elbow joint.

Occasionally also the nerve is anchored so insecurely in the post-condylar groove that it can slip backwards and forwards with each movement of flexion and extension. This instability often results in neuritis, with pain, and weakness of the fingers.

CLINICAL FEATURES

In lesions above the post-condylar groove, the paralysis affects the flexor carpi ulnaris and the medial half of the flexor digitorum profundus, the hypothenar muscles, the interossei and the medial two lumbricals, the adductor of the thumb and sometimes the deep head of the flexor pollicis brevis. Abduction and adduction movements of the fingers are lost and also adduction of the thumb, so the patient is unable to grasp a pencil placed crosswise between the thumb and the index finger. In paralysis of the dorsal interossei, abduction of the fingers can be carried out only by the extensor digitorum longus but this produces also hyperextension of the metacarpophalangeal joints. The most precise method of testing for motor deficiency in the ulnar nerve is to force the patient's index finger into adduction against resistance, while the examiner palpates the muscle mass of the contracting first dorsal interosseous muscle.

The muscular atrophy gives the familiar flattening of the hypothenar eminence, the depressed interosseous spaces, and the prominence of the metacarpal heads in the palm. A claw-like deformity, most marked in the ring and little fingers, develops – the metacarpophalangeal joints are extended, and the interphalangeal joints are flexed, while the little finger is usually abducted (Figure 12.12). As time goes on, this contracture becomes more and more marked, and the little and ring fingers gradually assume a fixed attitude.

Sensation is lost over the ulnar border of the hand, the entire little finger and the ulnar half of the ring finger on both extensor and flexor surfaces. If the lesion is below the origin of the dorsal cutaneous branch, which arises from the main trunk, a variable distance above the wrist in the distal forearm, sensation is retained on the dorsum of the hand.

Functional disability following division of the ulnar nerve relates principally to the loss of the intrinsic muscle function and consequent diminution of dexterity and inability to achieve fine manipulative manoeuvres. In high ulnar nerve lesions, where the flexor carpi ulnaris and the ulnar half of flexor digitorum profundus are also paralysed, there is a concomitant substantial loss in power grip which further reduces the functional capacity of the hand.

Traumatic ulnar neuritis

Like the median nerve, the ulnar nerve is liable to a temporary or permanent neuropathy as it traverses confined spaces in the arm and forearm. At the elbow compression occurs behind the medial epicondyle or immediately distal as the nerve passes under an aponeurosis between the two heads of flexor carpi ulnaris (Osborne, 1959). At the wrist it is liable to compression as it passes deep to the muscles of the hypothenar eminence (through Guyon's canal), sometimes due to a ganglion (Seddon, 1954) or a tight pisohamate ligament.

As with median nerve compression, the symptoms are those of pain and paraesthesia in the appropriate fingers, plus weakness of the hand due to interosseous muscle palsies. Diagnosis of these syndromes is achieved by careful assessment of the history and physical findings, plus electrophysiological studies which will show slowing of nerve conduction over the zone of nerve pressure.

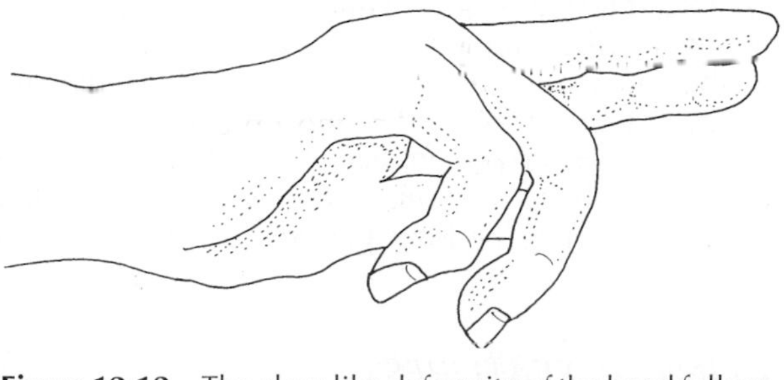

Figure 12.12 The claw-like deformity of the hand following ulnar nerve division due to paralysis of the small muscles of the little and ring fingers.

TREATMENT

The treatment is surgical, consisting of decompression by division of the constricting bands or muscles, or by transposition of the nerve anteriorly. Such an anterior transposition of the ulnar nerve at the elbow may also be utilized in order to gain length for a nerve suture in the arm or forearm. Simple decompression of the nerve around the medial epicondyle and as it passes between the heads of flexor carpi ulnaris is a simple and safe procedure and consequently should be recommended in most cases of simple ulnar nerve compression. When the palsy is due to osteophytic lipping around the joint or follows injury with subsequent deformity, anterior transposition into a subcutaneous or submuscular (Learmonth, 1944) position, which decreases tension during flexion, should be undertaken (Figure 12.13). Dellon (1989), in reviewing the results of published series of the treatment of ulnar nerve compression, concluded that for minimal symptoms, any one of the surgical procedures was effective. For moderate symptoms, anterior transposition was advisable and when the symptoms were severe, anterior submuscular transposition in association with an internal neurolysis should be undertaken.

Other entrapment syndromes, e.g. in Guyon's canal, lateral popliteal nerve in the neck of the fibula, tarsal tunnel syndrome, etc., will be dealt with in the appropriate chapters.

Reconstruction following ulnar nerve injury

Following ulnar nerve palsy multiple tendon transfer procedures can be undertaken to correct the deficits that occur as a consequence of the intrinsic muscle paralysis. A careful assessment of the functional deficit must be undertaken to determine the requirement and tailor the appropriate transfer to achieve optimum results.

Following a lesion of the ulnar nerve below the innervation of the long flexor muscles, the principal muscle loss is that of the small muscles in the hand. Power of thumb adduction is lost as is intrinsic function of the little and ring fingers. These functions may be replaced by tendon transfers, supplemented on occasions by fusion of the thumb MCP joint. A

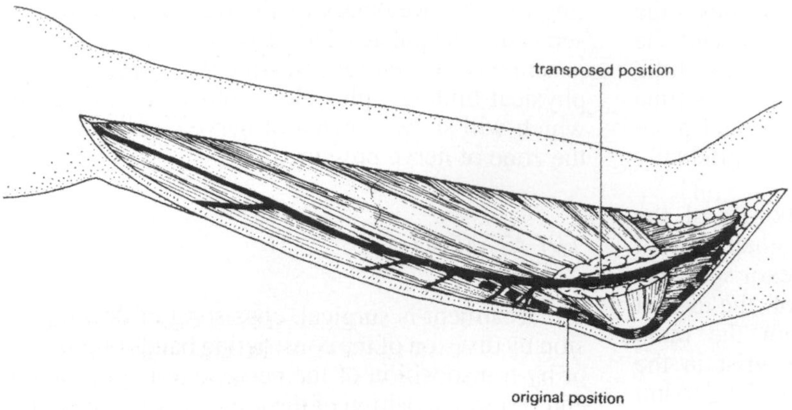

Figure 12.13 Anterior submuscular transposition of the ulnar nerve. Proximal dissections with division of the medial intermuscular septum and distal dissection to free the nerve between the two heads of flexor carpi ulnaris is undertaken.

satisfactory motor in such lesions is the ring finger superficialis. The radial slip of the tendon is transferred behind the flexor tendons of the index and ring fingers to insert into the tendon of the abductor pollicis brevis or the abductor tubercle. The ulnar half of the tendon is split into two, passed volar to the transverse metacarpal ligament and inserted into either the A2 pulley over the proximal phalanges or into the central slip of the extensor tendon over the middle phalanx of the ring and little fingers (Littler, 1949; Omer, 1971, 1980; Brooks and Jones, 1975; Doyle and Blythe, 1975). This transfer does not significantly increase the power of flexion of the fingers, which can, however, be improved by introducing an extrinsic tendon such as the extensor carpi radialis longus elongated with a free tendon graft (Brand, 1970; Burkhalter and Strait, 1973). An alternative method of controlling MCP joint hyperextension is by utilizing the superficialis to each finger and forming a lasso around the proximal phalanx (Zancolli, 1978).

With a more proximal ulnar nerve palsy the flexor digitorum superficialis to the ring or little fingers must not be sacrificed because of the loss of function of the flexor digitorum profundus. Appropriate motors under these circumstances are the extensor carpi radialis longus and the brachioradialis, which may be transferred with a free graft to provide thumb adduction (Boyes, 1964), and tenodesis of the ring and little flexor digitorum profundus tendons to the long finger tendon.

Cubital tunnel syndrome

Gelberman *et al.* (1993) have described in detail the various lesions affecting the ulnar nerve above, in and below the elbow – i.e. the cubital tunnel syndrome.

This recently described syndrome is distinct from the tardy ulnar palsy associated with cubitus valgus deformity. Above the cubital tunnel the ulnar nerve is rarely compressed at the arcade of Struthers about 8 cm above the medial epicondyle. Below this the thickened medial intermuscular septum can cause problems when the nerve subluxes. In the actual tunnel consisting of the medial epicondyle and the proximal part of the ulnar bone there is the fascial sheet of Osborne. It is the change in size and shape during flexion and extension with inflammation which produces the compression and actual attenuation of the ulnar nerve. Below the tunnel there is a gap between the flexor carpi ulnaris head and the pronator teres which can become inflamed and scarred, leading to compression. Within the muscle substance surrounding the ulnar nerve, scarring or fascial bands can obstruct the normal migration of this nerve.

The radial nerve

The radial nerve is one of the most frequently injured of all nerves. Its intimate relation to the humerus explains its common association with lesions, especially fractures, of that bone. If it escapes injury after the actual fracture is sustained, it may later become involved in the scar contracture of the soft tissues or in callus formation at the site of the fracture. The nerve may be injured also by pressure of a crutch in the axilla, and it may be contused when the arm is left hanging over the back of a chair for long periods, as in a drunken sleep.

CLINICAL FEATURES

The paralysis affects the extensor group of muscles –

the brachioradialis, the radial and ulnar wrist extensors, and the extensor of the thumb and fingers – so there at once results a characteristic drop-wrist. Paralysis of the triceps is very rare, as all the branches supplying it arise before or just as the main trunk enters the radial groove.

The sensory signs are trivial. When the lesion is in the upper third of the arm there is a small, ill-defined, triangular zone of anaesthesia on the dorsum of the hand over the first web space.

DIAGNOSIS

The diagnosis is rarely in doubt. It should be remembered that the interphalangeal joints of the finger are extended by the interossei and lumbricals, and that it is principally the metacarpophalangeal joints which are extended by the muscles supplied by the radial nerve. The lumbricals and interossei consequently have an unopposed action of flexion on the metacarpophalangeal joint in radial nerve lesions. The grip is very materially weakened in radial paralysis because the flexors of the fingers are placed at a mechanical disadvantage due to the loss of the synergistic function of the radial wrist extensors which are utilized in stabilizing the carpus in dorsiflexion whilst making a power grip.

PROGNOSIS

The results of suture of this nerve may be better than others, and some recovery in all the muscles usually occurs; sensory function is unlikely to return but the loss causes no handicap. Repair of the radial nerve probably produces good results because the nerve is almost entirely motor with a small sensory component and the regenerative motor axons do not have very far to travel to their appropriate muscles.

TREATMENT

Closed injury to the radial nerve in association with fractures of the humerus are commonly axonotmesis or neurapraxia and only rarely neurotmesis. A conservative policy of expectant treatment is therefore reasonably pursued for a number of months. Only if the anticipated recovery does not occur is exploration later indicated. It is, however, in this later situation that neurolysis may have an important place, particularly in relation to humeral shaft fractures.

If there is loss of length of the nerve as a consequence of the severity of the injury, it is possible to mobilize the nerve by anterior transposition and thus gain several centimetres in length. It is, however, probably preferable to achieve repair with nerve grafts rather than perform an extensive mobilization of both ends of the nerve with the consequent risks of devascularization.

Reconstruction following radial nerve injury

In a patient with unrecoverable radial nerve palsy, considerable improvement in the function of the forearm and hand may be gained by transferring median and ulnar nerve innervated muscles from the anterior compartment of the forearm to replace the missing extensor function in the wrist and hand.

Loss of function of the triceps rarely occurs unless the injury occurs as part of a brachial plexus palsy. Consequently the functional loss is largely restricted to the wrist and fingers. The requirements for reconstruction are wrist extension, finger (metacarpophalangeal joint) extension, and thumb extension and abduction. Various transfers have been recommended to achieve this motor reconstruction.

Flexor carpi ulnaris transfer

The three transfers used are pronator teres to extensor carpi radialis brevis; flexor carpi ulnaris to extensor digitorum communis; and palmaris longus to a rerouted extensor pollicis brevis (Green, 1988).

Superficialis transfer

In this reconstruction the pronator teres is transferred to both the extensor carpi radialis longus and extensor carpi radialis brevis; the flexor digitorum superficialis to the ring finger is transferred to the extensor digitorum communis; the flexor digitorum superficialis to the little finger is transferred to extensor indicis proprius and extensor pollicis longus; and the flexor carpi radialis is transferred to the abductor pollicis longus and extensor pollicis brevis.

This group of tendon transfers (omitting the pronator teres transfer) is of particular value in posterior interosseous nerve palsy where the preservation of the radial extensors of the wrist may result in unacceptable radial deviation following utilization of the flexor carpi ulnaris as a motor.

See Boyes, 1960; Chuinard *et al.*, 1978.

Flexor carpi radialis transfer

This transfer uses the flexor carpi radialis to motor the extensor digitorum communis rather than the flexor carpi ulnaris as in the first transfer described.

This also has the effect of reducing the resultant radial deviation of the wrist that occurs when the powerful flexor carpi ulnaris is sacrificed.

See Starr, 1922; Tsuge and Adachi, 1969; Brand, 1975.

Radial tunnel syndrome

Radial tunnel syndrome or resistant tennis elbow was first described by Roles and Maudsley in 1972. This results from the compression with pain of the posterior interosseous nerve within the radial tunnel, by fibrous bands, recurrent radial blood vessels, the muscles – supinator or extensor carpi radialis brevis and the arcade of Frohse – a fibrous proximal border of the supinator. Compression without pain but measurable motor weakness can also occur, i.e. the posterior interosseous nerve syndrome. This latter syndrome can be produced by rheumatoid synovitis or nodular formation, lipoma, dislocation of the radial head, Monteggia fracture, local injection, iatrogenic after operation, and various radial tunnel abnormalities. Treatment is by careful dissection and resection (Gelberman *et al.*, 1993).

The axillary nerve

The axillary or circumflex nerve may be injured in dislocations of the shoulder and in fractures of the neck of the humerus, and inadvertently divided in exposing the shoulder joint.

CLINICAL FEATURES

The axillary nerve supplies the deltoid and teres major muscles as well as the shoulder joint and the skin over the deltoid. Paralysis of the muscle is therefore the main result of a lesion of the nerve. The patient is unable to abduct the arm at the shoulder joint, while there is diminution in the power of flexion and extension, these movements being to a considerable extent initiated by the deltoid.

Sensation is decreased in the skin over the middle of the deltoid; the loss is seldom complete, there being only hypoaesthesia over the lateral surface of the shoulder.

In the majority of cases, the nerve suffers only an axonotmesis or a neurapraxia, and operative repair is indicated only if the nerve has been inadvertently divided during shoulder joint surgery. A conservative and expectant policy should therefore be pursued with passive movements of the shoulder joint being maintained until recovery occurs.

If the nerve has been lacerated it may be exposed in the axilla or at the level of the surgical neck of the humerus, according to the site of injury.

RECONSTRUCTION

Following unrecoverable axillary nerve injuries the shoulder may be stabilized by fusion of the joint or the trapezius may be transferred to insert into the upper end of the humerus.

Brachial plexus lesions

The brachial plexus is formed by the anterior primary rami of the fifth, sixth, seventh and eighth cervical and first thoracic nerves, which join and then subdivide according to a constant plan. The plexus may be reinforced by contribution of the fourth cervical, when it is known as pre-fixed plexus; or a reinforcement may be present from the second thoracic, in which case it is known as a post-fixed plexus.

The plexus may be injured directly by a incised wound, by bony callus in fractures of the first rib or clavicle, or by scar contraction. It may also be affected by the forcible traction of the arm, by extreme lateral flexion of the head, or by violent downward pressure of the shoulder (Figure 12.14).

ROOT SUPPLY OF THE PLEXUS

Many of the large muscles are innervated from several segments. The following list gives the commonest effects of section of the individual roots in terms of paralysis (Figure 12.15).

- C5 Rhomboids, deltoid, supraspinatus, biceps, brachialis, clavicular head of pectoralis major.
- C6 Sternal head of pectoralis major and triceps.
- C7 Extensors of wrist and fingers.
- C8 Flexors of wrist and fingers.
- T1 Intrinsic muscles of hand (and cervical sympathetic)

The lowest root of the plexus carries in it for a short distance some of the sympathetic fibres that have left the cord in the anterior roots of the first and second thoracic segments. Rupture of the first thoracic root will therefore be accompanied by Horner's syndrome (see p. 883) as well as by paralysis of the small muscles of the hand. Lesions must be close to the spine to affect the sympathetic fibres as these leave the nerve after a very short course.

Injury may affect the nerve roots proper, their

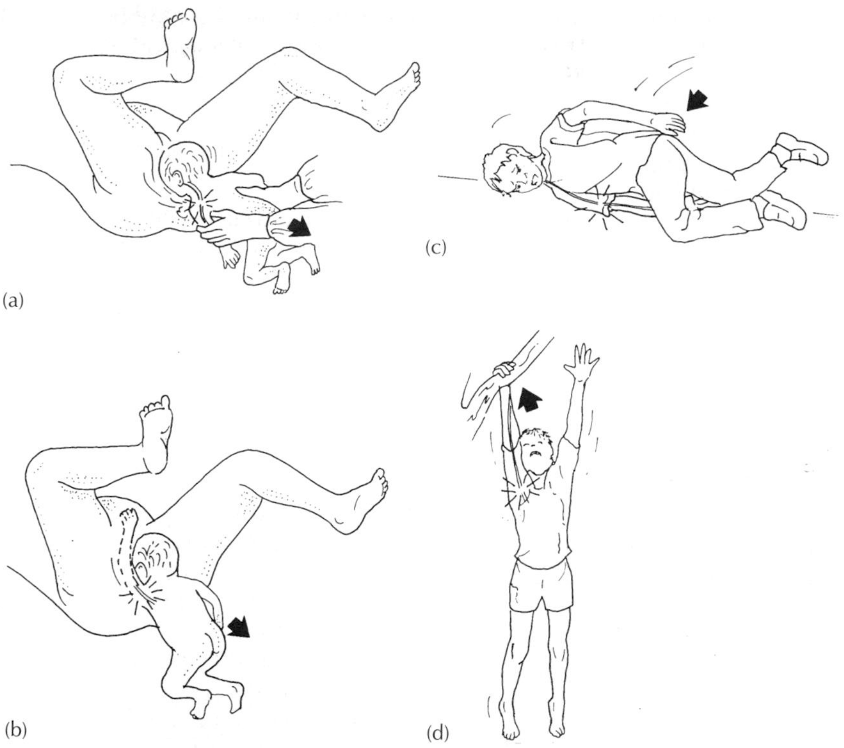

Figure 12.14 Brachial plexus injuries: (a) and (b) birth injuries of the plexus during delivery; (c) a direct fall from a motorcycle onto the neck and shoulder area injuring the upper trunks of the plexus; (d) a hyperflexion/abduction injury when falling from a tree, injuring the inferior trunks of the plexus.

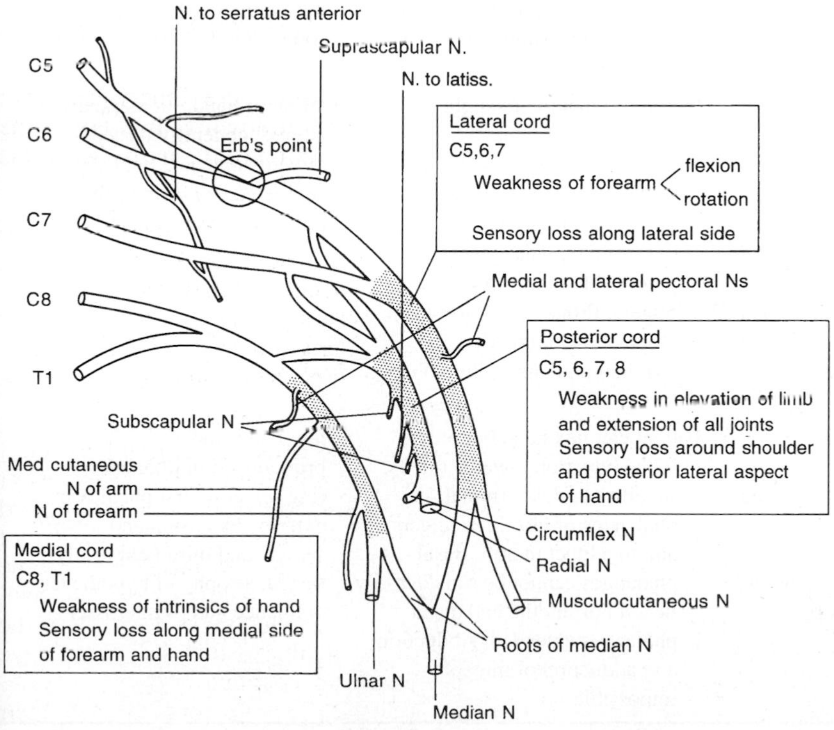

Figure 12.15 The brachial plexus.

anterior primary rami, the trunks, cords or branches of the plexus itself, either separately or in combination. The injuries are commonly grouped on a topographical basis as supraclavicular and infraclaviular lesions. Goldie and Coates (1992) have described about 350 cases of complete or incomplete supraclavicular injuries each year in the UK and about 150 severe infraclavicular injuries. In this series, 30% of the patients had associated head, chest or visceral injuries with rupture of the subclavicular artery in 15% supraclavicular, and 30% infraclavicular lesions. It is important to differentiate between preganglionic lesions – about 25% in the supraclavicular group in which the presence of early and severe pain is found – and the postganglionic type in which there is a strong Tinel sign radiating downwards to the appropriate dermatome.

Supraclavicular lesions are caused by:

- traction lesions
- penetrating wounds
- frictional compression lesions associated with rudimentary cervical ribs.

Infraclavicular lesion are produced by:

- contusion or compression lesions, associated with shoulder joint dislocation
- penetrating injuries

These lesions are divided into three groups according to their clinical features – the lesion of the complete plexus, the upper arm and the lower arm syndromes (Table 12.7).

Table 12.7 Injuries to nerves of the upper limbs

Nerve roots	Muscles supplied	If paralysed	Deformity produced
Musculocutaneous/ C5.6	Coracobrachialis Biceps Brachialis	Forearm flexed with difficulty, especially in supinated position	Characteristic depression on outer surface of upper arm between insertion of deltoid and origin of supinator
Circumflex/C5.6	Deltoid Teres minor	Arm cannot be abducted or elevated backwards or forwards	Change in the shape of the shoulder: relaxation of shoulder joint develops later
Radial/C6–T1	Triceps Anconeus Supinator Extensor carpi radialis longus Brachialis	Elbow, wrist and basal phalanges of fingers cannot be extended; grip weakened; impaired flexion of forearm if supinator is involved	'Wrist-drop', fingers flexed at metacarpophalangeal joints; thumb opposed to fingers and somewhat depressed downwards
Median/C6–T1	Pronator teres Palmaris longus Flexor carpi radialis Flexor digitorum sublimis Flexor pollicis longus Opponens pollicis Abductor pollicis First and second lumbricals Parts of flexor pollicis brevis and flexor digitorum profundus	Flexion of hand with slight force and with ulnar deviation. Fingers cannot be properly flexed at first phalangeal joint, whilst flexion of terminal phalanges only practicable in last three fingers. Pronation of arm lost. Opposition and flexion of terminal phalanx of thumb lost	Position of hand not markedly altered, generally turned towards ulna and held slightly supinated. Wasting of thenar muscles conspicuous
Ulnar/C8–T1	Flexor carpi ulnaris Adductor pollicis Muscles of ball of little finger Interossei Last two lumbricals Part of flexor pollicis brevis and flexor digitorum profundus	Patient can flex hand but only with abduction towards radius. Inability to flex terminal phalanges of last three fingers and to adduct thumb. Basal phalanges cannot be satisfactorily flexed nor middle and distal phalanges extended. Abduction and adduction of fingers impossible	'Claw-hand' most pronounced in little and ring fingers. First phalanx in extreme extension and second and third held firmly flexed, atrophy of hypothenar eminence and of interossei

COMPLETE PLEXUS SYNDROME

Commonly caused by violent trauma producing a traction lesion, the characteristic clinical appearances are bruising and abrasions over the malar region and the ipsilateral shoulder region, with fullness in the supraclavicular fossa and total paralysis of the arm. It is important to palpate and auscultate the supraclavicular swelling to exclude a concomitant vascular injury. It is also important to inspect the face for an ipsilateral Horner's syndrome and to examine the lower extremities as root avulsion may have caused local cord damage.

Motor signs

There is complete paralysis of all the muscles of the hand, forearm and upper arm. It is important to examine the more proximally innervated muscles – suprascapularis, serratus anterior and the rhomboids to determine the proximal extent of the injury.

Sensory signs

There is a wide zone of anaesthesia involving the hand, forearm and the upper part of the arm. Frequently sensation over the inner aspect of the arm and the axilla is spared due to a communication from the intercostobrachial nerve.

Sympathetic signs (Horner's syndrome)

When the eighth cervical and first thoracic nerves are injured close to the intervertebral foramina, or the nerve roots are avulsed, the oculopupillary and other sympathetic fibres which run with them are implicated, causing Horner's syndrome, which has the following features:

1. Drooping of the upper lid.
2. Narrowing of the palpebral fissure.
3. Retrogression of the eyeball (enophthalmos).
4. Contraction of the pupil.
5. Loss of the ciliospinal reflex: normally the pupil dilates when the skin of the neck is pinched, but when the sympathetic is paralysed the reflex is lost.
6. Absence of sweating in the whole of the upper limb, the upper part of the chest, neck and half of the face, the area being accurately delimited by the midline.

UPPER ARM SYNDROME (ERB–DUCHENNE TYPE)

This syndrome is probably the most common brachial plexus palsy that is now seen, particularly following motorcycle accidents. There is evidence of a combined lesion of the upper two cervical nerves or the upper trunk.

Motor signs

There is paralysis of the deltoid, teres minor, supraspinatus, infraspinatus and the clavicular head of pectoralis major. Innervation of the serratus anterior and rhomboids is frequently preserved. The arm is therefore rotated internally by the latissimus dorsi and the sternal head of pectoralis major. The biceps and coracobrachialis are paralysed and the brachialis is weakened; the elbow is extended by the triceps. The supinators of the forearm are affected and the forearm is pronated by the pronator quadratus alone (pronator teres being supplied by C6). The radial extensors of the wrist and brachioradialis are paralysed, resulting in ulnar deviation of the hand.

Sensory signs

These are minimal if the lesion is confined to the anterior primary ramus of C5 but if C6 is affected there is loss of sensation on the lateral aspect of the arm, forearm and thumb.

LOWER ARM SYNDROME (ARAN–DUCHENNE)

This is most commonly seen in obstetrical paralysis. The lesion usually affects the first thoracic nerve but may involve the whole lower trunk (C8 and T1).

Motor signs

The intrinsic muscles of the hand are paralysed and a claw-hand deformity results, interphalangeal joints being flexed and the metacarpophalangeal joints hyperextended. Paralysis of the flexors and extensors of the fingers follow lesions of the entire lower trunk.

Sensory signs

The zone of anaesthesia includes the ulnar side of the hand and forearm and a narrow strip of the upper arm.

Sympathetic signs

When the first thoracic nerve is injured proximal to the point of origin of its white ramus communicans, oculopupillary symptoms are a characteristic feature and the paralysis is known as Klumpke's paralysis.

Acute brachial plexus injury

In the adult, acute plexus injuries following major trauma must be assessed carefully to determine the extent and level of the lesion. This includes taking an adequate history in order to get some idea of the circumstances, velocities and mechanism which pertained at the moment of trauma. It is also important to exclude previous neurological disease.

On initial examination, the face and lower extremities must be included and the cervical spine should be examined for local bony tenderness, range of motion and function of the paravertebral muscles. The supraclavicular fossa must be palpated and auscultated to exclude a concomitant vascular injury. A detailed MRC-type muscle and sensory chart should be documented to determine the nature of the lesion and to act as a base line for further examinations.

The psychological, social and vocational assessment should not be overlooked as this provides useful guidance as to how the patient will react to any future disability.

Electrophysiological assessment is of limited value in dealing with a fresh injury though valuable in providing a baseline for further studies. Wallerian degeneration occurs following axonotmesis or neurotmesis within a few days but these two injuries, one of which requires surgical exploration and the other of which does not, cannot be differentiated in this manner.

Electromyography should include examination of the paravertebral muscles, paralysis of which almost certainly indicates nerve root avulsion from the cord.

RADIOGRAPHIC EVALUATION

Anteroposterior and lateral views of the cervical spine should be taken on arrival. These serve to exclude a concomitant cervical spine fracture-dislocation but, more importantly, may reveal a scoliosis away from the side of the lesion, indicating that the ipsilateral cervical musculature may have been torn or denervated by the traction violence. Ipsilateral avulsion of the cervical transverse process by the levator scapulae muscle indicates severe local violence.

Computerized axial tomography with myelography is also particularly useful in delineating proximal lesions and demonstrating nerve root avulsion from the cervical spinal cord, and has probably replaced myleography because of its false-positive and false-negative results.

AXON REFLEX TEST

The prognosis for recovery and the potential operative methods are considerably different depending upon the level of the brachial plexus injury. Where nerve root avulsion has occurred from the spinal cord no local surgical procedure can be undertaken with any hope of producing reinnervation. Conversely, ruptures of the plexus distal to the dorsal root ganglion are amenable to surgical exploration and nerve grafting. The signs that are indicative of nerve root avulsion are:

1. Paralysis of proximally innervated muscles – posterior paravertebral muscles, rhomboids, serratus anterior and suprascapularis.
2. Horner's syndrome.
3. A positive axon reflex test (Bonney, 1954).

This test is based upon the preservation of the axon reflex via the dorsal root ganglion when the lesion is due to nerve root avulsion. If histamine is applied to the skin a triple response is evoked-red reaction, flare and weal. The red reaction and weal are local responses of the skin to the applied histamine, but the flare is mediated by an axon reflex which stops short of the spinal cord at the posterior root ganglion.

THE NATURAL HISTORY OF UNTREATED BRACHIAL PLEXUS LESIONS

A quarter of the upper trunk lesions recover spontaneously and half of the C5, 6, 7 supraclavicular lesions spontaneously recover wrist and finger extension. Of lower lesions, 70% recover median and ulnar intrinsic activity (Seddon, 1963). Two-thirds of complete plexus lesions recover pectoralis major function, 20% recover wrist flexion, and 12% recover deltoid and biceps activity.

TREATMENT OF BRACHIAL PLEXUS INJURIES

Following a postganglionic lesion, expectant conservative treatment used to be routine, followed by exploration in the absence of recovery at a period up to 6 months following injury. However, early exploration has been undertaken more regularly (Burge *et al.*, 1985). Birch (1993) emphasized the importance of repairing the subclavian artery for survival of limb as well as improving the nerve regeneration as soon as possible. Nerve repair should also take place promptly – after 6 months it is not worthwhile, between 3 and 6 months over half the repairs will fail. Stab wounds with involvement of artery and C5, 6 and 7 roots when repaired urgently will give almost normal function. The results for closed traction lesions are not so good but there is significant gain in shoulder and elbow function in 80% of patients with repair by graft or transfer within 3 weeks of injury. Postganglionic lesions can be treated by neurolysis, neurorrhaphy or nerve grafting. Preganglionic lesions are best treated by nerve transfer operations.

Early exploration has the advantages of allowing identification and grafting of ruptures with probable minimal increased damage being caused to lesions in continuity. Early exploration is furthermore technically very much simpler because of the absence of scar tissue and permits a more accurate prognosis to be determined. Murase *et al.* (1993) have described the safe use of evoked spinal cord potentials for the intraoperative diagnosis in 17 patients with brachial plexus injuries, as well as simultaneous observed somatosensory evoked potentials. These tests provided useful information for the particular lesions, to show whether neural continuity to the spinal cord had been preserved and that the damaged neural stumps were usable for nerve repair.

Exploration should be undertaken through an extensive incision allowing adequate exposure and, if necessary, extension down from the supraclavicular fossa into the arm, thereby exposing both the supra- and infraclavicular portions of the plexus. The sural nerve is probably the most valuable donor material, up to 40 cm in length being obtainable from either leg. In future, other graft materials, such as denatured pectoralis major, may be appropriate (Glasby *et al.*, 1986). Hems and Glasby (1992) have shown good regeneration in sheep by using muscle grafts in experimental repair of cervical roots preganglionic lesions. From this same group Glasby *et al.* (1992) have found good regeneration using freeze-thawed skeletal muscle grafts in brachial plexus repair in primates.

Infraclavicular injuries are the most amenable to surgical repair and demonstrate the best results. Of 54 cases described by Millesi (1977), 70% achieved useful movements in at least one distal articulation following interfascicular nerve grafting. Of 164 cases reported by Narakas (1978), 85% of the distal lesions, but only 50% of the supraclavicular lesions, showed recovery. These results, using interfascicular nerve grafting techniques, are a great improvement on the uniformly bad results achieved by traditional epineurial repair where very little improvement was achieved in large numbers of cases (Brookes, 1949).

Narakas and Millesi have also utilized intercostal nerves as a new motor supply. This is perhaps potentially most useful in proximal upper root avulsions, where distal function remains. The musculocutaneous nerve may be reinnervated in this manner providing elbow flexion.

Late reconstruction following brachial plexus palsy

When it is apparent that the return of muscle function is either not possible because of root avulsion or such time has elapsed that no further recovery is anticipated, late reconstructive procedures should be considered.

In the shoulder stabilization may be achieved either by arthrodesis or tendon transfers, utilizing the posterior deltoid, the latissimus dorsi and teres major (L'Episcopo, 1939) or trapezius transfer (Bateman, 1955; Ariz *et al.*, 1990). When the upper part of the brachial plexus is irretrievably damaged, shoulder stabilization and elbow flexion are of prime importance in improving function in the arm.

Elbow flexion may be achieved by transfers such as the Steindler transfer in which the common flexor origin is moved proximally on the humerus to improve its leverage, a Clarke transfer in which the sternocostal portion of pectoralis major is swung down, leaving its neurovascular pedicle intact, to be attached to the biceps tendon (Clarke, 1945); a triceps transfer which has the disadvantage of sacrificing active elbow extension, may be acceptable in a severely deficient limb where gravity can thereafter be used for extension and the transferred triceps may be used to place the hand in functional positions (Bunnell, 1951; Carroll and Hill, 1970); or the sternocleidomastoid transfer which will produce elbow flexion at the price of a cosmetically unpleasing web in the neck (Bunnell, 1951).

At the wrist the choice of procedure depends on the number of tendons that are available to provide adequate motor function. If possible, flexion and extension at the wrist should be preserved by appropriate transfers in order to maximize the benefit obtained from function of possibly weaker finger flexors and extensors. If this is not possible, arthrodesis of the wrist is appropriate in order to stabilize the joint and allow the residual motors to be utilized exclusively for finger flexion and extension.

In selected cases amputation may be the procedure of choice. This was recommended by Yeoman and Seddon (1961) but Ransford and Hughes (1977) found that many of the amputees did not use their prostheses. They therefore recommended reserving amputation until at least 1 year after injury and then only if the flail limb caused revulsion, or if the patient was having difficulty in using his remaining arm.

Berger *et al.* (1991) have reviewed their multidisciplinary approach of using nerve repair, transfers, muscle tendon transfers and free muscle transfers in 193 patients. They achieved a 60% useful function in all these patients, but nearly 50% required additional procedures of tendon and muscle transfers and an arthrodesis. Their goals were to obtain active control of the shoulder, active elbow flexion, function of the arm and hand as a supporting extremity, no pain and a simple sensitivity to prevent trophic ulcers.

Gu *et al.* (1991) have described their unique and satisfactory results transferring the contralateral normal side C7 cervical root in the presence of root avulsions.

Accessory nerve injury

Damage to this nerve can result from injuries or surgical procedures such as a radical dissection operation on the neck, particularly in the vicinity of the posterior triangle. Some patients present with disability involving the ipsilateral shoulder joint – abduction is limited, there may be sensory disturbance and an obvious scar is seen. Obvious wasting of the trapezius, with positional deformity of the body of the scapula can be found, with absence of active elevation of the involved shoulder girdle.

Hoaglund and Duthie (1966) recommended stabilization of the scapula with strands of fascia lata passed from the medial margin to the spinous processes of T2 and T3 in association with a transfer of the levator scapulae insertion to a more lateral and superior position as described by Dewar and Harris (1950).

Thoracic outlet syndrome

This condition is characterized by vague and often diffuse arm and shoulder pain, sometimes in association with vascular symptoms and signs. The cause of the symptoms is compression of the lowest trunk of the brachial plexus and the subclavian artery.

Multiple causes for this compression have been described as follows.

CERVICAL RIB

An accessory rib arising from the seventh transverse process may extend laterally and then turn forwards and downwards between the scalenus anterior and scalenus medius muscles to join the costal cartilage of the first rib. The 'rib' may be partially or completely represented by a fibrous band. As it turns downwards, the brachial plexus passes over it; and, on its downward course, the subclavian artery arches backwards and laterally across it. Usually the scalenus anterior acquires some attachment to the cervical rib, and separates it from the subclavian vein. Above the vein and close to the rib, the transverse scapula and transverse cervical branches of the thyrocervical trunk pass across the root of the neck. Above, and almost parallel to them, is the posterior belly of the omohyoid muscle.

When the rib is incomplete, the scalenus anterior is less likely to be attached to it. Murphy stated that, if the rib is long enough, the space between the cervical and the first thoracic rib is occupied by intercostal muscles and by an intercostal vein and artery, in exactly the same manner as in normal thoracic intercostal spaces.

As the lowest cord of the brachial plexus and the subclavian artery arch upwards and over the cervical rib, the abnormally long course may produce compression of the structure.

SCALENUS ANTERIOR SYNDROME

An abnormally positioned or abnormally large scalenus anterior muscle may cause compression of the brachial plexus as it runs between it and the posteriorly lying scalenus medius (Figure 12.16).

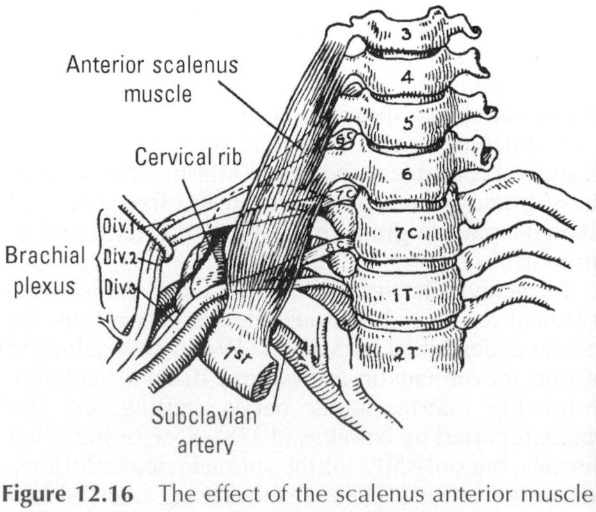

Figure 12.16 The effect of the scalenus anterior muscle on the lower cords. (After Adson and Coffey, 1927)

COSTOCLAVICULAR COMPRESSION

Walshe *et al.* (1944) suggested that compression might also occur where the thoracic outlet was normal but with an altered topographical relationship between it and the shoulder girdle. The normal dropping back of the shoulder girdle and the upper extremity which occurs in adolescence, and is particularly noticeable in women, will reduce the space between the clavicle and first rib.

The vascular symptoms are more difficult to explain than the neurological symptoms. At first it was thought that the circulatory disturbances were causes by stretching, or kinking, of the subclavian artery over the rib or by thrombosis of the artery, or a combination of these factors. They were explained on the basis of pressure or friction on the sympathetic fibres occasionally situated in the lowest trunk of the plexus in contact with the rib. It was suggested that the irritation produced spasm of the vessel wall, obliteration of the vasa vasorum, and eventually thrombosis and occlusion. Walshe *et al.* (1944) considered, however, that long-standing irritation should lead to structural impairment with paralysis and vasodilatation, increased warmth, redness and sweating.

CLINICAL FEATURES

Symptoms may occur at any age, with the average age being about 30 years, women more than men. Clinical features of the thoracic outlet syndrome may be grouped as neurological, vasomotor and local. It is rarely bilateral and usually these patients have had their symptoms for several years.

NEUROLOGICAL FEATURES

Sensory

The patient often complains of pain and paraesthesia along the medial aspect of the forearm and into the little and ring fingers. The symptoms are sometimes relieved by raising the arm and shoulder. The usual distribution is that of the lower trunk of the brachial plexus, the eighth cervical and first thoracic roots. There may be diffuse pain felt elsewhere around the shoulder, the scapula and upper arm.

Sympathetic

A cervicothoracic ganglion effect may be observed as a Horner's syndrome of the eye, flushing of the face with anhidrosis due to a fasciopupillary sympathetic paralysis.

Motor

In the early stages, clumsiness of the hand and inability to perform fine movements is described followed by increasing weakness. Wasting may be slight or absent and usually affects the small muscles of the hand innervated by the first thoracic nerve.

Vasomotor features

Circulatory changes may produce a dusky discoloration of the affected arm and hand, associated with mild trophic changes in the tips of the fingers. Gangrene has occurred following obliteration of either the radial or ulnar artery, or both. Diminution in the volume of the radial pulse is common and may be precipitated by Adson's test (1947), in which the patient elevates the chin and rotates the head to the affected side during deep inspiration. Other subclavian artery compression tests, e.g. the Roos 'surrender' test, the hyperabduction opening and closing the hand tests, can reproduce the symptoms when positive.

Local features

There may be increased pulsation of the subclavian artery with a palpable thrill or audible bruit due to a narrowing above the constricting element and a distal post-stenotic dilatation. Distal emboli have been reported for an aneurysm, as well as Raynaud's vasospasm.

DIFFERENTIAL DIAGNOSIS

Similar symptoms may occur in patients with certain spinal diseases, such as syringomyelia, in lesions of the ulnar nerve and in cervical spondylosis. The possibility of a double crush compression syndrome must also be considered, which was found to occur in 44% of patients following thoracic outlet surgery examined by Wood and Biondi (1990). A Pancoast's tumour of the lung apex should be considered.

INVESTIGATIONS

A chest and a thoracic outlet radiograph should be routinely performed. Nerve conduction tests to exclude a 'double crush' syndrome are useful. Magnetic resonance imaging is now proving helpful for soft tissue compression.

Treatment

Surgical treatment of the condition is indicated when the symptoms are sufficient to incapacitate the patient, and also when there is evidence of circulatory disturbance such as obliteration or reduction of the pulse on extending the neck or rotating the head.

If a cervical rib is discovered accidentally and is causing no symptoms, surgical treatment is not indicated.

In many cases where the symptoms are slight, improvement results from the development of the trapezius and the levator scapulae muscles. Bracing up the shoulder relieves the constant strain on the nerve trunk as it crosses the abnormal rib and enlarges the costoclavicular space. This improvement is particularly seen in cases where there has been a recent illness with loss of muscular power. In some cases it may be advisable to change the occupation to one in which less strain is thrown on the affected arm.

In cases with severe symptoms, operation should be considered, as the condition can be cured by removal of the first rib or the fibrous band which may be causing abnormal pressure. Pain and circulatory disturbance are the principal indications for surgery, but when the condition has gone as far as muscular atrophy, operation is unlikely to be of benefit. Complications are frequent, e.g. pneumothorax 10%, damage to nerve, lymphatics and blood vessels.

Adson and Coffey (1927) believed that removal of an accessory rib or of the first rib was unnecessary, in as much as the subclavian artery and the brachial plexus are immediately removed from pressure and irritation by detaching the scalenus anterior from its

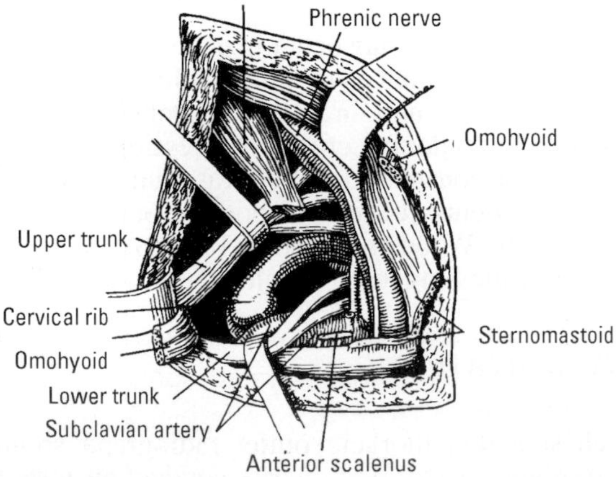

Figure 12.17 Adson's operation. The scalenus anterior is divided near its insertion and the pressure on the plexus removed. (After Adson and Coffey, 1927)

insertion (Figure 12.17). The operation, performed through an anterior incision, is not as predictable as resection of a rib in relieving the symptoms but has the advantage of greater simplicity and a lower complication rate.

Resection of a cervical rib can be performed through an anterior incision as for division of the scalenus anterior. The trapezius and the spinal accessory nerves are retracted and the plexus is exposed along the anterior surface of the scalenus medius muscle, between the lateral border of the scalenus anterior and the clavicle. The lower part of the scalenus medius muscle is reached by mobilizing the plexus, then retracting it downward and inward. The suprascapular nerve is found arising from the lateral border of the upper trunk of the plexus. The long thoracic nerve is carefully protected from injury in freeing the plexus from the scalenus medius. The scalenus anterior, which occupies the floor of the outer angle of the wound, is recognized by the transverse direction of its fibres. Should the cervical rib not be well developed, it will be found by dividing the fibres of the scalenus medius above the first thoracic rib. Stretching between the two ribs is a thin sheet of muscles fibres, the homologues of the thoracic muscles; they are divided close to the cervical rib, so as not to injure the pleura, and what corresponds to Sibson's suprapleural fascia is carefully divided along its inner border. Before this can be done, the lowest trunk of the plexus, which arches over the cervical rib, must be freed and retracted downward and inward. Before freeing the rib carefully from the cervical pleura it is divided at its junction with the tip of the transverse process of the seventh cervical vertebra.

In dealing with this condition the third part of the subclavian artery is exposed to the lower and inner angle of the wound, freed from its fascial sheath and retracted downward and inward. This allows the detachment of the insertion of the scalenus anterior from the tip of the cervical rib and also the removal of the outgrowth of bone which is sometimes thrown out to meet the cervical rib.

If the rib is rudimentary, it is completely embedded in the substance of the scalenus medius; in such cases a fibrous band frequently extends downward and forward like a bowstring, to be attached to the first rib at, or distal to, the scalene tubercle.

When first rib resection (Figure 12.18) is to be undertaken the transaxillary approach (Roos, 1966) has the advantages of leaving a cosmetically acceptable scar and affording excellent exposure of the rib prior to resection.

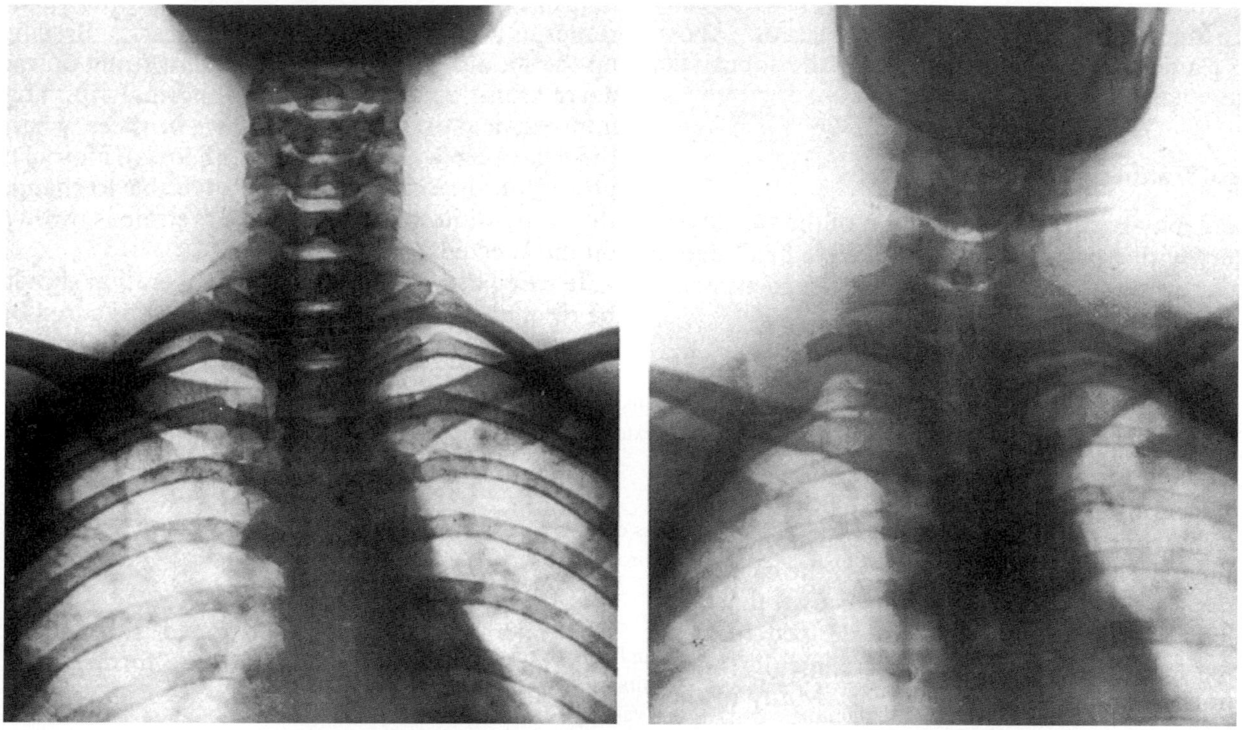

Figure 12.18 Radiographs showing bilateral cervical rib, with unilateral symptoms. The first rib appeared to be causing pressure also, so part of it was removed.

The sciatic nerve

The sciatic nerve may be injured in deep wounds of the thigh, especially gunshot wounds, and following acetabular fractures, in particular posterior dislocation of the hip (Table 12.8). Several reports of methacrylate cement burn of the sciatic nerves during total hip replacement are appearing. Birch *et al.* (1992) have reviewed the literature and reported on their patient who required a resection of the sciatic nerve 1 cm from either side of the cement bolus, with grafting to relieve the pain and restore some function, but the foot remained cold and swollen.

CLINICAL FEATURES

In a complete lesion of the sciatic nerve there is usually paralysis of all the muscles below the knee, but the hamstrings rarely suffer. In partial injuries, it is usual to find the common peroneal motor syndrome predominating. Sensation is abolished in the foot over a zone described as the 'slipper' area. With persistence of anaesthesia, ulceration frequently occurs from loss of trophic influences, the ulcers usually being under the fifth metatarsal head on the sole of the foot, or on the terminal phalanx of the great toe. Such ulcers are very intractable – they perforate deeply, and infection and necrosis of bone often follow. In partial lesions, the sensory phenomena are those of the irritation syndrome, and after gunshot wounds a true causalgia frequently develops.

TREATMENT

Clawson and Seddon (1960) reviewed the results of sciatic nerve repair and suggested that a gap of less than 12 cm may be closed by end-to-end suture. It would, however, appear preferable to use nerve grafts in order to avoid tension. They described that there is rarely any return of motor power in the long flexors or the intrinsic musculature of the foot, but that worthwhile function can be achieved, especially with the prevention of pressure sores. However, more than one-third of their cases had hyperalgesia or pain. These workers emphasized strongly the poor results of attempting to relieve this pain by amputation.

Table 12.8 Injuries to nerves of the lower limbs

Nerve roots	Muscles supplied	If paralysed	Deformity produced
Femoral/L2–4	Quadriceps femoris Sartorius Pectineus	Inability to extend lower leg. Absence of knee reflex. Paralysis of iliopsoas evident by inability to flex hip	Gait disturbed. Patient steps carefully, avoiding flexion of knee
Obturator/L2–4	Adductor longus Adductor brevis Adductor magnus Gracilis Obturator externus	Adduction and, to a slight extent external and internal rotation impaired	
Inferior gluteal/L5–S2	Gluteus maximus	Abduction and particularly extension at hip joint hampered	In walking leg swings too far inward; also excessive lifting and sinking and forward tilting of pelvis
Superior gluteal/L4–S1	Gluteus medius Gluteus minimus Tensor fasciae latae	Loss of abduction and circumduction of thigh	
Medial popliteal/L4–S2	Gastrocnemius Soleus Tibialis posterior Flexor digitorum Flexor hallucis longus	Loss of plantar flexion of foot and toes. Patient unable to lift himself upon tips of his toes. Walking difficult	Claw position of toe (*pied-en-griffe*). Pes calcaneus or valgus
Lateral popliteal/L4–S2	Tibialis anterior Extensor hallucis longus Extensor digitorum longus Peroneus longus Extensor digitorum brevis	Foot falls from its own weight, and cannot be raised nor can first phalanx be extended. Walking difficult; toes scrape the floor	'Foot-drop'. Foot remains in equinovarus position

The lateral popliteal nerve

The lateral popliteal nerve may be injured in comminuted fractures of the head of the fibula, severe varus injuries of the knee, wounds in this area, due to external pressure, as from application of a tight plaster cast, or as a complication of surgical procedures such as high tibial osteotomy.

The nerve supplies the tibialis anterior, the extensor digitorum longus, the extensor hallucis longus, the extensor digitorum brevis, and the long and short peroneal muscles. Paresis of these muscles results in plantarflexion and inversion of the foot, along with a certain degree of flattening of the longitudinal arch, which is normally maintained to some extent by the tibialis anterior and peroneus longus. The patient walks with a high-stepping gait, the foot being elevated to allow the dropped toes to clear the ground. Anaesthesia is noted over the dorsum of the foot.

The nerve may be ruptured in the course of a major knee ligament injury involving disruption of the lateral structures. Following this or incision of the nerve, repair is indicated, if necessary with nerve grafts. Sedel and Nizard (1993) have reported on their results of treating 17 patients by grafting of the lateral popliteal nerve following severe traction injuries. Their indications were complete palsy, failing to show any clinical or electrophysiological evidence of recovery 3 months or more after the injury. The delay was between 3 and 15 months. The nerve gap ranged between 7 and 20 cm. A functionally satisfactory result was achieved in 37.5% and a fair result also in 37.5%, i.e. dorsiflexing the foot to neutral. These authors emphasize that excision of all fibrous tissue is essential and that the use of vascularized nerve grafts would improve results. Vascular damage, even though repaired, appeared to be a contraindication to the operation of grafting.

Whilst recovery is awaited, provision of a foot-drop splint, either in the form of a simple plastic support posteriorly which is inserted within the shoe, or a sprung calliper, may improve gait.

Late reconstruction following lateral popliteal nerve injury

If the nerve does not recover and function is sufficiently impaired, a worthwhile procedure is a transfer of the tibialis posterior through the interosseous membrane and insertion of the tendon into the medial cuneiform on the dorsum of the foot as described by Barr (1947). The tendon of the tibialis posterior is freed from its insertion into the medial cuneiform and other bones. This will provide active dorsiflexion of the ankle joint to a right angle and improve gait. In the presence of inversion and eversion weakness in addition to the above, it is necessary to stabilize the hindfoot by triple arthrodesis.

Tarsal tunnel syndrome

Like carpal tunnel syndrome in the hand, this consists of a compression neuropathy but involving the posterior tibial nerve within the fibro-osseous tunnel under the flexor retinaculum of the ankle joint (Lam, 1967).

The clinical features consist of a burning pain or paraesthesia in all the toes and along the sole of the foot. The symptoms are often worse at night. Sensory loss in the distribution of the medial and lateral plantar nerves may be found, and also a positive Tinel's sign over the posterior tibial nerve at the level of the compression under the flexor retinaculum. Electrodiagnostic tests of conduction velocities and electromyographic studies will aid in confirming the diagnosis and the site of compression.

Differential diagnosis is usually more difficult than in the hand since there are numerous local foot conditions such as Morton's metatarsalgia, peripheral vascular disease and peripheral neuritis, that may mimic the condition.

Nerve compression may also arise from local pressure on the nerve as a consequence of a ganglion, scar formation, bony irregularities after fracture or dislocation, or poor foot posture and external pressure by shoes.

Surgical decompression by wide excision of the flexor retinaculum and removal of any compressing structures may be undertaken. Operative treatment is most successful when it is undertaken early and a specific compression lesion is identified (Takakura *et al.*, 1991).

The (medial) popliteal nerve

This branch of the sciatic nerve supplies the posterior muscles of the leg, and all the plantar muscles, so that, when divided, there is complete inability both to plantar flex the foot and to flex the toes. Walking is not grossly interfered with by this paralysis it may, therefore, easily pass unnoticed. The patient puts his foot down flat and does not lift his heel from the ground. He walks with a splay foot, without spring or elasticity. The anaesthesia affects the sole and the dorsal surface of the lateral four toes, and this lesion is, more frequently than the peroneal, followed by trophic disturbances – cyanosis of the foot, hyperaesthesia and, especially, ulceration.

The healing of a trophic ulcer is often prevented by hard thickened skin around it. This obstructs the circulation so must be removed to allow the formation of granulation tissue. Accordingly excision is the best form of treatment.

MISCELLANEOUS NEUROLOGICAL CONDITIONS

Causalgia

The term 'causalgia' is used to describe a bizarre syndrome resulting from injury to peripheral nerves. Its cardinal features are the subjective complaint of intense burning pain in association with trophic and vasomotor changes in the injured extremity. Its cause is unknown, though it invariably follows an injury to a major nerve, most usually of an incomplete nature. It has similarities to other painful neurological conditions such as reflex sympathetic dystrophy and phantom limb pain and may represent the most extreme end of a spectrum of conditions of similar aetiology and nature.

Devor (1983) suggested that most of the features of causalgia could be explained by sproutings from the injured terminal nerve endings which would be mechanosensitive. Axonal sprouts can produce abnormal upward current conductances and excess number of δ-adrenergic receptors. Catecholamines released in the area of injury, and spontaneous afferent discharges would produce spontaneous pain and increase sympathetic activity. α-adrenergic blocking agents may be effective and Ghostine *et al.* 1984) have described them in causalgia secondary to nerve injury.

Roberts (1986) proposed that with traumatic nerve injury, the increased nociceptive activity would sensitize other multi-receptive neurons to all afferent inputs. This chronic sensitization would be interpreted as pain when mechanoreceptors (A fibres) were stimulated (allodynia) by sympathetic efferent action or via direct ephaptic coupling within the trauma neuroma.

The pain is usually in the distal part of an extremity, either the palm of the hand or the dorsum of the foot, but not confined to the autonomous zone of the injured nerve. The burning pain usually comes on within a few hours of the injury. It is of an intense burning nature and the intensity varies with emotional stimuli such as anxiety, anger or fear. Noises such as the scraping of a chair, tearing of paper or loud music cause intense suffering. Lighting the room without warning often provokes a severe paroxysm of pain. The patients usually exercise great care to prevent the part being touched, particularly by rough objects.

This severe type of causalgia, caused by injury to a major nerve, is frequently a consequence of major limb injuries as sustained in warfare. It is consequently now more common to see a less severe form associated with injury to a more peripheral nerve branch.

The history seems to suggest that the disorder might be entirely psychogenic in character. The motor and sensory losses are difficult to determine for usually the patient refuses to move the part or permit it to be touched. In addition, there is usually marked stiffness of the joints, probably due to disuse.

In some cases the skin is cold, thin and glistening. The superficial layers are denuded and sweating is profuse. With this there is loss of hair, tapering of the digits and a tendency for the nails to curl. In other cases the skin of the painful part is warmer than that of the opposite side and the hair long and coarse. The skin is relatively dry in these cases and at times actually scaly. The severity of the trophic changes increases with the duration of symptoms. Radiography shows spotty osteoporosis of the small bones of the hands and feet.

TREATMENT

Success has been reported with many forms of treatment though none is universally satisfactory. Direct surgical attack on the nerve trunk above, below and at the level of the injury is reported to relieve the syndrome at times. Varying degrees of success have been reported with drugs and physiotherapy. Interruption of the sympathetic chain has consistently been the most efficacious procedure and the results of preganglionic section are superior to those of postganglionic sympathectomy. Interruption of the appropriate sympathetic chain by block, sometimes repeated several times, is followed by dramatic relief. It is instantaneous and absolute. This is a definite indication for surgical sympathectomy; in the case of the leg, the second, third and fourth lumbar ganglia are removed and usually the patient is free of pain on waking, and remains so. Similarly, in the arm an appropriate preganglionic resection is followed by dramatic relief. The operation should be done early to prevent the crippling deformity of the joints which follows prolonged voluntary immobilization of the painful limb. Doupe and his co-workers (1944) found that temporary sympathetic block gave immediate relief from pain, even in patients demoralized by long-standing severe pain, and sympathectomy gave permanent relief.

In phantom limb pain the futility of repeated amputation is widely realized. If simple retrimming fails to relieve the pain, sympathetic block with local anaesthetic should be tried. One or more injections of the local anaesthetic or an appropriate sympathectomy may be successful, but if these fail the contralateral spinothalamic tract should be divided well above the level at which the plexus from the limb joins the cord. This cordotomy should not be unduly delayed in cases in which the symptoms are severe lest pain fixation becomes a cerebral condition for which such procedures as post-central cortical ablation or frontal leucotomy may have to be considered. Success with such measures has been reported. Transcutaneous electrical nerve stimulation (TENS) has been applied with good results, although rarely of any duration. Finsen *et al.* (1988) have studied the effect of TENS on stump heal in, postoperative and late phantom pain after major amputations. Greater and rapid stump healing occurred among the below-knee amputees who had received active TENS. There was considerable placebo effect on pain on using sham TENS. Phantom pain was significantly lower after 4 months with active TENS but not after more than 1 year. Nashold *et al.* (1982) have reported better pain control with the use of implanted electrodes for prolonged stimulation of injured peripheral nerves. They have obtained relief of pain in 50% of patients in the upper extremity (mainly in the median nerve) but in only 31% in the lower extremities.

HIV infection of peripheral nerves

The human immunodeficiency virus (HIV) has been cultured from brain, spinal cord, cerebrospinal fluid and from peripheral nerves (Bailey *et al.*, 1988). Peripheral neuropathy makes up 20% of all the neurological complications of HIV infection and accounts for up to 52% of all symptomatic neuropathies in patients with HIV infection or AIDS disease (de la Monte *et al.*, 1988). It is usually an inflammatory demyelinating polyneuropathy which can occur at the time of seroconversion in the early stages of HIV infection through to full blown AIDS disease.

The presenting feature is generalized weakness of the limbs, hypoflexia and often sensory loss. On lumbar puncture the protein levels in the cerebrospinal fluid are increased, nerve conduction studies show prolonged latencies and marked velocity slowing. A biopsy of the sural nerve shows intense inflammation and demyelination (Connolly and Manji, 1991). The clinical course is variable, some showing spontaneous improvement. Corticosteroids in heavy dosages, e.g. 60 mg/day for 2 weeks, can lead to improvement and plasma exchange is also recommended.

A distal symmetrical peripheral neuropathy is seen, particularly in AIDS patients and associated with severe weight loss. Painful or burning dysaesthesia of the feet with sensory loss is common. The outcome is poor with steady progression in spite of steroids and plasma exchange. Ankle foot orthoses may be required.

Progressive radiculopathy of the lumbosacral roots is uncommon and the cytomegalovirus is implicated. An insidious cauda equinus syndrome with pain, paraesthesiae, sensory loss, distal weakness, urinary retention and back pain are all clinical features.

Primary muscle involvement is relatively uncommon but presents as a progressive proximal muscle weakness with or without muscle pain.

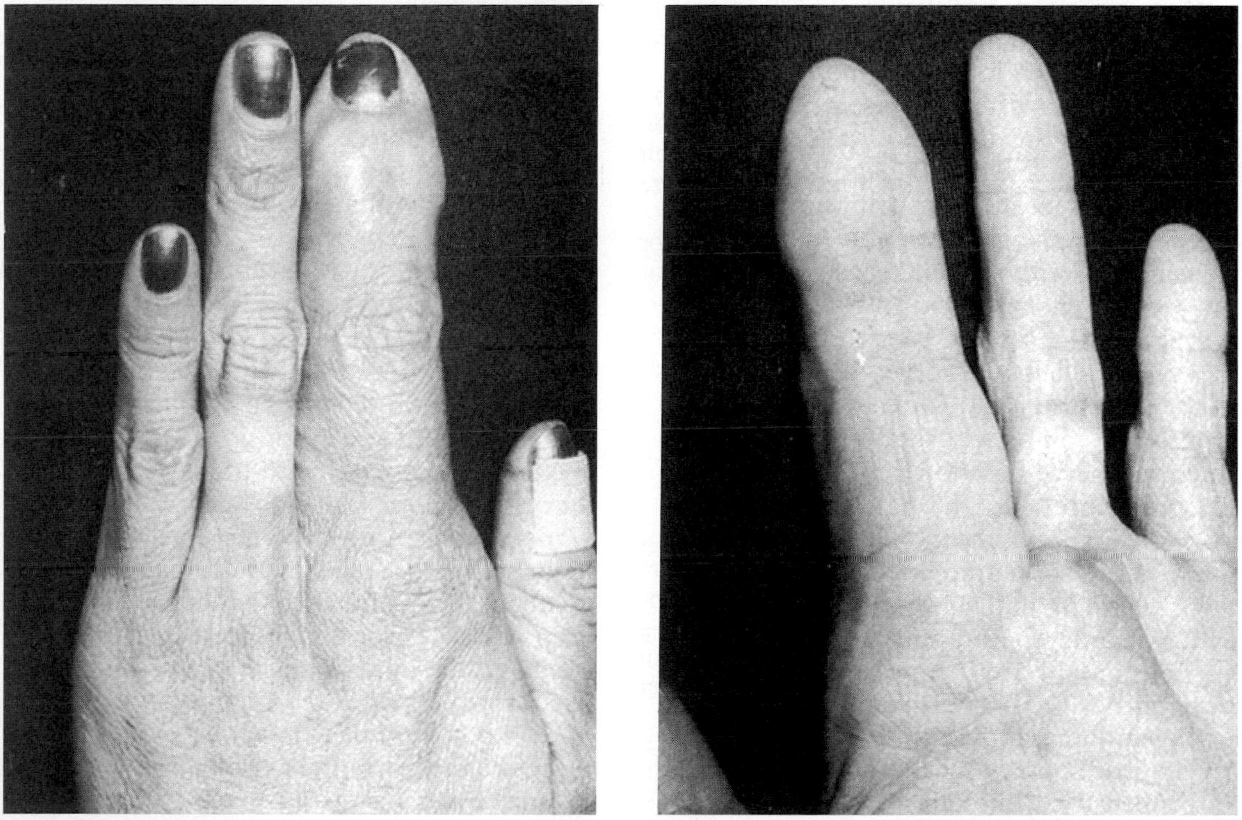

(a) (b)

Figure 12.19 (a) The back and (b) front of the hand which had a plexiform neurofibromatosis of the palmar structures, producing gigantism of the middle finger. The index finger had been amputated.

Neurofibromatosis – von Recklinghausen's disease

This is an inherited disease involving ectodermal as well as mesodermal structures – e.g. skin, soft tissues, nerves and bones. Hunt and Pugh (1961) reviewed 192 cases in which 51% had various bone defects – e.g. tumours around the eye, growth and developmental defects of long bones, and cystic areas of bone – all produced by adjacent neurofibromatous tumours. There may be osteoporosis, hyperostosis, subperiosteal cysts of bone with scoliosis, pseudarthrosis and gigantism of digits (Figure 12.19).

There is proliferation of the cells of the Schwann sheath to give thickening of the nerve in an irregular fashion or bulge, with the perineurium being unusually vascular. Its relationship to the nerve fibres is variable, from displacing them to one side or to growing within them. The tumour cells are similar to the Schwann cells, with long, narrow hyperchromatic nuclei, arranged in rows among connective tissue fibres.

One or more nerves may be involved in any tissue or site in the body, with or without local gigantism (see page 896).

Skin manifestations present early as pigmentation from *café-au=lait* spots, to complete pigmentation involving a segment or even the whole limb as well as numerous neurofibromata subcutaneosly (Figure 12.20).

Treatment is usually surgical excision for pain, for pressure effect within a confined space or for sarcomatous change (see Chapter 3).

Motor neuron disease (progressive muscular atrophy)

This condition, of unknown aetiology, causes progressive atrophic paralysis as a consequence of a gradual degenerative loss of the ganglionic cells in the anterior horn of the spinal cord, the motor nuclei of the cranial nerves and the corticospinal tracts.

SYMPTOMS

The disease most commonly occurs between the ages of 50 and 70 years and begins insidiously, usually with weakness or wasting of some of the muscles in the hand, especially those of the thenar eminence and of the interossei. The atrophy gradually increases in extent, involving the more proximal muscles and subsequently the leg muscles until paralysis intervenes. A characteristic deformity is soon produced by the weakness of the interossei, for the flexor muscles of the fingers flex the interphalangeal joint whilst the long extensor muscle hyperextends the metacarpophalangeal joint; hence the claw-hand, or *main-en-griffe*, appearance results. The weakness and wasting is not symmetrical and progresses from distal to proximal in the limbs. When the forearm is affected the flexors suffer first and as a consequence the claw-shaped appearance of the hand may disappear. At a later period the deltoid, the upper part of the pectoralis major, the biceps, the brachialis and other muscles in the proximal limb may become atrophied.

The cranial nuclei are also frequently affected, resulting in bulbar palsy causing dysarthria and dysphagia.

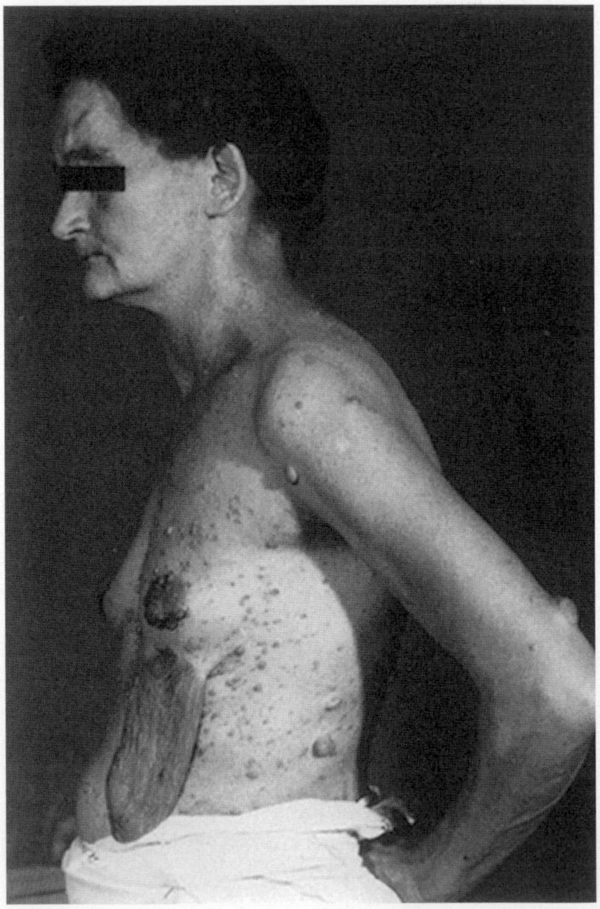

Figure 12.20 Lesion of neurofibromatosis involving the skin.

The lower motor neuron loss in the anterior horn cells usually predominates over the corticospinal tract loss, consequently, the neurological findings indicate a lower motor neuron lesion in the majority of cases. Subsidiary types in which the upper motor neurons are affected (amyotrophic lateral sclerosis, pseudobulbar palsy) may occur.

There is no specific treatment, symptomatic measures being used as indicated.

Syringomyelia

Syringomyelia is a very chronic and irregularly progressive affection of the nervous system, which is probably congenital in origin although it is rarely noticed before the age of 15 years. The cord on section shows a central gelatinous mass of glial tissue containing an irregular cavity, usually in the cervicodorsal and lumbar enlargements. The surrounding structures are compressed – well demonstrated by CT or MR investigations.

A patient presenting with the disease is usually a young adult who has a wasted hand with dissociated anaesthesia. Although commonly a painless disease, dull aching pains and lightning pains may occur. The disease is slowly progressive, with intermissions, and extends over many years.

There are five chief areas of presentation:

1. *Sensory changes*. 'Dissociated anaesthesia' arises from interruptions of the nerve fibres supplying pain, temperature and tactile cutaneous sensibility. Over the affected area the patient is unable to detect pinpricks and hot objects, yet he may be able to feel light touch with cotton wool. Joint vibration senses are normal. In later stages, however, all forms of sensibility may be impaired.
2. *Motor symptoms*. Muscular atrophy occurs frequently in the intrinsic muscles of hand and forearm on one side or both. Claw-hand may be produced or contractures occur in relation to degeneration in the wasted muscles. Spastic paralysis of the legs is a late and inconstant feature due to compression of the pyramidal tracts as these traverse the affected cord segments.
3. *Trophic and vasomotor phenomena occur.*
   (a) Bulbous oedema of the hands with diffuse thickening of the subcutaneous tissue is found.
   (b) The fingers are often scarred, necrosed, blistered or ulcerated.
   (c) Trauma to the joints leads to the production of painless arthropathies of the Charcot type.
4. *Skeletal deformities* are common such as kyphosis, pes cavus or cranial asymmetry.
5. *The cervical sympathetic* may be involved, with enophthalmos, myosis, ptosis and narrowing of the palpebral fissure.

The diagnosis depends on the finding of dissociated anaesthesia with muscular wasting and skeletal deformity. When, in a patient presenting with symptoms suggestive of thoracic outlet syndrome, any physical sign is found outside the arm and neck, the diagnosis is probably syringomyelia.

The disease runs a very slow but progressive course; the patient may live to an old age or may die of some intercurrent disease.

TUMOURS OF PERIPHERAL NERVES

The peripheral nerve tumours which are encountered in orthopaedic practice are in fact lesions of the supporting tissues of the nerve, the Schwann cell system, and fibrous elements. Tumours of the axons are represented by the neuroectodermal tumours of childhood, the neuroblastoma and the ganglioneuroma, and by the phaeochromocytoma of the adrenal medulla.

The simple term 'neuroma' is generally taken to mean any non-specific swelling of a nerve, and the commonest examples are a terminal neuroma in an amputation stump, or the neuroma-in-continuity following partial nerve damage or a nerve repair. Such a swelling is generally firm or even hard to the touch. It is composed largely of scar collagen, although considerable numbers of axons may have found their way across the fibrous barrier. A mature neuroma is generally painless and non-tender, but frequently a patient presents with an acutely tender swelling of a nerve, usually at the site of previous trauma, surgery or amputation. Histological examination will reveal a bizarre profusion of nerve endings bound up in scar tissue. When amputating a limb or a finger various methods have been recommended to minimize the formation of a terminal neuroma. The simplest method is to cut the nerve cleanly across and allow the end to retract proximally so that the neuroma will not lie in the immediate area of the amputation stump. Particularly painful or recurrent neuromata may be dealt with by capping the nerve with silastic or by dissecting the nerve and the terminal neuroma free and burying the neuroma in adjacent fat or bone.

Morton's neuroma

This is the name applied to a tender and painful thickening of the common digital nerve between the toes (commonly the third and fourth toes), often presenting in middle aged women. The aetiology is obscure and histology reveals peri- and endoneurial fibrosis, with considerable demyelination of the nerve fibres. Treatment consists of simple excision of the neuroma and adjacent nerve via either a dorsal or plantar interdigital incision.

Neurofibroma

This is a rare tumour which occurs on the trunk of peripheral nerves and is composed of masses of fibrous and fatty tissue that are intimately mixed with nerve fasciculi and axons. It is therefore impossible to dissect such a tumour free from its parent nerve, and it should usually be left in place, unless there is evidence of recent rapid growth that might suggest malignant change. Neurofibromata occur most commonly as part of the syndrome of neurofibromatosis although they may occasionally occur singly.

Schwannoma

This is a specific type of benign nerve cell tumour, and has a number of synonyms: neurilemmoma, neurinoma, perineurial fibroblastoma, solitary nerve sheath tumour. It may occur along the course of any peripheral nerve, although the eighth cranial nerve is probably the commonest site. When the tumour occurs proximally on an intercostal nerve it may assume a 'dumb-bell' character, with part of its mass lying in the spinal canal and part lying through the intervertebral foramen.

In orthopaedic practice these tumours usually present as mildly tender masses along the course of a peripheral nerve, and the patient may have sensory or motor changes apparent in the distribution of the nerve. At operation the schwannoma presents a classic appearance, with normal nerve fasciculi spread out over an encapsulated firm mass in the nerve, although in the case of larger tumours the mass may lie to one side of the nerve. A longitudinal incision in the epineurium of the nerve, preferably carried out under microscopic control, allows the neuroma to be shelled out with sacrifice only of the single fascicle from which it arises. Histologically a schwannoma has a characteristic appearance consisting of columns and whorls of cells, interspersed with rather degenerative areas. The tumour mass does not contain axons and is probably derived from Schwann cells although this origin is not universally agreed. Solitary schwannomas have no malignant propensity, although an acoustic nerve tumour may be fatal due to its enclosed and dangerous position anatomically. Multiple schwannomas may occur in von Recklinghausen's neurofibromatosis, and it is believed that in this condition they may occasionally progress to a malignant sarcomatous lesion.

CIRCULATORY DISTURBANCES OF THE EXTREMITIES

Lesions of the peripheral vessels may cause pain and fatigue in both the upper and lower extremities, and frequently require the attention of an orthopaedic surgeon. Advances in our knowledge of the structure and function of the autonomic nervous system, based largely on the results of surgical procedures in human subjects, have resulted in a clearer understanding of the mechanisms underlying many of the disturbances of the peripheral circulation.

THE CIRCULATION OF THE EXTREMITIES

Since Claude Bernard first postulated the preservation of the *milieu intérieur* as the determining factor in the freedom and independence of warm-blooded animals, evidence has accumulated regarding the important part played by the peripheral circulation in the maintenance of the necessary constancy of internal conditions. The circulation of the extremities subserves such purely local functions as the transport of the metabolic requirements and the products of the tissues, the production of an inflammatory defence in response to injury, and the maintenance of local temperature at a suitable level. In addition, it plays an important part in the regulation of the body core temperature. The surface area of the extremities is about 65% of that of the whole body, and as the limbs are usually lightly clad a large proportion of heat loss occurs from the skin of the limbs. The capacity of the vascular bed is greater than the total volume of blood contained therein, and therefore at all times active vasoconstriction must be present in a large part of the circulatory system to ensure that vital organs receive an adequate blood supply. Unusual demands for blood in one organ are met by local vasodilatation, associated with vasoconstriction in other parts of the body. The most common vasoconstrictor stimulus is cold. Other factors that produce intense constriction in the extremities are fear, pain, anger, asphyxia, haemorrhage or dehydration. Such constriction may be so intense that the cutaneous circulation may temporarily cease. Vasomotor reactions are most intense in the distal part of the extremities. Constriction is most marked in the arterioles but also occurs in the capillaries and veins.

Sympathetic control

The peripheral vessels are controlled by the autonomic nervous system. Preganglionic sympathetic neurons pass out in the anterior spinal root, which they leave as a white ramus communicans to the sympathetic chain, and thence postganglionic fibres run in a grey ramus communicans to reach a spinal nerve and to be distributed segmentally with the branches of that nerve to hair follicles, sweat glands and vessels. Other postganglionic fibres run directly to form periarterial plexuses around the large arteries of the trunk (e.g. aorta, iliac, subclavian and carotid). Such plexuses pass into the limb for a short distance only, stopping just beyond the groin or the axilla. For the remainder of its course the artery is surrounded by a periarterial plexus derived from fibres which travel with the spinal nerves, and are distributed according to a segmental plan at local level.

By stimulation of the anterior spinal roots on the operating table it has been shown that the constrictor fibres in the arm arise in the third to the seventh thoracic segments (Foerster, 1939); those to the leg arise from the eleventh thoracic to the second or third lumbar segments.

The chemical mediator at the nerve endings of the autonomic system contain noradrenaline (norepinephrine) on the vessels and acetylcholine on the sweat glands. Following section, the nerve fibre degenerates and hypersensitivity of the neuroeffector mechanism occurs, resulting in a greatly increased and exaggerated response to the appropriate chemical mediator in low concentration. Incomplete denervation of a structure controlled by the autonomic nervous system thus results in little loss of function, since the chemical mediator diffuses from cells with an intact nerve supply to those denervated and consequently sensitized.

Vasodilatation

Knowledge of the vasodilator mechanism is less complete. The inability of the peripheral arteries of a limb to dilate further after sympathectomy may be evidence of the presence of sympathetic dilator fibres in the rami divided. It is believed that other dilator fibres exist in the posterior roots of the spinal nerves, and that these fibres are part of an axon reflex stimulated through the spinal sensory fibres.

Sudomotor and pilomotor fibres are associated with those of vasoconstriction. In the hands and feet there are numerous arteriovenous anastomoses – the digital glomal system of Popoff – by means of which, in response to nerve impulses, the blood flow through the part, and hence the rate and amount of heat lost, may be varied very rapidly. For this reason, among others, vasospasm is more evident in the hands and feet than in other parts of the body. Vasoconstriction results in pallor and coldness and is associated with sweating. Vasodilatation is followed by heat, redness and dryness of the part.

The capillary bed

The capillary bed of the peripheral circulation is the site of the main physiological activity where interchange of oxygen, carbon dioxide and of nutritive and waste material, between the blood and the tissues takes place through the delicate endothelium of the capillary tubes. Interference with blood flow in this area is likely, therefore, to lead to profound changes in local tissue metabolism, temperature and health.

Classification of vascular disturbances

An arbitrary division may be made between the disturbances that are chiefly of function, the anatomy of the vessels remaining relatively normal, and those in which there are early organic changes (Table 12.9). It must be remembered that anatomical changes will be found in the late stages of the former and that often vasospasm is an important factor in the latter group.

1. *Primary vasomotor lesions*
   - Vasoconstrictor disturbances – Raynaud's disease and acrocyanosis.
   - Vasodilator disturbances – erythromelalgia.

Table 12.9 Differential diagnosis of vascular diseases affecting the extremities

	Raynaud's disease and similar conditions	Acrocyanosis	Primary erythromelalgia	Thromboangiitis obliterans	Arteriosclerotic disease
Pulsation of arteries	Normal	Normal	Normal	Pulseless 50% Diminished 45% Normal 5%	Pulseless 50% Diminished 45% Normal 5%
Excessive rubor with dependency	Absent	Absent	Present	Present	Present
Excessive pallor with elevation	Absent	Absent	Absent	Present	Present
Claudication	Absent	Absent	Absent	Usually present	Usually present
Gangrene	Rare	Never	Never	Common	Common
Rest pain	Usually absent	Absent	Usually mild	Usually very severe	Usually mild
Type of rest pain	Absent	Absent	Burning	Sharp stinging	Aching
Appearance of gangrenous ulcers	Small punched out areas	None	None	Moist inflamed; discharging	Usually dry
Superficial phlebitis	Absent	Absent	Absent	30% of cases	Absent
Age	Mostly between 18 and 30 years	Mostly between 30 and 50 years	Mostly between 30 and 50 years	Mostly between 25 and 45 years	Mostly between 55 and 85 years
Sex	Females 95%	Females 70%	Females 70%	Males 99%	Males 90%
Colour changes following exposure to cold	Always	Always	Always	30%	15–20%
Oedema	Absent	Present during attacks	Absent	Frequent	Infrequent

- Peripheral vasoneuropathy after chilling – immersion foot and immersion hand, diabetic foot and frostbite.

2. *Primary obliterative lesions*
   - Mechanical – embolism and thrombosis.
   - Inflammatory – thromboangiitis obliterans.
   - Degenerative – arteriosclerosis and atherosclerosis.

Raynaud's disease

Raynaud's phenomenon is defined as an episode of constriction of the small arteries and arterioles in the periphery of the extremity, resulting in intermittent changes in the colour of the skin, such as pallor or cyanosis or both. Following the constrictive episode, hyperaemia may produce redness. When these signs occur primarily without associated or contributing conditions, it is called Raynaud's disease. It may, however, occur in association with a number of contributing conditions, including occlusive arterial disease (arteriosclerosis, thromboangiitis); with embolism and thrombosis; with intoxication by heavy metals such as lead; ergot poisoning; and with collagen vascular diseases such as scleroderma, lupus erythematosus and dermatomyositis.

Raynaud's disease is five times more common in women than in men and usually occurs after puberty and before the menopause. Its effects are most marked in the peripheral exposed parts of the limb. It is often symmetrical in distribution and may involve any or all four extremities in any combination. Typical attacks of Raynaud's disease may be initiated by exposure to cold, by excitement or embarrassment. The first sign is pallor of the tips of the affected digits, followed by transient greyness as the remaining blood gives up its oxygen. Initially the pallor may be patchy or intermittent, but if the initiating factor continues, spasm increases and the digits appear more and more pallid, waxen and numb, and no fine movements can be carried out. Following relaxation of the spasm, the circulation slowly returns to the digits, their colour becomes bright red and capillary pulsation may be noticed. The digits swell and tingle, there may be an intense sensation of 'pins and needles' or severe pain after a prolonged attack; these symptoms are intensified by rapid warming.

If the episodes continue and extend more proximally as far as the wrists and ankles, they are more readily provoked. Recovery occurs only following prolonged warming. Secondary changes may appear in the digits; the pulp of the finger atrophies, its skin becomes smooth and glistening, and the finger tapers towards the tip over which the nail curves. Small areas of thickened skin appear on the fingertips – especially under the nails, which may separate, leaving small painful areas with a prolonged healing time. Ulceration, infection or frank dry gangrene are uncommon, but the pain may be so intense that the digit or even the extremity becomes useless. These changes are usually more marked in the upper limb.

PATHOLOGY

There is an intermittent flow of blood through the constricted arterioles during the state of pallid asphyxia. The colour depends on the amount of blood flow into the part and the temperature of the part. The rate of dissociation of oxyhaemoglobin and tissue metabolism are markedly reduced at low temperature. Thus hands dipped in ice cold water may remain pink, while at a higher temperature there may be marked vascular spasm combined with ready dissociation of oxyhaemoglobin, resulting in cyanosis. Rapid warming causes abolition of spasm with increased rate of flow, increased metabolism and increased dissociation of oxyhaemoglobin, leading to deep cyanosis, which may be associated with severe pain. When the vasospasm is relieved, the reactive hyperaemia with vasodilatation may well result from the accumulation of toxic metabolites.

The late stages of Raynaud's disease are commonly associated with secondary changes, particularly in the skin and subcutaneous tissues, giving rise to the condition of sclerodactyly. At first the digits are swollen and firm and the skin is smooth (stage of oedema). Later they become stony hard and tense, the skin is glistening and fixed and may appear varnished (stage of induration). Finally there is wasting and the skin becomes thinned and there may be brown pigmentation (stage of atrophy). These changes have been recorded in the ears and nose. There is often associated ulceration and reduced growth of nails and hair.

TREATMENT

Ulceration of fingers may well require the administration of methyldopa or intra-arterial reserpine. However, cervicodorsal sympathectomy is the most efficacious therapy, although relapses have been reported. It is essential in the case of a particular patient to assess the relative importance of the factors concerned before deciding the most suitable form of treatment. For each individual there is a critical temperature below which vasospasm occurs. The higher the temperature the more severe and disabling the disease: recovery from an attack is correspondingly longer and changes in the vessel walls are usually more marked. In most cases some improvement will follow the wearing of warm woollen socks and gloves and the avoidance of extreme cold. In the early stages, where there are no detectable changes in the vessels or soft tissues, and full vasodilatation follows heating, the results of preganglionic sympathetic denervation are excellent. Where there are slight changes in the digits and reflex vasodilatation is slow and incomplete, the progress of the disease may be arrested and the frequency and severity of the attacks reduced by preganglionic denervation. Where the disease is in an advanced stage and there is little local reflex response to heating other parts of the body, preganglionic denervation is useless because any response is slight and usually transitory. If a lower limb is affected, the second and third lumbar ganglia and intervening trunk are removed (in females the first may also be included). In the upper limb the trunk is divided below the third thoracic ganglion and all the rami to and from the second and third ganglia are divided.

Acrocyanosis

This condition is characterized by painless and persistent coldness and cyanosis of the distal parts of the extremities. It most commonly affects the female sex. The fingers and the toes become cold, the movements of the part are impaired, and the finer adjustments of co-ordinated movements are sluggish and awkward. A peculiar hypoaesthesia seems characteristic. This diminished sensibility does not appear to be of an hysterical nature. The cyanosis is often bilateral and in such cases roughly symmetrical, although there may be slight differences in the intensity of the colour. The condition is usually most severe in the hands, probably because as a rule the feet are more adequately protected against low temperature.

Acrocyanosis resembles Raynaud's disease in its location, but the two may be distinguished by the persistent nature of the colour changes in acrocyanosis and by the absence of pain and blanching as compared with Raynaud's disease.

PATHOLOGY

It was pointed out by Lewis (1938) that the clinical picture of acrocyanosis resembles the changes which appear with a normal hand when it is subjected to a low temperature. He suggested that there is a peculiar sensitivity of the cutaneous arterioles to the effects of cold in those individuals who suffer from the disease. There is slowing of the cutaneous circulation due to arteriolar spasm with secondary dilatation in the capillaries and venules. This leads to anoxia, increased plasma outflow and, therefore, local swelling. The dilated capillaries packed with red cells impart a deep red colour which turns blue as the oxyhaemoglobin becomes reduced; the intensity of the colour depends on the quantity of blood contained in the part.

TREATMENT

Avoidance of cold is of paramount importance but if the condition is sufficiently severe, sympathectomy may be of value.

Erythromelalgia

This condition was first described in 1878 by Weir Mitchell, who believed it to be a rare vasomotor neurosis involving the extremities. It is characterized by redness, burning pain, and swelling of the hands and feet brought on by heat, exercise or the dependent position. During at attack the hands and feet become intensely warm and the skin acquires a bright red colour. When the parts are warmed, a feeling of swelling, fullness and throbbing is experienced. Burning pain may be induced by cold, friction, tension or elevation of the temperature of the limb to a certain critical point which varies with each individual. Pain is brought on by such a rise of temperature irrespective of whether the rise is due to the application of external heat or to increase in blood supply produced by other means. There may be great disability, the patient being unable to tolerate any covering or pressure on the affected part. The vessels are dilated with full bounding pulses, and capillary pulsation may be present.

Sympathectomy may be of value in the treatment of this condition (the vessels of a sympathectomized limb are incapable of dilatation as well as of constriction), following such operation pain is abolished and the circulation returns to normal.

Anterior tibial syndrome

This syndrome, occurring in fit young men and consisting of acute ischaemic necrosis of the muscles of the anterior tibial compartment of the leg, is not uncommon. The symptoms usually follow exertion involving strenuous use of the leg muscles.

Clinically intense pain commences in the front of the leg shortly after exercise, followed by signs of tension within the anterior compartment and paresis of the dorsiflexors of the foot and toes. The peroneal muscles are not involved and foot-drop is minimal because of contracture of the ischaemic muscles. Rest does not improve the pain, as it does that arising from 'shin splints', a stress fracture of the tibia, or thrombophlebitis. In the pathogenesis of the syndrome the sequence of events is: unaccustomed exercise – muscle trauma – pressure increase within the anterior tibial compartment obstructing venous outflow – impaired inflow as a consequence of the obstructed venous outflow to the affected muscles – ischaemic necrosis. Spasm of the anterior tibial artery may occur and the common peroneal nerve is involved either by compression (in which case it recovers rapidly following decompression) or by ischaemia (in which case the loss of function may be permanent). The condition can be prevented by graduated physical training. When the full blown syndrome occurs, surgical decompression of the anterior tibial compartment as an emergency measure is essential by carrying out a wide fasciotomy. This permits the oedematous swelling of the muscle bellies to be accommodated. If necrotic muscle tissue is found, thorough debridement is necessary.

Immersion foot (trench foot)

This disturbance, for which Ungley and Blackwood (1942) suggested the alternative name of 'peripheral vasoneuropathy after chilling', results from prolonged exposure to cold which is not so severe as to cause frostbite. Most subjects have been the survivors of shipwreck, but the condition has followed exposure without immersion. When due to exposure in open lifeboats the most important causal factors are the duration of exposure and the temperature of the sea; sea water at temperatures of 5–8°C may produce nerve damage in 22 hours. Any factors which impair the circulation, such as constricting boots, socks or other clothing, immobility, chilling of the trunk, starvation or seasickness, will increase the severity of the disturbance. Distinction should be made from frostbite, in which the superficial tissues are frozen, and the oedema without nerve lesions which follows prolonged immersion in sea water at colder temperature.

There are three clinical stages. At first in the *pre-hyperaemic* stage the cold swollen limbs are pale, mottled or blue in colour, numb and anaesthetic, and pulsation is absent in the main vessels. After several hours the picture changes suddenly to that of the *hyperaemic stage* with pain, heat, redness, increased swelling and full arterial pulsation. The normal skin temperature gradient of the limb is abolished and procaine block produces slight, if any, rise in temperature. When the limb is horizontal, the foot or hand is red; if dependent, the colour becomes a deep purple and blanching rapidly follows elevation. In the more severe cases blisters appear after about 3 days, especially in areas which are to become gangrenous. Healing of blistered areas may take from 1 to 6 months. Pain, tingling, 'pins and needles' or burning appear early, may be very severe, and are made worse by warmth, cold, dependency and exercise. There is weakness and wasting of the muscles in the affected areas, leading to later disturbances such as flat feet. Sweating, at first absent, later returns rapidly and may ultimately be excessive. The hyperaemic stage may last from a few hours or days up to 3 months. In the *post-hyperaemic stage* inflammation subsides, vascular tone and skin temperature return to normal, but the state of 'cold sensitivity' may develop in which, after cooling the limb, there are attacks of Raynaud's phenomenon or delay in warming in spite of attempts at reflex vasodilatation. A similar disturbance, the so-called 'algid state', may occur during the latter part of the hyperaemic stage; both are probably due to partial interference with sympathetic innervation with sensitization to adrenaline.

The lesions were classified by Ungley and Blackwood (1942) into four grades according to their severity. Those with minimal lesions without interference with nerve function have swollen feet for a few days and transient tingling, but symptoms subside within a week. Mild cases with reversible nerve lesions have symptoms for from 3 to 6 weeks with slight weakness of the intrinsic muscles of the feet; later there may be excessive sweating or cold sensitivity. Of moderately severe cases with severe (degenerative) nerve lesions, 50% have blistering and a few superficial gangrene, anaesthesia extends nearly to the ankle joint, and muscle wasting is more marked. Symptoms may last for 3 months and functional return may be delayed for 6 months. Very severe cases with irreversible (degenerative) nerve lesions, usually with gangrene, have loss of sensation above the ankle, gangrene of the toes or distal half of the foot, infection may occur and amputation be necessary. Symptoms may last 6 months or more and late complications are frequent.

TREATMENT

The principles of treatment will vary with different phases of the disease.

In the hyperaemic phase, cooling the affected limbs while warming the rest of the body should be carried out. At no time should the affected areas be wrapped or heated. The extremity should be elevated and precautions taken to give chemotherapy against any secondary infection of ulcerated or gangrenous areas. The patient should remain in bed until all swelling has subsided and walking is painless.

During the late vasospastic or ischaemic phase, the extremities and body should be protected from cold and given passive exercises and mildly heated. Treatment will include any measures used in any post-traumatic vasospastic state including sympathetic ganglion blocking agents, with sympathectomy being indicated in some cases.

Frostbite

This is usually defined as a condition in which freezing of the tissues occurs as a result of exposure to cold. There is still uncertainty as to whether frostbite effects are due solely to freezing of the tissues or of the cellular fluids, or due to the changes which occur in the blood vessels. The first sign of frostbite is pallor resulting from the subsequent vasoconstriction. Sensation may be lost, but if freezing is temporary and there is vasodilatation, rapid recovery will result.

PATHOLOGY

Peripheral vasoconstriction occurs immediately on exposure to the cold, and in mild frostbite there is a low-grade vasculitis and inflammatory reaction of all the affected tissues. With severe or prolonged exposure to cold, and a persistent vasoconstriction, there is marked vasculitis of the smaller arteries and arterioles, and this may be accompanied by increased permeability of the capillary walls. Thrombosis may occur in the arterioles and capillaries.

First-degree frostbite consists of a white or yellow patch involving the outer layers of skin, but no blistering or peeling is present. Second-degree frostbite is severe enough to produce blistering or peeling, but without affecting the deeper layers of skin or subcutaneous tissue. Third-degree frostbite produces death of a thick layer of skin and subcutaneous tissue. Fourth-degree frostbite causes gangrene, with the loss of the extremity or some part of it.

In mild frostbite there is an associated numbness and prickling sensation which disappears within an hour or two after adequate treatment, but even in the milder forms of frostbite the affected region may remain hypersensitive to temperature change for many months or years.

In severe frostbite there may be complete insensibility to touch in the affected extremities. The tissues feel hard and it may not be possible to move the fingers or toes. When the extremity is thawing, reactive hyperaemia will develop with a red weal surrounding the frozen tissues, and this gradually spreads over the ischaemic and pallid skin until the entire part becomes red, this being accompanied by tenderness and blistering pain. Blisters and oedema will occur rapidly; some areas may become gangrenous, but it is usually difficult to evaluate the depth of the necrotic tissue. Therefore, debridement and amputation should be delayed as long as possible.

TREATMENT

If at all possible frostbite should be prevented when in cold climes by the wearing of adequate clothing and footwear for warmth and dryness whilst avoiding constriction. Daily washing and careful drying of the feet and even gentle rubbing with a coating of oil increases the phenomenon of supercooling and allows exposure of the skin to much lower temperatures.

Treatment of mild frostbite is aimed at returning the natural warmth to the skin as quickly as possible. If the hand is involved, it should be placed inside the clothing against the skin of the chest or abdomen. The affected part should never be rubbed vigorously as this may traumatize the sensitive skin.

In severe frostbite the same principles of avoidance of trauma, maintenance of asepsis and rewarming are followed. Experimentally it has been shown that rapid thawing increases the survival of this tissue as opposed to slow thawing. However, this should not begin until the individual is in a place where he will not have to be moved again until healing is complete. For example, a mountaineer with a frozen foot should be evacuated to his base camp or to a place where treatment can be completed before rewarming is begun. A sympathetic block or an intravenous injection of a solution of papaverine may be helpful in the early stages. Systemically administered heparin has been shown to be helpful in the prevention of gangrene in the experimental animal and this may be indicated in the treatment of clinical frostbite. After the rewarming has been completed, the patient will progress through a stage of blistering, oedema and perhaps gangrene. Antibiotics during this stage are important. Amputation or even debridement of the necrotic parts should be postponed until autoamputation occurs or there is absolutely no question about the line of demarcation.

Intra-arterial reserpine has been shown to produce rapid relief of vasospasm. Indeed, early sympathectomy (i.e. within 3 days after exposure) reduces the amount of oedema formation and tissue necrosis.

Diabetic foot

Although the middle-aged and diabetic patient may have atherosclerosis, especially of the femoral vessels, he may also develop a specific type of arterial occlusive disease affecting the terminal arterioles. Not only is there a poor blood supply to the tissues but there is also loss of sensation due to the diabetic neuropathy and the well known susceptibility to rapid, fulminating infections with necrosis of soft tissues.

The aim of treatment is to control the diabetes, and to control the infection by suitable antibiotics and radical debridement of all wet necrotic tissue. Arterial reconstruction may be necessary to save the foot or digits and amputation is frequently required, i.e. 75% of all non-traumatic major amputations occur in diabetes, Christensen *et al.* (1988). If the gangrene is dry, conservative treatment with local antibiotic powder and protection of the digit allows the development of a collateral circulation with, perhaps, autoamputation. Trophic ulceration should be treated with cleansing and protection from mechanical trauma of compression and shear. Laing *et al.* (1991) have emphasized the great morbidity in diabetic patients resulting from ulceration of the insensitive foot. By applying total contact plaster-of-Paris casts with padding and rocker, they achieved healing in most neuropathic ulcers within 6 weeks, but not when the ulcers were due to ischaemia. After the cast, immobilization rocker shoes with contact insoles are prescribed.

Primary obliterative disturbances – general effects

The general clinical manifestations of occlusion of limb arteries are the same whatever the aetiological factors involved and depend upon:

1. The size of the artery involved.
2. The rate of occlusion – gradual or sudden.
3. Availability of a collateral blood supply.
4. Metabolic demands upon the tissues distal to the block.

Sudden occlusion of a large peripheral artery, due to ligation, embolism or injury, is followed by pallor of the skin distal to the block, and motor and sensory paralysis of a varying degree. Interruption of blood flow in a main vessel may be followed by generalized spasm of all the vessels distal to the obstruction, and if the collateral circulation is insufficient for the needs of the limb, gangrene will follow.

If the arterial occlusion is gradual, or if the limb has survived a sudden major occlusion, the blood supply, while sufficient to maintain the nutrition of the skin, may not be sufficient to allow the increase necessary for exercise, and the patient may present with the complaint of cramp-like pain in muscles on exercise (intermittent claudication) which is quickly relieved by rest. In the leg the calf is most commonly affected, but Leriche (1938) pointed out that in cases of aortic thrombosis and/or thrombosis of the common iliac or internal iliac arteries, the initial complaint may be of pain in the hip or buttock or of

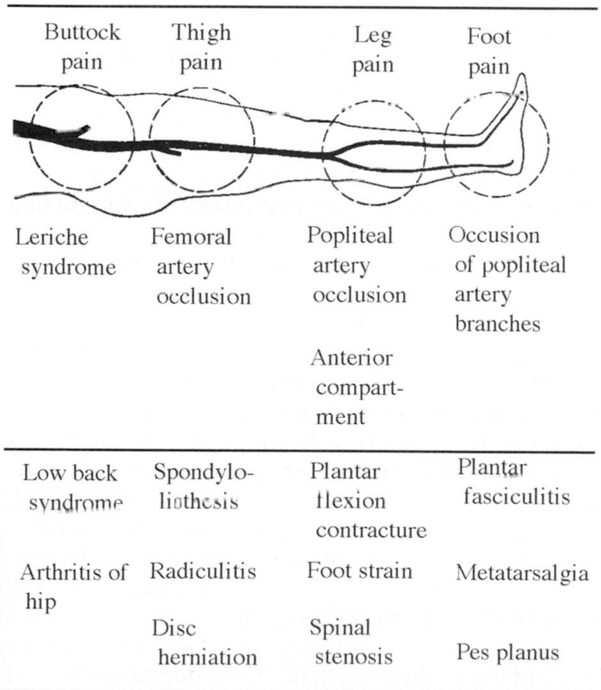

Figure 12.21 Diagram relating the primary obliterative level to the symptoms, which have to be differentiated from various orthopaedic conditions.

general tiredness of the limb on exercise that is relieved by rest. In some cases where the block is short and the collateral circulation good, the peripheral pulses may be present but may disappear on exercise. This condition may occasionally be confused with pain due to arthritis in the hip (Figure 12.21).

Embolism and thrombosis

When large peripheral vessels are occluded suddenly by injury or ligation there is marked danger of the subsequent onset of gangrene, particularly in the leg where the collateral circulation is poorer than in the arm. Ninety per cent of all cases of occlusion result from emboli arising in the heart due to mitral stenosis, myocardial infarction or atrial fibrillation.

Surgical exploration to relieve the obstruction should be undertaken as an emergency by an arterial surgeon. Investigation by Doppler will give the position of the obstruction.

Thromboangiitis obliterans

The classic description of this disease was made in 1908 by Buerger (1924) and his name is still associated with the condition. The disease affects males almost exclusively and is associated with heavy smoking. The symptoms usually begin with pain and cramp in the foot which is brought on by exercise and relieved by rest. As the arterial obstruction progresses symptoms of Raynaud's phenomenon may occur and trophic changes ultimately appear in the form of localized superficial ulcers that will not heal, and subsequently dry gangrene. In the severe late forms of the condition there is intense pain which is unrelieved by rest.

The condition is due to progressive obliteration of the large vessels of the lower limb, the veins being affected as well as the arteries. Intimal proliferation and adventitial thickening of the vessels occur followed by thrombosis and occlusion of the vessels.

No specific treatment is available, though smoking should clearly be avoided.

Arteriosclerosis and atherosclerosis

Degenerative arteriopathy is based upon hypertension, age-related changes and the deposition of lipids within the intima as causes of vascular insufficiency and occlusion resulting in limb ischaemia, cardiovascular and cerebrovascular incidents.

Multiple aetiological factors are involved including diabetes, cigarette smoking, hereditary disposition, diet and exercise. The prevention of these conditions is of great economic importance since men of working age are primarily affected.

There are at least four different types of degenerative arteriopathy on the basis of different anatomical features with perhaps different causes, all of which are included in the broad category of 'arteriosclerosis'.

1. *Hypertensive arteriopathy*. This is a widespread lesion found primarily in arterioles and small arteries, being characterized by hypertrophy of the medial coat of the vessel. It is associated with arterial hypertension.
2. *Medial wall sclerosis*. This is a lesion of large and medium-sized vessels, characterized by inflammation and degeneration of the elastic fibres of the media with fibrosis and deposition of calcium in this layer.
3. *Cystic medial wall necrosis*. This is a lesion of the aorta and its larger branches, characterized by cystic accumulations of mucoid material in the media and frequently associated with dissecting aneurysm.
4. *Atherosclerosis*. This is a lesion of the aorta and of large and medium-sized arteries, characterized by focal plaque-like thickenings of the intima, containing cholesterol, other lipids, fibrous tissue and blood pigment. The intimal plaques are associated with changes in the medial wall and may be complicated by a thrombotic occlusion of the lumen. Measurements of cholesterol, lipid survey for triglyceride, 24-hour blood pressure are all essential.

Arteriosclerosis

Arteriosclerotic vascular occlusion is an accompaniment of old age. The vascular involvement may be patchy in the early stages, as it is in Buerger's disease, but later tends to be diffuse, so that when occlusion becomes manifest there are no entirely healthy alternative channels which can dilate to maintain the circulation. The margin of safety is therefore small. The process is slow and the duration of symptoms from the onset to the development of serious surgical situations necessitating amputation is very long except when occlusion is accelerated by infection or thrombosis. Apart from these accidents, proper care may postpone the necessity for amputation by 5 or 10 years.

LERICHE SYNDROME

Pain in the hip on exercise may be a sign of aortic, common iliac or internal iliac artery occlusion. In the two latter the peripheral pulse may be present and the condition may simulate or be confused with arthritis of the hip – or both may be present.

There is no significant difference between the lesions produced in the diabetic and the non-diabetic subjects. There is doubt as to whether vascular spasm is the initial factor giving rise to changes in the arterial wall, or whether spasm results from these changes. A significant degree of spasm is found in some patients, especially in the earlier stages. Pain is a prominent symptom, largely because of the severe degree of circulatory insufficiency, and alone may be sufficient indication for amputation. The blood supply may be worse in a painful though non-gangrenous leg than when gangrene is actually present.

METHODS OF INVESTIGATION TO DETERMINE COMPETENCE OF ARTERIES

In addition to the history and physical examination with specific reference to condition of the skin, hair pattern, colour, ulceration, etc., the most important examination is the determination of arterial pulsations by Doppler investigation. In the lower extremity, an accurate evaluation must be made with grading of arterial pulsations using the scale of 0 to 4 for the femoral, popliteal, dorsalis pedis and posterior tibial arteries. In the upper extremity this will include brachial, radial, ulnar and digital arteries. In addition to palpating the arteries at rest, such determinations should be carried out after exercise, for any indication of vascular insufficiency. An estimate of temperature change in the extremity and change of temperature in contralateral extremities should be obtained by testing the skin with either the back of the examiner's hand or the dorsal surfaces of the fingers. In the past, more refined temperature testing was carried out in controlled temperature rooms, but the information obtained was not sufficient to justify their use.

Doppler ultrasound is now the required investigation to determine both angle and multiple level blockage.

Arteriography/angiography

Normal arteries cast no shadow on the radiograph only the main vessels of the arteriosclerotic limb can be directly visualized. The arterial tree can be demonstrated by injecting some opaque substance into the main vessel in the proximal part of the limb. An 85% solution of sodium diatrizoate (Hypaque) is commonly used. It is commonly recommended that closed arterial puncture be performed, but exposure of the vessel under local anaesthesia is easily carried out and is more accurate. The vessel is compressed proximally during the injection and a film is taken after momentary release of compression. The method is of use in localizing the level of blockage of a vessel and gives valuable information regarding the collateral circulation.

It is sometimes necessary to test the vasomotor responses after sympathectomy to show that denervation is complete or to detect regeneration. Any of the methods already described for inhibiting constriction or producing dilation by heat or procaine block may be used; the most convenient is peripheral nerve block. In addition, the presence or absence of sweating may be demonstrated by the presence of moisture giving a deep blue-black colour with quinizarin compound when dusted onto the skin. Dry skin is a poor conductor of electricity and after sympathectomy the resistance of the skin to passage of a small electric current is therefore increased and can be measured.

Treatment of peripheral vascular disease

Therapeutic measures available are:

1. Local and general measures to improve the circulation.
2. Surgical treatment:
   (a) sympathetic denervation;
   (b) thromboendarterectomy;
   (c) bypass arterial transplants;
   (d) neurectomy or tenotomy of the tendo calcaneus;
   (e) amputation.

LOCAL AND GENERAL MEASURES TO IMPROVE THE CIRCULATION

The broad principles of the treatment of early peripheral vascular disturbances may be stated shortly as the prevention or abolition of vasospasm where this is present, combined with the protection of areas with an impoverished blood supply from trauma of all kinds. In the later stages, palliative procedures, designed to relieve pain, and amputation may be necessary.

A period of complete rest in bed is always beneficial but should not be prolonged as this may result in undue loss of mobility in elderly subjects. Vasodilation is marked during sleep and persists for some time after waking if the extremities are kept warm. For this reason many of these patients immerse their unaffected extremities in hot water on rising which produces a lasting vasodilation, especially if combined with warm gloves and socks. There is no doubt that excessive smoking has an adverse effect on peripheral vascular disturbances, and in many subjects even slight indulgence is followed by an evident increase of spasm. Indeed, abstinence is now regarded as mandatory. Alcohol, by producing vasodilation, is of benefit but subsequent excessive cooling may result in intense spasm, and alcoholic drinks should be consumed only in warm surroundings or before going to bed. Such measures as active and passive exercises, dry heat and hot baths may be employed to improve collateral circulation. In Buerger's exercises the patient lies on his back and raises the limb to an angle of 60° with the horizontal for 3 minutes, then lowers it to hang in a vertical position for 3 minutes and finally it is raised to the horizontal for 5 minutes. The cycle is then repeated. Long-term anticoagulants are useful to prevent the spread of thrombosis. Syphilis, diabetes or bad teeth should be treated by suitable measures and any infections controlled by suitable chemotherapeutic agents. Reducing hypertension and triglycerides by drug therapy is indicated.

General directions for patients suffering from vascular disturbances of the feet

In addition to the above, great care must be taken of the affected part and the following rules will be found invaluable. The feet should be washed each night with warm water and soap and dried with a soft towel. Methyl or ethyl alcohol should be applied and allowed to dry, after which the skin may be anointed gently with hydrous lanolin to keep the skin soft, supple and free from scales. The feet should always be kept warm. Woollen socks or wool-lined shoes in the winter and cotton socks in warm weather are satisfactory, and where possible a fresh pair of socks should be used each day. Loose-fitting bed socks should be used in preference to hot-water bottles or other mechanical heating devices. Walking shoes should be loosely fitting and of soft leather. Very great care should be exercised when the toenails, corns or callous skin are being cut, and if the nails are dry and brittle they should be softened in warm water nightly and lanolin generously applied on, about and under the nail. Circular garters and strong antiseptic drugs should be avoided. The appearance of blisters on the feet should be the signal for careful treatment. The blisters should be snipped, the skin removed and a dry dressing applied. Regular exercises, short of fatigue, should be prescribed. The extremities should be carefully protected from trauma since mild abrasions frequently initiate gangrene. The patient should be warned of the danger of injury to his extremities and the reasons for the precautions enjoined should be explained to him in order to secure his co-operation.

THROMBOENDARTERECTOMY

This concept in the surgery of peripheral arterial disease is based upon the finding that the thrombosis of arteriosclerosis often involves a localized segment of a major artery and that it is technically possible to restore normal arterial flow through the segment by surgical resection of the diseased intima.

The criteria for the selection of suitable cases for operation include:

1. The presence of disabling symptoms.
2. The radiographic demonstration of segmental occlusion of a large artery.
3. Relatively good physical status.

The contraindications to operation are:

1. Debility of advanced age.
2. The presence of serious concomitant disease in other organic systems.
3. The arteriographic demonstration of the diffuse form of arteriosclerosis.

In addition to their use during the operation, anticoagulants are employed as a long-term measure in patients with obliterative vascular disease.

ARTERIAL RECONSTRUCTION

Arteriosclerosis being a general disease, this type of surgery is justified only when the local manifestation predominates to an unusual extent.

An artery may be repaired by end-to-end anastomosis – not very likely in limited arteriosclerosis – by the interposition of an autogenous vein graft, a homologous arterial transplant, or by some plastic or other artificial prosthesis. It may also be repaired by a bypass or end-to-side anastomosis, particularly in the larger vessels.

Relatively high failure rates are reported for arterial transplants inserted by an end-to-end technique and record the better early results when end-to-side technique is used, though longer-term results have still to be proved.

Surgery

There are two types of reconstructive procedures. The first is the end-to-end procedure, where the diseased segment is removed and a prosthetic graft inserted. In the past, homografts were used, but this is now rare because of occasional early failures with this procedure and because of the improvement of prosthetic grafts (i.e. woven Teflon and knitted Dacron). This prosthetic replacement is even applicable to aortoiliac occlusions.

The second type of procedure is the bypass graft in which the existing obstructed segment of vessel is left in place, but is bypassed by connecting a Teflon graft or the autologous long saphenous vein proximal and distal to it. This has the added advantage of maintaining all possible collateral circulation from the patient's artery. This type of reconstruction is used particularly in femoral and popliteal occlusions.

AMPUTATION

Amputation is most commonly required in obliterative conditions affecting the legs. The digits are supplied by end arteries and their collateral circulation is poor. Conservative treatment should always be tried when gangrene is localized to one toe and there is a good line of demarcation, absence of lymphangitis, cellulitis and osteomyelitis, and no generalized toxaemia. Early amputation of a single toe is dangerous and often results in a further spread of gangrene, and healing is usually delayed. The patient is put to bed with the affected part covered with a light dry gauze dressing. The remainder of the body is warmed and chemotherapy is given. In the presence of mild local infection, a localized debridement of the gangrenous area should be carried out as a preliminary step to lessen toxaemia and lower the temperature and pulse rate. In such cases it may be permissible to wait for local healing where the first step has been a limited procedure, but if it has been at all extensive amputation should be carried out as soon as the patient's condition permits. In diabetic gangrene, inability to control glycosuria even with large doses of insulin is an indication for immediate amputation, following which control of the diabetes is usually readily effected. When a limb is useless, intractably painful or endangering life, amputation is necessary. Amputations through the foot or ankle region are seldom successful; transmetatarsal amputation has been suggested in certain cases with success, but the indications are not easy to define. More commonly the level of amputation is below or above the knee. Great care must be taken with the handling of the tissues which may be of dubious viability even at the level of amputation. Atraumatic technique, with great care to protect the wound margins from injury and meticulous haemostasis to prevent formation, is essential to ensure good results (see Chapter 18).

The stroke syndrome

A sudden neurological deficit can result from cerebral vascular disease producing reduction in the circulation to any part of the brain. This may arise from: abnormality of the vessel wall (e.g. atherosclerosis); an occlusion by thrombosis or embolism; a rupture of a saccular aneurysm in the circle of Willis; a sudden reduction in the cerebral blood flow due to hypotension, injury to the carotid artery, acute blood loss, Stokes–Adams syndrome, or increased viscosity of the blood.

The orthopaedic management of stroke syndrome has been largely neglected in the past and requires the same type of team approach to the problem as has been used with good effect in rehabilitation following poliomyelitis, and following the more aggressive surgical treatment of meningomyelocele and rheumatoid arthritis.

EARLY TREATMENT

Rehabilitation of the patient should begin early following the acute event. In the flaccid state the patient is in urgent need of external stimuli, to replace the proprioceptive impulses produced by movement of the limbs. This deficiency of motion may be replaced by a trained physiotherapist, and as soon as the general condition of the patient improves every effort should be made to remove the sickroom atmosphere and encourage the patient to fend for himself as much as possible.

In the early stages the quality of nursing care is of vital importance in the prevention of deformity: correct positioning in bed by the use of a foot board to prevent equinus; and a rolled blanket beneath the greater trochanters to internally rotate the legs to prevent external rotation deformity at the hip and flexion deformity of the knee; correct support of the upper limb by the use of a pillow in the axilla to maintain shoulder abduction and to prevent a frozen shoulder. Frequent change of position is of vital importance, both for the prevention of hypostatic pneumonia and pressure sores, as well as for the prevention of deformity. At each change of position the joints of the limbs are placed through a range of motion passively and positioned to maintain or increase their range of movement for about thirty minutes per day. When the lateral position is used, good pelvic and shoulder alignment are maintained using pillows, and the upper leg is held in an abducted position to prevent hip strain. The prone lying position should also be used to provide good drainage of secretions and to prevent hip flexion and knee flexion deformities. In this position there should be a gap between the end of the bed and the footboard.

ASSESSMENT

In the early stages following a stroke, accurate assessment of recovery is difficult but certain factors are helpful. Age by itself is not a major determinant of recovery. Enlargement of the communicating arteries in the circle of Willis in the older patient who has had previous small strokes accounts for this better prognosis as compared with the younger person who has had a massive cerebral infarction. Assessment of pseudomotor changes is of value in the assessment of motor control deficits; it may be possible by these to predict whether the involvement is bilateral or not.

The extrapyramidal system may be involved and assessment of this is important in determining the potential for improvement by the use of antirigidity drugs.

Difficulties in balance are often overlooked and it is essential to evaluate the patient in the upright position when attempting to assess his ability to walk. Only very occasionally does a stroke disturb the central control of balance, more frequently the inability to stand erect is related to disturbance of the patient's body image, resulting from a lesion in the non-dominant hemisphere of the brain.

A normal person is well aware of his body image and automatically adjusts the alignment of his extremities to maintain the centre of gravity over its base of support. Patients with motor deficits, but an intact body image, guard against falling by reaching out for available support. The patient with a distorted body image is unaware of the problem and will make no attempt to support or otherwise accommodate the weight of that side and thus falls towards the involved side. Techniques to stimulate body awareness, walking aids and braces are possible means of overcoming this inadequacy.

It is important in assessing a deformity to find the degree caused by structural contracture and the amount due to unopposed excessive muscle tone or spasticity. Unrelieved, a spastic deformity will gradually develop into a structural contracture. Another important point in the evaluation is the effect of functional position upon the deformity. It is essential to examine patients in the postures of standing and walking to note the effect of postural reflexes upon lower extremity deformities.

Whilst surgical release of spasticity provides a most reliable method of controlling deformity it has the disadvantage of causing associated muscle weakness and consequently non-invasive methods of control should be considered.

Peripheral nerve blocks, if shown to be successful with local anaesthetic, can be prolonged for 2–3 months by injecting a 2% phenol solution (Mooney *et al.*, 1969) although this can cause troublesome hyperanaesthia or causalgia.

A simpler technique for the reduction of spasticity using alcohol injection at the approximate locus of the motor point has been described by Tardieu *et al.* (1971). The results of injecting a 45% alcohol solution are comparable to those obtained using phenol and the effect lasts on average 3 months without any significant complication. The value of these injection techniques has been the predictable ability to reduce spasticity, allowing the physiotherapist to teach and retrain the patient in movements and patterns of movement at an early stage.

Drugs may have a part to play; however, the presence of structural contractures, the effects of environmental temperature and the mood of the patient, the balance between muscle weakness and spasticity and the presence of natural remissions and exacerbations create major problems in such therapy.

SURGICAL CORRECTION OF DISABILITIES

Lower limb problems

The most common site of deformity in the stroke patient is the foot and ankle. Fortunately, surgical correction of these deformities often results in great functional improvement. Walking ability after a stroke can be expected in over 60% of patients, because the sensory component is less important and the muscle power recovery is often sufficient for weight-bearing and taking some steps.

Primitive reflex patterns commonly emerge after the flaccidity has been replaced with spasticity; e.g. a primitive flexor pattern, in which there is synergistic flexion of the hip and knee and dorsiflexion with inversion of the foot, or a primitive extensor pattern consisting of extension of hip and knee and plantar flexion of the foot. However, failure of primitive reflexes to appear with some motor power by 6 weeks after the stroke onset is a poor sign for the likelihood of being able to walk, as are the loss of proprioception and of the body image.

A scissoring gait due to spasticity of the adductors can be improved by adductor tenotomy and anterior obdurator neurectomy.

A reliable standing base is most important. Even a patient with very minimal motor control can achieve stability of the knee and hip, provided a stable plantigrade position is obtainable. The most common disability is an equinus deformity due to uncontrolled tone in the gastrocnemius–soleus group. This deformity, whether due to actual contracture or to spasticity, is relieved by elongation of the tendo Achillis. This may be carried by the heel-cord lengthening technique described for use in cerebral palsy by Banks and Green (1958). It is, however, possible to perform elongation with less morbidity by carrying our percutaneous elongation. The distal incision is always carried out on the medial aspect of the tendo Achillis and correction is achieved just to a neutral position and no more than this, and then a short below-knee plaster cast is applied. The patient is encouraged to walk and stand from 3 to 5 days following surgery. By this means a stable stance phase becomes available. It has not been found necessary to carry out a capsulectomy of the ankle joint.

Inadequate dorsiflexion of the foot because of motor power loss can be controlled by an orthotic device made from plastic materials and applied to wear within the shoe or slipper, or even a double iron brace with a ankle stop. This orthosis is difficult to replace by a surgical reconstruction procedure, and will give knee control.

In order to control the varus deformity of the foot which is frequently associated with spasticity or contracture of the gastrocnemius–soleus, the tibialis anterior tendon transfer is a useful adjunct. The technique of splitting the anterior tibialis tendon and transferring the split portion to the lateral cuneiform bone was described by Mooney and Goodman (1969). They found that all patients showed improvement following this procedure and that 10 out of 65 patients were eventually free of all appliances. Following the procedure the secondary excessive toe flexor spasticity is often brought to light and now a toe flexor release is carried out at the same time as the split anterior tibialis transfer.

Knee flexion deformity is favoured by a persistence of the primitive flexor pattern and lack of early stimulation of extensor patterns. Usually the flexed knee deformity is equally accountable to lack of quadriceps muscle tone as to excessive hamstrings spasticity. Release of the hamstrings by sectioning the musculotendinous junction enables correction of this deformity. However, where the deformity has been long standing and severe, the shortening of the neurovascular bundle and tightness of the skin usually allow only 50% improvement at the time of surgery and the additional contracture must be gradually reduced by serial plaster casts. Long leg bracing to stabilize the knee for weight-bearing is not practical because of difficulty in putting the brace on, and inability to rise from the sitting position due to hip extension being too poor for the push-off (McCullough, 1975).

Persistent knee extension due to spasticity of the quadriceps muscle may be improved by division of one of the heads of the quadriceps muscles.

Disability at the hip joint may arise from three causes:

1. Abductor and extensor weakness.
2. Persistent hip flexion deformity.
3. Excessive adductor motor tone.

Abductor and extensor weakness may often be improved by the use of a walking stick carried in the opposite hand. The transfer of the greater trochanter distally on the femur would seem to be the logical procedure to improve this, but Mooney and Goodman carried this out only once with a poor result.

Hip adduction contracture may be released by a adductor division, or, in the case of spasticity, by obturator neurectomy.

Hip flexion deformity can be released but it is important in considering this to demonstrate that the spasticity is so severe with the contractual deformity so marked, that subsequent weakness of hip flexion will be a less marked problem than the pre-existing one. The technique advocated is that of an intrapelvic iliopsoas myotomy as described by Michaelis (1964).

Upper limbs

The recovery of normal upper extremity function is poor, with only 30% achieving sufficient use of the involved limb to assist the contralateral limb. This results from the loss of proprioception, astereognosis, two-point discrimination, vision disturbances in perception of spatial and geometric relations, and actual loss of part of the visual field. These, added to inco-ordination of muscle activity – let alone any muscle weakness or spasticity – make recovery of useful function following a dense hemiplegia most unlikely.

Surgical procedures in the upper limb are usually carried out for problems of painful contracture, hygiene, severe spasticity or mechanical impairment of function. In many cases the surgery must be carried out before a full occupational therapy programme can benefit the patient.

Shoulder

A passive range of at least 45° of abduction at the shoulder should be maintained at all costs in order to assist dressing. The wearing of a hemiplegic sling, supporting the downward subluxing shoulder, is of value as soon as the patient sits up or stands.

A painful frozen shoulder is a major impairment to the rehabilitation of the patient. Mild spasticity in the internal rotation adductor group of the shoulder is noted frequently in the third and fourth months following a stroke. Active exercises combined with a positioning programme may maintain or regain a good range of shoulder movements. Repeated injections of steroid into the joint may be necessary for pericapsulitis. Should the shoulder pain be severe, with marked limitation of movement and increased spasticity, the surgical procedure devised at Rancho los Amigos Hospital, releasing the subscapularis tendon from the humerus, can be carried out. Since this shoulder spasticity is frequently associated with elbow flexor spasm, resection of the coracobrachialis and biceps insertion is carried out at the same time and the musculocutaneous nerve injected with 2% phenol. Following this an active exercise programme is instituted to retain the movement obtained by this procedure.

Severe spasticity of the flexors of the elbow does not respond to exercising or positioning programmes and may result in a flexion contracture. The deformity is unsightly and prevents the patient from positioning his hand. As stated previously, the spastic elbow flexion contracture is frequently associated with a symptomatic adducted shoulder and simultaneous operative treatment in both areas may be accomplished during shoulder release surgery. Release procedures in the antecubital fossa are seldom necessary but the surgeon must be prepared to release or lengthen the biceps tendon, brachialis, brachioradialis, the forearm flexor muscles and the elbow joint capsule. The result is frequently compromised by shortening involving the nerves and major blood vessels.

Forearm and hand

Spasticity and poor motor control are common in the hemiplegic flexed forearm and hand. Procedures to improve these may be considered when the general state of the patient is good and there is intact sensation associated with some selective motor control in the arm. Occasionally the younger patient may require cosmetic improvement or the deformity of the clawed fingers may be so severe that hygiene of the palm becomes a problem. Initial evaluation using phenol nerve blocks or alcohol muscle injections may be extremely helpful in the assessment of hand function. If a patient with an apparent flexion deformity of the wrist and fingers is able to extend the wrist and fingers selectively following a nerve block, then a flexor slide procedure will be of value to weaken the spastic flexor pronators. However, when there is significant fixed flexion contracture of the wrist and fingers, a simple muscle origin release procedure will not be sufficient. An extended procedure that releases and elevates all forearm muscles from the bone and interosseous membrane usually allows enough functional lengthening of the musculotendinous unit to enable dynamic splinting to bring the wrist and fingers to the neutral position.

It will be seen that the management of stroke requires a combined multidisciplinary approach. The place of surgery in the management is limited and when required, it is carried out in conjunction with a total planned programme for the individual patient which requires intensive treatment by the physiotherapist and occupational therapist, both before and after surgery.

References

Adson, A.W. (1947) Surgical treatment for symptoms produced by cervical ribs and the scalenus anterior muscle. *Surgery, Gynecology and Obstetrics* **85**, 687

Adson, A.W. and Coffey, J.R. (1927) *Annals of Surgery* **85**, 839

Albert, E. (1885) Einige Operationen an Nerven. *Weiner Medizinische Presse* **26**, 1285

Attardi, D.G. and Sperry, R.W. (1963) Preferential selection of central pathways by regenerating optic fibres. *Journal of Experimental Neurology* **7**, 46

Aziz, W., Singer, R.M. and Wolff, T.W. (1990) Transfer of the trapezius for flail shoulder after brachial plexus injury. *Journal of Bone and Joint Surgery* **72B**, 701–704

Bailey, R.O., Baltech, A.L., Verikatesh, R. *et al.* (1988) Sensory motor neuropathy associated with AIDS. *Neurology* **38**, 886–889

Ballance, C. and Duel, A.B. (1932) The operative treatment of facial palsy by the introduction of nerve grafts in the fallopian canal and by other intratemporal methods. *Archives of Otolarangology* **15**, 1–70

Banks, H.H. and Green, W.T. (1958) The correction of equinus deformities in cerebral palsy. *Journal of Bone and Joint Surgery* **40A**, 1359–1379

Barr, J.S. (1947) *Journal of Bone and Joint Surgery* **29**, 429

Bassett, C.A.L. and Campbell, J.B. (1960) Calcification in millipore in vivo. *Transplantation Bulletin* **26**, 132

Bateman, J.E. (1955) *The Shoulder and Environs*. C.V. Mosby: St Louis

Berger, A., Schaller, E. and Mailander, P. (1991) Brachial plexus injuries: an integrated treatment concept. *Annals of Plastic Surgery* **26**, 70–76

Birch, R. (1993) Surgery for brachial plexus injury – editorial. *Journal of Bone and Joint Surgery* **75B**, 346–348

Birch, R. and Raji, A. (1991) Repair of median and ulnar nerves. *Journal of Bone and Joint Surgery* **73B**, 154–157

Birch, R., Wilkinson, M.C.P., Vijayou, K.P. and Gschmeissner, S. (1992) Cement burn of the sciatic nerve. *Journal of Bone and Joint Surgery* **74B**, 731–733

Bolesta, M.J., Garrett, W.E. Jr, Ribbeck, B.M., Glisson, R.R., Seaber, A.V. and Goldner, J.L. (1988) Immediate and delayed neurorrhaphy in a rabbit model: a functional, histologic, and biochemical comparison. *Journal of Hand Surgery* **13A**, 352–357

Bonney, G. (1954) The value of axon responses in determining the site of lesions in traction injuries of the brachial plexus. *Brain* **77**, 588–609

Bonney, G., Birch, R., Jamieson, A. and Eames, R. (1984) Experience with vascularized nerve grafts. *Clinics in Plastic Surgery* **11**, 137–142

Boyes, J.A. (1976) *On the Shoulders of Giants*. J.B. Lippincott: Philadelphia

Boyes, J.H. (1960) Tendon transfers for radial palsy. *Bulletin of the Hospital for Joint Diseases Orthopaedic Institute* **21**, 97–105

Boyes, J.H. (1964) *Bunnell's Surgery of the Hand*, 4th edn, p. 514. J.B. Lippincott: Philadelphia

Brand, P.W. (1970) Tendon transfers for median and ulnar nerve paralysis. *Orthopedic Clinics of North America* **1**, 446–454

Brand, P.W. (1975) Tendon transfers in the forearm. In: *Hand Surgery*, 2nd edn. Edited by J.E. Flynn. Williams & Wilkins, Baltimore

Brookes, D.M. (1949) Open wounds of the brachial plexus. *Journal of Bone and Joint Surgery* **31B**, 17–33

Brooks, A.L. and Jones, D.S. (1975) A new intrinsic tendon transfer for the paralytic hand. *Journal of Bone and Joint Surgery* **57A**, 730

Buerger, L. (1924) *Circulatory Disturbances of the Extremities*. W.B. Saunders: Philadelphia and London

Bunnell, S. (1938) Opposition of the thumb. *Journal of Bone and Joint Surgery* **20**, 269–284

Bunnell, S. (1951) Restoring flexion to the paralytic elbow. *Journal of Bone and Joint Surgery* **33A**, 566–571

Burge, P., Rushworth, G. and Watson, N. (1985) Patterns of injury to the terminal branches of the brachial plexus. The place for early exploration. *Journal of Bone and Joint Surgery* **67B**, 630–634

Burkhalter, W.E. (1974) Tendon transfer in median nerve paralysis. *Orthopedic Clinics of North America* **5**, 271

Burkhalter, W.E. and Strait, J.L. (1973) Metacarpophalangeal flexor replacement for intrinsic paralysis. *Journal of Bone and Joint Surgery* **55A**, 1666–1676

Camitz, H. (1929) Uber die Behandlung der oppositionslahmung. *Acta Chirurgica Scandinavica* **65**, 77

Campbell, J.B. and Luzio, J. (1960) Facial nerve repair: new surgical techniques. *Transactions of the American Academy of Ophthalmology and Otolaryngology* **68**, 1068

Carroll, R.E. and Hill, N.A. (1970) Triceps transfer to restore elbow flexion: a study of 15 patients with paralytic lesions and arthrogryposis. *Journal of Bone and Joint Surgery* **52A** 239–244

Christensen, K.S., Falstie-Jensen, N., Christensen, E.S. and Brochner-Mortensen, J. (1988) Results of amputation for gangrene in diabetic and non-diabetic patients. Selection of amputation level using photoelectric measurements of skin-perfusion pressure. *Journal of Bone and Joint Surgery* **70A**, 1514–1519

Chuinard, R.G.A Boyes, J.H., Stark, H.H. and Ashworth, C.R. (1978) Tendon transfers for radial nerve palsy: use of superficialis tendons for digital extension. *Journal of Hand Surgery* **3**, 560–570

Clarke, J.M.P. (1945) Reconstruction of biceps brachiae by pectoral muscle transplantation. *British Journal of Surgery* **34**, 180

Clawson, D.K. and Seddon, H.J. (1960) *Journal of Bone and Joint Surgery* **42B**, 205

Connolly, S. and Manji, H. (1991) AIDS and the peripheral nervous system. *Hospital Update* **1**, 474–485

Cragg, B.G. and Thomas, P.K. (1961) Changes in conduction velocity and fibre size proximal to peripheral nerve lesions. *Journal of Physiology* **157**, 315

Dekel, S., Papaioannou, T., Rushworth, G. and Coates, R. (1980) Idiopathic carpal tunnel syndrome caused by a carpal stenosis. *British Medical Journal* **280**, 1297

de la Monte, S.M., Gabuzda, D.H., Ho, D.D. *et al.* (1988) Peripheral neuropathy in the acquired immunodeficiency syndrome. *Annals of Neurology* **23**, 485–492

Dellon, A.L. (1989) Review of treatment results for ulnar nerve entrapment at the elbow. *Journal of Hand Surgery* **14A**, 89

Devor, M. (1983) Nerve pathophysiology and mechanisms of pain in causalgia. *Journal of the Autonomic Nervous System* **20**, 335–353

Dewar, F.P. and Harris, R.I. (1950) Restoration of function of the shoulder following paralysis of the trapezius by fascial sling fixation and transplantation of the levator scapuli. *Annals of Surgery* **132**, 1111–1115

Dickson, R.A., Dinley, J., Rushworth, G. and Colwyn, A. (1977) Delayed (degenerate) interfascicular nerve grafting: a new concept in peripheral nerve repair. *British Journal of Surgery* **64**, 698–701

Doupe, J., Cullen, C.H. and Chance, C.Q. (1944) *Journal of Neurology, Neurosurgery and Psychiatry* **7**, 33

Doyle, J.A. and Blythe, W. (1975) The finger flexor tendon sheath and pulleys: anatomy and reconstruction. In: *AAOS Symposium on Tendon Surgery in the Hand*, pp. 81–87. Edited by J.M. Hunter. L.H. Schneider. C.V. Mosby: St Louis

Ducker, T.B., Kempe, L.G. and Hayes, G.J. (1969) The metabolic background for peripheral nerve surgery. *Journal of Neurosurgery* **30**, 270

Eckman-Ordeberg, G., Salgeback, S. and Ordeberg, G. (1987) Carpal tunnel syndrome in pregnancy. A prospective study. *Acta Obstetrica et Gynecologica Scandinavica* **66**, 233–235

Finsen, V., Persen, L., Lovlien, M. *et al.* (1988) Transcutaneous electrical nerve stimulation after major amputation. *Journal of Bone and Joint Surgery* **70B**, 109–112

Flatt, A.E. (1980) Digital artery sympathectomy. *Journal of Hand Surgery* **5**, 550–556

Foerster, O. (1939) *Zeitschrift für die Gesamte Neurologie und Psychiatrie* **167**, 439

Gelberman, R.H., Pfeffer, G.B., Galbraith, R.T., Szabo, R.M., Rydevik, B. and Dimick, M. (1987) Results of treatment of severe carpal tunnel syndrome without internal neurolysis of the median nerve *Journal of Bone and Joint Surgery* **69A**, 896–903

Gelberman, R.H., Eaton, R. and Urbaniak, J.R. (1993) Peripheral nerve compression. *Journal of Bone and Joint Surgery* **75A**, 1854–1878

Gellman, H., Gelberman, R.H., Tan, A.M. and Botte, M.J. (1986) Carpal tunnel syndrome. An evaluation of the provocative diagnostic tests. *Journal of Bone and Joint Surgery* **68A**, 735

Gersh, I. and Bodian, D. (1943) Some chemical mechanisms in chromatolysis. *Journal of Cellular and Comparative Physiology* **21**, 253

Ghostine, S.Y., Comair, Y.G. and Turner, D.H. (1984) Phenoxybenzamine in the treatment of causalgia – report of 40 cases. *Journal of Neurosurgery* **60**, 1263–1268

Giddins, G.E., Wade, P.J. and Amis, A.A. (1989) Primary nerve repair: the strength of repair with different gauges of nylon suture material. *Journal of Hand Surgery* **14B**, 301–302

Glasby, M.A., Gschmeissner, S.E. Huang, C.L.-H. and De Souza, B.A. (1986) Degenerated muscle grafts used for peripheral nerve repair in primates. *Journal of Hand Surgery* **11B**, 347–351

Glasby, M.A., Gilmour, J.A., Gschmeissner, S.E., Hems, T.E.J. and Myles, L.M. (1990) The repair of large peripheral nerves using skeletal muscle autografts. *British Journal of Plastic Surgery* **43**, 169–178

Glasby, M.A., Carrick, M.J. and Hems, T.E.J. (1992) Freeze-thawed skeletal muscle autografts used for brachial plexus repair in the non-human primate. *Journal of Hand Surgery* **17B**, 526–535

Goldie, B.S. and Coates, C.J. (1992) Brachial plexus injury: a survey of incidence and referral pattern. *Journal of Hand Surgery* **17B**, 86–88

Green, D.P. (1988) In: Green, D.P. (Ed). *Operative Hand Surgery*, 2nd edn, pp. 1486–1490. Edited by D.P. Green. Churchill Livingstone: New York

Grundberg, A.B. (1983) Carpal tunnel decompression in spite of normal electromyography. *Journal of Hand Surgery* **8**, 348–349

Gschmeissner, S.E., Peveira, J.H. and Cowley, S.A. (1991) The rapid assessment of nerve stumps. *Journal of Bone and Joint Surgery* **73B**, 688–689

Gu, Y.D., Zhang, G.M., Chen, D.S. *et al.* (1991) Cervical nerve root transfer from the contralateral normal side for treatment of brachial plexus root avulsion. *Chinese Medical Journal* **104**, 208–211

Hems, T.E.J. and Glasby, M.A. (1992) Repair of cervical roots proximal to the ganglia: an experimental study in sheep. *Journal of Bone and Joint Surgery* **74B**, 918–922

Highet, W.B. and Holmes, W. (1943) Traction injuries to the lateral popliteal nerve and traction injuries to peripheral nerves after suture. *British Journal of Surgery* **30**, 212–233
Hoaglund, F.T. and Duthie, R.B. (1966) Surgical reconstruction for shoulder pain after radical neck dissection. *American Journal of Surgery* **112**, 522–526
Hoen, T.I. and Brackett, C.E. (1956) Peripheral nerve lengthening. *Journal of Neurosurgery* **13**, 43–62
Huber, E. (1921) Hilfs operation bei median Uslahmung. *Deutsche Archiv fur Klinische Medizin* **136**, 271
Hunt, J.C. and Pugh, D.G. (1961) Radiology **76**, 1
Koshima, I. and Harii, K. (1985) Experimental study of vascularized nerve grafts: multifactorial analyses of axonal regeneration of nerves transplanted into an acute burn wound. *Journal of Hand Surgery* **10A**, 64–72
Laing, P.W., Cougley, D. and Klenerman, L. (1991) Neuropathic foot ulceration treated by contact casts. *Journal of Bone and Joint Surgery* **74B**, 133–135
Lam, S.J.S. (1967) Tarsal tunnel syndrome. *Journal of Bone and Joint Surgery* **49B**, 87–97
Learmonth, J.R. (1933) The principal of decompression in the treatment of certain diseases of peripheral nerves. *Surgical Clinics of North America* **13**, 905–913
Learmonth, J.R. (1944) *Proceedings of the Royal Society of Medicine* **37**, 553
L'Episcopo, J.B. (1939) Restoration of muscle balance in the treatment of obstetrical paralysis. *New York State Journal of Medicine* **39**, 357–363
Leriche, R. (1938) *Journal International de Chirurgie* **35**, 584
Lewis, T. (1938) *Clinical Science* **3**, 287
Littler, J.W. (1949) Tendon transfers and arthrodesis in combined median and ulnar nerve palsies. *Journal of Bone and Joint Surgery* **31A**, 225–234
Liu, C.T., Bender, C.E. and Sanders, F.K. (1948) Tensile strength of human nerves. *Archives of Neurology and Psychiatry* **59**, 322–336
Low, P., Marchand, G., Knox, F. and Dyck, P. (1977) Measurement of endoneurial fluid pressure with polyethylene matrix capsules. *Brain Research* **133**, 373
Lytton, B. and Murray, J.G. (1954) Effects of the peripheral pathway on the regeneration of nerve fibres. *Journal of Physiology* **126**, 626–636
McCullough, C.J., Gagey, O., Higginson, D.W., Sandin, B.M., Crow, J.C. and Sebile, A. (1984) Axon regeneration and vascularization of nerve grafts. An experimental study. *Journal of Hand Surgery* **9B**, 323
McCullough, N.C. (1975) *AAOS Instructional Course Lectures* **24**, 29–40
Mackenzie, I.G. and Woods, C.G. (1961) *Journal of Bone and Joint Surgery* **43B**, 465
Marmor, L. (1967) *Peripheral Nerve Regeneration using Nerve Grafts*. Charles C Thomas: Springfield, IL
Marsh, D. and Barton, N. (1987) Does the use of the operating microscope improve the results of peripheral nerve suture? *Journal of Bone and Joint Surgery* **69B**, 625
Marshall, R.W. and De Silva, R.D.D. (1986) Computerised axial tomography in traction injuries of the brachial plexus. *Journal of Bone and Joint Surgery* **68B**, 734
Matsuda, Y., Oki, S., Kitaoka, K. *et al.* (1988) Scanning electron microscope study of denervated and reinnervated neuromuscular junction. *Muscle and Nerve* **11**, 1266–1271
Michaelis, L.S. (1964) Ilopsoas myotomy for spastic flexion-contracture at the hip. In: *Orthopaedic Surgery of the Limbs in Paraplegia*. Springer-Verlag: Berlin
Millesi, H. (1968) Zum Problem der Uberbruckung von Defekten peripherer Nerven. *Wiener Medizinische Wochenschrift* **118**, 182–187
Millesi, H. (1977) Interfascicular grafts for repair of peripheral nerves of the upper extremity. *Orthopedic Clinics of North America* **8**, 387–406
Moberg, E. (1958) Objective methods for determining the functional value of sensibility of the hand. *Journal of Bone and Joint Surgery* **40B**, 454–476
Mooney, V., Frykman, G. and McLamb, J. (1969) Present status of the intra-neural phenol injections. *Clinical Orthopaedics and Related Research* **63**, 122–131
Mooney, V. and Goodman, F. (1969) Clinical lower extremity disabilities due to strokes. *Clinical Orthopaedics and Related Research* **63**, 142–152
Murase, T., Kawai, H., Masatomi, T., Kawabata, H. and Ono, K. (1993) Evoked spinal cord potentials for diagnosis during brachial plexus surgery. *Journal of Bone and Joint Surgery* **75B**, 775–781
Myers, R.R., Powell, H.C., Costello, M.L., Lambert, P.W. and Zwerfach, B.E. (1978) Endoneurial fluid pressure: direct measurement with micropipettes. *Brain Research* **148**, 510
Narakas, A. (1978) *Clinical Orthopaedics and Related Research* **133**, 71
Nashold, B.S., Goldner, J.L., Mullen, J.B. and Bright, D.S. (1982) *Journal of Bone and Joint Surgery* **64A**, 1–10
Nicolle, F.V. and Woodhouse, F.M. (1965) New compression syndromes of the upper limb. *Journal of Trauma* **5**, 313–318
Norris, R.W., Glasby, M.A., Gattuso, J.M. and Bowden, R.E.M. (1988) Peripheral nerve repair in humans using muscle autografts. *Journal of Bone and Joint Surgery* **70B**, 530–533
Ochoa, J., Fowler, T.J. and Gilliatt, R.W. (1972) *Journal of Anatomy* **113**, 433
Ochs, S., Sabri, M.I. and Ranish, N. (1970) Somal site of synthesis of fast transported materials in mammalian nerve fibres. *Journal of Neurobiology* **1**, 329–344
Omer, G.E. Jr (1971) Restoring power grip in ulnar palsy. *Journal of Bone and Joint Surgery* **53A**, 814
Omer, G.E. Jr (1980) Tendon transfers for reconstruction of the forearm and hand following peripheral nerve injuries. In: *Management of Peripheral Nerve Problems*, pp. 817–846. Edited by G.E. Omer and M. Spinner. W.B. Saunders: Philadelphia
Osborne, G. (1959) *British Medical Journal* **1**, 98
Paget, J. (1865) In: *Lectures on Surgical Pathology*, 3rd edn. Lindsay and Blakiston: Philadelphia
Phalen, G.S. (1966) The carpal tunnel syndrome: 17 years experience in diagnosis and treatment of 644 hands. *Journal of Bone and Joint Surgery* **48A**, 211–228
Phalen, G.S. and Millar, R.C. (1947) Transfer of wrist extensor muscles to restore or reinforce flexion power of the fingers and opposition of the thumb. *Journal of Bone and Joint Surgery* **29**, 993–997
Phillipeaux, J.M. and Vulpian, A. (1870) Note sur des essais de greffe d'un tronçon de nerf lingual entre des deux bouts nerf hypoglasse, après excision d'un segment

de ce dernier nerf. *Archives du Physiologie normale et pathologique* **3**, 618

Pho, R.W.H., Lee, Y.S., Rujiwetpongstorn, V. and Pang, M. (1985) Histological studies of vascularized nerve graft and conventional nerve graft. *Journal of Hand Surgery* **10B**, 45

Pollard, J.D., Gye, R.S. and MacLeod, G.J. (1966) An assessment of immunosuppressive agents in experimental peripheral nerve transplantation. *Surgery, Gynecology and Obstetrics* **132**, 839–845

Ransford, A.D. and Hughes, S.P.F. (1977) *Journal of Bone and Joint Surgery* **59B**, 417

Riordan, D.C. (1964) Tendon transfers for nerve paralysis of the hand and wrist. *Current Practice in Orthopedic Surgery* **2**, 17

Roberts, W.J. (1986) A hypothesis on the physiological basis for causalgia and related pains. *Pain* **24**, 294–311

Roles, N.C. and Maudsley, R.H. (1972) Radial tunnel syndrome. Resistant tennis elbow as a nerve entrapment. *Journal of Bone and Joint Surgery* **54B**, 499–508

Roos, D. (1966) Transaxillary approach for first rib resection to relieve thoracic outlet syndrome. *Annals of Surgery* **163**, 354

Royle, N.D. (1938) An operation for paralysis of the intrinsic muscles of the thumb. *Journal of the American Medical Association* **111**, 612

Sanders, F.K. and Young, J.Z. (1942) The degeneration and reinnervation of grafted nerves. *Journal of Anatomy* **76**, 143–166

Schneider, L.H. (1969) Opponensplasty using the extensor digiti minimi. *Journal of Bone and Joint Surgery* **51A**, 1297–1302

Seddon, H.J. (1949) *Proceedings of the Royal Society of Medicine* **42**, 427

Seddon, H.J. (Ed.) (1954) *Peripheral Nerve Injuries.* Medical Research Council Report No. 282. HMSO: London

Seddon, H.J. (1963) Nerve grafting. *Journal of Bone and Joint Surgery* **45B**, 447–461

Seddon, H.J. (1972) *Surgical Disorders of the Peripheral Nerves.* Williams and Wilkins: Baltimore

Sedel, L. and Nizard, R.S. (1993) Nerve grafting for traction injuries of the common peroneal nerve. *Journal of Bone and Joint Surgery* **75B**, 772–774

Semple, J.C. and Cargill, A.O. (1969) Carpal tunnel syndrome: results of surgical decompression. *Lancet* **1**, 918–919

Skie, M., Zeiss, J., Ebraheim, N.A. and Jackson, W.T. (1990) Carpal tunnel changes and median nerve compression during wrist flexion and extension seen by magnetic resonance imaging. *Journal of Hand Surgery* **15A**, 934

Smith, P.J. and Mott, G. (1986) Sensory threshold and conductance testing in nerve injuries. *Journal of Hand Surgery* **11B**, 157

Soderfelt, B., Olsson, Y. and Kristensson, K. (1973) The perineurium as a diffusion barrier to protein tracers in human peripheral nerve. *Acta Neuropathologica* **25**, 120

Starr, C.L. (1922) Army experience with tendon transference. *Journal of Bone and Joint Surgery* **4**, 3–21

Steindler, A. (1918) Orthopaedic operations on the hand. *Journal of the American Medical Association* **71**, 1288

Sunderland, S. (1968) *Nerves and Nerve Injuries.* Livingstone: Edinburgh and London

Sunderland, S. and Bradley, K.C. (1949) The cross-sectional area of peripheral nerve trunks devoted to nerve fibres. *Brain* **72**, 428

Takakura, Y., Kitada, C., Sugimoto, K., Tanaka, Y. and Tamai, S. (1991) Tarsal tunnel syndrome. *Journal of Bone and Joint Surgery* **73B**, 125–128

Taleisnik, J. (1973) The palmar-cutaneous branch of the median nerve and the approach to the carpal tunnel. An anatomical study. *Journal of Bone and Joint Surgery* **55A**, 1212–1217

Tardieu, C., Cockin, J., Hamilton, E.A., Nichols, P.J.R. and Price, D.A. (1971) Preliminary report on the treatment of spasticity with 45% ethyl alcohol injection into the muscles. *British Journal off Clinical Practice* **25**, 73–75

Taylor, G.I. and Ham, F.J. (1976) The free vascularized nerve graft. A further experimental and clinical application of microvascular techniques. *Plastic and Reconstructive Surgery* **57**, 413

Thompson, T.C. (1942) A modified operation for opponens paralysis. *Journal of Bone and Joint Surgery* **24**, 632–640

Tinel, J. (1917) *Nerve Wounds.* Baillière, Tindall and Cox: London

Tricker, J., O'Hara, J.P., Rushworth, G. and Dixon, R.A. (1979) The influence of tension on nerve anastamoses. *Journal of Bone and Joint Surgery* **61B**, 380

Tsuge, K. and Adachi, N. (1969) Tendon transfer for extensor palsy of forearm. *Hiroshima Journal of Medical Science* **18**, 219–232

Ungley, C.C. and Blackwood, W. (1942) *Lancet* **2**, 447

Upton, A.R.M. and McComas, A.J. (1973) The double crush in nerve entrapment syndromes. *Lancet* **2**, 359–361

Van Beek, A. and Kleinert, H.E. (1977) Practical microneurorrhaphy. *Orthopedic Clinics of North America* **8**, 377–386

Walshe, F.M.R., Jackson, H. and Wyburn-Mason, R. (1944) *Brain* **67**, 141

Weiss, P. (1944) The technology of nerve regeneration. *Journal of Neurosurgery* **1**, 400

Wood, V.E. and Biondi, J. (1990) Double-crush nerve compression in thoracic outlet syndrome. *Journal of Bone and Joint Surgery* **72A**, 85

Woodhall, M.B. and Beebe, G.W. (1956) *Peripheral Nerve Regeneration. A Follow-up Study of 3,656 World War II Injuries.* Veterans Administration Medical Monograph. US Government Printing Office: Washington, DC

Yeoman, P.M. and Seddon, H.J. (1961) Brachial plexus injuries: treatment of the flail arm. *Journal of Bone and Joint Surgery* **43B**, 493–500

Young, L., Wray, R.C. and Weeks, P.M. (1981) A randomized prospective comparison of fascicular and epineural digital nerve repair. *Plastic and Reconstructive Surgery* **68**, 89–92

Zachary, R.B. (1954) In: *Peripheral Nerve Injuries. Edited by H.J. Seddon. Medical Research Council report No. 282. HMSO: London*

Zancolli, E.A. (1978) Structural and Dynamic Bases of Hand Surgery, 2nd edn, p. 168. J.B. Lippincott: Philadelphia

CHAPTER 13

Affections of the Spine

ROBERT B. DUTHIE

Anatomy of the lumbosacral region

The lumbar spinal column, during its development into a secondary curvature (i.e. the lumbar lordosis), has become adapted to transmit and support enormous biomechanical loads resulting from transference of the body weight of the trunk down through the pelvis into the lower extremities. It also provides mobility of flexion, extension, lateral flexion and rotation and posture. It is made up of basic units which Schmorl called 'vertebral motor units', and they consist of two adjacent vertebral bodies separated by the intervertebral disc anteriorly but supported posteriorly by the diarthrodial facet joints. Maintaining and supporting these structures are the anterior and posterior longitudinal ligaments, the annulus fibrosus which is in physical continuity with these ligaments but also with the nucleus pulposus of the disc, and the articular structures of joint capsular ligament, infra- and supraspinous ligaments and intralaminar ligaments over the ligamenta flava. Covering these structures posteriorly, there are the imbricated supraspinal muscles, deep fascia, fat and skin. Contained within these units is the lower end of the spinal cord – i.e. the conus medullaris (at the lower border of the first lumbar vertebra), the filum terminale to the coccyx, surrounded by the lumbosacral nerve roots down to S2 and 3 level, making up the cauda equina. Surrounding these structures bathed with cerebrospinal fluid is the dura mater or theca, which is separated from the bony, ligamentous column by the extradural space. This contains fat and a plexus of veins, and is now important for epidural anaesthesia injection.

Leaving the cauda equina at successive levels are the motor and sensory roots which have joined up as a peripheral nerve root before penetrating the dura. The peripheral nerve root is surrounded by a sleeve or sheath of dura which can be as long as 5, 7 mm and continues as the epineurium. It should be noted that in the lumbar region, the peripheral nerve root usually leaves the dural sheath opposite a disc level (e.g. L3/4) and then passes distally within the canal to leave it through the intervertebral foramen one segment lower (e.g. L4/5). Between the dural sheath and the foramen the root lies in the lateral recess, covered over by the thickened lateral part of the ligamentum flavum, attached to the posterior facet joint capsular ligament. This means that the peripheral nerve root can be involved by a pathological process (e.g. disc protrusion at one or other levels), lateral recess bony disease (e.g. tumour) or osteophyte formation from posterior facet arthritis.

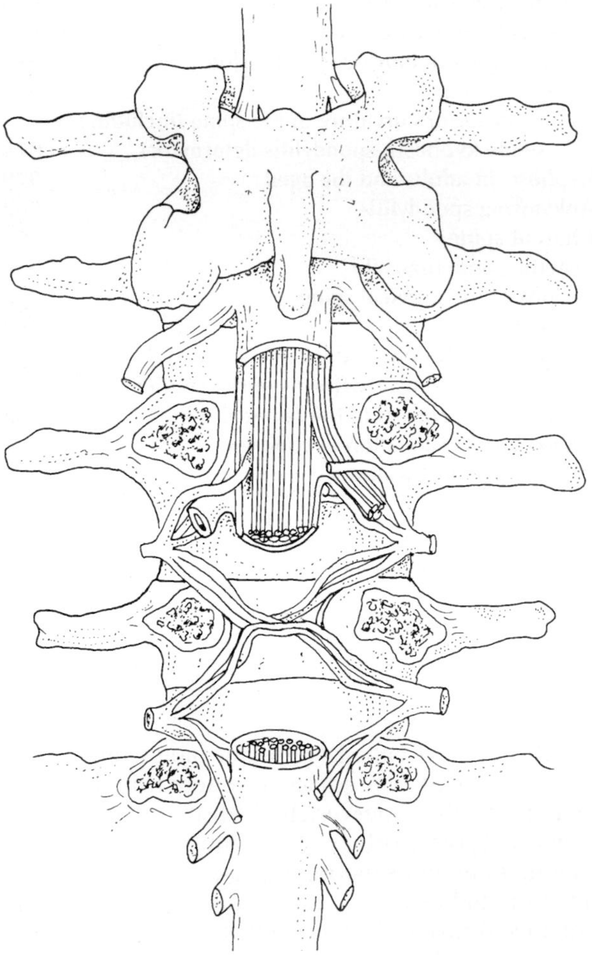

Figure 13.1 Diagrammatic representation of the cauda equina with the peripheral nerve roots coming out into the intervertebral foramina, close to the sulcar arteries and veins which anastomose with each other. (Designed by Farquharson-Roberts)

The sympathetic and parasympathetic outflow in the lower lumbar and upper sacral regions lies anteriorly, forming the presacral plexus or nervi erigentes.

All these structures are supplied by blood vessels arising from the lumbar aortic branches, the lateral sacral arteries from the internal iliac arteries. These give off feeder spinal arteries – both posterior and anterior – which enter through the intervertebral foramina to accompany the nerve roots and to join up with named anterior and two posterior spinal arteries. These segmental horizontal feeder arteries anastomose with paired radicular tributaries but infrequently with each other. However, they are connected longitudinally especially distally around the cauda equina. The most important feeder or anastomosing artery is that of Adamkiewicz between D8 and L4 since there are no other segmental arteries between these levels. The anterior spinal arteries are the most important, giving off sulcar arteries which are very numerous in lumbar regions and supply most of the spinal cord structures in the anterior two-thirds (Figure 13.1).

Venous drainage in the main corresponds to the arteries but is very large in the extradural spaces and in the intervertebral foramina in which there are large anastomosing branches from cord, roots and the paravertebral venous plexus.

Contained within these vascular walls there are free nerve endings and a plexus of non-myelinated nerve fibres, subserving pain sensations. Wyke (Molina *et al.*, 1976), who contributed greatly to this subject, described similar nerve endings in the capsule of the posterior facet joints and in the periosteum of vertebrae as well as in the tendinous and fascial attachments, in the spinal longitudinal ligaments (especially in the posterior where its fibres mingle with the annulus fibrosus), in the dura mater and in the epidural fat. Neither the disc nucleus pulposus nor the deeper annulus fibres contain nerve endings.

Stimulation of these free nerve endings by inflammatory reactions with oedema and swelling, release of pain-producing substances, increased vascularity with increase in tissue pressure, mechanical stress of distortion or deformations of surface planes, if not frank tears of fascia, tendon, capsule, ligaments, muscle, or fractures of bony trabecula, subchondral plate, etc., must all be considered when pain is experienced in this region.

The late Carl Hirsch (1959) studied several patients with low back pain and found that saline injected under pressure into the suspected disc would produce the characteristic pain and this was relieved by a local anaesthetic injection. Injection of the annulus with hypertonic saline produced deep-seated low back pain, but superficial ligaments when injected gave rise to local pain. Injections to the posterior facet joints gave rise to buttock radiation.

Recently Konttinen *et al.* (1990) using neuroimmunochemical labelling techniques have shown abundant neural filaments in the posterior longitudinal ligament and in the peripheral annulus fibrosus, which contain neuropeptides, substance P or calcitonin gene-related peptides. They suggest that the pressure and chemical irritation of nociceptive nerves excite sensory neural elements of the posterior ligament and possibly of the peripheral annulus fibrosus. The normal disc unless penetrated by vascular granulation tissue is painless because it does not contain any neural elements.

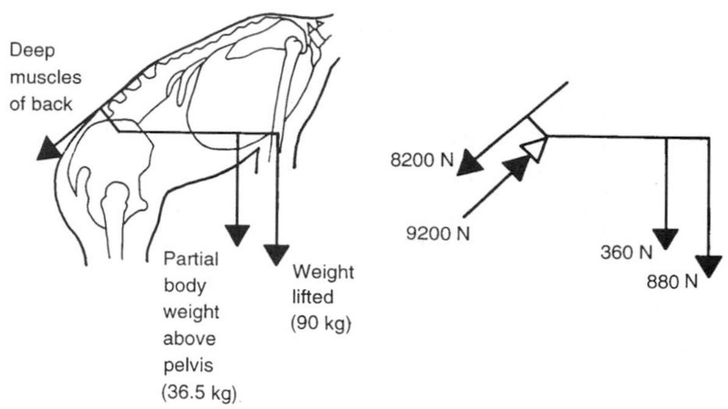

Figure 13.2 Bending forwards and lifting weights produces moments of force tending to flex the spine still further. These moments must be counteracted by tensions in the back muscles to provide the opposing extension moment required for equilibrium. Both sets of forces act on the trunk, and must be resisted by forces in the spine. Hence very high compressive loadings on the spine can be produced in lifting. These are minimized by keeping the lifted weights close to the spine. (Adapted by I.A.F. Stokes from Morris, J.M., Lucas, D.B. and Bresler, B. (1961) *Journal of Bone and Joint Surgery* **43A**, 327–31)

Mechanical factors affecting the spine

High loadings can be imposed on the spine by the back muscles, as shown in Figure 13.2. Ultimately compressive loads on the spine can produce crushing injuries in vertebrae or rupture of a disc through the vertebral end plate (Schmorl's node). However, the onset of painful conditions of the spine is not always associated with any abnormal traumatic event. Such painful lesions are apparently the product of chronic degenerative processes in which mechanical loading plays a part.

Painful conditions of the spine have been associated with abnormal movements of intervertebral joints. Hypermobility (Froning and Frohman, 1968), reduced movement (Mensor and Duvall, 1959), axial rotation abnormalities (Farfan *et al.*, 1970) and displacement of the centre of rotation (Pennal *et al.*, 1972) have been observed in degenerative intervertebral joints. Such movement abnormalities may result from muscle imbalance or spasm, structural changes in the joint or a manoeuvre used by the patient to avoid a painful range of movement. Demonstration of such abnormalities by radiology is often difficult because of the three-dimensional geometry and motion of the spine. Biplanar radiography is a technique which has been used to measure the three-dimensional movements of the lumbar joints (Stokes *et al.*, 1981). Asymmetries of movement were found in spines affected by herniated nucleus pulposus. These asymmetries suggested that the patients had developed a finely tuned ability to restrict painful movement at a particular joint.

The loading on the component parts of the spine is a product of external forces, especially that of gravity, the position adopted by the body and its muscular activity. The position of the body is particularly important because this determines the degree of stretch of passive structures such as ligaments, and also the magnitude of the muscle forces required to maintain the equilibrium of the body segments (Figures 13.2 and 13.3).

INTERVERTEBRAL DISC

The nucleus pulposus and the surrounding annulus behaves as an elastic hydrostatic structure to take loads of up to 70 kg in a 70 kg person on standing – at the third level. This compression loading is reduced by half when supine, is decreased during walking and side flexion and is increased by jumping and by lifting weights with straight knees. Stiffness of disc material is a non-linear curve which increases with compression loading. The creep behaviour can

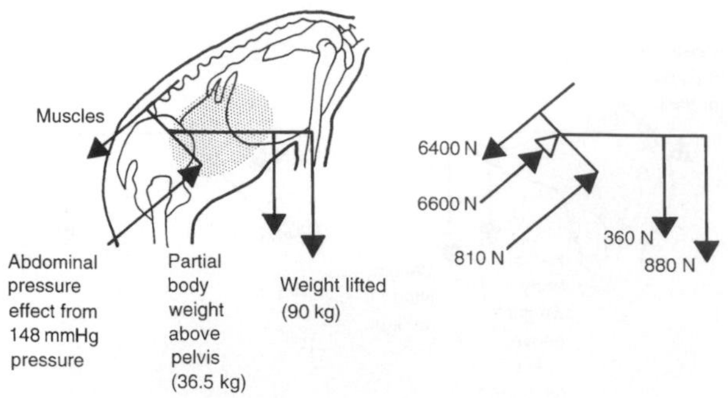

Figure 13.3 Forces on the spine are modified from those in Figure 13.2 by the effects of intra-abdominal pressure. This produces forces on the pelvic floor and on the diaphragm which have an extension moment about the spine. These pressures are normally contained by tensions in the abdominal muscles, which also have a counterproductive flexion moment about the spine. In this example, however, the abdominal pressure has reduced the compressive force in the spine by about one-third. Wearing a corset promotes this effect, but may harm abdominal muscle tone by partially replacing the activity of these muscles. (Adapted by I.A.F. Stokes from Morris, J.M., Lucas, D.B. and Bresler, B. (1961) *Journal of Bone and Joint Surgery* **43A**, 327–31)

be observed by applying and maintaining sudden loads. Higher loads have faster rates of creep with greater deformation.

The annulus fibrosus with its complex orientation of collagen bundles receives the compressive forces transmitted from the disc. The annulus does not bulge when both structures are normal, but reduction, in the nucleus pulposus material will result in bulging on extension – posteriorly – and on flexion anteriorly. Many of these observations on bulging, displacement of disc walls and indeed mechanical stresses and strains have been made in vitro, in cadaveric studies. MRI studies are giving much better and realistic data.

During the day with differing changes in the loading of the spine, there is change in the water content and height of the disc with secondary effects upon the posterior longitudinal ligament, the adjacent facet joints and the segmental nerves. Adams *et al.* (1990) in a cadaveric study have demonstrated with creep loading of 700–1000 N over a period of time up to 6 hours, that lumbar intervertebral discs lose height and bulge more and become stiffer in compression and more flexible in bending. The disc tissue on losing water becomes more elastic with prolapse less likely, but there is an increased loading of compression and bending stresses on the other spinal structures.

These observations have been confirmed by direct transducer measurements. A newly developed instrument when inserted into the disc recorded compressive stress components under compressive loads of 500–2000 N, and for creep with loads of 1200 N for 3 hours. In the latter study the sagittal diameter was increased up to 13%. Changes were found in the stress gradients of the normally constant levels around the posterior and anterior annulus fibrosus during flexion and extension loading. The sagittal diameter of the disc was increased to 12% during full flexion. Such measurement *in vivo* will add greatly to our knowledge of disc function and pathology (McNally and Adams, 1992).

The capsule resists flexion of the lumbar spine – making up almost 40% against full flexion, with 30% contribution by the intervertebral disc, 20% by the supraspinatous and interspinous ligaments and about 10% by the ligamentous flava. Its tensile strength is about 600 N. During axial loading, extreme torsion of the lumbar spine is prevented by the facet joints which becomes compressed. Beyond 1–2° of rotation the posterior facet joint will fracture in the presence of a normal disc. When there is annular fibrosus damage with narrowing of the disc material, this will result in decrease in the ability of the disc material to handle the rotationary forces (Farfan *et al.*, 1970).

Measurement of the pressures in intervertebral discs (Nachemson, 1972) has helped to explain their function. It has been confirmed that a healthy disc has a hydraulic function, with high pressure in the nucleus being contained by 'hoop' stresses in the annulus which itself carries a smaller pure compressive load. The pressure in the nucleus resulting from compressive load on an intervertebral disc is about 1.5 times the average pressure over the whole of the healthy disc. An older or degenerative disc does not display this differentiation so clearly. Disc pressures measured during various activities and in various postures can be used to estimate the magnitude of the compressive force imposed on the disc. The lumbar disc pressure is higher in seated positions compared with standing. This increase in pressure correlates with increased muscular activity in the back in sitting. However, the provision of a lumbar support minimizes this effect. This suggests that increasing the lordosis reduces the tension in the posterior structures and helps to unload the disc (Andersson *et al.*, 1974).

Spinal biomechanics is a recent science and is still developing its vocabulary for use both by the clinician and the bioengineer. White and Panjabi (1990) have described the functional spinal unit within an XYZ orthogonal co-ordinate system placed in the centrum of the vertebral body. Load, either as a force *F* or a moment *M*, is applied from the upper to the lower vertebra. This results or translates in a resultant motion of the functional spinal unit in six

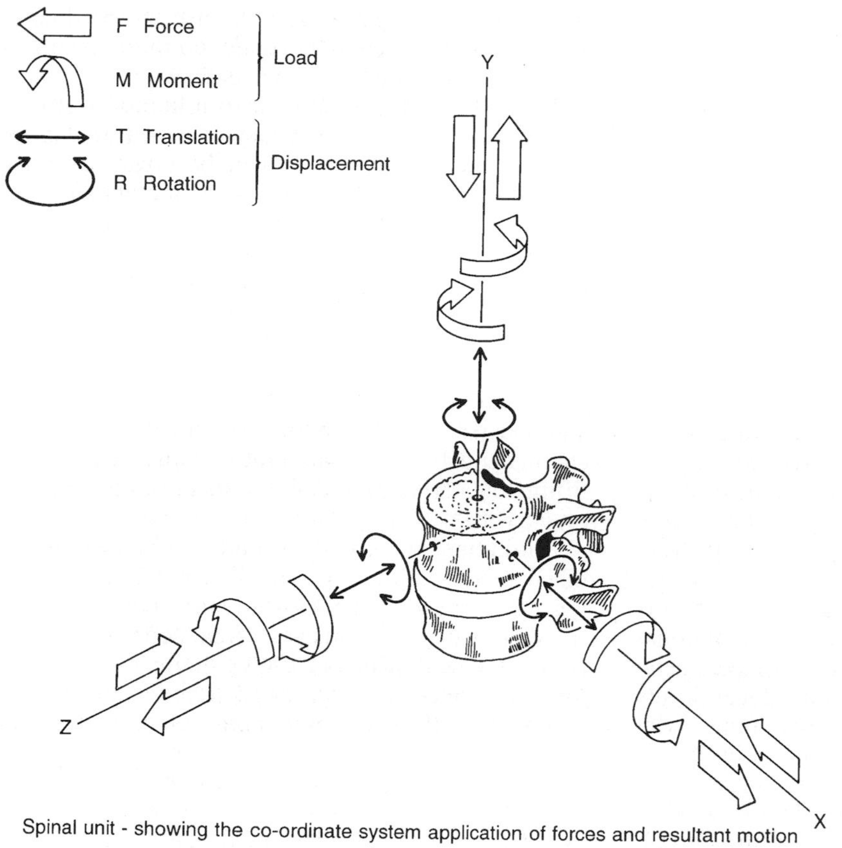

Figure 13.4 The functional spinal unit within an orthogonal co-ordination system, placed in the centrum of the vertebral body and showing the loading, the displacement with the resultant motion. (Reproduced, with permission, from White, A. and Panjabi, M.M. (1990) Clinical *Biomechanics of the Spine* pp. 53–54. Philadelphia: J.B. Lippincott Co.)

parameters or degrees of freedom, i.e. three translations with motion parallel to the axis and three rotations generating motion centred around the axis (Figure 13.4). Measuring all of these is difficult, although loading of the spine can result in motion of the spine in one of all of these parameters – especially from stress (force per unit area) or strain (change in unit length or angle).

The mechanics of the spine in the sagittal plane are the most easy to visualize, but the importance of forces and movements in other directions has been recognized. Torsion and rotation forces in particular have been shown to produce posterior disc lesions in tests on cadaver specimens (Farfan *et al.*, 1970).

FACET JOINTS

The posterior facet joints contribute about half of the resistance to anteroposterior and to rotational forces acting on the intervertebral joints (Farfan *et al.*, 1970). Thus the mechanical consequences of loss or impairment of function in these joints is very significant. Such impairment of function can result from asymmetrical facets, neural arch defects and spondylolysis, surgical removal of lamina, congenital abnormalities of the neural arch, and muscle and ligament attachments.

The facet joint in the lumbar spine is a load-bearing structure and requires its capsule to undergo extensive stretching during physiological loading. Auramou *et al.* (1992) have studied *in vitro* the responses of afferent units of spinal sensory nerves around the lumbar spinal unit.

The first type of response measured was in the phasic type mechanoreceptors, responding to movement regardless of direction or initial position and were velocity detectors. The second type was seen in slowly adapting, low threshold mechanoreceptors in the muscles and tendons inserted into the facet joint of a low 0.3–0.5 k range. The third type were slowly adapting, high threshold mechanoreceptors, triggered by 3–5 k in the capsule – signalling noxious mechanical stimulation comparable to that associated with pain in humans.

Yang and King (1984) emphasized how load transmission through the facet joints and the spine as a whole may exceed 400% of the body weight without producing pain. However, minor pathological changes of loss of disc height or segmental instability may give rise to high loading and stretching of the facet joint capsule with pain.

Lumbosacral junction

This most important joint is prone to congenital anomalies and acquired disorders because of its anatomical arrangement both in development and in use. The iliolumbar ligament, which develops from the quadratus lumborum muscle, appears after the second decade of life. It arises from the top and lower anterior parts of the transverse processes of the fifth lumbar vertebra and runs distally and laterally to the iliac crest on two separate bands with the quadratus sandwiched in between. It has the fifth lumbar root running across with the iliolumbar vein and artery. Chow *et al.* (1989) have studied this important restraining ligament in flexion, extension and lateral bending of L5 upon S1. Their subsequent studies have shown that this ligament was also important in maintaining torsional stability, contributing 35% of the normalized elastic strain of the junction. The posterior facet joints also play an important role in restraining axial rotation of the spine and the intervertebral disc contributes with its annulus fibrosus. From their measurements this group described the iliolumbar ligament as contributing to 14.6% of the failure torque, the facet joints 35% and the disc 50%.

Although work and physical activity are often described as causing low back pain and disability, there are very few direct correlative studies available for such a conclusion. Videman *et al.* (1990) examined 86 male cadavers for symmetrical disc degeneration, annular ruptures and plate defects, osteophyte formation and posterior facet joint arthritis for whom there were occupational, physical loading and back pain histories. History of back injury was related to the presence of disc degeneration, annular ruptures and vertebral osteophytes. Sedentary work was associated with disc degeneration and heavy work was associated with disc degeneration and vertebral osteophyte formation. The least pathologies were related to moderate physical loading and the least back pain was associated with sedentary work.

Bartolotti's syndrome describes the association of low back pain and a transitional lumbosacral vertebrae. From CT and MR imaging studies Elster (1989) found that the overall incidence of structural pathology was not any higher, but the distribution of the associated lesions differed. Bulging or herniation of the disc lesion was nine times more common at the interspace immediately above the transitional vertebra than at the other levels. Spinal stenosis and nerve root canal stenosis was also more common at the above interspace. He described the hypermobility and altered stresses above the transitional vertebra producing secondary pathologies.

Methods used in treatment to influence loadings on the spine include the supply of corsets, prescription of muscle-relaxing drugs, bed, rest, exercise regimens, recommendations about methods of lifting, types of chair and mattress to be used, and surgery. These can be characterized according to their effects on body habitus, especially the lumbar lordosis, limitation of motion of the spine and direct unloading effects. Corsets can have this latter effect in that they increase intra-abdominal pressure, which has an unloading effect on the lumbar spine (Grew and Deane, 1982). Abdominal pressure is raised spontaneously in many activities, especially weight-lifting, by activity of the abdominal muscles (Morris *et al.*, 1961).

Limitation of movement and bed rest of recognized benefit, although restriction of motion by a corset or brace can be disadvantageous in some activities such as transfers from beds and chairs (Lumsden and Morris, 1968). Increasing lumbar lordosis reduces tension on posterior ligaments but compresses the posterior parts of intervertebral discs, while straightening the back has the opposite effect.

Low back pain with or without leg pain

The variable character of low back pain, its multiplicity of causes and the difficulties in its treatment render this affection one of the most perplexing, and also one of the most frequent, problems that confront an orthopaedic surgeon. Moreover, the condition has important industrial and economic aspects, and in this connection the advice of the surgeon is often sought. Many individuals habitually assume, at work or otherwise, positions of great mechanical disability, and sooner or later under the stress and strain, backache results. Industry, both heavy and light, therefore, suffers a severe drain on its manpower from this type of affection, since slight traumata may throw on the disabled list for very long periods those whose bodies have been repeatedly insulted by postural errors and the consequent mechanical strain. Patients with affections of the spine make up a very significant proportion of those permanently disabled for work. Fewer than 50% returned to work again if they had been out of work for over 6 months, no matter what treatment they had received (Wood, 1976).

Low back pain arises from disease, disorder or injury of the lumbosacral spine. Because of the anatomical components making up the motor spinal unit of the spine, pain may be described as:

1. *Local pain* – felt at the site of pathological processes in superficial structures and is usually associated with local tenderness on palpation or percussion.
2. *Diffuse pain* – appears to be more characteristic of deep-lying tissues and has a more or less segmental distribution.
3. *Radicular pain* – as seen in sciatica and brachalgia, and is characterized by its radiation from the centre to the periphery in a strict anatomical sense. It is often associated with paraesthesia and tenderness along the nerve root with neurological signs. Clinical examination frequently reveals neurological deficits such as sensory loss, reflex depression and muscle paresis or paralysis.
4. *Referred pain.*

The nature of referred pain

Kellgren (1937) showed experimentally that distribution of referred muscle pain is difficult to determine because of its diffuse nature and its individual variation.

Pain arising from muscle may not be recognized and is thought to arise from joints, teeth, testes, etc., whereas fasia and tendon sheath give a sharply localized pain. When saline is injected into muscle, pain is referred into the spinal segments from which its motor innervation arises, but does not correspond to the sensory segmental patterns of the skin (Figure 13.5). Tenderness is present in the region in which the pain is felt.

Pain arising in deep fascia, periosteum, ligament or tendon sheath, when these are situated subcutaneously, is localized accurately, but when situated deeper there is a more diffuse pain of a more or less segmental distribution. When arising from interspinous ligaments or intercostal space tissues, it is fully segmental in distribution (Figure 13.6). Therefore, pain from deeper somatic structures can present as a localized and deep pain or as a diffuse pain which may be of a fully segmental distribution, but also can give some form of false localization. This form of pain cannot be distinguished in character from that which arises from visceral disease (Lewis and Kellgren, 1939).

Feinstein *et al.* (1954) injected paravertebral muscles and the intervertebral articulations and demonstrated a gripping, boring pain, somewhat associated with autonomic reflex changes in blood pressure.

The reflex radiation from stimulation of the intervertebral joints is shown in Table 13.1.

ORIGIN OF LOW BACK PAIN

The symptoms may arise from:

1. Bone pain.
2. Muscle and tendon pain.
3. Joint pain.

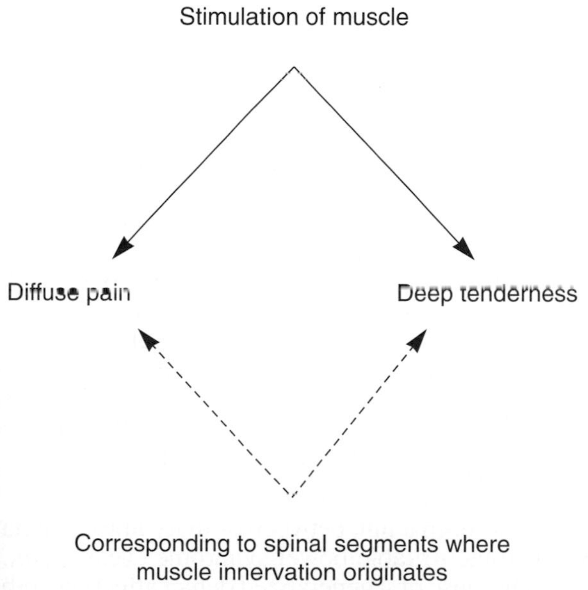

Figure 13.5 Showing the effect of stimulation of muscle. (After Kellgren, J.H. (1939) *Clinical Science* **4**, 35)

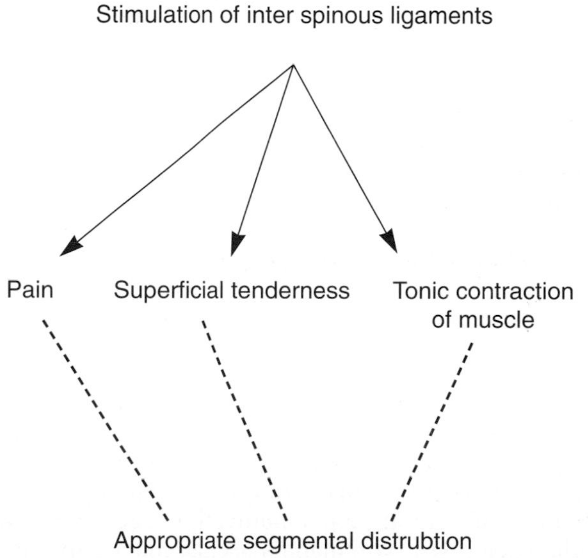

Figure 13.6 Showing the clinical features after stimulation of the intraspinous ligament. (After Kellgren, J.H. (1939) *Clinical Science* **4**, 35)

Table 13.1 Cervical spine

C1	Occipital pain, radiation to forehead
C2–4	Posterior aspect of neck
C3–5	Shoulder region
C6	Arm and forearm
C7, 8	Ulnar side of arm and forearm
Thoracic spine	
T1–10	Thoracic vertebrae: chest and abdomen
Lumbosacral spine	
L1	Groin
L2, 3	Groin and outer side of thigh
L4	Posterior, buttocks, lateral and anterior thigh
L5	Buttocks, anterior, lateral and posterior thigh, lateral leg
S1	Buttocks, posterolateral and anterior thigh, posterior and lateral leg
S2	Buttocks, anterolateral and posterior thigh, lateral and anterior leg
S3	Buttocks, posterior thigh, lateral leg

4. Neurogenic pain – intermittent pseudoclaudication.

Bone pain

Pain, originating in bone is carried by small myelinated and unmeylinated fibres from the periosteum and small blood vessels. It has a characteristic deep, boring quality usually attributable to the stimulus of internal tension. The deep, boring night pain of osteoarthritis is probably of vascular origin. Pain of a similar boring nature but of a somewhat diffuse character occurs in generalized osseous diseases such as osteomalacia, osteoporosis, hyperparathyroidism and metastatic lesions. Bone pain associated with fracture has quite a different character. It is often described as sharp or piercing and is characteristically relieved by rest.

Muscle and tendon pain

Muscle pain may be the result of direct injury or the effects of chemical irritants such as lactic acid and other products of tissue anoxia. When due to direct injury, it is usually described as 'tearing' and is followed by a soreness aggravated by movement, whereas the pain from anoxia is described as a 'cramp-like' pain. Such 'cramp-like' pain is characteristic of intermittent claudication secondary to atherosclerosis, Volkmann's ischaemia or the anterior tibial syndrome. The pain is aggravated by muscle movement. Muscle spasm refers to sustained muscular contraction and is felt as deep, diffuse, persistent pain. Characteristically, in sciatica it produces a scoliosis and in brachalgia a torticollis due to lumbar and cervical nerve root irritation. It is accompanied by local tenderness and a feeling of hardness or spasm of the muscles.

Paroxysmal cramp-like pain accompanied by rigidity or excessive muscle spasm is seen in tetany, which is due to increased sensitivity of the neuromuscular unit consequent upon hypocalcaemia or alkalosis. Muscle cramps are also noted with sodium depletion due to hypermotility of muscle cells, a condition rapidly reversed by restoration of the electrolyte balance. Peripheral neuritis may also present as cramping of muscle masses as well as paraesthesia. Pain is rare in muscular dystrophies and myotonic disorders but is common in the inflammatory myopathies. The pain and accompanying tenderness of fibrositis are related to a specific muscle group, but the pathology is not understood. Morgan-Hughes has emphasized how rare muscle pain is in the muscular dystrophies and in myotonic disorders. Pain is common in the inflammatory myopathies such as polyarthritis nodosa or in polymyalgia rheumatica where there is rapid destruction of muscle cells, involvement of intramuscular blood vessels and defects in the muscular energy metabolism.

Myalgia or pain in a muscle or muscle groups can be differentiated into:

1. Localized myalgia after heavy or unaccustomed exercise, usually resolves quickly with or without treatment. Local acute pathology, e.g. infection, haemorrhage in the haemophiliac, tumour, e.g. sarcoma, myositis ossificans, etc., will have focal signs and positive investigations.
2. Generalized myalgia, secondary to serious pathology, e.g. collagen disease, hypothyroidism, osteomalacia and drug toxicity.
3. Idiopathic chronic myalgia, e.g. primary fibromyalgia syndrome and chronic fatigue syndrome. In primary fibromyalgia syndrome there is diffuse muscle pain and tender areas, but no supportive laboratory or clinical findings. Psychological testing has shown that only 27% were characterized as having a normal personality profile, 52% having a chronic pain profile personality and 24% as having a psychological disturbance profile, but the authors concluded that the features of fibromyalgia are independent of psychological status (Yunus *et al.*, 1991).

There has been a link between primary fibromyalgia and chronic irritable bowel syndrome (Veale *et al.*, 1991) because of a generalized defect affecting both smooth and striated muscle. It is not believed to be an autoimmune disorder.

Tricyclic agents, e.g. amitryptyline or cyclobenaprine may be of use as are anti-inflammatory agents and hypnosis.

Chronic fatigue syndrome is even more indefinite a syndrome. It was called neuraethesia over a hundred years ago, or post-infection fatigue after influenza or infectious mononucleosis disease. Many viruses have been considered as possible agents, or a primary neuromuscular disease, but none has been proven to be causative. Byrne (1992), in reviewing this complex subject, especially when it comes to treatment states one must consider:

1. Background factors, e.g. personality or immunogenetic factors.
2. Trigger factors, i.e. physical or emotional.
3. Enhancing factors, e.g. psychiatric illness.

Joint pain

Joint pain may be attributable to a number of factors:

1. Hyperaemia, of both the synovium and bone.
2. Joint effusion, producing capsular distension and ligamentous laxity.
3. Joint instability, producing traction on capsular structures.
4. Asymmetry of the joint surfaces, particularly in the presence of exposed subchondral bone or cyst formation with tension, i.e. osteoarthritis.
5. Muscle spasm.

Cartilage is avascular and aneural and therefore insensitve to injury.

Neurogenic pain in spinal stenosis

Several spinal studies have demonstrated bilateral nerve root impingement in extension which is relieved in flexion. Penning and Wilmink (1987) performed post-myelographic CT in flexion and extension on patients with spinal stenosis and showed concentric narrowing of the canal in extension, with widening and relief of nerve root involvement in flexion. In extension, bulging of the disc towards the hypertrophic facets caused a pincer action at the anterolateral angles of the spinal canal, which, aggravated by marked dorsal indentation of the dural sac because of anterior movement of the dorsal fat pad. Herzog *et al.* (1991) found that over 50% of patients, with acquired spinal stenosis secondary to facet arthrosis, had posterior compression by epidural fat.

Arterial obstruction, venous hypertension and pressure or traction on the sinuvertebral nerves of Luschka and posterior primary rami have been cited as possible causal factors (Moreland *et al.*, 1989). Venous hypertension within the spinal column is also an important cause. Ooi *et al.* (1990) performed dynamic myeloscopy on 25 patients with lumbar stenosis and 13 patients with disc prolapse. They found transient constriction followed by persistent dilatation of the blood vessels on the cauda equina in only the stenosis patients and postulated that this microcirculatory disturbance might play an important role in the development of neurogenic claudication. Similar evidence by Yazaki *et al.* (1988) relating measuring venous pressure in the ascending lumbar vein, found higher values both at rest and during a Valsalva manoeuvre but a slower recovery in patients with spinal stenosis compared with controls. They suggest that the increased lumbar vertebral venous plexus pressure may be part of the pathogenesis of cauda equina claudation. Although describing a rather different symptom complex known as 'Vesper's curse' LaBan and Wesolowski (1988) reported a series of patients with spinal stenosis whose back and leg pain with neurological symptoms is worse at night and related to their degree of heart failure. They suggest that right heart failure can induce a sufficient increase in pressure and volume in Batson's prevertebral plexus to bring on the symptoms.

Kondo *et al.* (1989) examined somatosensory evoked potentials (stress SEPs) and nerve action potentials (stress NAPs) before and after walking stress. The stress SEPs became abnormal immediately after walking in 31 of 37 patients. Possible causes for the amplitude reduction include blockade of impulses, temporal dispersion and a rise in thresholds. These dynamic studies show that the neural conduction block is caused by stress due to walking in lumbar stenosis. These authors suggest that the pathogenesis of this neural conduction block is due to relative ischaemia of the nerve roots rather than to mechanical compression.

It seems that both mechanical compression and ischaemia are involved concurrently. Indeed, in a post-mortem study of 83 degenerate human lumbar spines that were frozen *in situ* after injection of contrast medium into arteries, Rauschning (1988) showed that in extension and rotation there was significant encroachment on both the nerve root complex and the radicular blood vessels.

CHARACTERISTICS OF LOW BACK PAIN

1. *The situation.* Pain may be described as diffuse, poorly localized, deep-seated or localized to an anatomical area, or radiating, lancinating, and so on.
2. *The reference.* The pain may be referred to a variety of areas.

3. *The duration*. It is important to know how long the pain has been present, and so determine whether the condition is acute or chronic or intermittent.
4. *The mode of onset*. It is essential to know how the condition started, and particularly whether trauma preceded its onset. If there is a history of anything in the nature of an accident, a careful statement should be obtained. Was there a direct injury to the part, or was there a twisting form of violence liable to cause a strain or sprain of some of the joints? Does the history fit in with a diagnosis of a ruptured muscle, or of certain fibres of a muscle, or of ligaments? When the patient is a woman, the history of previous pregnancies should be considered.
5. *What relieves the pain?* Is the pain relieved by resting? Drugs?
6. *What makes it worse?* In the above cases, and in tuberculosis and neoplasm, exercises and unguarded movements cause acute pain. Any awkward, stooping position while at work increases the ache in strains. Coughing, sneezing and straining at stool aggravate the pain in sciatica due to radiculitis or to an intervertebral disc.
7. *Is it worse in the morning?* In organic inflammatory diseases of the spine the pain is worse.
8. *Stiffness*. Does the patient complain of stiffness, and if so where is the stiffness? When is it most noticeable? Stiffness usually indicates some arthritic change, and is therefore most marked in the morning, the site depending on the joint or joints affected.

ACCOMPANYING COMPLAINTS IN OTHER PARTS OF THE BODY

1. *The joints*. If the patient complains of pain in the joints, rheumatoid arthritis may be considered.
2. *Neurological symptoms*, such as paraesthesiae altered sensation and imbalance.
3. *Genitourinary symptoms*. If there is any frequency of micturition, dysuria or obstruction, a careful urological investigation should be carried out.
4. *Gynaecological history*. In women, the condition of the reproductive organs should be the subject of inquiry, and a gynaecological opinion sought. Pain which is increased during menstruation suggests a chronic ligamentous strain, as the ligaments of the pelvis are congested at that time.
5. *History of other diseases*. Osteomyelitis, arthritis, gonorrnoea, typhoid fever, tuberculosis, syphilis and secondary neoplasm should be excluded.

EXAMINATION OF THE PATIENT

The patient is examined in both the erect and recumbent positions.

Standing

The general posture, weight, muscular development and tone are noted. Careful observation is necessary for some minor abnormality of posture which the patient adopts.

The spinal curves are examined and any deviation from the normal noted. A slight tilt of the pelvis which has resulted from the shortening of one limb and which has caused a compensatory scoliosis may be the error of posture responsible for the symptoms.

The movements of flexion, extension and lateral flexion are carried out and abnormalities such as rigidity, muscle spasm or the production of pain noted (Figure 13.7).

Aird (1955) emphasized a test for spinal movements much used in medical tribunals to diagnose a case of hysterical limitation of movement or even malingering. Flexion of the spine is first examined with the patient standing and thereafter on the examination couch. On the couch he is invited to sit up and bend forward while a show is made of palpating his spine from behind. It is sometimes quite remarkable how differently the spine flexes in the two methods. This forward flexion movement to touch the toes, with the knees extended, is also a means to confirm the straight leg raise test.

Sitting

Movements of the spine, both active and passive, are investigated in the manner indicated above.

The reflexes are tested, the condition of the circulation observed and blood pressure recorded.

Lying

Measurement of the length and girth of the limbs is carried out. Demonstrable wasting of calf or thigh is important since it is an objective finding.

The contour and range of movement of the joints of the legs are observed.

Abdominal palpation is carried out.

Points of tenderness are sought, although they are rarely useful.

Rectal and prostatic examinations are made.

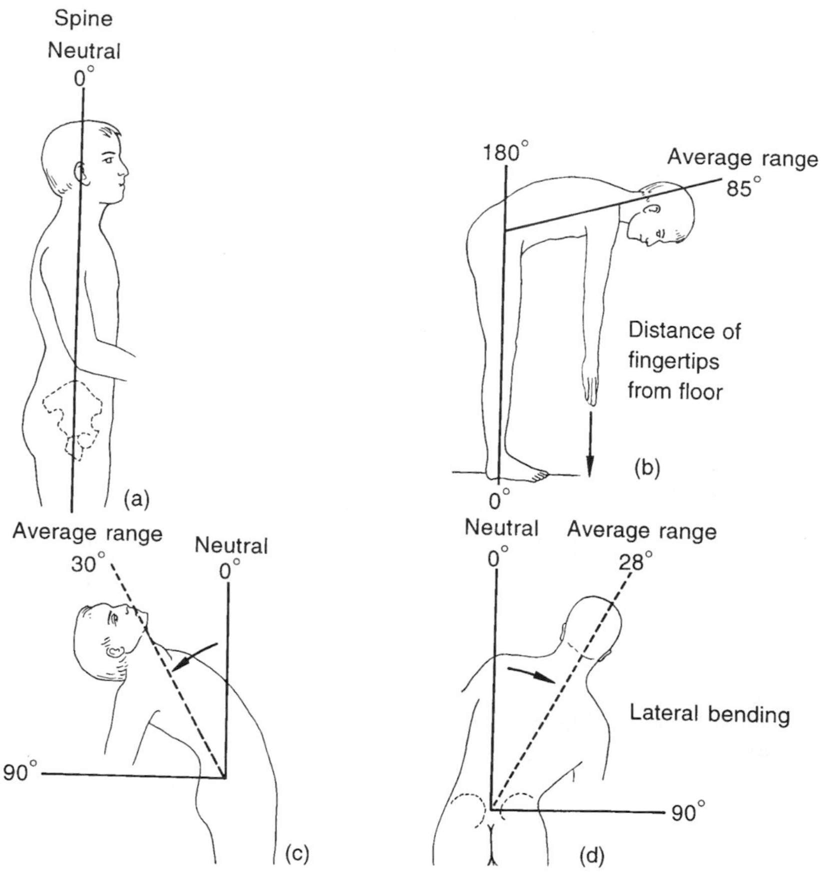

Figure 13.7 (a) Neutral position (0°) of the spine from the side. (b) Forward flexion of the spine with an average range of 85° or by measuring distance of fingertips from the floor. (c) Extension of lumbar spine to an average range of 30° from the neutral plane of 0°. (d) Lateral flexion of an average range of 28°.

Straight leg raising test

Although accredited to Lasègue who had written on sciatica in 1864, it was Forst who first described it in 1881 and dedicated it to Lasègue and to his parents. However, Forst wrongly described it as resulting from compression of the nerve by the hamstrings. It was De Beurmann in 1884 who redescribed the test and wrote that it was due to stretching of the sciatic nerve, after Lazarenic's description in 1880 of the effect of straight leg raising in six patients. Inman and Saunders (1942) demonstrated in cadavers the radiographic migration of lumbar roots, and Falconer *et al.* (1948) demonstrated these root excursions at the time of surgery with straight leg raising and crossed straight leg raising.

Lasègue's sign (straight leg raising test) is carried out with the patient supine on a couch. The straight leg is flexed at the hip and usually it can be lifted to 90° or more, the distance depending on the tautness of the hamstrings. Limitation of movement and pain are usually present in low back pain and sciatica. When the leg is flexed, dorsiflexion of the foot increases the pull on the sciatic nerve without altering the tension of the hamstrings and this increases sciatic pain but not pain from other causes. O'Connell (1950) pointed out that there is a 2 cm excursion on straight leg raising of the L4, 5 and S1 and 2 nerve roots, which is readily obstructed or hindered by adhesion formation or prolapse of disc material.

Well leg raising test

Fajersztajn described in 1901 the cross-sciatic reflex test or well leg raising test. Woodhall and Hayes (1950) demonstrated that the third of their patients with disc prolapse and a positive well leg raising test had a large protrusion affecting the medial aspect of the nerve root.

Fajersztajn also added the foot dorsiflexion and neck flexion tests which are performed with the leg elevated and are positive when pain on straight leg raising is aggravated.

Femoral stretch test

The patient should be placed in the prone position and then the lower extremity with the knee straight is lifted at the hip. This produces tension on the upper three lumbar roots in the back and the femoral nerve in the thigh. If there is any deformation of these structures, pain may be experienced in the thigh. This test is of doubtful clinical value.

Neurological examination

Power, tone, reflexes, sensation, posterior column function and balance should be tested.

Radiographic examination

Anteroposterior and lateral views of the spine, extending well above and well below the suspected site, should be taken. It is important, in cases of doubt, to take an oblique view in order to get a view of the pars interarticularis (Figure 13.8).

Plain films

These cannot produce conclusive diagnosis of lumbar disc protrusion, but a single narrowed disc space in a patient of less than 40 years with associated loss of lordosis, is very suggestive. They are helpful to exclude other conditions (e.g. malignant disease) and to assess spinal stenosis, facet joints, spondylolisthesis, etc. Flexion and extension views are often helpful to demonstrate instability.

Myelography

Myelography in which contrast media is injected is still very helpful in some cases, especially using water-soluble materials – e.g. metrizamide (Amipaque), iohexol (Omnipaque). Some reported adverse effects are:

1. Headache, nausea, vomiting.
2. Spasms, seizures and interaction with epileptogenic drugs (phenothiazines, cytotoxics, etc.).
3. Others:
   (a) short term: areflexia, numbness, pain increase, voiding disturbances;
   (b) long term: arachnoiditis.

Myelography is most useful in determining the level of pathology when it is not clear from MRI or CT scanning.

MRI

Magnetic resonance imaging (MRI) can show significant signs associated with arachnoiditis, i.e. central roots within the thecal space are adherent and

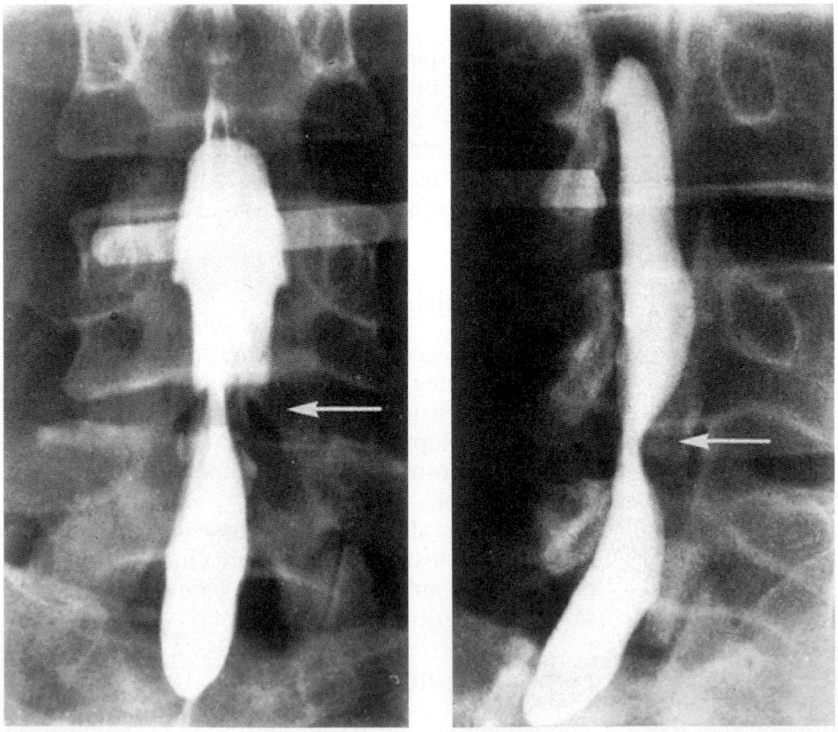

(a) (b)

Figure 13.8 Radiographs with radiopaque dye *in situ* to show a filling defect of L4/5 level due to disc protrusion: (a) anteroposterior view and; (b) lateral–oblique view.

clumped together, peripherally the roots are thickened and in severe cases a soft tissue mass replaces the subarachnoid space. Johnson and Sze (1990) did not believe that gadolinium enhancement significantly improved the diagnosis.

Arachnoiditis may also be caused by misplaced catheters during epidural anaesthesia as well as chemically induced arachnoiditis by higher concentration of the local anaesthetic agent. Sklar *et al.* (1991) have described the MR imaging appearances as subarachnoid cyst formation, loculations and spinal cord surface irregularities.

Discography

Discography is indicated when there had been a previous negative myelogram, or previous surgery or the possibility of vertebral fusion – probably now the only valid indication. There may be pain reproduction, or a normal disc outline assessed by appearance on screening and 'hydraulic' sensation on injection, or pathological findings (e.g. fissuring with leakage).

Discography is still controversial with strong supporters on either side. Schecter *et al.* (1991) used this technique to evaluate patients with low back pain, but without disc herniation, stenosis or instability, to select levels for fusion with 89% good or excellent results.

Simmons *et al.* (1991) have used 'awake' discography with MR imaging in patients with low back pain with or without radicular symptoms, to differentiate symptomatic from asymptomatic degenerative discs.

High false-positive rates have been reported but a more recent study by Walsh *et al.* (1990) of normal human volunteers who received a discographic injection showed 17% of the 30 discs were abnormal; no significant pain response occurred. However, in the symptomatic group 65% of the discs were abnormal and typical pain was induced in 8 discs in 6 patients. Therefore the false-positive rates were low.

^{99}Tc-diphosphonate bone scan

^{99}Tc scanning is most useful as an indicator of inflammation or tumour in the spine. It is thus very useful in spinal pain of unclear cause to exclude malignancy and in young people to indicate conditions such as osteoid osteoma or ankylosing spondylitis.

The principles of MR imaging have been discussed in Chapter 1. However, it is now imperative to consider all these techniques for various back problems and to use them appropriately where indicated.

Spinal imaging for back pain with or without leg pain

Plain radiology

Valid clinical indications, i.e. intractable pain, progressive neurological deficit and failed conservative therapy, are essential for all x-ray examinations. The doses received by patients in the UK during diagnostic medical radiographic examinations make up 87% of the total collective dose to the whole population, i.e. 15% of this coming from lumbar spinal radiographs. Plain x-rays for diagnosing the pathology of herniated disc are of little value. There is no correlation between back pain and transitional vertebrae, spina bifida, lumbar lordosis or Schmorl's nodes.

Plain x-rays have a very limited role in diagnosis of pathologies associated with low back pain, except to demonstrate spondolisthesis and congenital defects, spondylosis, ankylosing spondylitis, pedicular metastases and other neoplasms, and infection.

Most radiologists now do not recommend using routine AP, lateral and oblique views of the lumbar or lumbosacral spine. No significant diagnostic information is lost by only examining a single film view – either AP or lateral. Indeed, most just recommend a single lateral view in patients with symptoms of back pain but without apparent or suspected cause (Padley *et al.*, 1990) especially if a subsequent CT examination is planned (Tress and Hare, 1990).

A comparison of MRI, CT, discography and myelography techniques in spinal imaging

Many clinicians now have ready access to those investigative modalities which have high sensitivity and specificity but are expensive and time-consuming. Therefore, their selection for being most appropriate must be based upon knowing their advantages and disadvantages. The advantages of MR imaging are in not requiring any radiation, being non-invasive, having excellent simultaneous axial and sagittal images of soft tissues, disc structure, ligaments, muscles, joints and bone marrow (Figure 13.9). CT imaging with or without enhancement gives excellent bone and joint structural images, but at a price of some radiation.

False-positive findings are common with these techniques, and highlight how their results must be strictly correlated with the clinical picture and the suspected pathology before any treatment is initiated.

CT, particularly contrast-enhanced, is well estab-

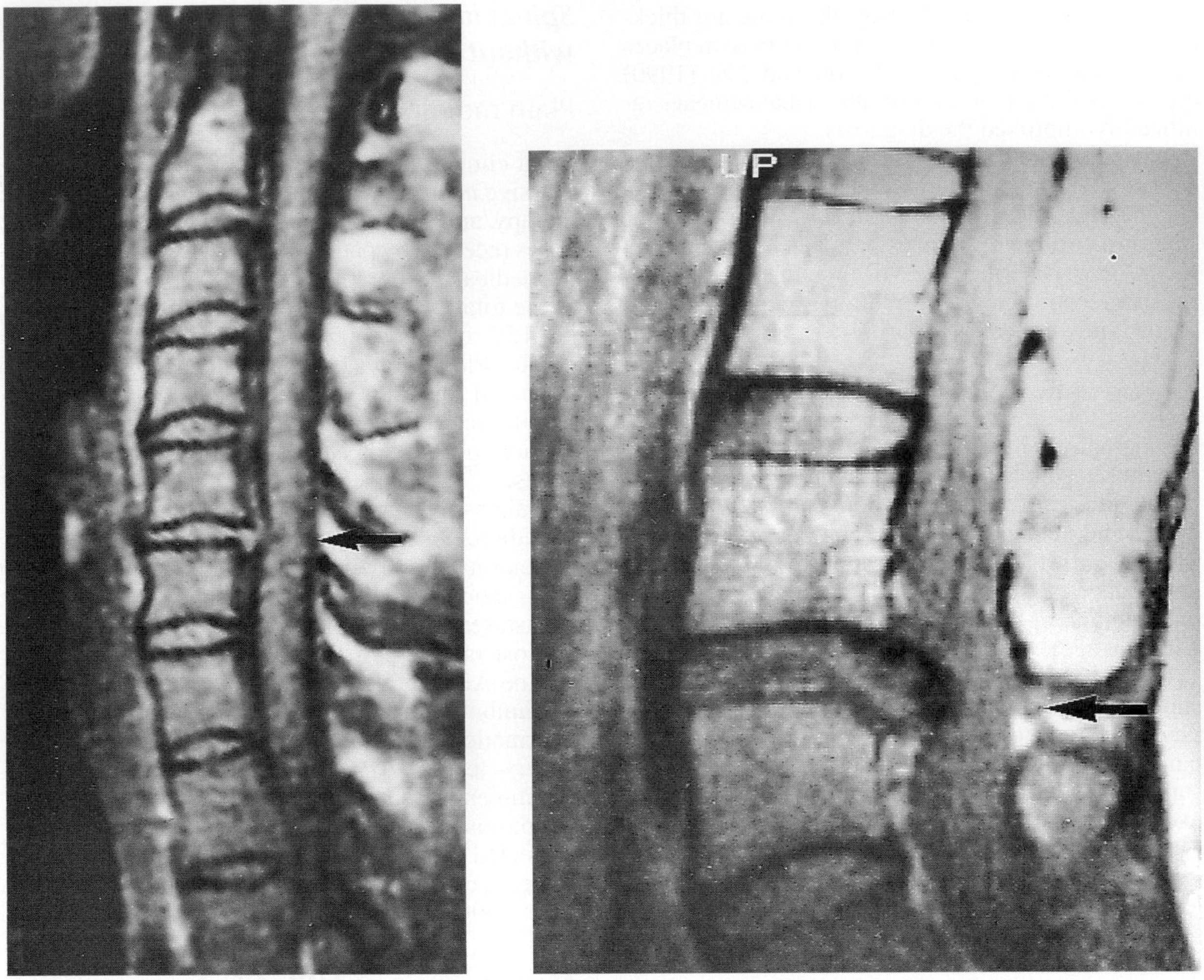

(a) (b)

Figure 13.9 (a) MRI of cervical spine in lateral projection (T1 weighted image). Dorsal discal prolapse with displacement of posterior longitudinal ligament and indention of the theca at the C5/6 level (arrow). (b) MRI of lumbar spine in lateral projection showing a prolapsed and degenerate lumbar disc associated with marked narrowing of the spinal canal (T1 weighted image).

lished as a useful technique, as also is myelography followed by CT (Moreland *et al*., 1989). It demonstrates the configuration of the lateral recesses better than myelography as even water soluble contrast agents rarely diffuse that far laterally. It has also been invaluable in visualizing levels below a myelographic block. Schnebel *et al*. 1989) compared MRI with contrast CT in 41 patients (123 segments) and found a 96.6% agreement in the diagnosis of spinal stenosis. MRI is more sensitive in diagnosing disc degeneration, showing it in 74 of 123 segments compared with 27 by CT.

MRI is becoming the modality of choice in imaging following surgery in patients with recurrent symptoms as it can differentiate scar from disc and show haematoma, infection or even fat graft compression on the thecal sac (Djukic *et al*., 1990). Care must be taken to correlate both these techniques with the clinical picture. Wiesel *et al*. (1984) found CT abnormalities in 50% of asymptomatic patients over 40 years of age and Boden *et al*. (1990) found MRI abnormalities in 57% of asymptomatic patients over 60 years of age. Thus both techniques have high sensitivity but relatively low specificity.

A few authors still believe myelography to be the investigation of choice as it can be performed sitting or even standing and can exclude tumour of the conus medullaris. Chevrot *et al*. (1988) studied lateral images in the sitting and standing positions in 150 myelograms in patients with disc prolapse or spinal stenosis. Twenty-three per cent had an AP dural sac measurement of 10 mm or less in the standing position, due in 65% of cases to an isolated or predominant posterior impression, the latter appearing only in the standing position in 55% of cases. They suggested that only myelography can be performed standing and should be used in suspected spinal stenosis even if CT or MRI performed lying, showed normal canal dimensions.

Laboratory examination

This should include haemoglobin, ESR and full blood count, and urine, blood calcium, phosphate, alkaline and acid phosphatases, sugar, serum protein immuno-electrophoresis and SGOT titres.

The low back syndrome

By 'low back syndrome' is meant either disease or injury of the lumbosacral spine with or without an underlying predisposing condition. This can be acute or become chronic with definite increasing frequency, longer duration and eventual deterioration of the physical condition (Table 13.2). Such a syndrome has increasing importance in our middle-aged and ageing populations, particularly in relationship to industry and work, since it is the greatest cause of loss of work and permanency in compensation cases. Varying conditions can produce such a syndrome. These are seen in Table 13.3, but referred lumbosacral pain from intra-abdominal or pelvic causes, and any psychosomatic condition are also important.

The low back syndrome usually occurs in the third, fourth and fifth decades of life as an acute low back pain and spasm. This is aggravated by coughing, sneezing or defaecation, but rarely has any true radicular nature and is relieved by lying with flexion of the knees. On examination, there may be tenderness in the lumbosacral angles or along the spinous processes of the ligaments between. There is some limitation of vertebral movement with spasm of the paravertebral muscles.

Table 13.2 The various factors making up the low back syndrome

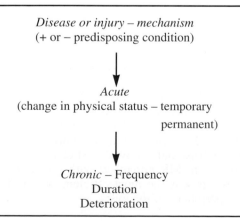

Disease or injury – mechanism
(+ or – predisposing condition)

↓

Acute
(change in physical status – temporary
permanent)

↓

Chronic – Frequency
Duration
Deterioration

Sciatica may be present and x-rays frequently show non-specific disc space narrowing or early osteophytes. The vast majority of cases are simply strains of the ligaments or protrusion from spinal joints and settle rapidly (Nachemson, 1985). Low back pain in children and adolescents is often serious and should be investigated thoroughly (Figure 13.10).

Treatment is conservative with adequate bed rest, sedation and some form of superficial heat to help the muscle spasm.

Rowe (1960) emphasized the concept of degenerative disc disease as being one of the explanations for the commonly recurring acute low back pain. During the normal ageing process – when the mechanical stresses in the lower lumbar spine fall primarily on the posterior aspects of the annulus fibrosus, particularly at the fourth and fifth lumbar levels – multiple, but minor, traumata will produce gradual loss of disc material. This may result in irritation of the adjacent nerve root to give the clinical diagnosis of a 'lumbosacral strain' or a 'lumbago', or a 'myositis' or a 'sacroiliac strain'. Narrowing of the intervertebral space may progress so that the neural foramen becomes small and distorted, and spondylosis or a reverse spondylolisthesis may occur with further narrowing of the intervertebral foramen (Figure 13.11). Involvement of the nerve root results in a pain-spasm reflex which may produce some degree of ischaemia of the muscle tissue and, hence, further pain.

Posterior facet joint disease

As the intervertebral discs narrow with age and degenerative changes, the posterior facet joints, which are synovial, develop greater or lesser degrees of osteoarthritis. Symptoms may predominate from these joints, producing the posterior facet joint syndrome. Experimental studies in which hypertonic saline was injected into these joints caused severe local back pain and some referred pain into the buttocks and posterior thigh (McCall *et al.*, 1979).

The nerve supply to these joints comes from the posterior primary rami at the same level and from above. This fact has given rise to the treatment of injecting the lumbar facet joints for low back pain with local anaesthetic agents and cortisone. However, Lilius *et al.* (1989), in a carefully carried out randomized trial, showed that a significant

Table 13.3 Causes of low back pain

Structural defects of bone
Segmentation defects
1. 6 lumbar vertebrae
2. 4 lumbar vertebrae
3. Transitional lumbosacral junction (Bertolotti's syndrome)
Ossification defects
1. Spina bifida
2. Spondylosis
3. Spondylolisthesis
Facet abnormalities
1. Asymmetry (tropism)
2. Anteroposterior lumbosacral facets
3. Increased lumbosacral angle
Functional defects
Lateral imbalance (leg length discrepancy, scoliosis, postural attitudes, etc.)
Anteroposterior imbalance (pregnancy, pot belly, flexion contracture of hips and knees)
Infections
Bone and joint
1. Staphylococcal, streptococcal
2. Tuberculosis
3. Brucellosis
4. Salmonella (in sickle-cell disease)
5. Spondyloarthropathies, e.g. spondylitis, ankylosis and Reiter's syndrome
Soft tissue – muscle and fascia
1. Myositis
2. Fibrositis
Degenerative processes
Osteoarthritis
Postmenopausal osteoporosis
Degenerative disc disease
Neoplastic processes
Primary
1. Multiple myeloma
2. Haemangioma
3. Giant cell tumour, eosinophilic granuloma, osteoid osteoma (Figure 13.10)
Metastatic
1. Prostate and breast
2. Lung, kidney, thyroid, gastrointestinal tract
Traumatic
Compression fracture
Vertebral process fracture (facet, transverse and spinous process) and subchondral plate
Sprain and strain
Ruptured disc – herniation – tear of annulus fibrosus

improvement was achieved in work attendance, pain and disability scores, but this was independent of whether physiological saline or local anaesthetic agents were used with cortisone, or when injections were given intracapsularly or pericapsularly. They concluded their good results came from a non-specific method of treatment and depended upon a spontaneous regression tendency and to the psychosocial aspects of back pain.

Synovial cyst formation can occur around degenerative lumbar joints. These are usually extraspinal but Silbergleit *et al.* (1990), using myelography, axial CT, MR imaging and pathology, have described intraspinal synovial cyst causing nerve root compression. MR enhanced with gadolinium contrast agents was the most efficient in outlining the rim or periphery of the cysts.

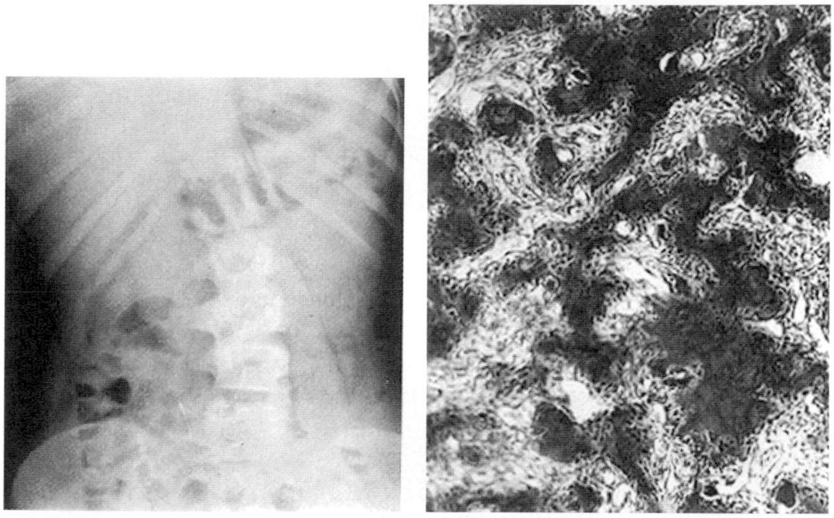

(a) (b)

Figure 13.10 (a) Osteoid osteoma of the third lumbar vertebra with sclerosis and enlargement of the bone of the transverse process. A protective scoliosis is secondary to muscle spasm. (b) Photomicrograph of osteoid material removed from lesion.

Low back pain and congenital developmental errors

There are numerous minor developmental abnormalities seen in radiographs of the lumbar spine but very few have been shown to produce pain. It is important to look for other abnormalities when such changes are seen.

THE VERTEBRAL BODY

The bodies of the vertebrae ossify from two separate centres, which may be alongside each other, be superimposed or even be one behind the other. When the two centres of ossification do not develop properly, or fail to fuse, the radiographic appearance is that of a split body, and there is often some separation between the two halves. The appearance has no clinical significance, and is thought to be due to delayed union of the notochordal segments. A split

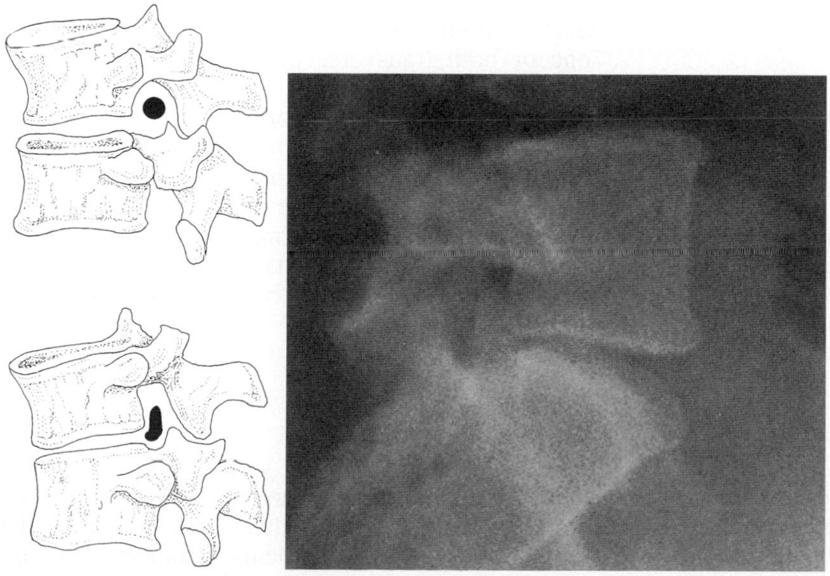

(a) (b)

Figure 13.11 (a) Diagram of two adjacent lumbar vertebrae showing how narrowing of the intervertebral disc space and reduction in the foramen may produce deformity of the nerve (after Rowe, M.L. (1960) *Journal of Occupational Medicine* **2**, 219). (b) Lateral radiograph of the lumbar spine, showing some disc space narrowing between L5 and S1 vertebrae with a reverse spondylolysis.

body does not give rise to deformity, but if one of the true centres actually fails to appear, a hemivertebra is produced and leads to a spinal curvature, usually a scoliosis. The balance of the erect posture is then altered and compensating secondary lateral curvatures arise.

Intraspinal abnormalities occur particularly when congenital spinal deformities are present. Bradford *et al.* (1991) found, by MR scanning, 38% of patients with such deformities, usually a congenital scoliosis, have also tethered cord (10), diastomatomyelia (4), diplomella (3) and syringomyelia (4). Therefore they recommend routine MR scanning in preparation for any spinal stabilization procedure.

Sometimes two vertebral bodies may be fused together, but this condition is usually symptomless.

THE ARTICULAR PROCESSES

The articular facts of the lumbosacral joints show great variations in shape and in the plane of their surfaces. Normally the articular processes are vertical, and the facets lie in the sagittal plane, but on one or both sides the processes may show the characteristics of the thoracic region, where the facets face forward and backward respectively; in other cases, one facet may be directed backward and the other medially.

When the facets are thus asymmetrical, abnormal movements may occur. Brailsford (1929) found that the articular facets of the fifth lumbar vertebra were directed in various ways: 57% backward; 12% medially; and 31% mixed, the directions on the two sides being different.

THE NEURAL ARCH

The principal anomaly in this region is a lack of fusion between the two halves of the arch. The condition occurs either in the fifth lumbar or in the first sacral vertebra, and the defect is situated in the midline, thus constituting a spina bifida occulta. The only evidence of such an error may be a small lipoma, a tuft of hair or a dimple in the skin of the lumbosacral region. There may be no symptoms, although frequently there are coexisting deformities of the lower limb (e.g. pes cavus). Instability in the lumbosacral region and low back pain are common accompaniments.

In addition to this central defect, there may be anomalies in the attachment of the laminae to the body on one or both sides. These may be found along with the commoner central defect. All varieties of congenital error in this situation are more common in males (Figure 13.12).

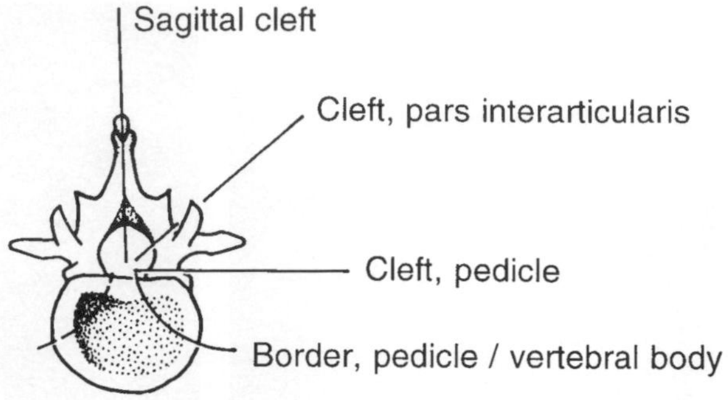

Figure 13.12 The various anatomical sites in which lack of fusion can be found in the developing vertebrae.

TRANSVERSE PROCESSES OF THE LUMBAR VERTEBRAE

Most of the anomalies of transverse processes concern the fifth lumbar vertebra, of which they comprise by far the most variable components. Variation in the size and shape of the transverse processes of the remaining vertebrae, such as may be seen in the third lumbar vertebra especially in women, is of little clinical significance.

Sacralization of the transverse processes of the fifth lumbar vertebra

Sacralization is a developmental anomaly in which one or both transverse processes of the vertebra become abnormally large and strong. They may become so large that they form a connection with the base of the sacrum or ilium, and by this union a foramen forms between the lower margin of the transverse process and the upper free edge of the sacrum instead of the normal broad and irregular cleft. In such cases the transverse process often has the appearance of a butterfly's wing (Figures 13.13 and 13.14).

PATHOLOGY

The so-called transitional vertebrae are vertebrae which, by transition from one segment of the vertebral column to another, have acquired the characteristics of both segments. Instances of this are seen in the so-called cervical rib which is really a dorsalization of the seventh cervical vertebra.

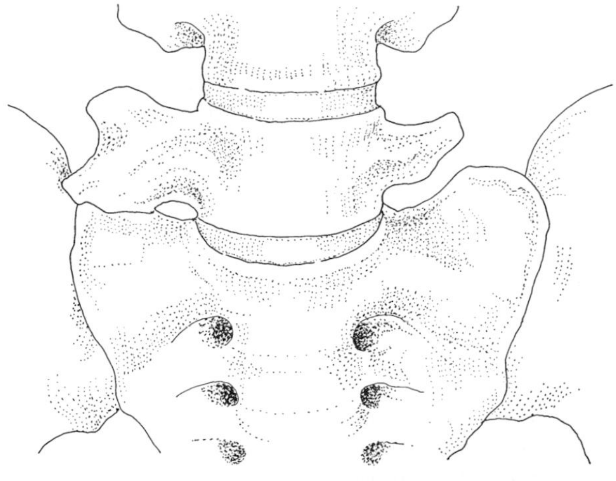

Figure 13.13 Sacralization of the transverse process of the fifth vertebra.

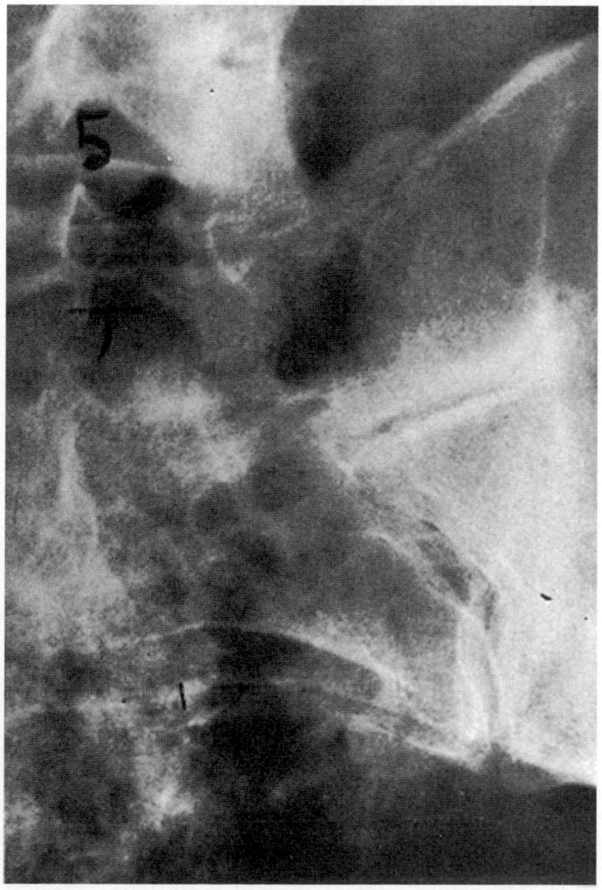

Figure 13.14 An enlarged anteroposterior radiograph showing a transitional lumbar vertebra with sacralization. There is also an abnormal joint formation in the left sacroiliac area with sclerosis and irregularity of the anomalous joint.

Ossification of the sacral vertebrae proceeds from three centres of ossification – one in the body and one in each of the two lateral processes – but in the first, second and third sacral vertebrae there appears, ventral to the centre of ossification in the lateral process an extra centre of ossification.

Various theories have been put forward to explain local pain in such. It has been suggested that it might be due to arthritis of the new joint, while many have suggested that it is due to compression or stretching of nerve fibres where they leave the column. The fourth lumbar nerve is said to be occasionally stretched over the large transverse process. The posterior branch of the fifth lumbar nerve comes out in front of the transverse process of the fifth lumbar vertebra which, even in its worst form, appears to leave sufficient room for the branches of this nerve.

It is generally agreed that this congenital anomaly produces symptoms only when it is unilateral and, hence, preventing normal lateral flexion. The fifth root is particularly vulnerable during excision.

TREATMENT

Treatment, if necessary, is usually conservative with physiotherapy and support. Rarely is an excision indicated.

Low back pain following trauma: lumbosacral strain

Under this heading come an assortment of clinical presentations which are characterized by a history of trauma and absence of nerve root symptoms and signs. The diagnosis is therefore to be used with caution.

AETIOLOGY

In the embryo of 9 weeks the sacrum is nearly straight and forms a direct continuation of the lumbar region. From this time onward the sacrum alters its direction and the lumbosacral angle begins to form. In the adult the average angle is 120°, but variations are common. In addition to the great variations in the angle, this region is unstable for the following reasons:

1. It is the junction of a mobile and a fixed part of the spinal column.
2. It is developmentally designed for the four-footed position and hence is at a disadvantage in the upright position.

3. It is the site of a rotatory and shearing strains which are often asymmetrical.

Structural abnormalities in the lumbosacral region render this part of the spine more vulnerable to mechanical stress and strain than is normal. This does not imply that all individuals with anomalies in this area have symptoms in consequence, but it does mean that if an individual with symptoms referable to the lower part of the back is found to have some anatomical variation in the lumbosacral region, this anomaly should be borne in mind as a cause of symptoms until or unless another cause can be demonstrated.

Lumbosacral strain occurs in both acute and chronic forms. The acute form may be caused by a sudden blow forcing the joint into positions beyond the normal range of movement, by an effort to prevent a heavy article falling or by a sudden body movement while attempting to regain lost balance. The spinal muscles are caught off guard and thus the ligaments are assumed to sustain the full force of the injury.

The chronic form is usually insidious in onset but may follow an acute strain which has been unrecognized or untreated. It occurs in the back with poor musculature and an increase of the normal lumbar lordosis or in a type of patient whose increase of weight in recent years takes the form of a pendulous abdomen. The maintenance of the body balance necessitates an exaggeration of lumbar lordosis with consequent increase of the shearing strain at the lumbosacral angle. In some cases, narrowing of the intervertebral disc space is noted. As the bodies approximate, there may be encroachment on the intervertebral foramen with root pressure.

SYMPTOMATOLOGY

In acute cases with a history of recent trauma the pain and tenderness are situated at the lumbosacral junction and the movements of the spine are restricted in all directions.

In chronic cases the symptoms vary, some patients merely complaining of a 'weak back' which tires easily, while others suffer very acute pain and real disability. Often there is a history of intervening periods of comfort lasting several years, between attacks of pain, but gradually the attacks become more and more frequent or the pain may become constant as age advances. Sciatic pain and sciatic scoliosis may be present if there is root pressure, but neurological signs are not present and radiographs usually are normal.

TREATMENT

In the acute stage, rest in bed for a short period of 1–2 weeks may be necessary. The patient should lie in a bed fitted with fracture boards, and pillows are placed beneath the knees. When the acute symptoms have subsided and, as improvement takes place, graduated spinal and postural exercises are instituted. Anti-inflammatory agents are useful.

Chronic lumbosacral strain presents a more complex problem and dramatic results are not to be expected. Thereafter exercises designed to flatten the lumbar curve, increase muscle tone and improve posture form the essential local treatment. The fitting of a back brace is rarely necessary or desirable, but those patients with pendulous abdomens frequently benefit from weight loss or occasionally the support of a lumbosacral corset.

Low back pain following trauma: injuries to intervertebral joints, ligaments and muscles

These injuries are produced by such external violence as overstretching of the spinal column and are thus common in the mobile areas of the cervical, thoracolumbar and lumbar regions. The pain is sudden and, although increased by certain movements, it is constantly present during the acute stage and is only partly relieved by rest.

Considerable violence is needed to produce ligamentous injury and is certainly present if fractures of the lumbar transverse processes are seen on radiographs. Sporting injuries are increasing and the use of MRI and CT for stress fractures in the pars interarticularis of the L5 vertebra is very valuable (Hardcastle *et al.*, 1992). Muscle injuries also undoubtedly occur, but are usually due to a voluntary action which presumably produces rupture of some muscle fibres with consequent bleeding into the tissues.

TREATMENT

In severe injuries the treatment is initially bed rest and analgesics, followed by rapid mobilization in an appropriate brace until the pain is controlled. It is vital to encourage the patient to be as active as possible and physiotherapy, especially trunk and back exercises, should begin within a few days.

In some cases, particularly those who apply for treatment only at a late stage, the symptoms will persist or even become worse. The patient, consciously or unconsciously, exaggerates his symptoms. When it is suspected that the patient is exaggerating his disability, or that a frank neurosis has developed, the services of a psychiatrist should be considered, as the treatment of the mental condition is of more importance than that of the back.

Psychological aspects of back pain

The understanding of specific problems of back pain requires an appreciation of pain in general.

NEUROPHYSIOLOGICAL ASPECTS OF PAIN

Weddell (1962) and Noordenbos (1959) suggested that when peripheral stimuli are great enough to threaten the integrity of tissues, they are transferred via nerve terminals into a pattern or code which, when conducted to the neuraxis and thence to the thalamus and higher brain centres, may be interpreted as 'pain'. This process of interpretation is made mentally, and hence by definition is always a psychological process. Also, the higher nervous system representation of such coded impulses allows for the possibility of pain experience which is not necessarily induced by any new impulse from peripheral sites.

For further discussion of this topic see Chapter 1.

PSYCHOLOGICAL ASPECTS OF PAIN

The psychological and developmental significance of pain was thoroughly reviewed by Engel (1962), who made the following points:

1. Pain is an intimate part of the warning systems of the body which serve to signal the presence of danger. Accordingly, in infancy it is initially part of the process whereby the child learns about the environment and its dangers, as well as about the body and its limitations. Early experiences of pain may be recorded in the individual's 'memory'.
2. The infant responds to pain by crying (a communication to another person), and the cry evokes a response from the other person – usually an effort to relieve the infant's distress. In this manner, pain begins to assume value in relationship to another person; and, since the other person's response relieves the pain and expresses love, pleasure begins to be associated with pain.
3. Later, in the process of disciplinary training, the child is taught that being 'bad' will often bring him pain, and pain can become associated in such a manner that it may come to mean, 'I am bad'. He is also taught that suffering pain is a means of expiating guilt, gaining forgiveness and regaining a pleasurable reunion with another person.
4. Aggression and power become associated with pain because the child learns that he can impose his will on others by inflicting (or threatening to inflict) pain, and others can control his aggressive impulses by the same device. He may incorporate this device into his own intrapsychic mechanisms and come to either experience pain or expose himself to painful injuries as a means of controlling his own aggressive impulses.

THE 'CHOICE' OF PAIN AS A SYMPTOM

A patient may complain of many symptoms, but the sensation of pain begins early in life and in the course of development comes to subserve many important intrapsychic functions of which the invariable factor is conscious or unconscious guilt. In addition, the complaint of pain is effective as a means of communicating with others for the purposes of gaining attention, protection, love or forgiveness.

Clinical experience reveals that certain individuals have a predilection towards pain as a symptom. This pain is described as a somatic symptom, but it is derived mentally to serve psychological needs. By and large, these are mediated through unconscious mental mechanisms. It is these 'pain-prone' patients and their psychogenic pain which are important clinically.

THE 'CHOICE' OF BACK PAIN

A patient may complain of pain in any part of his body, but there are certain regions for the complaint of pain, which include the back and in particular the lower back.

Special meanings of the back

These relate to certain unique aspects of the anatomy, function and location of the back. The back is used to support other portions of the body and loads which may be placed upon it for transportation.

Being located posteriorly, it is the part of the body not visible to us without the aid of some mechanical device; so to observe one's own back, some sort of reflector becomes necessary.

Both in the impulse to take aggressive action against someone else and in the fear of being attacked, the back again figures prominently.

Special meanings of the back to a particular individual

Besides the general symbolic meanings of the back noted above, it may come to have special significance to a given individual. To understand these it becomes necessary to learn more about the individual patient's life experiences, attitudes and interpersonal relationships because the back may be 'selected' (unconsciously) as the site of symptom formation through two particular mental mechanisms:

1. *Identification*, in which the patient identifies himself with someone else and assumes the other person's symptom, or what he *believes* the other person's symptom to be, or what he *wishes* the other person to have.
2. *Somatic compliance*. In this unconscious process the patient re-experiences a back pain which he had once before experienced in a setting which provided some type of secondary gain. Thus, the person who at some earlier time in his life had a back injury which was painful and gained him protection, help and certain pleasurable associations may unconsciously reproduce the same symptom at a time of crisis later on. Clinically, one sees also a modification of this process in situations where a patient sustains an injury (either mild or severe) resulting in objective pathological changes which are known to be reversible. But often this patient continues to complain of pain after the objective signs of injury have been resolved.

THE 'PAIN-PRONE' PATIENT – CLINICAL CATEGORIES

The implication is that the patient, at the time of his illness, is especially vulnerable to the establishment of a severe or prolonged painful syndrome. This attitude of 'pain-proneness' may be a long-standing one or it may be a relatively recent development for the patient, and patients may be arbitrarily subdivided on this basis into several categories as follows.

The chronically pain-prone patient

Patients who come under this designation are those whose histories reveal that problems involving the symptom of pain or painful experiences have occurred with a high incidence in the patient's past history. Such patients may be further subdivided into two groups:

1. *The constant sufferer*. This is the patient whose pain-proneness has been a *prevailing or predominant theme throughout his lifetime*. For example, he might describe a childhood in which there was continual strife within the family, frequent episodes of harsh, punitive, sadistic treatment, poverty and deprivation. Relationships between the parents themselves and between the child and one or both parents will have been characterized by violent outbursts, tantrums and other expressions of uncontrolled anger with mutual inflictions of pain (physical or psychic). He may describe, during the childhood or adolescent periods, painful illnesses. He may describe failure or early dropout from school, a variety of unsuccessful and unpleasant job experiences, one or more unhappy marriages, and frequent accidents, injuries or illnesses characterized by prolonged periods of pain. *It should be clearly understood that such patients do not consciously wish to have pain, nor do they get pleasure from their pain.* Furthermore, the expression (communication) of their painful (penitent) state to others may hold for these patients the hope of obtaining a comforting and loving relationship with someone.
2. *The intermittent sufferer.* This patient will not present a past history of constant pain or other problems as described above, but he will have a history of frequent episodes of pain. These are related to conflicts of guilt, aggression and the potential or actual loss of someone or something important to him. Such events are so commonplace and 'normal' that we tend to overlook the degree of stress and the amount of adaptation and conflict that may be involved. In the case of the 'intermittent sufferer', one would, in trying to assess the symptoms of the present painful illness, look carefully for some stressful situation which would help to explain why the patient is having pain at this particular time. *However*, in the case of the 'constant sufferer', *the exact*

reverse is true; that is, these patients tend to develop pain at a time when everything is *going well* for them.

The acutely pain-prone patient

This group includes patients who do *not* give past histories which include frequent previous experiences of illness or pain. They can be subdivided further into four general categories:

1. *Patients with isolated or single events mediating strong guilt feelings*. Here previously healthy persons may have given in to an impulse to act out some forbidden or criminal activity, such as stealing money from their employer or having an extramarital affair. These patients generally have unremarkable past histories, but are heavily burdened by guilt for this indiscretion.
2. *Depressed patients*. Like the group above, past histories may be essentially negative; but some significant event which can be described as a real, threatened or fantasized loss of someone or something of great value to him has resulted in the patient's becoming depressed. Examples include the patient who has learned that his mother has cancer, or who has substantiated the rumour that the factory in which he works is going to be closed down.
3. *Elderly patients*. Elderly people who have been healthy all their lives and who have been characterized as being independent and self-sustaining are threatened greatly by their waning physical capacities and the awareness that they are unlikely to continue to enjoy the health and vigour necessary to maintain their independence. They tend to fear disability even more than death itself. They may not appear to be significantly depressed, but if some sort of illness episode or an accident occurs, they are particularly predisposed to depression and excessive or prolonged pain. The initiating episode commonly will be a very minor one, such as a thrombosed and inflamed haemorrhoid, a minor musculoligamentous strain of the lower back or a fall.
4. *The excessively independent self-sustaining patient of any age*. There are certain patients who not only enjoy good health and other successes, but who make it clear that, for them, this is an absolute necessity. They avoid doctors and are inordinately stoical when they have symptoms. They generally work for themselves, or occupy supervisory or executive positions if they are employed by someone. In general, they follow the pattern of doing things by themselves or in a position of leadership. These are people whom we do not ordinarily expect to develop psychogenic pain.

   They actually have an excessive fear of illness or injury, since either threatens them with the possibility of having to be dependent upon others. Although they deal very well with most illnesses or injuries, they tend to fall victim to more serious episodes in which their façade of invincibility and self-sufficiency becomes shattered.

The psychotic patient

There are a number of patients who are psychotic who complain of backache which, in fact, may represent a somatic delusion. The nature of the psychosis involved may vary and their identification is beyond the scope of this discussion. In general these patients will be characterized by:

1. their difficulty relating to the physician and others;
2. an attitude of suspiciousness towards doctors who have treated them, people they work with, or their families; and
3. litigation minded.

Careful attention to their words in describing their problem may suggest:

4. that they are not so much expressing bodily discomfort as a fixed belief that something is wrong inside them; or
5. that they are being persecuted by their pain; or
6. that their description is bizarre (e.g. the belief that the pain is being caused by electrical waves from the radio).

The malingerer

This patient may be very difficult to differentiate from some of the patients previously described – especially those who have psychogenic pain, who often very naively present themselves with symptoms clearly out of proportion to the degree of injury or disability. The diagnosis can only be established by 'detective work', including observing the patient at home, socially, etc. Observation of these patients during a long stay in the hospital and alerting interested third parties to the possibility of the deception will usually clarify the situation.

'Compensation neurosis'

This term is ambiguous since it implies a conscious attempt to defraud, while at the same time implying a psychological disease. It is a term which is used freely in 'scientific' papers but seldom in patients' charts. It is almost always used to depreciate either the patients or the agencies which provide the compensation.

Careful and unbiased observation of these patients will usually make it evident that they are not enjoying themselves, but put their families to considerable distress and have poor incomes. Many who have given up their alleged 'good life' return to work, normal social functions and the gratification of earning their own way; and many continue to be disabled after their claim has been settled with or without monetary gain.

DIAGNOSIS

The history

As with other diagnoses in the practice of medicine or surgery, the diagnosis of psychogenic back pain must be established on a sound basis of positive findings – not simply because of a lack of physical or laboratory findings.

Meaningful, historical data relating to previous illnesses, the precise attitude and events at the time of onset of the present illness, and pertinent family and social data are best obtained in the initial contacts with the patient. The possibility of psychogenic pain should be included among, and explored with, other diagnostic possibilities at the time of initial evaluation – not weeks or months later when things have not gone well.

Two commonly seen and helpful clues in the history are:

1. Vagueness in description of symptoms and defensiveness in giving details of the setting of the onset of the pain or other aspects of the history.
2. Emphasis by the patient on blaming someone else for his plight (e.g. the supervisor didn't heed his warning about the hazard of faulty equipment).

Positive findings

Positive findings in the examination (which begins with observation of the patient in the waiting room or when he enters the consultation room and continues through the period of history-taking, as well as during the more formal examination) may include the following:

1. The facies and posture and voice of a depressed patient.
2. Inappropriate affect:
   - (a) he complains of severe pain while not actually appearing to be in pain;
   - (b) he can be easily distracted from his allegedly severe pain;
   - (c) he may describe his terrible plight in a boastful manner even with evident pleasure.
3. Histrionic displays of the degree of suffering out of proportion to the evident injuries or lesions.
4. Little evidence of discomfort or limitation of motion while reciting the history, dressing or undressing, etc., but marked display of these during the more formal examination.
5. Distribution of pain which does not follow a logical anatomical distribution.

Finally, it is important to point out that in most cases the issue is not a simple one of whether there is a pathological tissue defect *or* a psychological problem, but, rather, a question of how much of each. It should be borne in mind that the presence of positive signs of physical injury or disease does not rule out significant psychological factors.

TREATMENT

In most instances the proper diagnosis can be established early in the course of illness, and this is the keystone of good treatment. Difficulties occur when the physician is unsure of the nature of the problem, as the patient quickly senses this. He is likely then to become more concerned and more disabled, since he cannot perform with confidence in the manner the physician requests.

Conservative therapy with a minimum of diagnostic studies, hospitalization and treatment is in itself reassuring to most patients. However, this does not mean that necessary studies should be omitted because of the vague notion that they will upset the patient, and it is best to do all studies necessary to clarify the diagnosis expeditiously. For example, an elderly patient who falls and sustains a simple contusion, but who is depressed and apprehensive, may require hospitalization for the latter reasons. A brief hospitalization may prevent a prolonged illness.

The initial contacts in which diagnostic studies and conservative measures are being instituted should be utilized by the physician to establish a doctor–patient relationship in which the physician establishes himself as a person of integrity. When a patient does not respond to conservative measures, it becomes necessary in many cases to discuss some of the psychological factors involved and the role they play in the illness. This should be done with an attitude of sympathy and the constructive wish to help the patient, not in a derogatory manner nor with an attitude of accusation.

If the steps outlined cannot be carried out or fail to help the patient, a psychiatric consultation should be considered. Before making this suggestion to the patient, however, the problem should be discussed with a psychiatrist who may be able to advise as to the appropriateness of the referral as well as its timing and manner. When the referral is proposed to the patient, it will generally be best to advise it for purposes of 'advice' rather than 'treatment', leaving this question to be discussed between the psychiatrist and the patient. The referral should be made with some indication that the doctor is not just trying to get rid of the patient and with the same attitude of dignity and respect and no more defensively or apologetically than a referral to any other colleague.

Some patients with a great deal of guilt or excessive needs to be dependent, as well as almost all patients in the 'constant-sufferer' group described earlier, are not likely to become asymptomatic, no matter how capably they are treated. These patients will often do better if the physician is willing to accept less than a complete recovery and to tolerate the patient's return visits for a prolonged period of time (sometimes for years). In this way many will be helped to return to useful function even though still complaining of their pain. Others may indicate a need to be intermittently disabled, and a few unfortunately may remain totally disabled, but the overwhelming majority will utilize the physician's skills and interest to achieve a return to good health.

Low back pain associated with pathological changes

This is discussed in the following sections on: osteoarthritis of the spine; other pathological conditions of the spine; fibrositis; pyogenic osteomyelitis of the spine; and pyogenic infection of the intervertebral discs.

Osteoarthritis of the spine (spondylosis deformans)

There are two main types of this condition:

1. polyspondylitis marginalis osteophytica; and
2. osteoarthritis of the spinal apophyseal joints.

MARGINAL POLYSPONDYLITIS

This is the condition usually referred to as osteoarthritis of the spine. It is characterized clinically by pain in the back for which other causes have been excluded, and radiographically by lipping of the vertebral bodies at or near the site complained of. 'Osteophytes' appear on the lateral and anterior aspects of the vertebral bodies and not from the posterior aspect. They are broad at the base and taper off. It is unusual to have them formed on a single vertebra. The 'osteophytes' arise from the short deep fibres of the anterior common ligament where they are firmly attached to the edges of the body. They lie, therefore, a little below the outer edge of the epiphyseal ring and proliferate so as to overlap the intervertebral space until eventually 'osteophytes' from neighbouring vertebrae may fuse together. The 'osteophytes' arise principally at the junction points of the anteroposterior curves of the spinal column; i.e. about the fifth to sixth cervical, eighth to ninth dorsal, and fourth to fifth lumbar region. At these points the vertebrae are more mobile and are prone to slide and rotate on one another, while at other parts the bodies are held firmly in place by the direct strain which they take. Degeneration of the discs and loss of elasticity in the nucleus pulposus are often precursors of polyspondylitis and this forms a typical feature of this form of the disease. Spinal deformity, with loss of movement, takes place.

OSTEOARTHRITIS OF THE APOPHYSEAL ARTICULATIONS

The dorsal arch of each vertebra provides a superior and an inferior articular process. These form movable synovial joints and are frequently the seat of osteoarthritis. This occurs where the joint balance is upset, as in scoliosis on the concave side, in disc degeneration with loss of the intervertebral space, and also following the collapse of a vertebral body from disease or injury (e.g. osteoporosis, spondylolisthesis). The sites of lesions in this type of disease are C6–T1, T2–5 and L2–4. The typical changes of articular cartilage fibrillation, erosion, subchondral bone sclerosis and osteophyte formation occur, and there may be encroachment into the foramen or spinal canal producing most pain in the legs.

Ankylosing spinal hyperostosis is characterizied by the hyperostosis pathology being accompanied by ossification of the posterior longitudinal ligament, often accompanied by a severe neurological deficit. It is common in Japan, especially in the cervical spine (Hattori *et al.*, 1976; Matsuzaki,

1993) and affects the lower thoracic spine in middle age with a compression myelopathy. This presents gradually with motor weakness in the legs and urinary incontinence. Decompression laminectomy and resection of the ossified ligaments may only partially relieve the myelopathy and spread of ossification can occur.

Miyamota *et al.* (1992) have produced in mice a similar clinical picture and neurological deficit by administering the bone morphogenetic protein (BMP) of Urist. This substance produces bone formation in ectopic sites by endochondral ossification.

Other pathological conditions of the spine

Specific infections of the spine (e.g. tuberculosis, syphilis and osteomyelitis) are considered in other chapters. Cases of spinal metastases, from carcinoma of the breast, are quite common. Other neoplasms are rare but should be considered, e.g. haemangiomata.

Fibrositis (lumbago)

Fibrositis is a vague diagnostic label applied to some cases of back pain which are almost certainly due to muscle strain or degenerative change in the posterior spinal joints. Treatment is of the primary cause.

Pyogenic osteomyelitis of the spine

In the acute and fulminating types, diagnosis is not often made of the osteomyelitis since it is only an incident in the course of the general disease; but in the less acute conditions, where the condition is limited to an affection of a region of the spine, the diagnosis is straightforward.

The lumbar region is most frequently involved, and the bodies of the vertebrae are generally affected, usually as a metastatic phenomenon, the primary focus being recognizable in about half the cases as a typical infection, such as a boil, septic wound, urinary or respiratory infection.

There is an increasing incidence of spinal infections due to improved clinical and laboratory diagnoses, increased intravenous drug use and immunodeficiency states and antibiotic-resistant organisms. For tuberculosis of the spine see Chapter 9.

Infants and children can develop spinal infections, particularly from *Staphylococcus aureus* pyaemia, and present in a general way with irritability, back pain, reluctance to walk or stand. The pyrexia is usually low grade with an elevated ESR and CRP measurements. Either the disc or the vertebral body is infected and can be visualized by plain radiography or ^{99}Tc bone scans (or enhanced by indium-111 leucocytes or gallium) and MR imaging. Treatment is usually conservative with immobilization, appropriate antibiotics over a prolonged period and careful monitoring of the serological and radiographic progress of healing.

In adults *Staphylococcus aureus* still predominates in over 60% of cases, but there is an increasing incidence of *Pseudomonas aeruginosa* (5–10%) in intravenous drug users. Gram-negative organisms, e.g. *Eschericha coli* (10–20%) and *Proteus* in patients with genitourinary infections and diabetes, and *Streptococcus pneumonia* and *pyogenes* in patients with respiratory infections. Tuberculosis is increasing and has to be differentiated from fungal infections, candidiasis, cryptococcus, blastomycosis and brucellosis. Salmonella in sickle-cell disease is fairly common. Back pain at rest, toxicity and fever are the presenting features.

In the elderly, i.e. over 65 years of age, misdiagnosis is common because of degenerative changes – spinal stenosis or even tumours obscuring the diagnosis. Secondary paralysis can result because of the instability and movement of the vertebrae, compromising the spinal cord or cauda equina. Diabetes, rheumatoid arthritis and old age all tend to give rise to these complications, especially with a failed diagnosis of an epidural abscess. Technetium-99 bone scanning and MR imaging are necessary to delineate multiple levels of infections.

Epidural abscess formation must be considered in the elderly patient with back pain, systemic evidence of infection and sensory/motor deficit. *Staphylococcus aureus* is the most common organism. Treatment is by open decompression with appropriate antibiotics. CT and myelography are non-specific and MR imaging is now the diagnostic investigation of choice.

Salmonella spondylitis is very rare, especially in immunologically normal patients and in the absence of sickle-cell haemoglobinopathy. However, Miller *et al.* (1988) have reported on two cases. Both children had insidious onset of low back pain, pyrexia and radiographic evidence of erosion of bone between L4 and L5. Blood cultures and biopsy of the involved areas were positive for Salmonella B, sensitive to ampicillin and cephalothin. With bracing and antibiotics, relief of symptoms with spontaneous fusion occurred by 4 months.

PATHOLOGY

In the early stages there is a destructive lesion with a tendency to spread to adjacent segments because of the fact that the vertebral bodies lack a compact bony layer thus allowing the intervertebral discs to become involved and rapidly destroyed by the proteolytic enzymes of the pyogenic exudate. In tuberculous infection the disc substance is not so readily destroyed and the route of spread to adjacent segments is under the anterior common ligament. These changes are of value in the differential diagnosis, as in pyogenic osteomyelitis early narrowing or disappearance of the intervertebral space is evident on radiographs. Although narrowing of the space is seen in tuberculous disease it is neither so early nor so marked a feature as in the pyogenic form. The abundant blood supply with the local excess of calcium results in early new bone formation, giving rise at first to beaking of the lower and upper margins of adjacent vertebral bodies and later to a fusion of adjacent vertebrae by means of these bony outgrowths. The free blood supply and the cancellous nature of the bone make the formation of visible sequestra unlikely.

This early subperiosteal new bone formation is important in the diagnosis. In pyogenic osteomyelitis, collapse of the bodies and gibbus formation are not common because the severity of the symptoms, particularly the pain, leads to the patient seeking advice at an early stage. Suppuration is common and abscess formation often occurs. These enlarge, usually forward, and are guided in their course by normal cleavage planes – forming psoas, perinephric, pelvic or pelvirectal abscesses. An epidural abscess may form with compression meningitis or vascular disturbances in the cord. The onset of spinal symptoms is rapid compared with the more usual slow and gradual appearance in tuberculous disease.

CLINICAL FEATURES

The onset is usually acute but in some cases it may be more insidious. In the more acute type of case toxaemia and general malaise may completely override the local signs. There is always a spontaneous intense lumbar pain which is usually severe enough to confine the patient to bed. Spasm of the erector spinae is present and all movements of the spine are limited and painful. At a later date there is a localized tenderness over the affected area, and where the posterior processes are involved oedema and tenderness of the area may be present, to be followed by palpable abscess formation.

In the early stages a blood culture may be positive. Pyrexia and leucocytosis are present in varying degrees, but signs of an acute and severe systemic upset may not be prominent. ESR and CRP are raised. In all cases of obscure deep-seated pus, pyogenic osteomyelitis of the spine should be considered. The progress of the disease is rapidly limited in most cases and in 2 or 3 months after the onset an x-ray will show firm bony union.

DIAGNOSIS

The radiological findings are of great importance. It has also to be remembered that in some cases the bone focus is minimal so that it may never be evident. When the disease attacks the body it may be a month or two before changes are seen on x-ray examination. There is a marked narrowing of the disc space and a moth-eaten irregularity of the bodies bounding it. The affected vertebrae show an increased density with some areas of mottled bone density loss (Figure 13.15). This is in marked contradistinction to the osteoporosis/demineralization of tuberculosis. At about the same time, subperiosteal new bone is formed at the margins of contiguous vertebrae, leading to 'beaking'. In the early cases the diagnosis rests, therefore, on severe backache, pyrexia, leucocytosis, elevated ESR and CRP, with possibly rigors in the history. There is often a primary focus (e.g. boils, tonsillitis, chest or urinary infection). The diagnosis may not be complete until a later stage when x-ray changes are evident or when a needle biopsy of the infected material is obtained under radiographic control (Table 13.4).

Magnetic resonance imaging has proved to be most valuable in evaluating spinal infection. Sharif *et al.* (1990) described the use of MRI in evaluating granulomatous spinal infection in 81 patients with proven disease and blinded interpretations were correlated with the clinical, microbiological and surgical findings. MRI enabled the prediction of the presence of neurological complications in 93% of patients and diagnosis of the type of infection in 94%. It also correlated well with surgical findings in 24 of 27 patients. The value of enhancement with gadolinium diethylenetriamine pentaacetic acid was noted; these paramagnetic contrast-enhanced studies showed well vertebral intraosseous abscesses, meningeal involvement, subligamentous spread and paraspinal abscess location. In addition high signal intensity on T1 weighted images of previously affected vertebrae suggested healing and correlated well

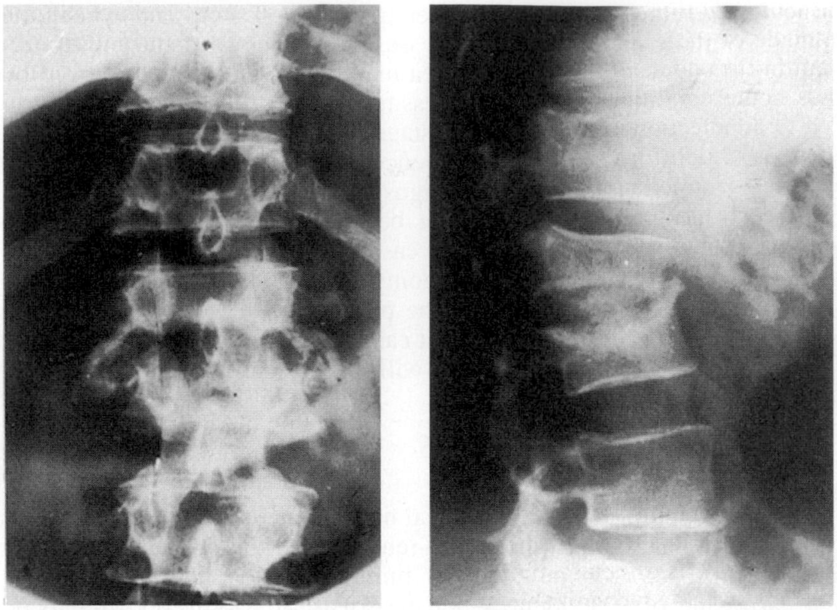

(a) (b)

Figure 13.15 (a) Anteroposterior radiograph of thoracolumbar spine, showing new bone formation between L1 and 2 with some obliteration of the normal vertebral outline. (b) Lateral view, showing loss of bone substance, some degree of sclerosis from new bone formation and a very mild kyphosis being present. Spontaneous fusion is taking place. The intervertebral disc spaces above and below are normal in width.

with symptoms. The authors concluded that MRI is the method of first choice for the initial assessment and also for further follow-up post-surgery of patients with granulomatous spinal infection. Post *et al.* (1990) also looked at gadolinium – enhanced MRI in spinal infection and showed it to provide excellent anatomical delineation of all epidural abscesses, routinely differentiating them from the adjacent thecal sac even when this was not possible by non-contrast MRI, It also increased observer confidence in the diagnosis of disc space infection and osteomyelitis in patients with equivocal non-contrast MRI and localized those portions of paraspinal masses most likely to yield a positive percutaneous biopsy. In addition, it was possible to identify active infections from those that had responded adequately to antibiotic therapy. Bell *et al.* (1990) reported the exact anatomical localization of vertebral and paravertebral tuberculous abscesses provided by MRI in multiple planes which were not previously available with more conventional diagnostic methods and are therefore very helpful for the planning of the surgical approach to these patients.

An important and critical differentiation in diagnosis is between infection and tumour. An *et al.* (1991) have defined the characteristic findings of

Table 13.4 Main features of pyogenic and tuberculous spinal osteomyelitis

	Pyogenic osteomyelitis	Tuberculosis
Site of disease	Body usually; often appendages	Body almost invariably
Primary focus	Typical pyogenic infection 50%	Often TB distance foci
Onset	Usually sudden; sometimes gradual	Gradual
Pyrexia	Often marked	Seldom marked
Pain	Intense	Aching
Leucocytosis	May be marked	Not a feature
Vertebral collapse	None	Usual
x-Ray	Increased density	Decreased density, with collapse
	New bone	No new bone
	Spread through disc	Spread under anterior common ligament
Cord involvement	Rare and acute onset	Common and gradual onset
Course	Short to bone fusion	Prolonged to recalcification and fusion
		? Fibrous fusion

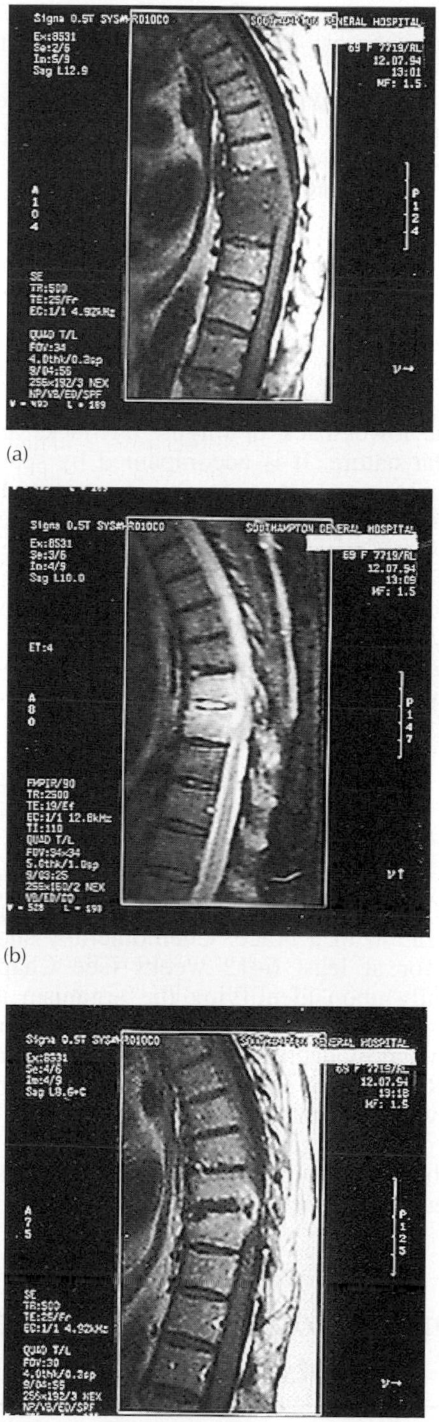

(a)

(b)

(c)

Figure 13.16 Infection affecting the vertebral column, demonstrated by MR scanning, with T1 (a) and T2 (b) weighting. Gadolinium enhancement (c) shows the abscess more clearly invading the spinal canal with cord compression. (Kindly supplied by Dr Richard Blaquiere, Consultant Radiologist at Southampton University Hospitals)

infection involving the disc by MR imaging as an increased signal density on T2 near the end plate, with loss of vertebral end-plate definition, fluid collections, obscured fat planes by oedema and a soft tissue mass surrounding the disc and vertebrae (Figure 13.16). With tumour there is an increased T2 signal of the vertebral body and none of the above findings.

TREATMENT

This consists of immobilization of the spine in a plaster jacket until the disease process is over and bony fusion is complete. Abscesses are evacuated, and appropriate antibiotics both locally and systemically play an important part in the treatment. Fusion is usually unnecessary, as bony ankylosis is an early constant feature. For systemic treatment by antibiotics see Chapter 9.

In the treatment of chronic infective lesions of the spine, the organisms and their sensitivities, as well as pathological material, must be obtained. In lesions located in the cervical spine, an anterior approach is carried out; in the thoracic, a transthoracic rather than a costotransversectomy approach; and in the lumbar spine, loin, anterior and transversectomy approaches are used. Indications for operation, particularly in the tuberculous cases, are:

1. Disease of adjacent vertebrae with concomitant mechanical instability.
2. Paraplegia.
3. Failure to respond quickly to conservative treatment.
4. Where the bacteriological diagnosis is in doubt.
5. Disease affecting the cervical and thoracic spine, especially in children.

Brucella spondylitis

The incidence of bone and joint complications of brucellosis is said to be about 30–40%. Back pain may be the presenting symptom or it may accompany or follow a febrile illness. This may be associated with loss of weight, feverishness, and sweating at night for several weeks. Abscess formation in the shape of an ill-defined swelling in the iliac fossa may be palpable. Spinal movements may be full and painless when the spine is involved. Radiographic examination of the spine may show marginal erosion of the body, narrowing of the disc space and bulging at the psoas shadow. The ESR is increased.

Brucellosis should be considered as a possible aetiological factor in chronic spinal lesions. Brucella agglutinations are raised significantly: *Brucella abortus* 1 : 3840, and *Brucella melitensis* 1 : 3960. A blood culture may grow the organism after 2–3 weeks. The organism is sensitive to penicillin, streptomycin, chloramphenicol or chlortetracycline. Tuberculosis can be excluded by repeatedly negative cultures and guinea-pig inoculations, by the absence of tuberculous changes in the sinus biopsy and by repeated negative Mantoux tests.

Persistent local pain is the main symptom, accompanied by local tenderness and muscle spasm.

Cordero and Sanchez (1991) have compared a group of 19 patients with brucellar spondylitis and 15 with tuberculous spondylitis from the Mediterranean area. They found that brucellar spondylitis is typically a disease involving the lumbar spine of middle-aged men who were at risk occupationally. Signs and symptoms of brucellosis were usually present. Tuberculous spondylitis occurred in both sexes of varying age groups – 16–78 years of age – with isolated signs and symptoms involving the thoracic spine and no prodomal clinical signs of earlier tuberculous lesions. The final diagnosis required bacteriological testing.

Treatment should be conservative in the absence of abscess formation. Complete rest in bed is beneficial initially followed by brace support. Abscess formation may be treated by aspiration initially and, if necessary, later by surgery. Antibiotic treatment should be started as early as possible and be prolonged for 6–12 weeks or, if there are bone complications, for even longer.

Pyogenic infection of intervertebral discs

This follows surgical intervention such as a lumbar puncture, myelography, discography or disc removal (when the organism is usually a staphylococcus), or may occur by a bacteraemic process (when the organism is usually of a Gram-negative type) via blood vessels entering the vertebral bodies and lying in close proximity to the discs. Batson (1942) and other workers described vertebral infections secondary to pelvic or genitourinary infections by spread along the pelvic veins to the paravertebral plexus.

More than one disc space may be involved and, therefore, radiographs of the entire spine should be carried out. It is of importance that there may be at least 6–12 weeks before there is any radiographic evidence of disease or even the clinical presentation. The typical x-ray changes are narrowing of the disc interspace and irregular destruction of the adjacent bone surfaces (Figure 13.17), and intradural abscess formation with sinus tracts have been reported.

MR imaging with gadolinium enhancement has aided greatly in diagnosing the actual soft tissue extent and involvement as well as spread through the vertebral end plates.

CLINICAL FEATURES

The patient may or may not give the history of a previous operation or infection. Pain is localized around the involved vertebral area; it may radiate into the lower back or thighs, but lacks any true radicular nature. It is accompanied by spasm and can progressively become more severe. Pyrexia may or may not be present, but usually there is a leucocytosis with an increase in the sedimentation rate. The differential diagnosis is from an early ankylosing spondylitis or a degenerative disc with spondylosis.

Every attempt must be made to obtain the bacterial organism, and hence its sensitivity, by needle aspiration of the involved intervertebral space.

TREATMENT

This is usually conservative with complete immobilization in a plaster jacket, followed by gradual mobilization in a brace. Chemotherapy should be given for at least 6–12 weeks (see Chapter 9), especially upon identifying the organism and the sensitivity. Successful treatment is followed by relief of pain and by decrease in the white cell count and ESR. Radiographs show the progressive narrowing, and new bone formation with eventual fusion in up to 1 or 2 years. Surgery is indicated only when fever and other signs progress to suggest the formation of paravertebral abscess.

Compression of the spinal cord and its roots

This can be produced by disease or deformity in:

1. the vertebral column, such as intervertebral disc protrusion, tuberculous osteitis with abscess formation, secondary carcinoma, primary malignancy of the vertebrae (e.g. osteosarcoma, multiple myeloma), or
2. the soft tissues around the spinal cord such

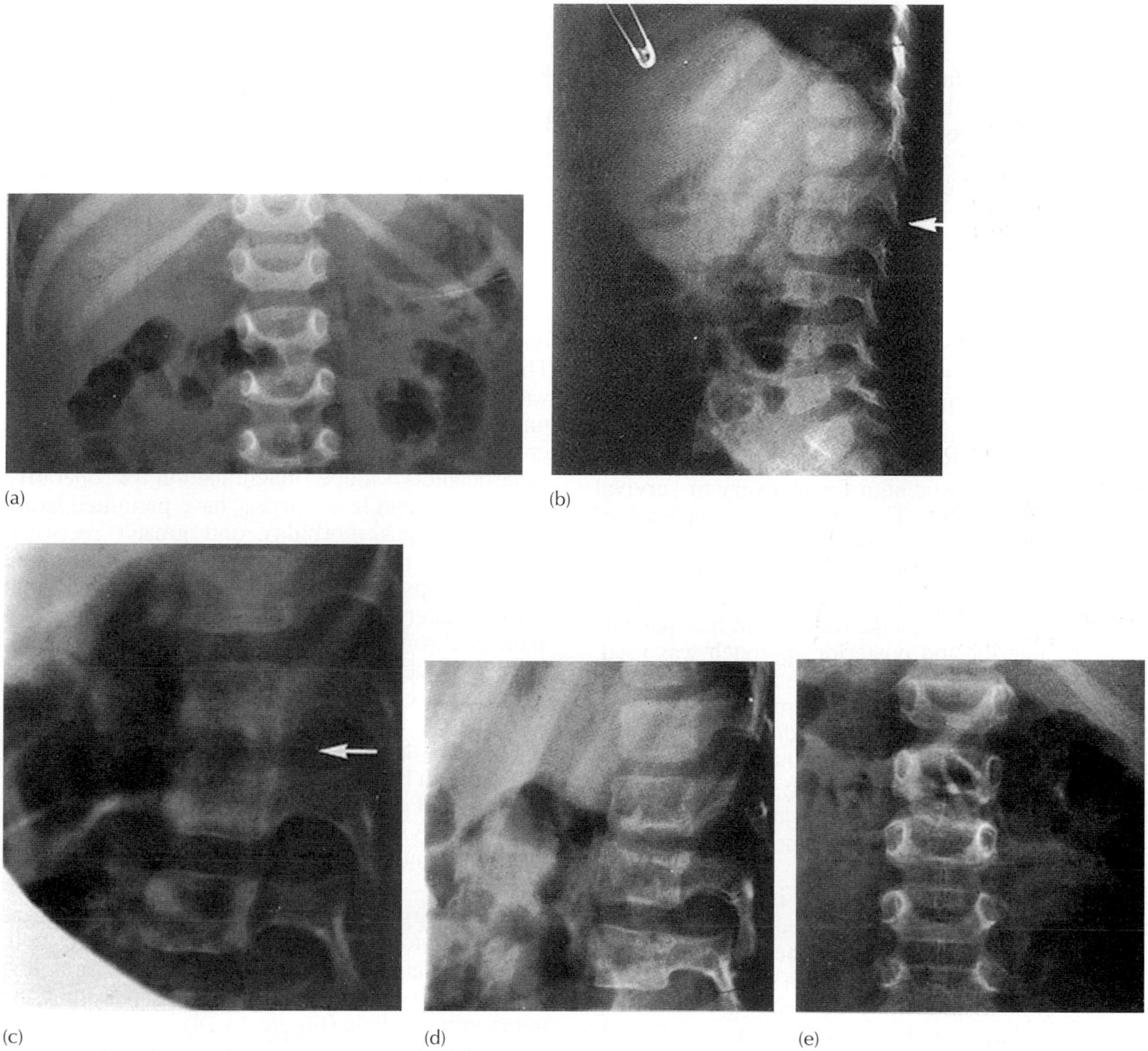

Figure 13.17 (a) Anteroposterior and (b, c) lateral views of the thoracolumbar spine of a young boy who developed narrowing of the L2 and intervertebral disc space and adjacent body destruction, following a lumbar puncture of a meningitis 1 month before. (d) Anteroposterior and (e) lateral views 15 months later, showing the present position with some wedging of the bodies, sclerosis of adjacent surfaces and bony union anteriorly.

as inflammation (e.g. tuberculosis), extradural spinal tumours (e.g. meningioma, neurofibromatosis or chordoma) and intramedullary tumours such as spongioblastomata or angiomata.

The most common region of the cord affected by tumour is in the thoracic area, although it is recognized that a prolapsed or protruded disc occurs more commonly in the lower lumbar spine or cervical spine.

Tumours of the vertebral column

These can be either extradural and arising in bone or from the vascular tissues in the extradural space, which are usually malignant, or intradural, being usually benign and arising from the meninges or from nerve tissue (e.g. meningioma, ependymoma, neurofibroma).

EXTRADURAL TUMOURS

Malignant extradural tumours of the spine may present with back pain or signs of spinal cord compression or both. Spinal symptoms may be the first indication of disease with the primary tumour being unrecognized. In a series by Turner *et al.* (1988) this presentation made up 31% of their patients; 10% were myeloma, 2% giant cell tumour and chordoma with the remainder being made up of metastases from the breast (38%), from the prostate (12%), hypernephroma (12%), lung, bladder, mesothelioma, leiomyosarcoma and adenocarcinoma of unknown origin. The lesion was found in the cervical spine (12%), the thoracic spine (78%) and lumbar spine (12%). The majority of the patients had partial to complete paralysis with incontinence; the latter was a bad prognostic sign for recovery or survival following treatment. Their treatment consisted of anterior decompression, especially as in most cases the site of the cord compression is anteriorly, with the establishment of anterior stability by acrylic block, rib grafts and Zielke rodding. In four patients both an anterior and posterior approach was used. Relief of back pain was good and most of the patients regained mobility and improved sphincter control. Adjuvant treatment of radiotherapy or drugs depends upon the sensitivity of the tumour. Four of their patients died early with 23 dying from disseminated disease after a mean survival of 4 months, but 14 patients were still alive 14 months after undergoing spinal surgery.

Giant cell tumour of the spine is rare, commonly arising in the vertebral body, advancing into the posterior arch. It occurs during the second and third decades of life, most frequently in women. Selective arterial embolization may be necessary when the tumour is large, highly vascular and in difficult operative sites. It can be used to control or assist in haemostasis. If possible, curettage with N_2O ice or phenol covering is carried out and followed by an anterior stabilization procedure.

INTRADURAL TUMOURS

Primary tumours involving the meninges, nerve roots, spinal cord are rare – about 2 per 100 000 population. The most common are *intramedullary*, of which half are glial in origin (e.g. osteocytomas, glioblastomas) and others (e.g. oligodendrogliomas or ependymomas, haemoglobastomas, lipomas and dermoid tumours) make up the rest. *Extramedullary* tumours are meningiomas, neurofibromas, epidermoids, angiomas and lipomas.

Astrocytomas are found uniformly distributed, but ependymomas are seen most commonly in the region of the filum terminale – distally in the cauda equina. Meningiomas can be found in the foramen magnum and thoracic spinal areas, as are neurofibromata.

All present with pain – particularly at night in bed but some with sphincter loss of control and saddle anaesthesia. Spinal tract syndromes can be found or radicular cord deficiencies and syringomyelic syndrome with muscle atrophy and weakness, tendon reflex loss and dissociated sensory loss of pain and temperature. North and North (1993) have reviewed this subject and have emphasized the value of MR imaging to differentiate between solid and cystic tumours with enhancement by gadolinium DPTA. This can distinguish the tumour growth on the wall of a cyst, vascular lesions and intramedullary tumours. These authors have outlined how the great improvement in surgical techniques of bipolar electrocautery, loupe magnification or operative microscopy, and laser surgery have permitted larger resections, less morbidity and greater recovery. Radiation is recommended after subtotal resection, or after biopsy of low-grade tumours, with careful dosage patterns to prevent radiation myelopathy – acute or chronic – acute transient myelopathy, motor paralysis due to infarction of blood vessels, anterior horn cell damage and chronic progressive myelopathy.

Survival depends upon the malignancy of the tumour with both local recurrence as well as further neurological damage.

In the cervical spine neoplasms are less frequent. One of the most common is the benign extramedullary tumour – the neurinoma or neurofibroma. These can grow large enough to produce root, as well as cord, symptoms and signs. They may be both intraspinal and extraspinal through the foramina, forming the typical hourglass shape and eroding the intervening pedicle (Figure 13.18).

Alteration of the spinal cord contents results from direct pressure onto the tissues or secondarily by a change in the blood supply to produce oedema, haemorrhage and degeneration.

The most common presenting feature is radicular pain in the distribution of one or more spinal roots. This can be of slow onset in severity, may be associated with stiffness and is aggravated by jarring movement of the spine or anything increasing the intradural pressure, such as coughing, sneezing or defaecation. Night pain in the back is progressive and rarely remits. Motor symptoms of long tract involvement, such as weakness, stiffness and ataxia, develop later and can involve one or both limbs. Sphincter disturbances will appear late and indicate either a cord or cauda equina lesion. Paraesthesia in and around the perineum is a most critical symptom, requiring detailed investigation. On examination there may be evidence of the *lower motor neuron*

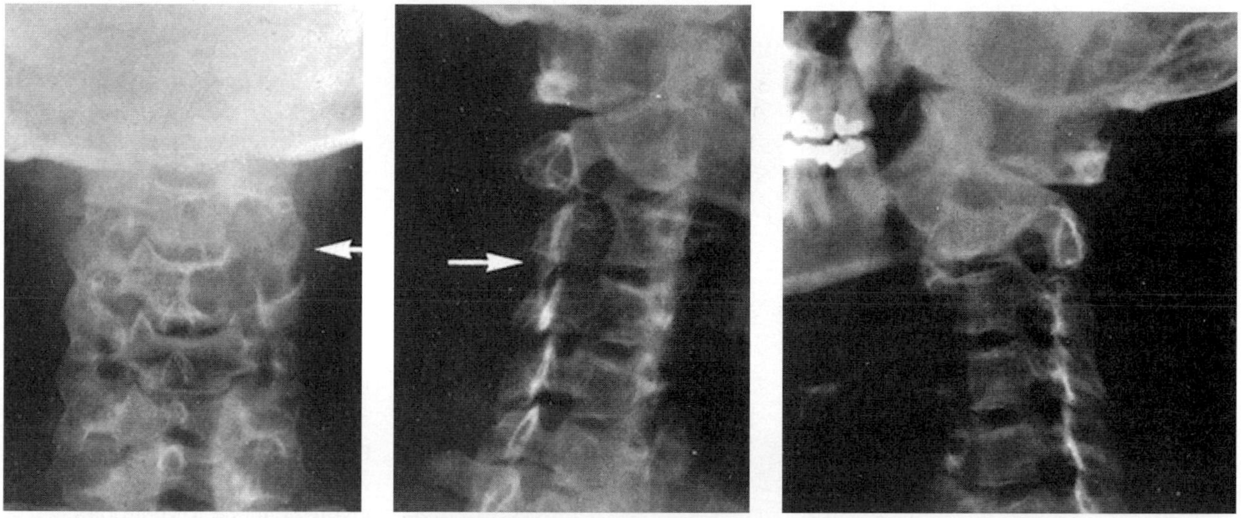

Figure 13.18 Anterolateral radiographs of the cervical spine in a young male, showing destruction of the pedicles of the third and fourth cervical vertebrae due to a neurofibroma.

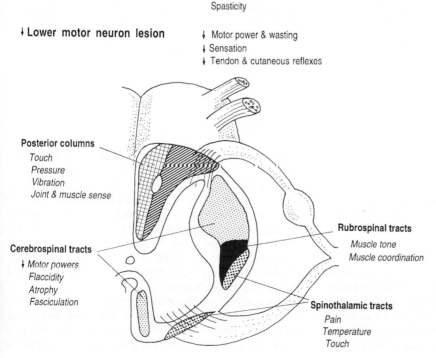

lesion, such as weakness or paralysis of individual muscles, decrease in muscle tone and reduction in tendon, and cutaneous reflexes, and wasting of muscle – all of which help to delineate the level of involvement – or it may be of an *upper motor neuron disease* of the pyramidal tract with loss of voluntary movement accompanied by spasticity, increased tendon reflexes, sensory changes and a positive Babinski sign. Involvement of the posterior columns, of the posterior nerve roots or of the peripheral nerve can also occur (Figure 13.19).

On examination of the spine, there may be

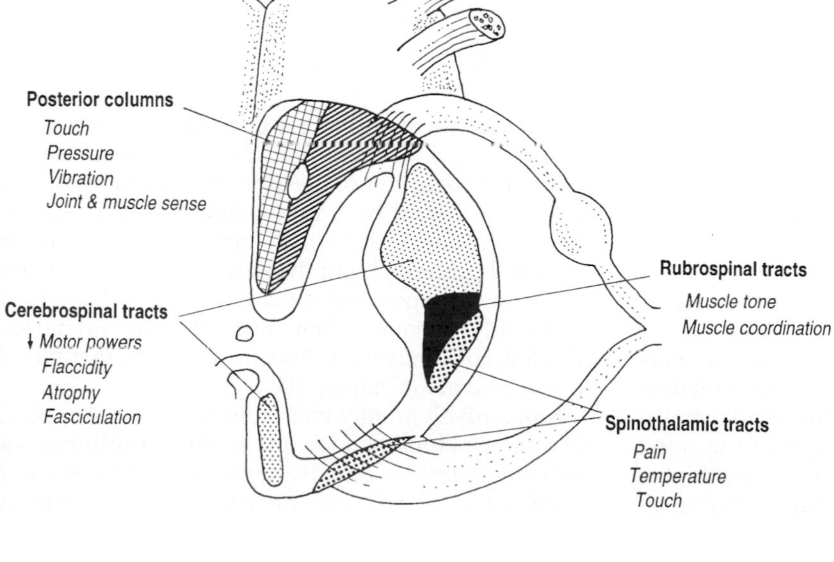

Figure 13.19 The clinical features of upper and lower motor neuron lesions and of the more common tracts in the spinal cord.

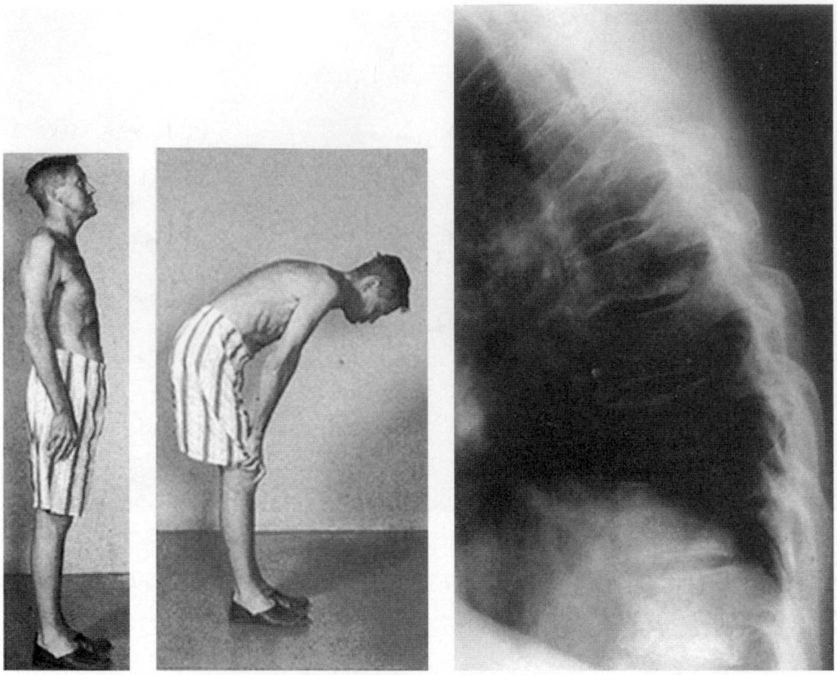

(a) (b) (c)

Figure 13.20 (a) An elderly male who had a malignant lymphoma involving thoracic vertebrae. (b) and (c) On forward flexion, there is straightening of the thoracolumbar spine and he is supporting his painful spine by placing his hands on his knees.

tenderness on deep pressure in the area in which the disease process is present, or there may be limitation of movement or aggravation of the symptoms when the spine is actively moved (Figure 13.20). The function of the sphincters must be carefully examined since incontinence or retention of urine, constipation or incontinence of faeces may be present. A rectal examination will often demonstrate sphincteric weakness with a patulous anus, and loss of sensation will be noted by the patient.

Autonomic system involvement may be seen by increased sweating with vasomotor and pilomotor reactions as well as a Horner syndrome when the inferior cervical ganglion is involved.

Radiography may show the destruction of the body of the vertebra or 'erosive' hollowing out of the posterior surface. Myelography may demonstrate a complete block with enlargement of the venous channels and the smooth scalloped upper surface (Figures 13.21 and 13.22). Bone scanning with technetium-99 is now always indicated to demonstrate whether or not the lesion is multiple. CT imaging as well as MRI are being used for greater detail.

In the involvement of the cauda equina, particularly by prolapse of the L5/S1 intervertebral disc or by a chordoma, the pain is usually localized as a dull, aching sensation in the lower part of the spine with some radiation into both buttocks and thighs. Paralysis of muscles may occur with alteration in the reflexes. There may be saddle-shaped areas of anaesthesia over the buttocks and back of the thighs, but if there is involvement of the fifth lumbar roots, such change can extend down the leg to the lateral malleolus and over the dorsum of the foot. Disturbance of function of the bladder and bowel are late, but are an important feature. Of 70 patients reviewed by Fearnside and Adams (1978) in Oxford, 57 presented with backache or sciatica and many had their symptoms from 2 to 5 years before any tumour was discovered.

SPINAL CORD COMPRESSION BY METASTASES

Metastases to the vertebral column will present in almost 50% of cases with a spinal or radicular pain without recognition of the primary carcinoma. This is often followed by a motor function and sensory defect and sometimes a disturbance of sphincter control. Radiography of the vertebrae may show destruction, collapse, and a paravertebral mass which is usually smaller than one due to infection. Myelography may well show the invading extradural lesion. See also Chapter 10.

Since myelography can include the whole spine, thoracic and lumbar, etc., it is useful in outlining not only single lesions but also separate lesions. Van der Sonde *et al.* (1990) investigated over 100 patients

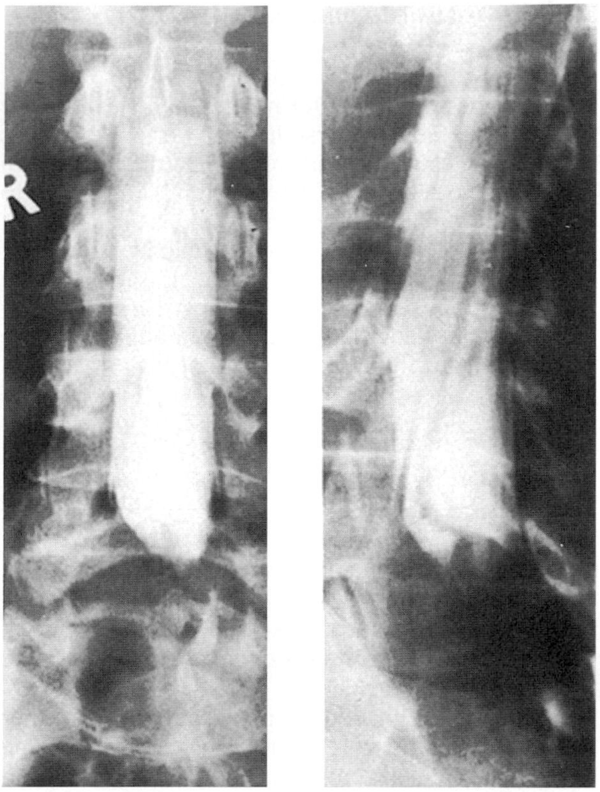

(a) (b)

Figure 13.21 Myelograms showing an extradural neurofibroma: (a) anteroposterior view; (b) oblique view.

who were symptomatic and with back pain but not suspected of having spinal epidural metastases. Over 50% had one epidural metastasis, 12% two separate lesions and 4% had three.

However, MR imaging is proving to be much more sensitive, particularly in the extradural space, for involvement of the vertebral bodies and also for intramedullary space lesions (Sze, 1991). Computed tomography is important for anatomically detailing the severity of bone destruction.

Colletti *et al.* (1991) have compared bone scanning, spinal MR imaging, CT scanning, myelography and radiography and demonstrated the presence of spinal lesions in 88% of patients who had malignant disease and suspected spinal metastases. MR imaging was particularly sensitive of lesions showing subtle marrow changes with less cortical bone involvement.

TREATMENT

Treatment (see also Chapter 10) is primarily directed towards the relief of pain and the restoration of spinal

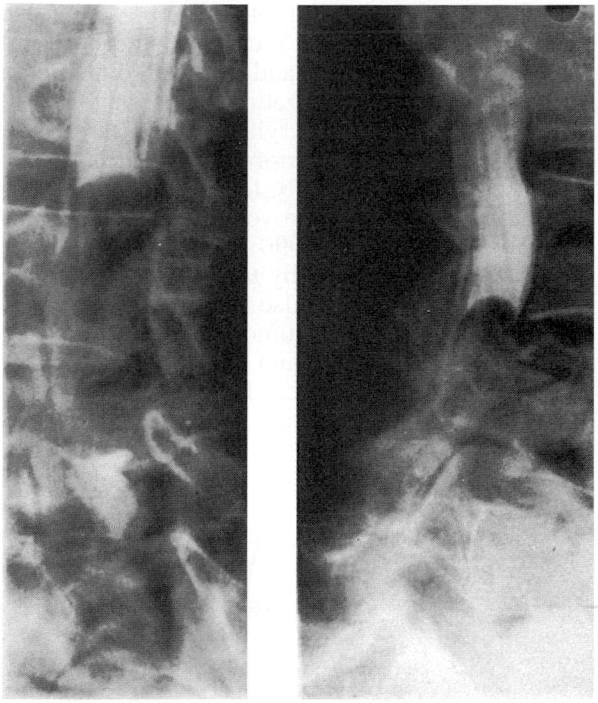

(a) (b)

Figure 13.22 Myelograms to demonstrate an intradural ependymoma: (a) oblique view of the lumbar spine; (b) lateral view, showing the complete smooth cut-off on the dye pattern.

stability so that the patient can regain some form of physical independence and mobility. Radiotherapy versus other therapy still remains controversial because of the numerous pathologies being reported and how early diagnosis has been made. Metastatic cancer of the breast and of the kidney are radiosensitive and do well. Marazano *et al.* (1991) have described their results from a prospective study in which 90% of their patients received radiotherapy alone and the remainder received surgery for diagnosis and stabilization combined with radiotherapy. Of their patients, 80% had improvement in back pain, 48% with motor dysfunction and 31% had no deterioration in motor function. The mean survival time was 7 months and improvement in clinical picture was 8 months.

Histological diagnosis can be made by percutaneous biopsy with CT scanning and has proven to be most useful in differentiating metastatic lesions, infections and primary bone tumours.

Surgery is now widely practised and consists of anterior approach with decompression and stabilization when there are no spinal cord lesions nor epidural spread. Combined anterior and posterior procedures are also necessary with or without radiotherapy or chemotherapy. Galasko (1991) has described complete relief of pain in 90% of his patients, 70% with major recovery of neurological function of the cord or cauda equina compression lesions. Segmental stabilization by instrumentation, insertion of methylmethacrylate infills is necessary.

Arterial embolization prior to tumour resection of involved bone, particularly for vascular renal carcinoma metastases, has proved to be most successful. Broaddis *et al.* (1990) have described the beneficial effects treated by this means not only in renal cancer patients but also for metastatic thyroid, melanoma and giant cell tumours.

The prognosis for life and function is very poor, especially if the neurological defect develops rapidly and when the primary cancer is bronchial in origin (prostatic or mammary cancer have a better outlook because of their radiosensitivity and hormonal control).

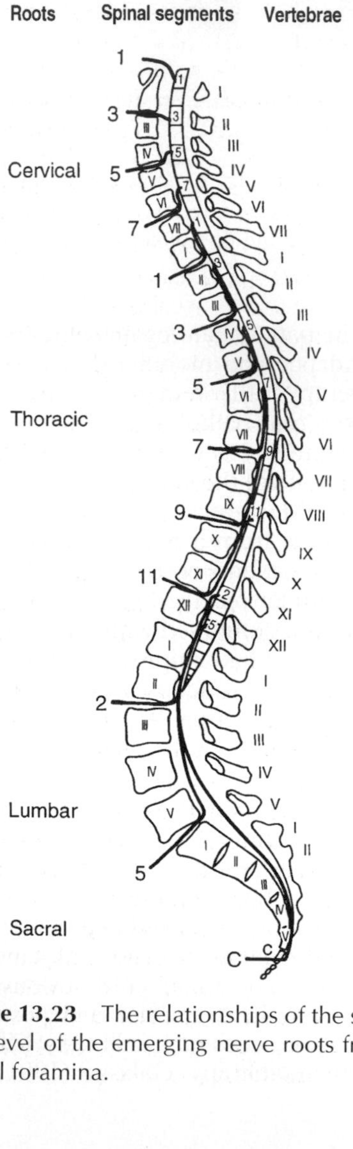

Figure 13.23 The relationships of the spinal segments to the level of the emerging nerve roots from their intervertebral foramina.

Relationship of spinal segments to vertebrae

Because the spinal cord terminates at the level of the lower border of the first lumbar vertebra, nerves forming the cauda equina are peripheral in type with the ability to regenerate. However, it is important to identify the spinal segment involved, one can relate it back to its particular vertebra and its level of segmental origin (Figure 13.23). It is seen that the cervical roots pass out above their corresponding vertebrae, the other roots below, although they rise far up the cord from their segments.

Sciatica

Sciatica signifies sciatic pain without connoting any particular pathogenesis. It is a symptom not a disease. Essential sciatica, or sciatic neuralgia, should be differentiated from a sciatic neuritis or a true inflammation of the nerve.

An inflammation of the sciatic nerve may be either primary or secondary. Primary sciatic neuritis is due to a generalized toxaemia, as from alcoholism or lead or arsenic poisoning, or it may be the result of systemic disease, such as diabetes or syphilis. The secondary form is likewise a peripheral neuritis, but it is due to pressure on the nerve, usually before it leaves the pelvis, as from a spinal cord tumour that exerts pressure within the canal, or metastatic tumours that press on the root, plexus or trunk. Pelvic tumours may give unilateral pain from pressure on the plexus or nerve.

The chief symptom is pain, either sudden or gradual in onset. It is gnawing or burning and may be continually present or occur in paroxysms. It is often extremely severe, especially at night. It is worse in any position that causes pressure on the nerve, such as sitting. The patient in bed lies on his side with the hip and the knee bent and the ankle plantar flexed. The pain begins in the lumbar region or in the buttock area and tends to spread downward. It may never reach below the knee and is generally worse at the back of the hip and thigh, but it may involve any or all branches of the nerve in its course. Special points of tenderness, known as Valleix's points, are found on the nerve and its branches: between the ischial tuberosity and the greater trochanter, at the centre of the posterior aspect of the thigh, just lateral to the middle of the popliteal space, the middle of the calf and, lastly, just behind the medial malleolus.

Lasègue's sign is present in all cases. If the knee is kept in full extension and the foot dorsiflexed, the hip cannot be flexed to any extent without causing great pain, this being brought about by the direct stretching of the nerve.

To avoid stretching the nerve, the patient in a severe case walks on the toes of the foot of the affected side with a plantar flexed ankle, the hip and knee being kept flexed. The knee jerk may be diminished or absent. Scoliosis is often produced and there may also be paraesthesia or hyperaesthesia. Gluteal atrophy is often present, and x-ray frequently reveals arthritic changes.

DIAGNOSIS

In all forms of sciatic pain a full investigation should be carried out. Where a tumour is exerting direct pressure onto the cauda equina (i.e. in the spinal canal) a bilateral sciatica may develop. This is rare in other circumstances. Secondary carcinoma subsequent to a breast or thyroid gland operation has a special predilection for this site and inquiries should always be made with regard to previous operations. Diseased kidneys or prostate gland, ovarian or fibroid tumours, or infected sacroiliac joints and lumbar spondylitis may not infrequently give rise to a form of sciatica to be diagnosed only by a thorough examination, including rectal and x-ray examinations. It is wise also to exclude the lightning pains of tabes and transverse myelitis before embarking on treatment.

Differential diagnosis of radicular pain into legs

1. Tabes dorsalis: spontaneous lancinating pains into the trunk and extremities may give the impression of following true nerve root segments, as in sciatica. 'Gastric crises', ocular changes of an Argyll Robertson pupil, as well as depressed reflexes aid the clinical diagnosis. The blood and CSF serology are positive.
2. Syringomyelia and diabetic neuropathy – varying severity and patterns of pain – often aggravated by rest and accompanied by marked hyperaesthesia, paraesthesia, loss of vibration and proprioceptive sense, etc.
3. Poliomyelitis and Guillain–Barré syndrome – both produce lancinating pains with deep muscle aches, particularly in the back and legs.
4. Tumours – usually the pain is more continuous, can be bilateral; sensory loss can be marked, as can visceral dysfunction.

TREATMENT

If any specific cause can be discovered, the primary treatment will naturally be directed towards this.

Lesions of the lumbar intervertebral disc

ANATOMY OF THE DISC

The intervertebral disc consists of three histologically different components: the cartilage plate, annulus fibrosus and nucleus pulposus. The cartilage plate is a thin layer of hyaline cartilage adherent to the trabeculae of cancellous bone of the vertebral body through a thin layer of calcified cartilage at the junction – thus the plate comes into contact with marrow between trabeculae from which it receives its nutrition (Figure 13.24). The vascular channels are said to be present in cartilage plate extending from marrow but disappear before the third decade. The cartilage plate peripherally fades into the annulus fibrosus. The latter structure consists of dense fibrous tissue in concentrically arranged lamellae – the outer attached to the epiphyseal ring by Sharpey's fibres, the inner derived from the cartilage plate surrounding and merging into the nucleus pulposus. The nucleus pulposus, which lies a little posteriorly to the central axis of the vertebrae, is composed of whitish, glistening, semi-fluid material which is composed principally of glycosaminoglycans (GAGs). Microscopically it reveals fine fibrillar structure, with clear stroma, resembling connective tissue, mucin, and fibroblastic cartilage and rarely, notochordal cells. The borders of the nucleus are not distinct, as they gradually merge into the annulus fibrosus. The nucleus pulposus is enclosed in its fibrocartilage capsule under considerable tension – it amounts to 15 kg in the lumbar region in a supine position, being, naturally, very much higher during spinal movements.

The turgor of the disc is dependent on high osmotic pressure of the nucleus pulposus, drawing fluid from the spongiosa of the vertebrae; the nucleus, being non-compressible, transmits the pressure against the cartilage plate and annulus fibrosus, the latter with other ligamentous structures of the spine being responsible for the resilience and flexibility of the vertebral column. The diurnal variations in height – being up to 1.5 cm taller in the morning than in the evening – are mostly due to alterations in water content of the nucleus, as the annulus fibrosus is only very slightly elastic.

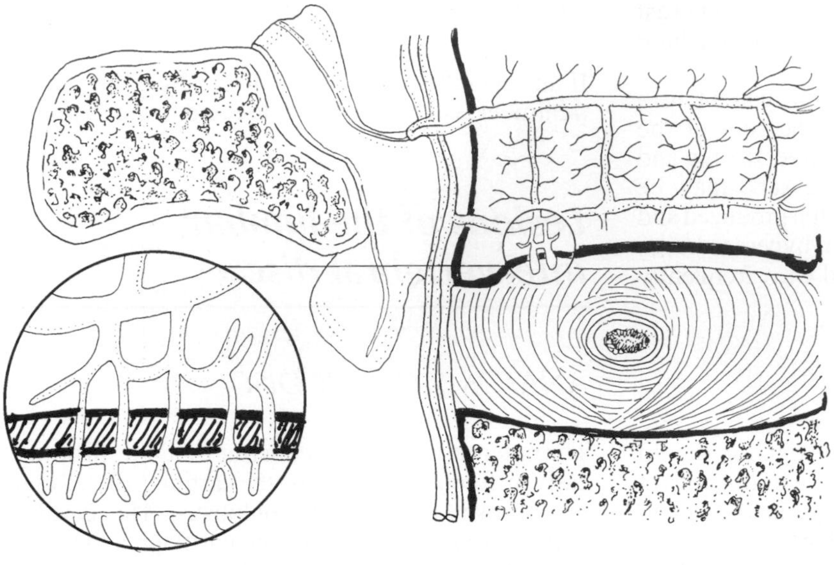

Figure 13.24 The vascular channels penetrate the subchondral bone and calcified plate as far as the annulus fibrosus. (Redrawn by Farquharson-Roberts, with permission of the authors, editor and publisher, from Crock, H.V. and Yoshizawa, H. (1976) *Clinical Orthopaedics and Related Research* **115**, 19; J.B. Lippincott Co., Philadelphia and Toronto)

The annulus is made up of collagen, giving the appearance of lamellar layering of fibre sheets, so that it can withstand very large pressures from within the nucleus pulposus as well as from horizontal rotation, but less from extension or flexion. It is described as being thinnest and therefore weakest at its posterior aspect. Another weak area is opposite the cartilage end plate where small defects are common because of pre-existing fetal blood vessel channels. With movement of gel material through these defects, Schmorl's nodes are formed. These are commonly discovered at routine autopsies and are usually asymptomatic.

The nucleus is entirely avascular. Fine unmyelinated nerve fibres have been found in the posterior longitudinal ligaments and in lesser number in the annulus fibrosus. The ligamentous and articular structures of the vertebral column have sensory innervation from the nervus sinuvertebralis (von Luschka) – a recurrent branch arising just distally to the ganglion of the posterior nerve root.

PATHOLOGY

Although in 1930 Mixter and Barr first described the successful removal of disc material for sciatica, Middleton and Teacher in 1911 described the first pathological traumatic (heavy lifting injury) rupture of a thoracolumbar disc into the lumbar cord with subsequent paralysis and death. Both macroscopic and microscopic findings showed that the structure was characteristic of the pulp of the intervertebral disc. Experimentally they attempted to reproduce such a lesion in the cadaveric lumbar spine and with applied pressure demonstrate disc bulging between the first and second lumbar spine.

Intervertebral discs are one of the most 'hard-worked' structures in the body, particularly in the lower lumbar region, and the majority begin to show evidence of senescence in the third decade. The function of the disc may be disturbed in a twofold manner – either by alteration of the water content of the nucleus pulposus or 'wear and tear' changes in the annulus fibrosus leading to partial or complete extrusion of its interior.

The water equilibrium may be destroyed by changes in the cartilage plate with escape of disc material into the spongiosa of the vertebrae with subsequent formation of granulation tissue and vascularization. Desiccation of the nucleus may occur through fissural tears in the annulus fibrosus – degenerative or traumatic. Due to these changes, the disc space becomes diminished, bulging of the annulus ensues – in any direction – followed by proliferation of collagenous tissue, and its calcification at the edges of the vertebrae may occur resulting in so-called osteophyte formation. Bulging, whether anteriorly or laterally, does not give rise *per se* to any appreciable symptoms.

The fibres in the lamellae of the annulus fibrosus may give way gradually, usually the internal layers first, thus attenuated annulus may protrude more or less prominently either due to turgor of not entirely degenerated nucleus or simply due to mechanical pressure in weight-bearing position. The name protrusion, or herniation, is generally given to the lesion in which some form of capsule still limits the nucleus pulposus. The protrusion may eventually rupture completely and extruded material lies free in the epidural space. This lesion is termed a ruptured disc or prolapse. Probably in the earlier stages the nucleus is capable of being displaced inwards from a posterior herniation by alteration of the spinal curve or may protrude more, for instance in hyperextension of the spine.

Apart from the minor repeated trauma, an injury such as a fall or lifting heavy weights is the precipitating factor in over half of the cases. It is possible that only excessively severe trauma may produce acute herniation of a normal disc. Penetration of the disc with a lumbar puncture needle has resulted in a herniation in a few reported cases.

The disturbance of disc function leads to some derangement of interdependent structures of the spine (e.g. articular facets and ligaments). The secondary changes of strains or arthritis may be the source of some of the backache in disc herniations. Males are affected twice as frequently as females. The age of incidence is fairly evenly distributed in the three decades between the ages of 20 and 50.

There is a three-stage cycle of pathological change which commonly affects the lower lumbar discs. The first stage, a progressive degeneration associated with disturbance of water content and actual sequestration, starts in the nucleus pulposus, spreads to the posterior annulus and ends with annular rupture. The second stage, that of nuclear escape, is characterized by episodic extrusion of sequestrated nuclear fragments through the annular defect. The final stage, that of fibrosis or repair, overlaps the second and progresses over a period of years until the abnormal disc is replaced by fibrous tissue.

Osti *et al.* (Osti and Fraser, 1992; Osti *et al.*, 1992) from a post-mortem study of 135 discs from subjects averaging 31.5 years of age found peripheral tears were most frequent in the anterior annulus (except in the L5/S1 disc) and circumferential tears were equally distributed front and back with radiating tears mainly involving the posterior annulus (and closely related to severe nuclear degeneration). They thought that peripheral tears were due to trauma rather than biochemical degeneration and were independent of nuclear change of dehydration and fraying. They may well influence the degeneration of discs and produce discogenic pain.

This same group describe that discography is more accurate than MR imaging for the detection of annular pathology and hence in diagnosing a cause of low back pain.

From material obtained at operation and from autopsy specimens Yasima *et al.* (1990) have described the histology of ageing lumbar intervertebral discs. They found, in patients over the age of 60 years, that changes in the annulus fibrosus were more extensive in prolapsed discs than protruded, e.g. myxomatous degeneration, fibrosis and swollen annular fibres, with cyst formation. In this age group they also observed reversal of the orientation of the inner fibre bundles of the annulus so that they bulged outwards with atrophy of the nucleus and narrowing of the disc space, bizarre giant cells. In the young age group – from 20 to 59 years of age – these changes were less pronounced.

In the older patients, because of decrease in the water content of the nucleus gel, the stromal atrophy and the formation of a gap in the nucleus, the disc rarely protrudes. At this age it is the rarer bulging of the annulus fibrosus which predominates.

BIOCHEMICAL AND BIOMECHANICAL FACTORS ASSOCIATED WITH DISC PROTRUSION

Nachemson (1966) carried out a study of loading in lumbar discs as well as the distribution of stress within these structures in different body positions. Using *in vivo* disc pressure measurements and electromyographic techniques, he showed that, when anaesthetized and supine, a patient weighing 70 kg has a loading of 20 kg in his L3 disc. This increases to a maximum loading of 270 kg when the individual is sitting and leaning forwards with an additional 20 kg in his hands. Standing it was 100 kg. The psoas major muscle acts as a very important stabilizer of the lumbar spine in the erect position and contributes to the compression loading on the discs. With the intradiscal pressure increasing with bending, he described the expansion of the annulus on its concave side with simultaneous reduction on the convex. but not any movement of the nucleus pulposus which has been described by others.

Farfan *et al.* (1970) postulated the biomechanical theory that *in vivo* disc degeneration is associated with imposed torsional strains rather than compressive loads. They also felt that any impairment of facet joint function might put the disc at risk.

Occupational hazards may be relevant. Intradiscal pressures, myoelectric activity and intra-abdominal pressure measurements have demonstrated that the distance between the weight and the body influences the stress on the back much more than the method used to lift (Andersson *et al.*, 1976).

Myoelectric activity is about the same in standing and in relaxed unsupported sitting. Disc pressures have been found to be considerably higher in unsupported sitting than in standing.

Disc pressures and myoelectric activity are highest in an anterior unsupported position and lowest when sitting straight. The addition of a back support to a chair decreases both parameters. The inclination of the back rest is most important; as it increases, the disc pressure and myoelectric activity decrease. They are also reduced by the addition of a lumbar support and arm rests.

Measurements of these parameters in several occupational situations have shown that they are lowest in writing, higher in typing and still higher in lifting. Disc pressure and myoelectric activity increase in the car driver's seat when the gear is shifted and disc pressure rises when the clutch is depressed (Andersson *et al.*, 1975). However, many workers feel that there is an inherent biochemical defect in the disc which makes it susceptible to trauma.

Naylor (1970) carried out an extensive review of the fine structure and biochemistry of the disc and its surrounding annulus. Disc degeneration is characterized by:

1. Reduction in the amount of glycosaminoglycans.
2. Increase in the lower molecular weight glycoproteins.
3. Increase in fibrillation, fissuring and precipitation of collagen.

These changes result in decrease of the disc's gel properties, and disturbance of their normal function of absorption and stress absorption. In nuclear herniation the changes were:

1. Fall in total protein polysaccharides, with increased fibrillation and precipitation of collagen content.
2. Increase in the less mature and degraded collagen.
3. Increase in the lower molecular glycoproteins.

With an unequal stress or trauma on the annulus in the presence of these changes in collagen, in protein polysaccharides and in the fluid content, increase in the interdiscal pressure will lead to protrusion or prolapse of the nuclear content.

SITES

Strain and stress being obviously important factors in degenerative change of the disc and its frequent outcome – posterior herniation or rupture – it is natural to find it most commonly in segments of the spine most liable to chronic or acute trauma: lower lumbar and lower cervical spine. Multiple protrusions frequently occur.

A very helpful pathological staging of disc herniation has been presented by Eismont and Currier (1989):

- Stage 1 – dehydration, desiccation with early degeneration of the disc material.
- Stage 2 – prolapse of disc material within the annulus.
- Stage 3 – extruded disc material through the annulus, but not through the posterior ligament.
- Stage 4 – sequestrated disc material through both the annulus and the posterior ligament, free to move within the spinal canal.

As one moves down through these stages, signs and symptoms become more severe, conservative treatment less likely to succeed and surgery is required. The authors emphasize that 75% of all patients with acute sciatica will improve on conservative treatment within 30 days.

Mechanism of production of symptoms

The common site for a posterior herniation of a disc is just lateral to the posterior longitudinal ligament; it may start more or less gradually through a fissure, and it is probable that at this stage it may be a source of backache even before there is any demonstrable disturbance of spinal mechanics (Figure 13.25). With or without undue stress the herniation may enlarge and impinge on a neighbouring nerve root, thus producing symptoms and signs similar to any other space-occupying lesion in this area. Whatever is the ultimate explanation – irritation of the root due to compression, stretching, friction, occlusion of vasa nervorum, degeneration of nerve fibres, or a combination of any or all of these factors – the result is the same – interference with its function. The compressed nerve root becomes oedematous, enlarged and often adherent to the protrusion. The extruded material from a ruptured disc appears to be more prone to irritate the tissue and set up an inflammatory reaction, with oedema and increased redness of the dural sheath as well as of the epineurium.

Jensen *et al.* (1991) have studied by CT scanning, postoperative findings at 3 months. Although 88%

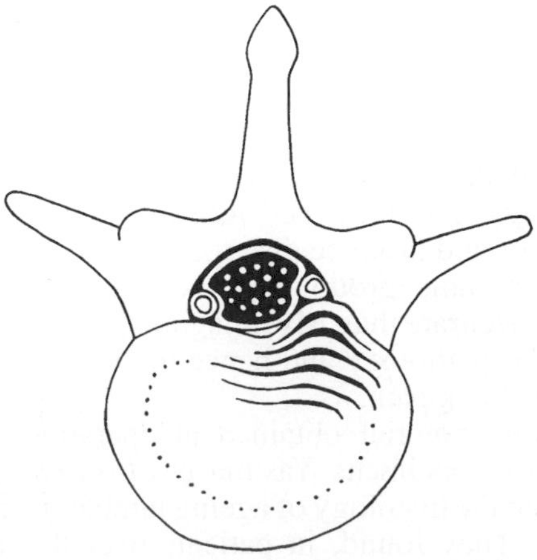

Figure 13.25 Diagrammatic representation of the common type and site of disc protrusion displacing the nerve root posteriorly.

showed dural or radicular scarring, and 9% persistent disc herniation, there was no correlation of the pathological findings to the clinical outcome. The only correlation to persistent symptoms was the presence of posterior facet joint arthritis. They believe that it is not the mechanical effects of disc herniation, but the symptoms and even signs are due to inflammatory pressure or chemical effects upon the nerve roots.

It should be noted that a study by Houghton (personal communication, 1984) showed that there was no abnormal amount of prostaglandin E or F within the vicinity of the inflamed nerve roots or dura.

Obviously, histological examination of these tissues is rarely possible. The extradural veins become engorged due to obstruction, often having the appearance of extensive varices, and undoubtedly add to irritation of the root. In the chronic phase of sciatica the root is usually seen embedded in fibrous tissue and stretched over a protrusion.

Pain is produced by the prolapse or actual protrusion of disc material consisting of fibrocartilage debris. The nerve root is stretched tautly over this in close proximity to the ligamentum flava. Therefore, with the compression or irritation, congestion, oedema and adhesion formation occur around the peripheral nerve and its dural sheath. Direct pressure from a tumour on the peripheral nerve impairs conductivity, whereas the posterior nerve root fibres, which are proximal to the ganglion, have less insulation and also lack the property to regenerate.

The first sensation of pain accompanied by muscle spasm or what is called low back pain or 'lumbago' is produced by the tearing of the annulus fibrosus containing sensory nerves. Further deterioration occurs with the development of pain due to root compression.

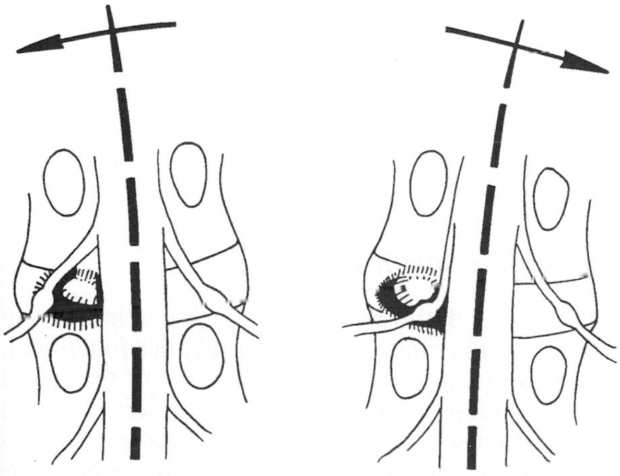

Figure 13.26 The direction of tilt, depending on the relation of nerve root to protrusion: (a) nerve root displaced laterally, (b) nerve root displaced medially.

Types and sites of protrusions

The commonest type of protrusion is a fairly well circumscribed bulging of the disc, yellowish or white, glistening attenuated annulus fibrosus, with soft elastic summit. Less often there is rupture of the capsule with the extruded degenerated material lying in the epidural space embedded in dense fibrous tissue. Occasionally the herniation extends centrally right across the vertebral canal in the form of a firm ridge. An important variety of protrusion which occurs, though infrequently, is the 'intermittent herniation' of Falconer, or the 'concealed disc' of Dandy. This herniation is not obvious from the position of flexion on the operating table, but the abnormality may be betrayed by softness and thinness of the annulus fibrosus and the bulging can be reproduced by hyperextension of the spine.

Apart from the type of protrusion, its situation in relation to nerve root and/or thecal sac is of great importance both clinically and operatively. The protrusion may be central, paramedian or lateral, the commonest site being lateral to the posterior longitudinal ligament which means usually under the nerve root (Figure 13.25) and, depending on its size, the root may be compressed backwards and medially (Figure 13.26b) or the protrusion may displace the root laterally and present itself in the angle between the theca and root (Figure 13.26a). The paramedian type of protrusion quite often affects two nerve roots – one in its extradural course, the other intradurally. The laterally situated herniation may affect two nerve roots, both *extradurally*.

Unusually, a sequestrated piece of disc material may become displaced into the foramen of the existing root.

CLINICAL FEATURES

Pain

A careful and detailed history is essential in the diagnosis of a protruded intervertebral disc, and often it may be the only guide to the localization of the lesion since the other signs may not be conclusive.

A typical syndrome consists of low backache followed by radicular sciatic pain. This sequence occurs in half of the cases; about a third of patients give a history of sciatica preceding backache; in the remainder, both sciatica and backache ensue simultaneously. It is debatable how often a herniated disc is the cause of low backache only.

The onset may be acute, following a trauma – a fall in a sitting position, lifting weights in a stooping position, etc. Not infrequently there is a latent period of hours, days or weeks between the trauma and the beginning of pain. Still further, in patients subjected to habitual back strain, the onset may be chronic – patients complaining of intermittent, gradually increasing backache, starting as lumbar 'tiredness' or 'aching stiffness'.

A characteristic feature of a disc syndrome is the intermittency (or fluctuation) of symptoms. The backache or sciatica comes on in the form of attacks – lasting days or months. The attacks commence usually fairly rapidly and may incapacitate the victim totally in the course of a few days – the slightest movement in bed may cause excruciating pain; then gradually in a few weeks the pain fades away. The remissions may be complete, but more often there is either slight ache remaining or a sense of 'back awareness'. The explanation of spontaneous remissions is not clearly understood. Regression of herniation probably may occur only in the very early stages. Degeneration of compressed nerve fibres, adjustment of the nerve root into its displaced situation, diminution of the swelling of the herniation, disappearance of the oedema of the nerve root, subsidence of central excitatory state, etc., have been offered as possible causes of retrogression of symptoms.

The pain is usually described as a dull ache, or 'like toothache', 'dragging', 'ache with stabbing jars', 'shooting pain', etc. The lower lumbar region is usually indicated as the site of pain and, though not well defined, it is generally in the midline. The pain may be referred to the sacroiliac joint on one or both sides, to the buttock, and further distally to the lower limb. The radiation of pain may descend, gradually affecting the lower levels of the extremity successively – buttock, thigh, etc. – or it may be referred to any one part of the leg leaving the proximal parts apparently unaffected. The pain is referred to the sclerotome of the involved nerve root – therefore detailed note of it should be taken. The aggravating factors are, as a rule, straightening up from a stooping position far more than bending down, lifting weights, coughing, sneezing and straining at defaecation. Amelioration of pain is usually brought about by recumbency, the position of greatest ease varying with each patient.

Paraesthesia

Paraesthesia, most often described as 'pins and needles', is present at one time or another in the majority of cases. They can be localized by the patient, thereby assisting in the identification of the nerve root involved.

Sensation

In well over half of the cases with protruded intervertebral disc affecting a single nerve root, there is a sensory depression in a given dermatome. The loss is rarely complete and not often in the entire dermatome. Some patients are aware of numbness, subjectively; in others the deficit is found only on objective and careful examination. Loss of other modalities – cold and warmth – although often demonstrable, is difficult to define.

Muscle wasting

In muscle groups innervated chiefly by the affected nerve root, some degree of wasting is quite frequently observed, but the diminution of motor power is not always demonstrable clinically, especially in the flexor group, since the muscles of the lower limbs are very powerful and minor degrees of weakness are difficult to appreciate. Occasionally, various degrees of drop-foot are present. Rarely, flaccid paraplegia is encountered. Weakness of extensor hallucis longus with its single fifth root supply is helpful in determining the level involved.

Tendon reflexes

The tendon reflexes – knee (L3–4) or ankle jerks (L5–S1) – may be depressed depending on the root and the severity of the compression. Occasionally, the ankle jerk may be totally absent but even a slight reduction in the response of the threshold stimulus may be of significance.

Sphincteric disturbance

Urinary retention is found in cases with paraparesis due to central disc prolapse. In milder degrees of compression there is sometimes difficulty in initiation of voiding or incomplete emptying of the bladder.

Postural deformity

The postural deformities of the lumbar spine seen in each case of herniated disc are mostly of a functional, but not organic, nature. The alteration of the spinal curves, limitation of movement and rigidity (spasm) of spinal muscles are part of the protective mechanism adopted subconsciously to prevent, or ameliorate or abolish pain.

The commonest change in the lumbar spine is flattening of the lumbar curve, quite frequently

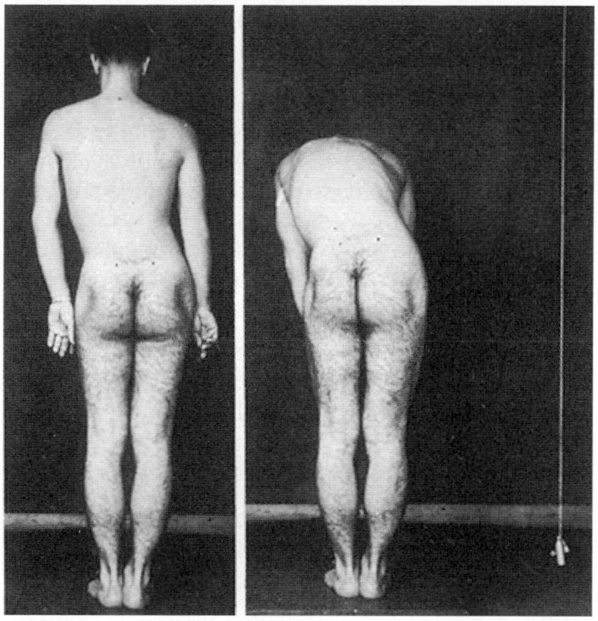

Figure 13.27 A young man with an acute disc prolapse and sciatica, showing a typical scoliotic tilt of the lumbar spine.

noticeable even in relatively mild cases or during remissions. Very rarely, there may be an increase of lumbar lordosis.

The tilt of the trunk is very often observed, either towards or away from the affected side (Figure 13.27). At times it may be present only on bending forward, in others only in the upright position. The term 'tilt' is preferred to scoliosis, as the latter in the lower lumbar region is not always clearly discernible, commonly being missed owing to the presence of a more evident compensatory scoliotic curve higher up in the vertebral column.

When the tilt is absent or indefinite, the relationship between the nerve root and protrusion may at times be ascertained by a circumduction test. Standing firmly, the patient performs half of a circle movement of the trunk in flexion – e.g. bending to the left side, then carrying on circumduction with the spine flexed in the lumbar region forward and then to the right side. If in any particular direction a referred pain may be induced or there is distinct exacerbation of the present sciatic pain in some of the sectors, the test is positive and may be helpful in defining the position of the affected nerve root in relation to the protrusion (Figure 13.28).

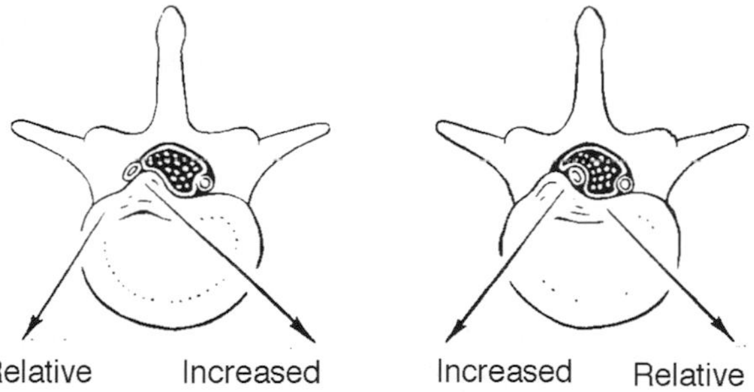

Figure 13.28 Circumduction test. Forward flexion of spine (arrows) or circumduction away from the affected side may produce increased pain. This suggests lateral displacement of the nerve root. Flexion towards affected side does not stretch the root and is a movement of relative ease. The reverse results from medial displacement of the root. A root stretched over the summit of the protrusion would give pain on flexion straight forwards. The more lateral the angle of flexion which causes pain, the more reliably the test indicates sideways displacement of the root.

Some degree of restriction of mobility of the spine is another frequent sign in disc syndrome. Limitation of forward flexion is usually complained of; hyperextension of the spine, relatively speaking, may be more affected but this movement is seldom called for and, being of limited range, difficult to judge. Flexion of the spine improves with the patient in a sitting position. The pain is the limiting factor of spinal movements; the stiffness found in a sense is a voluntary effort, and to some extent a 'reflex' mechanism. The tenderness of muscles may be a referred phenomenon from the affected root or due to localized muscle spasm brought about by irritation of the root, or any source of irritation (e.g. overactivity).

The limitation of forward flexion is best measured by the distance of the fingers from the floor on attempts to reach it. Palpation of the spine is then carried out. Local tenderness over the interspinous ligament or just laterally to the spinous process over the interspace is found in a great majority of cases, and if, on pressure with the examiner's thumb over the suspected level, pain is referred to the buttock, thigh or more distally, a diagnosis of herniated disc may be made with considerable confidence. The sacroiliac joints and the hip joints should be examined.

Straight leg raising test

This test produces an aggravation of pain or reference to the extremity. The greater the restriction of straight leg raising, the larger the protrusion. By the same mechanism, dorsiflexion of the foot in this position (Bragard's sign) often causes increase of pain and possibly more distal reference – e.g. to some of the toes – thus identifying the nerve root involved. The test, however, has no differential value as it is merely indicative of lumbosacral radiculitis from whatever cause.

Radiography

Plain films, anteroposterior or lateral views of the whole lumbar spine and sacrum should be taken routinely. The radiographs have chiefly a twofold value – the possibility of the presence of bone pathology, and they may have disc diagnostic significance. The lumbar disc spaces, as is evident in true lateral radiographs, normally show progressive widening in caudal directions (L2–3 disc space being wider than the one above, etc.) except the lumbosacral interspace which as a rule is narrower than the higher one. Therefore, slight narrowing of L4–5 space, or even its being equal in width to L3–4 disc, can be accurately estimated and it may have a diagnostic value. Recognition of pathological narrowing of the lumbosacral disc is less certain, and in only about one-third of the cases of herniation at this level are x-ray signs considered positive. Various developmental errors in the lumbosacral skeleton are frequently discovered on routine radiography, some of them (e.g. spina bifida occulta) generally are of no importance and have no bearing on the disc syndrome. The presence of a transitional vertebra may lead to diagnostic errors of localization and is probably responsible for some 'negative' explorations. There are relatively frequent variations in the number of lumbar vertebrae. If the number is increased it may be due either to the absence of the twelfth rib or to complete lumbarization of the first sacral piece. This condition may be misinterpreted or overlooked, as frequently, for economic reasons, one plate is used for the x-ray of the sacrum and lumbar spine, and the latter is not fully shown. In cases of lumbarization of sacral vertebrae, if overlooked, the exploration will be carried out at too low a level. If six lumbar vertebrae are present, unassociated with absence of the twelfth rib, the twelfth thoracic vertebra is counted as the first lumbar; consequently, the exploration will be undertaken cephalad to the lesion. Whenever there is any suspicion of an abnormality, a lateral radiograph of the entire spinal column should be taken, and the vertebrae counted downwards from the first cervical to settle the issue.

Myelography

The materials employed are water-soluble compounds (e.g. Omnipaque); 3–5 ml of the solution is injected slowly into the epidural space, followed by x-ray screening on a tilting table. In positive films shadow defects of the column in the thecal sac are seen. Deflection or abolition of small subarachnoid pouches at and below the origin of the nerve root is also of diagnostic significance. The method is recommended to differentiate from a tumour of cauda equina or possibly in some obscure cases of backache. It has been shown that certain cauda equina tumours are clinically indistinguishable from disc lesions, the tumours representing about 4.5% of all surgically treated low back lesions. The procedure is also of value in cases of multiple disc protrusion. It should be stressed, however, that negative myelography does not rule out the presence of disc protrusion.

The typical myelographic appearances of disc lesions were described by Lansche and Ford (1960):

1. Lateral indentation and deformation of the contrast column by a posterolateral disc.
2. Hourglass deformity from a midline herniation.
3. Root pouch filling defects.
4. Complete or partial blocks at the level of the disc or, rarely, opposite a vertebral body.

Although up to 25% of errors of diagnosis have been reported using oil-soluble myelography, with water-soluble myelography using Omnipaque the accuracy has been greatly improved.

Electromyography

Electromyography has become better understood and therefore is now contributing more in diagnosing the causes and levels of root pain, in differentiating between neurapraxia lesions (physiological interruption but intact anatomy) and those of irreversible axonotmesis, and in calculating the duration of the lesion. Johnson and Melvin (1971) described in detail the background behind carrying out the electromyogram in five phases:

1. Muscle at rest exhibits fasciculation potentials (spontaneous discharges from motor units) and fibrillation (electrical discharges from individual muscle fibres).
2. Insertional activity from injury potentials, which stops when the movement of the electrode stops; but when there is muscle cell instability, sharp positive waves continue.
3. Minimal contraction of the muscle under test gives rise to distinct wave patterns as well as motor unit polyphasic potentials.
4. Maximal contraction – similar patterns but greater and more frequent.
5. Distribution differences in anatomical segments and in peripheral nerve innervated areas are explored. The distribution of the posterior primary rami into the paraspinal muscles and in such muscles as extensor hallucis longus and anterior tibialis (for L5) and medial head of gastrocnemius and gluteus maximum (Sl root) for the anterior primary rami.

Johnson and Melvin also described how, 72 hours after the injury, electrical stimulation of the appropriate muscle will give a proportional reduction in the evoked potentials due to Wallerian degeneration of the axon. After 14–28 days, fibrillation potentials appear with the axon undergoing Wallerian degeneration. In a review of 314 electromyograms, the L5 root was most commonly involved and one-third of all patients had abnormalities only in the paraspinal muscles via their post-primary ramus distribution – particularly in acute radiculopathy of 7–14 days. Although other workers had reported that electromyography results are of no value in patients having had previous surgery of laminectomy, Johnson and Melvin, by studying the paraspinal muscles at least 3 cm from the middle and 3 cm deep into the muscle, identified characteristic evoked potentials in the muscles of the extremities.

Leyshon *et al.* (1981) have described how, by measuring fibrillation potential, H-reflex latencies, electronic-triggered patellar response and the Sl root ankle reflex latencies, they obtained 90% accuracy in diagnosing nerve root lesions – against myelographic ‘positives’ of 52% and clinical ‘positives’ of 40%. However, the correct identification of specific roots were reduced to 76%, 33% and 24%, respectively.

Cerebrospinal fluid

Lumbar puncture, to test the dynamics of the CSF as well as its contents, is rarely indicated.

CT and MRI scanning

The diagnosis of both level and degree of the protrusion or prolapse of the nucleus pulposus based upon clinical findings can now be substantiated by numerous scanning methods of varying accuracy, sensitivity and specificity.

In 1984, Bell *et al.* published a comparison of metrizamide water-soluble myelography and computed tomography in the diagnosis of herniated lumbar disc and spinal stenosis. Included were 122 patients with surgically confirmed pathology of either disc herniation or spinal stenosis and each of them had had preoperative myelography and non-contrast CT. On analysis myelography was more accurate than CT in the diagnosis of prolapsed disc at 83% versus 72%. In the diagnosis of spinal stenosis myelography was slightly more accurate than CT at 93% versus 89%. The authors concluded that metrizamide myelography is more accurate than CT in these conditions and remains the diagnostic study of choice. They also pointed out that myelography can visualize the thoracolumbar junction and thus afford the opportunity to diagnose occult spinal tumours. CT was becoming popular then and its proponents pointed out the better visualization of lateral pathology, the absence of adverse reactions and the use of less radiation with CT resulted in lower cost because hospitalization was not required. MRI has overcome some of the criticisms of CT particularly in its definitions of soft tissue and its ability to give a myelographic type of sagittal plane image. A number of papers have been published confirming that MRI is superior even to contrast CT in the diagnosis of intervertebral disc disease. In particular Jackson *et al.* (1989) compared the accuracy of CT, myelography, CT-myelography and MRI for the diagnosis of prolapsed lumbar interbertebral disc prospectively in 59 patients all of whom underwent surgical exploration. The accuracy of each of the four techniques was similar with MRI 76.5%, myelo-CT 76%, CT 73.6% and myelography 71.4%. False-positive rates varied from 13.5% for MRI to 21.1% for myelo-CT. The false-negative rate was lowest for myelo-CT at 27.2%, followed by MRI at 35.7%, CT at 40.2% and myelography at 41%. They concluded that MRI compared very favourably with other currently available imaging modalities, was painless with no known side-effects, was non-invasive with no radiation exposure. It therefore was the procedure of choice in the diagnosis of disc disease (Figure 13.29).

The question of the far lateral disc herniation does not appear to be resolved. Maroon *et al.* (1990) present a series of 25 patients with far lateral lumbar disc herniations and report that myelography was uniformly normal and high quality MRI was often not helpful. They recommend discography with enhanced CT as the best investigation or failing that, high resolution CT. However, for far lateral disc herniations and lateral recess stenosis CT-myelography is particularly valuable.

The question whether intervertebral disc degeneration occurs before facet joint degeneration was studied by Butler *et al.* (1990) using MRI to determine disc degeneration and CT to determine facet joint arthritis. From 68 sets of scans they found 144 degenerated discs and 41 levels with facet osteoarthritis. Disc degeneration without facet osteoarthritis was found at 108 levels. All but one of the 41 levels with facet degeneration also had disc degeneration; the exception occurred in a patient with advanced Paget’s disease. Both conditions increased with increasing age. They concluded that disc degeneration occurred before facet joint osteoarthritis which may arise secondary to abnormal loading of the facet joints.

Discography

Milette *et al.* (1990) compared high resolution CT with discography in 100 patients with symptoms suggestive of prolapsed disc but without objective

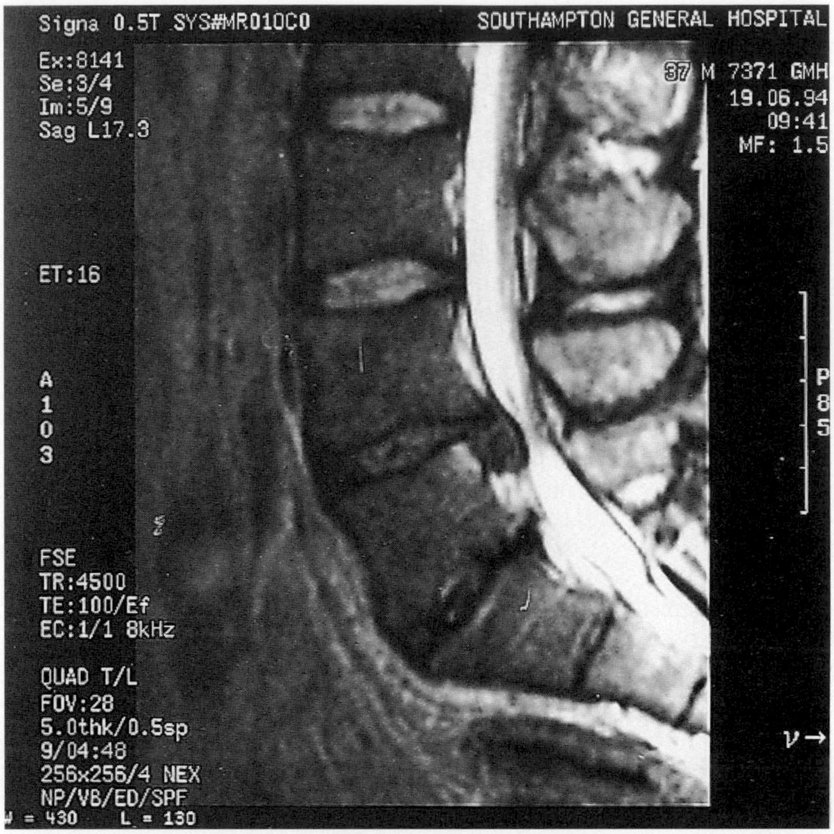

Figure 13.29 A prolapsed intervertebral disc with clear thecal impingement. Axial views will give further information with regard to the site and size of the protrusion. MRI is superior to CT scanning in assessing the magnitude of the protrusion. (Films kindly supplied by Dr Richard Blaquiere, Consultant Radiologist at Southampton University Hospitals)

neurology and thought CT to be inadequate, thus justifying discography before undertaking surgery; once again this was a non-contrast CT study. Bernard (1990) used discography followed by CT in 250 patients and found this a very valuable technique in correctly predicting the disc herniation as protruded, extruded, sequestrated or internally disrupted in 94% of the patients who had surgery. He suggested that discography CT may be more sensitive than MRI in the early stages of disc degeneration because 18 of 177 with a normal T2 weighted image were discographically abnormal with the CT discogram revealing annular tears or radial fissuring. The complications following 750 discograms were only one case of urticaria and one disc space infection. He concluded that, even with the availability of high resolution CT and MRI, lumbar discography remained the only pain provocation challenge to the lumbar disc.

Frocrain *et al.* (1989), in studying particular patients with recurrent postoperative sciatica, found that intravenous enhanced CT only gave an accuracy of 42% when the recurrent disc material was frequently misdiagnosed as only fibrosis. MR with gadolinium was much more accurate, i.e. 97.8%.

Discography to determine disc pathology and symptomatology particularly as a preoperative diagnostic test is becoming popular. However, Nachemson (1989) has recently warned about excessive treatment being carried out because of the use of this test, particularly as an indication for spinal fusion.

Localizing features of intervertebral disc collapse

Central disc:

1. Asymmetrical muscle weakness and wasting in legs.
2. Radicular sensory loss over sacrum, perineum and back of thigh.
3. Impotence, urinary frequency and/or retention.

Saddle anaesthesia, gluteal wasting and patulous anal sphincter on digital examination are often found. The differential diagnosis of a tumour must be contemplated.

Peripheral disc:

1. Segmental root pain.
2. Corresponding segmental muscle weakness and wasting in legs.
3. Absent segmental reflexes.
4. Late development of sphincter disturbance and bilateral signs.

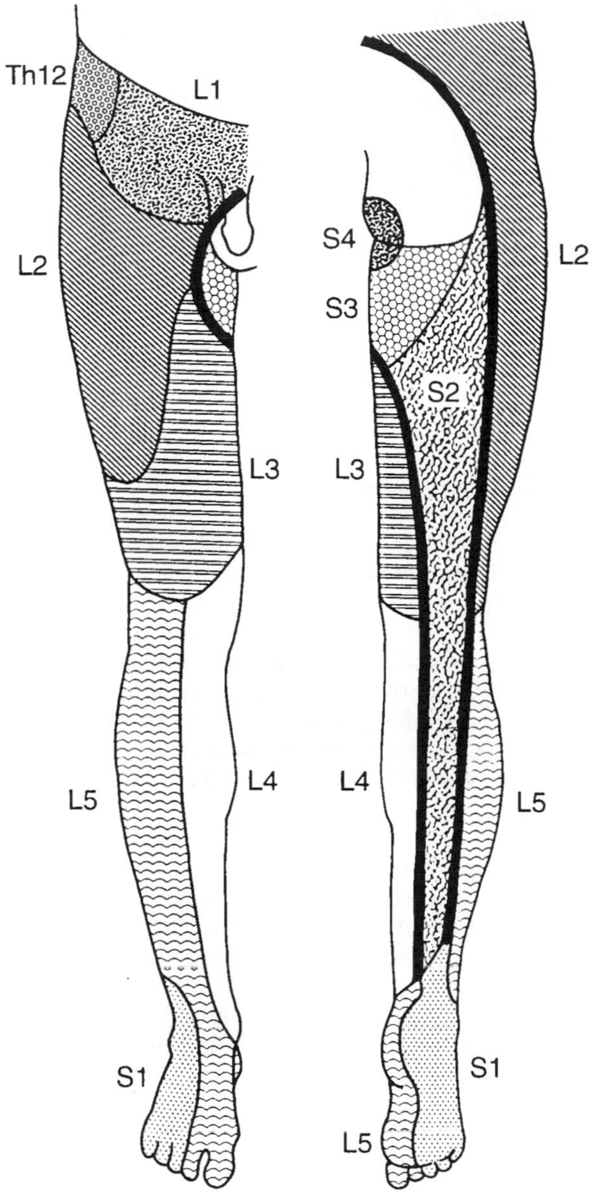

Figure 13.30 Keegan's dermatomes. A possible modification is to include the big toe in L4 dermatome entirely. The L5 dermatome usually terminates on the medial aspect of the foot.

Compression of the L4 nerve root may result in weakness of the quadriceps muscle and diminution of knee jerk. The dermatome extends along the anterolateral aspect of the thigh, front of the knee, medial aspect of the ankle joint, and the medial aspect of the foot, not reaching the great toe (Figure 13.30).

The L5 nerve root involvement leads to some wasting of the glutei and dorsiflexors of the foot. Inversion and dorsiflexion of foot and toes are weakened. Knee and ankle jerks are normal. The L5 dermatome traverses the lateral aspect of the thigh, anterolateral aspect of the leg and dorsum of the foot, and covers the big toe and one or more adjacent toes – never the little toe.

The SI root affection shows wasting of the glutei, hamstrings and calf muscles; weakness of eversion and plantar flexors of the foot and toes is found. The ankle jerk is reduced or absent. The first sacral dermatome occupies the posterolateral aspect of the thigh, lateral or posterolateral aspect of the leg, lateral border of the foot and little toe; two adjacent toes may also be included – never the big toe.

Naturally, not all symptoms are necessarily present in every case. Furthermore, in polyradicular syndromes, the symptoms or signs referable to one root may differ from those of another.

Vesical sphincteric dysfunction

(Crosbie Ross and Jameson, 1971)

Single root lesions are unlikely to cause bladder dysfunction. Massive blockage due to central protrusion or multiple disc lesions are more likely to result in disturbance of voiding. Higher lesions also are most likely to cause symptoms. However, it can exist without typical back or leg pain. Three types have been described:

1. Temporary:
   (a) relieved by conservative measures;
   (b) transient postoperative symptoms.
2. Occult – insensitive bladder with minimal back or leg pain.
3. Permanent – bladder function not improved by disc surgery.

The occult variety described by Emmett and Love (1968) occurred in obese women with childhood neurosis and an injury antedating the symptoms, which consisted of frequency, nocturia and urgency without evidence of infection.

DIFFERENTIAL DIAGNOSIS

Among many pathological conditions which theoretically could come into differential diagnosis, there are only a few which may resemble closely prolapsed disc syndrome and which from a practical point of view need be considered.

Tumours

Tumours of the cauda equina, such as ependymoma of filum terminale or conus medullaris, meningioma or neurinoma, are common in this region. The last-named is most likely to simulate prolapsed intervertebral disc. Arising from any of the nerve roots, it may attain a very large size before it begins to give rise to other than monoradicular symptoms. Pain may be agonizingly severe, especially on coughing or sneezing – the increased CSF pressure displacing the tumour distally like a piston with a sudden drag on the nerve root. There is no such conditioning of pain on spinal movements as there is in a disc syndrome. Bladder disturbance may occur early. Paraplegia of flaccid type, with marked muscular wasting and trophic and sensory changes, supervenes. The course is slowly progressive without remissions. x-Rays may show increase in interpediculate measurements. Manometry and the protein content of CSF settle the diagnosis. Myelography and MRI scanning are often necessary for the exact localization.

Spondylolisthesis

This condition may closely resemble prolapsed disc syndrome. The sciatic pain may be unilateral or bilateral and is apt to be less affected by postural changes; backache, which not infrequently is a less prominent feature than one would anticipate, is relieved by rest. Forward flexion of the spine is often surprisingly good. Major degrees of slipping of the vertebrae are obvious on clinical inspection. Radiography settles the diagnosis (Figure 13.31). The sciatic symptoms are commonly produced by stretching of the nerve roots over the upper posterior margin of the prominent lower vertebral body. Independently herniations of a disc may occur immediately above the level of spondylolisthesis, and be wholly responsible for any symptoms present, the latter being entirely symptomless.

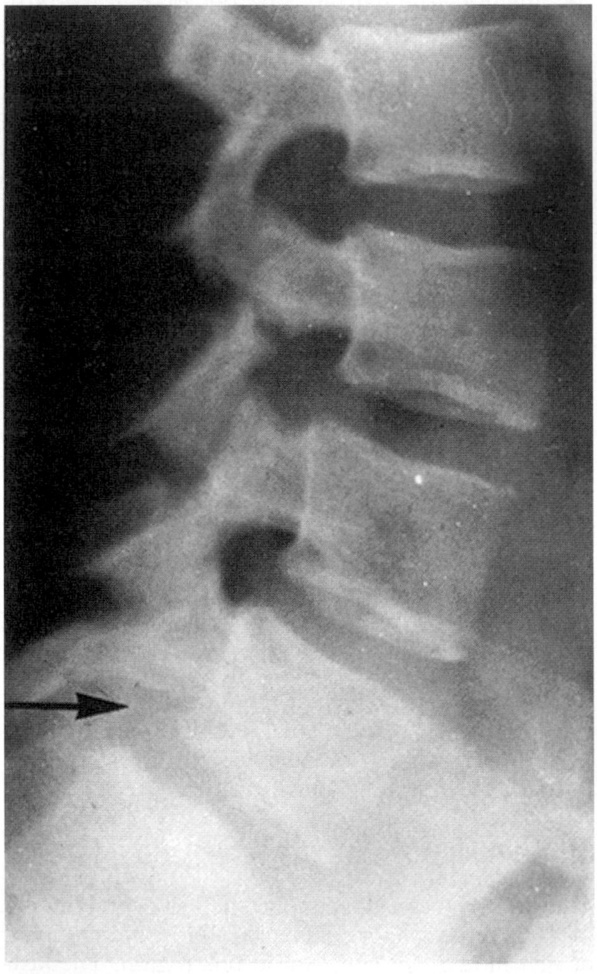

Figure 13.31 Spondylolisthesis of L5 without any defect of the pars interarticularis but with abnormal facet motion.

Radiculitis (primary)

Diagnosis of this condition is difficult to make and usually is arrived at by exclusion, since radiculitis is commonly secondary to some other lesion in the vicinity of the roots. The aetiology of primary radiculitis is unknown but in some virus infection is generally accepted. A history of preceding generalized or local infection may be present. The disease may affect one or several roots of cauda equina, sacral ones being most affected; consequently sphincteric disturbance of the bladder and rectum as a rule is present. The disease begins with sudden acute pains in the lower extremities; paraesthesia, sensory deficit and increasing muscular weakness soon follow. Unlike the disc syndrome, there is distinct tenderness of muscles and rest in bed for a week or two does not appear to have any effect on the pain. CSF in some cases shows slight lymphocytic pleocytosis. There is no history of previous recurrent attacks. Very rarely, exploration may be necessary to establish the diagnosis, as differentiation from massive disc protrusion or tumour compressing cauda equina is obviously difficult.

Other conditions

Granulomatous lesions, gynaecological or genitourinary conditions, etc., should not prove difficult to differentiate if sufficient attention is paid to detailed history and careful examination.

CONSERVATIVE TREATMENT

With few exceptions, conservative treatment is recommended initially in all cases of prolapsed intervertebral disc. In many cases this may effect a complete and permanent relief.

The cardinal features in conservative treatment are rest of the lumbar spine with heavy doses of non-steroidal anti-inflammatory agents (e.g. indomethacin, ibuprofen) as well as a muscle relaxant (e.g. diazepam) and night sedation. Strict recumbency for a few weeks brings about some measure of relief even in the most acute cases. This really can be enforced only under hospital regimen. Immobilization in a plaster-of-Paris jacket is frequently recommended, either instead of bed rest or to follow it, depending on the severity of the sciatica. A plaster-of-Paris jacket extending from immediately above the pubis to the nipples, after correction of scoliosis (or without it, on the assumption that abnormal curvatures of the spine express optimal position for relief of pain), is applied and is usually followed by prompt alleviation of sciatica. Naylor *et al.* (1977) reported this as being successful in 90% of cases. This treatment should be followed by mobilization within a lumbosacral support to maintain the lumbar lordosis and increase the intra-abdominal pressure. The patient should be advised to avoid high disc pressure postures – i.e. anterior sitting posture (Andersson *et al.*, 1975) and disadvantageous bending and lifting.

Doran and Newell (1975), in a poorly organized multi-centre trial which included 456 selected patients, showed that only a few responded to manipulation and such patients were difficult to identify in advance. They concluded that although the response to a corset was slow it was effective. Patients treated with analgesics alone fared slightly worse than others; manipulation was not cost-effective and should not be pursued if response was not seen in the early stages. Resisted spinal and abdominal wall exercises were of some value.

To substantiate the value of non-operative treatment Saal *et al.* (1990) have followed up 11 non-operated upon disc herniations with positive neurological signs, e.g. motor weakness, a positive straight leg sign and a positive CT scan. After 25 months all had resolution of their signs and symptoms and MR imaging showed the majority had disc material resorption without perineural or peridural fibrosis.

Epidural injection

Because the inflammatory changes around the affected nerve root may be important in producing the sciatic symptoms in lumbar disc prolapse, an extradural injection is the safest way to place steroid material in the immediate vicinity of inflamed tissue. Methylprednisolone suspension is known to persist in the intrathecal space at therapeutic levels for 3 weeks. But this route of injection is not safe whereas the epidural is safer and easier to perform.

A low-volume, high-steroid dose is now most commonly used (e.g. methylprednisolone) and is indicated in the following:

1. Patients with acute symptoms including:
   (a) painful straight leg raising or femoral stretch test;
   (b) sciatic scoliosis;
   (c) an appropriate neurological deficit.
2. Patients with acute-on-chronic attacks, with long symptom-free intervals before presenting.
3. Patients with acute-on-chronic symptoms, with a different level of disc pathology (e.g. after previous surgery).

Dilke *et al.* (1973) reported that, of 100 patients from a double-blind study, the treated group returned to work earlier with less pain at a 3-month follow-up and there were fewer referrals for surgery.

Complications noted were low pressure headaches, sciatic pain reproduced during injection and a transitory muscle weakness lasting 15–20 minutes following epidural injection of local anaesthetic.

Chemonucleolysis

Chymopapain was first introduced into the clinical situation by Dr Lyman Smith who, in 1964, reported the use of chymopapain in 10 patients with good response in seven.

Chymopapain is a heat labile cystine proteinase which is produced from the papaya fruit *Carica papaya* as papain. It acts in the clinical situation by degrading the proteoglycans of the nucleus pulposus when injected directly into the intervertebral disc. The proteoglycan is split into its components glycan and protein, the water holding property of the disc is decreased, and the disc shrinks. The effect is maximum at 4–8 days. However, breakdown products of the proteoglycans can be detected in the blood almost immediately after injection. Chymopapain itself is rapidly inactivated (30–60 s).

The drug is also extensively used in the food and drug industry, particularly for clearing cloudy contact lenses, as a meat tenderizer and as an additive in beer and toothpaste manufacture.

Chymodiactin, a related proteinase extracted from the papaya, is replacing chymopapain as it is less heat labile and easier to produce.

Patient selection for chemonucleolysis

Chemonucleolysis should be considered as an alternative form of management for the prolapsed intervertebral disc, as well as a formal discectomy, microdiscectomy and percutaneous nucleotomy. Its use should be restricted to lumbar disc herniations, preferably at one level, and the patient should have failed to respond to standard conservative measures.

Herniation should be confirmed by MRI/CT examination which allows better differentiation of the sequestrated disc, free disc fragment and spinal stenosis or later recess syndrome.

The patient should have a classical history of sciatica, preferably with a straight leg raising, a dermatomal sensory loss, or motor weakness and reflex changes.

Contraindications for the use of chymopapain

1. Known papaya sensitivity and demonstrated papaya sensitivity.
2. Disc protrusion with sphincter disturbance and/or rapidly progressive severe neurological disturbance.
3. Pregnancy.
4. Previous lumbar surgery at the intended level of injection.
5. Ongoing litigation or compensation case.
6. Demonstrated associated spinal stenosis or lateral recess syndrome.
7. Long-standing symptomatology.
8. Sequestrated or free disc fragment.
9. Strong history of previous allergic or anaphylactic reactions.

Practical use of chemonucleolysis

It is now generally accepted that local anaesthesia is preferable to general anaesthesia for three reasons:

1. It allows early recognition of an allergic response by the patient.
2. The patient can report any neurological symptoms produced during the procedure.
3. Halothane is hepatotoxic and in combination with the drugs used to treat anaphylaxis appears to contribute to the deaths reported.

The patient should be medically fit and be negative when tested by chymopapain interdermal skin testing. In the USA, but rarely in the UK, premedication is used in association with an antihistamine 50 mg i.v., cimetidine 300 mg and frequently the use of steroids.

Full operating room precautions are taken with a large intravenous entry for management of any anaphylactic response. The patient is placed in the right or left lateral position. For the L4/5 disc space a posterolateral or lateral approach is used.

For the L5/S1 level a similar needle and lumen is used, and in addition to the 45–60° sagittal angle, a 30° caudal angle is selected to allow entry into the disc space. A pre-bent needle tip technique is used by some operators.

After entry into the intervertebral disc, discography is performed using a non-ionic contrast medium. This excludes the very rare instances of direct communication between the site of disc rupture and the intrathecal space. There is no evidence that modern contrast media inactivate chymopapain/chymodiactin and may in fact act synergistically to enhance the disc breakdown. The total dose of chymopapain used varies between 1000 and 4000 units. A test dose of 400 units or 0.2 ml is given and if there is no allergic response then the remaining 1.2 ml is injected.

After injection close observation of the patient is required. Most anaphylactic responses occur within 5 minutes, but there have been reports of severe reactions up to 4 hours after injection. Any anaphylaxis is treated in the standard way relying mainly on large volume fluid replacement. Postoperatively the main problem is muscle spasm, sometimes severe, occurring in at least 50% of patients. Average hospital stay is 4 days. Patients can then be allowed to increase activity gradually, but should probably empirically avoid any heavy activity for 6 weeks.

The incidence of anaphylaxis with chymopapain is variously reported at between 0.44 and 2% of patients treated, with a mortality of 0.01–0.2%. This compares with a known surgical mortality of 0.1–0.14%. Initial attempts to avoid anaphylaxis centred around avoiding those individuals with known sensitivity or exposure to chymopapain or its products, avoiding hypersensitive individuals and pretreatment of patients with steroids, cimetidine and antihistamines. More recently, specific testing has been introduced for chymopapain allergy.

Transverse myelitis following an injection of chymopapain has been reported in 1:18 000 injections, compared to a natural incidence of this problem of 1:100 000. The mechanism for this response is not known, although it is suspected that some cases have resulted following intrathecal leakage or injection of the chymopapain.

There have been several studies reporting repeat chymopapain for recurrent intervertebral protrusion. However, the sensitization to chymopapain after a first injection is approximately 36%; 50% of those then react with anaphylaxis to further injections.

CT evaluation and further surgery after chymopapain confirms the expected causes for failure, namely extruded and sequestrated discs in approximately 50% with the remainder due to a combination of spinal stenosis and lateral recess stenosis, epidural cysts, etc. Thus the failures in chymopapain appear to be due almost entirely to inadequate patient selection.

Studies of the success rate of surgery after chymopapain show a satisfactory outcome in approximately 87%.

In summary, chemonucleolysis has stood up well with the passage of time. Unlike so many new medical procedures, it offers a definite alternative for the management of the prolapse or the herniated intervertebral disc. Future advances will probably come in the area of alternative human proteinases for injection and/or further sophistication in the detection of the hypersensitive individual.

OPERATIVE TREATMENT (OPEN DISCECTOMY)

Disc excision with exposure adequate to preserve the neural tissue and to visualize the disc is essential. There is no place for routine spinal fusion in the majority of patients undergoing disc excision (Cauchoix and Giraud, 1978).

Indications

1. Paraplegia or acute bladder paralysis due to cauda equina compression.
2. Severe peripheral neurological defect, e.g. foot-drop.
3. Failure of conservative treatment to relieve pain and neurological symptoms and signs.
4. Severe, persistent pain.

Operations

The laminectomy exposure has become less extensive, and has been improved by an interlaminar approach with excision of the ligamentum flavum and little, if any, of parts of the adjacent laminae – the so-called 'fenestration' operation. Although laminectomy does not really jeopardize the stability of the spine, it is unnecessary to employ the major procedure if the minor interlaminar exposure proves adequate; if need be, it may easily be enlarged into hemilaminectomy.

Indications for fusion after laminectomy and/or disc removal are:

1. An associated spondylolisthesis.
2. A congenital malformation.
3. Advanced intervertebral arthritis.
4. Instability due to bone removal (i.e. by the laminectomy).
5. Need for a return to heavy manual work.

McNab (1975) considered that an accompanying fusion is necessary in:

1. A patient under 50 years with normal disc heights and root entrapment associated with changes in the posterior facet joint necessitating extensive joint excision.
2. A patient with progressive history of backache culminating in backache associated with severe sciatic pain and nerve root irritation. In this case mechanical instability is the main problem.
3. Emotionally stable patients who are unable to restrict work or when, despite doing so, are disabled by recurrent episodes of incapacitating low back pain.

Spinal fusion is becoming more popular but the results are unimpressive. If fusion is required, which is rarely the case, an interlaminar fusion is the simplest and most effective method. Although internal fixation devices, including pedicle screw fixation, are being proposed, there is little evidence of their value.

Operative technique

The patient is placed prone on the operating table with the spine moderately flexed by the aid of a bridge or pillows. The weight should be taken by the iliac spines because compression of the abdomen, apart from its interference with respiration, tends to produce an engorgement of the epidural veins.

A midline incision, centred over the affected interspace, is used. A length of 8–10 cm is usually adequate. The lumbodorsal fascia is divided in the midline and the muscles are separated with diathermy close to the bone on one or both sides. The spinous processes and the laminae adjacent to the suspected space are exposed. Frequently the lower border of the higher lamina, partly overlapping the ligamentum flavum, is nibbled away with a bone rongeur. The ligamentum flavum is then incised longitudinally near the midline. A pledget of wool is inserted underneath it for the protection of the theca and roots, and the excision of the ligamentum flavum is completed. Care should be taken while excising it laterally, as not infrequently the nerve root is displaced right up against it. The small square window usually needs enlargement by nibbling with angled punches, as a rule in an upward (cephalad) direction, since it is preferred to identify the root above the disc. Alternatively, a satisfactory exposure without removal of any bone may sometimes be achieved by division of the interspinous ligament and ligamentum flavum and wide retraction (spreading) of the spinous processes. The enlarging of the 'window' laterally, if necessary, should be done carefully to avoid injury to the nerve root and also to avoid damage to the intervertebral joint.

The theca and nerve root may be immediately evident upon opening the epidural space, or may be hidden under a layer of epidural fat traversed by numerous veins. The nerve root being fully exposed, vessels coagulated and divided, its position in relation to the protrusion is verified; it is gently mobilized by blunt dissection if adherent to the protrusion, and retracted medially. If the protrusion lies medially to the root, and the latter cannot be 'slipped' over the summit medially without undue stretching, the protrusion should be partly removed and then the root retracted medially as this is the safest and most convenient position during removal of the disc. The acute angle between theca and root contains as a rule a rich network of vessels which bleed easily when disturbed and are difficult to control. The protrusion usually is evident as a white or yellowish glistening bulge with the root stretched over it; its abnormal consistency is obvious on pressure with the tip of the forceps. Having the protrusion exposed and the root safely guarded with the retractor, a circular incision is made with a pointed knife in the capsule of the herniation. The extruding material is removed, the opening, if necessary, being enlarged further, and the space is first cleared with end-cutting punches.

Mobility of the nerve root should be gently ascertained – with a little experience it is possible to tell if it is free or fixed by a herniation outside the exposed area. A probe is passed along the root into the intervertebral foramen and diameters of its lumen are ascertained; a probe is passed under the theca medially in search of a central or paramedian protrusion. A search should also be made over the vertebral bodies adjacent to the disc, as sometimes the nucleus pulposus may 'dissect' upwards under the capsule, or a loose fragment of ruptured disc may become displaced. In the latter case, an opening in the annulus fibrosus is found only in recent ruptures.

If no herniation is found, the next space should be opened, either by making a separate interlaminar opening or by extending the already made exposure by removing the remaining bridge of lamina and so converting it into a hemilaminectomy exposure.

The wound is closed in layers with Vicryl and the patient nursed free in bed for 24 hours. He should then be mobilized, avoiding deep flexion of the spine for 10–14 days. Postoperative back exercises are taught, which the patient must continue.

Complications

Wound infection very occasionally occurs and as a rule is superficial. Treatment with appropriate antibiotics for a week is usually successful.

Very rarely, CSF leaking from a cut or tear in the dura may find its way into the subcutaneous tissues. Aspiration should be carried out followed by a compression bandage. Repeated leakage is effectively treated by reopening the wound, excising the lining of the tract, but making no attempt to close it specifically. Closure of the wound then follows.

Occasionally weakness such as drop-foot may be accentuated by surgical interference. The weakness is as a rule temporary, though it may take months to recover. A drop-foot appliance may be recommended.

Rehabilitation by physiotherapy and occupational therapy is an important part of treatment, and should be controlled by experienced physiotherapists under hospital conditions. Graded exercises of the spinal muscles and lower limbs should restore the patient's confidence as well as his spinal mobility.

Patients returning to sedentary work may be allowed to do so in 3–4 weeks; those in more active types of work, in 2 months. Patients whose work involves heavy back strain should be employed at a light type of work for at least 3 months from the date of operation prior to the return to their normal employment.

Operation results and prognosis

The surgical treatment of backache and sciatica due to protruded intervertebral disc fulfils its purpose – the abolition or relief of pain – in the vast majority of cases – 75% on average. As a rule, sciatic pain is abolished or improved in a much greater proportion of cases than is backache. When the improvement in the severity of symptoms brought about by an operation is taken into account, about 80% or more cases show benefit derived from surgery.

Abramovitz and Neff (1991) have described the following preoperative features which are associated with a good outcome after discectomy:

1. Absence of any work related injury and likelihood of compensation.
2. Absence of back pain.
3. Radicular pain with a positive straight leg raise test.
4. Absence of back pain or straight leg raise test.
5. Asymmetric loss or decreased reflexes.
6. Presence of sensory deficit.

Obesity, age or motor loss did not appear to have any predictive value. Good results were obtained in over 80% of their multicentre series.

Causes of failure

Rosen *et al.* (1991) have studied the perioperative complication of facet fracture as a cause of back pain. They found that removal of more than 25% of the lamina predisposes to fracture and this can clearly be demonstrated by CT scanning.

Failed disc surgery with persistent clinical features is usually due to recurrent or persistent disc herniation, epidural fibrosis, adhesive arachnoiditis, but, most importantly, lateral canal stenosis.

Intra- or extraforaminal herniation should be

obvious preoperatively by modern diagnostic technology and requires resection of the pars and part or whole of the inferior facet, followed by fusion.

Arterial or venous laceration or fistula formation has been reported when the anterior annulus is perforated. Full and postoperative blood and cramping abdominal pain are common features requiring immediate diagnosis and operative treatment. Dural tears and lacerations are common. Disc space infection occurs in 1–5% of all operations as does systemic reaction but ESR or CR protein tests only become indicative 2 weeks or more after surgery.

Factors predisposing to failure of discectomy with persistent low back pain were patients receiving workman's compensation, heavy smokers and patients over 40 years of age (Hanley and Shapiro, 1989).

Tregonning *et al.* (1991) have compared the chemonucleolysis procedure with discectomy – carried out in the 1970s and therefore a 10-year follow-up. With surgery there were significantly more excellent results and relief of pain. Of the chemonucleolysis group 23% required revision surgery against 10% of the discectomies due to recurrent herniations or scarring. Revision surgery results were fair or poor in 60% of the lysis group and 54% in the surgical group.

They emphasize that the presence of workman's compensation leads to worse results in both groups – but higher with chemonucleolysis. The authors reported a 1.5% anaphylaxis rate and 1.5% fewer allergic reactions.

Nucleotomy: percutaneous aspiration discectomy

Currently this procedure is considered as an alternative to formal discectomy. Onik and Helms (1991) have described the indications for this procedure as well as using automated lumbar discectomy:

1. Primary complaint of incapacitating, radicular leg pains, especially those made worse by standing and sitting and eased by lying as the herniation is still within the disc.
2. Failure of conservative treatment for 6 weeks or more.
3. Positive sciatic stretch test.
4. Myelographic, CR or MRI evidence of subannular disc herniation consistent with patient's symptoms and signs.
5. At least two of the following:
   - weakness of plantar flexors or extensors;
   - wasting of plantar flexor or extensors;
   - lost or diminished reflexes; and
   - loss of diminished sensation in a specific dermatome distribution.

Contraindications are:

1. Acute disc prolapse with sphincter disturbance.
2. Sequestered or free disc fragment.
3. Massive disc herniation with more than 50% compromise of thecal sac as 90% of these have a free fragment.
4. Association spinal stenosis or nerve root stenosis.
5. Osteophytes or developmental abnormalities causing nerve root compression.
6. Compensation claim.
7. L5/S1 level – although there is now new instrumentation available which is able to curve over iliac crest and enter this disc space. Onik also excluded patients who had had:
   - previous lumbar surgery,
   - previous chymopapain injection, or have degenerative disc disease,
   - nerve compression due to scar formation.

Mink (1989) has usefully defined disc herniations as a:

1. Simple herniated disc (subannular herniation): a portion of the annulus and the entire posterior longitudinal ligament (PLL) are intact and contain the nuclear material.
2. Extruded herniation (subligamentous herniation): the annulus is completely torn, but the post-longitudinal ligament (PLL) remains intact
   (a) without migration
   (b) with migration
      - in continuity with the disc space
      - without continuity with the disc space (sequestrated fragment).
3. Free fragment: the annulus and the PLL are torn, and the disc material lies free in the epidural space
   (a) without migration
   (b) with migration
      - in continuity with the disc
      - without continuity with the disc (sequestrated fragment).

In 1990 Maroon *et al.* reported results of the first 50 patients having received a nucleotomy who were examined at 1 month, 2 months and at 6 months. About 37/50 = 75% excellent or good results were found.

Most patients have returned to work in 5 weeks, but 10/50 required a formal operation and 7 of these 10 were found to have extruded fragment or migrated fragments under posterior longitudinal ligament.

Bonneville *et al.* (1989) reviewed 40 patients at 3 months postoperatively and found 40% had a good result, 30% had a fair result and 30% had a bad result. In the Bonneville study, clinical results were better for the patients complaining of chronic low back pain with multiple blockages due to mild subligamentous median disc bulges, rather than for true radicular pain. Twenty-five per cent required a further operation.

Complications described were:

- Transient pain for 2–5 days at insertion site noted.
- Transient ipsilateral thigh paraesthesia in patients under general anaesthetic.
- Paravertebral muscle spasm.
- Vasovagal syncope.
- Discitis.
- Haematoma causing temporary hypalgesia in lateral femoral cutaneous nerve.

The advantages were:

- Shorter hospital stay under a local anaesthetic procedure.
- There was reduced morbidity especially with obese patients and absence of scar tissue and adhesion formation.

Percutaneous discectomy using a nucleotome is a new technique with great potential. It has many advantages over open procedures. The exact role needs to be more clearly defined. This will require more accurate diagnosis of disc pathology (e.g. sequestered, free fragment, mushroom shaped herniations); CT discography and high resolution MRI using surface coils may be useful for this.

Although more surgeons are practising percutaneous discectomy techniques which are proving effective, there is still no clear evidence that the clinical success rates are better than that for the classical open procedure. Kahanovitz *et al.* (1990) from a multicentre trial found that after 17 months only 55% of their patients had returned to work and that 34% required a secondary open procedure for continuing pain, weakness and numbness. Barrios *et al.* (1990), in a retrospective, comparative study between these two procedures, found that in 85% good or excellent results were obtained. There was a higher recurrence rate and need for operation in those patients who had a percutaneous microdiscectomy procedure.

Failed back surgery syndrome

This is an area of constant difficulty for the practising clinician. Djukic *et al.* (1990) states that MR imaging is rapidly becoming the imaging modality of choice in the assessment of patients with recurrent symptoms following spinal surgery. They claim it can differentiate persistent or recurrent disc herniation from postoperative scar formation with a greater degree of confidence than other imaging modalities and can determine clinically important functional instability when CT and plain films are inconclusive. They have also found MRI useful in showing the presence of other causes of failed back surgery such as lateral spinal stenosis, arachnoiditis, fat graft compression of the thecal sac and the presence of haematoma or infection. Ross *et al.* (1990) looked at 193 postoperative patients who had MR imaging of the lumbar spine: 27 had repeat surgery at 31 levels and the surgical diagnoses differed from the MR diagnoses in two patients at two levels. Over all they found a 96% accuracy on MR in differentiating scar from disc in 44 patients at 50 reoperated levels.

For studying the bony problems CT scanning should be used. Two- and three-dimensional scanning can display well the surgical procedure and its extent, lateral neural foraminal narrowing and fractures of the posterior elements. Ross *et al.* (1990) demonstrated fusion or pseudarthrosis formation and the degree of incorporation of transverse processes and facet joints. Delamarter *et al.* (1990) evaluated 24 cases of lumbar arachnoiditis with MRI and compared them in 20 cases with CT myelography and plain myelography. Three anatomical groups were identified, one with conglomerations of adherent nerve roots centrally within the thecal sac, another with nerve roots adherent peripherally to the meninges and a third with a soft tissue mass replacing the subarachnoid space. There was excellent correlation between the different imaging methods.

Cauda equina syndrome

Cauda equina syndrome resulting from a disc herniation is uncommon – about 2.2% of patients admitted for laminectomy (Kostuik *et al.*, 1986), but is more commonly seen in trauma, metastatic lesions, infections – pyogenic osteomyelitis, and spinal stenosis. Its importance lies in the involvement of the sympathetic outflow, i.e. the presacral plexus with bowel and bladder disturbance, saddle anaesthesiae, motor weakness of the lower extremities as well as low back pain. Paraplegia can result rarely with bilateral sciatica. Similar to spinal stenosis syndrome, it results from both compression as well as vascular ischaemia and it is this later pathology which is responsible for the severity and permanency of the lesion, particularly of visceral function. Delamarter *et al.* (1991) have produced an experimental model in dogs of this lesion which had a much better recovery rate after decompression even although delayed up to 1 week more than that found in humans.

Diagnosis is based upon the three classical features of sciatica, a saddle sensory deficit and urinary retention with or without overflow incontinence. Delay in diagnosis and in the decision for surgery must be avoided. Rapid onset even without sciatica has a poor prognosis.

Disc prolapse in the young adult or adolescent (see Chapter 8)

Stamm (1962) drew attention to this comparatively newly recognized clinical entity. A young adult or adolescent presents with a history of minor injury such as lifting or a strain at athletics, and this is followed by the gradual onset of severe pain and spasm in the lumbar area. On examination, straight leg raising is greatly reduced with cross-leg irritation. Radiographs do not usually show narrowing of the disc space, but MR imaging is the investigation of choice, showing the protrusion.

Massobrio (1991) has reported upon a series of adolescent–teenage–young adult lumbar disc herniations, age range 13–20 years. The incidence in the west is low – up to 3.8% – compared with Japan where it has increased from 7.8% to 22.9%. They most commonly presented with back stiffness, decreased lordosis and often a secondary scoliosis. Over 50% had some anomaly of the lumbar spine. No disc degeneration or sequestration was found at operation. Conservative treatment was not successful and the best results were obtained by early surgery. Chemonucleolysis and percutaneous nucleotomy were also successful.

Thoracic disc syndrome

Although this is a very rare condition (less than 0.5% of all discs coming to surgery), its results are catastrophic unless recognized early and treated promptly. Most commonly affected are the T9/10 and T10/11 levels – this being the level at which the artery of Adamkiewicz supplies the cord. Therefore, ischaemia of the cord may easily follow, rather than deformation or compression only of the cord, by the protruded disc material.

The clinical features are very variable but appear in two groups – first, those who appear with upper backache and a very slowly progressive cord compression with unpleasant paraesthesia, loss of sensation particularly to pain, and occasional loss of power in the lower extremities; and, second, those in whom the symptoms and signs of acute cord compression appear within days or weeks, with marked numbness and weakness in the legs.

As in the cervical and lumbar spine, thoracic disc degeneration or herniation can present in one of two forms or, indeed, a mixture.

THORACIC DISC DEGENERATION WITHOUT A NEUROLOGICAL DEFICIT

The pain can be radicular or radiating anteriorly around the chest, local or referred – midscapular or through the chest. It may or may not be related to activity and has to be differentiated from intrathoracic, or intra-upper abdominal disease and from other pathologies, e.g. spondyloarthropathies, tumours, infections, herpes zoster, etc.

Careful history-taking and physical examination and radiography should determine how far the diagnostic examination should extend but delay is to be avoided. Therefore CT scanning with myelography or MR imaging should be carried out when the symptoms persist. Because of the sensitivity of these procedures it is sometimes difficult to localize the level.

When a diagnosis of 'benign' thoracic pain syndrome is made, conservative treatment with nonsteroidal anti-inflammatory drugs, physical therapy and a thoracic support can be given. Surgery is only indicated in a very few patients after thorough exclusion of psychological and other such features. Discography should be used to 'localize' the level and an anterior thoracic discectomy with fusion carried out.

THORACIC DISC DEGENERATION WITH A NEUROLOGICAL DEFICIT

Pain as a presenting features can vary as described above. Neurological symptoms of weakness in the legs, numbness, spastic ataxia, bladder and bowel disturbances can be subtle and varying in intensity or severity. Delay in diagnosis can occur but must be avoided. Careful examination will reveal the neurological deficiencies, with the condition of the spinal cord being determined by prompt CT scanning with enhancement by myelography or MR imaging. The latter is particularly useful in giving details of compression of the spinal cord by herniations. However, because of their sensitivity rather than specificity, these investigations can uncover asymptomatic herniated discs as false positives in up to 1–14%. This increases with age as elsewhere in the spine.

Skubic and Kostvik (1991) and Skubic (1993)in excellent reviews have described the surgical treatment of this condition when signs and symptoms of myelopathy are found. Laminectomy is no longer carried out because of a high risk of neurological injury. They recommend, with good results, a transthoracic–transpleural approach for central or centrolateral herniations with fusion by rib or iliac crest grafts, or a transpedicular–transfacetal approach for lateral disc herniation and a posterolateral–extrapleural approach for centrolateral discs.

Lumbar canal stenosis

The first description of spinal stenosis is accredited to Portal who, in 1803, described the stenosis found in patients with chondrodystrophia fetalis. Parker and Adson in 1925 described spinal stenosis and reported eight further cases; 9 years later, Mixter and Barr (1930) produced their classic paper which focused on the lumbar disc as being the chief cause of back pathology. Following this there were many isolated reports of spinal stenotic conditions in the literature, but these were never considered a common cause of back pain until Verbiest (1954) re-described this clinical syndrome with his operative studies, showing bony changes producing a narrowed spinal canal particularly in the sagittal plane.

To appreciate this syndrome the anatomy of the nerve root and spinal column must be understood. The clinical findings and the therapy are based on the pathological changes in this normal anatomy.

1. The spinal canal is found behind the articulated vertebral bodies between which are the annulus fibrosus and its disc, the posterior longitudinal ligament, and the posterior elements, made up of the pedicles, the facet joints, the lamina and spinous processes and their ligaments especially ligamentum flavum. Normally it is circular in the upper lumbar spine and triangular or trefoil in the lower lumbar spine, and is smallest opposite L4.
2. The nerve root canal is part of the spinal canal. The roof of this canal is formed by the ligamentum flavum and the superior articular facet and its adjacent lamina. The floor is formed by the annulus fibrosus and the posterior surface of the vertebral body. The medial wall is the dural sac; the lateral wall is formed first by the medial side and then by the inferior aspect of the pedicle (Figure 13.32). The lateral recess is the most lateral aspect of the spinal canal. Specifically it is the space bounded by the medial portion of the superior articular facet and lamina above the pedicle laterally and by the vertebral body, its superior lip and the disc below.
3. The intervertebral foramen has the shape of an inverted teardrop. The superior border is the pedicle, the anterior wall being formed by the posterior vertebral body and the disc. The inferior border is the pedicle of the vertebral body below, and the posterior wall is composed of the pars interarticularis and the superior facet.

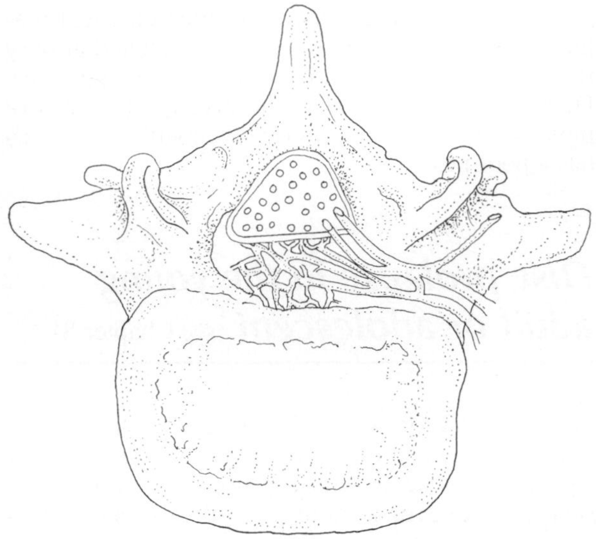

Figure 13.32 The boundaries of the nerve root canal. (By Farquharson-Roberts)

The term 'stenosis' implies constriction of a tube. In this sense a spinal tumour or a herniated nucleus pulposus clearly can produce a spinal stenosis. However, lumbar canal stenosis is cauda equina compression in which the lateral or anterior posterior diameter of the spinal canal is abnormal, with or without a change in the cross-sectional area.

Spinal stenosis is usually classified into one of four aetiological patterns:

1. Congenital or developmental stenosis.
2. Degenerative stenosis.
3. Spondylitic stenosis.
4. Iatrogenic or traumatic stenosis.

CONGENITAL OR DEVELOPMENTAL STENOSIS

There is a uniform narrowing throughout the lumbar canal, more marked in the anteroposterior than in its transverse diameter. The lower limit of the normal anteroposterior diameter of the canal is variously reported as being between 10 and 15 mm. This diameter can be reduced in an achondroplastic dwarf, rickets, mucopolysaccharidoses, spondylolisthesis, scoliosis, Down's syndrome, dysplasias, acromegaly, renal osteodystrophy and osteoporosis with fractures.

In the population there is great variation in the dimensions of the spinal canal. At one end of the scale there can be an enlarged canal in which even a herniation of the lumbar disc would not necessarily precipitate symptoms. On the other hand, a spinal canal might be very narrow and any slight change in its diameter secondary to degeneration may well precipitate severe symptoms.

The main pathology is an abnormal neural arch. The lamina are heavy and often exceed 10 mm in thickness, whereas the normal laminar thickness is from 4 to 5 mm. They may be foreshortened and overlap. In addition, they end in enlarged articulations at the facet. The intraluminal space is often obliterated and the dural sac commonly bulges into the laminectomy site with the dural fat being markedly reduced in amount, making dissection difficult (Schatzker and Pennal, 1968).

DEGENERATIVE SPINAL STENOSIS

This is basically an arthropathy with degenerative changes which impinge on either the intervertebral bony foramen or the lateral recess (Figure 13.33). As the disc degenerates and loses its elasticity and height, the annulus fibrosus bulges inwards into the canal and the vertebral bodies approach one another with osteophyte formation at their margins. Because of the articular surface shape and inclination the upper vertebral body slides downwards and backwards with the facets overriding and subluxing (Figures 13.34 and 13.35). The nerve root, as it emerges through the intervertebral canal, can be trapped between the pedicle and the superior articulating facet. Osteophytic outgrowth from the superior facet often adds to the compression (McNab, 1971; Kirkaldy-Willis and McIvor, 1976). It can also occur postoperatively after laminectomy or fusion.

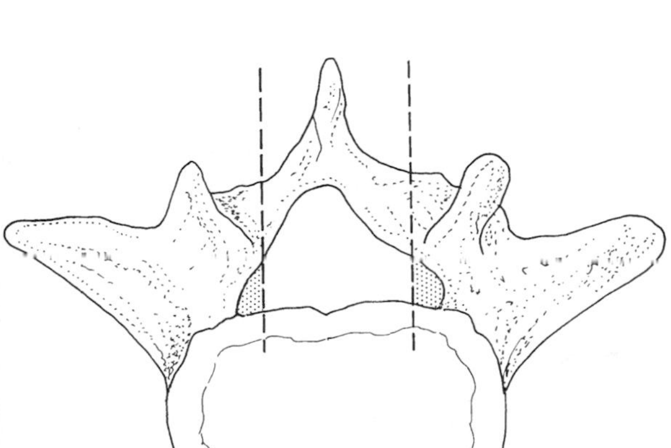

Figure 13.33 The lateral recesses which can be narrowed by degenerative changes of the posterior facet joints in spinal stenosis. (By Farquharson-Roberts)

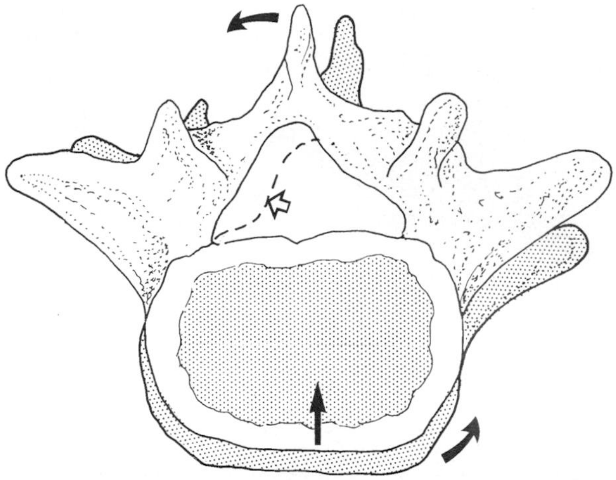

Figure 13.34 The narrowing and reaction to the subluxation of the facet joints with degenerative changes. (By Farquharson-Roberts)

SPONDYLITIC STENOSIS

While isthmic defect spondylolisthesis can occasionally entrap a nerve root, degenerative or pseudospondylolisthesis produces a picture of spinal stenosis. This condition was first described by Junghanns in 1930 and later in detail by McNab (1950). It is a backward slip allowed by a poorly developed posterior facet with an intact neural arch. It is much more commonly seen in females after the age of 40 and usually affects the L4–5 level. The slip is usually less than 1 cm; surgical specimens have revealed that the orientation of the L4–5 facet joint, instead of being at 90° to the pedicle, is actually parallel to it – allowing the forward subluxation to take place. Once this subluxation has taken place, the superior facet of L5 tends to hypertrophy with osteophytic formation in order to provide a support for the inferior facet of L4. It is this mass of fibrocartilage which usually entraps the nerve root. In addition, as a result of the slip there is a large step in the canal, often resulting in marked stenosis (Figure 13.36).

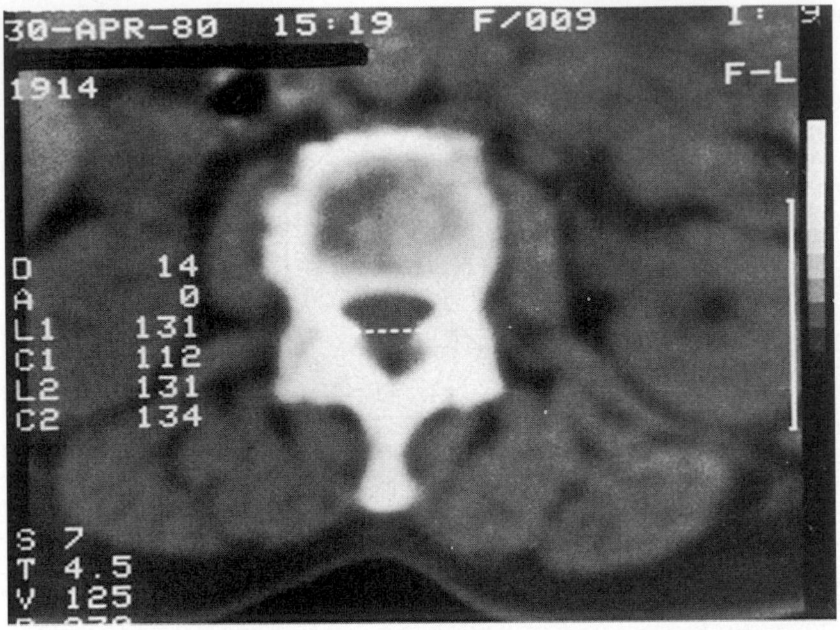

Figure 13.35 CT scan showing the stenotic narrowing of the interlaminar distance by arthritis.

IATROGENIC STENOSIS

Several authors have reported spinal stenosis as a complication of spinal surgery (Schatzker and Pennal, 1968; Brodsky, 1976). It is unclear if this condition is due to, say, hypertrophy of a posterior bone graft or to incomplete treatment of the stenotic condition with a recurrence of the original symptoms. Brodsky reports that the most common stenosis is due to an infolding of the ligamentum flavum just superior to the fusion mass in association with a disc herniation. Langenskiöld and Kiviluoto (1976) inserted a free fat transplant in the epidural space to protect against epidural scar formation.

CLINICAL PRESENTATION

The varied clinical presentation of spinal stenosis is well recognized but is most commonly seen in males over the age of 40 years. Some degree of spinal stenosis is probably quite common in the ageing population. Only those with severe symptoms are seen by doctors.

There is no uniform clinical picture applicable to all cases of spinal stenosis. Indeed, it can exist with no physical findings at all. A classic symptom pattern of stenosis is that of cauda equina claudication (see beginning of chapter for explanation of neurogenic pain). In this the patient presents with pain in the buttocks or lower extremities after walking, which is relieved by sitting forward or lying for 20 minutes or so. The patient may adopt the so-called 'simian' (monkey-like) stance to obtain relief (Simkin, 1982). Hypoaesthesiae or paraesthesiae are often precipitated by exercise and persist longer. Walking up hill is usually done with ease and a bicycle can often be ridden a long distance with no

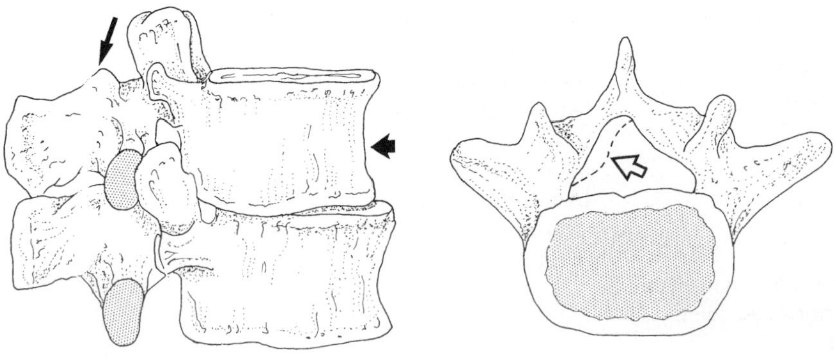

Figure 13.36 The spondylitic stenosis lesion with a backward slip, with intervertebral narrowing and osteophyte formation. (By Farquharson-Roberts)

discomfort at all. Spontaneous erections, urinary and even faecal incontinence on walking have been reported (Ram *et al.*, 1987). Neurological findings are not consistent but often include muscle weakness, areas of sensory loss and imbalance. These can often be aggravated by exercise.

Dong and Porter (1989) examined the walking and cycling tolerance of patients with neurogenic and vascular claudication in the upright position and in 30° of flexion. They concluded that although some patients with neurogenic claudication could increase their walking distance by flexing forward, these posture-related walking and cycling tests are insufficiently sensitive to distinguish the types of claudication. It has also been said that in neurogenic claudication the patient will prefer walking uphill rather than downhill with lordosis. Again these authors found this not to discriminate the pathologies.

Physical findings are often minimal and non-specific at rest, the most common being decreased lumbosacral motion. Nerve root tension signs, if found, usually indicate lateral recess stenosis. Neurological findings may be detected more readily if the patient is examined shortly after performing exercise. MR scanning will show accurately the amount of stenosis and its source (Figure 13.37).

The natural history of patients without surgery is important. Porter (1988) reported on a series of 249 patients diagnosed clinically as having root entrapment syndrome on the basis of severe constant pain in the lower limb unrelieved by rest, minimal tension signs, over aged 40 years and with ultrasound as the only investigation. Forty-two per cent had no neurological signs. No active treatment was given in 81% of the patients. Twenty-four patients (9.6%) subsequently had surgery. Of 169 (75%) of the remainder when followed for between 1 and 4 years by questionnaire, 78% still had some root pain, although the majority did not seek further treatment and their symptoms were manageable.

Johnsson *et al.* (1989) reported that 30% of patients with central spinal stenosis experience remission of their symptoms and suggested that the natural tendency of the degenerative spine to stabilize with time may explain this observation.

Nixon (1991) prospectively reviewed 221 patients with the symptoms of spinal stenosis and reported the following results at the end of treatment. Some of the patients had more than one modality of treatment and 72 (33%) patients went on to surgery.

With bed rest and traction, a Spencer corset or plaster-of-Paris jacket and non-steroidal anti-inflammatory tablets or epidural and physiotherapy, between 41 and 61% improved.

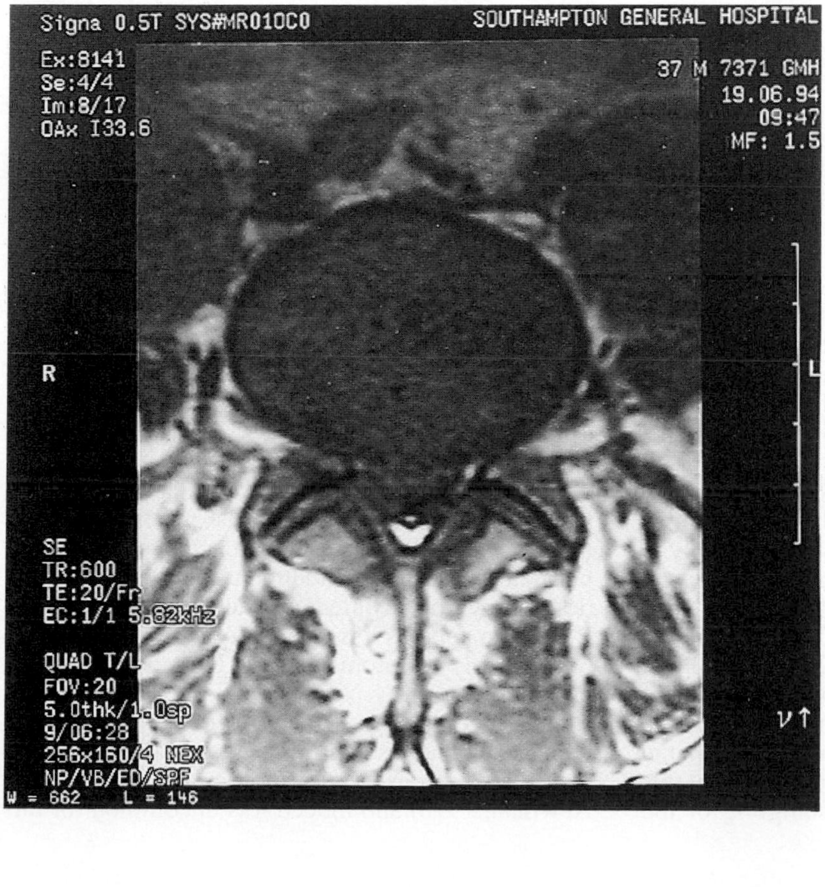

Figure 13.37 Spinal stenosis clearly shown on an axial section of the lumbar spine by MR scanning. (Films kindly supplied by Dr Richard Blaquiere, Consultant Radiologist at Southampton University Hospitals)

Calcitonin or diphosphonates have been described for patients with Paget's disease and impending paraplegia but in spinal stenosis cases the beneficial effect is likely to be due to a central analgesic.

Differentiation from ischaemic, vascular claudication is obviously most important. Ischaemic claudication usually appears more quickly and disappears on rest in a much shorter time (in minutes). There are rarely neurological signs but there are usually absent femoral, popliteal and dorsalis pulses, bruits may be present, nutritional changes in the foot or toes may be seen and any sensory loss is not segmental in type.

In some cases where there is nerve root entrapment in the lateral recess the clinical picture is one of claudication with sciatica. The sciatica is often bilateral but even so the neurological signs tend to be minimal. The explanation for how the claudication is relieved by sitting or leaning forward was given by Breig (1960) from his cadaveric studies. When the spine moves from flexion to extension, with an increase in lordosis, the lumbar canal shortens by 2.2 mm and the contained nerve tissue also shortens. The fibres of the ligamentum flavum become slack and their cross-sectional area increases, but the intravertebral foramen narrows with the lumbar disc protruding slightly into the spinal canal. He described how all these changes interfere with the microcirculation to the nerve roots and hence their interruption.

INVESTIGATIONS AND DIAGNOSIS

From the history and examination it is essential to request anteroposterior and lateral views of the lumbar spine. The interpedicular distance is of little importance unless the patient is achondroplastic. Of particular importance are the anteroposterior or midsagittal diameter and the degree of facet sclerosis and hypertrophy (Sheldon *et al.*, 1976). Transitional vertebrae and particularly unilateral sacral articulations of the lowest lumbar vertebra have been associated with gross facet arthritis and nerve root entrapment (Epstein *et al.*, 1972).

The presence of a spondylolisthesis – either degenerative or spondylitic – should be sought, for even a relatively slight slip (e.g. 25%) can produce stenotic symptoms in the adult. This is most likely to be seen at the L4–5 level but it may be seen above or, less commonly, below this level (Wiltse *et al.*, 1976). Associated with degenerative spondylolisthesis are gross facet sclerosis and hypertrophy (Sheldon *et al.*, 1976). The sclerosis and hypertrophy at the level of an isthmic defect may indicate hypertrophy of the fibrocartilaginous repair mass associated with the defect, and the nerve root may be entrapped by this tissue. Disc space narrowing and shingling of the laminae (i.e. loss of the normal interval between the laminae) are commonly observed. Foraminal narrowing due to facet subluxation is also observed; the subluxation may precede facet arthritis and, as arthritic changes advance, greater foraminal stenosis results. The features mentioned are largely degenerative and may be implicated in either central or lateral stenosis.

Myelography was essential in confirming the clinical diagnosis. However, it is now combined with CT for even greater detail. MR imaging is proving to be most helpful in determining the soft tissue components (see beginning of chapter) (Figures 13.38 and 13.39).

Ultrasound scanning

This safe, non-invasive technique was developed by Porter *et al.* (Porter *et al.*, 1978; Porter, 1981; Porter and Miller, 1988) to give an oblique measurement of the normal spinal canal as well as in various pathological conditions. They have demonstrated the stenotic lesion and have applied it clinically, but other workers have not found it helpful.

Electromyography

Electromyography is abnormal in some 80% of patients with spinal stenosis and helps provide confirmatory evidence of the level of nerve root involvement. Findings of coexistent myelopathy and radiculopathy may suggest tandem spinal stenosis, i.e. concurrent stenoses of the cervical and lumbar spines, a not uncommon situation which was present in 19 out of 100 patients in one series of Moreland *et al.* (1989).

TREATMENT

There is little doubt that patients in whom claudication is the dominant feature respond well with surgery and that they fare poorly with conservative treatment (Hasue *et al.*, 1977). The expectations of patients with a neurological deficit should not be encouraged because full recovery does not occur frequently; only about half of the patients operated upon with a neurological deficit achieved full relief, but with conservative treatment there is little prospect of any improvement and deterioration is likely. Back pain appears to respond poorly to surgery, and relief of this symptom seems to be unpredictable. It has been stated by Verbiest (1977), however, that surgery does not predispose to or aggravate back pain. Back pain seems to be comparatively well controlled by conservative measures (Fitzgerald and Newman, 1976) and indeed it is uncommon for this

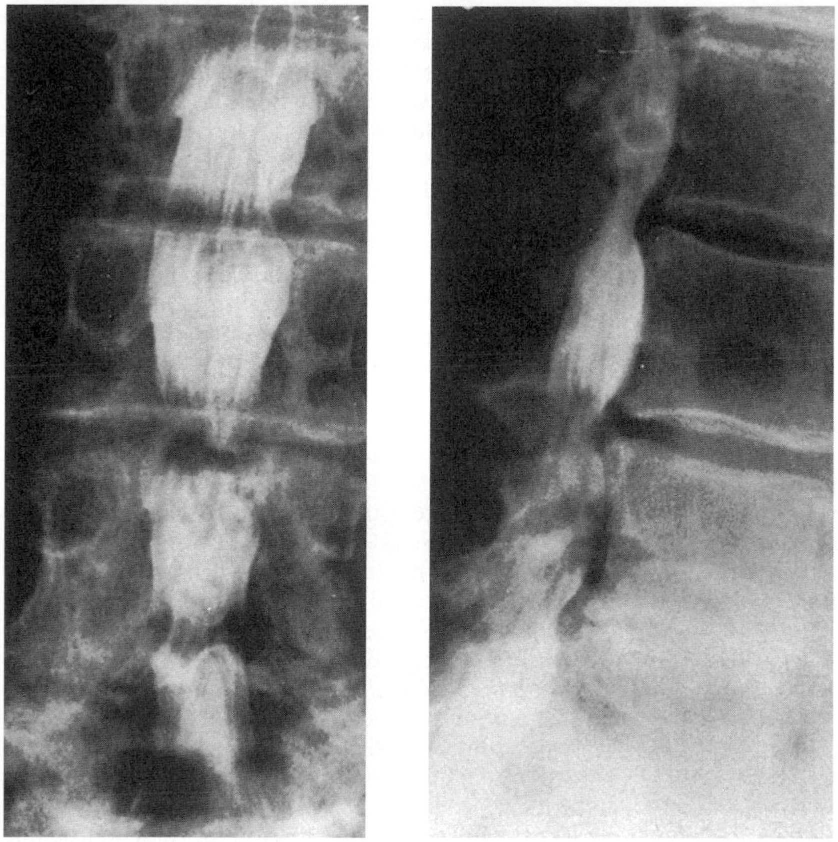

(a) (b)

Figure 13.38 Myelograms of a two-level degenerative stenotic lesion: (a) anteroposterior plane; (b) lateral view, showing the indentation of the contrast column both anteriorly as well as posteriorly.

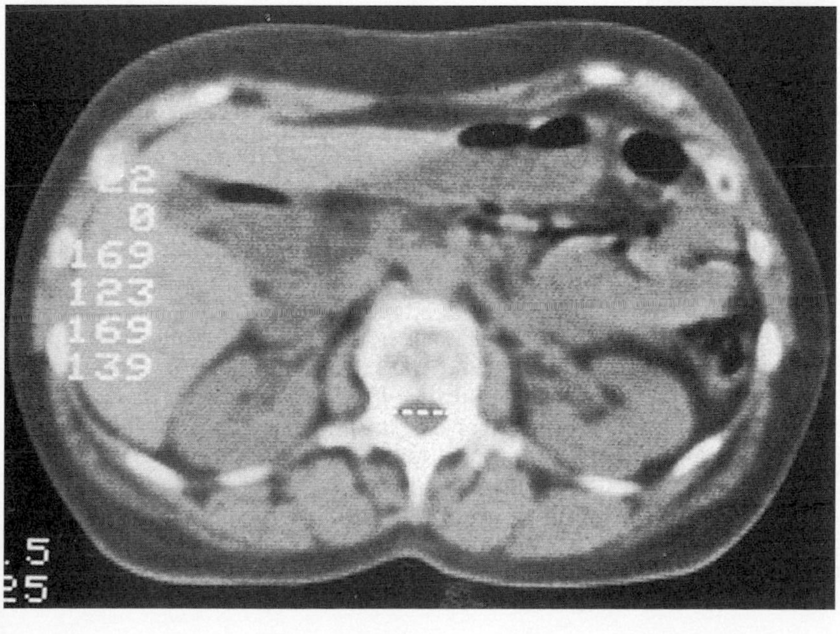

Figure 13.39 A CT scan of the patient in Figure 13.37 showing the direct measurement of the cross-section of the intraspinal canal.

symptom alone to be disabling enough to warrant surgery. Sciatic pain, however, is poorly controlled by conservative measures and seems to respond well to surgery. In summary, it may be stated that the presence of objective neurological signs is a strong indication for operative intervention, as are the symptoms of cauda equina claudication or sciatic pain.

Operative treatment

Several principles emerge from the literature and McNab (1971) has emphasized that the nerve roots must be freed from pressure throughout their course. The cauda equina also should be decompressed completely.

Where the stenosis is central, little controversy is present regarding decompression. Laminectomy until the canal depth is of near-normal dimensions proximally and distally is necessary. Kirkcaldy-Willis *et al.* (1974) recommend that the canal width should be 2 cm after laminectomy. To obtain atraumatic access into the spinal canal it is advised that the laminectomy is commenced either proximally or distally where the stenosis is not marked. Care needs to be taken in removing the ligamentum flavum in the vicinity of the stenosis, as the dura is often adherent and the epidural fat absent. The inferomedial aspect of the inferior articular processes frequently require osteotomy to excise this hypertrophied osteophytic element. Verbiest (1977) has given a good description of the technique for this part of the procedure. Where central stenosis is the main feature it should be possible to retain sufficient of the facet articulations to prevent the need for any stabilization procedure (Figure 13.40).

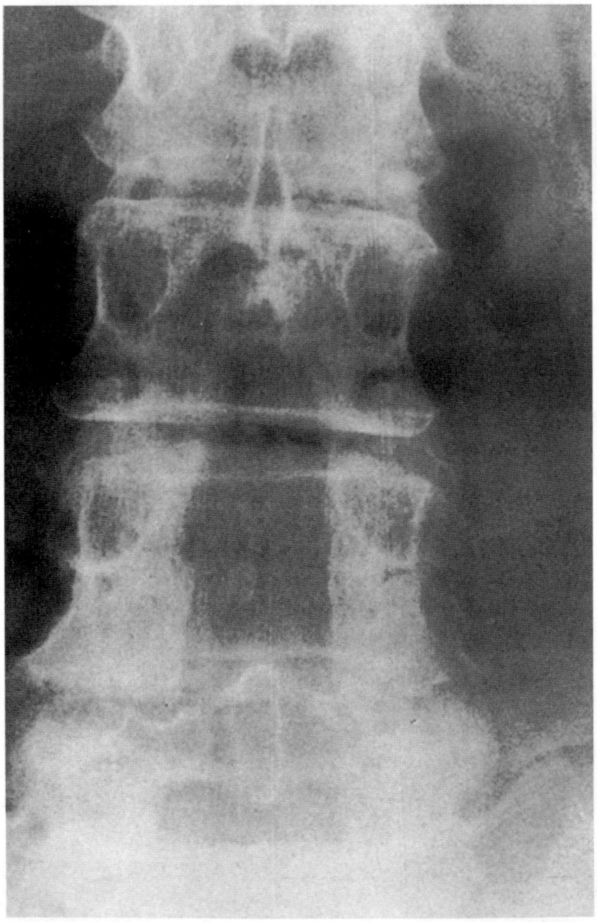

Figure 13.40 Anteroposterior radiograph showing the bilateral laminectomy at two levels but retaining the facet articulations.

Patients with lateral stenosis are more difficult to deal with surgically, as foraminotomy and/or facetectomy are usually required.

Wiltse *et al.* (1976) advocated removal of the laminae and medial part of the facets for the treatment of central spinal stenosis with neurogenic claudication. Wiltse stated that in the presence of anterior disc narrowing and osteophyte formation iatrogenic slippage seldom occurs even with very radical posterior decompression. Segmental decompression and excision of the medial portion (one-third) of the facet joints is possible without removing the laminae.

The results of decompression for both neurogenic claudication secondary to central canal stenosis and root canal entrapment are generally reasonable. Most studies focus on the resolution of leg symptoms and signs only. Nasca (1989) performed laminectomy (unilateral) and medial facetectomy for lateral recess stenosis and had resolution of leg pain and neurological signs in 80% of patients, and with bilateral laminectomies for central stenosis, found resolution of signs and symptoms in 82%.

Johnsson *et al.* (1989) noted that women did significantly less well following decompression for central stenosis than men. Radical facetectomy slipped more often and had significantly more patients with a poor result. Preoperative instability, as revealed by functional myelography, was associated with a poorer prognosis for the results of decompression.

Multiple level laminectomies and decompression are effective in relieving the symptoms from central stenosis, with good relief of symptoms and return to work. Watanabe (1989) observed that patients who underwent wide decompression with total laminectomy were likely to have residual back symptoms and neurological symptoms. He introduced a technique of spinous process flap removal and demonstrated a reduction in these symptoms.

The role of fusion in the treatment of patients with spinal stenosis is still being defined. It is rarely required after unilateral decompression for root canal stenosis (Nasca, 1989). Instability demonstrated preoperatively by functional myelography (Johnsson *et al.*, 1989) or by flexion/extension translation (Nasca, 1989) is associated with a poorer result from decompression and may be a relative contraindication. Iatrogenic operative instability is suggested by some to be an indication for fusion and Nasca (1989) recommends intertransverse fusion without instrumentation.

Other indications in spinal stenosis for fusion suggested are isolated disc resorption with degenerative facet joints and a degenerative scoliosis with multidirectional instability (Nasca, 1989).

Fusion of the lumbar spine

Fusion of the lumbar spine has enjoyed vogues for the past 50 years in the treatment of back pain but is rarely indicated unless there is definite evidence of spinal instability. There has been dispute regarding the relative merits of posterior and anterior fusion but, although anterior fusion gives a higher fusion rate, neither gives 100% and the anterior method is prone to more complications because of the possible effects of vascular damage, sympathetic plexus injury with impotence in men, and incisional hernia. Recently lumbar fusion has increased in popularity with the refinement of pedicle screw fixation techniques, which are more rigid than screws, plates or wiring, but the long-term results are as yet unknown. The most promising results appear to be those of West *et al.* (1991) who described high fusion rates after pedicle screw fixation in painful degenerative disc disease (90%), for spondylolisthesis (93%) and for failed surgery with pseudoarthrosis (65%). Over 60% of all patients returned to work. Others (Horowitch *et al.*, 1989) have reported problems with this demanding technique including 7% major perioperative complications, 7% major metal fixation failure, and 32% non-union.

Lumbar spine fusion is indicated for:

1. Spondylolisthesis.
2. Infections (e.g. tuberculosis) with bone destruction and deformity.
3. Tumours with bone destruction, deformity and neurological compression.
4. Trauma – some fractures and fracture dislocations with neurological compression and deformity.
5. Some cases of disc degeneration and posterior facet joint arthritis with backache but no neurological signs.

Many methods have been described of which the Wiltse *et al.* (1968) posterolateral fusion is reasonably reliable for grade I–II spondylolisthesis and disc degeneration with posterior facet joint arthritis.

Infections, tumours and trauma to the spine usually require anterior stabilization with bone grafting from pelvis and/or ribs together with such devices as the Moss cage for fractures and tumours.

RESULTS

Results of spinal fusion are extremely difficult to assess in chronic low back pain but the newer techniques certainly require long-term evaluation. A major problem is that even if fusion of the spinal segment or segments is proven by CT, there is no definite correlation between fusion and pain relief which may mean that pain relief is due to denervation of the posterior spinal joints rather than bone fusion. In general, unless there are definite indications, fusion of the lumbar spine should be avoided.

Bone grafting in lumbar spinal fusion

As in scoliosis surgery, autogenous bone is used, usually cancellous taken from the iliac crest since it is the most osteogenic. The complications associated with removal of autogenous bone are few if care is exercised. Allograft bone and bone substitutes are not required usually in lumbar spine fusion because the quantity needed is small. The poor performance of allograft bone in producing fusion and the potential risks make its use unnecessary (West *et al.*, 1991).

Coccygodynia

This is pain in the vicinity of the coccyx which may arise because of congenital deformity, injury, infection, tumour or arthritis of the sacrococcygeal joint. Protrusion of a disc between L5 and S1 vertebrae has to be excluded. There may be abnormality in the size, shape and direction of the coccygeal fragments. However, in the majority of patients no pathology can be demonstrated i.e. the condition is idiopathic. Pain is the usual presenting feature and is aggravated by sitting, sometimes by defaecation, and tends to be relieved by standing or lying down. The patient may prefer to sit on one or the other buttock, or use a special cushion. The majority of patients are between the ages of 30 and 50 years.

On examination *per rectum*, there may be localized tenderness, particularly on movement at the sacrococcygeal joint. x-Rays are usually of little use because of the frequent anatomical variations which occur here, although marked displacement – because of fractures or dislocations, or osteoarthritis of the sacrococcygeal joint – may be seen.

Differential diagnosis consists of such conditions as rectal abscess or fistula formation, tumours of the cauda equina, and the condition of proctalgia.

Treatment is palliative by prescribing a proper form of cushion. Local injections of hydrocortisone with a local anaesthetic such as 1% procaine are quite helpful in certain cases as is manipulation under general anaesthesia.

In a prospective study of 50 patients with full investigation including CT scans, ^{99}Tc bone scans and comprehensive personality, behavioural assessment, Wray *et al.* (1991) found that only 16% were cured by physiotherapy or ultrasound followed by short wave diathermy, 38% with local injection of methylprednisolone acetate and bupivacaine, and 71% with an injection and manipulation under general anaesthesia. In an extended further study of 120 patients 30 patients began symptoms after a fall, or after parturition and 15 after repetitive injury and 6 after an operation. The psychiatric/psychological assessment did not reveal any hysterical or neurotic condition and their profile was similar to other groups of patients. Although CT scans suggested that the pain was caused by a lumbar sacral disc prolapse, not only is this a common finding in many asymptomatic patients over the age of 30 years but the majority of the patients in this series were cured by treatment localized to the coccyx. There was a 20% relapse rate which responded to re-injection and manipulation. Of all patients, 20%, i.e. 23 patients, came to coccygectomy – and 21 of these patients had an excellent result with complete relief of symptoms and no recurrence. No reasons could be found for the two failures. Histological examination of the coccyx and joint showed no abnormality.

Coccygectomy

The operation consists of a skin incision to one side of midline with careful subperiosteal dissection off the ligamentous attachments. The coccyx can be removed at the sacrococcygeal joint and the soft tissues are carefully closed together to avoid leaving any dead space.

Anteroposterior curvature of the spine (including senile kyphosis, spondylitis deformans)

The fetal vertebral column possesses two *primary curves*, both convex dorsally. The upper of these extends from the head to the pelvis; the lower affects the sacral region.

After birth, two *secondary curves* develop. As soon as the child begins to hold the head erect a cervical curve appears, its concavity directed backwards; and on the assumption of the erect attitude, a lumbar curve appears which is also concave backwards. The object of these secondary curves is to bring the centre of gravity directly above the stance of the body.

The primary curvatures are dependent on the shape of the vertebral bodies; the secondary curves, on the other hand, are the result of the special shapes of the intervertebral discs, which are wider in front than posteriorly in the cervical and lumbar regions.

In addition to the shapes of the bodies and of the intervertebral discs, normal spinal curvature depends to some extent on the long spinal muscles and on the ligaments binding the individual bony segments together.

Alterations in the normal anteroposterior curvatures of the spinal column are frequently met with in the young and the old, and many erroneous ideas as to their mechanism and cause have sprung up. In general it may be said that deformed anteroposterior posture of the spine must follow interference in one of the factors producing the normal curves:

1. *The bones* – this form is seen in tuberculosis, rickets, Kümmell's disease, etc.
2. *The discs.*
3. *The long spinal muscles* – the type commonly seen in debilitated children with flabby muscles.

PATHOLOGY OF THE DISCS

Developmental and degenerative changes

The common changes in the cartilage range from localized bulgings towards the spongy tissue of the vertebral body, to complete collapse and rupture. In old spines such changes are the result of senile degeneration of the cartilage itself, or of the deprivation of support that follows senile osteoporotic processes in the body of the vertebra. The generalized collapse is seen in the increased biconvexity assumed by the disc at the expense of the bone, and the stretching of the cartilage accelerates the degenerative processes. It is probable that some slight shock is the cause of the final rupture or fracture.

Schmorl (1932) drew attention to the frequency of congenital errors in the intervertebral discs (Figure 13.41). These are of great importance in predisposing to pathological errors in the young. Perhaps the commonest of these developmental anomalies is the presence of localized herniations in the nuclear regions of the discs – the-so-called 'nuclear expansions'. They occur mostly in the lower thoracic and lumbar regions, and consist of small hemispherical protrusions of disc tissue into the substance of the vertebral spongy tissue. The cartilage over these expansions is very much weaker and thinner, and represents an area of diminished resistance where even the slight trauma of incessant functional activity is likely to lead to rupture or fracture of the cartilage.

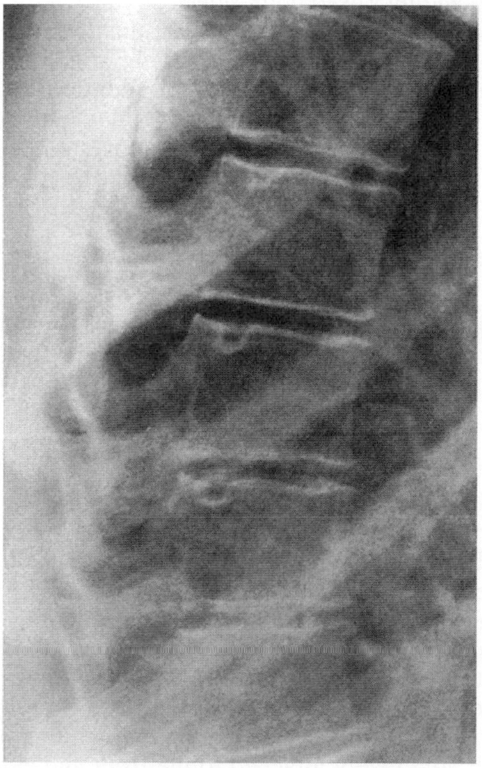

Figure 13.41 Schmorl's nodes – a failure of conversion of cartilage to bone. Note the square edges and flat bottom of the defect consistent with growth rather than invasion of disc material. The narrowed cartilage disc space and the irregularity of the subchondral plate accompany the other manifestations of this growth abnormality.

Fracture of the cartilage plates; prolapse of the disc

Apart from the developmental and degenerative changes described above, Schmorl (Schmorl, 1932; Schmorl and Junghanns, 1971) showed that the cartilaginous plate is extraordinarily resistant to severe trauma and to those diseases which affect the vertebral body.

The predisposing causes of rupture are:

1. Nuclear expansion of the disc – a developmental error.
2. Senile degeneration of the cartilage.
3. Loss of support to the cartilage through osteoporosis of the vertebral body.

The result of rupture is the prolapse or protrusion of the disc tissue into the spongiosa – a phenomenon the recognition of which we owe to Schmorl and the Dresden school of spinal pathologists. The frequency of the condition may be gauged from the fact that these observers found it in 30% of all spines examined, and in all cases of juvenile and senile anteroposterior spinal curvatures.

Kyphosis in adults and the aged

Increasing spinal deformity commonly accompanies advancing years, and is associated with a variety of pathological changes in the spinal components. Many of these cases have hitherto been classed as osteoarthritic, and certainly the vertebral changes often bear a close resemblance to the manifestations of this disease in larger joints, such as the hip or the knee. Other cases have been ascribed to occupation, the demands of which have led to certain adaptive changes which are rendered permanent as the years go on. When such a group of cases is analysed critically, it appears that several distinct types may be distinguished.

TRUE SENILE KYPHOSIS

The whole spine appears remarkably well preserved, but the vertebral bodies are somewhat wedge-shaped. In their major portion the discs appear relatively normal, but there are constant changes at their anterior edges, varying from patches of necrosis or fibrosis to total disappearance. In the latter event, the adjacent vertebral bodies may be joined at their anterior edges by bands of spongy bone (Figure

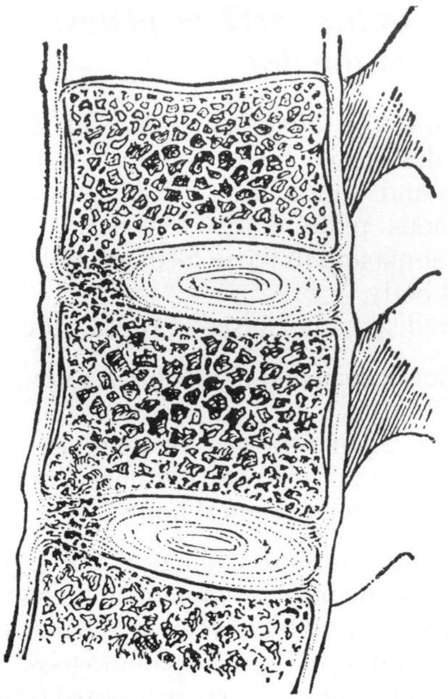

Figure 13.42 Senile kyphosis: the bodies joined to their anterior edges by spongy bone.

13.42). The changes are most marked in the upper and middle thoracic regions.

Schmorl demonstrated beyond doubt that the earliest phenomenon is the necrosis of the anterior part of the disc, resulting from the strain exerted on this area of the disc, especially in those whose occupation is heavy and demands continual stooping. The 'necrosis' leads to tears in the annulus, and finally to the complete dissipation of the disc, as a result of which the anterior ends of the two opposing bony surfaces are forced into contact. Long-continued pressure of this kind leads to bone absorption, and the body of the vertebra gradually assumes a wedge shape. If the anterior ends of the cartilage plates are at the same time destroyed, the adjacent bodies may become ankylosed by bridges of new bone.

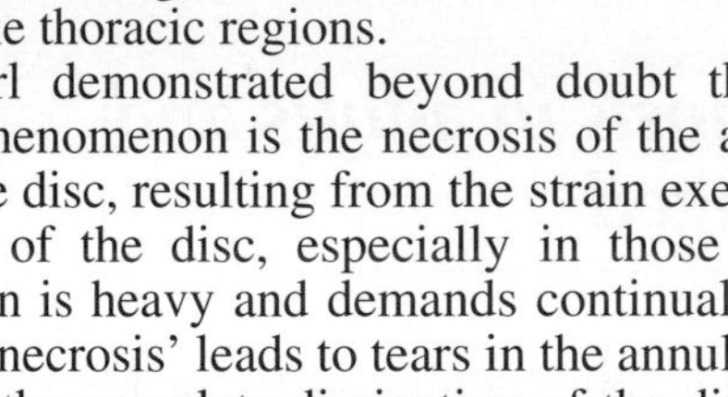

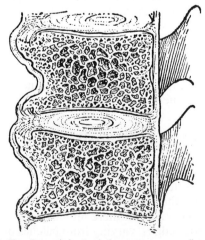

Figure 13.43 Spondylosis deformans: some flattening at the discs and osteophytic outgrowths in front of the bodies a little distance from the upper and lower edges.

SPONDYLOSIS DEFORMANS

The most typical feature of this form of disease is the generalized degeneration of the intervertebral discs. In many cases the disc is prolapsed and invaded by granulation tissue, so that it is present only as an inert fibrous nodule.

The shape of the actual vertebral body is usually unchanged, but the epiphyseal rings may be flattened out. Characteristically there are osteophytes of varying size on the anterior and lateral edges of the vertebral body. These lie a little below the outer edge of the epiphyseal ring, and proliferate so as to overlap the intervertebral space until eventually osteophytes from adjacent vertebrae may fuse together (Figure 13.43). These osteophytes tend to be arranged in rows, and adjacent nodules are usually connected by raised bony ridges on the anterolateral surface of the body. It seems clear that this marginal bone proliferation is the result of abnormal tensions on the fibres of the anterior longitudinal ligament, and the bony ridges actually reproduce with accuracy the direction of the ligamentous strands. The condition therefore has been called polyspondylitis marginalis.

The sequence of events

These changes were carefully worked out by Schmorl, and described by Beadle. Formerly, this condition was referred to as osteoarthritis, or as spondylitis deformans. Since the bulk of the changes affect the discs and the vertebral bodies, where there are no joints in the true sense of the word, the former term should be discarded. In the absence of evidence of an inflammatory process, the term spondylitis should also be avoided, and hence Schmorl (1932) coined the term 'spondylosis'.

The essential factor in the process is obviously the degeneration in the discs. As these waste, there results an increased mobility of the vertebrae one on the other, and the consequent continuous tugging on the fibres of the anterior longitudinal ligaments, which are closely attached to the front and sides of the vertebrae, leads to the production of bony exostoses or osteophytes. The looser attachment of the posterior ligament prevents the gross changes seen anteriorly, but occasionally small osteophytes are found on the posterior surface of the vertebral bodies as well.

The occasional absence of kyphotic deformity is

due to the fact that the disc degeneration, being diffuse and the posterior intervertebral articulations looser than in youth, the bodies of the vertebrae sink together more or less squarely.

OSTEOPOROSIS OF THE SPINE

The commonest form of spinal osteoporosis is that following the menopause in women. The condition may occur much less commonly in men. In this form of 'senile spine' an osteoporosis of marked degree is evenly distributed throughout the spine. The bone trabeculae are largely absorbed and replaced by marrow. The discs are usually in a state of excellent preservation and bulge markedly into the atrophied spongy tissue of the vertebral body (Figure 13.44). Viewed as a whole, the spine is grossly deformed, owing to the softened vertebral bodies being unable to withstand the superincumbent weight.

It seems that this type of spinal deformity is common in those who, through the light nature of their work or profession, or through the inherent strength of their constitution, escape the common stresses of advancing age – namely, degeneration of the discs or senile kyphosis (see Chapter 5).

RHEUMATOID SPONDYLITIS

Rheumatiod spondylitis is clearly differentiated from ankylosing spondylitis and can produce kyphosis/scoliosis in adults and the elderly. It involves the thoracolumbar vertebrae in patients with rheumatoid arthritis. Plain radiography shows erosive arthritis of the facet joints with often major displacement in sacral direction of the vertebral bodies upon each other. The vertebral end plates are also involved with erosions. These changes are much more clearly defined by CT scanning. One of the difficulties of pathogenesis is that these patients have often been on long-term corticosteroids with their secondary osteoporotic effect. Heywood and Meyers (1986) have reported on four cases with histological positive findings. They described this condition as beginning with synovitis, subchondral erosions, subchondral bone loss, all resulting in anteroposterior and even lateral instability and then loss of disc substance and invasive erosion of the subchondral plates. Costovertebral joints were also involved.

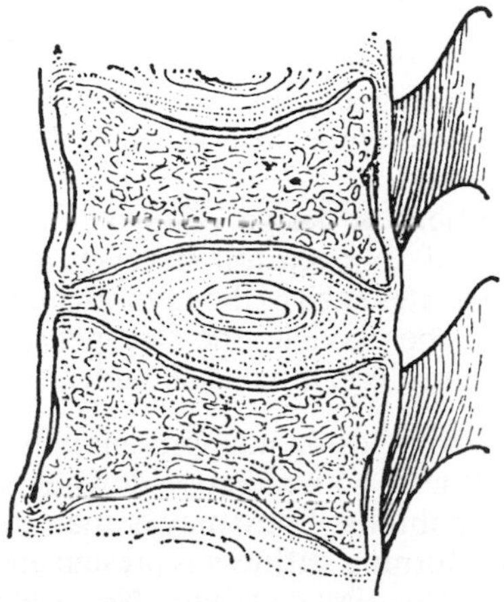

Figure 13.44 Senile osteoporosis: the 'fish-tailing' and porosis of the vertebra and the bulging of the discs.

CLINICAL FEATURES

Spondylosis deformans, the so-called osteoarthritis of the spine, occurs in the lumbar spine, an area which is mobile and therefore most liable to the trauma of overexertion. It is seen most commonly in patients whose occupation, such as coal-mining and dock-labouring, has incurred strain over a period of many years.

In the earliest phase the patient is conscious of his back and has difficulty in carrying out certain movements. There is frequently a history of attacks of 'lumbago'. At a later stage the pain never completely disappears, one attack merging into another. With each successive attack the spinal symptoms become more marked and movements more limited. Pain is present particularly in the morning when the patient straightens up after bending. The pain and stiffness progress, with remissions, until eventually the whole spine is involved.

Sensory symptoms become prominent later, and are due to pressure on the nerve roots as they leave the spinal foramina. They may occur before any radiological evidence of the disease is apparent. Motor root symptoms are uncommon.

When osteophytes are present, the x-ray picture is characteristic. In the degenerative form the vertebrae are atrophied and the vertebral shadow is uneven. In the more advanced cases a mottling or stippling of the vertebral shadow is evident.

The remaining forms of senile kyphosis are evidenced by a change in the figure. The individual reduces in stature, and carries himself with a pronounced stoop with the head and shoulders apparently thrust forward.

DIAGNOSIS

Senile kyphosis must be distinguished from those diseases of the vertebral body which result in deformity. These are mainly tuberculosis – rare at this age – Paget's disease, Kümmell's disease and secondary malignant deposits.

TREATMENT

The treatment of spondylosis may be considered under two headings:

1. *General*:
   (a) correction of postural defects;
   (b) reduction of weight;
   (c) the possibility of a change to a less arduous occupation should be considered.
2. *Local*. The common physiotherapeutic measures of short-wave diathermy and local heat are of service in relieving pain and accompanying muscle spasm. When the acute phase has passed, to these methods of producing local heat are added graduated exercises to maintain the maximum range of mobility. In more advanced cases recumbency on a firm bed may be necessary to reduce the deformity prior to the fitting of a spinal support.

The remaining conditions in this series are seldom amenable to active treatment, but if pain is a prominent feature the use of a spinal brace will afford a considerable measure of relief.

Ankylosing spondylitis

There is increasing evidence that ankylosing spondylitis is a separate entity from the lesions produced by rheumatoid arthritis. Rommanus (1953) stated that in the majority of the patients the onset of joint symptoms followed a urogenital infection, and that in 37 cases an exacerbation of such an infection was followed by exacerbation of this arthritis. He suggested that the infections from the prostate and vesicular spaces spread to the sacroiliac joints via the lymphatics, and to the spine by the vertebral venous system of Batson (1942). A real difficulty has been in trying to identify non-gonococcal organisms in the urogenital infections, since they may be abacterial in type.

Ankylosing spondylitis is no longer grouped with the rheumatoid arthropathies, but rather within the 'seronegative spondyloarthropathies'. Moll *et al.* (1976) defined the criteria for inclusion as:

1. Negative rheumatoid factor serology.
2. Absence of subcutaneous nodules.
3. Inflammatory peripheral arthritis.
4. Radiological sacroilitis – classical ankylosing spondylitis.
5. Clinical overlap, e.g. skin or nail lesions, ocular inflammation (conjunctivitis or ureitis), bowel ulceration, genitourinary infection (urethritis, prostatitis), thrombophlebitis.
6. Familial aggregations – increased prevalence of associated disease in first-degree relatives, e.g.
   - idiopathic ankylosing spondylitis – uncomplicated psoriasis,
   - uncomplicated psoriasis – arthritis, ankylosing,
   - Reiter's disease – psoriasis, ankylosing,
   - ulcerative colitis – ankylosing polyarthritis,
   - Crohn's disease – ankylosing polyarthritis, colitis.

It has, in the past, been called Marie-Strümpell disease and its incidence is about 1% of patients presenting in rheumatological clinics with equal distributions in males and females.

The HLA B27 genetic marker is commonly found in patients with ankylosing spondylitis and the risk factor for the disease is less than 10% of individuals who are positive for this histocompatibility complex antigen. Unfortunately, the discovery of the marker HLA B27 has not led to any improvement in diagnosis or treatment as yet.

The expression of the clinical features of ankylosing spondylitis is now thought to arise in genetically predisposed hosts, triggered off by some environmental agent, e.g. postvenereal infection in Reiter's disease and post-enteric (*Salmonella, Shigella* and *Klebsiella* organisms).

Although preliminary results suggested that ankylosing spondylitis was associated with a high incidence of the homozygous MN blood group, this was not substantiated by Mathiesen and Haar (1986). They found a normal distribution and the MN blood type was of no use in screening for ankylosing spondylitis.

There are three main areas of involvement:

1. Sacroiliitis or arthritis.
2. An ankylosing arthritis involving the apophyseal joints of the spine with secondary metaplastic ossification.
3. Involvement of the pelvis, spine, and the costovertebral and costotransverse articulations and other sites such as the sternomanubrial joint, joints of the clavicle, the calcaneus, and other major joints, e.g. hip and shoulder.

The sacroiliitis lesion may present with low back pain and stiffness, with radiation down the posterior aspect of both thighs. There may or may not be local tenderness. Morning stiffness is present and tends to improve with the day's activity. Non-specific poor health symptoms of anorexia, fatigue and low-grade pyrexia may present.

Earliest x-ray changes are bilateral arthritis of the sacroiliac joints which present as decalcification, resorption with lytic defects, destruction, ossification and sclerosis and synostosis formation. There may or may not be progressive narrowing of one or more of the intervertebral spaces, particularly in the lumbar spine. Complete paravertebral ossification around the whole periphery of the vertebral bodies may occur in the annulus fibrosus with reduction in height of the disc spaces, to give bony bridging and involvement of the ligamentum flavum and the posterior vertebral ligaments. Ossification is not primary in these ligaments, but more likely to occur in the fibrous and poorly vascularized neighbouring areolar tissues, between the ligaments and the margins of vertebral bodies (Figures 13.45 to 13.48).

Seaman and Wells (1961) described 11 cases of destructive lesions involving the adjacent surfaces of contiguous vertebrae in radiographs of 110 patients with ankylosing spondylitis. These workers emphasized that this sudden collapse of the vertebrae has to be differentiated from osteomyelitis due to tuberculosis, brucellosis or typhoid fever, in which the presence of paravertebral masses will be helpful. The actual pathological changes involved are not known.

Engfeldt *et al.* (1954) described the histological changes of the condition they called 'pelvo-spondylitis ossificans'. There is small artery pathology with thickening of the vessel walls to give the appearance of an endarteritis obliterans. Hyperplasia of small round cells occurs particularly around small vessels, these cells being diffusely distributed in connective and fatty tissues and muscles. New bone formation with osteoblastic activity and osteoid tissue formation may be present as well as localized destruction of articular cartilage and bone.

Peripheral major joint arthritis can occur soon after the clinical features of axial skeletal disease. It has been reported that over 25% of all patients with ankylosing spondylitis have involvement of the hip – of two distinct types – a unilateral destructive type and a bilateral type with sclerosis but no destruction (Forestier and Lagier, 1971). Involvement of the shoulder is also common (Emery *et al.*, 1991). These authors have described 52 Chinese patients with symptomatic shoulder girdle lesion of three major types – limitation of scapulothoracic motion, acute inflammatory arthropathy of the sternoclavicular and acromioclavicular joints and severe glenohumeral disease. They found radiographic changes similar to those described by Resnick (1979) – erosive change and osseous proliferation, intra-articular osseous ankylosis and the absence of periarticular or widespread osteoporosis. There was narrowing of the glenohumeral joint space with upward displacement of the humeral head. A characteristic finding was the presence of enthesophytes (osteophytes arising at the attachments of tendon, muscle and

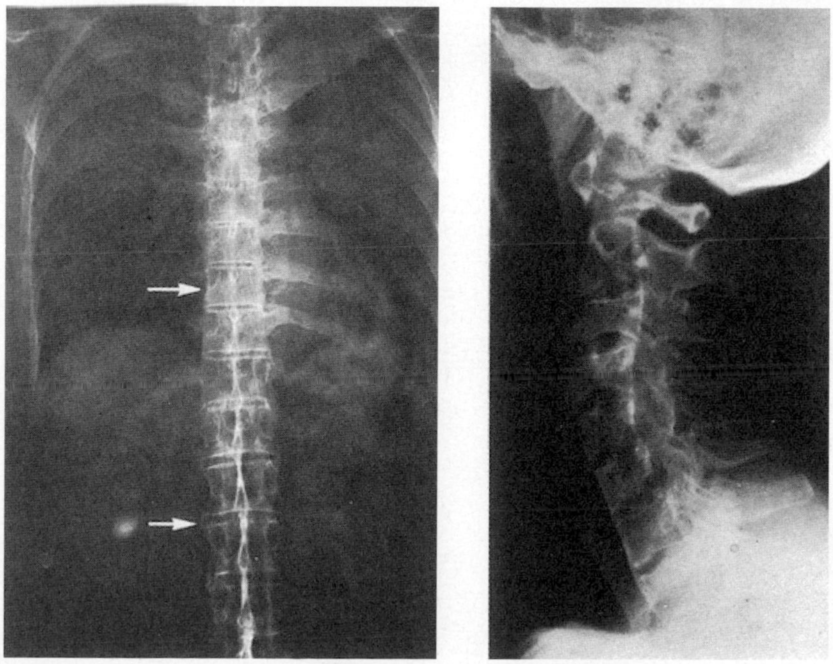

(a) (b)

Figure 13.45 (a) Radiograph of the thoracolumbar spine, showing the fairly early 'squaring' of the vertebral bodies of an elderly ankylosing spondylitis. Some osseous continuity between the lumbar spine is seen. (b) Radiograph of the cervical spine, showing the anterior longitudinal ligaments' ossification with squaring.

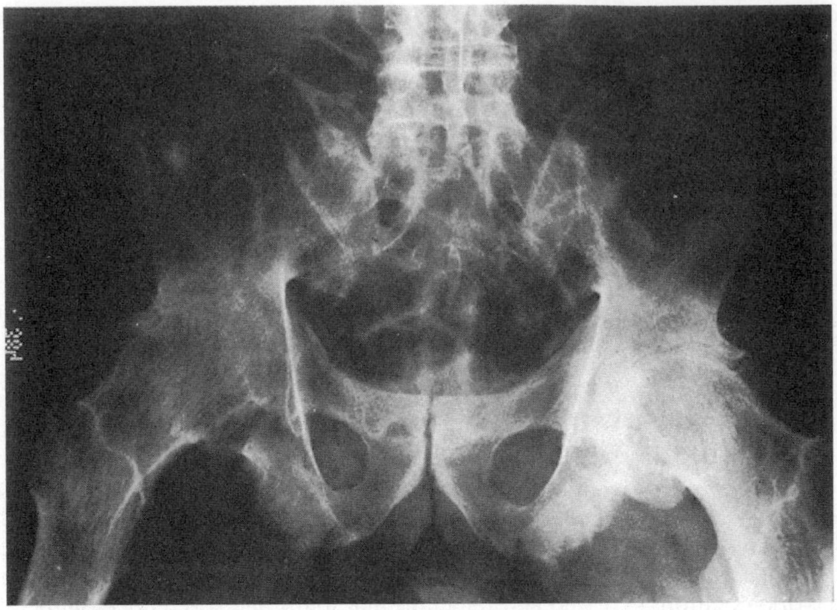

Figure 13.46 A more advanced case of ankylosing spondylitis with more new bone formation at the margins of adjacent vertebrae. In the pelvis there is obliteration of the sacroiliac joints as well as a bony ankylosis of the right hip joint with arthritis on the left.

capsule) – which are also commonly seen around the calcaneus, in psoriasis and hyperostosis.

Fong *et al.* (1988) have reviewed 40 extensive destructive lesions of ankylosing vertebrae – e.g. united fractures through either ankylosed discs (37) or vertebral bodies (3), with corresponding fractures

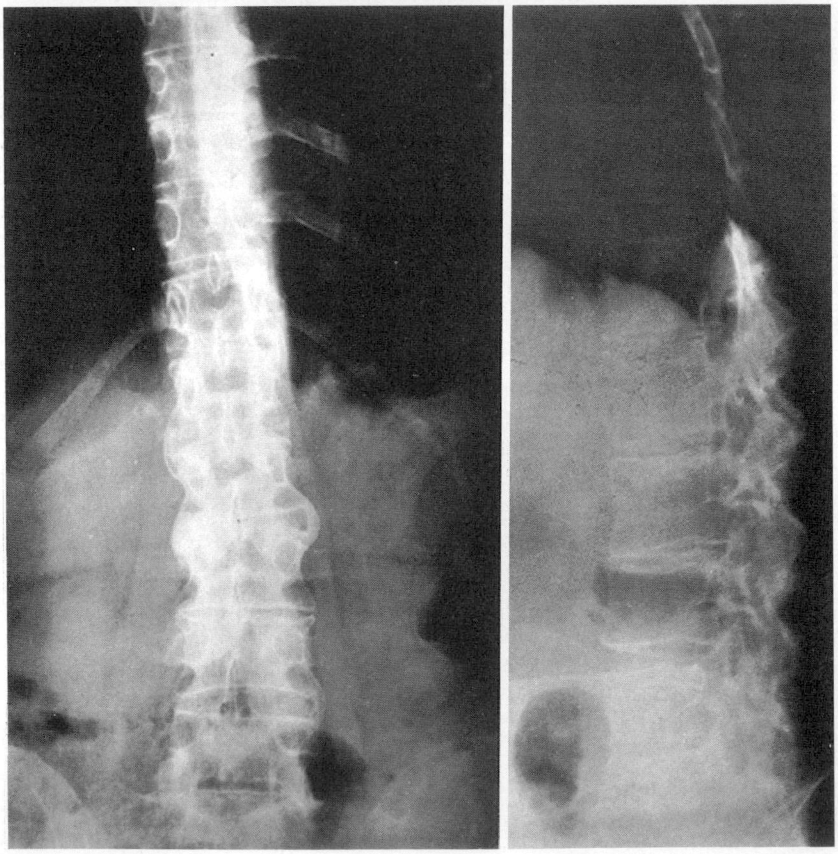

(a) (b)

Figure 13.47 Radiographs of the lower thoracolumbar spine showing the typical 'bamboo spine' with marked new bone formation joining the lumbar spine together.

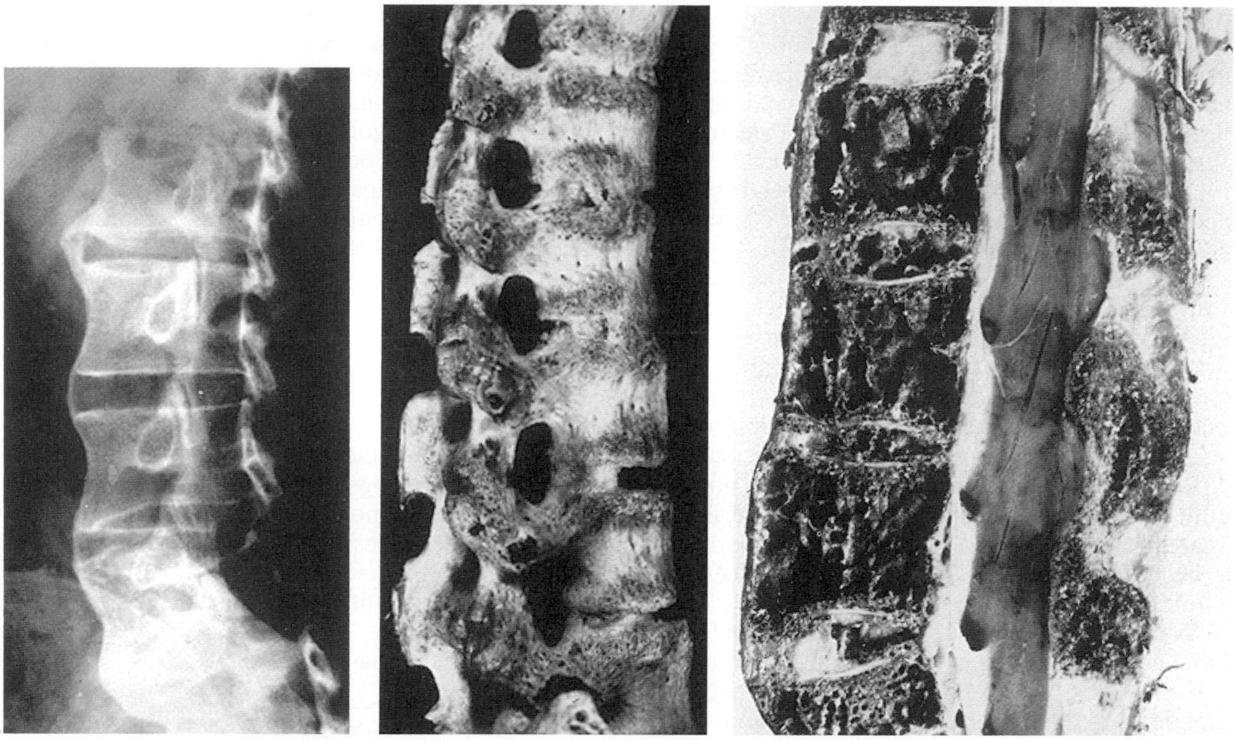

(a) (b) (c)

Figure 13.48 Ankylosing spondylitis with ligament calcification and ossification and an isthmic defect visible at L5. (a) Oblique radiograph of lumbar spine. (b) Post-mortem specimen. (c) Sagittal section of (b), showing the spinal canal.

in the posterior column in 34 patients. Pain was the most common feature and three had a neurological deficit – paraparesis in 2, and one patient with motor weakness and hypoaesthesia. Of these patients 16 had significant hip disease. Sixteen of their patients underwent anterior spinal fusion and pseudoarthrosis was consistently proven by histopathology. Two went on to non-union, one requiring an additional posterior fusion.

Trauma was recorded in about 10% of these cases. They believe that the mechanical stresses of a stiff kyphotic spine result in fatigue fractures through the ankylosed disc which offers less resistance than the vertebral body. Another cause may be that the segment which 'fractures' may have escaped, becoming incorporated into the non-ossified fusion mass.

DIAGNOSIS

Recognition of advanced cases with gross spinal deformity, forward craning of the neck, ankylosis of the hips and fixed flexion deformities at the knees is not difficult. Similarly, radiographic features such as fusion of the sacroiliac joints, calcification in the anterior spinal ligament and the classic 'bamboo' spines, do not provide diagnostic difficulties. Such diagnosis is of little value because, by the time such features are apparent, little can be done to improve the patient's lot, and the prognosis is poor. The need for early diagnosis has been met by two groups of criteria:

1. *The Rome criteria* (Kellgren *et al.*, 1963) – ankylosing spondylitis is diagnosed if bilateral sacroiliitis is seen on radiographs with any one of the following:
   (a) low back pain and stiffness of 3 months' duration and not relieved by rest;
   (b) pain and stiffness in the thoracic spine;
   (c) limited lumbar spinal movement;
   (d) limited chest expansion;
   (e) history or evidence of iritis or its sequelae.
2. *The New York criteria* (Bennett and Wood, 1968):
   (a) limitation of lumbosacral movement in three planes;
   (b) history and/or presence of pain at the dorsolumbar junction, with or without lumbar spine pain;
   (c) limited chest expansion of 2.5 cm or less at the fourth intercostal space.

Anterior spinal movement can be measured by a

modification of Schober's method, which assesses the distraction of a segment of the lumbar spine, by using fixed points at the level of the sacroiliac joints and 10 cm above it in extension and then remeasuring the segment in maximal flexion (Macrae and Wright, 1969). Chest expansion measured in the fourth intercostal space is known to decrease with age, but in established spondylitis it is often markedly decreased (Moll and Wright, 1972).

The distance between the occipital eminence and a wall or other upright plane against which the heels are pressed, maintaining the mandible parallel to the floor, is a measure of cervical flexion.

Measuring the shortest finger-to-floor distance may well aid assessment of lumbar flexion but can easily be confused if good hip movement is retained.

Routine laboratory tests frequently are non-specific for any inflammatory process. There is mild anaemia, an elevated ESR, but the rheumatoid factor is negative and HLA B27 typing has no diagnostic significance.

Systemic bone scanning with techneteum-99 will indicate the widespread joint involvement and the earlier lesions. The specificity of response of the pain arising from the sacroiliitis, to a dose of non-steroid anti-inflammatory drug, e.g. indomethacin or, before it was banned, phenylbutazone, is striking.

DIFFERENTIAL DIAGNOSIS

Radiographic abnormalities may cause difficulties in differentiating between ankylosing hyperostosis and ankylosing spondylitis (Forestier and Lagier, 1971) (Table 13.5).

ASSOCIATED DISORDERS

From early times ankylosing spondylitis has been recognized as having an association with acute anterior uveitis. Careful studies suggest an incidence of 20% of uveitis in known cases of ankylosing spondylitis, and it is usually unilateral. It may precede spinal symptoms and is more common in patients with peripheral joint involvement.

There has been described an incidence between 2 and 7% of ankylosing spondylitis in Crohn's disease (or regional ileitis), with radiographic sacroiliitis being found in 16.4% of a Leeds series (Moll, 1978).

In ulcerative colitis, ankylosing spondylitis has been shown to vary from 1.6% to 25.6% in various groups.

The prevalence of psoriasis in the general population has varied between 2.6 and 7%. The most recent British series suggests 4.5% of the population have or have had the disease. Psoriatic spondylitis has only been recognized since the mid-195Os and the incidence of spondylitis in the psoriatic population has been assessed at 2–5%.

Sacroiliitis is increasingly common in the population who have suffered Reiter's disease, with a 50–70% incidence where symptoms have been present for more than 5 years.

The human leucocyte antigen

The human leucocyte antigen (HLA) system is a major and complex antigen of which over 30×10^6 variants are possible. The determinants are found on the surface of leucocytes, platelets, spermatozoa and other cells. In transplantation they have become known as tissue-typing or histocompatibility antigens. Antigenic variants can be defined by serological or by leucocyte cytotoxity tests. The latter test requires blood collected into citrate and the live lymphocytes can be removed and studied in culture, but it is laborious and expensive (Brewerton, 1974). The antigens of the HLA system are glycoproteins with a molecular weight of 50 000–55 000, and are found on the short arm of chromosome 6 near to the centromere.

Table 13.5 Differential diagnosis between ankylosing hyperostosis and ankylosing spondylitis

	Ankylosing hyperostosis	Ankylosing spondylitis
Age	Elderly	Adolescent, young adult
Pain	Mild dorsolumbar pain; root pain rare	Night pain; frequent 'root' pain
Kyphosis	Normal/slight	Pronounced
Spine	Stiff dorsal spine	Rigid spine
Chest expansion	Normal (for age)	Progressive decrease
ESR	Normal	Raised in 80% of patients
Vertebral changes	Continuous and thick outgrowth extending over vertebral bodies; no osteoporosis	Squaring of vertebrae; osteoporosis; syndesmophytes
Apophyseal joints	Normal	Joint space partly/completely obliterated
Sacroiliac joints	Normal	Bilateral erosions leading to ankylosis

Ankylosing spondylitis was first demonstrated as having a close correlation with a certain HLA grouping (Brewerton *et al.*, 1973) when 72 of 75 cases were shown to have the HLA-B(W)27 antigen, which was present in only 3 of 75 controls. The prevalence of B27 varies between population groups, as does the percentage of B27 in spondylitis. Examples of the varying prevalence of HLA-B27 in different populations are:

- Caucasians: 8%
- American negroes: 4%
- African negroes: 0%
- Japanese: 1%
- Pima indians: 100%

The strong family history of ankylosing spondylitis has been confirmed by tissue typing the parents of these patients: approximately 50% are B27-positive. By HLA typing patients with diseases associated with spondylitis (Brewerton *et al.*, 1973), the close inter-relationship between these conditions has been confirmed. The prevalence of B27-positive individuals with ankylosing spondylitis and related diseases is:

- idiopathic ankylosing spondylitis: 90%
- Reiter's disease: 90%
- psoriasis, spondylitis and sacroiliitis: 90%
- inflammatory bowel disease with ankylosing spondylitis: 80%
- Behçet's disease: 27%

It should be noted that a significant increase in B27 is found in anterior uveitis (50%) and in juvenile chronic polyarthritis (25%) as well as in 'reactive arthritis' associated with *Salmonella/Shigella/Yersinia* infections.

The mechanisms of B27 association are thought to arise from:

1. Molecular mimicry by the HLA molecule reacting with a virus or other foreign particles.
2. Linkage disequilibrium in which the HLA molecule is associated with a 'disease susceptibility gene'.
3. Shared antigenic determinants in which there is antigenic similarity between the B27 molecule and some infecting agent, resulting in an autoimmune process.

Some support in understanding the B27 reactions comes from a combination theory of a susceptible population and an otherwise common infecting agent – e.g. an increase in the isolation of *Klebsiella* from the stools of patients with 'active' ankylosing spondylitis as opposed to those with inactive disease or controls (Ebringer *et al.*, 1978).

TREATMENT

Gradual reduction of the spinal deformity by pillows on a bed fitted with a fracture board is instituted. The patient is encouraged to lie on his back for increasing periods each day so that in a short time the improvement in the back deformity becomes obvious even to the patient. Occasionally a spinal support may help in relieving pain (Figure 13.49). Recording the distance between the occiput and the mattress on which he lies allows measurement of his progress and is encouraging to the patient. Because of the occasional spread to the hips and shoulders, one should be on guard to see that these joints retain their full range of mobility. Where the neck movement is limited, a Glisson sling with traction from the head of the bed helps greatly. Sometimes it is useful in reducing the deformity to suspend the body by a series of transverse slings hung on horizontal bars at either side of the bed. In the interim, suitable exercises are given. Breathing exercises are important and are done in various positions.

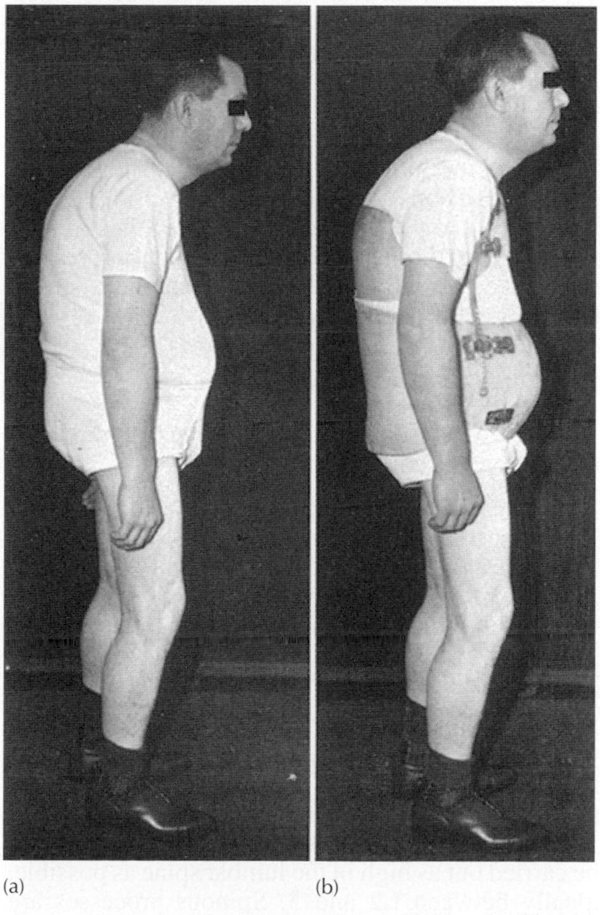

(a) (b)

Figure 13.49 (a) Ankylosing spondylitis with shortness of breath, (b) relieved by hyperextension brace.

The results seem reasonably good for, following supervision of the treatment for about a year, it is rare to have them report unless it is to advise that they are proceeding satisfactorily.

Non-steroidal anti-inflammatory agents (e.g. indomethacin) have proved useful for symptomatic relief. Although radiotherapy gives definite relief and improvement in the stiffness, it is not used now because of the likelihood of these patients developing leukaemia in later life.

A new drug, sulphasalazine, has been introduced but unfortunately, although it improved symptoms of peripheral joint pain at 4 weeks, it did not improve the long-standing disease (Corkill *et al.*, 1990). Improvement in chest expansion, a drop in ESR and serum IgA, and improvement in pain and spondylometry measurements have been reported (Corkill *et al.*, 1990).

Osteotomy of the spine

For the flexion deformity of the spine produced by ankylosing spondylitis and also in rheumatoid arthritis, Smith-Petersen *et al.* (1945) described an operation of osteotomy of the spine to correct the serious deformity. The operation is confined to the laminae and articular facets and does not involve the vertebral bodies. The operation is not undertaken until all conservative measures have failed. It is performed in the lumbar region at levels showing the minimum of bone bridging. Such bony bridging may be expected to yield after osteotomy of the articular facets. The thoracic region commonly presents ankylosed costovertebral joints which make correction difficult if not impossible.

Lumbar spinal osteotomy

Law (1959) described the objectives of this procedure for this condition:

1. To improve the erect position and thereby to balance the effect of gravity and decrease the progressive plature of the deformity.
2. To increase the respiratory function by lifting the thoracic cage, and allowing greater excursion of the diaphragm.
3. To increase the gastrointestinal function.

His technique was based upon Smith-Petersen's in which, through posterior oblique osteotomies, the bones are divided with eventual breaking of the anterior longitudinal ligament by manipulation under control. He recommended that the osteotomy should be carried out as high in the lumbar spine as possible, ideally between L2 and 3. Spinous processes are divided, and, because the ligamenta flava and interspinous ligaments are usually ossified, these are removed by rongeurs. The osteotomes are passed across the articular processes at an angle of 45° to the frontal plane and usually enter the intervertebral foramina above each cut. Immobilization is carried out in plaster for at least 6 weeks to 3 months.

Law (1969) reviewed his experience of 120 lumbar osteotomies and 20 cervical operations. In these there were 8 deaths – 3 due to shock or cerebral anoxia; 2 to spinal cord damage; 2 to perforated peptic ulceration or gastric erosion; 1 to acute psychosis. Other, non-fatal, complications were 2 paraplegia (spastic and flaccid); a superior mesenteric arterial thrombosis; and several paralytic ileus problems.

Goel (1968) performed a lumbar osteotomy on 15 patients, 11 of whom had ankylosing spondylitis or osteomalacia. He performed the osteotomy at one level in the lumbar spine and the correction obtained in these patients ranged between 25° and 60°. Three patients who had had a correction of 25° developed abdominal distension, and two patients root irritation. There were no other complications.

In these cases a correction of 20–25° would lift the chin off the sternum so the patient could see ahead more easily. In addition, swallowing and breathing became easier and the danger of subluxation from the weight of the head being thrust forward was lessened considerably.

Spinal correction osteotomy for progressive kyphosis has been reported on by Styblo *et al.* (1986) who carried out 22 such procedures with a mean correction of 44° in the thoracic region. Loss of correction was reduced greatly by the use of internal fixation and postoperative support for 3–6 months by a plaster-of-Paris jacket with leg extension. There were no fatalities and few complications, but there were three cases of retrograde ejaculation which has not been previously reported. They also noted that 75% of these patients had involvement of the hips.

In summary, it can be stated that osteotomy of the spine is a dramatic operation, not without risk, but which, performed at the right time, can both prevent and overcome serious disabling deformity and thus render the life of the unfortunate patient much more worth while.

Management of involved hips

When the hips are involved in bony ankylosis with the spine, and particularly if there is accompanying flexion deformity, some mobilizing and corrective procedure should be carried out prior to the spinal osteotomy. Mobilizing the hips before spinal osteotomy makes it easier to determine the desired degree of correction in the spine. Mobilization also reduces the effects of leverage in a rigid system at the time of operation (see Chapter 12).

May and Yeoman (1986) have reported from a small series of 36 patients receiving 54 total hip replacements with very successful results. The average age at the time of operation was 39 years with 81% becoming excellent with an average follow-up of 5 years. Ectopic bone formation was 18% but of these only 2.6% was significant. They recommended early and extending physiotherapy and hydrotherapy with concentration on the range of extension, to produce the best results.

Indications for cervical osteotomy

1. To correct deformity by elevating the chin from the sternum, thus enabling the patient to see ahead more easily.
2. To prevent atlantoaxial subluxation and dislocation resulting from the weight of head being carried forward.
3. To relieve tracheal and oesophageal kinking accompanied by dyspnoca or dysphagia.
4. To prevent kinking of the spinal cord or undue traction on the nerve roots that might result in neurological disturbance.

Postoperative care

With internal fixation the patient may become ambulant in 2–3 days otherwise it is preferable to wait 6 weeks before the thigh is freed from the plaster or before an ordinary plaster jacket is applied. Fusion is usually consolidated in 3–4 months and, since the bone is likely to be vascular and soft, a neck support is worn for 6 months. Frequently, ossification occurs in the gap created between the vertebral bodies, thereby providing sound fusion and a correction which is likely to be permanent.

Charcot spine

As well as involving joints of the lower extremities, this condition can also be seen in contiguous vertebrae of the thoracic and lumbar segments of the spine. It is characterized by areas of disintegration, bone sclerosis and large, but irregular, amounts of new bone formation at the margins of articular surfaces, with much fragmentation (Figure 13.50). This usually produces a sharp scoliosis involving two or three vertebrae. It arises by extensive damage to the articular cartilage, as well as to the subchondral bone layers, and consists of a mixture of proliferation and fragmentation of vertebral bodies. Although about 15% of the patients may present because of low back pain, in the majority of cases this is more often a coincidental radiographic finding, as are the deposits of radiopaque metallic salts in the buttock areas. Treatment is usually directed

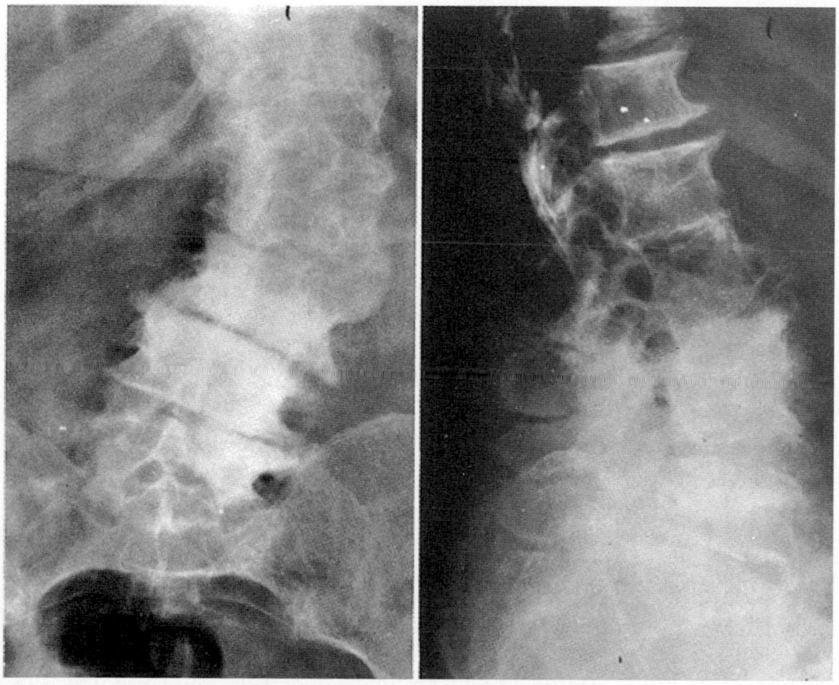

(a) (b)

Figure 13.50 (a) Anteroposterior and (b) lateral radiographs of thoracolumbar Charcot spine of a middle-aged woman, showing a sharp scoliosis with destruction of bone and new bone formation, sclerosis and loss of intervertebral disc spaces.

towards physiotherapy and the wearing of an adequate lumbosacral support.

Osteitis condensans ilii

Usually a woman between the ages of 20 and 40 years complains of a recurrent low back pain with occasional radiation down into both buttocks and thighs, but not usually of a true radicular type. It tends to be aggravated by movement of the lower lumbar spine. Often there is a history of recent childbearing, It is important to appreciate that this is a true self-limiting disease because radiographically it is rarely seen in later life, even as a coincidental finding. The typical x-ray appearances are of sclerosis in the ilium adjacent to the sacroiliac joint and usually involving the distal half (Figure 13.51). It may be bilateral. It may be a reaction of bone to the effect of the hormone relaxin on the pelvic joints just before her delivery. Treatment is usually palliative by such measures as short-wave diathermy, salicylates and the wearing of a firm corset. The condition has to be distinguished from osteoarthritis, tuberculosis and osteomyelitis of the sacroiliac joint, which are rarely bilateral.

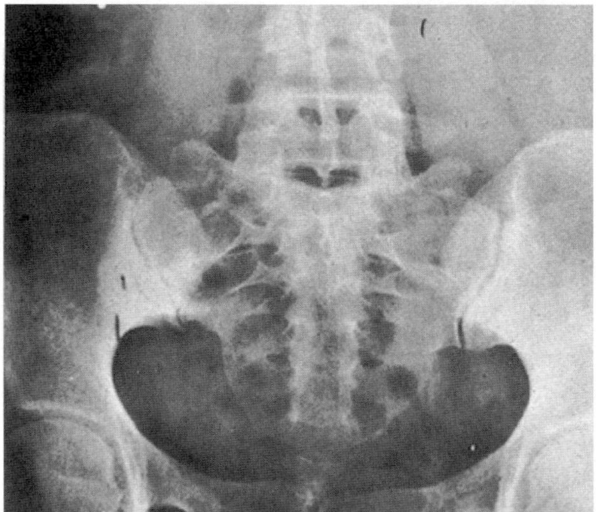

Figure 13.51 Anteroposterior radiograph of the pelvis of a young woman post-partum, showing sclerosis of bone in the lower aspect of the right and left ilium adjacent to the sacroiliac joints, of an osteitis condensans ilii.

Lesions of the cervical spine

These are discussed below, in sections on: brachialgia; cervical disc lesions and spondylosis; spondylosis and osteoarthritis of the cervical spine; rheumatoid arthritis of the cervical spine; and atlantoaxial dislocation in children.

Brachialgia

Typical features are:

1. Pain radiating into the upper extremity or the occipital area of the skull, with fairly accurate referral to one or more dermatomes and/or pain, with or without tenderness, in muscles of the involved root. Often the patient is unable to find a comfortable position in bed when spasm is severe and has to lie prone with the head resting on the hands.
2. Paraesthesiae, which may or may not be localized to a particular dermatome, with numbness and sensory loss.
3. Disturbance of appropriate reflexes of the upper extremity.
4. Muscle weakness. Accompanying the muscle weakness there may be wasting with or without fibrillation. More often these features are seen in only one arm, but it can occur in both.
5. Involvement of the vertebral artery or, rarely, the sympathetic plexus – giving rise to giddiness, 'drop attacks', tinnitus or visual disturbance (Figure 13.52).

It is important to determine the site of the disease process – which may be due to disturbances in the pyramidal tract, the motor neuron, the root or in the surrounding vertebrae. If the main complaint is muscle pain and this can be relieved by various

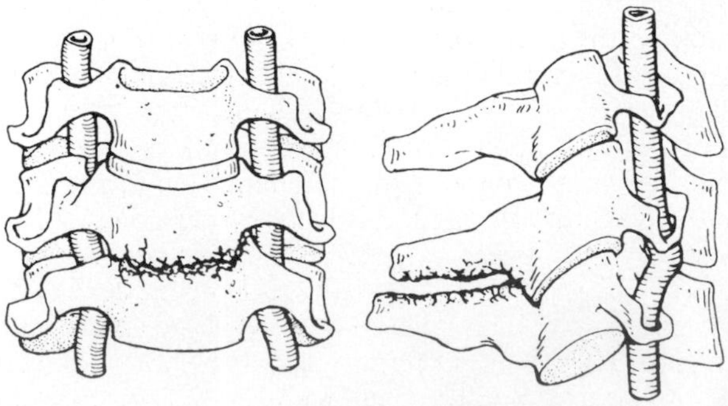

Figure 13.52 An intervertebral disc prolapse which involves the vertebral artery on one side.

palliative physiotherapy procedures, it is unlikely to be due to true nerve root involvement. It is important to remember that involvement of the spinal cord may occur, and this may be manifested by alteration of trunk sensation and reflexes and alteration of muscle tone, vibration sense and proprioception in the lower limbs.

Differential diagnosis of brachialgia consists of:

1. Tumours of the cord and its membranes or the bony vertebral column.
2. Infections, such as acute osteomyelitis, tuberculosis and actinomycoses.
3. Prolapsed intervertebral disc.
4. Cervical spondylosis.
5. Cervical rib or 'thoracic outlet syndrome'.
6. Neuralgic amyotrophy or Spillain's syndrome.
7. Pancoast's tumour.
8. Congenital abnormalities of the cord (e.g. syringomyelia).
9. Atlantoaxial dislocation or subluxation.

Cervical disc lesions and spondylosis

ANATOMY AND PATHOLOGY

The anatomy and pathology of cervical intervertebral discs are similar to that of lumbar disc herniations and the reader is referred to their description on p. 951 et seq.

The principal differences between the lumbar and cervical regions in relation to protrusions are those of contents and function. The cervical spine is subjected to strains of mobility much more than weight-bearing compared to the lumbar. These strains are greatest at the very mobile lower segment; consequently disc herniations and spondylosis are commonest at C5–6 and C6–7 levels. The cervical canal, though quite capacious, contains a relatively immobile and thick cord anchored to the meninges by the denticulate ligament and to some extent by the short, almost transversely running, nerve roots. These roots pursue their short horizontal course outside the thecal sac, though still intradural, into the intervertebral foramina, clinging quite closely to the vertebral bodies at the level of the intervertebral discs, and add to the relative fixation of the cord and its coverings. The anteroposterior diameter of the intervertebral foramina in the lower cervical region is fairly small, and may be narrowed still further by arthritic changes in the posterior facet joints and in the joints of Luschka. The anterolateral margins of the upper surface of a cervical vertebra possess an upward bony lip-like projection, arising just at the base of the pedicle, which embraces the lower anterolateral margins of the upper vertebra, forming a small joint with a synovial lining. The resulting 'concave–convex' fitting prevents lateral displacement of one vertebra upon the other, a displacement prevented chiefly in the lumbar region by the arrangement of the posterior articular facet joints. Compere *et al.* (1959) described the anatomy, physiology and pathology of the *Luschka joints* which have been termed 'neurocentral' are found in the posterolateral areas between two vertebrae. They are anteromedial to the nerve roots, but posteromedial to the vertebral arteries and veins, so that the artery is immediately adjacent to the outer side of the Luschka joint. Being vertical in shape, they tend to prevent posterolateral prolapse of the intervertebral discs as well as lateral shift of the vertebral bodies.

As a result of this anatomical structure the potentialities of the protrusion of a cervical intervertebral disc involving neural structures is of a far more serious nature, the differential diagnosis is often more complicated, and the surgical approach more hazardous than it is in the case of the lumbar spine.

The exact situation in the horizontal plane of a protruded cervical intervertebral disc is therefore of greater and potentially graver importance than in the lumbar region:

1. A *laterally placed* herniation – the commonest – will give rise to purely a root syndrome.
2. A *paramedian* protrusion may also impinge upon the spinal cord, thus producing the mixed syndrome of cord and root compression, sometimes starting with root symptoms and progressing to cord compression or *vice versa*.
3. A *more centrally placed* protrusion may involve the entire width of the cord or only its ipsilateral columns, causing clinical features of an extramedullary intradural pressure on the cord.

The protrusions in the cervical region are usually of small dimensions, but the relative fixation of the cord increases the severity and often the rapidity of onset. The short horizontal course of roots, unlike those in the lumbar spine, does not permit any play and is mostly responsible for the greater persistence of symptoms.

The types of herniation are similar to those in the lumbar region except that protrusions in the form of a transverse ridge or bar across the spinal canal are commoner. The most frequent type is the posterolateral protrusion producing nerve root symptoms and signs in the arms together with neck spasm and severe pain. Although the nucleus pulposus may protrude through the annulus into the epidural space, this is less common than in the lumbar region; more often, the pathology is that of a thinned annulus fibrosus bulging but intact. There is also in later life a tendency for the formation of a more rigid type of prolapse which may become calcified and be associated with osteophytes. Multiple protrusions may occur in the cervical region, though their incidence is not established.

With increasing age, gradual degeneration of the intervertebral discs occurs. The glycosaminoglycan of the intervertebral disc diminishes. This results in a reduction of the water content of the disc, especially in the nucleus pulposus. The effect is a gradual collapse and narrowing of the intervertebral disc space and the stretching of the annulus fibrosus, which therefore protrudes at its periphery. The annulus lifts off the margins of the vertebrae and as a result new bone is formed, producing 'osteophytes' more correctly termed 'bony outgrowths'. Posteriorly these impinge into the spinal canal and laterally into the intervertebral foramina. The posterior spinal facet joints are placed under increasing load by the narrowing of the intervertebral disc space, and consequently degeneration of the articular cartilage occurs. This results in secondary osteoarthrosis of posterior facet joints, with formation of marginal true osteophytes which narrow the intervertebral canal space from behind. Thus the nerve roots become pinched behind the two bony projections and only minor trauma is required to produce nipping and neck and nerve root pain. At any time during this process minor trauma, which may occur during sleep, may cause an acute prolapse of the nucleus pulposus through the annulus fibrosus posteriorly, laterally or centrally. If this is a minor prolapse then the individual simply feels pain in the neck and spasm; if greater then there will be either spinal cord compression or, much more commonly, nerve root compression with obvious root symptoms and signs. As the nerve root is nipped repeatedly during neck movement, it becomes more inflamed and oedematous and will continue so until some measure is taken to either reduce the movement (for example, by the wearing of a collar or by performing cervical spine fusion at that level) or the space from the nerve root is increased by surgical removal of the osteophytes or removal of a prolapsed intervertebral disc.

O'Connell (1956) considered that the gradual-onset myelopathy resulted not from any sustained compression of nerve or neural tissue but rather from repeated movements of the neck causing pressure by the intervertebral disc on the anterior spinal arteries, particularly between C5 and 6, and C6 and 7.

Brain *et al.* (1952) described how multiple disc degeneration might involve the medulla of the cord so that there was motor disturbance due to pyramidal tract involvement in both the lower extremities with hyperspasticity, hyper-reflexia and extensor plantar responses.

CLINICAL FEATURES

Trauma to the neck as a precipitating factor in the aetiology of prolapsed intervertebral disc is not always definite. More severe trauma, such as that caused by an abrupt forward movement to the head in a motor car accident or sudden extension of the neck occurring from a rear-end collision in a motor car producing the so-called 'whiplash', may be more definite in the history.

Whiplash injury usually results in long-term disability with a history of hyperextension of the cervical spine against a head rest during a rear-end collision. Objective diagnostic criteria are usually poor with restriction of range of all movements of the cervical spine with pain and spasm, but rarely radicular signs. Response to treatment is prolonged and demanding. Radiographs of the cervical spine are most commonly normal except for reduction in forward flexion – in four distinct patterns. Bohrer *et al.* (1990) from an extensive study found that in about 25% of patients no flexion at any level was seen; a single flexion angle was seen in another 25%, with two (30%) or more (20%) flexion angles in the remaining 50%. Soft tissue abnormality of ligament, muscle or soft tissue was diagnosed in the first two groups. Davis *et al.* (1991) have reported the results from MR scanning of patients sustaining a 'whiplash' injury within 4 months of the time of injury, with normal cervical radiographs but persisting chronic pain. The scans showed up anterior, vertebral end-plate fractures, anterior annular ligamentous tears, disc separation from the vertebral end plate, and anterior longitudinal ligamentous tears. If no pathology is found, 75% will have resolution of signs and symptoms by 2 years.

Pain

The onset is often quite gradual but frequently the patient awakes from sleep with pain suggesting some inadvertent trauma. The pain may be in the form of neck stiffness, with or without an ache on head movement. In others pain is referred to the shoulder girdle and may precede pain in the neck and frequently runs posterolaterally across the shoulder and down the outer aspect of the arm and forearm involving the fingers and thumb. Less often, paraesthesia in the fingers may be the precursor of pain. The discomfort and ache of the early stages may often progress rapidly to marked stiffness of the neck, with or without a lateral tilt. All movements are frequently restricted by spasm and aggravate the pain in the upper limb. The pain is usually of a dull and gnawing character, not strictly localized but very persistent and with superimposed lancinating pains especially on head movements. It is frequently aggravated by coughing or sneezing and by jolting of the body. The distribution of the pain gives a clue to its origin.

Paraesthesiae

These almost invariably occur in the cervical herniations at a very early stage of the disease, indicating irritation of the nerve root. They usually occur distally to the pain areas in the affected dermatome. Commonly they take the form of a feeling of numbness, tingling or deadness and are usually referred to the fingers and thumbs. Like the pain, they are aggravated by neck movements and, not infrequently, by increase of intraspinal pressure.

Sensory depression

Sensory depression in the affected dermatome is a frequent accompaniment of cervical herniation, though often in the more advanced stages of the syndrome. Sensory deficit in a dermatome as opposed to that of a peripheral nerve area simplifies the differential diagnosis. The posterior column sensation such as proprioception and vibration sense are usually normal.

Reduction in motor power

Reduction in motor power is evident in the great proportion of cases, and muscle wasting is often obvious even in cases of relatively recent standing. It is important in examination to test root function rather than muscle groups.

The tendon reflexes of biceps (C5–6) and triceps (C6–7)

These are sometimes depressed or absent and help to localize the level of the lesion. The reflex changes with muscle weakness and sensory depression indicate some degree of organic change in the fibres of the affected group. The extent to which these are reversible depends on the duration and severity of compression. Sensory depression, if due to degeneration in the sensory fibres, is not recoverable since the lesion is proximal to the ganglion.

The syndrome, whether mild or severe, has a marked tendency to a protracted course. Intermittent pain may continue for several months and be provoked by movements of the neck. Gradual subsidence of symptoms and signs is the rule.

CLINICAL PRESENTATION

The majority of cases show some degree of limitation of head or neck movement due to pain and muscle spasm. In severe cases the restriction may be in all directions but frequently it is in one direction only, particularly of rotation and lateral flexion on the affected side. Extension of the neck towards the affected side is often the most painful manoeuvre. It may also be increased by downward traction of the shoulder girdle on the affected side. Whilst neck compression downwards may aggravate the pain, suspension by the head may relieve it. Localized tenderness to palpation of the spinous processes at the affected level may be found, and muscle tenderness in the shoulder girdle is not infrequent.

Neurological examination will reveal wasting, weakness, sensory loss and reflex changes as indicated in Table 13.6. It must be emphasized that the examination of the lower limbs and the abdomen is essential to exclude the onset of long tract signs.

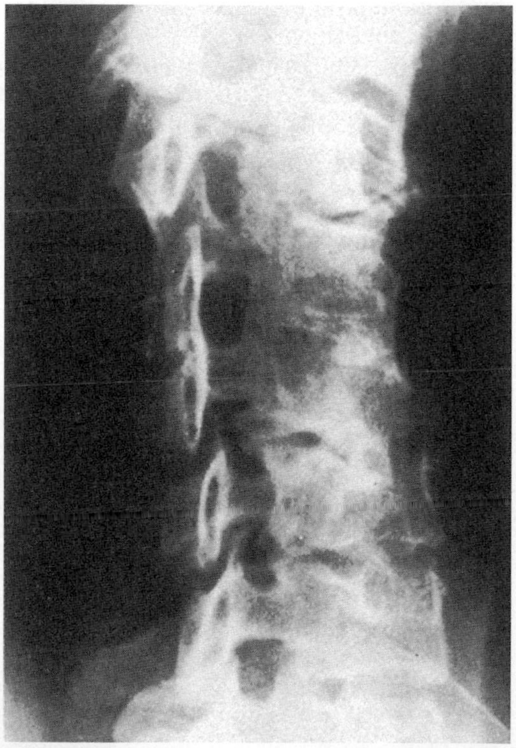

Figure 13.53 Oblique radiograph showing the narrowing of the anteroposterior diameter of the intervertebral foramen at C5–6 level.

Table 13.6 Symptoms and signs of prolapsed cervical intervertebral disc

	C5–6 (C6 nerve root)	C6–7 (C7 nerve root)	C8–T1 (C8 nerve root)
Pain	Neck, shoulder, medial border of scapula. Occasionally anterior chest, lateral aspect of arm and dorsum of forearm	Same as for C6	Neck, medial border of scapula, anterior chest, medial aspect upper arm and forearm
Numbness	Thumb and index finger	Index and middle fingers	Little and ring fingers
Weakness	Biceps (mild)	Triceps (marked)	Wrist and hand (marked)
Reflexes	Biceps ↓ or absent	Triceps ↓ or absent	Triceps occasionally ↓ or absent

RADIOGRAPHIC EXAMINATION

Radiographs in the lateral view may show absence of normal lordosis of the cervical spine. Narrowing of the suspected intervertebral space is often revealed and, with the clinical findings, is positive evidence of a cervical disc degeneration or prolapse. Negative x-rays, however, as in the lumbar spine, do not exclude the possibility of disc herniation. Oblique views of the cervical spine are taken routinely to demonstrate any narrowing of the anteroposterior diameter of the intervertebral foramina by osteoarthritic changes or by a laterally placed protrusion (Figure 13.53). It should be remembered that the lumen of the intervertebral foramina in the cervical spine diminishes in size from above downwards.

Myelography is not usually required unless there is evidence of cervical spinal cord pressure. A partial or complete block may be seen in severe cases with metrizamide radiculograms (Figure 13.54). An opportunity is taken to examine the cerebrospinal fluid content and pressure at the time of the myelogram. The myelogram is also useful for identifying the level of any obstruction of the spinal canal (Figure 13.55).

MR scanning will indicate the involved level more accurately than myelography without CT imaging. This investigation will differentiate and outline soft and calcified discs, as well as osteophytes, deforming the adjacent soft tissues (Neuhold *et al.*, 1991).

Discography is relatively simple to perform in the lower cervical region but its value is disputed. When performed under sedation, injection of a saline solution into a pathological disc may reproduce the symptoms complained of by the patient. Perhaps more valuable is a demonstration of disc distortion and leakage of radiopaque dye (Figure 13.56), which, if very definite and correlating closely with

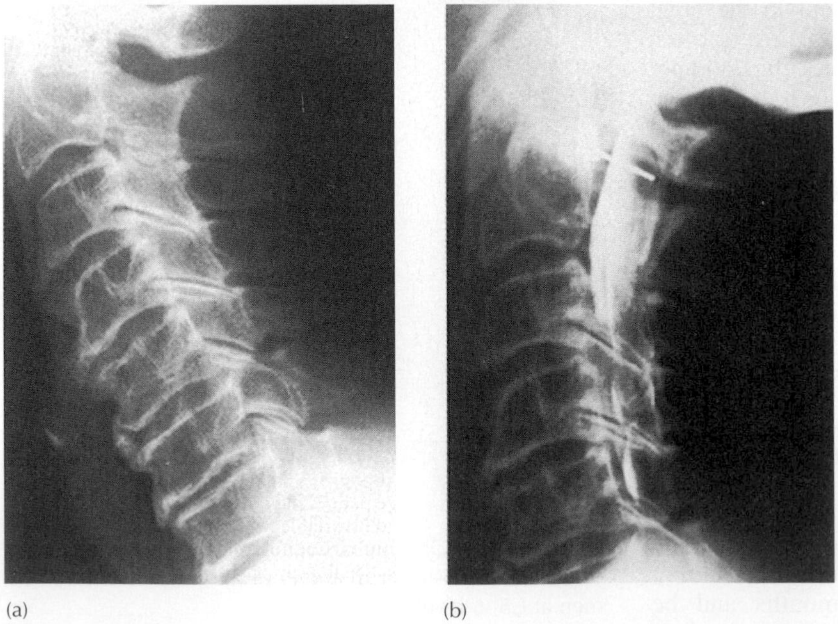

(a)

(b)

Figure 13.54 (a) Radiograph and (b) myelogram of the patient in Figure 13.53, showing marked cervical spondylosis complicated by cervical spinal stenosis.

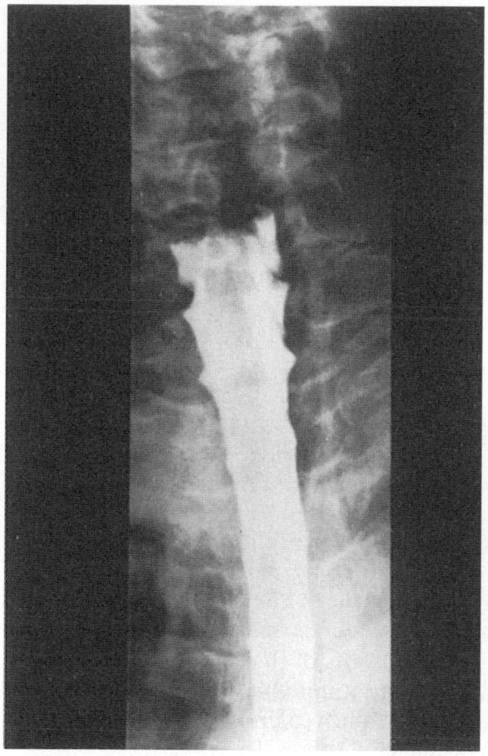

Figure 13.55 Myelogram of the cervical spine, showing a complete block at C5–6 level in a patient with a cervical spondylosis and a central cord syndrome.

the clinical findings, may be useful in localizing the level of disc degeneration. Jeffreys (1980) points out that a normal disc will accept up to 0.2 ml of contrast medium such as sodium diatrizoate (Hypaque). Radiological control with an image intensifier is required to ensure that the tip of the needle is in the disc space when performing discography. If the injection produces the pain the patient complains of, this is valuable information – but injection by error into the annulus is painful also.

We consider that discography gives useful additional information for the C4–5, C5–6, C6–7, discs in localizing pathology and corroborating clinical impressions in about 50% of cases only (Figure 13.57). It is most useful in the investigation of cervical spondylosis but is not indicated for patients in whom an acute prolapse is diagnosed clinically.

DIAGNOSIS

The diagnosis of cervical protrusion of an intervertebral disc remains primarily clinical, and relatively simple with the aid of detailed history and physical examination. Well over half of the cervical herniations occur at C6–7 level and the majority of the remainder at C5–6. It is important to bear in mind pre- and post-fixation of the brachial plexus.

DIFFERENTIAL DIAGNOSIS

There are several conditions which may be confused with the syndrome of cervical disc herniation.

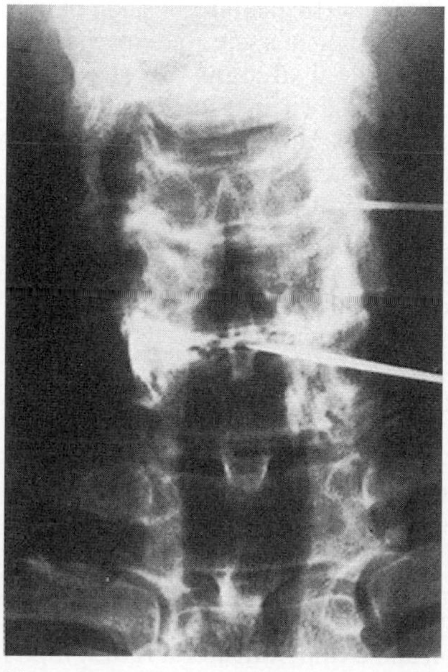

(a)

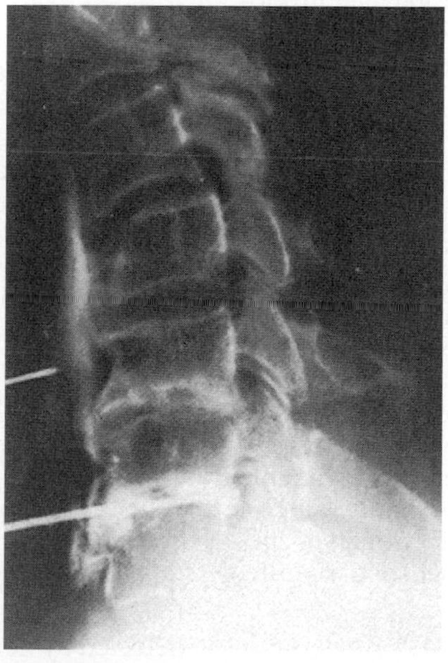

(b)

Figure 13.56 (a) Anteroposterior radiograph of the cervical spine, showing the marker needle at the C4–5 level and the discogram at the lower level. (b) Lateral radiograph of the same patient, showing the degeneration lesion of the C5–6 level with extension of the radiopaque dye.

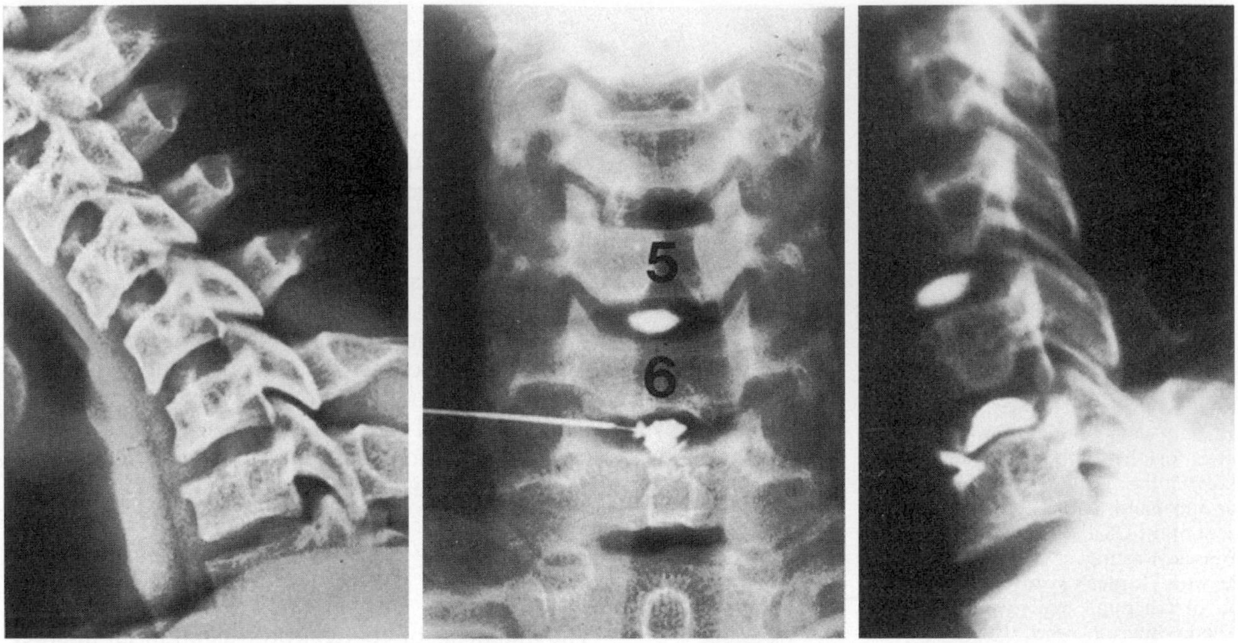

(a) (b) (c)

Figure 13.57 (a) Lateral radiograph following injury, showing subluxation due to interspinous ligamentous rupture. (b) Anteroposterior discogram of the same patient, showing an abnormal appearance at C6–7 level. (c) Lateral discogram of same patient, illustrating the intraosseous leakage of the radiopaque material.

Spinal cord tumours and syringomyelia

This may be considered in cases of prolapsed cervical disc with some element of cord compression. In the former, absence of trauma in the history, a slow progressive unremitting course, negative clinical and radiological investigations for protrusion, and myelography will lead to its recognition. In the latter the characteristic dissociated sensory loss is obvious.

Radiculitis

A history of a preceding virus infection with pain in nerve root distribution is often attributed to a radiculitis with inflammation of the nerve root. This is a rare syndrome, if it ever occurs, but should be borne in mind in exceptional circumstances. Wasting is reported as being rapid in onset, with pronounced tenderness of muscles and nerve on palpation. A more specific condition is neuralgic amyotrophy, or Spillain's syndrome, in which there is severe pain in the upper limb with marked weakness and invariable recovery over the course of several months. Careful examination reveals that this usually affects a specific peripheral nerve, especially that supplying the nerve to serratus anterior.

Cervical spondylosis or osteoarthritis of the cervical spine

This occurs in the older age group in the fourth and fifth decades and affects the spine over more than one segment. It has a slow chronic course with neck stiffness and sometimes diffuse tenderness on palpation of the cervical spine. Muscle spasm may be present but often neurological signs are absent. In some instances however, severe muscle wasting may occur without any pain. Radiographs will show the well known features of osteoarthritis at the posterior joints with osteophytes protruding into the intervertebral foramina and bony lips on the posterior margins of the vertebral bodies which are responsible for radicular pain and paraesthesia. These are readily seen on an oblique radiograph.

Laminar fractures

Laminar fractures in the cervical region may occasionally simulate cervical herniation, both conditions having a history of trauma and symptoms and signs of neck irritability. Therefore, radiography (including tomography) is required to exclude the injuries. Lateral instability due to old subluxation may be detected by flexion and extension lateral radiographs (Figure 13.58).

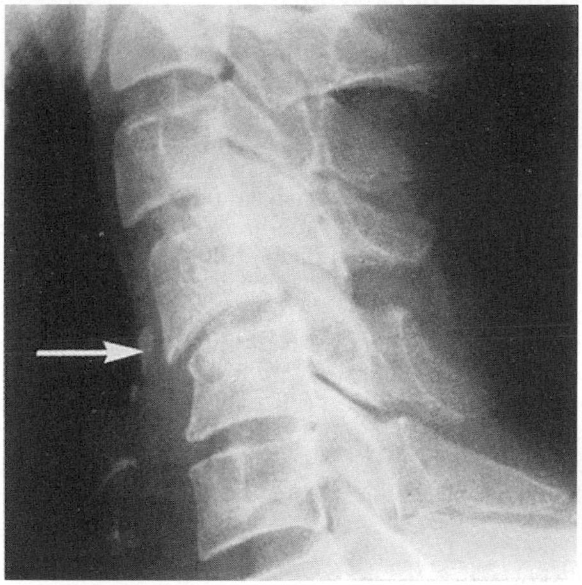

(a)

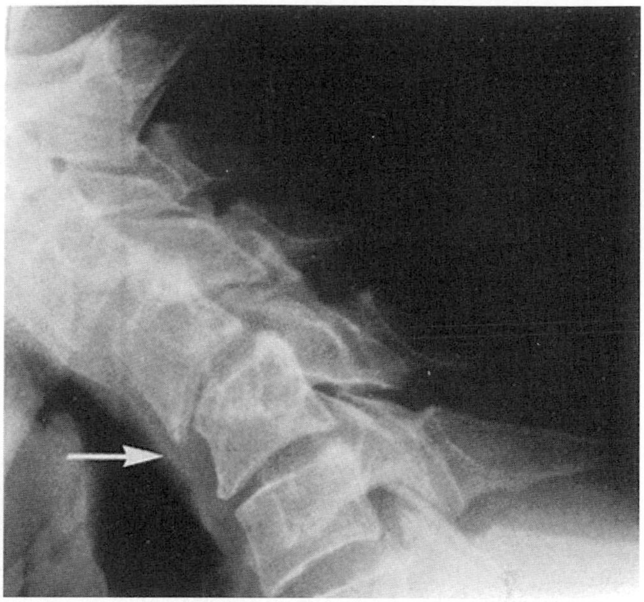

(b)

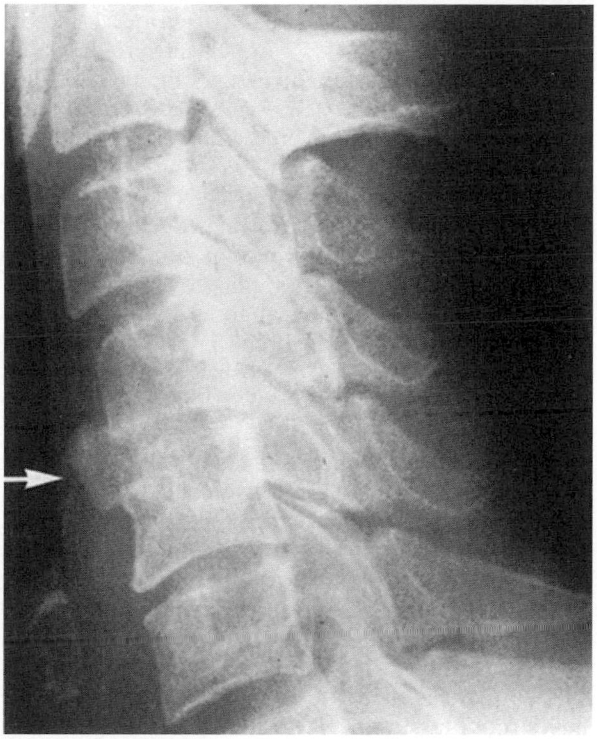

(c)

Figure 13.58 Lateral radiographs of a patient with brachialgia: (a) showing malalignment of C4 on 5; (b) in forward flexion, showing instability at the same level; (c) after anterior fusion with iliac bone grafting to achieve stability and relief of symptoms.

Scalenus anterior or 'thoracic outlet syndrome'

The lower nerve roots of the brachial plexus, particularly T1, may be compressed at the thoracic outlet as they emerge behind scalenus anterior and in front of scalenus medius, and cross the first rib. When there is an extra rudimentary rib or band rising from the C7 vertebra, the T1 nerve root and the subclavian artery are lifted upwards and subjected to pressure inferiorly. Symptoms in such a patient are usually gradual in onset without remissions or exacerbations.

The patient complains of pain and sensory loss in the medial side of the lower arm and sensory blunting may be present in the C8 or T1 dermatome. Although it was considered that such an abnormality was always associated with vascular symptoms, it is apparent from the work of Bonney (1964) that a cervical rib or, more commonly, a band can cause pressure on the Tl nerve root without causing vascular symptoms. Furthermore, Bonney demonstrated that excision of the rib or band may relieve symptoms. Others have recommended excision of the first rib to relieve nerve root pressure by a transaxillary route, but Hamblen (1979) concluded that this was not necessary in most cases and that removal of a band or the rib produced relief of symptoms. This has been our experience also.

Acromioclavicular arthritis

Disorders of the acromioclavicular joint and conditions such as subacromial bursitis and capsulitis of the shoulder, including ruptures of the supraspinatus, can be confused with pain due to cervical disc prolapse. However, the freedom of the neck from pain and limitation of shoulder movement together with negative radiography clarify the situation in most cases.

Pancoast tumour (superior pulmonary sulcus tumour of Pancoast)

This rare condition (Pancoast, 1932) occurs when a pleomorphic adenocarcinoma involves the apex of the lung parenchyma in the supraclavicular area. The patient then presents with radicular pain running down into one of the extremities together with paraesthesia and sensory loss involving the dermatomes of C5 and C6 in the forearm and hand. More commonly, there is involvement of the C8 and T1 nerve roots resulting in small muscle wasting in the hand, and this may coincide with Horner's syndrome (ptosis and constriction of the pupil due to involvement of the sympathetic inferior cervical ganglion). Radiographically the tumour may be seen as an opacity in the apical area of the lung, but there may also be destruction of the ribs particularly the second or the vertebral column itself. Treatment is usually palliative.

Acute stiff neck syndrome

Acute painful stiff neck frequently occurs in young adults who are often active but in whom there is no definite history of injury. Characteristically the pain is severe, the head is held fixed, frequently with a torticollis, and there is tenderness over the lower cervical spine and the paraspinal muscles. Movement is usually restricted in one direction only and there is no radiation of pain or neurological signs in the upper limbs. Radiographs are normal. The clinical picture is one of acute muscle spasm and the cause is unknown. Frequently this condition settles with the wearing of a supportive collar for 3–4 days, or in some cases by gentle neck traction. Although this condition is very common, the association with the cervical disc pathology or posterior facet joint pathology has not been established.

TREATMENT

The treatment of cervical herniated disc is essentially conservative, except in cases complicated by cord compression when surgery is necessary. The neck is rested with the patient in bed with a suitable arrangement of pillows, or in very severe cases, by means of halter traction. Generally the patient finds most comfort with the head slightly flexed forward. Within a few days the severe pain is usually reduced and the patient can mobilize with a well-fitting plastic collar. Adequate analgesics are required, and it is important to emphasize that, during and after treatment, repeated examinations are necessary to exclude the possibility of spinal cord involvement. Manipulation of the cervical spine is strongly contraindicated. After the acute pain has subsided, physiotherapy methods such as short-wave diathermy, heat treatment and resisted neck exercises are useful.

In some instances acute pressure on the cervical spinal cord makes surgery necessary. Whilst it is generally agreed that decompression of the cervical spine is necessary following myelopathy, there is some dispute as to the value of attempted discectomy in the acute prolapse. Brink and Edmonson (1980) recommend transdural removal of the affected prolapsed vertebral disc where the prolapse is central. Where there is a lateral prolapse producing acute nerve root pressure, an expectant policy is generally carried out, though Brink and Edmonson report excellent results from operative removal by laminectomy, traction of the nerve root upwards and removal of the disc by a posterior approach.

Anterior cervical disc

Bohlman *et al.* (1993) reported from a large series of 122 patients who had received the Robinson operation of disc excision and arthrodesis for brachialgia (over 95%) motor power deficient (over 60%) and/or sensory loss (over 80% of all patients). Duration of follow-up was 6 years and the majority had no neck pain and only four patients had mild radicular pain. Less than 10% had any functional impairment of daily living activities. There was a pseudarthrosis at 24 of 195 operated upon segments with 16 being symptomatic, particularly when more than one level had been 'fused'. These authors point out that this is a safe and very successful procedure.

Spondylosis and osteoarthritis of the cervical spine

Spondylosis of the cervical spine should be regarded as a clinical syndrome resulting from degeneration of the intervertebral disc and consequent pressure on the cervical nerve roots or cervical spinal cord.

The pathology is essentially an aggravation of changes in fluid content of the disc, collapse of the disc space, protrusion of the nucleus pulposus and stretching of annulus fibrosus and secondary formation of bony lips on the vertebral bodies. This is accompanied by secondary osteoarthritis in the posterior facet joints of the spine, producing osteoarthritic lips which also narrow the intervertebral foramina, posteriorly compressing the nerve roots. The protruding invertebral disc and osteophytes produce two clinical syndromes depending on their effects: spinal cord pressure or myelopathy, and spinal nerve root pressure or radiculopathy.

CERVICAL MYELOPATHY

A significant number of patients who develop degenerative changes in the cervical spine as described above will develop a slowly progressive pressure syndrome affecting the cervical spinal cord. This is characterized by a lower motor neuron lesion in the upper extremities which is frequently bilateral, together with an upper motor neuron lesion in the lower limbs producing spasticity, hyper-reflexia and extensor plantar responses in the lower limbs. In addition, there may be visceral disturbances of bladder and bowel, producing degrees of incontinence.

The radiographs show severe narrowing of the intervertebral disc and changes at many levels in the cervical spine with lipping of the vertebral bodies, osteophytes from the posterior spinal joints, and sometimes ossification of the posterior longitudinal ligament which occurs most frequently in Japanese patients. Hughes (1966) reported a series of 20 autopsies and described the bulging of the intervertebral discs to form transverse bars extending across the whole transverse diameter of the spinal canal. The spinal cord showed indentation at the levels of intervertebral discs, and impingement on the vertebral arteries laterally was also present due to the malalignment of the spine. Histologically, Hughes found:

1. Posterior and lateral columnar long tract degeneration.
2. White cell destruction – necrosis of myelin.
3. Grey matter destruction with loss of neurons.

Murone (1974) found a reduction in the average sagittal diameter of the cervical spinal canal in patients with myelopathy compared with controls, thus explaining the presence of symptoms with only small osteophytes or mild intervertebral disc protrusion. He considered that the risk of myelopathy was high where the average spinal canal diameter was less than 12 mm. Chakravorty (1969), in studying the blood supply of the cervical cord in autopsy specimens of man, emphasized that below the level of C3 the small radicular arteries maintain the blood supply. Fewer but larger ones accompany the C4–6 roots and they also can be compressed by osteophytes to produce the myelopathy. Most of the compressive lesions, e.g. disc protrusion or spondylitic ridging, lie anterior to the cervical cord, where they can easily produce an interruption of the flow through the anterior spinal artery or its intramedullary branches. The corticospinal tracts within the grey matter of the cord structure are particularly sensitive to vascular ischaemia (Zeidman and Ducker, 1992) to produce the lower motor neuron syndrome. Because of this involvement there is cerebellar dysfunction as a stiff hyper-reflexive gait.

Immobility due to fibrosis of the root sleeves may predispose to damage during neck movements, particularly by the ligamentum flavum bulging anteriorly during extension of the neck. It is notable that patients with these changes are extremely susceptible to central spinal cord injury due to hyperextension. This syndrome of partial or total tetraplegia, which has a poor prognosis, is characterized by the history of a trivial injury to the neck in a patient with severe spondylotic changes and myelographic evidence of compression of the spinal cord in the cervical region.

In 1972 Nurick described a most useful clarification grading the severity:

- Grade 0 – root involvement or radiculopathy without spinal cord disease.
- Grade 1 – some stiffness and hyper-reflexion in gait.
- Grade 2 – numbness, intrinsic muscle atrophy and loss of manual dexterity of the hands with increasing gait problems but employable.
- Grade 3 – more difficulty in walking requiring a cane and in 25% of this group of patients the hands become unco-ordinated and are unable to carry out many tasks about the house.
- Grade 4 – require a walker and assistance for everyday living activities.
- Grade 5 – chair bound or bedridden with bowel and bladder incontinence.

Although clinical bowel and bladder dysfunction occurs late in this disease process, with improved dynamic urological pressure studies, evidence of early dysfunction can be found and followed.

Zeidman and Ducker have emphasized that this is a progressive disease and that in over 70% of patients a significant progression occurs within a year of diagnosis – many necessitating operative intervention.

A Brown-Séquard syndrome can occur unusually, produced by a large disc protrusion.

RADICULOPATHY

Radiculopathy of the spinal nerve roots by spondylotic protrusions, either in the lateral part of the spinal canal or in the intervertebral foramina, is common. Hughes (1966) described how radiculopathy often accompanies myelopathy with Wallerian degeneration in the posterior column, through the effect upon the radicular nerve and posterior root ganglion but sparing of the anterior root.

CLINICAL FEATURES

The clinical symptoms and signs are similar to those in acute cervical intervertebral disc protrusion but more chronic. Stiffness of the neck is complained of, particularly in rotation, and radiating pain into the arm is troublesome. Also pain may radiate up into the occipital region, causing distressing headaches, and patients may complain of altered sensation when brushing their hair. Physical examination reveals the restriction of lateral bending and rotation, muscle tenderness over the lower cervical spine and peripheral neurological abnormalities in the upper limbs according to the level of the nerve root compression. The differential diagnosis is the same as that for cervical disc prolapse but includes amyotrophic lateral sclerosis, syringomyelia, spinal cord tumours and multiple sclerosis. Oblique radiographs will show the appearances of osteophytes and bony lips impinging on the intervertebral foramina, and radiographs in flexion and extension viewed from the lateral aspect will demonstrate instability of the spine. Occasionally, destruction of the vertebral bodies may be considerable and cause confusion with the diagnosis of tumour or infection.

For multilevel pathology, CT scanning with myelography is necessary to determine the size and shape of the spinal canal for any compromise in capacity and for bony deformation by ridging and osteophyte formation. If plain radiographs are normal MR imaging is necessary to delineate spinal cord structure and for soft tissue disc protrusion.

Electromyelography is of value particularly for the 'myelopathic hand' lesion of a lower motor neuron type and fasciculation in the intrinsic muscles.

Multiple sclerosis requires examination of the cerebrospinal fluid by electrophoresis and determination of the IgG component.

CONSERVATIVE TREATMENT

Certain patients are improved by conservative treatment involving support of the neck in a collar or, if the pain is severe, by a period in hospital on light traction employing a halter. This is accompanied by heavy analgesia as well as non-steroidal anti-inflammatory agents. After several weeks, gentle active movements and other physiotherapy methods such as heat and massage are helpful, and gradually the patient improves over the course of 1 or 2 months.

OPERATIVE TREATMENT FOR DISC PROTRUSION

If conservative treatment fails to relieve pain or if the pain is repetitive and severe, surgical treatment should be considered. It is now established that posterior exposure of the spine in an attempt to remove the degenerated disc is not only ineffective but also harmful. Anterior interbody fusion as described by Cloward (1962) or Smith and Robinson (1958) consists of removing the disc through an anterior sternomastoid incision, excision of osteophytes and the insertion of an iliac bone graft between the two vertebral bodies. No decompression of the intervertebral foramina is possible but removal of the osteophytes from the posterior aspect of the vertebral bodies appears to have similar results. Certainly fusion of the affected level causes reduction of symptoms in the majority of patients. White *et al.*

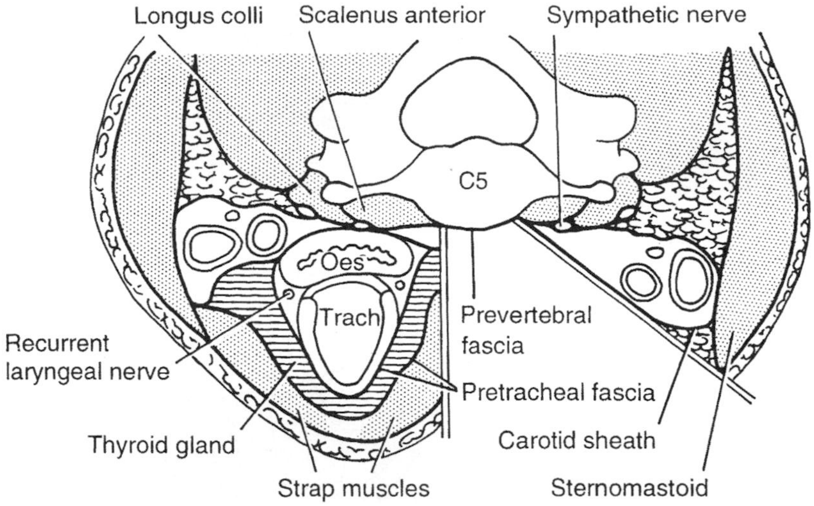

Figure 13.59 Transverse section through the neck at the level of C5 vertebra, showing the anterior approach to the anterior longitudinal ligament. (Reproduced, with permission, from Hamblen, D.L. (1979) *Operative Surgery*, 3rd edn, vol. *Orthopaedics*, pp. 347–354. Edited by G. Bentley. Butterworths: London and Boston)

(1973) reported the results in 65 patients treated by total anterior removal of the intervertebral disc with curettage of the osteophytes from the posterior aspect of the vertebral body. They found the following favourable prognostic factors:

1. Presence of radicular symptoms preoperatively.
2. Presence of radiographic changes at one level only.
3. Presence of myelographic defects which correlated with the levels operated upon.
4. Achievement of solid union without interspace collapse.

The presence of long tract signs and preoperative vertebral subluxation were unfavourable prognostic signs.

Operation

The patient is under general anaesthesia and should be intubated. The supine position is used with a sandbag under the neck and with the latter in slight hyperextension, and usually with slight traction on the head by means of a halter or halo.

A vertical incision is made in front of the sternomastoid on the left side, as there is less likelihood of traction on the recurrent nerve on this side. The carotid sheath is retracted laterally and the middle thyroid vein ligatured. This appears under cover of the anterior belly of the omohyoid and enters the internal jugular vein after piercing the anterior aspect of the carotid sheath. This allows the cervical spine to be rendered visible when the sternohyoid, sternothyroid and omohyoid muscles, the oesophagus, trachea and thyroid gland are retracted medially (Figure 13.59).

When osteophytic spurs are present they can be palpated through the anterior ligament. A needle may now be placed in the suspected disc space and a confirmatory lateral x-ray taken (Figure 13.60). The space is then approached by turning back a flap of the anterior ligament (Figure 13.61a). Through this aperture the disc is removed with pituitary rongeurs and curettes (Figure 13.61b). The osteophytes may have to be pared to allow good access, but the cortical edges of the adjacent vertebrae should be retained to hold the bone block in place when the neck is brought to the normal neutral position. The

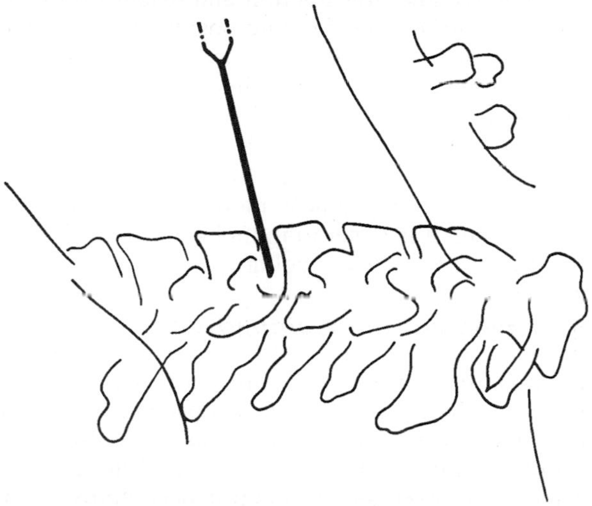

Figure 13.60 Diagram of a marker needle placed into C4–5 intervertebral disc level as seen on a lateral radiograph. (Reproduced, with permission, from Hamblen, D.L. (1979) *Operative Surgery*, 3rd edn, vol. *Orthopaedics*, pp. 347–354. Edited by G. Bentley. Butterworths: London and Boston)

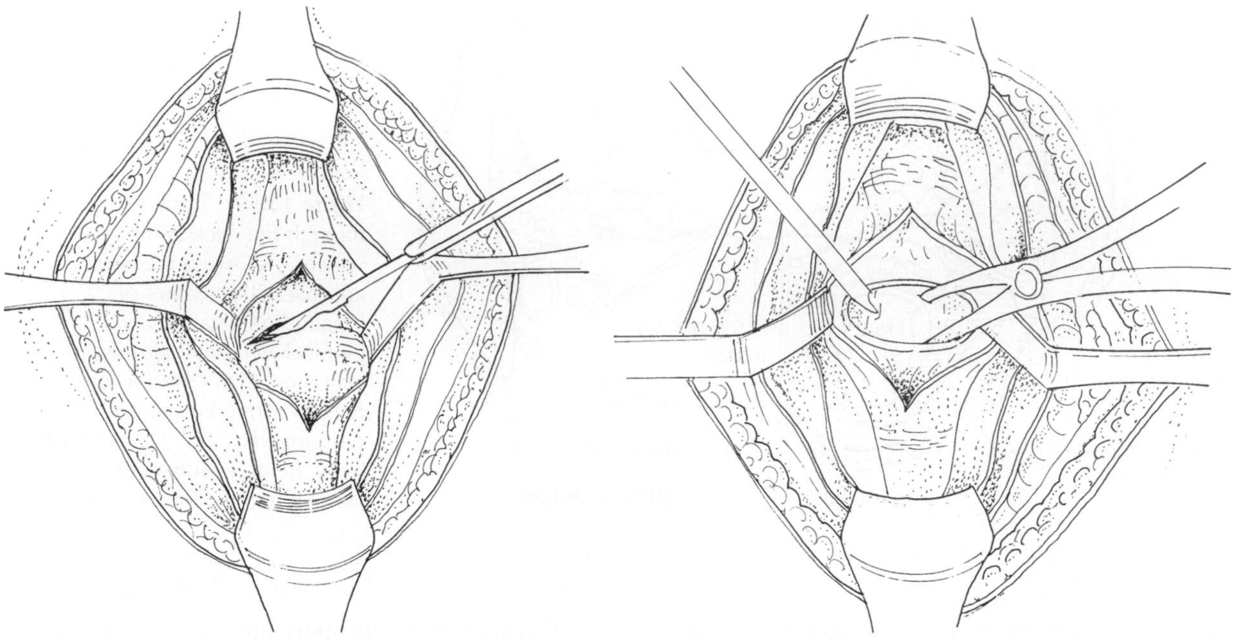

(a) (b)

Figure 13.61 (a) Incision of the annulus fibrosus after laterally retracting the bisected anterior longitudinal ligament. (b) Removal of the intervertebral disc material by rongeur and curette. (Reproduced, with permission, from Hamblen, D.L. (1979) *Operative Surgery*, 3rd edn, vol. *Orthopaedics*, pp. 347–354. Edited by G. Bentley. Butterworths: London and Boston)

bone of the vertebra is then exposed by removal of the cartilage plates and subchondral bone (Figure 13.62). The space is then measured and a piece of iliac bone removed with a sharp osteotome. The space is widened by traction and extension of the neck. The graft is tapped into position and countersunk (Figure 13.63). When seated, it should be very stable. The flap is stitched into position, the soft tissues are allowed to fall together, and the skin is sutured. The neck is placed in a felt collar and the patient begins walking after 48 hours. No immobilization is necessary unless more than one space is fused, when it is wiser to immobilize the neck for 3 months in a four-poster collar.

Management of myelopathy

Zeidman and Ducker (1992) in their excellent review have described how 80% of their patients have been improved by suitable operations and that there should be improvement of at least one Nurick grade. Their indication for an anterior decompression is anterior and focal pathology, e.g. large anterior disc herniation with rapid cord compression or permanent focal kyphotic deformity. When there are focal indentations at several levels, corpectomy or body excision with graft reconstruction is required. Posterior decompression, i.e. laminectomy, is required for multilevel spinal stenosis and a coexisting lordotic spinal curvature. Anterior plating with locking screws is a new addition to provide additional stabilization especially when there are two or more vertebral bodies removed.

Rheumatoid arthritis of the cervical spine

The cervical spine is commonly involved in rheumatoid arthritis and in recent years the clinical consequences have been better recognized. As early as 1890 Garrod noted that 36% of patients with rheumatoid arthritis had involvement of the cervical spine. After the metatarsophalangeal joints, the most common region to be involved is the neck and the metacarpophalangeal joints.

The pathology of this condition in the neck consists of rheumatoid granulomata involving all the diarthrodial joints, including those of Luschka – particularly the upper 4–5 segments. Attenuation, with laxity of such ligaments as the transverse ligament and of the anterior atlanto-occipital ligaments, is marked. Cavitation by invasion of granulo-

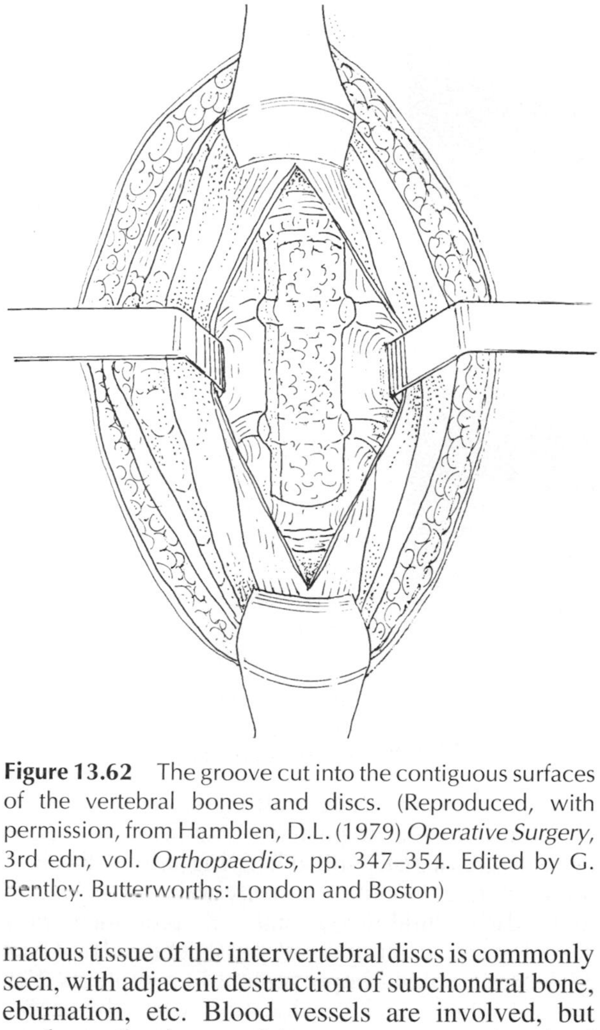

Figure 13.62 The groove cut into the contiguous surfaces of the vertebral bones and discs. (Reproduced, with permission, from Hamblen, D.L. (1979) *Operative Surgery*, 3rd edn, vol. *Orthopaedics*, pp. 347–354. Edited by G. Bentley. Butterworths: London and Boston)

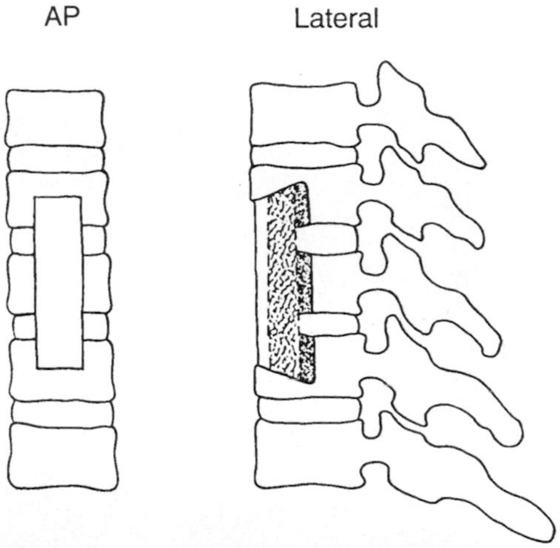

Figure 13.63 The position of the countersunk bone graft. (Reproduced, with permission, from Hamblen, D.L. (1979) *Operative Surgery*, 3rd edn. vol. *Orthopaedics*, pp. 347–354. Edited by G. Bentley. Butterworths: London and Boston)

matous tissue of the intervertebral discs is commonly seen, with adjacent destruction of subchondral bone, eburnation, etc. Blood vessels are involved, but rarely are the tissues of the nervous system involved directly.

MR imaging has been used by Glew *et al.* (1991) in a comparative study of patients with neurological symptoms and of a matched group with cervical spondylosis. The classical pathological change of rheumatoid arthritis, i.e. bone destruction, subchondral bony erosions (especially at C1 and 2 levels with subluxation) and soft tissue synovitis and pannus formation, were commonly seen in the first group but not in cervical spondylosis. In both groups the spinal cord or brain stem was compressed – in rheumatoid patients by subluxation and synovitis and in cervical spondylitic patients by disc material and/or osteophyte formation.

The natural history of rheumatoid arthritis involving the cervical spine has only recently been described. Rana (1989) has followed 41 patients by radiography with atlantoaxial disease over a 12-year period and found that over 60% of patients remained unchanged with 27% progressing and 12% decreasing, all with increase in occipital eventration. Two patients had died because of neurological disease; the degree of subluxation did not appear as a significant factor, but the upward suboccipital eventration was much more serious. Surgery was indicated when neurological signs – period of unconsciousness, gait disturbances, loss of manual dexterity – were progressive, with unremitting suboccipital pain and when the subluxation or dislocation at the C1 and C2 junction was greater than 10 mm.

Dvorak *et al.* (1989) have emphasized that dynamic scanning will show significant narrowing of the upper cervical spinal canal occurring with flexion when there is atlantoaxial subluxation as well as suboccipital upward translocation. More than one-third of their patients had a myelopathy proven by intracranial brain stimulation with delay in the cerebral motor latency.

Zdeblick (1991) also agrees that MR scanning is most important in evaluating the rheumatoid patient with upper cervical spinal disease. It shows clearly cord compression either from instability in flexion, or from the granulation/pannus formation behind the odontoid peg or from suboccipital cranial translocation on the brain stem.

Radiology is best defined as multiple disc space narrowing with little osteophyte formation and erosion of adjacent and osteoporotic vertebrae. Multiple subluxation at all levels can occur and there may be atlantoaxial subluxation of more than 2.5–3.0 mm (Figure 13.64) in over 25% of patients, with obvious erosion or absorption of the odontoid process. Widening posteriorly between the posterior arches of the atlas and the axis may be seen, and narrowing between the posterior arches of the atlas and the occiput ('platybasia' similar to acetabular

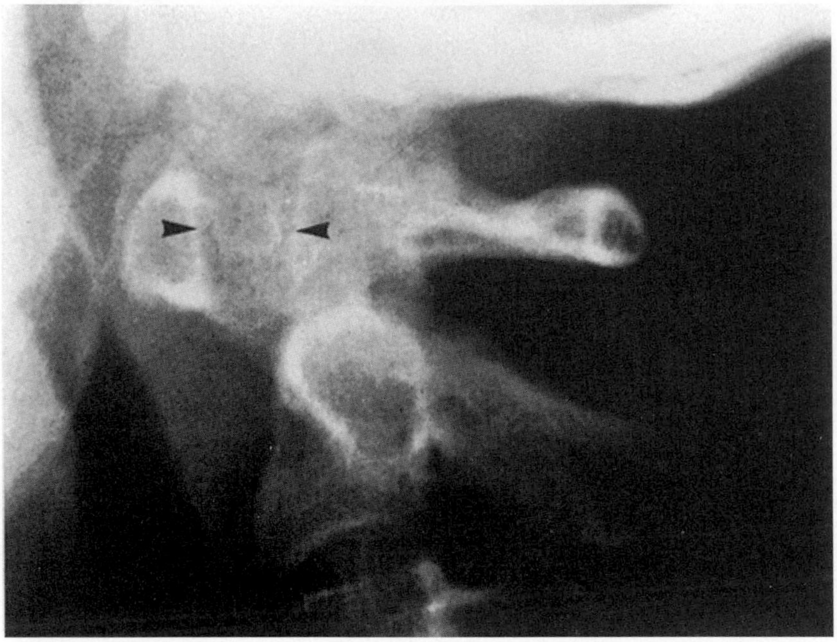

Figure 13.64 Lateral radiograph of an upper cervical spine, showing the posterior dislocation of the odontoid process with widening anteriorly.

protrusio). Subaxial dislocation of C4–5 occurs less frequently than in degenerative cervical spondylosis but it is more likely to be associated with neurological complications.

Clinical features are variable but pain is common, particularly in the cervical and occipital areas – as a deep-seated, persistent pain which may radiate as an occipital headache, or into the temporal regions. Importantly, these pains may be made worse by cervical traction. Rarely is there a true brachialgia with paraesthesia, weakness and/or wasting of the limbs and muscles, and/or loss of deep tendon reflexes. Arterial insufficiency syndromes of the cerebrum (vertigo, eye change) or spinal cord (pyramidal tract changes) by involvement of the vertebral or anterior spinal arteries are unusual. Severity of neurological symptoms or signs cannot be correlated to the severity of pathological changes as seen on radiography – and indeed are not any more common than found in degenerative cervical spondylosis.

Treatment is usually conservative in the form of an immobilization by a collar made of plastic material. Physiotherapy in the form of traction, heat and exercises usually aggravates the symptoms.

Surgical treatment is indicated as described by Rana (1989) but also in those patients in which there is a spinal cord diameter of less than 6 mm in flexion on MR imaging and a delay in the central motor latency on transcranial stimulation, as proposed by Dvorak *et al.* (1989).

Crockard *et al.* (1990) have described a one-stage transoral decompression with posterior element sublaminar wire fixation for irreducible anterior neuroaxial compression. Bone grafting was not necessary to achieve fusion or posterior stabilization. These patients are at risk with 6% dying within the first postoperative month, 3% vertebral artery lacerations, 10% dural leaks and 5% presented with neurological deterioration postoperatively. Over 33% had a striking improvement in symptoms. For upward suboccipital translocation it may be necessary to stabilize by fusion from the occiput down to the laminae of C2 vertebrae without evidence of compression, but with significant instability and/or atlantoaxial subluxation the C1 and C2 level can be fused with intralaminar wiring posteriorly (Figure 13.65).

Atlantoaxial dislocation in children

This may follow a definite injury or disease, such as rheumatoid arthritis or ankylosing spondylitis (Martel, 1961). It has been described in children and in adolescents, when it is associated with infection in the posterior pharyngeal region with a hyperaemia softening the ligaments, particularly the transverse ligament, which holds this joint in position (Watson-Jones, 1934; Werne, 1957). The child usually pre-

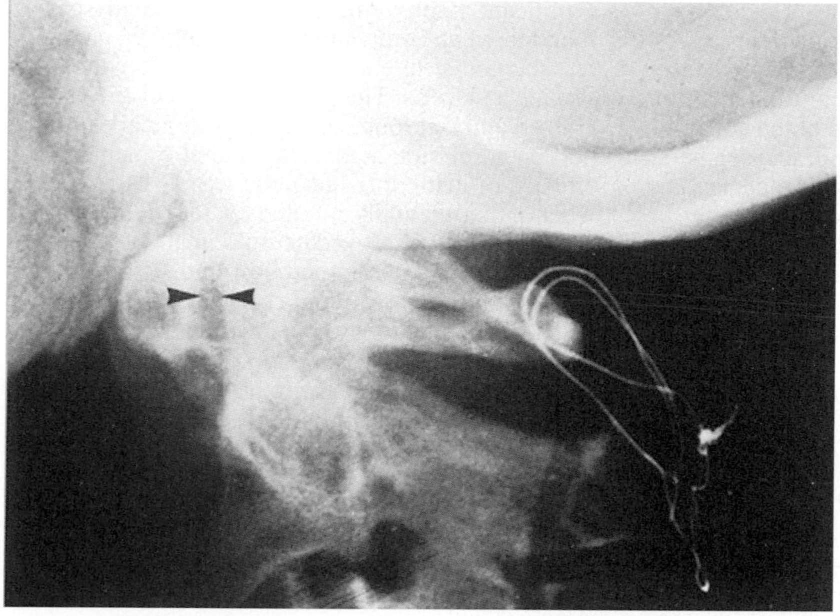

Figure 13.65 Lateral radiograph of same patient as in Figure 13.64, showing reduction with posterior fusion and wire internal fixation.

sents after the sore throat has subsided, with abnormal rotation of the head in a mild spasmodic torticollis, but pain may not be a prominent feature. Radiographs show the abnormal separation of the odontoid process from the arch of the atlas (Figure 13.66), and there may be erosion of adjacent bone or rarefaction. Treatment usually consists of light halter traction in extension of the neck, in bed, with adequate treatment of infection. Following this, ambulation begins with support of the head in a collar until the ligaments have consolidated again.

Pain in the chest wall

Such pain may be referred or may arise from local disease of the thoracic cage. The differential diagnosis is important since the pain can rise in the spinal cord and its membranes from tumours or inflammation; or in the posterior root ganglion from herpes zoster or tabes dorsalis; or from disease of the vertebrae, such as tumour, tuberculosis, spondylosis, osteophyte formation; or from peripheral nerve lesions; or from visceral disease of underlying lung,

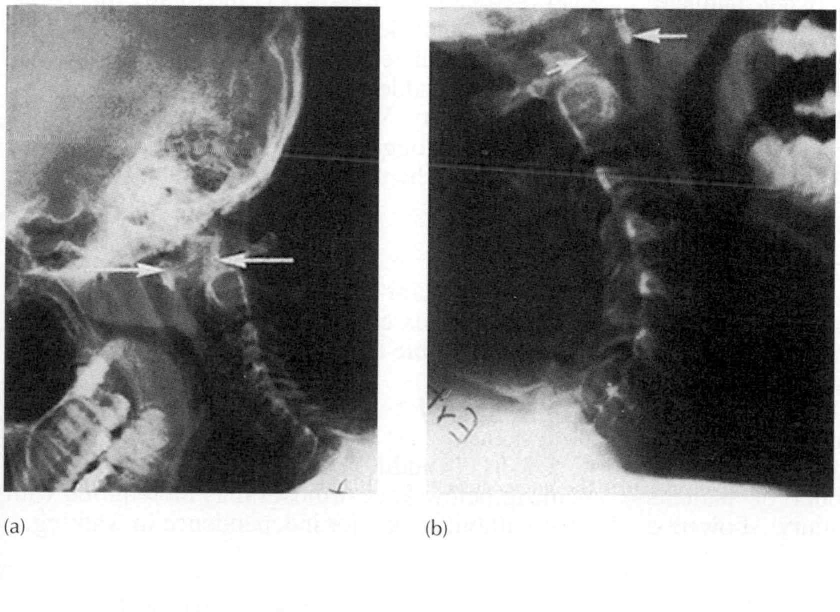

(a) (b)

Figure 13.66 Lateral radiographs of the cervical spine in (a) flexion and (b) extension of a young boy who one month after an attack of tonsillitis developed a painful and spasmodic torticollis. The x-rays show a widening between the anterior surface of the odontoid process and the ring of the atlas. With chemotherapy and immobilization, this distance gradually disappeared, with the relief of the clinical features.

pleura, mediastinum, heart; or from Tietze's syndrome involving the costochondral junctions.

Motor paralysis involves either the intercostals or the diaphragm, but there may be an upper motor neuron lesion involving the muscles of the abdomen or lower extremities. In the lower thoracic segments there may be paralysis of the abdominal muscles, and again an upper motor neuron lesion involving the lower extremities. The first thoracic segment enters the upper extremity via the posterior cord as the ulnar nerve producing disturbance in the little finger and ulnar border of the hand and forearm. The second thoracic segment leaves the second space as the intercostobrachialis, to supply sensation to the upper inner aspect of the arm.

Paraplegia

Although literally meaning a stroke on one side – i.e. a hemiplegia – 'paraplegia' is now used to indicate a paralysis of the lower limbs and trunk. Its causes are many: *traumatic* with increasing civil violence and war, road traffic accidents, *infective* from tuberculosis, polyneuritis, transverse myelitis, syphilis; *vascular* with infarction or malformation; *congenital* (e.g. myelodysplasia): *tumours* either primary or secondary from metastases; *intervertebral disc lesions* and *multiple sclerosis*.

Acute traumatic spinal cord injury is now the most common cause of paraplegia and has been studied extensively. The primary injury obviously is mechanical and due to contusion, compression, laceration or traction with immediate damage to the cord structures and their supporting blood supply. However, secondary mechanisms are now recognized as sustaining or producing further neurological damage, e.g. oedema, haemorrhage, ischaemia and the release of cytotoxic substances such as free oxygen radicals, opioids such as dynorphin which secondarily reduces the microcirculation blood flow, prostanoids (prostaglandins and other arachidonic acid metabolites, e.g. thromboxane), proteases and other amino acids (Tator, 1991).

Experimentally Giulian and Robertson (1990) from a rabbit lumbosacral cord model have suggested that the ischaemia, mediated by inflammatory phagocytic cells derived from circulating macrophages and microglial cells, destroy nervous tissue by direct cell–cell contact of released toxins.

Clinically, Bracken *et al.* (1990), from a multicentre randomized controlled trial in 10 centres, have shown that large doses of methylprednisolone when given intravenously within 8 hours of patients sustaining an acute spinal cord injury, showed a significant improvement in motor and in sensory function when compared with those given naxolone (an antagonist to endogenous opioids) or those receiving a placebo. The patients had received a standardized and rigorous clinical neurological examination on admission at 6 weeks and at 6 months. The efficacy of methylprednisolone was dose dependent when experimentally studied in rats. The animals had showed an improved neurological outcome with increased spinal cord blood flow and a reduced lipid peroxidation in the injured cord segments.

The complications of being paraplegic are also numerous but in the main can be prevented or treated effectively. They should not be permitted to add to the already overwhelming burden of these patients who, depending upon the causative pathology, can now be expected to live for years.

The evaluation of the functional disabilities must be realistic and is strictly related to the level of pathology as described by Bedbrook and Sedgley (1980) as follows.

Cervical

- (C5) All patients require assistance for all activities. Living alone is not possible.
- (C6) At this level some assistance is required for all activities except eating and communication. It may be difficult to propel a wheelchair manually, so electric wheelchairs are useful.
- (C7–T1) The bladder becomes even more reflexic in activity and incontinence is a problem. Patients rely on a wheelchair but almost all can be completely independent in all activities of daily living.

Thoracic

- (T2–6) Patients always become totally independent in a wheelchair with plenty of training in dressing, transfers and driving.
- (T4–12) Bladder and bowel are evacuated by reflex activity. Walking is strenuous, but can be achieved in long-leg orthoses. Complete independence in a wheelchair is always to be expected.

Lumbar

- (L1–3) If sacral reflexes are present these may be used for reflex emptying of the bladder. Walking is also possible in long-leg orthoses.

Lumbosacral

- (L4–S1) In addition to bladder and bowel impairment, below-knee orthoses may be required with or without sticks, for independence in walking.

Sacral

- (S2–4) Bowel and bladder function are impaired. The bladder may be emptied by strain.

There has always been controversy over the merits of surgery in the treatment of spinal cord injury. Sir Charles Bell in 1807 wrote on the conservative management whilst Sir Astley Cooper was advocating surgical intervention in 1824. This controversy continues, with proponents of internal fixation using the Harrington and Luque rods (Dickson *et al.*, 1978) against others (Burke and Murray, 1976; Bedbrook, 1979) who believe there is little or no place for surgery. It is, however, agreed that surgery does not result in any greater return of neurological function than that seen in patients treated by postural reduction, but it can improve nursing and mobilization, and perhaps reduce the factors responsible for the secondary changes.

COMMON COMPLICATIONS

Genitourinary

One of the major advances in the treatment of spinal paralysis has been the improvement in the management of infection. Indwelling catheters will become infected within 96 hours and intermittent catheterization is indicated for the entire duration of treatment. Strict aseptic technique with perhaps the instillation of an antiseptic will further reduce the presence of bacteriuria.

Stones are liable to form in the bladder and kidneys of these patients. They are, however, more common in those with indwelling catheters and ileal conduits.

Detrusor urethral sphincter dyssynergia

The synergistic action is altered in upper motor neuron lesions, and a poor detrusor may be opposed by a sphincter that fails to relax or contracts clonically. This problem is now more apparent as more patients are catheter-free. Although the sphincter can be released surgically, it can also be relaxed by anal stretch or a pudendal nerve block.

Deep vein thrombosis

An increased incidence of deep vein thrombosis is present and appears to follow complete lesions more than incomplete. Prophylactic heparin is used in some units as well as the normal preventive measures of elevation, support stockings and physiotherapy.

Hypotension

The sympathetic nervous system leaves the spinal cord between Tl and L2, and high paraplegics are left with incomplete innervation. Subnormal blood pressures are therefore seen in these patients, and orthostatic hypotension may be profound due to the lack of reflexes.

Osteoporosis

Recumbency, immobilization and paralysis all contribute to osteoporosis and hypercalciuria. Osteopenia seems to involve trabecular bone more than cortical. Mobilization may at least partially reverse the osteoporosis, but does not seem to lower the increased urinary calcium output.

Spasticity

Two types of reflexes appear after the initial period of 'spinal shock' has disappeared:

1. Stretch reflexes – primarily extensor muscle activity.
2. Nociceptive reflexes – primarily flexor, and are activated by painful cutaneous stimuli.

Therapy to control spasticity consists of drugs (e.g. diazepam) or surgery such as tenotomy of hyper-reflexic muscles, peripheral nerve division (Stöffel's) or rhizotomies.

Pain

Pain after that resulting from the original injury has settled is quite frequent, and is of four main types:

1. Mechanical – in muscle, ligament, bone and joints.
2. Radicular – from some form of irritation of a nerve root.
3. Phantom pain – mostly seen in cauda equina lesions.
4. Visceral – ill-defined and has no physiological explanation.

Skin ulcers

Skin ulcers comprise one of the most common complications and are the cause of most hospital admissions. Prevention is the key, and the patient and attendant must always be alert and carry out the necessary preventive routine.

Factors causing these trophic lesions are ischaemia, oedema, anaemia and venous thrombosis.

When an ulcer has developed, conservative treatment consisting of complete relief of weight-bearing along with a check on the nutritional status of the patient, ultraviolet light and the application of zinc-containing ointments all have a role.

Full-thickness ulcers usually require surgery, which takes the form of flap repair once infection has been eradicated.

Because of the loss of motor power and sensation, regular turning 2-hourly is essential to prevent the development of pressure sores. Regular chest physiotherapy with postural drainage is also essential, because of the likely impairment of the muscles of respiration. Tracheostomy, either temporary or permanent, may be necessary. With time, the accessory muscles of respiration and diaphragmatic function will improve in the majority of cases, and one can anticipate improvement in ventilatory function.

LATER MANAGEMENT

Further problems in the management and rehabilitation of the paraplegic patient relate to bladder and kidney function. In the phase after injury a period of spinal shock may persist for up to 18 months. It is now recommended that the most effective treatment for bladder management is intermittent catheterization to encourage full bladder emptying, and a reduction in residual urine volume to prevent the development of infection and bladder fibrosis. Thereafter, those with spastic bladder function may be expected to develop a reflex bladder, and those with a hypotonic bladder may achieve satisfactory emptying with manual pressure. There may be outlet obstruction at the bladder neck which may require surgical resection, or inhibition of the α-adrenergic smooth muscle fibres with phenoxybenzamine. If the external sphincter is affected, a sphincterotomy or pudendal nerve block may help. Sometimes spasmolytics such as baclofen or dantrolene may also improve bladder emptying. The single most important innovation in recent years has been the abandonment of indwelling catheterization, which inevitably results in bacteriuria within 48 hours. With intermittent catheterization in the acute phase, 50% of cases retain sterile urine. Stones are far more likely to develop in those with infected urine.

Bowel management should be started early and a regular pattern of emptying encouraged.

Alterations of muscle power and tone require early physiotherapy to prevent the formation of contractures, and those muscle groups which retain useful function should be exercised so that they may be used in the patient's rehabilitation. Spasticity may be reduced by centrally acting drugs such as baclofen and diazepam or those acting at the periphery such as dantrolene sodium.

Pressure sores are a cause of great morbidity and eventual mortality. Healing of an established sore is related to the thickness; if a sore is of full thickness, and involving underlying bone, surgery will be necessary in the majority. Urinary incontinence and excessive sweating will exacerbate the tendency to pressure sores, and a depressed patient who is insufficiently motivated to lift himself periodically from his wheelchair will be at particular risk. It has been shown that regular follow-up and good access to a unit with an interest in the treatment of sores help in the patient's management.

Each patient must be assessed individually for his specific needs by the occupational therapist. Some patients will require wheelchairs, while those with thoracic and lumbar spinal lesions may be able to walk short distances with the aid of crutches and calipers. Those with tetraplegia will require electric wheelchairs and the advantages of a modern controlled environment.

References

Abramovitz, J. and Neff, S. (1991) Lumbar disc surgery. *Neurosurgery* **29**, 301–308

Adams, M.A., Dolan, P., Hutton, W.C. and Porter, R.W. (1990) Diurnal changes in spinal mechanics and their clinical significance. *Journal of Bone and Joint Surgery* **72B**, 266–270

Aird, I. (1995) *British Medical Journal* **2**, 1110

An, H.S., Vaccoro, A.R., Dolinska, C.A. *et al.* (1991) Differentiation between spinal tumours and infections with MR imaging. *Spine* **16**, 334–337

Andersson, B.J., Ortengren, R., Nachemson, A. *et al.* (1974) Lumbar disc pressure and myoelectric back muscle activity during sitting. I. Studies on an experimental chair. *Scandinavian Journal of Rehabilitation Medicine* **6**, 104–114

Andersson, B.J.G., Ortengren, R., Nachemson, A.L., Elfstrom, F. and Broman H. (1975) The sitting posture: an electromyographic and discometric study. *Orthopedic Clinics of North America* **6**, 105–120

Andersson B.J.G., Ortengren, R. and Nachemson, A. (1976) Quantitative studies of back loads in lifting. *Spine* **1**, 178–185

Auramou, A.I., Cavanaugh, J.M. Ozaktay, C.A. *et al.* (1992) The effects of controlled mechanical loading on Group II, III, IV afferent units from the lumbar facet joint and surrounding tissue. *Journal of Bone and Joint Surgery* **74A**, 1464–1471

Barrios, C., Ahmed, M., Arrotegui, J. *et al.* (1990) Microsurgery versus standard removal of herniated lumbar disc. *Acta Orthopaedica Scandinavica* **61**, 399–343

Batson, O.V. (1942) *Annals of Internal Medicine* **16**, 38

Bedbrook, G.M. (1979) Spinal deformities with tetraplegia and paraplegia. *Journal of Bone and Joint Surgery* **61B**, 267

Bedbrook, G.M. and Sedgley, G.I. (1980) The management of spinal injuries past and present. *International Journal of Rehabilitation Research* **2**, 45–61

Bell, G.R., Rothman, R.H., Booth, R.E. *et al.* (1984) A study of computer-assisted tomography. Comparison of metrizamide myelography and computed tomography in the diagnosis of herniated lumbar disc and spinal stenosis. *Spine* **9**, 552–556

Bell, G.R., Stearns, K.L., Bonutti, P.M. and Boumphrey, F.R. (1990) MRI diagnosis of tuberculous vertebral osteomyelitis. *Spine* **15**, 462–465

Bennett, P.H. and Wood, P.H.N. (1968) In: *Population Studies of the Rheumatic Diseases*, p. 456. Proceedings of the Third International Symposium, New York, 1966. Excerpta Medica: Amsterdam

Bernard, T.N. (1990) Lumbar discography followed by computed tomography. Refining the diagnosis of low back pain. *Spine* **15**, 690–707

Boden, S.D., Davis, D.O., Dina, T.S. *et al.* (1990) Abnormal magnetic resonance scans of the lumbar spine in asymptomatic subjects. *Journal of Bone and Joint Surgery* **72A**, 403–408

Bohlman, H.H., Emery, S.E., Goodfellow, D.B. *et al.* (1993) Robinson anterior cervical discectomy and arthrodesis for cervical radiculopathy. *Journal of Bone and Joint Surgery* **75A**, 1294–1307

Bohrer, S.P., Chen, Y.M. and Sayers, D.G. (1990) Cervical spine flexion patterns. *Skeletal Radiology* **19**, 521–525

Bonneville, J.F., Runge, M., Catin, F., Tang, T.S., Paris, D. and Boulard, D. (1989). Computed tomography of the lumbar intervertebral disc after automated percutaneous discectomy. *Orthopedic Transactions* **13**, 648–649

Bonney, G.L.W. (1964) The cervical rib syndrome. *Journal of Bone and Joint Surgery* **46B**, 780

Bracken, M.B., Shephard, M.J., Collins, W.F. *et al.* (1990) A randomized controlled trial of methyl prednisolone or naloxone in the treatment of acute spinal cord injuries. Results of the Second National Spinal Cord Injury Study. *New England Journal of Medicine* **322**, 1405–1411

Bradford, D.S., Heithoff, K.B. and Cohen, M. (1991) Intraspinal abnormalities and congenital spine deformities: a radiographic and MR study. *Journal of Pediatric Orthopedics* **11**, 36–41

Brailsford, J.F. (1929) *British Journal of Surgery* **16**, 562

Brain, W.R., Northfield, D. and Wilkinson, M. (1952) *Brain* **75**, 187

Breig, A. (1960) *Biomechanics of the Central Nervous System*. Almqvist and Wiksell: Stockholm

Brewerton, D.A. (1974) The inherited antigen (HL-A27) and arthritis. *Reports on the Rheumatic Diseases* **55**, 1

Brewerton, D.A., Coffrey, M., Hart, D., James, D.C.O., Nicholls, A. and Sturrock, R.D. (1973) Ankylosing spondylitis and HL-A27. Lancet **1**, 904–907

Brink, K.D.V. and Edmonson, A.S. (1980) In: *Campbell's Operative Orthopaedics*, 6th edn, vol. 2, pp. 1939–2155. Edited by A.J. Edmondson and A.H. Crenshaw. C.V. Mosby: St Louis, Toronto, London

Broaddis, W.C., Grady, M.S. and Delashaw, J.B.J. (1990) Preoperative superselective arteriolar embolisation: a new approach to enhance respectability of spinal tumours. *Neurosurgery* **27**, 755–759

Brodsky, A. (1976) Post-laminectomy and post-fusion stenosis of the lumbar spine. *Clinical Orthopaedics and Related Research* **115**, 130–139

Burke, D.C. and Murray, D.D. (1976) The management of thoracic and thoraco-lumbar injuries of the spine with neurological involvement. *Journal of Bone and Joint Surgery* **58B**, 72–78

Butler, D., Trafinow, J.H., Andersson, G.B., McNeill, T.W. and Huckman, M.S. (1990) Discs degenerate before facets. *Spine* **15**, 111–113

Bryne, E. (1992) Chronic myalgia: facts and fallacies. *Current Science. Current Opinion in Orthopaedics* **3**, 229–235

Cauchoix, J. and Giraud, B. (1978) Repeat surgery after disc excision. *Spine* **3**, 256–259

Chakravorty, B.G. (1969) Arterial supply of cervical spinal cord and its relation to the cervical myelopathy in spondylosis. *Annals of the Royal College of Surgeons of England* **45**, 232

Chevrot, A., Dupont, A.M., Vallec, C. *et al.* (1988) The dural sheath in the sitting and standing position during saccoradiculography. *Journal de Radiologie* **69**, 397–403

Chow, D.H.K., Luk, K.D.K., Leong, J.C.Y. and Woo, C.W. (1989) Torsional stability of the lumbo-sacral junction. Significance of the ilio-lumbar ligament. *Spine* **14**, 611–615

Cloward, R.B. (1962) New method of diagnosis and treatment of cervical disc diseases. *Clinical Neurosurgery* **8**, 93

Colletti, P.M., Dang, H.T., Deseran, M.W. *et al.* (1991) Spinal MR imaging in suspected metastases: correlation with skeletal scintography. *Magnetic Resonance Imaging* **9**, 349–355

Compere, E.L., Tachdjian, M.O. and Kernahan, W.T. (1959) *Orthopedics* **1**, 159

Cordero, M. and Sanchez, I. (1991) Brucellar and tuberculous spondylitis. *Journal of Bone and Joint Surgery* **73B**, 100–103

Corkhill, M.M., Jobanputra, P., Gibson, T. and MacFarlane, D.G. (1990) A controlled trial of sulphasalazine treatment in chronic ankylosing spondylitis. *British Journal of Rheumatology* **29**, 41–45

Crockard, H.A., Calder, I. and Ransford, A.O. (1990) One stage transoral decompression and posterior fixation in rheumatoid atlanto-axial subluxation. *Journal of Bone and Joint Surgery* **72**, 682

Crosbie Ross, J. and Jameson, R.M. (1971) Vesical dysfunction due to prolapsed disc. *British Medical Journal* **3**, 752–754

Davis, S.J., Teresi, L.M., Bradley Jr, W.R. *et al.* (1991) Cervical spine hyperextension injuries: MR findings. *Radiology* **180**, 245–251

Delamarter, R.B., Ross, J.S., Masaryk, T.J., Modic, M.T. and Bohlman, H.H. (1990) Diagnosis of lumbar arachnoiditis by magnetic resonance imaging. *Spine* **15**, 304–310

Delamarter, R.B., Sherman, J.E. and Carr, J.B. (1991) Cauda equina syndrome: neurologic recovery following immediate early or late decompressions. *Spine* **16**, 1022–1029

Dickson, J.M., Harrington, P.R. and Erwin, W.D. (1978) Results of reduction stabilization of the fractured thoracic and lumbar spine. *Journal of Bone and Joint Surgery* **60A**, 799–815

Dilke, T.W.F., Burry, H.C. and Grahame, R. (1973) Extradural corticosteroid injection in management of the lumbar nerve root compression. *British Medical Journal* **2**, 635–637

Djukic, S., Lang, P., Morris, J., Hoaglund, F. and Genant, H.K. (1990) The postoperative spine. Magnetic resonance imaging. *Orthopedic Clinics of North America* **21**, 603–624

Dong, G.X. and Porter, R.W. (1989) Walking and cycling tests in neurogenic and intermittent claudication. *Spine* **14**, 965–969

Doran, D.M.L. and Newell, D.J. (1975) Manipulation in treatment of low back pain; a multicentre study. *British Medical Journal* **2**, 161–164

Dvorak, J., Grob, D., Baumgartner, H. *et al.* (1989) Functional evaluation of the spinal cord by magnetic resonance imagining in patients with rheumatoid arthritis and instability of upper cervical spine. *Spine* **14**, 1057–1064

Ebringer, R.W., Cawdell, D.R., Cowling, P.P. and Ebringer, A. (1978) Sequential studies in ankylosing spondylitis. Association of *Klebsiella pneumonia* with active disease. *Annals of the Rheumatic Diseases* **37**, 146–151

Eismont, F. and Currier, B. (1989) Current concepts review: surgical management of lumbar intervertebral disc disease. *Journal of Bone and Joint Surgery* **71A**, 1266–1271

Elster, A.D. (1989) Bertolotti's syndrome revisited. Transitional vertebrae of the lumbar spine. *Spine* **1**, 1373–1377

Emery, R.J.H., Ho, E.K.W. and Leong, J.C.V. (1991) The shoulder girdle in ankylosing spondylitis. *Journal of Bone and Joint Surgery* **73B**, 1526–1531

Emmett, J.L. and Love, J.G. (1968) Urinary retention in women caused by asymptomatic protruded lumbar disc. *Journal of Urology* **99**, 596–606

Engel, G.L. (1962) *Psychological Development in Health and Disease*, p. 375. Saunders: Philadelphia and London

Engfeldt, B., Rommanus, R. and Yden, S. (1954)*Annals of the Rheumatic Diseases* **13**, 3

Epstein, J.A., Epstein, B.A. and Rosenthal, A.D. (1972) *Journal of Neurosurgery* **36**, 584–589

Falconer, M.A., McGeorge, M. and Begg, A.C. (1948) *Journal of Neurology, Neurosurgery and Psychiatry* **11**, 13–26

Farfan, H.F., Cossette, J.W., Robertson, G.H., Wells, R.V. and Kraus, H. (1970) The effects of torsion on the lumbar intervertebral joints. The role of torsion in the production of disc degeneration. *Journal of Bone and Joint Surgery* **52A**, 468

Fearnside, M.R. and Adams, C.B.T. (1978) Tumours of the cauda equina. *Journal of Neurology, Neurosurgery and Psychiatry* **41**, 24–31

Feinstein, B., Langton, J.N.K., Jameson, R.M. and Schiller, F. (1954) *Journal of Bone and Joint Surgery* **36A**, 98

Fitzgerald, J.A. and Newman, P.H. (1976) Degenerative spondylolisthesis. *Journal of Bone and Joint Surgery* **58B**, 184–192

Fong, D., Leong, J.C.Y., Ho, E.K. *et al.* (1988) Spinal pseudarthrosis in ankylosing spondylitis. *Journal of Bone and Joint Surgery* **70B**, 443–447

Forestier, J. and Lagier, R. (1971) *Clinical Orthopaedics and Related Research* **74**, 65–83

Fraser, S.M. and Sturrock, R.D. (1988) Spinal pseudarthrosis in ankylosing spondylitis. *Journal of Bone and Joint Surgery* **73A**, 1526–1531

Frocrain, L., Duvauferrier, R., Husson, J.L., Noel, J., Ramee, A. and Pawlotsky, Y. (1989) Recurrent postoperative sciatica: evaluation with MR imaging and enhanced CT. *Radiology* **170**, 531–533

Froning, E.C. and Frohman, B. (1968) Motion of the lumbosacral spine after laminectomy and spine fusion: correlation of motion with the result. *Journal of Bone and Joint Surgery* **50A**, 897–918

Galasko, C.S. (1991) Spinal instability secondary to metastatic cancer. *Journal of Bone and Joint Surgery* **73B**, 104–108

Giulian, D. and Robertson, C. (1990) Inhibition of mononuclear phagocytosis reduces ischaemic injury in the spinal cord. *Annals of Neurology* **27**, 33–42

Glew, D., Watt, I., Dieppe, P.A. and Goddard, P.R. (1991) MRI of the cervical spine: rheumatoid arthritis compared with cervical spondylosis. *Clinical Radiology* **44**, 71–76

Goel, M.K. (1968) Vertebral osteotomy for correction of fixed flexion deformity of the spine. *Journal of Bone and Joint Surgery* **50A**, 287

Grew, N.D. and Deane, G. (1982) The physical effects of lumbar spinal supports. *Prosthestics and Orthotics International* **6**, 79–87

Hamblem, D.H. (1979) Operation for cervical rib and scalene syndrome. In: *Operative Surgery*, 3rd edn, vol. *Orthopaedics*, pp. 344–347. Edited by G. Bentley. Butterworths: London and Boston

Hanley, E.N. and Shapiro, D.E. (1989) The development of low back pain after excision of a lumbar disc. *Journal of Bone and Joint Surgery* **71A**, 719–721

Hardcastle, R., Annear, P., Foster, D.H. *et al.* (1992) Spinal abnormalities in young fast bowlers. *Journal of Bone and Joint Surgery* **74B**, 421–425

Hasue, M., Kida, H., Inoue, K. and Awano, N. (1977) Lumbar spinal stenosis. A clinical study of symptoms and therapeutic results. *International Orthopaedics* **1**, 133–137

Hattori, A., Endoh, H., Suzuki, K. and Daneda, M. (1976) Ossification of the thoracic ligamentum flavum with compression of the spinal cord. *Journal of the Japanese Orthopaedic Association* **50**, 1141–1146

Herzog, R.J., Kaiser, J.A., Saal, J.A. and Saal, J.S. (1991) The importance of posterior epidural fat in lumbar central canal stenosis. *Spine* **16** (Supplement), 227–233

Heywood, A.W.B. and Meyers, O.L. (1986) Rheumatoid arthritis of the thoracic and lumbar spine. *Journal of Bone and Joint Surgery* **68B**, 362–368

Hirsch, C. (1959) *Journal of Bone and Joint Surgery* **41B**, 237–243

Horowitch, A., Peek, R.D., Thomas, J.C. *et al.* (1989) The Wiltse pedicle screw fixation system: early clinical results. *Spine* **14**, 461–467

Hughes, J.T. (1966) *Pathology of the Spinal Cord*. Lloyd-Luke: London

Inman, V.T. and Saunder, J.B. (1942) *Radiology* **38**, 669–678

Jackson, R.P., Cain, J.E., Jacobs, R.R. *et al.* (1989) The neuroradiographic diagnosis of lumbar herniated nucleus pulposus. A comparison of computed tomography (CT), CT myelography and magnetic resonance. *Spine* **14**, 1362–1367

Jeffreys, E. (1980) *Disorders of the Cervical Spine*. Butterworths: London and Boston

Jensen, T.T., Overgaard, S., Thomsen, N.O.B. *et al.* (1991) Postoperative computed tomography three months after lumbar disc surgery. *Spine* **16**, 620–622

Johnson, E.W. and Melvin, J.L. (1971) *Archives of Physical Medicine and Rehabilitation* **52**, 239–243

Johnson, C.E. and Sze, G. (1990) Benign arachnoiditis MRI imaging with gadopentate dimeglumine. *American Journal of Roentgenology* **155**, 873–880

Johnsson, K.E., Redlund-Johnell, I., Uden, A. and Willner, S. (1989) Preoperative and postoperative instability in lumbar spinal stenosis. *Spine* **14**, 591–593

Kahanovitz, N., Viola, K., Goldsten, T. and Dawson, E. (1990) A multicentre analysis of percutaneous discectomy. *Spine* **15**, 713–715

Kellgren, J.H. (1937) *Clinical Science* **3**, 175

Kellgren, J.H., Jeffrey, M.R. and Ball, J. (eds) (1963) *The Epidemiology of Chronic Rheumatism*, vol. 1, p. 326. Blackwell Scientific: Oxford

Kirkcaldy-Willis, W.H. and McIvor, G.W.O. (guest editors) (1976) Symposium 'Spinal Stenosis'. *Clinical Orthopaedics and Related Research* **115**, 1–144

Kirkcaldy-Willis, W.H., Paine, K.W.E., Cauchoix, J. and McIvor, G. (1974) Lumbar spinal stenosis. *Clinical Orthopaedics and Related Research* **99**, 30–50

Kondo, M., Matsuda, H., Kureya, S. and Shimazu, A. (1989) Electrophysiological studies of intermittent claudication in spinal stenosis. *Spine* **14**, 862–866

Konttinen, Y.T., Gronblad, M., Anti-Pocka, I. *et al.* (1990) Neuroimmunohistochemical analysis of peridiscal nociceptive elements. *Spine* **15**, 383–386

Kostuik, J.P., Harrington, I., Alexander, D. *et al.* (1986) Cauda equina syndrome and lumbar disc herniation. *Journal of Bone and Joint Surgery* **68**, 386–391

LaBan, M.M. and Wesolowski, D.P. (1988) Night pain associated with diminished cardiopulmonary compliance. A concomitant of lumbar spinal stenosis and degenerative spondylolisthesis. *American Journal of Physical Medicine and Rehabilitation* **67**, 155–170

Langenskiöld, A. and Kiviluoto, O. (1976) Prevention of epidural scar formation after operations on the lumbar spine by means of free fat transplants. A preliminary report. *Clinical Orthopaedics and Related Research* **115**, 92–95

Lansche, W.E. and Ford, L.T. (1960) *Journal of Bone and Joint Surgery* **42A**, 193–206

Law, W.A. (1959) *Journal of Bone and Joint Surgery* **41B**, 271

Law, W.A. (1969) *Clinical Orthopaedics and Related Research* **66**, 70–82

Lewis, T. and Kellgren, J.H. (1939) *Clinical Science* **4**, 47

Leyshon, A., Kirwan, E.O.G. and Parry, C.B. (1981) Electrical studies in the diagnosis of compression of the lumbar root. *Journal of Bone and Joint Surgery* **63B**, 71–75

Lilius, G., Laasonen, E.M. and Myllynen, P. (1989) Lumbar facet joint syndrome. *Journal of Bone and Joint Surgery* **71B**, 681–684

Lumsden, R.M. and Morris, J.M. (1968) In vivo study of axial rotation and immobilization at the lumbosacral joint. *Journal of Bone and Joint Surgery* **50A**, 1591–1602

McCall, I.W., Park, W.M. and O'Brien, J.P. (1979) Induced pain referral from posterior lumbar elements in normal subjects. *Spine* **4**, 441–446

McNab, I. (1950) *Journal of Bone and Joint Surgery* **32B**, 325

McNab, I. (1971) *Journal of Bone and Joint Surgery* **53A**, 891–903

McNab, I. (1975) In: Surgical treatment of degenerative disc disease of the lumbar spine. *Recent Advances in Orthopaedics – 2*, pp. 1–33. Edited by B. McKibbin. Churchill Livingstone: Edinburgh, London, New York

McNally, D.S. and Adams, M.A. (1992) Internal intervertebral disc mechanisms as revealed by stress profilometry. *Spine* **17**, 66–73

Macrae, I.F. and Wright, V. (1969) Measurement of back movement. *Annals of the Rheumatic Diseases* **28**, 584

Marazano, E., Latini, P., Checcagini, F. *et al.* (1991) Radiation therapy in metastatic spinal cord compression. A prospective analysis of 105 consecutive patients. *Cancer* **67**, 1311–1317

Maroon, J.C., Kopitnik, T.A., Schulhof, L.A., Abla, A. and Wilberger, J.E. (1990) Diagnosis and microsurgical approach to far-lateral disc herniation in the lumbar spine. *Journal of Neurosurgery* **72**, 378–382

Martel, W. (1961) *American Journal of Roentgenology* **86**, 223

Massobrio, M. (1991) Herniation of the lumbar intervertebral disc in teenagers. *Italian Journal of Orthopaedics and Traumatology* **17**, 5–21

Mathiesen, F.K. and Haar, D. (1986) MNS genotypes in ankylosing spondylitis. *Journal of Bone and Joint Surgery* **68B**, 656–657

Matsuzaki, H. (1993) The Japanese approach to ossification of the posterior longitudinal ligament. *Current Science. Current Opinion in Orthopaedics* **4**(2), 69–77

May, P.C. and Yeoman, P.M. (1986) Hip arthroplasty in ankylosing spondylitis. *Journal of Bone and Joint Surgery* **68B**, 669

Mensor, M.C. and Duvall, G. (1959) *Journal of Bone and Joint Surgery* **41A**, 1037

Middleton, G.S. and Teacher, J.H. (1911) Injury of the spinal cord due to rupture of an intervertebral disc during muscular effort. *Glasgow Medical Journal* **76**, 1–7

Milette, P.C., Raymond, J. and Fontaine, S. (1990) Comparison of high-resolution computer tomography with discography in the evaluation of lumbar disc herniations. *Spine* **15**, 525–533

Miller, M.E., Fogel, G.R. and Denham, W.K. (1988) Salmonella spondylitis. *Journal of Bone and Joint Surgery* **70A**, 463–466

Mink, J.H. (1989) Imagining evaluation of the candidate for percutaneous lumbar discectomy. *Clinical Orthopaedics and Related Research* **288**, 83–91

Mixter, W.J. and Barr, J.S. (1930) Rupture of intervertebral disc with involvement of the spinal canal. *New England Journal of Medicine* **211**, 210–215

Miyamoto, S., Takoha, K., Yoneobu, L. and Ono, K. (1992) Ossification of the ligamentum flavum induced by bone morphogenetic protein. *Journal of Bone and Joint Surgery* **74B**, 279–283

Molina, F., Ramcharan, J.E. and Wyke, B.D. (1976) Structure and function of articular receptor systems in the cervical spine. *Journal of Bone and Joint Surgery* **58B**, 255–256

Moll, J.M.H. (1978) Ankylosing spondylitis. In: *Copeman's Textbook of the Rheumatic Diseases*, 5th edn, pp. 511–536. Edited by J.T. Scott. Churchill Livingstone: Edinburgh, London, New York

Moll, J.M.H. and Wright, V. (1972) An objective clinical study of chest expansion. *Annals of the Rheumatic Diseases* **31**, 1–8

Moll, J.M.H., Haslock, I., McCrae, I.F. *et al.* (1976) Associations between ankylosing spondylitis, psoriatic arthritis, Reiter's disease, arthropathies and Beckett's disease. *Medicine* **53**, 343–364

Moreland, L.W., Lopez-Mendez, A. and Alarcon, G.S. (1989) Spinal stenosis: a comprehensive review of the literature. *Seminars in Arthritis and Rheumatism* **19**, 127–149

Morris, J.M., Lucas, D.B. and Bresler, B. (1961) *Journal of Bone and Joint Surgery* **43A**, 327–331

Murone, I. (1974) The importance of sagittal diameters of the cervical spine canal in relation to spondylosis and myelopathy. *Journal of Bone and Joint Surgery* **56B**, 30–36

Nachemson, A. (1966) The load on lumbar discs in different positions of the body. *Clinical Orthopaedics and Related Research* **45**, 107–122

Nachemson, A. (1972) The mechanical properties of the lumbar intervertebral discs and their clinical implications. *Journal of Bone and Joint Surgery* **54B**, 195

Nachemson, A.L. (1985) Advances in low back pain. *Clinical Orthopaedics and Related Research* **200**, 266–278

Nachemson, A. (1989) Lumbar Discography: where are we today? *Spine* **14**, 555–557

Nasca, R.J. (1989) Rationale for spinal fusion in lumbar spinal stenosis. *Spine* **14**, 451–454

Naylor, A. (1970) Studies of the function of the intervertebral disc. *Orthopaedics* **3**, 7–22

Naylor, A., Flowers, M.W. and Bramley, J.E. (1977) The value of dexamethasone in the postoperative treatment of lumbar disc prolapse. *Orthopedic Clinics of North America* **8**, 3–8

Neuhold, A., Stiskal, M., Platzer, C. *et al.* (1991) Combined use of spinal-echo and gradient-echo MR imaging in cervical disc disease. *Neuroradiology* **83**, 422–426

Nixon, J. (1991) *Spinal Stenosis*. Edward Arnold: London

Noordenbos, W. (1959) *Pain*. Elsevier: New York and London

North, C.A. and North, R.B. (1993) Neurogenic spinal tumours. *Current Science. Current Opinion in Orthopaedics* **4**, 186–191

Nurick, S. (1972) The pathogenesis of the spinal cord disorder associated with cervical spondylosis. *Brain* **95**, 87–100

O'Connell, J.E.A. (1950) *Annals of the Royal College of Surgeons* **6**, 403

O'Connell, J.E.A. (1956) *Proceedings of the Royal Society of Medicine* **49**, 202

Onik, G. and Helms, C.A. (1991) Automated percutaneous lumbar discectomy. *American Journal of Roentgenology* **156**, 531–538

Ooi, Y., Mita, F. and Satoh, Y. (1990) Myeloscopic study on lumbar spinal cord stenosis with special reference to intermittent claudication. *Spine* **15**, 544–549

Osti, O.L. and Fraser, R.D. (1992) MRI and discography of annular tears and intervertebral disc degeneration. *Journal of Bone and Joint Surgery* **74B**, 431–435

Osti, O.L., Vernon-Roberts, B., Moore, R. and Fraser, R.D. (1992) Annular tears and disc degeneration in the lumbar spine. *Journal of Bone and Joint Surgery* **74B**, 678–682

Padley, S., Gleeson, F., Chisholm, R. and Baldwin, J. (1990) Assessment of a single lumbar spine radiograph in low back pain. *British Journal of Radiology* **63**, 535–536

Pancoast, H.K. (1932) *Journal of the American Medical Association* **99**, 1391

Pennal, G.F., Conn, G.S., McDonald, G. *et al.* (1972) Motion studies of the lumbar spine: a preliminary report. *Journal of Bone and Joint Surgery* **54B**, 442–452

Penning, L. and Wilmink, J.T. (1987) Posture-dependent bilateral compression of L4 or L5 nerve roots in facet hypertrophy. A dynamic CT-myelographic study. *Spine* **12**, 488–500

Porter, R.W. (1981) MD Thesis, University of Edinburgh

Porter, R.W. and Miller, C.G. (1988) Neurogenic claudication and root claudication treated with calcitonin. A double-blind trial. *Spine* **13**, 1061–1064

Porter, R.W., Wicks, M. and Ottewell, D. (1978) Measurement of the spinal canal by diagnostic ultrasound. *Journal of Bone and Joint Surgery* **60B**, 481–484

Post, M.J., Sze, G., Quencer, R.M., Eismont, F.J., Green, B.A. and Gahbauer, H. (1990) Gadolinium enhanced MR in spinal infection. *Journal of Computer Assisted Tomography* **14**, 721–729

Ram, Z., Findler, G., Spiegelman, R., Shacked, I., Tadmoor, R. and Sahar, A. (1987) Intermittent priapism in spinal canal stenosis. *Spine* **12**, 377–378

Rana, N. (1989) Natural history of atlanto-axial subluxation in rheumatoid arthritis. *Spine* **14**, 1054–1056

Rauschning, W. (1988) Normal and pathologic anatomy of the lumbar root canal. *Spine* **12**, 1008–1019

Resnick, D. (1979) Radiology of sero-negative spondyloarthropathies. *Clinical Orthopaedics and Related Research* **143**, 38–45

Rommanus, R. (1953) *Acta Medica Scandinavica* **145**, 162

Rosen, C., Rothman, S., Zigler, J. and Capen, D. (1991) Lumbar facet fracture as a possible source of pain after lumbar laminectomy. *Spine* **16**, S234–238

Ross, J.S., Masaryk, T.J., Schrader, M., Gentili, A., Bohlman, H. and Modic, M.T. (1990) MR imaging of the postoperative lumbar spine: assessment with gadopentate dimeglumine. *American Journal of Neuroradiology* **11**, 771–776

Rowe, M.L. (1960) *Journal of Occupational Medicine* **2**, 219

Saal, J.A., Saal, J.S. and Herzog, R.J. (1990) The natural history of lumbar intervertebral disc extrusions treated nonoperatively. *Spine* **15**, 683–686

Schatzker, J. and Pennal, G.F. (1968) Spinal stenosis – a cause of cauda equina compression. *Journal of Bone and Joint Surgery* **50B**, 606–618

Schecter, N.A., France, M.P. and Lee, C.K. (1991) Painful internal disc degeneration of the lumbo-sacral spine: discographic diagnosis and treatment by posterior lumbar interbody fusion. *Orthopaedics* **14**, 447–449

Schmorl, G. (1932) *Archiv für Klinische Chirurgie* **172**, 240

Schmorl, G. and Junghanns, K. (1971) *The Human Spine in Health and Disease*. 2nd American edition. Translated by E.F. Besemann. Grune & Stratton: New York and London

Schnebel, B., Kingston, S., Watkins, R. and Dillin, W. (1989) Comparison of MRI to contrast CT in the diagnosis of spinal stenosis. *Spine* **14**, 332–337

Seaman, B. and Wells, J. (1961) *American Journal of Roentgenology* **86**, 241

Sharif, H.S., Clark, D.C., Aabed, M.Y. *et al.* (1990) Granulomatous spinal infections. MR imaging. *Radiology* **177**, 101–107

Sheldon, J., Russin, L.A. and Gargano, F.P. (1976) Lumbar spinal stenosis. Radiographic diagnosis with special reference to transverse axial tomography. *Clinical Orthopaedics and Related Research* **115**, 53–67

Silbergleit, R., Gebarski, S.S., Brunberg, J.A. *et al.* (1990) Lumbar synovial cysts: correlation of myelographic, CT, MR and pathological findings. *American Journal of Neuroradiology* **11**, 777–779

Simkin, P.A. (1982) Simionstance: a sign of spinal stenosis. *Lancet* **2**, 652–653

Simmons, J.W., Emery, S.F. McMillan, J.N. *et al.* (1991) Awake discography: a comparison study with MR imaging. *Spine* **16**, 216–219

Sklar, E.M.L., Quencer, R.M., Green, B.A., Montalvo, B.M. and Post, M.J. (1991) Complications of epidural anaesthesia: MR appearance of abnormalities. *Radiology* **181**, 549–552

Skubic, J.W. and Kostvik, J.P. (1991) Thoracic pain syndromes and thoracic disc herniation. In: *Adult Spine. Principles and Practice*, pp. 1444–1461. Edited by J.W. Frymoyer. Raven Press: New York

Skubic, J.W. (1993) Thoracic disc disease. *Current Science. Current Opinion in Orthopaedics* **4**, 96–103

Smith, G.W. and Robinson, R.A. (1958) *Journal of Bone and Joint Surgery* **40A**, 607

Smith-Petersen, M.N., Larson, C.B. and Aufranc, O.E. (1945) *Journal of Bone and Joint Surgery* **27**, 1

Stamm, T.T. (1962) *British Medical Journal* **1**, 190

Stokes, I.A.F., Wilder, D.G., Frymoyer, J.W. and Pope, M.H. (1981) 1980 Volvo award in clinical sciences. Assessment of patients with low-back pain by biplanar radiographic measurement of intervertebral motion. *Spine* **6**, 233–240

Styblo, K., Bossers, G.T.M. and Scot, G.H. (1986) Spinal correction osteotomy of progressive kyphosis caused by ankylosing spondylitis. *Journal of Bone and Joint Surgery* **68B**, 679–680

Sze, G. (1991) Magnetic resonance imaging of spinal metastases. *Cancer* **67**, 1229–1241

Tator, C.H. (1991) Pathophysiology of acute traumatic spinal cord injury. *Current Science. Current Opinion in Orthopaedics* **2**, 269–274

Tregonning, G.D., Transfeld, E.E., McCulloch, J.A., Macnab, I. and Nachemson, A. (1991) Chymopapain versus conventional surgery for lumbar disc herniation. Ten-year results of treatment. *Journal of Bone and Joint Surgery* **73B**, 481–486

Tress, B.M. and Hare, W.S.C. (1990) CT of the spine: are pain radiographs necessary? *Clinical Radiology* **41**, 317–320

Turner, P.L., Prince, H.G., Webb, J.K. and Sokal, M.P. (1988) Surgery for malignant extradural tumours of the spine. *Journal of Bone and Joint Surgery* **70B**, 51–56

Van der Sonde, J.J., Kroger, R. and Boogerd, W. (1990) Multiple spinal epidural metastases in unexpected frequent finding. *Journal of Neurology, Neurosurgery and Psychiatry* **53**, 1001–1003

Veale, D., Kavanagh, G., Fielding, J.F. and Fitzgerald, O. (1991) Primary fibromyalgia and the irritable bowel syndrome: different expressions of a common pathogenic process. *British Journal of Rheumatology* **30**, 220–222

Verbiest, H. (1954) *Journal of Bone and Joint Surgery* **36B**, 230–237

Verbiest, H. (1977) Results of surgical treatment of idiopathic developmental stenosis of the lumbar vertebral canal. A review of twenty-seven years. *Journal of Bone and Joint Surgery* **59B**, 181–188

Videman, T., Nurringen, M. and Troup, I.D.G. (1990) Lumbar spine pathologies in cadaveric material in relation to history of back pain, occupation and physical loading. *Spine* **15**, 728–738

Walsh, T.R., Weinstern, J.N. Spratt, K.F. *et al.* (1990) Lumbar discography in normal subjects. *Journal of Bone and Joint Surgery* **72**, 1081–1088

Watanabe, H. (1989) [A new surgical treatment for lumbar spinal canal stenosis]. [Japanese] *Nippon Seikeigeka Gakkai Zasshi* **63**, 728–740

Watson-Jones, R. (1934) *Journal of Bone and Joint Surgery* **16**, 30

Weddell, A.G.N. (1962) 'Activity pattern' hypothesis for sensation of pain. In: *Neural Physiopathology*, p. 134. Edited by R. Grennell. Hoeber: New York

Werne, S. (1957) *Acta Orthopaedica Scandinavica* **Supplement 23**

West, J.L., Bradford, D.S. and Ogilvie, J.W. (1991) Results of spinal arthrodesis with pedicle screw-plate fixation. *Journal of Bone and Joint Surgery* **73A**, 1179–1184

White, A. III and Panjabl, M.M. (1990) *Clinical Biomechanics of the Spine*. J.B. Lippincott Co.: Philadelphia

White, A.A., Southwick, W.O., Deponte, R.J., Gainor, J.W. and Hardy, R. (1973) Relief of pain by anterior cervical spine fusion of spondylosis. *Journal of Bone and Joint Surgery* **55A**, 525–534

Wiesel, S.W., Tsourmas, N., Feffer, H.L., Citrin, C.M. and Patronas, N. (1984) A study of a CAT. i. The incidence of positive CAT scans in an asymptomatic group of patients. *Spine* **9**, 549–551

Wiltse, L.L., Kirkcaldy-Willis, W.H. and McIvor, G.W. (1976) The treatment of spinal stenosis. *Clinical Orthopaedics and Related Research* **115**, 83–91

Wiltse, L.L., Bateman, J.G., Hutchinson, R.H. and Nelson, W.E. (1968) *Journal of Bone and Joint Surgery* **50A**, 919–926

Wood, P.H.N. (1976) The epidemiology of back pain. In.: *The Epidemiology of Back Pain*, pp. 13–27 Edited by M.I.V. Jayson. Grune & Stratton: New York/Sector Publishing Limited: London

Woodhall, B. and Hayes, G.J. (1950) The well-leg raising test of Fajersztajn in the diagnosis of ruptured lumbar intervertebral disc. *Journal of Bone and Joint Surgery* **32A**, 786–792

Wray, C.C., Easom, S. and Hoskinson, J. (1991) Coccydynia. Aetiology and treatment. *Journal of Bone and Joint Surgery* **73B**, 335–338

Yang, K.H. and King, A.I. (1984) Mechanism of facet load transmission as a hypothesis of low back pain. *Spine* **9**, 557

Yazaki, S., Muramatsu, T., Yoneda, M. and Fujita, K. (1988) Venous pressure in the vertebral venous plexus and its role in cauda equina claudication. *Nippon Seikeigeka Gakkai Zasshi* **62**, 733–745

Yasima, T., Koh, S., Okamura, T. and Yamenichi, Y. (1990) Histological changes in ageing lumbar intervertebral discs. *Journal of Bone and Joint Surgery* **72A**, 220–229

Yunus, M.B., Ahles, T.A., Aldag, J.C. and Masi, A.T. (1991) Relationship of clinical features with psychological status in primary fibromyalgia. *Arthritis and Rheumatism* **34**, 15–31

Zdeblick, T.A. (1991) Conditions comprising neural structures in the vertebral column. *Current Science. Current Opinion in Orthopaedics* **2**, 212–216

Zeidman, S.M. and Ducker, T.B. (1992) Cervical disc disease I. Treatment options and outcomes. *Neurosurgery Quarterly* **2**, 116–143

CHAPTER 14

The Shoulder and Elbow Joints

JOHN R. SHEARER AND ARESH HASHEMI-NEJAD

THE SHOULDER JOINT

Injuries in the region of the shoulder are common and the effects of trauma are demonstrable in all the components of the shoulder. The major injuries such as dislocations and fractures will not be discussed here.

The minor injuries, however, are of great importance. Damage to soft tissues, to the joint surfaces in the absence of dislocation, and to the bony components in the absence of actual fracture, have all to be considered. Watkins, from a consideration of the comparative anatomy of the joint, suggested that the slow or incomplete return of function could be explained by its recently acquired capabilities. He pointed out that, despite the gradual evolution of orthograde man, there had been no development of new muscles. Those which were adapted to plantigrade action (i.e. with the body held horizontally) merely had orthograde functions superimposed on them. Man's ability to raise and maintain his arm above his head is thus a late acquisition in the evolution of his muscular apparatus and is therefore correspondingly unstable. It follows that whenever the limb is disabled, this most recent function is the first to be affected and the last to recover. Probably the most important of the movements of the shoulder, at least in its relation to trauma, is that of abduction. Basmajian (1969) carried out an electromyographic analysis of function around the shoulder joint, and showed that the deltoid muscle, as well as initiating abduction, is also most active at 90–180° of abduction. In elevation of the scapula with upward rotation of the glenoid, the upper trapezius, the upper serratus anterior and the levator scapulae are most active.

Mechanics of the shoulder

Many complex movements contribute to motion in the shoulder, and most of these are important to function. Saha (1978) has described these movements in three phases. In phase one the first 60° of flexion or 30° of elevation of the humerus involves about 15° of movement of the clavicle at the sternoclavicular joint. The scapula does not elevate significantly, but rotates to allow the elevation of the clavicle. Phase two consists of subsequent movement to 90° of flexion or abduction. At this time the scapula and clavicle elevate about 5° for every 10° of glenohumeral movement. Phase three completes the movement of the humerus to the fully elevated position (Figure 14.1). Elevation of the scapula is now twice that of the glenohumeral joint, but without further elevation of the clavicle. The clavicle rotates about its long axis to permit elevation of the scapula. Poppen and Walker (1976) observed elevation of the shoulder during the second phase in patients with abnormalities of the shoulder, and found abnormal

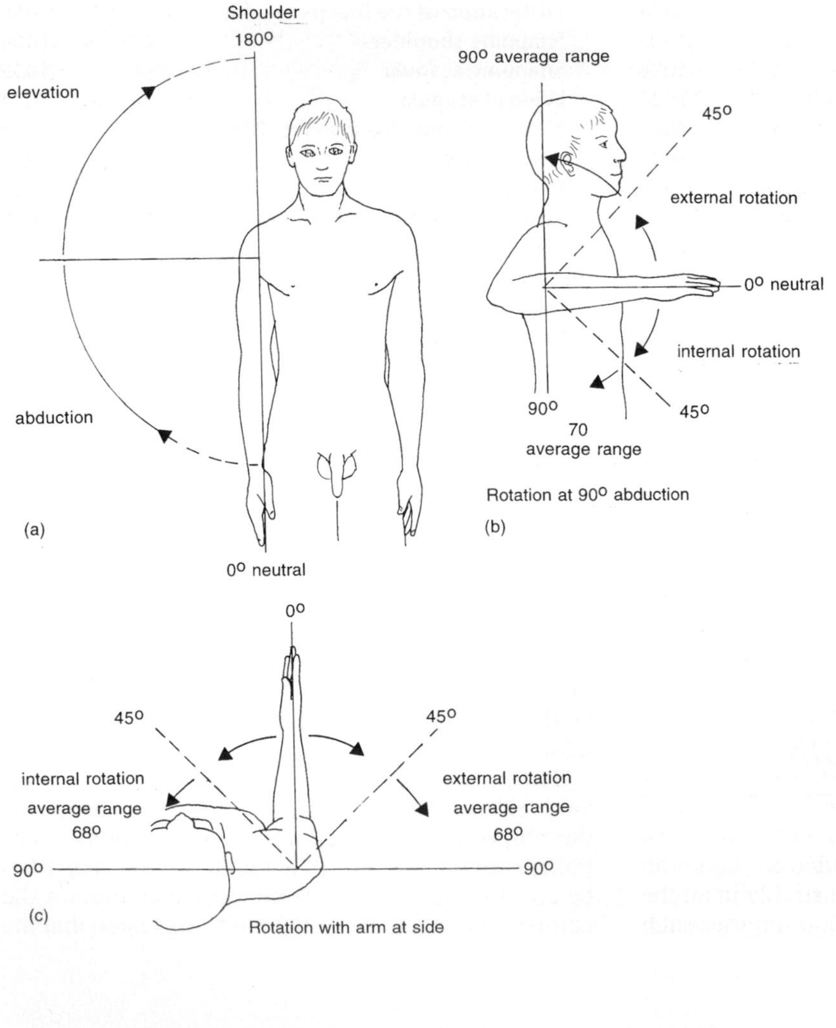

Figure 14.1 (a) The movement of abduction to 90° and elevation to 180°. (b) Rotation with the shoulder at 90° to show average range of 70°. (c) External rotation of average 68° and internal rotation of 68°.

ratios of glenohumeral/scapulothoracic movement, along with an abnormal amount of vertical displacement of the humeral head.

Maximum humeral elevation takes place in a plane anterior to the scapular plane and requires external axial rotation. Elevation posterior to the scapular plane requires internal rotation (Ann *et al.*, 1991).

RESTRAINTS TO SCAPULOHUMERAL MOVEMENT

There are, of course, passive as well as active restraints of scapulohumeral joint movement. Terry *et al.* (1991), evaluated the stabilizing function of static restraints of the scapulohumeral joint in cadavers. They found that the coracohumeral ligament presented a primary restraint function in flexion and extension, whilst restraints in extension, abduction and external rotation comprised the anterior glenohumeral ligaments, with the posterior capsule providing stability in flexion, abduction and internal rotation.

It has been suggested that negative intra-articular pressure in the shoulder joint contributes significantly to maintaining glenohumeral stability. Howell and Kraft (1991) studied the stabilizing role of supraspinatus and infraspinatus in 13 unstable shoulders by inducing a supracapsular nerve block. They found that normal glenohumeral kinematics persisted despite a dysfunctional rotator cuff and concluded that normal kinematics was due to a socket mechanism which contributed to function despite labral lesions. Division of the rotator interval of the capsule significantly impairs passive glenohumeral joint stability (Harryman *et al.*, 1992).

Increasing interest in the coracoacromial arch and its influence in rotator cuff tears has resulted in a number of studies. Zuckerman *et al.* (1991) demonstrated in cadaver shoulders that in 20% of cases a full thickness rotator cuff tear was present and was significantly more frequent in patients of 60 years or older. They investigated the role of the position of the humeral head in contributing to the availability of the subacromial space within the coracoacromial arch. The group of cadavers with rotator cuff tears had a significant anterior projection of the acromion and a reduced supraspinatus outlet.

Saha (1969) also studied the shapes of the articulating surfaces of the glenoid and humerus, and how these contributed to the movement and stability of the joint. He concluded that in some cases the surfaces are congruent, in some cases the radius of the humerus is the greatest, and in some cases the glenoid has the greater radius. He considered that the glenoid is potentially unstable because of the direction of the force transmission through the joint and the rolling motion between the two surfaces permitted by this type of joint. Movement between two articulating surfaces can be classified as sliding, rolling or pivoting about a point. This last is in fact a combination of sliding and rolling. The direction of the joint force, and hence the shape of the glenoid surface, is important for the stability of the joint (Figure 14.2).

Walker and Poppen (1977) have estimated the magnitude and direction of the glenohumeral joint force during abduction. They concluded that between 30° and 60° of elevation the direction of the joint force is closest to the superior margin of the glenoid, but stability is increased by external rotation of the humerus (Figure 14.3). Saha (1969) stressed the importance of the latissimus dorsi and subscapularis for maintaining this stability. In a mathematical analysis of the glenohumeral joint, Saha (1978) considered the actions of eight muscles and the force of gravity which produces moments of force about the joint. The vector total (allowing for magnitude and direction) of these moments determines the resultant motion of the joint in terms of instantaneous rotations and translations. If this resultant is zero, then the joint comes to rest because of friction and soft tissue resistance to motion. Of the eight muscles, the innermost group were considered to be 'steerers' which are almost tangential to the spherical joint surface and thus produce mainly pure couples in horizontal and vertical planes. The 'inter-

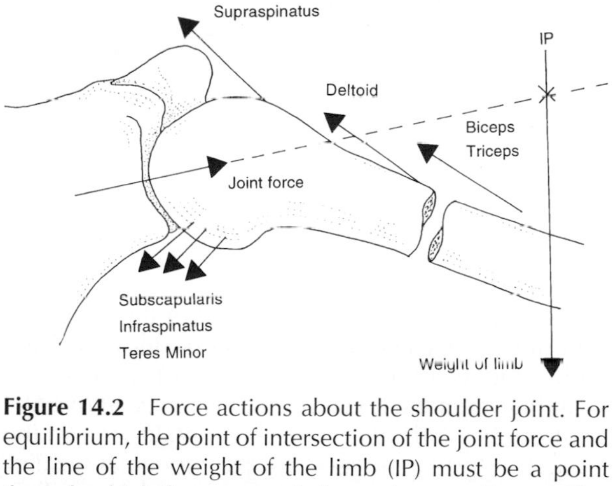

Figure 14.2 Force actions about the shoulder joint. For equilibrium, the point of intersection of the joint force and the line of the weight of the limb (IP) must be a point through which the net muscle force also acts. For stability, the joint force must act within the margins of the glenoid. These requirements may demand tensions in the depressor muscles to maintain stability of the joint (After Saha, A.K. (1978) *Proceedings of the Indian National Science Academy* **44**, 195–201)

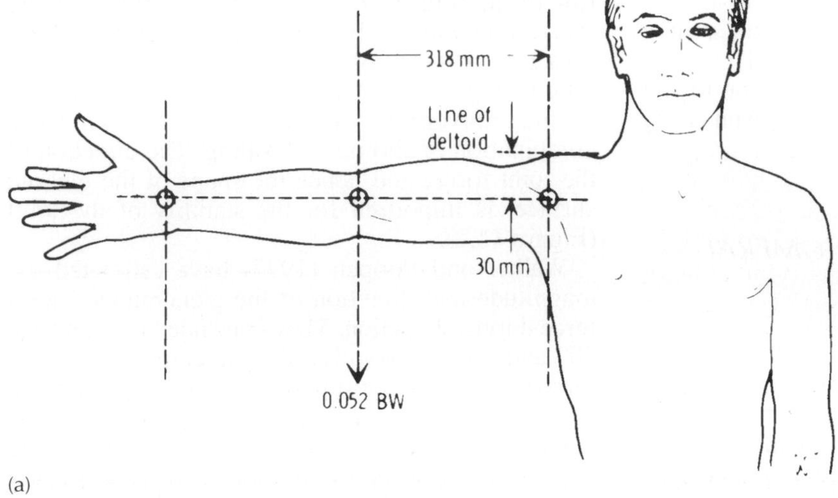

(a)

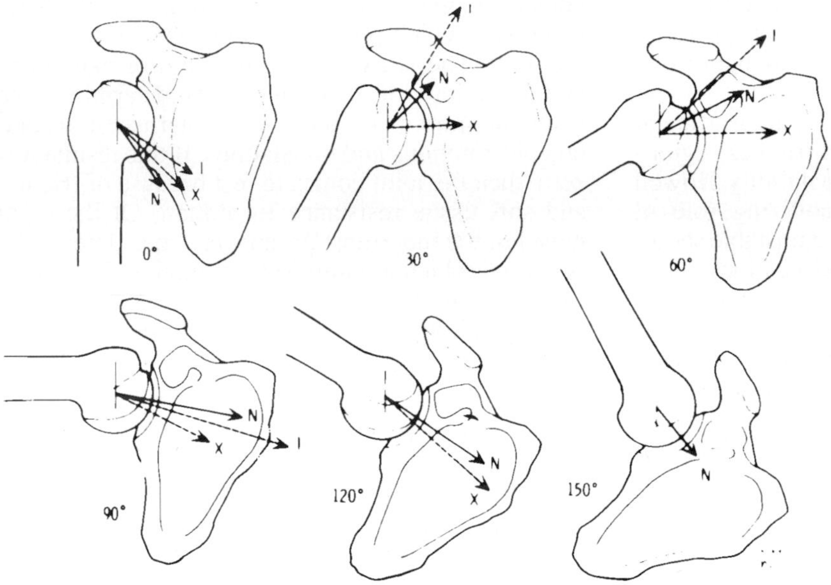

(b)

Figure 14.3 (a) Arm held at 90° of abduction. Weight of the arm is 0.052 times body weight at a centre of mass 318 mm from the centre of the humeral head. Deltoid force at 30 mm from the centre of the humeral head gives a joint force of approximately 10 times the weight of the arm of one-half body weight (see text). (b) Resultant glenohumeral joint force vectors at varying degrees of abduction with the arm in neutral (N), internal rotation (I), and external rotation (X). (Reprinted, with permission from Poppen, N.K. and Walker, P.S. (1978) *Clinical Orthopaedics* **135**, 165–170)

mediate' group of muscles consisted of three muscles anteriorly, opposed by teres minor posteriorly. They initially give rolling and slipping in the joint, and spinning when the humeral shaft is raised above 60° to align the shaft axis with the contact area in the joint. The 'prime movers' are the clavicular head of pectoralis major and the deltoid, which produce desired movements of the joint, along with rolling and slipping of the surfaces. These mechanical principles can be incorporated into the design of surgical procedures for stabilization of the shoulder (Saha, 1969).

Attention may be drawn to the wide range of movement in the joint, and the fact that the attachment of the arm to the body is effected principally by muscles. The importance of carefully applying the principles of muscle balance when treating injured shoulders is thus apparent. The location of the subdeltoid bursa, and the relationship of the circumflex nerve to the surgical neck of the humerus, in which situation it is peculiarly exposed to injury, should also be borne in mind.

Anatomical basis of shoulder pain

Injury to the shoulder is constantly followed by pain, limitation of movement and muscular atrophy. Pain in this region, however, may be produced by lesions other than in the shoulder itself (Figure 14.4). Various cervical, thoracic and abdominal lesions may be responsible, and it is important to realize that such referred pain may lead to actual limitation of movement and stiffness of the joint. The pain is referred through the phrenic nerve, and Cope attempted to localize the causal lesions by mapping out the exact site of the referred shoulder pain. Thus pain in the clavicular area (i.e. over the front of the shoulders) is referred from a lesion in the anterior part of the diaphragm. Pain over the supraspinatus muscle follows a lesion of the posterior part of the diaphragm. In lesions affecting the dome of the diaphragm the area of reference is over the acromioclavicular joint. When both shoulders are painful the lesion is usually situated in the central tendon of the diaphragm.

Diagnosis of shoulder disorders

The diagnosis of shoulder disorders may present great difficulty. The patient's history should be carefully elicited and too much attention should not be paid to the occurrence of minor trauma, as most can recall some previous injury.

Every investigation of shoulder symptoms should conclude with a radiographic examination of both

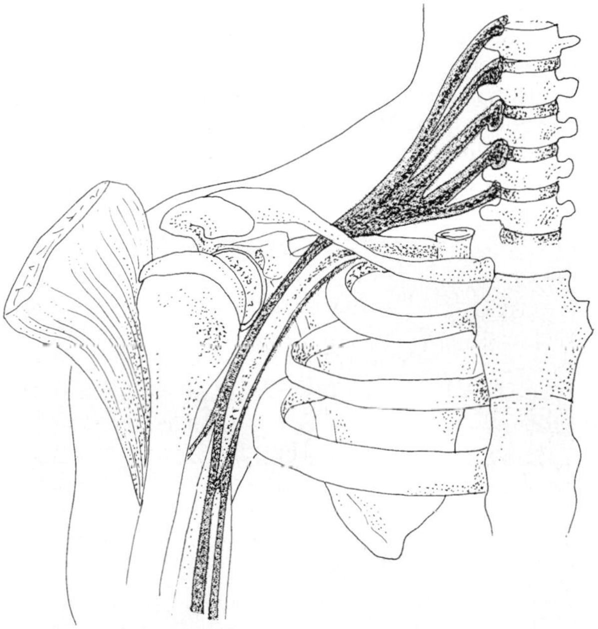

Figure 14.4 The various anatomical components in the vicinity of the shoulder joint which when diseased produce shoulder pain.

Diseases of the vertebral column
Neoplasm
Spondylitis
Cervical disc lesion

Diseases of the spinal cord
Tumour
Syringomyelia
Progressive muscle atrophy
Syphilis
Herpes zoster

Diseases of the brachial plexus
Cervical rib and scalenus anterior syndrome
Pancoast's tumour
Shoulder–hand syndrome

Diseases of peripheral nerves, shoulder and acromioclavicular joints
Rotator cuff – calcification and rupture
Tendinitis and calcification
1. Supraspinatus tendon
2. Biceps tendon

Bursitis – acute, chronic and calcification
1. Subacromial
2. Subdeltoid
3. Subcoracoid

Subluxations and arthritis

Referred pain
Diaphragm and diaphragmatic hernia
Pleura
Heart
Gall bladder
Vascular
Thrombotic
Arteriosclerotic
Autonomic

shoulders, including anteroposterior, lateral rotation, and axial views. In this way lesions such as myositis ossificans, loose bodies, traction osteophytes of the acromion and small fractures involving the articular surfaces may be revealed. But it is also important to examine and x-ray the cervical spine, as it is notable that in arthritis of this area the main symptom may be pain in the shoulder region.

CT SCANNING, MR SCANNING AND ARTHROGRAPHY

Many shoulder joint lesions affect the rotator cuff and soft tissues of the shoulder rather than the bony anatomy. MRI scanning has proved to be a valuable tool in both the diagnosis of rotator cuff tears and in the diagnosis of subacromial impingement syndromes. In the case of rotator cuff tears, it has been estimated to give a positive diagnosis in over 90% of cases, and it is often possible to estimate the size and site of the rotator cuff tear which is an advance in preoperative planning (Figure 14.5). This technique is also valuable in diagnosis of subacromial impingement syndromes, giving a satisfactory estimate of the degree of subacromial impingement and of the severity of the local abrasion of the rotator cuff. CT scanning can be valuable in the assessment of bone stock around the shoulder, which is particularly important in preoperative planning for total shoulder replacement. Three-dimensional studies of the anatomy of the shoulder joint by CT scanning is also helpful in preoperative planning in recurrent dislocations of the shoulder.

Iannotti *et al.* (1991) were able to check the MR imaging diagnosis at surgery and introduced a scoring system for the status of the cuff evaluated by MR imaging. They found a 100% sensitivity and a 97% specificity in full tears of the cuff.

The differentiation of tendinitis and degenerative cuff lesions give a sensitivity of 82% and a specificity of 87%, whilst these figures for labral pathology were 88% and 93% for sensitivity and specificity respectively.

Vellet *et al.* (1991) reviewed common sports shoulder injuries diagnosed by MR imaging and ultrasound and concluded that MR imaging was an excellent method of demonstrating even minor pathological changes. They suggest the addition of contrast agents to enhance the MR imaging together with kinematic studies to evaluate shoulder pathology further.

Nelson *et al.* (1991) reviewed painful shoulders by ultrasonography, MR scanning and CT arthrography and compared the results of investigation with the pathology identified at surgery. They concluded that

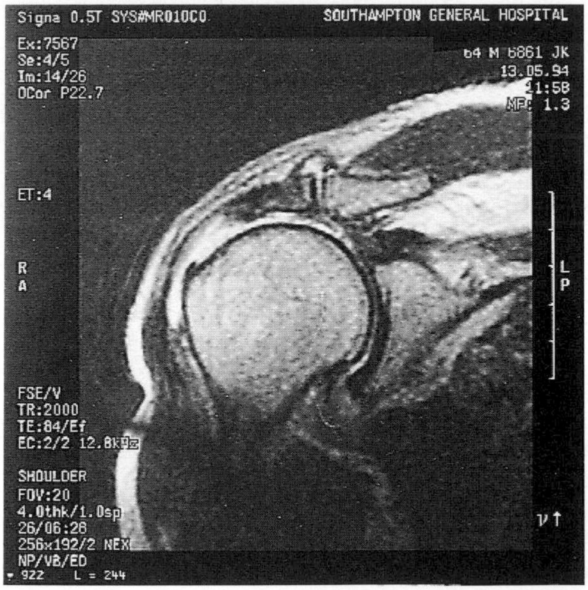

(a)

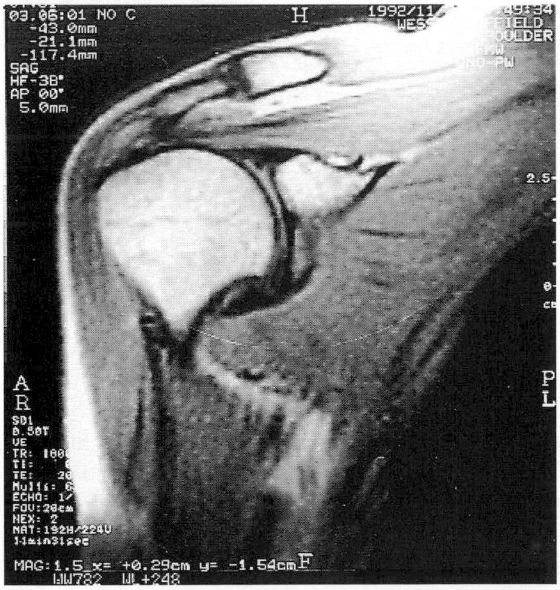

(b)

Figure 14.5 (a) A complete rotator cuff tear on MR scan. There is loss of subacromial space and the clear appearance in the subacromial space indicates a large tear of the rotator cuff extending almost from the acromioclavicular joint to the insertion of supraspinatus. (b) This patient had a subacromial compression syndrome due to a cartilaginous spike extending from the edge of the acromion impinging on the subacromial space. At operation this was confirmed, although the tendon itself was intact. MRI is the investigation of choice for rotator cuff problems. (Films kindly supplied by Dr Richard Blaquiere, Consultant Radiologist at Southampton University Hospitals)

MR imaging was more accurate in the finding of rotator cuff pathology than was ultrasonography or CT arthrography, whilst in defining pathology around the labrum MR imaging was also equal in quality and accuracy to CT arthrography. It had the advantage of being non-invasive.

Misamore and Woodward (1991) compared the accuracy of arthrography and ultrasonography in diagnosing rotator cuff tears. The subsequent surgical exploration allowed comparison of the accuracy of the two techniques. Arthrography was accurate in 87% of the cases and ultrasonography in 37%.

ARTHROGRAPHY

The normal arthrographic anatomy was described by Nelson and Burton (1975) as a smooth round outline parallel to the humeral head, with contrast medium passing into the subscapularis bursa but not into the subdeltoid bursa. Often there is a redundant axillary fold and lax anterior capsule in neutral position when tight in abduction. The passage of contrast along the biceps tendon is limited by its synovial reflection (see Figure 14.19).

In rotator cuff tears, if the contrast medium enters the subdeltoid bursa this indicates a complete (i.e. full thickness) tear. Incomplete tears may show an 'ulcer' appearance in the cuff surface but no subdeltoid extravasation.

With recurrent dislocation there is usually no difficulty in determining the direction of dislocation by the history, the apprehension test and the site of Hill–Sachs lesion. However, if doubt exists, especially in recurrent subluxation, arthrography is usually diagnostic because of the position of the redundant joint capsule and the stripping of the capsule from the scapular neck.

In a frozen shoulder, there is seen a reduced joint volume, loss of normal axillary pouch and absence of dye in the biceps tendon sheath. After a manipulation, arthrography reveals some rents in the inferior capsule and therefore occasionally is useful to exclude frozen shoulder in a hysterical patient (Neviaser, 1975).

Arthroscopy of the shoulder

Arthroscopy is now established not only for diagnosis but also for operative procedures. Loose body or calcium deposit removal, acromioplasty for rotator cuff impingement, drainage of septic arthritis and latterly labral lesions repairs are now performed arthroscopically.

Standard knee arthroscopic equipment is used. There is abundant space in the glenohumeral and subacromial space to accommodate the arthroscope. General anaesthesia is usually employed although the operation can be performed under supraclavicular or interscalene block. The patient is either positioned in the lateral decubitus or beach chair position. Five pounds of traction are applied to the arm but care should be taken to minimize the tendency for excessive distraction and risk of injury to the brachial plexus and peripheral nerves. An absolute contraindication to shoulder arthroscopy is any infection in the skin or soft tissues in the shoulder area.

A small skin incision is made 1 cm inferior and 1 cm medial to the posterolateral corner of the acromion. Through this incision posterior or posterolateral portals to the joint can be made (Figure 14.6). The subacromial bursa is inspected initially. The bursa,

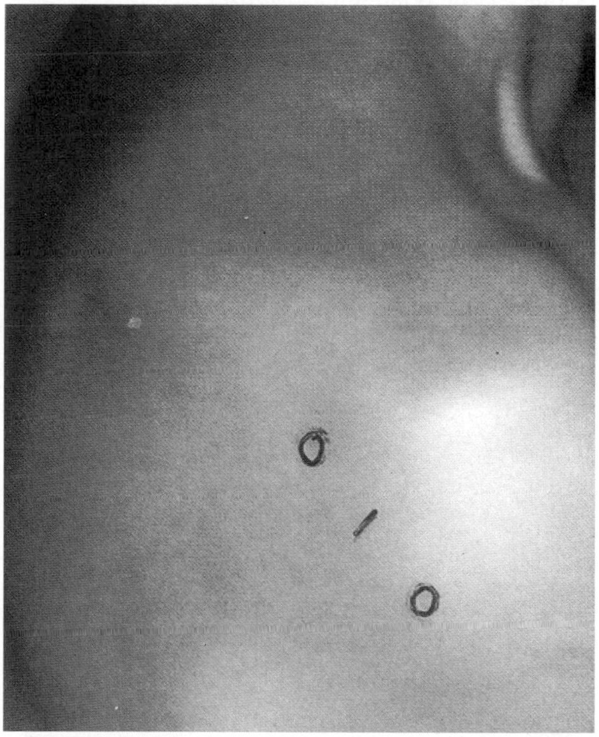

Figure 14.6 *Top circle*: posterior portal for glenohumeral arthroscopy; *middle line*: skin incision to create either portal; *bottom circle*: posterolateral portal for subacromial space. Anteriorly, skin incision is likewise placed between anterior glenohumeral portal and anterolateral subacromial portal, thus achieving 4 or more portals with 2 incisions.(Reproduced, with permission, from Watson, M.E., ed. (1991) *Surgical Disorders of the Shoulder.* Churchill Livingstone: London, Edinburgh, New York)

cuff, undersurface of acromion and coracoacromial ligament are inspected.

The glenohumeral joint is next visualized systematically, beginning with the biceps tendon (Figure 14.7). The tendon is followed to its exit through the rotator cuff. This is the most anterior part of the supraspinatus. Then the tendons of infraspinatus and teres minor, the superior, middle, inferior glenohumeral ligaments, the subscapularis tendon and recess (Figure 14.8) are inspected.

The condition of the labrum is noted circumferentially (Figure 14.9). If the posterior aspect of the joint is not well visualized or instrumentation is needed, an anterior portal is established (Figure 14.10).

In the hands of skilled shoulder arthroscopists, shoulder arthroscopy is employed in the management of unidirectional recurrent dislocations, decompression acromioplasty for stage II subacromial impingement and massive irreparable rotator cuff tears and has a limited role in the management of smaller complete tears where pain control is the primary issue (Gartsman, 1990).

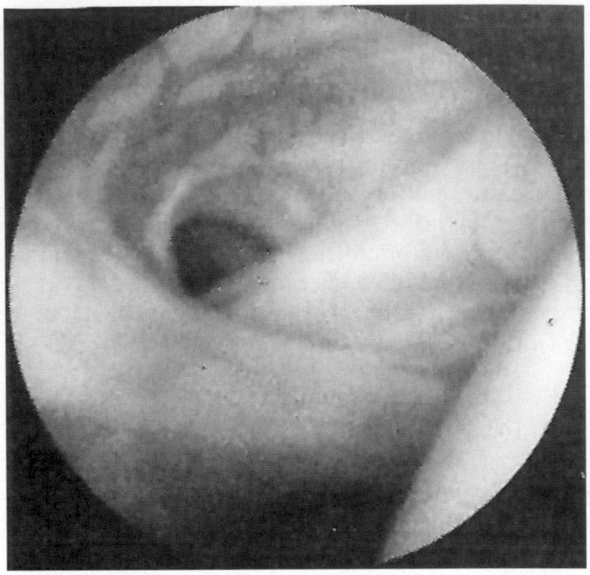

Figure 14.8 Advancing the arthroscope shows the subscapularis bursa above the subscapularis tendon and the middle glenohumeral ligament below this.

Sprain of the shoulder joint

A sprain or strain results when the shoulder joint capsule is wrenched and the normal limits of its movement are exceeded. Owing to the shallowness of the glenoid cavity, two abnormal movements may be produced at this joint – forward and backward movement of the humeral head in the glenoid cavity. These displacements may be caused by falls on the back or front of the shoulder, or upon the elbow or hand when directed backwards or forwards. The capsule, the synovial membrane or the ligaments may be stretched or torn, either alone or in combination. There is usually an extravasation of blood into the periarticular tissues, and occasionally the effusion may involve the tendon sheaths, especially of

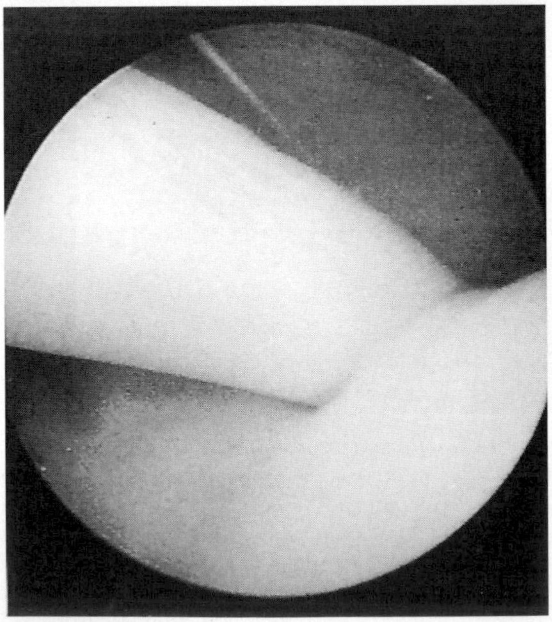

Figure 14.7 Right shoulder showing the long head of biceps entering the bicipital groove in the humeral head.

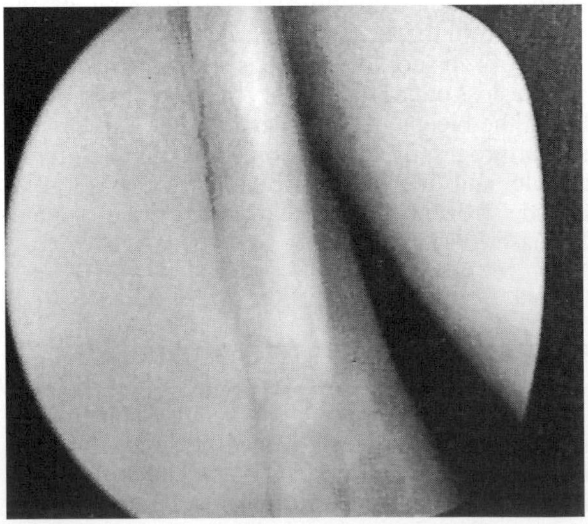

Figure 14.9 A normal labrum seen between the convex humeral head and the flatter glenoid surface.

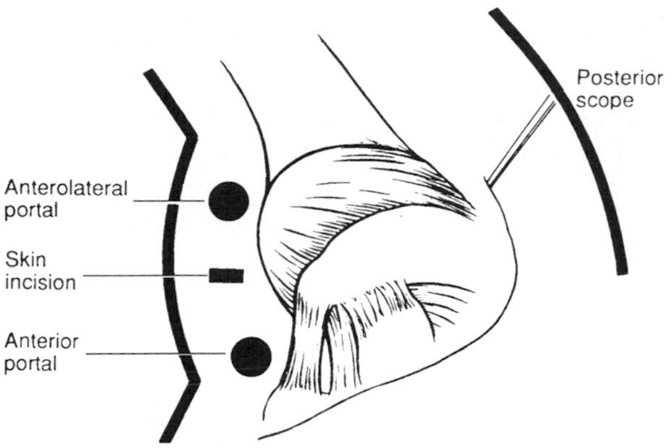

Figure 14.10 *Top left*: anterolateral portal for subacromial instruments; *middle*: skin incision to allow portal creation above and below; *bottom*: anterior portal for glenohumeral instruments; *top right*: the scope is posterior.

long heads of biceps, so that sprains of the shoulder are likely to be followed by periarticular fibrosis or adhesions. The shoulder region is swollen and painful, the pain being most intense when the patient attempts to move the joint in the direction which produced the injury.

Bloch and Fischer (1960) described 'scapulo-humeral periarthritis' as arising from:

1. Acute and chronic inflammatory processes, such as a bursitis, a bicipital tendovaginitis, tendinitis, calcareous deposits or rheumatic shoulder disease.
2. Trauma, contusions, sprains, fractures, dislocations, ruptures of the rotator cuff or of the long biceps tendon and tears of the capsule.
3. Extensive immobilization for fracture, infection or dislocation.
4. Referred pain from lesions elsewhere such as myocardial infarction, cervical spine disease, shoulder–hand syndrome and pulmonary lesions.

In arriving at a diagnosis, radiography and arthrography should be employed to exclude bone damage. Sprains of the shoulder may be incidental to some other more serious injury, such as Colles' fracture, and may pass unnoticed at the time.

In treating shoulder strains and contusions the troublesome complication is the formation of adhesions from prolonged immobilization. In the acute stage the arm is best rested in a triangular sling to give some support to the shoulder and to reduce movement. As soon as the acute pain has settled, however, active movement should be commenced initially for ordinary daily activities and, if stiffness persists, with the aid of physiotherapy including heat treatment.

Muscular strains in the shoulder region

It is difficult to distinguish the capsular strains from specific injuries to muscles about the shoulder. Injuries of the supraspinatus tendon are fairly common and will be dealt with later in this chapter. Injuries to the deltoid muscle, the biceps, the medial rotators and the lateral rotators are much less common.

DELTOID

When the deltoid muscle is partially torn, active abduction is either greatly restricted or painful. This is particularly so against resistance, whereas passive abduction is carried out painlessly. The lesion is usually the rupture of a few muscle fibres and settles rapidly spontaneously.

THE BICEPS

The main function of the biceps is to supinate the forearm and flex the arm at the shoulder joint with flexion of the elbow as an accessory movement. Bicipital lesions may take the form of a complete division of one of the muscles bellies, which is easily recognized. On contraction of the muscle an excessive swelling is seen in the belly of the muscle, which disappears during relaxation. When the tendon of the long head is injured, pain is experienced at the shoulder joint when the forearm is actively supinated, and there is tenderness over the tendon in the bicipital groove.

RUPTURE OF THE LONG HEAD OF THE BICEPS

This injury may follow violent activity in a young person but generally occurs in older individuals associated with spontaneous degeneration of the tendon together with a possible attrition of the tendon against osteophytes at the margin of the glenoid. It is a feature of the late stages of the shoulder impingement syndrome.

The clinical features are characteristic in that the patient may or may not have felt the tendon rupture but often observes that the biceps appear to have increased in size. This is most obvious when he flexes the elbow, as seen in Figure 14.11. Treatment is almost always conservative; in the older patient it

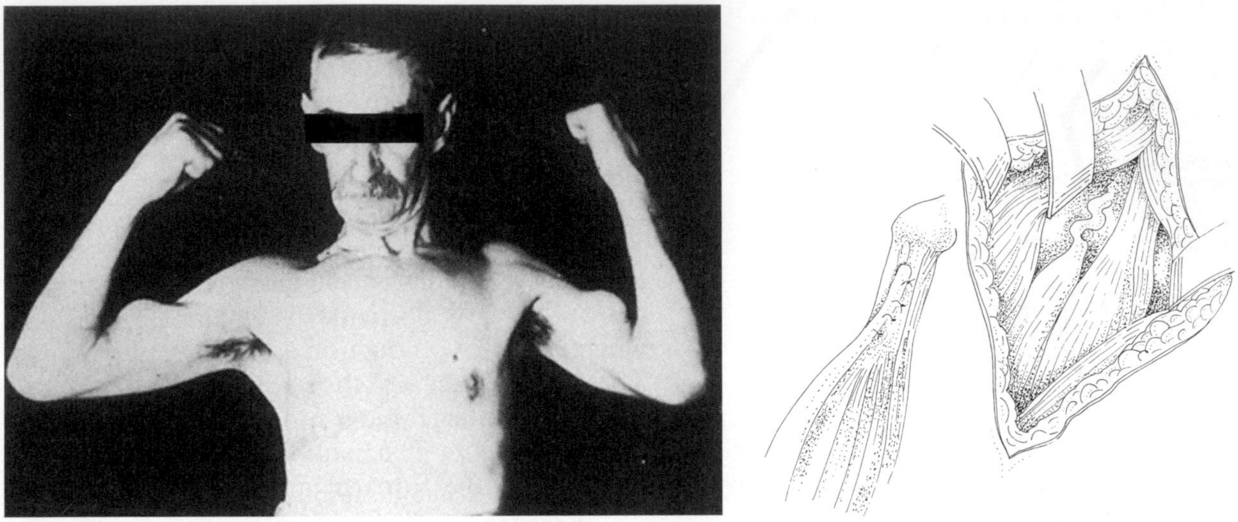

(a) (b)

Figure 14.11 (a) Bilateral rupture of the biceps through the long head, with the deformity being aggravated by forced flexion of the elbow joints. (b) The simple method of treatment of rupture of the long head of biceps by suturing the tendon to the short head. (b reproduced with permission from Helal, B. and Chen, S.C. (1979) Rupture of the biceps. In: *Operative Surgery*, 3rd edn, vol. *Orthopaedics*. Edited by G. Bentley. Butterworths: London and Boston

is difficult, if not impossible, to achieve repair of the tendon but the weakness is not considerable. Occasionally it may be worthwhile carrying out repair in the young patient; if repair cannot be achieved, then suture of the long head of the biceps into the bicipital groove under an osteoperiosteal flap is satisfactory (Figure 14.11).

Rarely, there may be avulsion of the distal end of the biceps from its insertion into the tubercule of the radius. Recurrent dislocation of the long head of the biceps may follow tearing of the bicipital fascia.

THE MEDIAL ROTATORS

Intermittent strain of the medial rotators (i.e. pectoralis major and the subscapularis) is probably very common. Total rupture, however, is extraordinarily rare, if it ever occurs. A period of reduced activity is all that is required to treat these injuries. Similarly, strain of the infraspinatus and the teres minor is rare since forcible internal rotation of the shoulder is rare, and requires simple rest.

Acute synovitis of the shoulder

Synovitis of the shoulder is less common than in the knee, but once present is very painful and sometimes difficult to treat. It may be caused by a contusion, or in association with inflammatory conditions such as rheumatoid arthritis and pseudogout or due to an acute staphylococcal infection. Chronic infections such as tuberculosis and osteoarthritis also may produce synovitis. The bicipital sheath is involved in such inflammation and, occasionally, the subdeltoid and subacromial bursae.

CLINICAL FEATURES

The joint will appear slightly swollen and movements in all directions are painful. The swelling tends to present anteriorly in the deltopectoral groove.

TREATMENT

Treatment of irritable shoulder follows the same principles as in other joints. Aspiration of the joint and arthroscopic washout is advisable in most cases to allow examination of the fluid for micro-organisms, crystals, etc. If clinically the shoulder is infected, the best treatment is immediate surgical drainage, leaving the capsule open but closing the overlying muscle and skin. Postoperative drainage is to be avoided due to the strong tendency of the shoulder to develop an open sinus. Following the aspiration or surgical drainage, the arm is supported in a triangular sling and anti-inflammatory drugs or antibiotics are given as required. When wound healing has occurred and irritability of the shoulder is absent on attempted active movement then progressively increased activities are allowed, including active movements under the supervision of a physiotherapist.

Bursitis

SUBDELTOID OR SUBACROMIAL BURSITIS

The subacromial bursa lies under the upper part of the deltoid muscle and extends upwards underneath the acromion process. It separates the greater tuberosity of the humerus from the deltoid muscle, the acromion process and the coracoacromial ligament (Figure 14.12). This bursa serves to reduce friction and to permit the greater tuberosity of the humerus to rotate inwards under the acromion process in movements of abduction and rotation of the shoulder.

The peripheral portions of the bursa are loose and redundant, and this permits the floor of the bursa to glide under the roof during movement. The layers of the bursa are normally approximated but enough fluid is secreted to keep them moist and lubricated.

Inflammation of the bursa occurs practically always as a consequence of a lesion involving neighbouring structures. Codman (1934) said that to describe subacromial bursitis as an entity would be equivalent to describing peritonitis as an entity. It is not a structure where disease starts, so much as a structure which limits disease in the adjacent structures by temporary adhesions causing fixation of the parts. In the bursa the source of most of the pathological changes is the structure forming the larger part of its floor, particularly the supraspinatus element of that structure. Owing to the peculiar mechanics of the shoulder joint, the relatively avascular and inert supraspinatus tendon is the most vulnerable part of the joint. Inflammation in it may be painless until the adjacent bursa is involved which, being abundantly supplied with vessels and nerves, produces the symptoms of which the patient complains.

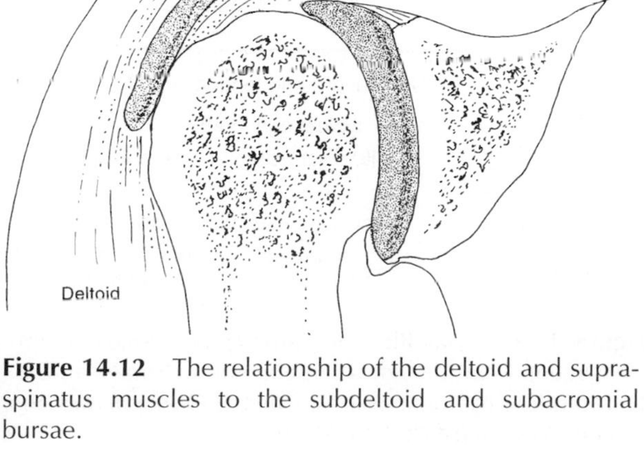

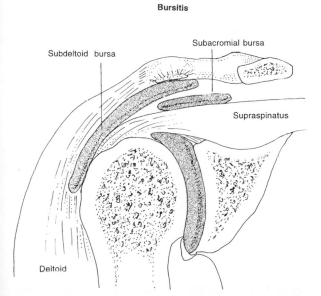

Figure 14.12 The relationship of the deltoid and supraspinatus muscles to the subdeltoid and subacromial bursae.

CLINICAL FEATURES

Pain in the shoulder is felt on abduction and internal rotation of the humerus, with severe aching at night and tenderness over the anterior aspect of the humeral head. Pain on movement may be of all grades of intensity, and is usually felt near the insertion of the deltoid muscle rather than in the joint itself, although it may radiate widely.

Usually there is a point of tenderness on the greater tuberosity, disappearing under the acromion on abduction (Dawbarn's sign). This tenderness may be absent or it may be widespread over the deltoid region.

In some cases the patient gives a history of an injury to the shoulder. This usually takes the form of a fall on the outstretched arm or the point of the shoulder (stubbed shoulder). When the pain follows an injury there is usually an interval of a few days before it manifests itself.

x-Rays may also show calcareous deposits in the supraspinatus tendon.

SUBCORACOID BURSITIS

The subcoracoid bursa is situated between the tip of the coracoid process and the capsule of the shoulder joint: it extends up to and even over the lesser tuberosity of the humerus. Normally the humerus and the coracoid are closely applied to each other, the tip of the latter resting against, or being opposite, the lesser tuberosity of the humerus. It follows that though this bursa is not particularly exposed to external violence, it is distinctly liable to suffer derangement through irritation from the pressure of the lesser tuberosity against the coracoid when the arm is used a great deal.

The patient complains of pain in the region of the

coracoid and there is definite tenderness over the interval between the two bones. Late cases, in which adhesions are present, have marked limitation of lateral rotation and abduction. A diagnostic injection of 5 ml of 1% lignocaine with hydrocortisone into this area may be of considerable help, by producing relief from pain.

TREATMENT

In an acute case, rest of the shoulder in a triangular sling together with anti-inflammatory drugs such as aspirin will effect relief, in many cases, over the course of a week. In cases which fail to settle, the injection of 1% lignocaine plus hydrocortisone solution into the tender bursa is helpful. This, of course, should not be carried out if any question of infection exists. In cases of persistent bursitis, exploration and excision of the inflamed bursa may be carried out and any associated calcified deposits in the supraspinatus tendon are removed.

Lesions of the supraspinatus tendon

The superior and the posterior portions of the capsule of the shoulder joint are strengthened by the incorporation of the flat expanded tendons of the supraspinatus, the infraspinatus and the teres minor. These tendons form a thick continuous fibrous sheet fused with the underlying capsule of the shoulder joint and separated from the deltoid and the acromion process by the subdeltoid and subacromial bursae.

The supraspinatus lies superiorly, and forms the roof of the joint as well as the floor of the subacromial bursa. Complete rupture of its tendon occurs usually in close proximity to the greater tuberosity. The muscle then retracts, leaving a direct communication between the bursa and the joint. The gap between the edges varies. There are, as a rule, degenerative changes in the intact portion of the supraspinatus and in the infraspinatus tendon.

In addition to such extensive ruptures, it is probable that smaller tears occur frequently, involving only a few of the tendon fibres.

AETIOLOGY

With every abduction movement of the shoulder there is friction and contact of the supraspinatus tendon against the acromion process. The subcoracoid bursa from its position minimizes this friction. As age advances, the bursal protection becomes inadequate and degenerative changes occur from the constantly repeated trauma. The fibres become worn, and rupture of 'tendinitis' results. As the tendon is avascular, calcareous deposits may occur and produce calcification. When either of these conditions occurs, a partial or complete rupture may easily result.

Rockwood (1981) has emphasized that a sequence of changes occurs, resulting in the 'shoulder impingement syndrome' which produces tendinitis and rupture of the supraspinatus tendon. With increasing age there may be formation of a traction osteophyte on the anteroinferior border of the acromion. During flexion and abduction of the shoulder the greater tuberosity and its overlying supraspinatus tendon impinge on the coracoacromial ligament and the osteophyte.

Three progressive stages of the impingement syndrome are described (Neer, 1983) (Figure 14.13):

1. In stage I reversible oedema and haemorrhage are present in a patient under the age of 25 years.

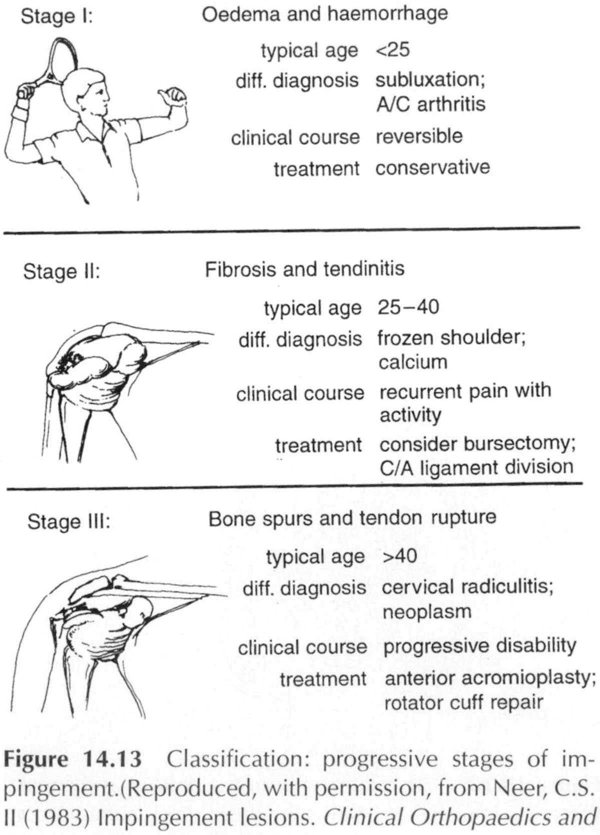
Stage I:
Oedema and haemorrhage
typical age <25
diff. diagnosis subluxation; A/C arthritis
clinical course reversible
treatment conservative
Stage II:
Fibrosis and tendinitis
typical age 25–40
diff. diagnosis frozen shoulder; calcium
clinical course recurrent pain with activity
treatment consider bursectomy; C/A ligament division
Stage III:
Bone spurs and tendon rupture
typical age >40
diff. diagnosis cervical radiculitis; neoplasm
clinical course progressive disability
treatment anterior acromioplasty; rotator cuff repair

Figure 14.13 Classification: progressive stages of impingement.(Reproduced, with permission, from Neer, C.S. II (1983) Impingement lesions. *Clinical Orthopaedics and Related Research* **173**, 70–77)

2. In stage II fibrosis and tendinitis affect the rotator cuff of a patient typically 25–40 years of age and this may settle with conservative treatment (not more than two to three steroid injections) or may require surgical decompression.
3. In stage III bone spurs and tendon ruptures are present in a patient over the age of 40 and surgical decompression with cuff repair is usually indicated.

Rarely the tendon of the long head of biceps may be impinged upon and ruptured at a later stage.

Tendinitis of the supraspinatus tendon

Those affected are in the age range 20–40 years and are frequently athletic.

The symptom complex often follows a history of a minor sprain, and the patient presents complaining of pain in the outer aspect of the shoulder and over the deltoid insertion. There is tenderness over the greater tuberosity at the insertion of the supraspinatus tendon. Movements are usually not limited but there is an arc of abduction between 60° and 120° which is acutely painful and apparently is at the point where the tender area impinges against the margin of the acromion (Figure 14.14). There is again sharp pain through the same arc from 120° to 60° on lowering the arm from the abducted position. There is no abnormality on x-ray. In true capsulitis or arthritis the pain continues throughout the movement as well as during rotation.

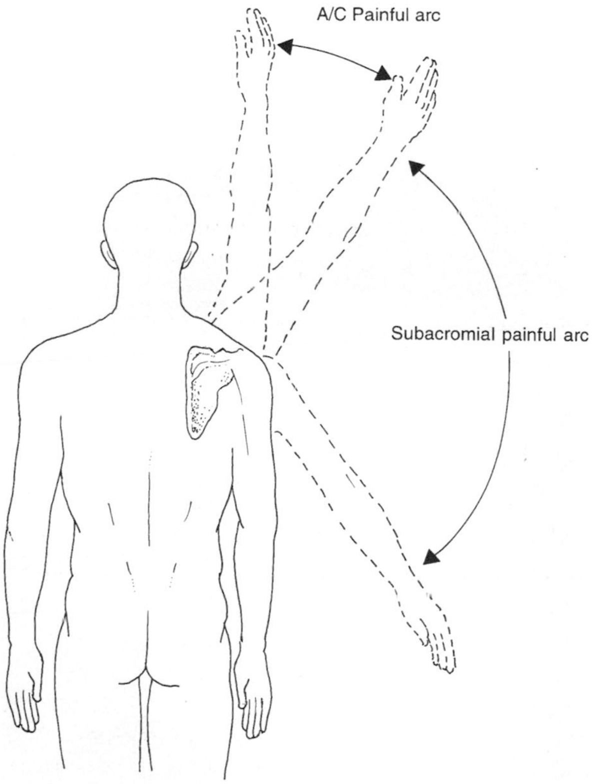

Figure 14.14 The painful arcs associated with subacromial pathology and acromioclavicular joint pathology. (Reproduced, with permission, from Kessel, L. and Watson, M. (1977) *Journal of Bone and Joint Surgery* **59B**, 166–172)

TREATMENT

In the early stages when the shoulder is painful it is best to rest it in a triangular sling and to administer anti-inflammatory drugs such as aspirin. In addition, the injection of 1% lignocaine plus hydrocortisone solution into the tender area frequently relieves pain over the course of a few days. It is argued that such treatment may weaken the tendon and precipitate rupture, but the disability from such treatment has not been proven. When the acute pain has subsided over the course of 2 weeks gentle active exercises of a pendulum type may commence with progressive reduction in the use of the sling. The condition may take 6–18 months to settle and further injections may be required, but complete resolution is the rule with only terminal loss of movement. If the shoulder is stiff when the pain has subsided, careful manipulation under general anaesthetic, and under the cover of non-steroidal anti-inflammatory agents, is useful.

Calcification of the supraspinatus tendon

The formation of calcareous deposits overlying the tip of the greater tuberosity of the shoulder has long been recognized. The deposits almost invariably originate in the tendocapsular structures and in the supraspinatus tendon near its insertion. Whether or not the deposit gives rise to painful symptoms would seem to depend upon its having reached the tissue layer beneath the bursal wall which, being richly supplied with nerves and vessels, is capable of reacting in the usual manner and of transmitting painful stimuli. When the deposit lies deep in the tendinous structure, it causes no symptoms.

The condition occurs in adults of all ages, and

there is usually a history of injury. The condition may pursue an acute course, the trauma being followed by severe and constant pain, or the injury may recover from and be so mild that it causes nothing more than a transient pain and stiffness. Later the patient may develop gradually increasing stiffness, with pain on abduction to a right angle and a constant ache over the greater tuberosity.

The radiographic appearances are characteristic. There is a small, rather discrete, uneven and irregular shadow over the greater tuberosity in the region of the supraspinatus tendon, though there is some variation in the location of the shadow (Figure 14.15). This can be distinguished from a loose body in the joint because it lies too far out to be intra-articular. In addition to the shadow, the greater tuberosity shows a greater or lesser degree of osteoporosis.

PATHOLOGY

The material is composed of non-crystalline calcareous matter embedded in a mass of inflammatory cells containing foreign body giant cells. In older cases well formed fibrous tissue is present. Cultures taken at the time of operation are sterile, and the biochemical examination of the contents shows the presence of amorphous calcium carbonate and phosphate. Cholesterol also may be present but the test for uric acid is negative. The material in the early stage is creamy in consistency, then like toothpaste, and only finally frankly calcareous.

The deposits are probably the result of degenerative changes in the dense avascular fibrous tissue from preceding tendinitis and not unlike that seen in arteriosclerosis. Biochemically there appears to be some relationship between the seeding of the calcium complexes and the avascularity and the degenerative changes within the tendon, as suggested in 1910 by Wells. However, this metaplastic calcification mechanism is ill-understood.

TREATMENT

In acute cases, immobilization in a simple triangular sling to prevent dependency of the limb and aspirin therapy are sometimes associated with disappearance of the deposit and the subsidence of the inflammatory process. At the same time, short-wave therapy or radiant heat are of benefit. Active exercises are encouraged as soon as possible.

The results of surgical excision of the deposits are definite and the relief conferred upon patients with the acute type of symptoms is so immediate and so

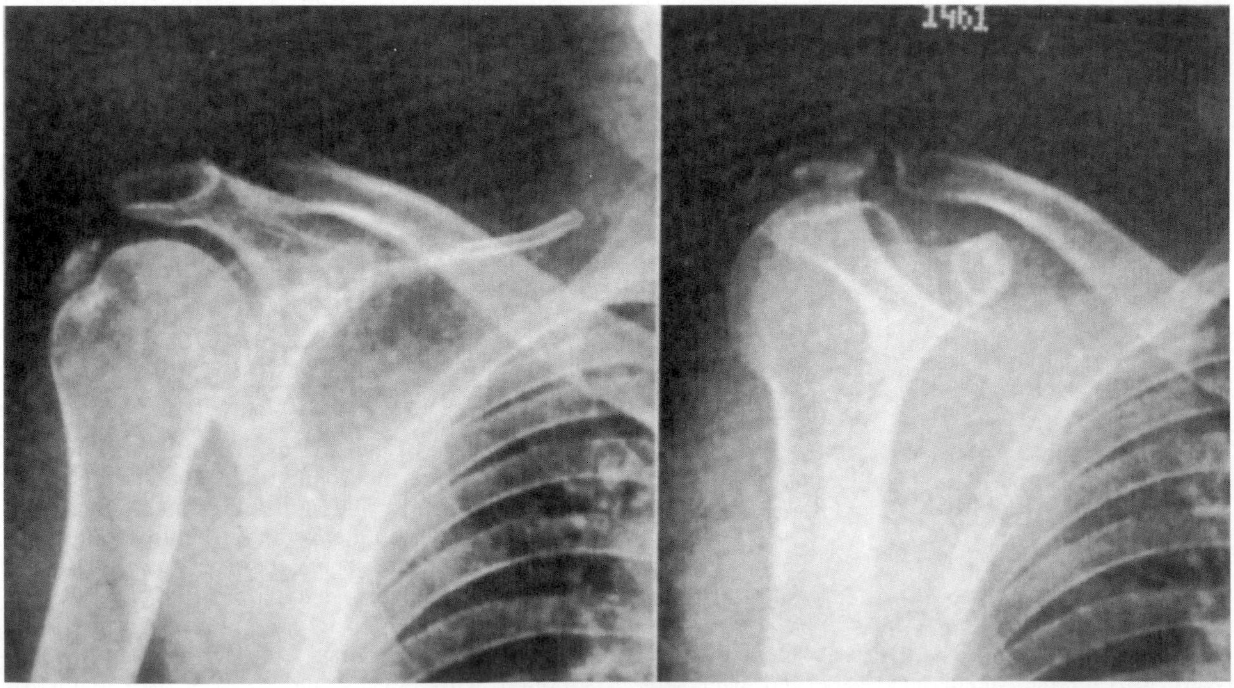

(a) (b)

Figure 14.15 (a) Calcified supraspinatus tendinitis just above the insertion of the tendon, with some underlying bone reaction of the humerus. (b) Adduction and rotation of the shoulder, showing how the calcified area has moved under the acromion process, where it is masked.

great that there is much to recommend it.

The material is usually too thick to be removed by aspiration. The tendon is exposed by an anterior incision, and the deposit removed with a sharp curette. There is immediate relief from the pain and full active exercises can be practised as soon as wound healing has occurred.

Types and incidence of cuff tear

Rotator cuff tears are uncommon before the age of 40. The vast majority of tears are the chronic attritional type. Cuff tears occurring as a direct result of a specific injury are unusual. They may occur as a part of anterior dislocation in patients over the age of 40 (Neviaser, 1975). There is frequently no traumatic cause the patient can remember, although acute extension of a chronic tear can occur after trauma. Chronic tears are also a feature of rheumatoid disease.

Those tears with a communication between the bursa and the joint are called complete tears, and those with no communication as incomplete tears which are further subclassified into bursal, intratendinous and joint side tears (Fukuda, 1990) (Figure 14.16). Complete tears are divided into various sizes, measured in its longest diameter; a small tear is defined as less than 1 cm, a medium size tear as 1–3 cm, a large tear 3–5 cm and a massive tear as more than 5 cm usually with retraction of the torn cuff.

The incidence of rotator cuff tears in cadavers has been variously reported with a range of 6–19% for complete tears and 6–33% for incomplete tears. Neer (1983) reported the incidence of complete tears in a 500 cadaveric study to be 5%. In 122 autopsy dissections with an average age of 79 Jerosch *et al.* (1991) reported that the incidence of partial rotator cuff tears was 28.7% and complete tears 30.3.%. The incidence increased with age and women had a higher prevalence. Fukuda (1990) showed that of the incomplete tears intratendinous tears were the most frequent followed by joint side followed by bursal side tears. There is therefore a significant proportion of the population over the age of 50 with compensated asymptomatic rotator cuff tears which with minor trauma may become decompensated or convert into a larger tear.

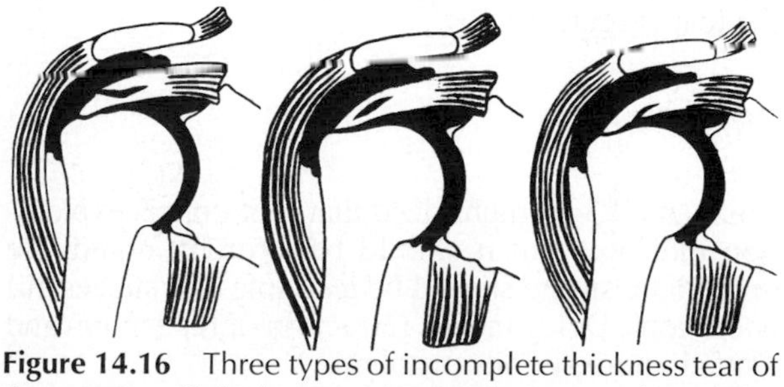

Figure 14.16 Three types of incomplete thickness tear of the rotator cuff; the bursal side tear, the intratendinous tear and the joint side tear (rim rent).(Reproduced, with permission, from Fukuda, H. (1990) *Current Orthopedics* **4**, 225–232)

Partial rupture of the supraspinatus tendon

An incomplete rupture of the tendon is a common sequel to tendinitis, though often not diagnosed. It is said to be present in no less than 30% of all cadavers.

Pain is complained of over the shoulder and radiates down the circumflex nerve to the deltoid insertion. Tenderness is present over the insertion of the tendon. Abduction is usually possible though there is pain when the torn fibres impinge under the acromion. Abduction can easily be prevented by resistance.

TREATMENT

Immobilization in an abduction splint may be tried in the early stages for 2 weeks. If no symptomatic improvement is produced, the tendon is exposed by operation and the tear repaired as in complete rupture (see below). If there is little evidence of a tear, the subdeltoid bursa is fully explored and any hyperaemic fringes and the bursal wall removed. If nothing more than tendinitis is found then the tendon is scarified to attempt to produce revascularization, and this usually relieves the symptoms.

Rupture of the supraspinatus tendon and the rotator cuff

The actual tear may be associated with only slight pain, but there is immediate weakness of the arm and the patient is unable to abduct the shoulder. Occasionally a definite 'crack' in the shoulder accompanies the pain at the moment of injury. Localized tenderness can be elicited over the tip of the greater tuberosity, or just medial to it, but it disappears when the arm is abducted because the tuberosity then passes beneath the acromion. Attempts at active movement may be accompanied by coarse crepitation in the region of the bursa, and by a characteristic 'abduction' painful arc syndrome. After complete rupture, the patient sometimes cannot voluntarily perform the first 15° of abduction but can complete the movement if the first stage is performed for him or if he leans towards the affected side. However, he cannot abduct beyond 60° and, when attempting to do so, there is marked elevation of the whole shoulder girdle.

When the patient is inspected as he stands with his arms at the sides and elbows pulled backwards, the tuberosity of the humerus may appear unduly prominent on the injured side and a sulcus may be seen proximal to the tuberosity where the tendon should be. In the sulcus there is usually a tender spot which rotates with the humerus and disappears under the acromion when the humerus is abducted.

DIAGNOSIS

The primary diagnostic sign is a greater limitation of active (60°) than of passive abduction in the presence of a normally contracting deltoid. Normal abduction cannot be carried out by the deltoid alone; the supraspinatus is an essential synergist. If the supraspinatus is inactive, strong contraction of the deltoid pushes the humeral head up towards the acromion (Figure 14.17) and holds it there while the scapula rotates. Scapular movement accounts for some 50° of abduction, but there is no true abduction at the shoulder joint. The deltoid can be felt strongly contracting, thus excluding circumflex paralysis, and since passive movement is possible adhesions cannot be the cause. The wince of pain at 90–100° abduction as the limb is raised or lowered passively, and the tenderness on pressure over the insertion of the supraspinatus, clinch the diagnosis (Figure 14.18).

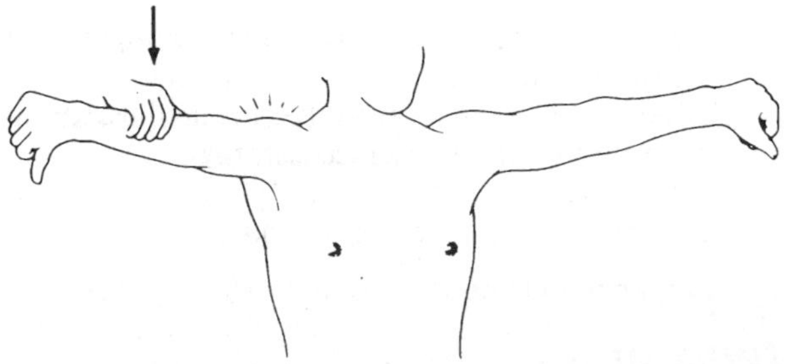

Figure 14.17 Jobe test: in impingement the patient will signal pain when the arm is depressed from 90° of abduction and 30° of forward flexion (Reproduced, with permission, from Watson, M. (1991) *Surgical Disorders of the Shoulder.* Churchill Livingstone: Edinburgh, London, New York

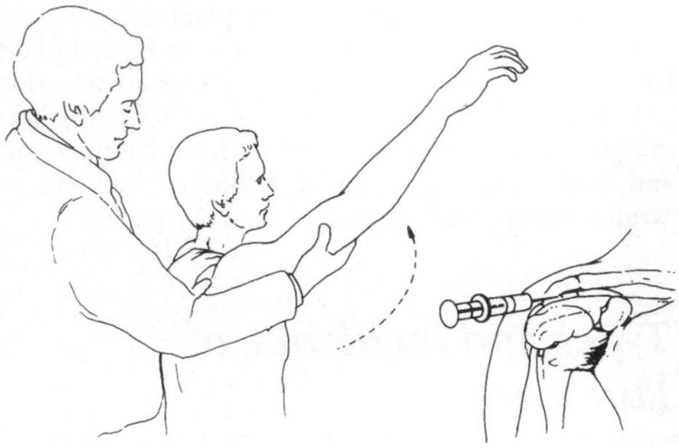

Figure 14.18 Diagnosis of impingement lesions. (Reproduced, with permission from Neer, C.S. II (1983) Impingement lesions. *Clinical Orthopaedics and Related Research* **173**, 70–77)

The 'impingement sign' is elicited with the patient seated and the examiner standing. Scapular rotation is prevented with one hand while the other hand raises the arm in forced forward elevation, causing the greater tuberosity to impinge against the acromion. This manoeuvre produces pain in patients with impingement lesions of all stages. It also causes pain in many other shoulder conditions. In the case of the impingement lesions, however, the pain caused by this manoeuvre is relieved by the injection of 10.0 ml of 1.0% xylocaine beneath the anterior acromion. The test is useful in separating impingement lesions of all stages from other causes of shoulder pain. See Figure 14.18.

Arthrography, by injecting a radiopaque substance, may aid in outlining the severity of the rupture by demonstrating the spillage of dye through the tear (Figure 14.19).

TREATMENT

Codman (1934) emphasized that 'not only is exploration indicated but it should be strongly urged, for immediate suture should be a simple and successful operation'. Delay means retraction of the tendon and a much more serious problem.

The conservative treatment for rotator cuff disease is effective in relieving inflammation in all stages. However, if the cuff is torn, satisfactory results can be expected in only approximately 50% or less of

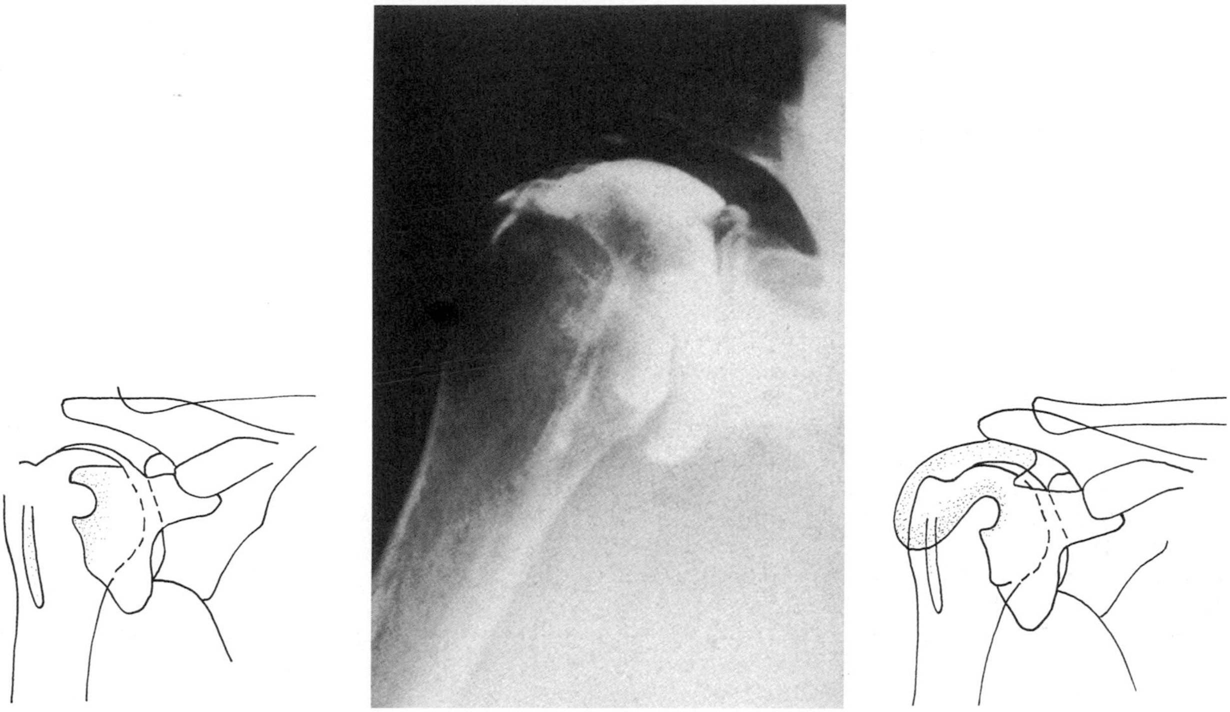

(a) (b) (c)

Figure 14.19 (a) Diagrammatic representation of a normal shoulder arthrogram. (b) Radiograph of normal arthrogram. (c) Diagram demonstrating the leakage of dye from the main shoulder joint cavity through a tear in the supraspinatus into the subacromial bursa. (Reproduced, with permission, from Kessel, L. (1979) Rotator cuff injury of the shoulder. In: *Operative Surgery*, 3rd edn, vol. 1. *Orthopaedics*. Edited by G. Bentley. Butterworths: London and Boston)

such patients as spontaneous healing of the torn cuff tendon has not been substantiated (Fukuda, 1990).

Conservative treatment consists of rest and avoidance of harmful or provocative motions but not inactivity. In tendon or bursal inflammation, rest, cold or heat, massage, non-steroidal anti-inflammatory medication, modification of activity, gentle exercises for maintaining and increasing range of motion and later muscle strengthening are methods of treatment. The judicious use of no more than three or four steroid injections into the subacromial space can be useful.

Itoi and Tabata (1992), however, reported their results in 54 patients with full thickness rotator cuff tears treated conservatively. They concluded that conservative treatment is effective when applied early. Short- and mid-term results were satisfactory, but the long-term results were likely to be less satisfactory.

Surgical treatment historically consisted of complete or lateral acromionectomy. These procedures weakened the deltoid and in 1972 Neer described anterior acromioplasty for chronic impingement problems with the objective of increasing the space for the supraspinatus tendon. In this procedure the anterior edge of the acromion and its undersurface are removed with an osteotome as a wedged-shaped piece of bone including the entire attachment of the coracoacromial ligament (Figure 14.20).

Resection of the acromioclavicular joint was added in three situations:

1. When the acromioclavicular joint is arthritic and symptomatic.
2. When more exposure of the supraspinatus is needed for mobilization and repair.
3. When the acromioclavicular joint is enlarged and impinges on the supraspinatus.

In the management of rotator cuff tears the best long-term pain relief and return to function are seen following tendon repair following adequate decompression of the subacromial space. Small and medium size tears are managed by debridement and direct tendon repair to bone. A trough is made in the sulcus between the head and the tuberosity, sutures are placed through drill holes and the cuff is reattached. A watertight anastomotic repair which

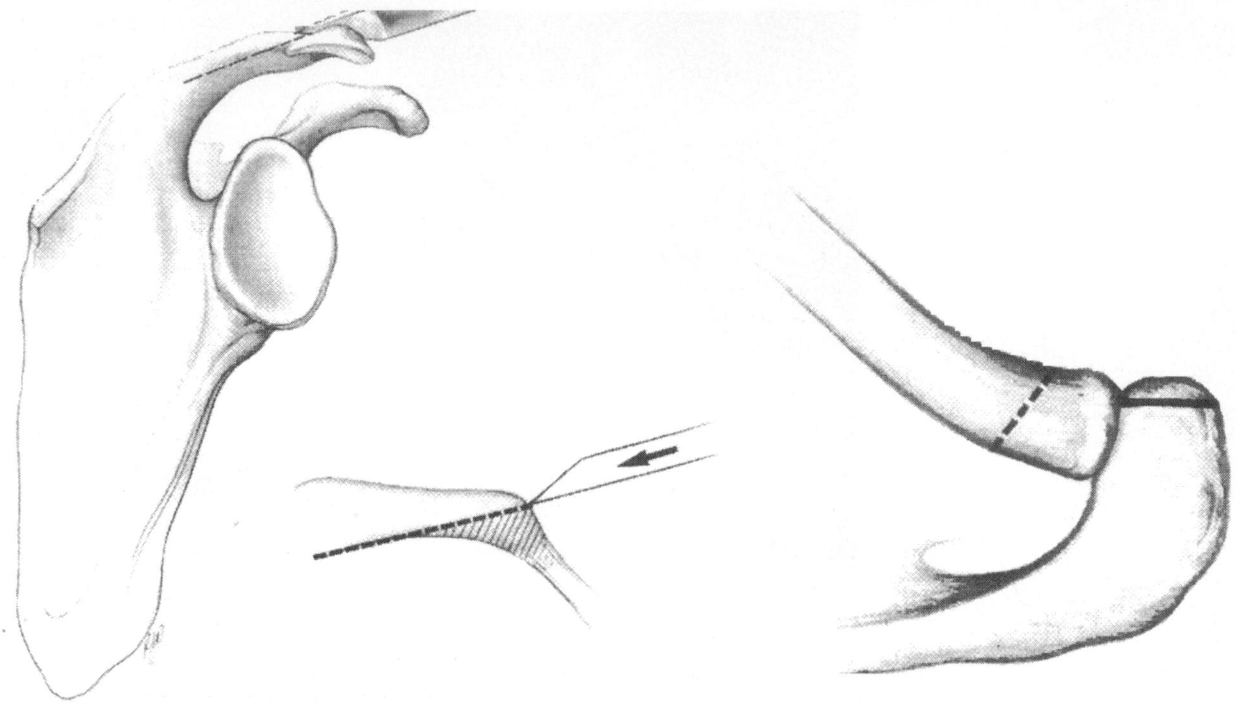

Figure 14.20 Depicting the removal of anterior lip and undersurface of acromion. (Reproduced, with permission, from Neer, C.S.J. (1983) *Clinical Orthopaedics and Related Research* **173**, 70–77)

provides maximum restoration of dynamic rotator cuff function and contains the synovial fluid for adequate joint cartilage nutrition is best. Arthroscopic debridement versus open repair for this group of tears (1–4 cm) showed the open repair group to have much better function but arthroscopic debridement was useful in low demand patients for pain relief and improved range of movement (Ogilvie-Harris and Demazière, 1993). Arthroscopic assisted rotator cuff repair has been reported (Snyder, 1993) for small tears where arthroscopic debridement is followed by cuff release and the use of special suture passers to get a purchase on the cuff and then a small incision is made and a suture anchoring device screwed in. Long-term results are awaited.

In 1985 Ellman reported 88% good to excellent results in his initial 50 arthroscopic acromioplasties. Arthroscopic acromioplasty has proven to be comparable to open acromioplasty particularly in stage II lesions with the added advantage of shorter hospital stay and the quicker postoperative rehabilitation (Gartsman, 1990). Gartsman reported 94% satisfactory results for arthroscopic acromioplasty in stage II (at 32 month follow-up), 82% with partial tears and 56% with complete tears.

Large and massive tears where there is scarring, retraction and possible loss of substance are more complex but less complicated repair techniques are used whenever possible. Sometimes releasing the scarred tendons (with division of the coracohumeral ligament) is adequate for direct repair. If anastomotic repair is not possible after mobilization then a McLaughlin V-Y repair is used. Occasionally the long head of biceps tendon or the upper half of the subscapularis tendon is incorporated into the repair followed by rehabilitation in an abduction brace. Fascial grafts, muscle transfers, freeze dried rotator cuff and synthetic materials have been described for repair of massive defects but the results have not been predictable and the follow-up short.

Even in the case of rotator cuff tears which are impossible to repair because of their size and/or a degree of attrition of the rotator cuff, subacromial decompression will give the patient significant symptomatic relief, although the patient may not recover substantial amounts of movement.

Postoperatively, in the case of rotator cuff tears, a sling should be used for the first 4 weeks to allow daily mobilization of the elbow, wrist and hand whilst resting the shoulder joint. Thereafter, active mobilization together with hydrotherapy should be used to regain movement. Passive and resisted movements of the shoulder should be avoided.

In the case of subacromial decompression alone, active movement should be encouraged from the start.

Results of rotator cuff repairs are generally good. Essman *et al.* (1991) describe 91% satisfactory outcomes in 66 of 72 tears. In this series 17 of 72 tears were rated as 'massive', but only 4 were irreparable. Three of these four achieved excellent results with one good result.

Pigliani *et al.* (1992) reported their results in 23 tennis players. In all cases the dominant shoulder was involved and up to surgery all were unable to play tennis. By 42 months postoperative 83% achieved good results with pain-free shoulders and were able to play tennis at presymptomatic competitive level. Three cases (13%) had massive tears with satisfactory results, being able to return to tennis at a lower competitive level. These workers concluded that subacromial impingement may account for shoulder pain in active tennis players especially over 40 years of age. To return to sport at a high competitive level may require a prolonged and intensive rehabilitation programme.

Harryman *et al.* (1991) correlated functional results with cuff integrity in 105 rotator cuff repairs. If the tear is restricted to the supraspinatus, 80% of repairs are intact at 5 years, but if more than the supraspinatus tendon had been involved in the original tear, more than 50% had recurrent defects, although most of the patients were comfortable and satisfied with the results of operation. Provided that a large tear repair remains intact, the result is comparable to the result following the repair of a small tear.

Uhthoff and Sarkar (1991) emphasized the importance of retaining as much of the subacromial bursa as possible. Warner *et al.* (1992) warned against trying to mobilize too much of the rotator cuff in order to effect a repair, and that this may prejudice the suprascapular nerve on its neurovascular pedicle.

Prosthetic replacement for cuff tears

Arantz *et al.* (1991) described humeral head replacement by a Neer prosthesis for patients with preserved passive movement, normal deltoid function, loss of glenohumeral joint surface and sculpting of the coracoacromial arch. In patients with irreparable tears of the rotator cuff and irreparable deltoid muscle deficiencies, they recommended shoulder arthrodesis.

Laurence (1991) described a semi-constrained arthroplasty for patients with rotator cuff tears and glenohumeral joint damage. Complete pain relief was achieved in 31% of patients of those followed up, and minor discomfort in over half. Of 72 patients, 56 regained active use of the arm and 26 returned to gainful employment.

Gerber (1992) described latissimus dorsi transfers for patients with irreparable massive rotator cuff tears and reported 94% satisfactory pain relief at rest and 81% on exertion.

Subscapularis tears

This is a rare condition caused either by forceful hyperextension of the arm or external rotation of the adducted arm.

Patients describe anterior shoulder pain and weakness, but no instability. A 'lift-off test' is described. MRI scanning or ultrasonography may confirm the diagnosis. Gerber and Krushell (1991) described the repair of this condition as being difficult because of adhesion of the tendon to the brachial plexus.

Bicipital tendinitis

The long tendon of biceps is a very intimate component of the articular capsule of the shoulder joint and therefore is frequently involved by the inflammatory processes which affect this joint, particularly capsulitis. It also has a synovial sheath continuous with the shoulder and contained within the transverse ligament, and this in itself can undergo inflammatory change. Hyperaemia, oedema, cellular infiltration and finally fibrosis may go on to produce a marked thickening of the synovial membrane and adhesion formation.

The symptoms are of pain in the shoulder joint which can usually be differentiated by its localization in the vicinity of the bicipital groove. It can also be aggravated by forced resistance to flexion of the elbow joint and supination of the forearm. There is rarely any painful abduction arc present. The pathological process may go on so that the tendon becomes atrophied and necrotic enough to rupture. Usually the treatment consists of the injection of hydrocortisone and lignocaine, and rest by the use of a triangular sling for 2–3 weeks. It has a much better prognosis than the chronic inflammations involving the shoulder joint itself. Occasionally, it may give rise to persistent symptoms necessitating operation.

Crenshaw and Kilgore (1966) reviewed the surgical treatment of this condition and found that over 80% had gross changes in the tendon at the time of the operation. They emphasized that Speed's test of forward flexion of the shoulder against resistance with the elbow extended and the forearm supinated was often positive, with pain over the biceps tendon proximally. The basic operation was to fix or anchor the tendon within the bicipital groove or into the humeral head. Relief of severe pain was dramatic – often leaving a nagging pain – but 6 months were required to regain maximum shoulder motion.

'Frozen shoulder' or adhesive capsulitis

This condition accounts for far more cases of shoulder disability than does supraspinatus tendinitis. It affects males and females equally, over the age of 40 years. It is frequently accompanied by bicipital tendinitis.

The patient gives a history of having noticed a slight painful catch in the region of the shoulder and upper arm for several months. Gradually he has become aware of an inability to perform certain tasks or to participate in certain sports because of stiffness of the arm. Night pain, often awakening him from sleep, is a common complaint. Frequently it radiates down the arm to the hand but without being localized to any nerve distribution. Stiffness of the shoulder increases until all movement may be lost (i.e. 'frozen shoulder').

On examination there is a generalized tenderness about the shoulder and marked restriction of all movements but especially abduction and rotation, with pain if force is used. The x-ray examination is negative except for some osteoporosis.

This is one of the least understood syndromes, causing pain in the shoulder.

One of the earliest descriptions of the pathology of a frozen shoulder was by Neviaser (1945), who found thickened contracted capsule around the humeral head. Histology of the capsule showed fibrosis and inflammatory cells. DePalma (1953) considered that bicipital tenosynovitis played an important part because of the frequency of tenderness over the bicipital groove. This tenosynovitis has long been known – usually following a strain injury – and it responds usually to conservative treatment. DePalma operated on 42 such patients and found in each case that every tissue around the shoulder was implicated in a low-grade inflammatory process. This inflammatory process was of varying intensity and involved the gliding mechanism of the tendon. The adhesions within the sheath ranged from filmy, frail haemorrhagic adhesions to firm, dense bands of fibrous tissue binding the tendon firmly to the bicipital groove and to the undersurface of the rotator cuff. In such cases there was dramatic relief when the tendon became firmly attached to bone by strong fibrous adhesions. It is suggested also that in cases where there is a sudden cessation of symptoms, this occurs because the tendon ruptures.

McNab (1973) found alteration in the microvascular supply of the supraspinatus tendon, with changes in the infarcted tendon. Bulgen *et al.* (1976, 1978) found lowered immunoglobulins, reduced transformation of lymphocytes by phytohaemagglutinin, and an increased incidence of HLA B27 antigen.

Thompson and Compere (1959) wrote on 'iatrogenic stiff shoulders' and pointed out that, when the arm is held in adduction, there is a great tendency for the redundant shoulder capsule to become adherent. Reeves (1966a) demonstrated the reduced capacity of the shoulder with failure to fill the subcapsular bursa, bicipital tendon sheath and axillary pouch by arthrography, and the converse in post-traumatic shoulders. This results from immobilization in a sling for too long a period without adequate instruction to the patient to carry out shoulder exercises. It is seen frequently in older patients with Colles' fractures who have not been instructed to exercise the shoulder. In a survey of 130 patients with arm or hand injuries, 11 who had suffered no known injury to the shoulder were found to have less than normal motion of the shoulder. Pain results from the limitation of motion and, as attempts are made to stretch the frozen shoulder, further pain is produced. Therefore, there is much resistance by the patient to achieving greater movement.

Frozen shoulder is usually self-limiting but symptoms can persist for 6 months or more, and it takes many more months for all ranges of movements to return to normal.

TREATMENT

A frozen shoulder is apt to pass through three stages during its resolution. The first is the acutely painful phase when the best treatment is rest in a triangular sling plus injections of hydrocortisone and local anaesthetic into the most tender area. When the pain has subsided the second stage begins which is a period of stiffness and reduced pain. At this stage more active treatment may begin and we favour the use of manipulation under a general anaesthetic. This should be carried out carefully, with flexion first followed by gentle abduction. It is helpful to immobilize the shoulder in abduction post-manipulation and then to commence active physiotherapy movement after 4 or 5 days when all irritability has ceased. In the acutely painful stage the use of anti-inflammatory and analgesic drugs such as aspirin, flurbiprofen, etc., is also helpful.

In almost every case the pain of acute capsulitis disappears over the course of 12–18 months but in some patients residual terminal restriction of movement by about 20% is present. This rarely constitutes a severe disability.

Hsu and Chan (1991), in a prospective study for treatment of frozen shoulder by manipulation and physiotherapy, arthroscopic distension and physiotherapy, and physiotherapy alone, found the first two gave better results and recommended arthroscopic distension as a good alternative to manipulation.

Chronic disability is usually caused by degenerative arthritic change, either in the shoulder or in the acromioclavicular joint.

Milwaukee shoulder

The patient is usually elderly – over 65 years – with a long history of painful shoulders, limitation of movement and an occasional obvious swelling.

Radiography shows periarticular calcification, and exceptionally marked degenerative changes in the glenohumeral joint. McCarty and his co-workers (Garancis *et al.*, 1981; Halverson *et al.*, 1981; McCarty *et al.*, 1981) on aspirating the synovial fluid, found it to be viscous, with a low cell count of predominantly mononuclear distribution – a so-called 'non-inflammatory' effusion. In addition, these workers found spheroid-shaped masses of hydroxyapatite crystals, and collagenase and neutral protease activities were very high with floating collagen fibrils and degradation products. A synovial biopsy specimen showed evidence of osteochondromatosis with crystals in superficial areas and evidence of crystal phagocytosis within cells. It was this combination of a destructive arthritis in the presence of hydroxyapatite deposition and activated collagenase and neutral proteases which gave rise to this syndrome which they termed 'Milwaukee shoulder'.

Activated collagenase and neutral protease are thought to produce degradation of the articular cartilage by the crystal phagocytosis which triggers their release. See Chapter 11 for further discussion of this condition.

Recurrent dislocation of the shoulder

This is discussed in the following sections on: recurrent anterior dislocations; habitual anterior dislocation of the shoulder; recurrent posterior dislocation; recurrent dislocation of the acromioclavicular joint; and dislocations of the medial end of the clavicle.

Recurrent anterior dislocation of the shoulder

MECHANISM OF INJURY

The type of initial injury which is responsible for recurrent dislocation of the shoulder has been the subject of debate for years.

In 1926 and in 1938, Bankart stated: 'Recurrent dislocation has nothing whatever to do with ordinary traumatic dislocation. It is from the first an entirely different injury condition.' He described two types of injuries:

- *Type I* – following a fall on the abducted arm, the head is forced through the lowest weak part of the capsule. After reduction, the capsule heals rapidly and soundly, and dislocation never recurs.
- *Type II* – direct injury on the back of the shoulder or a fall on the elbow directed backward and outward. The humeral head is forced forward and shears the capsule from the scapular neck. This lesion rarely heals and is responsible for recurrent dislocation (Bankart lesion).

Other more recent studies have disproved these views. In only 29% of recurrent dislocation cases could a direct injury be recalled; in 30% a combined abduction and external rotation injury was responsible, flexion and external rotation in 24%, and a fall on an outstretched hand in 16% (Rowe, 1956).

Gallie and Le Mesurier (1948) stated rightly therefore that the mechanisms of injury causing recurrent dislocation are indistinguishable from those of ordinary traumatic dislocation.

Reeves (1968), in experimental studies on the tensile strength of the anterior capsule, described that in young people the weakest point was in the glenoid labral attachment but in the elderly the capsule and the subscapular muscle were the weakest points. He concluded that the age of the patient is important and not the mechanism of injury.

Hawkins and Mohtadi (1991) describe different clinical stages in recurrent anterior instability. They describe an initial dislocation followed by further dislocations, although between dislocations shoulder function is normal. In a second group they describe recurrent subluxation with intervening episodes of subluxation, and in a third group they describe recurrent subluxation with no previous documented anterior dislocation. The 'essential lesion' in recurrent instability continues to be a matter of debate and various studies have been carried out investigating the role of various different soft tissues and ligaments in glenohumeral instability (Howell and Kraft, 1991; Terry *et al.*, 1991; Harryman *et al.*, 1992).

A family history is present in 8–27% of the cases and only 30% are females (Rowe *et al.*, 1978). One cannot avoid the conclusion that hereditary anatomical variations are the basis of this atraumatic recurrent dislocation group, which may explain why these cases are frequently bilateral. In this group of atraumatic initial dislocation, a very high incidence of recurrent dislocation was observed (86%). In comparison, in traumatic dislocation the recurrence rate was only 57%.

AGE AT ONSET

Young athletic people aged 15–25 are most commonly involved. While acute dislocation of the shoulder was equally distributed, with small peaks at the ages of 10–20 and 50–60 (i.e. a mean age of 48), the mean age of patients with recurrent dislocation was 23 (Rowe, 1956). McLaughlin and MacLellan (1967) showed 96% of patients with recurrent dislocation below 30 and 90% of non-recurrent dislocations above 30. The age of first dislocation is therefore an important prognostic sign (Table 14.1).

Tsai *et al.* (1991) described 26 consecutive patients with unoperated anterior shoulder instability; 58% had occurred during sports activity, at an average of 23 ± 8 years. None had undergone a supervised rehabilitation programme. The average time lapse between initial dislocation and presentation was 7 years. Fifty-nine per cent of patients had restricted ability in sport because of impairment of instability, strength and range of movement.

PATHOLOGICAL BASIS

Although Bankart described the 'essential' lesion as stripping of the fibrocartilaginous labrum from the glenoid which did not heal and bone changes did not play a significant role in the causation of recurrent dislocation, very few investigators now agree with these views. Soon it was evident that in spite of meticulous search for this lesion during operation, there was a significant proportion of patients (85%) in whom it was not found (Rowe *et al.*, 1978).

Reeves (1966b), in an arthrographic study, demonstrated that after acute dislocation two different pathologies could be seen:

1. Rupture of the anterior or anteroinferior capsule.
2. Detached glenoid labrum and filling of the area beneath the subscapularis.

When the arthrogram was repeated after 10 days, no more leaking was observed in the first group. In the second group a repeat arthrogram was normal in 50% after 10 days and an additional 30% showed a normal arthrogram after 3 weeks. Two patients with abnormal arthrograms had a recurrent dislocation later. These findings supported Bankart's views that capsular ruptures heal quickly but detachment of the labrum and capsule from the glenoid does not heal in some cases.

Table 14.1 Differences between recurrent and non-recurrent dislocations

	Recurrent	Non-recurrent
Mean age	Early 20s	Late 40s
Mechanism of injury	No significant difference	
Pathology		
Bankart's lesion	Common (50–100%)	Uncommon (20–30%)
Hill–Sachs lesion	Common (50–100%)	Uncommon (20–30%)
Rupture of anterior capsule	Uncommon	Common
Rotator cuff injury	Rare	4–10%
Nerve injuries	2%*	10.5%†
Fracture of tubercle	0–7%	20–28%
Fracture of neck of humerus	Rare	8.9%
Fracture of coracoid	Rare	2%

* Morrey and Janes (1976)
† McLaughlin and MacLennan (1967)

HILL–SACHS LESION

Hill and Sachs (1940) emphasized the frequent occurrence of bone changes in the head of the humerus in the posterolateral aspect of its articular surface (Figure 14.21). That this can lead to dislocation has been described by several observers.

Nevertheless, the frequency and significance of these changes did not receive general recognition for many years because the defect is not shown on anteroposterior radiographs: serial radiographs in 60–80° of internal rotation are necessary. It is difficult to demonstrate the defect during operation.

Palmer and Widen (1948) found Hill–Sachs lesion in 60 patients with recurrent dislocation. Bankart's lesion was observed in 80%. They stated that Hill–Sachs lesion deserves the name 'essential lesion' and suggested reconstruction of the humeral head. As this procedure is not practical, however, one should reinforce the anterior part of the joint.

Rowe (1956) pointed out that the Hill–Sachs lesion is found in 10% of any trauma to the shoulder without dislocation, in 38% after initial dislocation and in 57% of the recurrent dislocations. His conclusions were that Hill–Sachs lesion contributed significantly to the instability of the joint and that the lesion increased in size with every recurrent dislocation.

ABNORMALITIES OF SUBSCAPULARIS AND OTHER MUSCLES

Defects of the subscapularis muscle have long been considered an important factor in the pathogenesis of recurrent shoulder dislocations.

Magnuson and Stack (1943) pointed out the importance of the muscle as a major defence against anterior dislocation.

Symeonides (1972) found, in 39 out of 46 patients, major damage to the subscapularis (displaced 5, narrow 4, signs of damage 30). The role of the capsule, subscapularis, glenoid labrum and Hill–Sachs lesion was examined in 180 cadaveric shoulders. Capsular damage of Hill–Sachs lesion was found not to affect the force required to dislocate the shoulders. Symeonides concluded that Hill–Sachs lesion does not produce instability as long as the subscapularis is intact. This lesion increases the instability once the subscapularis is divided. Finally, good results are achieved in any operation which shortens the subscapularis (Bankart, Putti–Platt, Magnuson–Stack, etc).

Despite this evidence, there is still debate on the incidence of the lesion and the method of examination of the subscapularis. In the work of Rowe *et al.* (1978) subscapularis attenuation was found in only 10% and rupture in 7%. Other muscle abnormalities, however, were also reported, including absence of pectoralis major and pectoralis minor arising from the lesser tuberosity.

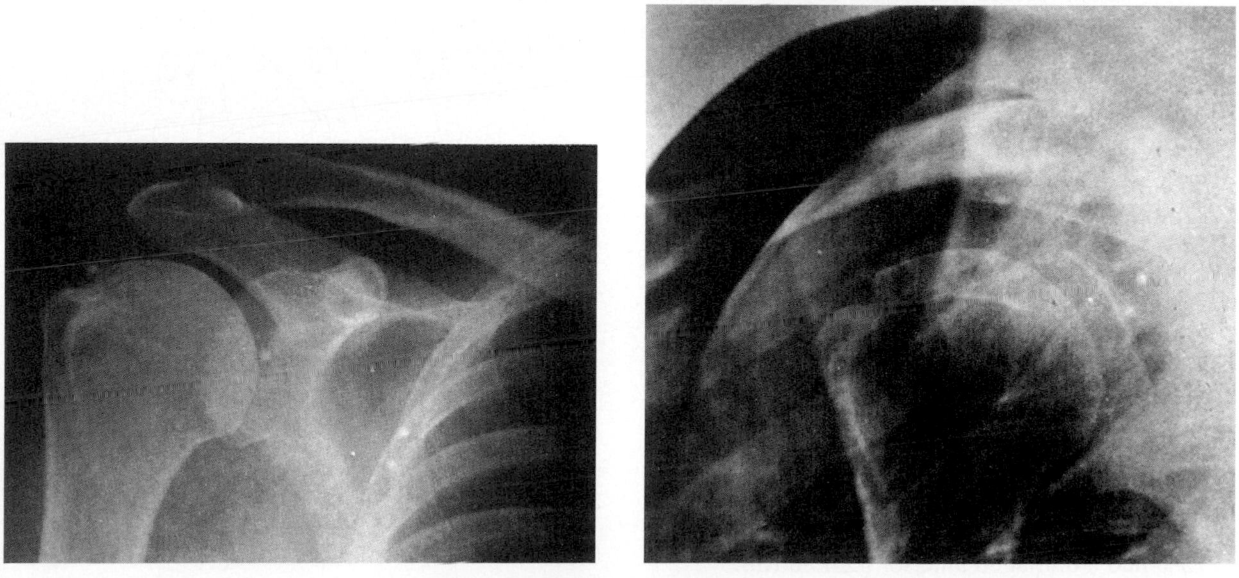

(a) (b)

Figure 14.21 (a) Anteroposterior radiograph and (b) a transthoracic view with the typical defect of a recurrent anterior dislocation of the right shoulder joint in the posterior aspect of the humeral head.

A loose capsule is a common finding. This may result from recurrent dislocation rather than the result of a healed ruptured capsule.

LABRUM AND GLENOID

The labrum and the glenoid can either be fractured or eroded, contributing to the instability. Erosion of the labrum was found in 73%, displacement of the labrum as a bucket-handle tear in 14% and the labrum was found to be intact but separate in 13% in Rowe's series (Rowe *et al.*, 1978). Fracture of the glenoid was found in 44% in this series, but other series reported have a lower incidence (e.g. 18%, Symeonides, 1972).

The most common operations now performed fall into four groups:

1. Repair of the Bankart lesion.
2. Reefing of subscapularis.
3. Repositioning of the coracoid process.
4. Bone grafting anteriorly.

Two important aspects are common to all these procedures – the first being a thorough inspection of the joint for loose bodies and the presence of degenerative changes, and the second division and repair of subscapularis.

Repair of Bankart lesion

The lesion was first described by Bankart in 1938, as was his operative repair. He reattached the labrum to the glenoid and reefed the lateral capsule onto the labrum under the medial capsule, merely resuturing subscapularis on top.

In a review of 161 patients operated upon over a 30-year span, Rowe *et al.* (1973) set down some valuable statistics:

- 86% of their patients had had a traumatic dislocation.
- 14% were atraumatic.
- 12% were bilateral, only 1 being repaired.
- 3.5% overall had a recurrence.
- 70% had complete external rotation and full abduction.
- 21% had 75% of full range of movement; there was no increased incidence of recurrence or instability with increased range of movement.
- 86% of their patients had separation of the anterior glenoid rim.
- 77% had Hill–Sachs lesion.
- 73% had a damaged anterior glenoid rim.
- 14.2% did not have a Bankart's lesion.
- 17% showed subscapularis laxity and/or rupture.

They concluded that the strongest reinforcement of the capsule was along the glenoid rim and this was the first line of defence against a recurrence.

Bankart operation

Since the dislocation is due to the wide detachment of the glenoid labrum from the anterior margin of the glenoid cavity, the operation is directed to the repair of this defect.

The incision is made from the clavicle above the coracoid and extends 12 cm down the anterior border of the deltoid muscle. This muscle is separated from the pectoralis major, avoiding the cephalic vein and exposing by retraction the coracoid and the muscles inserted into it. The coracoid process is now divided with an osteotome in a downward direction at its tip and the attached muscles are displaced forwards. On lateral rotation of the humerus the subscapularis is exposed and its tendon divided about 2 cm from its insertion into the lesser tuberosity. The anterior margin of the glenoid cavity will be found to be rounded, smooth and free of any attachments, and a blunt instrument can be freely passed inwards over the bare bone on the front of the neck of the scapula. If the capsule

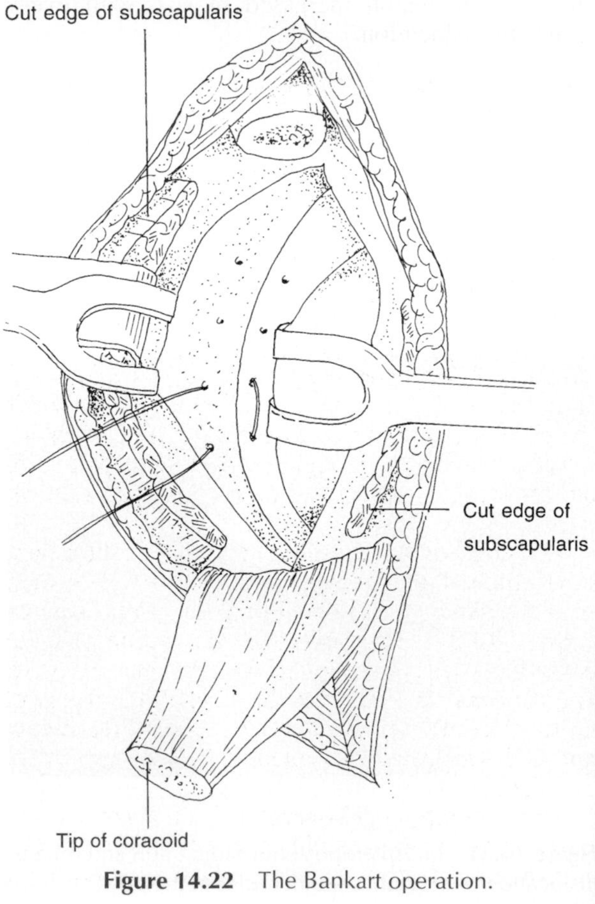

Figure 14.22 The Bankart operation.

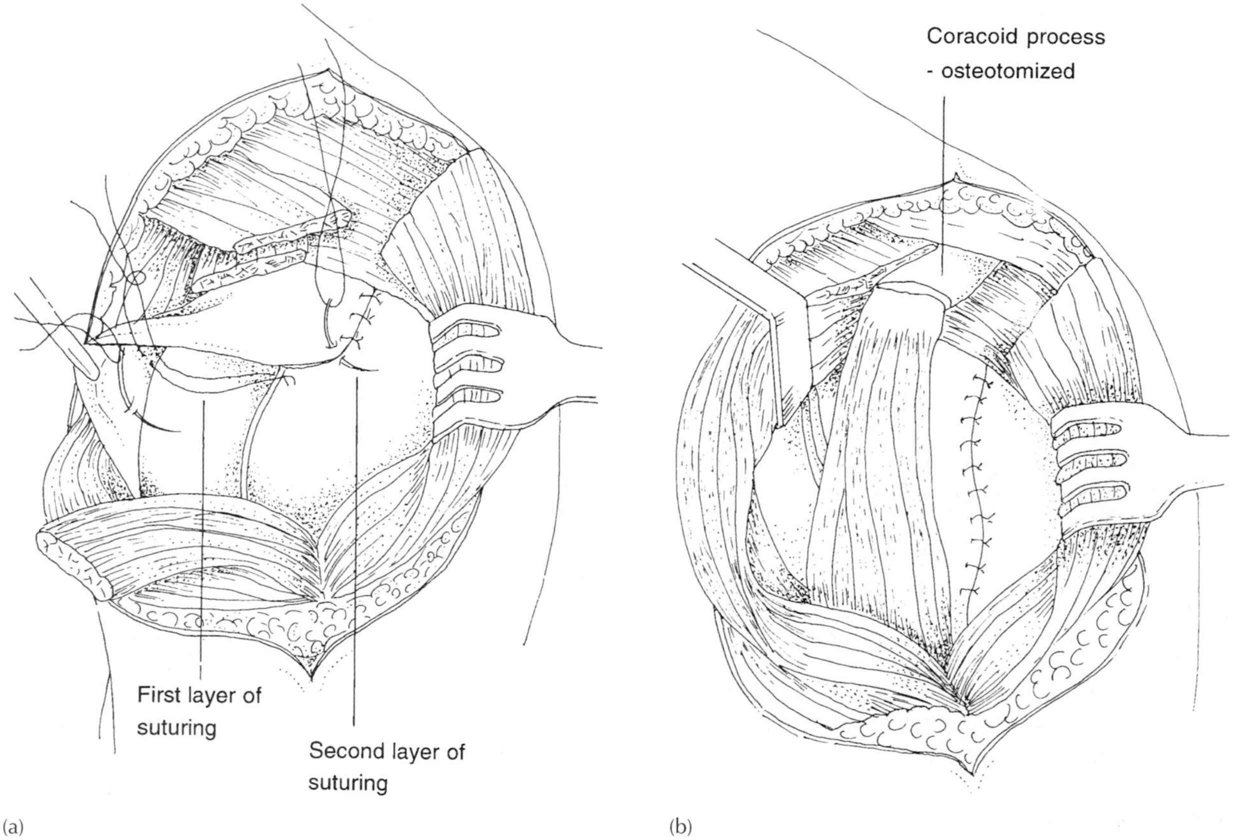

Figure 14.23 Putti–Platt reconstruction. (a) Suturing of subscapularis to the anterior aspect of the glenoid, and the second layer in which the remaining portion of the subscapularis tendon is sutured laterally with the arm internally rotated. (b) Reconstruction of the coracobrachialis and short head of biceps to the tip of the coracoid process, which has been osteotomized and 'bent' downwards.

appears to be intact, it should be incised near the glenoid margin and the narrow portion on the inner side of the incision raised. The outer cut edge is fixed to the glenoid margin. Before fixation, a thin shaving of bone is raised by an osteotome from the front of the glenoid and neck of the scapula. While the humerus is drawn away from the glenoid, holes may be perforated through the glenoid margin with an angled drill, sharp vulsellum forceps or towel clips.

The edge of the capsule and glenoid labrum are now stitched to the perforation in the bare area over the glenoid edge using non-absorbable sutures (Figure 14.22). The subscapularis tendon and the coracoid process are reconstituted, the skin is closed and the arm is bandaged to the side. The arm is kept so for 3 weeks. Active movements are then begun and a full range of movement should be present in another month.

The difficulty in this operation is drilling the holes transversely on the glenoid edge, situated as it is at a considerable depth in the wound, and the Putti–Platt procedure is a technically less demanding procedure. However, full abduction and external rotation of the shoulder is lost so the procedure cannot be used in athletes.

Jobe *et al.* (1991) described 68% excellent results with capsular labral reconstruction. Of their patients, 96% were satisfied with overall results. Modifications of the Bankart procedure are described by Richmond *et al.* (1991) and Altchek *et al.* (1991).

Reefing of subscapularis

This procedure gained wide acceptance with uniformly good results in early series. Adams (1948) reviewed 37 cases with one dislocation (95% success rate). He considered it easy to do and that it got to the point of weakness of the capsule at the anterior glenoid margin. The resulting limitation of motion was not considered a problem. Recent studies have shown that the procedure is not satisfactory alone but is an essential part of most anterior repairs.

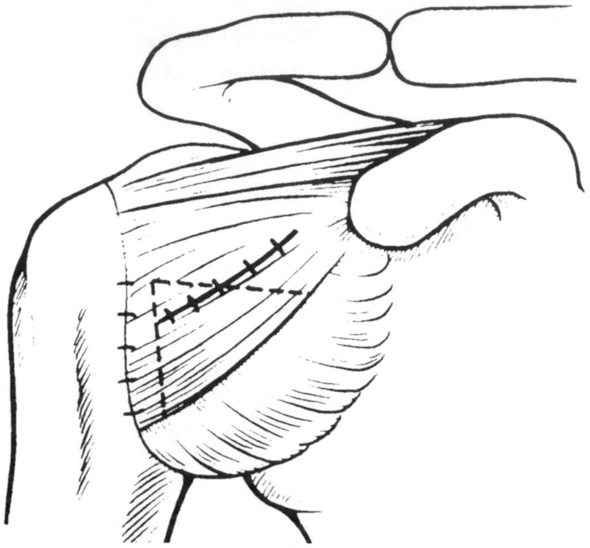

Figure 14.24 Neer reinforced repair operation. The inferior flap is sutured first and the superior flap drawn down over it to reinforce the middle glenohumeral ligament and the capsule anteriorly.(Reproduced, with permission, from Watson, M. (1991) *Surgical Disorders of the Shoulder.* Churchill Livingstone: Edinburgh, London, New York

Putti–Platt repair

A modification of this operation as used by Putti and Platt was reported by Osmond-Clarke (1948). (The method was first used apparently by Codivilla.) In this operation the exposure is substantially the same as in the Bankart. The subscapularis is divided about 2.5 cm from its insertion and the capsule deliberately opened. In the repair, the anterior surface of the neck of the scapula from which the periosteum has been stripped is rawed thoroughly so that eventually the sutured tendon and capsule will adhere to it. The distal cut end of the scapularis is attached to the most convenient soft tissue structure – often the labrum itself – along the anterior rim of the glenoid cavity, by means of four sutures tied while the limb is internally rotated (Figure 14.23). The medial part of the capsule is now drawn out to overlap this and stitched to the distal part. Further overlapping is provided by suturing the muscle belly of the subscapularis to the scarified tendinous cuff which overlies the greater tuberosity, but should not involve the biceps tendon. This last overlap shortens the subscapularis and prevents a full range of external rotation by about 15°. The tip of the coracoid is replaced and the wound closed. The arm is fixed in internal rotation and abduction for 3 weeks by a collar-and-cuff sling and body bandage and thereafter movement is restored by graduated exercises.

Leslie and Ryan (1962) described an anterior axillary exposure to the shoulder joint in order to prevent the usual widening and keloid formation following the standard deltopectoral approach. With the arm supported in 90° of abduction and external rotation, an incision is made from the midpoint of the anterior axillary fold, over pectoralis major, to another point 6 cm posteriorly in the axilla. Because of the mobility of the skin, it is readily reflected outwards and upwards to show the deltopectoral groove and the cephalic vein which is retracted. The tendon of pectoralis major is partially or completely detached from its insertion and retracted downwards and inwards, to expose the structures over the front of the joint. Bleeding and the subsequent scarring are much less; therefore this approach is preferred in women.

The Bankart repair and the Putti–Platt procedure have been combined frequently. Morrey and Janes (1976) reported 183 procedures in 176 patients with a mean follow-up 10 years. They carried out 132 Putti–Platt, 35 combined and 16 Bankart procedures. Their overall dislocation rate was high at 11%, all occurring within 2 years after surgery.

Capsular reefing and advancement

Lebar and Alexander (1992) reviewed results of a capsular shift procedure in 10 patients. One patient required further surgery for recurrent instability. Patients with generalized ligamentous laxity had less pain and more posterior instability than those without laxity. In six cases a previous instability repair had been carried out, and this gave the least improvement after a further procedure. This suggests that inferior capsular shift (Figure 14.24), described by Neer for multi-directional instability, is successful in improving pain and stability with minimal functional loss of movement.

Bristow procedure

This procedure depends on the transfer of the tip of the coracoid process with its attached pectoralis minor and coracobrachialis muscles to the anterior aspect of the glenoid where they can act as a support to the head of the humerus during abduction of the shoulder without restricting external rotation or abduction. It is important to expose the bony surface of the scapula and to raw the surface of the bone and then to secure the tip of coracoid process at the 4 o'clock position on the right and at the 8 o'clock position on the left by passing a screw through the fragment and through both cortices of the scapula. In this way avulsion of the fragment will be prevented (Figure 14.25). Lombardo *et al.* (1976) reported the

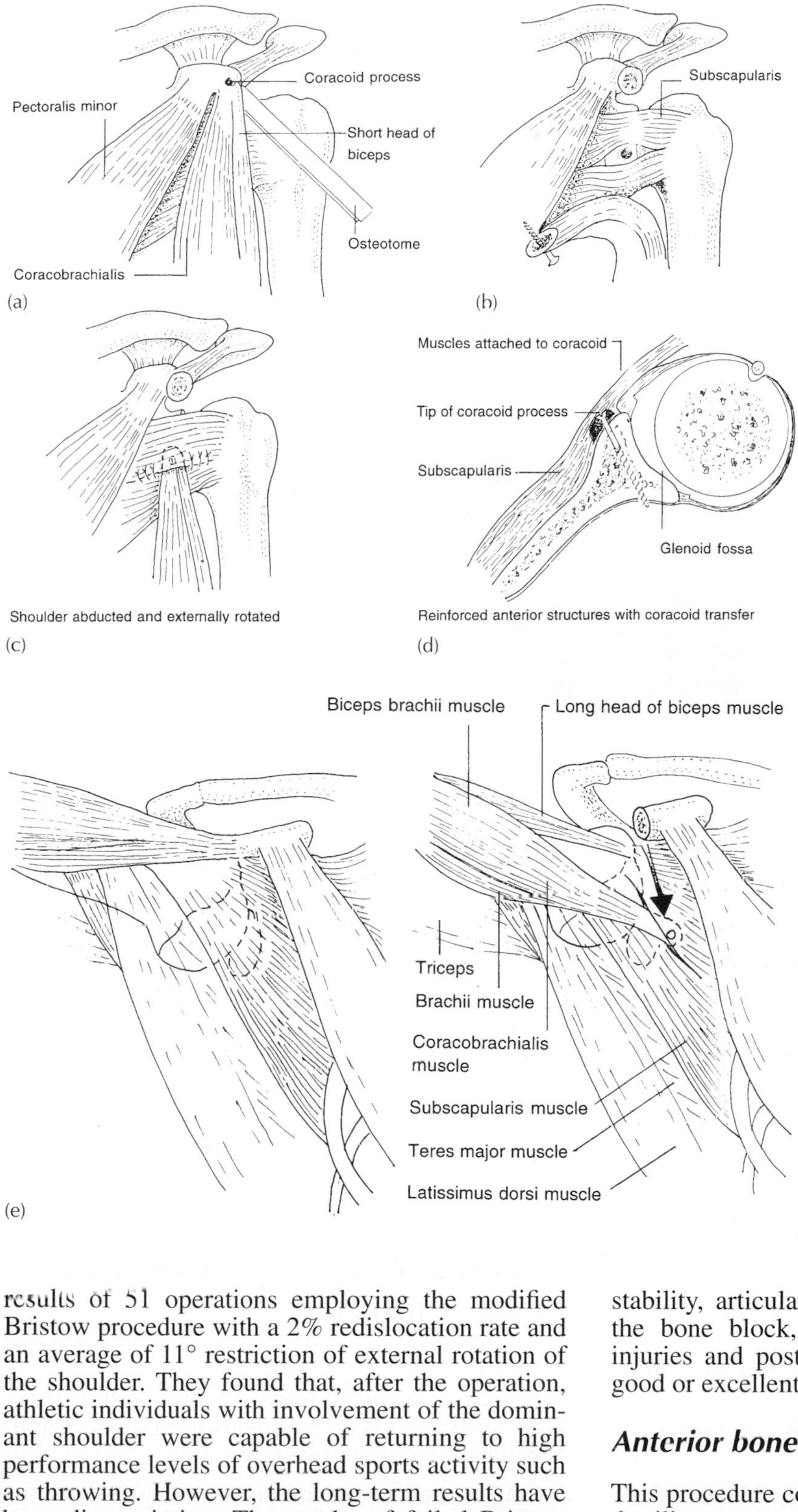

Figure 14.25 The Bristow procedure. (a) Separation of short head of biceps and coracobrachialis from the coracoid process. (b) A lag screw is passed through the top of the coracoid and a drill hole is made at the 8 o'clock position just proximal to the glenoid margin. (c) The tip of the coracoid, with the attached short head of biceps and coracobrachialis, is screwed into position. (d) Showing the lag screw passing through both anterior and posterior cortices of the scapula to give security to the transfer. (e) Illustrating the support given to the head of the humerus by short head of biceps and coracobrachialis. (Reproduced, with permission, (a–d) from Helfet, A.J. (1958) *Journal of Bone and Joint Surgery* **40B**, 198; (e) from Lombardo, S.J., Kerland, R. K., Jobe, F.W., Canter, M.E., Blazina, M.E. and Shields, C.L. (1976) *Journal of Bone and Joint Surgery* **58A**, 256)

results of 51 operations employing the modified Bristow procedure with a 2% redislocation rate and an average of 11° restriction of external rotation of the shoulder. They found that, after the operation, athletic individuals with involvement of the dominant shoulder were capable of returning to high performance levels of overhead sports activity such as throwing. However, the long-term results have been disappointing. The results of failed Bristow procedures are described by Young and Rockwood (1991) and include recurrent painful anterior instability, articular cartilage damage, non-union of the bone block, screw loosening, neurovascular injuries and posterior instability. They reported a good or excellent outcome in only 50% of patients.

Anterior bone block

This procedure consists of taking a bone graft from the iliac crest and placing it on the anteroinferior aspect of the glenoid. It is intended to allow the anterior capsule and other soft structures to become

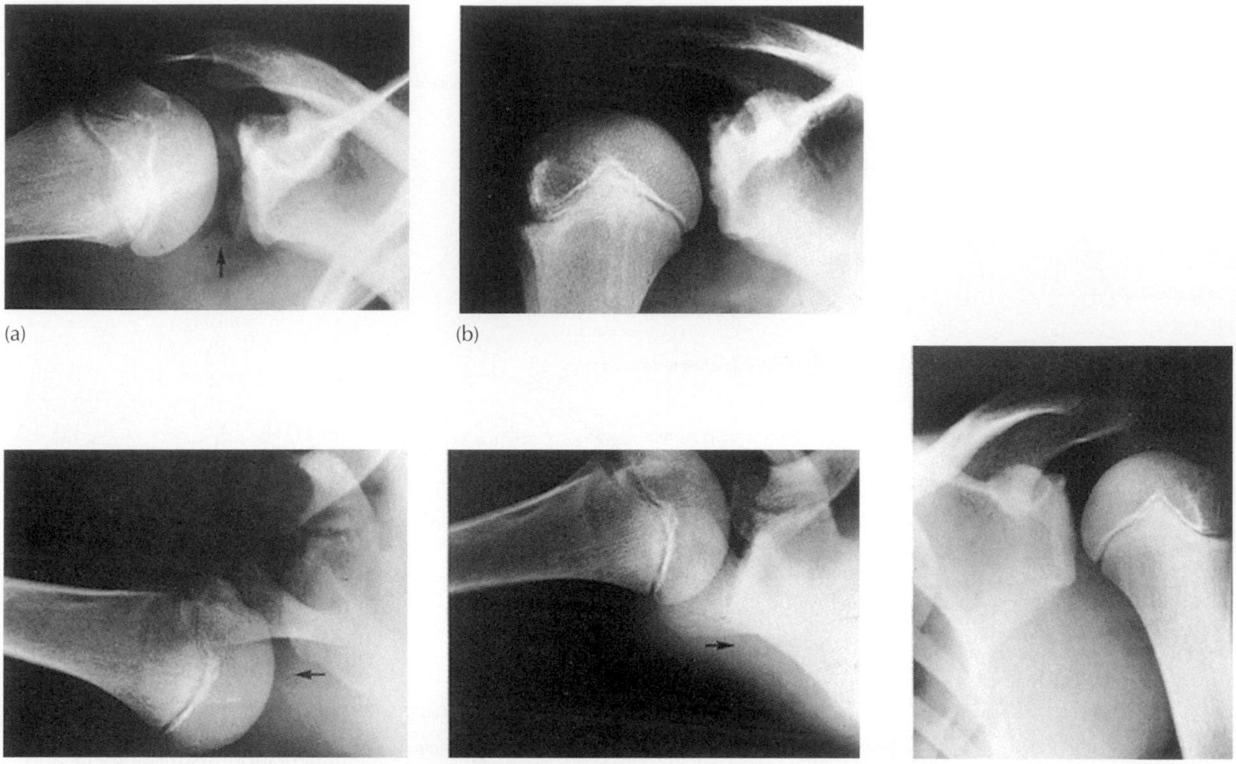
(a) (b) (c) (d) (e)

Figure 14.26 (a,b) Radiographs of the right shoulder joint, showing bony irregularity and deformity of the glenoid surface and a gas shadow after reduction of a recurrent dislocation. (c–e) Radiographs of the left shoulder joint showing a posterior dislocation (c), the reduction appearance (d) and the standard anteroposterior view (e).

attached to the glenoid. Recurrent dislocation follows frequently and the procedure has largely been abandoned.

Habitual anterior dislocation of the shoulder

This condition is characterized by the ability of the patient to dislocate at will. There is usually no history of trauma. The precise pathology underlying this condition is not always evident. In some cases a combination of a lax capsule and muscle abnormality were found. Rowe *et al.* (1973), in a clinical electromyographic and psychiatric study on 26 patients concluded:

1. The syndrome begins in early childhood or adolescence.
2. The displacement of the humeral head anteriorly, posteriorly or inferiorly is usually painless and is produced atraumatically by voluntary muscle action.
3. Intra-articular injury as a result of the repeated voluntary dislocation is rare.

Surgical treatment is often unsuccessful so that treatment is based on physical therapy and muscular autofacilitation techniques.

Recurrent posterior dislocation of the shoulder

Because this lesion comprises 1–3% of all dislocations, many reports are based on only a small sample of patients. There are two types:

1. A traumatic recurrent dislocation giving rise to a posterior Bankart lesion.
2. An atraumatic or habitual dislocation or sub-

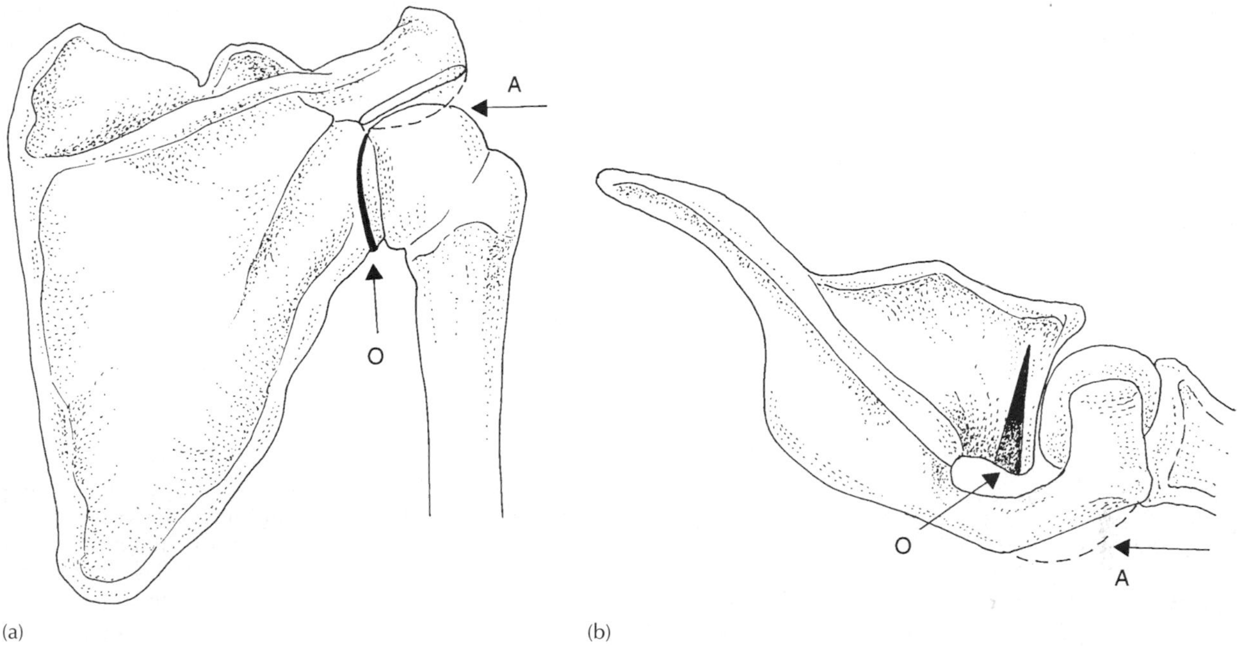

Figure 14.27 The Scott procedure for recurrent posterior shoulder dislocation. (a) Line of osteotomy (O) of glenoid neck which is also inclined slightly medially above. (b) The opened osteotomy and the site of removal of bone graft from the acromion (A) which holds the osteotomy in position. (Reproduced, with permission, from Scott, D.J. (1967) *Journal of Bone and Joint Surgery* **49A**, 471–476)

luxation associated with a lax capsule, epileptic fits and generalized joint laxity (Figure 14.26).

McLaughlin (1962) advocated posterior capsular plication and a bone block whilst Eyre-Brook (1973) advocated McLaughlin's revised method for persistent traumatic dislocation but did not advise surgery for the atraumatic dislocation. He felt that surgery was indicated only when failure of adequate conservative therapy and a large posterior pouch (shown on an arthrogram) existed. He proposed a generous extracapsular graft fixed across the infraspinous fossa posteriorly.

Scott (1967) and English (1973) advocated a glenoid osteotomy with posterior glenoplasty to antevert the glenoid fossa. English reported on all 11 dislocations in 9 patients treated this way with reefing of infraspinatus as in the Putti–Platt procedure. The results of these procedures still are not well established (Figure 14.27) but the authors have used the Scott technique with success in a small number of cases.

Derotation osteotomy of the humerous for recurrent dislocation of the shoulder

Saha (1978) commented on retroversion of the humerus reversing into antitorsion with abduction of the humerus. Clinically, when the shoulder is elevated to 120°, the head of the humerus can be felt more easily beneath the anterior axillary wall in cases with enhanced retrotorsion. He demonstrated excessive external rotation and a corresponding diminution of internal rotation with the arm by the side of the chest.

His indications for derotation osteotomy in patients with anterior dislocation were exaggerated retrotorsion of the humerus above 35° and no reduced anteversion of the glenoid cavity. The operation is successful only where habitual dislocation of the glenohumeral joint is due to insufficiency of the horizontal steering muscles from paresis and there is

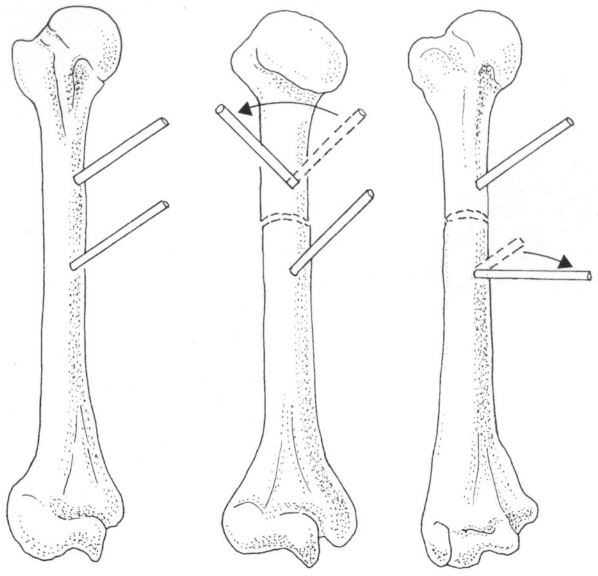

Figure 14.28 Derotational osteotomy of humerus (After Saha, A.K. (1969) *Recurrent Anterior Dislocation of the Shoulder: a New Concept.* Academic Publishers: Calcutta)

no muscle sufficiently strong to transfer as a posterior horizontal steerer.

The operation consists of carrying out a derotation osteotomy of the humerus at a level just above the deltoid muscle insertion. A small plate is used as internal fixation (Figure 14.28).

The 11 operations done in 10 cases had follow-up periods of from 6 months to more than 3 years. None of the cases had any apprehension or recurrence. Some of the cases showed slight temporary restriction of the external rotation with a corresponding increase of the internal rotation in the immediate postoperative period. There was no disturbance of scapulohumeral rhythm, and in the 'zero position' the reciprocal glenohumeral joint articular surfaces were exactly the same as in the normal. The increase of stability is obvious from the identical axial radiographs of the shoulder taken at 120° elevation in the coronal plane. In this position the centre of the articular surface of the head of the humerus is seen to articulate with the depth of the glenoid cavity, abolishing the asymmetry of the articular surface leading to the critical stage of stability.

Duthie has now used the Saha technique for posterior recurrent dislocation on five patients with, after 2–5 years, no recurrence and excellent function.

Krönberg and Broström (1991) describe results of a proximal humeral rotational osteotomy in patients with traumatic or non-traumatic anterior instability. Eleven patients with small humeral head retroversion angles had the abnormal anatomy corrected by humeral osteotomy extracapsularly, although in three patients some reefing of the subscapularis muscle was also carried out. One year after surgery shoulder function was excellent in all shoulders with good stability and an average 10° reduction in external rotation range.

Recurrent dislocation of the acromioclavicular joint

The clavicle may be dislocated either upwards or downwards at the acromioclavicular joint, the upward dislocation being more common. The displacement results from a blow on the back of the acromion or from a fall on the tip of the shoulder. When the upward dislocation is complete, the acromioclavicular ligament and the conoid and trapezoid ligaments which hold the clavicle down to the coracoid are ruptured and the lateral end of the clavicle slides upwards and projects. As a result, there is considerable deformity, some difficulty in lifting the arm and limitation of certain of the shoulder movements.

If reduction has not occurred spontaneously, it can be secured easily by raising the arm and manipulating the joint. However, the reduction, though easily obtained, may be difficult to preserve, especially if coracoclavicular ligaments are ruptured. If there is a subluxation only, the best immediate measure is by means of a brachioclavicular sling. Broad strips of adhesive plaster are passed round the elbow and over the top of the shoulder, medial to the acromioclavicular joint. The arm is supported by a separate triangular sling.

If the dislocation is complete, operative treatment should be performed. The best procedure is to attempt to repair the coracoclavicular ligaments with sutures and transfixion of the acromioclavicular joint with heavy Kirschner wires which are left *in situ* for 6 weeks (Figure 14.29).

A lag screw can be inserted downwards through the clavicle to engage the superior cortex of the coracoid process, but this frequently loosens (Figure 14.30).

Excision of the outer aspect of the clavicle for about 3 cm (i.e. up to the trapezoid and conoid ligament) may be helpful in symptomatic late acromioclavicular dislocation. This was initially described by Mumford (1941) and he emphasized the suturing together of the trapezius and deltoid insertions into the gap left by the excision of bone. It should be considered only as a last resort.

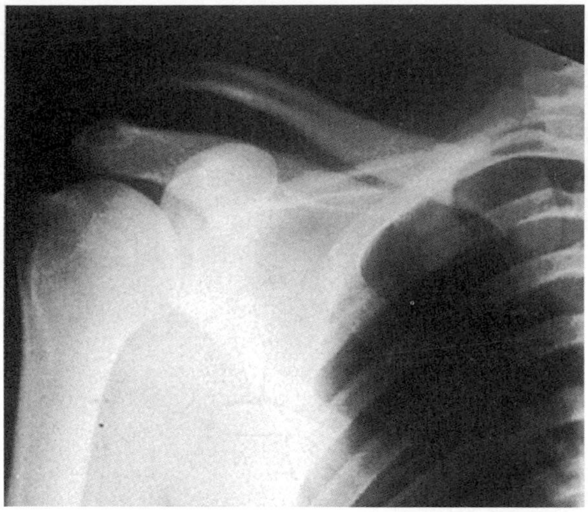

(a)

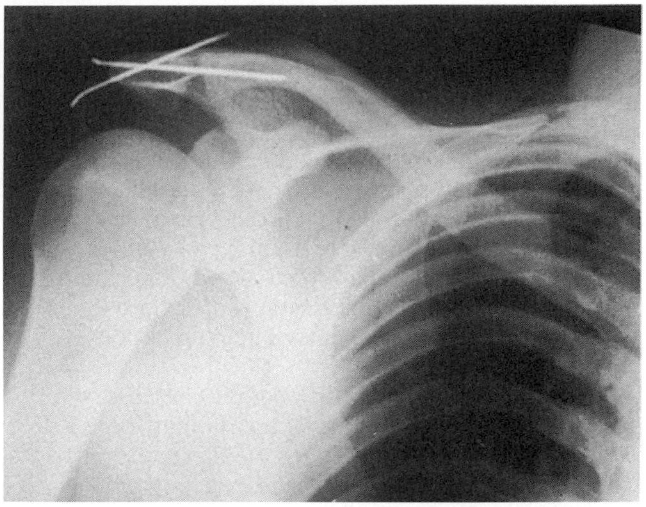

(b)

Figure 14.29 (a) Radiograph showing dislocation of the acromioclavicular joint. (b) Postoperative radiograph showing the reduction secured after repair of conoid and trapezoid ligaments by crossed Kirschner wires (Courtesy of Mr G.S.E. Dowd)

Dislocations of the medial end of the clavicle

Dislocations of the medial end of the clavicle are rare, as the bone breaks easily and the ligaments supporting the articulation are strong. In particular, the rhomboid ligament (costoclavicular ligament) stretching from the clavicle to the front of the costal cartilage is very strong, and resists the tendency of the clavicle to slip upwards, medially and forwards in the line of slope of the joint cavity. The dislocation is usually an anterior and medial one on this account, and when complete there must be rupture of the costoclavicular ligament. Subluxation may occur if the capsule and ligaments stretch without completely breaking.

Posterior dislocation may be caused by direct violence, but is fortunately rare, as the displaced clavicle in this case may injure the large vessels in the superior mediastinum or produce tracheal compression.

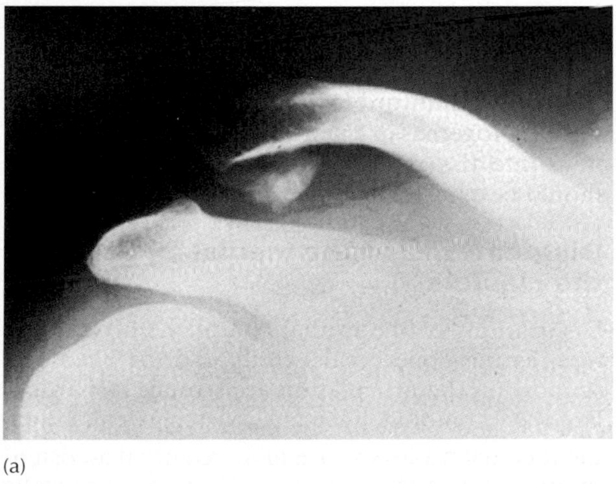

(a)

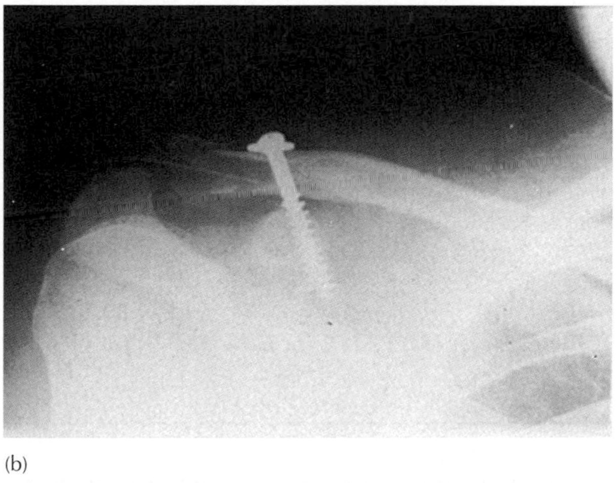

(b)

Figure 14.30 (a) Dislocation of acromioclavicular joint with healing ossification. (b) Lag screw with reduction.

Subluxation can usually be reduced by direct pressure over the clavicle while the shoulder is simultaneously pulled upwards and outwards. It is difficult to maintain the reduction.

In the posterior dislocation, manipulation is usually ineffective, and the reduction must be made by open operation, the clavicle being replaced by the use of some form of lever. In this case some means of fixing the clavicle must be employed. Thin metal removable intramedullary pins or fascial sutures may be used, or the meniscus may be stitched to the front of the capsule, or the clavicle to the first costal cartilage.

If a recurrent anterior dislocation causes severe symptoms, which is unusual, a similar type of operation may be employed, or the clavicle may be sutured to the first costal cartilage by a loop of fascia lata in a way similar to that employed in recurring acromioclavicular dislocation. In this method the fascial suture replaces the costoclavicular ligament.

Bankart (1938) described an operation which he stated had been very successful in his experience. By means of a 10 cm incision along the inner end of the clavicle and over the sternum, the dislocated bones are exposed. A flake of bone about 0.75 cm long is raised by a periosteum elevator from in front of both bones and turned downwards. After the insertion of the sternomastoid is freed, the posterior aspect of the joint is exposed by blunt dissection and protected by a broad spatula while two holes are drilled in an anteroposterior direction through both bones. A strip of fascia lata is now threaded through the clavicular holes from behind, leaving the two loose ends in front. These ends are now taken through the joint in a backward direction and brought through the sternal holes from back to front. The dislocation is now reduced and the fascia pulled tight, tied in a single knot, stitched with suture and then the reef knot in the fascia completed. By further sutures and replacement of the bone flakes a secure fixation is obtained. The arm is kept bandaged to the side for 1 month.

Resection of the inner end of the clavicle has been carried out for relief of symptoms with little residual disability. However, heterotopic ossification in young people may result.

Rheumatoid arthritis of the shoulder

Rheumatoid arthritis frequently affects the shoulder. The synovial membrane of the main cavity is first affected, followed by the subacromial bursa which communicates with the joint and the tendon sheath of the long head of biceps which is an extension of the synovial cavity. Involvement of the subacromial bursa may lead to a large swelling which restricts movement and activities and is obvious at the anterior aspect of the joint.

Pain in the shoulder with restriction of movement, especially abduction, is the first symptom but is frequently overshadowed by elbow joint pain. Pain is usually intermittent and relieved by reduced activity but late in the disease may be a serious problem. Bilateral shoulder involvement often calls for operative treatment on one shoulder at least.

For further discussion of this topic see Chapter 11.

TREATMENT

In the unusual situation of a painful shoulder with stage 1 rheumatoid arthritis with or without involvement of the subacromial bursa which has failed to respond to systemic medical therapy and rest in a sling for 3 weeks, injection of the joint with a local anaesthetic and hydrocortisone is a logical and useful device. Such treatment will relieve pain by reducing synovial inflammation without damaging the articular cartilage (Bentley *et al.*, 1973). Injections may be repeated up to six times, preferably spaced at monthly intervals, but if these fail to relieve symptoms synovectomy of the joint is indicated.

Synovectomy is performed from an anterior approach via the deltopectoral groove and as much as possible of the membrane is removed with knife and bone nibblers. Often the subacromial bursa is involved also and this should be removed. This procedure will give relief from pain in the majority of cases and appears to slow down progression of the disease as in the knee and the metacarpophalangeal joints of the hand.

Usually, however, the joint is more extensively involved with stage 2 or stage 3 changes before serious disability and symptoms ensue. Fortunately, the simple use of a triangular sling, to support and rest the shoulder for a period of 3 weeks, often produces relief of symptoms, thus making surgical procedures unnecessary. When symptoms persist, the following operative procedures must be considered.

Arthrodesis

Arthrodesis has little to offer the rheumatoid patient since it involves a long period of splintage, both internal and external, for success. It is true that the rheumatoid joints fuse more readily than osteoarthritic or post-traumatic joints, but the same results can be achieved by a sling supporting the arm for 3–4 weeks, when often a painless fibrous ankylosis results. Indeed, this may progress to bony ankylosis. The disability is slight because the scapulothoracic movement is retained in rheumatoid arthritis and the resultant total shoulder movement is quite adequate for most patients.

Excisional arthroplasty

Wainwright (1974) has described glenoidectomy, which is effectively an excisional arthroplasty of the shoulder joint. This procedure produces acceptable stability, mobility and pain relief. It is indicated in those patients in whom pain is a predominant problem, particularly if there are contraindications to replacement arthroplasty due to poor bone stock in the glenoid. Wainwright (1977, personal communication) reported good results, with relief of pain and maintenance of a satisfactory functional range of movement in eight of nine patients followed up for 6 years.

Glenoidectomy is also valuable in stage 3 disease, especially when the patient is osteoporotic, making replacement procedures difficult, and if there is any question of low-grade infection within the shoulder joint when replacement arthroplasty is contraindicated.

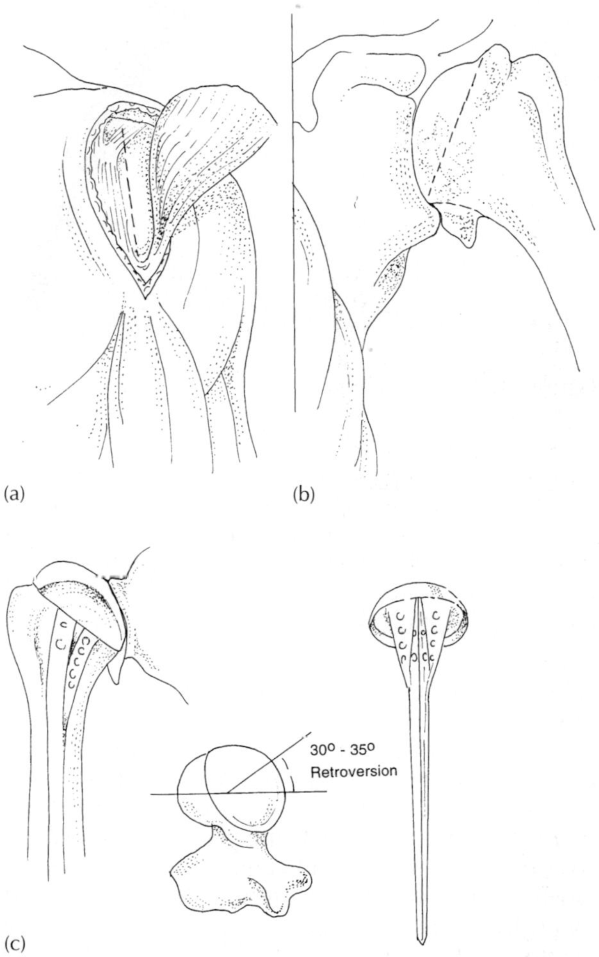

Figure 14.31 The Neer humeral head replacement prosthesis. (a) Line of muscle – splitting incision between deltoid and pectoralis major and (b) line of excision of humeral head. (c) The prosthesis. (Reproduced, with permission, from Neer, C.S. (1974) *Journal of Bone and Joint Surgery* **56A**, 1–13)

Arthroplasty

Humeral head replacement arthroplasty

Neer (1955) described a stainless steel humeral head replacement prosthesis similar to the Moore prosthesis used for femoral neck fractures (Figure 14.31). This prosthesis has been used extensively in the treatment of severe fractures of the humeral head and neck, and has been applied sporadically in rheumatoid arthritis with varying results. From individual reports it appears that pain is usually relieved and stability maintained but movement is little improved. It is probably indicated only when total replacement arthroplasty is not available or contraindicated due to technical difficulties of implantation in the osteoporotic scapula and humerus.

Total prosthetic replacement of the shoulder

Loss of glenohumeral movement is a relatively minor disability as scapulothoracic movement is still possible under these circumstances. Nevertheless, in most shoulder movements the glenohumeral joint does participate to some extent, even in small amounts of movement, so that glenohumeral joint disease, usually due to rheumatoid arthritis or to primary or secondary degenerative arthritis, may cause patients severe symptoms of pain and discomfort. Although scapulothoracic movement is still possible, the loss of glenohumeral joint movement is part of an arthritic process. It does cause significant loss of upper limb mobility and therefore upper limb function. Total shoulder replacement therefore is becoming a more common procedure. Under these circumstances, that is in older patients with arthritic glenohumeral disease, there is often an associated rotator cuff problem. Wholly unconstrained total shoulder replacements therefore, although they may relieve the pain arising from the arthritic process itself, may in fact contribute to pain arising from the degenerate rotator cuff.

There is therefore less controversy now regarding the results of total shoulder replacement.

The most widely used unconstrained total shoul-

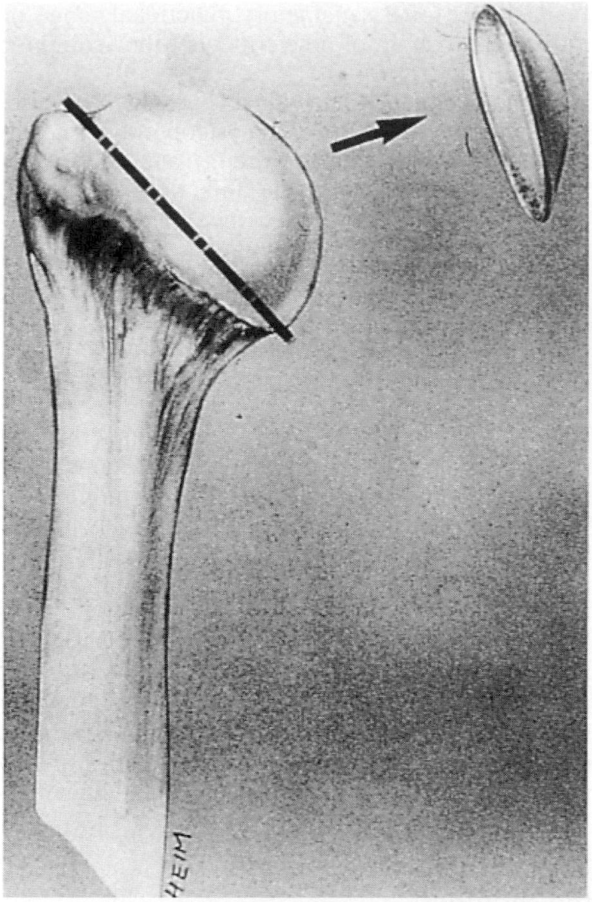

Figure 14.32 The level of the humeral head is critical. To prevent impingement and to maintain the length of the myofascial sleeve of the deltoid and rotator cuff, the osteotomy must be done above the tip of the greater tuberosity. In reality, only a very small portion of the articular surface is removed. A trial component is held over the bone to determine the proper angular orientation. (Reproduced, with permission, from Watson, M. (1991) *Disorders of the Shoulder*. Churchill Livingstone: Edinburgh, London, New York)

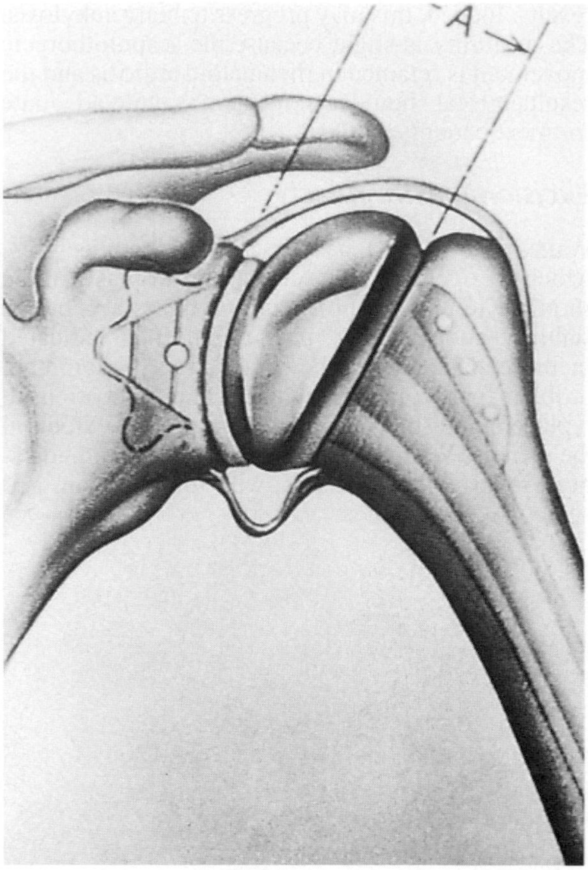

Figure 14.33 The humeral component acting as a spacer in shoulder replacement. The distance from the glenoid to the neck of the humerus (A) must be maximized to tighten the supraspinatus with the arm in the resting position. If this muscle tendon unit is too loose, when the muscle contracts little energy will be transferred to movement of the arm (Reproduced, with permission, from Watson, M. (1991) *Disorders of the Shoulder*. Churchill Livingstone: Edinburgh, London, New York)

der replacement is the Neer prosthesis (Figure 14.32). The outcome after this procedure is often excellent in patients with osteoarthritis without rotator cuff problems but is less certain in cases with rotator cuff involvement particularly with rotator cuff tears (Figure 14.33). A reverse-anatomy unconstrained prosthesis preventing rotator cuff impingement by the prosthesis may give a better outcome in such patients. The results of a reverse anatomy unconstrained prosthesis (Shearer, 1994, unpublished observations), in 26 patients with equal numbers of rheumatoid and osteoarthritics showed a 73% good or excellent result. All patients achieved substantial pain relief and 50% increased their range of movement.

A prosthetic shoulder made of polyethylene has been described by Mathys and Mathys (1977), and used by Duthie for tumour excision and for severe traumatic arthritis. Its advantages are in its screw fixation into bone without cement and in its design which allows interlocking through the humeral head by the long head of biceps to provide greater stability (Figure 14.34).

Although, like the hip, the shoulder is surrounded by powerful muscles, the biomechanics of the shoulder is more complex and movement after total shoulder replacement in abduction especially is not good, usually because of the poor mechanical adaptation of the shoulder abductor muscles. Furthermore,

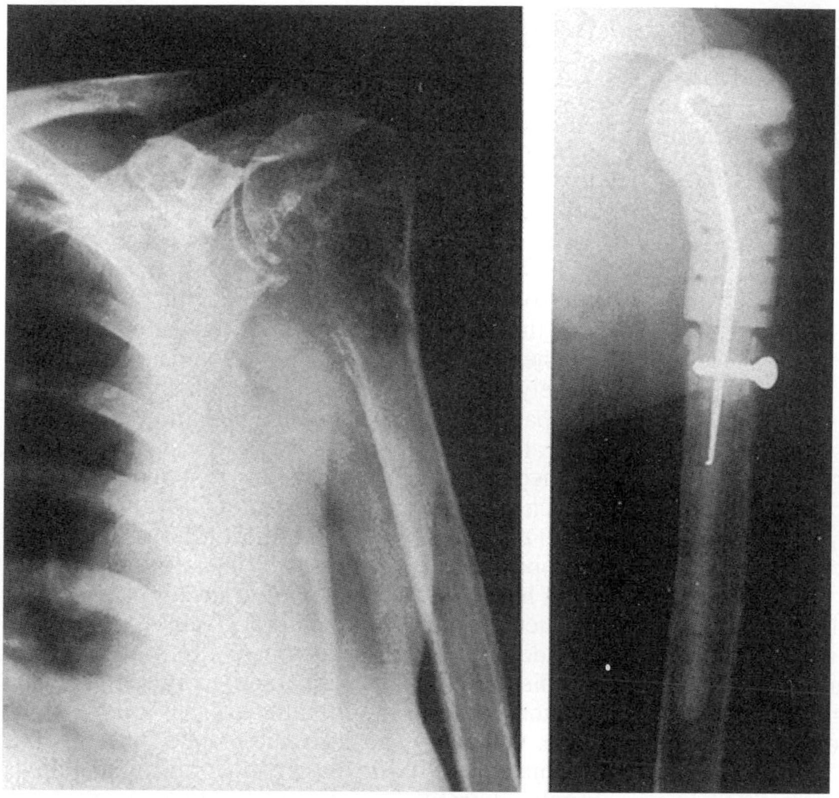

(a) (b)

Figure 14.34 Radiographs showing (a) a melanotic secondary lesion in the upper end of the humerus and (b) replacement of the tumour with a Mathys prosthesis.

fixation of the prosthesis in the thin bone of the scapula presents problems which have not yet been solved completely. Whilst methylmethacrylate bone cement is adequate for fixation for hip prostheses, which are loaded primarily in compression, shoulder and upper limb joints are frequently loaded in tension making methylmethacrylate less satisfactory as a fixing agent. Nevertheless, the relief of pain produced by replacing the arthritic joint surfaces is very valuable especially in bilateral disease.

Total shoulder replacement may also be undertaken for trauma, although it is commoner to use the Neer as a hemi-arthroplasty prosthesis in this situation.

Thomas *et al.* (1991) described 30 shoulder replacements in 23 patients with rheumatoid arthritis with a minimum 2-year follow-up. Of their patients, 40% had significant rotator cuff tears. Superior subluxation of the humeral head component relative to the glenoid occurred in only 15 of the 30 shoulders, indicating that the rotator cuff is not functioning properly, which is of concern, as cuff malfunction may contribute to glenoid loosening. Two glenoid components required revision for loosening (7.7%) and one in four hooded components (25%) required revision for late acromial failure.

In rheumatoid patients with an intact rotator cuff and satisfactory bone stock a total shoulder arthroplasty offers excellent relief of pain and improvement in function, but in the presence of rotator cuff deficiencies or poor bone quality, many problems remain, particularly for the glenoid component. Hemi-arthroplasty may be indicated in these patients or, alternatively, the use of a total shoulder replacement with protection for the rotator cuff in the subacromial space.

Osteoarthritis of the shoulder

Osteoarthrosis of the shoulder is rare, and primary osteoarthrosis probably never occurs. Due to the relative instability of the shoulder, however, secondary osteoarthrosis may occur in various circumstances, especially when the shoulder is called upon to take over weight-bearing function. Thus patients with paraplegia from trauma or from spinal diseases who employ crutches for walking for many years may develop painful osteoarthrosis of the shoulder due to the increased usage joint.

Secondary osteoarthrosis of the shoulder occurs following intra-articular fractures and in conditions such as haemophilia, sickle-cell disease, and following avascular necrosis of the humeral head from causes such as diving, steroid therapy and metabolic disorders (e.g. gout, pseudogout, porphyria and haemochromatosis).

The treatment is conservative in the first instance but severe pain may result in the necessity for shoulder fusion in the younger patient. Arthroplasty should be preserved for the older age groups who place less physical stress on the shoulder (Neer, 1974)

Dislocation of the biceps brachii

This condition has been recognized since the time of Hippocrates. The tendon of the long head is retained in position mainly by the attachment of the articular capsule in the region proximal to the lesser tuberosity and by the medial ridge of the bicipital sulcus which is often very deep. It is not believed that the transverse ligament is important in retaining position. The capsule of the joint may stretch and allow the tendon to slip over the lesser tuberosity and, since the tuberosity is rough, wear of the tendon and even rupture may ensue. It is probable that violent muscular action may dislocate the tendon. When the tendon slips over the lesser tuberosity, the tension of the muscle is immediately lessened and the classic bicipital syndrome results.

The symptoms in most cases are similar to those of a ruptured biceps tendon, and the onset is acute. There is pain in the region of the bicipital groove, which may radiate down the muscle. The pain is increased on external rotation and overhead extension while weakness in the arm is marked and function impaired. The muscle belly is flabby and lower than the normal position.

Diagnosis is not always easy, but in any disability of the shoulder brought on by a sudden movement or by movement of external rotation and overhead extension, and continued over a long time, the possibility should be considered. The patient can often produce the dislocation by bringing his extended arm to overhead extension and external rotation holding a 3 kg weight in the hand. The observer puts his finger on the tendon and may feel the snap and often hear it.

Treatment is by anchoring the tendon by sutures in its grooves or medial to the groove if degenerate.

Snapping shoulder

An audible click or snap may be produced by certain movements of the shoulder joint, or be due to a tendon slipping over a bony prominence (e.g. the long tendon of biceps over the lesser tuberosity). The sound occurs usually when the joint is voluntarily brought to an abnormal position; in two recent (personal) cases the head of the humerus subluxed into the edge of the glenoid, pulled there apparently by the pectoralis major. The phenomenon may ultimately become habitual or involuntary. Sometimes the patient can reproduce the condition on request, and, following the audible snap, the shoulder is immediately painful. Bristow reported a case in which he found abnormal muscular fibres arising from the lateral side of the short head of the biceps, and passing downwards and laterally towards the long head. He was to demonstrate at operation that abduction and rotation of the arm caused these fibres to ride over the lesser tuberosity. Removal of a part of this muscle, which apparently corresponds to the rotator humeri of lower mammals, was followed by a cure. Generally speaking these syndromes resolve spontaneously with reassurance, and operation is rarely advisable.

Snapping scapula

Scapular grating or snapping, the expression of some anomalous condition between the ribs and the undersurface of the scapula, is a tactile-acoustic phenomenon which has been observed in varying intensity in different persons. In some there may be a loud snap, while in others there is only a fine grating barely perceptible to the touch. It appears that the causes of these sounds may be divided into three main groups, as discussed below.

BONY CAUSES

In the category of cases due to changes in the bony structure of the undersurface of the scapula or the chest wall, a number of subgroups have been denoted:

1. The tubercle of Luschka – a small bony or fibrocartilaginous elevation located on the anterior aspect of the superior angle of the scapula, at its largest the size of a pea, usually covered by a bursa – was first described by Luschka. It appears to be a matter of doubt whether this is ever a cause of scapular snapping.

2. Abnormal curvature of the superior angle of the scapula. This is apparently of congenital origin.
3. Scapular snapping has been noted in the presence of exostoses on the ribs or on the undersurface of the scapula. The exostoses may be found at either the superior or the inferior angle of the scapula and may vary in size from osteocartilaginous nodules to relatively large mushroom-shaped masses.
4. Tumours of the ribs or scapula, fracture of either, angulation or buckling of the ribs, as in scoliosis, are all possible causes in the osseous group.

MUSCULAR CAUSES

The second main group is that associated with changes in the muscles lying between the scapula and the ribs. Voelcker (1922) suggested that a lesion in the muscles similar to tendinitis might be responsible for this type of snapping.

BURSAL CAUSES

The third main group is that in which scapular snapping has been attributed to the presence of normal or adventitious bursae. Normally, two are present beneath the scapula; one at the upper angle, situated in the depth of the serratus anterior muscle, is present in about one in every eight persons. The other, somewhat rarer, is found in the connective tissue between the serratus anterior and the upper part of the lateral wall of the chest.

For the most part only a short period of rest is required, but when there are definite bony changes (e.g. exostoses), surgical removal of these should be undertaken.

Winged scapula

Unusual winging of the scapula is a deformity which is fairly well recognized as secondary – usually to paralysis of the serratus anterior muscle though some authors favour the view that the disability is due to a traumatic rupture of the muscle at its scapular insertion.

The serratus anterior arises from the lateral surfaces of the upper eight ribs a short distance in front of the mid-axillary line. Its fibres pass backwards, closely applied to the chest wall, and are inserted into the ventral aspect of the medial border of the scapula but mostly to the inferior angle.

The long thoracic nerve arises from the fifth, sixth and seventh cervical nerves, the upper two piercing the scalenus medius and that from the seventh root passing in front of this muscle. The three roots unite at the level of the first rib to form a single trunk which descends along the inner wall of the axilla behind the brachial plexus and axillary vessels and upon the lateral aspect of the serratus to which it is distributed.

The function of the serratus anterior is mainly to aid in fixing the scapula to the thorax when the arm is elevated, particularly anteriorly, and also to rotate the scapula in abduction and during forward elevation of the arm at the shoulder.

The nerve is liable to damage:

1. In the suprascapular region from sudden or protracted trauma – e.g. carrying heaving weights on the shoulder.
2. In the axilla from direct force or from the pressure of enlarged lymphatic glands.
3. At the level of the union of the three roots, from abnormalities of the first rib.
4. From violent contractions of the scalenus medius muscle, as in swimming, a vigorous swing at a punching-bag which misses, a violent pull up when hand starting an engine, or the excessive use of muscular movements of the arm, as after prolonged elevation of the arms such as from painting a ceiling or hanging from a cross-bar.
5. Following radical neck gland resection for tumour.

There also exists a group of cases following poliomyelitis, typhoid, measles, influenza and other virus infections and injection of antitetanus serum.

The earliest symptom is pain along the base of the neck and downward over the scapula and deltoid. A common symptoms is the patient's fatigue on elevating the arm or the inability fully to do this. The weakness may pass unnoticed by the patient himself. Abnormal prominence of the scapula is a sign more frequently noticed by others than by the patient himself. The time of onset of the pain is usually immediately after acute trauma, but is variable in the toxic or repeated minor trauma cases. Weakness of abduction only begins at once when the cause is acute trauma.

On examination of the patient the principal clinical observations are weakness of the pushing power of the affected shoulder and weakness of abduction power of the arm above the horizontal plane. Winging of the scapula is always present. Some winging also occurs in many instances in which the arm is dependent. Tenderness may be present over the course of the long thoracic nerve, the maximal point being the mid-axillary line in the fourth intercostal space. The affected scapula is nearer the midline and may overlap the vertebral column when the arm is abducted. In trapezius paralysis the scapula is further from the midline.

Treatment is usually conservative. The shoulder is supported in a triangular sling during the painful stage, after which active movement is begun. Usually, whether recovery occurs or not, functional activity returns to the shoulder and the various operative methods are not now employed.

In poliomyelitis patients, very real improvement in upper extremity function (e.g. hand-to-mouth feeding) can be achieved by an intra-articular arthrodesis (Figure 14.35a,b). The acromion is osteotomized and held down to the humeral head by a compression screw. The intra-articular surfaces are excised and cancellous bone graft material is inserted with a large bone screw to maintain position until union has taken place (Figure 14.35c). It is essential that the trapezius and rhomboid muscles have good innervation and function.

Neuralgic amyotrophy (shoulder girdle syndrome)

Parsonage and Turner (1948) described a syndrome comprising pain and flaccid paralysis of the muscles round the shoulder girdle, occurring frequently during World War II though apparently previously it had been rare.

They described 136 cases, and quoted several articles where cases have been described under different names. Most of the cases showed some precipitating cause. Many of them had been in hospital with other conditions, some of them for simple operations, others with infections. Some had serum injections and, in a few cases, there was a history of trauma.

Johnson and Kendall (1961) reported 13 cases of isolated long thoracic nerve of Bell paralysis, 6 cases of axillary or circumflex nerves and 2 cases of accessory nerve paralysis – which occurred suddenly without any recognizable cause. Recovery to 70–80% of normal power occurred, but only if stretching from gravitational forces of the involved muscles was prevented.

AETIOLOGY

This remains obscure. A virus has been suggested but, in the absence of constitutional symptoms, seems unlikely. A similar condition occurs following serum injection, and it is possible that the two are related, resulting in a perineural oedema of the affected roots and peripheral nerves.

CLINICAL FEATURES

The onset is usually not accompanied by any constitutional symptoms whatever. Pain locally is almost always the presenting symptom. The pain is localized across the back of the scapula and may go down the arm or up into the neck. It is generally a constant severe ache, and lasts for a few hours to 14 days. Thereafter it seems to stop fairly suddenly and muscular paralysis then appears.

A striking feature of the syndrome is the rapid development of muscle weakness after the variable period of pain. This weakness is of the lower motor neuron type, with flaccidity of the affected muscles, and often rapid wasting. Fasciculation is never seen. Bilateral cases occur but there is usually an interval between the involvement of the two sides. The muscles involved show that in many cases the pathological process is in one or more peripheral nerves, while in others it must have been in the nerve root. In some cases, however, a lesion in the spinal cord must be assumed.

The nerves frequently affected are the long thoracic, the supracapsular and the circumflex. The common nerve roots to be affected are the fifth and sixth cervical, with the weakness of the spinati, deltoid, supinator longus and, at times, the clavicular head of the pectoralis major. Impairment of the biceps and supinator jerks and sensory impairment over the strip of skin on the outer side of the arm and forearm occur. Both anterior and posterior roots are therefore involved.

In a high proportion of cases there is patchy muscle wasting and weakness not corresponding to a nerve or nerve roots, and a spinal cord involvement is assumed. Practically every muscle in the arm may be involved, together or separately. Sensory changes occur in half the cases. The cerebrospinal fluid is normal, as are the radiographs.

DIFFERENTIAL DIAGNOSIS

The differential diagnosis of this condition will include anterior poliomyelitis, prolapsed cervical disc, brachial neuritis and progressive muscular atrophy.

Anterior poliomyelitis may be excluded from the fact that the CSF is normal, there are no constitutional upsets and sensory changes are present.

Prolapsed cervical disc affects only one root. The profound weakness and atrophy of the shoulder

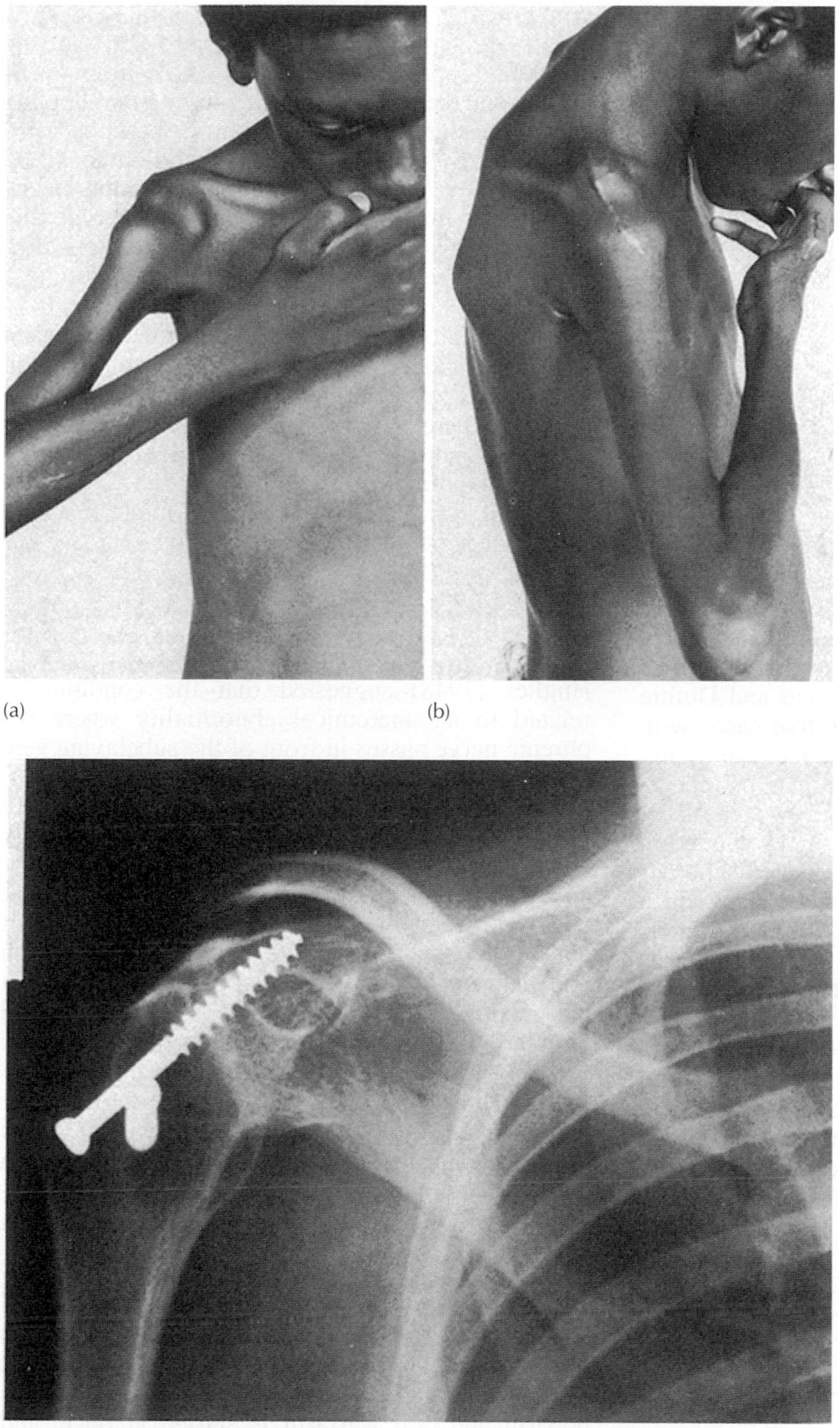

(a) (b) (c)

Figure 14.35 (a) and (b) The hand-to-mouth position. (c) Radiograph of same shoulder arthrodesed.

girdle syndrome do not occur, however. Localized paralysis and wasting of muscles are not features of brachial neuritis.

Progressive muscular atrophy may be excluded because of the acute onset with pain, the rapid development of wasting, the absence of fasciculation and the non-progressive course of the disease, as well as by the sensory changes that are often present.

The prognosis of cases seen in the early stages is

as difficult as in anterior poliomyelitis, and similar principles apply.

TREATMENT

No specific treatment for the condition is known and it may be managed as poliomyelitis – with analgesics, and splints to rest muscles. It is important to put the shoulder joint through its full range of movements at least twice a day to prevent stiffness.

Dropped shoulder

Injury to the spinal accessory nerve producing paralysis of the trapezius muscle is seen as the result of direct trauma, traction lesions, its use as a nerve pedicle transfer for facial paralysis or after operation on the posterior triangle or during radical neck dissections for cancer. Hoaglund and Duthie (1966) described this syndrome in five cases with their treatment. Patients may complain of a dragging sensation about the shoulder girdle or in the operative scar area, with a generalized weakness of the shoulder, including loss of shoulder abduction beyond 90°. On examination, the affected shoulder will have dropped, with the clavicle taking up a horizontal position. The scapula is displaced laterally and inferiorly as well as being rotated outwards away from the midline. Conservative measures are attempted first; if they are not successful, treatment consists of an operation described by Dewar and Harris (1950) which utilizes a tensor fascia lata sling of the medial region to the spinous processes of T1 and 2 vertebrae and the outward transfer of levator scapulae muscle to the lateral portion of the scapular spine.

Spontaneous axillary vein thrombosis

This condition may suddenly arise in an otherwise healthy individual – often a young man – in whom the upper arm becomes diffusely swollen and discoloured. About 80% of the cases are males, and in 70% the right arm is involved.

The condition is often ascribed to trauma, as in a man vigorously scrubbing his back while in a bath, or in another case where the patient strained his arm jumping from a tractor. The initial injury is usually accompanied by acute pain, and the arm becomes limp and useless. The whole limb swells rapidly and there is difficulty in moving the shoulder and to a lesser degree, the elbow. Superficial veins of the arm become very distended and obvious, and there is often a curious tingling sensation in the fingers. At first the pain is stabbing in type and later it changes to a dull intermittent ache aggravated by use of the arm. The hand and arm assume a faintly dusky hue.

On examination the veins of the hand and arm and pectoral region are prominent and engorged in appearance, particularly at the acromiothoracic anastomosis. There is marked tenderness of the axillary veins. No motor or sensory changes occur. Radiographs are normal.

Venography, carried out via the median cubital vein, may show the site of the obstruction.

AETIOLOGY

Hughes (1948) suggested that the condition is related to an anatomical abnormality where the phrenic nerve passes in front of the subclavian vein and so may obstruct the vessel by pressure against the tendon of the scalenus anterior almost as effectively as a ligature. That such an abnormality occurs has been shown by Hovelacque who discovered it in 10 out of 138 anatomical dissections, and Schroeder in 4% of cases. This theory of a prevenous phrenic nerve obstruction offers an adequate explanation of an apparently permanent obstruction. Recovery depends on the collateral circulation and this in turn depends on whether the nerve passes medial or lateral to the external jugular vein and the thrombus formation. It may be that after anticoagulant treatment is instituted the simple operation of section of the phrenic nerve might be a wise procedure.

TREATMENT

The patient is treated in bed with the arm elevated and exercises are instituted, graduated by the limits of comfort. Anticoagulant therapy by intravenous heparin and oral warfarin is started at once, and warfarin continued for 8 weeks.

Tumours of the shoulder

Tumours around the shoulder region may require extensive surgical procedures. Malawer *et al.* (1991) have developed a comprehensive unified classification system based on anatomical and functional structures removed during surgery. The procedures are classified into six types:

- *Type 1* – intra-articular proximal humeral resection allowing the retention of the abductors (type A), and resection of the abductors (type B).
- *Type 2* – partial scapulectomy may be undertaken, again allowing retention (type A), or resection (type B), of the shoulder abductors.
- *Type 3* – intra-articular total scapulectomy is required. This again is subdivided into abductor-retaining and abductor resecting operations.
- *Type 4* – extra-articular scapular and humeral head resection, again retaining or resecting the abductors.
- *Type 5* – extra-articular humeral and glenoid resection is undertaken.
- *Type 6* – extra-articular humeral and total scapular resection.

Types 1, 2 and 3 resections usually involve retention of the abductor mechanism and are therefore applicable to benign or low-grade lesions of the proximal humerus and scapula. In types 4, 5 and 6 the abductor mechanism usually requires removal; these types are therefore usually reserved for treatment of malignant sarcomas.

Reconstruction using a titanium modular spacer is described by Frassica *et al.* (1991).

Kocialkowski *et al.* (1992) reports four cases of localized metastatic renal cell carcinoma in the proximal humerus treated successfully by massive surgical *en bloc* resection, with reconstruction using a long stem Neer humeral head replacement prosthesis.

For further discussion of this topic see Chapter 10.

THE ELBOW JOINT

The elbow is the key joint in the upper limb, combining with the shoulder, forearm and wrist to place the hand in almost any position on the surface of the body. In particular it is vital for feeding, washing and toilet care, through not only its hinge function but its collateral stability. The loss of collateral stability in, for example, rheumatoid arthritis causes great disability, and it is the ability to provide this rather than hinge movement which is the major problem of prosthetic joint replacements. The superior radioulnar joint is an extension of the elbow and the synovial cavities are continuous. Both are affected simultaneously in rheumatoid arthritis and osteoarthritis, and it is the pain of forearm rotation felt at the radiohumeral joint which is a major cause of disability in arthritic states. Stability of the joint is provided mainly by the articular congruity between the humerus and the ulna but also by the thickening of the capsule forming the medial and lateral collateral ligaments (Bentley, 1978).

Flexion movement is produced by brachialis, supplemented by biceps, which is chiefly a supinator of the forearm, together with the forearm flexors. Extension and some posterior stability are provided by the triceps. The normal range of movement in the elbow is from 0° to 146° of flexion (Figure 14.36). There is a valgus angle at the elbow between the axis of the forearm and the axis of the humerus called the 'carrying angle' which normally measures 10–15° but may reach up to 20° in women. Slight hyperextension of the elbow is seen frequently in women and also in connective tissue diseases, such as congenital ligament laxity, Marfan's syndrome, Ehlers–Danlos syndrome, etc. Bilateral elbow stiffness is a great disability and is one of the major indications for surgical treatment.

Pronation and supination are performed by a combination of rotation on the radius around the ulna at the superior and inferior radioulnar joints with abduction and adduction of the ulna on the humerus when the elbow is flexed. The pronated forearm with the semi-flexed elbow gives the working position of the hand. Restriction of pronation and supination of the forearm which prevents the palm being turned horizontally upwards (e.g. to hold money) is a great disability.

Malalignment of the elbow is particularly prone to occur following injuries, especially in children, such as supracondylar fractures which results in cubitus varus (reduced carrying angle) and more rarely cubitus valgus (increased carrying angle). Cubitus valgus may very well be complicated by ulnar nerve neuritis caused by pressure and tension as the nerve passes along the medial side of the elbow in the groove behind the medial epicondyle of the humerus.

Mechanics of the elbow

The motion of the elbow joint during flexion, pronation and supination of the forearm has been

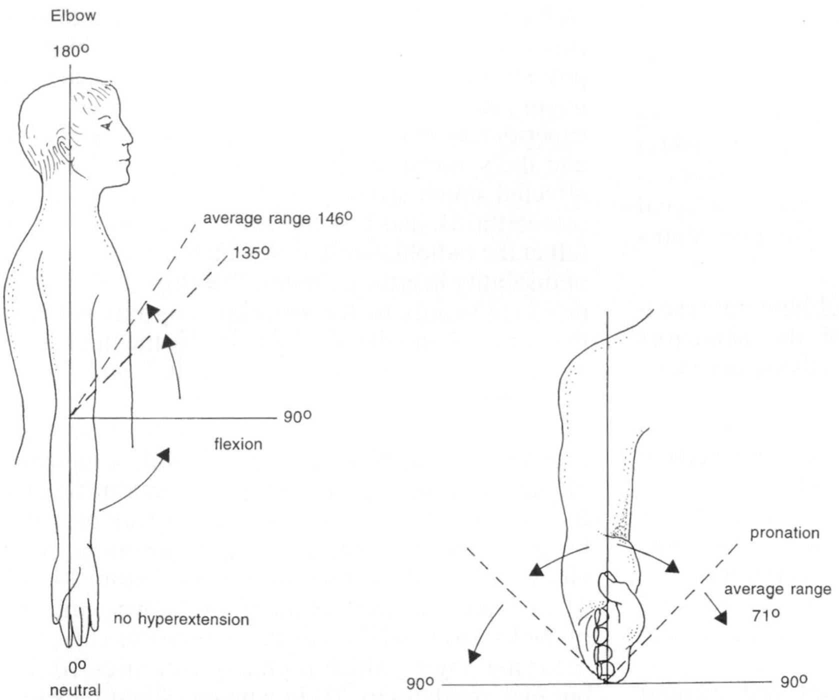

Figure 14.36 Average ranges of (left) flexion (146°) from 0° neutral and (right) supination (84°) and pronation (71°) of the elbow joint.

studied radiographically in cadaver specimens by Morrey and Chao (1976). They confirmed that the centre of rotation remained very close to the trochlear centre during flexion, and also found internal rotation of the ulna during this flexion which is associated with a change in the carrying angle. The carrying angle varied linearly between about 10° positive and negative, and this was almost independent of the degree of pronation or supination. This is consistent with there being a fixed relationship of the ulna to the humerus during pronation and supination. During active pronation and supination in the living, the motion is usually somewhat different, in that motion of the ulna occurs to give an axis of rotation through the middle of the hand.

The force transmitted through the elbow when lifting 1 kg in the hand was estimated by Walker (1977) to be about 450 Newtons or 46 times the lifted weight at 45° of flexion and 200 Newtons or 20 times the lifted weight at 90° of flexion, with the forearm horizontal in both cases. Amis *et al.* (1979) made a more complex analysis of force actions by including muscles of the forearm which are used to grip in the hand and stabilize the wrist. The forces in the humerocoronoid and humeroradial joints were each found to be about 12 times the force at the hand at 45° of flexion, and about eight times the force at the hand at 90° of flexion. This analysis indicated that excision of the radial head may more than double the force on the trochlea while imposing high stresses on the medial ligament of the elbow and the interosseous membrane of the forearm. Migration of the radius and instability of the wrist are possible complications of radial head excision. However, in a clinical and biomechanical study of patients between 11 and 28 years after this procedure (for traumatic injury to the radial head), Morrey *et al.* (1979) found only minor functional impairment. There was minimal loss of movement, although moderate loss of strength especially in pronation, supination and gripping. Functional impairment did not correlate with the degree of migration of the radius.

Ewald (1975), from a basic biomechanical study, showed that the elbow is not a simple hinge joint with the instant centre of rotation changing during flexion and extension. Because the trochlea is nearly a perfect circle with a single centre of rotation, and the capitulum being more hinged, the overall motion of the elbow is eccentric. He also showed that, by loading the forearm with a force of 4.5 kg, two-thirds of this force is transmitted across the radiocapitulum joint and the remaining one-third across the ulnar-trochlear joint.

Lifting an 0.454 kg (1 lb) weight through 90° of flexion by a 70 kg person produced a 3.175 kg (7 lb) reactive force with 0.562 kg/cm^2 (8 lb/in^2) across a prosthesis. A 22.68 kg (50 lb) weight produced a 167.829 kg (370 lb) reactive force with 32.3 kg/cm^2

(458 lb/in²) across the prosthesis. These severe forces highlight the need for greater knowledge in engineering design and material as well as in the biological demands on this joint.

Prosthetic replacement of the elbow has been complicated by the lack of soft tissue covering, and by loosening. The mechanical demands of this joint require that a prosthesis have strong attachment to bone over a wide range of its movement, and especially when the arm is extended and the muscles act nearly in line with the joint. The direction of the joint forces depends on the balance of tensions between muscles of the forearm and those of the upper arm. This ratio is quite variable with the activity of the arm.

Bursitis of the elbow

Inflammation of the bursae in the vicinity of the elbow is relatively common. The olecranon bursae and the radiohumeral bursa are involved.

OLECRANON BURSITIS

The upper olecranon bursa separates the tendon of the triceps muscle from the posterior ligament of the elbow joint, and from the olecranon process, at which point it facilitates the movement of the triceps tendon over the bone. The bursa is usually so small that its presence is not evident. Under the stimulus of repeated trauma, however, it may become distended and appear as a rounded swelling.

The lower olecranon bursa lies between the fascial expansion from the triceps tendon and the subcutaneous triangular area on the dorsum of the ulna. It is large and important. It is frequently the site of pyogenic infection, and of traumatic or trade bursitis, the latter condition being often known as miner's, or student's elbow. A rounded, fluctuating tumour appears over the olecranon about 4 × 2.5 cm in size. The distended bursa is not tender, nor does it interfere with the movements of the joint, unless it is severely traumatized or infected. Bursitis is sometimes difficult to differentiate from cellulitis of the elbow or acute arthritis of the elbow joint. Usually, however, there has been a swelling over the olecranon before any question of infection arose. Septic infection often supervenes and may cause superficial necrosis of the bone but it is unlikely to spread to the joint.

TREATMENT

The primary attack usually responds to aspiration followed by firm compression by bandages or strapping. If the swelling reappears, the sac should be dissected out and completely removed. It is wise to splint the elbow with a light plaster back-slab following the operation as this materially aids healing and prevents recurrence. Acute infections are drained surgically and treated with local rest in a sling and antibiotics until the wound is healed. Excision may be required later.

Tennis elbow

This troublesome and crippling affection of the elbow has been considered by some to be due to a radiohumeral bursitis, but is probably a strain of the extensor origin (Figure 14.37). It masquerades under a variety of names. Thus it is also known as epicondylitis or epicondylalgia. The condition is rare in tennis players but is usually seen in active individuals.

CLINICAL FEATURES

Rarely, it has a sudden onset and is accompanied by a definite swelling over the origin of the extensor tendons. More frequently it appears after prolonged and constant exercise, which has necessitated continuous flexion and extension of the elbow, and pronation and supination of the forearm. Following

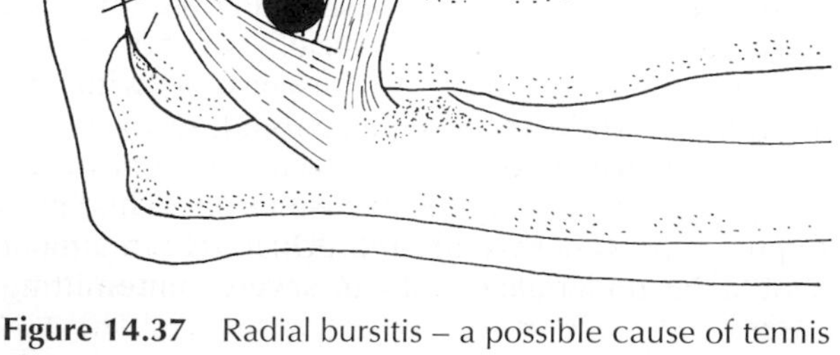

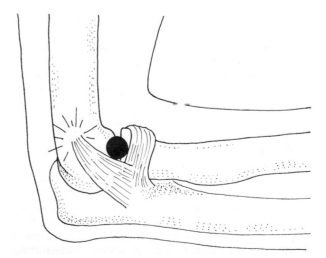

Figure 14.37 Radial bursitis – a possible cause of tennis elbow.

exercise, discomfort amounting to acute pain is felt in the outer aspect of the elbow. Tenderness is present on the lateral or anterior aspect of the lateral epicondyle of the humerus. The pain is very persistent and gives rise to continuous annoyance; it radiates down the forearm. There is a sense of weakness when attempts are made to perform lifting movements.

Examination shows little more than an area of definite tenderness over the extensor origin. On active movement, with the wrist palmar flexed, there is pain at the site of the lesion, particularly when the forearm is pronated and the elbow extended. x-Rays of the elbow are, of course, normal.

Bosworth (1941) believed that the orbicular ligament was important in the production of pain in the tennis elbow. Resection of this ligament gave relief in many cases. At the same time he sometimes divided the common origin of the extensor muscles. Compere frequently found a buttonhole slit in the ligament at operation and usually he, too, resected it.

TREATMENT

It is commonly agreed that in the acute case rest from the causative factor will bring immediate relief and ultimate cure always occurs. This is, however, slow. Various types of physical treatment – short-wave therapy, radiant heat, etc. – may be combined with rest in a wrist splint but the beneficial effect of this is probably just supportive.

Mills pointed out that many patients with tennis elbow had been relieved by osteopaths and bonesetters. He also observed that in patients with tennis elbow, when the forearm was fully pronated and the wrist and fingers were flexed, there was considerable limitation in extension at the elbow. By manipulating the elbow into complete extension, and keeping up pressure over the medial epicondyle with the hand and forearm in the above position, so producing a certain amount of adduction, he was able to relieve the symptoms in every case. Where the symptoms were of long standing, he advocated the use of an anaesthetic. In the typical successful case the manipulation is accompanied by an audible click.

We have found that the best results are obtained from an injection subperiosteally of 50 mg of hydrocortisone in a 2 ml suspension with the addition of 1000 units of hyaluronidase to ensure maximum dispersion and contact. These are used along with a 2% lignocaine solution. This may require repeating several times. Operative treatment should be undertaken only in severe, unremitting cases.

Operative treatment

When the condition is unremitting, operation may produce relief. The operative procedure consists in cutting down to the bone and raising the origin of the common extensor tendon together with the periosteum. In exceptional cases an adventitious bursa or a hypertrophied synovial fringe from the radiohumeral joint is found and this should be removed. The annular ligament can also be divided if tight.

A similar condition presenting with pain on the inner aspect of the elbow after a lot of use is 'golfers' elbow' which is due to strain of the flexor muscle origin. Like tennis elbow, it responds to prolonged reduction in activity and to injections of hydrocortisone and local anaesthetics. Surgical treatment by release of the origin from the medial humeral condyle is rarely required.

Malalignment of the elbow

CUBITUS VALGUS

Cubitus valgus is present when the carrying angle is greater than the normal. It is usually associated with fractures of the lateral condyle of the elbow, but may rarely follow inadequate reduction of supracondylar fractures. It may be due to asymmetrical bone growth following infection in the lower end of the humerus. It may also be associated with syndromes such as the nail-patella and Turner's syndrome.

In cases of late cubitus valgus deformity caused by non-union or malunion of the lateral condylar fractures, it is probably better not to treat the condylar fracture but to wait until bone growth is nearly complete and then perform a supracondylar osteotomy (Blount, 1955; Jakob *et al.*, 1975). The deformity may be associated with tardy ulnar neuritis which may develop many years later in adult life. This should be treated by anterior transposition of the nerve.

CUBITUS VARUS

Cubitus varus is a deformity in which the forearm is adducted when the elbow is extended. The deformity cannot be seen with the elbow flexed.

Most cases of cubitus varus are due to inadequate reduction of supracondylar fractures (Figure 14.38), although it may occasionally be due to alternation in

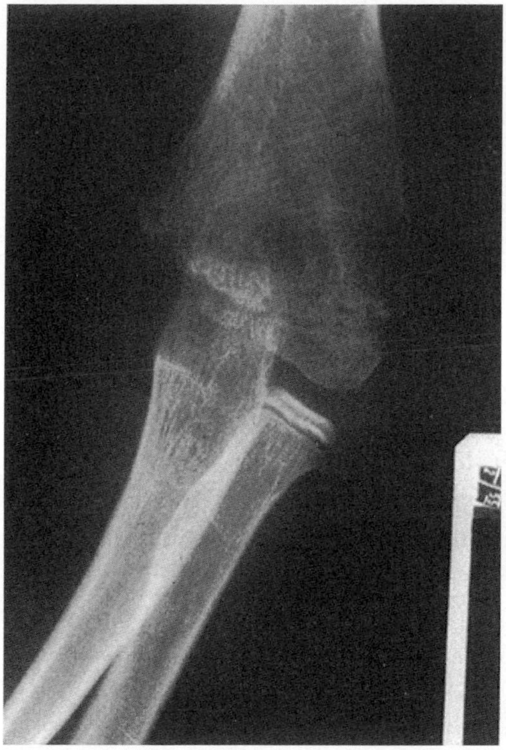

Figure 14.38 Anteroposterior radiograph 3 years after a supracondylar fracture, showing cubitus varus deformity.

epiphyseal growth of the distal humerus following trauma or infection.

Loss of carrying angle following supracondylar fracture may occur in as many as 30% of displaced fractures (Smith, 1960). The most probable cause of the deformity is residual medial tilt and rotation of the distal fragment following reduction (Wainwright, 1962; Dowd and Hopcroft, 1979). The deformity is a cosmetic rather than functional problem (Figure 14.39). If the deformity is severe and requires treatment, a supracondylar osteotomy will correct the angulation (French, 1959) as well as the rotational deformity (Figure 14.40).

Rheumatoid arthritis of the elbow

In rheumatoid arthritis the elbow frequently becomes extensively involved by the disease process so that proliferation synovium erodes the articular cartilage not only by formation of pannus and interference with articular cartilage nutrition but also by the release of proteolytic enzymes into the joint which

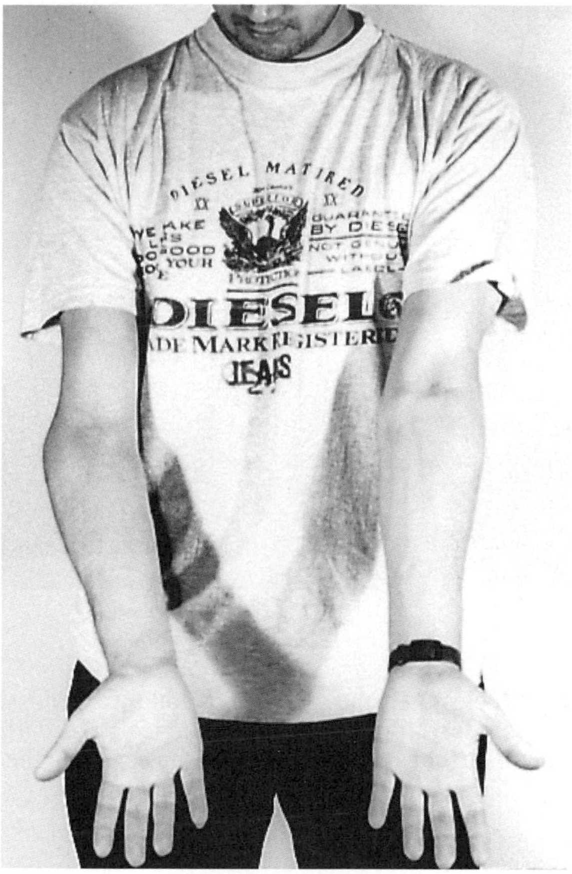

Figure 14.39 Cubitus varus right elbow following supracondylar fracture at age 5.

damage the cartilage. The bulkiness of the synovial membrane together with changes in the collagen structure and cross-linking of the capsule and ligaments of the joint cause laxity of the ligaments and loss of the stable hinge articulation. This results in a loss of the unique function of the elbow to provide flexion and extension through not only a vertical plane but also a horizontal plane under load, allowing the vital movement of lifting food and drink to the mouth. Thus all treatment is aimed at relieving pain and stiffness but at the same time maintaining collateral ligament stability (Bentley, 1978).

In early stage 1 disease (Barron, 1969) quite frequently the acute inflammation of the joint is controlled by splintage with the elbow in a back- slab at 90° for a period of 2–3 weeks combined with correct systemic therapy. When pain persists in the absence of articular cartilage damage in stage 1, it is useful to inject the joint with local anaesthetic solution and hydrocortisone; these injections may be repeated at monthly intervals up to a total of six. Beyond this time further injections probably will

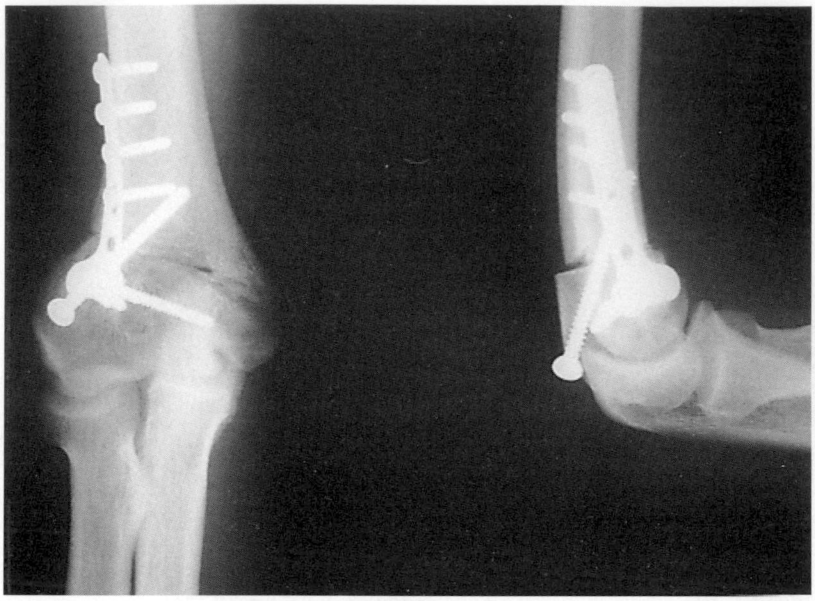

Figure 14.40 Immediate postoperative radiographs of patient in Figure 14.39 following closing wedge supracondylar osteotomy showing restoration of carrying angle.

be valueless. If the patient fails to respond to these conservative methods then surgical procedures should be considered, but they must be applied according to the staging of the disease process.

For further discussion, see Chapter 11.

SYNOVECTOMY

Synovectomy of the elbow joint is useful in stage 1 disease for relieving pain and also restoring mobility and function. However, it is rare to find totally normal articular cartilage at operation. More frequently, by the time the patient has reached the point of requiring surgical treatment the staging of the disease is more severe and more radical treatment is required.

SYNOVECTOMY AND DEBRIDEMENT OF THE ELBOW WITH EXCISION OF THE RADIAL HEAD

Experience has shown that the operation of synovectomy and debridement of the elbow with excision of the radial head will relieve pain and retain a good range of movement in a high percentage of patients with stage 2 and even stage 3 rheumatoid arthritis. It appears to arrest the progress of the disease and also to preserve collateral ligament stability (Stein *et al.*, 1975). The patients present with pain in the elbow joint during flexion and extension but also pain from the superior radioulnar joints during rotation of the forearm. The crepitus from the joint is easy to feel during movement and the crepitus from the radioulnar articulation during pronation and supination of the forearm. Thus, removal of the head of the radius with simultaneous synovectomy of the main joint and the superior radioulnar joint produces a combination of an excisional arthroplasty and synovectomy.

The operation is best carried out through a lateral (Kocher) approach, which gives excellent exposure to the whole joint. The proliferative synovium, any loose bodies and fragments of bone are moved from the joint by a combination of sharp dissection and bone nibblers. The head of the radius is then removed, care being taken to avoid damage to the posterior interosseous nerve by not placing bone levers around the neck of the radius. Following closure of the joint the arm is placed in a supporting sling for 10 days until the wound heals, when active mobilization of the elbow may commence. Figure 14.41 demonstrates the pre- and postoperative radiographs following a satisfactory synovectomy and excision of the head of the radius. It can be seen that the disease process has been arrested and the osteoporosis and cyst formation have diminished.

RADIAL HEAD REPLACEMENT FOR RHEUMATOID ARTHRITIS

Swanson and Herndon (1982) have emphasized how, when a radial head is excised, there is stretching of the interosseous membrane and the annular

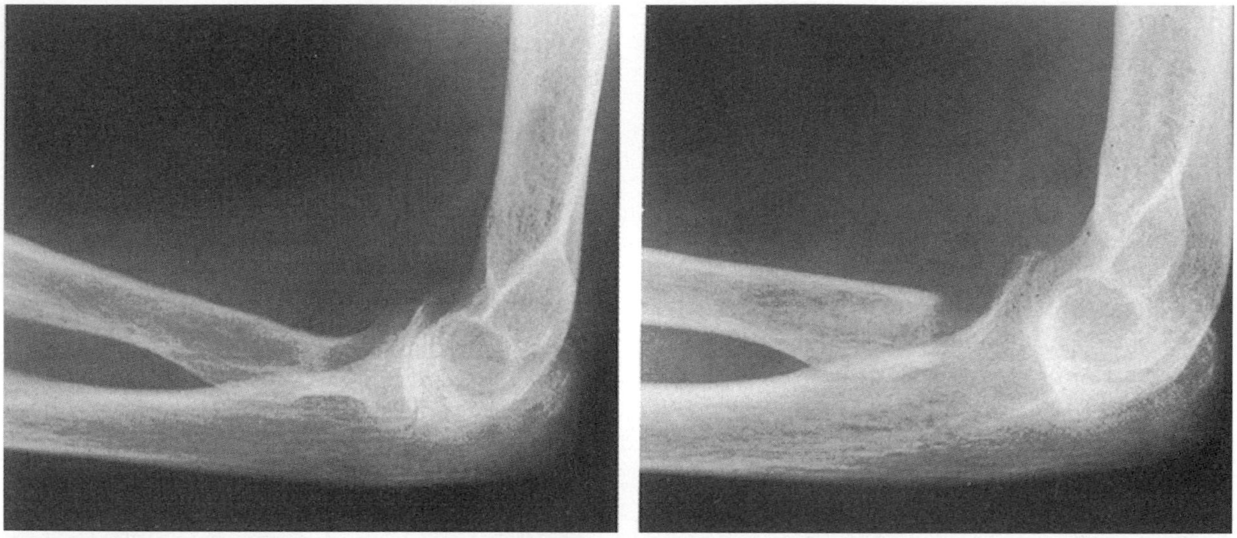

Figure 14.41 (a) Preoperative lateral radiograph of elbow with rheumatoid changes. (b) Postoperative radiograph following a successful synovectomy and excision of the head of the radius.

and quadrate ligaments, with upward migration of the radial bone. This will produce disruption of the inferior radioulnar joint with pain and limitation in pronation and supination as well as instability. There may well be an increase in the normal valgus angulation of the elbow joint. Because of this, Swanson inserted a silicone rubber implant. He strongly recommended this procedure in order to maintain the length of the radius, stability, the joint space and its mobility with improved rehabilitation. In a review of 53 elbows, there was only one case of bone resorption with loosening of the implant and no incidence of infection or implant fracture. Long-term results proved disappointing and this procedure has now been abandoned.

ARTHROPLASTY OF THE ELBOW JOINT

Total replacement arthroplasty

When the joint damage is very advanced, as in stage 3, producing pain and collateral ligament instability, or if the elbow is so stiff the normal activities of daily living cannot be performed, replacement arthroplasty must be considered. Generally speaking, if the opposite elbow has good function and if the other joints in the upper limbs are not seriously affected, replacement arthroplasty is contraindicated. If the patient is severely disabled with a stiff, painful elbow and bilateral involvement, and if synovectomy and excision of the head of the radius have failed, replacement arthroplasty may be performed. The problems with this procedure are:

1. Restoration of hinge stability.
2. Provision of adequate range of motion.
3. Counteraction of tension and rotation stresses which tend to loosen the prosthesis when fixed with methylmethacrylate bone cement in the osteoporotic humerus and ulna.

There have been many types of implants designed and inserted into patients – flexible implants, flexible hinges, hemiarthroplasty of the humerus, hinged implants of Dee (1972), McKee, Shiers, Stanmore, etc., unrestrained surface replacement implants of Imperial College, Lowe–Miller, Souter and Wadsworth – some with cement and others without. Unfortunately the long list of complications (e.g. infection, skin loss, loosening, or fracture, nerve injury and heterotopic ossification) indicates that this type of surgery is still experimental and that the likelihood of restoring a long-lasting painless, stable and mobile joint is remote.

Street and Stevens (1974) listed the requirements of a successful prosthesis:

1. To leave as much bone stock as possible for a possible arthrodesis.
2. Stability of fixation to the bone ends as well as in the joint.
3. Few moving parts.
4. Durable, inert materials.
5. Technically easy to insert.
6. Pain-free and mobile.

The experience with hinge prostheses (Souter,

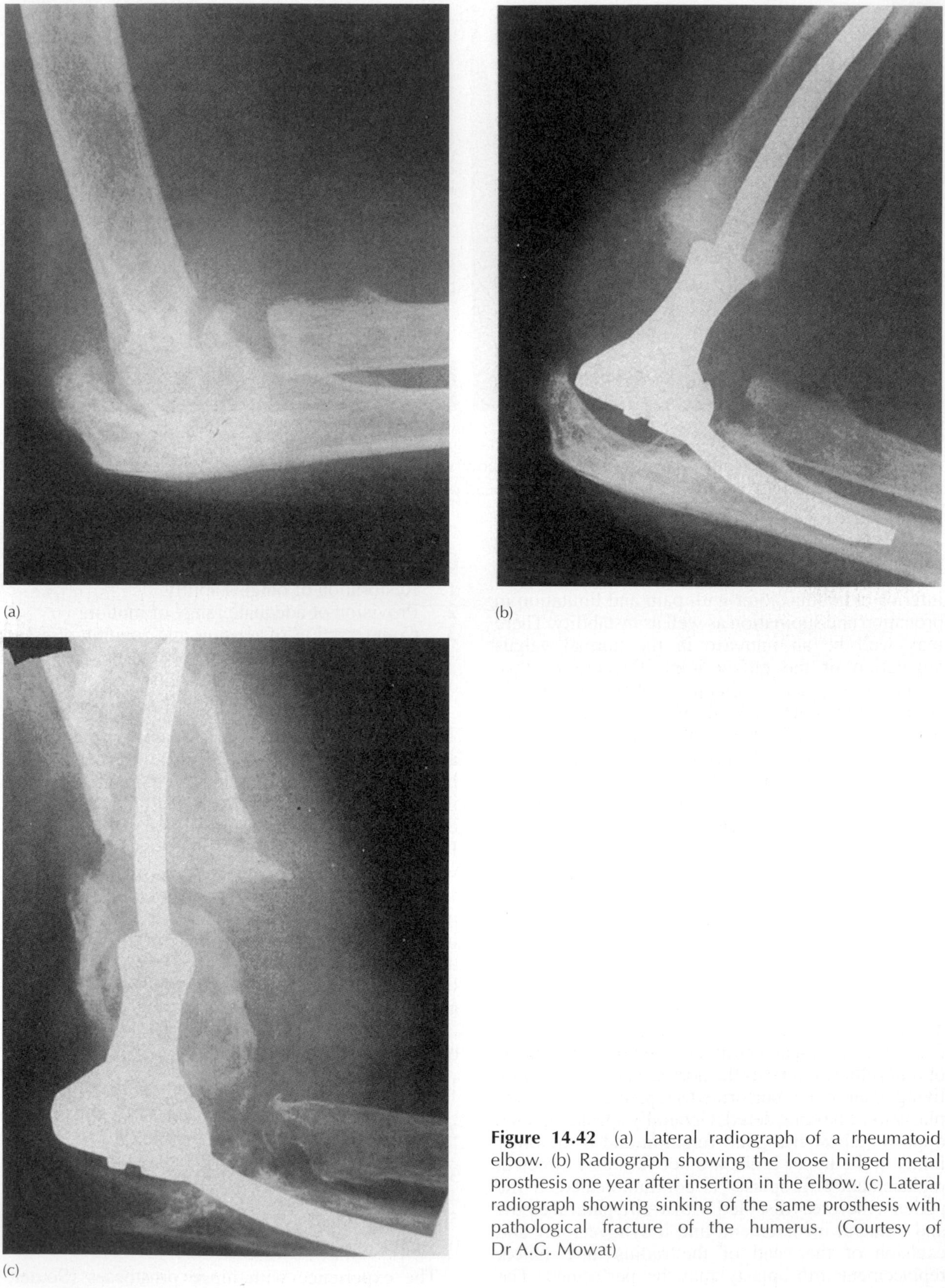

(a) (b) (c)

Figure 14.42 (a) Lateral radiograph of a rheumatoid elbow. (b) Radiograph showing the loose hinged metal prosthesis one year after insertion in the elbow. (c) Lateral radiograph showing sinking of the same prosthesis with pathological fracture of the humerus. (Courtesy of Dr A.G. Mowat)

(a)

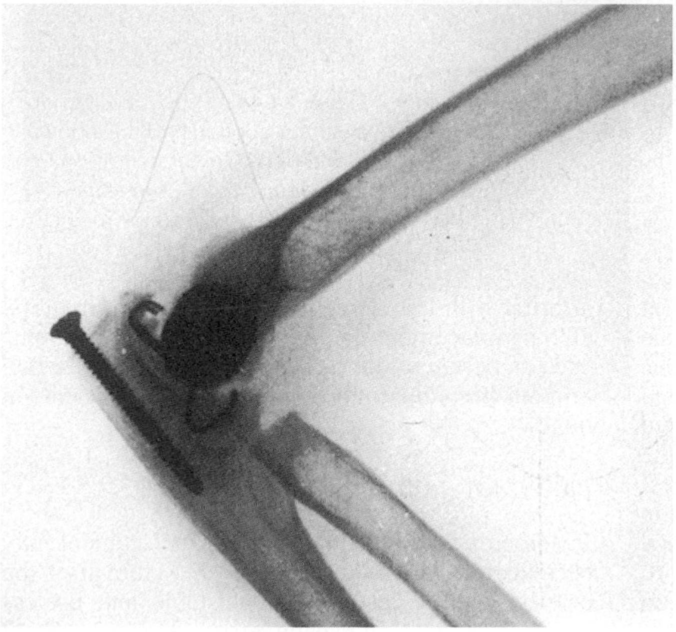

(b)

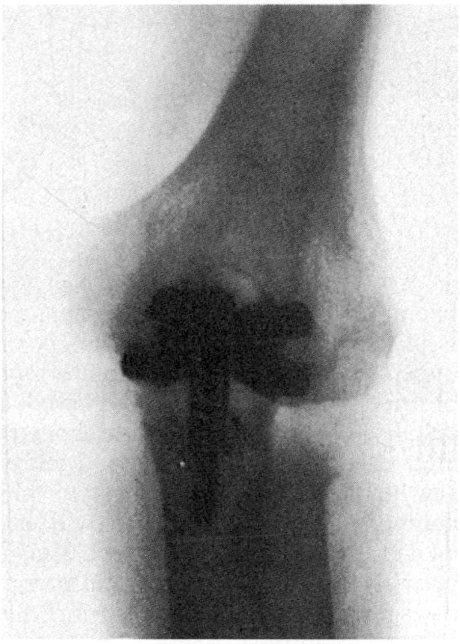

(c)

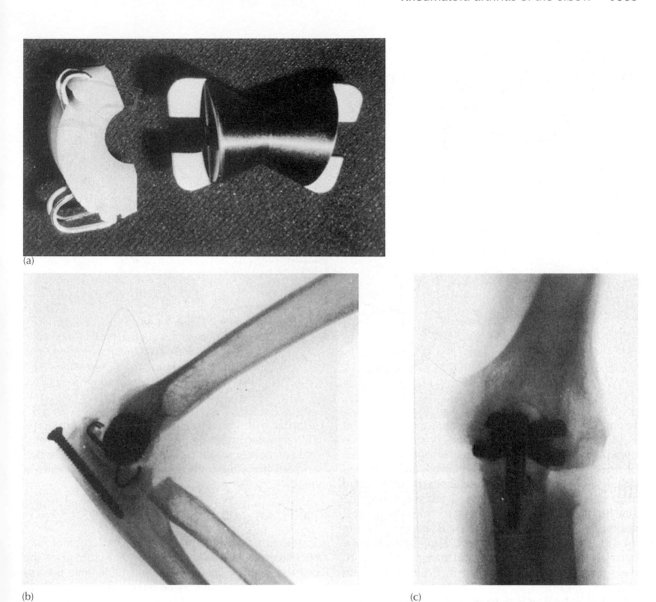

Figure 14.43 The Liverpool prosthesis. (a) The bobbin shaped stainless steel humeral component with its stabilizing pins and the high density polyethylene ulnar component. (b) and (c) Postoperative radiographs showing the prosthesis *in situ*. (Reproduced, with permission, from Cavendish, M.E. and Elloy, M.A. (1976) *Journal of Bone and Joint Surgery* **58B**, 253)

1978) has been disappointing, with a high proportion of failures due to loosening of the prosthetic stems in the humerus (Figure 14.42). Cavendish and Elloy (1976) reported the use of a prosthesis (the Liverpool prosthesis) which does not employ stems within the humerus or ulna. It also has a fail-safe device such that the prosthesis dislocates rather than becoming loose when placed under excessive stress (Figure 14.43). Reduction of the joint may be performed in such circumstances, also without loosening of the prosthesis.

Recent reports show that the results of elbow replacements are improving. The two problems of mechanical loosening of constrained (hinged) prostheses and dislocation of non-constrained designs have been overcome largely by semi-constrained designs.

Unconstrained prostheses are still used rarely in patients with early rheumatoid arthritis. Intact collateral ligaments (particularly the medial collateral ligament) are necessary for a successful result. At the present time it is difficult to obtain a stable unconstrained elbow replacement and achieve full extension. Perfect balancing of soft tissues and appropriate bone cuts are essential.

The most common approaches are the posterior or

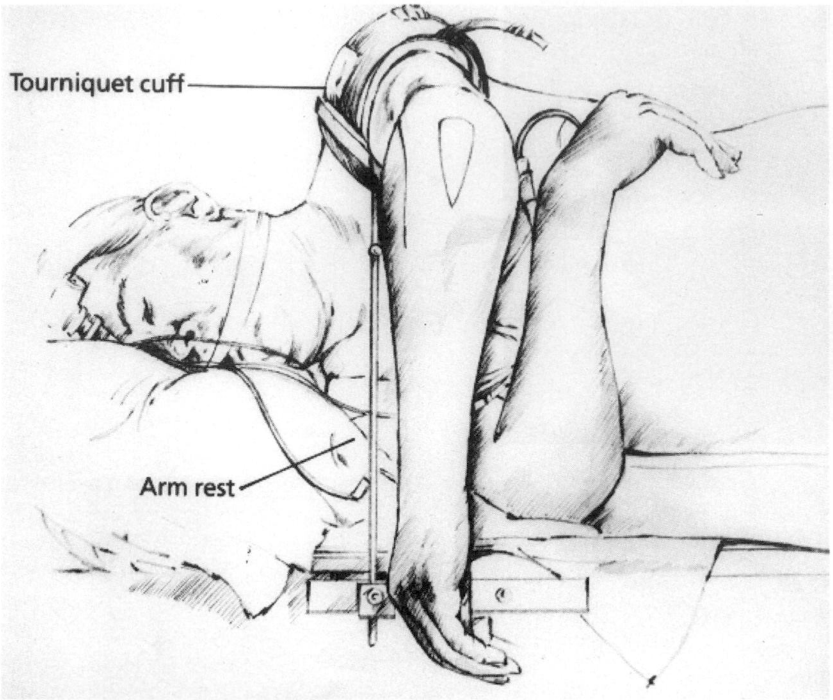

Figure 14.44 Patient position for posterior approach to the elbow. (Reproduced, with permission, from *Souter Elbow Surgical Technique Booklet*, Howmedica)

lateral Kocher. For the posterior approach the patient is placed in the lateral decubitus position with the upper arm placed on a rest (Figure 14.44). A tongue of triceps aponeurosis is preserved and reflected distally. The radial head is dislocated and resected after adequate lateral soft tissue release. Using the saw guide the humerus is cut to take the largest component which the bone will accept (Figure 14.45). The ulna is then prepared using a ball-headed burr. The aim is to insert the ulnar stem in line with the shaft of the ulna, and not in a flexed position (Figure 14.45b).

A trial reduction is performed to ensure adequate movement is possible and the humeral and ulnar prostheses are then cemented in place (Figure 14.46). Following release of the tourniquet and haemostasis the wound is then closed in layers.

RESULTS

At least 90% of patients are highly satisfied with pain relief at 5–10 year review. Some improvement in flexion, pronation and supination is seen although extension strength remains unchanged. The average arc of movements are 100° of flexion–extension and 130° of pronation–supination (Souter, 1992).

Careful patient selection is essential in elbow replacement. Prosthetic replacement is indicated for the physiologically older patient with relatively low demand. Selected young patients with rheumatoid arthritis with low demands also benefit from a total elbow replacement. In young, high-demand patients such as post-traumatic osteoarthritis the failure rate remains high due to loosening of the components in bone.

Failed total elbow replacements

In some cases a loose total elbow replacement may be retained. This is rare, however. Removal of the prosthesis may result in an unstable and useless elbow. The situation may be retrieved to some extent by recessing the semilunar fossa in the residual humeral epicondyle (Figgie *et al*., 1987).

Revision of a total elbow arthroplasty can give satisfactory results, although in the absence of sufficient bone stock this may be impossible. A semi-constrained prosthesis is usually indicated in these cases.

Goldberg *et al*. (1988) and Figgie *et al*. (1987) have described up to 85% satisfactory results in this situation. In infected cases, replacement of the infected prosthesis still results in a high infection rate and this remains unacceptable.

Excisional arthroplasty

Until total replacement of the elbow becomes a more reliably successful procedure, excisional arthroplasty retains a place in the surgical armamentarium. This procedure will give an excellent range

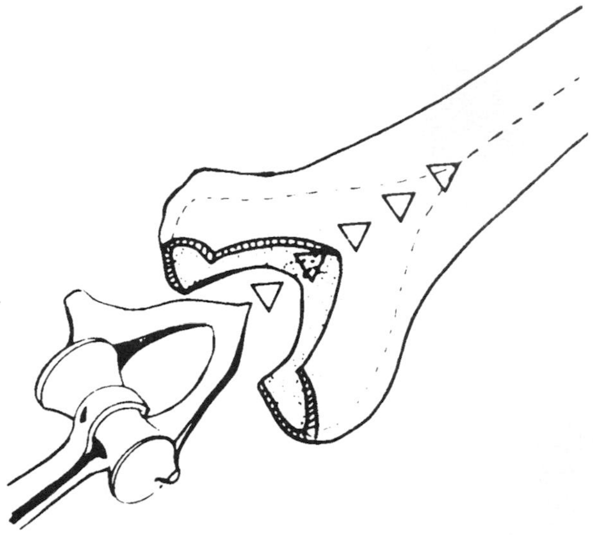

(a)

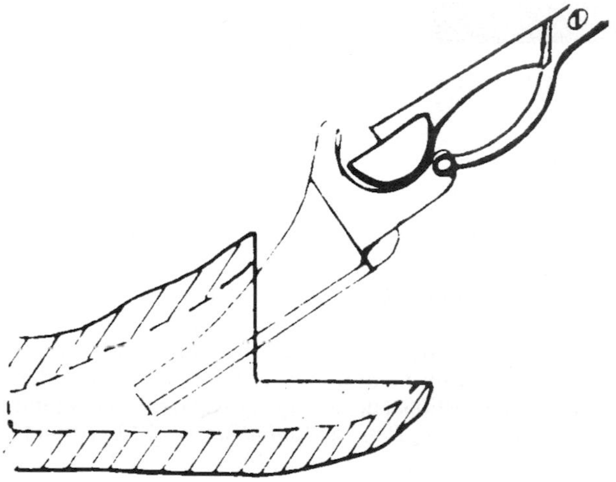

(b)

Figure 14.45 (a) Humeral preparation and (b) ulnar preparation. (Reproduced, with permission, from *Souter Elbow Surgical Technique Booklet*, Howmedica)

of movement but normally lacks the collateral stability so vital in elbow function. In a long-term review, Dickson *et al.* (1976) reported good relief of pain and a useful increase of hinge motion and of forearm rotation in 12 patients. Instability was not a serious problem unless the patient had to bear weight on crutches. To increase stability after arthroplasty it appeared that Kirschner wire fixation with two crossed wires traversing the joint was advisable postoperatively as well as a supporting posterior plaster slab (Goodfellow, 1975, personal communication). It was important to retain the position of the elbow in splintage for 6 weeks postoperatively before the wires and the cast were removed. It was concluded that, for advanced rheumatoid disease, unilateral excisional arthroplasty had definite value and especially so in patients who were confined to wheelchairs and were therefore particularly dependent on the mobility of the upper limb joints for feeding and toilet purposes.

Osteoarthritis of the elbow

Osteoarthritis of the elbow is rare, and primary osteoarthritis probably occurs except rarely as part of generalized osteoarthrosis in association with Heberden's nodes when involvement is bilateral. Certain occupations are said to be associated with secondary osteoarthritis, especially those involving vibrating tools such as pneumatic drills. Osteochondritis dissecans of the capitellum may precede osteoarthrosis but takes many years to develop. However, it may give rise also to loose bodies in the elbow which require removal due to painful locking. For a reason which is not very clear, haemophiliacs tend to bleed frequently into the elbows, a surprising fact since the joint is relatively stable. Fractures into the joint of the humerus, ulna and radial head may predispose the joint to osteoarthrosis also.

TREATMENT

Generally, the patient with osteoarthrosis of the elbow does not have serious problems unless he is involved in heavy physical work, so the treatment is usually conservative based on periods of reduced activity and anti-inflammatory analgesic drugs such as aspirin. If pain becomes severe and intolerable, conservative surgery such as articular drilling of denuded areas and removal of loose cartilage and bony fragments can give relief. This procedure is best performed through a lateral Kocher's approach.

Generally, removal of the head of the radius should be avoided unless there is severe pain from this joint and the articular cartilage is seriously damaged. Fusion of the elbow at 90° of flexion is a very disabling operation which should be performed only in the presence of a normal contralateral elbow and after very careful consideration. Arthroplasty is less successful than in rheumatoid arthritis due to the problem of collateral ligament stability and loosening after operation. In carefully selected cases it can be useful (Souter, 1992).

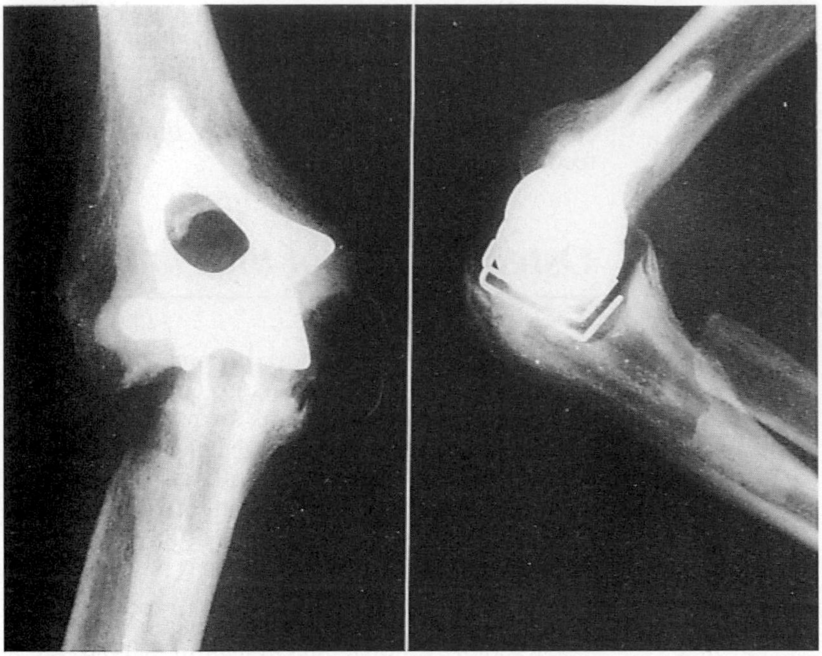

Figure 14.46 Anteroposterior and lateral radiographs of the Souter-Strathclyde prosthesis after successful revision of a previous arthroplasty.

The stiff elbow

Morrey *et al.* (1981, 1985) have suggested that fixed flexion deformity of 30° in the elbow with flexion to 130° and a range of rotation from 40° of pronation to 40° of supination allows performance of 90% of activities of daily living. Elbow stiffness may be intrinsic or extrinsic to the joint. Intrinsic causes are usually post-traumatic or inflammatory and are usually associated with secondary extrinsic contractures. Primary extrinsic contractures are often isolated and include heterotopic ossification. Excision of the relevant structure may result in significant improvement in elbow movement (Roberts and Pankratz, 1979; Shahriaree *et al.*, 1979; Cooney, 1985; Seth and Khurana, 1985; Morrey, 1990).

In intrinsic contractures, provided the joint surfaces are satisfactory, debridement of the joint and its margins, removal of loose bodies and excision of the joint capsular contractures may produce a satisfactory result (Volkov and Oganesian, 1975; Deland *et al.*, 1987; Morrey, 1990).

Excision arthroplasty may restore satisfactory range of motion in up to 80% of patients, although results are unpredictable and the loss of stability may be unsatisfactory from a functional point of view (Shahriaree *et al.*, 1979). This is not recommended except in exceptional bilateral cases where some mobility is essential.

References

Adams, J.C. (1948) Recurrent dislocation of the shoulder. *Journal of Bone and Joint Surgery* **30B**, 26–38

Altchek, D.W., Warren, R.F., Skyhar, M.J. and Ortiz, G. (1991) T-plasty modification of the Bankart procedure for multidirectional instability of the anterior and inferior types. *Journal of Bone and Joint Surgery* **73A**, 105–112

Amis, A.A., Dowson, D. and Wright, V. (1979) Muscle strengths and musculoskeletal geometry of the upper limb. *Engineering in Medicine* **8**, 41–48

Ann, K.N., Browene, A.O., Korinek, S., Tanaka, S. and Morrey, B.F. (1991) Three dimensional kinematics of glenohumeral elevation. *Journal of Orthopaedic Research* **9**, 143–149

Arantz, C.T., Matsen, F.A. and Jackins, S. (1991) Surgical management of complex irreparable rotator cuff deficiency. *Journal of Arthroplasty* **6**, 363–370

Bankart, A.S.B. (1938) The pathology and treatment of recurrent dislocation of the shoulder. *British Journal of Surgery* **26**, 23–29

Barron, J.N. (1969) *Annals of the Rheumatic Diseases* **28**, Supplement 74

Basmajian, J.V. (1969) Recent advances in functional anatomy of the upper limb. *American Journal of Physical Medicine* **48**, 165–177

Bentley, G. (1978) Wrist, elbow and shoulder surgery in rheumatoid arthritis. *Clinics in the Rheumatic Diseases* **4**, 385–402

Bentley, G., Krentner, A. and Ferguson, A.B. Jr (1973) The effect of hydrocortisone on synovial regeneration and on

articular surfaces following synovectomy in rabbits. *Journal of Bone and Joint Surgery* **56B**, 572
Bloch, J. and Fischer, F.K. (1960) *Acta Rheumatologica* **2**, 11
Blount, W. (1955) *Fractures in Children*. Williams & Wilkins: Baltimore, Maryland
Bosworth, B.M. (1941) *Surgery, Gynecology and Obstetrics* **73**, 866
Bulgen, D.Y., Hazleman, B.L. and Voak, D. (1976) HLA-B27 and frozen shoulder. *Lancet* **1**, 1042–1044
Bulgen, D.Y., Hazleman, B., Ward, M. and McCallum, M. (1978) Immunological studies in frozen shoulder. *Annals of the Rheumatic Diseases* **37**, 135–138
Cavendish, M.E. and Elloy, M.A. (1976) A simple method of total elbow replacement. *Journal of Bone and Joint Surgery* **58B**, 253
Codman, E.A. (1934) *The Shoulder: Rupture of Supraspinatus Tendon and Other Lesions on or about the Subacromial Bursa*. Thomas Todd: Boston
Cooney, W.P. III (1985) Contractures and burns. In: *The Elbow and its Disorders*, pp. 433–451. Edited by B.F. Morrey, Philadelphia: W.B. Saunders
Crenshaw, A.H. and Kilgore, W.E. (1966) Surgical treatment of bicipital tenosynovitis. *Journal of Bone and Joint Surgery* **48A**, 1496–1502
Dee, R. (1972) Total replacement of the elbow for rheumatoid arthritis. *Journal of Bone and Joint Surgery* **54B**, 88–95
Deland, J.T., Garg, A. and Walker, P.S. (1987) Biomechanical basis for elbow hinge-distractor design. *Clinical Orthopaedics* **215**, 303–312
DePalma, A. (1953) *Bulletin of the Hospital for Joint Diseases* **14**, 35
Dewar, F.P. and Harris, R.T. (1950) *Annals of Surgery* **132**, 111
Dickson, R.A., Stein, H. and Bentley, G. (1976) Excision arthroplasty of the elbow in rheumatoid disease. *Journal of Bone and Joint Surgery* **58B**, 227–229
Dowd, G.S.E. and Hopcroft, P. (1979) Varus deformity in supracondylar fractures of the humerus in children. *Injury* **10**, 297–303
Ellman, H. (1985) Arthroscopic subacromial decompression. A preliminary report. *Orthopedic Transactions* **9**, 49
English, E. (1973) Recurrent posterior dislocation of the shoulder. *Orthopedic Clinics of North America* **6**, 685–696
Essman, J.A., Bell, R.H. and Askew, M. (1991) Full-thickness rotator-cuff tear. *Clinical Orthopaedics* **265**, 170–177
Ewald, F.C. (1975) Total elbow replacement. *Orthopedic Clinics of North America* **6**, 685–696
Eyre-Brook, A. (1973) Posterior dislocation of the shoulder. *Journal of Bone and Joint Surgery* **55B**, 441
Figgie, H. E. III, Inglis, A., Ranawat, C.S. and Rosenberg, G.M. (1987) Results of total elbow arthroplasty as a salvage procedure for failed elbow reconstructive operations. *Clinical Orthopaedics* **219**, 185–193
Frassica, F.J., Chao, E.Y., Shives, T.C. and Sim, F.H. (1991) Resection of malignant bone tumours about the shoulder. *Clinical Orthopaedics* **267**, 57–64
French, P.R. (1959) Varus deformity of the elbow following supracondylar fracture of the elbow in children. *Lancet* **2**, 439–441
Fukuda, H. (1990) Shoulder impingement and rotator cuff disease. *Current Orthopedics* **4**, 225–232
Gallie, W.E. and Le Mesurier, A.B. (1948) Recurring dislocation of the shoulder. *Journal of Bone and Joint Surgery* **30B**, 9–18
Garancis, J.C., Cheung, H.S., Halverson, P.B. and McCarty, D.J. (1981) Milwaukee shoulder III. Morphologic and biochemical studies of an excised synovium showing chondromatosis. *Arthritis and Rheumatism* **24**, 484–491
Gartsman, G.M. (1990) Arthroscopic acromioplasty for lesions of the rotator cuff. *Journal of Bone and Joint Surgery* **72A**, 169–180
Gerber, C. (1992) Latissimus dorsi transfer for the treatment of irreparable tears of the rotator cuff. *Clinical Orthopaedics* **275**, 152–160
Gerber, C. and Krushell, R.J. (1991) Isolated rupture of the tendon of the subscapularis muscle: clinical fractures in 16 cases. *Journal of Bone and Joint Surgery* **73B**, 389–394
Goldberg, M., Figgie, H.E. III, Inglis, A.E. and Figgie, M.P. (1988) Current concepts review: total elbow arthroplasty. *Journal of Bone and Joint Surgery* **70A**, 778–783
Halverson, P.B., Cheung, H.S., McCarty, D.J., Garancis, J. and Mandel, N. (1981) Milwaukee shoulder II. Synovial fluid findings. *Arthritis and Rheumatism* **24**, 474–483
Harryman, D.T., Mack, L.A., Wang, K.Y., Jackins, S.E., Richardson, M.L. and Matsen, F.A. (1991) Repairs of the rotator cuff: correlation of functional results with integrity of the cuff. *Journal of Bone and Joint Surgery* **73A**, 982–989
Harryman, D.T., Sidles, J.A., Harris, S.L. and Matzen, F.A. (1992) The role of the rotator interval capsule in passive motion and stability of the shoulder. *Journal of Bone and Joint Surgery* **74A**, 53–66
Hawkins, R.J. and Mohtadi, N.G.H. (1991) Controversy in anterior shoulder instability. *Clinical Orthopaedics* **272**, 152–161
Hill, H.A. and Sachs, M.D. (1940) Grooved defect of the humeral head. *Radiology* **35**, 690–700
Hoaglund, F.J. and Duthie, R.B. (1966) Surgical reconstruction for shoulder pain after radical neck dissection. *American Journal of Surgery* **112**, 522–526
Howell, S.M. and Kraft, T.A. (1991) The role of the supraspinatus and infraspinatus muscles in glenohumeral kinematics of anterior shoulder instability. *Clinical Orthopaedics* **263**, 128–134
Hsu, S.Y. and Chan, K.M. (1991) Arthroscopic distension in management of frozen shoulder. *International Orthopedics* **15**, 79–83
Hughes, C.S.R. (1948) *British Journal of Surgery* **36**, 158
Iannotti, J.P., Zlatkin, M.B., Esterhai, J.L., Kressel, H.J., Dalinka, M.K. and Spindler, K.P. (1991) Magnetic resonance of the shoulder. *Journal of Bone and Joint Surgery* **73A**, 17–29
Itoi, E. and Tabata, S. (1992) Conservative treatment of rotator cuff tears. *Clinical Orthopaedics* **275**, 165–173
Jakob, R., Fowles, J.V., Rang, M. and Kassab, M.T. (1975) Observations concerning fractures of the lateral humeral condyle in children. *Journal of Bone and Joint Surgery* **57B**, 430–436

Jerosch, J., Muller, T. and Castro, W.M. (1991) The incidence of rotator cuff rupture: an anatomic study. *Acta Orthopaedica Belgica* **57**, 124–129

Jobe, F.W., Giangarra, C.E., Kvitine, R.S. and Glousman, R.E. (1991) Anterior capsulolabral reconstruction of the shoulder in athletes in overhand sports. *American Journal of Sports Medicine* **19**, 428–434

Johnson, J.T.H. and Kendall, H.O. (1961) *Clinical Orthopaedics* **20**, 151

Kessel, L. and Watson, M. (1977) The painful arc syndrome. *Journal of Bone and Joint Surgery* **59B**, 166–172

Kocialkowski, A., Romberg, P.H. and Wallace, A. (1992) The treatment of localized metastases in the proximal humerus from renal cell carcinoma. *Journal of Shoulder and Elbow Surgery* **1**, 56–62

Krönberg, M. and Broström, L.A. (1991) Proximal humeral osteotomy to correct the anatomy in patients with recurrent shoulder dislocations. *Journal of Orthopaedic Trauma* **5**, 129–133

Laurence, M. (1991) Replacement arthroplasty of the rotator cuff deficient shoulder. *Journal of Bone and Joint Surgery* **73B**, 916–919

Lebar, R.D. and Alexander, A.H. (1992) Multidirectional shoulder instability: clinical results of inferior capsular shift in active-duty population. *American Journal of Sports Medicine* **20**, 193–198

Leslie, J.T. and Ryan, T.J. (1962) *Journal of Bone and Joint Surgery* **44A**, 1193

Lombardo, S.J., Kerlan, R.K., Jobe, F.W., Carter, V.S., Blazina, M.E. and Shields, C.L. (1976) The modified Bristow procedure for recurrent dislocation of the shoulder. *Journal of Bone and Joint Surgery* **58A**, 256–261

McCarty, D.J., Halverson, P.B., Carrera, G.F., Brewer, B.J. and Kozin, F. (1981) Milwaukee shoulder. I. Clinical aspects. *Arthritis and Rheumatism* **24**, 464–473

McLaughlin, H.L. (1962) Posterior dislocation of the shoulder. *Journal of Bone and Joint Surgery* **44A**, 1477

McLaughlin, H.L. and MacLellan, D.I. (1967) Recurrent anterior dislocation of the shoulder. A comparative study. *Journal of Trauma* **7**, 191–201

McNab, I. (1973) Rotator cuff tendinitis. *Annals of the Royal College of Surgeons of England* **53**, 271–287

Magnuson, P.B. and Stack, J.K. (1943) Recurrent dislocation of the shoulder. *Journal of the American Medical Association* **123**, 889–892

Malawer, M.M., Meller, I. and Dunham, W.K. (1991) A new surgical classification system for shoulder-girdle resections – analysis of 38 patients. *Clinical Orthopaedics* **267**, 33–44

Mathys, R. and Mathys, R. Jr (1977) In: *Endoprostheses and Alternatives for the Arm Shoulder Joint*, p. 5. Edited by C. Burri, J. Coldewey and A. Ruter. Hans Huber: Bern, Stuttgart, Vienna

Misamore, G.W. and Woodward, C. (1991) Evaluation of rotator cuff lesions. *Journal of Bone and Joint Surgery* **73A**, 704–706

Morrey, B.F. (1990) Post-traumatic contracture of the elbow. *Journal of Bone and Joint Surgery* **72A**, 601–618

Morrey, B.F. and Chao, E.Y.S (1976) Passive motion of the elbow joint. *Journal of Bone and Joint Surgery* **58A**, 501–508

Morrey, B.F. and Janes, J.M. (1976) Recurrent anterior dislocation of the shoulder. *Journal of Bone and Joint Surgery* **53A**, 252–256

Morrey, B.F., Chao, E.Y.S. and Hui, F.C. (1979) Biomechanical study of the elbow following excision of the radial head. *Journal of Bone and Joint Surgery* **61A**, 63–68

Morrey, B.F., Askew, L.J., An, K.N. and Chao, E.Y. (1981) A biomechanical study of normal functional elbow motion. *Journal of Bone and Joint Surgury* **63A**, 872–877

Morrey, B.F., An, K.N. and Chao, E.Y.S. (1985) Functional evaluation of the elbow. In: *The Elbow and its Disorders*, pp. 73–91. Edited by B.F. Morrey. Philadelphia: W.B. Saunders

Mumford, E.B. (1941) *Journal of Bone and Joint Surgery* **23**, 799

Neer, C.S. (1955) Articular replacement for the humeral head. *Journal of Bone and Joint Surgery* **37A**, 215–228

Neer, C.S. II (1972) Anterior acromioplasty for the chronic impingement syndrome in the shoulder, a preliminary report. *Journal of Bone and Joint Surgery* **54A**, 41–50

Neer, C.S. (1974) Replacement arthroplasty for glenohumeral osteoarthritis. *Journal of Bone and Joint Surgery* **56A**, 1–13

Neer, C.S. II (1983) Impingements lesions. *Clinical Orthopaedics and Related Research* **173**, 70–77

Nelson, C.L. and Burton, R.I. (1975) Upper extremity arthrography. *Clinical Orthopaedics and Related Research* **107**, 62–72

Nelson, M.C., Leather, G.P., Nirschl, P.R., Pettrone, F.A. and Freedman, M.T. (1991) Evaluation of the painful shoulder. *Journal of Bone and Joint Surgery* **73A**, 707–716

Neviaser, J.S. (1945) Adhesive capsulitis of the shoulder. A study of the pathological findings in periarthritis of the shoulder. *Journal of Bone and Joint Surgery* **27**, 211–222

Neviaser, J.S. (1975) *Arthrography of the Shoulder*. Charles C Thomas: Springfield, Illinois

Ogilvie-Harris, D.J. and Demazière, A. (1993) Arthroscopic debridement versus open repair for rotator cuff tears. *Journal of Bone and Joint Surgery* **75B**, 416–420

Osmond-Clarke, H. (1948) Habitual dislocation of the shoulder. *Journal of Bone and Joint Surgery* **30B**, 19–25

Palmer, I. and Widen, A. (1948) The bone block method for recurrent dislocation of the shoulder joint. *Journal of Bone and Joint Surgery* **30B**, 53–58

Parsonage, M.J. and Turner, W.A. (1948) *Lancet* **1**, 973

Pigliani, L.U., Kimmel, J. and McCann, P. (1992) Repair of rotator cuff tears in tennis players. *American Journal of Sportsmen* **20**, 112–117

Poppen, N.K. and Walker, P.S. (1976) Normal and abnormal motion of the shoulder. *Journal of Bone and Joint Surgery* **58A**, 195–201

Reeves, B. (1966a) Arthrographic changes in frozen and post-traumatic stiff shoulders. *Proceedings of the Royal Society of Medicine* **59**, 827–830

Reeves, B.(1966b) Arthrography of the shoulder. *Journal of Bone and Joint Surgery* **48B**, 424–435

Reeves, B. (1968) Experiments on the tensile strength of

the anterior capsular structures of the shoulder in man. *Journal of Bone and Joint Surgery* **50B**, 858–865

Richmond, J.C., Donaldson, W.R., Fu, F. and Harner, C.D. (1991) Modification of the Bankart reconstruction with a suture anchor. *American Journal of Sports Medicine* **19**, 343–346

Roberts, J.B. and Pankratz, D.G. (1979) The surgical treatment of heterotopic ossification at the elbow following long-term coma. *Journal of Bone and Joint Surgery* **61A**, 760–763

Rockwood, C. (1981) The shoulder impingement syndrome and its relationship to lesions of the rotation cuff. Lecture to British Orthopaedic Association, 1st October 1981

Rowe, C.R. (1956) Prognosis in dislocation of the shoulder. *Journal of Bone and Joint Surgery* **38A**, 957–977

Rowe, C.R., Pierce, D.S. and Clarke, J.G. (1973) Voluntary dislocation of the shoulder. *Journal of Bone and Joint Surgery* **55A**, 745–760

Rowe, C.R., Patel, D. and Southmayd, W.W. (1978) The Bankart procedure. *Journal of Bone and Joint Surgery* **60A**, 1–16

Saha, A.K. (1969) *Recurrent Anterior Dislocation of the Shoulder: a New Concept*. Academic Publishers: Calcutta

Saha, A.K. (1978) *Proceedings of the Indian National Science Academy* **44**, Part A, 195–201

Scott, D.J. (1967) Treatment of recurrent posterior dislocations of the shoulder by glenoplasty. *Journal of Bone and Joint Surgery* **49A**, 471–476

Seth, M.K. and Khurana, J.K. (1985) Bony ankylosis of the elbow after burns. *Journal of Bone and Joint Surgery* **67B**, 747–749

Shahriaree, H., Sajadi, K., Silver, C.M. and Sheikholeslamzadeh, S. (1979) Excisional arthroplasty of the elbow. *Journal of Bone and Joint Surgery* **61A**, 922–927

Smith, L. (1960) Deformity following supracondylar fractures of the humerus. *Journal of Bone and Joint Surgery* **42A**, 235–252

Snyder, S.J. (1993) Evaluation and treatment of the rotator cuff. *Orthopedic Clinics of North America* **24**, 173–192

Souter, W.A. (1978) Arthroplasty of the elbow with particular reference to metallic hinge arthroplasty in rheumatoid arthritis. *Orthopedic Clinics of North America* **4**, 395–413

Souter, W.A. (1992) Souter-Strathclyde arthroplasty in the management of the rheumatoid elbow. Results at five and ten year follow-up. *Journal of Bone and Joint Surgery* **74B**, Supplement III, 268

Stein, H., Dickson, R.A. and Bentley, G. (1975) Rheumatoid arthritis of the elbow. Pattern of joint involvement and results of synovectomy with excision of the radial head. *Annals of the Rheumatic Diseases* **34**, 403–408

Street, D.M. and Stevens, P.S. (1974) A humeral replacement prosthesis for the elbow. *Journal of Bone and Joint Surgery* **56A**, 1147–1158

Swanson, A.B. and Herndon, J.H. (1982) *The Elbow*. Churchill Livingstone: Edinburgh, London, New York

Symeonides, P.P. (1972) The significance of the subscapularis muscle in the pathogenesis of recurrent dislocation of the shoulder. *Journal of Bone and Joint Surgery* **54B**, 476–483

Terry, G.C., Hammon, D., France, P. and Norwood, L. (1991) The stabilizing function of passive shoulder restraints. *American Journal of Sports Medicine* **19**, 26–34

Thomas, B.J., Amstutz, H.C. and Cracchiolo, A. (1991) Shoulder arthroplasty for rheumatoid arthritis. *Clinical Orthopaedics* **265**, 125–128

Thompson, R.G. and Compere, E.L. (1959) *Journal of the American Medical Association* **2**, 11

Tsai, L., Wredmark, T. and Johansson, C. (1991) Shoulder function in patients with unoperated anterior shoulder instability. *American Journal of Sports Medicine* **19**, 469–473

Uhthoff, H.K. and Sarkar, K. (1991) Surgical repair of rotator cuff ruptures: the importance of the subacromial bursa. *Journal of Bone and Joint Surgery* **73B**, 399–401

Vellet, A.D., Munk, P.L. and Marks, P. (1991) Imaging techniques of the shoulder: present perspectives. *Clinical Sports Medicine* **10**, 721–756

Voelcker, J. (1922) *Klinische Wochenschrift* **37**, 1838

Volkov, M.V. and Oganesian, O.V. (1975) Restoration of function in the knee and elbow with a hinge-distractor apparatus. *Journal of Bone and Joint Surgery* **57A**, 591–600

Wainwright, D. (1962) Fractures involving the elbow joint. In: *Modern Trends in Orthopaedics 3. Fracture Treatment*. Edited by J.M.P. Clark. Butterworths: London

Wainwright, D. (1974) Glenoidectomy – a method of treating the painful shoulder in severe rheumatoid arthritis. *Annals of the Rheumatic Diseases* **33**, 110

Walker, P.S. (1977) *Human Joints and their Artificial Replacements*. Charles C Thomas: Springfield, Illinois

Walker, P.S. and Poppen, N.K. (1977) Biomechanics of the shoulder joint during abduction in the plane of the scapula. *Bulletin of the Hospital for Joint Diseases* **38**, 107–111

Warner, J.J.P., Krushell, R.J., Masquelet, A. and Gerber, C. (1992) Anatomy and relationship of the supra-scapular nerve: anatomic constraints to mobilization of the supraspinatus and infraspinatus muscles in the management of massive rotator cuff tears. *Journal of Bone and Joint Surgery* **74A**, 36–45

Watson, M.S. (1991) *Surgical Disorders of the Shoulder*. Churchill Livingstone: Edinburgh, London and New York

Young, D.C. and Rockwood, C.A. (1991) Complications of a failed Bristow procedure and their management. *Journal of Bone and Joint Surgery* **73A**, 969–981

Zuckerman, J.D., Leblanc, J.M., Choveka, J. and Kummer, F. (1991) The effect of arm position and capsular release on rotator cuff repair. A biomedical study. *Journal of Bone and Joint Surgery* **73B**, 402–405

CHAPTER 15

Affections of the Wrist and Hand

R.I. BURTON, J.P. CULLEN AND S.H. DOERSCHUK

Introduction

The hand is the primary means through which human beings physically interact with the environment around them. In order to fulfil this crucial and varied role, the human hand has remarkable sensibility, in the form of pain, light touch, vibration, temperature recognition, and proprioceptive input. This sensory end organ is combined with a complex tool capable of performing a wide variety of co-ordinated motions and tasks with precision, speed, and strength.

Because of the resultant diversity of function, the hands are used for nearly all physical tasks. Further, because of this dependence on our hands for both proprioception and physical interaction, any condition which affects the hand will have a profound effect on overall function.

In order to appreciate how the hand functions and how various conditions may affect that function, it is important to understand some of the basic anatomy. This initial section on anatomy of the hand and wrist is an overview. The anatomical details of each condition will be addressed in subsequent sections.

Functional anatomy

The radius and ulna rotate around each other in order to allow pronation and supination. As a result, there are two articulations between these bones – the proximal and distal radioulnar joints.

The radiocarpal articulation consists of the distal radius articulating with the scaphoid and lunate distally. The distal carpal row consists of the distal pole of the scaphoid, trapezium, trapezoid, capitate, and hamate. These bones are held in alignment by volar, dorsal, and intercarpal ligaments. The pisiform is a sesamoid bone within the flexor carpi ulnaris tendon which articulates with the triquetrum and hamate (Figure 15.1)

The ulnocarpal articulation is formed by the triangular fibrocartilage complex (TFCC), which originates from the most ulnar distal aspect of the radius and attaches to the ulnar styloid and the base of the fifth metacarpal. It consists of the dorsal and volar radioulnar ligaments, the articular disc, the meniscus homologue, and the ulnar collateral ligament. It articulates with the triquetrum and lunate of the proximal carpal row (Figure 15.1).

Each of the fingers (digits II–V) consists of a metacarpal and three phalanges (Figure 15.2). The secondary ossification centres are distal in all of these bones. Minimal motion is present at the carpometacarpal (CMP) joints of the index (II) and long (III) digits but some flexion and extension is possible at the carpometacarpal joints of the ring (IV)

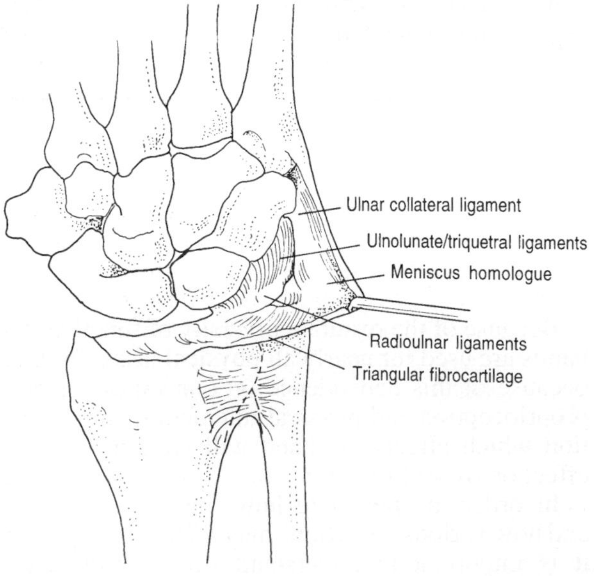

Figure 15.1 A dorsal view of the wrist, showing the triangular fibrocartilage complex and the carpal bones. (After Dell, P.C. (1987) *Hand Clinics of North America* **3**, 563)

and small (V) fingers. The volar plates limit extension in the metacarpophalangeal (MCP), proximal interphalangeal (PIP), and distal interphalangeal (DIP) joints. The collateral and accessory collateral ligaments limit varus/valgus motion. The MCP joint collateral ligaments are lax in extension, allowing a 60° arc of varus/valgus motion, and tight in flexion, essentially eliminating varus/valgus motion. The collateral ligaments of the PIP and DIP joints are relatively lax in flexion, allowing a small amount of varus/valgus motion, and tight in extension. The normal active ranges of extension/flexion for the MCP, PIP, and DIP joints of the fingers (digits II–V) are 0–90°, 0–100° and 0–90° respectively.

The thumb consists of a metacarpal and two phalanges. The secondary ossification centre of the thumb metacarpal is proximal. The carpometacarpal articulation is saddle-shaped, allowing flexion, extension, abduction, and adduction along with limited rotation, which allows the thumb to oppose the other digits. The MCP and interphalangeal (IP) joints are similarly constrained by the collateral and accessory collateral ligaments along with the volar plate (Figure 15.2).

The muscles which power the hand and wrist consist of the extrinsic flexors, the extrinsic extensors, and the intrinsics. The extrinsic muscles have their muscle bellies in the forearm whereas the intrinsic muscles are contained completely within the hand. The extrinsic wrist flexors (Figure 15.3) consist of the flexor carpi radialis (FCR) and flexor carpi ulnaris (FCU). The FCR inserts into the base of the second metacarpal. It is innervated by the median nerve and acts to flex and radially deviate the wrist. The FCU inserts into the pisiform and the base of the fifth metacarpal. It is innervated by the ulnar nerve, and functions primarily to flex and ulnarly deviate the wrist. The extrinsic wrist extensors (Figure 15.4) consist of the extensor carpi radialis longus (ECRL), extensor carpi radialis brevis (ECRB), and extensor carpi ulnaris (ECU). The ECRL and ECRB insert into the bases of the second and third metacarpals respectively. The ECU inserts into the base of the fifth metacarpal. In addition to extending the wrist the ECRL also radially deviates the wrist, while the ECU also ulnarly deviates the wrist. The ECRL and ECRB are innervated by the radial nerve and the ECU is innervated by the posterior interosseous nerve.

The extrinsic finger flexors (Figure 15.3) consist of the flexor digitorum superficialis (FDS) and the flexor digitorum profundus (FDP). The FDS attaches to the palmar aspect of the middle phalanx of digits II–V and acts to flex the PIP joints. It is innervated by the median nerve. The FDP attaches to the palmar base of the distal phalanx of digits IV–V and acts to flex the DIP joints. The FDP to digits II and III are

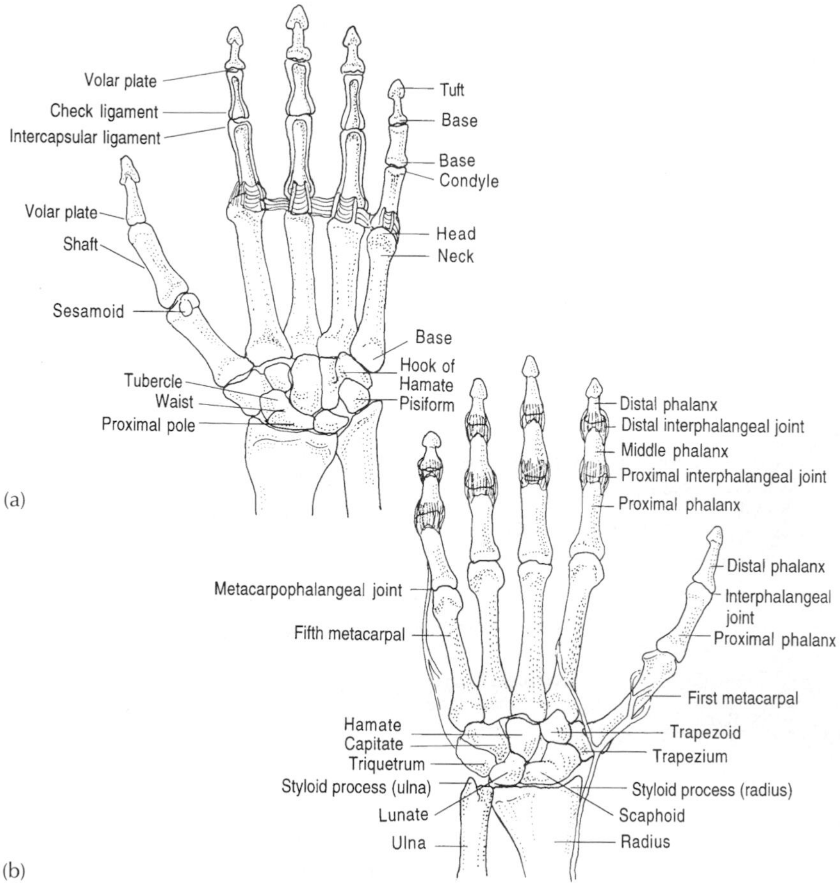

Figure 15.2 The bony anatomy of the hand and wrist. (a) Volar view. (b) Dorsal view. (After Beasley, R.W. (1981) *Hand Injuries*, W.B. Saunders: Philadelphia)

innervated by the median nerve and the FDP to digits IV and V are innervated by the ulnar nerve. The extrinsic flexor tendons pass through a fibro-osseous tunnel from the metacarpal head level distally along the digit. The volar portion is formed by five annular and three cruciate pulleys (A1-5 and C1-3). These pulleys, especially A2 and A4, prevent bowstringing of the tendons as the finger flexes and thereby maintain mechanical advantage.

The extrinsic finger extensors (Figure 15.4) consist of the extensor digitorum communis (EDC), extensor indicis proprius (EIP), and extensor digiti quinti (EDQ). The EDC is a single muscle which extends the MCP joints of digits II–V. The EIP and EDQ are similar muscles which allow isolated extension of digits II and V. These three muscles are innervated by the posterior interosseous nerve (PIN), a branch of the radial nerve in the forearm.

The extensor mechanism of the finger (Figure 15.5) is quite complex, and has contributions from both the extrinsic extensors (EDC, EIP, EDQ) and from the intrinsic musculature (interossei and lumbricals). The extrinsic extensor tendon (EDC) has four insertions into each digit. The first is into the volar plate and transverse metacarpal ligaments through the sagittal fibres of the extensor hood at the level of the MCP joint. These fibres run in a volar and distal direction around the metacarpal head into the volar plate at the level of the base of the proximal phalanx, causing MCP extension as the muscle contracts. The second insertion is into the base of the proximal phalanx, a very weak insertion which is often missing. At the level of the proximal phalanx, the tendon splits into three slips. The central slip inserts into the base of the middle phalanx while the two lateral bands coalesce to form the terminal insertion into the base of the distal phalanx. The interossei and lumbricals insert into the lateral bands and extensor hood. They function to flex the MCP joints and extend the interphalangeal joints.

The intrinsic muscles to the fingers consist of the dorsal interossei, volar interossei, and lumbricals (Figure 15.6). The interossei act to flex the MCP joints and extend the interphalangeal (PIP and DIP) joints of the fingers. The four dorsal interossei also abduct the digits with the MCP joints in extension,

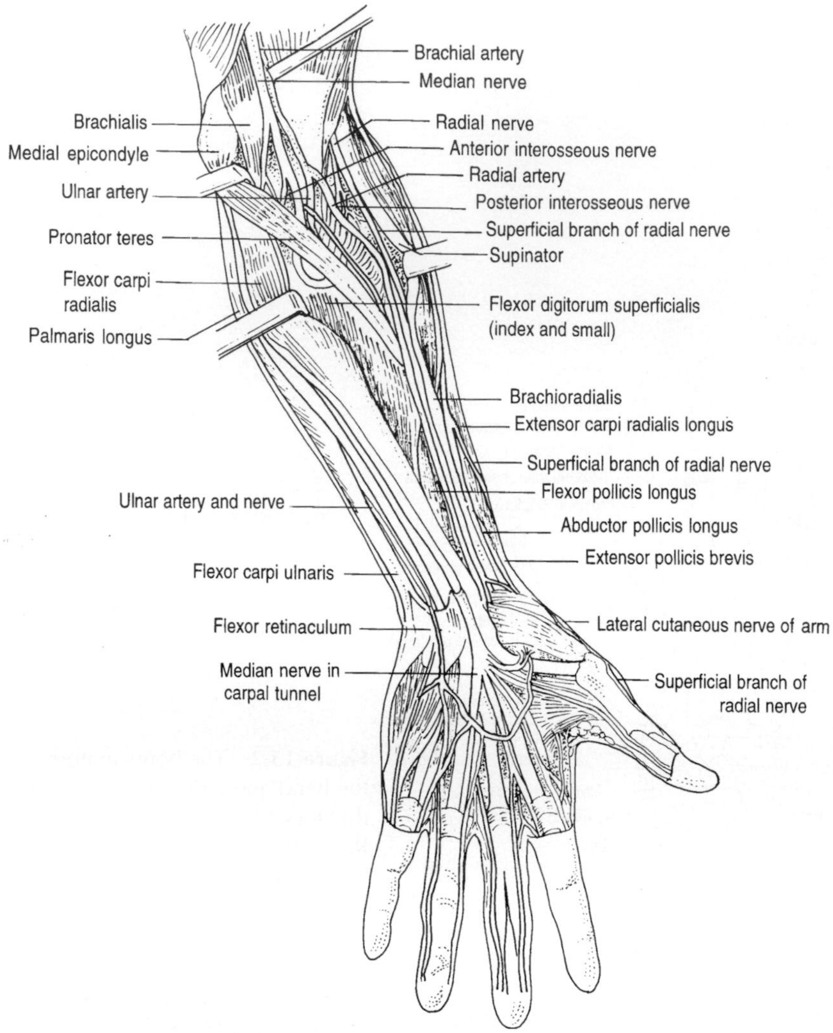

Figure 15.3 The essential longitudinal structures of the volar forearm and palm. (After Beasley, R.W. (1981) *Hand Injuries*, W.B. Saunders: Philadelphia)

while the three volar interossei adduct the digits with the MCP joints in extension. The dorsal interossei originate from adjacent metacarpals and insert into the extensor apparatus at the level of the proximal phalanx. The three volar interossei originate from the second, fourth, and fifth metacarpals. They insert into the extensor apparatus of the same digit. The four lumbricals originate on their respective FDP tendons I–V and insert into the radial lateral bands of the same digit. The line of pull of all these intrinsic muscles is palmar to the axes of the MCP joints, causing MCP flexion, and dorsal to the axes of motion of the PIP and DIP joints, resulting in PIP and DIP joint extension. As the PIP extends, the DIP is also passively extended through the pull of the oblique retinacular ligaments. All of the interossei are innervated by the ulnar nerve. The lumbricals are innervated by the median (II, III) and ulnar (IV, V) nerves.

The extrinsic flexor of the thumb (Figure 15.3) is the flexor pollicis longus (FPL) which inserts into the palmar aspect of the distal phalanx. It functions primarily to flex the thumb IP joint and is innervated by the anterior interosseous nerve, which is a branch of the median nerve in the forearm.

The extrinsic extensors of the thumb (Figure 15.4) include the abductor pollicis longus (APL), extensor pollicis brevis (EPB), and extensor pollicis longus (EPL). The APL passes through the first dorsal compartment of the wrist and inserts into the base of the thumb metacarpal. It functions to abduct and extend the thumb at the CMC joint. The EPB also passes through the first dorsal compartment and inserts into the dorsal base of the proximal phalanx. It primarily extends the thumb MCP joint although it is also an efficient abductor of the thumb. The EPL passes through the third dorsal compartment and inserts into the dorsal base of the distal phalanx. It

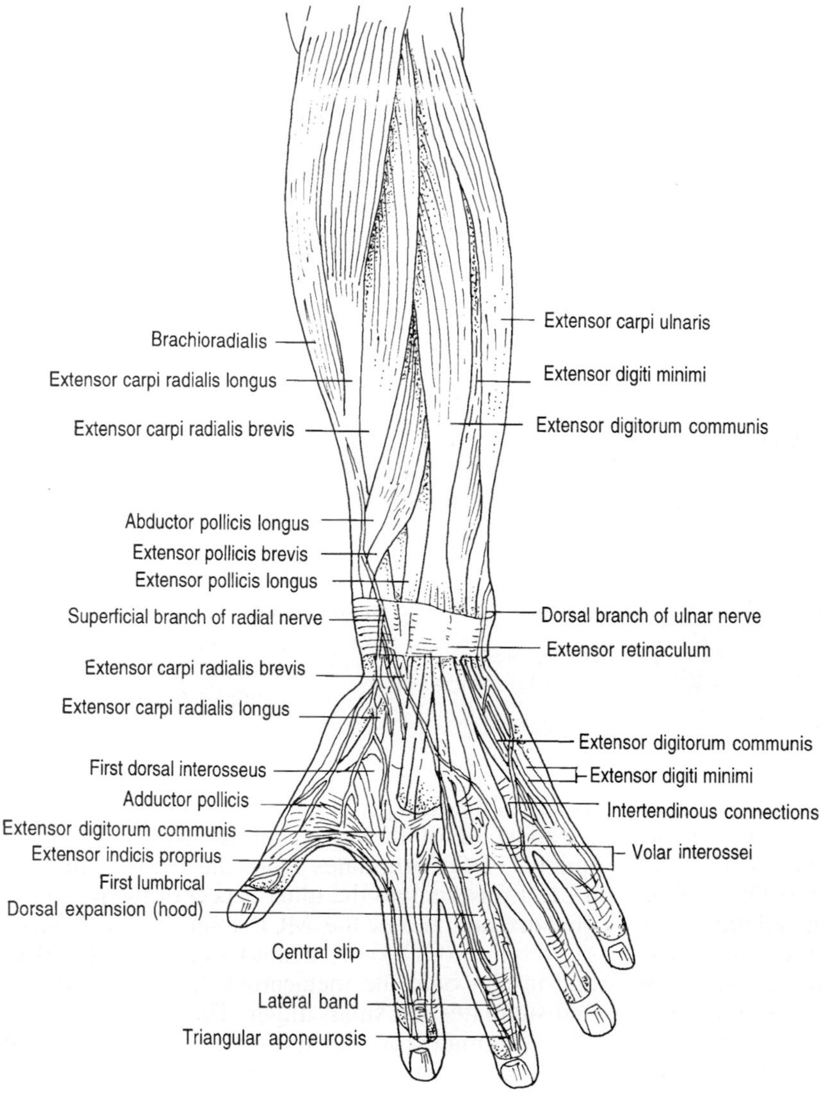

Figure 15.4 The dorsal forearm and hand. (After Beasley, R.W. (1981) *Hand Injuries*, W.B. Saunders: Philadelphia)

extends the IP joint, extends the MCP joint, and adducts the thumb. All of these muscles are innervated by the posterior interosseous nerve.

The intrinsic musculature of the thumb consists of the abductor pollicis brevis (APB), flexor pollicis brevis (FPB), opponens pollicis (OPP), and adductor

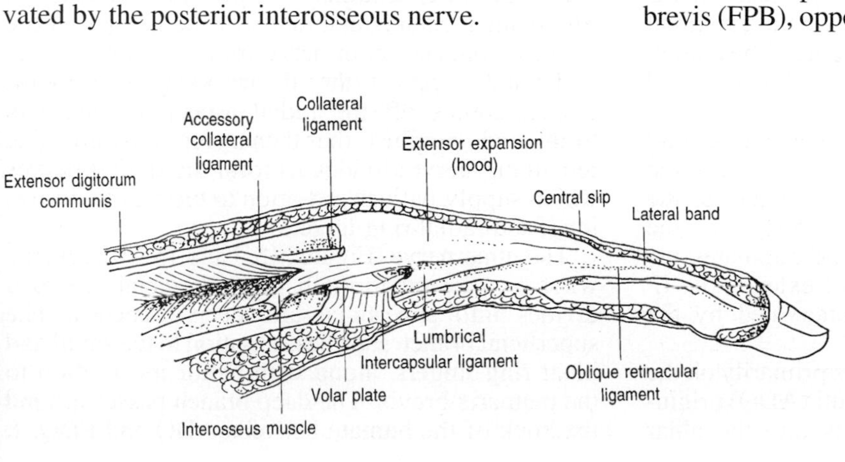

Figure 15.5 The digital extensor mechanism (see also Figure 15.4). (After Beasley, R.W. (1981) *Hand Injuries*, W.B. Saunders: Philadelphia)

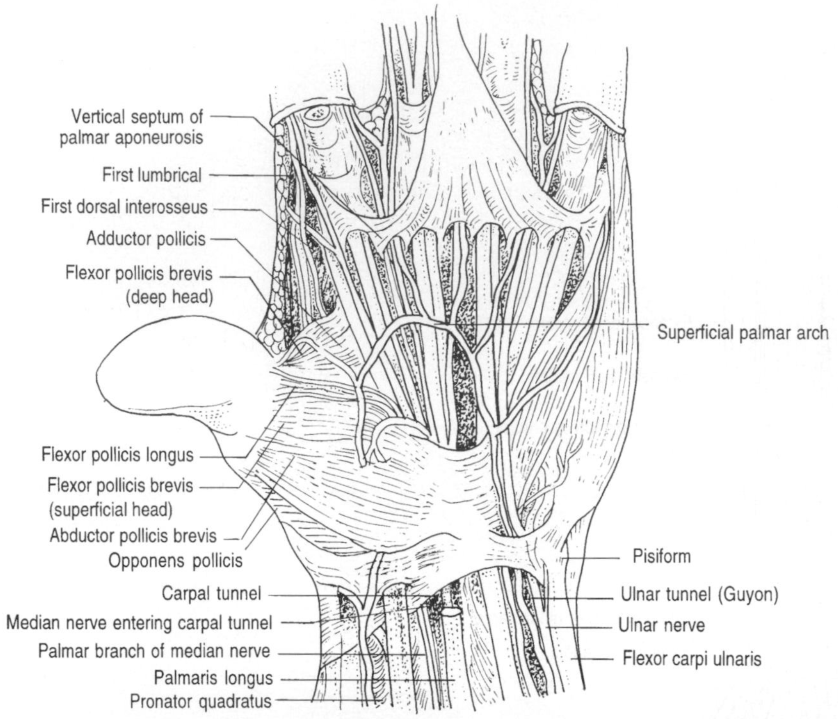

Figure 15.6 The intrinsic muscles of the hand. (After Beasley, R.W. (1981) *Hand Injuries*, W.B. Saunders: Philadelphia)

pollicis (ADD). The FPB is divided into a superficial head radial to the FPL tendon and innervated by the median nerve, and a deep head ulnar to the FPL tendon and innervated by the ulnar nerve. Opposition of the thumb allows palmar abduction and pronation of the thumb such that it is parallel to the plane of the palm and the other digits. This motion, which is crucial for grasping and pinching activities, is carried out by the median innervated thenar musculature – the APB, superficial head of FPB, and the OPP. The APB originates from the scaphoid and trapezium. It inserts into the base of the proximal phalanx and the extensor hood on the radial aspect. As a result, it abducts and pronates the thumb, extends the MCP, and extends the IP joint. The superficial head of FPB also inserts into the radial aspect of the proximal phalanx and thereby abducts and pronates the thumb. The OPP inserts on the metacarpal and is considered the weakest muscle of opposition.

The adductor pollicis originates on the second and third metacarpals. It inserts into the base of the proximal phalanx and the extensor hood on the ulnar side. As a result, this muscle, along with the deep head of the FPB, adducts and supinates the thumb. It also flexes the MCP and extends the IP joint. The adductor pollicis is innervated by the ulnar nerve.

The hypothenar musculature acts primarily on the small digit. The abductor digiti quinti (ADQ) originates from the pisiform and inserts into the ulnar aspect of the fifth proximal phalanx and functions as an abductor of the small finger. The flexor digiti quinti (FDQ) originates from the hamate and the TCL. It inserts into the ulnar aspect of the proximal phalanx and flexes the MCP joint. The opponens digiti quinti (ODQ) has a similar origin as the FDQ and inserts onto the metacarpal. It flexes, abducts, and supinates the small finger. The palmaris brevis (PB) originates on the transverse carpal ligament (TCL) and inserts into the hypothenar skin; it acts to retract the palmar skin. All of these muscles are innervated by the ulnar nerve.

The median nerve enters the wrist beneath the transverse carpal ligament along with the FDS, FDP, and FPL tendons (Figures 15.3 and 15.6). The palmar cutaneous branch of the median nerve divides from the main nerve trunk proximal to the TCL and supplies the thenar skin. The motor branch comes off the radial aspect of the main trunk and supplies the thenar musculature. The remaining nerve divides to form the digital nerves which supply palmar sensation to the thumb, index, long, and radial ring fingers.

The ulnar nerve (Figures 15.3 and 15.6) enters the wrist by passing through Guyon's canal where it divides into superficial and deep branches. The superficial branch supplies sensation to the small and ulnar ring fingers, along with motor innervation to the palmaris brevis. The deep branch passes around the hook of the hamate between ADQ and FDQ. It supplies all of the ulnar innervated intrinsic muscles. The dorsal cutaneous branch of the ulnar nerve comes off the main nerve in the distal half of the forearm. It pierces the deep fascia and travels ulnar and dorsal to supply the dorsal–ulnar skin of the hand including the small and ring fingers.

The radial sensory nerve (Figure 15.4) branches from the posterior interosseous nerve in the proximal forearm to travel beneath the brachioradialis muscle. In the distal forearm, approximately 3 cm above the radial styloid, the nerve pierces the deep fascia after passing between the brachioradialis and extensor carpi radialis longus tendons. It then divides into the dorsal digital nerves which supply sensation to the thumb, index, and long fingers. This nerve has multiple branches which lie just beneath the skin which are subject to damage during relatively minor procedures; this can lead to painful neuroma formation.

The radial artery lies deep to the brachioradialis and FCR in the forearm. At the wrist, the artery is radial to the FCR tendon and divides into superficial and deep branches. The superficial branch passes over or through the thenar musculature radial to the scaphoid tuberosity and then anastamoses with the ulnar artery to form the superficial arch. The deep branch passes deep to the first dorsal compartment tendons (APL, EPB) to enter the anatomical 'snuff box'. It then passes between the two heads of the first dorsal interosseus muscle to enter the palm, and forms the deep palmar arterial arch by anastomosing with the deep ulnar artery.

The ulnar artery enters Guyon's canal just radial to the ulnar nerve. It then gives off its deep branch which passes between the ADQ and FDQ along with the deep motor branch of the ulnar nerve. These structures then pass in the plane between the metacarpals and interossei dorsal, and the flexor tendons and lumbricals palmar. Ultimately, the deep ulnar branch of the ulnar artery anastomoses with the radial artery to complete the deep palmar arch. The main or superficial ulnar branch parallels the superficial ulnar nerve into the palm. These structures lie deep to the palmar fascia but superficial to the flexor tendons and lumbricals. This main branch of the ulnar artery anastomoses with the superficial radial artery to form the superficial palmar arch.

It should be noted that the anatomy of the hand is extremely variable in terms of sensory distribution (median, radial, and ulnar nerves) as well as vascular supply (superficial and deep palmar arches). This must be borne in mind during evaluation of patients and surgery.

Functions of the hand

MOTOR POWER

In everyday use there are three basic types of work carried out by the hand (Figure 15.7). as described by Schlesinger in 1919:

1. To grasp – cylindrically or spherically.
2. To pinch – by tip pressure, by pulp pressure or by lateral pressure.
3. To hook.

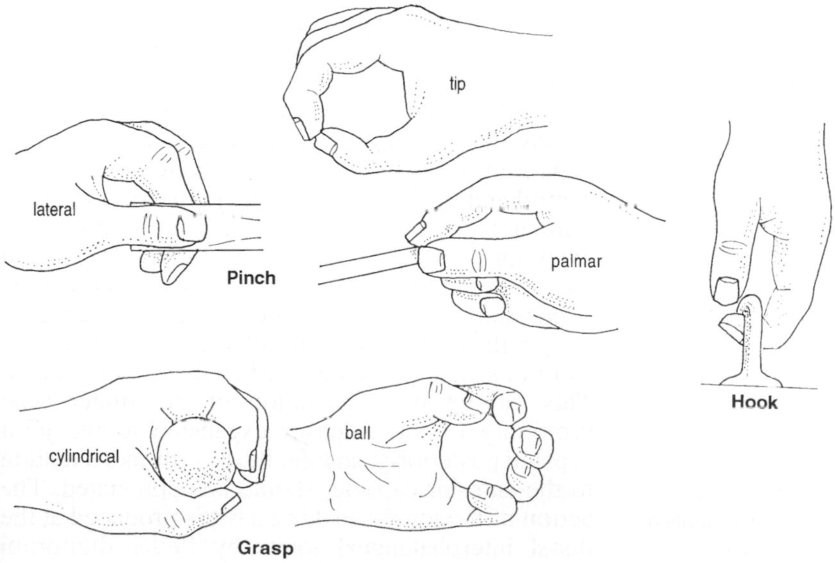

Figure 15.7 Shows the three basic types of work carried out to pinch, to grasp, and to hook (as described by Schlesinger in 1919).

The fingers

Three main groups of muscles act on the fingers. Their contribution to finger movements were worked out by the work of Long and colleagues (1970) using multiple channel electromyography.

1. *Long extensors*. These position the fingers and clear them outwards from the palm. They can also abduct the extending fingers when flexed at the metacarpophalangeal joints. Their main function is to extend the metacarpophalangeal joints, and to give final extension of the distal interphalangeal joints.
2. *Intrinsics*. The interossei abduct and adduct the extended fingers (Figure 15.8). They also participate in metacarpophalangeal flexion to an extent not previously appreciated. The lumbricals contribute to all movements of interphalangeal extension regardless of the position of the metacarpophalangeal joints. They are active in precision handling but not in power grip, and they are always inactive when the flexor digitorum profundus is contracting. One of their functions may be to pull the tendons of the deep flexors distally during fast extension of the fingers under small loads. The rich proprioceptive nerve supply of these slender muscles should also be noted.
3. *Long flexors*. These provide most of the power for pinch and grasp as well as adducting the flexing fingers, when extended at the metacarpophalangeal joints (Figure 15.9).

Unlike the long flexors, the extensor digitorum tendons act *en masse*. However, both the index and

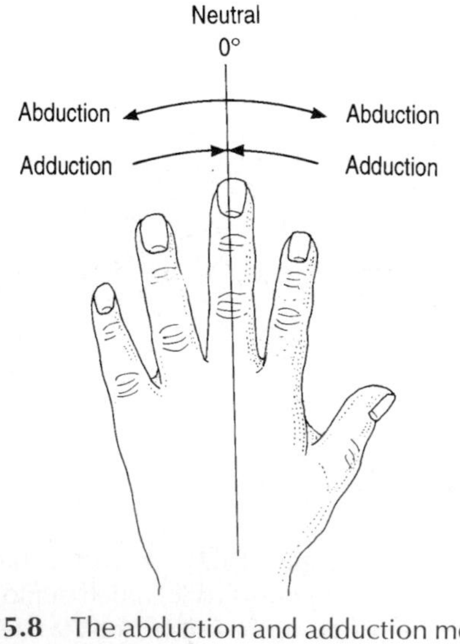

Figure 15.8 The abduction and adduction movements of the extended fingers.

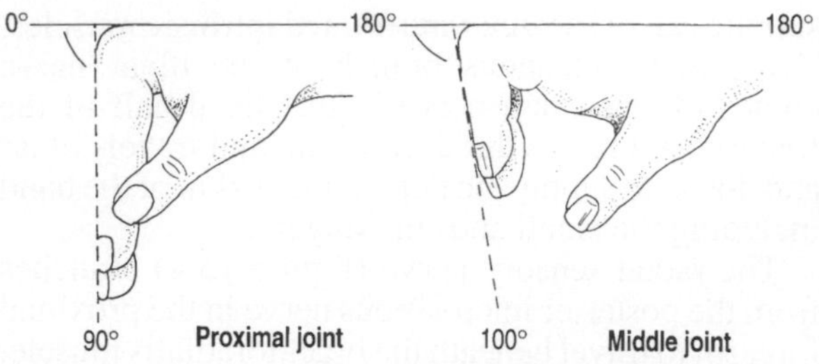

Figure 15.9 The average range of flexion at the metacarpophangeal joint (90°) and the proximal interphalangeal joint (100°).

little fingers have separate extensors, which means they can function individually.

Considerable force is needed to separate two congruous surfaces sealed from the atmospheric pressure, and this may play a part in maintaining joint stability. Semlak and Ferguson (1970) found that sudden separation of the metacarpophalangeal joint occurred with appearance of a gas bubble in the joint when a distraction force of over 3.2 kg (8 lb) was applied. As tension along the finger was increased, further separation took place due to stretching of the ligaments. This stabilizing effect of atmospheric pressure may be abolished by lax ligaments, joint effusion or incongruous joint surfaces – all of which may be present in rheumatoid arthritis.

Bowden and Napier (1961) classified these functions further into non-prehensile actions, in which no seizing is involved, and prehensile movements in which objects are held within the compass of the hand. Prehensile movements include precision handling between the finger pulp and the opposed thumb, mainly executed by muscles supplied by the median nerve; and power grip between the fingers and the palm, mainly performed by ulnar-nerve-innervated muscles with stabilization of the wrist by radial-nerve-innervated groups. However, both the index and little fingers have separate extensors, which means they can function separately. The extensor expansion consists of two main components – the central and the lateral or peripheral bands which are intimately joined by the oblique and transverse fibres extending into the expansion and give insertion to the lumbrical and interossei muscles. Division of the expansion at one side of the metacarpophalangeal joint will produce slipping of the extensor tendon from this side, particularly when the joint is flexed. This can produce deviation of the finger. The proximity of the extensor expansion to the joint capsule posteriorly, and the flexor profundus tendon to the anterior capsule, should be appreciated. The action of flexion for making a fist is produced at the distal interphalangeal joints by flexor digitorum profundus and at the proximal interphalangeal joints by flexor digitorum sublimis. The lumbrical muscle is the primary flexor of the metacarpophalangeal joint as described by Kaplan (1959).

During flexion of the fingers to make a fist there is convergence, but also there is an adaptation to hold a sphere-like object.

The thumb

The long and short flexors, and the extensors, position the thumb with stabilization of its joints. The abductors clear the thumb away from the palm or palmar abduction, with the nail vertical to the palmar surface (Figure 15.10). The adductors bring the thumb towards the palm and fingers in order to pinch and grasp, with the nail being vertical to the palmar surface. The opponens rotates the thumb so that the thumb nail becomes parallel to the palmar surface, particularly for pinching and grasping or locking the hook position (Figure 15.11).

In the thumb, the abductor pollicis longus stabilizes the carpometacarpal joint in extension, with the abductor brevis stabilizing the metacarpophalangeal joint in flexion.

The wrist

Extensors and flexors give the forearm–hand relationship of maximum stability and strength with functional position for finger movements, at about 35° dorsiflexion (Figure 15.12). The rotation at the inferior radioulnar joint is also important to position the hand around the articular disc mechanism. The movement of supination is initiated by the biceps muscle and completed by the supinator muscle as well as brachioradialis. Pronation is by pronator teres and quadratus.

For adequate joint function there must be mobility of the joint itself, which depends upon articular cartilage, capsular laxity, stability of the collateral ligaments and, finally, adequate muscle power through gliding tendons. This function of glide is produced by the tendons lying within synovial sheaths or a loose elastic tissue called paratenon. Hence these

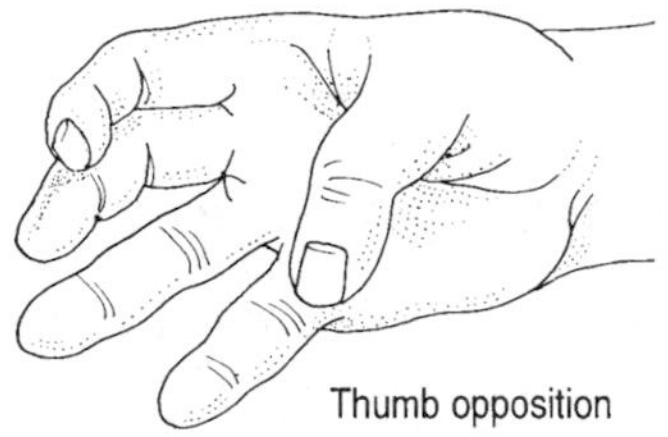

Figure 15.11 Opposition of the thumb.

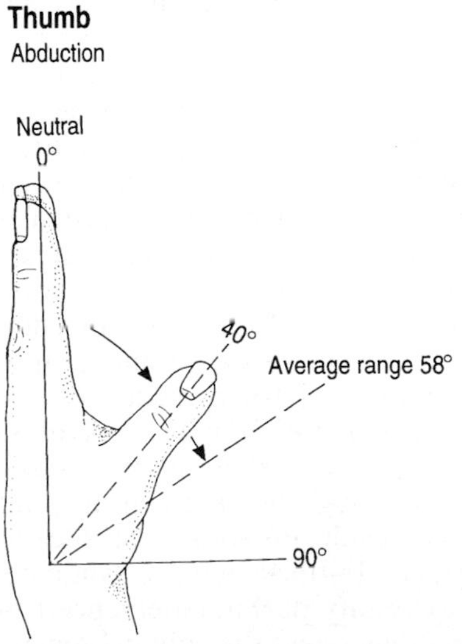

Figure 15.10 The abducted thumb showing the average range of 58°.

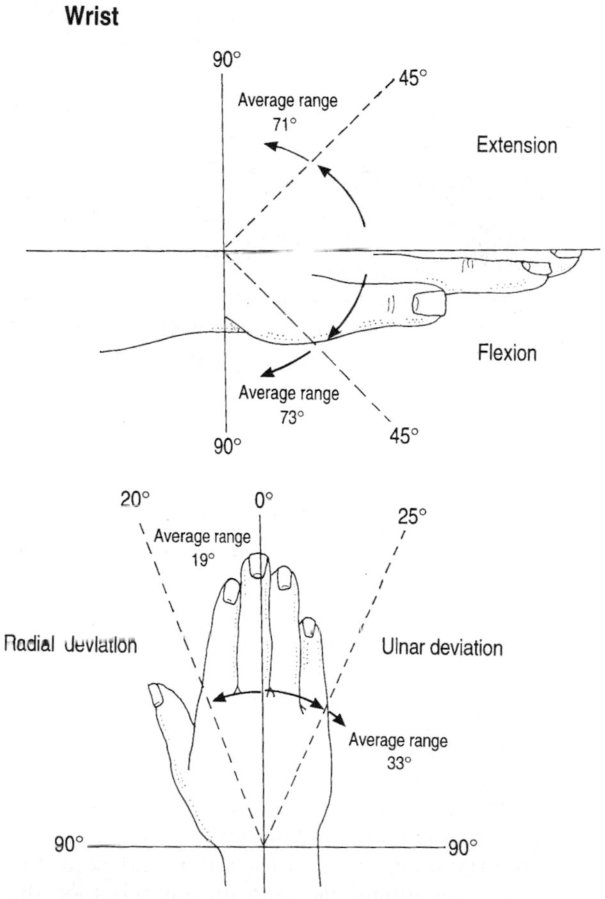

Figure 15.12 (a) The average range of extension (71°) of the wrist joint and of flexion (73°). (b) Radial deviation (19°) and ulnar deviation (33°).

must be preserved and cicatricial fibrosis prevented so that glide is maintained.

Functional axis of the forearm bones

In longitudinal rotation of pronation and supination it is no longer acceptable to think that the radius simply rotates around the lower end of the ulna. The latter remains as a fixed point with the axis being a straight line joining the head of the radius to the pit at the base of the ulnar styloid process. Rotation occurs through the centre of the radial head at its proximal aspect but distally it can be at any point between the radial and ulnar styloid processes. This is particularly true when we look at the lateral and radial deviation movements of the radiocarpal and mid-carpal joints, particularly on ulnar deviation of the hand. At this distal point the axis lies near the centre of the ulnar border of the carpal capitulum bone. There is also an anteroposterior sliding rotation movement around the transverse axes of the radiocarpal and mid-carpal joints.

SENSATION

Sensation is seen as:

1. Information of position, size, shape and weight of objects or measurements of distance. Moberg (1958) described this as 'tactile gnosis' or a complex sensibility that gives 'grip sight' – i.e. a precision-sensory grip. When such sensation is lost, it is usually accompanied by loss of sudomotor function of perspiration. This can be tested for by staining methods using ninhydrin and iodine starch powders. It is of interest that on skin grafting, although the sudomotor function may return, the tactile gnosis may not.
2. Sensibility for gross grip.
3. Protective sensibility.

EXPRESSION AND COMMUNICATION OF MOOD, SIGN LANGUAGE, ETC.

Seddon (1956) and his colleagues, from their vast experience in peripheral nerve surgery, emphasized the importance of distinguishing between academic recovery and functional recovery as these apply to functions of the hand. Academic recovery is measured by conventional tests for touch and pain, but these are inadequate in determining whether the hand is able to perform certain precision-sensory movement.

PREHENSION

This is concerned with the performance of the more intricate movements and functions, mainly by the median nerve innervation.

General operative considerations

ANAESTHESIA

Although general anaesthesia remains the anaesthetic of choice for children, regional anaesthetics provide a number of distinct advantages in the adult population undergoing elective or emergent hand surgery. Axillary blocks are the anaesthetic of choice at our institution. They are relatively safe and are successful in over 90% of our upper extremity procedures.

Underlying medical conditions are much easier to control using regional anaesthesia because, although somewhat altered by the stress of surgery, the patient's own homoeostatic regulatory systems are essentially intact. Certainly, this is the method of choice for patients with serious pulmonary, cardiac, or endocrine abnormalities because they have a quicker anaesthetic recovery and fewer postoperative complications. This is not to say that regional blocks are without risk. One must be aware of the toxic and allergic side-effects of the medications used for regional anaesthesia (lignocaine, mepivacaine, bupivacaine). Any patient receiving a regional block must have an intravenous line, and the appropriate resuscitative equipment must be available.

Other advantages of regional anaesthesia include better initial postoperative pain control. Regional blocks also cause a sympathectomy which can be of vital importance in providing maximal blood flow following trauma, reimplantation, or the treatment of vascular disorders and reflex sympathetic dystrophy. There is less risk of postoperative bleeding or stress at the surgical site because the arm is initially paralysed with a gradual return of function. In contrast, with extubation in a non-paralysed patient, there is a definite increase in venous pressure secondary to coughing and Valsalva manoeuvres which may result in additional bleeding at the operative site. Further, muscle contraction in the operated extremity during emergence from general anaesthesia may stress the surgical repair.

Other forms of anaesthesia for hand procedures include wrist and digital blocks which are valuable for distal procedures. They have the advantage of maintaining active motor function. As a result, motor function can be tested intraoperatively which may be beneficial in certain situations (e.g. trigger digit). Adrenaline (epinephrine) should never be used for digital, wrist, or intravenous blocks because of the risk of vascular spasm and possible necrosis.

Intravenous blocks (Bier blocks) provide adequate anaesthesia for relatively short procedures but they have a number of disadvantages when compared with regional blocks. They are intimately dependent on a functional tourniquet. If the tourniquet fails early in the procedure seizures and cardiac arrhythmias may result. Further, once the tourniquet is released all anaesthetic effect is lost within a few minutes. Finally, tissue oedema may obscure tissue planes.

Local anaesthetic infiltration is valuable in isolated circumstances. Its major disadvantage is that it requires infiltration into the area of trauma or pathology, and it leads to significant tissue oedema which may obscure the pathological anatomy. However, it is often used to supplement regional anaesthetic blocks.

TOURNIQUET

The use of a tourniquet is of critical importance in the majority of hand procedures because of the need for adequate visualization of intricate anatomy. Despite its widespread use, a number of complications have been reported following tourniquet use. These include tissue necrosis, nerve damage, paralysis, venous thrombosis, and death. It is clear that metabolic changes do occur during ischaemia and that many of these changes persist long after the limb is reperfused. As a result, great care is needed when using tourniquets.

The most common cause of tourniquet-related problems is inaccurate tourniquet pressure. As a result, the pressure gauge should be checked for accuracy before every use. The tourniquet should be placed high on the arm with adequate padding beneath it. A 46 cm (18 inch) tourniquet fits most adults, and should be placed over two to four layers of smooth cotton. The arm is exsanguinated with a Martin rubber bandage unless one is treating either an infectious or a neoplastic condition. In that case, the arm is elevated above the heart for a period of 2 minutes prior to tourniquet inflation. Tourniquet pressure should be set at approximately 100 mmHg above the systolic pressure and should not exceed 300 mmHg. Tourniquet time should not exceed 2 hours. If additional time is needed to complete the procedure, the tourniquet is released for 10 minutes and then reinflated. Total tourniquet time should not exceed 3 hours.

INCISIONS

Care must be taken in designing skin incisions for hand procedures. The goals are to provide adequate exposure with the minimal residual scar disability (Littler, 1974). The volar aspect of the digits is best exposed using a zig-zag incision. The apices should be at the axes of joint motion (Littler, 1974), and the apical angle should be no less than 60° to prevent apical necrosis. No incision should fall perpendicular to a flexion crease because this may lead to a flexion contracture (Figure 15.13).

The carpal tunnel should be approached through a curved incision parallel and just medial to the thenar eminence. It should be medial to the axis of the ring finger to avoid the palmar cutaneous branch of the median nerve (Figure 15.13).

Incisions on the dorsum of the wrist should be longitudinal or bayonet in shape for best exposure. The bayonet incision is contraindicated in the rheumatoid arthritis patient because of the increased risk of skin necrosis in the distally-based flap. Digital incisions over the DIP and PIP joints are often curved bayonet shape or, for the best exposure, triradiate type. This is generally safe because of the excellent blood supply to the digits (Figure 15.13).

In those situations in which there is a contracture preoperatively, such as in patients with Dupuytren's contracture or burns, Z-plasty incisions are often helpful in reducing the contracture while maintaining local skin coverage.

DRESSINGS AND SPLINTS

Hand dressings should absorb any drainage from the wound, control oedema formation, and provide support for the affected area. The dressing should be limited to those areas which must be immobilized while allowing active motion in those joints where motion is safe. In general, no hand should be completely immobilized for more than 2 weeks. When immobilized, the hand should be in the 'safe position' with the metacarpophalangeal joints in 70° of flexion and the interphalangeal joints fully extended (Figure 15.14). This position maintains the collateral ligaments of the MCP, PIP, and DIP joints at maximal stretch, preventing contracture. Unless contraindicated by the condition, the wrist should be immobilized in slight extension.

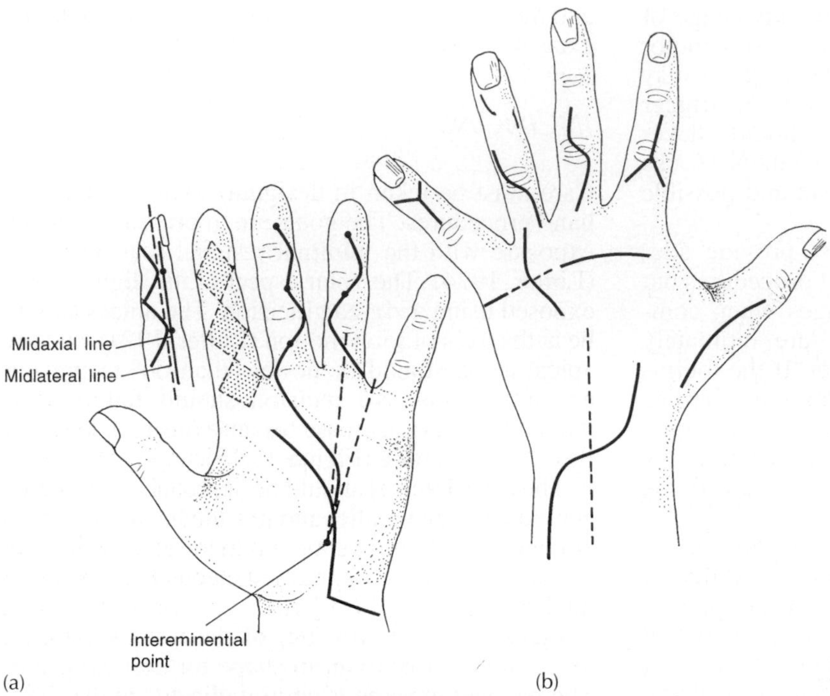

Figure 15.13 Suggested incisions in the hand and wrist. (a) Volar incisions. The shaded area shown should be avoided to prevent scar contracture. Incisions on the side of the digit should be on the midaxial line rather than midlateral.
(b) Dorsal incisions. The curved or bayonet incision may lead to skin slough in the rheumatoid patient; therefore a straight incision is preferred in that instance. (After Burton, R.I. (1991) *Atlas of Orthopaedic Surgery*. Edited by L.A. Goldstein. C.V. Mosby: St Louis, p. 138)

TENDON CONDITIONS

Tenosynovitis

Inflammation of the tenosynovial sheath can be caused by a number of pathological conditions. These range from acute infectious tenosynovitis, which will be addressed in the section of this chapter on infection, to chronic inflammatory tenosynovitis. Treatment must address the aetiology rather than the tenosynovitis itself.

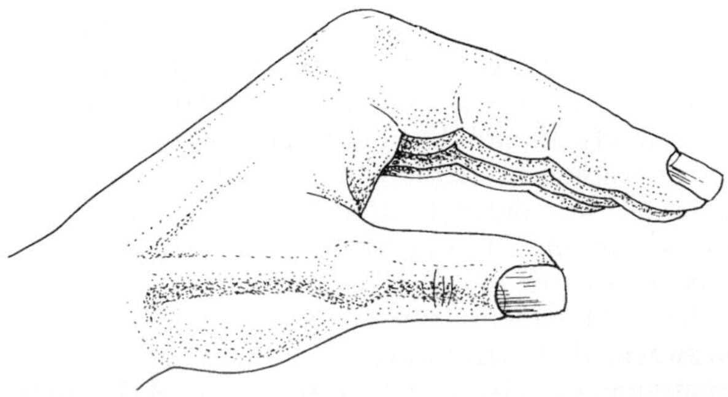

Figure 15.14 The 'safe' or 'intrinsic plus' position of hand immobilization. (After Stern, P.J. (1993) *Operative Hand Surgery*. Edited by D.P. Green. Churchill Livingstone: New York, pp. 695–758)

TRAUMATIC TENOSYNOVITIS

Traumatic tenosynovitis is a condition which presents primarily with pain, swelling, and stiffness localized to a specific tendon or group of tendons. It is most often unilateral, and is usually related either to an acute injury, or to a change in work activity or intensity. The wrist flexors (flexor carpi radialis more than flexor carpi ulnaris) are commonly involved tendons. Treatment generally begins with non-steroidal anti-inflammatory agents, rest, and splinting of the affected area. If the condition persists despite rest, a steroid injection into the tendon sheath is often helpful, taking care to avoid intratendinous injection. Surgical intervention is rarely required, although job modification is often necessary in those performing repetitive tasks.

The FCR tendon lies in its own separate tunnel at the wrist, covered by the transverse carpal ligament. The tendon passes over the scaphoid tubercle and the trapezial crest before inserting into the base of the second metacarpal. Surgical intervention for persistent FCR tenosynovitis involves releasing this 3 cm tunnel with or without resecting the scaphoid tubercle and trapezial crest.

CHRONIC INFLAMMATORY TENOSYNOVITIS

Chronic inflammatory tenosynovitis is most commonly caused by rheumatoid arthritis. The most commonly affected areas are the dorsal wrist, volar wrist and digital flexors. If left untreated, this condition may lead to tendon attenuation, weakness, and ultimate rupture. Patients with this condition will have pain, swelling and stiffness of the involved area, and better passive than active range of motion.

Dorsal wrist tenosynovitis is heralded by swelling over the dorsum of the wrist with associated pain and weakness. The thin skin over the dorsum of the wrist makes the fullness easily recognized. Volar wrist tenosynovitis is generally localized within the carpal canal which contains nine digital flexor tendons and the median nerve. Because the carpal canal is a non-distensible fibro-osseous tunnel, the swelling is not as notable. Instead, these patients often present with symptoms of median nerve compression. Digital flexor tenosynovitis presents with swelling of the finger, pain, and more passive than active motion of the affected digit. These patients may also present with triggering from the synovitis or a tendon nodule.

Treatment of early rheumatoid tenosynovitis is medical through the use of various pharmacological agents (see Chapter 11). If it persists despite 6 months of appropriate medical management, synovectomy should be considered to prevent further tendon damage. This will be addressed further in the section on rheumatoid arthritis.

STENOSING TENOSYNOVITIS

Stenosing tenosynovitis is a group of conditions in which there is a mismatch between the size of the tendon sheath and the tendon which passes through it. It may result from enlargement of the tendon as seen in trigger finger, or from narrowing and fibrosis of the tendon sheath seen in de Quervain's tenosynovitis.

The trigger finger, or stenosing tenosynovitis, is caused by a nodule or thickening of the flexor tendon which catches on the proximal edge of the first annular pulley (A1) when the finger is actively flexed. Sampson *et al.* (1991) from detailed immunohistochemical and electron microscope studies, found fibrocartilage metaplasia on the inner surface of the A1 pulley which was the cause of the triggering. When severe, the finger may lock in flexion, requiring the patient to use the other hand to release the finger. The catching and locking is often painful and interferes with activity.

The aetiology of stenosing tenosynovitis is unclear, but repetitive trauma does appear to play a role. It is most common in the ring and long fingers and rare in the index finger. If a patient presents with multiple or recurrent trigger digits a systemic cause such as rheumatoid arthritis should be considered.

Treatment of trigger digits depends on the aetiology. In non-rheumatoid patients, a steroid injection into the flexor tendon sheath is very effective. Anderson and Kaye (1991) from a prospective study found that 61% responded to a single injection of steroids, 27% recurred and only 12% required surgical release. No cases became infected or suffered tendon rupture; 6% presented with subcutaneous fat atrophy and this should be explained to the patient beforehand. The steroid is injected at the level of the A1 pulley; care is taken to avoid an intratendinous injection which may lead to tendon rupture. Some patients will require a second injection; the majority of patients will have lasting relief of their symptoms. In those who have persistent triggering despite two steroid injections, surgical release of the proximal portion of the A1 pulley should be performed under tourniquet control (Figure 15.15). It is best performed under wrist block so that the patient can actively flex and extend the affected digit once the release is performed. The A2 pulley must be preserved.

In rheumatoid patients, the underlying problem is synovitis within the flexor tendon sheath, which weakens both tendons and surrounding synovial sheath. Therefore, medical management should first be tried to control the synovitis along with a programme of active assisted exercises and splinting. Steroid injections should not be used because there is a real risk of tendon rupture in these patients. If the synovitis and triggering persists despite the

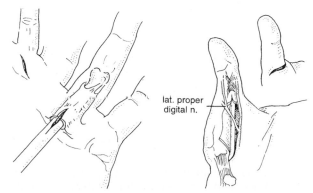

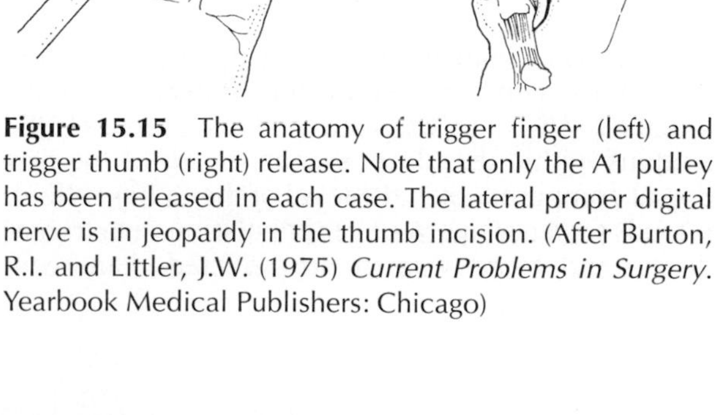

Figure 15.15 The anatomy of trigger finger (left) and trigger thumb (right) release. Note that only the A1 pulley has been released in each case. The lateral proper digital nerve is in jeopardy in the thumb incision. (After Burton, R.I. and Littler, J.W. (1975) *Current Problems in Surgery*. Yearbook Medical Publishers: Chicago)

above therapy, then surgical synovectomy should be performed without releasing the annular pulleys. Release of the A1 pulley has been associated with ulnar subluxation of the tendon, leading to further deformity.

In the thumb, the flexor sheath is much tighter than in the fingers. As a result, it is more difficult to inject the tendon sheath without injecting into the tendon. As a result, many surgeons proceed to operative intervention if a single injection is ineffective. Surgical release requires retraction of the radial digital nerve which crosses directly over the A1 pulley. Excellent visualization is crucial when performing this procedure.

Congenital trigger thumb usually presents with the digit in a position of flexion. Although usually present at birth, it is often not appreciated until months later. As with adult trigger digits, the anomaly is usually secondary to either sheath stenosis, a tendon nodule, or both. According to Dinham and Meggitt (1974), spontaneous resolution will occur in 30% of those with trigger thumbs noted at birth, and in 12% of those with trigger thumbs noted between 6 months and 3 years of age. Further, there appears to be no long-term deformity or functional deficit if this condition is treated before the age of 3 (Dinham and Meggitt, 1974; Ger *et al.*, 1991). A period of observation with or without splinting and stretching is warranted in the child less than 6 months of age. The condition is less likely to resolve in the older child, so surgery is recommended. The surgical approach and procedure are very similar to that in the adult. The proximal edge of the A1 pulley should be released. Care must be taken to avoid the digital nerves in small children. These nerves are placed on the volar aspect of the thumb.

If left untreated, the older child may develop a fixed flexion deformity and joint contractures. This condition is generally painless, and the thumb is functional. As a result, many will leave the condition untreated. In the older child who presents for evaluation and treatment, not only the trigger thumb but also the secondary joint contractures must be corrected.

DE QUERVAIN TENOSYNOVITIS

De Quervain tenosynovitis is a painful condition caused by compression of the abductor pollicis longus (APL) and extensor pollicis brevis (EPB) tendons within the fibro-osseous sheath of the first dorsal compartment at the level of the radial styloid. It tends to occur in a younger population than trigger digits, and more women are affected than men. Patients present with a complaint of pain localized to the region of the radial styloid which radiates up the forearm and is aggravated by use of the thumb. Classically, the patient has a positive Finkelstein test, i.e. pain over the first dorsal compartment when the thumb is flexed in the palm and the wrist is ulnarly deviated.

De Quervain tenosynovitis may be confused with symptoms of trapeziometacarpal instability or arthritis. Trapeziometacarpal arthritis pain and tenderness should be localized more distally at the thumb basal joint. Further, the axial compression–adduction test and the axial compression–rotation test (crank and grind) should differentiate these two conditions (Burton, 1986). In these tests, the thumb is axially loaded and the thumb metacarpal is then passively adducted and rotated which causes pain in those with basal joint pathology. Both de Quervain tenosynovitis and basal joint arthritis may be present in a single patient.

Most patients with de Quervain tenosynovitis are successfully treated non-surgically. The initial treatment for these patients is a cortisone injection into the fibro-osseous tunnel followed by a splint with the wrist in neutral and the thumb in ‘fist projection’. Most patients will have a lasting response to one or two injections combined with splinting and activity modification. In those with persistent symptoms, surgical release should be performed.

Surgical release is best performed through a 2–3 cm longitudinal slightly curved incision which will allow more extensile exposure if needed (Figure 15.16). Multiple branches of the radial sensory nerve are located in the subcutaneous tissue. Great care should be taken to preserve these branches because, if cut, they often lead to very painful neuromata. Once the sheath is identified and clear visualization is achieved, a dorsally based longitudinal cut is made in the sheath. This will expose the EPB tendon. In 20–30% of cases, a longitudinal septum will separate the smaller EPB tendon from the larger, and often multislipped, APL tendon. Care must be taken to release all slips of the APL to prevent recurrence. The radial artery passes deep to these tendons at the level of the anatomical ‘snuff box’ and must be protected. After release, the wrist is splinted for 7–10 days with the wrist extended 30° and the thumb mildly abducted. The long volar flap is made to prevent volar subluxation of the APL and EPB tendons with wrist flexion and thumb palmar abduction.

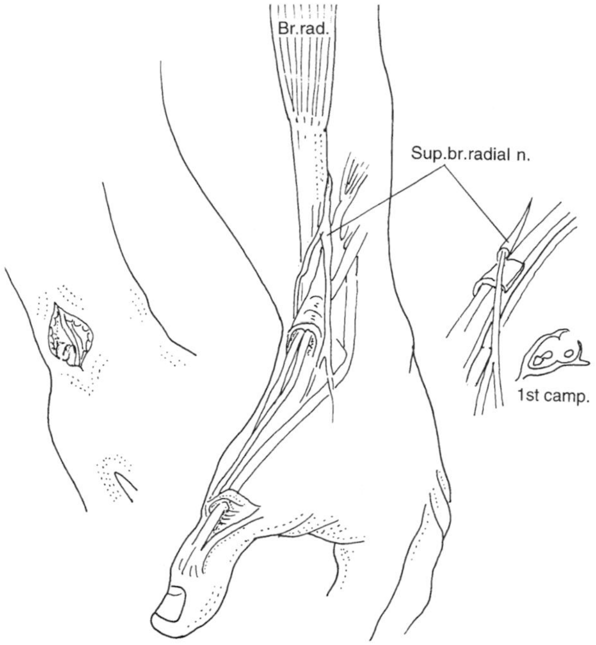

Figure 15.16 Surgical release in de Quervain's tenosynovitis requires complete decompression of the tendon sheaths of both abductor pollicis brevis and extensor pollicis longus. Care must be taken to avoid injury to branches of the radial sensory nerve. (After Burton, R.I. (1991) *Atlas of Orthopaedic Surgery*. Edited by L.A. Goldstein. C.V. Mosby: St Louis, p. 138)

OSTEOARTHRITIS OF THE HAND AND CARPUS

The aetiology of osteoarthritis is unclear; it is, a slowly progressive disorder presenting later in life and affecting the large weight-bearing joints as well as the hands. It tends to be polyarticular, and presents with pain, stiffness, and gradual deformity. Osteoarthritis of the hands is most common in postmenopausal women who have a positive family history. Increasing age, female gender, and a positive family history are the three most important risk factors in the development of this disease. Osteoarthritis can be primary and idiopathic, or secondary to trauma, avascular necrosis, infection, and metabolic disorders such as pseudogout. Although most patients have a slowly progressive form of the disease which develops over many years, some patients have a very aggressive form of primary osteoarthritis which has been termed erosive osteoarthritis. These patients present with the acute onset of pain and swelling involving the interphalangeal joints of the hands. Erosions are seen early, and joint deformity rapidly develops.

The joints most commonly affected in the hand are the interphalangeal joints of the fingers and the trapeziometacarpal joint of the thumb. The MCP joints are generally spared. Pathologically, there is articular cartilage destruction with underlying bony erosion and cyst formation. Once the articular cartilage has been destroyed, the bony surface becomes eburnated with subchondral sclerosis and peripheral osteophyte formation.

Most patients with osteoarthritis of the hands are treated conservatively with good results. Education about the disease process often reassures the patient. Non-steroidal anti-inflammatory agents are generally effective in pain control. Steroid injections may be beneficial. Physical therapy using intermittent splinting, activity restrictions, specific exercises, and other modalities is often helpful. If the above interventions fail to control the patient's symptoms, then surgical treatment must be considered.

DISTAL INTERPHALANGEAL JOINT

In osteoarthritis at the distal interphalangeal joint (DIP), three pathological problems may arise. Generalized joint destruction and peripheral osteophyte formation may lead to areas of enlargement along the joint margin. These localized areas have been termed Heberden nodes and, unless painful, they represent primarily a cosmetic deformity. Over time, the joint may become severely deformed and functionally unstable. This condition is best treated, if necessary, by fusion of the affected DIP joint which leads to little functional deficit provided the other joints remain mobile. Fusion is performed through a dorsal approach (Figure 15.17). Any remaining articular cartilage and the sclerotic subchondral bone should be removed to promote fusion. The DIP joint should be placed in 10–15° of flexion and held using crossed K-wires, a screw, or a tension band device. Fusion usually occurs in 6–8 weeks.

The third condition which may develop is a mucous cyst, which is an outpouching of joint fluid around a peripheral osteophyte usually over the dorsal–lateral aspect of the DIP joint just proximal to the nail. Because it is close to the nail matrix, nail ridging and deformity are common. In addition, the skin over these cysts is often thin and may erode. If the cyst ruptures, a secondary infection may develop which can ultimately result in osteomyelitis of the distal phalanx or septic arthritis of the DIP joint. Therefore, leakage of a mucous cyst is an indication to excise both cyst and underlying osteophyte. The

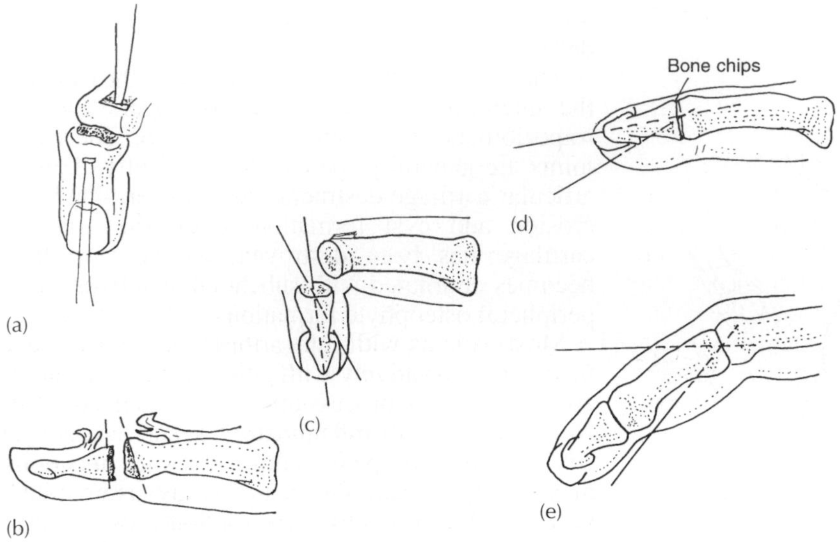

Figure 15.17 The technique for small joint fusion in the hand. (a) Exposure. (b) Resection of joint to medullary surface at desired angulation on each side. (c) Distal insertion of crossed K-wires. (d) and (e) Coaption of bony surfaces and advancement of K-wires. (After Burton, R.I. *et al.* (1986) *Journal of Bone and Joint Surgery* **11A**, 687)

osteophyte must be removed to prevent recurrence. If severe joint destruction and instability are present, then DIP arthrodesis should be considered. This should be performed as a secondary procedure if the cyst appears to be superinfected at the time of initial treatment. Because of the close proximity to the nail matrix, care should be taken to protect the matrix during operative excision or arthrodesis.

PROXIMAL INTERPHALANGEAL JOINT

The proximal interphalangeal joint (PIP) is similarly affected by osteoarthritis. Peripheral osteophytes at the PIP joints are called Bouchard nodes. Pathologically, they are identical to Heberden nodes at the DIP joints and do not warrant operative treatment unless pain, stiffness, or instability develops which is unresponsive to conservative therapy. Although stiffness often develops at the PIP joints, it rarely warrants surgical treatment. The most common indication for operative treatment is progressive joint destruction with instability.

Treatment of osteoarthritis of the PIP joints varies depending on the finger involved, the overall alignment, and the bone stock. Surgical treatment consists either of PIP arthrodesis or implant arthroplasty. The index finger (and to a lesser degree the long) functions primarily as a post for tip and lateral pinch activities. Lateral pinch exerts a great deal of ulnarly directed force on the radial collateral ligament and the accessory radial collateral ligament of the PIP joint, which leads to instability. Because PIP joint stability is necessary for the index finger to function as a post for lateral pinch, stability takes precedence over motion when treating osteoarthritis of the index (and possibly long) PIP joints. As a result, osteoarthritis of the index PIP joint is usually treated by fusion to provide a stable 'pinch post'.

In contrast, the ulnar digits (ring and small) are used for power grip. For this reason, motion is the most important goal in the treatment of the ring and small finger PIP joints. These fingers are generally treated with PIP joint arthroplasty which maintains motion, yet relies on the collateral ligaments and volar plate for stability. In order for arthroplasty to be successful, the patient must have reasonable finger alignment, good bone stock, and intact motor function.

The long finger is important for both lateral pinch and grip activities. The best treatment, arthroplasty or arthrodesis, must be individualized according to disease pattern and functional needs.

PIP joint fusion is performed through a dorsal bayonet incision (Figure 15.17). A longitudinal approach through the extensor tendon is made, taking great care to preserve both lateral bands. The central slip is excised and the collateral ligaments are released to aid exposure. Once the articular cartilage and subchondral bone are removed, the joint should be fused in a position of 40–55° of flexion (Urbaniak, 1990). The index and long fingers are fused in 40–45° of flexion because of their primary roles as posts for lateral pinch. The ring and small fingers are fused in 50–55° of flexion because of the role of these fingers in power grip. Just as with the DIP joint fusion, numerous devices can be used for stabilization until fusion occurs. Stabilization with crossed

K-wires has been shown to result in a 99.4% interphalangeal joint (DIP and PIP) fusion rate by Burton *et al.* (1986).

PIP arthroplasty can be performed through either a dorsal bayonet incision (most common) or volar approach. Collateral ligament integrity, especially on the radial side, is crucial. The extensor mechanism is split longitudinally from the mid-proximal phalanx to the central slip insertion on the base of the middle phalanx. The extensor mechanism is then elevated in a subperiosteal fashion in both the radial and ulnar directions. The collateral ligaments are preserved to provide stability. The head of the proximal phalanx is then excised, and the canals are broached for subsequent prosthesis placement. After placement of the prosthesis, the extensor mechanism is re-approximated centrally. If the central slip is detached from its insertion into the base of the middle phalanx, it should be reattached through bone holes, taking care to maintain proper length and tension.

Postoperatively, the fingers are splinted in extension for 10 days. Active flexion and active assisted extension are then started under direct supervision three times a day. The PIP joints are splinted in extension at all other times, and the DIP joints are splinted or pinned in full extension for 8 weeks. This is to prevent a mallet deformity and also to concentrate active motion at the PIP joints. Potential complications include stiffness, instability, boutonnière deformity, swan-neck deformity, synovitis, infection, and fracture.

TRAPEZIOMETACARPAL JOINT

The trapeziometacarpal joint (TMJ) of the thumb is also a common site of primary osteoarthritis. The trapeziometacarpal joint is an inherently incongruous double saddle joint with different radii of curvature between the articular surfaces of the trapezium and the metacarpal. The two main planes of motion based on the bony contour are flexion–adduction to extension–abduction and palmar abduction and adduction. Some rotation is allowed because of the incongruous nature of the joint.

The main ligamentous supports of the joint are the palmar oblique or palmar beak ligament which originates on the palmar ulnar trapezium and inserts into the volar metacarpal beak and the dorsal expansion of the abductor pollicis longus. The palmar beak ligament is the primary stabilizer of the joint in preventing dorsal subluxation during lateral pinch. Further, this ligament is stressed when the thumb is pronated and thereby stabilizes the joint during lateral pinch. The dorsal expansion of the APL does not prevent dorsal subluxation but tightens with supination of the thumb.

Women are more commonly affected than men. Patients present with pain which is exacerbated by attempts to pinch or grip objects. The pain is sometimes difficult to localize to the TMJ because of the number of overlying structures which may also be a source of pain. These include branches of the radial sensory nerve or palmar cutaneous branch of the median nerve, tendinitis of the FCR or first dorsal compartment tendons (de Quervain), scaphoid fracture, or wrist instability. Differentiation of basal joint osteoarthritis from de Quervain tenosynovitis may be difficult, and the two conditions may coexist. Carpal tunnel syndrome may also coexist. Florack *et al.* (1992) have shown that 43% of patients undergoing surgery for basal joint arthritis also had carpal tunnel syndrome (CTS). If a patient has a history suggestive of CTS or has signs consistent with CTS on physical examination (positive wrist flexion test, positive tinel over the median nerve, decreased sensation in the median nerve distribution, or thenar atrophy), then nerve conduction studies should be considered preoperatively the better to assess the clinical situation.

A strong link between palmar oblique ligament laxity and trapeziometacarpal joint arthritis has been established (Eaton and Littler, 1973; Eaton *et al.*, 1984; Pellegrini, 1991a, b). Eaton and Littler (1973) were the first to implicate ligamentous laxity as a major factor in the aetiology of idiopathic osteoarthritis of the trapeziometacarpal joint. They developed a procedure to reconstruct the palmar oblique ligament using one-half of the flexor carpi radialis (FCR) tendon. Long-term follow-up suggests that ligament reconstruction can effectively prevent or delay the onset of degenerative change in those with early disease (Eaton *et al.*, 1984). The relationship between ligamentous laxity and degenerative arthritis in the TMJ has been further supported by studies in a cadaveric model as well as observations in surgical specimens (Pellegrini, 1991a, b). Further, some feel that the articular surfaces of the trapeziometacarpal joint are shallower in women, allowing less inherent bony stability and more translation with motion (Eaton and Littler, 1973).

As the palmar oblique ligament attenuates, the joint subluxates and instability develops. The resulting shear forces lead to cartilage loss and ultimate degenerative arthritis with peripheral osteophyte formation. With progressive joint instability, a secondary metacarpal adduction contracture develops with a narrowing of the first web space. This results from the combined pull of the abductor pollicis longus (APL) and the adductor pollicis (ADD) on the distal aspect of the first metacarpal leading to dorsal–radial subluxation of the metacarpal base and flexion–adduction contracture of the distal metacarpal. A compensatory MCP joint hyperextension deformity often develops and, less frequently, the ulnar collateral ligament becomes unstable.

On physical examination, the patient will often have a 'shoulder sign' secondary to metacarpal subluxation at the trapeziometacarpal joint. Further, the 'crank and grind' test will often elicit pain, crepitis, and palpable instability at the TMJ in those with basal joint arthritis. Pain is also elicited by rotating the first metacarpal while distracting the TMJ, as described by Eaton and Littler (1973).

Radiographs in basal joint arthritis (Figure 15.18) will often show subluxation, narrowing of the joint space, subchondral sclerosis, osteophytes, loose bodies, and finally pantrapezial involvement. Eaton and Littler (1973) and Eaton *et al.* (1984) have developed a staging system for TMJ arthritis based on posteroanterior (PA), lateral and stress radiographs of the basal joint. At the authors' institution, the stress view has been modified by taking a 30° oblique view with the radial aspect of the thumbs pressed together.

Four stages of radiographic findings are described. In stage I, articular contours are normal, there is less than one-third subluxation in any projection, and there is no evidence of joint degeneration. The joint space may be widened secondary to an effusion or synovitis. In stage II, slight narrowing of the joint space and at least one-third subluxation is noted on stress radiographs. The articular contours remain normal and any joint debris, if present, is smaller than 2 mm in size. In stage III, significant joint destruction is evident with sclerotic and cystic changes noted. Osteophytes and joint debris are larger than 2 mm. The scaphotrapeziotrapezoidal (STT) joint remains normal without evidence of degeneration. In stage IV, the degenerative process now involves the STT joint as well as the TMJ, resulting in pantrapezial disease (Eaton and Littler, 1973; Eaton *et al.*, 1984).

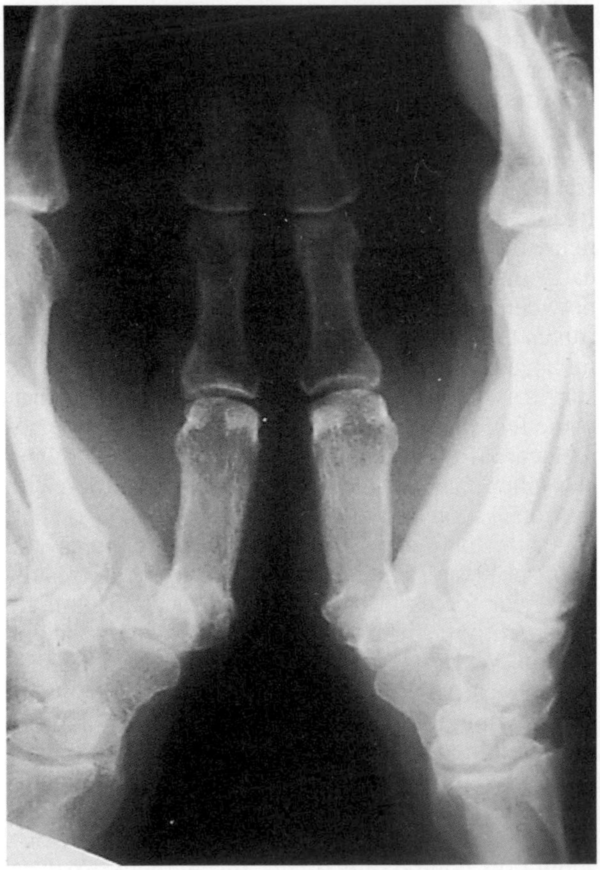

Figure 15.18 Radiograph of hand with severe (stage III) basal joint arthritis.

Conservative therapy for basal joint arthritis includes splinting and non-steroidal anti-inflammatory agents to help control symptoms. Thenar cone (abductor pollicis brevis, flexor pollicis brevis, opponens pollicis) strengthening exercises are also helpful in strengthening the 'secondary or dynamic restraints' to dorsal subluxation. Although these measures are often helpful in controlling symptoms, they have not been shown to alter the disease process. With time, many patients progress with pain, deformity and functional limitation.

The goals of operative intervention are to restore stability and strength, decrease pain, and to provide a functional range of motion. The two components to basal joint arthritis, ligament instability and joint degeneration, may each be present to varying degrees. Four types of intervention are possible: fusion of the trapeziometacarpal joint; palmar oblique ligament reconstruction to provide stability to the joint; resurfacing arthroplasty to allow relatively pain-free motion of the joint; and finally, some combination of the above.

Ligament reconstruction alone is indicated in those with symptomatic trapeziometacarpal joint instability and subluxation without joint degeneration. This procedure was described by Eaton and Littler in 1973 and uses one-half of the FCR tendon to reconstruct the palmar oblique ligament and restore joint stability (Figure 15.19). It was initially used in those with all stages of TMJ arthritis; yet a long-term evaluation of these patients (Eaton *et al.*, 1984) revealed that only those with early disease (radiographic stages I and II) had reliably good results. With an average 7-year follow-up, those with radiographic stage I or II disease had 95% good or excellent results. Further, all of the stage I cases and 82% of the stage II cases were free of radiographic degeneration on follow-up radiographs, suggesting that this procedure effectively prevents the development of degeneration in those with early symptomatic instability.

Resurfacing arthroplasty is indicated either alone or in combination with ligament reconstruction in

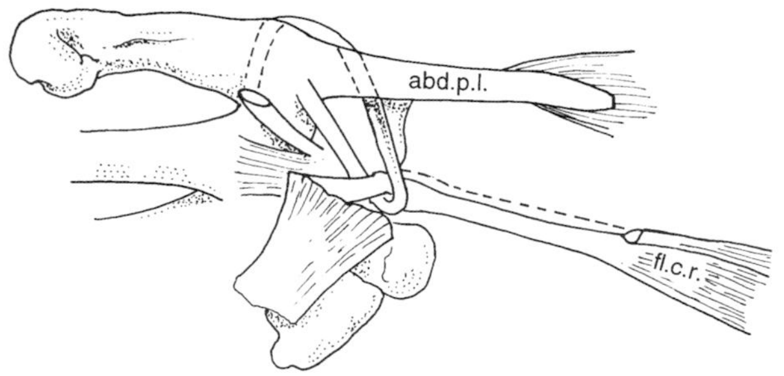

Figure 15.19 Volar ligament reconstruction in the trapeziometacarpal joint using one half of the flexor carpi radialis tendon. (After Eaton, R.G. and Littler, J.W. (1973) *Journal of Bone and Joint Surgery* **11A**, 687)

those with degenerative disease. This can be performed using either foreign or biological materials. As popularized by Swanson, who began using these implants in the TMJ in 1965 (Swanson, 1972, 1973a, b), silastic implants of various designs have been used extensively. They can resurface the trapezial articular surface, resurface the metacarpal articular surface, or resurface both surfaces (metatarsophalangeal implant design). In addition, some designs allow simultaneous ligamentous stabilization (Eaton, 1979). Despite the advantages of less extensive dissection and an easier early postoperative course, there are many problems when using these prostheses for basal joint osteoarthritis. Instability of the trapezial implant, resulting in pain and loss of grip strength, has been reported in 10–32% of cases (Kessler, 1973; Haffajee, 1977; Weilby and Sondorf, 1978; Eaton, 1979; Brannohler and Waddel, 1982). Eaton's design of a cannulated trapezial implant allowing ligament reconstruction improved stability yet led to an increase in wear, fragmentation, and 'cold flow' secondary to the increased stresses on the implant (Eaton, 1979; Pellegrini and Burton, 1986a, b). These prostheses have fallen out of favour for the above reasons, and because of concern about giant-cell silicone synovitis. The inflammatory nature of the reaction combined with radiographic erosion have led to a drastic drop in the use of these prostheses. Pellegrini and Burton (1986a, b) found reactive synovitis and bone resorption around the silicone implants with an increased incidence of revision when compared to ligament reconstruction and tendon interposition arthroplasty. They concluded that the silicone implant is not indicated in the osteoarthritic hand and should be reserved for use in the low-demand rheumatoid patient.

Biological material can also be used to resurface the trapeziometacarpal joint with or without ligament reconstruction. The distal half of the trapezium is removed and the space is then filled with either the palmaris longus (PL) or one-half of the FCR tendon. A secure dorsal capsuloplasty must be performed to prevent subluxation or dislocation of the tendon spacer. This procedure is analogous to the silicone implant arthroplasty, with the advantage of using the patient's own tissue. However, because ligament laxity has not been corrected, this procedure may fail due to recurrent instability and loss of spacer height.

At our institution, the procedure of choice for idiopathic osteoarthritis of the trapeziometacarpal joint has been ligament reconstruction combined with tendon interposition (LRTI) arthroplasty which effectively addresses both the palmar oblique ligament instability and the articular surface degeneration. By restoring ligamentous stability, both dorsal subluxation and flexion–adduction of the first metacarpal are corrected. This restores the first web space and allows better positioning of the thumb for pinch and grip activities. The fascial arthroplasty provides relatively pain-free motion at the trapeziometacarpal joint.

The basal joint is exposed through a dorsal–radial incision taking care to protect any branches of the radial sensory nerve. After making a dorsal capsulotomy, both the TMJ and the STT joints are inspected. The condition of the STT joints will determine how much of the trapezium should be removed. If the STT joints are involved, then the entire trapezium must be excised. Otherwise, only the distal half of the trapezium is removed. The procedure is performed using one-half of the FCR tendon. Proximally, the tendon is divided at the musculotendinous junction and distally it is left attached to the base of the second metacarpal. A hole is made at the base of the thumb metacarpal perpendicular to the plane of the nail. The FCR tendon is then brought through the hole from palmar to dorsal. The thumb metacarpal base is held reduced with the thumb in the 'fist position' of metacarpal abduction and pronation. The FCR tendon is secured to the dorsal metacarpal periosteum as well as folded back and attached to itself, effectively to produce a suspension sling. A K-wire is used to hold the metacarpal in proper position and protect the ligamentous reconstruction during early healing. The remaining FCR tendon is folded onto itself to make a 'soft tissue spacer' which is placed within the gap left by the missing trapezium, and then secured to the deep capsule to maintain its position. A dorsal capsuloplasty is performed to prevent dislocation of the spacer. The EPB tendon is usually tenodesed to the base of the thumb metacarpal to aid in metacarpal abduction and decrease extension stress at the thumb MCP joint. If unstable, the MCP joint is fused with crossed K-wires. Further, if there is documented carpal tunnel syndrome, a carpal tunnel release is performed.

LRTI arthroplasty has resulted in up to 95% excellent results with an average of nine years follow-up in one series (Tomaino, Pellegrini and Burton, 1995). When compared with silicone arthroplasty, it was found to improve pinch strength more consistently, improve grip strength, and restore the first web space. Proximal migration of the metacarpal was only 11% of the initial arthroplasty space compared with 50% in the silicone implants. Subluxation was 7% of the width of the metacarpal base compared with 35% in the silicone arthroplasty group (Pellegrini and Burton, 1986a, b). The LRTI arthroplasty is reliable and of sufficient durability for use in the high-demand osteoarthritic hand.

Fusion is the final option in treating arthritis of the trapeziometacarpal joint. This is often indicated in a young patient who has post-traumatic osteoarthritis and heavy functional demands. Because additional stress and compensatory motion develop at other joints, the procedure is contraindicated in those patients with either scaphotrapezial arthritis or MCP abnormality. If a patient's occupation requires palmar adduction of the thumb, another option must be chosen.

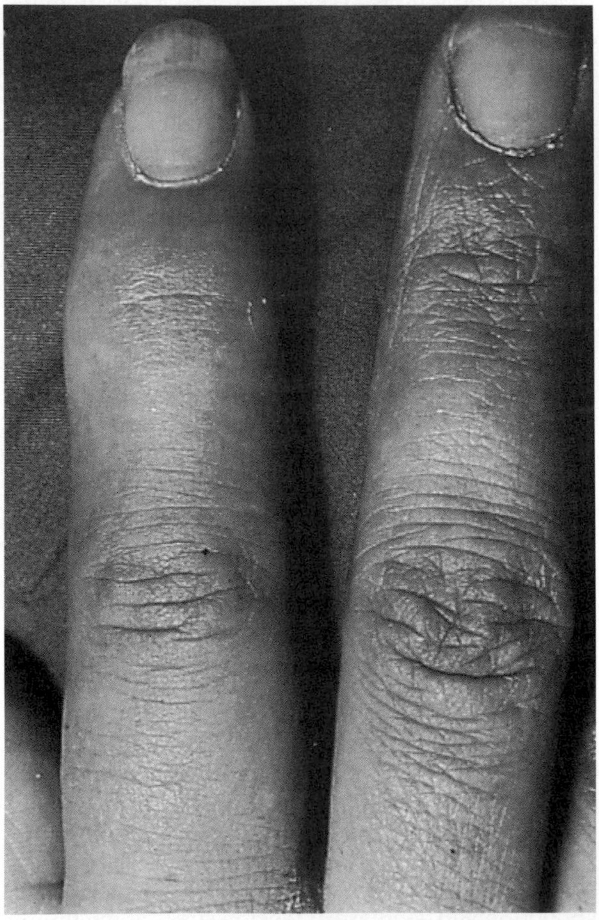

Figure 15.20 Clinical appearance of psoriatic arthritis with fusiform swelling of the distal interphalangeal joint and nail irregularities.

Fusion is performed with the thumb metacarpal in the 'fist position' (Eaton and Littler, 1973). The base of the metacarpal is removed perpendicular to its long axis. Once placed in the 'fist position', a parallel cut is made in the trapezium. The articular surfaces are held with two or three K-wires. The TMJ must then be immobilized for a period of 3–4 months. In a series of 20 patients, all had 'markedly improved hand function' and only one had pain. All those with degenerative arthritis were able to oppose the thumb to small finger. They did not use bone graft and two patients had painless fibrous unions (Eaton and Littler, 1973).

INFLAMMATORY ARTHRITIS

See Chapter 8.

Rheumatoid arthritis

The most common form of inflammatory arthritis is rheumatoid arthritis (RA). Other forms which may affect the hand are systemic lupus erythematosis (SLE), dermatomyositis, scleroderma, psoriatic arthritis (Figure 15.20) and gouty arthritis (Figure 15.21). Although the presentation of each of these may differ from RA is some ways, the general approach to evaluation and treatment is the same for all. Only in patients who have persistent problems despite adequate medical management should surgical intervention be considered.

Rheumatoid arthritis is a systemic condition. In addition to the musculoskeletal system, it affects the cardiac, pulmonary, renal, gastrointestinal and vascular systems. Medications including steroids may reduce the patient's ability to respond to the stresses of surgery. As a result, those on long-term systemic steroids with adrenal suppression may require relatively high doses of systemic steroids during the perioperative period.

General principles of orthopaedic care for this problem consist of:

1. Maintaining position and function of all joints by physiotherapy and splintage.
2. Treating the soft tissue and joint processes as they develop by injections, by the principles of rest and, where necessary, by early surgery.
3. Correcting established deformity and attempt-

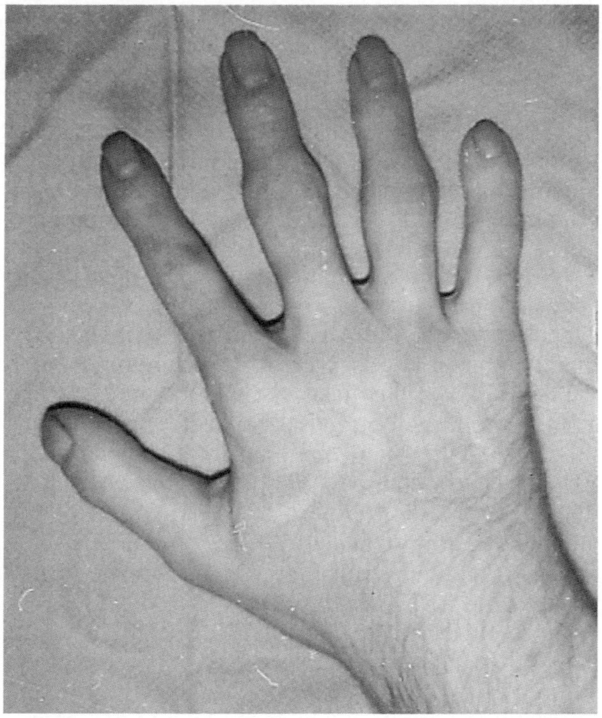

Figure 15.21 A man's hand showing the typical appearance of a gouty arthritis involving the proximal interphalangeal joints of all fingers and the interphalangeal joint of the thumb.

ing to restore function – but this does not mean the severely deformed 'burned out' *rheumatoid* hand in which there is little motor power left.

Another consideration in the surgical treatment of rheumatoid arthritis is the risk of anaesthesia. Most hand and wrist procedures can be performed under regional anaesthetics which are generally safer, allow a quicker recovery, and provide better postoperative pain relief than general anaesthesia. If a general anaesthetic is considered, then lateral flexion and extension radiographs of the cervical spine must be obtained to rule out C1–C2 instability.

Rheumatoid arthritis results from a proliferation of the synovium of the joints and tendons. Synovial hypertrophy or inflammatory synovitis is felt to cause damage through two basic mechanisms. The first is mechanical wear caused by the bulk of the synovium in areas of limited space, and the second is chemical via inflammatory cells and lysosomal enzymes which destroy articular cartilage. These two mechanisms destroy joints by mechanically stretching the capsule and surrounding ligamentous supports while weakening them with lysosomal enzymes and other chemical agents. Similarly, tendons can be infiltrated and weakened to the point of attenuation or rupture. Secondary disuse osteoporosis softens the bones, making surgical techniques more difficult and demanding than usual.

These changes produce the characteristic features of swelling and stiffness of joints, tendon drifting or subluxation (particularly at the metacarpophalangeal joints on the ulnar side), subluxation and dislocation of the metacarpophalangeal joints to give the classic features of ulnar deviation, flexion deformities and 'concertina' collapse of the hands and digits. Invasion by rheumatoid tissue into the tendons produces rupture of the tendon with loss of function, and contraction of the fibrotic muscles produces the characteristic intrinsic-plus deformity of recurvatum at the proximal interphalangeal joints. Tendons which most commonly rupture are the extensor pollicis longus, the extensor and the flexor indicis. Changes of the wrist characteristic of this disease process are as already stated, but there may be actual bone destruction or loss of bone substance, particularly of the ulna. One of the characteristic features of instability at the inferior radioulnar joint is seen on tapping the ulnar styloid which produces a definite bounce sensation because of the presence of an effusion and ligamentous instability. Accompanying these local manifestations, the general health appears poor with loss of weight, and investigations of the systemic disease reveal an increased ESR, a positive latex fixation test, etc. These have been described in detail in Chapter 11.

The aims of treatment are to provide improvement of muscle tone as well as circulation, to prevent joint contractures with adhesion formation or frank subluxation or dislocation, and to restore the functions of stability and power, particularly for pinch and grasp.

FLEXOR TENOSYNOVITIS

Flexor tenosynovitis was discussed briefly in an earlier section and is common in rheumatoid arthritis. In the region of the wrist and palm it often causes pain and symptoms of median and/or ulnar nerve compression due to the mass effect in the relatively rigid fibro-osseous carpal tunnel. The bulk of the synovium may cause compression of the nerves as well as ischaemic damage to extrinsic flexor tendons. Steroid injection is contraindicated because of the risk of weakening and rupture of the flexor tendons. In the digits, synovitis leads to decreased active range of motion and pain. The hypertrophic digital synovium may be palpable at the level of the proximal phalanx distal to the A2 pulley. Further, the bulk of the synovium along the tendons may cause triggering in either flexion or extension. This may occur at either the digital or wrist level. Ultimately, as the synovium infiltrates the tendons they may rupture, most commonly the FPL and the profundus to the small finger.

Surgical synovectomy is only considered if the patient does not respond after 6 months of medical management, or has a temporary response only. Flexor tenosynovectomy begins with a curved incision paralleling the thenar crease to the level of the wrist flexion crease where the incision passes proximally and ulnarly. The skin, subcutaneous tissue, palmar fascia, transverse ligament and antebrachial fascia are incised under direct vision to decompress the carpal canal. A careful synovectomy is then performed at the wrist level. Tension is then placed on each of the flexor tendons to ensure their integrity and to check range of motion. If there is any limitation of motion, then a distal palmar and digital synovectomy may be necessary.

The distal palm can be exposed through either a transverse incision or an extension of the digital incision, depending on the number of digits involved. Digital flexor tenosynovectomy is performed through the volar zig-zag incision described by Littler (1952) and Bruner (1967). Great care is taken to preserve the annular pulleys (especially A2 and A4) during synovectomy. The condition of the flexor tendons is then evaluated. If motion remains limited and there is severe flexor tendon involvement, then one of the flexor tendons is resected to provide more room for the less involved tendon. Preferably the superficialis tendon is removed to allow active flexion at both DIP and PIP joints, unless a swan-neck deformity would be exacerbated by removal of the FDS tendon.

Primary repair is generally not possible for flexor tendon ruptures in rheumatoid patients. Instead, if the rupture occurs at the level of the palm, it is repaired in a side-to-side fashion to an intact flexor tendon. If the rupture occurs at the digital level, then the superficialis tendon from another finger is used as a transfer.

EXTENSOR TENOSYNOVITIS

Extensor tenosynovitis is very common in the rheumatoid patient and presents with a mass over the dorsum of the hand with pain and limited motion. Tendon ruptures may be present. Surgical synovectomy is indicated after a failure of medical management and splinting. Steroid injections are contraindicated, and extensor tendon tenosynovectomy is often combined with wrist procedures.

The procedure is performed through a dorsal midline longitudinal incision. Bayonet incisions are contraindicated in the rheumatoid patient because of the risk of flap necrosis. The incision is taken down to the level of the retinaculum and full-thickness flaps are elevated, using care to preserve the dorsal veins as well as the sensory branches of the radial and ulnar nerves. The retinaculum is divided over the second or third compartment tendons and elevated to expose the second, third, and fourth dorsal compartments. The EPL is elevated out of its bed and Lister's tubercle is removed. A thorough tenosynovectomy is then performed. The fifth and sixth dorsal compartments are opened through separate incisions.

If a wrist joint (radiocarpal and intercarpal) synovectomy is to be performed, then the dorsal capsule is opened transversely. After synovectomy, the dorsal capsule is repaired through bone holes in the dorsal lip of the distal radius. In most cases, the distal radioulnar joint must also be dealt with at this time. Evaluation and treatment of the rheumatoid radiocarpal, intercarpal, and distal radioulnar joints will be discussed below. After completion of the tenosynovectomy (and any other procedures) the extensor tendons are placed in the subcutaneous tissue superficial to the extensor retinaculum. A drain is placed in the subcutaneous tissue, and the skin is then closed using interrupted vertical mattress sutures of 5–0 nylon. The drain is used to prevent haematoma formation which can lead to flap necrosis and a very difficult coverage problem. The wrist is splinted in 10–15° of extension for 3 weeks following isolated synovectomy. Active assisted range of motion of the fingers begins within 24 hours of surgery.

EXTENSOR TENDON RUPTURES

The diagnosis of extensor tendon ruptures is not always straightforward. The extensor pollicis longus is a common tendon rupture in the rheumatoid patient because of tension and friction as the tendon passes around Lister's tubercle. Rupture of the EPL does not lead to a complete lack of extension at the IP joint because of the attachments of the APB and adductor pollicis (ADD) tendons to the dorsal expansion. Instead, EPL rupture is best diagnosed by the inability of the patient to extend the thumb while the hand is held flat on a table, palm side down.

The extrinsic extensor tendons are the primary extensors of the MCP joints, whereas the intrinsics are the primary extensors of the interphalangeal joints. As a result, extrinsic extensor tendon ruptures only lead to a lag at the MCP joint level. If all four extensor digitorum communis tendons rupture, only the long and ring fingers will droop because of the intact EIP and EDQ tendons. Conversely, if EIP or EDQ is ruptured, only a small lag will be noted because of an intact EDC. As the rheumatoid process develops at the MCP level, the extrinsic extensor tendons often dislocate to the ulnar side of the metacarpal head, resulting in an extensor lag which may mimic an EDC rupture. This can usually be differentiated from a true rupture by palpating the intermetacarpal area during attempted active finger extension. The dislocated but intact tendon can be felt in the intermetacarpal groove.

As with flexor tendon ruptures, primary repair is not usually possible in the rheumatoid patient and tendon transfers need to be considered. Further, it is important to realize that finger extension is facilitated by wrist flexion, and finger flexion is potentiated by wrist extension. As a result, motion of the fingers following tendon transfer for ruptures may be limited after wrist fusion. EPL rupture is treated by transferring the EIP subcutaneously to the EPL stump. If this tendon is being used for another transfer, then palmaris longus (PL) is effective, although a tendon graft is necessary. PL to EPL transfer is valuable for IP extension and thumb abduction, yet it does not restore palmar adduction.

Rupture of a single EDC tendon is treated by side-to-side repair to an adjacent EDC tendon. Similarly, isolated EDQ rupture is treated by side-to-side repair to EDC. Rupture of both EDQ and EDC to small is best treated by EIP transfer to both tendon stumps. Rupture of EDC to ring and small is usually treated by side-to-side transfer of EDC long to EDC ring and transfer of EIP to EDC small. Rupture of EDC of long, ring, and small can be treated by side-to-side transfer of EDC long to EDC index, and EIP to EDC ring and EDC small. It can also be treated by EIP to EDC long and FDS ring to EDC ring and small. Rupture of all of the extrinsic finger extensors (II–V) is usually repaired using FDS tendons. FDS long is transferred to EDC index and FDS ring is transferred to EDC long, ring, and small.

The tension of the tendon transfers is critical for optimal function. The tendon transfer for finger extension is set with the wrist in maximal extension and the fingers in full flexion. This ensures that the transfer will not be too tight and thereby limit finger flexion. In those with a wrist fusion, the tendon transfer is set with the interphalangeal joints in full extension and the MCP joints flexed 25–30°. The functional results in those with wrist fusion is somewhat limited, because finger extension cannot be potentiated by simultaneous wrist flexion.

RHEUMATOID WRIST

Involvement of the rheumatoid wrist affects the function of the entire hand. In order to maximize hand function, the patient needs a stable, painless wrist in a functional position. Typically, the rheumatoid wrist develops progressive deformity as the disease process ensues. Wrist involvement classically leads to cartilage destruction, bony collapse, and loss of carpal height. Progressive anterior and ulnar translation of the carpus occurs, along with radial deviation and supination (Figure 15.22). This position leads to a relative dorsal prominence of the distal ulna and limited painful forearm rotation. Further, the relative prominence of the distal ulna can lead to extensor tendon ruptures (most commonly EDQ and EDC to ring and small).

Wrist alignment affects the alignment and function of the metacarpophalangeal joints. As the wrist collapses into radial deviation, the extrinsic flexor and extensor tendons approach these joints from the ulnar aspect and thereby exacerbate ulnar drift of the MCP joints. As a result, the wrist deformity must be addressed before more distal problems. Rebalancing of the MCP joints without correcting the wrist is doomed to failure.

Rheumatoid wrist disease can involve the radiocarpal, intercarpal and distal radioulnar joints. The

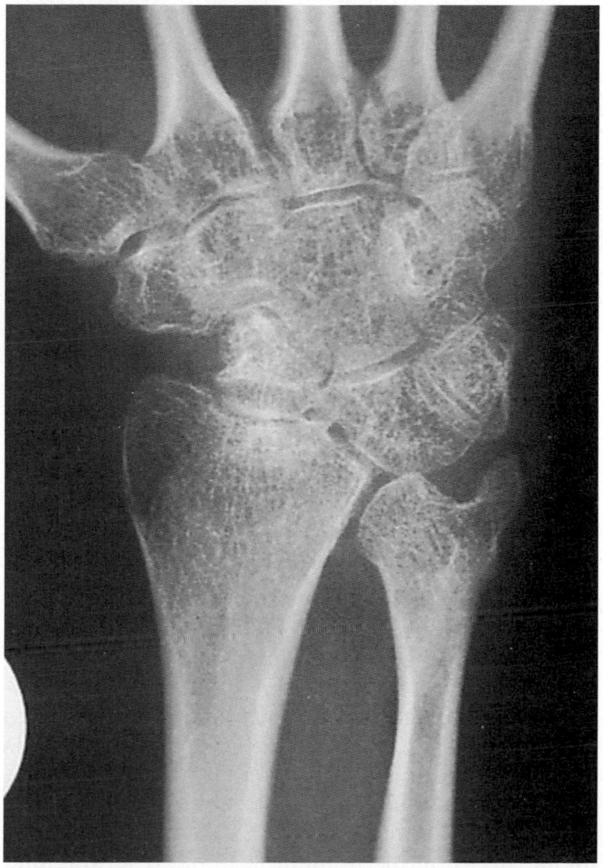

Figure 15.22 Radiograph of hand with severe rheumatoid arthritis.

surgical options for radiocarpal and intercarpal disease include synovectomy, arthroplasty and fusion. Synovectomy is only effective in those with early joint involvement. The main indication is synovitis and pain without bony destruction or malalignment. The procedure is usually done in conjunction with extensor tenosynovectomy. The carpus is exposed through a transverse dorsal capsulotomy and the synovectomy is performed. The capsulotomy is repaired primarily or through drill holes in the dorsal radius. The postoperative programme is the same as for isolated extensor tenosynovectomy, and includes early active assisted finger range of motion.

Wrist arthroplasty

Two types of wrist arthroplasty have been used in rheumatoid arthritis: resection arthroplasty with or without soft tissue interposition, and implant arthroplasty. Palmar shelf arthroplasty is a form of resectional arthroplasty described by Albright and Chase (1970) in which the distal radius is resected so that it is perpendicular to the longitudinal axis of the radius in both the anteroposterior and lateral planes. A shallow socket is then created in the distal radius with a small volar lip to keep the carpus from subluxating anteriorly. The carpus is reduced into this socket and held temporarily with K-wires. The volar capsule is detached proximally and sutured to the dorsal rim of the radius which creates a soft tissue interposition that discourages volar carpal subluxation. The dorsal capsule is repaired, any necessary extensor tendon procedures are performed, and the skin is closed over a drain.

Of numerous implants designed for the wrist, only the silicone wrist arthroplasty is appropriate for the rheumatoid patient. Resurfacing arthroplasties and 'total wrist' arthroplasties made of metal and polyethylene are associated with high rates of failure from loosening secondary to the underlying poor bone stock in rheumatoid patients. The silicone wrist arthroplasty functions as a soft tissue spacer and is indicated in those patients with relatively good bone stock both proximally and distally. Other prerequisites include intact wrist extensor tendons and independent ambulation without aids (Brase and Millender, 1986; Vicar and Burton, 1986). Adequate soft tissue rebalancing with good postoperative alignment are crucial to the success of this procedure. After arthroplasty, the patient is advised to wear a splint for all strenuous tasks, and the goal is 40–50° of motion. Implant failure is related to the time of follow-up and to the amount of motion (Brase and Millender, 1986). Excessive motion puts undue stress on the implant, leading to settling and fracture.

Although the early results with this form of arthroplasty are excellent, there is a relatively high rate of complications and failure. Brase and Millender showed a 25% failure rate of silicone wrist arthroplasty at an average follow-up of 67 months. Vicar and Burton reported a complication rate of 25% in their series of 37 arthroplasties at an average follow-up of 51 months. However, if this type of arthroplasty does fail, it can reliably be converted to fusion (Brase and Millender, 1986; Vicar and Burton, 1986).

Wrist fusion

Wrist fusion is a well accepted treatment for the rheumatoid patient with advanced wrist involvement. It reliably provides a painless, stable, well aligned wrist which allows better overall hand function (Carroll and Dick, 1971; Millender and Nalebuff, 1973; Clendenin and Green, 1981). However, the lack of wrist motion may be disabling in those patients with bilateral wrist disease and other upper extremity involvement. Finger flexion and extension cannot be augmented with concomitant wrist motion after a wrist fusion. Most authors feel that a neutral position is best for the rheumatoid patient (Flatt, 1963; Linscheid, 1968; Millender and Nalebuff, 1973; Vicar and Burton, 1986).

The method of fusion used at the authors' institution is that described by Millender and Nalebuff (1973). The wrist is exposed through a dorsal longitudinal incision (Figure 15.23). After extensor tenosynovectomy is performed, the radiocarpal joint is entered through a transverse dorsal capsulotomy. The distal radius is decorticated and the anterior lip is removed with care to protect the volar structures. If this volar lip of bone is left, it will leave a ridge at the base of the carpal canal which may lead to carpal tunnel syndrome or late flexor tendon ruptures. Care must also be taken to protect the first dorsal compartment tendons and radial nerve as the radial styloid region is decorticated.

Next, the carpus is decorticated while preserving as much bone as possible. The distal ulna must be resected to allow pronation and supination. This procedure is described below. The wrist is stabilized with a large, smooth Steinmann pin which is first inserted from proximal to distal through the capitate and then either into the shaft of the third metacarpal or between the second and third metacarpals. The pin is placed in the third metacarpal shaft if simultaneous MCP arthroplasties are to be performed, or between the second and third metacarpals, if MCP arthroplasties may be done at a later date. The carpus is then reduced onto the distal radius and the pin is then passed proximally into the medullary canal of the radius. Cancellous bone graft from the ulnar head or ilium is then packed around the carpus to facilitate

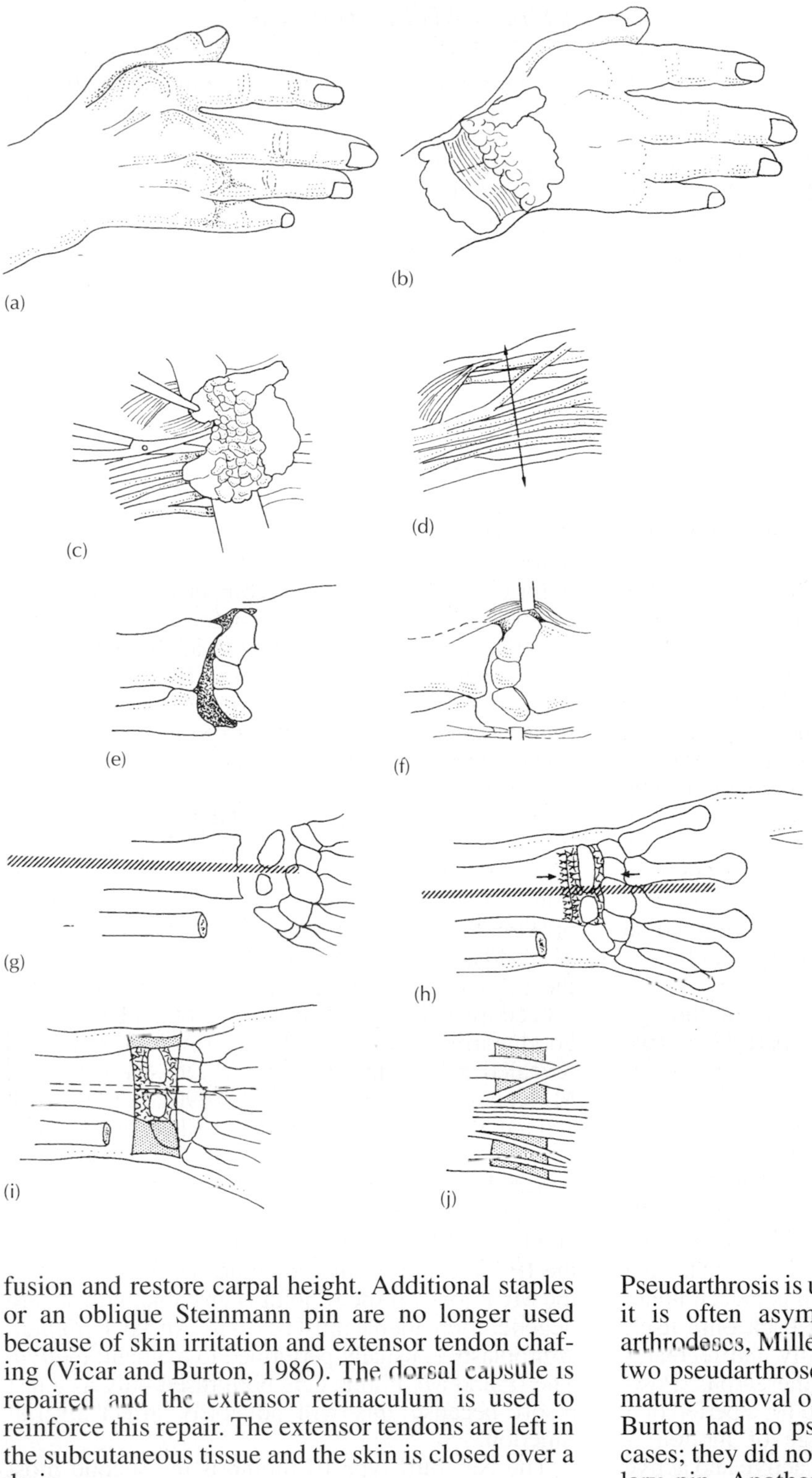

Figure 15.23 Arthrodesis of the wrist in rheumatoid arthritis. (a) Dorsal longitudinal incision. Curved or bayonet incisions are contraindicated in rheumatoid arthritis because of the high risk of skin slough. Full thickness flaps are created to the level of the extensor retinaculum, avoiding damage to the dorsal branches of the radial sensory and ulnar nerves. (b) Retinacular flaps are raised. (c) Tenosynovectomy of the second, third, fourth and fifth extensor compartments. (d) Extensor tendons retracted to expose the wrist capsule, usually between the fourth and fifth extensor compartments. (e) Distally based flaps raised from dorsal wrist capsule. (f) Areas of bony resection. The capsular incision is extended proximally along the ulnar margin to expose distal ulna, and 1–1.5 cm of distal ulna is resected. All bone is saved for later bone grafting. (g) Large, smooth Steinmann pin driven distally through base of capitate into the interval between the index and long metacarpals. The wrist is then aligned and the pin tapped retrograde into the shaft of the radius. (h) Bone graft packed in fusion site, which is then impacted tightly. Pin driven proximal to Index and long metacarpal heads. The rectangular capsular flap is closed. (i) Extensor retinacular flaps transposed deep to tendons and reapposed. (j) Extensor tendons now in subcutaneous plane. (After Burton, R.I. (1991) *Atlas of Orthopaedic Surgery*. Edited by L.A. Goldstein. C.V. Mosby: St Louis, p. 138)

fusion and restore carpal height. Additional staples or an oblique Steinmann pin are no longer used because of skin irritation and extensor tendon chafing (Vicar and Burton, 1986). The dorsal capsule is repaired and the extensor retinaculum is used to reinforce this repair. The extensor tendons are left in the subcutaneous tissue and the skin is closed over a drain.

Postoperatively, the patient's arm is placed in a below-elbow cast for 2 weeks followed by additional splinting for 4–6 weeks. Active assisted finger range of motion is begun in the first 24 hours after surgery.

Pseudarthrosis is uncommon, and when it does occur it is often asymptomatic. In their series of 70 arthrodeses, Millender and Nalebuff (1973) had just two pseudarthroses, both likely resulting from premature removal of the intramedullary pin. Vicar and Burton had no pseudarthroses in their series of 33 cases; they did not routinely remove the intramedullary pin. Another possible complication is carpal tunnel syndrome which may result from a lip of bone in the carpal canal or from postoperative swelling. If this persists, then flexor tenosynovectomy and carpal tunnel release should be performed.

CAPUT ULNAE SYNDROME

Involvement of the distal radioulnar joint (DRUJ) has been described by Blackdahl (1963) as the *caput ulnae syndrome*. It is characterized by a prominent appearing distal ulna. This develops as the supporting ligaments around the distal ulna deteriorate and the extensor carpi ulnaris subluxates anteriorly, causing flexion and supination of the carpus. In fact, the prominence of the distal ulna is, in part, secondary to the combined anterior subluxation and supination of the carpus. Patients with involvement of the DRUJ generally complain of pain over the ulnar border of the wrist which is aggravated by pronation and supination. On physical examination there is swelling and tenderness over the ulnar head. The combination of the prominence of the distal ulna and tenosynovitis often leads to rupture of the EDQ and the EDC tendons to ring and small.

Surgical treatment of the DRUJ depends on the degree of involvement. Although rarely indicated, synovectomy, reconstruction of the supporting ligaments, and ECU translocation alone can be performed if there is no evidence of articular cartilage destruction. Most commonly, destruction of the head of the ulna makes joint preservation impossible and the distal ulna is resected in conjunction with ligament reconstruction and ECU translocation. There is an increased risk of ulnar translocation, volar subluxation, and supination of the carpus after distal ulna resection. As a result, this procedure is often combined with other procedures aimed at stabilizing and realigning the radiocarpal and intercarpal joints.

The distal radioulnar joint is exposed through the floor of the fifth dorsal compartment. Two retinacular flaps are created for subsequent reconstruction, the first proximal and left attached to the ulna, and the second distal and left attached to the dorsoulnar radius. After excision of the distal ulna, the proximal ulnar based flap is sutured to the dorsoulnar aspect of the radius to stabilize the remaining ulna. The ECU tendon is then identified, mobilized, and brought dorsally. A sling is made out of the distal radial based flap which is placed under the ECU tendon and then sutured back onto itself which translocates the ECU dorsally and recreates its extensor and pronator pull on the carpus. Postoperatively, the wrist is immobilized for a period of 4 weeks and immediate finger range of motion is encouraged. After immobilization, active and active assist flexion, extension, pronation, and supination are initiated.

RHEUMATOID THUMB

Because of the importance of the thumb in all hand activities, it is crucial to attempt to provide the rheumatoid patient with a pain-free thumb that has both stability and adequate mobility. The three joints of the thumb, trapeziometacarpal, metacarpophalangeal and interphalangeal, may be involved individually, or more commonly in combination. As deformity of the wrist affects more distal disease, so trapeziometacarpal pathology may result in compensatory deformity at the MCP and IP joints, or primary MCP disease may lead to subsequent IP deformity. The most proximally involved joint must always be addressed first when treating these deformities.

Nalebuff has classified rheumatoid thumb deformity into five types. The two most common are the type I and type III thumbs. The type I thumb deformity is characterized by an MCP flexion deformity with a secondary compensatory IP hyperextension deformity. This deformity is felt to develop initially from synovitis at the MCP joint which causes attenuation of the EPB tendon and extensor hood, leading to an extensor lag at the MCP joint. The EPL tendon subluxates in an ulnar and volar direction functioning as an MCP flexor and IP extensor.

If addressed before any fixed deformity develops, the type I thumb can be treated by MCP joint synovectomy and extensor mechanism reconstruction by rerouting the EPL tendon to the base of the proximal phalanx. This increases MCP joint extension and allows IP extension through the insertion of the intrinsic muscles into the extensor hood. This procedure was described by Nalebuff (1968) with good early results, but long-term follow-up has revealed a high late recurrence rate (Terrono and Millender, 1989; Terrono *et al*., 1990). In those with a fixed flexion deformity at the MCP level and a passively correctable IP joint, MCP arthrodesis is generally recommended. The most difficult group to treat are those with fixed deformity at both the MCP and IP levels, with joint destruction. The treatment of the IP joint in this situation guides the treatment of the MCP joint. If the IP joint is unstable with severe degeneration, then it must be fused. An MCP implant arthroplasty is usually performed to maintain motion. The IP and MCP joints are both fused only as a last resort because this will adversely affect overall function.

The Nalebuff type III thumb is the second most common rheumatoid thumb deformity and is characterized primarily by instability at the TMJ followed by compensatory hyperextension deformity at the MCP joint. Synovitis at the TMJ leads to laxity of the palmar oblique ligament with dorsoradial subluxation of the metacarpal base. The combined forces of the APL and ADD lead to adduction of the first metacarpal and narrowing of the first web space. Hyperextension deformity at the MCP joint develops due to the first metacarpal adduction contracture. As the patient attempts to extend the thumb and grasp objects, extension force is transmitted to the MCP joint instead of the metacarpal which is fixed. Progressive volar plate laxity develops, leading to a MCP hyperextension deformity.

Treatment of the type III thumb is aimed primarily at the TMJ. Because TMJ disease is rarely an isolated process in the rheumatoid patient, some form of arthroplasty and ligament stabilization procedure is indicated, such as ligament reconstruction combined with either a silicone, fascial, or tendon interposition arthroplasty (see section on osteoarthritis of the thumb for a more complete discussion of the procedures available to treat the TMJ). Adduction contracture of the first metacarpal is treated by increasing the bone resection and if necessary a web space Z-plasty to allow abduction of the thumb. Indications for MCP fusion at the time of TMJ arthroplasty include either 20° of passive hyperextension or 30° of valgus instability. If the MCP joint is only mildly unstable, volar tenodesis or capsuloplasty may be considered instead of fusion.

The other thumb deformities classified by Nalebuff are rarer and will be discussed briefly. In the type II thumb deformity, there is primary TMJ disease with secondary IP joint hyperextension and instability. As with the type III deformity, the TMJ must be reconstructed, usually followed by IP arthrodesis. The type IV deformity is the same as the type III deformity except that the MCP joint develops valgus instability. Treatment is similar to that for the type III thumb discussed above. The type V thumb was not originally part of Nalebuff's classification, but was added later. It consists of volar plate laxity at the MCP joint and IP joint flexion deformity. The primary pathology is at the MCP joint. Treatment consists of stabilization of the MCP joint through capsulodesis or fusion.

Thumb IP arthrodesis is performed in an identical manner as DIP fusion of the other digits. The position of fusion is usually 0–10° of flexion, neutral abduction–adduction, and 5° of pronation (Burton, 1990). The position of MCP joint arthrodesis is controversial and must be determined in relation to the mobility of the trapeziometacarpal and interphalangeal joints. As a general guideline, Inglis *et al.* (1972) recommends 15° of flexion, 15° of abduction, and 15° of pronation. Others have recommended from 0 to 25° of flexion (Urbaniak 1990; Feldon *et al.*, 1993).

Thumb MCP arthroplasty is performed through a dorsal approach, taking care to preserve the collateral ligaments. The bone cuts are made, the canals are broached, and the implant is placed. Stability, especially to valgus stress, is crucial in this procedure and the ulnar collateral ligament may require reconstruction using local capsule or tendon graft such as a portion of the palmaris longus, adductor pollicis, or extensor pollicis brevis. After implant placement, a secure dorsal capsuloplasty must be performed such that the thumb rests with the MCP joint in neutral flexion–extension. The extensor mechanism must similarly be rebalanced, and the EPL may be rerouted to assist in MCP extension, if indicated. Both a K-wire and external splint are used to support the thumb postoperatively. The pin is removed at 4–6 weeks postoperatively and a supportive splint is worn with the thumb MCP and IP joints in neutral for a total of 8 weeks between exercise sessions.

Tendon ruptures may also affect thumb function. EPL rupture was addressed in an earlier section and generally presents not with loss of IP extension but instead weakness of thumb adduction. The FPL may also rupture in the rheumatoid patient at either the wrist level or within the fibro-osseous digital sheath. The two treatment options are arthrodesis or tendon transfer. If significant hyperextension deformity is present at the IP joint then arthrodesis is preferable. Otherwise, a FDS transfer can be used to restore IP flexion.

RHEUMATOID INVOLVEMENT OF THE FINGERS

The metacarpophalangeal joints

The metacarpophalangeal joints of the fingers characteristically develop an extensor lag and ulnar drift in rheumatoid arthritis. As the synovium proliferates, the radial sagittal fibres of the extensor hood attenuate, allowing the long finger extensors to subluxate in an ulnar direction into the cleft between metacarpals. This is further exacerbated by radial deviation of the wrist. Once they are no longer centred over the metacarpal head, the extrinsic extensors become ulnar deviators instead of MCP extensors. The extrinsic flexors also contribute to deformity at the MCP level. As the MCP joint synovitis leads to capsular attenuation and ligamentous laxity, the pull of the flexor tendons on the A1 pulley causes volar subluxation of the proximal phalanx at the MCP level. If the fingers remain in this position of MCP flexion and ulnar deviation, the intrinsic muscles (ulnar more than radial) shorten, accelerating the process. In advanced cases, the extrinsic extensor tendons pass volar to the axis of motion at the MCP joints, causing flexion.

Dysfunction at the MCP joint level may lead to deformity at the PIP joint. Once the extensor tendon is displaced off the metacarpal head, it loses its mechanical advantage at the MCP level and its power is diverted distally to the insertion at the base of the middle phalanx at the PIP joint. As a result, the force of both the extrinsic extensor tendons and the tight intrinsic musculature is focused on extension of the PIP joint. Volar plate laxity and PIP hyperextension then develop, leading to the so-called 'swan-neck' deformity.

Surgical treatment for MCP joint deformity must address primarily the soft tissue imbalance. The extrinsic extensor tendons are recentred over the metacarpal heads by releasing the ulnar sagittal bands and tightening the radial sagittal bands. The tight ulnar intrinsic musculature is released. Once these dynamic forces are balanced, the static deforming forces must be addressed. With prolonged positioning in flexion and ulnar deviation, MCP capsular contractures exist. These are corrected by releasing or lengthening the collateral ligaments (ulnar and possibly radial) and volar plate. Such soft tissue rebalancing must be considered whether one is performing synovectomy, resectional arthroplasty, or implant arthroplasty.

MCP arthroplasty

Metacarpophalangeal joint synovectomy is a procedure which has limited indications. It is not generally considered adequate treatment if there is significant joint destruction, instability, subluxation, or fixed deformity. Its benefits are temporary because a complete synovectomy is not possible, and scarring may make subsequent arthroplasty difficult.

Metacarpophalangeal joint arthroplasty can be of two basic types: excisional soft tissue arthroplasty and implant arthroplasty. One of the most common excisional arthroplasties is the Tupper arthroplasty (Weilby, 1977). Following synovectomy, the metacarpal head is resected with a slight volar angulation to the cut. After releasing the collateral ligaments and volar plate from their proximal attachment, the volar plate is brought through the joint and sutured into the dorsal rim of the remaining metacarpal neck. This provides a soft tissue interposition for pain relief and prevents recurrent volar subluxation. The radial collateral ligament is reattached snugly to help prevent recurrent ulnar deviation. The remainder of the soft tissue rebalancing is completed as described above.

In most hands, implant arthroplasty yields better results than excisional arthroplasty. The most common implant used is the Swanson silicone implant. As with other silicone implants, this truly represents an excisional arthroplasty with a silicone spacer. The soft tissue rebalancing, as described above, is still the most crucial aspect of this procedure. After placement of the implant, a pseudocapsule forms around the implant which, with surrounding ligamentous structures, provides the main support for the joint. Although implant fracture on radiographic follow-up is not uncommon, it usually does not affect motion or require replacement.

Although MCP implant arthroplasty improves finger function through realignment and correction of extensor lag, the total arc of motion after implant arthroplasty is not increased. Instead, the arc of motion is shifted to a more functional range. Similarly, grip strength is often unchanged postoperatively, yet the lack of pain makes the hand functionally stronger. Finally, because rheumatoid arthritis is a systemic problem, deformity may recur and require additional treatment.

MCP implant arthroplasty is performed through a dorsal exposure (Figure 15.24). Following synovectomy, the metacarpal head is resected at the level of the distal neck. The ulnar collateral ligament is released and the radial collateral ligament is left intact, especially in the index and long fingers, unless it prevents subsequent joint correction. In that case, it is released and later reattached through drill holes. An intrinsic release is then performed. If there appears to be too little space for the implant despite adequate bony resection, the volar plate is released. This allows inspection of the flexor tendons, and a limited tenosynovectomy can be performed if necessary. The canals of the metacarpal and proximal phalanx are then broached. The implant is sized so that it is able to slide in the medullary canals but still controls rotation. The capsule is then closed, and the extensor tendon is replaced over the metacarpal head by imbricating the radial sagittal band.

The postoperative therapy programme is extremely important in these patients and includes long-term static and dynamic splinting to prevent recurrence. Further, active assisted MCP flexion and extension exercises are taught and continued for a minimum of 6 months.

Interphalangeal joints

The interphalangeal joints are commonly affected in rheumatoid arthritis. The most common deformity is the swan-neck deformity which consists of hyperextension of the PIP joint and DIP flexion. This deformity is especially common in conjunction with extensor lag and ulnar drift at the MCP level as outlined above. PIP hyperextension leads to relative lengthening of the lateral bands, resulting in an extensor lag at the DIP joints. As with other

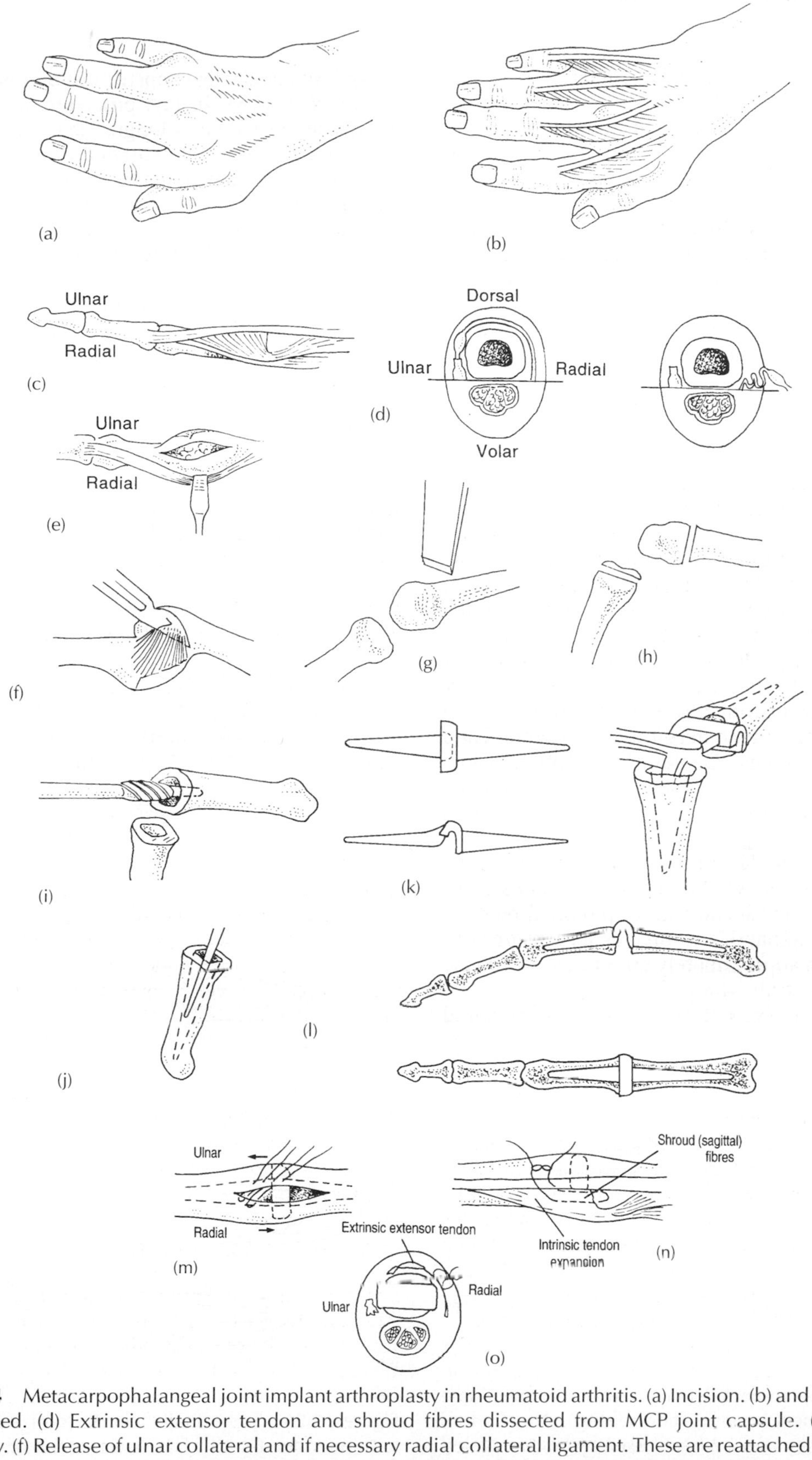

Figure 15.24 Metacarpophalangeal joint implant arthroplasty in rheumatoid arthritis. (a) Incision. (b) and (c) Ulnar shroud fibres released. (d) Extrinsic extensor tendon and shroud fibres dissected from MCP joint capsule. (e) Longitudinal capsulotomy. (f) Release of ulnar collateral and if necessary radial collateral ligament. These are reattached to bone through drill holes at closure. (g) and (h) Bony resection. (i) and (j) The canal is rasped to the appropriate size. (k) and (l) The implant is inserted. (m) The capsule is closed bringing the distal radial margin to the proximal ulnar margin. (n) and (o) The radial shroud fibres are imbricated to centralize the extrinsic extensor tendon dorsally. (After Burton, R.I. (1990) *Surgery of the Musculoskeletal System*. Edited by C.M. Evarts. Churchill Livingstone: New York, pp. 1087–1157)

rheumatoid deformities, it is crucial to treat the proximal joints, especially the MCP joints, before addressing the interphalangeal joint deformities. Volar plate laxity, which is central to the aetiology of the swan-neck deformity, must be corrected to prevent recurrence. The condition of the extrinsic flexors must be ascertained because tenosynovitis or rupture may contribute to PIP hyperextension.

Treatment of swan-neck deformities is difficult and varies according to the stage of the disease. In the early stage, the deformity is correctable with no fixed contractures and the patient has full active flexion. If the patient has intrinsic tightness on examination, this must be treated with stretching exercises or surgical release to decrease the deforming forces. In addition, the volar plate laxity must be treated by FDS tenodesis, oblique retinacular ligament reconstruction, or spiral oblique ligament reconstruction.

The oblique retinacular ligament reconstruction, originally described by Littler, is designed to correct both the PIP and DIP joint imbalances seen in the swan-neck deformity. The oblique retinacular ligament passes volar to the PIP joint axis and dorsal to the DIP joint axis. It tightens as the PIP joint actively extends both to prevent PIP hyperextension and to pull the DIP joint into extension. In the lateral band technique (Littler and Cooley, 1965; Littler, 1967, 1977), the ulnar lateral band is divided proximally. From its distal attachment, the lateral band is rerouted volar to Cleland's ligaments, deep to the neurovascular bundle. It then passes, anterior to the flexor sheath, obliquely across to the radial side of the digit where it is secured at the proximal phalanx level. The lateral band is secured under tension with the PIP joint in approximately 20° of flexion and the DIP joint in neutral.

This technique was later modified to the spiral oblique retinacular ligament reconstruction by Thompson *et al.* (1978). In this procedure a free tendon graft, usually palmaris longus, is used to construct the oblique retinacular ligament (Figure 15.25). The graft begins at the dorsum of the distal phalanx, passes anteriorly and proximally along the middle phalanx, passes obliquely across the anterior aspect of the PIP joint to the opposite side where it is secured to the base of the proximal phalanx through drill holes. Tension is set in the same fashion as the lateral band technique. The advantages of the free graft technique are the need for less dissection and better strength of the tendon distally where the lateral band insertion is often attenuated in the rheumatoid patient.

The superficialis tenodesis uses one or both slips of the flexor digitorum superficialis for tenodesis of the PIP joint to prevent hyperextension (Littler, 1952; Swanson, 1960; Curtis, 1964). The super-

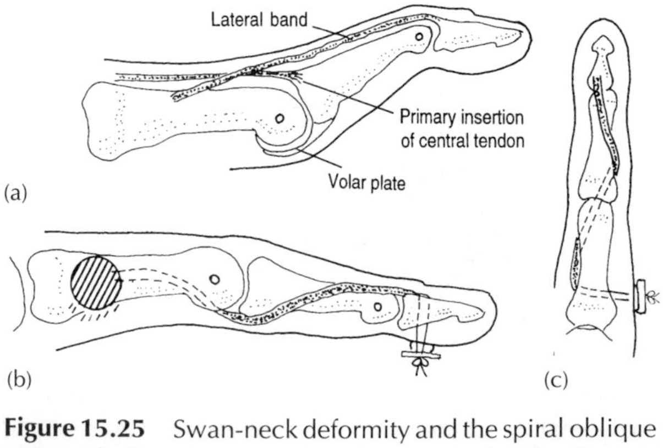

Figure 15.25 Swan-neck deformity and the spiral oblique retinacular ligament reconstruction (see text). (After Burton, R.I. (1990) *Surgery of the Musculoskeletal System*. Edited by C.M. Evarts. Churchill Livingstone: New York, pp. 1087–1157)

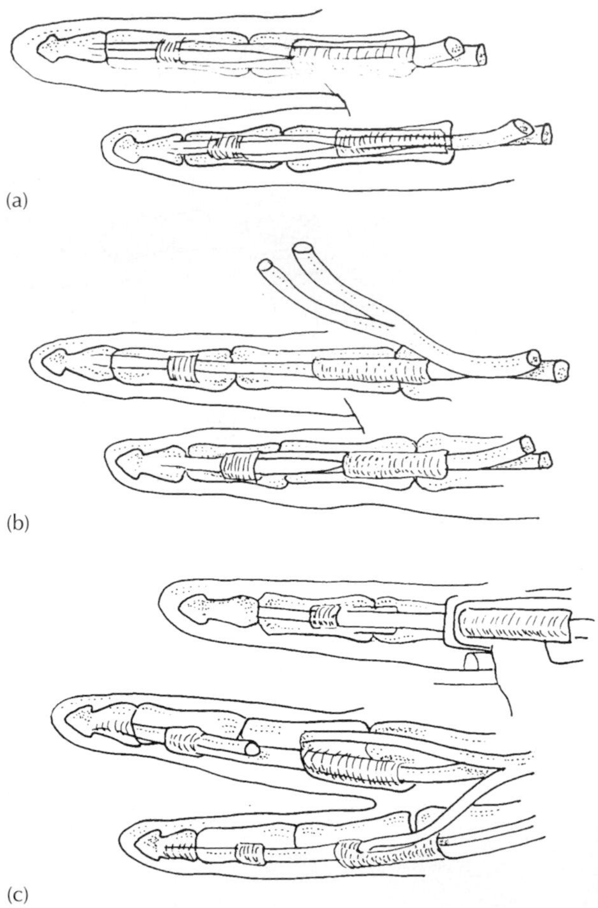

Figure 15.26 Superficialis tenodesis for swan-neck deformity. (After Burton, R.I. (1991) *Atlas of Orthopaedic Surgery*. Edited by L.A. Goldstein. C.V. Mosby: St Louis, p. 138)

ficialis tendon is cut at the proximal phalanx level and left attached distally (Figure 15.26). The free end is then passed from volar to dorsal through a drill hole in the proximal phalanx. The joint is stabilized in 20° of flexion. Because this procedure only corrects the PIP volar plate laxity, it may not fully correct the DIP joint imbalance. All of these procedures are initially stabilized by pinning the PIP joint at 20° of flexion and using a protective splint. The splint and K-wires are removed at 4 weeks and replaced with an extension block splint initially at 20° of flexion and ultimately decreasing to 5 or 10° of flexion by 8 weeks after surgery.

Mid-stage swan-neck deformity is characterized by limited active PIP motion in a finger which rests in the swan-neck position. Radiographs show a normal joint, which distinguishes this stage from the late deformity. In this situation, the lateral bands are adherent in a dorsal position, preventing flexion. In addition, the central slip has contracted along with the lateral bands. Treatment involves mobilization of the lateral bands to allow flexion of the PIP joint along with extension block splinting to prevent PIP hyperextension during the early healing phase. If significant volar plate laxity persists, then an anterior FDS tenodesis or ligament reconstruction is done.

Late-stage swan-neck deformity is a difficult problem to treat because there is significant joint destruction and often ankylosis of the joint. Treatment must be individualized. The two main surgical options are PIP joint arthrodesis and implant arthroplasty with soft tissue rebalancing. As discussed in the section on osteoarthritis, PIP fusion is usually performed in the index and long fingers to provide a stable post for pinch. Arthroplasty is often recommended in the ring and small PIP joints because these digits are necessary for power grip. If bony ankylosis is present then the only real option is arthrodesis.

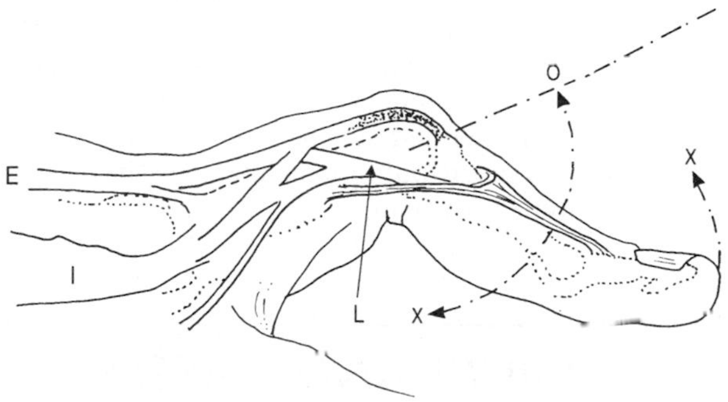

Figure 15.27 Established boutonnière deformity. Attenuation of extrinsic (E) and intrinsic (I) extensors, volar subluxation of lateral bands (L) due to unopposed flexor tone at PIP joint with secondary DIP hyperextension. (After Littler, J.W. and Eaton, R.G. (1967) *Journal of Bone and Joint Surgery* **49A**, 1268)

The boutonnière deformity is also common in rheumatoid disease and is characterized by flexion of the PIP joint and hyperextension of the DIP joint (Figure 15.27). This occurs from attenuation or rupture of the central slip of the extensor mechanism at its attachment at the base of the middle phalanx (Figure 15.28). This leads to an extensor lag at the PIP joint and volar subluxation of the lateral bands. Initially, this may be a dynamic imbalance but over time the lateral bands will become fixed volar to the axis of PIP motion. Unlike the swan-neck deformity which almost always requires surgical intervention, the boutonnière deformity can often be treated nonoperatively.

The early boutonnière is a dynamic imbalance in which the deformity is passively correctable, indicating that the lateral bands have subluxated anteriorly but are not adherent. This is best treated with splinting and specific exercises designed to regain both PIP extension and DIP flexion. The first step of the exercise involves active-assisted PIP joint extension which stretches the tight volar structures and simultaneously causes further hyperextension at the DIP joint. The second step involves forceful active

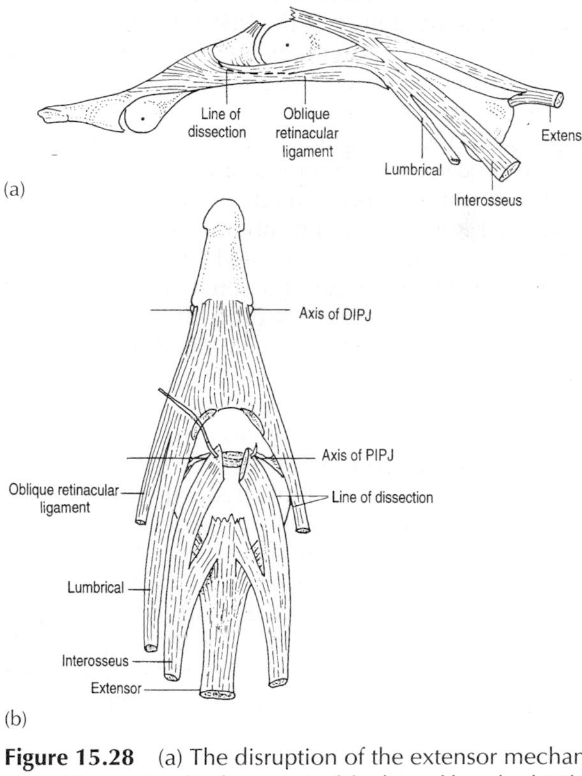

Figure 15.28 (a) The disruption of the extensor mechanism with anterior displacement of the lateral bands. (b) The operative correction of a boutonnière deformity by suturing the lateral bands to each other and to the central band. (After Littler, J.W. and Eaton, R.G. (1967) *Journal of Bone and Joint Surgery* **49A**, 1267–1274)

DIP joint flexion with the PIP joint extended which works to stretch gradually both the lateral bands and the oblique retinacular ligaments. A combination of dynamic and static splinting is also used to work on PIP extension, while allowing free motion at the MCP and DIP joints. This programme is generally successful in treating the early boutonnière deformity although it may need to be continued for an extended period to prevent recurrence.

The mid-stage boutonnière deformity is characterized by a PIP extensor lag of 30–60°, which is not passively correctable, indicating that the lateral bands are adherent in a volar subluxated position and the oblique retinacular ligaments are tight. An exercise and splinting programme is successful in treating this deformity, but operative intervention is indicated if a plateau in improvement is reached. A tenotomy of the extensor over the middle phalanx is performed, allowing the extensor mechanism to slide proximally, increasing the extensor tone at the base of the middle phalanx, allowing the lateral bands to slide proximally and dorsally, and decreasing the tone at the distal phalangeal insertion. After tenotomy, extension at the DIP joint depends on the integrity of the oblique retinacular ligaments.

The late stage boutonnière deformity consists of a fixed flexion deformity of the PIP joint of as much as 90°. The capsular structures are contracted and the PIP joint may show subluxation or ankylosis. The DIP joint may be fixed in hyperextension. Treatment of this late-stage deformity is difficult and results are limited. Because of the joint destruction, arthroplasty or fusion must be performed. As noted above, the index and long fingers are often fused whereas the ring and small fingers are treated by arthroplasty.

PIP joint arthroplasty in the setting of a swan-neck or boutonnière deformity is difficult because of the ligamentous and capsular contractures combined with severe bony destruction. The collateral ligaments are more important for stability in the PIP joints than in the MCP joints. In the advanced deformity with severe contractures, the volar plate and collateral ligaments must frequently be released to correct deformity which may lead to instability postoperatively. As with other procedures in the treatment of rheumatoid arthritis, the primary goal of the procedure is to rebalance the soft tissues in order to restore motion in a stable joint. If adequate soft tissue rebalancing and joint stability cannot be achieved, then arthroplasty is not an option.

Psoriasis and arthritis

Although psoriatic arthritis can involve larger joints, the more commonly involved are the distal interphalangeal joints of both hands, in an asymmetrical fashion suggesting a gouty arthritis rather than a rheumatoid arthritis. There is a fusiform swelling but no subcutaneous nodules. On x-ray there is massive destruction of the distal phalanges without the osteoporosis commonly seen in rheumatoid arthritis. The latex fixation or agglutination tests for the rheumatoid factor are, of course, negative. The psoriatic skin lesions are variable in appearance and in degree of severity but often appear as reddish, extensive and asymmetrical lesions which can be exudative or even pustular. Pitting and discoloration of the nails are common. Men are more commonly involved with this arthritis than women at any age group. The condition may appear early, and, if so, this has a serious prognosis. The psoriatic lesion tends to persist and resist most forms of treatment. Corticosteroids have been given in high dosages, and, although producing initial improvement, there may be little prevention of progression of the disease process.

Sarcoidosis

This condition can present as an arthritis, although more commonly it presents because of its pulmonary lesion. The arthritis is most common in the hands and fingers, but also occurs in the feet; radiographs show large cyst-like spaces in the phalangeal bones (Figure 15.29). Ocular manifestations have also been reported. Striated muscle biopsy has been advocated to demonstrate the presence of and confirm the diagnosis of a granuloma. Its aetiology is unknown and it is not now thought to be related to tuberculosis, but rather is thought to be another hypersensitivity state. Large epithelial cells and tubercle-like lesions are common (Figure 15.30). Treatment appears to be by steroids, which have only a temporary beneficial effect, but are particularly recommended when there is impairment of vision, advanced pulmonary changes, hypercalcaemia or hypersplenism.

TUMOURS AND MASSES

Tumours and masses of the hand constitute a wide range of conditions, and the treatment varies depending on the aetiology and natural history. In this section only the most common tumours and masses

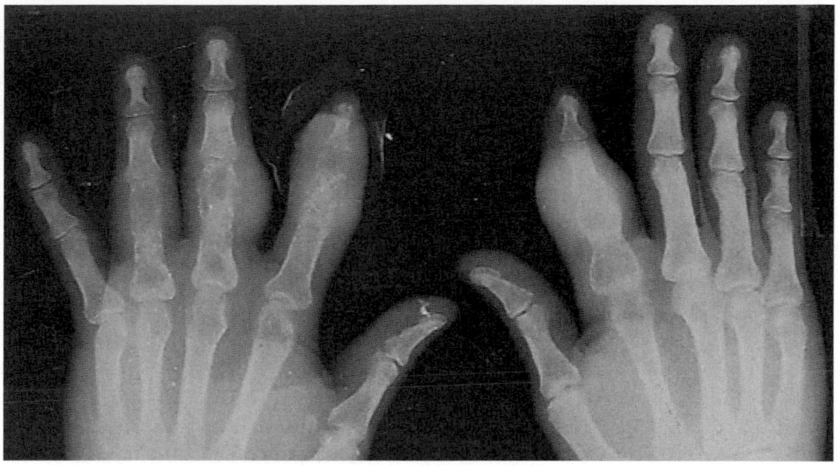

Figure 15.29 Radiographs of both hands to show the marked soft tissue as well as osseous changes associated with sarcoidosis. There is loss of trabecular structure of the short miniature bones which are also increased in width.

will be discussed. A complete history must be obtained to determine how and when the mass developed and any changes which may have occurred over time. Further, it is important to determine the symptoms related to the lesion and how these have progressed. Finally, a family history will determine if there is any hereditary component.

Physical examination should include a search for

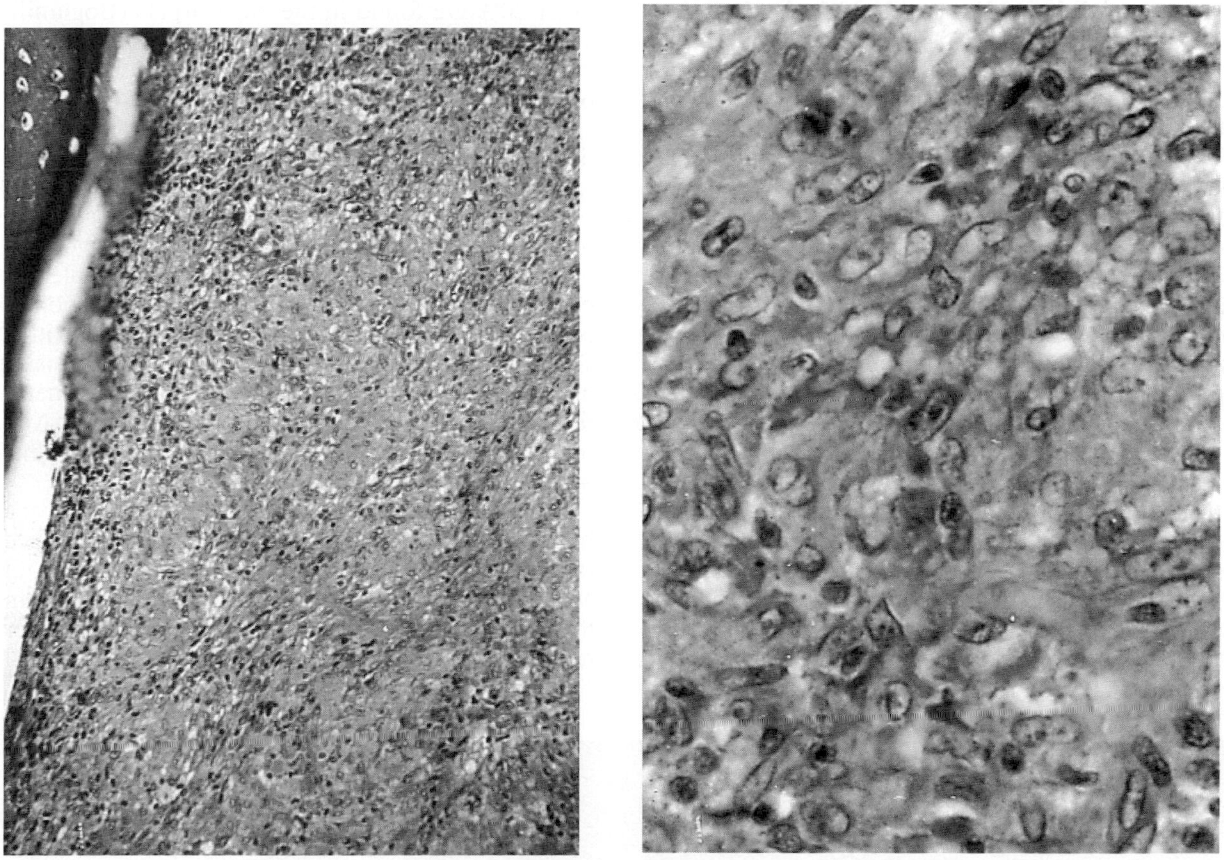

(a) (b)

Figure 15.30 (a) Photomicrograph showing the numerous epithelial cells adjacent to bone involved with sarcoidosis. (× 83). (b) Photomicrograph showing the large epithelial cells with relatively acellular stroma and a few blood vessels. (× 358).

similar masses or related skin lesions elsewhere. Axillary and epitrochlear lymph nodes are sought. Inspection of the skin may give valuable clues as to the aetiology, e.g. neurofibromatosis or psoriatic arthritis. The size, consistency, mobility, and tenderness of the mass are determined. The surrounding area is examined for oedema, swelling, atrophy, or lymphangitis. It is crucial to make accurate observations and measurements because many masses will be observed over a period of time to assess their behaviour. Clinical evaluation often includes laboratory studies including blood count and differential, erythrocyte sedimentation rate, calcium, phosphorus, alkaline phosphatase, acid phosphatase, and possibly urine or serum for protein electrophoresis. These vary depending upon the differential diagnosis and whether the lesion is likely to be neoplastic, inflammatory, metabolic, or infectious in nature.

Almost all masses, whether bony or soft tissue in origin, should be evaluated with plain radiographs. These are the most valuable imaging study in the evaluation of bony lesions. In soft tissue lesions they provide information about calcification, foreign bodies, and any reaction of the bone to the tumour. Other studies include the computed tomography (CT) scan which is very valuable in determining bony involvement and tumour extent, and the magnetic resonance imaging (MRI) study which is the study of choice in evaluating soft tissue lesions. MRI shows tumour extent and soft tissue oedema, especially with the use of surface coils which markedly enhance resolution. If a malignant or metastatic lesion is considered, then a plain chest radiograph or chest CT and bone scan or skeletal survey are indicated. The evaluation of a vascular lesion or considerations regarding reconstruction following excision may warrant the use of arteriography.

In many cases, the definitive diagnosis can not be made without a tissue diagnosis. As a result, biopsy is often indicated. Because of the uncertain nature of the process, the patient and his/her family must be counselled regarding the possibility of a change in the treatment plan depending on the intraoperative findings. With benign tumours, excision and definitive treatment are often completed at the time of biopsy. In suspected malignant lesions, it is often necessary to perform an incisional biopsy to obtain sufficient tissue for diagnosis. This is then followed by the definitive procedure.

Bone tumours

The most common bone tumour of the hand is the enchondroma (Figure 15.31). It is more common in males, and usually presents during adolescence or early adulthood. Diagnosis is commonly made either following pathological fracture through the lesion or following plain films taken for an unrelated injury. Pain is unusual if a pathological fracture is not present, and may represent malignant degeneration. Seventy per cent of the lesions are found in the proximal and middle phalanges of the fingers. Another 20% are found in the metacarpals (Bogumill, 1990). Plain radiographs reveal a lytic lesion with calcification. The cortex is expanded and thin, which often leads to pathological fracture.

Solitary enchondromas rarely undergo malignant degeneration, and treatment is curettage and bone grafting. Pathological fractures are allowed to heal before excision. Multiple enchondromatosis is a non-hereditary disorder which has been given the name Ollier's disease (Figure 15.32). Multiple enchondromas with associated multiple haemangiomas is termed Maffucci's syndrome. Unlike those with a solitary enchondroma, these patients develop significant hand deformities, and malignant degeneration has been reported in up to 50% of patients. Any increase in size or development of pain warrants treatment in these patients.

Depending upon its size curettage alone can give a high healing rate – 82% with only a 2% recurrence rate. However, it is claimed that curettage with autogenous bone grafting usually obtained from the iliac crest and its complications has a shorter radiographic incorporation of the bone graft material

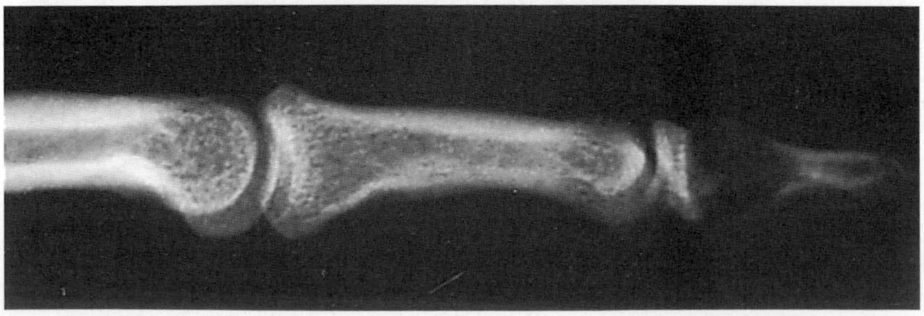

Figure 15.31 Radiograph of an enchondroma of the distal phalanx which presented as a pathological fracture.

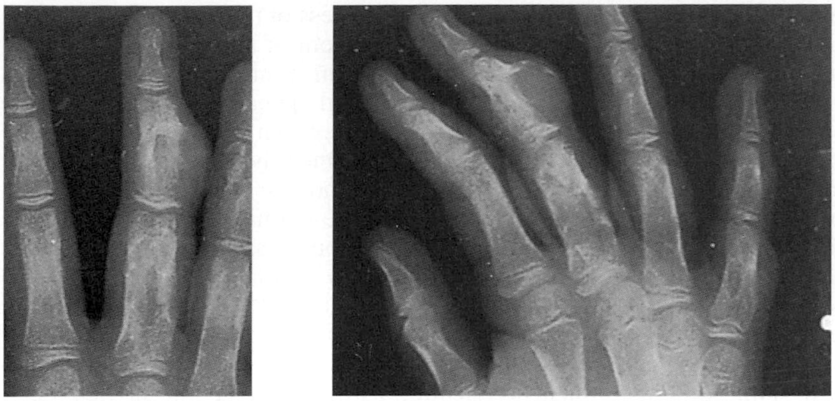

Figure 15.32 Radiographs of an 11-year-old girl with Ollier's disease, showing the cartilaginous tumours involving the shafts of the short miniature bones. There is an obvious soft tissue mass overlying the middle phalanx of the middle finger.

when compared with curettage and an allograft, i.e. 2–3 months shorter (Bauer *et al.*, 1988).

Osteochondromas of the hands are rarely solitary and are usually found in a patient with multiple hereditary exostoses. This condition is inherited in a dominant fashion, yet clinically affects males more than females. It generally presents as a bony lump discovered during the first or second decade. The lesions are found in the metaphyses of long bones, as well as in the vertebrae and pelvis. In the upper extremity, the distal radius and ulna account for approximately 80% of the lesions (Bogumill, 1990). These lesions may lead to bowing, angular deformity, or mechanical impingement.

Radiographically, these lesions appear as irregular bony protuberances from the metaphyseal region of the long bones. They may be either sessile or pedunculated in nature. The overlying cartilage cap may show areas of calcification. Because these lesions form a bony protuberance, they may interfere with function. Furthermore, overall growth of the affected bone may be altered by the presence of an osteochondroma, leading to deformity. Any of these problems are indications for excision which is curative.

Growth of these lesions should cease at skeletal maturity. Malignant degeneration of these lesions into chondrosarcomas is not uncommon in the hereditary disorder, and occurs in 10–25% of those affected. It is often heralded by pain or enlargement of a lesion after skeletal maturity and when it occurs in the upper extremity a biopsy should determine if sarcomatous change has occurred. Chondrosarcoma represents the most common malignant bone tumour of the hand and is best treated by amputation or *en bloc* excision.

Soft tissue tumours

The most common benign tumour and the second most common mass in the hand is the giant cell tumour of tendon sheath or fibroxanthoma. This is a slow growing benign tumour which is commonly found along the tendon sheath or joint synovium. It occurs most frequently along the palmar aspect of the digits, especially the index and long fingers and causes localized symptoms. Treatment is marginal excision. There is approximately a 10% recurrence rate.

Giant cell tumour is commonly found in the distal radius as are aneursymal bone cysts and chrondromyxoid fibroma. Investigations should include bone scintography for multicentric disease, and MR imaging for the intramedullary extent as well as any soft tissue involvement. Hackborth (1991) has described how resection of the distal end of the radius with involvement of the radiocarpal joint when indicated should be accompanied by either a non-vascular or vascular fibular graft to achieve an arthrodesis. He recommended, in addition, the use of a compression plate from the radial fragment, on to the graft and to the second metacarpal.

The glomus tumour is a benign, highly vascular tumour of the nail bed. Classically, it presents with a triad of symptoms which include pain, tenderness, and cold insensitivity. Physical examination reveals a dark or blue spot beneath the nail with secondary nail ridging. Radiographs may reveal a bony erosion in the dorsal aspect of the distal phalanx. The treatment of this lesion is excision which is curative.

Another fairly common benign soft tissue tumour of the hand is the lipoma. Lipomas are slow-growing painless hand masses which are non-tender and mobile. They are more common in women, often during middle age. Lipomas tend to develop in the subcutaneous tissue of palmar hand and forearm, especially in the thenar region. Malignant degeneration is very rare. Definitive treatment is excision, and recurrence is uncommon.

The most common malignant tumour of the hand is a squamous cell carcinoma which accounts for 70–90% of hand malignancies. Many patients have a history of long-term exposure to the sun, others exposure to radiation or arsenic. This lesion is most common in elderly males and is usually located on the dorsum of the hand. Usually, squamous cell carcinoma develops from a pre-existing hyperkeratotic lesion which shows signs of crusting, hyperaemia, ulceration, and growth. This tumour spreads through the lymphatic system and metastases are found in 5–15% of those with hand lesions. Treatment of local disease is through excision. The extent of the excision depends on the depth of the lesion. If the lesion is localized to the epidermis and dermis, then excision down to the subcutaneous tissue with a margin of 5–10 mm is usually sufficient. If the tumour is adherent to the deeper tissues, then a more extensive excision, including normal tissue deep to the lesion, must be performed. If the tumour extends down to bone, amputation should be considered. When localized to the skin, squamous cell carcinoma can be cured in approximately 90% of cases. With deeper involvement or metastatic spread, the prognosis is significantly worse.

Although it only represents 5% of all malignant hand tumours, malignant melanoma is the most aggressive skin cancer. It represents only 3% of all skin cancers yet is responsible for the majority of skin cancer mortality. Melanoma develops from the melanocytes of the epidermis; therefore it tends to be pigmented or arises from pre-existing pigmented lesions. Classically, these painless lesions develop in fair-skinned individuals. There are four types of melanoma: lentigo maligna melanoma, superficial spreading multiple melanoma, nodular malignant melanoma, and acral lentiginous melanoma. Acral lentiginous melanoma is the most frequent melanoma in the hands and presents on the palms and distal phalanges of the fingers. This darkly pigmented lesion can be subungual in location and may distort the nail. When localized to the epidermis it is a completely benign lesion. Later, as the depth increases, the prognosis worsens. Superficial spreading melanoma is the most common form and occurs in relatively young patients. In contrast, lentigo maligna melanoma occurs primarily in the elderly. Nodular malignant melanoma is the most aggressive form and tends to grow vertically instead of radially. As a result, the prognosis for this form of melanoma is the worst.

The therapy and prognosis of melanoma depend primarily on the thickness of the lesion and the depth of invasion. Management of a presumed melanoma should first include an excisional biopsy with a 5 mm margin of normal appearing tissue around the periphery, and taken down to the level of the subcutaneous tissue. Once the permanent histology has been reviewed and the depth of invasion is known, the appropriate definitive procedure can be carried out. For the subungual melanoma, treatment recommendations vary from PIP disarticulation to ray resection, depending on the level of invasion. Chemotherapy has only been used in palliation of metastatic disease. Clearly, the most effective treatment is education with early detection and treatment.

The most common hand mass (over 61% of all) is the ganglion cyst (Figure 15.33). It is most common in women in their third and fourth decades, and it is unclear whether there is an association with trauma. The majority occur dorsally over the scapholunate interval, and approximately 20% are found over the volar aspect of the wrist between the radial artery and the flexor carpi radialis tendon. The dorsal wrist ganglia are often painless masses but may be associated with pain. They are most commonly found between the EPL and EDC tendons. The mass does not move with finger flexion and extension. The volar wrist ganglia are commonly associated with basal joint arthritis or scaphotrapeziotrapezoid (STT) joint pathology. Although much less common, these cysts can also occur along the flexor tendon sheath, and are usually at the level of the proximal flexion crease. They are small and firm, producing symptoms with grip activities.

Microscopic findings show that the development of ganglia may be divided into three fairly definite stages. The first stage is characterized by a large number of spheroidal cells which are closely packed together and merged by insensible gradations into spindle cells of the periphery. The second stage may possess features of the first stage and present a central area which is beginning to take on the

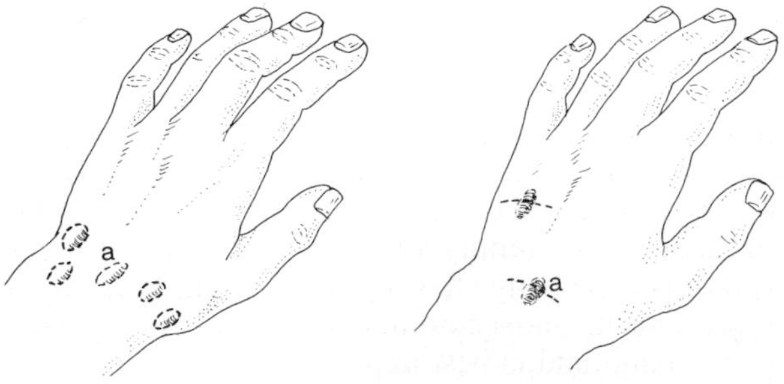

Figure 15.33 Ganglion cysts on the dorsum of the hand. (After Angelides, A.C. (1993) *Operative Hand Surgery*. Edited by D.P. Green. Churchill Livingstone: New York, pp. 2157–2172)

characteristics of a cavity filled partly with a secretion from those cells. Sometimes all of the spheroidal cells undergo the mucoid change at the same time, so that the mucoid material abuts on the spindle cell tissue. It is in the third stage that one finds the changes seen in the well developed ganglion. In this stage the wall is smooth and of variable thickness, and the lining membrane is similar to the synovial membrane of joints. The walls of the larger cysts are poorly supplied with blood vessels, and in many cases the vessels show a marked fibrosis of their wall and narrowing of their lumen. Indeed, it has been suggested that the vascular lesion is the real cause of the degeneration, the impoverished blood supply being supposed to induce a local impairment of nutrition.

Bundles of nerve fibres are frequently observed passing through the degenerated areas. These may account for the pain and tenderness which are so often associated with ganglion formation.

The most reliable form of treatment is excision. Rupture of a dorsal or volar wrist ganglion cyst is associated with recurrence rates of approximately 40%. Steroid injections have also been unsuccessful. Excision is performed under local or regional anaesthesia. The cyst is exposed, taking care to visualize and preserve the stalk which connects the cyst to the joint space or tendon sheath. Once exposed, the entire cyst, including the stalk and an area of surrounding capsule, is removed *en bloc*. Recurrence is uncommon (less than 10%) if the stalk and a portion of the capsule are removed. There is no need to close the capsule following excision. Complications of excision include recurrence, neuroma formation (radial sensory nerve or palmar sensory branch of the median nerve), or intercarpal instability if the intercarpal ligaments are excised with the capsule during cyst excision. Tendon sheath ganglia are also most reliably treated with excision, yet, unlike wrist ganglia, rupture may also be effective.

The mucous cyst is a common lesion which develops in patients with osteoarthritis involving the DIP joints of the fingers. For further discussion of the aetiology and treatment of this condition, please refer to the section on osteoarthritis.

The inclusion cyst results from the implantation of epithelial tissue beneath the skin due to trauma or surgery. The patient presents with a somewhat painful subcutaneous mass over the palmar aspect of the digit or hand. Excision is curative. Foreign body granulomas are firm fibrous lesions which develop in reaction to a foreign body. If symptomatic, they are best treated by excision.

OSTEOCHONDRITIS OF THE LUNATE

This rare condition was first described by Kienböck (1910) as an affection of the carpal lunate bone. Since that time a considerable volume of literature has accumulated, and many hypotheses have been advanced to explain its occurrence. It may affect many of the carpal bones in addition to the lunate – Buchman, for example, stated that it may also occur in the navicular, the trapezium and the hamate. So many of Buchman's cases gave a definite history of injury that he named it traumatic osteoporosis of the carpus. When it affects the lunate, however, the condition is usually called Kienböck's disease (also lunatomalacia), and, when the navicular is involved, Preiser's disease.

AETIOLOGY

There is usually a history of injury sustained while the hand is dorsiflexed, but the trauma may be a very insignificant one, and in some cases no history of injury can be obtained.

The condition usually begins with a primary total or partial, acute or chronic fracture which becomes pseudarthrotic and is accompanied by secondary changes in the spongiosa and the joint cartilage. Protracted use of the hand leads to further fragmentation. These characteristic secondary fractures are promoted by the perifractural osteolysis and osteosclerosis and develop into further pseudathroses. Complete recovery is possible with rest from the first but continued use leads to progressive atrophy of the semilunar bone.

Although the condition is usually compared with the various osteochondritides previously described, it differs very materially from them. It affects, for example, only fully formed tissue in which growth has been completed. It is, perhaps, more correct to compare it with Kümmell's disease of the spine, and with the absorption occasionally seen in certain fractures of the neck of the femur. These two conditions probably belong to the same group.

In 1928 Hulten described the increased incidence of ulnar negative variance as being increased by 1 mm in patients with Kienböch's disease. However, more recently Nakamura *et al.* (1991) have shown a positive correlation between ulnar variance and young age in normal wrists and therefore they point out the importance of careful selection of both age and sex matched controls in the limbs of Kienböch's patients in Japan.

CLINICAL COURSE

The course of the disease can be divided into three stages:

1. An acute stage, following injury, lasting some weeks.
2. A period without symptoms, sometimes lasting months.
3. A period of the actual disease, the symptoms of which may perhaps persist for years.

The trauma is not uncommonly a mild one, so the patient is often not disabled. It may be a simple strain, accompanied by swelling, pain and tenderness over the lunate, with limitation of the extremes of motion.

The painful period is followed by an interval of freedom from symptoms, which may last months or even years. The period of active disease then sets in. It is characterized by increasing disability, by swelling and tenderness over the lunate. In the early stages the pain is aching, present only on extreme exertion, and aggravated by excessive use of the wrist, but it gradually becomes more persistent, until, in the final stages, it is permanent and disabling.

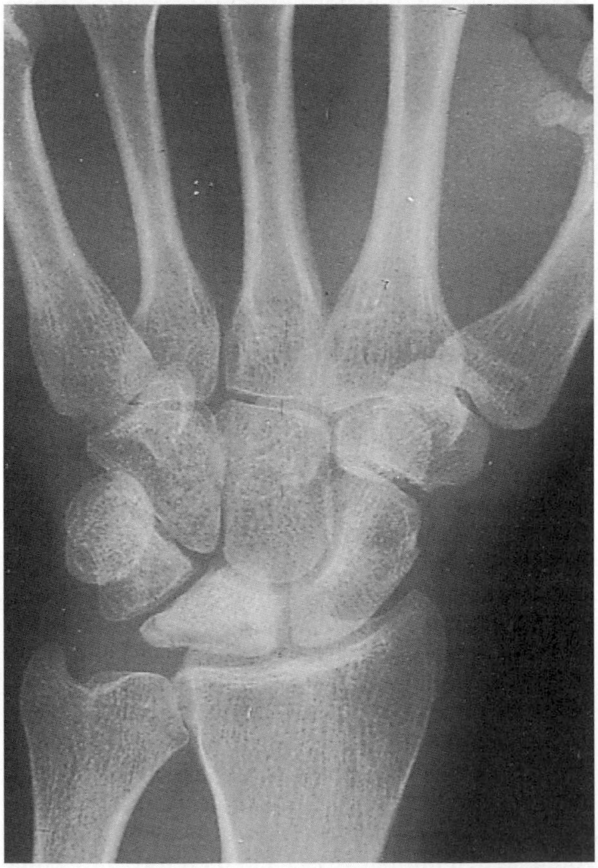

Figure 15.34 Radiograph of a young man's wrist, showing increased density of the lunate bone, which is abnormal in shape.

When the condition is well advanced, and destruction considerable, clenching of the hand fails to show the normal prominence of the head of the third metacarpal. This bone may even recede, because of shortening in the vertical axis of the affected lunate. This sign is known as Finsterer's sign and is said to be pathognomonic of Kienböck's disease. Percussion over the head of the third metacarpal also elicits tenderness, and pushing with the hand is painful. The depression normally situated just below the distal end of the radius is obliterated occasionally from the anteroposterior thickening of the lunate.

When the disease affects the navicular, the symptoms and signs are very similar. Pain is at first slight, and felt only on exertion, but it gradually becomes more and more severe and is finally present even when the hand is at rest. It may even become so excruciating that the patient is unable to sleep. Movement, especially dorsiflexion, is limited. There is usually slight swelling and tenderness over the navicular, and the anatomical snuff box may be obliterated.

RADIOLOGICAL APPEARANCES

In early cases there are no characteristic appearances, but later, areas of rarefaction and of increased density may be seen (Figure 15.34). The affected bone is denser than the others and is also wider in its anteroposterior axis, but thinned out in its short vertical axis. In the later stages, the proximal aspect may become fragmented, and areas may even disappear. Changes of an osteoarthritic character may also occur, so that the articular surface of the radius may show osteoporosis, and the points of insertion of the ligaments may become roughened.

The first radiological evidence of the condition may be one or more small circular or oval areas of absorption or rarefaction in the centre of the bone. These soon fuse into a large area of decreased density, and through this area the fracture occurs.

The histological findings in excised specimens vary with the extent and duration of the disease. but in general there is absorption of the bone lamellae with replacement by granulation tissue which goes on to form fibrous tissue instead of becoming calcified. This is a slow process and the deformity may be aggravated by fresh injuries.

In untreated cases the lunate bone continues to undergo collapse with movement of the adjacent scaphoid and the development of osteoarthritis with increasing signs of decreased mobility of the wrist, swelling, pain and local tenderness.

The ischaemia is thought to arise secondarily to a coronal stress fracture, caused by the compression forces applied through the capitate (Linscheid, 1992). Plain radiographs show the initial increased radiodensity or sclerosis, collapse and fragmentation. With CT scanning and MR imaging further information about the stage of the disease can be provided.

TREATMENT

Treatment before collapse with secondary osteoarthritic changes, i.e. early, is directed towards modifying the forces being applied to the lunate, i.e. intercarpal arthrodesis, arthrodesis of the scaphotrapeziotrapezoid (STT) joint or the scapulocapitate or capitohamate joints, or joint levelling procedures in which the length of the radius is equalized to the ulna – by lengthening the ulna or shortening the radius (Graham, 1933). Silicone implant arthroplasty is no longer indicated because of a destructive foreign body reaction to silicone fragments.

CARPAL INSTABILITY

Cooney *et al.* (1990), based upon an arthroscopic study, have defined carpal instability as 'the lack of ligamentous and skeletal support to maintain a stable wrist even under external forces of pinch and grasp'. This can be classified as static or dynamic and 'dissociative' in which ligaments are torn (carpal instability dissociative) or 'non-dissociative' in which the ligaments are intact but stretched (carpal instability non-dissociative).

The Darrach procedure is commonly performed for distal ulnar derangement. Nolan and Eaton (1992) have emphasized that only a minimal excision of the distal ulnar, about 6–8 mm, is required, leaving the interosseous membrane intact through an oblique cut. The dissection should be subperiosteal, leaving all ligaments in continuity. The more usual Darrach procedure with greater excision of bone and therefore greater disruption of ligaments and stability has not been too successful for rheumatoid or post-traumatic impingment syndromes.

Chronic disability, giving rise to wrist pain, is now more commonly being diagnosed accurately by wrist arthroscopy as carpal instability. Conyers (1990) has reported from a series of patients with scapholunate interosseous ligament disruption producing instability. These were treated by carpal reduction, stabilization and palmar ligament reconstruction with initial good results.

Viegas *et al.* (1990) have analysed the biomechanical efficiency of limited intercarpal fusions for treatment of scapholunate dissociation. With the decrease in lunate loading there was an increased scaphoid load. With scaphoid–trapezium–trapezoid fusion there was even greater decrease loading of the lunate fossa and increase in the scaphoid load. Obviously, shifting the load will result in new pathologies of degeneration with disability over time.

INFECTIONS OF THE HAND

Infections are relatively uncommon because of the excellent blood supply of the hand. When infections do occur, they generally result from bacterial inoculation or contamination through a cut or puncture wound. The risk of infection following an inoculum of bacteria into a wound can be increased with trauma, necrosis, or foreign material in the wound.

The principal pathogens in hand infections are the *Staphylococcus* and *Streptococcus* species. *Staphylococus aureus* has been shown in numerous studies to cause 50–80% of hand infections (Sneddon, 1969; Stone *et al.*, 1969; Eaton and Butsch, 1970). Gram-negative organisms are felt to cause less than 20% of hand infections (Linscheid and Dobyns, 1990). However, numerous organisms may be responsible for a given infection, and some infections are caused by multiple organisms.

The cornerstone to the treatment of any contaminated wound is copious irrigation and debridement of necrotic or grossly infected tissue followed by drainage. Similarly, any abscess or purulent collection must be drained. Antibiotics alone will not suffice.

Paronychia

The most common infection of the hand, the paronychia, develops beneath the eponychium of the digit. The patient presents with local pain and erythema with or without purulent discharge. When diagnosed early, oral antibiotics and soaks will usually be successful in clearing the cellulitic infection. If an abscess has collected, then formal drainage must be performed. The extent of the drainage procedure depends on the severity and time frame of the infection. Adequate drainage may be obtained early by lifting the eponychium off the nail. More commonly, an incision which parallels the eponychial fold is necessary for adequate drainage. This, along with antibiotics, is usually curative. In long-standing infections, the abscess may spread beneath the nail plate and a portion of the nail plate must be removed to allow adequate drainage.

Felon

A felon is a pulp space infection generally caused by a puncture wound which presents with severe pain, erythema, and swelling of the involved finger pulp (Figure 15.35). There may be skin necrosis or a sinus tract. The septated fascia of the pulp allows pressure to build with resulting loss of blood supply and necrosis. If chronic there may be associated osteomyelitis. Treatment includes drainage of the abscess through a longitudinal incision. It is then irrigated copiously, necrotic tissue is removed, and the wound is packed open to allow further drainage. Empirical intravenous antibiotics are started using a semisynthetic penicillin or cephalosporin. Antibiotics are later adjusted according to the specific organism responsible, based on culture results.

Fascial space infections

Fascial space infections include web space infections, midpalmar infections, thenar space infections, and less commonly hypothenar infections (Figure 15.36). All of these infections require adequate surgical irrigation and debridement followed by intravenous antibiotics.

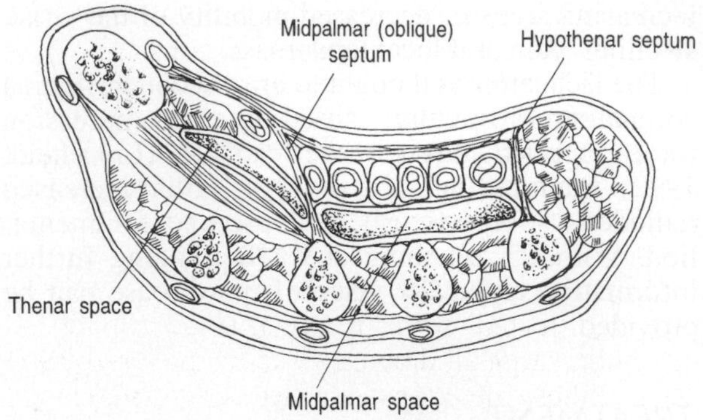

Figure 15.36 The potential fascial spaces in the hand. (After Neviaser, R.J. (1993) *Operative Hand Surgery*. Edited by D.P. Green. Churchill Livingstone: New York, pp. 1021–1038)

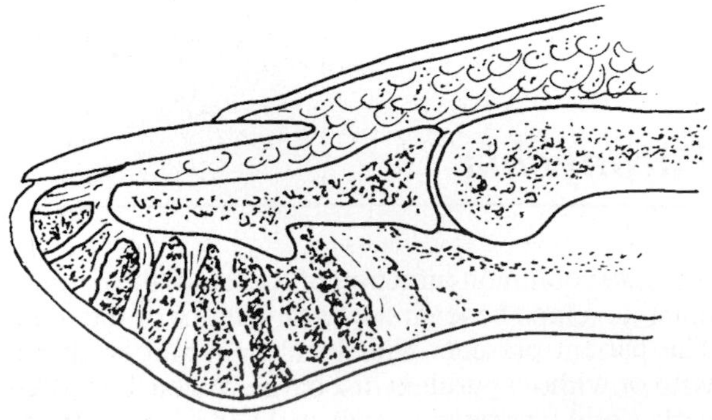

Figure 15.35 Diagram of a felon. (After Kilgore, E.S. Jr, *et al.* (1975) *American Journal of Surgery* **130**, 194)

The web space is defined by the dorsal skin, the vertical septae of fascia, and the transverse portions of the palmar fascia. A web space infection presents as a localized pain and swelling in the distal palm which points dorsally into one of the webs. As the abscess collects, the dorsum of the web swells markedly and the fingers are held apart by the collection. It has also been termed the collar-stud abscess. The transverse metacarpal ligament usually prevents proximal extension. The midpalmar space is defined radially by the vertical septum at the third metacarpal and ulnarly by the hypothenar fascia. The infection occurs through direct inoculation of the area or spread from a tendon sheath. The dorsum of the hand becomes markedly swollen, and there is pain with motion of the long, ring, or small fingers. Similarly, the thenar space includes the thenar area to the third metacarpal. Infection may be from direct inoculation or spread from the tendon sheaths of the thumb or index finger. Swelling is most notable in the thenar region with involvement of the first web space and dorsum of the hand. Pain is exacerbated by motion of the thumb or index finger. An isolated infection of the hypothenar space may also occur.

Infectious flexor tenosynovitis

Suppurative flexor tenosynovitis is an infection of the flexor tendon sheath which usually develops following direct inoculation. Classically, it presents with Kanavel's four cardinal signs which are a digit held in flexion, symmetric fusiform swelling throughout the digit, pain with passive extension, and tenderness along the flexor tendon sheath (Kanavel,

1925, 1935). The flexor tendon sheaths end at the distal palmar crease in the index, long, and ring fingers. The infection may spread into the thenar and midpalmar spaces from these tendon sheaths. The flexor tendon sheaths of the thumb and small fingers are continuous with the radial and ulnar bursae respectively. These bursae may communicate which leads to the so-called horseshoe abscess.

If caught very early, the tendon sheath infection may be treated with intravenous antibiotics. If in doubt surgical drainage should be performed because these infections, if inadequately treated, will lead to adhesions, stiffness, and marked disability in the affected digit. Further, non-surgical treatment may lead to suppression of the infection with the later development of a chronic infection and significant disability.

The tendon sheath is approached through a zigzag or midaxial incision. The tendon sheath is opened proximally and distally to allow adequate irrigation and drainage. Care is taken to preserve the A2 and A4 pulleys. A drainage or irrigation catheter may be left in for 48 hours postoperatively to assist in drainage. The patient is treated with intravenous antibiotics which are tailored according to the culture results. Motion and supervised hand therapy is begun early to prevent or limit permanent disability.

Lymphangitis

Lymphangitis, usually caused by streptococci, is an infection which spreads through the lymphatic system. Erythematous streaks develop along the lymphatic drainage system, and epitrochlear and axillary lymphadenopathy may be evident. Because there is rarely an abscess or fluid collection to drain, management involves aspiration of bullae for culture, intravenous antibiotics with good streptococci coverage, and local measures including immobilization, elevation, and warm compresses.

Necrotizing fasciitis

Necrotizing fasciitis is a severe and rapidly progressive anaerobic streptococcal infection. The involved area becomes erythematous, oedematous and painful with bullous formation and ultimate gangrene. The patient is systemically ill with overwhelming sepsis. Antibiotic treatment must be rapid and definitive based on Gram-stain results. Control of the local infection requires extensive surgical debridement and possible amputation. At the same time, the patient must receive systemic support and broad spectrum antibiotics consisting of a semi-synthetic penicillin and a broad spectrum cephalosporin.

Human bites

Human bites are common and may lead to severe infections. They most commonly occur during a fight when the fist strikes another person's teeth, leading to direct inoculation of the metacarpal head and/or MCP joint. Medical attention is often delayed. Typically, the patient presents 1–2 days after the injury with swelling, erythema, and sometimes drainage from a wound over the dorsum of the metacarpal. Late infections may present with joint destruction and osteomyelitis evident on radiographs.

The mouth contains numerous bacteria, including many anaerobic and Gram-negative species. As a result, these patients may develop a mixed infection with multiple organisms. Any patient with a wound about the MCP joint in the hand must be questioned about the possibility of a human bite. When seen acutely, these injuries may appear innocuous, but adequate evaluation, treatment, and follow-up must be ensured.

Following adequate anaesthesia, the wound is carefully extended to allow clear visualization of the injury. The wound is then copiously irrigated and the wound edges should be debrided. Adequate cultures must be obtained from the depths of the wound. The extensor mechanism must be inspected with the hand in the fist position because the extensor tendon will retract proximally as the fingers are extended. If the capsule has been violated, it is opened and the joint inspected and irrigated. Following appropriate irrigation and debridement, the wound should be left open and the hand should be immobilized in a bulky dressing in the intrinsic plus position.

Although *Staphylococcus aureus* is the most common organism in human bite infections, *Eikenella corrodens* should also be covered with penicillin, ampicillin, or penicillin with clavulanic acid. Broad spectrum antibiotics are started initially and then are modified based upon the culture results and clinical response. Active motion is encouraged at 24–48 hours, and the wounds are allowed to heal by secondary intention. Mennen and Howells (1991) from a large conservative series of 100 patients have described their antibiotic regimen of cloxacillin (intravenously 1 g every 6 hours). gentamicin (800 mg every 8 hours intramuscularly) and metronidazole (40 mg every 8 hours orally). Complications included 51% cellulitis, 50% septic arthritis and 22%

with osteomyelitis. Eighty-two per cent healed completely and 18% required amputation.

Animal bites

Animal bites can also lead to significant infections, and the treatment is essentially as outlined with human bites. Cultures from a high percentage of dog and cat bites reveal *Pasteurella multocida*, which is sensitive to penicillin. As a result, it is prudent to treat these patients with penicillin, ampicillin, or penicillin and clavulanic acid. As with human bites, appropriate exploration, irrigation, and debridement is crucial for successful treatment of these infections.

Viral infections

Herpetic whitlow is a viral infection seen most commonly in medical and dental personnel. It presents with pain, swelling, and a vesicular rash which may be in the pulp region of the finger or around the nail. It must be differentiated from a felon or paronychia. Unlike bacterial infections, irrigation and debridement are contraindicated in this condition and may cause the condition to spread. Treatment is supportive with splinting and elevation. Acyclovir may limit the course. The lesions will resolve in 10–14 days.

Mycobacterial infections

Musculoskeletal infections caused by tuberculosis and atypical mycobacterial infections are being recognized more frequently (Kelley *et al.*, 1967). The atypical mycobacterial infections seen clinically include *Mycobacterium kansasii, Mycobacterium avium*, and *Mycobacterium marinum. Mycobactedum kansasii* and *Mycobacterium avium* infections are most common in farmers, whereas *Mycobacterium marinum* infections occur in those working with water or fish (fishermen, pool workers, landscapers, and those with aquariums). These infections are generally indolent in nature and often involve either the tenosynovium or the wrist joint, causing chronic swelling; they may mimic rheumatoid arthritis.

Mycobacterial tenosynovitis often involves either the extensor or flexor compartments at the wrist. The condition may also present as carpal tunnel syndrome secondary to median nerve compression by the granulomatous tissue. Pathological specimens reveal granulomas, and cultures reveal the causative organism. Treatment is a combination of tenosynovectomy and systemic chemotherapy with rifampicin, isoniazid and/or ethambutol.

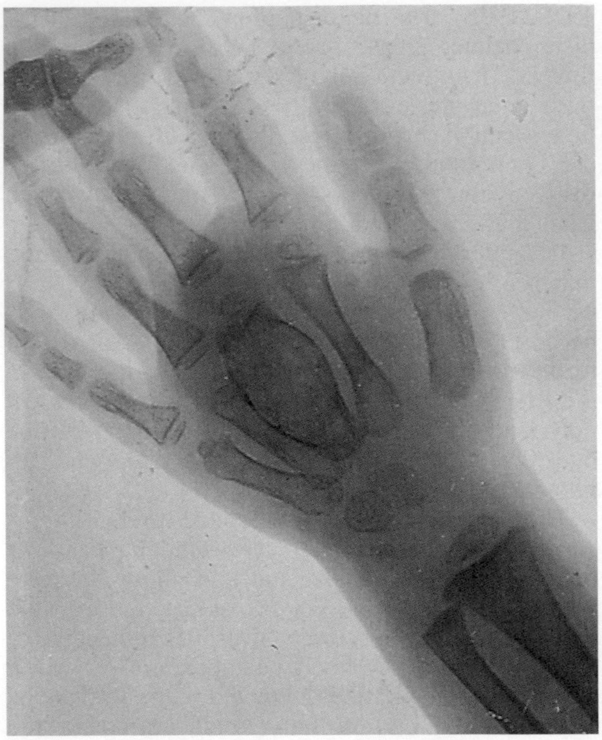

Figure 15.37 Tuberculous dactylitis of the third metacarpal.

Mycobacterial arthritis of the upper extremity often involves the carpus, with or without involvement of the overlying extensor compartments. Again, an indolent course with delayed diagnosis is characteristic. Radiographically, minimal changes are seen early. Late changes include erosions and generalized osteopenia due to carpal destruction. Treatment includes irrigation and debridement, aggressive synovectomy, and systemic chemotherapy as outlined above.

In children, tuberculous infection of the metacarpals or phalanges can lead to tuberculous dactylitis with cortical expansion (Figure 15.37) and bony dissolution. Treatment is usually curettage for culture material followed by chemotherapy and splinting.

PRINCIPLES OF TENDON TRANSFERS

General principles

Tendon transfers are used in hand surgery to replace deficient motor units and to restore function. Functional loss may occur secondary to tendon rupture, peripheral nerve injury, brachial plexopathy, stroke, or other problems. Tendon ruptures secondary to inflammatory arthritis have been discussed in an earlier section. This section will focus on tendon transfers used in restoring hand and wrist function or balancing deformity.

The functional tendon to be transferred is transected then transferred to another tendon or bone to restore function. The neurovascular supply of the donor unit is preserved, in contrast to a free tendon graft which functions primarily as a spacer or connection.

In order for a tendon transfer to function optimally, the soft tissue bed must be sufficient, the skeletal support must be stable, and the joints must be mobile. The transferred motor unit must have sufficient strength and excursion to restore function, and it must be expendable.

The strength of a muscle is proportional to its cross-sectional area and must be considered when choosing a donor. The transferred muscle loses about one grade of strength following transfer (grade 5 is normal, grade 4 is motion against resistance, grade 3 is motion against gravity, grade 2 is motion with gravity eliminated, grade 1 is trace motion or fasiculations, grade 0 is flaccid). Therefore, if a muscle was grade 5 (normal) it will be grade 4 (motion against resistance yet deficient strength) after transfer. Similarly, if the donor muscle is grade 3 (motion against gravity) before transfer, then it will be grade 2 (motion only with gravity eliminated) and non-functional after transfer. Ideally, transferred muscles should be of normal strength.

Excursion must also be considered when choosing a donor. Wrist flexors and extensors have approximately 3 cm of active excursion, finger extensors have 5 cm and the finger flexors have 7 cm of excursion. As a result, a wrist motor is not likely to function well as a finger flexor unless there is active wrist extension to help potentiate finger flexion.

Tendon transfers should pass in a straight line if possible to maximize strength. If a pulley is necessary it should be stable. Each transferred tendon should have only one function. Any joint that is crossed by the tendon transfer must be stable and have active control to avoid a collapse deformity. When evaluating a patient for tendon transfers, it is important to determine the functional needs of the patient, and the available motor units for transfer. In peripheral nerve injury, reinnervation occurs at a rate of 1 mm/day after an initial delay of approximately 1 month. As a result, 3 cm of nerve regeneration takes approximately 2 months. Although some advocate early tendon transfers to act as internal splints while awaiting the return of function, more commonly the tendon transfers are performed after the permanent motor deficit becomes clear based on clinical evaluation as well as nerve conduction studies and electromyography.

Radial nerve palsy

The radial nerve innervates the dorsal muscles of the forearm and hand. The deficit present in a radial nerve palsy includes the loss of wrist extension, finger extension, and thumb extension/abduction. The goals of tendon transfers are to restore these three functions (Figure 15.38). Wrist extension is generally restored using the pronator teres (PT) which is transferred to either the ECRL (Riordan, 1964), the ECRB (Beasley, 1970; Goldner, 1974; Brand, 1975) or both (Jones, 1921; Boyes, 1970). Thumb extension and abduction is usually restored using either palmaris longus (PL) to extensor pollicis longus (EPL) (Riordan, 1964; Brand, 1975) or flexor digitorum superficialis (FDS) of long or ring to EPL (Beasley, 1970; Boyes, 1970; Goldner, 1974). Finger extension has been restored using multiple tendons including flexor carpi ulnaris (FCU) (Jones, 1921; Riordan, 1964; Goldner, 1974); flexor carpi radialis (FCR) (Brand, 1975), and FDS (Beasley, 1970; Boyes, 1970) Each of these donors is transferred into the extensor digitorum communis (EDC) to restore finger extension. The Boyes transfer (1970) uses FDS ring to EPL and EIP, and FDS long to EDC, providing independent extension of the index finger. Transfers for posterior interosseous nerve palsy are identical to those described above except for the wrist extensors which are functional.

Median nerve palsy

The low median nerve palsy results in the denervation of the thenar musculature and the radial two lumbricals. No functional deficit is notable from

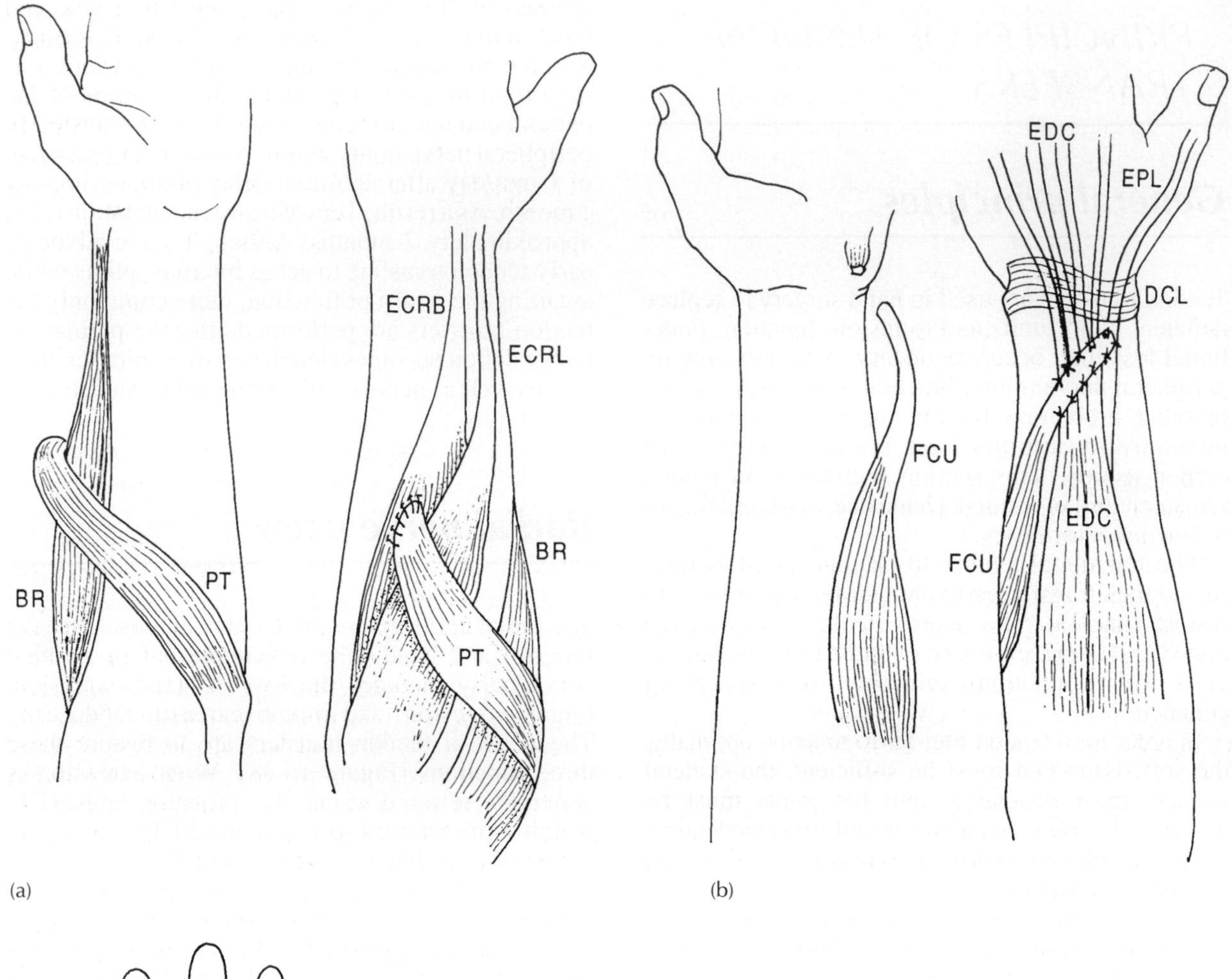

(a)

(b)

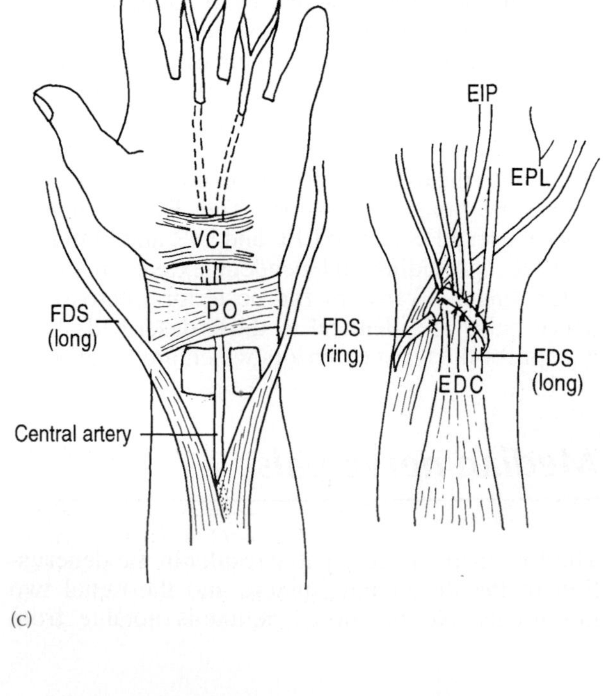

(c)

Figure 15.38 Tendon transfers for radial nerve palsy. Also see text. (a) Pronator teres (PT) to extensor carpi radialis brevis (ECRB). (b) Flexor carpi ulnaris (FCU) to EDC and EPL. (c) FDS of long and ring through interosseous membrane to EIP/EPL and EDC, respectively. (After Omer, G.E. (1980) *Management of Peripheral Nerve Problems*. Edited by G.E. Omer and M. Spinner. W.B. Saunders: Philadelphia) isolated lumbrical denervation. Thenar denervation leads to a deficiency in opposition and abduction of the thumb in approximately two-thirds of those with this injury (one-third of the patients will have adequate thumb opposition due to ulnar innervation). Tendon transfer to restore thumb opposition and abduction is called opponensplasty.

The classic Bunnell opponensplasty consists of the transfer of the FDS ring tendon through a pulley made from the distal FCU into the dorsal–ulnar base of the thumb proximal phalanx (Bunnell, 1938). Littler (1949) modified this transfer by inserting the FDS into the abductor pollicis brevis (APB). Riordan (1959) later modified the insertion site to include both the APB and the EPL. Another donor tendon is the extensor indicis proprius (EIP) which can be transferred around the ulnar border of the wrist and into the proximal phalanx or APB as described by Zancolli and Burkhalter (Figure 15.39). The abductor digiti quinti (ADQ) can also be effectively transferred to the APB without the need for a pulley or interpositional graft (Littler and Cooley, 1963). All of these transfers, with the exception of the intrinsic ADQ transfer, require a pulley, such as the FCU, carpal canal, Guyon's canal, palmaris longus, and the ulnar side of the wrist.

The high median nerve palsy leads to a loss of thumb opposition as well as FPL, FDS, FDP to index, pronator teres, and flexor carpi radialis. The deficits resulting from loss of FCR and pronator teres are small and do not warrant tendon transfers. Opposition is restored as described above. The additional deficits which must be addressed are the restoration of thumb interphalangeal (IP) flexion and index DIP flexion. Thumb IP flexion is usually restored by transferring the brachioradialis (BR) to the FPL (Burkhalter, 1974; Goldner, 1974); ECRL or ECRB have also been used (Boyes, 1970; Brand, 1975). The functioning FDP tendons (small, ring, and possibly long) can be transferred in a side-to-side fashion to the non-functioning FDP tendons (index and possibly long) as described by Brand in 1975. The ECRL can also be transferred to restore index and long DIP flexion (Burkhalter, 1974; Goldner, 1974).

Carpal tunnel syndrome

The incidence in the general population is about 1%. De Kom *et al.* (1992) from a random sample of the Dutch population found 5.8% in women and 0.6% in men with previously undiagnosed carpal syndrome. There was an increased incidence in factory workers and pregnant women. Although usually idiopathic, it can be seen rarely in association with rheumatoid tenosynovitis and in renal dialysis patients. Kerr *et al.* (1992) carried out biopsy of the tendon synovium and found an inflammatory synovitis, chronic in 4% and acute in 0.2% changes, but tensoynovectomy is rarely indicated. See also Chapter 12.

Phalen's test of acute flexion was only positive in 88% and Tinel's sign in 67%. The pressure provocative test of pressure as described by Durkan by pressure of both thumbs for 9 seconds was the most

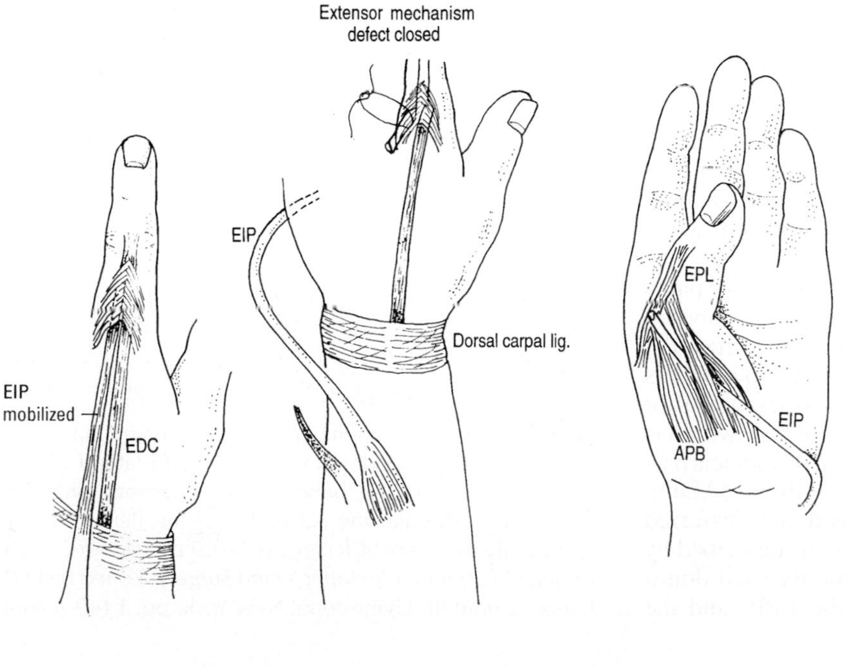

Figure 15.39 Opponensplasty in median nerve palsy using EIP transfer to insertion of APB. (After Omer, G.E. (1980) *Management of Peripheral Nerve Problems.* Edited by G.E. Omer and M. Spinner. W.B. Saunders: Philadelphia)

useful sign (Williams *et al.*, 1992). Serious complications of endoscopic carpal tunnel release have been reported, even in the hands of experienced endoscopic surgeons. These include laceration of the median and ulnar nerves, ulnar artery, and palmar vascular arch. Because of these infrequent but devastating complications endoscopic carpal tunnel release remains a controversial procedure.

Endoscopic release of the flexor retinaculum has been compared with open division, through a single portal and showed less scar tenderness and an earlier return to work (Agee *et al.*, 1992) for non-workers' compensation board patients. Interestingly there was no difference in return to work by either method in those patients receiving workman's compensation. Using two portals for entry is technically easier and has no added complications. Incomplete division can occur by this method in up to 15% of hands and surgical failure can be seen in 7–20% of patients.

Neurolysis is not indicated. Palmar cutaneous neuroma, painful scar, keloid formation, decreased grip strength have all been described. Recurrent carpal tunnel syndrome, especially in those carrying out repetitive work, all require open surgery and inspection with MR scanning if possible to show an incompletely divided transverse ligament.

Ulnar nerve palsy

Low ulnar nerve palsy from lesions of the peripheral nerve or roots at neck, elbow or wrist results in loss of most of the intrinsic muscles of the hand, i.e. loss of abduction and adduction of the digits as well as significant deformity. With loss of the ulnar-innervated thumb intrinsics, Froment's sign develops which consists of hyperflexion of the thumb IP joint with forceful pinch. The thumb MCP joint may also hyperextend with forceful pinch. Clawing develops in the ring and small fingers due to loss of lumbrical-powered MCP flexion and IP extension.

The goals in the treatment of low ulnar nerve palsy are to restore thumb adduction, restore index abduction (first dorsal interosseous), and to correct the claw deformity. Restoration of thumb adduction has been accomplished by Boyes, using either the BR or ECRL tendon with a graft as the donor unit which is threaded between the third and fourth metacarpals and inserted into the adductor pollicis (ADD). Another transfer uses an FDS tendon transferred across the palm and into the adductor as described by Zancolli in 1968. Other less commonly used donor tendons include the index EDC, the EPB, and the EDQ. Restoration of index abduction has been described using EIP, EPB, APL, EDQ, FDS, or ECRL with a graft to insert into the first dorsal interosseous tendon.

There are two approaches in tendon transfers for the correction of the claw deformity. The first is to transfer the donor tendon into the lateral bands which restores active MCP flexion and IP extension. Bunnell (1942) described the use of the FDS, EIP, or EDQ tendons to correct clawing. The donor tendon is split and inserted into the radial lateral bands of the affected digits. By splitting the donor tendon, a single donor can be used to treat multiple affected digits. The ECRL, ECRB, FCR and BR tendons have also been used as donors but require the use of a tendon graft for adequate length. The second approach involves inserting the tendon into the proximal phalanx (Burkhalter *et al.*, 1973) or looping it around the annular pulley (Zancolli, 1974) to restore active MCP flexion (Figure 15.40).

High ulnar nerve palsy, in addition to intrinsic muscle atrophy (Figure 15.41), also includes the loss

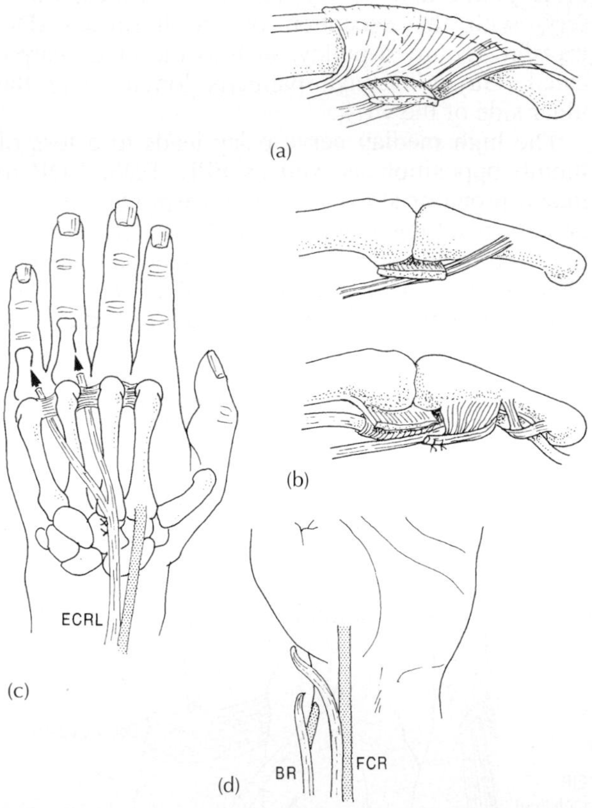

Figure 15.40 Correction of claw deformity in ulnar nerve palsy using ECRL tendon. (a) Insertion into lateral bands. (b) Insertion into the bone of the proximal phalanx. (c) Insertion through the A2 pulley of the flexor sheath. (d) Brachioradialis or FCR can also be used as donors. (After Omer, G.E. (1993) *Operative Hand Surgery*. Edited by D.P. Green. Churchill Livingstone: New York, pp. 1449–1466)

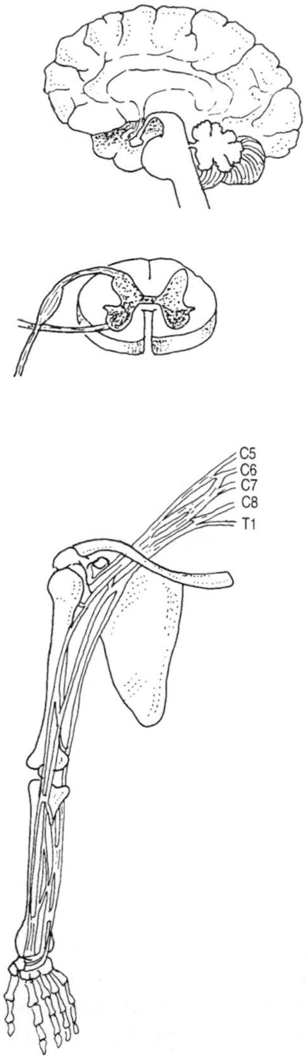

Figure 15.41 Lesions which can produce atrophy of the intrinsic muscles of the hand.

of FCU function and FDP function to the ring, small, and possibly the long fingers. Loss of FCU does not lead to a significant functional impairment. As a result, the goals of tendon transfer are the same as those for low ulnar nerve palsy, except that DIP flexion of the ring, small, and possibly long fingers must be restored. This is generally accomplished by performing a side-to-side transfer from the functioning FDP tendons.

Combined median and ulnar nerve palsy leads to marked sensory loss and motor deficiencies which include the loss of thumb opposition, thumb flexion, finger flexion, and clawing (Figure 15.42). The transfers which have been described for this condition follow the same principles; yet the number of possible donors is limited. Finger flexion is restored using ECRL to FDP (Littler, 1949; Riordan, 1964; Goldner, 1974; Brand, 1975). Thumb flexion is restored by transferring ECU (Riordan, 1964; Brand, 1975) or BR (Goldner, 1974) to the FPL. Thumb IP stability is achieved through IP fusion. Goldner (1974) then restored thumb opposition using ECU with a tendon graft to the thumb proximal phalanx. Index abduction is achieved by transferring the EIP to the first dorsal interosseous. Clawing is prevented by MCP volar capsulodeses.

Goldner (1953) described what is called 'the intrinsic negative or minus hand'. This results from a median and ulnar nerve lesion at the wrist with involvement of the interossei, lumbricals, thenar and hypothenar muscles. The thumb is in the characteristic position of external rotation, adduction and loss of opposition. The fingers are hyperextended at the metacarpophalangeal joint, but flexed at the distal and proximal interphalangeal joints. Because of contractures of soft tissues, particularly the collateral ligaments in this position, the dorsal interossei become extensors in function with aggravation of the extension at the metacarpophalangeal joints. Brand described the use of the extensor muscle as the motor with plantaris as grafts and carried as four separate strands anterior to the transverse ligaments, to be inserted into the extensor expansion over the proximal phalanx. This will give a mass action of flexion at the metacarpophalangeal joints, and is particularly indicated in a pure median nerve palsy lesion such as is seen in leprosy. However, Goldner emphasized that if there has been hyperextension of long duration in the metacarpophalangeal joints, in conjunction with absent intrinsic muscles, often a joint fusion is the more functional manoeuvre to carry out (Figure 15.43).

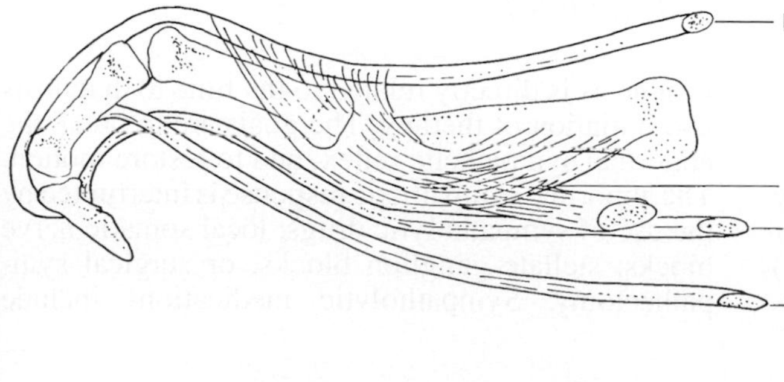

Figure 15.42 Typical claw deformity of the right ring finger with extension of metacarpophalangeal joint and flexion of the proximal interphalangeal joint, in the presence of soft tissue contractures anteriorly.

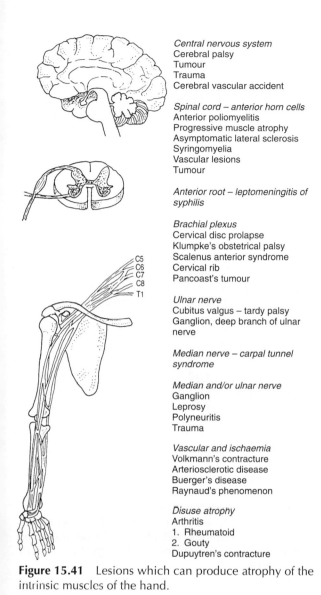

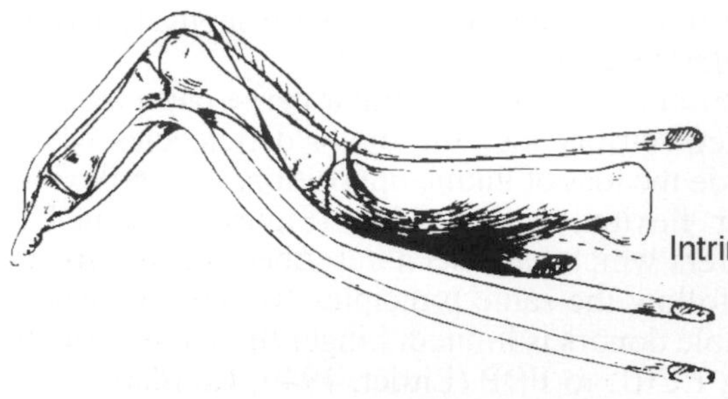

Figure 15.43 Intrinsic-minus deformity with hyperextension at the metacarpophalangeal joint, but flexion at the proximal interphalangeal joint and extension of the distal interphalangeal joint.

REFLEX SYMPATHETIC DYSTROPHY

Reflex sympathetic dystrophy (RSD) is a group of disorders in which there is a dysfunction in the normal injury and repair process leading to an exaggerated response to a noxious stimulus. It is characterized by pain, hyperaesthesia, swelling, stiffness, discoloration, and trophic changes which are out of proportion to the inciting event. Although these are characteristic findings in the injured extremity, the severity and time course are not. It is thought to result from an abnormality of the sympathetic nervous system as noted by Leriche (1939) and Spurling (1930). A high index of suspicion must be maintained because the prognosis for recovery relates directly to the speed of diagnosis and the initiation of therapy. See also Chapter 2.

The most characteristic symptom associated with this disorder is pain out of proportion to the inciting event in both severity and duration. It is often burning in character, hence the term 'causalgia' which means 'burning pain'. The pain may be intermittent at first but generally becomes constant over time. It is markedly increased with both active and passive motion. Hyperaesthesia to light touch is also common, and patients often withdraw when one attempts to examine the affected extremity.

Swelling is the most consistent physical finding with this condition. It often begins in the area of injury but spreads to involve a much broader area. Although soft initially, as the process continues, the oedema gradually becomes firm. Stiffness, another consistent finding, initially results from the oedema but later reflects soft tissue fibrosis.

Discoloration is considered another classic sign of RSD and three patterns are generally recognized. The red or erythematous phase is usually seen early in the course of this condition. Later, vasomotor instability leads to cyanosis from venous (outflow) constriction and pallor from arterial (inflow) constriction. All patterns may be seen simultaneously in a single extremity. Vasomotor instability may also lead to decreased capillary refill, cold intolerance, and temperature changes within the affected extremity. Increased sweating (hyperhidrosis) is also a common early finding; later, decreased sweating is seen.

The most common radiographic finding in patients with RSD is localized osteopenia of the affected extremity. It is felt to result from increased blood flow to the bone and may be noted as early as 3 weeks after the initial injury. Because osteopenia is not visible radiographically until 30–40% of bone mineral density is lost, this represents a fairly dramatic change. Atkins *et al.* (1993) have described by quantitative bone scintography the early changes of RSD after Colles' fracture, in particular the response of both cortical and trabeculae bone throughout the hand and wrist.

Trophic skin changes are characteristically seen late. The skin is shiny and thin with a loss of the normal skin wrinkles and creases. In addition, the subcutaneous tissue atrophies, leading to a loss of fingertip pulp.

The diagnosis of RSD is made when a patient experiences the four major signs and symptoms which are pain, swelling, stiffness, and discoloration out of proportion to the inciting event. Secondary signs include pseudomotor changes, temperature changes, demineralization, trophic changes, and vasomotor instability. The diagnosis is certain only after improvement is seen following a sympathetic block.

TREATMENT

Prognosis is directly related to the time to diagnosis and initiation of therapy. The goals are to break the abnormal sympathetic reflex, and to restore motion. The abnormal sympathetic response is interrupted by the use of sympatholytic drugs, local somatic nerve blocks, stellate ganglion blocks, or surgical sympathectomy. Sympatholytic medications include

α-adrenergic blocking agents such as phenoxybenzamine and prazosin hydrochloride. These medications decrease sympathetic tone; possible side-effects include dizziness, lightheadedness, and orthostatic hypotension. These agents are used in mild forms of RSD or in conjunction with other methods of sympathetic blockade.

Somatic nerve blocks (e.g. axillary block) affect motor, sensory, and sympathetic nerve fibres which may be helpful with mobilization of the affected extremity. Stellate ganglion nerve blocks selectively block the sympathetic chain without interfering with motor or sensory function. Surgical sympathectomy may be considered if a patient has a good initial response to stellate ganglion blocks but has a recurrence of symptoms despite several blocks. Adjunctive modalities which may be helpful are strict elevation to reduce swelling, transcutaneous electrical nerve stimulation (TENS), and carpal tunnel release if this appears to be the source of persistent pain. Acute carpal tunnel syndrome usually following wrist injury is the most common source of persistent pain in those developing major traumatic RSD (Lankford, 1990).

Physical therapy is of crucial importance. Active and passive range of motion should be performed to the level of discomfort but not pain. Massage, strict elevation, and a compressive glove all help control swelling. Intermittent splinting may be necessary to prevent or treat contractures and stiffness.

Koman *et al.* (1993) have emphasized that if left untreated, the dystrophic process persists with:

1. Irreversible damage to peripheral end structures, e.g. arteriovenous shunt mechanisms, development of arthrofibrosis.
2. Functional alterations in the neuropathy with alteration to the regulatory blood flow systems.
3. Central cortical pattern changes of pain syndromes.

DUPUYTREN'S CONTRACTURE

Dupuytren's contracture is seen most commonly in those over 40 years of age. It is more common in males, and in those of northern European descent. In patients of northern European descent, there is a familial tendency (Ling, 1963), though this is not the case in other groups who develop this condition. Risk factors include heavy alcohol intake, chronic liver disease, smoking, diabetes mellitis, and history of Epanutin therapy for epileptic seizures. Repetitive trauma has also been implicated.

Duthie and Francis (1988) have reviewed the possible role of oxygen free radicals (superoxides) in both health and disease – affecting the properties of cell membranes as well as controlling the flux of prostaglandin synthesis. The toxic substances are excessively formed during conditions of hypoxia, in ischaemia, radiation damage, during inflammation and by certain toxins, i.e. called 'oxidative stress'. Murrell *et al.* (1987) have demonstrated abnormal concentrations of hypoxanthine in Dupuytren's contracture and in other fibrotic tissues.

It is believed that the hypoxanthine reacts with the xanthine oxidase of the vessels' walls to release oxygen free radicals which damage perivascular connective cells which are repaired by fibrosis (Figure 15.44).

Pathologically, Dupuytren contracture is a form of fibromatosis which may be localized to the palmar fascia or part of a more generalized process. It is bilateral in approximately 45% of patients. Manifestations of a more generalized process include fibromatosis of the feet (Ledderhosen syndrome) which affects approximately 5% of those with Dupuytren's, as well as involvement of the penis (Peyronie's disease) which is less common. Locally, the process may also involve thickening of the skin over the dorsal proximal interphalangeal joints of the fingers, termed 'knuckle pads'. These do not appear to have a poor prognostic effect (Mikkelsen, 1977).

Histologically, the process appears to be an abnormality of fibroblasts in which the cells have developed contractile properties. These cells, called myofibroblasts, may represent the proliferation of a primitive mesenchymal cell with properties of both fibroblasts and smooth muscle (Gabbianni and Majno, 1972). The pathognomonic and earliest lesion of Dupuytren disease is a palpable nodular thickening of the palmar fascia along the pretendinous band. Histologically these nodules are very vascular and very cellular, consistent with this proliferative phase. Over time, fibrous bands and flexion contractures develop. In the end stage of this process, the nodules themselves disappear. Histologically, this stage reveals few cells which appear to be mature fibrocytes (McFarlane, 1990).

CLINICAL FEATURES

The first sign of the contracture is the appearance of a small hard nodule in the palmar fascia overlying the head of one of the metacarpals. Thereafter the patient notices a progressively increasing flexion contracture, most commonly of the ring finger or little

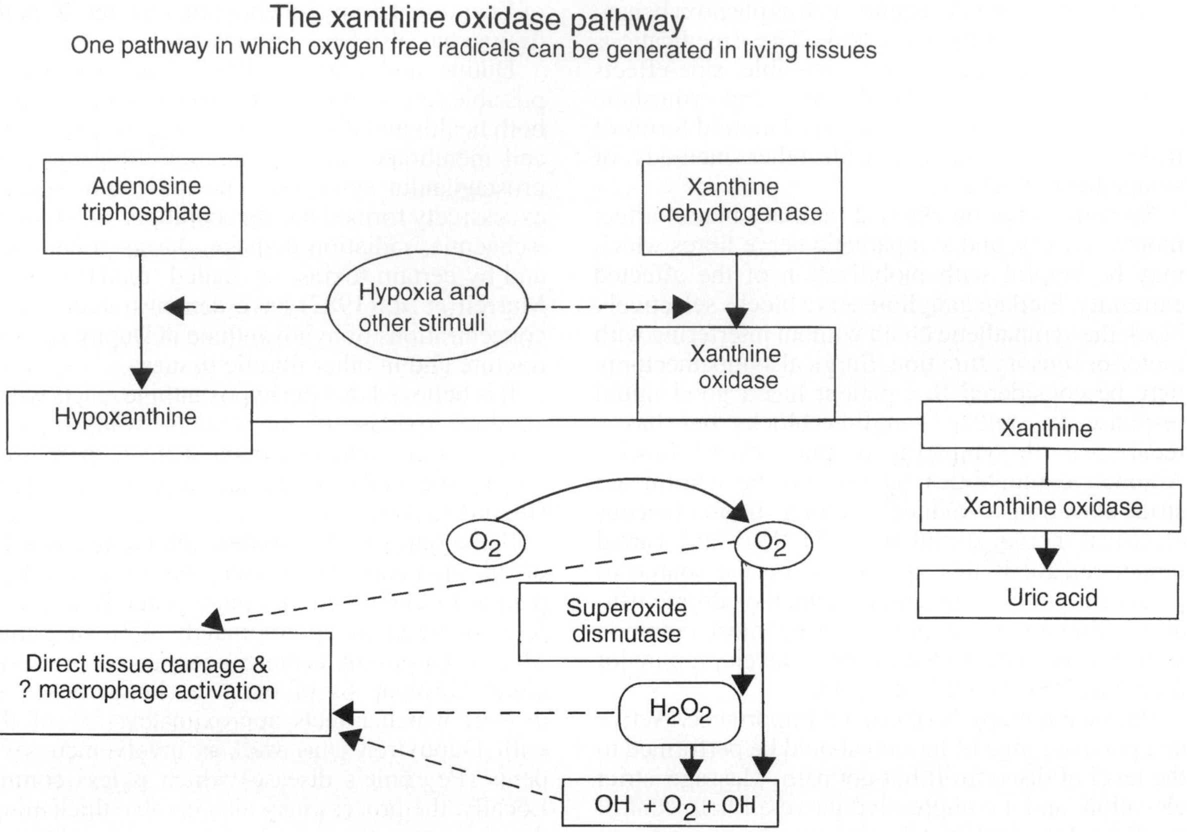

Figure 15.44 The xanthine oxidase pathway, to generate oxygen free radicals *in vivo* with direct tissue damage and fibrosis. (By M. Francis and G.A.C. Murrel, 1988)

finger. Eventually the nodule disappears, and is replaced by a narrow cord-like band of contracted fascia. Gradually other fingers may show some degree of flexion, and the overlying skin becomes puckered and bound down to the contracted fascia. The flexion of the fingers is due to the contraction of the slips or prolongations which pass from the main palmar fascia to the digits; these digital bands do not reach as far as the terminal phalanx, so the terminal interphalangeal joint remains extended.

Pain is uncommon. Occasionally a dull, aching sensation may be felt in the palm, and at times the nodules are distinctly tender.

Dupuytren's contracture must be distinguished from:

1. Contracture due to injury or infection.
2. Congenital contracture.
3. Spastic contractions.
4. Ulnar paralysis.

The first group can be readily recognized from the history, while in the spastic type the long flexor tendons are the structures principally involved, so that when the wrist is fully flexed, to relax the shortened tendons, the finger can be extended. The congenital type is usually bilateral. In both congenital and spastic contractures, too, the metacarpophalangeal joint may be fully or even hyperextended.

The proximal interphalangeal (PIP) joint contracture develops as a derangement of the normal fascial support structures of the digit (Figure 15.45). Normal structures have been termed 'band', whereas pathological structures seen in Dupuytren's contracture have been termed 'cords'. The most common 'cord' to develop in the digit is the spiral cord which develops as the pretendinous band, spiral band, lateral digital sheath, and Grayson ligament contract. This leads to flexion at the PIP joint and displacement of the neurovascular bundle in a proximal, central, and volar direction. The neurovascular bundle must be dissected throughout its course in the digit prior to excising the diseased fascia.

The thumb is sometimes involved in Dupuytren disease. The main functional pathology involving the thumb is usually contracture of the first web space which results from contracture within the natatory and superficial transverse ligaments.

TREATMENT

There is no proven non-surgical treatment for Dupuytren's contracture. Steroid injections into the

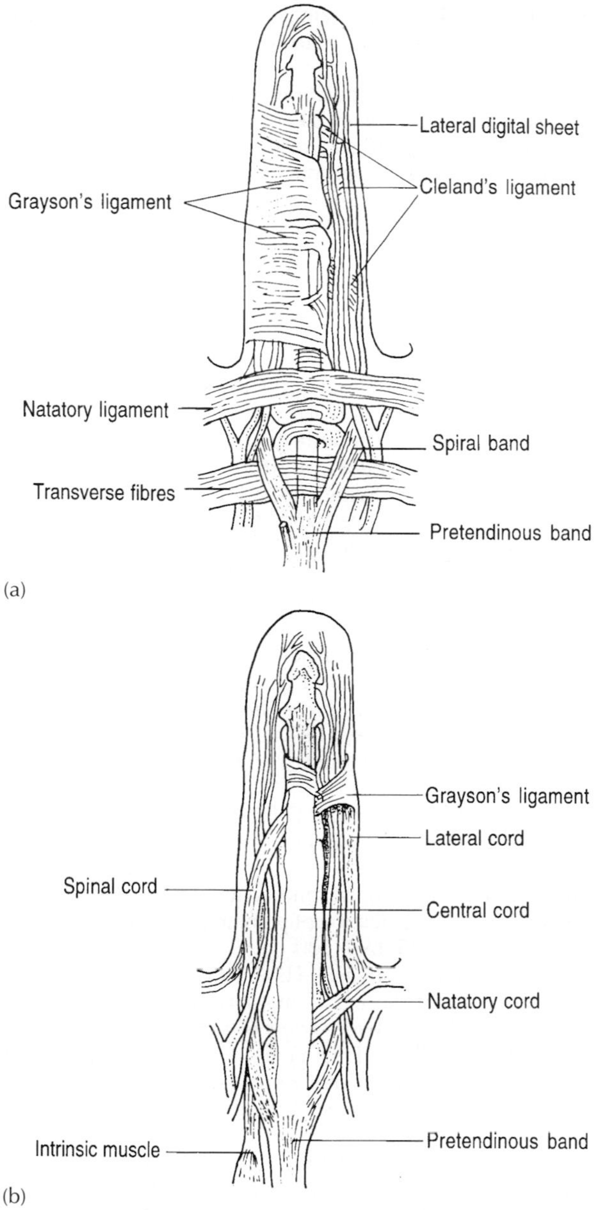

Figure 15.45 Dupuytren's disease. (a) Normal fascial structures. Cleland's ligaments, which are dorsal to the neurovascular bundle, do not become diseased. (b) Diseased cords which develop from normal fascial structures. (After McFarlane, R.M. (1974) *Plastic and Reconstructive Surgery* **54**, 31)

Dupuytren nodules have not been shown to alter the overall disease course. The nodule alone is not an indication for surgical excision unless painful, and most surgeons wait until flexion contractures develop. MCP flexion contractures are effectively treated surgically and can wait until the contracture is causing functional difficulties (30–45°). In contrast, PIP joint contractures are much more difficult to treat because of the distortion of the complex anatomy as the disease progresses. Furthermore, volar plate contractures and extensor mechanism imbalance may develop. For these reasons, most authors advocate surgical treatment as soon as any PIP joint contracture develops (McFarlane, 1990).

Surgical treatment of Dupuytren's contracture encompasses two areas: first, the treatment of palmar fascia and MCP contracture, and second, the treatment of digital involvement. Numerous procedures have been described for Dupuytren's contracture of the palm and MCP joints. These range from simple fasciotomies in which the fascial cords are cut (Luck, 1959), to total fasciectomies in which the entire palmar fascia is excised (McIndoe and Beare, 1958; McCash, 1964). Currently, the approach for palmar disease is the selective subtotal or regional fasciectomy in which the diseased fascia of the palm is removed and normal appearing fascia is left (Hueston, 1965). This is a compromise of the above two extremes which has resulted in fewer complications; yet there is the risk of recurrence as the disease progresses in previously uninvolved areas. Another issue concerns treatment of the skin wound. McIndoe advocates primary closure with or without local advancement flaps, Gonzales recommends full thickness skin grafts (FTSG) to hold the fascial ends apart, and McCash advocates the open palm technique in which the wound is allowed to heal by secondary intention. Our approach is individualized, based on the wound and the patient. If the skin is closed, it should be done without tension which may require multiple Z-plasties. With primary closure or FTSG, haemostasis is crucial to prevent haematoma formation and skin loss.

Digital fasciectomy is accomplished through wide exposure because of the complex anatomy and pathology. The skin incision may consist of the volar zig-zag, or a straight incision with multiple Z-plasties at the flexion creases to help correct the skin contracture. Surgery is carried out under loupe magnification with meticulous haemostasis. The neurovascular bundle is identified proximally and then followed distally. Because of the possible displacement of the neurovascular bundle by a spiral cord, the skin incision must be made with caution. The bundle may be directly beneath the skin at the level of the MCP joint. Once the neurovascular bundle is identified and mobilized throughout the length of the exposure, the diseased fascia may be removed, including the retrovascular tissue and natatory ligaments if they are involved. If the neurovascular bundle is damaged, it should be repaired. PIP joint contracture may not be fully correctable; however, little functional deficit will be seen if there is less than a 40° flexion contracture.

Treatment of the thumb is similar except one must be aware of the anatomical differences, especially the radial digital nerve over the volar aspect of the thumb at the level of the A1 pulley (MCP joint). Further, the web space contracture must be corrected through excision of the affected natatory ligament, pretendinous bands, and superficial transverse ligament as necessary.

Following surgery, the hand is splinted with the PIP joints extended to prevent recurrent contracture. The wrist should be in neutral or slight flexion as needed to relieve tension on the palmar incision. Motion is begun in 1–2 days unless a skin graft has been used, in which case gentle range of motion is initiated after approximately 7 days.

References

Albright, J.A. and Chase, R.A. (1970) Palmar shelf arthroplasty of the wrist in rheumatoid arthritis. A report of nine cases. *Journal of Bone and Joint Surgery* **52A**, 896

Agee, J.M., McCarrol, H.R. and Torosa, R.D. (1992) Endoscopic release of the carpal tunnel: a randomized prospective multicentre trial. *Journal of Hand Surgery* **17A**, 987–995

Anderson, B. and Kaye, S. (1991) Treatment of flexor tenosynovitis of the hand (trigger finger) with corticosteroids: a prospective study of the response to local injection. *Archives of Internal Medicine* **151**, 153–156

Angelides, A.C. (1993) Ganglions of the hand and wrist. In: *Operative Hand Surgery*, 3rd edn. Edited by D.P. Green. Churchill Livingstone: New York

Atkins, R.M., Tindale, W., Bickerstaff, D. and Kanis, J.A. (1993) Quantative bone scintography in reflex sympathetic dystrophy. *British Journal of Rheumatology* **32**, 41–45

Bauer, R.D., Lewis, M.M. and Posner, M.A. (1988) Treatment of enchondromas of the hand with allograft bone. *Journal of Hand Surgery* **13A**, 908–916

Beasley, R.W. (1970) Tendon transfers for radial nerve palsy. *Orthopedic Clinics of North America* **1**, 439

Beasley, R.W. (1981) *Hand Injuries*. W.B. Saunders: Philadelphia

Blackdahl, M. (1963) The caput ulnae syndrome in rheumatoid arthritis. A study of the morphology, abnormal anatomy and clinical picture. *Acta Rheumatologica Scandinavica* **5**, 1

Bogumill, G.P. (1990) Tumors of the hand. In: *Surgery of the Muscoskeletal System*, 2nd edn, pp. 1197–1250. Edited by C.M. Evarts. Churchill Livingstone: New York

Bowden, R.E.N. and Napier, J.R. (1961) The assessment of hand function after peripheral nerve injuries. *Journal of Bone and Joint Surgery* **43B**, 481–492

Boyes, J.H. (1970) *Bunnell's Surgery of the Hand*, 5th edn. J.B. Lippincott: Philadelphia

Brand, P.W. (1975) Tendon transfers in the forearm. In: *Hand Surgery*, 2nd edn. Edited by J.E. Flynn. Williams & Wilkins: Baltimore

Brase, D.W. and Millender, L.H. (1986) Failure of silicone rubber wrist arthroplasty in rheumatoid arthritis. *Journal of Hand Surgery* **11A**, 175

Bruner, J.M. (1967) The zigzag volar digital incision for flexor tendon surgery. *Plastic and Reconstructive Surgery* **40**, 571

Bunnell, S. (1938) Opposition of the thumb. *Journal of Bone and Joint Surgery* **20**, 269

Bunnell, S. (1942) Surgery of the intrinsic muscles of the hand other than those producing opposition of the thumb. *Journal of Bone and Joint Surgery* **24**, 1

Burkhalter, W.E. (1974) Early tendon transfers in upper extremity peripheral nerve injury. *Clinical Orthopaedics and Related Research* **104**, 68

Burkhalter, W.E., Christensen, R.C. and Brown, P.W. (1973) Extensor indicis proprius opponensplasty. *Journal of Bone and Joint Surgery* **55A**, 725

Burton, R.I. (1986) Basal joint arthrosis of the thumb. *Orthopedic Clinics of North America* **4**, 331

Burton, R.I. (1990) The arthritic hand. In: *Surgery of the Musculoskeletal System*, pp. 1087–1157. Edited by C.M. Evarts. Churchill Livingstone: New York

Burton, R.I. (1991) The hand. In: *Atlas of Orthopaedic Surgery*, 2nd edn. Edited by L.A. Goldstein. C.V. Mosby: St Louis

Burton, R.I. and Littler, J.W. (1975) Nontraumatic soft tissue afflictions of the hand. In: *Current Problems in Surgery*. Yearbook Medical Publishers: Chicago

Burton, R., Margles, S. and Lunseth, P. (1986) Small-joint arthrodesis. *Journal of Bone and Joint Surgery* **11A**, 687

Carroll, R.E. and Dick, H.M. (1971) Arthrodesis of the wrist for rheumatoid arthritis. *Journal of Bone and Joint Surgery* **53A**, 1365

Clendenin, M.B. and Green, D.P. (1981) Arthrodesis of the wrist – complications and their management. *Journal of Hand Surgery* **6**, 253

Conyers, D.J. (1990) Scapholunate interosseous reconstruction and imbrication of palmar ligaments. *Journal of Hand Surgery* **15**, 690–700

Cooney, W.P.M., Dobyns, J.H. and Lincheid, R.L. (1990) Arthroscopy of the wrist: anatomy and classification of carpal instability. *Arthroscopy* **6**, 133–140

Curtis, R.M. (1964) Treatment of injuries of proximal interphalangeal joints of the fingers. In: *Current Practice in Orthopaedic Surgery*. Edited by J.P. Adams. C.V. Mosby: St Louis

De Krom, M., Knipschied, P.G., Kester, A.D.M. *et al*. (1992) Carpal tunnel syndrome. Prevalence in the general population. *Journal of Clinical Epidemiology* **45**, 373–376

Dell, P.C. (1987) Distal radioulnar joint dysfunction. *Hand Clinics of North America* **3**, 563

Dinham, J.M. and Meggitt, B.K. (1974) Trigger thumbs in children: a review of the natural history and indications for treatment in 105 patients. *Journal of Bone and Joint Surgery* **56B**, 153–155

Duthie, R.B. and Francis, M.J.O. (1988) Free radicals and Dupuytren's contracture. *Journal of Bone and Joint Surgery* **70B**, 689–691

Eaton, R.G. (1979) Replacement of the trapezium for arthritis of the basal articulations. A new technique with stabilization by tenodesis. *Journal of Bone and Joint Surgery* **61A**, 76

Eaton, R.G. and Butsch, D.W. (1970) Antibiotic guidelines for hand infections. *Surgery, Gynecology and Obstetrics* **130**, 119

Eaton, R.G. and Littler, D.W. (1970) Ligament reconstruction for the painful thumb carpometacarpal joint. *Journal*

of Bone and Joint Surgery **55A**, 1655
Eaton, R.G., Lane, L.B., Littler, J.W. and Leyser, J.J. (1984) Ligament reconstruction for the painful thumb carpometacarpal joint: a long term assessment. *Journal of Hand Surgery* **9A**, 692
Feldon, P., Millender, L.H. and Nalebuff, E.A. (1993) Rheumatoid arthritis in the hand and wrist. In: *Operative Hand Surgery*, 3rd edn, pp. 1587–1690. Edited by D.P. Green. Churchill Livingstone: New York
Flatt, A.E. (1963) *The Care of the Arthritic Hand*, 4th edn, pp. 56–87. C.V. Mosby: St Louis
Florack, T.M., Miller, R.J., Pellegrini, V.D., Burton, R.I. and Dunn, M.G. (1992) The prevalence of carpal tunnel syndrome in patients with basal joint arthritis of the thumb. *Journal of Hand Surgery* **17A**, 624
Gabbiani, G. and Majno, G. (1972) Dupuytren's contracture: fibroblast contraction? *American Journal of Pathology* **66**, 131
Ger, E., Kupcha, P. and Ger, D. (1991) The management of the trigger thumb in children. *Journal of Hand Surgery* **16A**, 944–946
Goldner, J.L. (1953) Deformities of the hand incidental to pathological changes of the extensor and intrinsic muscle mechanisms. *Journal of Bone and Joint Surgery* **35A**, 115–131
Goldner, J.L. (1974) Tendon transfers in rheumatoid arthritis. *Orthopedic Clinics of North America* **5**, 425
Graham, B. (1993) Kienböck's disease. *Current Science. Current Opinion in Orthopaedics* **4**, 57–60
Hackborth, D.A. (1991) Resections and reconstructions for tumours of the distal radius. *Orthopedic Clinics of North America* **22**, 49–64
Haffajee, D. (1977) Endoprosthetic replacement of the trapezium for arthrosis of the carpometacarpal joint of the thumb. *Journal of Hand Surgery* **2**, 141
Hueston, J.T. (1965) Dupuytren's contracture: the trend to conservatism. *Annals of the Royal College of Surgeons of England* **36**, 134
Inglis, A.E., Hamlin, C., Sengelmann, R.P. and Straub, L.R. (1972) Reconstruction of the metacarpophalangeal joint of the thumb in rheumatoid arthritis. *Journal of Bone and Joint Surgery* **54A**, 704
Jones, R. (1921) Tendon transplantation in cases of musculospinal injuries not amenable to suture. *American Journal of Surgery* **35**, 333
Kaplan, E.B. (1959) Anatomy, injuries and treatment of the extensor apparatus of the hand and digits. *Clinical Orthopaedics and Related Research* **13**, 24–41
Kavanel, A.B. (1925) *Infections of the Hand: a Guide to the Surgical Treatment of Acute and Chronic Suppurative Processes in the Fingers, Hand and Forearm*, 5th edn. Lea & Febiger: Philadelphia
Kavanel, A.B. (1935) Hand infections in industrial accidents. *Surgery, Gynecology and Obstetrics* **60**, 568
Kelley, P.J., Karlston, A.G., Weed, L.A. *et al.* (1967) Infection of synovial tissues by mycobacteria other than *Mycobacterium tuberculosis*. *Journal of Bone and Joint Surgery* **49A**, 1521
Kerr, C.D., Syert, D.R. and Albarracin, N.S. (1992) An analysis of the flexor synovium in idiopathic carpal tunnel syndrome. Report of 625 cases. *Journal of Hand Surgery* **17A**, 1028–1030
Kessler, I. (1973) Silicone arthroplasty of the trapeziometacarpal joint. *Journal of Bone and Joint Surgery* **55B**, 285
Kienböch, R. (1910) Uber traumatische Malazie des Mondbeins und ihre Folgezustande: Entartungsformen und Kompressions-frakturen. *Fortschritte auf dem Gebiete Rontgenstrahlen* **16**, 77–103
Kilgore, E.S. Jr, Brown, L.G. and Newmeyer, W.L. *et al.* (1975) Treatment of felons. *American Journal of Surgery* **139**, 194
Koman, L.K., Smith, T.L., Poehling, G.G. and Smith, B.P. (1993) Reflex sympathetic dystrophy. *Current Science. Current Opinion Orthopaedics*
Lankford, L.L. (1990) Reflex sympathetic dystrophy. In: *Surgery of the Musculoskeletal System*, 2nd edn, pp. 1265–1296. Edited by C.M. Evarts. Churchill Livingstone: New York
Leriche, R. (1939) *The Surgery of Pain*. Edited by A. Young. Tindall & Cox: London
Ling, R.S.M. (1963) The genetic factor in Dupuytren's disease. *Journal of Bone and Joint Surgery* **45B**, 709
Linscheid, R. (1968) Surgery for rheumatoid arthritis – timing and techniques: the upper extremity. *Journal of Bone and Joint Surgery* **50A**, 605
Linscheid, R.L. (1992) Kienböck's disease. *AAOS Instructional Course Lecture Series* **41**, 45–53
Linscheid, R.L. and Dobyns, J.H. (1990) Bone and soft tissue infections of the hand and wrist. In: *Surgery of the Musculoskeletal System*, 2nd edn. Edited by C.M. Evarts. Churchill Livingstone: New York
Littler, J.W. (1949) Tendon transfers and arthrodeses in combined median and ulnar nerve paralysis. *Journal of Bone and Joint Surgery* **31A**, 225
Littler, J.W. (1952) The hand and wrist. In: *A Textbook of Orthopaedics*. Edited by M.B. Howorth. W.B. Saunders: Philadelphia
Littler, J.W. (1967) The finger extensor mechanism. *Surgical Clinics of North America* **47**, 415
Littler, J.W. (1974) Hand, wrist and forearm incisions. In: *Symposium on Reconstructive Hand Surgery*, vol. 9. Edited by J.W. Littler, L.M. Cramer and J.W. Smith. C.V. Mosby: St Louis
Littler, J.W. (1977) The hand and upper extremity. In: *Reconstructive Plastic Surgery*, vol. 6. Edited by J.M. Converse. W.B. Saunders: Philadelphia
Littler, J.W. and Cooley, S.G.E. (1963) Opposition of the thumb and its restoration by abductor digiti quinti transfer. *Journal of Bone and Joint Surgery* **45A**, 1389
Littler, J.W. and Cooley, S.G.E. (1965) Restoration of the retinacular system in hyperextension deformity of the interphalangeal joint. In: *Proceedings of the American Society for Surgery of the Hand. Journal of Bone and Joint Surgery* **47A**, 637
Littler, J.W. and Eaton, R.G. (1967) Redistribution of forces in the correction of the boutonnière deformity. *Journal of Bone and Joint Surgery* **49A**, 1268
Long, C., Conrad, P.W., Hall, E.A. and Furler, M.S. (1970) Intrinsic–extrinsic muscle control of the hand in power grip and precision handling. *Journal of Bone and Joint Surgery* **52A**, 853–867
Luck, J.V. (1959) Dupuytren's contracture: a new concept of the pathogenesis correlated with surgical management. *Journal of Bone and Joint Surgery* **41A**, 635
McCash, C.R. (1964) The open palm technique in Dupuytren's contracture. *British Journal of Plastic Surgery* **27**, 211
McFarlane, R.M. (1974) Patterns of diseased fascia in the

fingers in Dupuytren's contracture. *Plastic and Reconstructive Surgery* **54**, 31
McFarlane, R.M. (1990) Dupuytren's disease. In: *Surgery of the Musculoskeletal System*, 2nd edn, pp. 983–999. Edited by C.M. Evarts. Churchill Livingstone: New York
McIndoe, A. and Beare, R.L.B. (1958) Dupuytren's contracture. *American Journal of Surgery* **95**, 2
Mennen, U. and Howells C.J. (1991) Human fight-bite injuries of the hand. *Journal of Hand Surgery* **16B**, 431–435
Mikkelsen, O.A. (1977) Knuckle pads in Dupuyten's contracture. *Hand* **9**, 301–305
Millender, L.H. and Nalebuff, E.A. (1973) Arthrodesis of the rheumatoid wrist. An evaluation of sixty patients and a description of a different surgical technique. *Journal of Bone and Joint Surgery* **55A**, 1026
Moberg, E. (1958) *Journal of Bone and Joint Surgery* **40B**, 454
Murrell, G.A.C., Francis, M.J.O. and Granger, D.N. (1987) Free radicals and Dupuytren's contracture. *British Medical Journal* **295**, 1373–1375
Makamura, R., Tanaka, Y., Imalda, T. and Miura, T. (1991) The influence of age and sex on ulnar variance. *Journal of Hand Surgery* **16B**, 84–88
Neviaser, R.J. (1993) Infections. In: *Operative Hand Surgery*, 3rd edn. Edited by D.P. Green. Churchill Livingstone: New York
Nolan, W.B. and Eaton, R.G. (1992) Darrach procedure for distal ulnar pathology derangements. *Clinical Orthopaedics and Related Research* **27**, 85–89
Omer, G.E. Jr (1968) Evaluation and reconstruction of the forearm and hand after acute traumatic peripheral nerve injuries. *Journal of Bone and Joint Surgery* **50A**, 1454
Omer, G.E. Jr (1980) *Management of Peripheral Nerve Problems*. Edited by G.E. Omer Jr and M. Spinner. W.B. Saunders: Philadelphia, 817–846
Omer, G.E. Jr (1993) Ulnar nerve palsy. In: *Operative Hand Surgery*, 3rd edn. Edited by D.P. Green. Churchill Livingstone: New York
Pellegrini, V.D. Jr (199la) Osteoarthritis of the trapeziometacarpal joint: the pathophysiology of articular cartilage degeneration. I. Anatomy and pathology of the ageing joint. *Journal of Hand Surgery* **16A**, 967
Pellegrini, V.D. Jr (199lb) Osteoarthritis of the trapeziometacarpal joint: the pathophysiology of articular cartilage degeneration. II. Articular wear patterns in the osteoarthritic joint. *Journal of Hand Surgery* **16A**, 975
Pellegrini, V.D. Jr and Burton, R.I. (1986a) Surgical management of basal joint arthritis of the thumb. Part I. Long-term results of silicone implant arthroplasty. *Journal of Hand Surgery* **11A**, 309
Pellegrini, V.D. Jr and Burton, R.I. (1986b) Surgical management of basal joint arthritis of the thumb. Part II. Ligament reconstruction with tendon interposition arthroplasty. *Journal of Hand Surgery* **11A**, 324
Riordan, D.C. (1959) Surgery of the paralytic hand. *AAOS Instructional Course Lectures* **16**, 79
Riordan, D.C. (1964) Tendon transfers for nerve paralysis of the hand and wrist. *Current Practice in Orthopaedic Surgery* **2**, 17
Sampson, S.P., Badalamente, M.A., Hurst, L.C. and Seidman, J. (1991) Pathobiology of the human A1 pulley in trigger finger. *Journal of Hand Surgery* **16A**, 714–721
Seddon, H.J. (1956) *Journal of Bone and Joint Surgery* **38B**, 152
Semlack, K. and Fergusson, A.B. (1970) *Clinical Orthopaedics and Related Research* **68**, 294
Sneddon, J. (1969) *The Care of Hand Infections*. Williams & Wilkins: Baltimore
Spurling, R.G. (1930) Causalgia of the upper extremity: treatment by dorsal sympathetic ganglionectomy. *Archives of Neurology* **23**, 784
Stern, P.J. (1993) Fractures of the metacarpals and phalanges. In: *Operative Hand Surgery*, 3rd edn. Edited by D.P. Green. Churchill Livingstone: New York
Stone, N.H., Hursch, H., Humphrey, C.R. *et al.* (1969) Empirical selection of antibiotics for hand infections. *Journal of Bone and Joint Suraery* **51A**, 899
Swanson, A. (1960) Surgery of the hand in cerebral palsy and the swan-neck deformity. *Journal of Bone and Joint Surgery* **42A**, 951
Swanson, A. (1972) Disabling arthritis at the base of the thumb. Treatment by resection of the trapezium and flexible (silicone) implant arthroplasty. *Journal of Bone and Joint Surgery* **54A**, 456
Swanson, A. (1973a) Disabilities of the thumb joints and their surgical treatment including flexible implant arthroplasty. *AAOS Instructional Course Lectures*, p. 89. C.V. Mosby: St Louis
Swanson, A. (1973b) Flexible implant resection arthroplasty in the hand and extremities. *AAOS Instructional Lectures*, pp. 254–264. C.V. Mosby: St Louis
Terrono. A. and Millender, L. (1989) Surgical treatments of the boutonnière rheumatoid thumb deformity. *Hand Clinics* **5**, 239
Terrono, A., Millender, L. and Nalebuff, E. (1990) Boutonnière rheumatoid thumb deformity. *Journal of Hand Surgery* **15A**, 999
Thompson, J.S., Littler, J.W. and Upton, J. (1978) The spiral oblique retinacular ligament. *Journal of Hand Surgery* **3A**, 482–487
Tomaino, M.A., Pellegrini, V.C. Jr and Burton, R.I. (1995) arthroplasty of the basal joint of the thumb. *Journal of Bone and Joint Surgery* **77A**, 346
Urbaniak, J.R. (1990) Arthrodesis of the hand and wrist. In: *Surgery of the Musculoskeletal System*, 2nd edn, pp. 767–786. Edited by C.M. Evarts. Churchill Livingstone: New York
Vicar, A.J. and Burton, R.I. (1986) Surgical management of the rheumatoid wrist-fusion or arthroplasty. *Journal of Hand Surgery* **11A**, 790
Viegas, S.F., Patterson, R.M., Peterson, P.D. *et al.* (1990) Evaluation of the biomechanical efficacy of limited fusions for treatment of scapulolunate dissociation. *Journal of Hand Surgery* **15A**, 120–128
Weilby, A. (1977) Resection arthroplasty of the metacarpophalangeal joint using interpositions of the volar plate. *Scandinavian Journal of Plastic and Reconstructive Surgery and Hand Surgery* **11**, 239
Weilby, A. and Sondorf, J. (1978) Results following removal of silicone trapezium metacarpal implants. *Journal of Hand Surgery* **3A**, 154–156
Williams, T.M., McKinon, S.E., Novak, C.B. *et al.* (1992) Verification of the pressure provocative test in carpal tunnel syndrome. *Annals of Plastic Surgery* **29**, 8–11
Zancolli, E.A. (1968) *Structural and Dynamic Bases of Hand Surgery*. J. B. Lippincott: Philadelphia
Zancolli, E.A. (1974) Correccion de la 'garra' digital por paralisis intrinseca; la operacion del 'lazo'. *Acta Orthopaedica Latina* **1**, 65

CHAPTER 16

Affections of the Knee Joint

GEORGE BENTLEY

No other joint in the body so frequently suffers derangement of function and stability as the knee. Its complicated mechanism and intricate structure make accurate diagnosis of its many disabilities difficult. Manifestations of infection and fractures do not materially differ from those in other joints. When these are excluded there remain a series of conditions, chiefly mechanical, which interfere with the efficient action of the joint.

Some lesions are occupational – for example, meniscus injuries, once common in miners, occur in jobs involving kneeling and twisting such as carpet fitters, electricians, etc. The majority are associated with athletes and are now very frequent. Their importance to the orthopaedic surgeon is great, because accurate diagnosis and treatment in the early stages is often associated with complete relief and reduction of disability.

The development of new methods of investigation, notably arthroscopy, but also MRI, has made diagnosis and treatment much easier and more effective in the last decade.

Anatomy of the knee joint

The knee is the largest joint in the body and its security depends not so much on the intrinsic shape of its articular surfaces (as in the hip) but on the capsule and the powerful ligaments which bind the bones together, and on the muscles and tendons which surround it (Figure 16.1). It is, nevertheless, a relatively unstable joint, which explains the frequency of injuries and some of the problems of joint replacement.

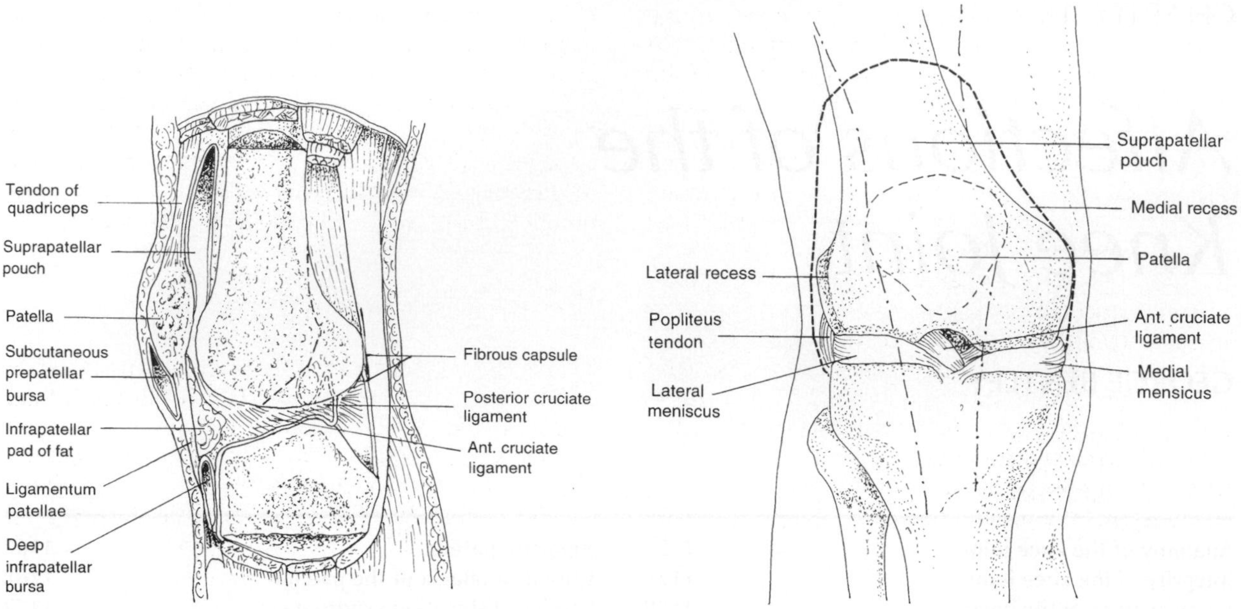

(a) (b)

Figure 16.1 (a) Lateral and (b) coronal sectional diagrams of the knee joint indicating the principal structures. (Reproduced, with permission, from Bentley, G. and Fogg, A.G. (1991) Diagnostic arthroscopy of the knee. In: *Rob & Smith's Operative Surgery, Orthopaedics.* Edited by G. Bentley and R.B. Greer. Butterworth Heinemann: London)

QUADRICEPS MUSCLE

The quadriceps is formed by the rectus femoris and the three vasti. It extends the knee joint and, to a lesser extent, flexes the hip joint, and is one of the most powerful muscles in the body. Any injury to the knee joint produces inhibition of this muscle and it quickly loses volume, tone and control, which is in itself a considerable disability.

The most important component of this muscle is the vastus medialis since it is responsible for the medial stability of the patella and also the 'screw home' movement of the femur on the tibia in the last 10° of extension. It is the first to waste following injury or disease and the last to recover. When the vastus medialis is weak or inactive the knee cannot be fully extended and in such a condition is vulnerable to stresses. The normal range of movement of the knee is seen in Figure 16.2 and is normally described as 0° (full extension) to 150° (full flexion).

HAMSTRING MUSCLES

Ordinarily the hamstring muscles act as flexors of the knee joint together with the gastrocnemius. The biceps femoris inserts into the fibular head where it surrounds the fibular collateral ligament. It has additional attachments to the iliotibial tract, the upper end of the tibia and deep fascia over the calf. It

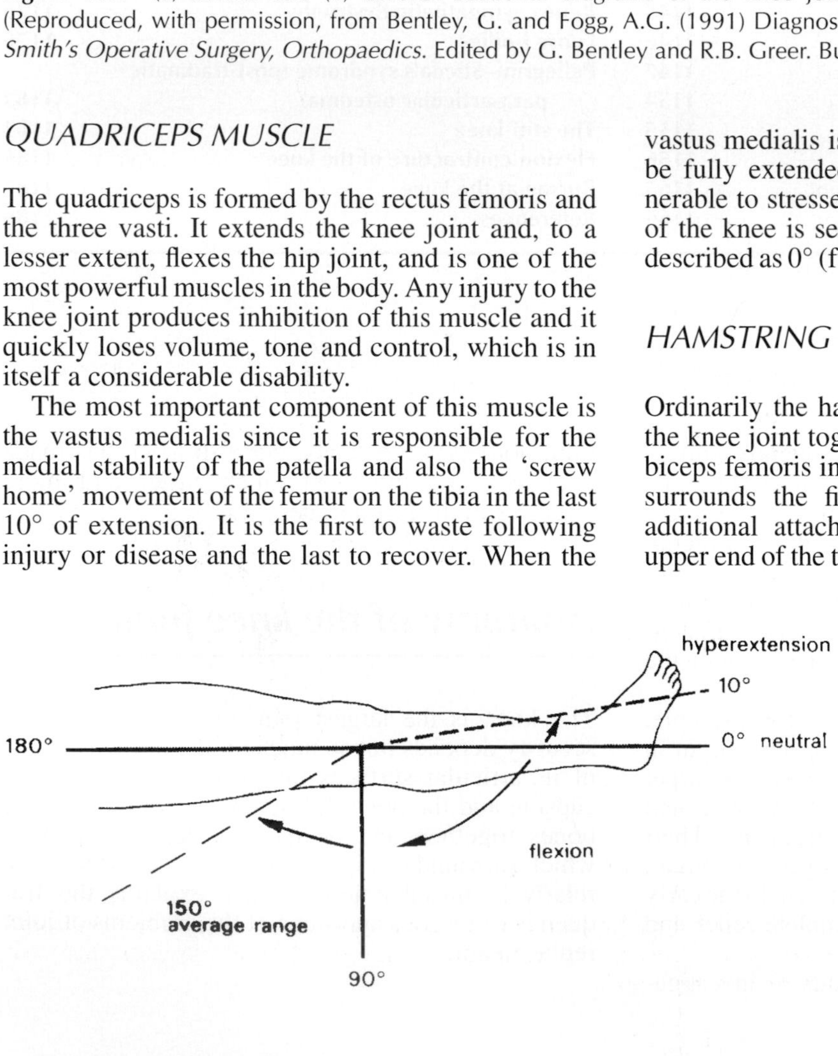

Figure 16.2 Full extension of 0° neutral with hyperextension of 10° and the average range of flexion to 150°.

provides dynamic support for the lateral side of the knee joint. The semimembranosus has an extensive insertion into the posterior and medial aspect of the medial condyle of the tibia and the posterior capsule of the knee joint (Figure 16.3a). This muscle is essential to the stability of the posterior and medial aspects of the knee joint and its tendon is extended across the posterior aspect from the medial tibial condyle upwards to the lateral femoral condyle as the posterior oblique ligament. The semitendinosus muscle joins the sartorius and gracilis in their insertion into the upper and medial surface of the shaft of the tibia (the pes anserinus). When the knee is extended, rotation is not possible. As soon as the knee is 'unlocked' and commences flexion, the tibia and femur may rotate on one another. The sartorius, gracilis, semitendinosus and semimembranosus medially rotate the knee whilst the biceps femoris laterally rotates the knee. The tensor fasciae latae through the iliotibial tract is also a very powerful lateral rotator of the tibia on the femur due to its attachment on the anterior aspect of the tibial condyle at Gurdy's tubercle. Therefore if the knee is retained in flexion for a period of time, for example, in rheumatoid arthritis, a characteristic lateral rotation deformity of the tibia on the femur occurs.

POPLITEUS MUSCLE

This is concerned particularly with rotatory stability of the knee joint. Its close proximity to the lateral meniscus should be noted since it can be damaged during lateral meniscectomy. Basmajian and Lovejoy (1971), in studying the function of the popliteus muscle in man, confirmed the descriptions of Last

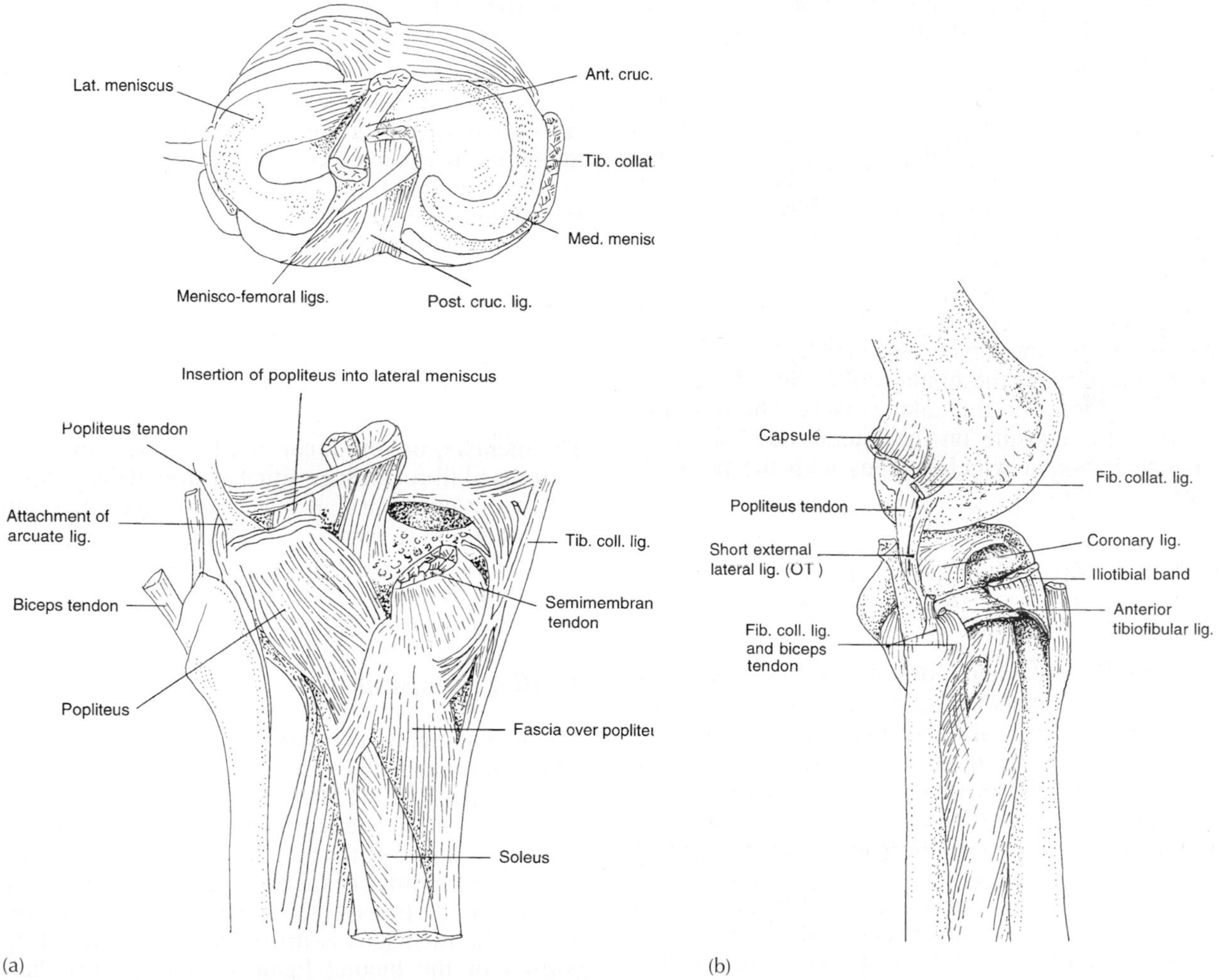

Figure 16.3 View of the partially dissected knee from (a) posterior and (b) lateral aspects to show the key muscle and ligamentous attachments. OT, old terminology. (Reproduced, with permission, from Last, R.J. (1966) *Anatomy: Regional and Applied*, 4th edn. Churchill Livingstone: Edinburgh, London)

(1973) who described the popliteus tendon as split into two, one inserted into the popliteus fossa of the lateral femoral condyle and one into the posterior margin of the lateral meniscus. Therefore, when the popliteus muscle contracts the tendon withdraws and protects the lateral meniscus by drawing it posterolaterally during flexion of the knee and medial rotation of the tibia. These workers have shown that the popliteus muscle is a medial rotator of the tibia on the femur. Mann and Hagy (1977) in a dynamic EMG study, confirmed that, during normal gait, the phasic activity of the popliteus coincides with medial rotation of the tibia on the femur.

FIBROUS CAPSULE

This is an extensive structure which is strengthened in parts by strong expansions from the tendon of the muscles which surround the knee joint. Anteriorly it blends indistinguishably with the expansions from the vastus medialis and vastus lateralis. On the medial side, the middle third of the capsule forms the medial capsular ligament which may be separated from the tibial collateral ligament by a bursa. The posterior third of the capsule on the medial side forms the posterior oblique ligament, as described by Hughston and Eilers (1973), and the posterior ligament reinforced by the insertion of the semimembranosus (oblique popliteal ligament). On the lateral side the middle third of the capsule forms the lateral capsular ligament, which is separated from the fibular collateral ligament by the lateral inferior genicular vessels. The posterior third of the capsule on the lateral side forms the arcuate ligament which merges with the posterior capsular ligament.

TIBIAL (MEDIAL) COLLATERAL LIGAMENT

The medial ligament consists of three portions; superficial, deep and oblique. The superficial (anterior) part is a vertical band with a distinct anterior edge extending from the medial femoral condyle distally and, in the extended knee, slightly forwards. It is attached to the tibia about as far as 4 cm distal to the joint line, and as the knee is flexed it glides posteriorly over the deep portion to a slight extent. The deep (posterior) part is derived from the joint capsule deep to the superficial and is attached to femoral and tibial condyles just beyond the articular cartilage. It is a thick, strong structure. The peripheral edge of the medial meniscus is firmly attached to it. It runs into the oblique part of the ligament.

The oblique part of the ligament is a fan-shaped structure arising from the medial femoral condyle behind the superficial part which extends distally and spreads out to be attached to the posterior half of the medial tibial condyle just distal to the joint line. The peripheral edge of the medial meniscus is attached to it. Anteriorly it blends completely with the superficial and deep parts. The posterior oblique edge blends with the posterior capsule which covers the back of the medial femoral condyle. It may be difficult to distinguish these two structures in the extended joint but in flexion the posterior capsule is very lax whereas the oblique part of the ligament is still tight.

Kennedy and Fowler (1971) showed that the tibial collateral ligament is the primary static stabilizing structure on the medial side of the knee.

FIBULAR (LATERAL) COLLATERAL LIGAMENT

The fibular, or lateral, collateral ligament is a strong rounded cord attached above to the lateral epicondyle of the femur and below to the head of the fibula. It is separated from the lateral meniscus by the tendon of the popliteus. The medial and lateral ligaments resist undue lateral movements of the joint when it is extended but are vulnerable to injury in flexion when severe rotational stresses are applied. See Figure 16.3(b).

THE MENISCI

The menisci, or semilunar cartilage, are crescentic portions of fibrocartilage situated around the periphery of the upper articular surface of the tibia. On cross-section the menisci are wedge shaped so that they match the adjacent articular surfaces of the femur and tibia and thereby increase the congruity of the joint.

Medial meniscus

The medial meniscus is larger and more oval than its fellow; it is attached by two horns to the anterior and posterior parts of the intercondylar area of the tibia. The horns of the lateral meniscus lie within the embrace of those of the medial, and occasionally the anterior extremities of the two menisci are united by the so-called 'transverse' ligament. The posterior half of the meniscus is firmly attached to the deep portion of the medial ligament, the anterior half being relatively mobile.

Lateral meniscus

The lateral meniscus is more circular than the medial, and its horns are attached to the intercondylar area of the tibia on either side of the tibial spine. The posterior horn has strong ligamentous attachment to the posterior cruciate ligament and may also be attached to the medial condyle of the femur by the anterior and posterior meniscofemoral ligaments. It is notable that the lateral meniscus is more mobile than the medial and has no weak point between a movable and relatively fixed point.

The peripheral one-third of each meniscus is relatively well vascularized, whereas the central zone is practically devoid of blood vessels and derives its nourishment from the synovial fluid. The avascular part of the meniscus increases both absolutely and proportionately during the growth period. Thus, in the mature individual healing of the body of the meniscus does not occur. Separation of the rim of the meniscus from the capsule of the joint may, however, result in healing and repair is feasible within the lateral third. Total removal of the meniscus at its attachment to the capsule is followed by the formation of an incomplete fibrocartilage replica.

The two menisci play an important part in the function of the joint. They slightly increase the stability of the knee and, by filling the space between the femur and tibia, to some extent restrict exaggerated lateral movement and facilitate the 'screw home' movement. They facilitate lubrication of the knee, acting as 'thrust pads', and play an important role in load-bearing. Seedholm *et al.* (1974) and Shrive (1974) have demonstrated that certainly in the extended position of the knee the menisci may transmit up to 70% of weight through the lateral side and 50% of weight through the medial side of the joint.

CRUCIATE LIGAMENTS

The articular surfaces are bound together by the two cruciate ligaments. The anterior cruciate ligament is attached to the tibia immediately behind the anterior horn of the medial meniscus and passes upwards, backwards and laterally to be attached to the posterior part of the medial surface of the lateral femoral condyle. The posterior cruciate ligament is attached to the tibia behind the posterior horn of the medial meniscus and the anterior cruciate ligament and passes upwards, forwards and medially to the posterior part of the lateral surface of the medial condyle. Its distal attachment also extends to the upper posterior surface of the tibia which is important in cruciate-retaining arthroplasty. Both cruciate ligaments are tense when the knee is fully extended. In other positions of the knee they help control anteroposterior displacement and rotation.

TIBIAL SPINE

The articular surfaces of the tibial condyles are separated from each other by the tibial spine, which corresponds to the intercondylar fossa of the femur. This spine consists of a smaller lateral tubercle separated by an anteroposterior groove from the larger medial tubercle. The lateral receives some of the fibres of the anterior extremity of the lateral semilunar cartilage. The medial receives fibres from the anterior cruciate ligament, and occasionally the posterior horn of the lateral meniscus is attached to it.

INFRAPATELLAR FAT PAD AND FOLDS

An intracapsular but extrasynovial pad of fat is situated behind the patellar tendon. From this pass extensions between the layers of a triangular synovial fold attached to the anterior end of the intercondylar notch of the femur. The synovial prolongation is known as the ligamentum mucosum or patellar synovial fold and its edges as alar folds or ligaments. The fatty extension is known as the alar pad. In addition, folds or plicae of synovium are present on the medial and lateral aspects of the joint extending into the synovial cavity. The infrapatellar fold and the medial and lateral plicae may become trapped during movements of the knee joint and give rise to painful symptoms which may be difficult to distinguish from meniscus injuries or chondromalacia of the patella. Variable folds have been observed separating the suprapatellar pouch which may cause anterior knee pain (Keene, 1992).

Integrity of the knee joint

Brantigan and Voshell (1941), from a study of amputation specimens, indicated that the integrity of the knee joint depends upon the muscles and tendons about the knee, the capsule, intrinsic ligaments of the joint and the bony and articular architecture of the tibia and femur. They established the following facts regarding stability by a series of classical observations:

1. Lateral motion of the knee joint in extension is controlled by the capsule, collateral ligaments and cruciate ligaments; in flexion, by the same structures minus the fibular collateral ligament.

2. Rotatory motion of the knee joint in extension is controlled by the capsule, collateral ligaments and cruciate ligaments; in flexion, by the same structures minus the fibular collateral ligament.
3. Forward gliding of the tibia on the femur is controlled by the anterior cruciate ligament and the quadriceps.
4. Backward gliding of the tibia on the femur is controlled by the posterior cruciate ligament and the posterior capsule.
5. Lateral gliding of the tibia on the femur is controlled by the tibia intercondylar spine and the femoral condyles with the aid of all the ligaments.
6. Hyperextension is controlled by both collateral ligaments, both cruciate ligaments, both menisci, the posterior aspect of the articular capsule, the oblique popliteal ligament, and the architecture of the femoral condyles.
7. Hyperflexion is controlled by both cruciate ligaments, both menisci, the femoral attachment of the posterior aspect of the capsule, the femoral attachment of both heads of the gastrocnemius muscle, and the bony structure of the condyles of the femur and the tibia.
8. The menisci cushion hyperextension and hyperflexion. The tibial collateral ligament is closely related to the medial meniscus, but there is no strong fibrous tissue attachment between them. The tibial collateral ligament glides forwards and backwards in extension and flexion.

Biomechanics of the knee

The biomechanics of the knee are most complex and, in trying to understand them, one must have some knowledge of the geometry, kinematics, joint loading and its stability.

GEOMETRY

In the coronal (frontal) plane a line joining the centres of the hip and ankle joints passes through the centre of the knee joint. This line represents the mechanical axis of the lower limb.

Therefore the long axis of the shaft of the femur is inclined at an angle to the long axis of the shaft of the tibia. This tibiofemoral shaft angle normally is 8° ± 3° and is the angle measured on anteroposterior radiographs of the standing knee joint. This angle has been termed physiological valgus.

In the sagittal plane the femoral condyles have a changing radius of curvature which decreases from before back. The shape of each condyle may equally well be described by two tangential circular arcs. In the transverse plane the condyles diverge from before back by an angle of 20°.

In general terms the articular surface of the upper end of the tibia is perpendicular to the long axis of the shaft of the tibia in both sagittal and coronal planes. In the sagittal plane the medial plateau is slightly concave while the lateral plateau is slightly convex. In the coronal plane both are slightly concave.

The menisci distribute load between the femur and tibia by increasing the area of contact. They are capable of changing their shape with knee movement to facilitate this load-bearing action. They are not efficient shock absorbers and act more like washers facilitating lubrication. The menisci seem almost dispensable, though their removal may predispose the knee to accelerated degenerative disease (Jackson, 1967) although this has recently been questioned (Reissis *et al.*, 1991).

The patella maintains the alignment of the quadriceps complex and patellar tendon and increases the mechanical advantage of the extensor mechanism by displacing its line of action further from the axis of movement of the knee. The patellofemoral joint is crucial for satisfactory function of the knee as a whole and its disorders lead to considerable disability.

KINEMATICS

Relative motion between two rigid bodies (bones) may be described in terms of translations along and rotations about a set of three orthogonal (mutually perpendicular) axes. The knee joint can be regarded as having six potential degrees of freedom.

If these axes coincide with standard anatomical planes the three rotations are:

- Flexion/extension – large available range
- Abduction/adduction range – increasingly available with knee flexion
- Rotation to 90° – 30–50° with knee flexed

and the three translations are:

- Compression/distraction – negligible
- Mediolateral translation – negligible
- Anterolateral translation – small available range except in extended knee.

The axes about which motion takes place are not fixed, and vary according to the magnitude and direction of the couples producing the movement (Figure 16.4). Frankel and Burstein (1984) introduced the concept of *instant centres of motion*, when all other movements except flexion and extension are ignored. They showed that the axis about which flexion and extension occur shifts backwards in relation to the tibia with increasing flexion. However, the instant centre pathway may be very variable even in normal knees but the axis about which flexion and extension occur lies approximately along the line joining the femoral epicondyles and the axis shifts backwards and forwards as the knee flexes and extends (Figure 16.4a and 16.4b).

Although superficially the knee appears as a simple hinge, it does not have a fixed axis of rotation since flexion and extension are accompanied by rotations in other senses. There is a 'screw home' external rotation of the tibia in the last 20° of extension, and internal and external rotation are permitted when the joint is flexed.

Gait analysis has provided information on the range of knee motion utilized during different activities. Kettlekamp and Chao (1972) described the range of movement in the knee joint required for common activities (Table 16.1).

The knee joint is maintained in an almost straight position during the support phase of normal walking. Small movements are used as a 'shock absorber' to minimize vertical movements of the pelvis. It is during the unloaded swing phase that flexion to about 40° is required to clear the foot from the ground. A good position for knee arthrodesis demands a compromise between these two requirements, i.e. 0–10° flexion.

The ligaments of the knee are required to restrain its motion to a well defined path (Figure 16.4c). Morrison (1968) estimated the forces in the cruciate and collateral ligaments during walking, and obtained tensions of around one-third of body weight. Injuries and ruptures of these ligaments are detected clinically by observing the associated joint laxity. However, quite considerable laxity was found to produce only small abnormalities of knee movements in walking (Tietjens, 1978). Division of the anterior cruciate ligament produces rapid degeneration of the knee joint in many species of animal, but more gradually in man in the case of untreated injuries. It appears that in man the other structures (ligaments and muscles) which cross the joint can compensate for the loss of this and other ligaments.

Table 16.1

	Flexion	Abduction/Adduction	Rotation
Level walking	70°	11°	13°
Climbing stairs	83°	–	–
Sitting and rising	93°	–	–

Painful conditions of the knee affect the passive (unloaded) and active ranges of movement of the joint, such as walking. Mukherjee (1976) observed considerable differences in the kinematics between the effects of rheumatoid arthritis and osteoarthritis of the knee. Patients with both conditions had reduced passive range of movement (about 90% of normal on clinical examination). Patients with rheumatoid arthritis used about 22% of the available range in walking and those with osteoarthritis about 39% compared with 40% of the available range in healthy subjects. The stride length used by the patients with rheumatoid arthritis was also reduced more than that of the patients with osteoarthritis.

During the support phase the limb is inclined forwards after heel strike and backwards before toe-off. The force transmitted to the floor acts in a similar direction, so the limb is retarded after heel strike and a propulsive force is provided before toe-off. This tends to minimize the flexion and extension movements at the knee by keeping the force in the limb close to the joint. These movements must be resisted by muscle forces to stabilize the joint. For most of the support phase of normal gait there is a flexion moment about the joint which must be resisted by the quadriceps group. Just after heel strike and just before toe-off there may be a small extension moment, so it is at these times that an unstable knee may tend towards a recurvatum position. This effect may be used by patients with quadriceps insufficiency, who may put their forefoot onto the ground early to increase the stabilizing effect.

Morrison (1968) made a study of the forces in the healthy knee during walking (Figure 16.4d). This showed that the tibiofemoral force reached a maximum of about three times body weight in the late stages of foot contact. Tensions developed in the gastrocnemius and quadriceps muscles at this stage of walking contributed significantly to this joint force. During foot contact, higher forces were transmitted through the medial than through the lateral condyle. This study indicated that the cruciate ligaments are subjected to loads of about 25% of body weight during walking. All the forces increased with walking speed.

The quadriceps muscle group is not altogether necessary for walking, since the leg can be straightened by a 'flick' of the thigh prior to heel strike and kept straight during the support phase of the limb, as is done by above-knee amputees with prostheses. However, rising from a chair and climbing stairs required good quadriceps function.

The knee flexors are used in walking for raising the foot from the ground, but EMG recordings demonstrate that they also function during the

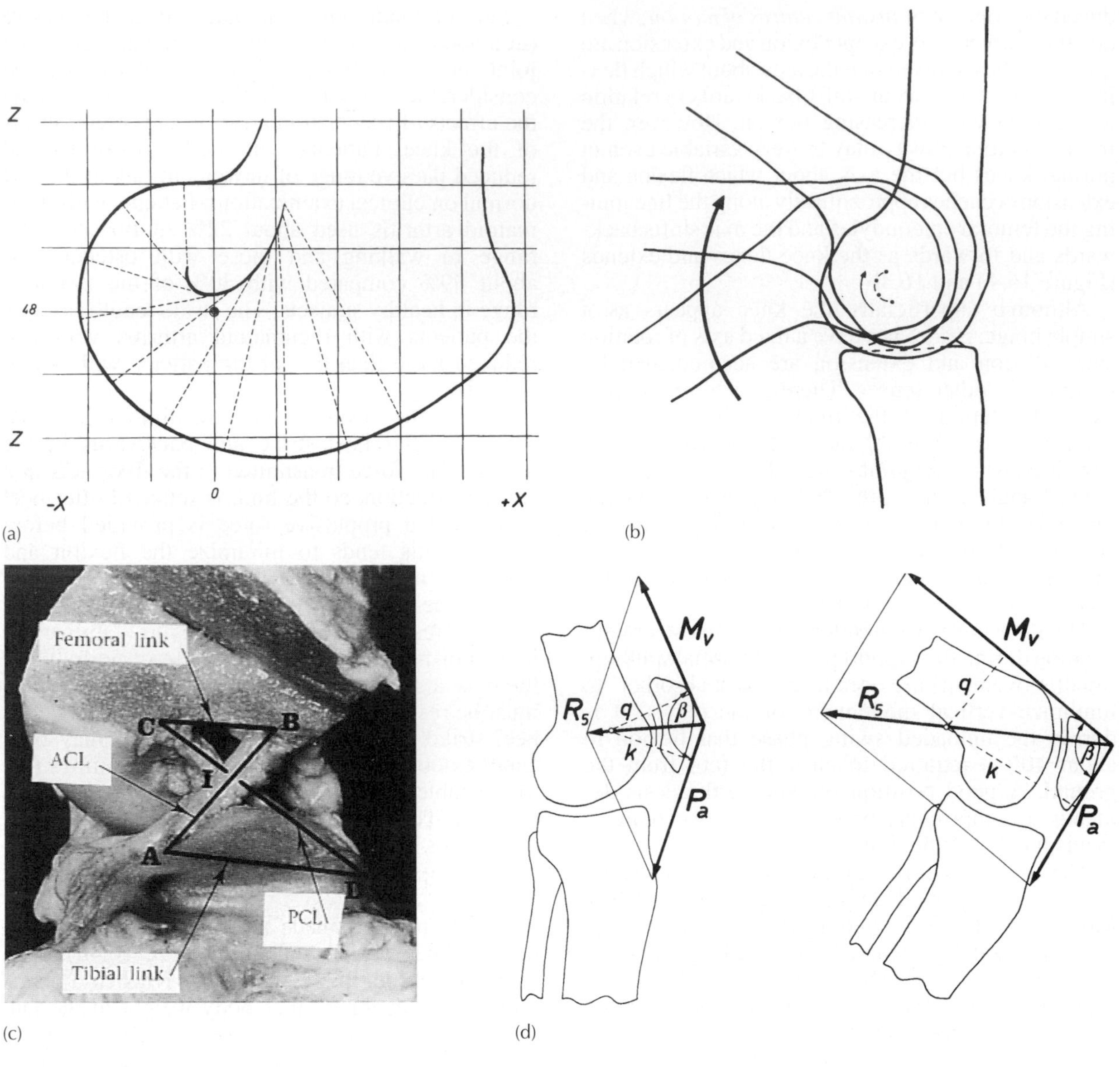

Figure 16.4

support phase, probably to help stabilize the joint against rotational forces.

The greater portion of the load is said to be transmitted by medial compartment but the centre of joint pressure oscillates between medial and lateral compartments. Kettlekamp and Chao (1972) described the medial compartment contact area as being 25% greater than the lateral (Figure 16.4e).

With varus or valgus deformity the distribution of load is obviously altered. Maquet (1984) described how a 10° deformity will double the load in the affected compartment.

McGrouther (1975) showed that, in patients with rheumatoid arthritis affecting the hip, the centre of knee pressure is displaced to the lateral compartment during stance phase due to the antalgic, moment-relieving gait.

In considering the contact areas, the tibiofemoral contact areas vary with joint loading and knee flexion.

Walker and Erkman (1975) described that, at 30° of flexion, there is two times body weight-loading and the contact area is 12 cm^2 with the menisci intact but only 3.5 cm^2 without menisci.

JOINT STABILITY

In the normal joint, stability is dependent on the geometry of articulating surfaces, the menisci, liga-

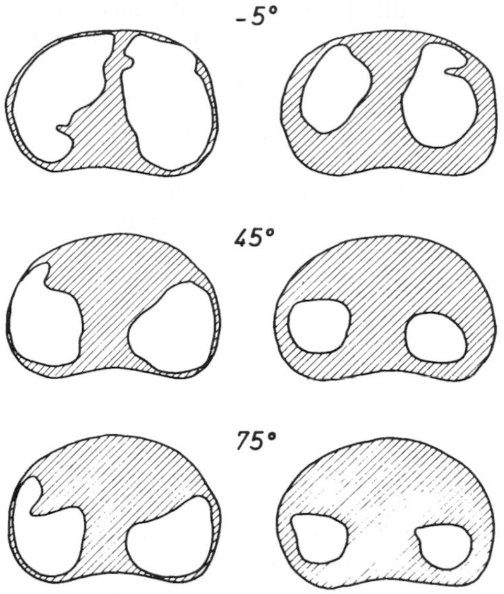

(e)

Figure 16.4 Diagrams demonstrating the instant centre of motion of the knee and its changes during movement. (a) According to Braune and Fischer. (Reproduced, with permission from Maquet, P.G. (1984) *Biomechanics of the Knee*. Springer-Verlag: Berlin, Heidelberg, New York, Tokyo) (b) Reproduced, with permission, from Nordin, M. and Frankel, V. (eds) (1980) *Basic Biomechanics of the Musculoskeletal System*, 2nd edn. Lea and Febiger: Philadelphia. (c) A human knee with the lateral femoral condyle removed, exposing the cruciate ligament. Superimposed diagram of a 4-bar linkage comprising the ACL (AB), the PCL (CD) joining the ligament attachment points on the femur and the tibial link (AD) joining their attachment on the tibia. (Reproduced, with permission, from O'Connor *et al.* (1990) Geometry of the knee. In: *Knee Ligaments – Structure, Function, Injury and Repair.* Edited by D. Daniel, W. Akeson and J. O'Connor. Raven Press: New York) (d) Diagram demonstrating the forces through the human knee in flexion. (Reproduced, with permission, from Maquet, P.G. (1984) *Biomechanics of the Knee*. Springer-Verlag: Berlin, Heidelberg, New York, Tokyo) (e) Contact areas of the knee in different positions of flexion. (Reproduced, with permission, from Maquet, P.G. (1984) *Biomechanics of the Knee*. Springer-Verlag: Berlin, Heidelberg, New York, Tokyo)

ments and the capsule. Muscle action stabilizes as well as producing acceleration and deceleration of body mass. Gravity and proprioceptive receptors in the capsule, cruciates and ligaments also play major roles.

Knee stability is provided by muscle and ligaments which act as:

1. Static stabilizers:
   - capsule and capsular ligaments;
   - extracapsular ligaments.
2. Dynamic stabilizers – musculotendinous units and their aponeuroses; but their protective reflexes act too slowly to prevent many injuries.

Hughston *et al.* (1976) and Slocum *et al.* (1976) divided the knee vertically in a sagittal plane in order to relate the anatomical structures to their function.

In the medial compartment, the anterior third is made up of a thin capsule which tightens in flexion and is reinforced by quadriceps aponeurosis. In the middle third the capsular ligaments are strong and supported superficially by the tibial collateral ligament. In the posterior third the capsule is thickened, and is called the posterior oblique ligament. Supporting this ligament is the semimembranosus tendon and aponeurosis. There is also dynamic support from pes anserinus and gastrocnemius muscles.

In the lateral compartment, in the anterior third there is a thin capsule. In the middle third the capsule is strengthened by the lateral capsular ligament, often misinterpreted as being insignificant. This is reinforced by the powerful iliotibial tract. In the posterior third is the arcuate complex, made up of the collateral ligament, arcuate ligament and aponeurotic tendon of popliteus. There is dynamic support from biceps femoris, popliteus and gastrocnemius muscles.

Nicholas (1973) introduced the concept of the flexible half-sleeve which encases the posterior halves of the femur and tibia and prevents hyperextension. It is made up of three complexes:

1. *Medial quadruple complex* – semimembranosus, oblique popliteal ligament, medial collateral ligament, tendons of pes anserinus.
2. *Lateral quadruple complex* – iliotibial tract, lateral collateral ligament, popliteus tendon and biceps tendon with aponeurosis including arcuate ligament.
3. *Central quadruple complex* – expansion of capsule into the joint including both cruciates and both menisci.

Anterior cruciate ligament (ACL)

From a cord-like origin on the anterior tibial plateau, fibres turn through 90° to a fan-like insertion on the inner aspect of the lateral femoral condyle. Furman *et al.* (1976) described it as two separate parts – anteromedial and posterolateral. Welsh (1980) considered it to be a continuum, part being in tension in any knee position. Grood (1992) has reviewed the biomechanics of the ACL and the optimal placement for knee ligament grafts. He noted that it is generally agreed that most of the isometric ACL fibres originate anteroproximally on the femur and insert anteromedially on the tibia. Disagreement exists over the remainder of the anatomy and function of the ligament. Most agree that the ACL fibres are recruited progressively with only the most anteromedial fibres being tight in full flexion. With extension the remainder of the fibres become progressively tense, starting with the most anterior and moving forwards to the posterior fibres which are only tense in full extension. Its mechanism is to stabilize internal rotation and extension of the tibia on the femur (Furman *et al.*, 1976). Its function is multiple in that it limits forward gliding of tibia on femur and limits hyperextension; it makes a significant contribution to lateral stability and limits anterolateral rotation of the tibia on the femur. Smillie (1978) stressed the role of the ACL in guiding the tibia in the 'screw home' mechanism, and blocks to this which may cause an 'isolated' tear.

Posterior cruciate ligament (PCL)

This is the stoutest ligamentous structure. Kennedy and Fowler (1971) showed it to be twice as strong as the anterior cruciate or the tibial collaterals. Isometrically it is under tension throughout the whole range of movement. Hughston *et al.* (1980) and Girgis *et al.* (1975) described it as two distinct bands.

Its functions are to limit backward glide of tibia on femur and hyperextension. It tightens in internal rotation of tibia on femur. Hughston *et al.* (1976) have stressed that it is the fundamental stabilizer of the knee, being at the axis of flexion–extension and rotation.

Injuries and displacements of the menisci

MECHANISM OF DERANGEMENT OF THE MEDIAL MENISCUS

Normally the medial meniscus or at least its anterior movable portion glides slightly backwards towards the interior of the joint as the knee is flexed. If the tibia is at the same time abducted and the medial compartment of the knee thus opened up, the mobility of the meniscus is still further increased. Sudden medial rotation of the femur on the fixed tibia forces the medial meniscus towards the back of the joint. The medial rotation causes the medial ligament to become taut, and the ligament at first steadies the posterior portion of the meniscus. If the ligament withstands this strain, the anterior movable part of the meniscus bears the brunt of the injury. It may either be detached at its junction with the fixed part or it may undergo a variety of transverse or oblique tears. The inner fragment slips into the interior of the joint, and when extension is attempted and the knee begins to 'screw home' the fragment is nipped between the condyles and the joint is 'locked', i.e. held in flexion.

When the rotatory strain is very severe the medial ligament may be so stretched that the connection between it and the meniscus is destroyed. Indeed, the ligament may be detached both from its tibial attachment and from the meniscus. In either event the whole meniscus or a large medial portion slips into the interior of the joint and, as extension occurs, is caught between the condyles, a longitudinal slit forming in the substance of the meniscus. This is the 'bucket-handle' tear. Smillie (1978) pointed out that if the tear involves the posterior third of the meniscus alone it springs back into place and locking does not occur. Displacements or splits of the posterior horn are caused by forcible lateral rotation of the femur on the fixed tibia, combined with flexion.

MECHANISM OF DERANGEMENT OF THE LATERAL MENISCUS

The lateral meniscus is injured less frequently than the medial, since it enjoys a greater range of movement and is not attached to the lateral ligament. The split tendon of insertion of the popliteus is inserted into the posterior horn as well as the femur and draws the meniscus out of the joint during rotation. Nevertheless, severe degrees of violence may result in tears or displacements.

The anterior horn may be torn if the femur is forcibly rotated outwards on the fixed tibia when the knee is flexed. Medial rotation of the femur on the fixed tibia, combined with or followed by violent flexion, is liable to cause a lesion of the posterior horn.

TYPES OF MENISCUS INJURY

Smillie (1978) described a simple classification of meniscus injuries (Figure 16.5) which is still useful:

1. Longitudinal tears:
   - peripheral detachments (10%);
   - complete (23%);
   - segmental – either anterior or posterior (2%).
2. Horizontal tears – posterior, middle or anterior (48%).
3. Cystic degeneration (12%).
4. Congenital abnormalities (5%).
5. Degenerative lesions.

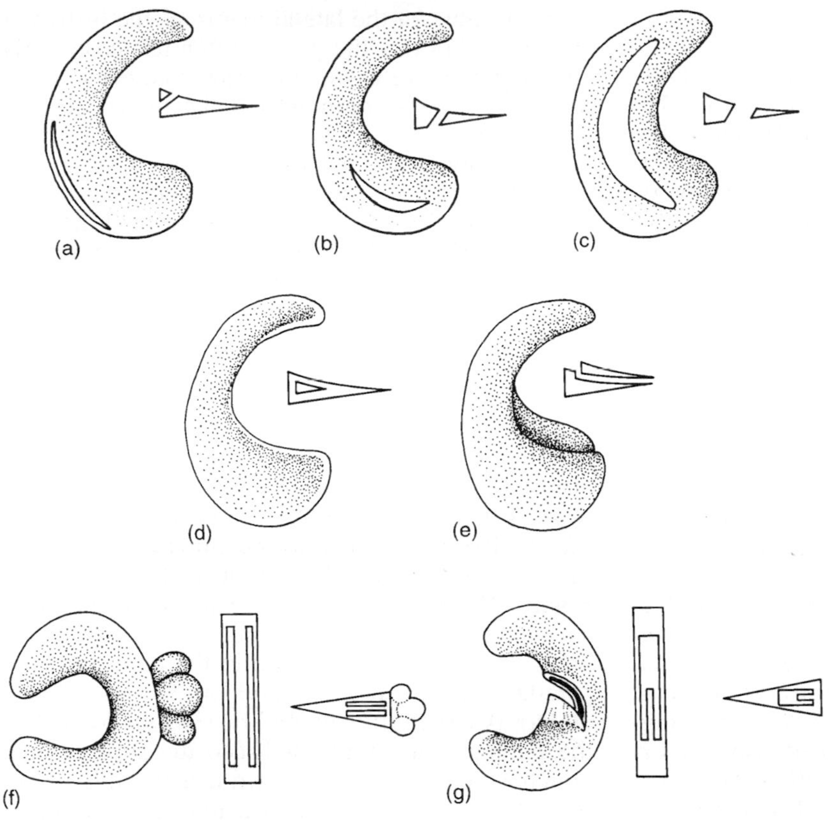

Figure 16.5 Smillie's classification of meniscus injuries: (a) peripheral longitudinal tear; (b) segmental posterior horn tear; (c) complete 'bucket-handle' tear; (d) horizontal mid-substance tear; (e) complete horizontal tear; (f) cystic degeneration; (g) cleft tear ('parrot-beak' or 'degenerative').

Acute traumatic tear

The commonest type of medial meniscus injury in a young adult is the bucket-handle tear. This is a longitudinal tear through the substance of the meniscus between the longitudinally arranged collagen fibres. The inner portion is displaced into the centre of the joint while anterior and posterior attachments remain intact. Almost all of the remaining lesions of the young meniscus consist of some form of bucket-handle tear with or without modifications caused by subsequent trauma (Figure 16.5).

The tear may begin in the anterior horn or in the posterior horn but usually follows the line of the collagen fibres regardless of its point of origin. Sometimes an anterior or posterior torn fragment may be further torn transversely, leaving a tag protruding into the joint from either horn. In the peripheral longitudinal tear the meniscus is separated from the capsule of the joint, and such a lesion is important since it may reattach to the capsule and heal. Furthermore, it may be amenable to repair by suture. Otherwise, meniscus injuries do not heal.

In Smillie's series of meniscectomies, 71% involved the medial meniscus and 5% of cases involved both the menisci.

PREDISPOSING FACTORS

Certain sports are commonly associated with meniscus injuries. Soccer players are particularly liable, especially when pivoting with all the weight on one leg with the knee flexed. Other sports such as hockey, tennis, badminton, squash and skiing all provide a number of meniscus injuries. It is important to remember that, with the increased involvement of the population in sporting activities, meniscus injuries are quite frequently associated with trauma to the medial collateral ligaments, capsule and cruciate ligaments and care must be taken to diagnose these injuries also.

Meniscus tears used to be common in coal miners. These men had to stoop or squat in narrow seams with the knee joints flexed. To clear away coal they emptied the shovel over the shoulder, imposing a severe rotational strain on the flexed knees.

Whilst meniscal injuries are less common in women, with the increasing involvement of women in sport the incidence is rising and the age of occurrence of meniscal injuries in women is falling.

CLINICAL FEATURES

An accurate detailed history is essential, and its importance is frequently greater than that of the clinical examination. The events from the time of the original injury should be carefully recorded in exact sequence. A description of the original injury is obtained: its mechanism, whether it was by external force or by rotation, whether there was immediate incapacity and whether there was a click, a snap or a feeling of tearing in the joint. Then the present complaints of locking, weakness, giving way or swelling are recorded.

A common history in a case of displacement of the medial meniscus is as follows: whilst involved in violent sporting activity or work with the knee in a position of flexion the patient suddenly sustains an outward twist of the foot or an inward twist of the femur on the fixed foot. He immediately feels acute pain on the anteromedial aspect of the joint so severe as to cause him to fall to the ground. He also feels a tearing sensation in the joint and a feeling as if there has been a displacement of an internal structure. On attempting to rise, straightening of the knee is usually not possible, depending on whether the meniscus has remained displaced or has slipped back into its normal position. The knee is usually locked at 20–30° short of full extension. Within a few hours of the injury the joint swells due to the development of an effusion. It is important to note whether swelling occurs immediately after the injury; this is due to haemarthrosis which may be caused by an injury to cruciate or collateral ligaments or by an osteochondral fracture. Over the course of the next two 2–3 weeks the swelling and the pain usually diminish and the knee joint becomes free again.

The pain is situated over the anterior horn of the meniscus and, frequently, also over the inner border of the tibia where the short deep fibres of the medial ligament are normally attached. If the injury is in the posterior horn the pain is felt posteriorly and towards the centre of the joint.

Often by the time the patient is seen the symptoms are less severe than those of the original injury. The common complaint is that the patient can walk and carry out normal activities but any twisting produces pain with giving way of the knee. Usually the knee is checked at a position of about 45° and the patient does not fall to the ground. Locking, i.e. inability to extend fully, also occurs from time to time and the patient may learn trick manoeuvres in order to release the knee, particularly by forcing the tibia into full flexion and rotating the foot. In addition to these locking episodes there may well be recurrent effusion of the knee and the patient may notice that the thigh muscle is wasted.

In an injury of the lateral meniscus the history is similar except that the pain is often felt posteriorly and may be more vague. Locking from tears of this meniscus is less common and the injury may be 'silent'.

It is unwise to make the diagnosis of a torn meniscus in a young person unless there has been a definite history of injury. However, degenerate tears of the meniscus do occur without severe injury in patients over the age of 40 years.

PHYSICAL EXAMINATION

The patient is examined with both legs fully exposed and the knees are inspected anteriorly and posteriorly in both the standing and recumbent positions. The affected joint may show an effusion, and the swollen appearance in the suprapatellar pouch may be accentuated by wasting of the quadriceps. Small effusions in the joint can be detected by stroking the fluid from one side of the joint to the other and noting the impulse in the opposite parapatellar hollow – the so-called 'stroke' test (Figure 16.6a). A larger effusion will be obvious by feeling the parapatellar hollow and also the suprapatellar pouch which extends for three finger-breadths above the patella. In addition, the effusion may be detected by the employment of the 'patellar tap' – where the synovial fluid is held under the patella by the left hand while the right hand taps the patella against the underlying femur with the knee in the straight position (Figure 16.6b). Quadriceps wasting will be present in most cases and this is measured at a point 6 cm above the patella. Where the difference is more than 2 cm compared with the opposite side, it is significant. Palpation over the joint line with the knee in a straight position may reveal some prominence of the anterior border of the meniscus, particularly in the presence of a posterior horn tear. If the meniscus or part of the meniscus is displaced into the centre of the joint, the joint will be 'locked'. This means that there is inability to extend the knee fully (Figure 16.7) and attempts to force the knee beyond this point will produce pain on the affected side. This is demonstrated more traumatically by the use of the 'bounce' test where the normal flexed knee is first allowed to snap into full extension while the leg is supported by the examiner. The repeating of this manoeuvre on the affected side produces severe pain and inhibition of the last few degrees of extension by muscle spasm.

While the knee is in the extended position it is advisable to test for retropatellar tenderness of the patella, particularly on the medial aspect which may indicate chondromalacia of the patella (Figure 16.8).

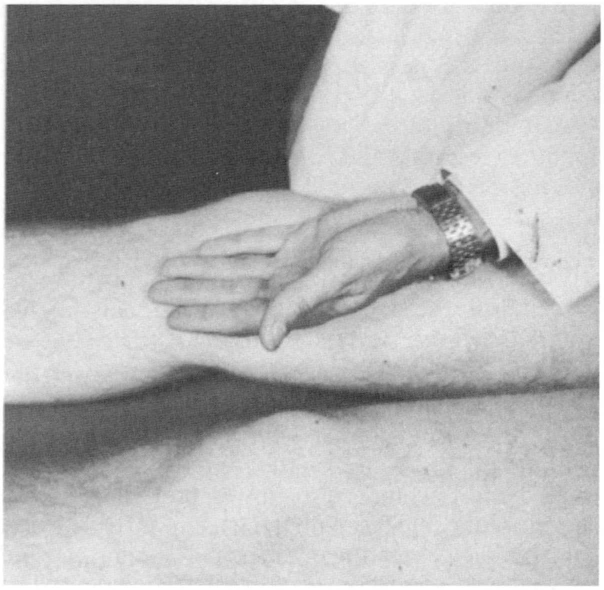

(a)

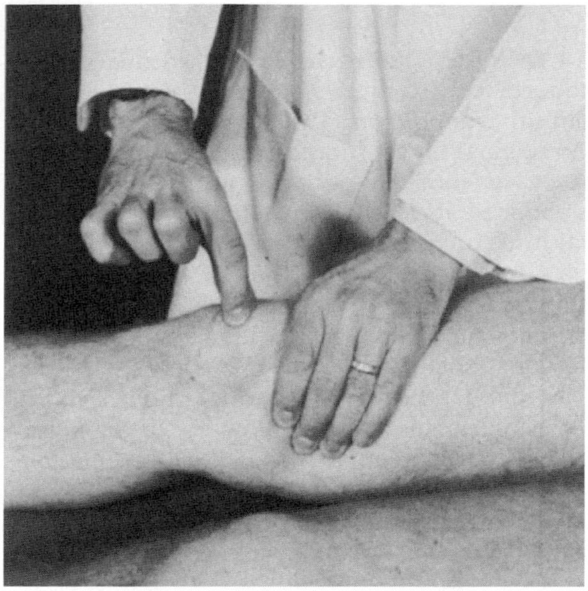

(b)

Figure 16.6 (a) 'Stroke test'. The fluid is stroked across the joint and can be seen on the opposite side in the presence of a small effusion. (b) Method of eliciting 'patellar tap' in the presence of a large effusion.

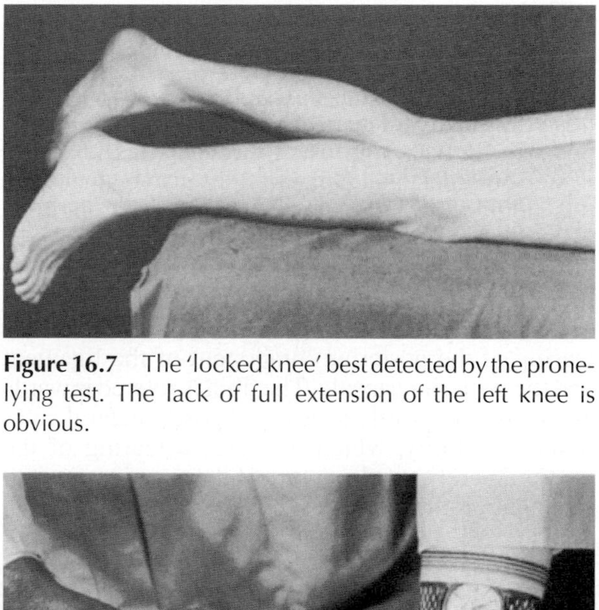

Figure 16.7 The 'locked knee' best detected by the prone-lying test. The lack of full extension of the left knee is obvious.

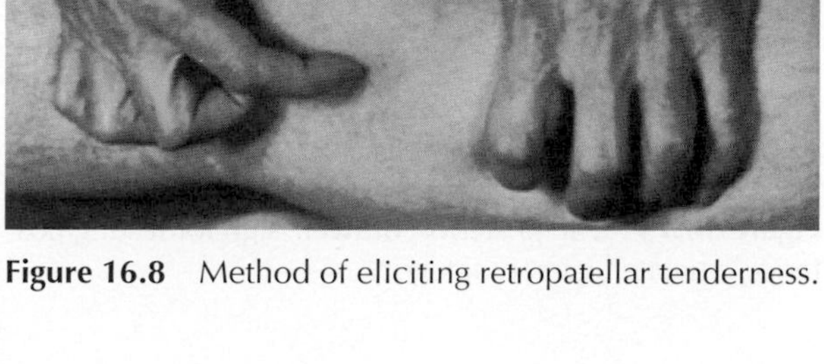

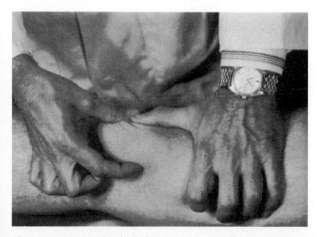

Figure 16.8 Method of eliciting retropatellar tenderness.

The knee is next examined in 90° flexion, where the medial femoral and tibial condyles are palpated and the medial joint line beginning anteriorly alongside the ligamentum patellae and progressing along the joint to the back. Tenderness localized to the joint line usually implies a torn meniscus (Figure 16.9). If the tenderness is above the joint line on the femoral condylar attachment of the medial ligament or below the joint line for a distance of up to four fingerbreadths then the medial ligament may be torn or strained (Figure 16.10). This may be confirmed if the medial ligament is stretched by valgus strain of the

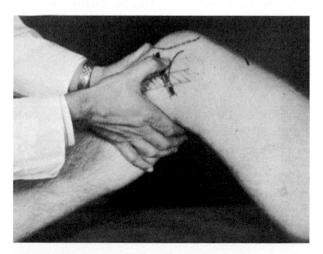

Figure 16.9 Tenderness localized to the joint line implies a torn meniscus.

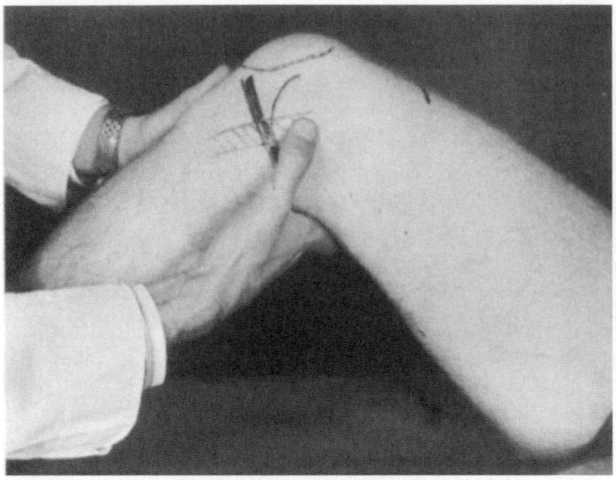

Figure 16.10 Tenderness over the medial ligament attachment to the femur indicates a partial tear.

knee with the joint in 10° of flexion (Figure 16.11). The pain produced by this manoeuvre is due to the partial tear of the medial ligament. The lateral aspect of the joint is then palpated, the femoral condyle, the tibial condyle, the lateral joint line and the attachment of the lateral ligament to the lateral condyle of the femur above and to the head of the fibula below, where it is embraced at its insertion by the insertion of the biceps tendon. Tears of the lateral ligament are unusual except following severe violence, but similarly the integrity of the ligament may be checked by flexing the knee to 10° and applying a varus strain. Tenderness over the lateral aspect of the medial femoral condyle in the semi-flexed position may indicate an area of osteochondritis dissecans. Also, tenderness over the infrapatellar fat pad would be obvious. Tenderness at the junction of the patella with the ligamentum patellae is usually due to a small prepatellar bursa or to a small tear of the ligament, the so-called 'jumper's knee'. The presence of an infrapatellar bursa will also be obvious over the lower end of the ligamentum patellae.

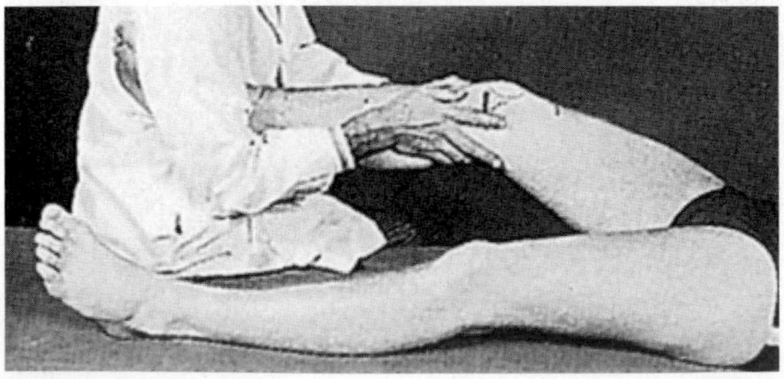

Figure 16.11 Testing the integrity of the collateral ligaments with the knee slightly flexed.

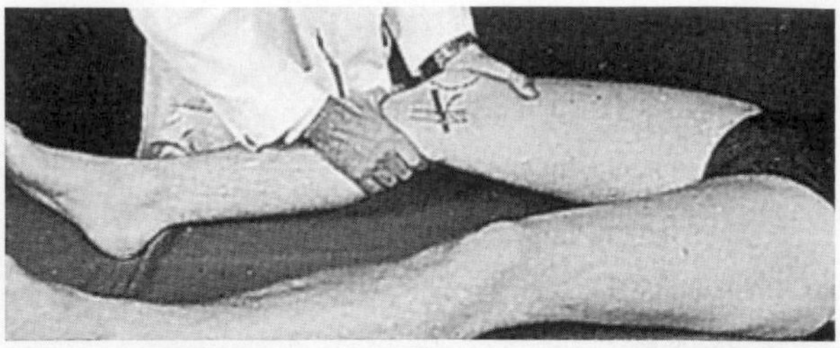

Figure 16.12 The Lachman anterior cruciate ligament test.

The cruciate ligaments are next tested. The anterior cruciate ligament is best tested with the knee flexed to 10° by grasping femur and tibia and attempting to pull the tibia forwards on the femur (Figure 16.12). Called the Lachman test, this is preferable to the anterior 'drawer' test with the knee in 90° of flexion which indicates tearing of the posteromedial capsule as well as a tear of anterior cruciate ligament. The posterior cruciate ligament is tested with the knee in 90° flexion (Figure 16.13). The alignment of the knee in relationship to the femur is noted to see if there is a posterior subluxation of the tibia, the 'sag' sign.

When the tibia is tested for subluxation, an apparent laxity of the anterior cruciate ligament on the anterior drawer sign may be due actually to a posterior ligament tear. In the flexed position the posterior drawer sign usually reveals laxity of the posterior cruciate ligament. It is also valuable at this point to test for medial and lateral rotational instability of the knee. This is carried out by externally rotating the tibia on the femur and performing the anterior drawer test. Movement anteriorly of the medial condyle of the tibia in this position indicates tearing of the posterior component of the ligament and the posterior capsule. The tibia is rotated inwards and drawn forwards to test for posterolateral rotational instability, which indicates a tearing of the posterolateral capsule. A tear of the anterior cruciate ligament producing anterior subluxation of the tibia

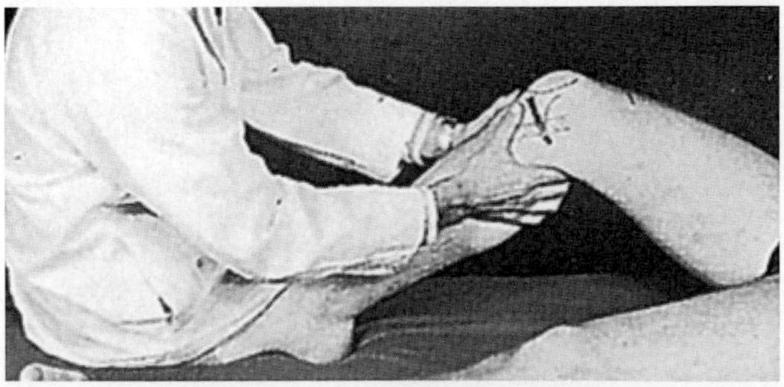

Figure 16.13 The posterior 'drawer' sign for testing posterior cruciate ligament integrity.

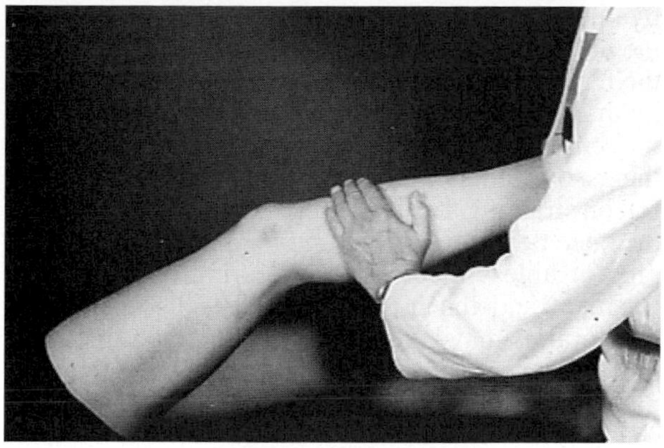

Figure 16.14 The McIntosh 'pivot shift' or 'jerk test'. With the knee fully extended and a valgus force applied the tibial condyle lies anterior to the femoral condyle. Gradual flexion produces relocation of the tibia on the femur with an obvious jerk.

on the femur can best be detected by McIntosh's 'jerk' test. The lower leg is supported by the examiner while a valgus strain is applied as the knee is flexed (Figure 16.14). As the tibia reduces into its correct position on the femur, sliding backwards, a jerk is clearly felt which is due to the reduction process. It is important to note that the tearing of both cruciate ligaments allows valgus and varus movement of the tibia on the femur with the knee completely straight. If either cruciate ligament is intact the knee is stable in full extension from the point of view of valgus and varus.

Rotational testing for meniscus injuries

If the knee is 'locked' in semi-flexion, it is useful to flex it to 90° and then rotate the foot and tibia medially and laterally on the femur. Frequently this produces discomfort on the affected side, lateral rotation causing pain on the medial side and medial rotation pain on the lateral side. On occasions this may be accompanied by a feeling of movement inside the joint or by a palpable 'click' or 'clunk'. The McMurray (1942) test is an extension of this, which is most easily carried out when the joint is slack and locking is not present. The knee joint is fully flexed with the heel placed almost on the buttock (Figure 16.15a). Abduction of the leg and lateral rotation of the foot will bring to bear on the medial semilunar cartilage a strain similar to that which produced the original lesion. With the foot and leg held in this position the leg is extended. If there is a lesion of the cartilage at any point from the level of attachment of the tibial collateral ligament to the posterior horn, a distinct clunk will be produced when the femur passes over the site of injury (Figure 16.15b). A similar procedure can be carried out with the foot now medially rotated. The patient may also complain of a pain or a clunk will be felt, as the leg is extended, over the lateral joint line with a lateral meniscus tear. In some cases simply a grating feeling will be felt on carrying out this manoeuvre, particularly when there is a horizon-tal tear associated with a degenerate meniscus.

The patient is then asked to squat and to walk in the squatting position (Payr's sign). If the meniscus

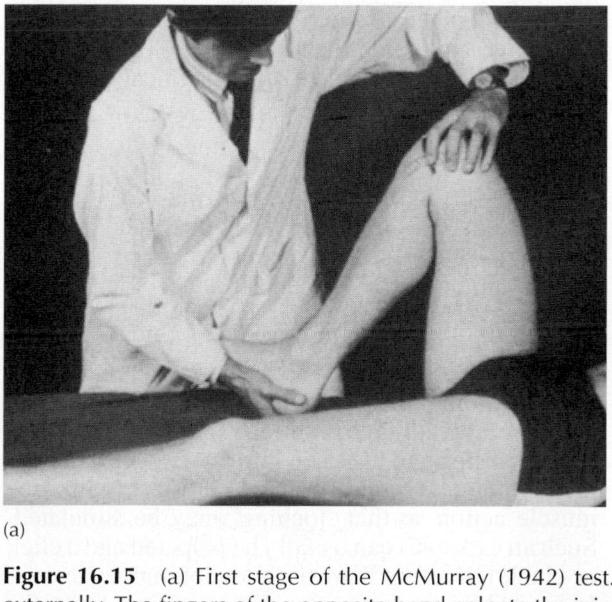

(a)

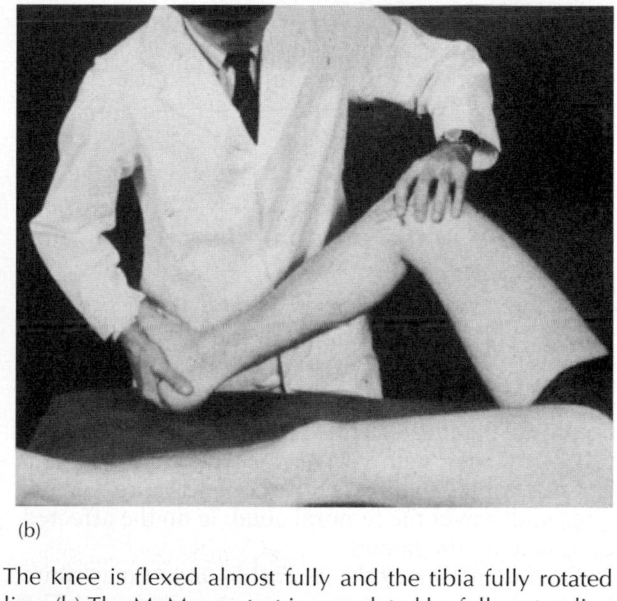

(b)

Figure 16.15 (a) First stage of the McMurray (1942) test. The knee is flexed almost fully and the tibia fully rotated externally. The fingers of the opposite hand palpate the joint line. (b) The McMurray test is completed by fully extending the knee with the tibia externally rotated. A 'clunk' felt over the joint line indicates a torn meniscus.

is displaced into the joint then full squatting will be impossible or extremely uncomfortable and pain will be felt over the affected side of the joint. It is useful to ask the patient if he can describe any manoeuvre which he carries out to relieve the pain in the joint or to release a locked joint. Any manoeuvre which involves flexion and rotation of the tibia usually indicates a genuine displacement. Finally, it is important to examine the posterior aspect of the joint for any tenderness or abnormal swellings which may be responsible for the symptoms.

RADIOGRAPHIC EXAMINATION

Anteroposterior and lateral radiographs are taken of both knees in the standing position. In addition tangential x-rays are taken of the patella at 30° of flexion. Radiographs of the femoral tunnel are taken to reveal osteochondritis dissecans of the medial femoral condyle or loose bodies. With these routine films it is usually possible to exclude other causes of symptoms. Radiography should eliminate such bony conditions as fracture of the tibial spine, loose bodies, exostoses, osteoarthritis, osteochondritis dissecans and intra-articular fracture. Double-contrast arthrography using contrast medium such as Hypaque is sometimes useful. Arthroscopy is, however, much the more useful procedure and is always performed prior to meniscectomy. A photographic record or videotape recording of the arthroscopic appearances is retained for reference purposes.

Magnetic resonance imaging (MRI) can give excellent images of the cruciate ligaments and menisci in 80–90% of cases but there is a small incidence of false positives for meniscus tears so that arthroscopy is still the most accurate diagnostic procedure, especially for articular cartilage injuries (Figure 16.16).

DIFFERENTIAL DIAGNOSIS

Contusion of the infrapatellar fat pad and plica syndromes

True locking is absent although full extension of the knee may be painful. Where the fat pad has been contused there is frequently tenderness over the pad below the patella. The plica syndrome is more likely to be confused with chondromalacia of the patella but sometimes there is a soft click to be felt as the plica slides over the femoral condyle on the affected side, usually the lateral.

Partial rupture of the medial ligament may quite frequently accompany a tear of the meniscus. The type of injury which causes tearing of the medial ligament is also that which causes the tearing of the medial meniscus. There is tenderness present over the femoral or tibial attachments or in the line of the ligament and there may be terminal restriction of movement as with a meniscus injury. This is due to the associated synovitis and effusion. Pain may be felt on straining the medial ligament into valgus with the knee flexed at 10° but undue mobility will not be present unless there is gross tearing of the medial ligament and the posterior cruciate ligament. The two injuries may well coincide and the trauma itself may not be apparent until examination under anaesthetic and arthroscopy is carried out.

Rupture of the cruciate ligaments

As indicated above, when the anterior cruciate ligament is ruptured, the tibia can be displaced forwards on the knee when it is slightly flexed; in the case of a ruptured posterior cruciate ligament, the tibia can be displaced backwards on the femur with the knee flexed to a right angle. In all these tests a careful comparison should be made with the sound side, especially in female patients who have more natural laxity of the knee ligaments. In cases of doubt, examination with full muscle relaxation under general anaesthesia is needed.

Fracture of the tibial spine

This injury is usually caused by severe violence resulting in detachment of one of the cruciate ligaments from the tibial spine, usually the anterior. Locking, if present, takes the form of a bony block to complete extension. It is important to look carefully for damage to the tibial spine, which may be easily overlooked on the radiographic examination, since it is very amenable to early surgical repair.

Loose bodies

Loose bodies in an otherwise normal knee usually result from osteochondral fractures. The locking produced by a loose body occurs at any point of the knee cycle of movement and it is accompanied by severe pain. Usually the pain is episodic and passes in a few minutes as the loose body disengages. The patient may also report a loose body which he feels moving around the joint. In most cases the radiograph will reveal the condition.

An exostosis at the knee joint, particularly on the medial femoral condyle, may interfere with free muscle action so that 'locking' may be simulated. Such an exostosis can usually be palpated and a click or clunk felt as the hamstring tendon moves over it. It is visible on the radiographs, arising from the metaphyseal portion of the bone.

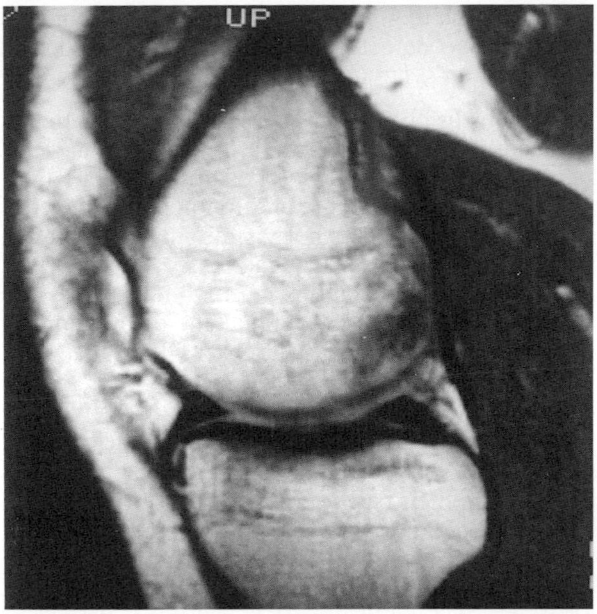

(a)

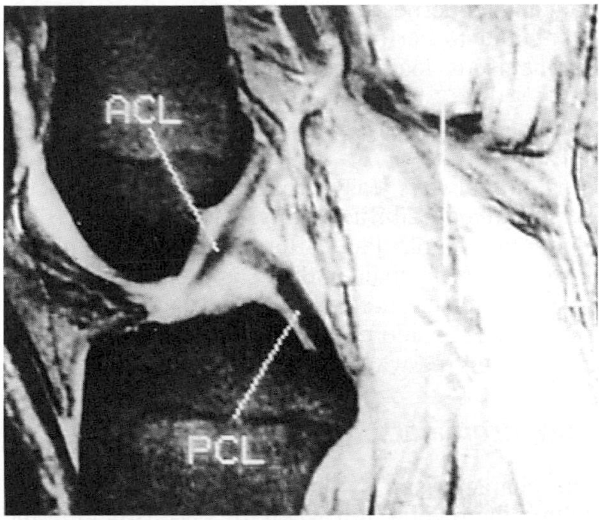

(b)

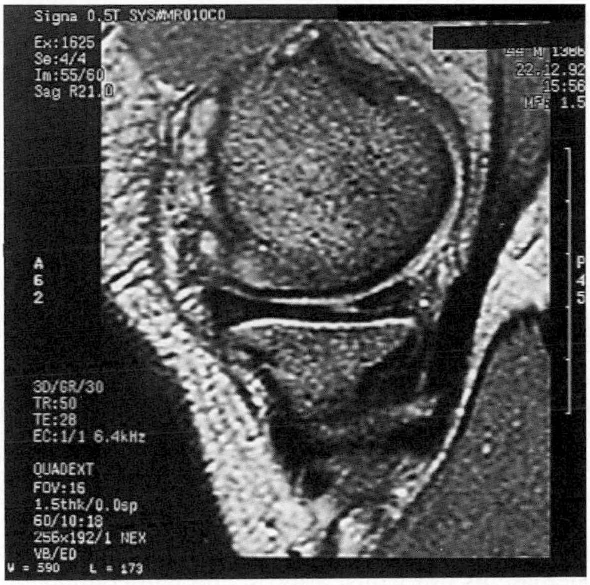

(c)

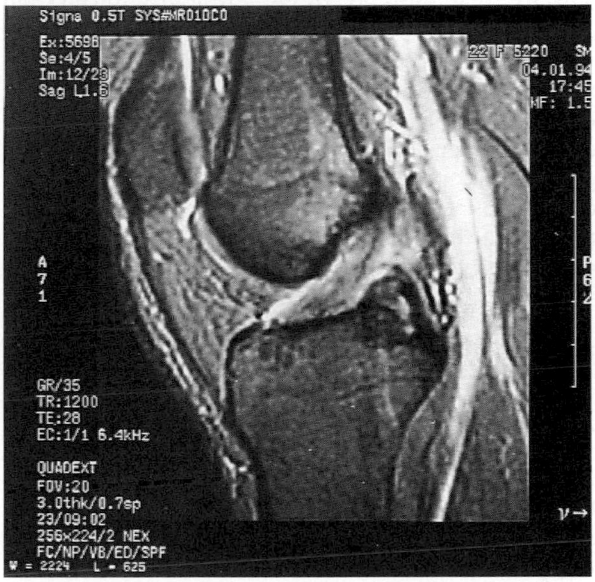

(d)

Figure 16.16 Magnetic resonance imaging of the knee. (a) Wedge-shaped sections of the menisci and (b) the anterior cruciate (ACL) and posterior cruciate ligaments are clearly seen. (Reproduced, with permission, from Stoller, D.W. (1991) in *Knee Surgery – Current Practice*. Edited by P. Aichroth, W.D. Cannon and D.P. Patel. Martin Dunitz: London) (c) A tear of the posterior horn of the medial meniscus clearly seen on MR scanning. (Films kindly supplied by Dr Richard Blaquiere, Consultant Radiologist at Southampton University Hospitals) (d) The anterior cruciate ligament in this patient is clearly abnormal with loss of signal and non-homogeneity of the ligament on MRI. Other sections showed a complete rupture. (Films kindly supplied by Dr Richard Blaquiere, Consultant Radiologist at Southampton University Hospitals)

Osteoarthritis

Here the onset is gradual with pain, stiffness and grating felt in the joint. These may be accompanied by tenderness due to synovial inflammation but generally tenderness is diffuse and the lipping of the articular margins can be recognized in the patient together with the crepitus from the joint surfaces on movement. Diagnosis is obvious from the radiographs. It is important to note that degenerative tears of the meniscus may arise in patients with osteoarthritis, but removal of these should be avoided unless severe locking occurs or there is marked focal pain and tenderness over the joint line. In such cases it is better to perform arthroscopic debridement of the meniscus, leaving a peripheral rim *in situ*.

Recurrent dislocation of the patella

It is not always easy from the history alone to exclude the possibility of this lesion. The joint is not tender but the patella is often smaller in size, placed higher than normal, and the apprehension test is positive (see Figure 16.46). The diagnosis should always be considered in female patients who complain of 'giving way' of the knee.

Chondromalacia patellae

The characteristic symptoms are pain and aching behind the patella, felt when the knee is held in the flexed position for a period of time and relieved by activity. It is unlikely to be confused with internal derangement of the knee. However, the synovitis which results from chondromalacia of the patella may cause an erroneous diagnosis of torn meniscus due to tenderness over the joint line. The patient will exhibit tenderness on the medial undersurface of the patella and possibly a small effusion as well as quadriceps wasting. Such knees should always undergo arthroscopy before any decision is made to carry out a meniscectomy.

INVESTIGATIONS

Radiographs

Anteroposterior and lateral radiographs should be taken in all cases to exclude an avulsion of the tibial spine or an osteochondral fracture with a loose fragment in the joint.

Arthroscopy

The indications for arthroscopy are:

1. Confirmation of clinical diagnosis (Jackson and Dandy, 1976).
2. Doubtful diagnosis, especially in women.
3. Therapeutic procedures (removal of menisci, loose bodies and repair of menisci and cruciate ligaments.
4. Early diagnosis of acute injury.
5. Detection of chondral defects.
6. As a diagnostic procedure (biopsy of synovium, rheumatoid or gouty arthritis).
7. Research (e.g. study of the natural evolution of articular defects, influence of intra-articular drugs on synovium).

The main disadvantages of arthroscopy are that it demands expertise (20–30 arthroscopies at least personally performed). The posterior cruciate ligament is not easily visible and the posterior horn of the medial meniscus is not visible in 10% of cases, which can result in false negatives.

However, complications are extremely rare, e.g. infection (less than 0.1%), breakage of instruments within the joint and haemarthrosis have been recorded.

False positives and false negatives can obviously be reduced with increasing experience. Jackson and Abe (1972) had 4.1% false negatives and false positives in their early series but missed injuries in experienced hands are very rare. In contrast to this, arthrograms in the same series were inaccurate in 31.8% of patients and have few applications today. However, it should be emphasized that arthroscopy does not replace the clinical examination and examination under anaesthesia which is extremely important in the diagnosis of cruciate ligament injuries and patellar instability (Dowd and Bentley, 1986).

Magnetic resonance imaging (MRI)

The MRI scan is becoming established as the most valuable non-invasive investigation for knee disorders. The menisci, cruciate ligaments, fat pads and plicae can be demonstrated with accuracy approaching that of arthroscopy but the assessment of articular cartilage defects is less reliable. MRI is especially accurate in revealing posterior horn tears of the medial meniscus which can be difficult to see arthroscopically and for visualizing the posterior cruciate ligament which is only partially accessible arthroscopically (see Figure 16.16). In future, the relative cost of MRI is likely to fall which will increase its use whilst arthroscopy will continue to be important where an operative arthroscopic procedure is likely to be required under the same anaesthetic.

DIAGNOSTIC PROBLEMS

Diagnostic problems have been greatly reduced with the use of arthroscopy and MRI. The major problem in the acutely injured knee is to assess the extent of damage to all structures because of bleeding but EUA (examination under anaesthesia) is very valuable. Acute arthroscopy of the knee has, in our view, limited value.

TREATMENT OF MENISCUS INJURIES

Treatment of the acute lesion

It is now generally agreed that forcible manipulation or attempts to reduce the displacement of the meniscus may be harmful to the joint by aggravating the injury to the meniscus or by stretching cruciate ligaments and damaging the articular cartilage. However, if a patient presents with an acute meniscus injury and if careful clinical and radiological examinations exclude any other diagnosis, such as a medial ligament disruption, the knee is placed in a well padded compression bandage and the patient encouraged to carry out quadriceps exercises. The patient is reviewed at 1 week and if the knee is still locked then a gentle flexion and extension of the knee under general anaesthetic is performed. Usually the administration of the anaesthetic and the consequent muscle relaxation allows the meniscus to reduce and the knee will fully extend. No force is employed and if the knee remains locked arthroscopy is performed and, if necessary, immediate meniscectomy. Full assessment of the collateral and cruciate ligaments is also performed.

After the general anaesthetic, the knee is placed in a compression bandage of wool and crepe and the patient commences isometric quadriceps exercises, weight-bearing as much as possible. If possible he attends physiotherapy three times a week for reinforcement of this discipline but must carry out the isometric quadriceps exercises regularly for four 15-minute periods each day.

After 2 weeks mobilization of the knee is commenced; if the patient is asymptomatic he is simply reviewed in the out-patient clinic at intervals. Arthroscopy is carried out at approximately 1 month after the acute injury, to clarify the diagnosis in doubtful cases.

Treatment of the late case

Frequently patients present at a later stage with a definite history of twisting injury of the knee, the gradual development of an effusion with inability to straighten the knee and pain over the medial joint aspect. By the time the patient is reviewed the history is one of ability to carry out many activities but not to twist the knee without pain, giving way or even locking on the medial side of the joint. Such patients are admitted as soon as possible for arthroscopy and meniscectomy. There is some doubt that a torn meniscus always requires removal, and with the knowledge that 20% of patients over a period of 25 years who underwent total meniscectomy developed osteoarthritis of the knee (Jackson, 1967), partial meniscectomy appears to be preferable.

Jackson and Dandy (1976), from a prospective 5-year study, proposed the criteria for partial meniscectomy as being cases with a vertical bucket-handle tear but in whom the peripheral rim, ligaments and capsule are intact or cases in which the flap tear occupies less than one-third of the total area of the meniscus.

McGinty *et al.* (1977) studied a group of 136 patients with meniscus injuries, with a short follow-up of average 5 years. They performed partial meniscectomies in bucket-handle and flap tears, and total meniscectomy in others. Short-term results were good in the partial group with a shorter hospital stay, fewer complications and less time on crutches postoperatively. At follow-up in all of the knees with partial meniscectomy there was a good result, but only 73% of knees were classified good after total meniscectomy. x-Ray degenerative changes were twice as common in the group who had had total meniscectomy, although this was not correlated fully with symptoms. Dandy (1978) also reported excellent results with arthroscopic partial meniscectomy.

It is now apparent that the approach to the torn meniscus should be much more conservative than was previously the case. The relatively high incidence of osteoarthritis following total meniscectomy suggests that partial meniscectomy is a preferable procedure but there are no long-term studies that actually support this view. The meniscus remnant remodels so that it assumes the shape of the original in most young knees but partial meniscectomy does not allow the regeneration of a replica fibrocartilage, as occurs following total meniscectomy, due to the avascularity of the body of the meniscus. Time will demonstrate which is best for the joint in the long term.

It is our custom to carry out partial meniscectomy arthroscopically and to remove only that part of the meniscus which is torn. It seems unlikely that this can be worse for the knee joint than total meniscectomy and the recovery of the patient from the operation is much more rapid due to the absence of the haemarthrosis which follows total meniscectomy.

Treatment of meniscus injuries can no longer be separated from total assessment of the injured knee since the injured meniscus may be only part of a complex of soft tissue injuries. Twenty years ago O'Donoghue (1973a,b) described the triad of torn meniscus, tear of the medial ligament and tear of the anterior cruciate ligament as the logical result of a medial rotation of the femur on the fixed tibia with the knee flexed. Although the details of injuries have been refined, the injured knee demands a thorough assessment based on history, physical signs, special investigations, examination under anaesthetic and arthroscopy to ensure that as few mistakes are made as possible.

In the acute case the management above takes account of the need to avoid precipitant action since assessment and acute meniscectomy of the knee early after injury is often difficult due to the presence of haemarthrosis, inflamed tissues or both. Thus, wherever possible, surgical treatment should be performed after 2–3 weeks when the acute inflammatory response has subsided. At this stage assessment of the knee by examination under anaesthetic and arthroscopy is relatively straightforward.

Examination under anaesthetic

This involves an assessment of collateral and cruciate instability and additional capsular damage. The collateral ligaments are best evaluated with the knee flexed at 10° and the anterior and posterior cruciates by the Lachman test at 10°. The 'pivot shift' or 'jerk' test is frequently only present under anaesthetic when the muscles are relaxed and is a strong indication for anterior cruciate ligament reconstruction. Rotational stability of the knee can also be assessed as indicated above. Finally, the stability of the patella should be assessed. Patellar instability only requires treatment when the patella can be locked over the margin of the lateral femoral condyle (Dowd and Bentley, 1986).

Arthroscopy

Arthroscopy is carried out through a standard lateral portal (Bentley and Fogg, 1991). The intra-articular structures are examined in turn. In the case of suspected torn meniscus it is vital to achieve a good view and general anaesthetic is best to achieve full relaxation. With care the whole of the lateral meniscus can be seen and most of the medial meniscus. Where access to the posterior horn is difficult the stability of the meniscus can be established by use of a hook placed over the meniscus. Probing beneath the meniscus is necessary to exclude a horizontal cleavage tear. Removal of such a damaged segment of the meniscus alone is all that is required (Stother, 1991) and this is achieved by instruments placed through one or more medial portals, the whole procedure being performed by direct visualization on the attached television camera and monitor (Figure 16.17). Rarely it is necessary to extend one of the portals to remove a large fragment but formal open meniscectomy is now no longer required. Where arthroscopic facilities are not available, formal arthrotomy can be performed but the rehabilitation programme takes much longer because the pain and reflex muscle inhibition produced by arthrotomy is far greater. Tears in the outer one-third or peripheral detachments are treated by repair following the 'inside-out' technique of Jackson and Kinkel (1991).

Postoperative management

Following removal of a meniscus fragment arthroscopically the patient experiences little pain whether or not bupivacaine (Marcain) is placed in the joint. The portals are closed with adhesive 'Steristrips' and a compression bandage of wool and crepe is applied from mid-calf to mid-thigh. Isometric quadriceps exercises commence as soon as consciousness is regained and the patient walks fully weight-bearing when comfortable, normally within 12 hours. It is important to perform isometric quadriceps exercises for four 10-minute periods during each day. After removal of the bandage at 24 hours and the Steristrips at 10 days, normal activities are allowed provided there is no effusion or pain, though sport should be curtailed for 6 weeks.

Prognosis after meniscectomy and incidence of OA

Many thousands of patients undergo meniscectomy but the incidence of osteoarthritis in patients who have previously undergone meniscectomy is small. Following the original observation by Fairbank in 1948, Jackson and Waugh (1967) reported an incidence of 20% over 25 years after total medial meniscectomy. This has recently been questioned by work in the author's unit (Reissis *et al.*, 1991) which showed that the incidence was no higher than that occurring in the average population at the age group reviewed and that, contrary to previous work, the incidence of osteoarthritis was related to delay in removal of the torn meniscus beyond 6 months.

No comparable data on the long-term results of partial arthroscopic meniscectomy exist but clinical experience thus far suggests that the incidence of late osteoarthritis is low.

The 'degenerate' meniscus

With ageing the structural integrity of the meniscus deteriorates so that tears may occur spontaneously or as a result of abrasion by the roughened articular cartilage of femur and tibia. The tears are not the longitudinal long tears caused by forcible splitting of the collagenous bands in the young knee, but short irregular tears which may be multiple so that the

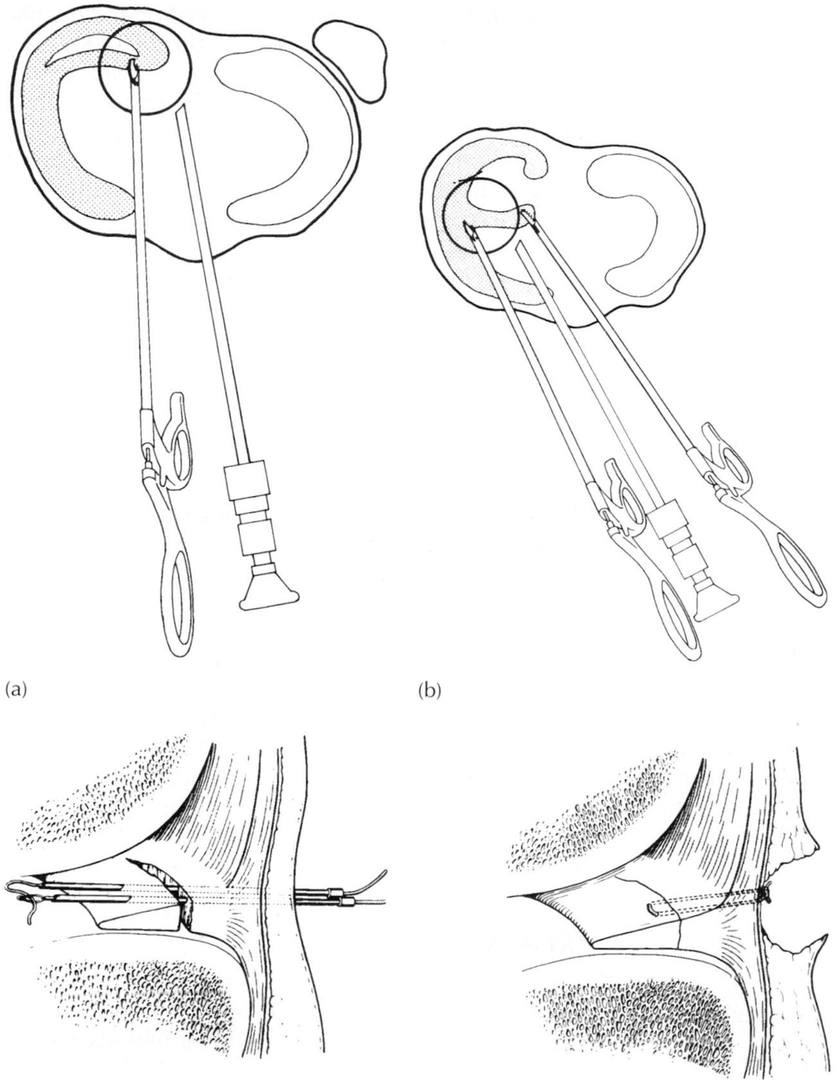

(a) (b) (c)

Figure 16.17 Arthroscopic removal and repair of the medial meniscus. (a) First the posterior end of the torn segment is divided with scissors. (b) The free end is then grasped whilst division of the anterior end of the torn meniscus is performed. The fragment is drawn from the joint through a slightly enlarged portal. ((a) and (b) (Reproduced, with permission,from Stother, I. (1991) Arthroscopic meniscectomy. In: *Rob & Smith's Operative Orthopaedics.* Edited by G. Bentley and R.B. Greer. Butterworth Heinemann: London, Boston, Sydney, Wellington, Singapore) (c) Repair of a peripheral one-third tear. (Reproduced, with permission, from Jackson, R.W. and Kinkel, S.S. (1991) In: *Rob & Smith's Operative Surgery: Orthopaedics* Edited by G. Bentley and R.B. Greer. Butterworth Heinemann: London, Boston, Sydney, Wellington, Singapore)

inner edge of the posterior horn is fragmented and fibrillated. Often such tears are asymptomatic (Noble and Hamblen, 1975) but if the patient with early osteoarthritis of the knee has a history of locking, giving way or focal joint line pain, the meniscus is responsible for the symptoms. If tenderness is felt over the joint line then arthroscopy is indicated and trimming of the degenerate meniscus will give gratifying relief of pain and mechanical symptoms. Such conservative treatment of the meniscus together with washout of the cartilage debris in the joint is adequate and total meniscectomy is contraindicated (Jones *et al.*, 1978; Lennox and Bentley, 1991).

Congenital discoid meniscus

Congenital discoid menisci are more liable to injury than a normal meniscus. In 10 000 cases Smillie (1978) recorded 7 discoid medial menisci and 467 discoid lateral menisci. The condition was previously thought to be an atavism but embryological studies of Kaplan (1955) have confirmed that the menisci show evidence of their adult shape when they first appear and that the discoid meniscus is a true congenital malformation. In an autopsy study, Noble (1977) found a 7% incidence of discoid lateral meniscus and implied that these are not always symptomatic.

CLINICAL FEATURES

The most characteristic sign of a discoid meniscus is undoubtedly the loud click or clunk, which is felt and heard when the knee joint is flexed or extended. This usually occurs in the first 30° of flexion and may be accompanied by pain on the other side of the joint and a feeling of weakness. Locking is most uncommon.

The condition frequently presents in early childhood but the diagnosis should be considered in all young patients reporting a loud clunk from the knee as the majority of cases in the literature have presented before the age of 18. The diagnosis is best confirmed by arthroscopy. Parental pressure to remove the meniscus must be resisted since symptoms and signs frequently subside over the course of a year. Only in very troublesome cases should the meniscus be removed.

Cysts of the meniscus

Cystic swellings in relation to the lateral meniscus are not uncommon. Only rarely are they seen in association with the medial meniscus. Although they often appear to follow an injury, their aetiology is disputed.

PATHOLOGY

Cysts of the menisci vary is size, are sometimes multiloculated and are usually situated on the peripheral aspect of the meniscus (Figure 16.18). The larger cysts possess a fibrous tissue wall which may or may not be lined by flattened cells. The origin and nature of these cells is disputed. Ollerenshaw originally thought them endothelial in nature, but other workers, notably King (1940), believed they were compressed synovial cells. They contain a thick mucoid meniscus resembling that found in ganglia, and indeed they may be regarded as comparable lesions. Cysts are often multiple but appear to occur in some cases as a solitary swelling associated with a longitudinal tear of the meniscus (Glasgow *et al.*, 1993).

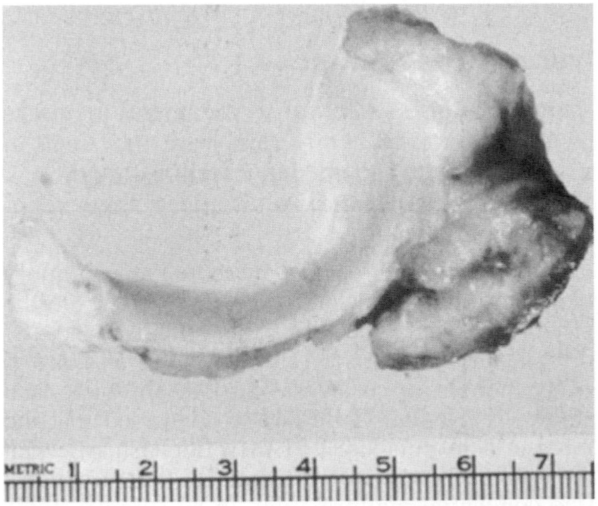

Figure 16.18 Lateral meniscus with a large cyst involving the posterior third extending outwards in a multilocular swelling.

CLINICAL FEATURES

The patient complains of aching pain and swelling usually on the outer side of the knee. In some there is a history of trauma in the past. The swelling is usually small and tense but may be fluctuant. The characteristic sign is that the swelling becomes more prominent when the knee is flexed at 45–50° but disappears in full flexion and full extension. Thus it is often missed (Figure 16.19). Tenderness is not always present. There may be symptoms and signs of an associated meniscal tear, particularly pain felt over the joint line on rotating the tibia or the femur. The doubtful case is often clarified by an MRI scan.

TREATMENT

It has been recommended in the past that the meniscus should be excised together with its related

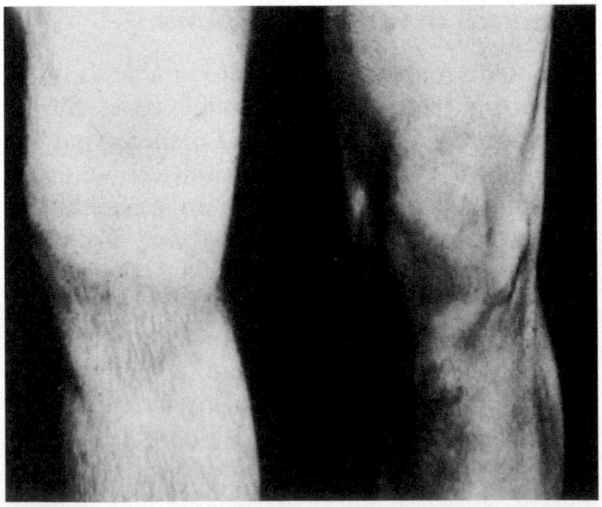

Figure 16.19 Photograph to show the lateral meniscus cyst present at 45–90° of flexion of the knee.

cysts. Local excision of the cyst may be followed by recurrence, and coexistent tears of the meniscus have been reported in 50% of cases.

Flynn and Kelly (1976) advocated local excision of cysts when there is no associated meniscal tear. In 12 patients no occurrence was seen after mean follow-up of over 7 years. This conservative approach is favoured unless the symptoms are severe and a tear of the meniscus is clearly demonstrable on arthroscopy.

Glasgow *et al.* (1993) reported that the cyst was, in their experience, frequently associated with a horizontal tear of the lateral meniscus and due to leakage of synovial fluid, from the joint through a tear, which became closed off (Figure 16.20). They therefore advocated opening the communication between the horizontal tear and the cyst after removing the former and thus draining the cyst into the joint by arthroscopy with a blunt-ended instrument such as a closed punch. They reported success in 62 of 72 patients.

In some cases there appears to have been a truly congenital cystic meniscus with multiple cysts and in these cases repeated meniscal tears occur. They can be treated by arthroscopic trimming and decompression initially but if they recur total meniscectomy is needed.

Ligamentous injuries of the knee

Injury to a knee ligament may be partial or complete. A *partial* tear (strain or sprain) of the medial collateral ligament can occur in isolation and is very painful. The stability of the ligament is undamaged and the treatment is pain relief and rehabilitation. Temporary splintage with a cylinder cast with full weight-bearing activity may be helpful for 2 weeks at the outset.

Complete tears of knee ligaments rarely occur in isolation since the knee is supported by the capsule, the collateral and cruciate ligaments and reinforcement from surrounding muscles as a complex whole. The most common serious injury is produced by internal rotation of the femur on the tibia combined with a valgus force. This produces some or all of the 'unhappy triad' of O'Donoghue (1955) of tears of the medial ligament, medial meniscus and ACL.

The major problem is accurate diagnosis since outcome is determined by the early diagnosis and treatment. In general the treatment of chronic instability is less good than acute treatment but experience has shown that certain injuries (e.g. medial ligament rupture) do very well with aspiration of the haemarthrosis and rapid rehabilitation alone (Mok, 1989), whereas the appropriate surgery for others (e.g. ACL rupture) is sometimes best delayed and then determined by the requirements of the patient.

DIAGNOSIS

It is important to take a careful history to determine, if possible, the mechanism of injury, and whether the patient was bearing weight on the affected limb. The onset of swelling is noted, whether it be immediate, as with a haemarthrosis, or delayed, as with an effusion associated with a meniscus injury. The site

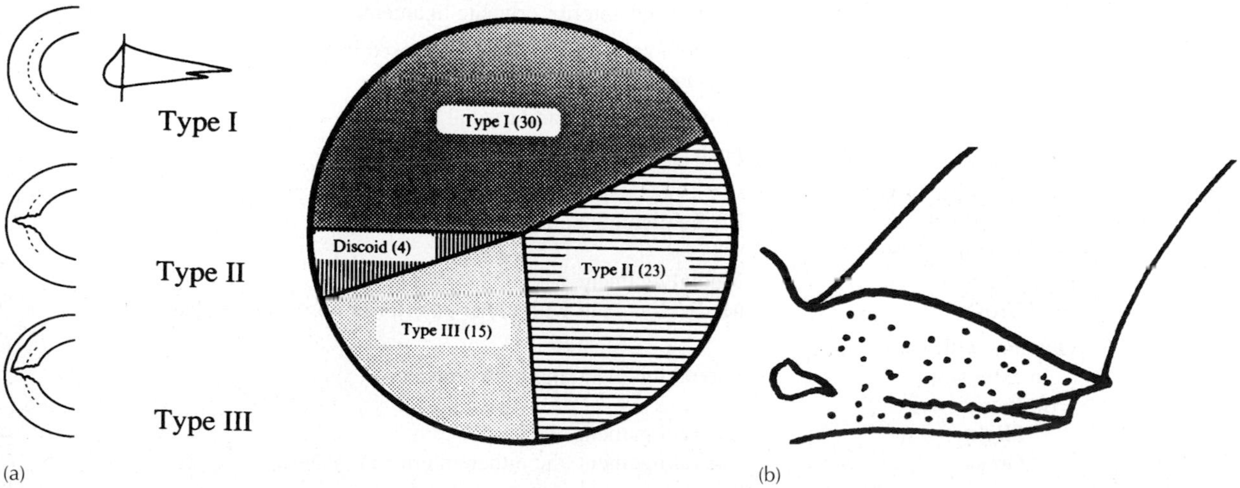

Figure 16.20 (a) Glasgow's classification of cystic lateral menisci. (b) Diagram illustrating the relationship between the cyst and the meniscus tear. (Reproduced, with permission, from Glasgow *et al.* (1993) *Journal of Bone and Joint Surgery* **75B**, 229)

of pain and the presence or absence of locking is noted. In all situations a knowledge of previous injury and treatment is essential.

Examination of the injured knee should include assessment of joint swelling. A complete ligamentous rupture with disruption of the joint capsule allows decompression of the joint with diffuse subcutaneous infiltration of blood and synovial fluid. Palpation of the points of attachment of the collateral ligaments may reveal local tenderness. The range of active joint motion should be measured. There may be a block to full extension when there has been an associated meniscal lesion but haemarthrosis also restricts full movement.

The most important part of the clinical assessment is the system of stress tests for instability (see Figures 16.11–16.14). Before examining the injured knee, the uninjured knee should be examined, provided this has not been subject to previous injury. This will provide a baseline for comparison. A relaxed, co-operative patient is essential. The original description of ligamentous instability by Brantigan and Voshell (1941) still provides a fundamental basis for diagnosis (Table 16.2).

Although most useful examinations of the knee are in the 10–20° flexed position, it must be remembered that with severe injuries, especially those involving the posterior cruciate and the posterior capsule, the knee will be unstable when fully extended or even hyperextensible. Therefore, examination of the collateral ligaments should be in slight flexion and extended positions.

Examination under anaesthesia is essential if there is any doubt, and arthroscopy has an important part to play. After washing out the knee thoroughly, careful examination of all the structures with a hook is required to assess stability of the ACL and menisci. The meniscal damage can be treated arthroscopically at this acute stage if it is slight, e.g. bucket-handle tear. The difficulty in evaluation is the masking of a rupture by secondary restraints too strong to be overcome in clinical examination (Butler *et al.*, 1980), especially in the athletic patient.

Valgus stress test

The abduction stress test is positive in extension when there is a posterior cruciate tear as well as the medial ligament. Being positive at 20° of flexion implies a medial collateral tear. See Figures 16.11 and 16.21.

Table 16.2 Assessment of knee ligament injuries

Abnormal movement	Cause
Anterior instability (anterior drawer)	Combined anterior cruciate ligament and posteromedial capsule
Positive Lachman	Anterior cruciate rupture
Posterior instability (posterior drawer)	Posterior cruciate ligament
Anteromedial instability	Medial and anterior cruciate ligaments
Anterolateral instability	Anterior cruciate ligament. Increased by posterolateral capsule disruption
Posteromedial instability	Posterior cruciate and medial ligaments
Posterolateral instability	Posterior cruciate and lateral ligaments
Opening with valgus strain	
In extension	Medial ligament and both cruciates
In flexion	
Slight	Medial ligament
Gross	Medial ligament with either anterior or posterior cruciate
Opening with varus strain	
In extension	Lateral ligament and both cruciates
In flexion	
Slight	Lateral ligament
Gross	Lateral ligament and either anterior or posterior cruciate
Lateral slide subluxation	Medial ligament and both cruciates
Medial slide subluxation	Lateral ligament and both cruciates

Modified from Brantigan and Voshell (1941).

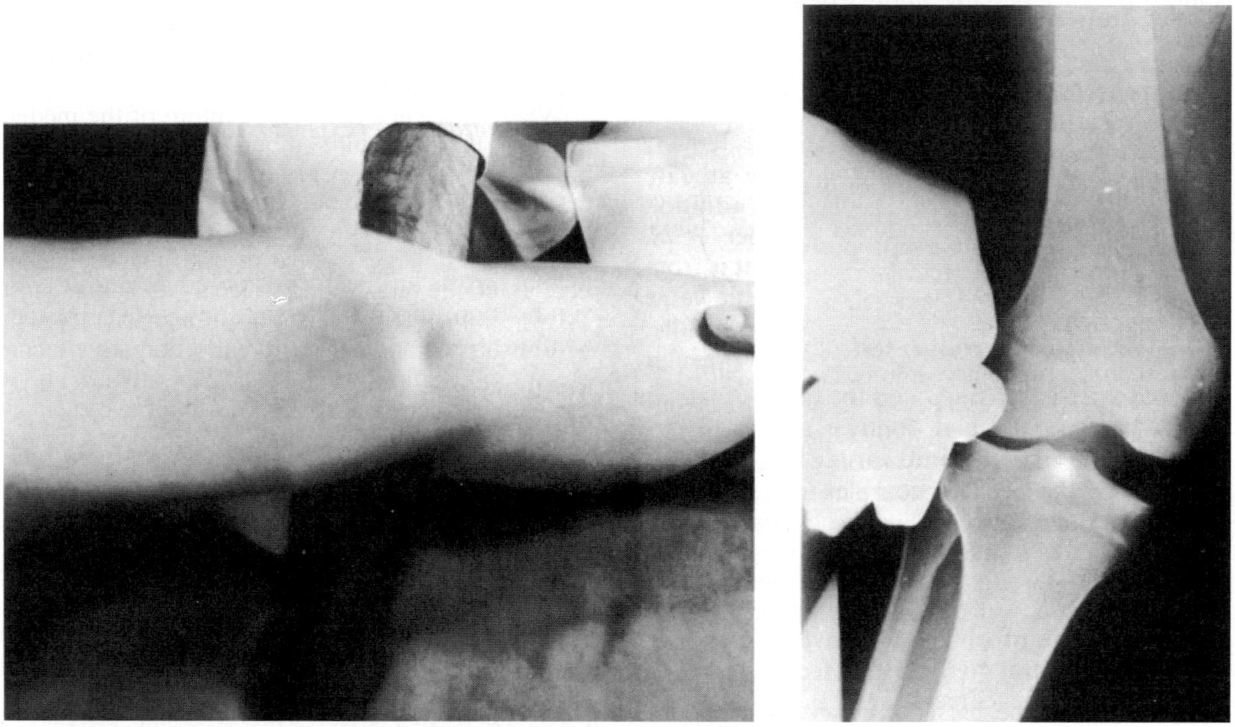

(a) (b)

Figure 16.21 (a) Knee undergoing a valgus stress, showing the dimpling over the medial joint line. (b) Anteroposterior radiograph of same knee showing the gross medial joint instability.

Varus stress test

This is carried out as above but on the lateral side. Instability at 20° flexion indicates a tear of the lateral collateral ligament which is rare in sport and is usually associated with severe trauma, e.g. pedestrian road traffic accident.

Cruciate ligament tests

The Lachman test (see Figure 16.12) is the best indicator of ACL rupture alone. The anterior cruciate ligament is tested with the knee flexed to 10° by grasping femur and tibia and attempting to pull the tibia forwards on the femur. The Lachman test is preferable to the anterior 'drawer' test with the knee in 90° of flexion which indicates tearing of the posteromedial capsule as well as a tear of anterior cruciate ligament. A tear of the anterior cruciate ligament producing anterior subluxation of the tibia on the femur can best be detected by MacIntosh's 'jerk' test or lateral pivot shift (Galway and MacIntosh, 1980). The lower leg is supported by the examiner in full extension while a valgus strain is applied as the knee is flexed. As the tibia reduces into its correct position on the femur, sliding backwards, a jerk is clearly felt which is due to the reduction process (see Figure 16.14).

The posterior cruciate ligament is tested with the knee in 90° flexion (see Figure 16.13). The alignment of the knee in relationship to the femur is noted to see if there is a posterior subluxation of the tibia, the 'sag' sign.

When the tibia is tested for subluxation, an apparent laxity of the anterior cruciate ligament on the anterior drawer sign may actually be due to a posterior cruciate ligament tear. In the flexed position the posterior drawer sign usually reveals laxity of the posterior cruciate ligament. It is also valuable at this point to test for medial and lateral rotational instability of the knee. This is carried out by externally rotating the tibia on the femur and performing the anterior drawer test. Movement anteriorly of the medial condyle of the tibia in this position indicates tearing of the posterior component of the ligament and the posterior capsule. The tibia is rotated inwards to test for posterolateral rotational instability, which indicates a tearing of the posterolateral capsule. It is important to note that the tearing of both cruciate ligaments allows valgus and varus movement of the tibia on the femur with the knee completely straight. If either cruciate ligament is intact the knee is stable in full extension from the point of view of valgus and varus.

External rotation – recurvatum test

The flexed knee is extended and the tibia externally rotated, the lateral tibial condyle subluxes posteriorly and the knee goes into varus which indicates disruption of the arcuate complex – posterolateral rotatory instability.

Arthroscopy

Arthroscopy of the acutely injured knee is controversial because the presence of haemarthrosis and inflammation of the soft tissues means that very abundant and persistent washout is required to provide a satisfactory view of the internal structures. Also, there is a risk of inducing acute posterior calf compression syndrome through loss of large quantities of saline through the damaged joint capsule. However, with proper technique it can be useful in providing:

1. Important information which may modify approach, e.g. the presence of an osteochondral fracture.
2. Definition of precise meniscal pathology.
3. Definition of isolated anterior cruciate tear.
4. Avulsion of one or other end of the anterior cruciate ligament which can be repaired immediately.

Radiography

Standard anteroposterior and lateral views should be taken, but these will usually show no abnormality unless there is an associated fracture. Stress films yield more information than can be obtained from physical examination but may be painful unless they are performed under anaesthesia. One unusual indication for stress x-rays is the young patient with open epiphyses whose knee is unstable on examination. Stress films will show whether the instability is occurring at the epiphyseal plate or at the joint line.

TREATMENT

Medial collateral ligament

A sprain of the medial collateral ligament with tenderness over either the ligament or its long attachments and pain on valgus testing should be treated conservatively. Support in a light cylinder cast reinforced with 'Scotchcast' for 2 weeks, followed by mobilization and physiotherapy for quadriceps and hamstrings, will usually result in a complete recovery in 6–8 weeks. If a haemarthrosis is present, aspiration will allow more rapid relief of pain and mobilization.

Where there is a complete rupture of the medial ligament this is usually associated with an anterior cruciate ligament injury and often a medial meniscus tear. Careful examination under anaesthesia is required in any knee with a history of severe rotational injury and a large haemarthrosis. The treatment here is controversial since recent studies suggest (Mok, 1989) that mobilization in a cast-brace will give results comparable with early operative repair or immobilization in a cast. Nevertheless it is preferable to perform arthroscopy to relieve haemarthrosis and examine the interior of the knee. When there is severe disruption of the medial structures they are explored and repaired as far as possible although often they are severely shredded. The associated ACL tear is not treated primarily unless there is avulsion from one or other end and the meniscus is repaired or reattached, when the tear is in the outer third or is a peripheral detachment. Following the repair the leg is rested in a cylinder cast for 3 weeks followed by 3 weeks in a mobilizing brace, after which full mobilization with quadriceps and hamstring exercises follow. The cruciate ligament rupture is repaired secondarily in athletes at 3 weeks and in others depending on the disability following a period of 3 months of conservative treatment.

Posterior oblique ligament

Hughston and Eilers (1973) considered this to be the keystone in the medial side of the joint. The ligament is made up of a thickening of the capsular ligament running from the adductor tubercle to the posterior capsule and posteromedial corner of the tibia. The semimembranosus insertion blends with the posterior oblique ligament, and at 60° of knee flexion, when semimembranosus is contracting, the posterior oblique ligament functions as a dynamic stabilizer of the knee, preventing anteromedial rotatory instability. Hughston and Eilers reported good results following repair. This detail in the anatomy is often difficult to identify in the acutely injured knee. If obvious, repair is made with the knee in 30° flexion, involving intra-articular procedures, this ligament and the medial capsular and tibial collateral ligaments.

Lateral collateral ligament

Injuries to the lateral soft tissue supporting structures are less common, as an adduction stress is unusual in sport. Such injuries usually occur from extreme violence such as road traffic accidents. The fibular collateral ligament is seldom torn in isolation and there is usually a combined lesion involving the fibular collateral ligament, lateral capsular ligament and biceps tendon. In addition, the popliteus tendon may be ruptured and sometimes the iliotibial band is torn. Furthermore, there may be injury to the lateral popliteal nerve – either a traction lesion, or, rarely, a complete disruption of the nerve.

Surgical exploration is indicated. The ligamentous structures are repaired and the lesion of the nerve dealt with according to the findings. Postoperative management follows the programme outlined for medial collateral ligament ruptures. Unfortunately, the results of treatment of the nerve lesion are often disappointing.

Posterior cruciate ligament

This is often an isolated injury classically caused by high velocity trauma with posterior dislocation of the tibia on a flexed knee as in a 'dashboard' impact in a motor car. Trickey (1968) described 17 cases with avulsion from the tibia treated by direct repair using either a screw if a bony fragment was involved or suture. However, when the part of a major injury involving the posterior capsule and other structures, as in a dislocation of the knee, it is often associated with neurovascular complications.

Posterior cruciate injuries often present late so that treatment is uncertain. It is vital to exclude an avulsion of the ligament from its bony attachment to the posterior tibial plateau on the lateral radiograph early because it is relatively simple to reattach surgically in the acute stage but very difficult after 3 weeks.

Treatment of chronic posterior cruciate ligament rupture is debated because some reports (Dandy and Pusey, 1981) considered that no disability results from its loss with no incidence of osteoarthritis. Others have challenged this view and it appears that the patient's demands on the knee determine the presence or absence of symptoms. No repair, be it by use of autologous or artificial materials, appears to be totally satisfactory and therefore surgical reconstruction is avoided unless the patient is athletic or disabled. In the latter case repair by use of the middle third of the patellar tendon is employed but the results are usually imperfect.

Anterior cruciate ligament

Reconstruction of the anterior cruciate ligament employing a portion of the patellar tendon has been demonstrated in numerous series to be a valuable procedure which abolishes instability and improves performance in 90% or more of patients over a 5-year period compared with no treatment (Jones, 1970; McDaniel and Dameron, 1980; Shelbourne *et al.*, 1990). Great motivation is required to build up the quadriceps and hamstring control following the operation so that only the most active individuals return to a pre-injury performance but the great majority find the relief of instability a great bonus. This also applies in knees with early degenerative changes although the knee rarely feels normal to the patient. Shortening of the period of immobility after operation and adoption of the fully extended knee to avoid fixed flexion deformity and the 'cyclops' lesion have also greatly improved results. In general, however, it is wise to avoid violent physical activity for 1 year after the repair which also appears to diminish the incidence of anterior knee pain. The earlier series using the 'over the top' technique for fixation of the replacement ligament to the femur were satisfactory but the use of a bony attachment in the 'isometric' position in the femoral condyle as well as in the tibia appears to be advantageous and allows earlier mobilization. The role of an additional extra-articular McIntosh tenodesis is debated though in high-demand patients with very slack knees this is employed also. The value of arthroscopic placement of the neoligament is not convincing whether using a patellar tendon repair, semitendinous or other tendon repair (Cho, 1975), but the reduced exposure speeds the early rehabilitation. In general, the surgery of anterior cruciate ligament and associated injuries has become more conservative and emphasis has shifted to rapid rehabilitation of the knee and the encouragement of proprioceptive recovery that appears to occur. Recent studies on proprioception show that knee proprioception is improved by ACL substitution using patellar tendon (Barrett *et al.*, 1991, 1992).

Anterolateral instability

Although this can occur as an acute phenomenon, most commonly it is a late development of progressive decompensation of other ligamentous supports in the anterior-cruciate-deficient knee. It is the most common form of disability in the athlete, and is associated with a high incidence of medial and lateral meniscus lesions. The patient gives a history of a twisting injury associated with haemarthrosis and inability to continue sport. The individual may recover to the extent of being able to run in a straight line but any attempt to twist or alter direction causes a feeling of the joint being unstable and the knee will 'give way'. The routine examination may show a small effusion with some tenderness over one or both joint lines, indicating a meniscus injury. The Lachman test is positive but the pivot shift test may only be obvious under the full relaxation of a general anaesthetic. Radiographs are usually non-contributory.

MRI scan may show a damaged anterior cruciate ligament but frequently is unnecessary since arthroscopy is required anyway. Diagnosis is by examination under anaesthetic and should always be accompanied by arthroscopy to assess the state of the anterior cruciate ligament and the menisci.

Treatment of anterolateral instability is dependent on the precise pathology but is usually reconstruction of the anterior cruciate ligament. Although Trickey and Patterson (1983) reported good relief of symptoms from meniscectomy where this coexisted for 5 years, the majority of patients have later problems and in those with symptomatic instability it is necessary to reconstruct the anterior cruciate ligament.

Jones repair of anterior cruciate ligament

The anterior cruciate ligament can be reconstructed using a strip of fascia lata as described by O'Donoghue (1973b) or, preferably, by the use of the middle third of the patella and quadriceps tendon as described by Jones (1970). A bony tunnel is drilled in the tibia so that the ligament replacement emerges at the site of the tibial attachment of the anterior cruciate ligament in front of the tibial spine. A similar tunnel is made through the lateral condyle of the femur and both ends are secured using interference screws with the knee in 15–20° of flexion and held in internal rotation (Figure 16.22). The use of specially designed jigs such as the Acufex greatly facilitates the placement of the ends of the graft in femur and tibia (Figure 16.23).

Extra-articular reconstruction

Extra-articular reconstructions were developed when intra-articular procedures were complicated by inadequate instrumentation, prolonged rehabilitation and complications such as stiffness, flexion deformity and anterior knee pain. The MacIntosh repair (Galway *et al.*, 1972; MacIntosh and Darby, 1976) was thought to have the advantages of a repair using autologous tissue (fascia lata) in a vascularized bed which avoided the extensive intra-articular assault. Also, by its position it was well placed to control anterior displacement of the lateral tibial condyle and give better support by being placed further away from the centre of rotation. See Figure 16.24.

However, experience has shown that in time such repairs stretch and results deteriorate so that the repair was employed to supplement an intra-articular repair in the athletic patient and only used alone in the more sedentary individual. This procedure also requires precise placement of the repair at the F9 position proximally (Grood *et al.*, 1992) (Figure 16.25). As the technique of reconstruction by the intra-articular route has become refined, the need for extra-articular procedures has declined. This method is recommended for the following indications:

- Children with proven instability and an open growth plate.
- Isolated partial anterior cruciate tears.
- Isolated anterior cruciate ligament tear in the non-athlete.
- ? Knees with less convex lateral tibial plateaux.

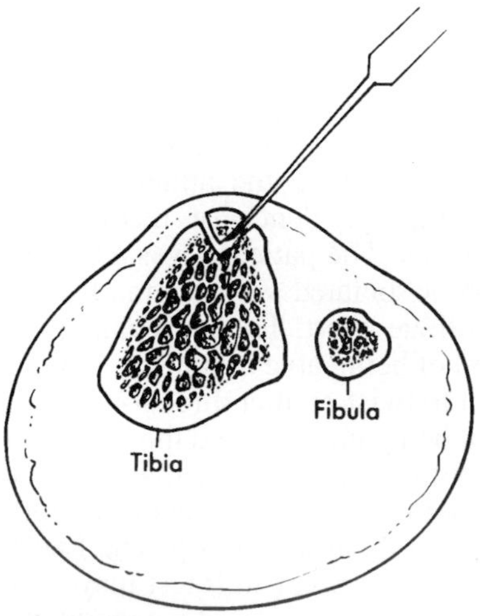

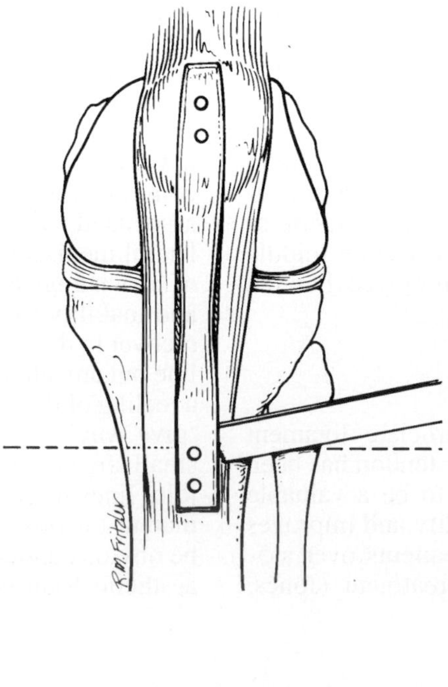

Figure 16.22 Diagram to show the taking of the middle third of the patellar tendon as a cruciate ligament replacement secured at each end by the bone blocks in tibial and femoral condyles. (Reproduced, with permission, from Crenshaw, A.H. (ed.) (1992) *Campbell's Operative Orthopaedics*, 8th edn, p. 1633. Mosby Year Book: St Louis)

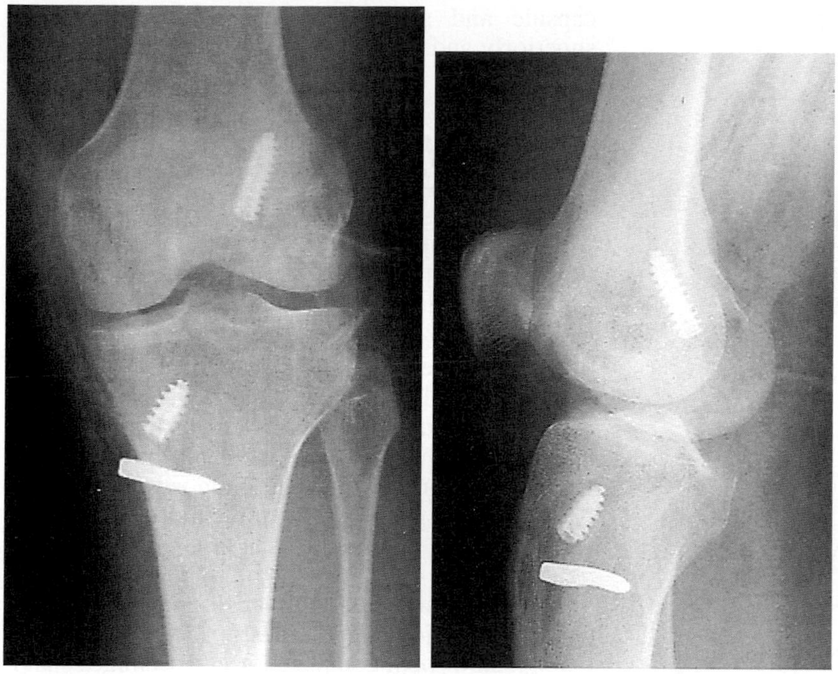

(a) (b)

Figure 16.23 (a) Anteroposterior and (b) lateral radiographs showing the fixation of the bone-patellar tendon – bone autograft fixed by interference screws in the femur and tibia.

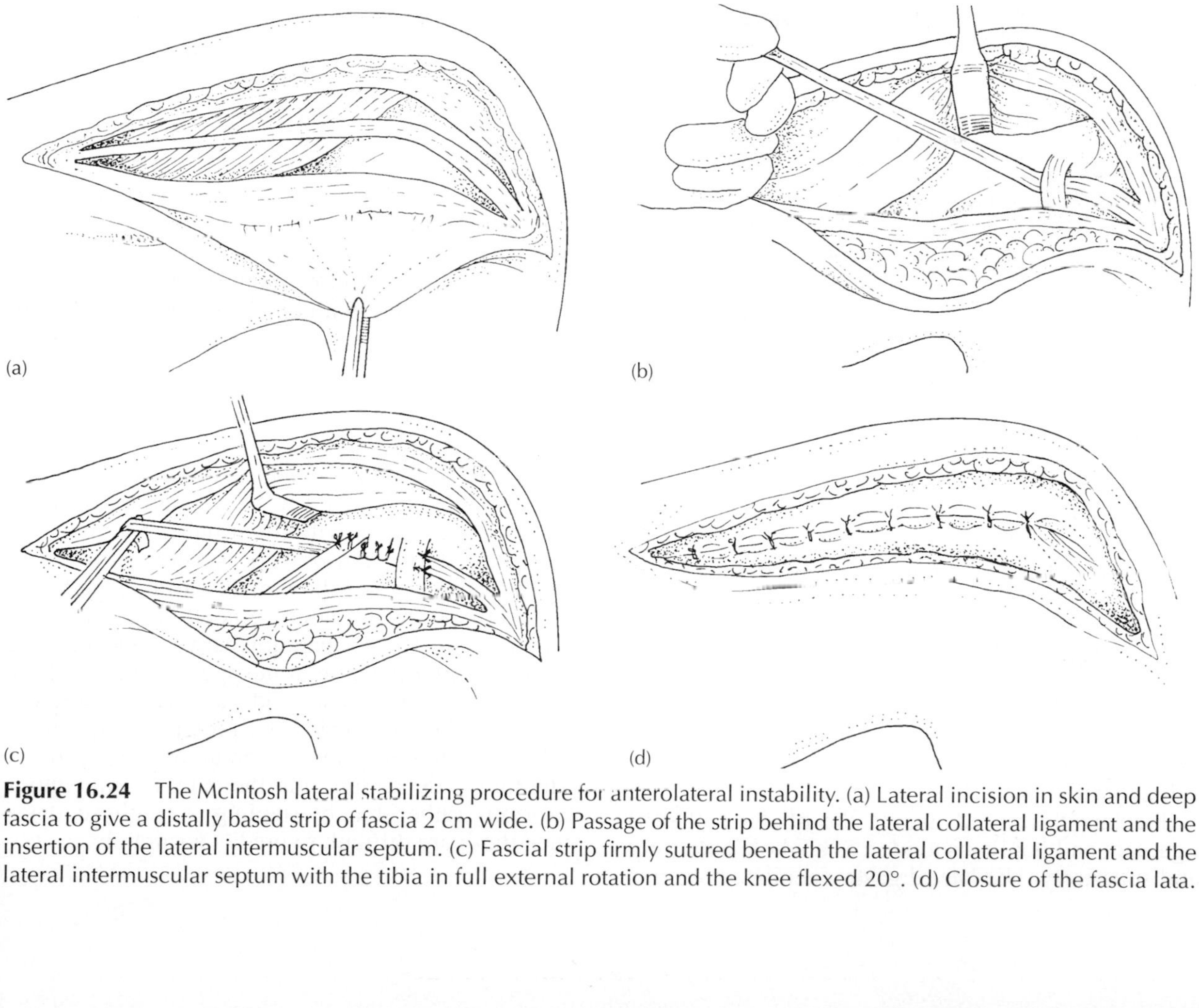

(a) (b) (c) (d)

Figure 16.24 The McIntosh lateral stabilizing procedure for anterolateral instability. (a) Lateral incision in skin and deep fascia to give a distally based strip of fascia 2 cm wide. (b) Passage of the strip behind the lateral collateral ligament and the insertion of the lateral intermuscular septum. (c) Fascial strip firmly sutured beneath the lateral collateral ligament and the lateral intermuscular septum with the tibia in full external rotation and the knee flexed 20°. (d) Closure of the fascia lata.

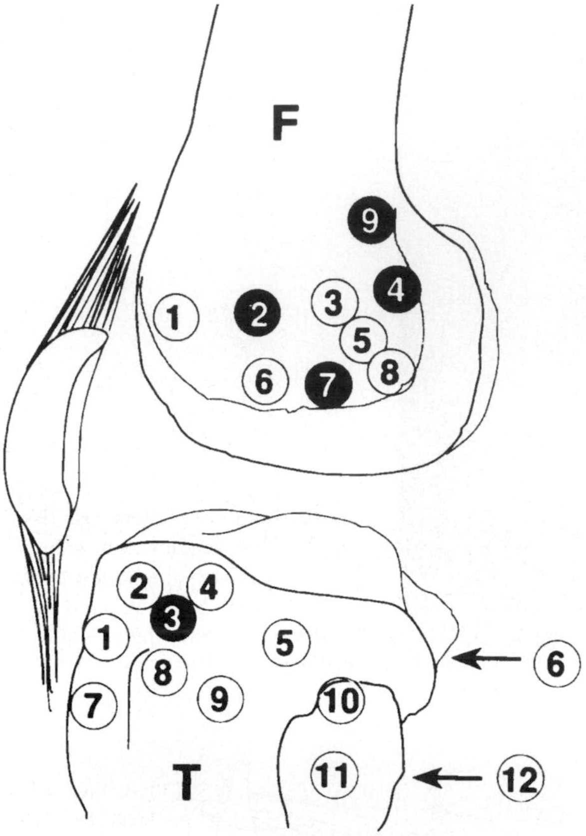

Figure 16.25 Diagram demonstrating the preferred site of fixation of the McIntosh tenodesis at the F9 position. (Reproduced, with permission, from Grood, E.S. (1992) Placement of knee ligament grafts. In: *Knee Surgery – Current Practice.* Edited by P.M. Aichroth, W.D. Cannon and V.P. Patel. Martin Dunitz: London)

Posterolateral instability

In posterolateral instability there is posterior subluxation and external rotation of the lateral tibial condyle on the femur. This is a rare but serious injury and treatment is often unsatisfactory since it is frequently part of a combination of injuries. It results from anteromedial varus and hyperextension injury with damage to the arcuate ligament complex (arcuate ligament, fibular collateral ligament, popliteus and lateral head of gastrocnemius). The patient complains of his knee giving way backwards, with difficulty on walking or climbing stairs, and avoids full extension of the knee.

Treatment is by advancing the fibular collateral ligament and popliteus tendon as a whole anteriorly and superiorly. The lateral gastrocnemius, posterior capsule and arcuate ligament all then advance superiorly and anteriorly (Larson, 1980).

Genu valgum

Bilateral knock knees are common during infancy but can hardly be regarded as an abnormality. Morley (1957) found that between the ages of 3 and $3^1/_2$ years, 22% of children have knock knee of 5 cm or more as measured by the distance between the medial malleoli with the extended knees just touching each other. The laxity of the medial collateral ligament commonly present in young children accentuates the deformity when the child is standing. This physiological genu valgum of childhood resolves spontaneously by the age of 7–8 years without treatment.

In determining the true angles of the weight-bearing knee joint it is necessary to take a frontal radiograph of both complete lower extremities standing so that the continuation of the tibial axis can be followed up to and through the centre of the femoral head.

Unilateral genu valgum or severe bilateral genu valgum, where the intermalleolar distance exceeds 10 cm, should be examined radiologically to determine whether there is any disturbance of epiphyseal growth. Rarely, this might be due to an epiphyseal dysplasia or to an endocrine or metabolic disorder such as rickets. Vitamin D deficiency is no longer common but occasionally a case of Fanconi's syndrome may present with knock knees. Unilateral knock knee may follow trauma or osteomyelitis which can interfere with epiphyseal growth (Figure 16.26).

TREATMENT

Knock knee in toddlers can usually be ignored and most patients are happy to be reassured that their child's deformity is within normal limits and will disappear. If the deformity is severe, particularly beyond the age of 6, follow-up is warranted until the deformity begins to regress. Knock-knee deformity of more than 10 cm separation between the malleoli in the standing position at the age of 10 is unlikely to correct spontaneously and may require surgical treatment. This is carried out preferably by supracondylar osteotomy of the femur or merely tibial osteotomy, depending on the site of maximum deformity rather than by stapling or epiphyseodesis since these are difficult to predict accurately.

Genu varum

Genu varum or 'bow leg' is a lateral curvature of the leg which involves either the tibia, the femur or both. When the leg is curved anteriorly the condition is termed anterior bow leg. A minor degree of the deformity is extremely common and may be regarded as normal in a child of 3 years of age or less. An excessive amount of bowing is often more apparent than real from internal rotation of the legs as occurs with persistent fetal anteversion of the femoral necks or from obliquity of the tibial epiphysis. The amount of bowing is measured in a similar way to knock knee, the internal malleoli being brought together and the distance between the knees measured. If bowing exceeds 5 cm separation of the knees or if it is unilateral, an underlying cause must be considered and appropriate investigations carried out. Childhood bowing can be divided into two groups.

PHYSIOLOGICAL BOWING

This type is bilateral and symmetrical and corrects with further growth after the age of 3 years. No treatment is necessary (Figure 16.27).

PATHOLOGICAL BOWING (TIBIA VARA)

Rickets used to be a common cause of genu varum. The anterior bow legs seen in rickets should not be confused with the sabre blade tibia of syphilis in which the tibia has always some periosteal thickening along the anterior border whereas in rickets the thickening is endosteal and more pronounced on the concave side of the curve. Typically, bowing due to rickets occurs in the distal third of the tibia and that due to Blount's disease in the proximal tibia. Trauma or infection may affect epiphyseal growth, as may benign tumours which involve the epiphyseal growth plate. In these instances realignment of the limb or closure of the unaffected side of the epiphysis may be necessary to limit the progressive deformity.

Blount's disease is a rare condition affecting the posteromedial part of the upper tibial epiphysis. It is most common amongst Afro-Caribbean children. A child may present in early infancy but usually not before the age of 2. The epiphysis is sloping and may be fragmented on the medial side, and is accompanied by a characteristic beak-like curving of medial metaphysis (Figure 16.28). Progressive deformity

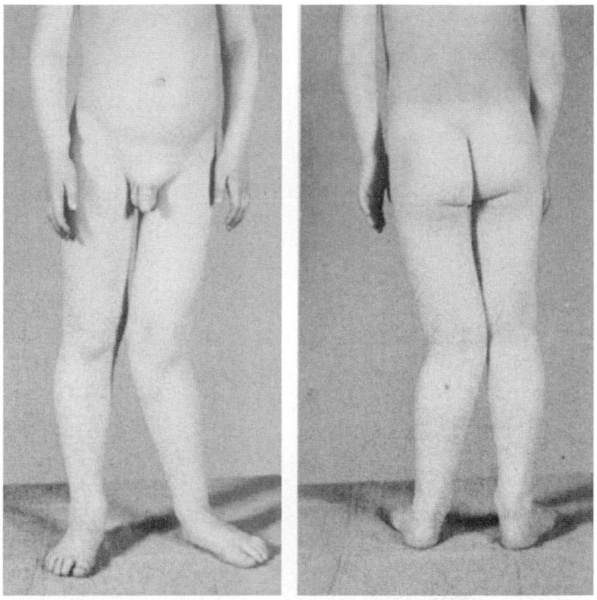

Figure 16.26 Photograph of a 6-year-old boy with a unilateral genu valgum of the left knee secondary to old epiphyseal injury.

may be accompanied by a shortening of the tibia, which is particularly important in unilateral cases.

In Blount's disease, or tibia vara, Langenskjöld (1975) divided the radiographic changes into various age groups:

- Up to the age of 3 years there is irregularity of the metaphyseal edge.
- Up to 6 years the epiphyseal plate is obviously abnormal, being widened and 'fragmented'.
- Up to 10 years the medial plate is growing inwards and downwards into the metaphysis.

At the age of 11–12 years this medial 'tongue' of cartilage divides off and finally unites with the tibia metaphysis on the medial side, leaving the lateral component still 'open'.

Rebouillat *et al.* (1978) described various surgical techniques of a curved osteotomy after epiphysiodesis of the lateral side, 'relèvement' of the medial half of the upper tibia, or excision of the medial bony bridge. Interposing an inert material such as fat has been described by Langenskjöld. However, osteotomy is frequently indicated to prevent a secondary pressure phenomenon on the joint cartilage and balancing of the knee with growth and in severe cases repeated osteotomy may be necessary.

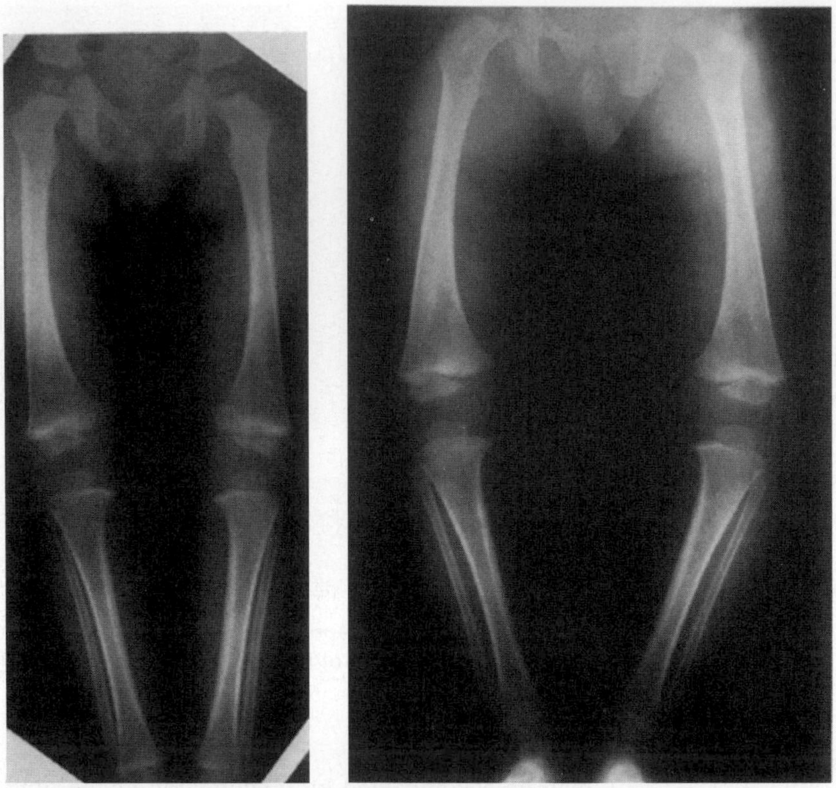

(a) (b)

Figure 16.27 Physiological bowing of the legs (a) recumbent and (b) standing. There is no abnormality of the femoral or tibial growth.

Osteoarthritis of the knee joint

The aetiology, pathology and treatment are discussed in Chapter 11.

Primary osteoarthritis affects the knee more frequently than any other joint and, unlike in the hip, all races are susceptible. The disease affects the older age group, women more frequently, and is associated in 90% of cases with a varus deformity of the knee (cf. rheumatoid arthritis – 90%, valgus deformity). Danielsson (1964) first reported a 40% incidence of osteoarthritis of the knee above the age of 40 years although only approximately half of these have disabling pain. Frequently the disease is primary but various predisposing conditions are recognized – especially trauma, including surgical trauma (e.g. meniscectomy). Although much is written on the prophylaxis of osteoarthritis by repair and reconstruction of ligaments, the incidence of osteoarthritis after untreated acute ligament injury appears to be small; this also applies whether the injury is of a stretching type following prolonged traction, for fractures of the femur (Rowntree and Getty, 1981) or a long-standing ligament injury (Pusey and Dandy, 1981). However, damage to the articular surfaces and incongruity do produce osteoarthritis and removal of the menisci produces at least 20% of osteoarthritis in the affected knee within 25 years (Jackson, 1967). Recent work (Reissis *et al.*, 1991) indicates that failure to remove the meniscus within 6 months after injury plays a part in the causation of osteoarthritis but otherwise the incidence of osteoarthritis was not greater than a control group.

Armstrong *et al.* (1993) felt that moderate exercise aggravated the changes in animals. The effect of closed arthroscopic meniscectomy on the subsequent incidence of osteoarthritis is as yet unclear.

The general clinical features are similar to those of the hip. The patient complains of pain, usually generalized at first, which appears with exercise but can be 'walked off'. The joint is often felt to creak and grate and swells from time to time, especially after any unusual activity involving a flexed position (e.g. kneeling and squatting). With the swelling and inflammation of the synovium the patient feels stiffness and tightness, especially at the back of the knee. Acute pain ensues if the joint is accidentally wrenched, and loose body locking may occur as fragments of cartilage and osteophytes become free in the joint. The patient may then complain of 'giving way', and this may occur also due to patellofemoral

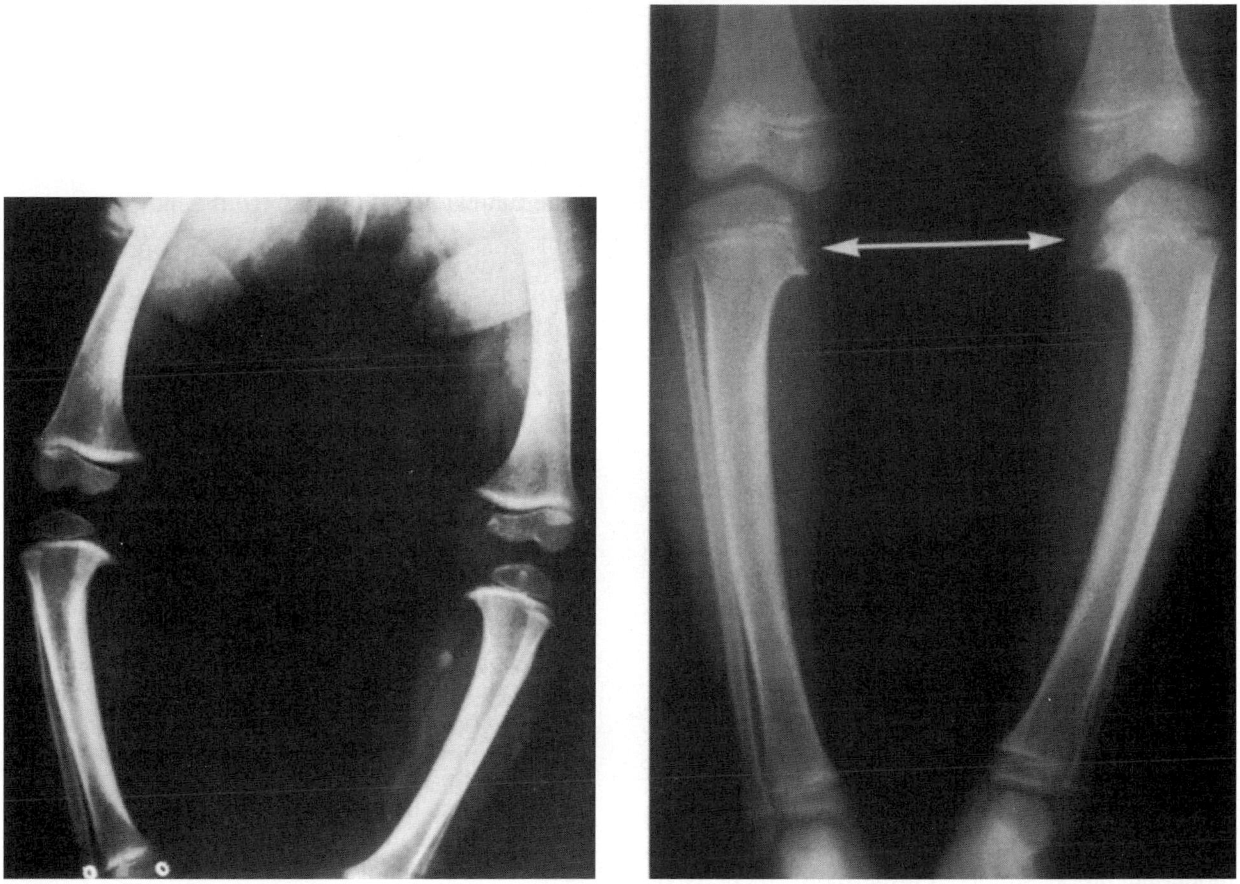

(a) (b)

Figure 16.28 (a) Radiograph of a 2-year-old child with marked genu varum involving both femoral and tibial epiphyses. (b) Blount's disease showing the typical growth disturbance of the medial proximal tibia affecting epiphysis and metaphysis.

joint involvement which frequently accompanies tibiofemoral changes. It may also be caused by tearing of a degenerate meniscus. The pain becomes more severe and of a near-constant type, and varus deformity gradually increases (Figure 16.29). Flexion deformity follows due to protective hamstring muscle spasm. The cause of the development of the varus deformity in osteoarthritis is not clear, but the articular cartilage of the medial tibial condyle is thicker than that on the lateral condyle and this may predispose it to relative nutritional deficiency.

Also, the mechanics of the joint, with the complicated movements involving an altered centre of rotation and 'screw home' of the medial femoral condyle during the last 20° of extension, may influence this predominance of medial joint compartment lesions.

Since the knee transmits forces of up to 3.03 times body weight (Morrison, 1968) and since up to 60% may pass through the menisci, the forces are greatly disturbed by angular deformity and by meniscectomy (Seedholm *et al.*, 1974).

As the disease progresses, the patient finds increasing difficulty in walking, in the activities of daily life, on stairs, and is unable to kneel or squat. Persistent rest pain, especially at night, compels surgical treatment.

TREATMENT

Whilst the common varus deformity is managed relatively successfully by surgical procedures, valgus deformity is a particular therapeutic problem. It should be emphasized that many patients can be managed by conservative means such as weight loss, isometric quadriceps exercises, use of a walking stick held in the ipsilateral hand and anti-inflammatory analgesic drugs such as aspirin in the early stages.

The predominant indication for surgical treatment

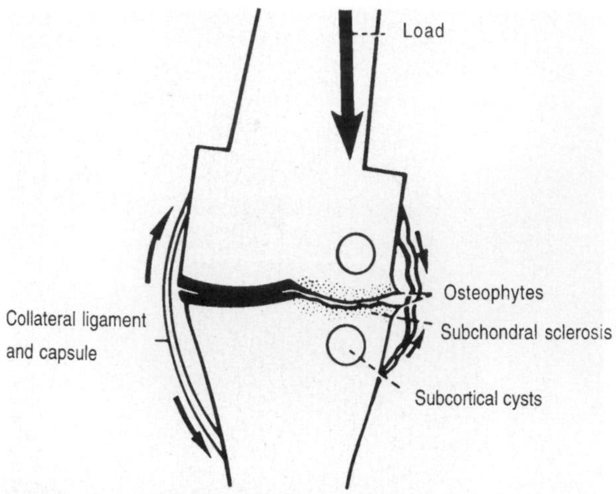

Figure 16.29 Loading on a varus unbalanced knee. Joint space loss, subchondral bone sclerosis, cysts and osteophytes are seen on the medial side of the joint. The medial ligament is slackened and the lateral ligament stretched. (Reproduced, with permission, from Coventry, M.B. (1973) *Journal of Bone and Joint Surgery* **55A**, 23–48)

is persistent pain felt especially at rest and disturbing sleep. The surgical problems of the osteoarthritic knee are much greater than that of the hip, primarily because of the inherent instability of the joint and poor coverage from the exterior by a capsule with moderate blood supply. Furthermore, there is no completely satisfactory salvage procedure in the event of surgical failure or infection.

Tibial osteotomy

This procedure has proved to be generally useful since its development for osteoarthritis by Jackson (1958). Jackson also advocated femoral supracondylar osteotomy but this procedure has not proved so successful except where the primary deformity is valgus. Garièpy (1964) made a significant advance by performing the osteotomy above the tibial tubercle in the cancellous bone 1 cm distal to the tibial articular surface. This added the advantages of easier correction, greater stability and more reliable union. He immobilized the knee in a plaster-of-Paris cast for only 12 days following operation, thus diminishing the problem of deep venous thrombosis and knee stiffness which had occurred with osteotomy below the tibial tubercle.

Osteotomy relieves pain in osteoarthritis by:

- Redistribution of loading, especially where the lateral joint surface is relatively normal on arthroscopy (Figure 16.30).
- Reducing tension on the lateral collateral ligament.
- Reducing the 'medial impingement' of the degenerate medial meniscus on the capsule.
- Reducing capsular stretching and tearing by correcting varus and flexion deformities.
- Altering of blood supply, especially reducing venous stasis.

Jackson *et al.* (1969) defined the indications as:

- Osteoarthritis with severe pain unrelieved by conservative treatment.
- Degenerative changes localized to the medial or lateral compartments.
- A flexion range of 90° with fixed flexion deformity no greater than 20°.
- Collateral ligament instability of only moderate degree.

The procedure is not successful in rheumatoid arthritis and may lead to avascularity of the head of the tibia (Bentley, 1981, unpublished observations).

The osteotomy is performed through the tibia above the tibial tubercle with excision of a wedge of bone. Anteroposterior radiographs are taken of the patient weight-bearing in order to assess the full degree of deformity as well as to measure the angle of intersection of lines drawn along the middle of the shaft of the femur and the middle of the shaft of the tibia. This radiography also indicates the presence of medial joint cartilage loss, which may only be obvious on a weight-bearing x-ray (Figure 16.30).

Technique

An anterior oblique incision is made over the patellar tendon as far as the head of the fibula and the upper end of the tibia is exposed. The lateral ligament of the knee is reflected upwards with a portion of the head of the fibula which is simply divided and reattached at the end of the procedure. It is not usually necessary or advisable to excise the whole fibular head.

It is advisable, however, to identify and protect the lateral popliteal nerve during the operation but to avoid traction. Under x-ray control, two Steinmann pins are placed across the tibia – the upper one being horizontal and parallel to the tibial plateau 1–1.5 cm below the articular surface, and the lower in the line of the wedge cut. The wedge is cut with a power saw but great care is needed to cut the posterior cortex under direct vision, with an osteotome and with the knee flexed, to avoid damage to the popliteal artery.

The medial tibial cortex is preserved and the osteotomy is closed on a medial hinge. If the osteotomy is not stable, it may be secured with one or two offset staples. The final femorotibial angle

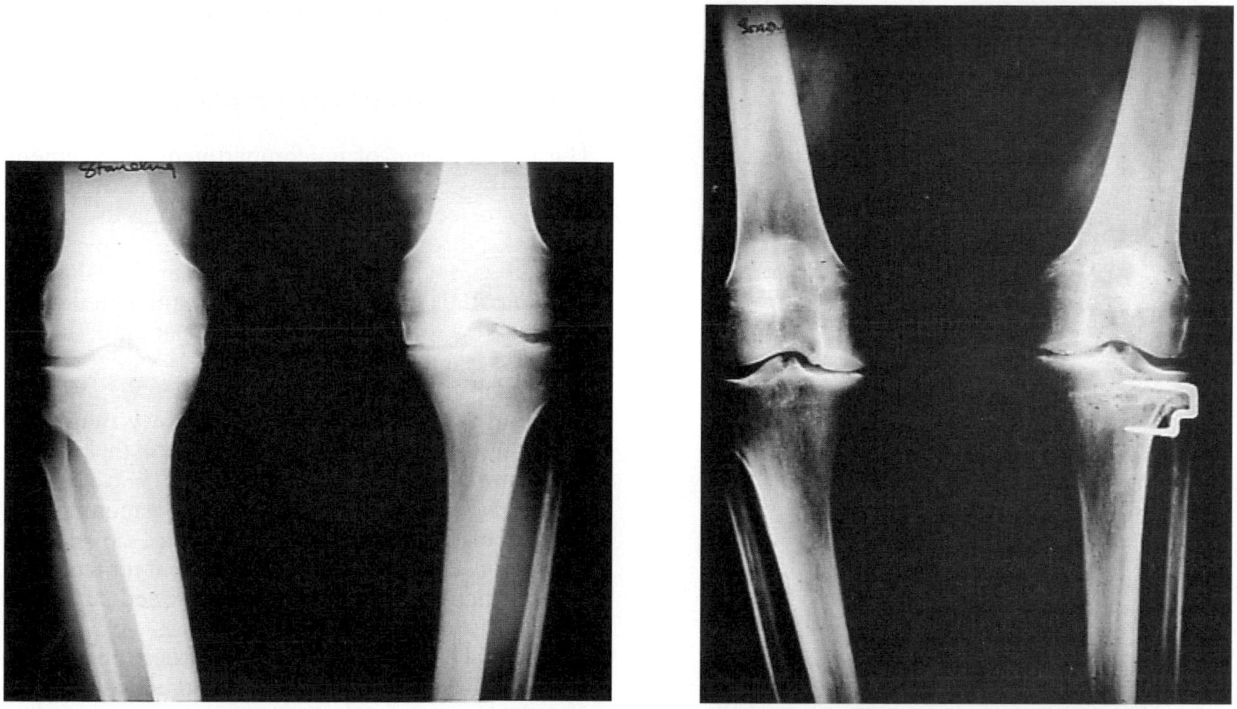

(a) (b)

Figure 16.30 (a) Anteroposterior weight-bearing radiograph of both knees showing classical varus deformity and medial compartment osteoarthritis. (b) Postoperative radiograph 3 years after successful high tibial valgus osteotomy.

should be one of slight valgus of 5–8° when correcting a varus deformity. Following closure of the wound, the limb is immobilized in a cylinder cast and the leg is elevated. The patient commences isometric quadriceps exercises as soon as consciousness is recovered, and begins to walk on the limb after 48 hours. At 2 weeks, the cast is removed and active flexion commences. As soon as quadriceps

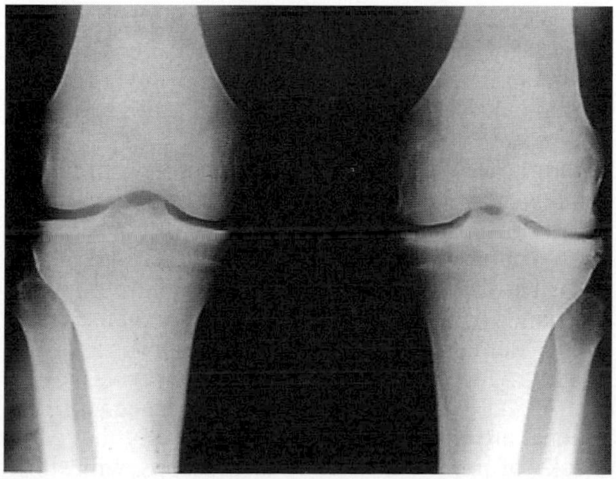

Figure 16.31 Anteroposterior weight-bearing radiograph of a 35-year-old man showing lateral compartment osteoarthritis with valgus deformity.

control is achieved, the patient may walk with the sole support of a walking stick until complete confidence is achieved.

Pain relief is reported as occurring in up to 80% of cases and was maintained for at least a 5-year period (Coventry, 1973). Insall *et al.* (1974) considered that osteotomy was indicated only if the varus or valgus deformity was 10° or less, i.e. when the joint damage was very early.

However, it is our experience and that of other authors that satisfactory relief of symptoms may follow osteotomy even with up to 25° of varus and even though the medial joint space is not opened up by the operation (Figure 16.30b).

Minor degrees of preoperative instability are acceptable and usually improve after osteotomy. There are several well documented studies showing that there is no radiographic evidence of improvement to the joint changes following tibial osteotomy unlike that seen in the hip.

Valgus deformity of the knee is not so effectively treated by a tibial osteotomy, and in our view it is better dealt with by a supracondylar wedge excision osteotomy (Figures 16.31, 16.32).

Complications such as the risk of infection are low but there is a definite incidence of partial lesions of the lateral popliteal nerve. Jackson *et al.* (1969) described eight such cases in 70 osteotomies. It has

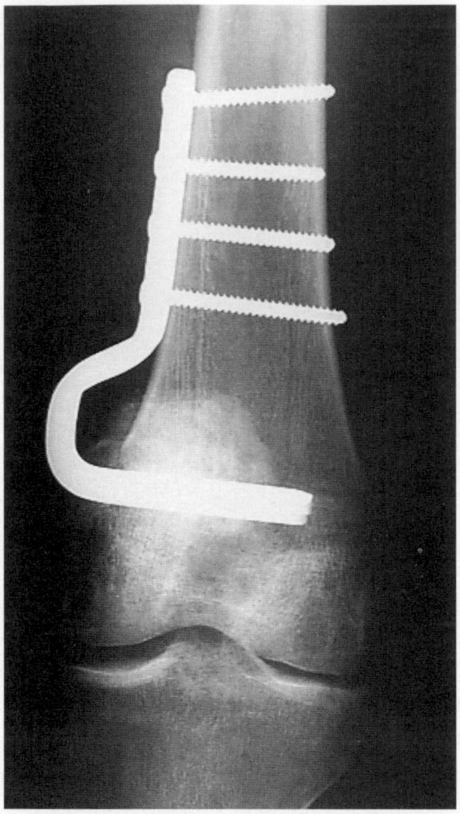

Figure 16.32 Postoperative radiograph showing correction of valgus deformity by supracondylar wedge osteotomy fixed with a blade-plate.

been shown that most of the unsatisfactory results of recurrence of pain and/or symptoms of instability were associated with undercorrection or occasionally overcorrection of the deformity at operation.

Although the presence of patellofemoral osteoarthrosis is not necessarily a contraindication, it is probably better not to perform intra-articular operations at the same time as the osteotomy, as there is a tendency to stiffness of the knee. Thus procedures such as patellectomy or debridement operations should be performed separately. Conversely, arthroscopic removal of loose bodies or trimming of a degenerate meniscus can be performed before the osteotomy under the same anaesthetic.

Recent studies have shown disappointing results over the longer term and our experience is that the results are very variable and unpredictable. The best results are, regardless of state of disease, in the 50+ active male who wishes to play sport. Unfortunately, the results are, as with the hip, never comparable with total knee replacement. Furthermore, the results of total knee replacement after high tibial osteotomy are disappointing, probably due to altered patellofemoral biomechanics, so that the procedure is losing ground to unicompartmental replacement and total knee replacement (Rorabeck and Bourne, 1989).

Unicompartment knee replacement

The development of unicompartment replacement, notably by Marmor (1988) and the unpredictability of tibial osteotomy has led to increasing use of this method.

Scott *et al.* (1991) reported 90% survivorship and 87% of patients with no significant pain in their 8–12 year review of 100 consecutive patients (Figure 16.33). Moreover, a prospective randomized comparison of unicompartment prostheses versus tibial osteotomy reviewed at 5–10 years showed a definite advantage of the unicompartment prosthesis with few complications (Broughton *et al.*, 1986).

Therefore we reserve high tibial osteotomy for patients of both sexes under the age of 60 who are very active and favour unicompartment replacement or total knee replacement for the more sedentary and 60-plus age group.

The final decision regarding the procedure is often dependent on the findings at operation since frequently the osteoarthritis is more extensive than expected, thus requiring a total knee replacement.

Joint surface allografting

In future it may be possible to predict before the event which individuals and which joints are likely to develop osteoarthritis, as knowledge increases of the relative contribution of meniscectomy, previous fractures, osteochondritis dissecans and ligament injuries to the development of deformity and osteoarthritis.

Since articular cartilage is privileged as an allograft material, it is logical to attempt replacement of early degenerative areas of cartilage with allografts. Extensive experimental studies have been carried out (Aston and Bentley, 1986) and have demonstrated successful incorporation of allografts and reconstitution of surface defects.

Similarly, the problems of rejection of the bony component of osteochondral allografts appear largely to have been overcome by the use of donor material from young knees and by transplantation of the grafts within 12 hours of death of the donor. Also, the avoidance of all methods of preservation of the grafts which damage articular cartilage, such as deep freezing, appears to reduce problems (Oakeshott *et al.*, 1988). Results from clinical experience with 108 patients are encouraging. It appears likely that early checks of joints 'at risk' by arthroscopy will allow very limited cartilage allografting with whole plugs in early cases to prevent the inevitable degeneration of joints which follows early articular cartilage loss.

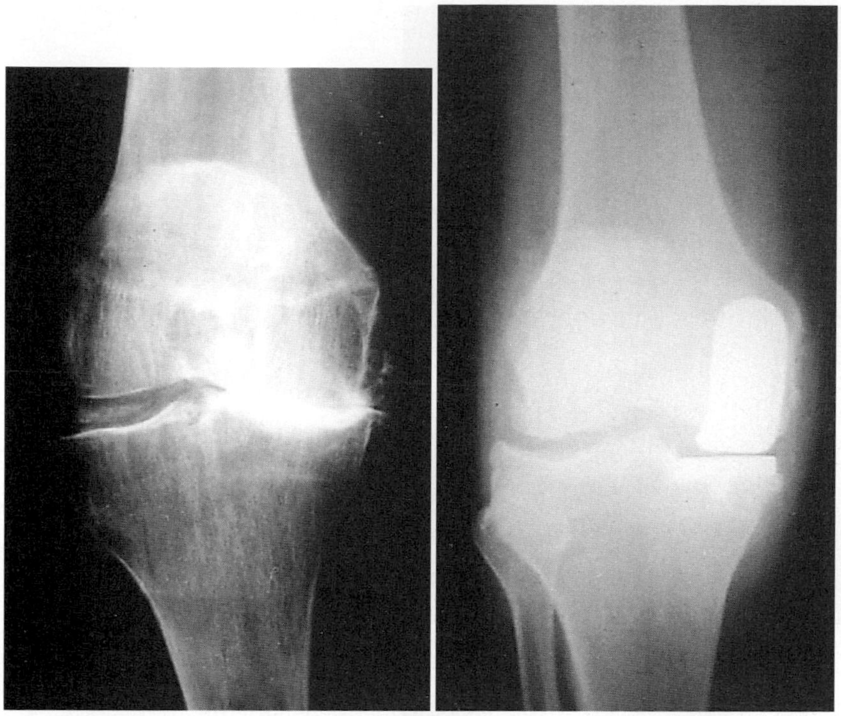

(a) (b)

Figure 16.33 (a) Preoperative and (b) postoperative radiographs of successful unicompartment knee replacement 5 years after operation.

Considerable promise is offered by the use of osteochondral grafts for more advanced lesions of the knee as an alternative to total joint replacement, especially in the younger patients where loosening of the prosthesis is such a problem (Figure 16.34).

Total prosthetic knee joint replacement

The situation regarding total knee replacement for advanced osteoarthritis or rheumatoid arthritis has changed dramatically in the last decade.

All the major centres have reported excellent results for relief of pain, range of movement of 90–110° and improved function which have been sustained for 10–15 years with prostheses such as the Insall Total Condylar (Scott and Volatile, 1986; Vince *et al.*, 1987; Ritter *et al.*, 1989; Ranawat *et al.*, 1993). The design of the successful total knee replacements have become remarkably similar with a metal condylar compartment with patellar flange and a metal-backed high-density polyethylene (HDP) tibial surface with a central keel for stability (Figure 16.35). Uncemented devices have been almost completely replaced by cemented. The sepsis rates with good technique, clean air theatres and antibiotics prophylaxis have dropped to an average of 1% and the major problems relate to the patellofemoral joint, wear of polyethylene and problems of revisions. Most total knee replacement systems involve intramedullary femoral jigs but tibial intramedullary jigs appear not so vital for achieving good alignment on the biomechanical axis, a point emphasized initially by Freeman, which is vital for success (Figure 16.36).

Problems have arisen because of patellar malalignment and patellofemoral pain, the commonest problem being to carry out insufficient removal of patellar bone in correct alignment (Kumar *et al.*, 1991). Realization that femoral rotational alignment of femur can give rise to patella instability has also reduced such problems. Whether or not to resurface the patella remains controversial. Levitsky *et al.* (1993) favoured non-replacement whilst our series showed marginally better results with replacement (Kumar *et al.*, 1991). Also 'proprioception' was improved with patella replacement (Warren *et al.*, 1993). However, generally we do not resurface the patella if there is maintenance of the shape of the articular surfaces. Similarly, there is no consensus on resection of the posterior cruciate ligament since the 10-year results show no obvious differences. However, 'proprioception' studies on a small number of cases showed improvement when the posterior cruciate ligament was retained so that long term this may be important (Warren *et al.*, 1993).

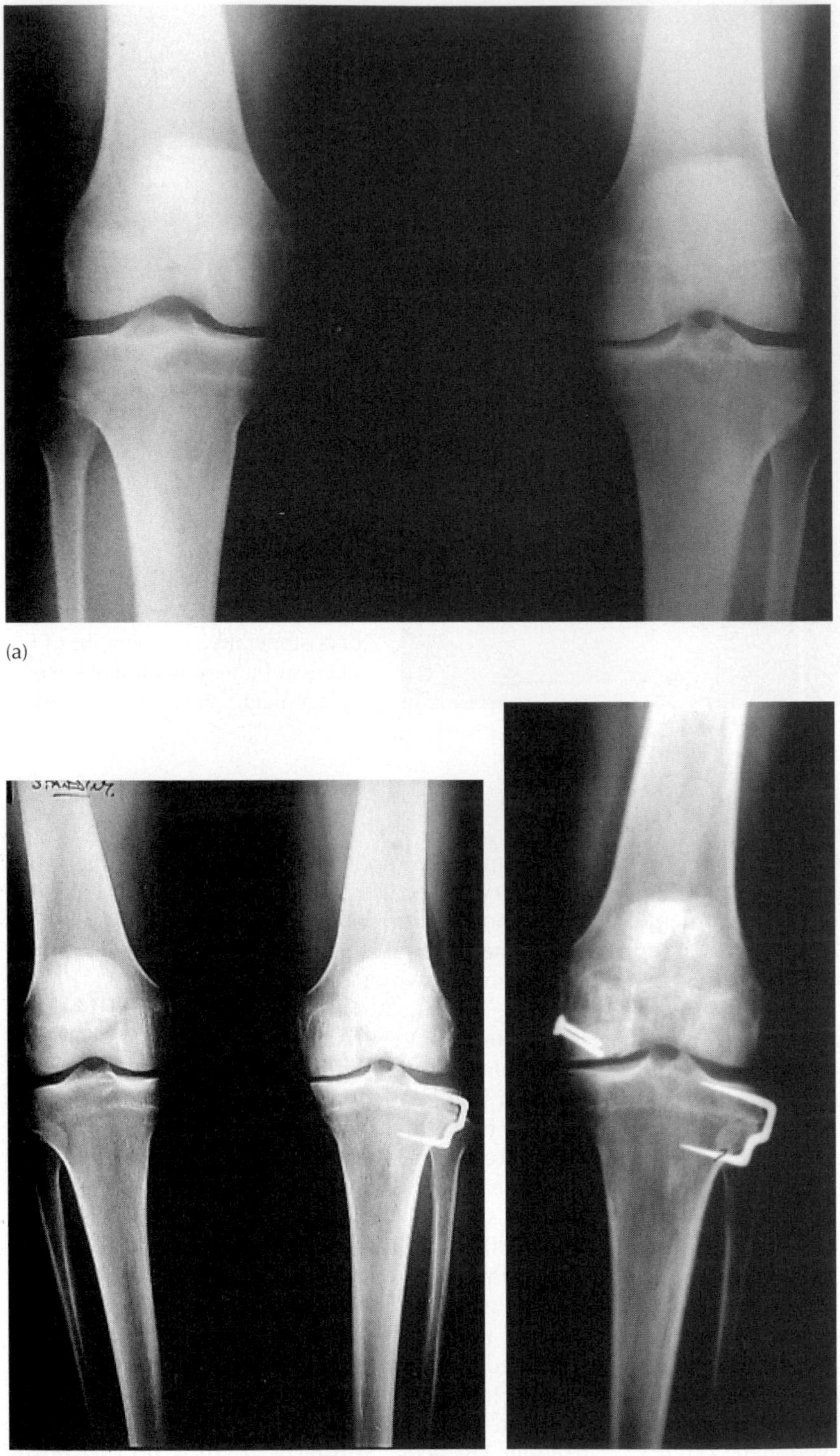

(a)

(b)

(c)

Figure 16.34 (a) Preoperative radiograph of 43-year-old man with early grade 2 osteoarthritis of the left medial femoral condyle and slight varus deformity. (b) Valgus tibial osteotomy was performed followed by an osteochondral allograft 3 months later. (c) At 6 years the graft is incorporated and the patient is asymptomatic.

Thus, it emerges that the total knee replacement arthroplasty is proving very satisfactory over 10–15 years (Figure 16.37). Precise placement of the components and contemporary cement techniques are essential for good results. Revision surgery is now yielding better results (Philips, 1993) so that, although infection and loosening are severe complications, they can be managed satisfactorily in a

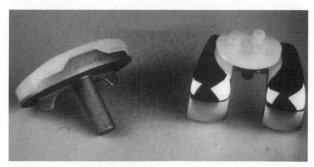

Figure 16.35 A typical contemporary total knee replacement prosthesis with a chrome-cobalt condylar component, a titanium tibial tray with a stabilizing keel and high density polyethylene insert and polyethylene patella button.

high proportion of cases (Figure 16.38).

However, the prosthesis should, in our view, generally be reserved for those over 60 years of age with severe, painful osteoarthritis and limited demands and those with physical restrictions such as rheumatoid arthritis and haemophilia.

With increased longevity of prostheses, a major concern is the high-density polyethylene (HDP) which is subject to wear. By considering wear characteristics of HDP and the loading of the prosthesis it is generally agreed that the most satisfactory type of articulation is one that avoids point loading and sliding of the metal surface on a relatively flat HDP tibial surface, thus reducing wear and particle formation. There is a balance to be struck between close fitting of the femoral condyles and the HDP of the tibial surface and the need to avoid constraint which may increase the incidence of loosening. Nevertheless, wear is a problem (Figures 16.39 and 16.40) and it is recommended that the polyethylene lining should be no less than 8 mm in thickness. New materials will be required to reduce friction and wear and, as in the hip, it may be that ceramics will be valuable. An alternative is to reduce point loading of the contributory surface by the use of a meniscus of HDP which slides on a metallic tibial tray (Bradley *et al.*, 1987).

Total knee replacement is indicated for painful osteoarthritis or rheumatoid arthritis involving all three compartments of the knee in patients aged 60 or older or who have physical disabilities which restrict the forces applied to the prosthesis.

Modern techniques of ligament balancing and soft tissue release allow correction of up to 50% of fixed flexion and 40° of varus or valgus deformity. Deficient bone stock can be treated by bone grafting and the use of a stemmed, modular prosthesis (see Figure 16.38). The use of cement means that osteoporosis should not be a problem. The extreme

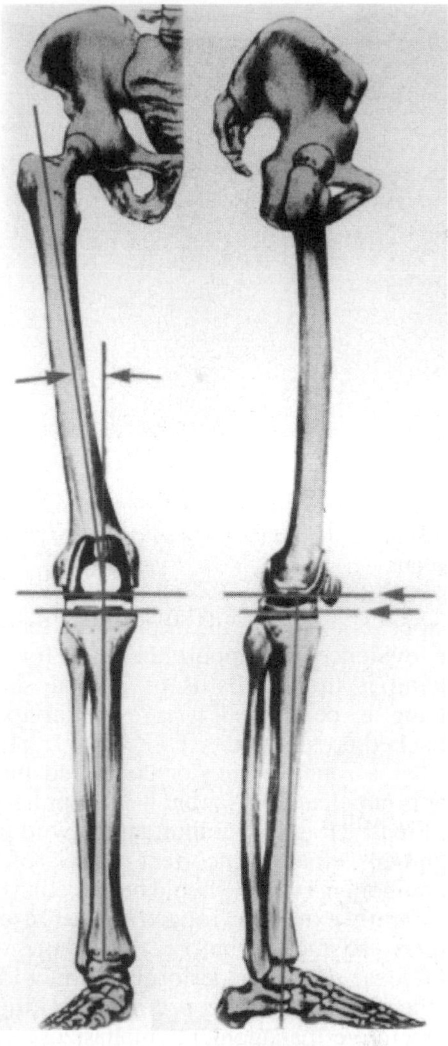

Figure 16.36 The biomechanical axis of the leg runs from the centre of the femoral head through the knee to the centre of the ankle. Total knee prostheses must be placed on this line and give a valgus alignment of the knee of 5–10°.

valgus knee over 25° is notoriously unstable and is probably best treated by a constrained hinge-type prosthesis such as the Stanmore.

Total knee replacement is contraindicated:

- In bony ankylosis with scarred and adherent quadriceps
- In the presence of active infection.

It is essential to remember that a good result for total knee replacement depends on a well functioning patellofemoral joint.

Although previous patellectomy will weaken the quadriceps, acceptable results can be achieved. Beuchel (1992) has described a technique of interpositional bone grafting to form a substitute patella

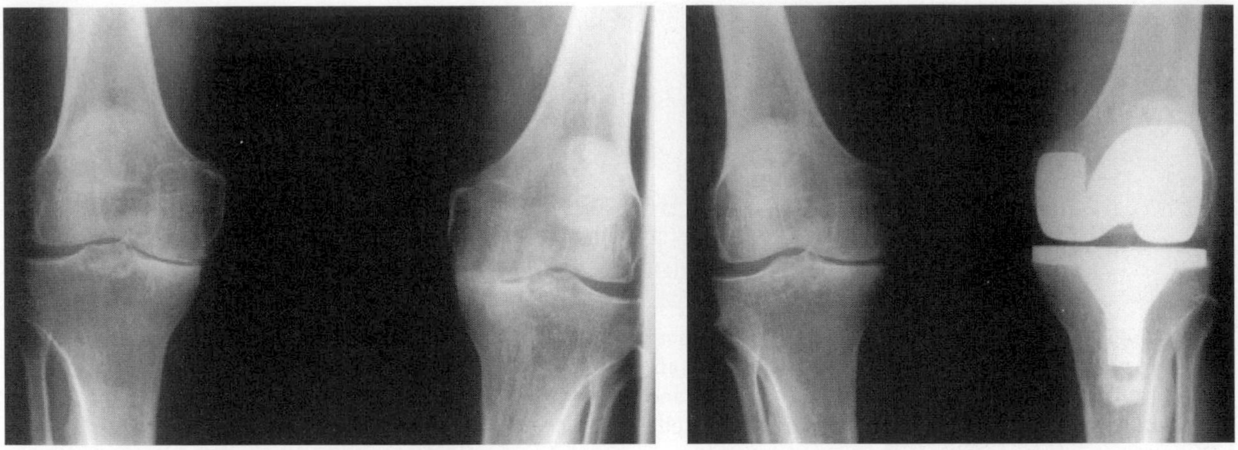

(a) (b)

Figure 16.37 (a) Preoperative weight-bearing x-ray of a 68-year-old man with medial compartment osteoarthritis of the knee and varus deformity. (b) Postoperative radiograph after insertion and fixation by cement of a condylar joint replacement.

which appears to be useful. In our view there is no definite evidence to support the case for patella resurfacing if the patella is of normal shape. If resurfacing is performed it is essential to avoid metal-backed prostheses.

Whether a round button or contoured button is superior is not clear thus far but we favour a rounded button. Finally, it is very important to avoid patellar malalignment either by incorrect rotation of the femoral component (which should be placed in neutral or very slightly externally rotated) and to ensure that tracking is satisfactory before closing the wound. Lateral release should be performed from within the joint if there is any doubt concerning tracking.

Postoperative management emphasizes rapid active mobilization after 48 hours and the use of continuous passive motion is unnecessary and may produce wound problems. It is our practice to use prophylactic antibiotics for 72 hours postoperatively and warfarin at a level to give an INR of 2 until the patient leaves hospital at 7–10 days.

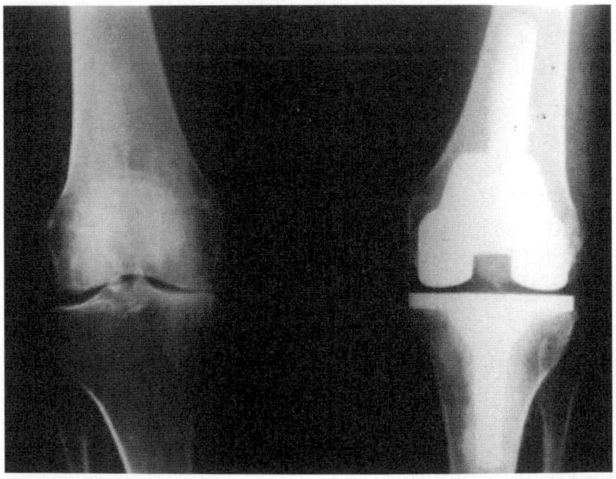

Figure 16.38 Postoperative radiograph following revision of an infected and loose knee replacement prosthesis. The use of extended stems and impacted cancellous bone grafts gives enhanced stability to the revision prosthesis.

Knee arthrodesis for osteoarthritis

Because osteoarthritis usually affects patients in middle age or beyond, treatment is aimed at maintaining mobility whilst relieving pain and deformity. Occasionally, following severe trauma to the knee and secondary osteoarthritis, compression arthrodesis of the knee in 10–15° of flexion is performed in younger patients who otherwise have normal joints.

Drilling and debridement

Magnuson (1941) described an operation to smooth roughened surfaces and remove debris and loose bodies in late osteoarthritis of the knee. Pridie (1959) foresaw the potential of early treatment by performing multiple drillings of the denuded articular surface of the femoral condyle and showed subsequently the formation of fibrocartilage on the surface, which he anticipated would fill the defects and form a new articulating layer. Insall (1967) followed 62 patients treated in this manner by Pridie for $6^1/_2$ years, and 77% considered the result to be good. Subsequent work has shown that, unlike in the hip, extensive repair and resurfacing of the joint with fibrocartilage does not occur and the matrix of the fibrocartilage is deficient in type II collagen which characterizes normal hyaline articular cartilage.

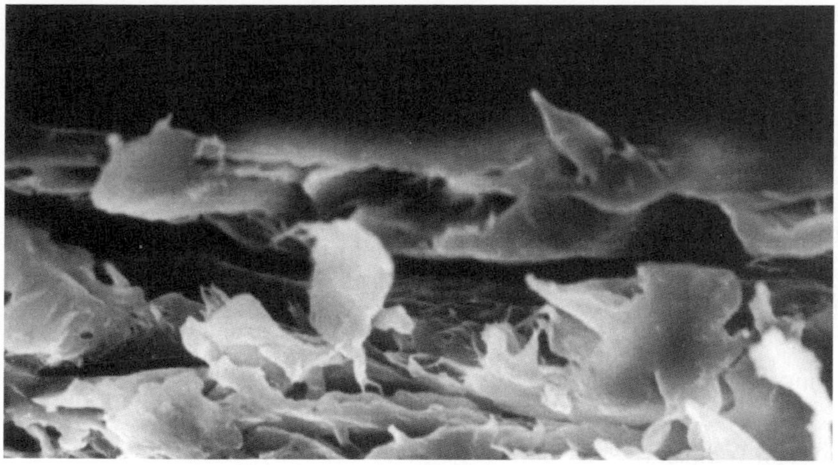

Figure 16.39 Scanning electron microscopy appearance of high density polyethylene showing early abrasion wear.

The authors have performed this procedure on a number of occasions but have not found it useful.

Arthroscopic washout of the knee

Following on from the debridement operation the advent of arthroscopy led to the use of saline washout to remove particulate debris of cartilage and bone from the knee.

This is firmly based on the observation by Chrisman in 1969 that articular cartilage matrix is irritant to the synovial membrane and the demonstration of the formation of marginal osteophytes in animal knees following injections of homogenates of cartilage. Several authors have reported the effectiveness of this method involving washout of debris together with arthroscopic trimming of degenerate meniscal tears and trimming of osteophytes by power shaving (Johnson and Rouse 1982; Patel *et al.*, 1992). Our own results in a series of 57 patients with grade II to IV osteoarthritis followed for 1–3 years showed 65% were good or excellent (Lennox and Bentley, 1991). Since this is a relatively minor procedure it is very worthwhile in the younger patient or in those who, on assessment, are not suitable for total knee replacement for local or general fitness reasons.

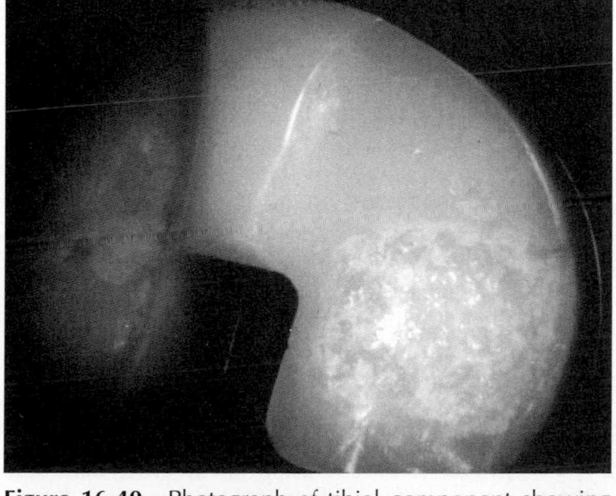

Figure 16.40 Photograph of tibial component showing wear of 'flat' polyethylene after 4 years.

Frequently a patient with osteoarthritis presents with focal pain and tenderness over the medial joint line and a history of locking or 'catching'. In this group arthroscopy normally reveals advanced osteoarthritis of the medial compartment and patellofemoral compartment or slight changes laterally with a degenerate or ragged medial meniscus.

Trimming of the meniscus and thorough washout of the knee will often give gratifying relief of pain. Total removal of the meniscus should be avoided since this increases instability and pain.

Osteoarthritis of the patellofemoral joint

Osteoarthritis of the patellofemoral joint may occur in isolation but more frequently in association with tibiofemoral osteoarthritis. It may follow recurrent dislocation or subluxation of the patella, traumatic articular cartilage fracture, fractures of the patella, osteochondritis dissecans and the excessive lateral pressure syndrome (ELPS) of Ficat (Ficat *et al.*, 1975). It has never been demonstrated that osteoarthritis follows chondromalacia patellae occurring earlier in life. In the majority of cases it is a primary disorder (Meachim and Bentley, 1979).

The patella is important in normal function of the

knee, and Stougard (1970) described the functions of the patella as follows:

1. During the movement of the knee it ensures that cartilage articulates with cartilage with a low friction effect, instead of between cartilage and the tendinous extensor expansion.
2. Increasing the power of knee extension by displacing the patellar tendon away from the axis of movement increases the moment of the quadriceps pull. The quadriceps strength is greater with than without the patella (Bentley, 1970).
3. The patella protects the knee joint from direct contusion.

Experimentally it was shown by Bruce and Walmsley (1942) in rabbits that, following patellectomy, degenerative changes occur in the femoral condyles and, later, throughout the knee joint; similar appearances were demonstrated by DePalma *et al.* (1960) in dogs. However, in man, where the knee is not in a flexed position, similar changes have not occurred (Bentley, 1978). The patella, therefore, has definite functions and its loss leads to weakness, especially in the last 30° of extension of the knee. However, the effect on function may be very small and allow high levels of athletic activity.

TREATMENT

As with main joint osteoarthritis, a good proportion of patients will be relieved by weight reduction, systematic and intensive isometric quadriceps exercises, anti-inflammatory drugs and avoidance of provocative flexion and kneeling activity.

Patellectomy

Patellectomy is an effective treatment of painful patellofemoral osteoarthritis with a normal or near-normal tibiofemoral joint (Lennox *et al.*, 1994).

It is best performed through a small (4 cm) lateral parapatellar incision to avoid disturbing the vastus medialis. The patient should have been prepared preoperatively with intensive quadriceps exercises, and the operation is designed to produce as little trauma as possible. The patella is removed through a longitudinal incision along the quadriceps expansion, leaving both retinacular expansions intact. No attempt is made to repair the extensor mechanism, the gap merely being closed with normal interrupted sutures. Postoperatively the limb is immobilized in a cylinder cast for 3 weeks and weight-bearing commences after 48 hours. The patient carries out isometric quadriceps exercises as soon as this is possible postoperatively and intensively at least three times a day whilst the limb is still in plaster. After 3 weeks the patient is readmitted to hospital for supervised mobilization and further quadriceps-building exercises.

Tibial tubercle advancement

Tibial tubercle advancement (Maquet, 1976) is a procedure with reported good results in patellofemoral osteoarthritis, as it is claimed to reduce the loading through the joint in flexion (Ferguson *et al.*, 1979). However, long-term experience with this procedure has been disappointing and we rarely perform the procedure except occasionally in post-fracture patients with high demands.

Prosthetic replacement

Prosthetic replacement of the patellofemoral joint has been reported and gives pain relief in the short term (Ackroyd, 1993, personal communication). Further evaluation of this procedure is required.

Affections of the infrapatellar fat pad

From the synovial membrane which covers the deep surface of the infrapatellar pad of fat a triangular fold passes upwards and backwards to be attached by its apex to the anterior extremity of the intercondylar fossa. This fold is called the infrapatellar synovial fold (ligamentum mucosum) and its free margins are known as the alar folds (ligamenta alaria). The pad of fat lies behind the patellar tendon and the part of it which is carried in between the synovial folds is frequently the site of hypertrophy (lipoma arborescens).

When the knee joint is extended the patella is drawn up by the contracting quadriceps, and the infrapatellar pad of fat is similarly pulled up to prevent its being caught between the tibia and the femur. When an excess of fat has been deposited in the pad, however, or when the quadriceps has lost its tone, the pad may not be drawn up sufficiently and is then liable to be nipped between the opposing articular surfaces. Repeated trauma of this nature is associated with haemorrhage into the pad, and further thickening (Smillie, 1978). This condition is also seen commonly in athletic individuals and is often known as Hoffa's disease.

In older subjects, the infrapatellar pad may be hypertrophied in association with intra-articular arthritic or secondary inflammatory changes, due to villous hypertrophy of the synovial membrane.

The knee is painful, but the pain – which is constantly situated immediately behind the patellar tendon – occurs only when the knee is used. The joint also tends to be stiff, and the patient may complain that it is weak and liable to recurrent attacks of swelling. From the interposition of the hypertrophied fat between the patellar tendon and the edges of articular surfaces there results a progressive limitation of extension which makes the patient walk with the knee partly flexed.

True locking does not occur, but at intervals the joint may appear to 'give way', or a sharp stabbing pain may occur which temporarily arrests the patient's activity.

The pad, on examination, is usually enlarged, and the swellings on either side of the patellar tendon are tender. This tenderness persists, or rather is more pronounced when the joint is fully extended, and this provides a characteristic sign. The quadriceps muscles constantly may show some atrophy.

Radiological examination is usually negative; occasionally, however, calcium is deposited in the hypertrophied fat and may give a radiodensity.

CONSERVATIVE TREATMENT

The symptoms are produced mainly when the knee is fully extended, so conservative measures should seek to limit this movement. In athletes some reduction of activity and of deep flexion exercises is effective. Robert Jones (1909) recommended the simple but effective device of raising the heel of the boot on the affected side; this prevents full extension, and may be followed by subsidence of swelling and disappearance of the symptoms.

Conservative measures should always be supplemented by exercises to strengthen the wasted quadriceps. When this fails an injection of local anaesthetic and hydrocortisone repeated several times may relieve the symptoms.

OPERATIVE TREATMENT

If conservative methods prove ineffective, the pad should be removed or reduced surgically. An incision is made on the lateral side of the lower part of the patella; the pad is found to be loosely attached to the posterior surface of the patellar tendon, about the upper end of the tibia, but firmly fixed to the articular capsule. This procedure may open the synovial cavity but no attempt is made to close it. After closure of the aponeurosis and skin the knee is supported in a cylinder cast for 2 weeks, and at the end of that time active movements are begun.

Bipartite patella

The patella, like other sesamoid bones, is subject to many anomalies of development which, though they have little or no clinical significance, are of great diagnostic importance.

The patella arises usually from a single centre of ossification, though occasionally two or even more centres are present. These several centres almost invariably fuse to form a single bone, but occasionally they remain discrete, giving the condition of bipartite or even multipartite patella. The importance of the condition lies in the fact that the unwary may confuse its radiographic appearance with that of fracture, particularly since it is usually first observed when the knee is x-rayed following injury.

RADIOLOGICAL APPEARANCES

The general contour of the patella is not grossly altered, but the bone is seen to consist of a larger and one or two smaller fragments, the latter situated usually at the upper outer quadrant (Figure 16.41). The structure of the smaller fragments is similar to that of the main part of the bone, consisting of a shell of cortical bone surrounding normal cancellous tissue. There is usually a definite radiological interval between the two fragments, but in the dissected specimen this apparent gap is occupied by cartilage.

In five out of six cases the condition is bilateral, while a similar condition is not uncommonly observed in the sesamoid bone beneath the head of the first metatarsal.

DIAGNOSIS

The condition has to be distinguished from fractures of the patella. These, however, are accompanied by a definite history of injury, and the usual clinical manifestations of trauma (i.e. swelling and tenderness) are present. The important points in the differential radiological diagnosis are:

- The margins of the fragments of bipartite patella are smooth and consist of cortical bone; fractured fragments show more or less serrated edges, and involve cancellous bone.
- The position of the intervening gap is also significant. Fractures rarely occur in the upper outer quadrant, but this is almost invariably the site of the congenital anomaly.
- The congenital error is frequently bilateral.

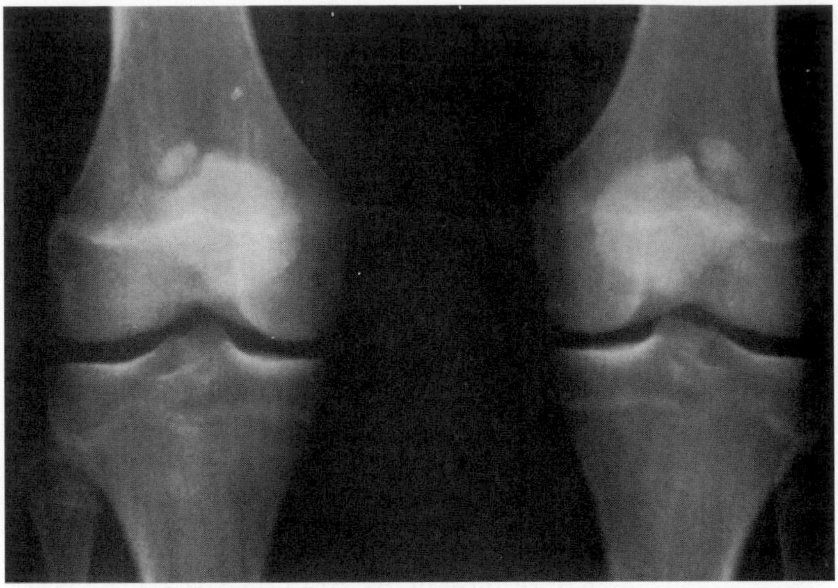

(a)

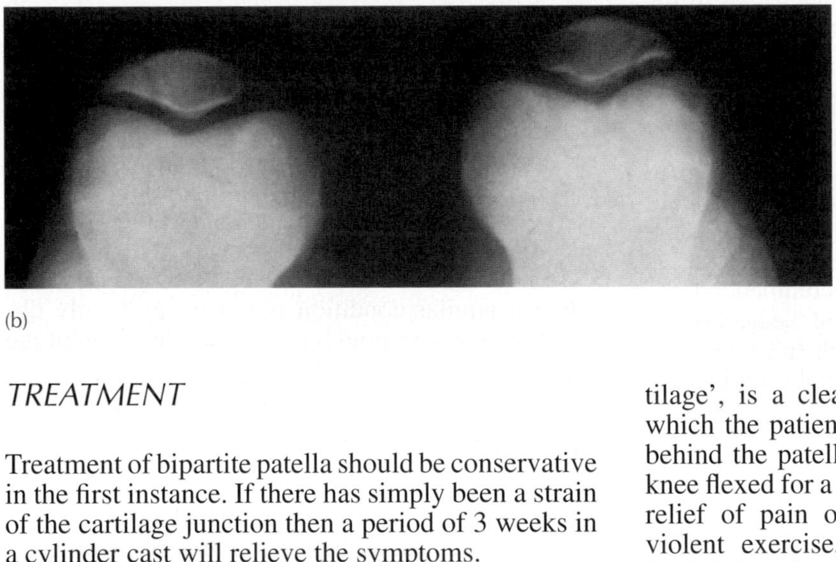

(b)

Figure 16.41 (a) Anteroposterior and (b) tangential radiographs showing bilateral bipartite patellae with clear demarcation of the fragments.

TREATMENT

Treatment of bipartite patella should be conservative in the first instance. If there has simply been a strain of the cartilage junction then a period of 3 weeks in a cylinder cast will relieve the symptoms.

If, however, there is chondromalacia of the bipartite fragment, excision may be necessary. This is carried out through a small transverse incision immediately above the patella; the fragment is enucleated and the defect closed with sutures. After support of the leg for 7 days in a Jones type of bandage, mobilization may commence freely and the symptoms usually subside.

Chondromalacia of the patella

This condition, which literally means 'soft cartilage', is a clearly defined clinical syndrome in which the patient complains of persistent pain felt behind the patella, especially after sitting with the knee flexed for a period of time. It is associated with relief of pain on movement but aggravation by violent exercise, particularly where the knee is loaded in a flexed position. The patients are often inactive, apparently introspective teenagers or very active athletes, but both groups can be very disabled. The microscopic findings are of roughened or frankly fibrillated articular cartilage, usually the latter (Figure 16.42), and the lesion begins most commonly at the junction of the medial and most medial or 'odd' facet of the undersurface of the patella. It was graded for convenience into four grades which simply indicate the extent of the involvement of the cartilage of the patella (Outerbridge, 1961) but is more precisely classified with regard to area and depth of cartilage exposure as follows (Bentley, 1992):

- Grade I (in an area <0.5 cm diameter)

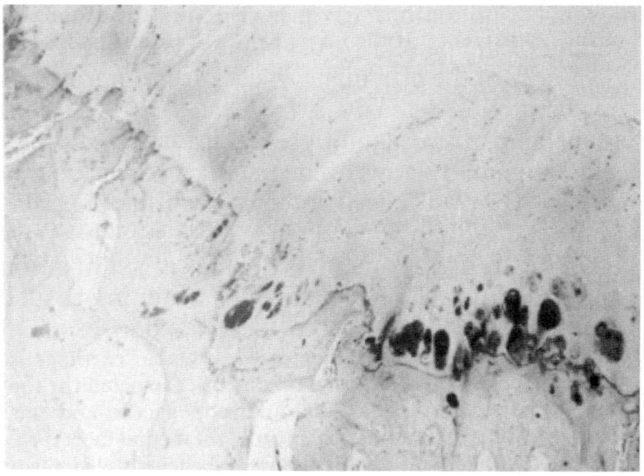

Figure 16.42 Early chondromalacia patellae showing fibrillation of the articular cartilage surface and loss of matrix staining in zones I and II. Small, heavily stained chondrocyte clusters are seen in the deep zone III which probably indicates a repair response (H&E × 72).

Ia – softening, swelling or fibrillation of cartilage
Ib – full thickness cartilage loss to bone

- Grade II (in an area 0.5–1.0 cm diameter)
  IIa – fibrillation of cartilage
  IIb – full thickness cartilage loss to bone
- Grade III (in an area 1–2 cm diameter)
  IIIa – fibrillation of cartilage
  IIIb – full thickness cartilage loss to bone

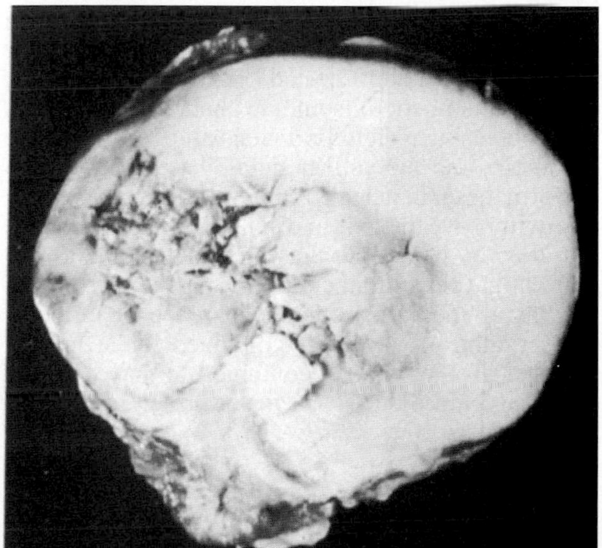

Figure 16.43 Undersurface of the patella showing grade IVa changes affecting the medial and odd facets and part of the lateral facet.

- Grade IV (in an area >2 cm diameter)
  IVa – fibrillation of cartilage
  IVb – full thickness cartilage loss to bone.

AETIOLOGY AND PATHOLOGY

The commonest lesion of the articular cartilage is fibrillation on the undersurface of the patella at the junction of the medial and 'odd' facets, and this may spread to involve most of the medial face (Figure 16.43). Ficat *et al.* (1975) described involvement of the lateral facet of the patella and defined a critical zone lateral to the median ridge of the patella. This is associated with a tightness of the lateral quadriceps expansion – usually congenital – which Ficat described as the excessive lateral pressure syndrome. This particular type of chondromalacia is rare in our experience and we have recorded it only once in a review of over 1000 cases. Similarly, the swollen appearance of articular cartilage on the medial and 'odd' facet described by Goodfellow *et al.* (1976) as a precursor of frank fibrillation of the articular cartilage was observed in only 5% of cases, though it is possible that this may represent the earliest stage of chondromalacia in a greater number. It is generally agreed that degeneration in the articular cartilage is the precipitating event; our early studies show fibrillation of the articular surface with death of superficial chondrocytes and at the same time proliferation of surrounding chondrocytes apparently in response to loss of cell matrix. There was no evidence in our study of a deep lesion such as that described by Goodfellow nor of a lesion of the subchondral bone as described by Darracott and Vernon-Roberts (1971). It is notable that the cartilage over the medial and 'odd' facets of the patella may be as thick as 0.8 cm (Hirsch, 1944), and the appearances suggest a mechanical breakdown of the surface skin of the articular cartilage due to constant and repetitive stresses after the manner described by Freeman (1974) for osteoarthritis.

Progress to osteoarthritis of the knee appears to be rare though there are few data available. Karlson (1940) followed a series of patients for 20 years and found no incidence of osteoarthritis. Furthermore, Meachim and Bentley (1977) have found that the typical distribution of osteoarthritis of the patellofemoral joint is principally on the lateral facet of the patella, which is not the area where chondromalacia most frequently occurs – suggesting a different aetiology and pathological process.

In a recent study of 100 patients with patellofemoral osteoarthritis (Bentley, 1988) 75 had extensive lateral facet involvement, 13 were medial and 12 had both facets involved. By contrast, a group of 102 young patients with chondromalacia patellae had involvement of the medial and odd facet in 94, with only 4 on the lateral facet and 4 involving both. Thus the two conditions appear to be different. However, the presence of lateral facet chondromalacia described by Ficat *et al.* (1975) in association with the excessive lateral pressure syndrome is almost certainly pre-osteoarthritic. This is the type of chondromalacia which is helped by lateral release and is indicated as a prophylaxis against later lateral facet osteoarthritis.

In patients with the common medial and odd facet chondromalacia patellae, it appears that the condition does not progress to osteoarthritis. In a review of 100 patients (Bentley, 1988) with patellofemoral and medial compartment osteoarthritis, none had a history of previous anterior knee pain or chondromalacia in their youth. Furthermore, in a review of patients followed for 3–30 years after treatment for chondromalacia patellae none showed osteoarthritis of the knee. Therefore the patient can be reassured about the long-term risk of osteoarthritis.

CLINICAL FEATURES

Two-thirds of the patients are female (Bentley, 1970) and typically the history is one of spontaneous onset of pain behind the patella which is aggravated by sitting with the knees flexed or by athletic activities or those which involve kneeling or squatting. Frequently there is no obvious malalignment of the leg and no obvious abnormality of the 'Q' angle. It has been suggested that the small, high patella is associated with the condition and that patella alta is also associated but Marks and Bentley (1978) found a correlation with patella alta only in the most severe degrees of chondromalacia.

Physical examination of the knee often reveals only tenderness on palpation of the medial undersurface of the patella (see Figure 16.8). If there is free fluid in the joint together with crepitus which can be palpated then these are valuable confirmatory physical signs. Rarely, there may be a large effusion into the joint but this is associated only with the more severe and advanced degrees of the condition where there is extensive breakdown of articular cartilage and reactive synovitis in response to the irritative effects of the cartilage matrix.

It should be emphasized, however, that the condition can be diagnosed only from direct inspection of the patella, by either arthroscopy or operation. Leslie and Bentley (1978) demonstrated that only 50% of patients who have the clinical syndrome actually have a demonstrable lesion of the articular cartilage.

Arthroscopy is the most valuable investigation; through the arthroscope it is possible to assess the presence and extent of a lesion and, by careful probing of the patella with a blunt probe, the degree of softness of the articular surface. Arthrography has been employed extensively by Ficat *et al.* (1975) but in our hands this has not proved useful. Radiology using tangential views of the patella as described by Ficat at 30°, 60° and 90° of flexion of the knee has not proved diagnostic and tends to be valuable only in demonstrating more gross degrees of subluxation or dislocation of the patella. MRI scanning is also helpful but localization of the defect and assessment of its size is still not accurate.

TREATMENT

The cause of pain in chondromalacia is not firmly established though it has been suggested that there is a vascular disturbance in the bone of the patella which is responsible for the symptoms. It appears more likely that the pain results from the stimulation of superficial bone nerve endings due, either to excessive loading where the articular cartilage is damaged or lost, or to reduction of pain threshold in bone by enzymatic action of lysosomal enzymes released from the articular cartilage.

Early on in treatment, reassurance that the condition is not serious and will not progress to osteoarthritis, with reduction of painful activities are often all that is required. The avoidance of kneeling and sports that involve deep knee bending and crouching are always helpful. In addition, it is useful to prescribe soluble aspirin for pain relief and reduction of synovitis although controlled clinical trials have demonstrated that there is no effect on the articular cartilage over a short period (Bentley *et al.*, 1981). The establishment of isometric quadriceps exercises with increasing weights is a vital part of conservative treatment, and the patient should be encouraged to perform these for at least 15 minutes four times every day to improve the tone and control of the quadriceps muscles. It is possible that such management also helps slight malalignment by increasing the tone of the vastus medialis component of the quadriceps. Conservative treatment is continued for at least 3 months; if the patient continues to have severe disabling pain arthroscopy is performed to confirm the diagnosis.

OPERATIVE TREATMENT OF CHONDROMALACIA PATELLAE

The choice of operative treatment is debatable though the presence of severe disabling pain makes this necessary in approximately one-third of patients.

Insall *et al.* (1976) attributed chondromalacia patellae to patellar malalignment and therefore recommend a procedure to realign the subluxed patella either by lateral release of the quadriceps expansion or by a transposition of the whole patellar apparatus. The major difficulty with this approach is that it is extremely difficult to demonstrate convincingly that subluxation of the patella is present with current methods of investigation (Dowd and Bentley, 1986). However, there is no doubt that, whilst lateral release alone appears to be of little value, lateral release of the quadriceps expansion together with a Goldthwait type of realignment of the patellar tendon and a generous medial reefing of the quadriceps expansion often effects good results even in patients with extensive lesions of grade 3 or more (Devas and Golski, 1973; Bentley, 1978). Whether this relief is due to the reduction of subluxation or simply due to the translation of stresses to a different area of the articular cartilage is debatable. The advantages of the procedure are that it requires very little disturbance of the knee mechanism and avoids the necessity for destructive operations such as shaving of the patella (Wiles *et al.*, 1960) or ridgectomy (Crookes, 1967), which in our long follow-up series proved to be valueless. In a follow-up series of 144 cases of chondromalacia patellae treated by four methods (i.e. shaving, excision of the defect and drilling of the subchondral bone; patellar tendon transfer with lateral release and medial reefing; and patellectomy), Bentley (1978) found that the best results were obtained with patellar tendon transfer and patellectomy, with overall good or excellent results in 60% and 77% respectively. As a result the authors' approach to this problem is to treat the patient intensively with conservative methods for a 3-month period including isometric quadriceps exercises, reduction of activities and aspirin therapy, and only to carry out surgery if this fails. Arthroscopy is then performed and where the patellar involvement is grade 1 or 2 then the patellar tendon transfer procedure is carried out. Where the changes in the articular cartilage are grade 3 or grade 4 the results to be expected from patellar tendon transfer are less good but Bentley favours tendon transfer as a primary procedure and performs patellectomy only if the patient is well motivated or has a large painful effusion and extensive cartilage damage.

Operative technique

Patellar realignment

In performing the realignment procedure a medial parapatellar incision is made, at least 2 cm medial to the patella to allow for the medial shift. The extensor apparatus of the knee is then exposed and the lateral retinaculum is completely released from the insertion of the patellar tendon into the tibia up to the vastus lateralis muscle fibres (Figure 16.44). It is important that the expansion be separated from the underlying synovium to which it is adherent. The lateral two-thirds of the patellar tendon are then separated and passed medially beneath the medial one-third of the patellar tendon and sutured with interrupted sutures to the periosteum and the medial ligament overlying the upper medial tibia. The medial retinaculum is then divided from the insertion of the patellar tendon up to the fibres of the vastus medialis and reefed by overlapping at least 1 cm and securing the overlap with mattress sutures and a reinforcing superficial layer of interrupted sutures. At the end of the procedure the knee should flex easily to 90°. Routine wound closure follows, and after the operation the patient is placed in a cylinder cast for a 3-week period. Walking commences after 48 hours and the patient is readmitted to hospital for supervised mobilization after 3 weeks. Throughout the preoperative and postoperative period emphasis is laid on isometric exercises and the patient's involvement in the result.

Patellectomy

This is performed through a small lateral parapatellar incision 2 cm long and a simple enucleation of the patella is carried out. No attempt is made to repair the patellar mechanism, the defect simply being closed with interrupted Vicryl sutures. The skin suture, as in all knee surgery, is of an intradermal atraumatic type. The leg is then enclosed in a cylinder cast for 3 weeks and walking commences after 48 hours. The patient is readmitted 3 weeks later for mobilization in hospital, which is supervised until a full range of movement is achieved.

Other procedures

Recent work on replacing the damaged area of the articular cartilage with a cartilage matrix support prosthesis of carbon fibre has been disappointing (Bentley *et al.*, 1992) but the use of another material or of a composite graft of fibres with living chondrocytes may prove useful in future (Hemmen *et al.*, 1991).

Some authors, notably Maquet (1984), emphasized the high loading of the patella, particularly of the 'odd' and medial facets, during flexion and weight-bearing – as for instance in sport or climbing stairs. Ferguson *et al.* (1979) confirmed this high loading by use of transducers implanted experimentally beneath the articular surface of the patella. Thus Maquet advocated tibial tubercle elevation by sup-

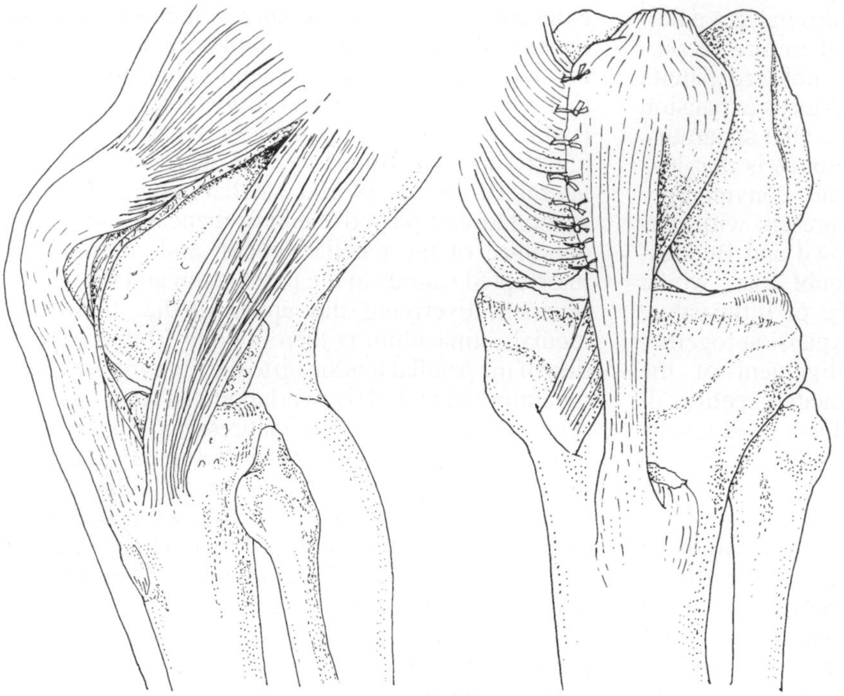

(a) (b)

Figure 16.44 Diagram to show (a) lateral patellar release with division of the retinaculum as far as the fibres of vastus lateralis and (b) medial transfer of the lateral part of the patellar tendon with medial reefing of the quadriceps to achieve patellar realignment. (Reproduced, with permission, from Aichroth, P.M. (1991) Recurrent dislocation of the patella. In: *Rob & Smith's Operative Surgery: Orthopaedics.* Edited by G. Bentley and R.B. Greer. Butterworth Heinemann: London, Boston, Sydney, Wellington, Singapore)

porting it with a corticocancellous graft as a means of reducing pressure on the patellar articular surface and hence symptoms of chondromalacia patellae. In some cases the results are encouraging but they have never been compared with the results of other types of treatment. Furthermore, the complications of the procedure include skin necrosis, fracture of the elevated tibial cortex, dislodgement of the graft and an uncomfortable prominence of the tibial tubercle.

In view of the benign nature of the condition conservative treatment should be pursued whenever possible. In patients with severe disability and an otherwise normal knee, who are well motivated and who are athletic, a distal quadriceps realignment is performed followed by 3 weeks' protection of the knee in a cylinder cast and vigorous rehabilitation. In older patients who are more sedentary and who have a healthy femoral groove, patellectomy is the procedure of choice followed by the same vigorous postoperative management. Successful patellectomy requires full commitment to rehabilitation by the patient and should not be employed otherwise.

Patellar dislocation syndrome

The patella, the largest sesamoid in the body, functions in a state of dynamic equilibrium between lateral forces, which consist of the lateral vectors of the 'Q' angle between the line drawn from the anterior superior iliac spine to the centre of the patella and the line of the patellar tendon, and medial forces made up of the medial capsule and vastus medialis insertion.

Lesions affecting the lateral structures – e.g. tightening of the iliotibial band, hyperplasia of vastus lateralis, abnormal fibrous insertion of vastus lateralis as well as abnormal bony relationship because of loss of trochlear depth, shallowness of the patella, external tibial torsion, femoral anteversion, lateral location of anterior tibial tubercle and genu valgum – have all been described as causes of lateral tracking of the patella.

On the medial side, ligamentous laxity (e.g. the familial joint laxity syndrome (Carter and Sweetnam, 1958), syndromes such as Ehlers–Danlos, Marfan's, osteogenesis imperfecta and vastus medialis insufficiency (e.g. in poliomyelitis, aberrant insertion or hypoplasia) are described causes. Most patients show none of these features and most authors now consider patella alta as being of primary importance (Ficat, 1977; Dowd and Bentley, 1986).

Patellar instability – habitual and recurrent subluxation/ dislocation of the patella

The patella may be displaced as a result of injury or congenital deformity. The displacement may be upward (patella alta), downwards (patella baja or patella infera), lateral or medial though clinically all except the lateral displacement are exceedingly rare (Figure 16.45a). Medial dislocation is even rarer and usually results from injury, but may occur in severe cases of genu varum. Occasionally, as a result of injury, the bone may rotate on its long axis, so that one of its borders engages between the condyles of the femur. This is a rare form of dislocation. The upward dislocation is also traumatic in origin, for there has usually been a neglected rupture of the ligamentum patellae.

The commoner lateral dislocation is the most important and also the type most liable to become habitual or recurrent; indeed, it is the lesion usually implied by the terms 'recurrent dislocation'. The condition is much more common in females. It may result from:

1. An abnormally high patella usually congenital or rarely after Osgood–Schlatter's disease.
2. Congenital causes – as in cases of poor development of the lateral femoral condyle, congenital anomalies of the patella, malattachment of the iliotibial tract, external rotation of the tibia and the nail-patella syndrome (Figure 16.45b, c).

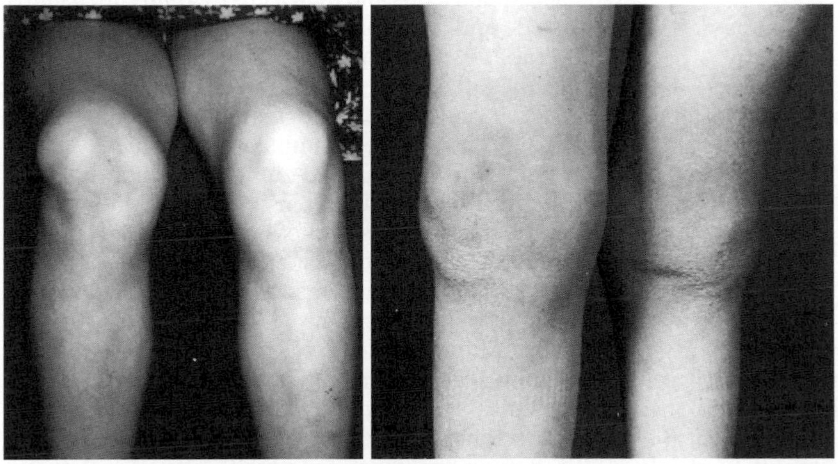

(a) (b)

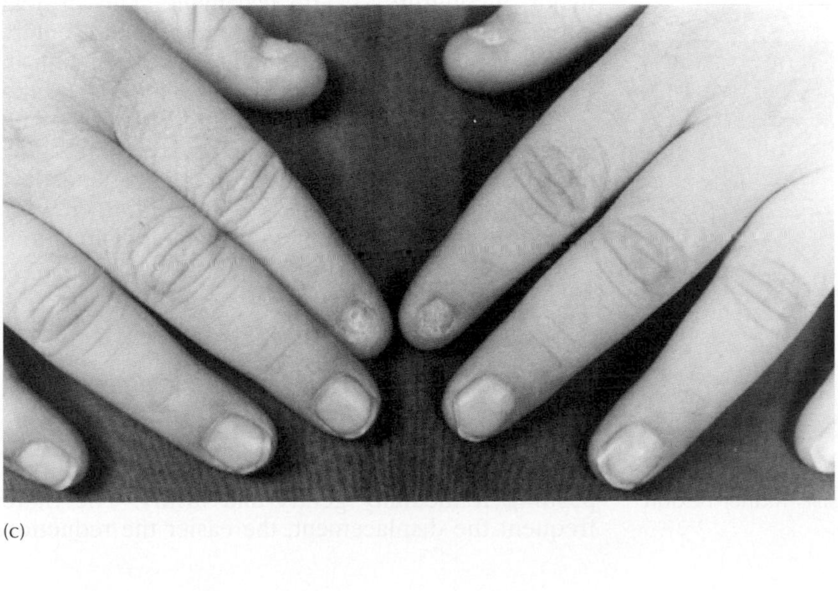

(c)

Figure 16.45 Flexion of the knee reveals obvious dislocation of the right patella. (b) Bilateral dislocation of patellae in a boy with the nail-patella syndrome. (c) The nail deformities – greatest in the thumb in a boy with the nail-patella syndrome.

3. Rachitic causes – lateral displacement of the patella may be associated with rachitic genu valgum. As the knock knee is flexed, the patella slips over the condyle, but at first complete reduction occurs when the leg is extended again. Later secondary changes may render the dislocation permanent.
4. Traumatic causes – this type usually occurs in females, often in adolescence, and it is often associated with a varying degree of genu valgum or with an extra-long ligamentum patellae producing patella alta. The patella is often small as well as high. Occasionally, too, the whole joint is of the loose relaxed type, and sometimes the lateral condyle is small. These conditions predispose to dislocation, since they all favour the outward pull of the quadriceps. The injury may be a blow or kick, but is commonly the result of muscular action.

CLINICAL FEATURES

Clinically there are three types of lateral patellar instability:

1. Habitual dislocation – which occurs every time the knee is flexed.
2. Recurrent dislocation, which is often post-traumatic and occurs at intervals.
3. Dislocation secondary to excessive lateral pressure syndrome (ELPS).

In mild cases the patella just slips momentarily over the condyle and the patient complains of the knee giving way and of the synovitis that follows the incident. Diagnosis in such cases is difficult. Fairbank (1933) pointed out that not uncommonly the patient will seize the examiner's hands to check a manipulation the sensation of which she immediately recognizes. This 'apprehension' sign, when present, is strong evidence in favour of recurrent dislocation (Figure 16.46). The possibility of a recurrent dislocation in a teenage female with a history of 'giving way' must always be considered and assessed to prevent long-term disability.

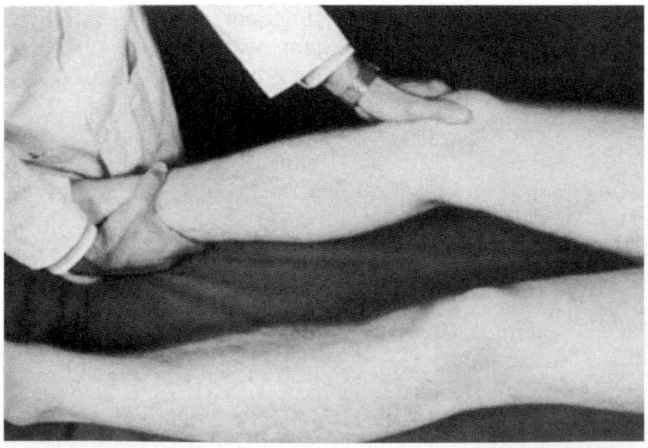

Figure 16.46 The apprehension test. The patella is pushed laterally during flexion. The patient resists further flexion because of pain.

Each recurrence is usually precipitated by a sudden contraction of the quadriceps when the knee is extended or semi-flexed and the foot and leg are everted, so that the insertion of the ligamentum patellae comes to lie more laterally, and the quadriceps is allowed to drag with increased force on the already unstable bone.

When the displacement is a frequent occurrence, little or no pain is experienced, but when longer intervals elapse between attacks, the incident is associated with considerable pain, disability and swelling of the joint.

The quadriceps and the vastus medialis are usually wasted and the patellar tendon is unduly lax. Lateral movement of the patella is sometimes more than the other side or appears more than normal. Observation of the knee movement with the leg over the end of the examination couch may show the patella moving in and out of the femoral groove either in flexion or in extension. The former occurs with the excessive lateral pressure syndromes (Ficat *et al.*, 1975) and the latter in cases of ligament laxity. Following trauma usually the dislocation occurs during flexion.

The radiological assessment consists of a standard anteroposterior film of both knees for patellar dysplasias, fragmentations, marginal defects and duplications, etc., and a lateral view with the knee in 30° flexion to assess for patella alta. Axial views taken at 30°, 60° and 90° of flexion may show up patellar dysplasias, trochlear dysplasias and any major incongruity or displacement. The critical angle is between 10° and 40° where the patella enters the trochlea. Lateral subluxation may be seen with an increase in the medial joint space or the loss of the lateral patellofemoral angle (Figure 16.47). The patella may be sitting astride the lateral trochlea facet. Retinacular calcification on the medial aspect of the patella seen on the 30° tangential view, if present, is diagnostic of previous lateral dislocation.

TREATMENT

Reduction is generally easy but may require general anaesthetic in the acute traumatic type. The knee is gently extended to relax the quadriceps. The kneecap is simultaneously manipulated into position by pushing it medially gently and firmly. The more frequent the displacement, the easier the reduction

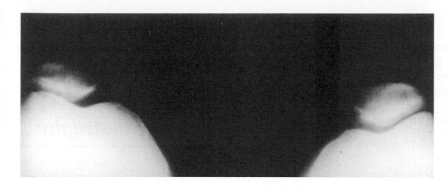

Figure 16.47 The 30° tangential radiograph confirms lateral displacement of the patella.

becomes; ultimately, indeed, the patient may learn to correct the dislocation herself. In time, however, the repeated recurrences result in a relaxed, weakened and unstable joint as well as growth disturbances, especially hypoplasia of the lateral femoral condyle, loose body formation and, in later years, osteoarthritis.

Occasionally, recurrence may be prevented by the use of a firm bandage, or knee cage, though as the condition is extremely disabling more radical measures are usually demanded.

Although it is often assumed that realignment of the patellar mechanism for recurrence dislocation is a routine and reliable procedure, necessary to prevent hypoplasia and maldevelopment of the femoral sulcus and possibly osteoarthritis, evidence contained in the literature does not support this assumption totally. Recent work suggests that some operations may not only fail to prevent osteoarthrosis, but may also hasten its development, especially those such as the Hauser procedure which overtighten the quadriceps apparatus.

Conservative treatment

In the management of established recurrent dislocation one tends to think immediately of operative treatment. There is, however, considerable variation in the frequency of dislocation and in the disability which it produces, and as the long-term results of operation are not always satisfactory, it is not indicated for patients whose symptoms are not disabling.

Intensive quadriceps exercises with taping will 'cure' a small percentage of patients (Heywood, 1961) but if there is dislocation more often than once per month and if there is lateral femoral condylar hypoplasia and permanent lateral positioning of the patella in the groove, then operation is indicated.

Operative treatment

Acute traumatic patellar dislocation

Recurrent dislocation frequently follows an injury in which the knee was twisted in flexion and locked in the lateral position. A history of requiring an anaesthetic to achieve reduction and a tangential radiograph showing ossification medial to the patella on the tangential view is very strong evidence of a traumatic dislocation. In cases of doubt an examination under anaesthetic in which the patella is pushed as far laterally as possible should be performed. There are a few cases of genuine instability in which dislocation cannot be achieved but generally the dislocation is easy to produce. Following the first acute dislocation some patients will recover but they need to tone-up their quadriceps by intensive isometric exercises. Where troublesome recurrence occurs, soft tissue realignment as a secondary procedure involving lateral release, medial reefing and transfer of the attachment of the patella tendon medially by the method described above which is similar to the Roux–Goldthwait is required (Figure 16.44).

The operation is performed by a medial parapatellar incision which is at least 2 cm medial to the patella at its centre to avoid its lying over the patella when medial realignment is completed. The extensor apparatus, i.e. patella, patellar tendon and medial and lateral capsule, are exposed subcutaneously. The lateral release is performed first with a knife and is carried upwards as far as the fibres of the vastus lateralis muscle, coagulating the lateral genicular vessel as necessary. The capsule is freed from the underlying synovium to allow the patella to move medially. The lateral 80% of the patellar tendon is cut from its insertion into the tibial tubercle and passed medial beneath the remaining 20% and secured under a flap of tissue on the medial tibia which is combined periosteum, medial ligament and pes anserinus with mattress sutures. The medial capsule is then divided as far as the upper margin of the patella and overlapped by 1–2 cm depending on the tracking of the patella required. This overlapping is secured with a double row of interrupted sutures. The knee is then flexed to 90° to ensure that the repair is not too tight and that the patella is stable. Wound closure follows and the leg is supported in a cylinder cast for 3 weeks after which vigorous mobilization exercises to strengthen quadriceps commence.

Recurrent patellar subluxation and dislocation

In a patient with a typical history either of an acute dislocation or of recurrent 'giving way' of the knee, appropriate radiographs are required to assess the presence of patella alta and/or a shallow femoral sulcus angle. This is because physical examination is often equivocal although the presence of small, high patellae and a positive apprehensive test are valuable indicators, especially if the patient has ligamentous laxity. Attempting to assess patellar tracking either clinically or arthroscopically has proved very difficult and much more emphasis is laid on the radiographs and the examination for patellar stability under general anaesthesia.

If the patella feels mobile but will not dislocate under general anaesthesia, a lateral release is performed arthroscopically and the patient performs vigorous quadriceps exercises postoperatively. When dislocation occurs easily a lateral release, medial quadriceps reefing and realignment of the patella tendon referred to above is performed. The use of bony operations such as the Hauser tibial tubercle transplant should be avoided except in cases of gross patella alta and always in patients prior to skeletal maturity to avoid damage and premature fusion of the tubercle growth plate, leading to patella infera or genu recurvatum. The long-term studies of the Hauser procedure indicate that there is a significant incidence of osteoarthritis, presumably due to overloading of the articular cartilage. With the soft tissue procedure described above it is possible to adjust the tension of the quadriceps at the time of operation so that the knee flexes to 90° on the operating table and thus excessive articular cartilage pressure and osteoarthritis are less likely. The biomechanics of the patellofemoral joint are complex in the normal joint (Goodfellow *et al.*, 1976). Alteration of these by any procedure may be painful unless performed before skeletal maturity when the cartilage as well as the bone has the capacity to remodel. Thus the results of different methods are very variable. It must be remembered, however, that the late, unreduced dislocated patella produces pain and disability due to secondary osteoarthritis which cannot be adequately corrected surgically because of the shortening of the quadriceps apparatus. Therefore everything must be done to avoid that situation since late quadriceps lengthening is an extensive and unpredictable procedure.

Reflex sympathetic dystrophy

The involvement of the knee and, in particular, the patella in the process of sympathetic dystrophy was popularized by Ficat and Hungerford (1977). They related the condition to Sudeck's atrophy in which there is a vasomotor disturbance in the blood supply to the patella and also in some cases to the femur and tibia associated with osteoporosis. The condition is initiated by injury and is interpreted as a failure of the normal vasomotor equilibrium such that the patient develops a syndrome characterized by pain, swelling, tenderness, stiffness, initial warmth and eventually sensitivity to cold. Clinically the patient complains of retropatellar pain, exquisite tenderness to touch and night pain. In the initial stages the discomfort is often accompanied by oedema and local heat and redness around the kneecap but later the local warmth is replaced by sensitivity to cold. The skin may demonstrate extreme hyperaesthesia, show definite decrease in skin temperature and appear cyanotic when exposed to cold. Another feature is stiffness of the knee joint with flexion only to 90° and induration of the capsule of the joint. The radiological features, when present, are striking with slight or gross osteoporosis which can be seen best on tangential views taken at 30° and 60° of flexion. Ficat (1977) found a rise in intramedullary pressure in the patella and the femur and occasionally the tibia, venostasis and a rise in blood flow as indicated by technetium-99 scintigraphy.

Treatment of this condition, which is difficult, involves gentle physiotherapy, aspirin therapy, sympathetic block and core decompression of the patella.

The authors distinguish between this syndrome and that due to long-standing disuse osteoporosis, though the differentiation in mild cases is not easy. It is a diagnosis worth considering in cases of unexplained patellofemoral pain.

Loose bodies

The occurrence in joints of a variety of types of loose body has long been recognized. Practically every

Table 16.3 Classification of loose bodies

Fibrinous loose bodies (composed of fibrinous material or of necrotic synovial membrane)	
Traumatic	
After haemorrhage	
Pathological	
In association with:	
Tuberculosis	
Rheumatoid arthritis	
Osteoarthritis	
Cartilaginous loose bodies (composed entirely of hyaline cartilage)	
Traumatic	
Clinical fractures	
Separation of whole or part of intra-articular fibro-cartilaginous meniscus	
Osteocartilaginous loose bodies	
Traumatic	
Osteochondral fractures of femoral condyles and patella	
Pathological	
Detachment of portion of articular surface from osteochondritis dissecans	
Synovial chondromatosis	
Detachment of osteophytes in:	
osteoarthritis	
neuropathic joints	
Separation of sequestra in tuberculosis	
Miscellaneous loose bodies	
Introduced foreign bodies	
Lipoma	
Angioma	
Secondary carcinoma, etc.	

joint in the body has been reported as containing such bodies, but they are most frequently found in the knee joint.

Table 16.3 outlines the classification of loose bodies according to composition but it should be understood that the majority of these are either rare or of little clinical significance as they are nothing more than a minor manifestation of some other disease. For practical purposes the differential diagnosis usually rests between osteoarthritic loose bodies, synovial chondromata and loose bodies associated with osteochondritis dissecans or osteochondral fractures.

FIBRINOUS LOOSE BODIES

Following intra-articular haemorrhage fibrinous loose bodies may arise in large numbers, formed from organized blood clot. In association with chronic synovitis loose bodies composed of fragments of hypertrophic synovial membrane may arise. They are seen in tuberculosis and rheumatoid arthritis and osteoarthritis.

CARTILAGINOUS LOOSE BODIES

Loose bodies composed of hyaline articular cartilage may arise following trauma to the joint or in osteoarthritis. Occasionally, torn fragments of the menisci may give rise to fibrocartilaginous loose bodies.

OSTEOCHONDRAL LOOSE BODIES

Osteochondral fractures

Osteochondral fractures may follow direct injury to the knee when a peripheral segment of cartilage and subchondral bone is sheared off. Often a large segment is involved and there is little doubt about the diagnosis. Osteochondral fractures may also arise indirectly as a result of combined rotation and compression forces. These injuries may produce centrally placed lesions in the lateral and medial condyles in adolescents. The role of the tibial spines in these injuries is unclear. Acute dislocation of the patella may result in a tangential osteochondral fracture of the patella or lateral femoral condylar groove, or both, either at the time of dislocation or on reduction.

Osteochondral fracture should always be considered following a knee injury associated with traumatic effusion or haemarthrosis and x-ray may reveal the fragment. The fragment is usually detached from the lateral margin of the femoral groove due to the pressure of the patella. Sometimes the fragment is off the patella and occasionally both surfaces are affected. In doubtful cases, arthroscopy of the knee in the acute stages will reveal a crater in the subchondral bone and the loose body.

Treatment

If small, <1.5 cm, the fragment is removed arthroscopically. The defect will fill with repair fibrocartilage. If larger, the joint is opened and the detached fragment is reduced and secured with Smillie pins or a Herbert screw. When the osteochondral fracture accompanies an acute dislocation of the patella, the associated capsular tear should be repaired to prevent further dislocation.

Osteochondritis dissecans

Osteochondritis dissecans is a condition in which a segment of subchondral bone and overlying articular cartilage becomes either partially or completely separated at characteristic sites on the articular surfaces of certain joints.

The joint most commonly affected is the knee, but similar lesions have been found in the elbow, ankle and hip. In some cases the condition is bilateral.

Typically the lesions involve convex surfaces in the various joints as follows: in the knee, the inner aspect of the medial femoral condyle (Figures 16.48 and 16.49); in the elbow, the capitellum; in the ankle, the outer trochlear surface of the talus; and in the hip, the superior aspect of the femoral head.

Originally it was believed that following trauma there developed a pathological process, 'quiet necrosis', which led to the gradual extrusion of part of the traumatized surface. This was the view of Paget (1870) and of König (1888), but both these observers agreed that by the time the body separated, all signs of the underlying pathological process had disappeared. It was this conception of the process that made König name it osteochondritis dissecans.

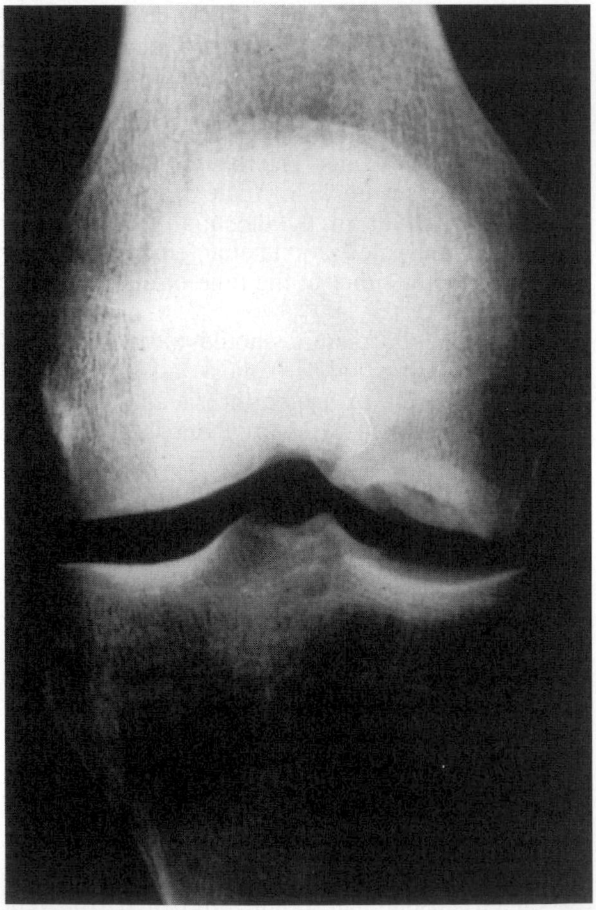

Figure 16.48 Anteroposterior radiograph of a 17-year-old male with an area of radiolucency in the medial femoral condyle containing an ossicle.

Many alternative explanations have been proposed. In the main, they may be grouped into those which attribute osteochondritis to trauma and those which postulate some primary disturbance of the subchondral bone. Among the possible sequelae of trauma are subchondral fracture with gradual separation of a fragment, damage to vessels supplying a portion of the subchondral bone, and a post-traumatic inflammatory condition. Observations on the patella (Edwards and Bentley, 1977) suggested that repetitive shearing stresses cause the gradual separation of the articular cartilage and subchondral bone fragment.

Trauma to the usual site in the medial femoral condyle may be caused by the medial tibial spine. The medial spine is often longer than the lateral, and it has been pointed out that in some cases of osteochondritis it appears hypertrophied. It is suggested that forced rotation of the tibia on the femur or forcible medial displacement of the tibia on the femur may cause the spine to impinge on the articular surface of the medial femoral condyle (Smillie, 1978).

Fairbank (1948) supported the view that the lesion is a fracture because:

1. It occurs most frequently in adolescents and young adults indulging in vigorous pastimes.
2. Typical lesions are seen on radiography, and are revealed by operation after definite and sometimes recent trauma.
3. A lesion at the typical site may involve the cartilage only, the detached fragment consisting of normal articular cartilage.
4. There is an entire absence of inflammatory changes in and about the lesion.
5. The gross appearances, when the operation is performed early, suggest nothing but a simple recent fracture. When sufficient time has elapsed for changes to occur, the only ones that do take place are those which would be expected from an effort on the part of the tissues to repair the damage.

Aichroth (1977) produced lesions indistinguishable from osteochondritis dissecans by creating unstable defects in animal knees. He attributed the condition to trauma also, but caused by direct impact of the medial articular facet of the patella on the outer aspect of the medial femoral condyle when the knee is flexed to 90° or more.

The aetiology of bilateral lesions is not so easy to explain and is best considered to be due to develop-

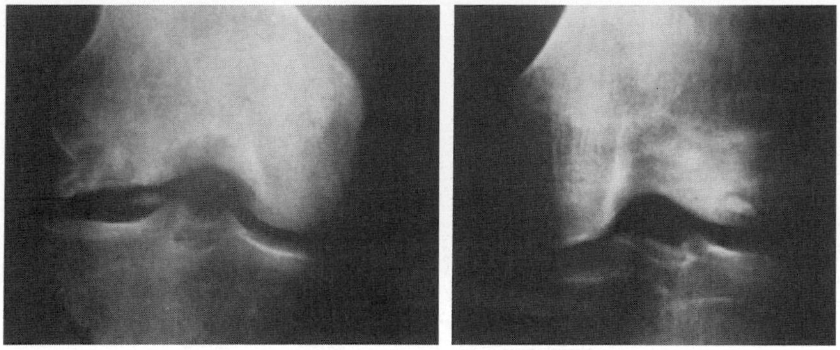

Figure 16.49 Anteroposterior radiographs of the knee of a 20-year-old male showing osteochondritis dissecans of the lateral femoral condyle with marked bony abnormality and separation of one fragment.

mental anatomical abnormalities of blood supply or articular congruence.

Pathology

The body may be lying quite free in the joint cavity, attached by a fibrous band in the intercondylar area or attached by a hinge of articular cartilage. In some cases the lesion is difficult to detect with the naked eye. The lesion is most commonly derived from the inner aspect of the medial femoral condyle. Less commonly, the central region of the femoral condyle is involved and, rarely, the lateral condyle.

The appearance of the body varies greatly according to the age of the lesion. The undersurface usually consists of cancellous bone, but when the body has existed in the joint for a long time the surface becomes smooth, rounded and covered with cartilage. Indeed, the cartilage may proliferate, nourished by synovial fluid, until the body acquires considerable proportions.

Symptoms and signs

Clinical presentation depends on the stage of the disease. At an early stage there may be little in the way of symptoms. It occasionally happens that an x-ray of the supposedly normal knee, taken for comparison, reveals a definite osteochondritic focus (see Figure 16.48). In other cases there may be mild discomfort after exercise with episodes of giving way. There may be persistent or recurrent effusion. In these patients the diagnosis may be overlooked for several years.

When the osteochondral fragment becomes detached, the symptoms are more definite. There is pain on weight-bearing, the episodes of giving way may be associated with intermittent 'loose body' locking and there is often quadriceps wasting. In some patients there is a definite history of trauma followed by disability and they present with a painful swollen locked knee. In the absence of a palpable loose body there may be no abnormality on examination in less severe cases. Sometimes there is tenderness on firm palpation of the affected area of the condyle with the knee flexed at 90°.

Radiography

The lesion may be overlooked on standard anteroposterior and lateral views and intercondylar ('tunnel') views of the knee should be taken if the diagnosis is suspected. MRI will reveal the osteochondritic area on the surface without difficulty in most cases. Loose bodies may be difficult to see when they contain very little bone.

Treatment

Smillie (1978) differentiated two main types of osteochondritis dissecans, and these are very useful in determining treatment:

1. *Juvenile osteochondritis dissecans*. If the child is below skeletal maturity it is very unusual for the osteochondritic fragment to separate into the joint and healing and incorporation occurs frequently. Therefore, treatment should be symptomatic with reduction of violent activities and the use of a cylinder cast for 3 weeks if there is an effusion.
2. *Adult osteochondritis dissecans*. In treatment of this condition it is important to remember that any incongruity of the articular surface will tend to predispose the joint to osteoarthritis in later life. Furthermore, the osteochondral fragment of osteochondritis should be regarded as being an autologous graft and should, with proper preparation, heal into the surface, thus restoring the articular congruity.

In the presence of persistent symptoms the joint should always be examined by arthroscopy to identify the area of damage and the nature of the lesion and to recognize any loose fragments in the joint.

When the articular surface is found to be unbroken but the site of the lesion is clearly indicated by a change in the colour or texture on probing the overlying cartilage, or the extent of the lesion is indicated by a groove (Figure 16.50), attempts should be made to determine whether this circumscribed area of cartilage is mobile or not. If it is fairly firm then it should be left in position and is best treated by multiple fine 1 mm drill holes through the articular surface into the subchondral bone. Although this damages the articular cartilage, the tiny holes produced will heal rapidly with fibrocartilage and the resulting surface will be satisfactory. If it is very mobile then it is probably better to perform a medial arthrotomy and lift the fragment by dividing the margins with a sharp knife, to drill and curette out the base of the defect of the femoral condyle and to replace the fragment. The fit of the fragment is important, and if necessary a small amount of cancellous bone may be taken from the outer aspect of the femoral condyle so that the surface fit is perfect. The fragment is then fixed with two Smillie pins driven beneath the articular surface or two Kirschner wires inserted retrograde into the fragment to avoid the cartilage surface (Figures 16.51 and 16.52). If the cartilage is extensively fibrillated and soft then it is better to excise it, to curette and drill

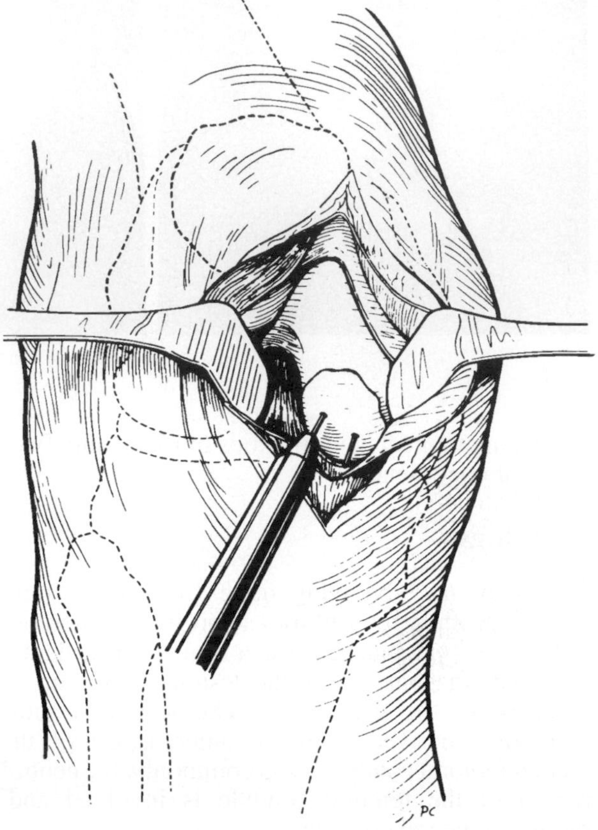

Figure 16.51 Diagram to illustrate pinning of loose osteochondritic fragment with 2 Smillie pins. (Reproduced, with permission, from Aichroth, P.M. (1991) Loose bodies in the knee. In: *Operative Surgery*, 4th edn. *Orthopaedics*. Edited by G. Bentley and R.B. Greer. Butterworth Heinemann: London, Boston, Sydney, Wellington, Singapore)

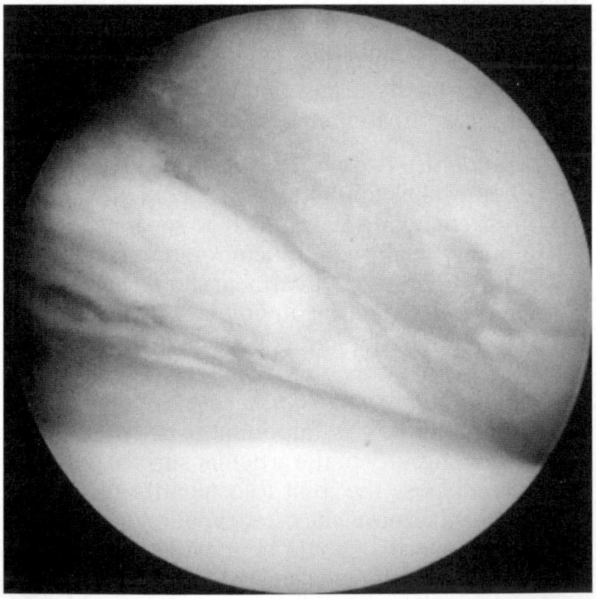

Figure 16.50 Arthroscopic view of a well-defined but stable osteochondritic fragment on the medial femoral condyle. (Reproduced, with permission, from Dandy, D.J. (1984) *Arthroscopy of the Knee*. Butterworths: London, Boston, Durban, Singapore, Sydney, Toronto, Washington)

the bed of the defect and to make the edges of the bed vertical to provide support to the fibrocartilage which will form in the defect of the surrounding cartilage. If the fragment is partially separated and hinged by an intact piece of cartilage then the bed should be curetted and drilled – if necessary, partially filled with cancellous bone – and the fragment replaced flush to the articular surface and fixed with two Smillie pins. The pins into the base of the articular cartilage are left *in situ*. Arthroscopy is performed at 1 year to check whether these pins are extruding into the joint and if so to remove them. Following this type of surgery the knee is immobilized in the fully extended position in a cylinder cast and the patient commences protected weight-bearing for 24 hours. The knee is retained in the cast for 4 weeks, after which gentle mobilization is commenced.

The long-term prognosis of osteochondritis dissecans has not been studied thoroughly but it is unusual to see older patients with osteoarthritis who

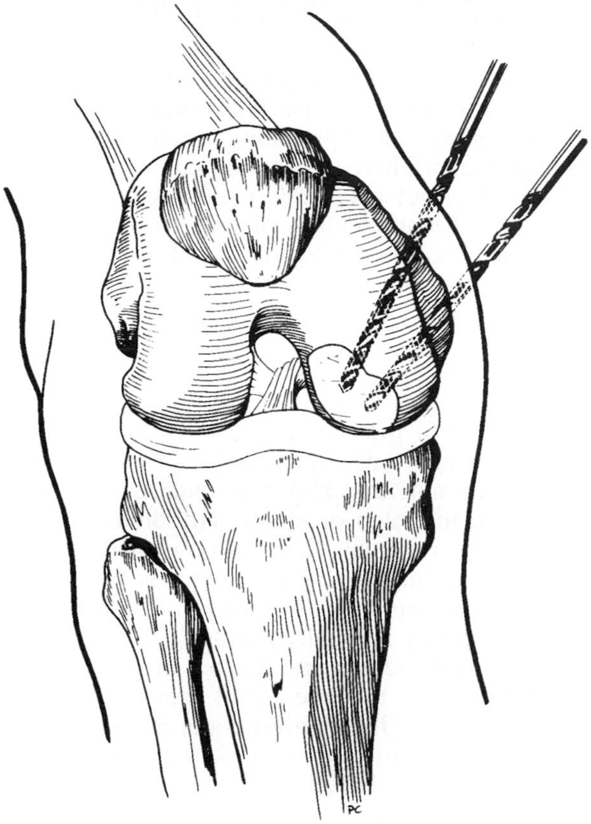

Figure 16.52 Alternative technique where the fragment is fixed by 2 Kirschner wires driven into the fragment retrograde to avoid the surface of the articular cartilage. (Reproduced, with permission, from Aichroth, P.M. (1991) Loose bodies in the knee. In: *Operative Surgery*, 4th edn. *Orthopaedics*. Edited by G. Bentley and R.B. Greer. Butterworth Heinemann: London, Boston, Sydney, Wellington, Singapore)

have a history of osteochondritis in earlier life, which suggests an overall benign process – particularly if treatment is correct. Linden (1977) reported that osteoarthrosis occurred in 80% of adult patients followed over 33 years after osteochondritis dissecans. The prognosis in osteochondritis beginning in childhood was excellent.

Synovial chondromatosis

Von Kolliker (1883) described the occurrence of cartilage cells in the villi of synovial membrane. Most observers agree that, under the influence of certain stimuli, connective tissue cells may undergo metaplasia to form specialized mesodermal tissue of the body such as bone or cartilage.

In the condition of synovial chondromatosis, innumerable small foci of hyaline cartilage and sometimes bone are formed as a result of metaplasia of the synovial and subsynovial connective tissues. The term 'osteochondromatosis' describes this condition. Cartilage fragments which have become detached and enter the joint cavity may increase in size since they are nourished by synovial fluid. The knee joint is the most commonly affected in young and middle-aged adults (Figure 16.53). The condition is usually monarticular, but sometimes both knees may be affected as well as such joints as the hip, elbow and wrist. The articular surface of the joint is not grossly altered, in contrast to other conditions which give rise to multiple loose bodies.

Malignant change has been reported but this is exceedingly rare. This condition should be thought of in the differential diagnosis of monarticular swelling since the ossification classically seen on the radiographs may occur late in the disease. In early cases the diagnosis is made by arthroscopy where the dramatic appearance of the joint full of cartilaginous loose bodies produces a 'snowstorm' appearance.

Osteoarthritis

In osteoarthritis, three forms of loose bodies may occur – synovial chondromata, detached osteophytes and detached fragments of articular cartilage. As with other cartilaginous loose bodies, they may increase in size while lying free in the joint and produce locking.

Neuropathic arthropathy

In tabes dorsalis, the hypertrophic form of Charcot's disease may be seen. The loose bodies that form in this condition are similar to the osteophytes of osteoarthritis, but are commonly bigger and much

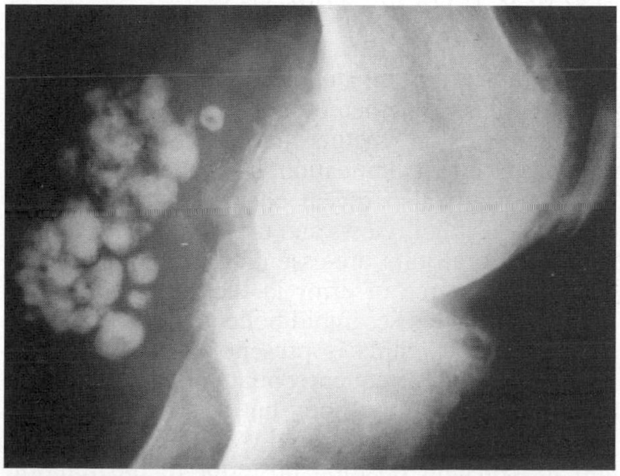

Figure 16.53 Lateral knee radiograph showing the multiple loose bodies of synovial chondromatosis.

more numerous owing to the extreme nature of the pathological process.

CLINICAL FEATURES OF LOOSE BODIES

Typically, the presence of a loose body in a joint is associated, sooner or later, with symptoms due to the impaction of the body between the opposing articular surfaces. While carrying out some movement, the patient experiences a sudden intense pain in the joint which may cause him to fall. He then finds that the limb is locked in the position of semi-flexion and neither extension nor further flexion is possible. This type of 'loose-body locking' occurring suddenly in mid-movement must be clearly differentiated from locking due to a torn meniscus.

There may be an obvious swelling at one part of the joint, pressure on which will release the joint and terminate the attack; or the body may become dislodged by some particular movement. Occasionally, however, an anaesthetic must be administered before the joint can be unlocked. After the attack there may be an effusion into the joint and in time a chronic synovitis may ensue.

An important point in the history is the variable site of the pain; in successive attacks, it may occur at widely differing parts of the joint, in contrast to meniscal lesions where the situation is usually constant. A most important diagnostic aid is that the patient may have palpated the loose body moving about the joint.

In some cases the symptoms are atypical and the usual history may not be forthcoming. The symptoms may be masked by those of underlying disease and the loose body may be overlooked in consequence.

RADIOGRAPHIC APPEARANCES

Radiographs are invaluable in the diagnosis of loose bodies. Whether or not they are visible on x-ray depends on whether there is an osseous component or any calcification has taken place, but the films will also reveal coexisting pathological changes. 'Tunnel' views and tangential views of the patellofemoral joint are essential. The fabella is an occasional source of error in the interpretation of radiographs. This sesamoid bone in the lateral head of the gastrocnemius is present in about 15% of individuals and is frequently bilateral. Its appearance may simulate a loose body but it is recognized by its regular sharply contoured oval or circular form and its constant position posterior to the femoral condyle.

TREATMENT OF LOOSE BODIES

A loose body which is giving rise to symptoms should be removed, and a loose body in a young person's joint should probably be removed even if asymptomatic. There may be difficulties in locating loose bodies but it is important to remember that following the application of an Esmarch type of tourniquet the loose body is usually found in the suprapatellar pouch. The simplest way of locating the loose body is to perform an arthroscopy with the knee filled with saline. Indeed, unless the loose body is very large it is usually quite simple to remove through the arthroscope (Figure 16.54). An examination of the remainder of the knee joint is carried out and a decision can then be made as to whether or not arthrotomy is required. In joints other than the knee or elbow, arthrotomy will be required for removal. In synovial chondromatosis of the knee, anterior synovectomy is performed, but in other joints – especially in the hip – an expectant policy is usually pursued.

When loose bodies are situated in the posterior compartment of the knee joint they may not be removable through the arthroscope, and if a definite cause of symptoms they may be removed by open operation. An S-shaped incision is made and the dissection is carried out medial to the popliteal nerve and vessel to expose the posterior aspect of the joint. This is much facilitated by the removal of the medial head of gastrocnemius from its attachment. For loose bodies in the posterolateral compartments the

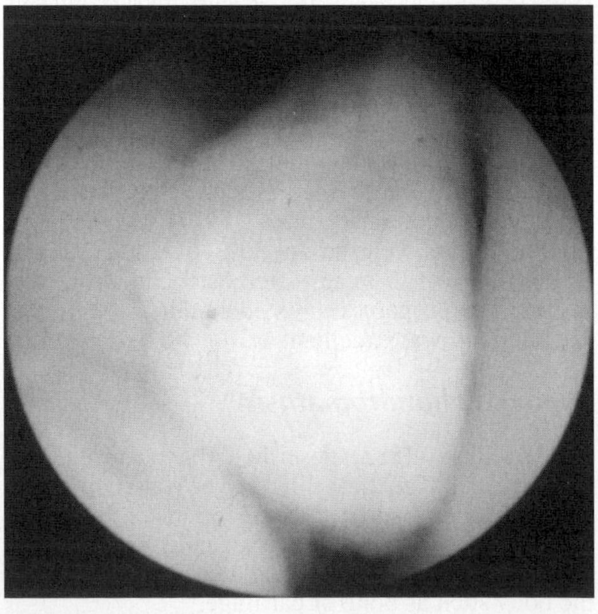

Figure 16.54 Arthroscopic appearances of a loose body in the suprapatellar pouch which is removed simply by a grasping forcep.

incision is parallel to the anterior border of the biceps tendon. The common peroneal nerve lies posterior to the biceps and is protected by it when this muscle has retracted backwards. The iliotibial band is divided longitudinally and the capsule opened either above or below the tendon of popliteus. The posterior horn of the lateral meniscus may also be explored through this incision.

When loose bodies are located in the posteromedial compartment, an incision may be made along the anterior border of sartorius. Muscle is retracted backwards and the capsule is opened behind the posterior margin of the tibial collateral ligament. There is a small recess behind the posterior horn of the medial meniscus in which a loose body may be trapped.

Pellegrini–Stieda's disease (post-traumatic para-articular osteoma)

This disease was first described by Köhler in 1903, although it is usually known by the names of the two authors who wrote about it 2 years later. The characteristic feature is the presence of new bone in the region of the medial ligament of the knee. A similar condition has been seen in the ankle and elbow joints. It occurs usually in adult males, and follows trauma. Following injury the earliest symptoms are those of a traumatic synovitis of the knee, followed by a period of improvement, though the knee never completely recovers; indeed, after 6 weeks or even months, pain and disability may increase until a point is reached at which they are stationary. Movement is then considerably limited with tenderness over the medial condyle, and often the condyle appears hypertrophied on palpation.

The symptoms are due to the interference with the function of the medial ligament, resulting in limitation of flexion from either adhesions or loss of elasticity associated with a partial tear of the attachment to the femoral condyle followed by ossification in the ligament.

An x-ray examination is essential for diagnosis and shows a bony shadow alongside the medial condyle, which may be uniform or composed of a series of separate small deposits (Figure 16.55). In the early stages the abnormal bone shadow is hazy and ill-defined, but when activity has ceased the edges are clear-cut. They are usually first seen about the level of the knee joint, and while in early cases they are quite separate from the condyle, in late cases the shadow may appear to be continuous with the condyle.

AETIOLOGY

By analogy with a similar disturbance – traumatic myositis ossificans – as a result of trauma, there is calcification of haematoma in the medial ligament at its site of attachment to the femoral condyle.

MANAGEMENT

The development of the ossification may be prevented by early recognition of the possibilities of the affection, and the injection of the area with hydrocortisone and local anaesthetic. A compression bandage is then applied. Passive movements should be prohibited as they so easily produce more bone and

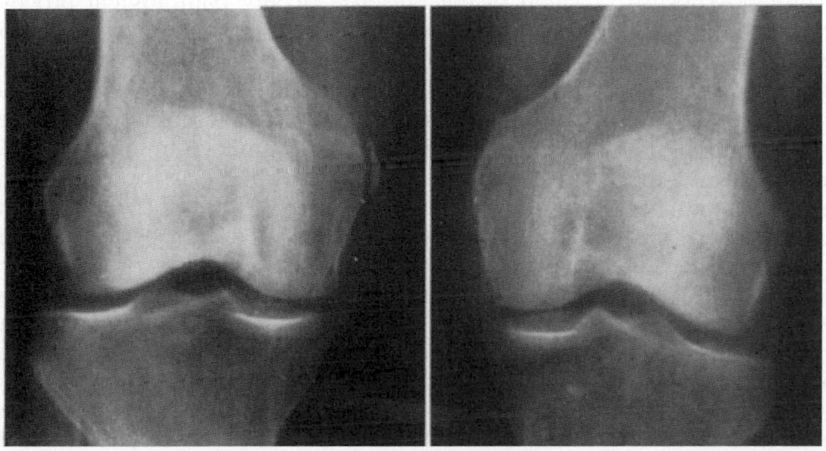

Figure 16.55 Anteroposterior radiograph of both knees of a middle-aged woman showing an area of radiodensity adjacent to the right medial femoral condyle at the site of attachment of the medial collateral ligament.

more stiffness, but isometric quadriceps exercises are maintained.

In established cases with a well marked area of calcification, an early restoration of full function must not be expected. The disease is self-limiting and, provided the case is not overtreated by vigorous movements, full recovery may be expected in 2–6 months. The slow return of flexion in such a case may provide the temptation to use passive movements or even manipulation. These forms of treatment are definitely detrimental. The patient's own active flexion to a point short of producing pain, together with quadriceps exercises, will eventually produce complete recovery.

The stiff knee

Free movement of the knee joint depends on the integrity of the various tissues surrounding it as well as the joint itself. The commonest factor interfering with movement is the presence of adhesions. They may occur within the synovial cavity, especially in the suprapatellar pouch, in the capsular and periarticular tissue between the quadriceps and the femur, and the fascia lata and the femur. Limitation of knee flexion is most commonly found after fractures in the vicinity of the knee, particularly the shaft of the femur and especially when these extend into the joint. It also occurs following infections in or about the knee joint, after operations where the knee is kept extended for long periods and in operations which have been badly planned with much damage to the soft tissue.

Most of these produce stiffness for clear reasons. When a fracture is slow in uniting, the knee is likely to be stiff afterwards. When union occurs without complications, knee stiffness is extraordinarily rare. The prevention is to secure union as quickly as possible. Therefore in cases necessitating exposure of the shaft of the femur, an anatomical approach should be used without division of muscle but passing between the muscle planes, as for example the posterolateral approach.

Knee stiffness may not only follow fracture of the femur, which results from the fragments entering the joint, but also from injudicious treatment. Skeletal traction through the femur, particularly if there is any pin tract infection and especially if the traction is fixed for too long with immobilization of the knee for periods of 8 weeks or more, also predisposes to stiffness. Conversely, a skeletal pin through the upper tibia allows some movement of the knee throughout the traction period. Knee stiffness can follow total knee arthroplasty especially if the knee was stiff beforehand and in elderly patients who are not motivated to do active exercises. This may largely be prevented by encouraging knee movements within 48 hours of operation using ice packs and under physiotherapy supervision. Occasionally continuous passive motion is useful but it must be used gently.

There can be limitation of knee movement either in extension or flexion.

LIMITATION OF MOVEMENT OF THE KNEE IN EXTENSION

This commonly may occur following total knee replacement or after fibrous ankylosis resulting from injury involving the quadriceps mechanism or the suprapatellar pouch, prolonged immobilization (particularly for delayed union or non-union of a fractured femur) or infection. It is of interest that the vastus intermedius is usually the most commonly affected by fibrosis, adhesion formation with rectus femoris or vastus medialis being rare although the whole quadriceps mass may be involved.

Fibrotic contracture of the quadriceps muscle mass produces restriction of both active and passive flexion of the knee, especially when the vastus intermedius is involved. The contraction may be congenital in infants. Gunn (1964) was the first to suggest that this condition was caused by repeated injection of antibiotics into the thighs in infants treated for infections which caused muscle fibrosis and contraction.

TREATMENT

Manipulation

Smillie (1978) stated that manipulation is contraindicated in the presence of any pathological process indicated by a 'hot joint', in the early stages of recovery from injury or operation, in the presence of any decalcification of the adjacent bones and in the presence of unsound union at a femoral fracture site. If the patella is relatively mobile, there is no fibrosis in the suprapatellar region and the resistance is elastic, manipulation may be successful. Manipulation is very useful following total knee replacement where the patient is not mobilizing progressively beyond 30° after 10 days. This should be performed under general anaesthetic with full muscle relaxation. As the manipulation proceeds the surgeon can feel the adhesions separating. Undue force should not be used since fracture of the lower femur or upper tibia is a major complication. Likewise, a fracture of the patella or femur is a very undesirable complication. It is useful to awaken the patient with the knee in the fully flexed position and to commence movement of the knee with ice-bag facilitation immediately on recovery of consciousness. Following any manipulation, supervised active exercises are carried out persistently and with vigour and determination by the patient and the physiotherapist from the earliest possible moment.

Quadricepsplasty

Quadricepsplasty is a major procedure and the patient should be warned that gaining flexion may result in permanent extensor lag. The procedure should be performed only after all conservative methods have been attempted and in the case of femoral fractures is best delayed for 18–24 months after injury since often knee flexion will improve even up to that time (Thompson, 1944).

In the *congenital* type of contracture, that following injection into the quadriceps in children, quadricepsplasty gives good results. Through a lateral approach the muscle is exposed and the tight compartment is divided, employing an inverted V, as in Bennett's operation (Figure 16.56). The knee is then simply immobilized in 90° of flexion for 2 weeks and active mobilization in hospital commences.

In the *adult*, e.g. following fracture of the femur, the classic procedure is performed by a lateral incision or one which avoids scarring. It extends from below the patella to the upper third of the thigh and the rectus is isolated and separated from the vasti lateralis and medialis. The anterior knee capsule is then divided transversely on both sides of the patella for a distance sufficient to overcome the capsular shortening. The vastus intermedius, which is usually a scarred band fixing the patella and rectus to the femur and obliterating the suprapatellar pouch, is excised completely, leaving a fibrous and periosteal covering on the anterior surface of the femur. The knee is then slowly flexed to 70°, releasing the remaining intra-articular adhesions. If the vasti are badly scarred then they are isolated from the rectus by suture of the subcutaneous tissue and fat to the anterior surface of the femur, thus creating an artificial intermuscular septum and eliminating all scarred muscle from the remaining quadriceps mechanism. If the vasti are relatively normal they are reunited to the rectus as far distally as the lower third of the thigh.

After operation the leg is placed on continuous passive motion beginning with a range of 0–40° and increasing this gradually over the course of the next 2 weeks. The patient also performs active exercises with the physiotherapist. When 90–100° have been achieved the passive motion is discontinued and active exercises continue.

Nicoll (1962) reported the results of 30 cases of quadricepsplasty with an average gain of 68° of flexion. Full extension was regained in all cases except the 4 in which lengthening of rectus femoris had been carried out. His results have not been bettered in the literature. Williams (1968) reported

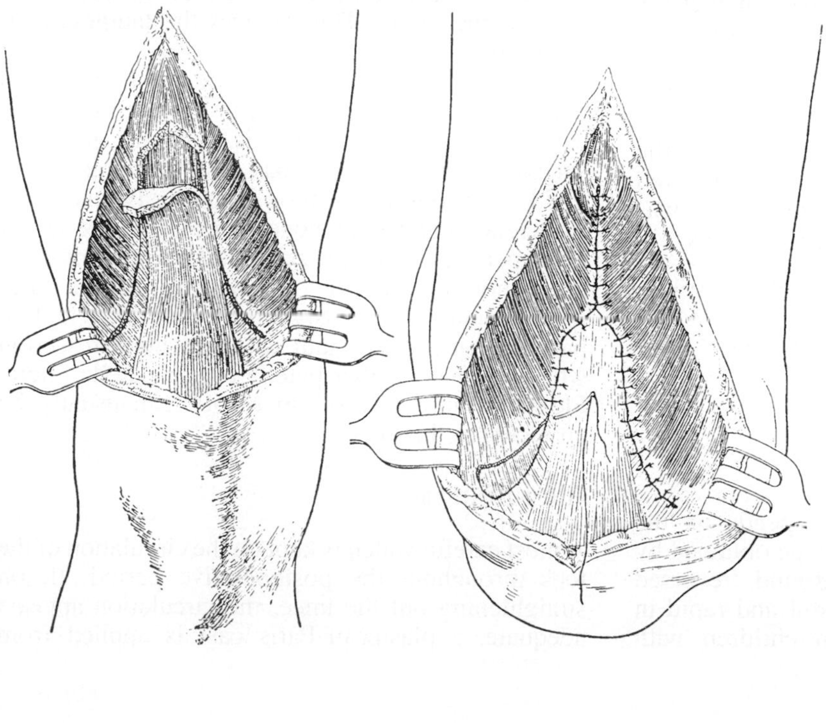

Figure 16.56 Diagrammatic representation of Bennett's operation of lengthening the quadriceps tendon for quadriceps adhesion.

his experience of 35 quadricepsplasties out of 47 cases with quadriceps contracture resulting from such causes as injections, arthrogryposis, recurrent dislocation of the patella or stiff knees. Five of these involved the rectus femoris muscle, which responded very well to simple lengthening of the tendon. This experience indicates that all parts of the quadriceps mass may be involved as well as the iliotibial tract excepting the vastus medialis. All of these may require correction to obtain reasonable flexion of the knee.

Flexion contracture of the knee

This is a common sequel of long-continued over-reaction of the hamstrings which became contracted. It is seen at its worst in a neglected tuberculous knee joint or haemophilia or in rheumatoid arthritis where, in addition to the contracture, a posterior and lateral rotation deformity of the tibia often occurs. The cases resulting from trauma and from neglect are more amenable to treatment. Somerville (1960) described two types of knee flexion contractures:

1. A simple contracture in which release of the tight posterior structures by division or stretching permitted the upper end of the tibia to glide around the femoral condyle into full extension.
2. A contracture in which even though there is division of the contracted posterior structures the upper end of the tibia, hinged at its anterior edge, instead of gliding around the femoral condyle subluxes posteriorly. He believed that this type was best treated by division of the anterior cruciate ligament so that the subluxed tibia could ride forward. This procedure was carried out in 12 patients with good results.

In current practice the commonest cause is osteoarthritis of the knee and correction of flexion as well as angular deformity is crucial for success of knee arthroplasty.

TREATMENT

Treatment of flexion contracture depends on the cause. In some cases correction may be obtained by conservative measures. We have found 'reversed dynamic slings' extremely successful and rapid in correction flexion contractures in children with haemophilia and rheumatoid arthritis even with posterior subluxation of the tibia and this is the preferred method of conservative treatment (Stein and Dickson, 1975). This method should be discontinued if no improvement is seen within 1 week.

Where conservative measures fail, certain operations have been used with success.

Posterior capsulotomy

A straight incision down the popliteal fossa is likely to produce a keloid scar with contracture, and so it is better to approach the area through two lateral incisions or an elongated S incision. These run from just above the condyles to below the joint line. On the outer side the iliotibial band is divided transversely and the peroneal nerve isolated. The biceps tendon is lengthened in a Z manner. The lateral condyle is now identified and the capsule incised and stripped upward from the posterior aspect of the femur, separating the outer head of gastrocnemius.

A medial incision is now made above the adductor tubercle to below the joint line. A similar stripping is carried out on this side. It is helpful to pass a retractor from side to side and so get a good view of the posterior aspect of the joint. With the knee in acute flexion and the posterior structures retracted, the tight capsular structures in the region of the intercondylar notch and the attachment of the inner head of the gastrocnemius are freed, divided or lengthened according to requirements. Manipulation should now produce a fairly straight knee. If the peroneal nerve appears stretched now it is carefully dissected free proximally and as far distally as the neck of the fibula. This reduces the tautness considerably.

In osteoarthritis the contracture can be managed during total knee replacement by release of the capsule from below upwards from the posterior surface of the femur. It may also be necessary to divide the popliteus tendon laterally. If this is not sufficient, removal of bone from the lower femur or upper tibia can be performed. Care must be taken not to alter the mechanisms of the knee replacement by excessive bone resection and in particular it is important to avoid bone resection which produces either patella alta or patella infera. Flexion contracture of up to 50° can usually be corrected in this way.

After-treatment

A most careful watch is kept on the circulation of the toes throughout the postoperative period. If, on straightening out the knee, the circulation appears adequate, a plaster-of-Paris cast is applied from ankle to groin with the knee in the fully extended position. Weight-bearing begins after 24 hours and intensive quadriceps exercises in the cast. This remains on for 2–3 weeks and then a posterior gutter splint is used and physiotherapy started. A removable polythene splint is fitted and used from the end of the second month and retained until the patient has muscular control of flexion and extension.

Femoral osteotomy

Where there is free movement of the knee from, say, a position of 30° of flexion up to 100°, a wedge osteotomy at the supracondylar level may be carried out. A wedge of bone with its base anteriorly is removed so that the 70° of movement is now from the straight position to 70° flexion. This is done only in the absence of any activity or disease in the knee joint. Internal fixation by a nail-plate allows early postoperative movement of the knee.

Bursae at the knee

Numerous bursae occur in the vicinity of the knee joint, in relation to the attachments of the various muscles and ligaments. Anteriorly there are the suprapatellar and the prepatellar bursae, a small subcutaneous bursa sometimes present in front of the tibial tuberosity, the infrapatellar bursa, and the deep infrapatellar bursa between the proximal extremity of the tibia and the deep surface of the ligamentum patellae (Figure 16.57).

Posteriorly there are two bursae, one between each head of origin of gastrocnemius and the capsule of the joint. They often communicate with the joint. The bursa between the medial head of gastrocnemius and the capsule sends a prolongation between the gastrocnemius and semimembranosus. This bursa is often enlarged, forming a swelling at the inner side of the popliteal space, which is the common semimembranosus bursa (Figure 16.58).

On the medial side there are three bursae. One separates the tendons of sartorius, gracilis and semitendinosus from the tibial collateral ligament as they cross it, the so-called 'anserine' bursa. The other two separate the tendon of semimembranosus from the tibial collateral ligament medially and the head of the tibia laterally, and serve to protect the tendon which is sandwiched between the ligament medially and the condyle of the tibia laterally.

On the lateral aspect of the knee joint there are

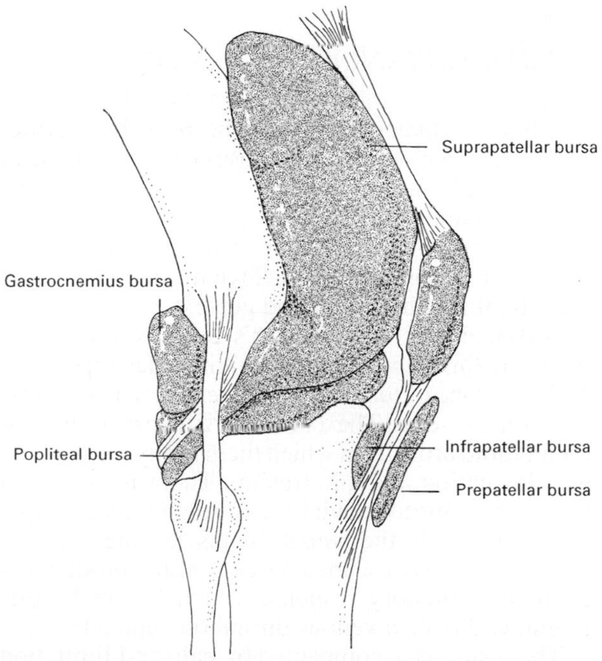

Figure 16.57 Lateral aspect of the knee showing the bursae.

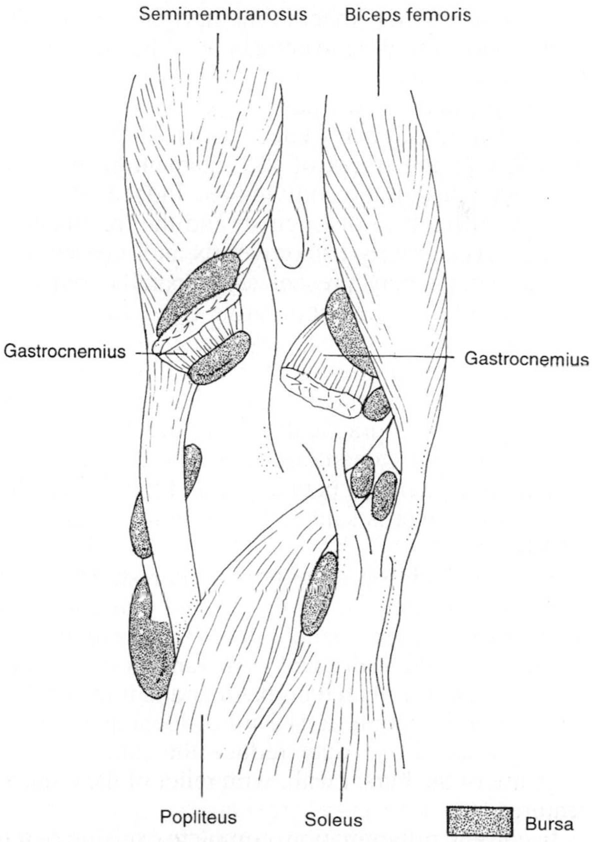

Figure 16.58 Posterior aspect of the knee showing the potential bursae which may become enlarged or inflamed.

three bursae – one between the biceps tendon and the fibular collateral ligament, one between the fibular collateral ligament and the popliteal tendon, and a third between the popliteus tendon and the lateral condyle of the femur. This last bursa is really a tube of synovial membrane round the popliteus tendon, like that round the long head of the biceps at the shoulder joint, and therefore communicates with the joint.

Symptoms arise most frequently in relation to the prepatellar and the infrapatellar sacs, in the bursa deep to the medial head of gastrocnemius and in those deep to the tendon of semimembranosus.

PREPATELLAR BURSITIS

The prepatellar bursa is subcutaneous, and is present in about 90% of people. It usually covers the lower half of the patella, and the upper half of the patella tendon. Bursitis is most common in those whose occupation demands prolonged kneeling, e.g. carpet layers. Indeed, effusions into the bursal sac are popularly known as 'housemaid's knee' because, in kneeling, the bursa comes into contact with the ground. Priests are said not to get prepatellar bursitis because when they kneel in the upright position the bursa is not brought into contact with the ground, but they are affected by infrapatellar bursitis!

Prepatellar bursitis has to be carefully distinguished from jumper's knee, which is an avulsion of a few of the fibres of the ligamentum patellae occurring in athletic individuals. Indeed, the two may be difficult to distinguish and the treatment is similar. Also, rarely osteomyelitis and tuberculosis of the patella may present as prepatellar bursitis. Occasionally, in the suppurative type, where there is also necrosis of the superficial aspect of the patella, it may be difficult to determine whether the bone or the bursal infection was the original lesion. The knee joint is practically never involved, owing to the dense ligamentous and fibrous structures which are interposed between it and the bursa. The prepatellar bursa is said to be liable to gummatous infiltration.

The treatment of acute bursitis is rest. The fluid may, in addition, be aspirated but the relief so obtained is not permanent. If the effusion suppurates, the bursa should be drained via a transverse incision.

In small non-infected prepatellar and infrapatellar bursitis, an injection of 1–2 ml of local anaesthetic and hydrocortisone may reduce the inflammatory response of the bursal wall, with relief of the clinical features.

In chronic inflammation, complete excision of the sac is the most successful method of treatment. The dissection is performed through a transverse incision and the knee should be immobilized for 10 days in a plaster cast following the operation, until the wound has healed to prevent recurrence. Thereafter, active function may be resumed.

DEEP INFRAPATELLAR BURSITIS

The infrapatellar bursa between the upper part of the tuberosity of the tibia and the ligamentum patellae is small, and separated from the synovial membrane of the knee joint by a pad of adipose tissue. When infected, there is pain and tenderness over the ligament, and the patient is unable to flex or extend the limb completely. The tibial tuberosity appears enlarged, and there is a fluctuating swelling on either side of the patella ligament, most marked when the knee is actively extended. This condition is exceedingly rare and treatment follows the same principles as for other bursae.

SUBCRURAL BURSITIS

This bursa beneath the quadriceps tendon usually communicates with the joint separated partially by a plica and shares in its diseases. When cut off from the joint it may be affected independently; when distended with fluid, it forms a horseshoe swelling around the patella. Keene (1992) considers that the plica or septum between the two spaces may be a cause of anterior knee pain and recommends excision.

SEMIMEMBRANOSUS BURSITIS

The bursa between the medial head of the gastrocnemius and the semimembranosus tendon is liable to become inflamed, especially in active individuals such as gamekeepers and shepherds. Its apparent predilection for the latter is said to be due to the increased amount of knee flexion necessitated by walking through heather and gorse!

Although the term 'Baker's cyst' is sometimes given to this type, Baker's original description in 1877 was one of tuberculous infection, which is now very rarely seen. The commonest cause is that of rheumatoid arthritis in which there is a synovitis with cyst formation and an effusion. There is a gradual build-up of intrasynovial pressure and a valve-like action through the small hiatus in the capsule posteriorly. The escaped viscous fluid produces a local inflammatory response which has to be differentiated from a venous thrombotic episode.

The lesion is accompanied by pain and limitation of movement at the knee joint. The swelling usually enlarges distally in the intermuscular interval deep to the medial head of gastrocnemius, and presents as an oval fluctuating swelling, limited on its outer aspect, but more free and less defined towards the inner aspect of the popliteal space. As in the majority of these periarticular swellings, it becomes tense on extension and flaccid on flexion of the knee. Such swellings are usually much larger than they appear and, since they lie under the deep fascia, they have been mistaken for varicose veins.

The treatment when the patient has symptoms depends on the cause. Simple removal if the cyst communicates with the joint as in osteoarthritis or rheumatoid arthritis results in recurrence. Often it is necessary to assess the interior of the joint by arthroscopy. If the patient has osteoarthritis or rheumatoid arthritis the treatment is of the primary pathology and the popliteal swelling is thereby dealt with. In early rheumatoid, where synovectomy is considered, removal of the anterior synovium, arthroscopically or open, results in resolution of the popliteal swelling unless it extends beyond the popliteal fossa when a separate incision and removal is required.

THE POPLITEUS BURSA

This arises from the synovial membrane of the knee joint surrounding the intra-articular portion of the popliteal tendon. It gives rise to a rounded swelling behind the external condyle of the femur deep to the biceps tendon and the iliotibial band. It has to be differentiated from a bicipital bursa, which lies lower down between the biceps tendon and the external lateral ligament, or a cyst of the lateral popliteal nerve which may or may not be producing a neurological deficiency. Both may be mistaken for a cyst of the lateral cartilage. Arthroscopy clarifies the diagnosis. Treatment is excision if there are symptoms from the bursa.

GANGLION OF THE SUPERIOR TIBIOFIBULAR JOINT

This is a swelling seen occasionally in children and may result in lateral popliteal nerve pressure and 'foot drop'. Treatment is by excision of the cyst.

References

Aichroth, P.M. (1977) Osteochondritis dissecans of the knee. *Journal of Bone and Joint Surgery* **59B**, 58

Armstrong, S.J., Read, R.A., Ghosh, P. and Wilson, D.M. (1993) Moderate exercise exacerbates the O/A lesion produced in cartilage by menisectomy: a morphological study. *Osteoarthritis and Cartilage* **1**, 89–96

Aston, J.E. and Bentley, G. (1986) Repair of articular surfaces by allografts of articular and growth plate cartilage. *Journal of Bone and Joint Surgery* **68B**, 29–35

Barrett, D.S., Cobb, A.G. and Bentley, G. (1991) Joint Proprioception in normal osteoarthritic and replaced knees. *Journal of Bone and Joint Surgery* **73B**, 53

Barrett, D.S., Brown, C. and Steiner, M. (1992) Proprioception determines the management of the cruciate deficient knee. *Journal of Bone and Joint Surgery* **75B**, Supplement 1, 39

Basmajian, J.V. and Lovejoy, J.F. Jr (1971) Function of the popliteus muscle in man. *Journal of Bone and Joint Surgery* **53A**, 557–562

Bentley, G. (1970) Chondromalacia patellae. *Journal of Bone and Joint Surgery* **52A**, 221–232

Bentley, G. (1978) The surgical treatment of chondromalacia patellae. *Journal of Bone and Joint Surgery* **60B**, 74–81

Bentley, G. (1988) Is chondromalacia patellae a precursor of osteoarthritis of the knee? *Journal of Bone and Joint Surgery* **70B**, 334

Bentley, G. (1992) Contemporary management of anterior knee pain. Guest Lecture, British Association for Surgery of the Knee. April 1992, Leicester

Bentley, G. and Fogg, A.J.B. (1991) Diagnostic arthroscopy of the knee. In: *Operative Surgery: Orthopaedics*, Edited by G. Bentley and R.B. Greer. 4th edn. Butterworth Heinemann: London, Boston, Sydney, Wellington, Singapore

Bentley, G., Leslie, I.J. and Fischer, D. (1981) Effect of aspirin treatment on chondromalacia patellae. *Annals of the Rheumatic Diseases* **40**, 37

Bentley, G., Cobb, A.C., Archer, C.W. and Hemmen, B. (1992) The cartilage matrix support prosthesis. An experimental and clinical study. *Journal of Bone and Joint Surgery* **74B**, Supplement 3, 267

Beuchel, F.F. (1992) Patella tendon bone grafting for patellectomized patients having total knee arthroplasty. *Clinical Orthopaedics* **271**, 72–78

Bradley, J., Goodfellow, J.W. and O'Connor, J.J. (1987) A radiographic study of bearing movement in unicompartmental Oxford knee replacements. *Journal of Bone and Joint Surgery* **69B**, 598–601

Brantigan, O.C. and Voshell, A.F. (1941) *Journal of Bone and Joint Surgery* **23**, 44

Broughton, N.S., Newman, J.H. and Baily, R.A. (1986) Unicompartmental replacement and high tibial osteotomy for osteoarthritis of the knee. A comparative study after 5 to 10 years' follow-up. *Journal of Bone and Joint Surgery* **68B**, 447–452

Bruce, J. and Walmsley, R. (1942) Excision of the patella. *Journal of Bone and Joint Surgery* **24NS**, 311–325

Butler, D.l., Noyes, F.R. and Grood, E.S. (1980) Ligamentous restraints to anterior-posterior drawer in the human knee. A biomechanical study. *Journal of Bone and Joint Surgery* **62A**, 259–270

Carter, C. and Sweetnam, R. (1958) Familial joint laxity and recurrent dislocation of the patella. *Journal of Bone and Joint Surgery* **40B**, 664–667

Cho, K. (1975) Reconstruction of anterior cruciate ligament by semitendinosus tenodesis. *Journal of Bone and Joint Surgery* **57A**, 608–612

Chrisman, O.D. (1963) Biomechanical aspects of degenerative joint disease. *Clinical Orthopaedics and Related Research* **67**, 77–86

Coventry, M.B. (1973) Osteotomy about the knee for degenerative and rheumatoid arthritis. *Journal of Bone and Joint Surgery* **55A**, 23–48

Crookes, L.M. (1967) Chondromalacia patellae: early results of a conservative operation. *Journal of Bone and Joint Surgery* **49B**, 495

Dandy, D.J. (1978) The early results of closed partial meniscectomy. *British Medical Journal* **1**, 1099–1100

Dandy, D.J. and Pusey, R.J. (1981) The late results of unrepaired rupture of the posterior cruciate ligament. *Journal of Bone and Joint Surgery* **63B**, 629

Danielsson, L.G. (1964) Incidence and prognosis of coxarthrosis. *Acta Orthopaedica Scandinavica Supplementum* **66**

Darracott, J. and Vernon-Roberts, B. (1971) The bone changes in chondromalacia patellae. *Rheumatology and Physical Medicine* **11**, 175

DePalma, A.F., Sawyer, B. and Hoffman, J.D. (1960) Reconsideration of lesions affecting the patellofemoral joint. *Clinical Orthopaedics* **18**, 63–85

Devas, M.B. and Golski, A. (1973) Treatment of chondromalacia patellae by transposition of the tibial tubercle. *British Medical Journal* **1**, 589–591

Dowd, G.S.E., and Bentley, G. (1986) Radiographic assessment in patellar instability and chondromalacia patellae. *Journal of Bone and Joint Surgery* **68B**, 297–300

Edwards, D.H. and Bentley, G. (1977) Osteochondritis dissecans patellae. *Journal of Bone and Joint Surgery* **59B**, 58–63

Fairbank, H.A.T. (1933) *Journal of Bone and Joint Surgery* **2**, 67

Fairbank, T.J. (1948) Knee joint changes after meniscectomy. *Journal of Bone and Joint Surgery* **30B**, 664

Ferguson, A.B. Jr, Brown, T.D., Fu, F.H.J and Rutkowski, R. (1979) Relief of patellofemoral contact stress by anterior displacement of the tibial tubercle. *Journal of Bone and Joint Surgery* **61A**, 159

Ficat, R.P. (1977) Excessive lateral pressure syndrome. In: *Disorders of the Patellofemoral Joint*, p. 127. Edited by R.P. Ficat and D.S. Hungerford. Masson: Paris

Ficat, R.P. and Hungerford D.S. (eds) (1977) *Disorders of the Patellofemoral Joint*. Williams & Wilkins: Baltimore, MD

Ficat, P., Ficat, C. and Boilleaux, A. (1975) Syndrome d'hyperpression externe de la rotoule (SHPE). *Revue de Chirugie Orthopédique et Reparatrice de l'Appareil Moteur* **61**, 39–59

Flynn, M. and Kelly, J.P. (1976) Local excision of cyst of lateral meniscus of knee without recurrence. *Journal of Bone and Joint Surgery* **58B**, 88–89

Frankel, V.H. and Burstein, A.H. (1984) *Orthopaedic Biomechanics*, 2nd edn, Lea & Febiger: Philadelphia

Freeman, M.A.R. (1974) Collagen fatigue as a cause of osteoarthrosis. In: *Normal and Osteoarthrotic Articular Cartilage*, p. 173. Edited by S.Y. Ali, M.W. Elves and D.H. Leabak. Pitman Medical: Tunbridge Wells

Furman, W., Marshall, J.L. and Girgis, F.G. (1976) The anterior cruciate ligament. A functional analysis based on postmortem studies. *Journal of Bone and Joint Surgery* **58A**, 179–185

Galway, H.R. and McIntosh, D.L. (1980) The lateral pivot shift: a symptom and sign of anterior cruciate ligament insufficiency. *Clinical Orthopaedics and Related Research* **147**, 45–50

Galway, R.D., Beaupré, A. and McIntosh, D.L. (1979) Pivot: a clinical sign of symptomatic anterior cruciate instability. *Journal of Bone and Joint Surgery* **54B**, 763

Garièpy, R. (1964) Genu varum treated by high tibial osteotomy. *Journal of Bone and Joint Surgery* **46B**, 783

Girgis, F.G., Marshall, S.L. and Monajem, A.N.S. (1975) The cruciate ligaments of the knee joint. Anatomical, functional and experimental analysis. *Clinical Orthopaedics and Related Research* **106**, 216–231

Glasgow, M.S., Allen, P.W. and Blakeway, C. (1993) Arthroscopic treatment of cysts of the lateral meniscus. *Journal of Bone and Joint Surgery* **75B**, 299

Goodfellow, J.W., Hungerford, D.S. and Zindel, M. (1976) Patello-femoral joint mechanics and pathology. 1: Functional anatomy of the patello-femoral joint. *Journal of Bone and Joint Surgery* **58B**, 287–290

Grood, E.S. (1992) Placement of knee ligament grafts. In: *Knee Surgery – Current Practice*. Edited by P.M. Aichroth, W. Dilworth Cannon and V.P. Patel. Martin Dunitz: London

Gunn, D.R. (1964) Contracture of the quadriceps muscle. Discussion on the aetiology and relationship to recurrent dislocation of the patella. *Journal of Bone and Joint Surgery* **46B**, 492

Hemmen, B., Archer, C.W. and Bentley, G. (1991) Repair of articular cartilage defects by carbon fibre plugs loaded with chondrocytes. *Transaction of the 37th Annual Meeting of the Orthopaedic Research Society*, vol. 16, Section 1, 278

Heywood, A. (1961) Recurrent dislocation of the patella. *Journal of Bone and Joint Surgery* **43B**, 508–517

Hirsch, C. (1944) *Acta Chirurgica Scandinavica Supplementum* **90**, 83

Hughston, J.C. and Eilers, A.F. (1973) The role of the posterior oblique ligament in repairs of acute medial (collateral) ligament tears of the knee. *Journal of Bone and Joint Surgery* **55A**, 923–940

Hughston, J.C., Andrews, J.R., Cross, M.J. and Moshi, A. (1976) Classification of knee ligament instabilities. Part 1: Medial compartment and cruciate ligaments. *Journal of Bone and Joint Surgery* **58A**, 159–172

Hughston J.C., Bowden, J.A., Andrews, J.R. and Norwood, L.A. (1980) Acute tears of the posterior cruciate ligament: results of operative treatment. *Journal of Bone and Joint Surgery* **62A**, 438–450

Insall, J.N. (1967) Intra-articular surgery for degenerative arthritis of the knee. *Journal of Bone and Joint Surgery* **49B**, 211–228

Insall, J.N., Shoji, H. and Mayer, V. (1974) High tibial osteotomy. *Journal of Bone and Joint Surgery* **56A**, 1397–1405

Insall, J., Falvo, K.A. and Wise, D.W. (1976) Chondromalacia patellae. *Journal of Bone and Joint Surgery* **58A**, 1–8

Jackson, J.P. (1958) Osteotomy for osteoarthritis of the knee. *Journal of Bone and Joint Surgery* **40B**, 826

Jackson, J.P. (1967) Degenerative changes in the knee after meniscectomy. *Journal of Bone and Joint Surgery* **49B**, 584

Jackson, J.P. and Waugh, W. (1967) Degenerative changes in the knee after meniscectomy. *Journal of Bone and Joint Surgery* **49B**, 584

Jackson, J.P., Waugh, W. and Green, J.P. (1969) High tibial osteotomy for osteoarthritis of the knee. *Journal of Bone and Joint Surgery* **51B**, 88

Jackson, R.W. and Abe, I. (1972) The role of arthroscopy in the management of disorders of the knee. *Journal of Bone and Joint Surgery* **54B**, 310–322

Jackson, R.W. and Dandy, D.J. (1976) Partial meniscectomy. *Journal of Bone and Joint Surgery* **58B**, 142

Jackson, R.W. and Kinkel, S.S. (1991) Arthroscopic meniscal repair. In: *Rob & Smith's Operative Surgery: Orthopaedics*, 4th edn, p. 1056. Edited by G. Bentley and R.B. Greer. Butterworth Heinemann: London, Boston, Sydney, Wellington, Singapore

Johnson, R.W. and Rouse, D.W. (1982) The results of partial arthroscopic meniscectomy in patients over 40 years of age. *Journal of Bone and Joint Surgery* **64B**, 481–485

Jones, K.G. (1970) Reconstruction of anterior cruciate ligament using the centralone-third of patellar tendon. *Journal of Bone and Joint Surgery* **52A**, 1302–1308

Jones, R. (1909) *Annals of Surgery* **43**, 969

Jones, R.E., Smith, E.C., and Reisch, J.S. (1978) Effects of medial meniscectomy in patients older than forty years. *Journal of Bone and Joint Surgery* **60A**, 783–786

Kaplan, J. (1955) The embryology of the menisci of the knee joint. *Bulletin of the Hospital for Joint Diseases* **16**, 111–124

Karlson, S. (1940) Chondromalacia patellae. *Acta Orthopaedica Scandinavica* **83**, 347

Keene, G. (1992) The role of suprapatellar plicae in anterior knee pain. *Proceedings of New Zealand Knee Society October 15, 1992*

Kennedy, J.C. and Fowler, P.J. (1971) Medial and anterior instability of the knee. *Journal of Bone and Joint Surgery* **53A**, 1257

Kettlecamp, D.B. and Chao, E.Y. (1972) *Clinical Orthopaedics and Related Research* **83**, 202

King, E.S.J. (1940) *Surgery, Gynecology and Obstetrics* **70**, 150

von Kolliker, A. (1883) *Manual of Human Histology*, vol. 1. Sydenham: London

König, F. (1888) *Dtsch. Z. Chir.* **27**, 90

Kumar, R.R., Cobb, A.G. and Bentley, G. (1991) The patella in knee replacement. *Journal of Bone and Joint Surgery* **73B**, Supplement II, 183–184

Langenskjöld, A. (1975) An operation for partial closure of an epiphyseal plate in children and its experimental basis. *Journal of Bone and Joint Surgery* **57B**, 325–330

Larson, R.L. (1980) Combined knee instabilities. *Clinical Orthopaedics and Related Research* **147**, 68–75

Last, R.J. (1973) *Anatomy: Regional and Applied*, 5th edn. Churchill Livingstone: Edinburgh, London

Lennox, I.A.C., Cobb, A.G., Knowles, J. and Bentley, G. (1994) Knee function after patellectomy. *Journal of Bone and Joint Surgery* **76B**, 485–488

Lennox, I.A.C. and Bentley, G. (1991) Is arthroscopic washout useful in the treatment of osteoarthritis in the knee? *Journal of Bone and Joint Surgery* **73B**, Supplement 1, 88

Leslie, I.J. and Bentley, G. (1978) Arthroscopy in the diagnosis of chondromalacia patellae. *Annals of the Rheumatic Diseases* **37**, 540

Levitsky, K.A., Harris, W.J., McManus, R. and Scott, R.D. (1993) Total knee arthroplasty without patellar resurfacing. *Clinical Orthopaedics* **286**, 116–121

Linden, B. (1977) Osteochondritis dissecans of the femoral condyles. *Journal of Bone and Joint Surgery* **59A**, 769–776

McDaniel, W.J. and Dameron T.B. (1980) Untreated rupture of the anterior cruciate ligament. *Journal of Bone and Joint Surgery* **62A**, 696–704

McGinty, J.B., Guess, L.F. and Marvin, R.A. (1977) Partial or total meniscectomy. *Journal of Bone and Joint Surgery* **59A**, 763–766

McGrouther, D.A. (1975) Load actions transmitted at the knee joint of the arthritic patient. In: *Total Knee Replacement*. A Joint Conference of the Tribology Group of the Institution and the British Orthopaedic Association, 16–18 September 1974, pp. 133–137. Institution of Mechanical Engineers: London

MacIntosh, D.N. and Darby, T.A. (1976) Lateral substitution reconstructions. *Journal of Bone and Joint Surgery* **58B**, 142

McMurray, T.P. (1942) *British Journal of Surgery* **29**, 407

Magnuson, P.B. (1941) Joint debridement. *Surgery, Gynecology and Obstetrics* **73**, 1

Mann, R.A. and Hagy, J.L. (1977) The popliteus muscle. *Journal of Bone and Joint Surgery* **59A**, 924–927

Maquet, P.G.J. (1976) *Biomechanics of the Knee with Application to the Pathogenesis and Surgical Treatment of Osteoarthritis*. Springer: Berlin

Maquet, P. (1984) *Biomechanics of the Knee with Application to the Pathogenesis and Surgical Treatment of Osteoarthritis*, 2nd edn. Springer-Verlag: Berlin

Marks, K.E. and Bentley, G. (1978) Patella alta and chondromalacia patellae. *Journal of Bone and Joint Surgery* **60B**, 71–73

Marmor, L. (1988) Unicompartmental knee arthroplasty: Ten to 13 year follow-up study. *Clinical Orthopaedics* **226**, 14

Meachim, G. and Bentley, G. (1977) The effect of age on the thickness of patellar articular cartilage. *Annals of the Rheumatic Diseases* **36**, 563–568

Meachim, G. and Bentley, G. (1979) Horizontal splitting in patella articular cartilage. *Arthritis and Rheumatism* **21**, 669

Mok, D.W.H. (1989) Non-operative management of grade III medial collateral ligament injury of the knee: a prospective study. *Injury* **20**, 277–280

Morley, A.J.M. (1957) *British Medical Journal* **2**, 976

Morrison, J.B. (1968) Bioengineering analysis of force actions transmitted by the knee joint. *Biomedical Engineering* **3**, 164

Mukherjee, A. (1976) DPhil thesis, University of Oxford

Nicholas, J.A. (1973) The five in one reconstruction for anteromedial instability of the knee. *Journal of Bone and Joint Surgery* **55A**, 899–922

Nicoll, E.A. (1962) *Journal of Bone and Joint Surgery* **44B**, 954

Noble, J. (1977) Lesions of the menisci. Autopsy incidents in adults less than fifty-five years old. *Journal of Bone and Joint Surgery* **59A**, 480–483

Noble, J. and Hamblen, D.L. (1975) The pathology of the degenerate meniscus lesion. *Journal of Bone and Joint Surgery* **57B**, 180–186

Oakeshott, R.D., Farine, I., Pritzker, K.P.I., Langer, F. and Gross, A.E. (1988) A clinical and histologic analysis of failed osteochondral allografts. *Clinical Orthopaedics* **233**, 283

O'Connor, J., Sherclift T. and Fitzpatrick, D. (1990) Geometry of the knee. In: *Knee Ligaments – Structure, Function, Injury and Repair*, pp. 163–199. Edited by D. Daniel, W. Akeson, and J. O'Connor. Raven Press, New York

O'Donoghue, D.H. (1955) *Journal of Bone and Joint Surgery* **37A**, 1

O'Donoghue, D.H. (1973a) Reconstruction for medial instability of the knee. *Journal of Bone and Joint Surgery* **55A**, 941–955

O'Donoghue, D.H. (1973b) Treatment of acute ligamentous injuries of the knee. *Orthopedic Clinics of North America* **4**, 617

Outerbridge, R.E. (1961) The etiology of chondromalacia patellae. *Journal of Bone and Joint Surgery* **43B**, 752

Paget, J. (1870) *St Bartholomew's Hospital Reports* **6**, 1

Patel, V.D., Aichroth, P.M. and Moyes, S.T. (1992) Arthroscopic debridement for degenerative joint disease of the knee. In: *Knee Surgery – Current Practice*. Edited by P.M. Aichroth, D.W. Cannon and D.V. Patel. Martin Dunitz: London

Philips, H. (1993) Revision knee replacement. Paper presented at Symposium – Controversies in knee replacement, London, September 1993

Pridie, K.H. (1959) A method of resurfacing osteoarthritic knee joints. *Journal of Bone and Joint Surgery* **41B**, 618

Pusey, R.J. and Dandy, D.J. (1981) The late results of unrepaired rupture of the posterior cruciate ligament. Paper presented to the Meeting of the British Orthopaedic Association, Norwich, 8 April 1981

Ranawat, C.S., Flynn, W.F., Saddler, S., Hansraj, K.K. and Magreed, M.J. (1993) Long-term results of the total condylar knee arthroplasty: a 15 year study. *Clinical Orthopaedics* **286**, 94–102

Rebouillat, J., Kohler, R., Jolivet, Y., Tiano, R. and Lerat, J.L. (1978) A propos de 7 cas de maladie de Blount ou tibia vara. *Lyon Chirurgical* **74**, 168–171

Reissis, N., Mitchell, R. and Bentley, G. (1991) Does meniscectomy cause osteoarthritis? *Journal of Bone and Joint Surgery* **74B**, Supplement II, 145–146

Ritter, M.A., Campbell, E., Faris, P.M. and Keatig, E.M. (1989) Long-term survival of posterior cruciate condylar total knee arthroplasty: a 10 year evaluation. *Journal of Arthroplasty* **4**, 293

Rorabeck, C.H. and Bourne, R.B. (1989) Total knee arthroplasty following high tibial osteotomy for osteoarthritis. *Journal of Arthroplasty* **4**, 511

Rowntree, M. and Getty, C.J.M. (1981) The knee after midshaft femoral fracture. Paper presented to the Meeting of the British Orthopaedic Association, Norwich, 8 April 1981

Scott, R.D. and Volatile, T.B. (1986) Twelve years' experience with posterior cruciate-retaining arthroplasty. *Clinical Orthopaedics* **205**, 100

Scott, R.D., Cobb, A.G., McQueeny, F.G. and Thornhill, T.S. (1991) Unicompartmental knee arthroplasty: eight to 12 year follow-up evaluation with analysis. *Clinical Orthopaedics* **271**, 96–101

Seedhom, B.B., Dowson, D. and Wright, V. (1974) Functions of the menisci: a preliminary study. *Annals of the Rheumatic Diseases* **33**, 111

Shelbourne, K.D., Whitaker, H.J. and McCaroll, J.R. (1990) Anterior cruciate injury. Evaluation of intra-articular reconstruction of acute tears without repair: two to seven year follow-up of 155 athletes. *American Journal of Sports Medicine* **18**, 841

Shrive, N. (1974) The weight-bearing role of the menisci of the knee. *Clinical Orthopaedics and Related Research* **131**, 279–287

Slocum, D.B., James, S.L., Larson, R.L. and Singer, K.M. (1976) Clinical test for anterolateral rotatory instability of the knee. *Clinical Orthopaedics and Related Research* **118**, 63–69

Smillie, I.S. (1978) *Injuries of the Knee Joint*, 5th edn. Churchill Livingstone: Edinburgh, London, New York

Somerville, E.W. (1960) *Journal of Bone and Joint Surgery* **42B**, 730

Stein, H. and Dickson, R.A. (1975) Reversed dynamic slings for knee flexion contracture in the haemophiliac. *Journal of Bone and Joint Surgery* **57A**, 282–283

Stother, I. (1991) Arthroscopic meniscectomy. In: *Operative Surgery: Orthopaedics*, 4th edn. Edited by G. Bentley and R.B. Greer. Butterworth Heinemann: London, Boston, Sydney, Wellington, Singapore

Stougard, J. (1970) Patellectomy. *Acta Orthopaedica Scandinavica* **41**, 110–121

Thompson, T.C. (1944) *Journal of Bone and Joint Surgery* **26**, 336

Tietjens, B. (1978) Knee joint instability. MSc Thesis, University of Oxford

Trickey, E.L. (1968) Rupture of the posterior cruciate ligament of the knee. *Journal of Bone and Joint Surgery* **50B**, 334–341

Trickey, E.L. and Paterson, F.W.N. (1983) Meniscectomy for tears of the meniscus combined with rupture of the anterior cruciate ligament. *Journal of Bone and Joint Surgery* **5B**, 388

Vince, K.G., Trusall, J.N., Kelly, M.A. and Silva, M. (1987) Total condylar knee prosthesis: 10 to 12 year follow-up and survival analysis. *Orthopaedic Trauma* **11**, 443

Walker, P.S. and Erkman, M.J. (1975) The role of the menisci in force transmission across the knee. *Clinical Orthopaedics and Related Research* **109**, 184–192

Warren, P.J., Alanakuhn, T.K., Cobb, A.G. and Bentley, G. (1993) Proprioception of the knee after knee arthroplasty: the influence of prosthetic design. *Clinical Orthopaedics* **297**, 182–187

Welsh, R.P. (1980) Knee joint structure and function. *Clinical Orthopaedics and Related Research* **147**, 7–14

Wiles, P., Andrews, P.S. and Bremner, R.A. (1960) Chondromalacia of the patella: a study of the latest results of excision of the articular cartilage. *Journal of Bone and Joint Surgery* **42B**, 65

Williams, P.F. (1968) Quadriceps contracture. *Journal of Bone and Joint Surgery* **50B**, 278

CHAPTER 17

The Foot and Ankle

GEORGE BENTLEY AND JOHN R. SHEARER

Foot disabilities are common in children and in adults. The proper conception of the mechanism of the foot in health and disease is therefore of great importance.

The human foot has become greatly specialized for the performance of two divergent functions:

1. In standing it must provide a stable support for the body weight – a passive function – balance.
2. In walking it must, in addition to supporting the body weight, provide a resilient spring or lever by which the body can be propelled forwards – an active function – propulsion.

These objectives are fulfilled by the architectural arrangement of a number of small spongy elastic bones grouped together in the form of a series of arches, for each of the functions muscular contractions are essential, their importance being greater in propulsion than in balancing.

In addition to conferring resilience on the foot, the arches serve for a dispersal of force applied to the plantar aspect of the foot, and they provide necessary space for the passage of nerves and vessels forward towards the toes.

The longitudinal arch extends from the calcaneus to the head of the first metatarsal, its summit being the midtarsal joint. The posterior pillar of the arch is short – from the calcaneus to the joint – whereas the anterior is long and its slope more gradual.

Variations in the height of the arch are achieved by lacerations in the position of the talonavicular joint, induced by contraction or relaxation of the tibial muscles. Despite this, the arches are to some extent permanent, and gross alterations in their position are to be regarded as pathological.

The transverse arch becomes apparent when the feet are placed together. It extends from the lateral border of one foot to the lateral border of the other and has no true summit because the medial malleoli prevent the absolute apposition of the medial borders of the feet.

The anterior metatarsal arch disappears with weight-bearing. It extends from the first to the fifth metatarsal head and its summit is placed opposite the heads of the second and third metatarsals. Normally the anterior arch has no great weight to sustain and it derives adequate support from the transverse inter-metatarsal ligament, which connects the plantar aspects of the heads of the bones.

The internal arch is sometimes referred to and is formed by the medial border of the foot with its concavity directed medially.

It is reasonably certain that the arches of the foot are present at birth, in that the cartilaginous skeleton of the foot has already assumed an arched formation. When the child begins to support the body weight, it will be seen that the foot becomes flat, and does not develop for some years an arch which persists during weight-bearing. In the foot of the orthograde primate the tibial muscles are concerned with active movement of the metatarsals on the tarsus and have no postural activity.

Mechanics of the foot

Rose (1979) has described the foot as being functionally divided at the subtalar joint into an inherently mechanical stable six-legged-stool-like structure distally with the talus balanced on it. Approximately one-third of the subtalar joint range is available for pronation and two-thirds for supination. The stool has one leg posteriorly – the os calcis – and five anteriorly – the metatarsal rays. It has the unique quality that, during standing, the articulations at the bases of the metatarsal rays are at the limit of one range of movement in extension (Figure 17.1a).

In the position of weight-bearing, the foot requires no muscular activity to maintain the posture. In supination of the foot there is a rotation outwards of the talus and the tibia, and a differential flexion of the medial metatarsal rays to maintain an even distribution of pressure under the metatarsal heads. Pronation reverses this situation and both these movements require muscular activity (Figure 17.1b).

In the static situation the weight passing down the tibia through the ankle and subtalar joint is distributed to the os calcis and the metatarsals more or less uniformly.

Hicks (1955) regarded the foot as being a balance between an arch, a truss mechanism and a beam

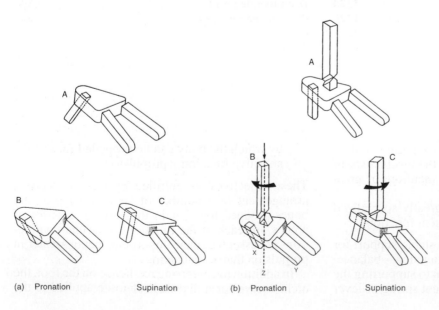

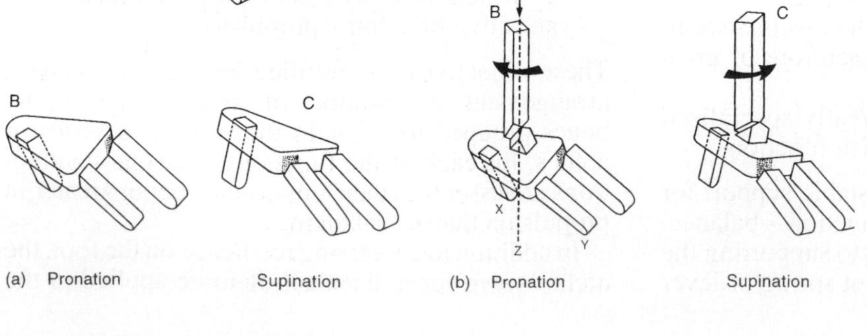

Figure 17.1 The foot represented as a six-legged stool with five legs anteriorly (the metatarsals) and one posteriorly (the os calcis) (a) the 'stool'; (b) the whole 'foot'; (Reproduced with kind permission from Rose, K.G. (1979) Soft tissue and bony operations for pes cavus and planus. In: *Operative Surgery*, 3rd edn, vol. 2, *Orthopaedics*. Edited by G. Bentley. Butterworths: London and Boston)

mechanism. An arch or a truss is a mechanical situation in which the ends can be thrust further apart when weight is applied vertically, whereas a beam is a mechanical situation in which the ends are prevented from being thrust apart. He emphasized the importance of the plantar aponeurosis and the five independent metatarsal rays. These rays under load are forced to the limit of extension, and share – though not necessarily equally – the total load of the body. If one metatarsal head is lower than the other, more load is transmitted through this joint. He described two positions of the foot:

1. While standing without activity there is flattening of the arch with the plantar aponeurosis taking stresses up to about twice that of body weight, but this is reduced by the beam mechanism.
2. On toe standing, as seen during walking, the arch mechanism takes over from that of the beam with extension of the toes at the metatarsophalangeal joints and compressive strains being exerted on all the bones as well as on the plantar aponeurosis.

Rose (1979) has emphasized the special role of the subtalar joint in the foot – leg linkage. Variations at one joint will cause modification of all others; e.g.

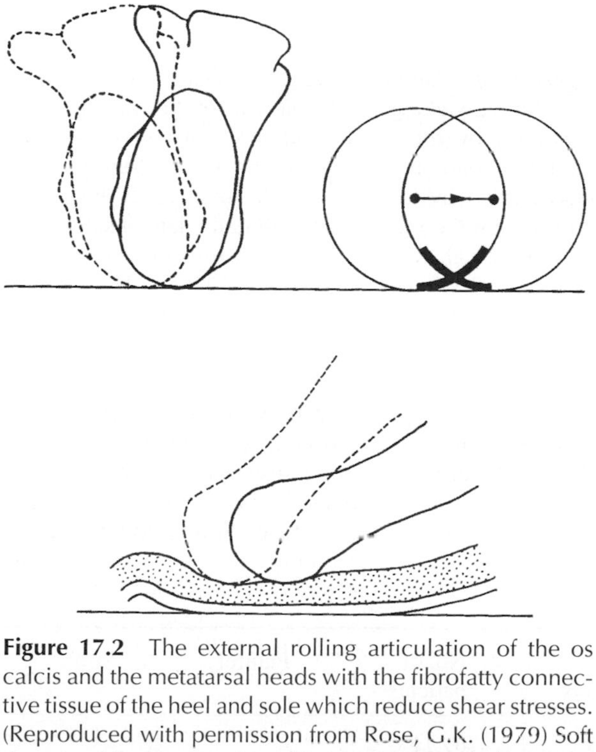

Figure 17.2 The external rolling articulation of the os calcis and the metatarsal heads with the fibrofatty connective tissue of the heel and sole which reduce shear stresses. (Reproduced with permission from Rose, G.K. (1979) Soft tissue and bony operations for pes cavus and planus. In: *Operative Surgery*, 3rd edn, vol. 2, *Orthopaedics*. Edited by G. Bentley. Butterworths: London and Boston)

pronation of the subtalar joint causes an inwards rotation of the metatarsophalangeal joint of the great toe. The axis of this joint, normally parallel with the ground, is now oblique and resolution of the forces at the end of the stance phase causes a valgus deformity component on the great toe.

In addition, extrinsic articulations exist between the undersurface of the os calcis and the metatarsal head and the fibro-fatty tissue lying between these and the skin (Figure 17.2). These are high-friction rolling types of articulations with movements in both the sagittal and coronal planes. Because the skin remains stationary in relationship to the ground these articulations have an important shear stress-relieving function. When subcutaneous tissue disappears, and particularly where skin becomes adherent to the underlying joint capsule, ill-effects become obvious.

The plantar aponeurosis is important functionally because of its attachment posteriorly to the os calcis and anteriorly by means of its slips to the proximal phalanges of all the toes. Extension of the proximal phalanx of a toe will cause tightness of the corresponding slip of the aponeurosis, shortening the distance between the base of the toe and the os calcis and flexing the corresponding metatarsal rays. To establish redistribution of weight under the metatarsal heads, pronation of the subtalar joint will occur provided the range exists for it to do so. The plantar aponeurosis is therefore vital in the interdependence of the hind- and forefoot.

Hutton *et al.* (1976) have reviewed the two complementary elements in the study of mechanics of the foot – kinematics of gait (i.e. information about the changing geometry of the lower limbs with respect to each other and to the ground) and kinetics (i.e. the analysis of forces exerted on the foot for the purpose of weight-bearing locomotion). It is only by considering these two together relative to the detailed anatomy of the foot that a comprehensive understanding of the mechanics can be achieved.

Kinematics of gait have usually been measured photographically whereas kinetics have been measured by the use of force plates and pressure transducers, with the aim of producing measurements of force distribution through the foot in standing, walking and running. With these methods it is possible to plot not only the line of distribution of load through the foot but also the relative pressures exerted on different parts of the foot, particularly the heel, the metatarsal heads and the toes.

The dynamic vertical force distribution during level walking under normal and rheumatic feet has been reported by Simkin (1981). The pressure distribution was measured with a footprint force plate incorporated into a walkway. A series of computer programs provided a graphical display of each footprint frame, a force/time curve for the whole foot or any chosen part of it, a trace of the movement of the centre of pressure of the force on a chosen area of the foot, and a list of the peak point forces and impulses, their location, magnitude and time.

In the results of parameters tested, force concentration was defined by Simkin as the ratio of the peak point force to the average force at the same instant. The mean force concentration factor was higher in the rheumatoid feet and in the third metatarsal head than the controls (Table 17.1).

The force concentration factor was described as a better indicator of the local stresses under the metatarsal heads than were the local forces and impulses. These were kept at a low level, as a result of the slower gait and the change of the velocity pattern of the centre of pressure.

In standing, Hutton *et al.* (1976) considered that the weight of the body was carried almost entirely by the heel and the forefoot and that very little load was carried on the midfoot. However, the distribution of the body weight was very variable from individual to individual and in most individuals the toes carried 5–10% of the forefoot load.

Distribution of the load during walking, as measured by force plate, is shown in Figure 17.3. The typical features of the normal pattern were the evenly distributed load on the forefoot, the absence of significant load carried by the midfoot, the moderately high load imposed on the toes and imposition of load on the medial rather than the lateral side of the foot.

Alexander *et al.* (1991) describe the evolution of current techniques with the assessment of dynamic foot to ground contact and plantar pressure distribution. The aim of gait kinematics is to produce figures of measurement of force distribution through the foot with standing, walking and running. With these methods it is possible to plot not only the direction of forces going through the foot, but also the relative pressures exerted in different parts of the foot, particularly the heel, metatarsal heads and the toes.

Zeitzelberger (1960) produced an excellent review of the mechanics of the foot, expressed as a statically

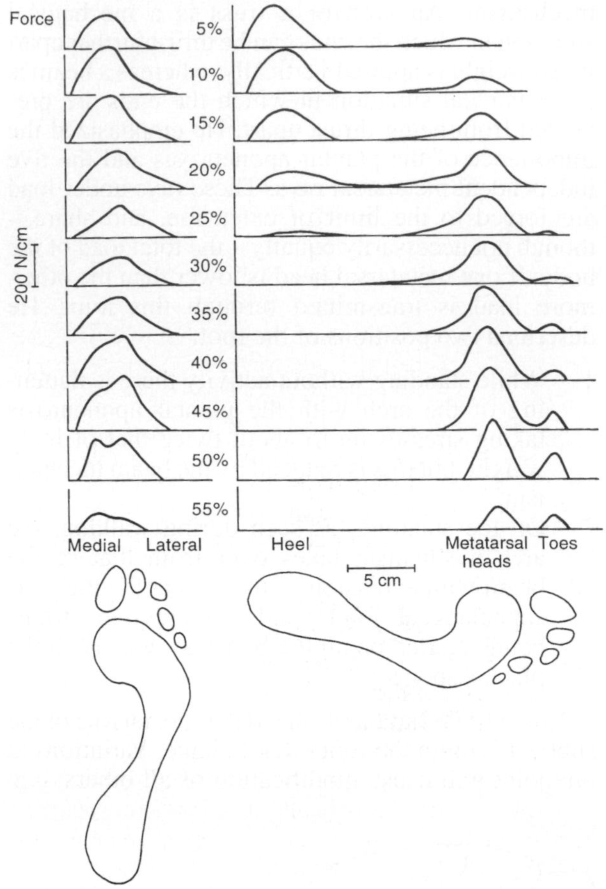

Figure 17.3 Pattern of load distribution on the normal foot during walking at 5% intervals of the walking cycle measured by the subdivided force plate. The smooth outline of load on the forefoot, the absence of significant load carried by the midfoot, the moderately high load imposed on the medial rather than the lateral side of the foot are typical. (Reproduced with permission from Hutton, W.C. Scott, J.R.R. and Stokes, I.A.F. (1976) In: *The Foot and its Disorders*. Edited by L. Klenerman. Blackwell Scientific: Oxford)

indeterminate spatial framework for analysis. He designed three main models with measurement of the short- and long-range stresses. The self-locking wedge mechanism through the naviculocuneiform bones with the forces of action coming down through

Table 17.1

Parameter	No. of controls	No. of patients	Painful	Stiff
Peak force on metatarsal heads (Newtons)	68.35	67.11	–	–
Force concentration factor – all metatarsal heads	5.01	5.63	–	–
Force concentration factor – third metatarsal head	4.31	5.62	5.85	5.21

the talus and the forces of reaction up along the metatarsals was emphasized. He believed that Hicks' concept of the plantar aponeurosis acting as a tie between the calcaneus and metatarsal heads should be expanded to include its being responsible for producing an effective interplay between the short- and long-range stresses. In his analysis he showed how forces are concentrated at one point or the centroid of the particular area, and between these centroids are the pathways of concentrated static forces. He related these forces to effects on the calcaneus of a fall from a great height, or from abnormal pressures being applied from the lateral to the medial side. The resilience and stability of the foot can be explained by such mechanical concepts, and it is better to regard the model of the foot not as an arch but as a dome-like structure.

By introducing alterations to the footwear Holmes and Tinnerman (1991) changed the distribution of the load along the foot.

Other factors may alter distribution of plantar pressures too. Zhu *et al.* (1991), using in-shoe transducers, compared volunteers with normal and shuffling gaits. Those with a shuffling gait had a longer period of flat foot and decreased peak plantar pressures compared to the normal population. Pressures were increased for the heel but decreased for the great toe and MTP joints. Floor-to-floor contact durations increased from 22% to 76%. The addition of a metatarsal pad reduced peak metatarsal pressure by 2–60% in women and 14–44% in men (Holmes and Tinnerman, 1991), whilst the provision of a rocker-bottom shoe reduced peak pressures in the medial forefoot by some 30%, but with an elevation of pressure in the heel, midfoot and lateral forefoot areas (Schaff and Cavanagh, 1991). Age, too, may alter the plantar pressure distribution patterns. Hennig and Rosenbaum (1991) compared early plantar pressures in 15 children and 111 adults. Peak pressures were lower in the children whilst the body weight-to-foot contact area was 1.5 times greater in children than in adults. In addition, children demonstrate a greater relative load through the midfoot, suggesting a relatively weak longitudinal arch.

More recently Kilmartin *et al.* (1991) measured the radiographs of the feet of school children. An increased angle between metatarsals 1 and 2 is present in the early stages of juvenile hallux valgus as well as in the feet of those at risk of developing that deformity. There was no overall congenital derangement of the forefoot, however, and no correlation between the metatarsus adductus and hallux valgus.

MOVEMENTS OF THE FOOT

It is usual to include the ankle in any consideration of movements of the foot. The main movements at the ankle joint are plantar flexion and dorsiflexion (Figure 17.4) but inversion and eversion are possible when the ankle is plantar flexed.

When the whole foot is rotated on an anteroposterior axis so that the sole faces medially, the foot is said to be inverted; the opposite movement is eversion. These actions occur mainly at the subtalar joint (Figures 17.5 and 17.6).

The anterior part of the foot is able to move on the posterior part on a vertical axis; when the forefoot is thus brought in towards the midline of the body it is said to be adducted. The counterpart of adduction is abduction, and these movements also originate at the talonavicular and calcaneocuboid joints which collectively form the midtarsal joint.

When the foot is in a position of abduction and eversion it is said to be pronated; supination similarly consists of a combination of adduction and inversion. In testing for movements of the subtalar joint it is important to dorsiflex the foot to 10° to lock the talus, which is widest in its anterior portion in the mortice of the ankle joint, before assessing inversion and eversion.

The normal neonatal foot can be dorsiflexed to 45° without any difficulty. Plantar flexion similarly is 50°.

KINEMATICS

The talus is described as forming a core within the body and trochlea, being wider anteriorly and laterally. Therefore the talus and fibula must rotate externally slightly on dorsiflexion. Ankle dorsiflexion and abduction are coupled movements in the ankle. Average range of movement in dorsiflexion is 25°, in plantar flexion 35° and rotation 5°.

In the subtalar joint the axis of rotation is 42° in the sagittal plane and 16° in the transverse plane. Its

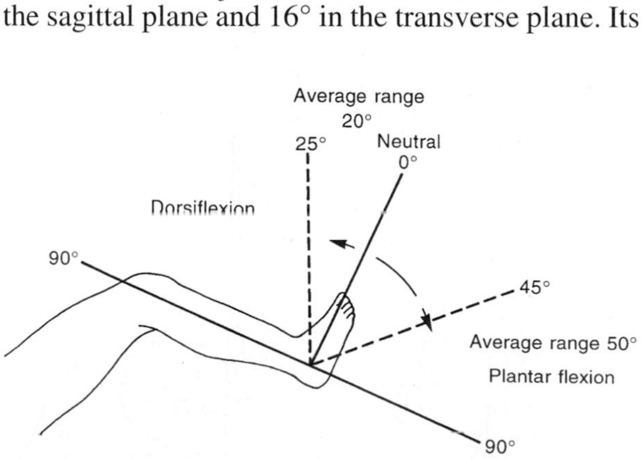

Figure 17.4 Ankle joint movements showing the average range of of dorsiflexion (20°) and plantar flexion (50°) from 0° neutral.

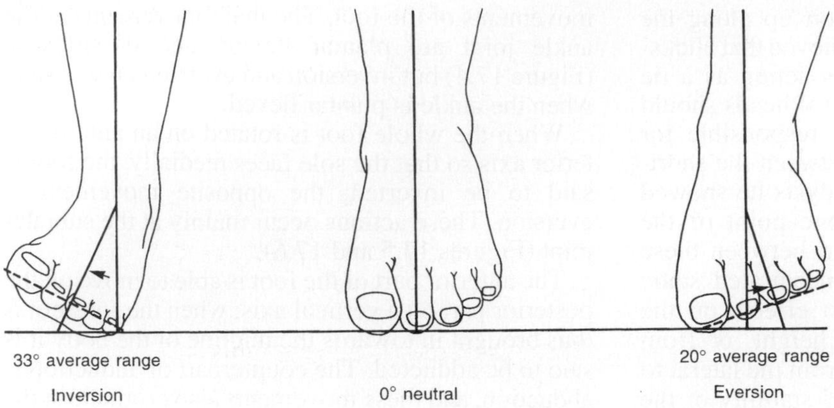

Figure 17.5 Forefoot movements showing the average range of inversion (33°) and of inversion (20°) from 0° neutral.

motions are also coupled with dorsiflexion, abduction and eversion (in pronation) and plantar flexion, adduction and inversion (supination) in the other. Average range of movement of pronation is 5°, that of supination 20°. The functional range of movement is 6°.

The flat foot

The factors which, in combination, preserve the long arch of the foot are the shape of the bony segments composing it, the plantar ligaments including the plantar aponeurosis and the activity of the posterior tibial group of muscles.

It follows therefore that flat foot may arise as either a congenital or an acquired deformity as a sequel to interference with one or other of these factors. Giannestras (1970) described two types of flat feet which should be identified at birth:

1. The calcaneovalgus foot, which is common and unimportant.
2. Congenital vertical talus (or rigid flat foot), which is rare and severely disabling if untreated.

The calcaneovalgus foot

This is a frequently seen infant foot disorder (incidence 1 per 1000 live births) and is thought to be the result of intrauterine positioning. They may also occur as a result of muscle imbalance.

The calcaneovalgus foot deformity is usually bilateral (90%) with an inherited predisposition of about 70%. The features are:

1. The foot is hyperextended and in valgus with the dorsum of the foot frequently touching the shin.
2. Tendo Achilles is not tight.
3. On attempting plantar flexion the anterior structures are tight and plantar flexion is possible to only 10°.
4. The talar head is palpable, pointing downwards and inwards, but it can be repositioned and the plantar arch reconstituted.

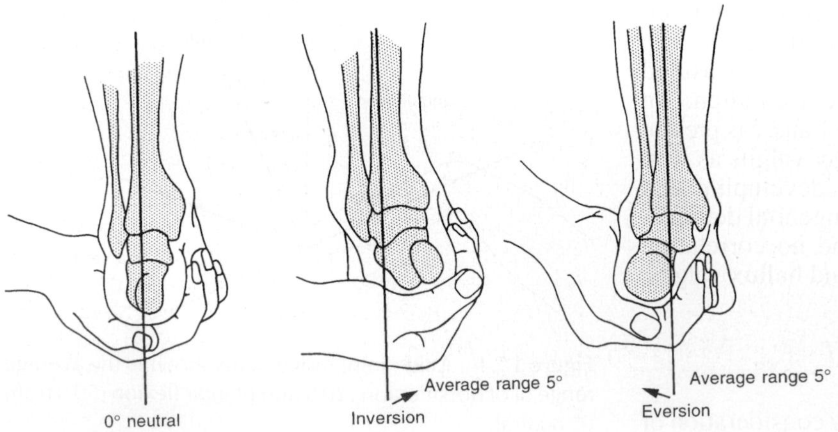

Figure 17.6 Hindfoot movements showing inversion (5°) and eversion (5°) from 0° neutral.

Usually the treatment of this deformity is adequate if manipulation of the foot into plantar flexion is carried out by the mother six times with every nappy change. Generally the correction occurs over the course of 2–3 months, and by the time the child walks the feet are normal. Occasionally the deformity may persist until walking occurs, in which case a medial type of arch support will be required. When there is muscle imbalance resulting from paralytic conditions, tendon transfers and occasionally subtalar fusion are needed.

Club foot (talipes equinovarus)

This has been covered largely in Chapter 3. Deformities of the foot in children and adults may be corrected by the use of ring fixators utilizing the principles of the Ilizarov technique. This has been described extensively but is not for the occasional user. Nevertheless, lengthening of the foot and progressive correction of deformities by gentle progressive stepwise distraction techniques have achieved considerable success in correcting otherwise recalcitrant deformities.

Vertical talus deformity

The characteristic features of this are:

1. Valgus position of the hindfoot at the midtarsal joint, resulting from dislocation of the talonavicular joint but the calcaneus is tilted downwards in plantar flexion rather than in much valgus (Figure 17.7).
2. Correction by inversion is difficult or impossible.
3. The talar head is prominent and easily palpable but cannot be manipulated back into position.
4. The tendo Achilles is tight.

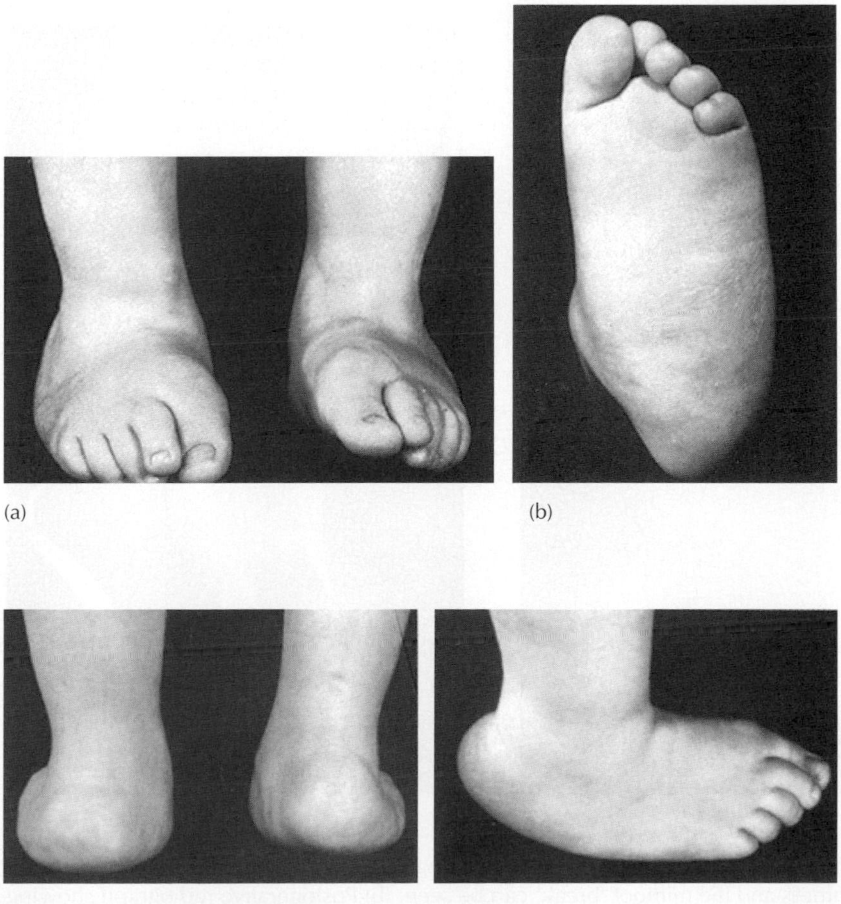

(a) (b) (c) (d)

Figure 17.7 (a) In 'vertical talus' deformity the forefoot has dislocated dorsally, bringing the medial projection of the talus into a weight-bearing position on the sole of the foot. (b) The medial projection of the talus is seen on the sole of the foot. (c) Viewing the foot from behind, the valgus of the heel and medial prominence of the foot are seen. (d) Top view of foot with a vertical talus, showing the convexity of boat-shaped foot.

At birth calcaneovalgus foot and vertical talus deformity appear similar except that there is no break of the foot and no tightness of tendo Achilles in the unimportant calcaneovalgus foot. In congenital vertical talus the talus is in a near-vertical position and lies anterior and medial to the os calcis, which is relatively laterally deviated. The talonavicular joint is dislocated and in some cases the navicular bone may be lying on top of the neck of the talus (Figure 17.8). Surprisingly, the calcaneocuboid joint remains almost normal, except for making up the convex deformity of the whole of the forefoot.

Patterson *et al.* (1968) found the talonavicular dislocation, but also abnormal tightness of the anterior muscle tendon structures which appeared normal except for a 'length deficiency'. The posterior tibial and peroneal tendons were displaced anteriorly over both malleoli. The head of the talus was oval rather than round and there was a reduction to two of the articular facets on the superior surface of the os calcis. The aetiology of the condition is not known but it is a severely disabling condition which must be treated promptly at birth. Rigid vertical talus rarely occurs as an isolated problem but is associated with various chromosomal disorders, neuromuscular defects, arthrogryposis and myelomingocele.

TREATMENT

Treatment of congenital vertical talus is difficult if delayed, but if the condition is recognized at birth and therapy begun early then the results can be very satisfactory. Conservative methods of corrective casting usually fail but attempted correction of equinus in a full leg cast may reduce the amount of surgery which is required subsequently.

Initially the foot is placed in full plantar flexion and check x-rays are carried out to see if reduction of the talonavicular dislocation has been achieved. If this is so then the conservative method may continue for 6–8 weeks after birth with the foot in full equinus and slight varus at the forefoot. Usually, however, this is sufficient only to stretch the anterior tissues and surgical treatment is required.

There are two components of the deformity which

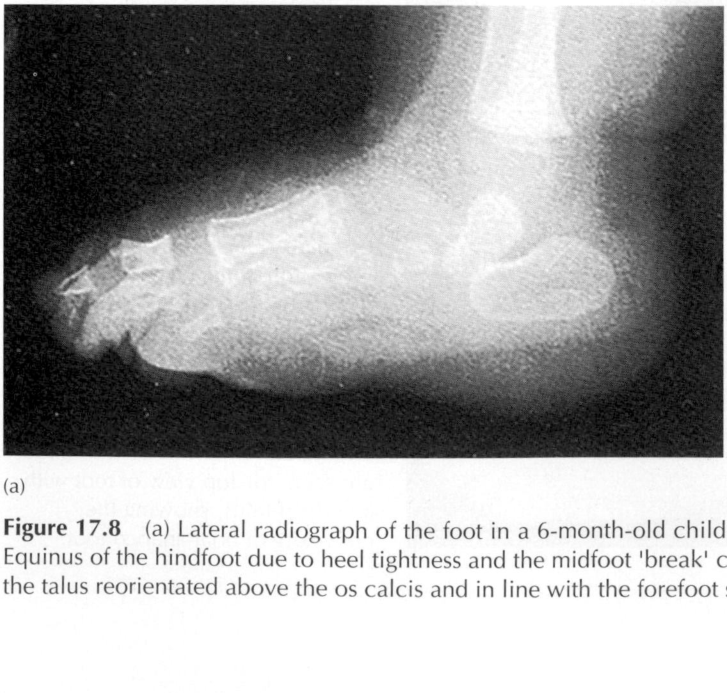

(a)

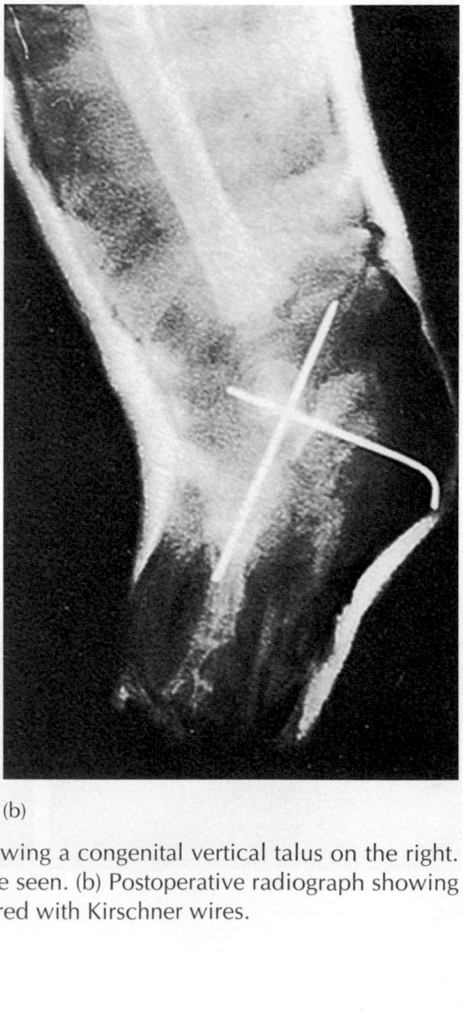

(b)

Figure 17.8 (a) Lateral radiograph of the foot in a 6-month-old child, showing a congenital vertical talus on the right. Equinus of the hindfoot due to heel tightness and the midfoot 'break' can be seen. (b) Postoperative radiograph showing the talus reorientated above the os calcis and in line with the forefoot secured with Kirschner wires.

must both be corrected surgically: equinus of the heel, and rotation and dislocation of the talus in relation to the calcaneus and forefoot. The first stage of the operation is capsulotomy of the talonavicular and calcaneocuboid joints with the division of the talocalcaneal intraosseous ligaments. The talus is reduced under direct vision into a normal position on top of the os calcis and the alignment is held by a Kirschner wire passed through the heel, os calcis and neck of the talus. Secondly, the navicular is reduced onto the anterior articular surface of the talus and its position is held by a second Kirschner wire placed longitudinally through the talonavicular joint. This procedure must be carried out by an open operation via a medial approach, and postoperatively the foot is held in plantar flexion in a full leg cast and the knee flexed to 20°(see Figure 17.8).

The second stage of the operation consists of lengthening the tendo Achillis and the posterior capsule of the ankle joint, which is performed 4 weeks after the first procedure with the wires remaining *in situ*. Following this operation the foot is placed in the neutral position and after a further 2 weeks the wires are removed. Mobilization of the foot may then be commenced with careful review of the child clinically and by x-ray until walking commences.

When the condition is diagnosed later, the Coleman two-stage procedure is carried out (Coleman *et al.*, 1970). This is preceded by 4–6 weeks of gradual casting into a fully plantar flexed position.

In the first stage of this procedure the tendons of the extensor digitorum longus, extensor hallucis longus and anterior tibial muscles are lengthened. The peronei require lengthening if they interfere with reduction. Capsulotomy of the talonavicular and calcaneocuboid joints together with their intraosseous ligaments is performed and reduction of the deformity is carried out as described previously, with the foot held in position by two Kirschner wires. An extra-articular bone block to the talonavicular joint may be required in children of 3 years or more. The second stage consists of heel cord lengthening and posterior capsulotomy and the advancement of the posterior tibial tendon to the plantar surface of the navicular. Following the operation the foot is maintained in the corrected position for a 6-week period and then active mobilization is commenced.

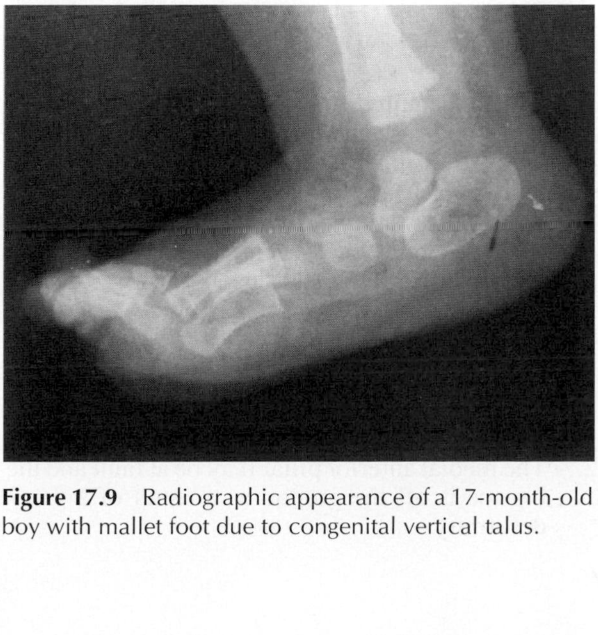

Figure 17.9 Radiographic appearance of a 17-month-old boy with mallet foot due to congenital vertical talus.

Outland and Sherk (1960) recommended a procedure similar to that described by Coleman *et al.*, but with a Grice extra-articular subtalar fusion as well as tendo Achillis lengthening (Figure 17.9).

It is important to remember that, as in other deformities of children, the earlier the commencement of treatment the better the results; in this condition, early recognition is the key to success. Children with recurrent deformity are treated with subtalar fusion. Triple arthrodesis is a salvage procedure reserved for the symptomatic adolescent foot.

Talocalcaneal bar

A further type of congenital flat foot occurs in the presence of a structural anomaly of the tarsus, known as a talocalcaneal bar. Harris (1955) described this as a bridge of bone joining the posterior aspect of the sustentaculum tali to the outer surface of the talus. It may be a complete or incomplete bridge and can be demonstrated by oblique x-rays. It prevents movement between the bones, and, though deformity is slight in childhood when the bones are still largely cartilaginous, with growth the calcaneus is forced into eversion. In adult life there develops an extreme valgus deformity. The child presents with a spastic flat foot. The only effective treatment in young children is excision of the bar of bone; in older children or adolescents the only effective treatment is triple arthrodesis. Olney and Asher (1987) reported excision of symptomatic coalition involving the middle facet of the talocalcaneal joint and interposition of an autogenous fat graft on ten feet with five excellent, three good, one fair and one poor result. They reported the procedure to be superior to triple arthrodesis in adolescents.

The results of surgical excision of symptomatic tarsal coalition of the talocalcaneal and navicular coalitions was reported by Jagannathan *et al.* (1994) who reported better results from calcaneonavicular excision than from talocalcaneal excision.

This condition will be dealt with in more detail below since it usually presents later in childhood.

Osteochondritis of the talus

Osteochondritis of the talus is rarely seen in the head of the talus as one of the osteochondroses – with minor repetitive trauma. However, it is more commonly the result of vascular damage after a fracture through the neck of the talus and will progress to osteochondrosis of the talonavicular joint (Figure 17.10).

See Chapter 3.

Congenital ligament laxity

Laxity of ligaments may be a congenital condition which presents with varying degrees of severity with no obvious cause or it may be secondary to such mesenchymal diseases as Marfan's syndrome and Ehlers–Danlos syndrome. In the idiopathic type no treatment is required if there is no disability, and frequently the flat foot improves with age and development. It requires 6-monthly review and if symptoms, especially pain, occur then surgical treatment by means of a Grice–Green extra-articular fusion may be required. The principles of treatment of secondary ligament laxity are the same but surgical treatment may be complicated by troublesome haemorrhage.

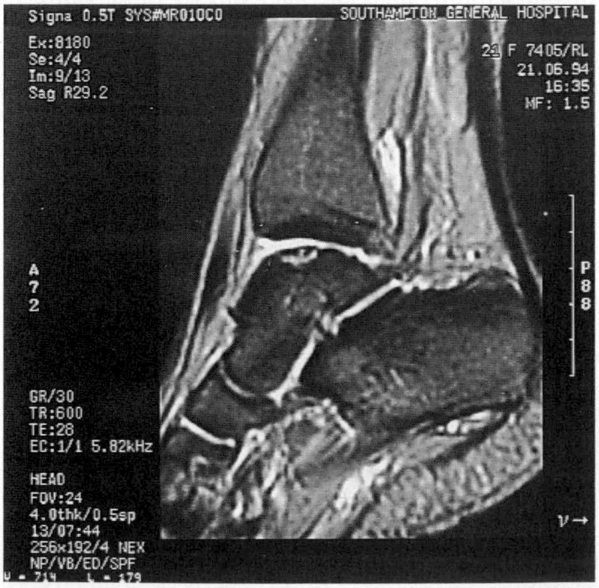

Figure 17.10 Osteochondritis dissecans affecting the head of the talus clearly shown in this sagital section MR scan. (Kindly supplied by Dr Richard Blaquiere, Consultant Radiologist at Southampton University Hospitals)

Acquired flat foot

This may be osseous, ligamentous, muscular-paralytic, spastic postural or static.

The osseous variety may result from trauma to the bones (e.g. in run-over fractures, fractures of the navicular or calcaneus) or from disease of the bones.

The ligamentous variety may follow rupture or avulsion of the plantar ligaments from their attachment.

In the paralytic and spastic muscular types the flattening of the arch is a secondary and late effect, resulting from weight-bearing on a foot whose position has been altered by muscular imbalance. They are considered separately in Chapter 7.

The static type of acquired flat foot is one of the most common and important of orthopaedic complaints.

AETIOLOGY OF STATIC FLAT FOOT

Flat foot arises when the postural muscles of the longitudinal arch become unable to fulfil their function. This arch transmits the body weight to the ground through a wide base of support. If the weight is passed normally through the subtaloid-midtarsal region the stress passes normally through the bones, but if a little further forward then the plantar and interosseous ligaments take the strain. This stretching of the ligaments calls into play the muscles which shift the strain back to the normal area. This is the balancing action of the foot, brought into play by the reflex postural activity of the muscles. This reflex is not present at birth but is gradually acquired in the first year or two of life. Balancing is gradually acquired and the flat foot deformity of infancy disappears. Perkins (1948) pointed out that once this postural activity has been acquired there can be only one reason for pes planus or instability of the long arch – that the foot when at right angles to the leg is not plantigrade, meaning that the three bearing points are not all equally on the ground. There are two common ways in which this may be so:

1. The calcaneus may be at fault and the heel is drawn up in an equinus deformity.
2. The medial anterior pillar may be at fault and the big toe is off the ground as a result of a varus deformity.

The equinus deformity is compensated for by dorsiflexion at the midtarsal joint and this is followed by eversion with a consequent malalignment of body weight. Varus deformity is compensated for by eversion at the subtaloid joint and similar malalignment of body weight. In the equinus foot the calf muscles do not grow as quickly as the tibia, and in the varus foot the bones outgrow the tibialis anterior. It appears, then, that the three main causes of foot strain are faulty postural activity of muscles, an equinus deformity of the foot and a varus deformity of the forefoot.

There are certain predisposing factors:

1. *General muscle hypotonus*. Convalescence after illness, for example, is apt to be associated with loss of muscular tone. Also when growth is rapid, the muscular development may lag behind the growth of the other tissues. Severe trauma to the leg complicated by muscular atrophy is also a cause.
2. *Excessive fatigue of normal muscles*. This may happen in occupations in which the individual has to stand or walk for hours at a time, and is common, for example, amongst nurses, policemen and soldiers; or it may follow excessive exercise after a period of relative disuse. Relative muscular insufficiency may be caused by a rapid increase in the body weight; this type of flat foot for which it is responsible is often found in conjunction with the rapid increase in the body weight of women at the menopause and is the explanation of the foot symptoms so often complained of at that time.
3. *Shoe wear*. It has frequently been implied that unsuitable footwear is a basis of many of our foot troubles in the presence of some inherent structural imperfection. On the other hand, it is commonly recognized that certain deformities arise among people who never wear shoes. Freebairn *et al.* (1959) carried out an extensive survey of school children's feet. They found that a greater number of girls than boys between the ages of 5 and 15 years had hallux valgus. In girls at the age of 5 years, 1.6% I were seen, whereas at 15 years, 54% of girls were involved. In boys, at 5 years 5.2% and at 15 years only 14.8% had a valgus deformity. Therefore, this marked difference must have begun before the age of 15 years, when there is practically no difference in the footwear of the two sexes. These workers pointed out that there was no simple correlation between foot defects and unsatisfactory footwear, but footwear of the proper size is essential for normal growth and development of the foot.

PATHOLOGY

In the earliest stages of flat foot there may be a few or no appreciable changes. As the calcaneonavicular ligament yields, however, the head of the talus is pressed forwards, downwards and medially and the body of the talus may glide forwards on the upper surface of the calcaneus. The calcaneus itself is deviated to the medial side, and its anterior end depressed, with the result that the sustentaculum tali, the head of the talus and the tuberosity of the navicular come to form prominences on the medial aspect of the foot. The long and short plantar ligaments also yield gradually and eventually the deltoid ligament of the ankle as well. When the foot is viewed from behind, the tendo calcaneus appears to be deviated laterally, the tibial tendons are seen to be overstretched, and the peroneal tendons adaptively shortened.

Jack (1953) reviewed the anatomical types of flat foot and pointed out that in the normal weight-bearing foot an axis through the talus, the middle of the navicular, the medial cuneiform and the metatarsals, formed a straight line on lateral radiographs taken with the patient standing. He described how a break would produce an unstable and everted foot, and usually occurred at:

1. the talonavicular joint, to give the perpendicular talus deformity (Figure 17.11a);
2. the naviculocuneiform (Figure 17.11b); and
3. both these joints as a combined break.

Dorsiflexion of the great toe will restore the arch by tightening of the plantar fascia, particularly in cases of naviculocuneiform break (Figure 17.11c) but not when the break occurs at other joints, although a tight tendo calcaneus may vitiate this test.

In neglected cases two further changes ensue. First, the displaced bones are gradually altered in shape, the navicular and medial cuneiform bones, for instance, becoming shaped like wedges with the apices situated dorsolaterally, and there is a permanent alteration in the position and shape of the tarsal bones, which amounts to subluxation at the tarsal joints. Second, portions of the joint surface now unused eventually show osteoarthrosis with marginal osteophytes.

SYMPTOMS

Initially the patient notices that the feet feel tired after use. Later the feet become stiff after sitting or resting, and are most uncomfortable when the patient rises in the morning. The gait becomes inelastic and clumsy, and there is a tendency to walk with the feet everted and not to rise on the toes.

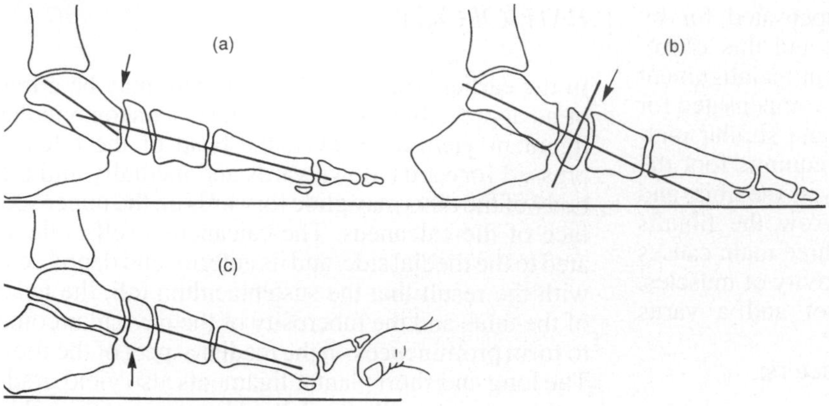

Figure 17.11 (a) A break at the talonavicular joint with a tilting of the talus and disruption of the normal longitudinal axis. (b) The break at the naviculocuneiform joint. (c) Reconstitution of the axis of the longitudinal arch by dorsiflexion of the big toe.

Pain

Pain is more severe when standing than when walking, since walking involves chiefly the use of muscles, whereas in standing the weak muscles relax and the while body weight is borne by the weakened ligaments.

Tenderness

The commonest areas of tenderness are over the navicular, the inferior calcaneonavicular ligament, the sole of the foot and, frequently, below the head of the first metatarsal.

Gait

In flat foot, raising of the heel is avoided, to prevent strain being put upon the tarsal and the metatarsal ligaments, and the patient carefully lifts the ball and the heel of the foot together. The toes are usually turned outwards – splay foot – and the gait is thus awkward and stiff, and without any spring.

Pressure symptoms

The medial part of the heel and sole of the shoe wears more quickly than the lateral. The skin along the medial border of the heel and foot is thickened and painful, and a callous ridge may form in this situation; painful callosities may form, too, in the weight-bearing areas, under the heads of the metatarsals. The lateral displacement of the foot often forces the little toe against the upper of the shoe, and induces the formation of a callosity or corn on its most prominent part. The toes are compressed laterally even when the shoe is not too narrow.

TYPES OF WEAK FOOT

It is useful to divide acquired flat foot into four classes:

1. *Foot strain, or incipient flat foot* – the earliest stage and corresponds to the period when pressure is first being exerted upon the ligaments. There is no evident deformity, but tenderness and pain.
2. *Mobile flat foot*
   (a) due to faulty postural activity of muscle. There is often a general postural defect and the foot is the most obvious element. It is also the obvious reason for examining every foot problem with the patient completely undressed. When the child stands there is flattening of the longitudinal arches but this disappears when he stands on his toes;
   (b) due to short tendo calcaneus. The malalignment of the body weight disappears on tip-toeing, but when the foot is correctly aligned it is in equinus. This limited dorsiflexion is common in women and a frequent cause of the valgoid mobile foot;
   (c) due to varus deformity of the forefoot;
   (d) due to persistent fetal alignment of the femora in an abnormal amount of internal rotation. This results in valgus deformities of the knees with the patellae pointing medially as well as the feet being 'flattened';
   (e) due to spinal dysraphism (e.g. spina bifida, diastematomyelia, lumbosacral lipomata).
3. *Rigid flat foot* – with secondary degenerative changes in the subtaloid and midtarsal joints (Figures 17.12–17.15) due to old club foot, old injury, rheumatoid arthritis or osteoarthritis.

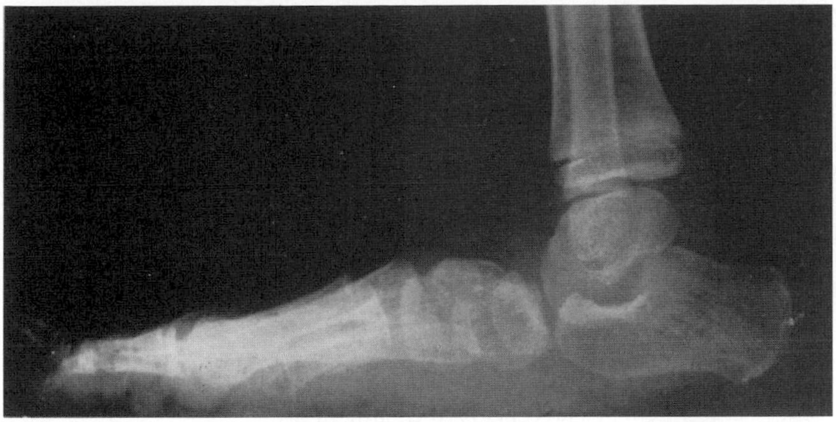

Figure 17.12 Depressed medial arch in a relaxed foot. Note, however, that the navicular remains related to the head of the talus.

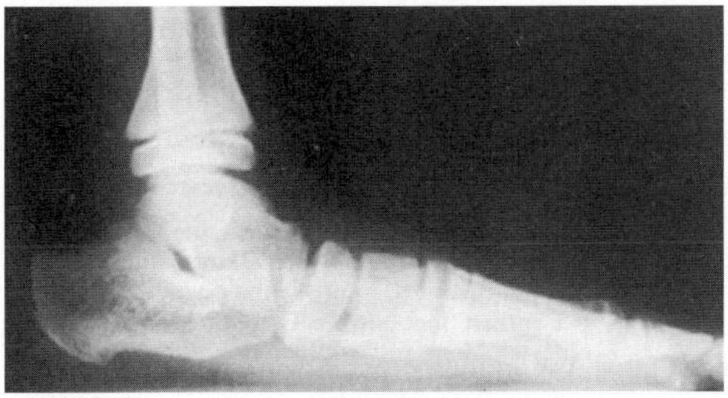

(a)

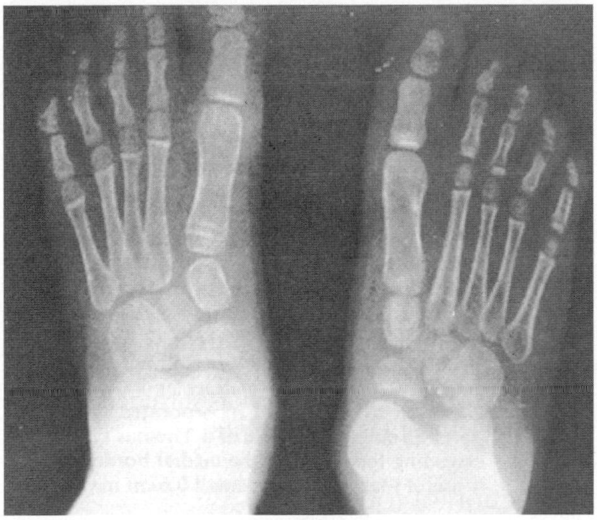

(b)

Figure 17.13 (a) Lateral radiograph of foot, showing a typical talonavicular break with vertical talus. (b) Antero-posterior view, showing the marked deviation of the talus medially with increase of the normal angle between the talus and the calcaneus.

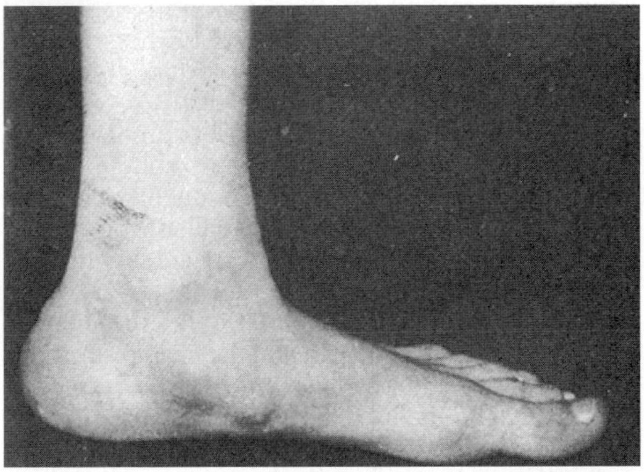

Figure 17.14 The rigid type of flat foot with dropped longitudinal arch and prominence of the navicular.

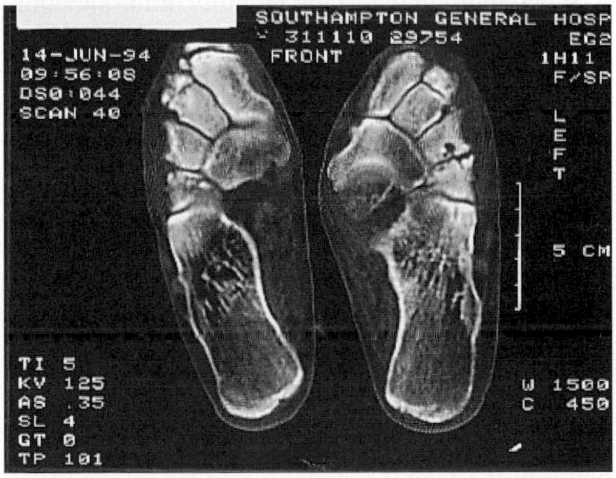

Figure 17.15 Transverse section of an MR scan showing osteoarthritis affecting the calcaneocuboid and cubocuneiform joints with loss of joint space, subchondral sclerosis and cyst formation mainly affecting the left foot. (Kindly supplied by Dr Richard Blaquiere, Consultant Radiologist at Southampton University Hospitals)

EXAMINATION OF THE FOOT

Inspection

The examination should commence by observing the manner of standing and walking. Any limp is noted, and the elasticity of the gait and the posture of the feet in walking are observed. Deformity of the shoes – excessive wearing away of the sole and heel on the medial side, bulging or the presence of localized prominences – is noted.

The patient now stands barefoot, and the attitude, the shape and the weight distribution of the foot are investigated. The line from the centre of the patella down the tibial crest should pass through the space between the second and third toes; in foot strain it constantly passes to the inner side of the great toe, and it also does so when the foot is externally rotated on the leg.

In slight cases the persistent eversion of the foot may not be pronounced from the front. In such a case, examination from behind frequently prevents error in diagnosis, as the medial malleolus is seen to be unduly prominent and there is marked valgus of the heel.

In addition, the medial border of the foot may be convex instead of concave, and the head of the talus or the navicular may stand out as a distinct bony prominence on the medial side of the foot.

If the stability of the longitudinal arch can be restored it can be most easily demonstrated by asking the patient to stand on his toes. If the deformity corrects fully it is of the mobile type, and is of no significance if painless.

It is important to test the mobility of the subtaloid joint. The heel is placed in a central or neutral position (i.e. neither varus nor valgus) and the forefoot placed so that the vertical line of the body weight passes through the second toe. If this cannot be done, the subtaloid and midtarsal joints have lost their mobility and the deformity is of the rigid type.

Palpation

The foot is now carefully palpated for evidence of abnormal tenderness. This is usually present on both medial and lateral aspects of the ankle, in the first instance because of ligamentous strain, and in the second from the compression of the soft tissues between the lateral malleolus and the everted foot. Tenderness is present on the sole, especially over the spring ligament.

DIAGNOSIS

The diagnosis of weak, or flat, foot should not be difficult. Certain conditions may sometimes have to be differentiated, and these are ligamentous and bony injuries, primary and secondary ligament laxity, infection, arthritis, synovitis, bursitis, tendinitis, paralysis, Köhler's disease and osteochondritis of the calcaneus.

TREATMENT

The objects of treatment are:

1. To correct the abnormal centre of gravity of the foot, so that the body weight is transmitted normally.
2. To remove external pressure symptoms.

The absolute indications for treatment are pain and impaired function. The existence of flat foot does not mean that treatment is required, as many people with perfectly flat and sometimes rigid feet have quite normal function.

Treatment of incipient flat foot (acute foot strain)

The most important factors in acute foot strain are to remove any obvious provoking painful activity and to attempt to improve the posture of the foot.

Electrical treatment

Faradic stimulation of the small muscles of the foot is effective in increasing their tone.

Exercises

Intrinsic foot exercises are often helpful in improving muscle tone generally in the feet, and the added stimulation may help in the early stages. Active exercises against resistance, initially supervised in the physiotherapy department, are useful for muscle groups at the ankle when pain has subsided. The use of a wobble-board is often helpful.

Correction of footwear

It is important that the patient wear well fitting shoes and these may be improved by the use of incorporated valgus supports. In children the use of a Thomas type of heel extending forwards on the medial border for 1 cm is useful together with a small 0.6 cm medial raise.

Treatment of mobile flat foot

This type of deformity requires treatment only if it is symptomatic. This condition has been treated by felt or sponge rubber supports or the use of Rose's shaped plastic heel cups for insertion in the shoes.

Wenger *et al.* (1989), in a prospective study to determine whether flexible flat foot in children can be influenced by treatment concluded that corrective shoes or inserts for 3 years does not influence the course of flexible flat foot in children.

Treatment of rigid flat foot

The body weight should be controlled, and with graduated active foot exercises and the use of a valgus insole in well fitting shoes, many patients can be relieved. If, however, the symptoms persist and if there is established osteoarthritis in the tarsus then operation may be required. Depending on the joints involved, fusion may be performed of the talonavicular joint or of the naviculocuneiform joint. In both instances a longitudinal incision is made over the joint, which is exposed and denuded of articular cartilage and then held with the foot in as near physiological position as can be achieved. Internal fixation with a staple may be required and also a corticocancellous bone graft which is placed in a slot across the joint. Following the operation the foot requires support in a carefully moulded above-knee cast for 2 months, but weight-bearing may begin as soon as the patient is comfortable.

Talocalcaneal extra-articular arthrodesis of the subtaloid joint as described by Grice is valuable in painful flat feet in children (Figure 17.16). In this procedure the sinus tarsi is opened and an extra-articular fusion is carried out by employing two corticocancellous grafts back to back placed into the sinus tarsi with the foot forced into slight varus. The grafts are then a tight fit and on load-bearing the longitudinal arch is supported. Following operation, immobilization in plaster is required for 12 weeks, 6 weeks in an above-knee and 6 weeks in a patellar-tendon bearing cast.

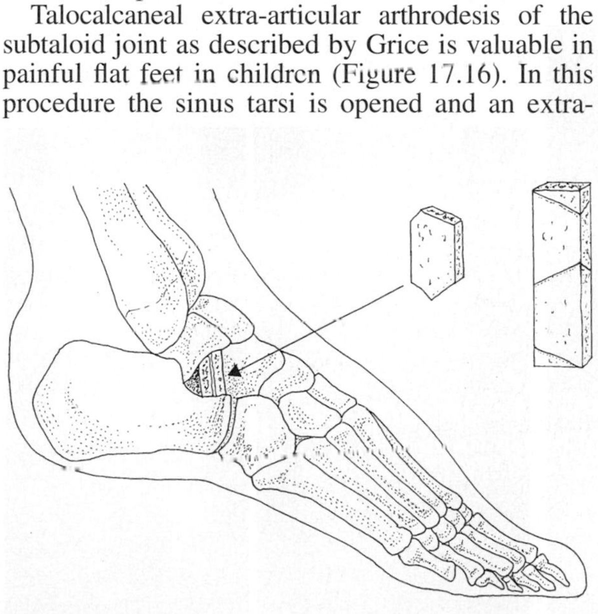

Figure 17.16 The Grice extra-articular arthrodesis for rigid and painful flat foot. The grafts are wedged into the sinus tarsi with the foot slightly inverted to allow for the slight bone resorption on impaction of the graft into the talus and os calcis.

Peroneal or spasmodic flat foot

In this acute condition which is commonly seen in young adolescents there is pain, tightness or spasm of the peroneal muscles and an eversion deformity of the foot. The onset is usually after starting work or changing to an occupation involving much standing, so that the complaint is known sometimes as 'apprentice's foot'.

Outland and Murphy (1960) reviewed the numerous conditions which can be implicated in this syndrome:

1. *Congenital:* tarsal anomalies and intertarsal bridges, e.g. calcaneonavicular (Figures 17.17–17.19), talocalcaneal and calcaneocuboid bars as described by Harris and Beath (1948), and anomalies of the navicular bone (Figures 17.20 and 17.21).
2. *Acquired:* in tuberculous lesions, rheumatoid arthritis, osteoarthritis, non-specific tarsal joint synovitis, trauma and occupational strains.

Outland and Murphy believed that it is important to distinguish between the rigid flat foot and the spastic flat foot. When the bar between the calcaneonavicular area is complete, it forms either a synchondrosis (by cartilage) or syndesmosis (by fibrous tissue). Ossification may be present, and when complete a synostosis of bone is formed. These workers believed that it is the degenerative changes in the talonavicular joint which produce pain and the spasm of the peroneals. The pathology of the peroneal spasm is probably that of a reflex muscle reaction, but as yet there is no established relationship between the sensory innervation of the talonavicular joint and that supplying the peroneal muscles. The spasm may also involve the extensor digitorum longus, especially in younger patients.

Braddock (1961) reviewed a series of peroneal spastic foot cases, and only 10% caused severe and persistent disability with the development of any symptomatic tarsal arthritis in subsequent years. He also stated that radiographs were of no use as a guide for prognosis or treatment.

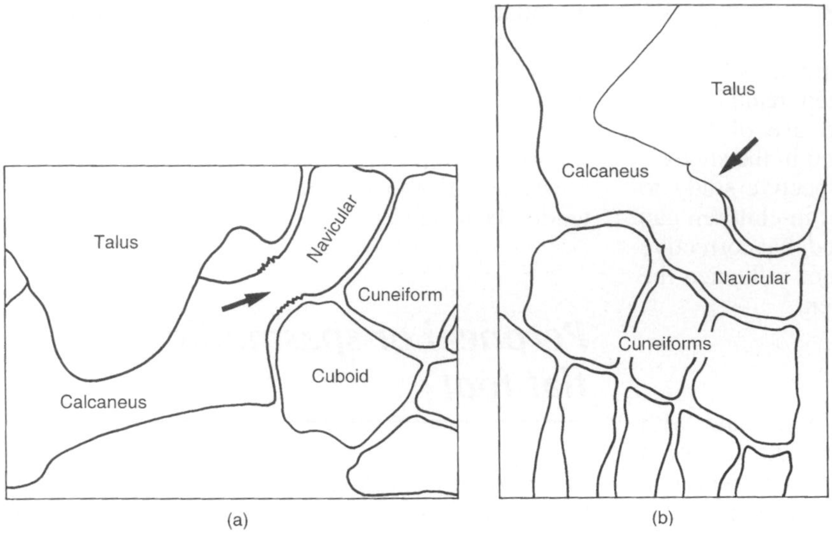

Figure 17.17 (a) The lateral appearance of the calcaneonavicular bar. (b) An oblique anteroposterior view showing the calcaneonavicular bar.

Tarsal coalition

Tarsal coalition is a congenital failure of segmentation of two or more of the tarsal bones and may be fibrous, cartilaginous or bony. It is thought to be inherited in autosomal dominant mode. The calcaneonavicular is the most common synostosis, followed by the middle facet of the talocalcaneal joint. Occasionally more than one condition is present in one foot and the condition is bilateral in 50%.

Typically, ossification occurs between 8 and 12 years of age for calcaneonavicular bar and between 12 and 15 for talocalcaneal conditions.

Jack (1954) reviewed the bone anomalies of the tarsus in this condition. The calcaneonavicular bar is a congenital anomaly in which the calcaneus and navicular bones are joined together by a complete or partial bridge of bone. It is not due to an unusual degree of development of an accessory bone, the os calcaneus secondarius. Trethowen (1930) pointed out how the strain of prolonged standing or unduly

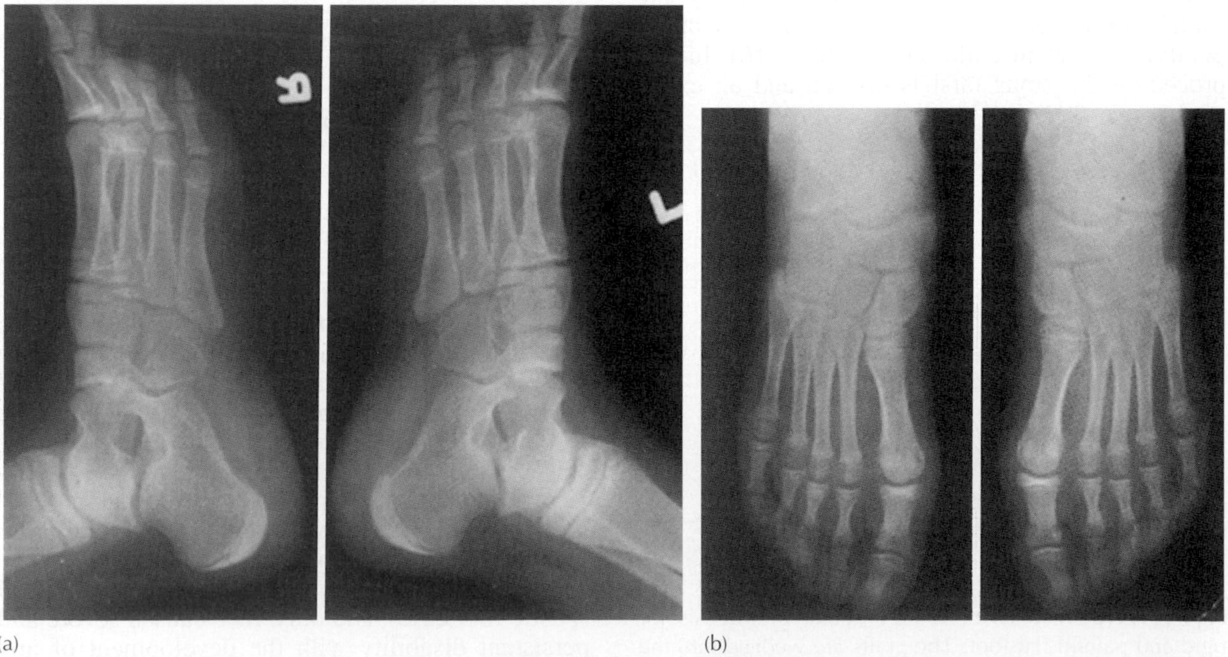

Figure 17.18 Radiographs showing an incomplete calcaneonavicular bar of both feet from (a) the lateral oblique view as well as from (b) the anteroposterior view.

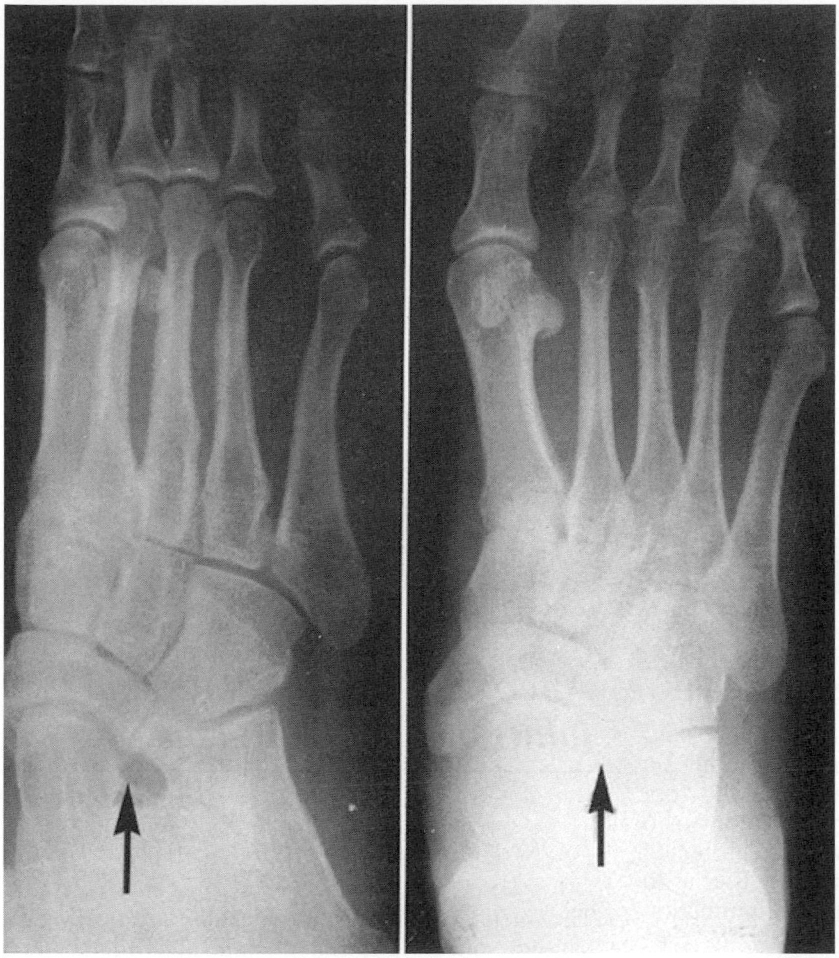

Figure 17.19 Apparent bar between navicular and os calcis, formed as result of reaction to foreign body.

heavy work in adolescents who had recently left school may be have a been factor in causing symptoms.

Special oblique and axial views on radiography are necessary to demonstrate the presence of the bony anomalies. Recently CT has become the investigation of choice to delineate the bony anomalies and the state of the joints.

TREATMENT

Mitchell (1970) described the treatment of spasmodic flat foot in two groups:

1. Those associated with a calcaneonavicular bar.
2. Those associated with early rheumatoid arthritis

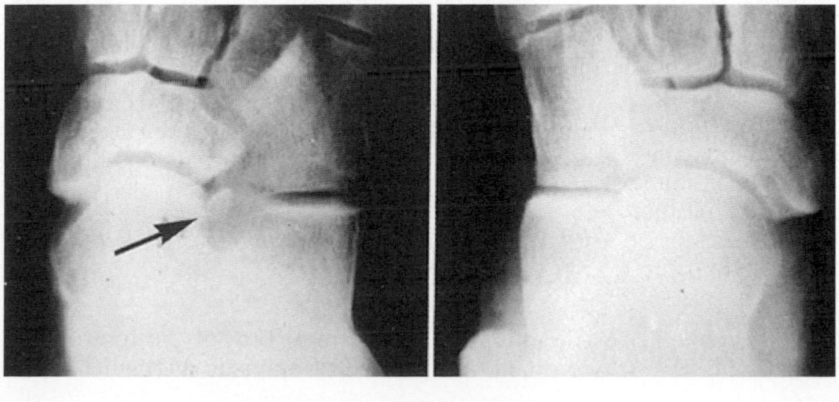

Figure 17.20 Separate ossicle in position of calcaneonavicular bar in 50-year-old male, causing peroneal spasm. The remainder of the bridge between the two was formed by fibrocartilage.

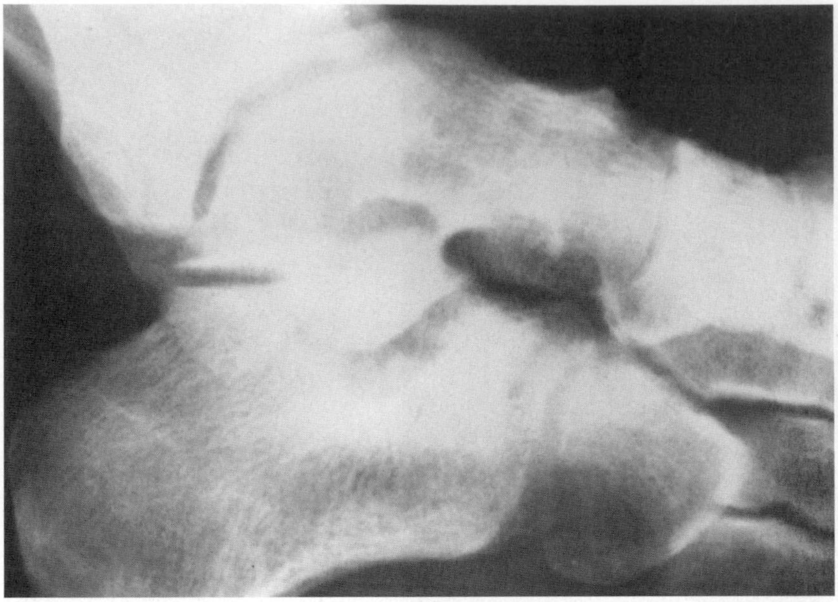

Figure 17.21 Beaking of the talus secondary to peroneal spasm.

or other causes of inflammation of the small foot joints.

For the latter, manipulation under anaesthesia will produce a more neutral position of the foot which can be held by plaster immobilization for 6 weeks. The foot thereafter may have to be protected by a double upright brace with an inner T-strap to prevent recurrence and to allow the inflammation to subside.

Patients with a calcaneonavicular bar usually present around 9 years of age and it is in this age group that the bar can be excised with good results. The incision is similar to that employed for a triple arthrodesis on the lateral aspect of the foot over the sinus tarsi exposing the tuberosity of the os calcis, the bar and the navicular. A generous portion of calcaneus and the navicular is removed with the osteotome. The foot is immobilized for 3 weeks in inversion and thereafter protected by a cast or brace for 3 months.

A subtalar arthrodesis may be required to restore the os calcis beneath the talus using a subtalar strut-graft when a talocalcaneal bony bar is present. Results of excision of the bar alone are not satisfactory. If the arch is restored and the grafts are correctly placed the midtarsal joints remain congruous and height is not lost in the subtalar joint area. In the older case a localized fusion of the talocalcaneal or the talonavicular joint is necessary, and if a rigid painful flat foot is present triple arthrodesis is carried out.

Affections of the bones and joints of the metatarsus

NORMAL FORM OF THE FOREFOOT

The metatarsal bones are usually arranged as a parallel series. The first metatarsal is thicker and stronger than the others, as it provides the weight-bearing foot with one of its three chief points of support. Furthermore, because it forms the fulcrum on which the body weight is swung forwards in walking, its head lies on a more anterior plane than the others. The other important weight-bearing points of the foot are the fifth metatarsal and the calcaneus; these, with the first metatarsal head, are usually regarded as forming the points of the tripod.

The intermediate metatarsal heads are sometimes said to form an arch – the anterior metatarsal arch – but the value of this observation is doubtful. It is likely that all the metatarsal heads are in contact with the ground in walking, but that, as a result of muscular and ligamentous support, they take a small part in weight-bearing under normal conditions.

DEVELOPMENTAL ANOMALIES OF THE METATARSUS

Alterations in the normal form of the forefoot are common, and consist of atavistic anomalies of the first metatarsal is gradually drawn laterally from an abducted position to become parallel to its neighbours. It loses the mobility it possesses in the primitive foot of the ape, and it grows in strength till it outstrips its fellows.

The common developmental errors which may occur are:

1. *Metatarsus primus varus*. Here the first metatarsal is distinctly abducted from the midline of the second and there is a palpable and radiologically demonstrable interval of more than 10° between the first and second shafts (Figure 17.22). Occasionally this wedge-shaped interval is occupied by an accessory ossicle – the os intermetatarseum.
2. *Metatarsus atavicus or brevis*. In this anomaly the first metatarsal bone is shorter than normal, and is situated behind the head of the second and commonly the third. The metatarsal is often abducted (primus varus).
3. *Metatarsus hypermobilis*. Here the first metatarsal is unduly mobile. This is the result of ineffectual fixation at its base, and can be demonstrated easily by taking the metatarsal head between the finger and thumb, and plantar and dorsiflexing it at its base while the tarsus is supported by the opposite hand. The normal range is 20° of plantar flexion and 90° of dorsiflexion of the hallux about the metatarsal axis.

CLINICAL EFFECT OF DEVELOPMENTAL ANOMALIES

In many people developmental errors are masked by efficient muscular support and by hypertrophy of the neighbouring bones, but it is obvious that certain effects may arise. In metatarsus primus varus, the first metatarsal is lying away from the long axis of the foot and fails to act as an effective fulcrum; its function, therefore, must in part be assumed by the second metatarsal, and possibly the third, and these – unless hypertrophied – are ill-adapted to fulfil its purpose. In metatarsus atavicus a similar effect obtains, while in metatarsus hypermobilis the first metatarsal, though it may act as a fulcrum quite effectively if fixed by the adductor muscle, without such fixation fails to form a stable weight-bearing point of the tripod, and becomes splayed out on long standing.

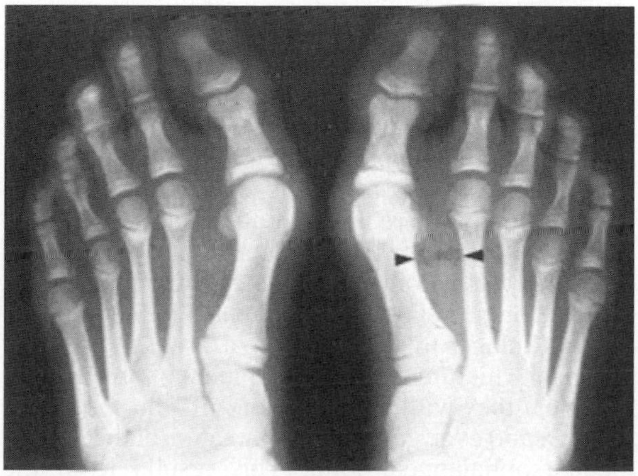

Figure 17.22 Metatarsus primus varus in a child with early hallux valgus deformity.

There is one further – and important – effect of metatarsus primus varus; the use of even ordinary footwear will cause the toe to become displaced, an effect that will be enhanced by the use of boots or shoes with abnormally pointed toes. The increased load thrown on the intermediate metatarsal heads is the factor underlying a series of interesting and important disturbances.

The following clinical conditions may arise in association with developmental anomalies:

1. Hallux valgus.
2. Metatarsalgia.
3. March foot or march fracture.
4. Köhler's disease of the metatarsal head (Freiberg's infraction).

Hallux valgus

The deformity of hallux valgus consists of abnormal adduction of the proximal phalanx of the great toe towards the midline of the foot and is associated, especially in the most extreme forms, with varying degrees of varus of the first metatarsal. It is present when the axis of the proximal phalanx of the great toe deviates laterally from the axis of the first metatarsal by more than 10° (Figure 17.23). Lake (1942) considered that the varus deviation of the first metatarsal, the cause of which is unknown, is the most important factor in the development of this lesion. Kaplan (1951) described a strong connecting band extending from the tendon of tibialis posterior muscle into the flexor hallucis brevis and adductor hallucis and regarded this as a contributory factor in producing this deformity. Lesser degrees of lateral deviation are not uncommon as a result of the prevalent use of badly designed and ill-fitting shoes even when the position of the metatarsal is normal.

The phalangeal deviation is progressively increased by the contracture and shortening of the adductor

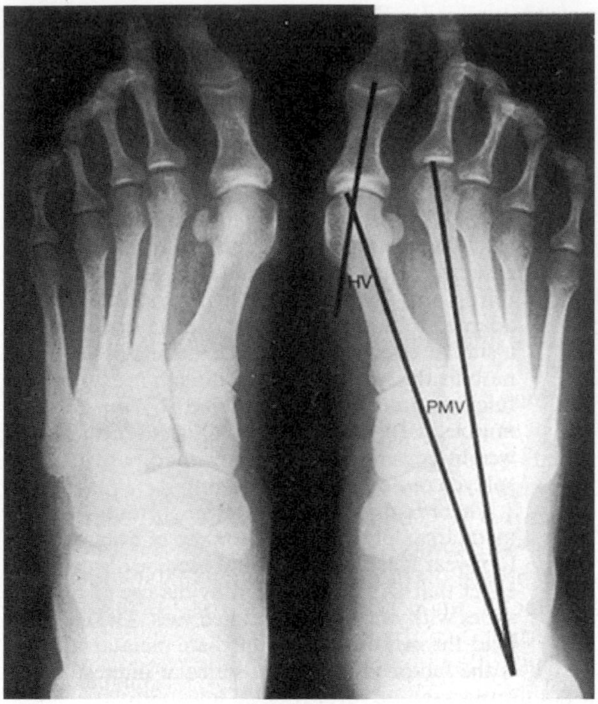

Figure 17.23 Standing anteroposterior radiograph of both feet of an adult, showing the primary metatarsus varus deformity (PMV) and valgus deformity of the hallux (HV).

hallucis and extensor hallucis longus, so that ultimately the base of the phalanx is displaced so far laterally that it articulates solely with the lateral condyle of the metatarsal head. The medial condyle of the metatarsal head remains as a prominence on the medial side of the foot and is subjected to friction and pressure from the shoe. An adventitious bursa is accordingly formed and a corn or callosity develops in the overlying skin. The projecting bone, together with the bursa and corn or callosity, are collectively known as a bunion.

Piggott (1960), writing on the natural history of this deformity in adolescents and early adult life, challenged the concept that metatarsus primus varus plays the primary role in the development of hallux valgus. There is not enough evidence at present to determine which is the primary deformity, but he considered that it is the lateral deviation of the great toe which occurs first. He pointed out that in many individuals there is an increase in the normal valgus alignment of the great toe. This normal variant has to be differentiated from the pathological valgus alignment in which the articular surfaces making up the first metatarsophalangeal joint are displaced on each other and are incongruent. He also described that in adolescents, even though hallux valgus may be present, if there is congruity of the articular surfaces, it is unlikely that this deformity will progress, and hence require any treatment. Hart and Bentley (1976), in a review of young adult patients with hallux valgus, found that 80% had metatarsus primus varus. It was not possible to establish in what proportion this was the primary deformity, but the absence of metatarsus primus varus in 20% indicates that it is not the invariable cause.

When the first intermetatarsal angle is increased beyond the normal 10°, there is a definite increase in the incidence of hallux valgus. This has been described as resulting from anomalies involving the first cuneiform-metatarsal joint.

Wilson (1980), in a very extensive review and a particular study of the static forces during walking barefoot and when shod, described how at 'toe off' in the barefoot the final force falls on the pulp of the big toe but in the shod foot this force is more lateral. This latter position produces a valgus movement at the metatarsophalangeal joint, throwing a strain on the medial capsule. When this becomes incompetent, the longitudinal force on the tip of the big toe produces the metatarsus primus varus deformity. Wilson also emphasized the importance of the fibrous plantar plate containing the embedded sesamoid bones, which forms a stationary articulating surface superiorly for the metatarsophalangeal joint whereas inferiorly it is in contact with the ground. This adapts to the transmission of weight-bearing forces from heel strike to toe push off.

With increasing valgus deformity the first metatarsal head displaces off the plantar plate and its sesamoid bones, and the abductor hallucis tendon moves inferiorly to act as a flexor with medial rotation of the first digit. This is particularly noticeable in the position of the big toenail.

PATHOLOGY

The tissues on the lateral side of the deformity – capsule, muscle tendons and ligaments – are adaptively shortened, while the capsule and ligaments on the medial side of the joint are stretched. The cartilage on the exposed part of the metatarsal head undergoes fibrillation and degeneration, and marginal osteophytes are thrown out, as in osteoarthritis. The functions of the intrinsic muscles of the foot are interfered with, contributing to anterior metatarsalgia. The bursa is liable to inflammatory changes and in its late stages the joint is osteoarthritic. A constant secondary feature is the development of an adjacent hammer toe with dorsiflexion of the proximal phalanx and even complete subluxation at the second metatarsophalangeal joint. This results from the body weight and 'take-off' a being displaced from the first metatarsal onto the head of the second metatarsal, causing arthritis and overlying callosity formation, with metatarsalgia. Hallux valgus commonly occurs in rheumatoid arthritis as part of a general forefoot deformity.

CLINICAL FEATURES

Many people with hallux valgus suffer relatively little trouble till osteoarthritis supervenes in later years. In others, pain may arise in association with the corn or callosity, or the bursa may become repeatedly or chronically enlarged, or even suppurate. In these individuals, pain is the result of pressure on the affected structures, and relief can be obtained by stretching the portion of the boot or shoe overlying the bunion. When the symptoms are due to arthritis, the range of movement of the joint is both limited and painful. The condition is often accompanied by symptoms of metatarsalgia, of foot strain or established flat foot.

The pain from hallux valgus is due to four causes:

1. Friction and pressure over the prominent head with production of a bursitis.
2. Osteoarthritis of the metatarsophalangeal joint of the hallux.
3. Involvement of the sesamoid bones in the arthritic process.
4. Callosities under the second and third metatarsal heads due to splaying of the transverse arch.

CONSERVATIVE TREATMENT

In mild cases the symptoms can be relieved by the provision of properly fitting shoes, and the upper may be stretched over the prominent metatarsal head. The fitting of a metatarsal bar on the sole of the shoe or a metatarsal insole is often a useful addition to reduce metatarsalgia.

OPERATIVE TREATMENT

Operative treatment may be regarded as prophylactic or curative.

Prophylactic operations

Hallux valgus in children or in young adults may present with only deformity and mild pain. It is important not to underestimate the cosmetic aspect of this deformity and also that progression of the deformity will lead to painful osteoarthritis

McBride operation

In this the lateral deforming forces of the conjoined tendons of adductor hallucis and the lateral head of the flexor hallucis brevis are transferred from the proximal phalanx into the lateral side of the head of the first metatarsal. The tendon is passed through a hole in the metatarsal and this releases the deforming force on the proximal phalanx and at the same time tends to correct any metatarsus primus varus. This operation is unpredictable, and sometimes a very ugly and painful metatarsus varus results.

Metatarsal osteotomy

This is indicated for hallux valgus when no arthritis is present in the metatarsophalangeal joint. It corrects deformity by shifting the axis of the metatarsal laterally towards the second metatarsal and is supplemented by the soft tissue procedures which involve tightening the medial capsule of the metatarsophalangeal joint to realign the toe in the correct position. We consider that the operation described by Mitchell *et al.* (1958) is a most valuable procedure in all age groups. The metatarsophalangeal joint is exposed by a dorsal incision and the small exostosis is removed from the medial aspect of the metatarsal head. Then osteotomy is made at the junction of the head with the neck of the metatarsal using parallel saw cuts, the distal one being incomplete. The effect of this is to leave a buttress of bone medially on the distal fragment so that the head may be pushed laterally towards the second toe and locked in position. It is also emphasized that the head should also be displaced downwards to ensure that it continues to be a weight-bearing bone with adequate length. The position is held by a suture passed through a drill hole in each fragment and finally the medial capsule of the joint is reefed to hold the corrected position of the toe (Figure 17.24). A plaster cast is applied which must embrace the great toe and is changed after 2 weeks, during which time the patient does not bear weight. The new cast is fitted in a similar way but the patient is then allowed to bear weight for 4 weeks before removal of the cast takes place.

Hart and Bentley (1976) reported the results of this operation in comparison with those of Reverdin, Hohmann, basal osteotomy and oblique osteotomy of the neck. They found that the number of good and fair results for the five types of osteotomy were as follows over a 6-year follow-up period:

1. Metatarsal neck wedge osteotomy (Reverdin) – 39%.
2. Basal osteotomy – 57%.
3. Hohmann's neck osteotomy – 68%.

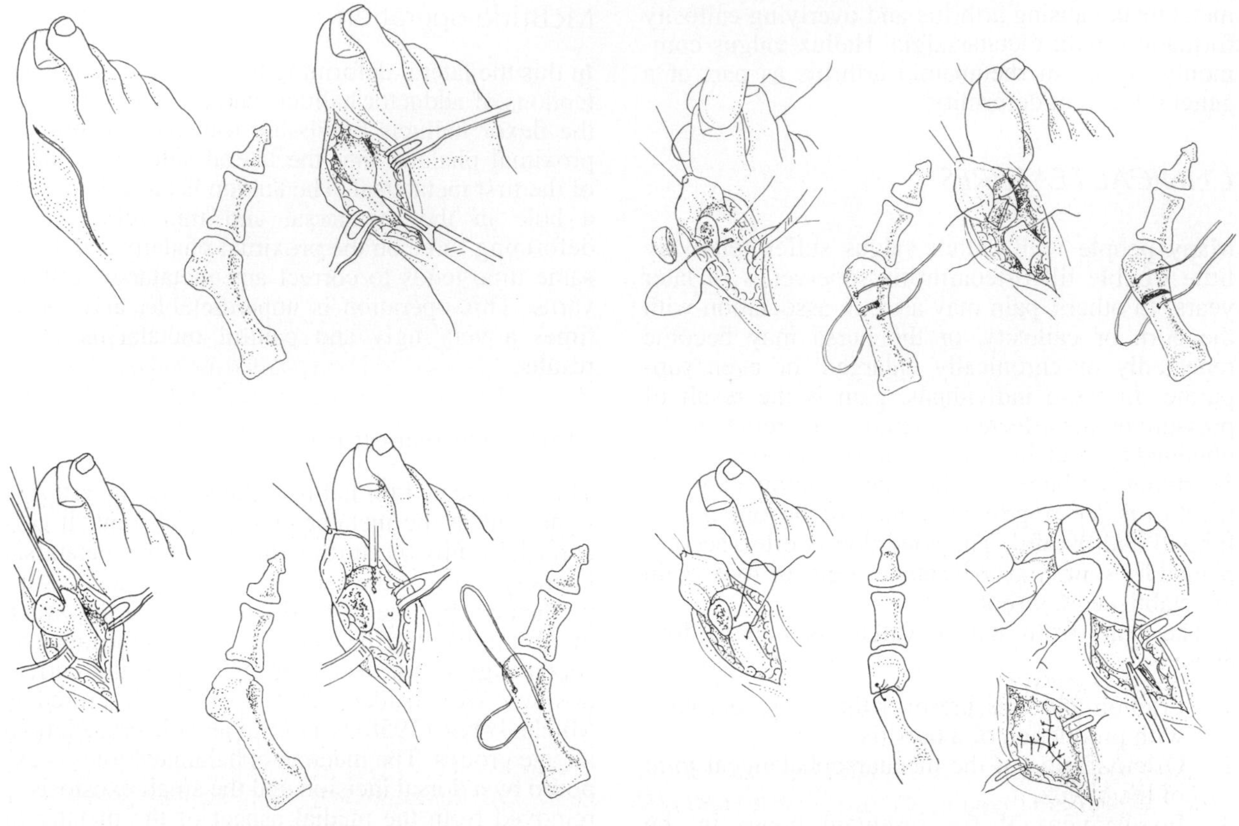

(a) (b)

Figure 17.24 The Mitchell metatarsal osteotomy (a) skin incision, fashioning of distally based capsular flap, removal of bunion and positioning of drill holes; (b) osteotomy of neck by two parallel saw cuts, the distal one being incomplete. The head is displaced medially, the suture tied and the medial capsule reefed.

4. Mitchell's neck osteotomy – 78%.
5. Oblique neck osteotomy fixed with a screw (Wilson) – 90%.

They favoured the Mitchell type of procedure because of its relative simplicity. The oblique osteotomy gave good results in 90% but produced an average 1 cm shortening of the metatarsal which was thought to be a disadvantage in the long term. The most common complication following correction of hallux valgus is recurrence. This is particularly true of adolescents who have reported recurrence rates of approximately 80%.

Mann *et al.* (1992) described the results of a distal soft tissue procedure together with a proximal metatarsal osteotomy. They achieved a 93% satisfaction rate in 109 feet, but described hallux varus in 12% and dorsiflexion malunion in 28% without any clinical problem.

Fixation of distal metatarsal osteotomies is reported more frequently now because of reported instances of loss of alignment (Hirvensalo *et al.*, 1991).

Borton and Stephens (1994) described a first metatarsal osteotomy of the chevron type with a bone wedge for severe hallux valgus with metatarsal primus varus. A prospective analysis of 1023 feet by McBride and Anderson (1994) emphasized the importance of a prospective analysis to assess symptomatic clinical and radiographic factors. Operative choices lay between a modified Wilson's realignment osteotomy with screw fixation, metatarsophalangeal joint fusion initially with K wires and subsequently using screw or power driven staple fixation, a combined basal wedge osteotomy of the first metatarsal with a double-stem silastic metatarsophalangeal spacer and Keller's excision arthroplasty with temporary wire fixation. Patient satisfaction in excess of 90% was reported with significant improvement in objective and radiographic data.

Other operations

Keller's operation (Figure 17.25)

When osteoarthritis is established in the metatarsophalangeal joint in an old patient then arthroplasty of the joint is sometimes indicated. The Keller's

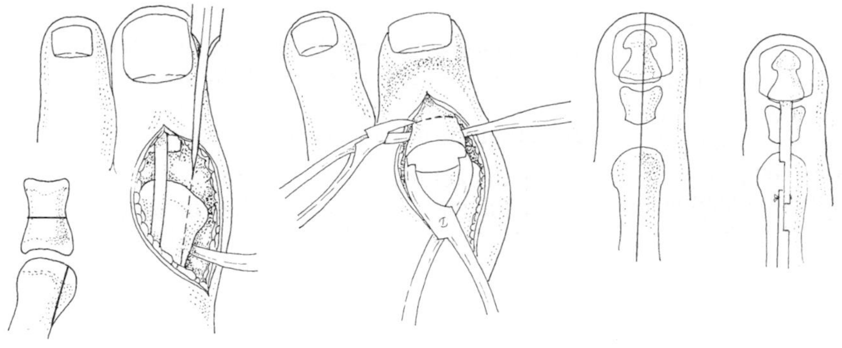

(a) (b) (c)

Figure 17.25 Keller's arthroplasty for hallux valgus: (a) removal of the osteophyte; (b) exposure and removal of the proximal half of the proximal phalanx; (c) optional stabilization of the hallux with intramedullary Kirschner wire and elongation of the extensor hallucis longus. (Reproduced with kind permission from Piggott, H. (1979) Hallus valgus and hallus rigidus. In: *Operative Surgery*, 3rd edn, vol. 2, *Orthopaedics*. Edited by G. Bentley. Butterworths: London and Boston)

arthroplasty, which involves the removal of the bunion and excision of the proximal half of the proximal phalanx of the great toe, is one solution but only in a patient with limited aspirations for walking to relieve pain. The shortening of the great toe produces great disability. An incision is made on the dorsum of the metatarsophalangeal joint, avoiding the medial side so as to prevent discomfort from the scar. The proximal half of the phalanx is denuded of soft tissue and the phalanx is divided halfway along its length and the proximal half removed. Care is taken throughout the procedure to prevent injury to the underlying flexor tendon. The head of the metatarsal is reshaped by removal of the exostosis and the flap of soft tissue medially is placed across the space and stitched into position. If the tendon of extensor hallux longus is contracted, it is lengthened. Following closure of the wound the position is maintained by careful bandaging of the great toe with wool and crêpe bandages secured with strapping holding the toe in slight plantar flexion and slight varus. The patient may commence weight-bearing 48 hours after the operation in a unilateral case and 1 week after operation in a bilateral case. The bandaging is retained for 2 weeks, after which stitches are removed and then a further bandaging is continued for at least another 2 weeks.

Arthrodesis of the first metatarsophalangeal joint

This operation was originally recommended by Ross-Smith (1952) to preserve the strength, function and length of the great toe. It is essential to have a mobile interphalangeal joint of the great toe in order to ensure the success of this operation, which should probably be restricted to the active young person who requires full power in the great toe. The base of the phalanx and the head of the metatarsal are denuded of articular cartilage and the osteophytes are trimmed. The joint is fixed in a position of 5° of dorsiflexion and held either by a transfixion screw or by a compression clamp. Immobilization in a plaster-of-Paris below-knee cast is required for a period of 8 weeks to allow fusion to take place (Figure 17.26).

Bunionectomy

This consists of removing the exostosis with a careful reefing and repair of the medial joint capsule. It is particularly indicated in the elderly patient with a slight valgus deformity. Occasionally it is of value in the young foot as a compromise between an osteotomy and a Keller's arthroplasty.

Kitaoka *et al.* (1991) reported the results of simple bunionectomy and medial capsulotomy in 37 patients. An overall dissatisfaction rate of 41% was reported so that they recommended this operation only for more elderly patients with prominent bunion but without significant degenerative arthritis or valgus deformity.

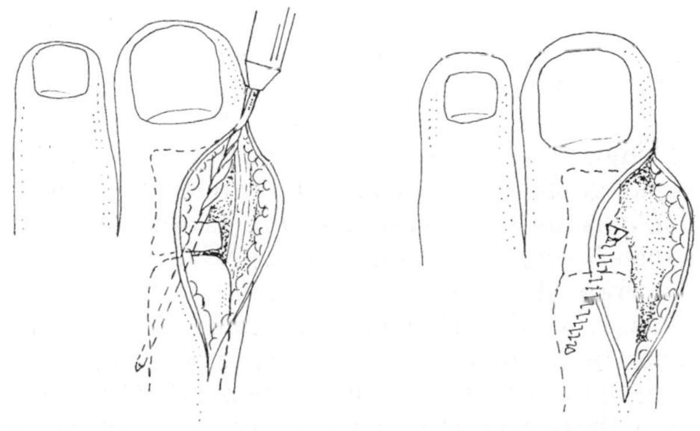

Figure 17.26 Arthrodesis of the metatarsophalangeal joint of the hallux by excision of the bone ends with a fine power saw and fixation with a countersunk screw. (Reproduced, with permission, from Piggott, H. (1979) Hallux valgus and hallux rigidus. In: *Operative Surgery*, 3rd edn, vol. 2, *Orthopaedics*. Edited by G. Bentley. Butterworths: London and Boston)

Hallux rigidus

Hallux rigidus is a condition of stiffness of the metatarsophalangeal joint of the great toe, especially characterized by absence of dorsiflexion, seen particularly in young men. In early cases, the power of plantar flexion is present, but in extreme examples all movement of the joint is abolished and a flexed position is gradually assumed – hallux flexus.

Rigidity of the joint may be associated with either inflammatory changes such as rheumatoid disease or a traumatic lesion, giving rise to contusion of the opposing cartilaginous surfaces of the joint and an intra-articular effusion. The limitation of movement in the first instance is the result of reflex muscle spasm to prevent movement at the painful joint, but secondary fibrosis in the capsule and ligaments renders the stiffness permanent.

In the static variety of hallux rigidus there is a concomitant flat foot. In the normal foot, the long axis of the first metatarsal is directed downwards and forwards from the summit of the arch, but when the arch is depressed, the base of the metatarsal sinks, its long axis becomes horizontally disposed and, in consequence, the head of the bone is rotated upwards and the dorsal portion of the articular surface ceases to be articular. The exposed area undergoes the usual changes of disuse – fibrillation and osteophytic outgrowth – so that any attempt to move the base of the phalanx over this degenerate surface is painful. Reflex spasm of the muscles ensues to prevent this, and the metatarsophalangeal joint is kept rigid.

In both varieties, the rigid joint in its later stages becomes the site of characteristic osteoarthritic changes.

CLINICAL FEATURES

In hallux rigidus, pain is experienced particularly on walking, and especially when attempts are made to dorsiflex the joint for the 'take-off' as in running; the pain is less severe on standing, unless there is severe flat foot. The joint is sometimes swollen from effusion, while a characteristic feature is the occurrence of a small marginal exostosis on the dorsal edge of the articular surface of the metatarsal head – i.e. at the degenerate area of the cartilage. The gait is shuffling and ungainly.

Attempts to move the joint cause great pain, but later, when the stiffness is permanent, ordinary passive attempts at motion are painless, and the condition may be masked by an abnormal degree of dorsiflexion acquired by the interphalangeal joint.

CONSERVATIVE TREATMENT

In the acute case rest by means of a below-knee walking plaster cast is indicated. In moderate degrees of the chronic type, relief may be obtained from restricting the movement of the joint:

1. by thickening the sole of the shoe,
2. by the insertion of a thin plate of tempered steel between the two layers of the sole, or
3. by the fitting of a metatarsal bar to the sole of the shoe.

In cases with a short history and in young people a cure may sometimes be effected by overcorrection of the deformity under anaesthesia and the application of a walking plaster cast to maintain the toe in dorsiflexion. The plaster cast should be retained for 4 weeks.

OPERATIVE TREATMENT

The large majority of cases eventually require operative intervention. The condition is treated in the same way as a hallux valgus, either by Keller's operation or by arthrodesis of the metatarsophalangeal joint (Figure 17.26). The latter operation has many advocates and seems to be very successful in the young active individual. It should not be carried out in the irritable phase and care should be taken not to dorsiflex the joint beyond 10° even in women who wear high heels.

Silastic implantation arthroplasty using Swanson's metacarpophalangeal joint component or a more specifically designed unicomponent (Figure 17.27) for the proximal third of the proximal phalanx is no longer used because of foreign-body reaction. Recently we have had good results from 20° extension osteotomy of the proximal phalanx which is fixed by a Kirschner wire for 4 weeks and protected in a below-knee walking cast for 6 weeks (Bentley, unpublished, 1995).

Hallux flexus

This is usually a static deformity which occurs initially during walking, but may become fixed and rigid. There is marked plantar flexion of the proximal phalanx of the big toe with some degree of dorsiflexion of the first metatarsal, resulting in dorsal bunion formation.

The normal longitudinal arch is lost and the talonavicular break is often present, with abnormality of the cuneiform which is tilted upwards

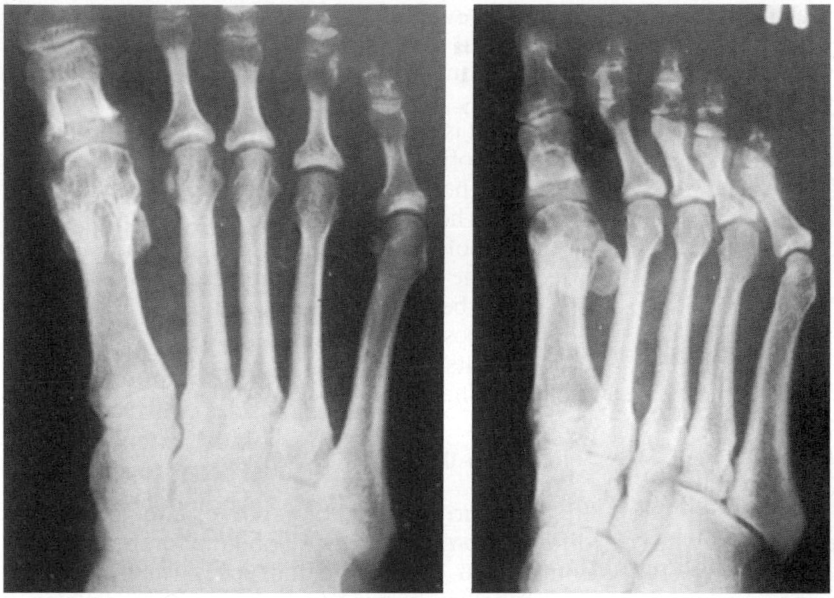

Figure 17.27 Radiographs showing a Silastic implant arthroplasty with metatarsal head changes of osteoarthritis.

(Figure 17.28). Soft tissue contractures occur, particularly of the capsule, the flexor hallucis longus and brevis tendons, so that there is loss of mobility of the first metatarsophalangeal joint. This condition occurs after:

1. poliomyelitis in which there is paralysis of all the foot muscle except for a normal gastrocnemius-soleus group posteriorly and normal flexors of the toes, as well as flexor hallucis brevis;
2. certain tendon transfer operations in which there is failure to achieve balance between the peroneus longus with its insertion into the lateral side of the medial cuneiform and first metatarsal base and the tibialis anterior muscle which is inserted into the medial surface of these two bones;
3. arthritic hallux rigidus with soft tissue contractures involving the plantar capsular structures; and
4. rocker-bottom deformity of a vertical talus or congenital flat foot. Walking is difficult because of pain over the bunion and also because of the inversion deformity of the forefoot.

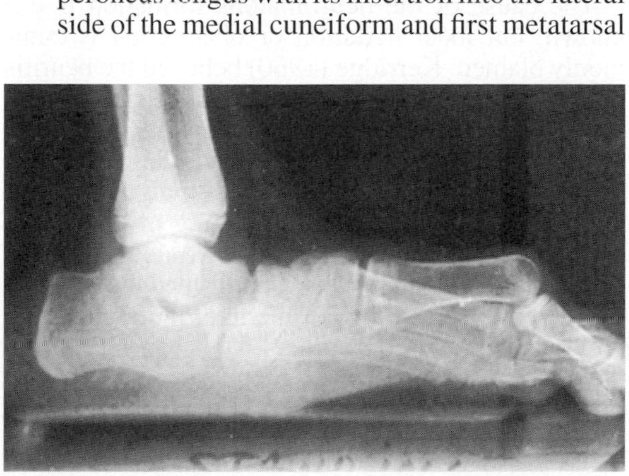

Figure 17.28 Radiograph of a standing foot to illustrate the typical deformities of a hallux flexus with plantar flexion of the proximal phalanx, dorsiflexion of the first metatarsal and some upward tilting of the medial cuneiform bone.

Duthie has used the Lapidus technique in which the insertion of tibialis anterior is transferred backwards, to be attached to the insertion of the tendon of tibialis posterior at the navicular tubercle. A wedge osteotomy is carried out at the naviculocuneiform-metatarsal joints. The flexor hallucis longus tendon is divided at its insertion and transferred proximally to be inserted through an oblique hole drilled in the shaft of the first metatarsal to become a plantar flexor of the first metatarsal. However, plantar capsulotomies may be necessary to relieve the flexion contracture of the big toe. The dorsal bunion and underlying exostoses are also excised.

Metatarsalgia

Pain beneath the metatarsal shafts or heads is commonly known as metatarsalgia, but it is important to discriminate between the different lesions which may give rise to it.

It has already been suggested that the anterior metatarsal arch, at least in the weight-bearing foot, does not exist, but under certain circumstances the intermediate metatarsal heads may be overloaded, and give rise to pain. Pain may also arise as a result of inflammatory affections (e.g. arthritis in the metatarsophalangeal joints) or as a sequel to using improper footwear.

Metatarsalgia, therefore, may be traumatic, inflammatory or static.

The static variety demands most consideration. It is frequently found in association with developmental anomalies, particularly metatarsus primus varus, hallux valgus and metatarsus hypermobilis, and commonly arises in those conditions where there is a rapid increase in body weight or a debilitating illness which renders the foot muscles atonic.

When the interosseous muscles contract they flex the metatarsophalangeal joints, extend the toe joints and draw the metatarsal heads together. Failure in these muscles allows splaying of the foot and curling up of the toes. The extra weight borne by the metatarsal heads throws a strain on the transverse ligaments of the metatarsal heads, and pain results, just as it does in longitudinal arch strain. This type of metatarsalgia is sometimes known as relaxation metatarsalgia.

When the metatarsal heads become crowded together as a result, for example, of the wearing of narrow shoes, the digital nerves passing forward to the toes between the heads of the metatarsals are liable to compression or irritation. This in time produces an interstitial neuritis which may be productive of agonizing pain and is known as compression metatarsalgia.

There are thus two main varieties of static metatarsalgia:

1. Relaxation metatarsalgia, due to overstretching of the plantar ligaments.
2. Compression metatarsalgia, or Morton's metatarsalgia, due to a neuroma of the digital nerves.

In addition, metatarsal pain is also a prominent feature of Köhler's disease and march foot.

CLINICAL FEATURES

Relaxation metatarsalgia

In the first of the static types – the ligamentous – the pain is situated beneath the metatarsal head and is of constant burning character. It may be relieved by lateral compression of the metatarsal heads, which relaxes the strain on the stretched ligaments. As it is so often a sign of overloading of the foot it may be associated with signs of foot strain related to the longitudinal arch. When the condition is acute there is not infrequently some oedema of the dorsum of the foot.

The foot is broader than normal – splay foot – and there are often obvious deficiencies between the metatarsal heads caused by atrophy of the interossei muscles. The clawing of the toes which arises is further proof of the occurrence of muscular atrophy affecting the lumbricals and interossei, the proximal phalanges becoming dorsiflexed as a result of the poorly opposed contraction of the extensor muscles of the digits. Often there are callouses under the metatarsal heads.

Morton's metatarsalgia

In the neuritic type, the foot usually presents a different form; it is narrow, and the forefoot appears compressed. The pain in this type is usually paroxysmal in nature, commencing beneath the metatarsal head and shooting forward toward the contiguous sides of two toes. It may affect any or all of the digital nerves, but is most common in relation to the third and fourth metatarsal spaces. The paroxysms may be so severe that the sufferer has to stop while walking and remove the shoe. In these cases the pain can sometimes be brought on, or accentuated, by side-to-side compression of the metatarsal heads. Pain is also produced by dorsoplantar compression of the intermetatarsal space at the level of the metatarsal heads. Paraesthesia with actual sensory loss may be present on the contiguous sides of the toes. In some cases, side-to-side compression of the foot causes a 'clink' the neuroma subluxes upwards.

The cause of the neuromatous formation is unknown, but local irritation or obstruction is commonly blamed. Kerridge (1960) believed the neuritis or neuroma formation to be secondary to an endarteritis obliterans of the accompanying metatarsal artery. Nissen, on the other hand, described the compression as resulting from a bulging of the intermetatarsal bursa with stretching of the dorsal communicating artery.

Shereff and Grande (1991) confirmed the electron microscopic appearance of the interdigital neuroma previously described by others. They considered that the neuroma formation is secondary to mechanical impingement.

TREATMENT

The object of the treatment must be to strengthen the muscles which support the forefoot, and to keep the forefoot in a corrected position while this is being accomplished. It is essential that the intrinsic muscles be strengthened by exercises and re-education. The patient should be taught to contract these muscles every time the forefoot touches the ground. Any coexisting defects in the mechanics of the foot should be treated, especially longitudinal arch strain and shortened tendo calcaneus.

The following measures may be employed.

Well designed shoe

In all types, the fitting of a shoe of rational design is essential for support. It should have a straight inner side, a broad thick sole, a low heel, and a metatarsal bar or crescent should be placed across the sole, well behind the heads of the metatarsals (Figure 17.29). Occasionally this simple method will effect a cure.

Pad and strapping

In more severe cases the support must be applied to the foot, and this may be most simply effected by means of a felt pad and adhesive strapping changed at intervals of 1 week.

An oval pad of felt with bevelled edges is placed under the metatarsal arch and secured immediately behind the metatarsal heads by adhesive strapping. In the splay foot, or ligamentous type, the strapping may be carried round the forefoot so that it produces slight compression only. The first felt pad is about 8 mm thick, but it is thickened each time the foot is restrapped until the symptoms disappear. Some experimentation may be required in order to determine the height of pad which produces complete relief of pain.

When the acute symptoms have been relieved, regular exercises – especially those designed to develop the lumbricals and interosseous muscles – should be practised.

Insole with pad

Few patients require some permanent means of supporting the anterior arch. A thin leather insole is cut to that it fits the shoe exactly. A resilient rubber pad of special shape is then securely fixed to the insole immediately behind the metatarsal heads.

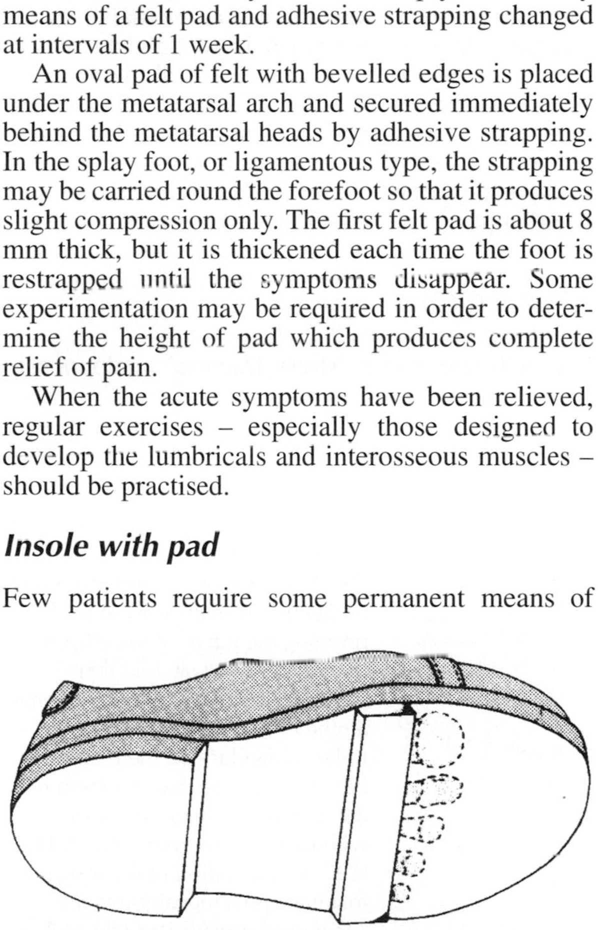

Figure 17.29 Type of external metatarsal bar sometimes used in metatarsalgia.

Operative treatment

Helal (1975) has developed an oblique osteotomy of the metatarsal necks for metatarsalgia associated with metatarsal head prolapse. The neck of the metatarsals is divided and the fragments are allowed to take up their own position. Early walking with protective dressing is allowed.

In cases resisting all other forms of treatment the question of resection of the head and neck of the affected metatarsal bone may arise.

When operation is considered essential, it is performed through a straight dorsal incision over the affected metatarsal, care being taken to see that no spicule of bone remains. At the termination of the operation the foot is put up in a light plaster cast moulded to the transverse arch but permitting plantar flexion at the metatarsophalangeal joints.

Walking is permitted after 3 weeks, with the type of pad and insole or strapping support described above, and shoes of sound design are fitted.

Plantar digital neurectomy

In those cases where the clinical diagnosis suggests a neuroma of the digital nerve, excision of the neuroma is the treatment of choice. A longitudinal incision is made on the dorsal aspect of the affected digital nerve. Dissection is carried down between the heads and necks of the metatarsal bone. The heads of the bones are retracted and the transverse ligament is incised, so producing adequate access to the floor of the incision. The neuroma usually then bulges into the wound (Figure 17.30) and is completely excised. The neuroma may also be approached by a plantar incision. It is well recognized that a Keller's arthroplasty for hallux valgus and metatarsalgia does not materially improve, and may aggravate the latter condition. The metatarsalgia usually results from metatarsophalangeal subluxation with clawing or hammering of the digits and callous formation, which require their own corrective operation.

Friscia *et al.* (1991), reported an 88% satisfaction rate in 259 patients undergoing excision of the neuroma through a longitudinal dorsal web space incision.

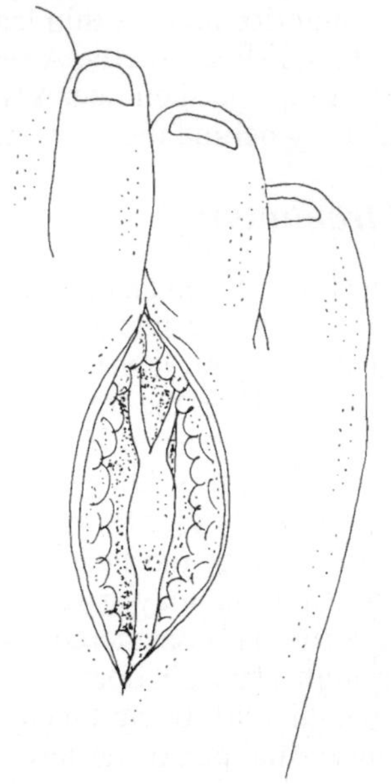

Figure 17.30 The exposure of a neuroma on the fourth metatarsal nerve.

Skin and soft tissue defects under the metatarsal heads

When there is a loss of the normal fibro-fatty supporting pad over the metatarsal heads associated with rheumatoid arthritis, with neurotrophic and vascular changes of diabetes mellitus or tabes dorsalis and with obesity, callosity formation occurs which, in the presence of infection, may ulcerate. Excision of the skin with the involved metatarsal head or heads will allow healing and comfort again. For marked clawing and contracture of the toes and painful callosity formation, the Fowler type of operation as originally described by Hoffman in 1912 is recommended; the toes will lie in a more extended position, with improvement in the dorsal callouses as well.

It is important to preserve the first metatarsal head and to achieve the excision arthroplasty by performing a Keller procedure on the hallux with excision of the heads of the lateral four metatarsals (Figure 17.31) through an elliptical plantar incision which can also remove the thickened callous skin and allow proximal advancement of the plantar skin under the metatarsal heads.

March foot or march fracture

This is a sequel to developmental anomalies of the forefoot. Deutschlander in 1925 reported a series of six cases of localized subperiosteal deposits of osteoid tissue on the shaft of one or other of the second, third or fourth metatarsal bones. He failed to recognize its relationship to the marching fracture of soldiers described about 70 years previously by Breithaupt.

AETIOLOGY

March fracture is a 'stress fracture' analogous to

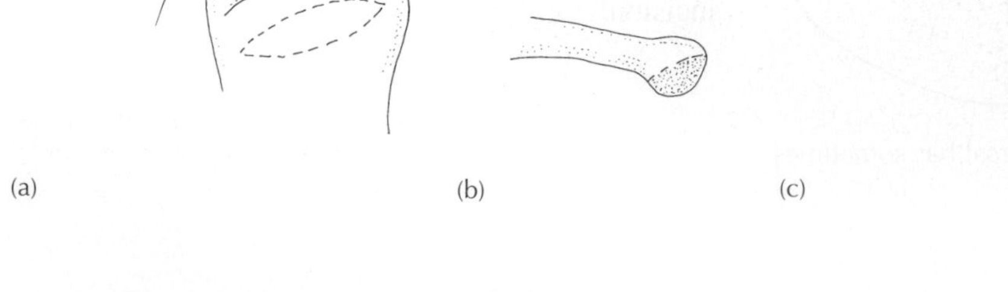

(a) (b) (c)

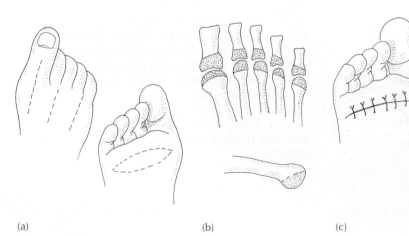

Figure 17.31 Forefoot arthroplasty (after Fowler): (a) incisions on the dorsal and plantar aspects of the foot with removal of ellipse of plantar skin; (b) line of excision of the metatarsal heads and proximal phalanges; (c) skin closure by bringing the edges of the ellipse together on the sole and then bringing the toes into more normal alignment. NB: Bentley finds a Keller procedure on the hallux a better procedure than excision of the metatarsal head. (Reproduced, with permission, from Piggott, H., (1979) Subluxation of the lesser metatarsophalangeal joints. In: *Operative Surgery*, 3rd edn, vol. 2, *Orthopaedics*. Edited by G. Bentley. Butterworths: London and Boston)

those which occur in the tibia end other weight-bearing bones.

It is now generally accepted that the primary factor is a developmental anomaly leading to a mechanical insufficiency of the first metatarsal (e.g. metatarsus primus varus or congenital short first metatarsal). In these conditions the longer second metatarsal must assume the role of the first, providing a fulcrum for the take-off in walking which may be quite efficient in ordinary circumstances. If, however, this foot of structurally weak type is suddenly subjected to the trauma of long marches, or to sudden change of employment demanding long hours of standing, the constant strain results in a 'stress' or 'fatigue' fracture.

CLINICAL FEATURES

The condition may begin insidiously, being obvious first as a puffy oedema of the forefoot when the foot is subjected to abnormal use – as in long marching. Sometimes the condition is associated with pain from the beginning. Radiography in the early stages shows no change in the bone, but in the course of time, if repeated examinations are made, there will become apparent a fusiform deposit of newly formed subperiosteal bone around the neck or adjacent part of the shaft of one or more of the metatarsals (Figure 17.32).

TREATMENT

Immobilization in a walking plaster is indicated to relieve acute pain and to promote healing. This is employed for 4–6 weeks and its use usually gives marked relief. A slip-in sole support of sponge rubber to the longitudinal arch helps to distribute the weight better. In cases seen at a late stage and with minimal symptoms the application of a metatarsal bar to the sole of the shoe in the position described previously, and institution of foot exercises, may constitute all the treatment required. When healed, the pain disappears, and the thickening of the metatarsal which results makes it capable of additional weight-bearing strain.

Köhler's disease of the metatarsal head (Freiberg's infraction)

In this condition there is great broadening of the metatarsal head – most frequently the second, less often the third, and rarely the others – and stiffness and pain at the metatarsophalangeal joint.

AETIOLOGY

Köhler compared the condition with other epiphyseal lesions such as Perthes' disease and Osgood–Schlatter's disease. Freiberg, on the other hand, interpreted the process in terms of trauma and supposed the primary condition to be a traumatic fracture of infraction of the articular surface, of the same nature as an osteochondritis dissecans.

There is no doubt, however, that the condition is associated with developmental anomalies which overload the middle group of the metatarsals. The dorsiflexed posture assumed by the toes as a result of the atrophy of the interossei and lumbricals has the

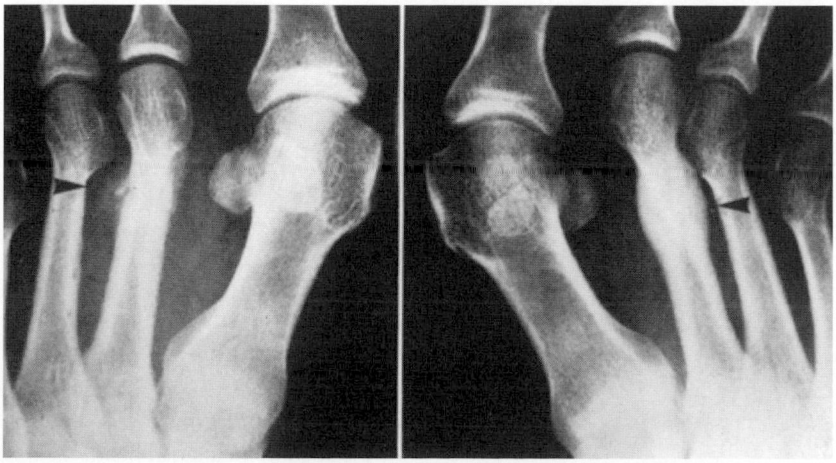

Figure 17.32 Radiographs showing bilateral march fracture – healed on the right.

effect of concentrating the effects of injury – single and repetitive – to the dorsal area of the articular surface.

There is often considerable thickening of the metatarsal shaft – a compensatory phenomenon designed to reinforce the second metatarsal for its undue proportion of functional stress.

PATHOLOGY

The sequence of changes occurring in this disease can be studied best radiologically. The earliest change is a slight subcapital osteoporosis, the porotic area being situated always in relation to the dorsal part of the articular surface, and the toe is usually clawed (i.e. the base of the phalanx is opposite the porotic area). The next stage is associated with increasing size of the rarified area, and indentation or collapse of the articular surface, which has now lost its normal trabecular support. Later the depressed area may become sequestrated and lie detached in the joint space as a loose body.

The histological changes are characteristic. The osseous trabeculae become progressively thinned out and replaced by granulation tissue.

CLINICAL FEATURES

The condition may arise at any age, and, as it is not confined to the period before the epiphysis is fused, Köhler's original conception is incorrect.

In the acute phase, while the articular surface is collapsing, there is extreme pain in the foot, movements are painful, and there may be considerable oedema of the forefoot, especially marked on the dorsum. Later, when the collapse is complete, the pain may subside, leaving a deformed joint which is also less capable of free mobility than before.

The x-ray changes (Figure 17.33) are characteristic:

1. There is broadening of the metatarsal head.
2. The head is irregular in contour and flattened.
3. The joint space is increased.
4. The shaft of the metatarsal is thick.
5. Detached portions of the articular surface may lie free in the joint.

TREATMENT

In the acute stages the application of a walking plaster cast will afford relief. In mild cases, the use of a metatarsal bar or pad may be all that is necessary.

If stiffness or pain persists when the cycle of pathology is complete, relief may be obtained by excision of the head, which, although it is more certain of relieving the immediate symptoms, may have the disadvantage of weakening the transverse arch.

Gauthier and Elbaz (1979) have described a wedge osteotomy of the head of the affected metatarsal which retains length and function for as long as 8 years. Of 53 patients who underwent the procedure, 52 obtained relief of pain and good mobility of the metatarsophalangeal joint (Figure 17.34).

Kinnard and Lirette (1991) described a dorsiflexion osteotomy of the head of the affected metatarsal with debridement of the joint to restore joint congruity in 15 patients, all of whom were able

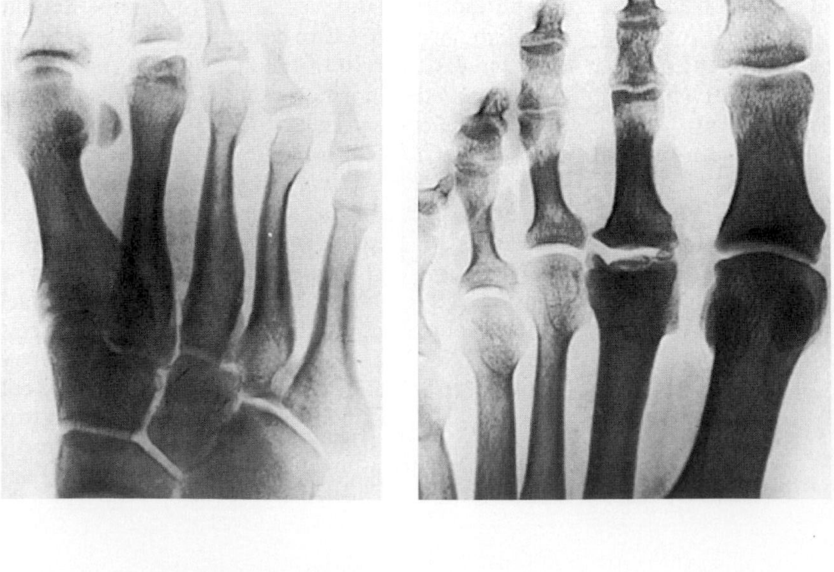

Figure 17.33 Köhler's disease of the second metatarsal head.

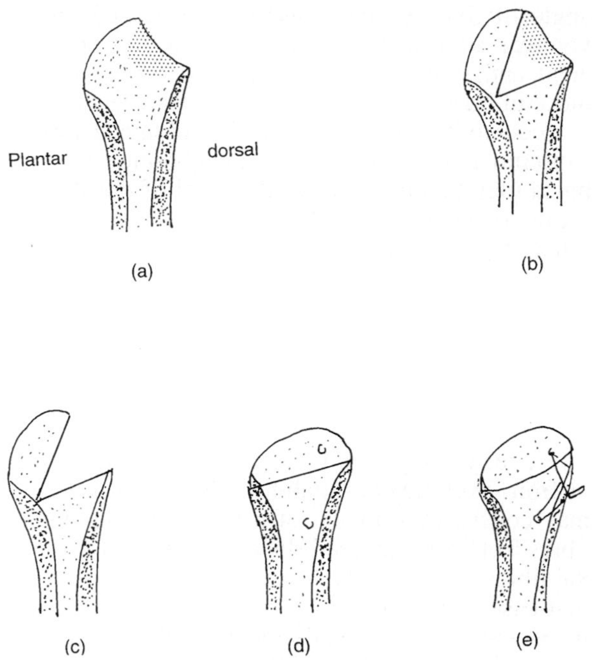

Figure 17.34 The osteotomy procedure for Freiberg's infraction: (a) shaded area represents region of sub-chondral osteonecrosis; (b) outline of bone wedge to be resected; (o) osteotomy of bone wedge; (d) closure of wedge osteotomy; (e) transfixation of osteotomy with wire. (Reproduced, with permission, from Gauthier, G. and Elbaz, R. (1979) *Clinical Orthopaedics and Related Research* **142**, 93–95)

to return to sporting activities whatever the stage of the disease at the time of operation.

Smith *et al.* (1991), described a diaphyseal shortening of the affected metatarsal with plate fixation. This encouraged bone remodelling in the metatarsal head but did not improve movement.

Painful conditions of the heel

Pain in the heel frequently occurs in people who stand or walk a great deal – hence the term 'policeman's heel' – but may also arise from other causes. Whatever the origin, the pain is usually aggravated by use, and may be entirely absent during rest. The painful area can always be found by digital pressure.

The causes of pain in the heel are:

1. traumatic disturbances,
2. developmental and pathological disturbances and
3. epiphysitis of the calcaneus, and are discussed in the main sections which follow.

Traumatic disturbances

Pain resulting from trauma may be at the back of the heel, around the insertion of the tendo calcaneus, or on the plantar aspect (Figure 17.35).

When situated in the region of the tendo calcaneus, the underlying conditions are tenosynovitis of the tendon sheath, the formation and irritation of enlarged bursae, and partial tears of the tendon. In all cases the pain is rendered worse by movement and may be completely relieved by rest. In tenosynovitis of the tendo calcaneus there is swelling from effusion, often accompanied by fine crepitus; when the condition is chronic there may be an actual deposit of fibrous tissue in and around the tendon, giving it an irregular form on palpation. When these fibrous deposits project backwards, the wearing of a boot is likely to entail discomfort. This condition was first described by Haglund and is often known as Haglund's disease, or 'winter' heel.

BURSAL ENLARGEMENTS

These may affect the bursa normally situated between the tendon and the calcaneus, or a subcutaneous adventitious bursa which occasionally develops over the most prominent part of the posterior surface of the bone. Attention has been drawn to the fact that this surface is often not flat but irregular, being more

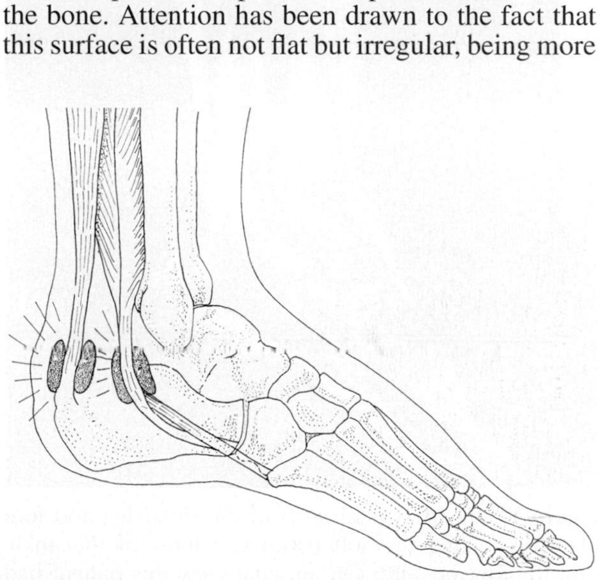

Figure 17.35 The areas of tenosynovitis and bursitis which can occur around the tendocalcaneus and peroneal tendons.

prominent on its lateral side at the lowest margin of the insertion of the tendon. This means that normally the part of the calcaneus projecting farthest back is not in the midline but lateral to that. Haglund found that in 39% of cases of pain in the heel, this prominence is marked and palpable as a tender hard lump, though as a general rule an x-ray examination does not reveal it. It is in this situation that the adventitious bursa forms, as a result of the rubbing of the shoe against the back of the heel, producing the common 'knobbly heels' seen in children and adolescents.

The deep bursa at the insertion of the tendon calcaneus is liable to inflammations from friction produced by ill-fitting footwear. As a result, there is localized tenderness at the site of the bursa, and occasionally a small area of fluctuation can be detected by lateral palpation anterior to the tendo calcaneus.

When the superficial adventitious bursa is enlarged, the swelling is situated lower down, and is usually larger, fluctuation is easily elicited, and the skin overlying the swelling is often red and oedematous.

Some surgeons deprecate operation in cases of prominent heel bone, believing that the symptoms produced by it may be obviated by beating out the lateral half of the counter of the shoe at the back of the heel to accommodate the enlargement. However, in most cases this conservative treatment fails and it is necessary to remove the prominent posterosuperior

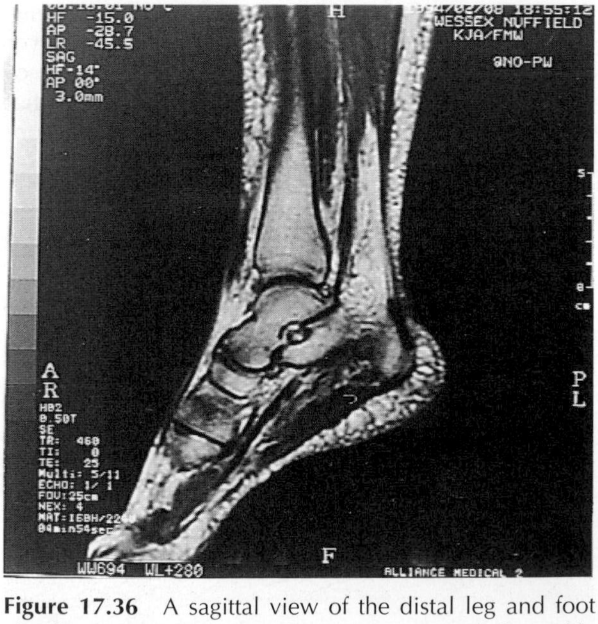

Figure 17.36 A sagittal view of the distal leg and foot clearly showing the soft tissue structures of the ankle and the foot on MRI. On an axial view this patient had tibialis posterior tendonitis. (Kindly supplied by Dr Richard Blaquiere, Consultant Radiologist at Southampton University Hospitals)

angle of the calcaneus and any exostoses. In the younger adolescent patient this may not be sufficient, and, in a few, excision of a large wedge-shaped piece of bone, the base uppermost, is necessary.

In acute bursitis, relief may be obtained by rest from movement. In subacute and chronic cases, the bursa may be raised above the level of the shoe by the use of an internal heel raise inside. In cases where relief of friction does not lead to resolution, the bursa and also the prominent bone should be excised.

PARTIAL TEARS OF THE ACHILLES TENDON

These result from forcible contraction of the tendon or from overstretching, and the lesion so produced may consist of avulsion of a few of the tendinous fibres from the bone, or of actual rupture of some of the fibres immediately above their insertion. In the first case, the disturbance of the periosteum results in periostitis, with relatively little or no swelling, but tenderness at the insertion of the tendon and exquisitely painful movements. Partial rupture of the tendon fibres may be associated, in the acute phase, with slight swelling from effusion of blood, and later with the formation of irregular masses of fibrous tissue in the tendon. MR scanning or ultrasonography is now very helpful in delineating the severity of the tear (Figure 17.36).

TREATMENT

In all cases, rest is essential. Relief is quickest if the limb is placed in a below-knee cast in full equinus for 3 weeks, followed by 2 weeks in the neutral position. If there is a history of a definite traumatic episode, operative inspection of any suspected tear or rupture is essential so that early suture can be carried out.

PLANTAR FASCIITIS

This condition causes pain and local tenderness just anterior to the calcaneal attachment of the plantar fascia. Treatment is usually conservative including steroid injection therapy or a heel wedge, or, alternatively and more recently, the provision of a night ankle/foot orthosis (Wagner and Sharkey, 1991). Rarely is subperiosteal elevation of the long plantar ligament by open operation necessary.

Pain in the plantar aspect of the heel may also be due to the formation of calcanean spurs, or to traumatic or inflammatory fibrositis at the insertion of the plantar fascia without spur formation.

Pain may arise at the insertion of the plantar fascia in association with metabolic disturbances such as gout, or rheumatoid arthritis or inflammatory conditions (i.e. gonorrhoea, Reiter's syndrome and ankylosing spondylitis).

CALCANEAN SPURS

The spike of bone at the anterior edge of the calcaneum on the medial aspect is otherwise called a calcaneal spur. It may be the sequel to repeated detachments of the plantar fascia, and does not give rise to symptoms *per se*, and that pain, when present, is due to the causative condition and not to the spur.

The characteristic features are pain in the ball of the heel (especially marked on long standing or walking), tenderness on the plantar aspect of the heel (most marked at the attachment of the plantar fascia to the medial tubercule of the calcaneus) and, occasionally, slight swelling at the attachment of the fascia.

x-Ray examination may or may not reveal the presence of a spur.

Conservative treatment

Any obvious cause, such as gonococcal infection, must be dealt with. If the pain is acute, the patient should be rested. After the pain and tenderness have disappeared, proper shoes should be ordered and felt or sponge-rubber pads inserted to relieve weight-bearing on painful areas. A rubber heel should be substituted for the heel of the shoe, with an area cut out below the tender area. Rose (1962) regarded the strain as being a longitudinal one along the plantar fascia and therefore recommended a complete insole with a convex wedge of sorbo rubber to support the entire length of the fascia.

In some cases, considerable relief may be afforded by the use of radiant heat or diathermy or by the injection of solutions of hydrocortisone acetate and lignocaine into the tender area (from the side and not through the sole).

Operative treatment

Operative treatment may be undertaken in resistant cases, and the spur, when present, removed; some observers think this unwise since they hold that the spur is never the cause of the symptoms *per se*.

The operation is performed through a transverse incision along the medial border of the foot, the spur being removed by means of an osteotome.

TRAUMATIC SUBTALOID ARTHRITIS

Fractures of the os calcis are usually caused by a fall on the feet from a height; as they may not produce any gross deformity at the time, they are liable to be overlooked unless the most careful x-ray, CT or MRI scanning is carried out (Figures 17.37, 17.38, 17.39). These undetected fractures may ultimately give rise to very troublesome pain and weakness of the foot which may constitute a grave and lasting disability for someone doing heavy manual work. The pain and weakness are due to a chronic subtaloid arthritis for which the only treatment likely to be of any benefit is fusion of the joint.

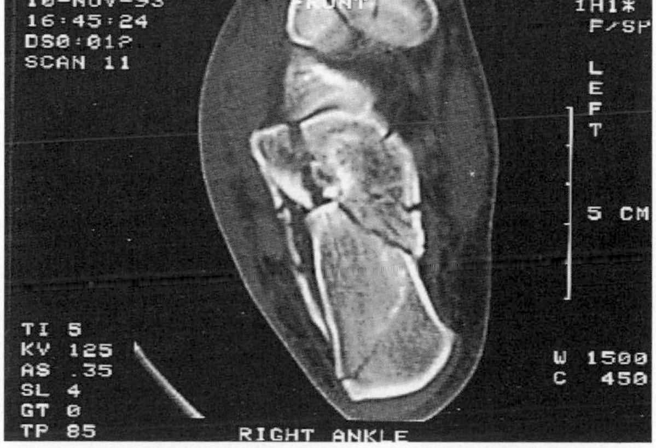

Figure 17.37 A fracture of the os calcis involving the calcaneocuboid joint on MR scan. (Kindly supplied by Dr Richard Blaquiere, Consultant Radiologist at Southampton University Hospitals)

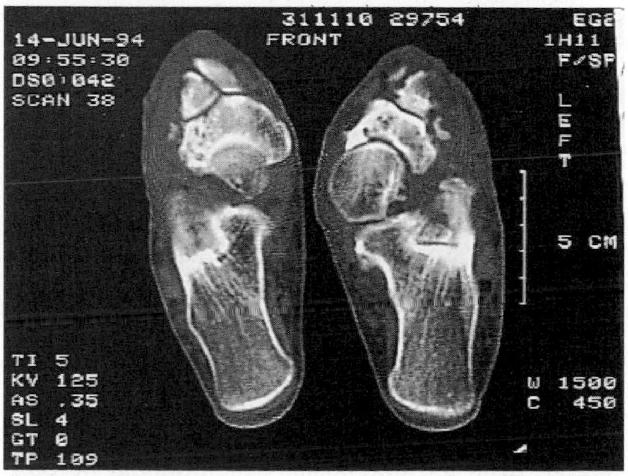

Figure 17.38 Talocalcaneal osteoarthritis affecting both feet on MR scan, although the loss of joint space is more severe on the right. (Kindly supplied by Dr Richard Blaquiere, Consultant Radiologist at Southampton University Hospitals)

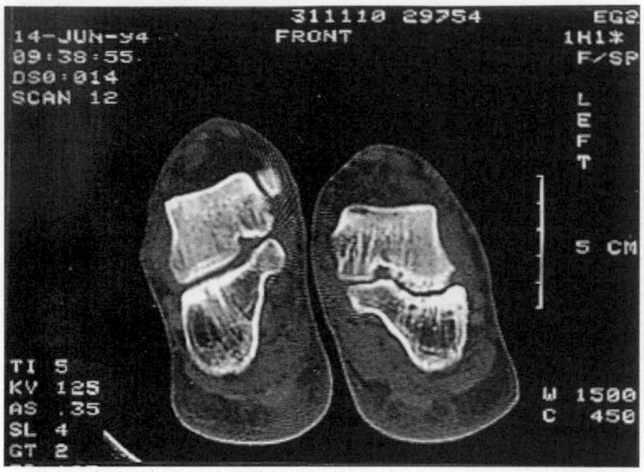

Figure 17.39 Coronal section showing the subtalar joint with osteoarthritis in the left side on MR scanning. (Kindly supplied by Dr Richard Blaquiere, Consultant Radiologist at Southampton University Hospitals)

Apart from trauma, pain in the heel may have its origin in organic disease of the bone or epiphysis, and the infection may be tuberculous, syphilitic, gonococcal or pyogenic or may follow a rheumatoid flare. Paget's disease must also be excluded.

Epiphysitis of the calcaneus

This condition is described in Chapter 6. It usually occurs in boys between the ages of 9 and 13, and in the differential diagnosis various conditions have to be borne in mind:

1. *Calcanean bursitis*. In this condition the inflammation is more superficial and localized. The x-ray is negative.
2. *Tenosynovitis of the tendo calcaneus*. This is characterized by pain referred to the tendon, and by palpable silky crepitus on movement. x-Ray examination is again negative.
3. *Bursitis*. Bursitis between the calcaneal tendon and the skin is a superficial inflammation, usually the result of pressure from the shoe, and is readily recognized.
4. *Calcaneal spurs*. These are rare in early adolescence and are usually found on the inferomedial aspect of the calcaneus. The area of sensitivity suggests the diagnosis, which should be confirmed by radiography.

Fibromatosis of the plantar fascia

Fibromatosis of the plantar fascia of the foot results in nodules which occasionally are large enough to become painful with pressure and weight-bearing. Their histopathology suggests a sarcomatous lesion with large active fibroblastic cells. The condition is similar to (and may coexist with) Duputren's contracture of the hand but is much rarer and occurs in much higher incidence in those having had anti-epileptiform drug regimens (e.g. phenytoin) over long periods. The nodules can be removed individually through an incision on the sole of the foot without untoward results. What should be avoided is placing the skin incision high on the medial side of the foot and undermining to expose the plantar fascia. Here one may lose the vascularity of the skin flaps, and weight-bearing on the side of the shoe becomes painful. In the arch area along the sole of the foot incisions are made directly over the fibrous nodule, avoiding dissecting underneath the flap where the area is extensive. There is a high recurrence rate and some surgeons advocate early radical excision and skin grafting.

Pes cavus – the claw foot

The term claw-foot, or pes cavus, is applied to a deformity in which clawing of the toes is combined with a raising of the long arch of the foot, and which

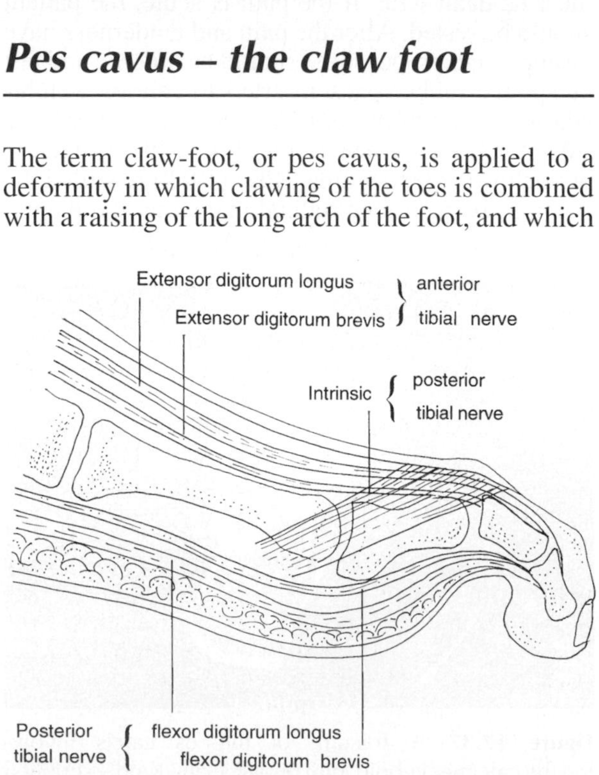

Figure 17.40 The tendons and intrinsic musculature involved in clawing of the toes and their nerve supply.

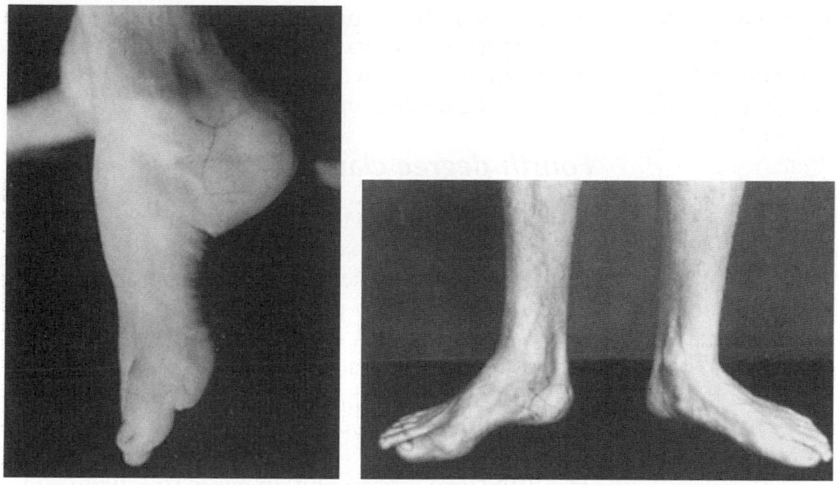

(a) (b)

Figure 17.41 (a) Cavus foot showing equinus of the forefoot in relation to the normal hindfoot. (b) Standing photograph showing claw toes on the right corrected by transplant of flexors into the extensors. Some calcaneous deformity of the os calcis remains.

may arise either as a congenital or as an acquired deformity (Figures 17.40 and 17.41).

AETIOLOGY

1. Congenital (e.g. Spina bifida or a myelodysplasia of the cord).
2. Idiopathic – the largest group.
3. Acquired.

Jones and Lovett divided the acquired type into two groups, as follows:

1. *Claw-foot in poliomyelitis*. Claw-foot frequently occurs after poliomyelitis, more especially where the paresis is almost negligible, and it is, in fact, frequently a characteristic deformity of the so-called 'sound leg'. Duchenne suggested that it was due to paralysis of the interossei and the lumbricals, thus bringing it into line with the *main-en-griffe* of ulnar paralysis.
2. *Claw-foot following inflammatory infections*. The deformity may be sequel to inflammatory contracture of the soft tissues of the sole of the foot.

There have been many suggested theories of the mechanism, e.g. Duchenne originally suggested that it was due to a weakness of the short muscles of the big toe as well as the interossei. Others have suggested a weakness of the extensor digitorum longus with weakness of the tibialis anterior, or an overaction of the intrinsic mechanism resulting from a shortened tendo calcaneus, or a loss of synergistic muscle control without specific weaknesses due to the effect of poliomyelitis on the spinal cord, and so on.

Brewerton *et al.* (1962), in a review of 629 cases of claw-foot, found that 25% of them had some degree of neurological involvement. In 79 cases, which had been investigated by electromyographic studies and biopsy, two-thirds of these had neurological involvement with 33% being due to progressive muscular dystrophy and 44% having a spina bifida.

Careful examination of the central nervous system must be made for wasting of musculature, any ataxia and any muscle power weakness, particularly of the long muscles of the foot such as the gastrocnemius or soleus group. The ability to walk on one's heels should be tested, as should the reflexes and sensation. Radiographs of the lumbar spine should be taken for any spina bifida deformity. Bladder symptoms (e.g. of enuresis), when present, may suggest a central nervous system lesion.

DEVELOPMENT OF THE DEFORMITY

The intrinsic musculature normally flexes the metatarsophalangeal joints and extends the interphalangeal ones. When the long flexor contracts on this straight digit it slings up the head of the metatarsals and prevents a drop of the forefoot on the hindfoot. In the absence of the lumbricals, the long flexor pulls the toes into flexion and no longer supports the metatarsal heads. The forefoot drops and the lax structures in the sole contract or 'take up the slack', with the formation of the typical claw-foot. The hindfoot in this deformity is normal – the condition being a dropping of the forefoot on the hindfoot followed by a contracture of the plantar fascia and a clawing of the toes (Figure 17.41).

There is, in addition to the pes cavus, some adduction of the forefoot from the beginning. An element of adduction and inversion appears in the late stage of the process, as well as some secondary contracture of the tendo calcaneus.

CLINICAL FEATURES

Great stress was formerly laid on the conventional division of the clinical features of claw-foot into a series of stages, but it is important to recall that the deformity is a progressive one. There is seldom pain in childhood but complaint may be made of the rapidity with which shoes are worn out.

First-degree claw-foot

At this stage the complaint is that the child is clumsy, and that, when running about, frequently falls without apparent cause, or catches his toes against low objects such as the edge of the carpet. Formerly attributed to contracture of the tendo calcaneus, the only physical sign at this stage is a slight extensor weakness which may be demonstrated by the inability to pull up the toes, or by slight difference in the circumference of the two calves. The tendo calcaneus is not shortened, and if the forefoot is covered, the posterior part of the foot looks normal.

Second-degree claw-foot

In addition to the slight flexion of the forefoot, there is dorsiflexion of the great toe at the metatarsophalangeal joint and flexion at the interphalangeal joint. The plantar fascia is felt to be tense and contracted, and there is visible deformity. A characteristic of the deformity at this stage is that clawing can be made to disappear by upward pressure on the ball of the great toe, showing that it is caused by a downward dropping of the metatarsal head. While a child may not complain of any pain, the older patient is apt to suffer some discomfort under the metatarsal heads after prolonged walking.

Third-degree claw-foot

The arch of the foot is markedly raised, and all the toes are clawed, while the tendo calcaneus may begin to appear contracted. The plantar structures are further shortened and all the toes are now dorsiflexed at the metatarsophalageal joints and flexed at the interphalangeal joints. These deformities are becoming rigid, and it is no longer possible to correct the deformity by finger pressure under the first metatarsal head. The chief complaint may be of painful corns which form on the dorsum of the flexed interphalangeal joints or on the points of the toes, but, in addition, such a foot is one which tires easily after much standing or walking (Figure 17.42).

Fourth-degree claw-foot

In addition to the cavus and the hammer toes, there is adduction at the tarsometatarsal joints, resulting in a varus deformity. The foot is now rigid and painful, tender callosities are present on the outer side and under the metatarsal heads, and walking becomes increasingly painful and difficult.

Fifth-degree claw-foot

The fifth stage is seen only in cases following some paralytic condition – usually poliomyelitis. The toes are blue and cold, and the whole foot is contracted into a rigid equinovarus, with a high arch. The patient is very disabled and exquisitely tender callosities are present (Figure 17.43).

TREATMENT

First-degree claw-foot

Progress may be arrested by re-educating the small muscle function by intrinsic exercises. If not, Girdlestone's flexor-to-extensor transfer is performed (see p. 1230).

Second-degree claw-foot

A shoe fitted with a metatarsal bar may give temporary relief, but adequate treatment of this stage is by operation. The plantar fascia is divided subcutaneously and the tendon of the extensor hallucis divided at its insertion and passed through the neck

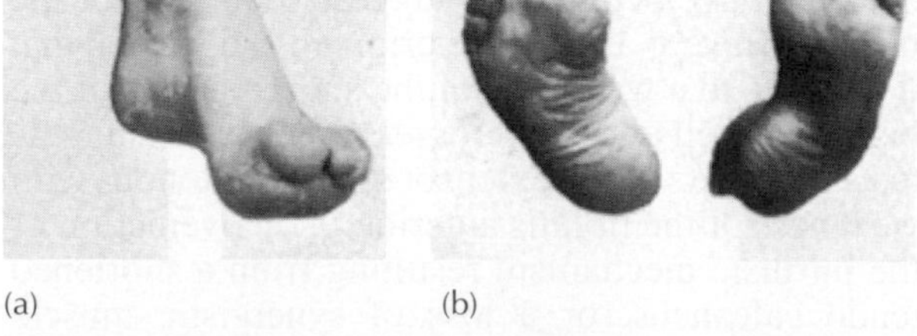

(a) (b)

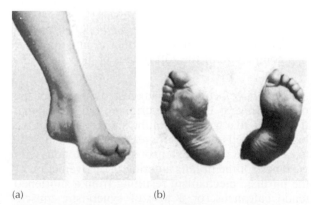

Figure 17.42 (a) Claw-foot of third degree with marked deformity of toes. (b) The plantar aspects of a claw-foot.

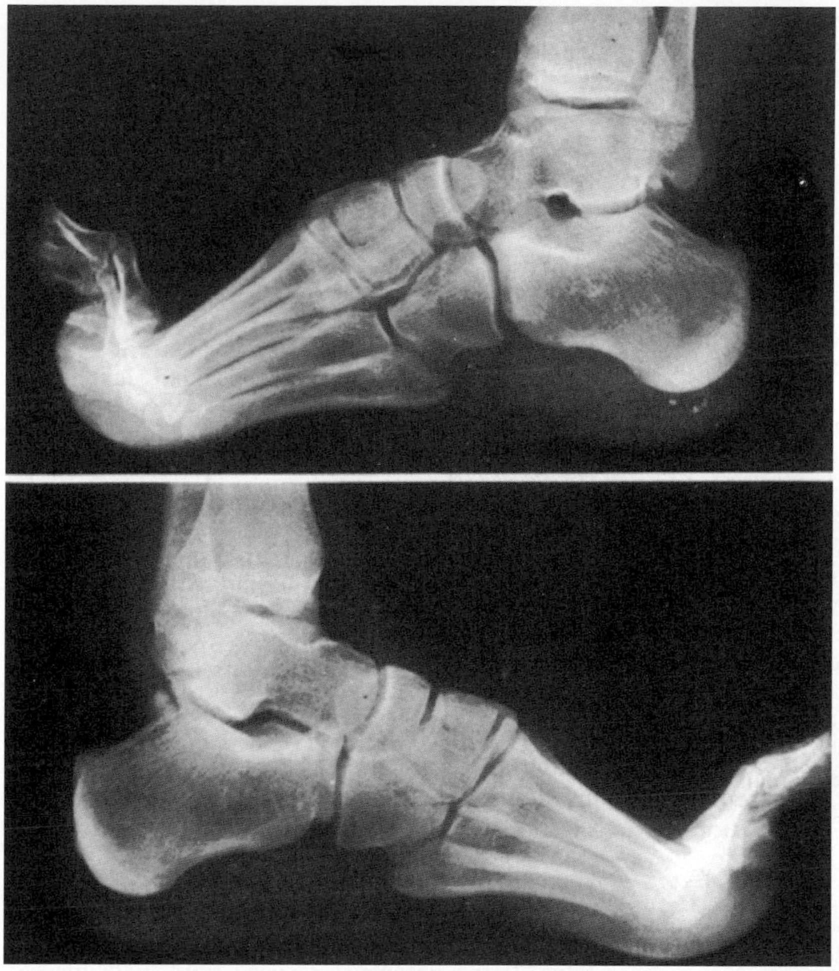

Figure 17.43 Radiographs of a young man, aged 18 years, showing fifth degree of claw-foot deformity involving particularly the longitudinal arch of the foot and the marked subluxation of the toes at the metatarsophalangeal joints.

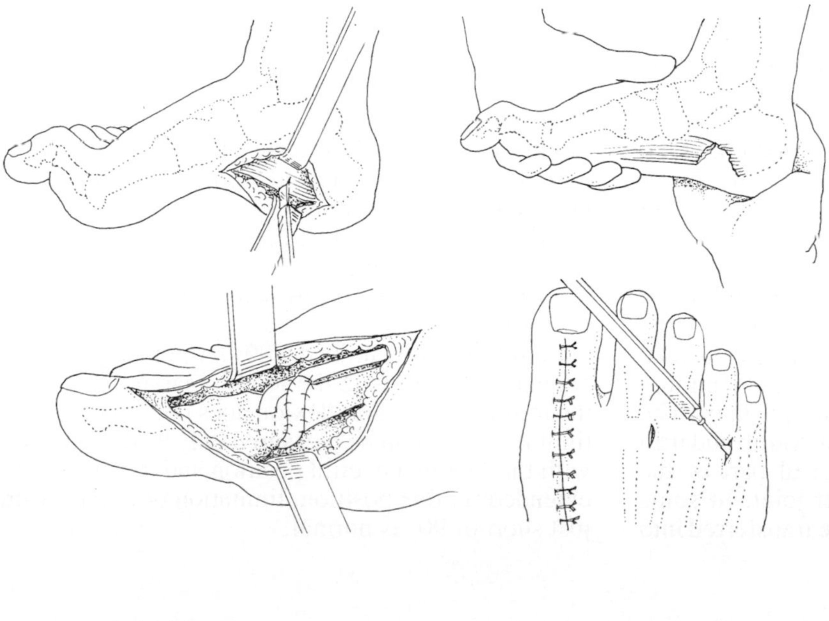

Figure 17.44 The treatment of a moderate degree of claw-foot by plantar fascia tenotomy and tendon transfer of extensor hallucis longus.

of the first metatarsal. Arthrodesis of the interphalangeal joint in a straight plane is then carried out to improve the function of take-off in walking. A below-knee plaster-of-Paris cast is then applied to the foot to maintain the corrected position for a period of 6 weeks. Afterwards a metatarsal bar may be fixed to the shoe temporarily (Figure 17.44).

Third-degree claw-foot

Treatment of the third-degree claw-foot is on the same lines as in second degree, but it is, of necessity, more thorough, more extensive and more drastic.

All the structures on the sole of the foot which arise from, or are attached to, the undersurface of the calcaneus are separated from that bone through an incision on the medial side of the heel. The structures are erased right forward to the calcaneocuboid joint on the lateral side, and to the talonavicular on the medial side where they take up a new attachment; the procedure is thus a 'muscle-slide' operation. The extensor tendons of the toes, which may lead to a relapse, may now be divided.

A horizontal osteotomy of the calcaneus with a slide forward of the lower half is a useful method used by the authors. It ensures a permanent forward displacement of the short structures which so often reattach themselves.

Lambrinudi's operation

Lambrinudi (1927) found that correction of the clawing of the toes causes not only considerable improvement of the deformity, and therefore reduction of symptoms from corns and callosities, but also a marked improvement of the general function of the foot. The principle underlying the operation is that, by arthrodesis of the interphalangeal joints, the long flexor muscles take up the function of the lumbricals and flex the toes at the meiatarsophalangeal joints and themselves sling up the metatarsal heads, tending to straighten out the foot.

Through lateral incisions along the dorsum of the toes or simple transverse incisions over the dorsal aspect of each joint the interphalangeal joints are exposed and their opposing surfaces excised. Arthrodesis may be achieved either by apposition of the apposed cut surfaces and a Kirschner wire through the joints or, in some cases, by carrying out the 'spike' operation which involves fashioning a spike from the head of the proximal phalanx and jamming it into a prepared slot in the middle phalanx. The extensor tendons of the second, third, fourth and fifth toes are tenotomized, as is the dorsal part of the capsule of the metatarsophalangeal joint. In some cases the extensor tendons should be transferred into their own metatarsal necks, though this is usually unnecessary since the flexor tendons act as slings to the metatarsal heads and hold them up. Interference with the fifth toe may be unnecessary. The procedure is tedious and time-consuming, but the results of this operation are good.

Girdlestone tendon transfer operation

(Taylor, 1951)

Through an incision on each toe, extending distally from the level of the metatarsophalangeal joint, the extensor expansion is outlined. A small blunt hook is passed underneath to pick up the long and short toe flexors, which are then brought round the lateral aspect of the proximal phalanx and sutured to the extensor expansion. A dorsal capsulotomy of the metatarsophalangeal joint may be necessary. A cast is applied, and is removed with the sutures after 6 weeks. This operation is particularly indicated in a child or young adult before there are fixed joint deformities and marked soft tissue contractures (Figure 17.45).

Fourth and fifth degrees of claw-foot

In the fourth stage, the high crooked arch can usually be corrected only by dividing the bones across at the level of the midtarsal joint by wedge tarsectomy (Figure 17.46). A wedge of bone has to be removed with its base at the dorsum of the foot, and including a considerable portion of the head and neck of the talus. If the deformity is very rigid, with marked bony deformation, a reconstruction and shortening of the foot such as the triple fusion of Naughton Dunn is required (Figure 17.47).

Shortening of tendo Achillis

Slight degrees of contracture of tendo Achillis are normal in many people, and women who habitually wear high heels may show this. In most cases it is not a source of discomfort. It may also be due to reflex spasm similar to that which occurs with subtalar disorders but mostly arises in association with other foot pathologies.

Tanz (1960) examined 200 normal subjects and emphasized that, with the foot in marked inversion, the movement of dorsiflexion does not test heel cord tightness. This can be measured only by dorsiflexion with the foot in a neutral position and the knee fully extended. In this position, limitation of dorsiflexion just short of 90° is normal.

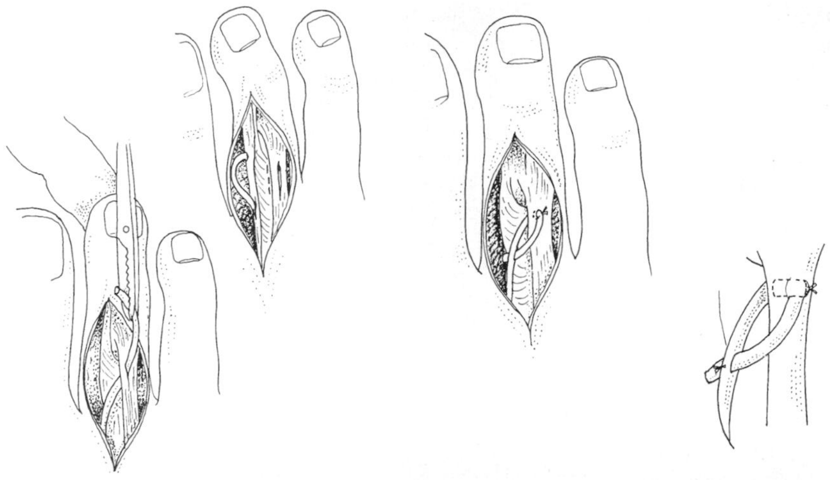

(a) (b)

Figure 17.45 (a) The first stage of the Girdlestone flexor-to-extensor transfer procedure – mobilization of the flexor tendon via a tibial incision and threading through the extensor. (b) The flexor is sutured to itself and the extensor tendon. (Reproduced, with permission, from Rose, K.G. (1979). Soft tissue and bony operations for pes cavus and planus. In: *Operative Surgery*, 3rd edn, vol. 2, *Orthopaedics*. Edited by G. Bentley. Butterworths: London and Boston)

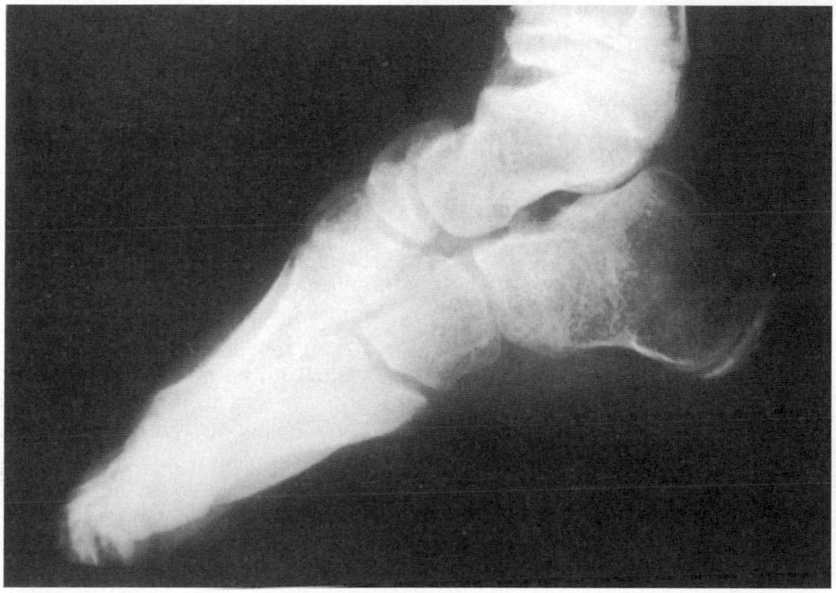

(a)

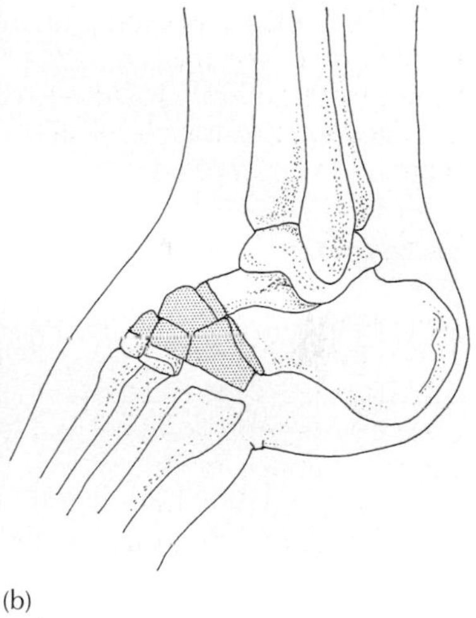

(b)

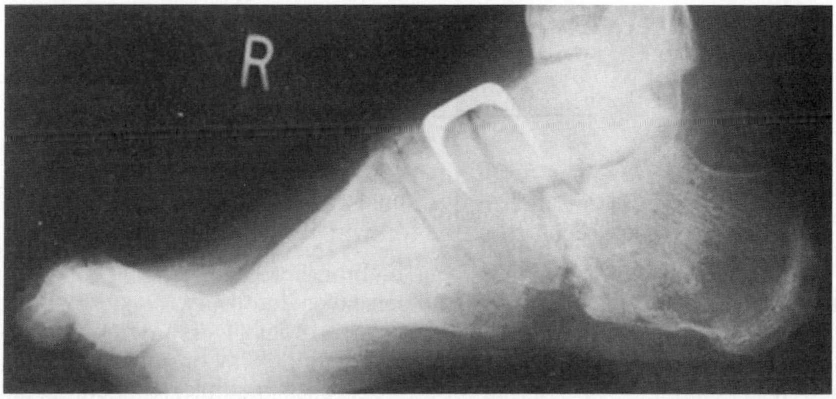

(c)

Figure 17.46 (a) Preoperative radiograph of the foot of a 16-year-old with severe idiopathic pes cavus. (b) Diagram of the bony resection required to correct such a deformity. (c) Postoperative radiograph showing the corrected foot (b reproduced, with permission, from Somerville, E.W. (1979) Wedge tarsectomy. In: *Operative Surgery*, 3rd edn, vol. 2, *Orthopaedics*. Edited by G. Bentley. Butterworths: London and Boston)

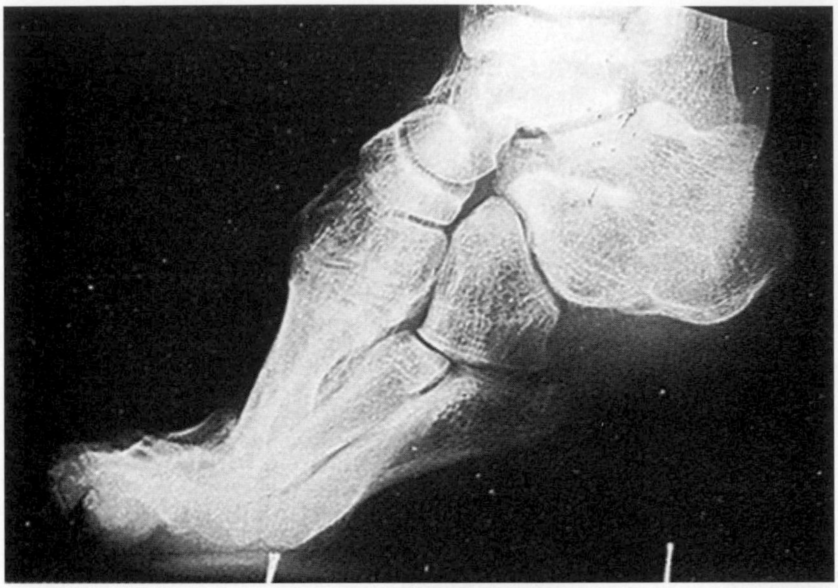

(a)

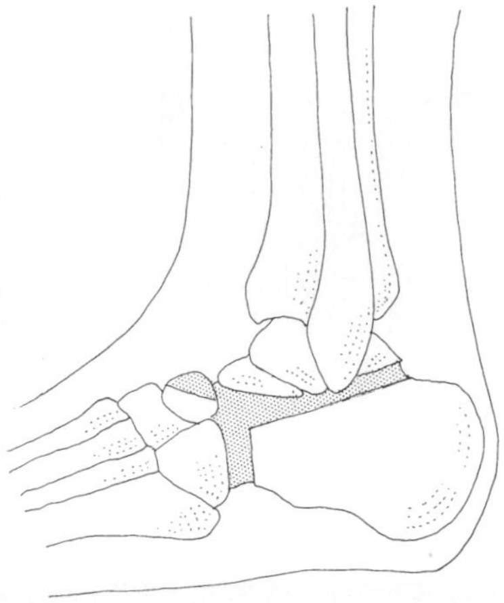

(b)

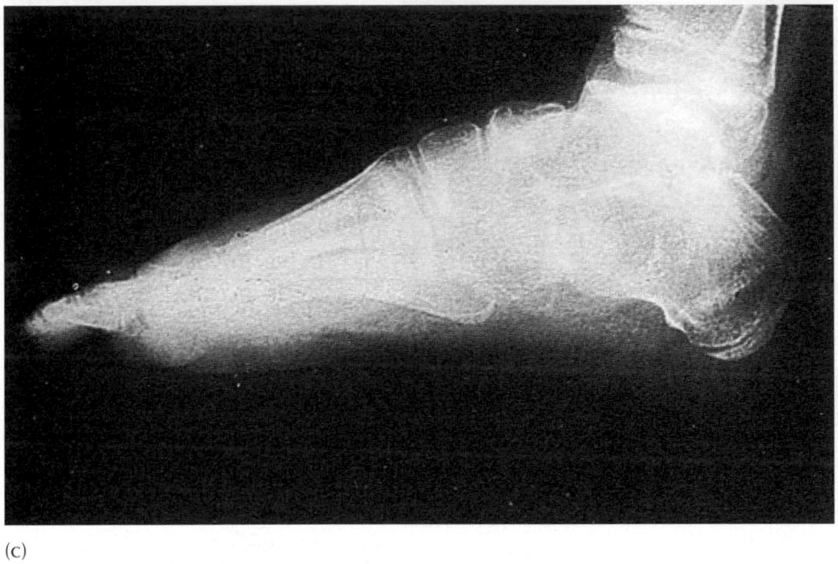

(c)

Figure 17.47 (a) Lateral radiograph of the foot showing an incompletely corrected pes cavus. (b) Diagram of the triple resection, talonavicular, talocalcaneal and calcaneocuboid joints involved in triple arthrodesis. (c) Radiograph 3 months postoperatively showing the correction of the pes cavus and commencing bony union. (b reproduced, with permission, from Somerville, E.W. (1979) Arthrodesis of the foot. In: *Operative Surgery*, 3rd edn, vol. 2, *Orthopaedics*. Edited by G. Bentley. Butterworths: London and Boston)

TREATMENT

Treatment of short tendo Achillis is part of the treatment of the disorder producing it. In the rare cases of idiopathic tightness, very satisfactory results are achieved by lengthening the tendon by the White procedure, diving the fibres at the upper end of the tendon medially and at the lower end of the tendon anteriorly and correcting the ankle just to 90° (Figure 17.48). Following the operation the foot is protected in a below-knee walking cast for a period of 4 weeks and then full activity is recommenced.

Varus deformity of the heel

This deformity is usually accompanied by an equinus deformity and is rarely present alone. It may result from the following:

1. an uncorrected or relapsed club foot,
2. as part of a pes cavus deformity,
3. as a result of neurological disorders such as spina bifida or cerebral palsy or poliomyelitis,
4. as part of arthrogryposis multiplex congenital, or
5. spastic hemiplegia.

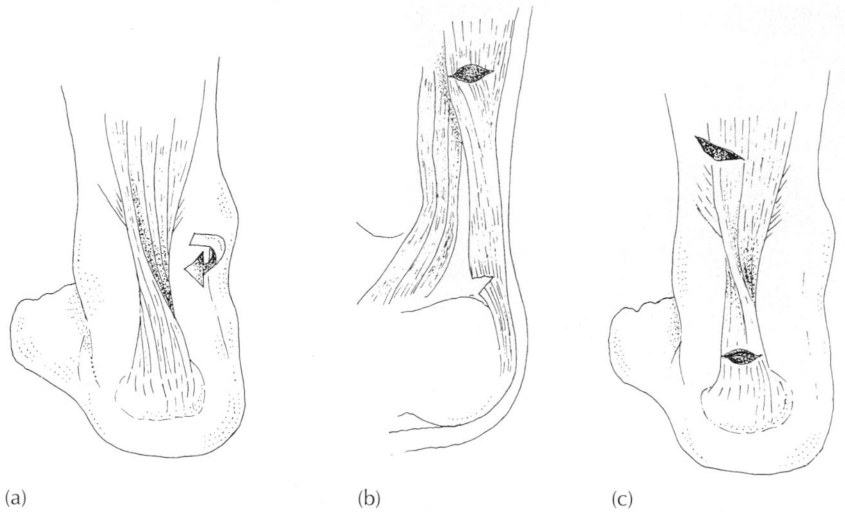

Figure 17.48 Tendo Achillis lengthening by the White technique: (a) lateral rotation of the fibres of the tendo Achillis from proximal to distal; (b) incision in the tendo Achillis above medially and anterior distally which divides opposite halves of the tendon. (Reproduced, with permission, from Helal, B. and Chen, S.C. (1979) Repair of the tendo Achillis. In *Operative Surgery*. 3rd edn, vol. 2, *Orthopaedics*. Edited by G. Bentley. Butterworths: London and Boston)

Management of the primary condition has been dealt with in Chapter 3. The later deformity presents as an inverted and small heel, a tight tendo calcaneus, forefoot abduction, and inversion-rotation at the midtarsal joint (Figure 17.49). There may also be some cavus deformity as well as clawing of the toes, and lateral torsion of the tibia due to muscle imbalance with the abnormal growth processes and weight-bearing.

Such a deformity resulting from poliomyelitis is usually fairly easy to correct. The gastrocnemius, soleus and tibialis posterior are often normal but the peroneals and tibialis anterior are weakened. In this situation the tibialis posterior muscle can be transferred through the interosseous membrane to the dorsum of the foot, and the tendo calcaneus is lengthened simultaneously. A Jones operation, in which the extensor hallucis longus is placed through the neck of the first metatarsal bone with fusion of the interphalangeal joint of great toe, is also carried out. If the tibialis anterior is normal it, too, may be transferred more laterally to provide greater balance.

In the early varus deformity of club foot, soft tissue stretching and splintage should be persisted with; where there is fixed deformity, however, operative reduction and stabilization are required. It is generally agreed that correction of the hindfoot in a young child will lead to subsequent spontaneous correction of the forefoot. Dwyer (1963) described in detail the deforming forces present in a relapsed club foot. The outer border of the foot strikes the ground first and, with contracture of the plantar fascia, the forefoot is adducted. At the same time the calcaneal tendon is directed towards the inner aspect of the small inverted heel, where it is in continuity with the medial part of the plantar fascia which therefore increases the varus deformity. The heel never touches the ground and so the adducted forefoot always strikes first in walking. Since the plantar fascia is not stretched by weight-bearing, it continues to contract and becomes yet another deforming force.

Dwyer described the operation, which was aimed at correcting varus of the hindfoot by increasing the medial height of the calcaneus and placing it directly under the line of weight-bearing. The calcaneal

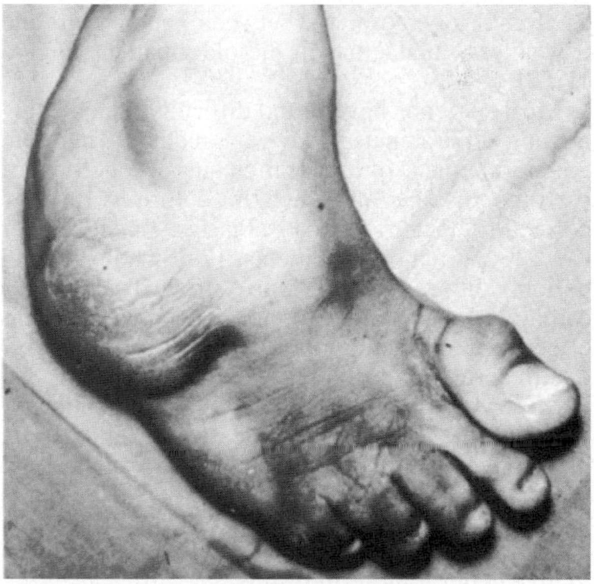

Figure 17.49 Uncorrected club foot in an adolescent boy, showing the marked inversion of the heel and the abnormal 'plantar' pad of hardened skin for weight-bearing beneath the lateral malleolus. There is marked inversion and rotation at the midtarsal joint area, with some clawing of the big toe.

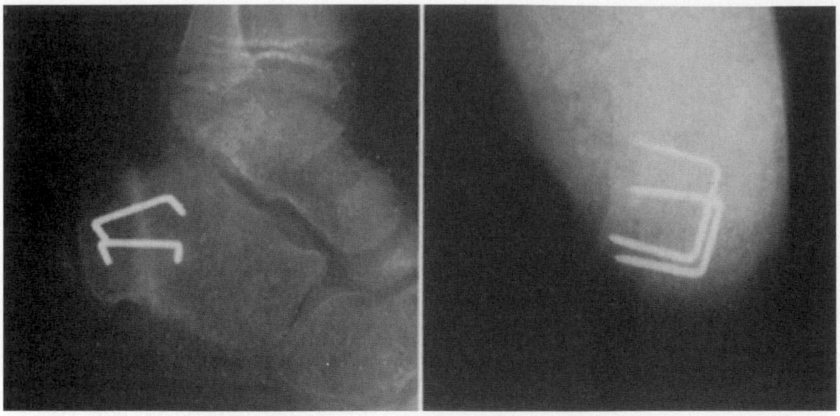

(a) (b)

Figure 17.50 (a) Lateral and (b) axial view of a cavus foot after Dwyer calcaneal osteotomy, showing the method of achieving correction by oblique osteotomy fixed with staples.

tendon is divided in the sagittal plane and the medial half is dissected from its insertion into the calcaneus. The plantar fascia is dissected from the surface of the calcaneus and the body of the calcaneus is divided in line with the groove for the flexor hallucis longus, leaving a small periosteal hinge anterolaterally. The distal fragment is tilted laterally and downwards and a small wedge of bone is taken from the tibia and placed into this wedge-shaped gap. The tendo Achilles is then sutured together with the foot in full dorsiflexion. Immobilization in a cast is continued for 10 weeks. Dwyer found that the best age for this operation was between 3 and 4 years and it was less satisfactory in the older patient (Figure 17.50).

Most surgeons have found difficulty in achieving healing of the skin using Dwyer's method. Therefore the employment of a lateral closing-wedge type of osteotomy is favoured when this deformity requires correcting (Figure 17.51). Fischer and Schaffer (1970) reported on 21 patients, 12 of whom had old poliomyelitis, 5 Charcot–Marie–Tooth disease and 4 cerebral palsy. They found the procedure was effective in correcting hindfoot varus but not effective in correcting forefoot adduction.

More recently, the Dilwyn Evans operation of extensive medial soft tissue release with lengthening of the tight tendons together with calcaneocuboid arthrodesis has been favoured for persistent varus foot. This has the advantage of correcting both hindfoot and forefoot in one operation and appears to give better long-term results.

As with all deformities in children, it is better to correct them surgically early than to undergo much soft tissue stretching and consequent damage to the architecture of the foot bones. If a satisfactory correction has not been achieved by the age of 10–12 years then triple arthrodesis is the best procedure. Hill *et al.* (1970) described the follow-up for 9 years of 43 triple arthrodesis procedures in 37 children between the ages of 5 and 8 years. The pseudarthrosis rate of 6% was acceptable and the average shortening was only 2 cm. It is, however, necessary to wait until the ossification centre for the navicular has appeared before carrying out this procedure.

It is important to stress that in club foot it is a matter of judgement to decide at which stage to apply surgical treatment and also what type of treatment to employ. Swann *et al.* (1969) emphasized the occurrence of late rotational deformity of the tibia in club foot, and in some instances this may need correction also.

In treating spastic varus foot, surgery similarly plays an important part. It must be remembered that osteotomies in general are more successful than tendon transfers in cerebral palsy because of the difficulty of predicting the function of muscles which are transferred in this condition. Nevertheless, lengthening of the tendo calcaneus by the White procedure together with tenotomy of the overacting tibialis posterior and flexor hallucis longus tendons is often valuable, followed by splintage in plaster and, if necessary, bracing.

Hammer toe

The deformity of hammer toe consists of dorsiflexion of the proximal, plantar flexion of the middle, and extension of the distal phalanx. It affects usually the second toe, though slighter degrees are not uncommon in the other toes. The head of the first phalanx is subjected to pressure by the upper of the shoe, and frequently shows a painful corn, beneath

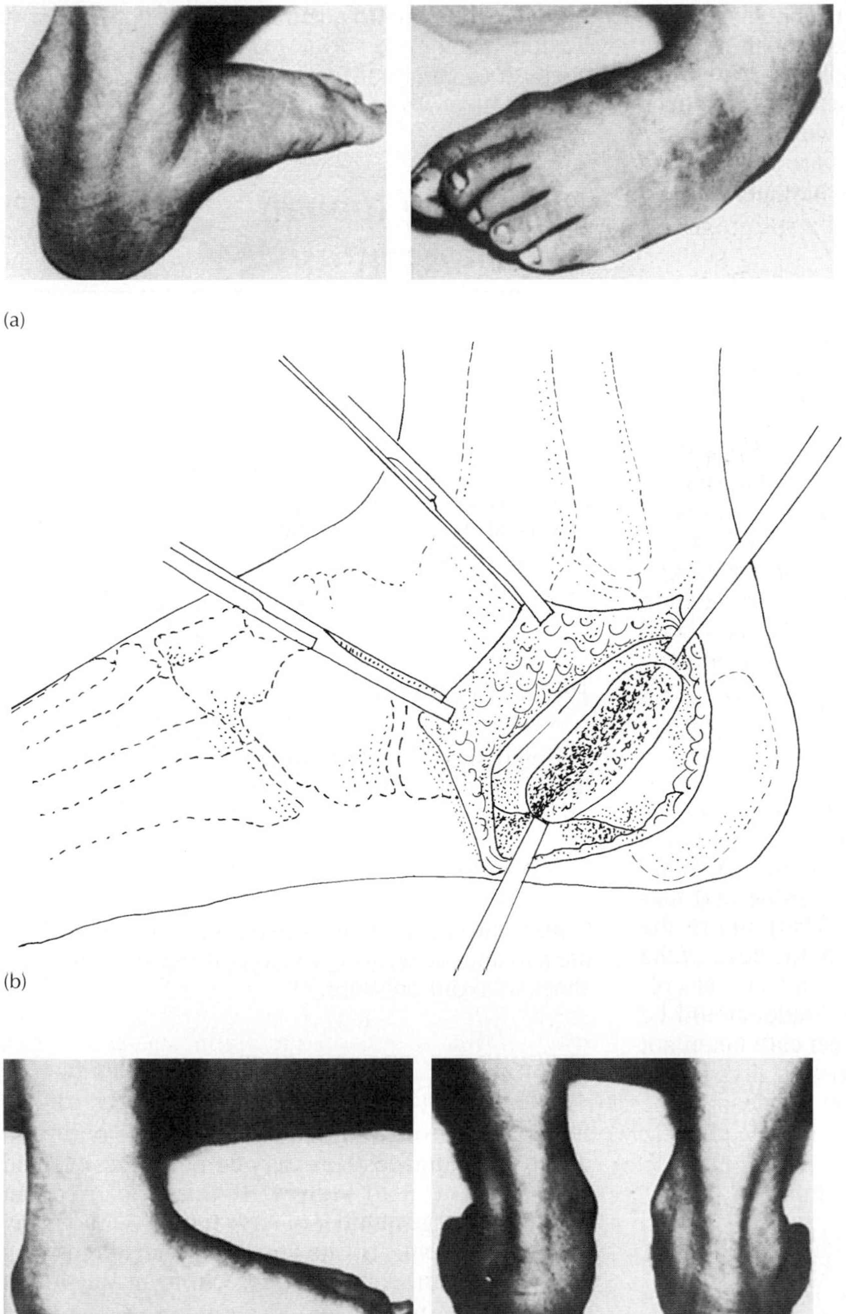

Figure 17.51 (a) Preoperative photograph showing severe varus deformity of heel and forefoot. (b) Dwyer lateral wedge excision osteotomy. (c) Postoperative appearance of the foot in (a), showing excellent correction of varus deformity.

which a bursa forms over the interphalangeal joint, and often becomes inflamed or even suppurates. The tip of the toe is pressed against the sole of the shoe, and a corn may also develop at this point, and make walking difficult or impossible. The compression by the adjoining toes and by the sole of the shoe produces a broadening and flattening of the tip of the terminal phalanx.

The condition is usually bilateral and is most commonly caused by crowding of the toes into ill-fitting and badly designed shoes. It is therefore commonly associated with hallux valgus, the displacement of the great toe forcing the second toe (which is the longest) into a flexed position. The condition usually begins in childhood, when the growth of the toes is rapid and when they are apt to be subjected to pressure by too-small shoes or socks.

The patient usually complains of a painful corn and bunion, and it is for this that treatment is sought rather than for the actual deformity.

TREATMENT

The chief obstacles to reduction are the contracted ligaments. In young children the distortion may be overcome by repeated manipulation, the corrected position being maintained by strips of adhesive plaster passing over and under the affected toe and its neighbours (Figure 17.52). The use of a digitated stocking and of wide footwear is also beneficial.

In adults, operation is indicated in order that recovery may be certain and quick. Amputation should never be carried out in view of the likelihood of a hallux valgus supervening – or, if already present, becoming more severe.

The operation (Figure 17.53)

A semilunar incision is made transversely over the dorsum of the affected joint and the corn and bursa are excised along with the ellipse of skin. A transverse incision is made across the capsule and tendinous expansion at the joint line. The point of the scalpel is now passed in both sides of the head of the proximal phalanx, and the medial and lateral collateral ligaments are divided. The blade should be kept parallel to the phalanx and great care taken not to divide the digital arteries. Following division of these tiny ligaments, access to both the head of the proximal phalanx and the base of the middle phalanx is excellent.

One of two procedures may be adopted:

1. The ‘spike’ operation. The head of the proximal phalanx is shaped to a point with the aid of a small pair of nibbling forceps. It is usually not necessary to reduce the length of the proximal phalanx. The bony point on the proximal phalanx is now inserted into the hole in the base of the middle phalanx, thus correcting the deformity.
2. Alternatively, the interphalangeal joint can be fused by clearing the articular surfaces of cartilage with an osteotome. Apposition of these surfaces is achieved and maintained by inserting a heavy Kirschner wire down through the phalanges.

In both operations it is necessary to tenotomize the structures on the dorsal aspect of the metatarsophalangeal joint to ensure correction of the dorsiflexion of the proximal joint and to hold the position of the joint by driving the Kirschner wire into the metatarsal head.

Ingrowing toenail (onychocryptosis)

Ingrowing toenail is a common and distressing complaint which is caused essentially by the pressure of the shoe against the toenail. The nail is driven into the soft part of the toe and considerable pain results. Normally the toe is protected to some extent from the nail by thickened skin in the groove at its edge but if the nail is cut back towards its base then the sharp corner may well be driven into and through the groove of skin, and cause infection and pain.

PROPHYLAXIS

The nail should be cut square at right angles to its long axis and not in a lunar shape.

CONSERVATIVE TREATMENT

Conservative treatment consists in correct cutting of the nail and the wearing of easy-fitting stockings and shoes to avoid pressure.

OPERATIVE TREATMENT

If the nail is grossly infected, it is better to remove it under general anaesthetic as gently as possible and then to allow it to regrow. If this is carried out carefully, a large number of nails regrow without any further problem. If, however, further ingrowing occurs with further pain and infection, an ablation of the nail bed is required.

The operation described by Zadik involves excision of all the nail bed, particularly that on the sides of the distal phalanx, and is much preferred to the more radical operation of amputation of the tip of the toe with removal of the nail bed. It is important to warn the patient that recurrence does arise in a few cases and a repeat operation may be required.

An alternative procedure is marginal nail avulsion and phenolization. There are no comparative studies of the effects of the relative merits of a Zadik’s procedure and marginal nail avulsion with phenolization available for comparison.

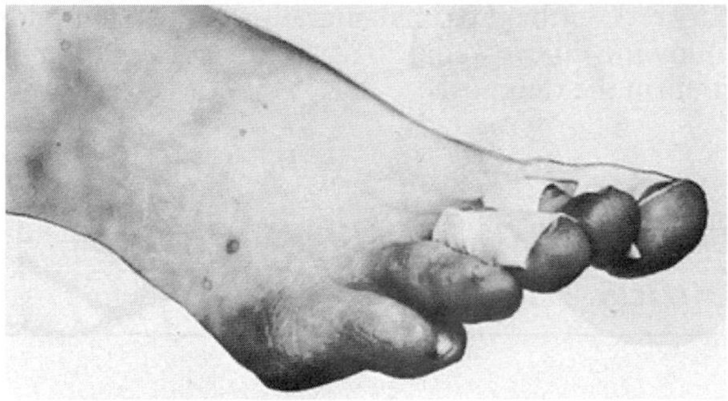

Figure 17.52 Method of correcting mild hammer toe with plaster strapping, passing the strapping under adjacent toes.

CONSERVATIVE TREATMENT

Ilfeld (1991) demonstrated a method of treating an incurvated nail with cotton with a collodion coating to separate the anterior tip and lateral edges of an ingrowing toenail from the adjacent soft tissues.

Subungual haematoma

This results from direct pressure on the toenail, and may be a small collection of blood or large haemorrhage which lifts the toenail from its bed. It is acutely painful at the beginning and may be treated by evacuation of the blood by drilling the nail carefully with a red-hot unfolded paper-clip.

Onychogryposis

This condition – sometimes called ram's horn nail or ostler's toe – usually affects the great toenail and is a response to trauma (Figure 17.54). The nail grows in an irregular fashion, curling with an appearance very much like that of a ram's horn. The tip of the nail may penetrate the pulp of the toe and produce an ulcer.

The most effective treatment is removal of the toenail under local anaesthetic; if it recurs, ablation of the nail bed is required, by the Zadik procedure.

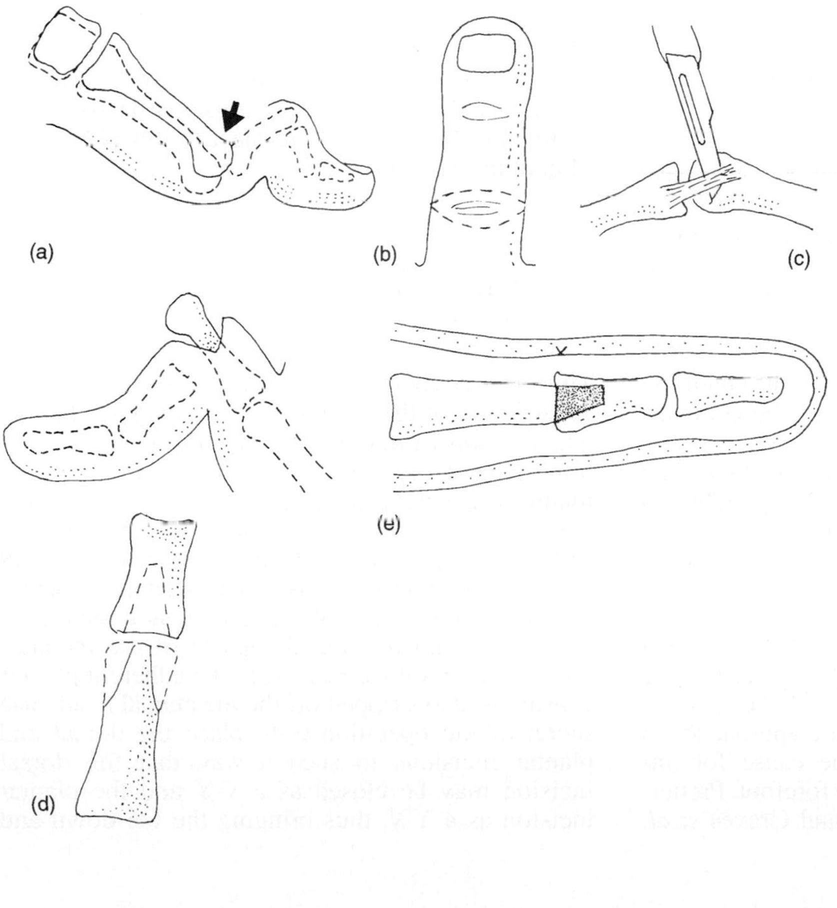

Figure 17.53 Spike arthrodesis for hammer toe: (a) the deformity; (b) elliptical skin incision over the dorsum of the proximal interphalangeal joint; (c) division of the collateral ligaments; (d) fashioning of the spike and socket by means of bone nibblers and awls; (e) the final position with the extensor tendon and skin firmly sutured over the dorsum. (Reproduced, with permission, from Piggott, H. (1979) Hammer and mallet toe. In: *Operative Surgery*, 3rd edn, vol. 2, *Orthopaedics*. Edited by G. Bentley. Butterworths: London and Boston)

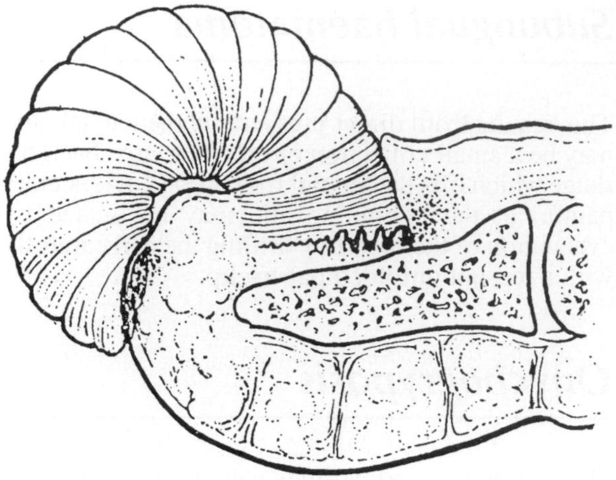

Figure 17.54 Onychogryposis. The nail eventually may grow into the pulp and produce an ulcer.

Subungal exostosis

A subungual exostosis may occur on the dorsum of the distal phalanx beneath the toenail due to old injuries or mild periostitis. Treatment is to raise the toenail and remove the exostosis, following which a normal nail will grow.

The sesamoid bones of the great toe

The cartilaginous precursors of the sesamoid bones appear in early fetal life but do not ossify until between the ages of 8 and 11 years. Ossification may occur from a single centre, or from several centres which are variable in position. In 10% of individuals these centres do not unite, constituting the condition of multiparite sesamoid – which may be confused with fracture.

Pain under the first metatarsal head or first MTP joint is often suspected of being attributable to pathology in and around the sesamoid bones.

Leventen (1991) reviewed most aspects of sesamoid pathology and concluded that excision of one sesamoid could be undertaken safely, but the excision of both would result in a claw-toe deformity and should be avoided. It has also been suggested that the arterial blood supply to the sesamoid bones may be damaged during the course of some approaches to the MTP joint. This may be one cause for unexplained postoperative pain in the forefoot. Pretterklieber and Wanivenhaus (1992) and Graves *et al.* (1991) describe proximal migration of the sesamoids following injury requiring careful investigation to confirm the diagnosis.

Fracture of the sesamoid bones

The sesamoid bones of the great toe are occasionally fractured, particularly the medial. Violence may be direct or indirect, but results usually from a fall on the forefoot. The symptoms are those of pain, and there is tenderness over the sesamoid and pain on movement of the metatarsophalangeal joint. Inge and Ferguson (1933) considered that the diagnosis should not be made unless a previous x-ray showed the affected bone to be complete or unless subsequent x-rays showed the appearance of callus. Differential diagnosis includes a bipartite sesamoid (25–30% incidence of which 85% are bilateral).

TREATMENT

The injured foot should be immobilized in a plaster-of-Paris cast for 2–3 weeks, and then mobilization may commence.

Rarely, osteoarthritis may occur in the joint between the sesamoid and the metatarsal head but this is always associated with osteoarthritis in the main joint. Treatment of the one is followed by relief of pain in the other.

Overlapping of the fifth toe

This is a frequent congenital lesion in which there is constriction of the tissues on the dorsum of the toe, which is drawn into a varus position with subluxation so that it lies above the fourth toe. Although it is mainly a cosmetic deformity, it does produce disability and discomfort which makes treatment necessary. Many operations have been recommended but the most reliable is the Butler procedure (Cockin, 1968). Through a dorsal racquet incision the extensor tendon and the dorsal capsule of the metatarsophalangeal joint are divided. The adherent plantar capsule is also stripped off the metatarsal head. The secret of the operation is to place the dorsal and plantar incisions in such a way that the dorsal incision may be closed as a V-Y and the plantar incision as a Y-V, thus bringing the toe down and

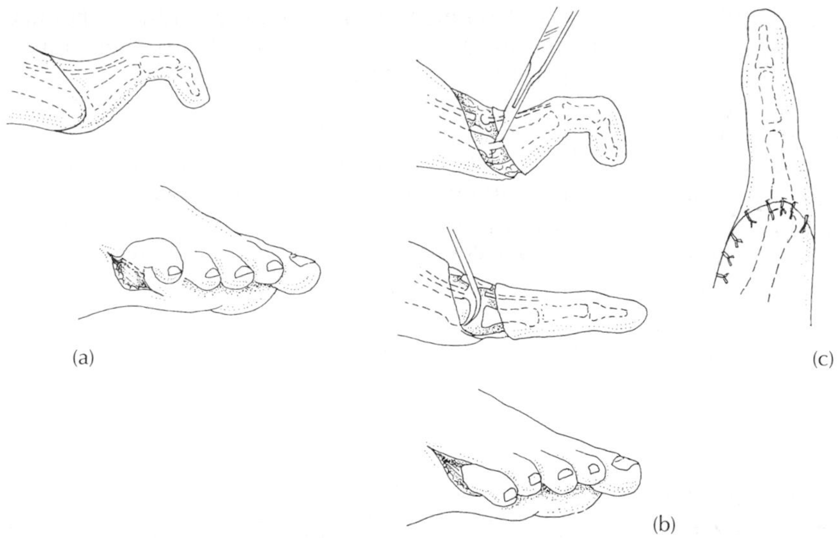

Figure 17.55 Butler's operation for over-riding fifth toe: (a) deformity and racquet incision; (b) division of dorsal capsule, extensor tendon and collateral ligaments of the metatarso-phalangeal joint, and correction of toe; (c) the plantar incision is closed as a V and the dorsal incision closed as a Y, allowing the toe to lie in a normal position. (Reproduced, with permission, from Piggott, H. (1979) Dorsally displaced fifth toe. In: *Operative Surgery*. 3rd edn, vol. 2, *Orthopaedics*. Edited by G. Bentley. Butterworths: London and Boston)

holding it in a satisfactory position. Apart from occasional problems with circulation of the toe due to dividing the skin and damaging the digital vessels, this is an excellent procedure.

See Figure 17.85.

Curly toe deformities

This term is used to describe a deformity in which the toes are medially rotated and in varus flexion. This may cause under-riding of the toes and pain.

TREATMENT

The condition is treated by Girdlestone's flexor-to-extensor tendon transfers, which derotates the toe and straightens it.

Henry and Zafiropoulos (1994) described persistent varus deformity after this operation, however, and described an alternative operation in which an osteotomy of the middle phalanx of the affected toe is carried out.

The ankle joint

This mortise joint is made up of the tibiotalar and fibulotalar joints and the inferior tibiofibular joint. Its excellent stability arises from the physical setting of its surfaces, the capsular, collateral and interosseous, talofibular and deltoid ligaments as well as the muscle restraints of gastrocnemius-soleus, tibialis anterior and posterior, peronei and extensor flexor tendons acting across it in four planes.

Inman (1976) has emphasized that the less stable talocalcaneal joint also has an important relationship to the ankle by providing the system with a type of rotational universal joint for weight distribution as well as movement. The movements of dorsi- and plantar flexion take place about a transverse axis slightly posterior in the sagittal plane as well as a few degrees of tilt. Around a longitudinal axis there may be a few degrees of rotation. Normal dorsiflexion is 10–20° and plantar flexion is 25–35°. These vary both in amount and in timing during the various phases of the gait cycle; e.g. at heel strike the ankle is in about 10° of plantar flexion, this smoothly passes into 10° of dorsiflexion in the flat foot position and back into plantar flexion during heel off and toe off (Murray *et al.*, 1964). At the actual surfaces, motions have been demonstrated by Sammarco *et al.* (1973). At the beginning there is some separation of the contact points, sliding then takes place and movement ends with compaction of the surfaces. This has been suggested as an important lubrication mechanism and obviously any minor instability or incongruence of the surfaces would disrupt the balance of transmitted stresses with resulting pathological changes.

Frankel and Nordin (1980) have argued that although the joint reaction forces acting on the ankle joints are equal to or greater than the forces across the hip or knee, because the ankle joint has a large weight-bearing surface area (about 1200 mm^2; Greenwald, 1977), lower loads per unit area (i.e. stress) are transmitted across them. When an individual stands, each ankle is receiving half the body weight as well as the gastrocnemius-soleus muscle force to give a joint reaction force. By constructing a triangle of forces, Frankel and Nordin have found that during stance the joint reaction force is about 1.2 times body weight. This can rise to 5 times body weight at the push-off phase of gait.

Painful conditions of the ankle

Pain around the ankle is a frequent complaint which may become chronic in nature, causing considerable disability. It arises commonly from:

1. Recurrent sprains and instability of the ankle.
2. Post-traumatic osteoarthritis.

Sprains of the ankle

These usually result from a twisting injury in which there is an inversion of the foot and a consequent external rotation Strain at the ankle joint itself, due to the torque-converting effect of the subtalar joint and the lateral pressure of the talus on the lateral ligament and lateral malleolus. The common injury is a partial tear of the lateral ligament of the ankle. If the injury is mild, only the anterior talofibular ligament is damaged; but the injury is more severe and is likely to become recurrent with instability if the calcaneofibular or posterior talofibular ligaments are divided also.

Buluco *et al.* (1991) demonstrated that all three parts of the lateral ligament complex contributed equally to stabilize the ankle, although the anterior talofibular ligament is said to be the weakest of the three.

There was also thought to be a reflex arc involved in controlling ankle stability (Freeman, 1965).

Ankle ligament sprains are more common in the presence of a previous medical history of ankle sprain and it is also commoner in patients who are tall or heavy. The use of boots as opposed to shoes does not alter the incidence of soft tissue ankle injuries.

After an acute injury it is important to assess the soft tissue bruising and tenderness around the ankle; usually it is easy clinically to assess how much of the lateral ligament has been damaged by the location of the tenderness. Also, it is necessary to check the state of the medial ligament though this is more rarely damaged.

Some 10–40% of acute sprains go on to become chronically unstable. Stress x-rays (Figure 17.56) showing a talar tilt of more than 7° in plantar flexion, demonstrate an anterior talofibular rupture. Stress x-rays are best interpreted in comparing two ankles. A tilt of greater than 15° demonstrates both an anterior talofibular and calcaneofibular ligament rupture. If the tilt on the injured side is 7° greater than that of the contralateral ankle, and injury to the anterior talofibular and calcaneofibular ligaments is demonstrated as well (Karlsson, 1989).

Two other stress tests are of use. The first is an anterior draw test, the talus being manually pulled forwards on the tibia. Rupture of the anterior talofibular ligament is demonstrated by 5 mm of forward movement of the talus on the tibia. The third and final test is a forced external rotation test in which more than 6 mm of widening of the tibia relative to the fibula in the mortise is indicative of a syndesmotic injury.

Under a general anaesthetic with full muscular relaxation, inversion of the ankle is performed on both the injured and the normal side and comparison is made. Ruben and Witten (1960) demonstrated, however, an average tilt of 3–27° during a survey of normal ankle joints but this was increased when there was ligamentous rupture or stretching (Figure 17.57).

It is important in such injuries to look for the appearance of a fracture of dome of the talus which may accompany the ligament injury. This osteochondral fragment may separate, forming a loose body inside the ankle and giving rise to 'loose body locking' subsequently. It should also be noted that osteochondritis of the dome of the talus may occur, giving rise to pain, instability and loose body, but this appears to be a separate pathology from the osteochondral fracture. The contribution of the subtalar and midtarsal joints must also be assessed.

TREATMENT

Where the injury is not severe then treatment with a below-knee walking cast for 2–3 weeks until the ankle is quite pain free is satisfactory followed by wobble-board exercise and normal usage. If there is pathological talar tilt then it is best to explore the ligament and to repair the torn component as an immediate procedure. Late symptoms of instability in the ankle are difficult to treat. Although talar tilt may be demonstrable and this may be corrected by a procedure such as the Watson-Jones tenodesis employing the tendon of peroneus brevis, the functional

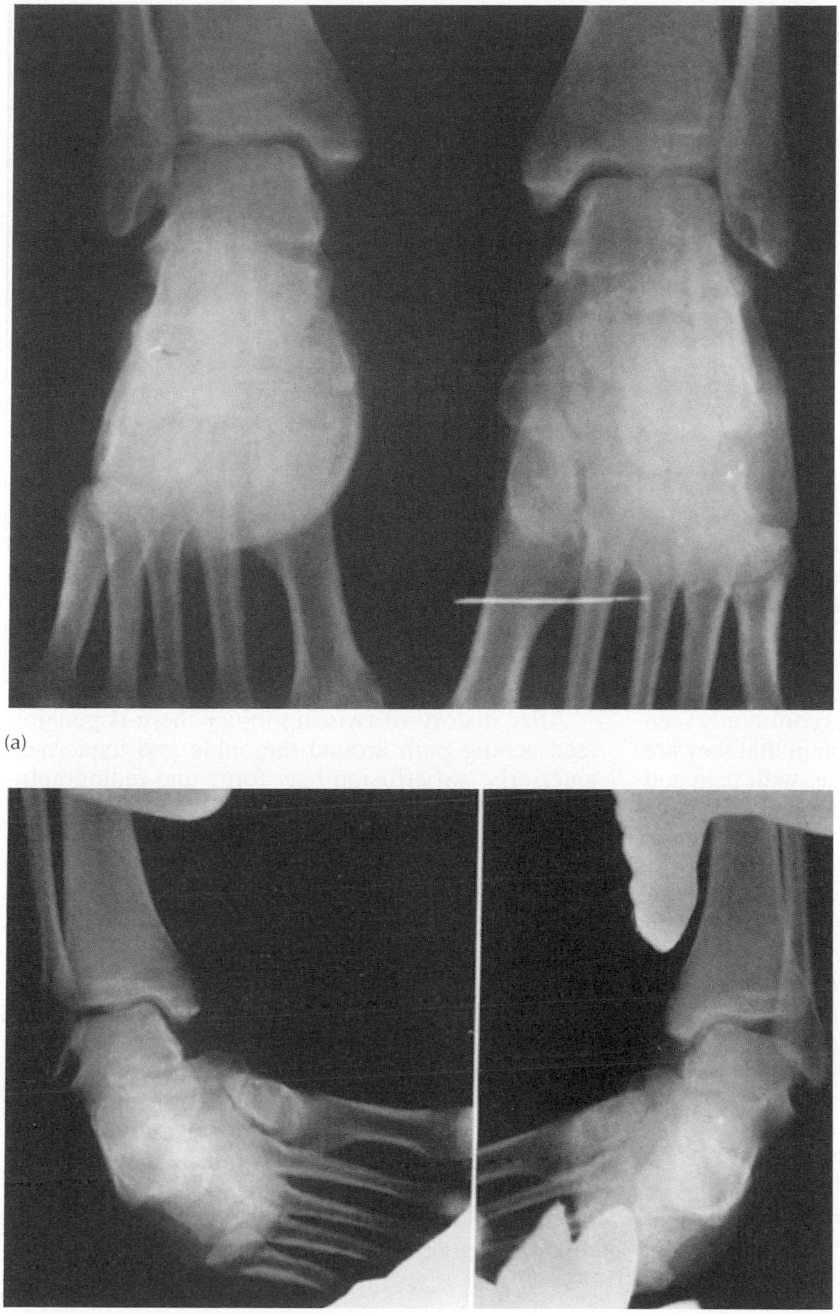

(a)

(b) (c)

Figure 17.56 Anteroposterior radiographs showing: (a) supposedly normal ankle joints and (b) a strong inversion force being applied to the right foot with very little increase in the talar tilt angle; (c) on the left side, there is marked opening of the talar tilt angle over to 25°.

results are not satisfactory in more than 50% of cases.

Leach *et al.* (1981) have emphasized that an increasing number of young people are presenting for surgical reconstruction of the lateral ligaments of the ankle following athletic injuries. They point out that the physical examination which includes measurement of the distance between the tip of the lateral malleolus to the prominence made up of the beak of the calcaneus when the foot is maximally inverted (i.e. more than 1 cm over the normal) and review of symptoms is often more helpful than the talar tilt radiograph. Those workers have described an efficient modification of the Elmslie procedure in which the anterior talofibular and calcaneofibular ligaments are replaced by the whole or split peroneus brevis tendon. This detached tendon is sutured to the repaired anterior talofibular ligament, through the

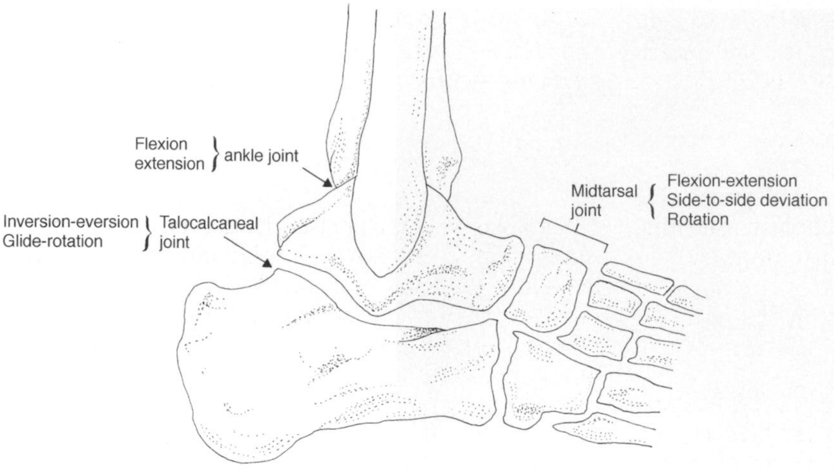

Figure 17.57 The movements of the ankle joint as well as the talocalcaneal joint.

bone of the lateral malleolus down behind the peronei tendons, stapled to the lateral wall of the calcaneus and finally back up to the anterior talofibular ligament.

Failure to treat the acute strains properly may result in the syndrome of the chronic strain of the external collateral ligament, which is commonly seen in middle-aged women. They complain that they are continually 'falling over' their ankle, with pain and swelling. On examination during an acute episode there is local tenderness and pain over the ligament on forced inversion of the foot. Radiographs for talar tilt are taken to exclude a complete rupture.

Treatment is aimed at preventing the twisting episodes by lowering the heel of the shoe and flaring out the lateral edge of the heel by 6 mm. The acute episode is treated by injecting procaine or hydrocortisone solutions and by bandaging.

Operative treatment

Part of the difficulty in achieving a satisfactory result in an operation may be the difficulty in obtaining a long enough length of tendon to complete the operation satisfactorily. The Evans procedure, adopting a similar principle, requires a shorter length of tendon to complete it, and the results are significantly better although no procedure is uniformly successful (Milgrem *et al.*, 1991).

Post-traumatic arthritis of the ankle

McMurray (1936) called this condition 'footballer's ankle' but it is seen in other athletes, particularly ballet dancers. McDougall (1955) considered it to be a result of minor trauma to the capsular attachments and repeated compression injury of the bones which are in contact during extreme dorsi- and plantar flexion. Bony exostoses are produced on the anterior tibial margin, on the malleoli and on the dorsum of the neck of the talus.

After history of twisting injury there is generalized aching pain around the ankle and tenderness anteriorly. An effusion may form, and radiographically the osteophytes can be seen.

TREATMENT

Treatment consists of resting in a walking cast for a period of 2–3 weeks and then graduated exercises before returning to full activity. Occasionally anterior cheilectomy with removal of the osteophytes, either open or arthroscopically, relieves pain and regains some range of movements, particularly dorseflexion. In advanced cases with severe unremitting pain arthrodesis of the ankle joint is required. The final position of the arthrodesis is neutral dorsiflexion, 5° of valgus hindfoot and 5° of external rotation (see below).

Rupture of tendo Achillis

Tendo Achillis rupture occurs predominantly in middle life and results from various types of indirect trauma. It is commonly found in badminton or tennis players and follows a sudden plantar flexion force of the foot (e.g. when leaping into the air).

Rupture is usually complete, the tendon separating about 4 cm above its insertion, and the line of separation is usually ragged, from the projecting bundles of tendon fibres. The sheath may or may not remain intact and the proximal end of the tendon retracts. Internally the sheath rapidly fills with blood, producing a swelling.

Incomplete ruptures are probably rare except at the musculotendinous junction. Calcified deposits may be present in the tendon as a degenerative phenomenon, or cholesterol in cholesterolaemia, producing weakening which results in rupture.

CLINICAL FEATURES

At the moment of rupture the patient experiences sharp pain as if he had been struck from behind on the heel. There is immediate disability and swelling, and tenderness follows shortly afterwards. The patient is unable to walk without severe pain.

In untreated cases the sheath may become adherent to the retracted ends of the tendon and act as a weak bond enabling a certain amount of calf contraction to move the foot. The calf muscles, however, remain shortened and plantar flexion is permanently weakened and diminished. Healing with heterotopic ossification may be discovered many years later because of ankle joint stiffness (Figure 17.58).

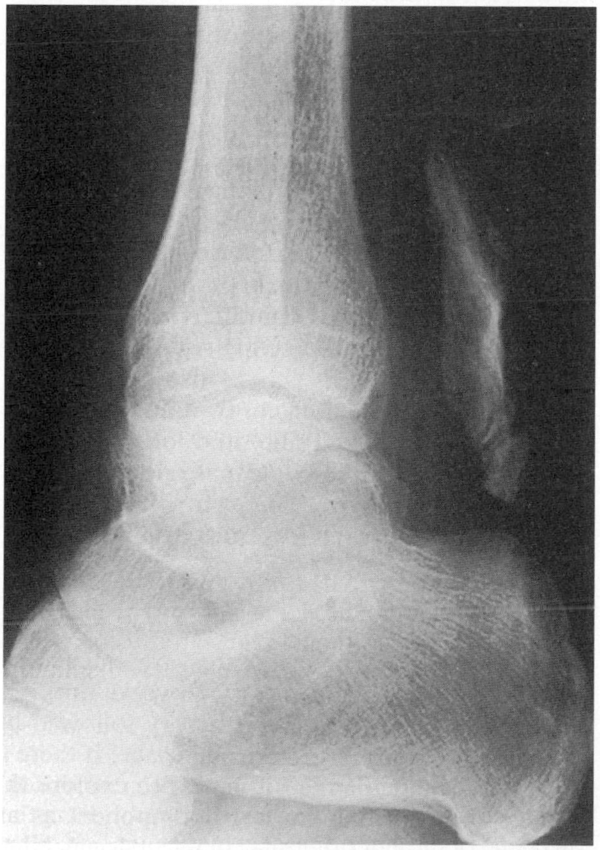

Figure 17.58 An old ruptured tendo Achillis containing a mass of heterotopic ossification.

DIAGNOSIS

Diagnosis is often missed by the unwary and it is important in dealing with ankle injuries to carefully examine the back of the ankle and tendo Achilles in all cases. After 24 hours from the time of the injury there is a filling of the defect by haematoma and it may be difficult to detect the gap between the separated ends. However, the following are diagnostic features:

1. Presence of a palpable gap in the tendo Achillis.
2. An abnormal range of passive dorsiflexion or the foot compared with that on the uninjured side.
3. Inability to perform, or marked limitation of, plantar flexion. Some plantar flexion may be achieved by the action of tibialis posterior and the long flexors of the toes but this is weak compared with the normal movement following active contraction of the calf muscle.
4. An unduly high level of the prominence of the bellies of the calf muscle may be detected in a thin leg.
5. Positive Thompson's test (1962). When the main mass of the calf muscle is compressed by the hand with the patient in the prone position and the foot free over the end of the table, passive plantar flexion of the ankle will occur. If there is a rupture of the tendo Achillis then there is no movement of the foot.
6. The use of a sphygmomanometer (Copeland, 1990) blown to 100 mgHg around the calf shows a rise in dorsiflexion of the foot if the tendo Achillis is intact.

DIFFERENTIAL DIAGNOSIS

Differential diagnosis consists of a localized thrombophlebitis of the saphenous vein or a rupture of a popliteal cyst into the calf which occurs in rheumatoid patients. An arthrogram will outline the leakage of the contrast medium down into the calf.

Ultrasound is more sensitive and specific than either CT scan or plain x-rays in detecting partial ruptures (Kalebo *et al.*, 1991).

MRI scanning can identify four types of lesion:

1. Inflammation and thickening of the tendon.
2. Degeneration of the tendon.
3. Incomplete rupture.
4. Complete rupture (Weinstabl *et al.*, 1991).

TREATMENT

There is still dispute about the best method of treatment of a complete rupture. Whilst there is no doubt that good results may be achieved by immobilization of the foot in plantar flexion for a period of 3 weeks and then gradual restoration to the plantigrade position (Gillies and Chalmers, 1970), there have been in all series of conservatively treated patients incidents of re-rupture. The re-rupture rate for surgical treatment is 2–7% and 8–35% for non-surgical treatment. Therefore, unless there is damage to the overlying skin, a recent complete rupture should be repaired as soon as possible by open operation. The tendon is exposed by a longitudinal medial incision. In a small number of cases there may be sufficient quality of tendon to allow apposition and suture with non-absorbable mattress sutures. Frequently, however, the quality of the tendon is poor and the defect requires filling – either with the plantaris tendon which is wound between the two ends or by bringing down superficial strips of tendon from the broad upper part. The superficial surface of both parts of the tendon is exposed, and the gap and the surfaces are cleared or clot and fibrous tissue. Two long strips of tendon 6 mm wide and 3 mm deep are divided above and downwards to within 1 cm of the upper end of the tendon rupture. These strips are then threaded through the upper tendon 1 cm above its rupture from back to front. The strips are then drawn through, pulled tight and fixed to the tendon inferiorly with mattress sutures of Prolene with the foot held in full equinus. A full-length plaster-of-Paris cast is applied with the foot in full plantar flexion and the knee flexed to 20°. The cast is retained for 4 weeks, after which it can be reduced to a below-knee cast with half correction of the equinus position. After a further 2 weeks the foot may be corrected to neutral and at this point the patient may begin active movements. Reduced activities continue for at least 3 months following the repair.

An alternative treatment is percutaneous repair. Bradley and Tibore (1990) compared percutaneous and open repair in a prospective study and found 5% higher re-rupture rate in the percutaneous group.

Late repairs or chronic ruptures present additional problems. End-to-end repair may not be possible and grafts using plantaris tendon, fascia lata or a strip of fascia from the proximal tendon may be used.

Rupture of the plantaris tendon

The existence of this entity is disputed and it appears likely that pains in the calf attributed to rupture of plantaris tendon are actually due to incomplete rupture of the tendo Achillis. The disability is slight and all that is required is for the patient to restrict his activities until the discomfort has subsided. It is vital to exclude rupture of the tendo Achillis.

Tibialis posterior tendon ruptures

The aetiology of this condition is unclear. Rupture of this tendon leads to development of a painful calcaneo-plano-valgus foot with midfoot abduction and forefoot varus supination deformities. According to Holmes and Mann (1992), the average age of this occurrence is 57 years.

In young patients, soon after rupture tendon reconstructions without or without tendon transfer may be undertaken, but patients with the condition established will require a triple arthrodesis. MR scanning may be useful in the confirmation of this diagnosis. See Figure 17.59.

Arthrodesis of the ankle joint

This is indicated when there are significant symptoms arising from the joint, particularly pain, limitation of movement and instability as well as cosmetic deformity. This may arise from trauma (e.g. an old Pott's fracture, with secondary osteoarthritis), haemophilic or pyogenic arthritis, tuberculosis and, rarely, from rheumatoid arthritis, paralytic drop-foot or bone tumours such as osteoclastoma of the talus.

Normally, the position of choice for fusion is 90°, which will allow the individual to walk with minimal limp and disability. Five degrees of plantar flexion may be the position of choice for women who wish to wear high-heel shoes habitually.

Various methods of fusion have been proposed. Watson-Jones cut a corticocancellous graft from the lower end of the anterior aspect of the tibia and, after turning this graft upside down, drove it into a pre-prepared socket in the talus (Figure 17.60). Adams

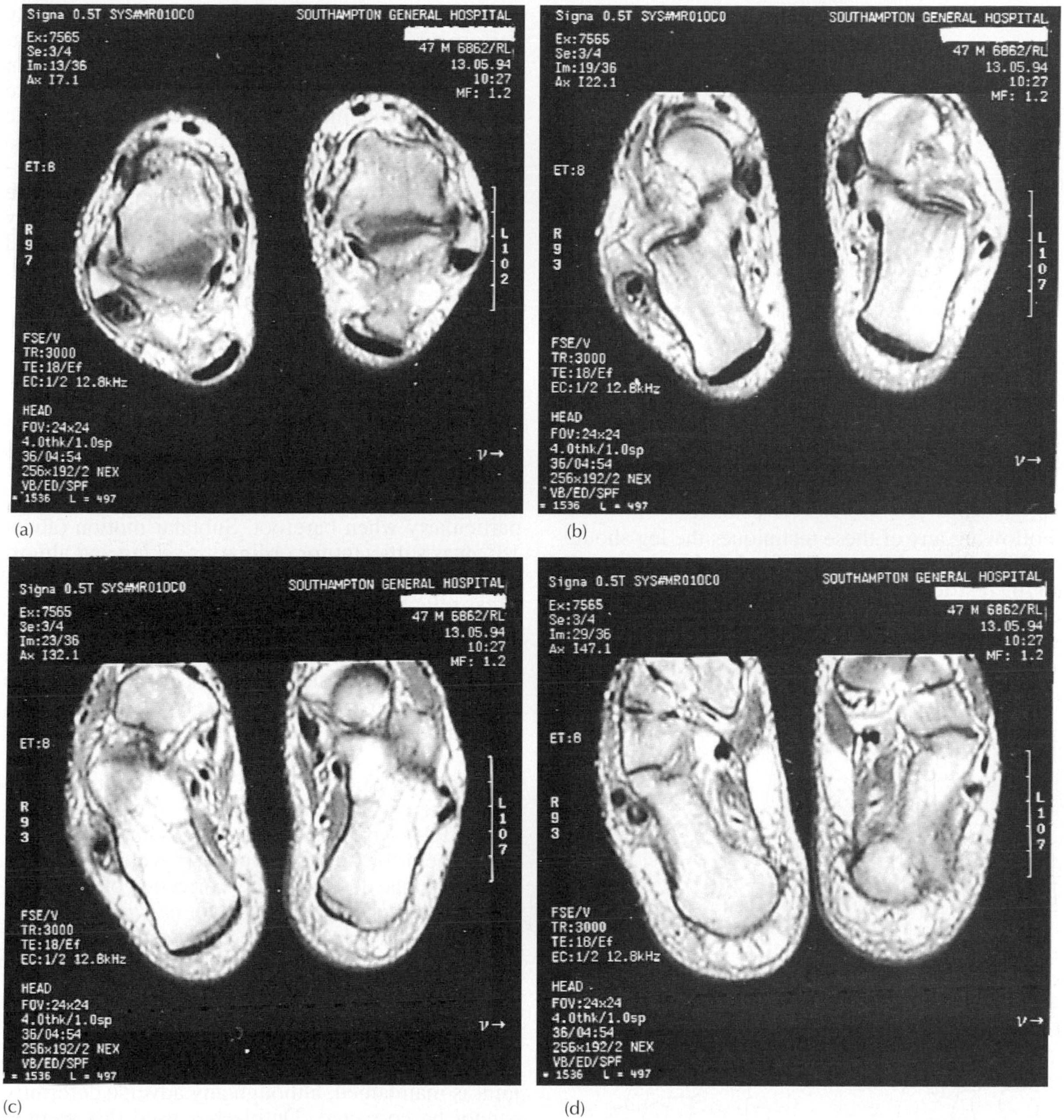

Figure 17.59 A rupture of the tibialis posterior tendon seen on MR scanning. In (a) the two tendons can be seen, one lying posterior to the other, the posterior one being non-homogeneous and with some loss of signal. In (b) only strands of the tendon are now visible. In (c) the tendon has disappeared completely, whilst in (d), a lower section, the distal part of the tendon can be seen again clearly indicating a rupture. (Kindly supplied by Dr Richard Blaquiere, Consultant Radiologist at Southampton University Hospitals)

(1948) reported the transfibular method, otherwise known as the RAF (Royal Air Force) fusion, in which the distal third of the fibula is removed subperiosteally and the ankle joint surface is excised from the lateral aspect (Figure 17.61). A bed is prepared for the fibular graft over the lateral surface of the tibia and talus, and the onlay graft is held to these two structures by screws. This is a very successful method of fusion, and Adams reported only two failures in 30 cases.

Alternatively, a compression arthrodesis method may be applied with compression clamps on the lower end of the tibia and in the talus (Figure 17.62).

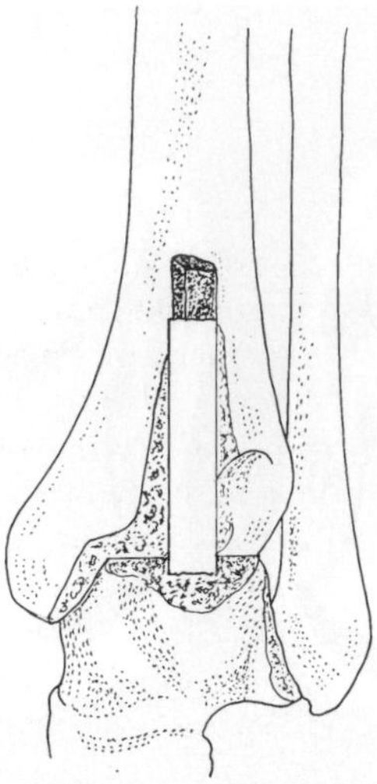

Figure 17.60 Arthrodesis of the ankle: Watson-Jones method.

Following any of these techniques the leg should be held in a Sarmiento-type of below-knee cast and walking restricted for 4 weeks. Following this period the plaster can be changed, the clamps removed and full weight-bearing allowed. Plaster protection is necessary for a period of 12 weeks.

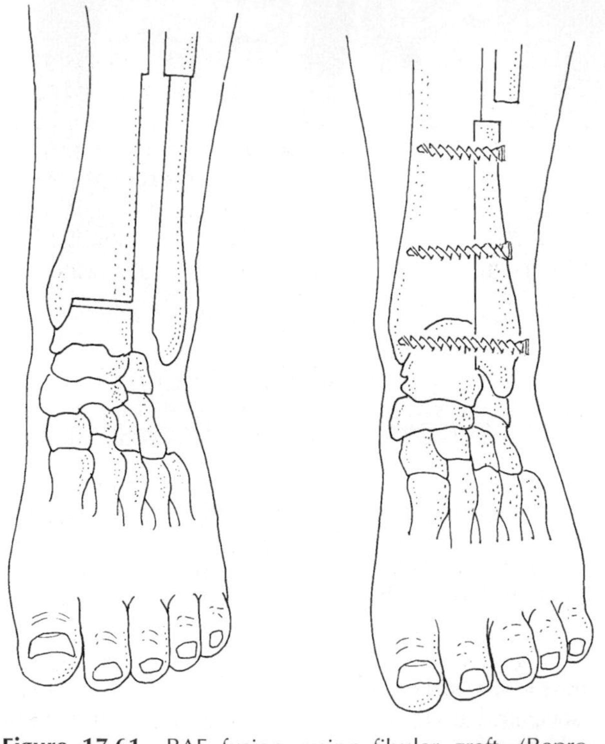

Figure 17.61 RAF fusion, using fibular graft. (Reproduced, with permission, from Somerville, E.W. (1979) Arthrodesis of the ankle. In: *Operative Surgery*, 3rd edn, vol. 2, *Orthopaedics*. Edited by G. Bentley. Butterworths: London and Boston)

It should be emphasized that when a properly performed arthrodesis of this joint for tibiotalar disease or paralysis is carried out, particularly in young or middle-aged persons, the complication rate is low and the improved function and cosmetic appearance are great with a high rate of return to former occupations. Failure to achieve an arthrodesis, which has been reported as high as 22% (with wound healing complications of 18%), usually results from poor technique, associated neurological or vascular problem or poor patient selection (e.g. involvement of other foot joints). Wagner (1982) described in detail a gait analysis study carried out upon himself with an arthrodesis for a post-traumatic fracture dislocation of the ankle. On comparison with his normal side there was no major difference in velocity, stride length, stance and swing phases during free or fast walking or running. There was some minor loss in flexion and extension at the knee joint, and obvious loss of plantar and dorsiflexion, particularly when barefoot. Subtalar motion (about 18°) was sufficient for ordinary walking and almost enough for barefoot running. He called this joint a stress reliever for the ankle joint.

Thordarson *et al.* (1990) have described an *in vitro* study of transarticular screws across the ankle joint and a lateral fibular strut graft. They confirm that this gives a very strong initial fixation consistent with a high rate of success, that is 90° or more in more recent clinical series.

Recently the possibility of undertaking ankle arthrodesis periarthrosopically has been explored (Patil *et al.*, 1994) Articular cartilage and joint debris is removed perarthrosocpically using power instruments. This technique does not allow correction of deformity however, and is only suggested for *in situ* arthrodesis.

Transmalleolar (O'Hara and Pearson, 1986) – usually via the fibula – using a large drill bit can expose the tibiotalar joint as well as the opposite malleolar surface. Removal of diseased surfaces is possible and bone graft material can be inserted and packed in. The integrity of the trimalleolar ankle joint is maintained, although any adverse deformity cannot be corrected. Duthie has used this method very successfully in haemophilic arthropathy of the ankle, and because of its minimal exposure and soft tissue dissection, little factor replacement is required (see Chapter 11).

Replacement arthroplasty of the ankle

Loss of movement at the ankle is, in normal circum-

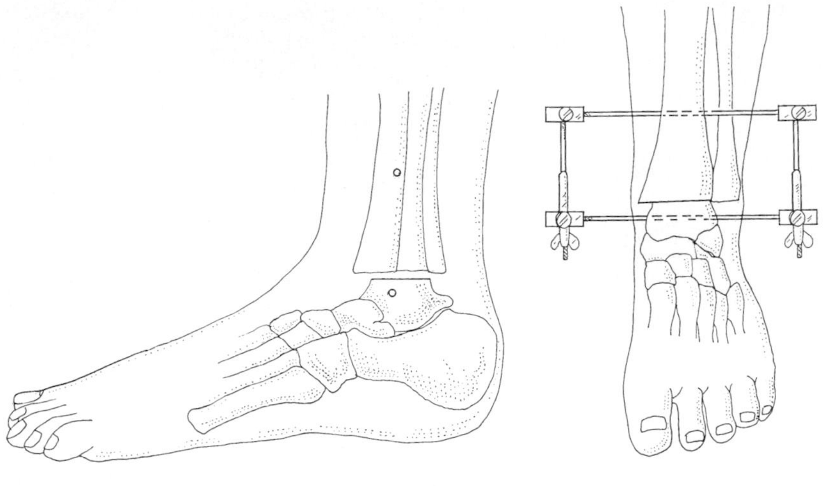

Figure 17.62 Charnley compression arthrodesis. Note the Steinmann pins placed slightly anterior to ensure that the arthrodesis does not open up anteriorly. (Reproduced, with permission, from Somerville, E.W. (979) Arthrodesis of the ankle. In: *Operative Surgery*, 3rd edn, vol. 2, *Orthopaedics*. Edited by G. Bentley. Butterworths: London and Boston)

stances, taken up by the subtalar and tarsal joints with very little disability, so arthrodesis is the operation of choice in most cases. However, some have pursued the use of a replacement prosthesis for the ankle. Most designs have a metallic dome for the talus and a high-density polyethylene concave component for the lower tibial replacement, providing a large area of contact. Stauffer and Segal (1981) have followed 102 cases for 4 years. They had complications in 41% of cases, including loosening and infection in 6.9% and 2.9% respectively. Impingement was a problem in 22%. They concluded that the high-density polyethylene-to-metal prosthesis secured by methylmethacrylate bone cement was most useful in patients with rheumatoid arthritis who had significant disability from involvement of many joints, and in post-traumatic osteoarthrosis only in those over the age of 60 years.

Total replacement of the ankle has been fraught with complications, usually with loosening of the tibial components, more frequently the talar component. Since arthrodesis of the ankle gives such good results, this still remains the treatment of choice for post-traumatic arthritis of the ankle or isolated osteoarthritis of the ankle joint. In patients with subtalar and/or midtarsal joint disease, however, ankle arthrodesis gives less satisfactory results, although a number of series have been reported in the past showing good results with an apparent talar arthrodesis in poliomyelitis. Some authors have reported satisfactory results in rheumatoid arthritis, that is in patients with subtalar or midtarsal joint disease, but who will be low-demand patients as far as ankle replacement is concerned. Kirkup (1990) reports two-thirds satisfactory results in this situation.

Disturbances of the peroneal tendons

PERONEAL NERVE SHEATH HAEMATOMA

About 30 years ago, Nobel (1966) emphasized the possibility of peroneal palsy being due to haematoma in the common peroneal nerve sheath after fibular fractures and inversion ankle sprains. Persistent pain, numbness and pain on movement may not be readily connected with the peroneal nerve. Sometimes a haematoma can be palpated or visualized on MRI scanning and in any event the nerve should be exposed and decompressed.

DISLOCATIONS OF THE PERONEAL TENDONS

Dislocation of the peroneal tendons longus and brevis upwards and forwards from their normal position behind the lateral malleolus is by no means rare, and is apt to recur. The condition normally occurs in older children and quite frequently a snap is felt at the time of dislocation. Most cases begin spontaneously but the snapping peroneal tendons may be a complication of talipes calcaneovalgus. The patient complains of the snapping sensation and some instability of the ankle and foot, and on careful examination of the peroneal tendon when the foot is being dorsiflexed against resistance the dislocation can be recognized (Figure 17.63).

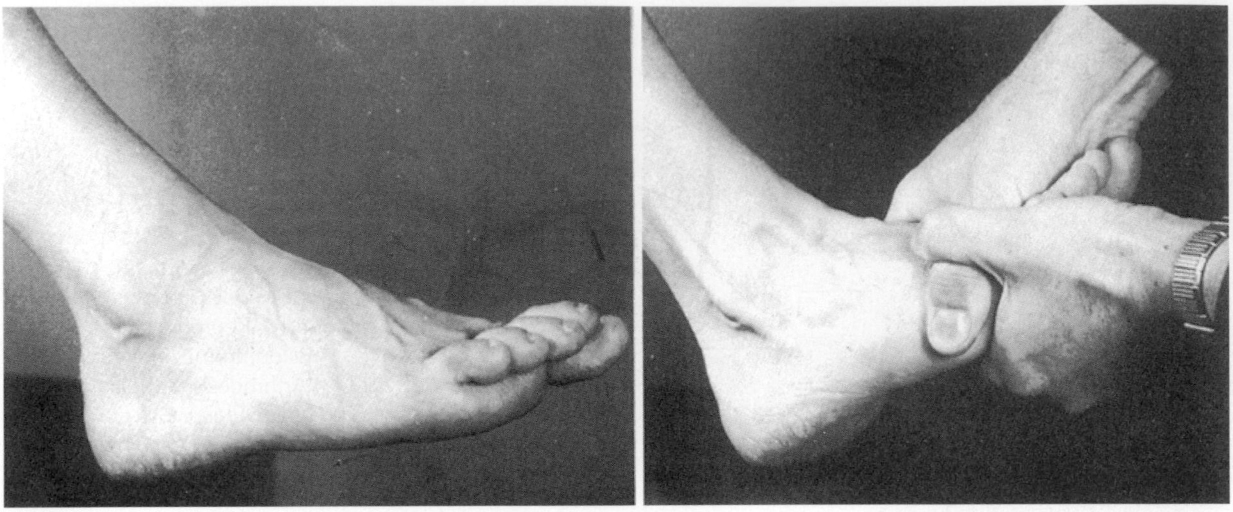

(a) (b

Figure 17.63 (a) The right ankle and foot beginning to dorsiflex. (b) When the resisted eversion of the forefoot is carried out, the peroneal tendons appear and ride forward over the lateral malleolus as a prominent ridge.

TREATMENT

If the condition is symptomatic then surgical treatment is required. The peroneal groove behind the malleolus may be deepened by a sliding graft of bone from the malleolus slid downwards. By means of an osteotome the lateral aspect of the malleolus is separated from the main bone in a vertical direction and then slid downwards about 1 cm and fixed by means of a screw. Watson-Jones described an operation in which the tendo Achillis is exposed and a strip 5 cm long and 1 cm wide is freed from the lateral aspect of the tendon from above downwards and left attached at its calcaneal insertion. The peroneal tendons are firmly retracted and a hole is drilled transversely through the fibula 1 cm above the tip of the malleolus. The tendon strip is passed from behind forward through the drill hole, looped and sutured on itself. This provides a substitute retinaculum for the tendons and prevents redislocation.

Tenosynovitis of the ankle

Tenosynovitis may occur in the dorsal and flexor tendon sheaths of the ankle, particularly in rheumatoid arthritis. It may also occur in tuberculosis but more commonly is of an idiopathic type which resembles de Quervain's stenosing tenosynovitis of the wrist (Figure 17.64).

As in de Quervain's stenosing tenosynovitis of the wrist, anatomical anomalies occur in the tendon masses of the posterior tibial compartment (Lipscomb, 1950). There is pain, swelling and local tenderness with occasional crepitus proximal to the calcaneal tubercle but below and behind the lateral malleolus. Resisted eversion movement will aggravate the symptoms. Parvin and Ford (1956) reviewed the literature on this condition and added two cases of their own with pathological description.

Treatment by injection of hydrocortisone into the sheath may be helpful but if the condition recurs surgical freeing of the tendons is required and, in the case of rheumatoid arthritis and tuberculosis, synovectomy, the latter with anti-tuberculous drug cover.

Drop-foot deformity

Paralysis of the dorsiflexors (tibialis anterior and extensors longus and brevis) and the evertors (peroneus longus and brevis) is common and very disabling. In the West this is mainly due to inadvertent pressure on the lateral popliteal nerve following fractures, dislocations of the knee, plaster pressure and operations on the hip with damage to the sciatic nerve. It is a common complication of leprosy.

In the child or young adult when the injury to the nerve is irrevocable then the transfer of tibialis posterior tendon through the intraosseous membrane to the dorsum of the foot is a very satisfactory procedure. However, this is not so successful in

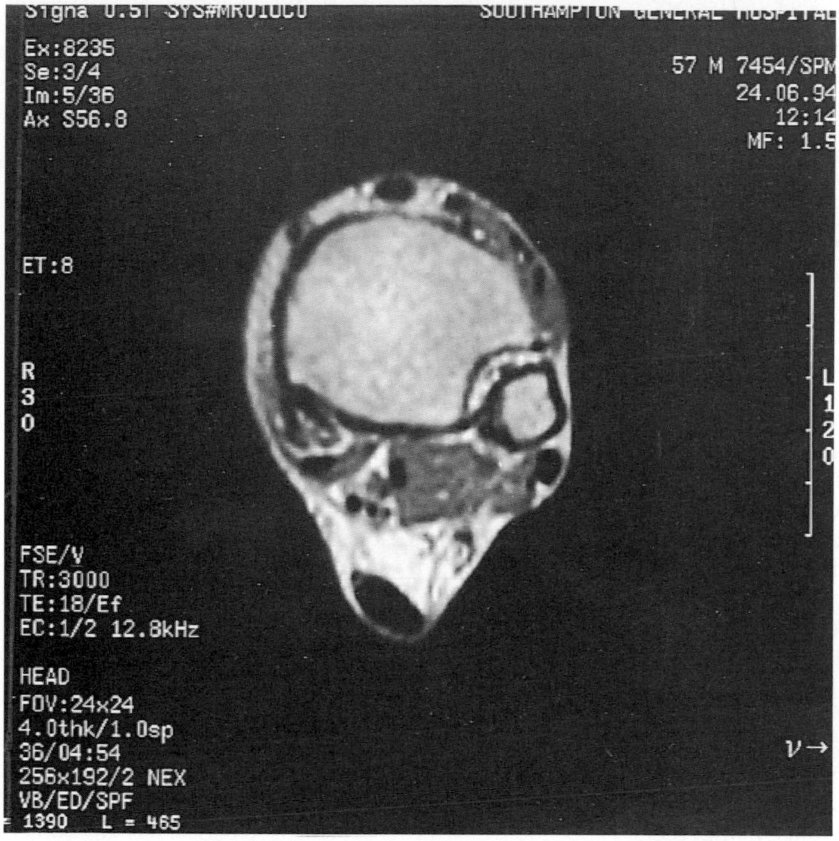

Figure 17.64 Tibialis posterior tendonitis on MR scan. Compared to the adjacent tendons which have a uniform black appearance, the affected tendon is oedematous and non-homogeneous and with a clear line round it indicative of an effusion surrounding the tendon. (Kindly supplied by Dr Richard Blaquiere, Consultant Radiologist at Southampton University Hospitals)

leprosy due to secondary contractures and deformities. Srinivasan *et al.* (1968) described splitting the distal end of the tibialis posterior into two halves and inserting half into the extensor hallucis longus tendon and the other into the extensor digitorum and peroneus brevis more laterally with the ankle held in at least 10° of dorsiflexion and the knee in at least 30° of flexion. They also recommended lengthening of tendo Achillis by Z-plasty. Walking commenced at 6 weeks, following removal of the plaster cast. Warren (1968) described a multiple tendon insertion procedure in which the tibialis posterior tendon is attached to the medial malleolus or just above; the tibialis anterior is then reinforced by the attachment of tibialis posterior to it at the junction of the distal and middle thirds of the leg anteriorly and this is reinforced further by a peroneal slip from peroneus brevis inserted into the tendon from the lateral side. Lengthening of tendo calcaneus may also be carried out.

Rheumatoid disease of the foot

Most patients with rheumatoid arthritis have some foot involvement and to a lesser extent ankle involvement too. It is important to integrate treatment of the foot with treatment of the ankle. The foot may either demonstrate metatarsophalangeal involvement or hindfoot involvement, the latter affecting mostly the subtalar and midtarsal joints. This will eventually lead to instability of the hindfoot with a calcaneovalgus deformity. This usually causes the patient to shorten his/her stride so that the gait is slow and painful.

In the ankle, involvement is less common. It is often accompanied by destructive bone changes. Arthrodesis is the common and recommended method of management, although in a few cases without bone destruction and with subtalar and midtarsal joint involvement total ankle replacement may still have a place.

Vainio (1991), in a seminal article has described foot involvement in rheumatoid disease. Keenan *et al.* (1991) have used the absence of valgus deformity to categorize patients, and to suggest that by preventing the development of calcaneovalgus deformity this will reduce pain and slow or arrest the developing planovalgus deformity.

Platto *et al.* (1991) and Freiberg and Moncur (1991) emphasized non-operative management of arthritis of the foot by orthotic means and braces, and have also suggested that preventative measures early in the course of the disease may delay the development of deformity.

Kirkup (1991) has suggested arthrodesis of the ankle in a neutral position for the painful rheumatoid ankle. He emphasized that surgery for the ankle joint is much less commonly required than surgery for the foot. He also discussed alternatives to arthrodesis in the earlier stages, including tenosynovectomy and tendon reconstruction. He described 57 cases of total ankle replacement with two-thirds satisfactory results.

In the forefoot, rheumatoid disease causes a characteristic deformity with reversal of the normal transverse arch and clawing of the toes, often leading to dislocation of the lateral four metatarsophalangeal joints. The increased height of the forefoot, because of the reversed arch and clawing of the toes, leads to development of callosities both under the metatarsal heads and over the proximal interphalangeal joints. The commonest operation undertaken for this condition is a modified Fowler's arthroplasty, together with a Keller's arthroplasty of the great toe.

An alternative operation is a Dwyer's forefoot arthroplasty. This involves surgical fusion of the metatarsophalangeal joint of the hallux and the proximal interphalangeal joints of the lateral four toes. The lateral four metatarsal heads are resected and the respective extensor tendons interposed to create a tenodesis effect. The results of this operation have been described recently by Rees *et al.* (1994). They reported 58% excellent or good results. A previous series by MacClean and Silver (1981) described an excellent outcome in 75% of cases.

Infections

Infection in the foot is commonly associated with diabetes mellitus and, in particular, diabetic neuropathy. Other neuropathies, too, may allow breakdown of the skin in aggressive infections. Infections may also occur in open injuries, particularly compound fractures treated by inappropriate internal fixation, although the diagnosis in the latter situation is less difficult. Adequate investigation, including MR scanning for bone marrow and joint involvement and nuclear isotope scanning, allows more accurate planning for the surgery, leading to less requirement for resecting bone and soft tissue. The results of investigation in these cases are, of course, very variable but a number of recent studies have emphasized the usefulness of these various means of investigation and some describe the outcome of more precisely planned forms of treatment (Wang *et al.*, 1990).

Pinzur *et al.* (1991) have reported on diabetic gangrene of the forefoot, Anderson *et al.* (1990) on osteomyeltiis of the calcaneum and Grattan-Smith *et al.* (1991) on osteomyelitis of the talus.

Faller *et al.* (1991) have described the primary presentation of Lyme's disease in the foot and ankle and the appropriate treatment.

References

Adams, J.C. (1948) *Journal of Bone and Joint Surgery* **30B**, 506

Alexander, I.J., Choey, S. and Johnson, K.A. (1991) The assessment of dynamic foot-to-ground contact forces and plantar pressure distribution: a review of the evolution of current techniques and clinical applications. *Foot and Ankle* **11**, 152–153

Anderson, R.B., Foster, M.D., Gould, J.S. and Hanel, B.P. (1990) Free tissue transfer and calcanectomy as treatment of chronic osteomyelitis of the os calcis: a case report. *Foot and Ankle* **11**, 168–171

Borton, D. and Stephens, M. (1994) Hallux valgus correction with basal metatarsal osteotomy. *Journal of Bone and Joint Surgery* **76B**, 35

Braddock, G.T.F. (1961) *Journal of Bone and Joint Surgery* **43B**, 734

Bradley, J.P. and Tibore, J.E. (1990) Percutaneous and open surgical repairs of Achilles tendon ruptures: a comprehensive study. *American Journal of Sports Medicine* **18**, 188–195

Brewerton, D., Sandifer, P. and Sweetnam, R. (1962) *Journal of Bone and Joint Surgery* **44B**, 741

Buluco, C., Thomas, K.A., Alverson, T.L. and Cook, S.D. (1991) Biomechanical evaluation of the anterior drawer test: the contribution of the lateral ligaments. *Foot and Ankle* **11**, 389–393

Cockin, J.C. (1968) Butler's operation for an overriding fifth toe. *Journal of Bone and Joint Surgery* **50B**, 78–81

Coleman, S.S., Sterling, F.H. and Jarrett, J. (1970) Pathomechanics and treatment of congenital vertical talus. *Clinical Orthopaedics and Related Research* **70**, 62–72

Copeland, S.A. (1990) Rupture of the Achilles tendon: a new clinical test. *Annals of the Royal College of Surgeons of England* **72**, 270–271

Dwyer, F.C. (1963) *Journal of Bone and Joint Surgery* **45B**, 67

Faller, J., Thompson, F. and Hamilton, W. (1991) Foot and

ankle disorders resulting from Lyme disease. *Foot and Ankle* **11**, 236–238

Fischer, R.L. and Schaffer, S.R. (1970) An evaluation of calcaneal osteotomy in congenital clubfoot and other disorders. *Clinical Orthopaedics and Related Research* **70**, 141–147

Frankel, V.H. and Nordin, M. (eds) (1980) Biomechanics of the ankle. In: *Basic Biomechanics of the Skeletal System*, 179, Lea & Febiger: Philadelphia

Freebairn, C., Scott, G.A. and Neil, R.E. (1959) *Medical Officer* **102**, 55

Freeman, M.A.R. (1965) Instability of the foot after injuries to the lateral ligaments of the ankle. *Journal of Bone and Joint Surgery* **47**, 669–670

Freiberg, R.A. and Moncur, C. (1991) Arthritis of the foot. *Bulletin of the Rheumatic Diseases* **40**, 1–8

Friscia, D.A., Strom, D.E., Parr, J.W., Saltzman, C.L. and Johnson, K.A. (1991) Surgical treatment for primary interdigital neuroma. *Orthopaedics* **14**, 669–672

Gauthier, G. and Elbaz, R. (1979) Freiberg's infraction in a subchondral bone fatigue fracture. *Clinical Orthopaedics and Related Research* **142**, 93–95

Giannestras, N.J. (1970) Recognition and treatment of flat feet in infancy; *Clinical Orthopaedics and Related Research* **70**, 10–29

Gillies, H. and Chalmers, J. (1970) The management of fresh ruptures of the tendo Achillis. *Journal of Bone and Joint Surgery* **52A**, 337–343

Girdlestone, G.R. (1937) *Journal of Bone and Joint Surgery* **19**, 30

Grattan-Smith, J.D., Wagner, M.L. and Barnes, D.A. (1991) Osteomyelitis of the talus: an unusual cause of limping in childhood. *American Journal of Roentgenology* **156**, 785–789

Graves, S.C., Prieskorn, D. and Mann, R.A. (1991) Post-traumatic proximal migration of the first metatarsophalangeal joint sesamoids: a report of four cases. *Foot and Ankle* **12**, 117–122

Greenwald, S. (1977) Unpublished data. Cited in Stauffer, R.N., Choa, E.Y.J. and Brewster, R.C. *Clinical Orthopaedics and Related Research* **127**, 189–196

Harris, R.I. (1955) *Journal of Bone and Joint Surgery* **37A**, 169

Harris, R.I. and Beath, T. (1948) *Journal of Bone and Joint Surgery* **30B**, 624

Hart, J.A.L. and Bentley, G. (1976) Metatarsal osteotomy in the treatment of hallux valgus. *Journal of Bone and Joint Surgery* **58B**, 261

Helal, B. (1975) Metatarsal osteotomy for metatarsalgia. *Journal of Bone and Joint Surgery* **57B**, 187–192

Hennig, R.M. and Rosenbaum, D. (1991) Pressure distribution patterns under the feet of children in comparison with adults. *Foot and Ankle* **11**, 306–311

Henry, A.P.J. and Zafiropoulos, G. (1994) Wedge osteotomy for curly toes gave better results than tendon transfer. *Journal of Bone and Joint Surgery* **76B**, 51

Hicks, J.H. (1955) *Anatomical Record* **96**, 313

Hill, N.A., Wilson, H.J., Chevres, F. and Swerterlitsch, P.R. (1970) Triple arthrodesis in the young child. *Clinical Orthopaedics and Related Research* **70**, 187–190

Hirvensalo, E., Bostman, O., Tomala, P., Vainionpa, S. and Rokkanen, P. (1991) Chevron osteotomy fixed with absorbable polyglycolide pins. *Foot and Ankle* **11**, 212–218

Holmes, G.B. and Mann, R.A. (1992) Possible epidemiological factors associated with rupture of the posterior tibial tendon. *Foot and Ankle* **13B**, 70–76

Holmes, G.B. and Tinnerman, L. (1991) A quantitative assessment of the effect of metatarsal pads on plantar pressures. *Foot and Ankle* **11**, 141–145

Hutton, W.C., Scott, J.R.R. and Stokes, I.A.F. (1976) In: *The Foot and its Disorders*. Edited by L. Klenerman. Blackwell Scientific: Oxford

Ilfeld, F.W. (1991) Ingrown toenail treated with cotton collodion insert. *Foot and Ankle* **11**, 312–313

Inge, G.A.L. and Ferguson, A.B. (1933) *Archives of Surgery* **27**, 466

Inman, V.T. (1976) *The Joints of the Ankle*. Williams & Wllkins: Baltimore, Maryland

Jack, E.A. (1953) *Journal of Bone and Joint Surgery* **35B**, 75

Jack, E.A. (1954) *Journal of Bone and Joint Surgery* **36B**, 530

Jagannathan, S., D'Souza, L., Masterson, E. and Stephens, M. (1994) Symptomatic tarsal coalition – its clinical significance and treatment. *Journal of Bone and Joint Surgery* **76B**, 353

Kalebo, P., Golssor, L.A., Sward, L. and Peterson, L. (1991) Soft tissue radiography, CT and ultrasound of partial Achilles tendon ruptures. *Acta Radiologica* **31**, 565–570

Kaplan, E.B. (1951) *Journal of Bone and Joint Surgery* **33A**, 270

Karlsson, J. (1989) Chronic lateral instability of the ankle joint. Dissertation: Goteburg, Sweden

Keenan, M.E., Peabody, T.D., Gronley, J.K. and Perry, J. (1991) Valgus deformities of the feet and characteristics of gait in patients who have rheumatoid arthritis. *Journal of Bone and Joint Surgery* **73A**, 237–247

Kerridge, G. (1960) *Journal of Bone and Joint Surgery* **42B**, 403

Kilmartin, T.E., Barrington, R.I. and Wallace, W.A. (1991) Metatarsus primus varus. *Journal of Bone and Joint Surgery* **73B**, 937–940

Kinnard, P. and Lirette, R. (1991) Freiberg's disease and dorsiflexion osteotomy. *Journal of Bone and Joint Surgery* **73B**, 864–865

Kirkup, J. (1990) Rheumatoid arthritis and ankle surgery. Annals of the Rheumatic Diseases **49**, 837–844

Kitaoka, H.B., Franco, M.G. and Weaver, A.L. (1991) Simple bunionectomy with medial capsulorrhaphy. *Foot and Ankle* **12**, 86–91

Lake, N.C. (1942) *British Medical Journal* **1**, 31

Lambrinudi, C. (1927) *British Journal of Surgery* **15**, 193

Leach, R.E., Osamu, N., Richard, P.G. and Stockel, J. (1981) *Clinical Orthopaedics and Related Research* **160**, 210

Leventen, E.O. (1991) Sesamoid disorders and treatment – an update. *Clinical Orthopaedics* **269**, 236–240

Lipscomb, P.R. (1950) *AAOS Instructional Course Lectures* **7**, 254

McBride, D.J. and Anderson, G. (1994) The surgical management of hallux valgus and rigidus – a prospective analysis of 1023 feet. *Journal of Bone and Joint Surgery* **76B**, 50

MacClean, C.R. and Silver, W.A. (1981) Dwyer's operation for the rheumatoid forefoot. *Foot and Ankle* **1**, 343–347

McDougall, A. (1955) *Journal of Bone and Joint Surgery* **37B**, 257

McMurray, T.P. (1936) *British Medical Journal* **2**, 218

Mann, R.A., Rudicel, S. and Graves, S.C. (1992) Repair of hallux valgus with a distal soft tissue procedure and proximal metatarsal osteotomy. *Journal of Bone and Joint Surgery* **74A**, 124–129

Milgrem, C., Shlamkovitch, N., Finestone, A. *et al.* (1991) Risk factors for lateral ankle sprain: a prospective study among military recruits. *Foot and Ankle* **12**, 26–29

Mitchell, G.P. (1970) Spasmodic flat foot. *Clinical Orthopaedics and Related Research* **70**, 73–78

Mitchell, L., Fleming, J.L., Allen, R., Glenney, C. and Sandford, G.A. (1958) *Journal of Bone and Joint Surgery* **40A**, 41

Murray, M.P., Drought, A.B. and Kory, R.C. (1964) Walking patterns in normal men. *Journal of Bone and Joint Surgery* **46A**, 335

Nobel, W. (1966) Peroneal palsy due to hematoma in the common peroneal nerve sheath and distal torsional fractures and inversion ankle sprains. *Journal of Bone and Joint Surgery* **48A**, 1484–1494

O'Hara, J.N. and Pearson, J.R. (1986) Arthrodesis of the ankle joint: a new technique. *Journal of the Royal College of Surgeons* **31**, 224–226

Olney, E.W. and Asher, M.A. (1987) Excision of symptomatic coalition of the middle facet of the talocalcaneal joint. *Journal of Bone and Joint Surgery* **69A**, 539–544

Outland, T. and Murphy, I.D. (1960) *Clinical Orthopaedics* **16**, 64

Outland, R. and Sherk, H.H. (1960) *Clinical Orthopaedics* **16**, 214

Parvin, R.W. and Ford, L.T. (1956) *Journal of Bone and Joint Surgery* **38A**, 1352

Patil, M., Dent, C. and Fairclough, J. (1994) Arthroscopic ankle arthrodesis. *Journal of Bone and Joint Surgery* **76B**, 51

Patterson, W.R., Fitz, D.A. and Smith, W.S. (1968) The pathologic anatomy of congenital convex valgus: post mortem study of a newborn infant with bilateral involvement. *Journal of Bone and Joint Surgery* **50A**, 458–467

Perkins, G. (1948) *Journal of Bone and Joint Surgery* **30B**, 211

Piggott, H. (1960) *Journal of Bone and Joint Surgery* **42B**, 749

Pinzur, M., Morrison, C., Sage, R., Stuck, R., Osterman, H. and Vrbos, L. (1991) Syme's two-stage amputation in insulin-requiring diabetics with gangrene of the forefoot. *Foot and Ankle* **11**, 394–396

Platto, M.S., O'Connel, P.G., Hicks, J.E. and Gerber, L.H. (1991) The relationship of pain and deformity of the foot to gait and an index of functional ambulation. *Journal of Rheumatology* **18**, 38–43

Pretterklieber, M.L. and Wanivenhaus, A. (1992) The arterial supply of the sesamoid bones of the hallux: the course and source of the nutrient arteries as an anatomical basis for surgical approaches to the great toe. *Foot and Ankle* **13**, 27–31

Rees, H., Yong-Hing, K. and Silver, W. (1994) The long-term results of Dwyer's forefoot arthroplasty. *Journal of Bone and Joint Surgery* **76B**, 24

Rose, G.K. (1962) *Journal of Bone and Joint Surgery* **44B**, 642

Rose, G.K. (1979) Soft tissue and bony operations for pes cavus and planus. In: *Operative Surgery*, 3rd edn, vol. *Orthopaedics*, p. 894. Edited by G. Bentley. Butterworths: London and Boston

Ross-Smith, N. (1952) *British Medical Journal* **1**, 1385

Ruben, G. and Witten, M. (1960) *Journal of Bone and Joint Surgery* **42A**, 311

Sammarco G.J., Burstein. A.H. and Frankel. V.H. (1973) *Orthopaedic Clinics of North America* **4**, 75

Schaff, P.S. and Cavanagh, P.R. (1991) Shoes for the insensitive foot: the effect of a rocker bottom shoe modification plantar pressure distribution. *Foot and Ankle* **11**, 129–140

Shereff, M.J. and Grande, D.A. (1991) Electron microscopic analysls of the interdigital neuroma. *Clinical Orthopaedics* **271**, 296–299

Simkin, A. (1981) The dynamic vertical force distribution during level walking under normal and rheumatic feet. *Rheumatology and Rehabilitation* **20**, 88–97

Smith, T.W.D., Stanley, D. and Rowley, D.I. (1991) Treatment of Freiberg's disease: a new operative technique. *Journal of Bone and Joint Surgery* **73B**, 129–130

Srinivasan, H., Mukherjee, S. and Subramaniam, R.A. (1968) Two-tailed transfer of tibialis posterior for correction of drop-foot in leprosy. *Journal of Bone and Joint Surgery* **50B**, 623–628

Stauffer, R.N. and Segal, N.M. (1981) Total ankle arthroplasty: four years' experience. *Clinical Orthopaedics and Related Research* **160**, 217–221

Swann, M., Lloyd-Roberts, G.C. and Catterall, A. (1969) The anatomy of uncorrected club feet. *Journal of Bone and Joint Surgery* **51B**, 263–269

Tanz, S.S. (1960) *Clinical Orthopaedics* **16**, 184

Taylor, R.G. (1951) *Journal of Bone and Joint Surgery* **33B**, 539

Thompson, S.A. (1962) *Acta Orthopaedica Scandinavica* **32**, 461

Thordarson, D.B., Markolf, K.L. and Cracchiolo, A. (1990) Arthrodesis of the ankle with cancellous-bone screws and fibular strut graft. *Journal of Bone and Joint Surgery* **72A**, 1359–1363

Trethowen, B. (1930) *Proceedings of the Royal Society of Medicine* **23**, 984

Vainio, K. (1991) The rheumatoid foot. *Clinical Orthopaedics* **265**, 4–8

Wagner, F.W. (1982) Ankle fusion: ask the man who owns one. In: *Controversies in Orthopaedics*. Edited by F.T. Hoaglund. W.B. Saunders: Philadelphia

Wang, A., Weinstein, D., Greenfield, *et al.* (1990) Magnetic resonance imaging and diabetic foot infections. *Magnetic Resonance Imaging* **8**, 805–809

Wapner, K.L. and Sharkey, P.F. (1991) The use of night splints for treatment of recalcitrant plantar fasciitis. *Foot and Ankle* **12**, 135–137

Warren, A.G. (1968) *Journal of Bone and Joint Surgery* **50B**, 629

Weinstabl, R., Stisk, M., Neuhold, A., Aamlid, B. and Hertz, H. (1991) Classifying calcaneal tendon injury

according to MRI findings . *Journal of Bone and Joint Surgery* **73B**, 683–685
Wenger, D.R., Mauldin, D., Speck, G., Morgan, D. and Lieber, R.L. (1989) Corrective shoes and inserts as treatment for a flexible flat foot in infants and children. *Journal of Bone and Joint Surgery* **71A**, 800–810
Wilson, D.W. (1980) *British Journal of Hospital Medicine* **24**, 548
Zeitzelberger, S. (1960) *Clinical Orthopaedics* **16**, 47
Zhu, H., Werstch, J.J., Harris, G., Loftsgaarden, J.D. and Price, M.B. (1991) Foot pressure distribution during walking and shuffling. *Archives of Physical Medicine and Rehabilitation* **72**, 390–397

CHAPTER 18

Amputations, Prostheses and Wheelchairs

J. DOUGALL MORRISON

AMPUTATIONS AND PROSTHESES

Introduction

It is important that both the surgeon and patient have a positive, and at the same time a realistic, approach to amputation. Amputation sometimes follows other procedures designed to save a limb, but should not be regarded as failure; it may be the treatment of choice to improve mobility, to relieve pain, or even to save life. It must be remembered, however, that even the best lower limb prosthesis will not restore entirely normal mobility, that the function of upper limb prostheses falls far short of that of the human hand, and that many elderly amputees are too frail (either physically or mentally) to benefit from an artificial limb.

Nowadays, in western Europe and North America at least, the great majority of amputations are carried out for vascular disease (Gregory-Dean, 1991), and this calls for some differences of surgical technique compared with limb ablation for trauma or malignant disease. There is a great difference between the rehabilitation goals and needs of young traumatic and old dysvascular amputees. Multi-disciplinary teams, of doctor, nurse, prosthetist, physiotherapist, occupational therapist, social worker, and sometimes psychologist, have evolved to cater for the physical, practical, social, and psychological needs of these disabled individuals.

Lower limb prosthetic design and prescription have changed dramatically in the last decade. The availability of lightweight composite materials, chiefly using carbon fibre, has resulted in the majority of limbs supplied in England now being of endoskeletal modular construction. This, plus the widespread use of thermoplastic materials such as polypropylene for sockets (the part of the prosthesis which contains the stump), means that limbs can now be assembled much more quickly, so temporary 'pylon' limbs are now rarely required. Figure 18.1 shows the internal structure of an above-knee prosthesis, and Figure 18.2 a completed endoskeletal limb.

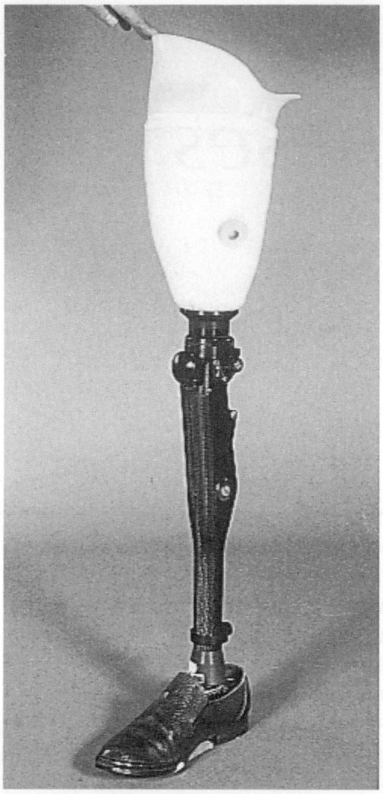

Figure 18.1 Endoskeletal above-knee prosthesis without cosmetic cover (note valve of suction socket).

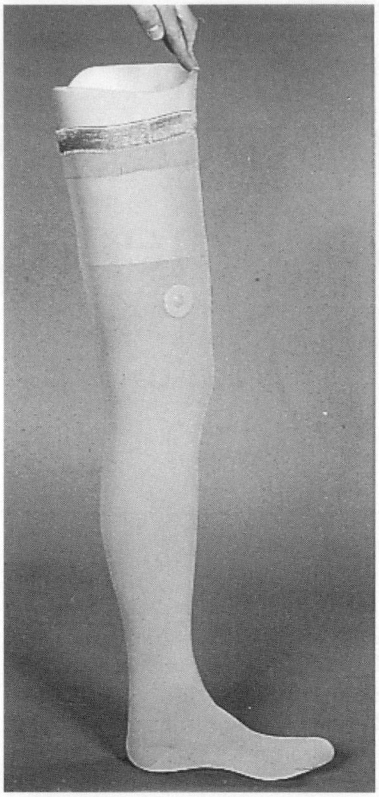

Figure 18.2 Completed endoskeletal above-knee prosthesis.

Indications for amputation

Limbs may require removal because they are non-viable, due to severe trauma or gangrene, or because of rest pain in severe ischaemia. Malignant disease, which is unsuitable for compartment resection, may necessitate amputation, and amputation may be the treatment of choice to eliminate chronic uncontrollable sepsis in some cases of osteomyelitis or neuropathic ulceration. Less clear-cut indications for amputation may occur with major limb deformity, either congenital or acquired, and certain congenital limb deficiencies will require prosthetic treatment in the absence of surgical amputation.

The most common causes of limb deficiency in patients referred to limb fitting centres in Great Britain (with approximate proportions) are:

- Peripheral vascular disease (mainly smokers with large artery disease. Embolism is not common, Raynaud's and Buerger's are rare) – 60%
- Diabetes mellitus (large and small artery disease plus neuropathy) – 20%
- Trauma (especially motorcyclists) – 10%
- Tumour (e.g. osteosarcoma) – <5%
- Congenital (e.g. transverse below-elbow loss) – <5%

In both the dysvascular and traumatic groups, there are about twice as many male as female amputees. Most of the patients in the dysvascular group are in their eighth or ninth decades, with the diabetics typically presenting in their 50s and 60s. These patients usually have multiple health problems, so their assessment and rehabilitation encompass much more than an evaluation of their stump and limb-fitting.

With the improvement in limb salvage techniques for compound open fractures of the tibia in young patients, there is an increasing emphasis on preserving the limb at all costs. However, although this may well be indicated in about half of such cases, amputation must be considered as primary treatment. Georgiadis *et al.* (1992), from a large series, have shown that amputees following severe open tibial fractures were hospitalized less often, had fewer operations and complications and higher rates of employment.

Before amputation

Preoperative counselling is particularly important for the prospective amputee; if the operation is elective, the patient should visit the limb-fitting centre before amputation. The prognosis for future mobility should be realistic, to avoid later disappointment, and the patient must be warned that he will experience 'phantom limb' sensation (feeling in the absent limb, which often appears to be in bizarre positions), and that the phantom limb is likely to be painful for the first few weeks. Unless patients are warned that this is normal, they may be frightened to mention it, and therefore not receive the necessary analgesia. A sense of grief or loss is also normal after amputation.

Joint movements, especially extension, should be noted and encouraged, and basic transfer and wheelchair techniques should be explained to the elderly. Unfortunately, many of these older patients, especially if diabetic, will be too toxic or in too much pain to comprehend more than simple advice.

General principles of amputation surgery

Performing an amputation should be thought of as constructing a new organ of locomotion, the stump (some prefer the term 'residual limb'). In most cases, the stump should be designed with the aim of powering a prosthesis, and the level, length, and shape are all important; it is not sufficient to produce a healed stump if its configuration makes it unsuitable for limb fitting. An extra 10 minutes in the operating theatre, carefully rounding the cut bone end(s) and removing excess muscle, to provide muscle cover of the bone end(s) but avoiding a bulbous soft tissue end to the stump, is time well spent; it can save the prosthetist hours of frustration and the patient years of discomfort. If the aim is clearly for wheelchair mobility only, for example in a patient with a profound neurological impairment, the ideal level and technique of amputation may well be different, as the stump will be used as a lever to help balance and transfers. Through-knee and Gritti–Stokes amputations, which provide better leverage than a mid-thigh amputation, are more tolerant of end pressure than a transtibial, and avoid the problems associated with fixed flexion of the knee which is likely to develop in a non-ambulant below-knee amputee, have a particular role in this situation.

Clearly the chosen level of amputation must eliminate the pathology and result in a healed stump, but when considering the subsequent function with a prosthesis, the preservation of joints is more important than the preservation of length. It is particularly important to preserve the knee joint, if at all possible; even a very short (9 cm or 3.5 inches) below-knee stump will allow much better function and comfort with a prosthesis than a through-knee or above-knee amputation. In the upper limb, it is equally vital to preserve the elbow joint. In younger patients it is worth considering whether plastic surgical techniques, such as myocutaneous flaps, could be employed (normally as a secondary procedure) to permit the retention of a below-knee or below-elbow stump. Split skin grafts, however, should in general be avoided if possible, except as a temporary measure; the resulting thin insensate skin is likely to result in recurrent skin breakdown when using a prosthesis.

The skin selected to cover the amputation stump should if possible have intact sensation. Stumps which lack pinprick sensation are prone to ulceration, because the patient is unaware of the effects of the inevitable minor trauma which the skin suffers within a prosthetic socket, particularly if the fit has deteriorated. Diabetic patients often have partial sensory loss over the anterior aspect of the tibia, a vulnerable area in a patellar tendon bearing below-knee prosthesis, but it is still usually worth preserving a below-knee stump in these people. Use of a supracondylar socket, which minimizes the movement of the stump within the socket, will often solve the problem for the elderly diabetic whose activity level will be low, and the more active younger diabetic can use a prosthesis with thigh corset, so that the loading on the skin below the knee is reduced, but the patient still has full use of his own knee joint.

With the provisos mentioned above, the amputation will normally be carried out at the most distal level which circumstances permit, but in cases of peripheral vascular disease the most distal level at which healing can be expected is not always obvious. Many methods, such as Doppler ultrasound measurement of the ankle systolic pressures, transcutaneous measurement of the skin oxygen level($TcPo_2$), skin thermography and xenon clearance measurement of skin blood flow have been suggested as aids to clinical assessment in predicting whether healing is likely at a given level. Clyne (1991) has recently reviewed these techniques, but concluded that although they can provide some helpful information, clinical judgement is the final arbiter to determine amputation level.

Joint mobility, particularly joint extension, is a prerequisite of good function with a prosthesis. It is important to aim for full extension of the knee and hip before lower limb amputation; indeed, more than 30° of fixed flexion at the knee usually contraindicates a below-knee amputation. Due to muscular imbalance, there is always a tendency to develop flexion contractures of these joints after amputation, and their avoidance is one of the most important aspects of post-amputation physiotherapy. Once established, it is usually impossible to eliminate such fixed flexion contractures after amputation.

Amputation stumps are fashioned by creating flaps of skin and muscle or skin and fascia, one or both of which extend distally beyond the point of bone section. It is essential to cut the flaps long enough to allow skin closure without tension, but it is also important to avoid excessive distal soft tissue as this can cause serious problems with limb-fitting. 'Guillotine' amputation, in which the limb is cut off in one transverse plane without the formation of flaps, is hardly ever indicated now. Major nerves should be cleanly cut with a sharp blade at a level sufficiently high that they retract into healthy muscle, so that the neuroma which inevitably forms as the nerve heals is not subject to pressure, as this can cause stump and phantom limb pain. Accompanying vessels may require precise ligation but the nerves themselves should not be tied. Major vessels should be individually double tied, using a suture-ligature. Suction drainage should be used. A tourniquet is helpful in cases where the blood supply is normal, but is contraindicated in ischaemic limbs.

Healing of amputation stumps is frequently precarious, because the blood supply is so often compromised, and infection is a common complication (Sethia *et al.*, 1986). The use of prophylactic antibiotics against both aerobic and anaerobic pathogens is advisable (e.g. a cephalosporin and metronidazole). Delicate handling of the tissues is essential, and is more important than the particular method of skin closure chosen; a non-absorbable monofilament suture material should be used, but both interrupted and subcuticular techniques are satisfactory. The latter is claimed to reduce local areas of high tension and thereby reduce the likelihood of skin necrosis, and gives better edge to edge apposition, but can impede the discharge of haematomas should they occur. The addition of adhesive skin closure strips may help to spread the tension more evenly. In cases of chronic infection, particularly osteomyelitis, or in a heavily contaminated traumatic amputation, wound infection is almost inevitable if it is sutured primarily, with consequent delay in rehabilitation; such cases should be dealt with by delayed primary closure, some 5–10 days later.

Postoperative management

In the initial postoperative period, the stump should be protected in a well padded wool and crepe bandage. A plaster of Paris dressing is an alternative but there is a risk of ischaemic or infective complications being overlooked. In the past, firm elastic stump bandages were employed, but their use is no longer recommended, as they are difficult to maintain at the correct tension, and if too tight can cause venous obstruction which will exacerbate the oedema they are intended to prevent, and in extreme cases can result in skin necrosis over bony prominences such as the tibial tubercle or the head of the fibula. Patients with peripheral vascular disease are at particular risk. It is recommended that a lightly elasticated tubular bandage, such as 'Tubifast' (Seton) is used for the first 2–3 weeks postoperatively, until healing is established. A shaped graduated compression elasticated stump sock of correct size, which will produce a pressure gradient with the greatest pressure distally, can then be employed if oedema is likely to be a problem. 'Tubigrip' (Seton) should not be used as it is too tight, and, being of uniform diameter and tension, is likely to cause a proximal constriction. Below- knee amputees who are mobilizing in a wheelchair in the early postoperative period, should keep the stump elevated to the horizontal on a stump board; this reduces oedema and encourages knee extension. Figure 18.3 shows a below-knee amputee using an elasticated sock and a stump board.

General principles of prosthetics

Prostheses may be classified into three main groups, according to which part of the prosthesis provides the structural strength of the limb. Endoskeletal limbs, the type now most widely used for the lower extremity in England (though not in all countries), have a central structural tube to which the socket and joints are attached, and this is usually covered with shaped foam to match the contour of the contralateral limb as closely as possible. The foam is in turn covered with a skin of silicone, PVC, or woven material. The load-bearing tubes are usually made of carbon fibre (graphite) or aluminium, which are lighter than steel. Aluminium is particularly suitable for children or upper limbs; when used for adult lower limb prostheses, aluminium tubes can be used in conjunction with titanium for highly stressed

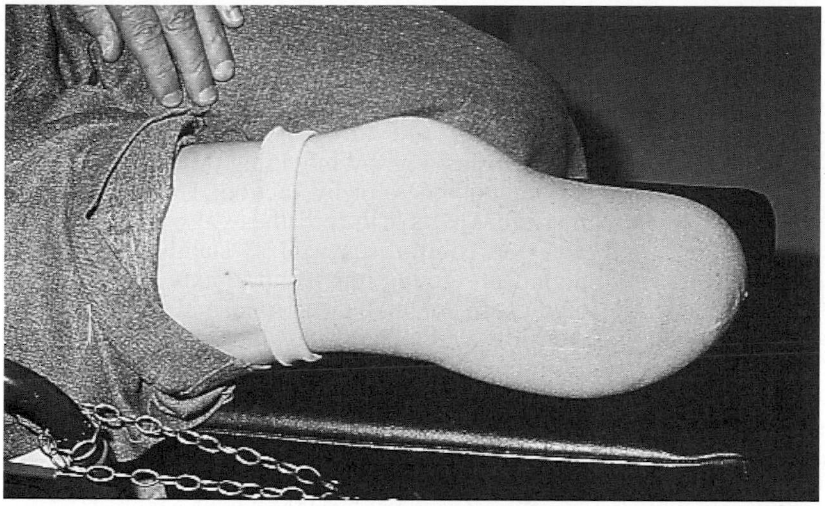

Figure 18.3 Below-knee amputee using a shaped elasticated stump sock and a stump board.

components, such as joints. Particularly in the United States of America, some young amputees prefer to wear their endoskeletal prostheses without the foam cosmesis; this may slightly improve the performance of an athletic above-knee amputee, and shows off the 'high-tech' components within! Endoskeletal limbs are usually referred to as 'modular limbs' because most of the components, except the socket, are prefabricated. Such limbs can be made and adjusted much more quickly than traditional designs. Figure 18.4 shows the component parts of a modular limb. The socket liner has already been formed, and the square on the left is a sheet of polypropylene from which the socket will be moulded.

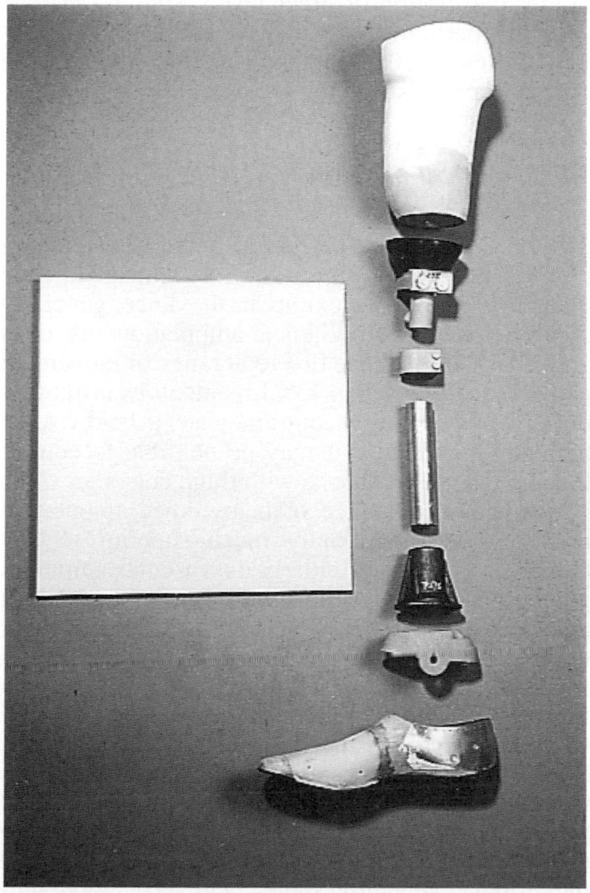

Figure 18.4 The components of a modular below-knee prosthesis.

In exoskeletal limbs (often referred to as 'conventional' limbs), by contrast, the outer visible 'skin' is the main structural element, and such limbs are hollow. The traditional material, willow, is rarely used now, having been replaced by the much lighter Dural (an aluminium alloy used in the so-called metal limbs), or plastic laminates (mainly glass fibre with acrylic or polyester resin). The majority of upper limbs are of plastic exoskeletal construction.

The third type of prosthesis is the temporary pylon, a simple device for the lower extremity with two self-locking jointed side struts ('steels'), resembling a traditional above-knee caliper. Because modular limbs can be made in a matter of days if necessary, temporary pylons are rarely used now, but two indications remain. The first indication is for the otherwise fit below-knee amputee whose stump is basically sound but slow to heal, because all the weight is taken on the ischial tuberosity and thigh (although the skin over the distal stump is still subjected to some traction in stance phase). The second indication is for the very frail above-knee amputee who can accept a poor cosmetic result, because, if fitted with a rocker base rather than a foot and shoe, the pylon is still the lightest possible type of limb (because of the leverage effect, minimizing the mass at the distal end of the prosthesis is particularly important). It should be noted that the word 'pylon' is also used, particularly in the USA, to describe the central structural tube of an endoskeletal prosthesis.

Prostheses are prescribed in the following way:

- Type
- Level of amputation
- Type of socket
- Material of socket
- Hip, knee or elbow mechanism (if any)
- Ankle/foot or hand/terminal appliance(s)
- Suspension
- Type of cosmesis.

In practice, trade names are often used to designate specific components, but using generic terms only, an example might be:

- Endoskeletal above-knee.
- Quadrilateral total contact polypropylene socket.
- Stabilized knee and pneumatic swing phase control.
- Multiaxial ankle and foot.
- Neoprene waist belt.
- One-piece silicone skin definitive cosmesis.

From the wearer's point of view, the socket is the most important part of the prosthesis, since this must transmit all the loads in both the swing and stance phases of walking between the prosthesis and the stump. If the socket is uncomfortable, even the most sophisticated prosthetic components will be to no avail. In general, women are more difficult to fit comfortably than men, because their stumps have less well defined muscles and more subcutaneous fat, and their stump volume may fluctuate due to hormonal changes during the menstrual cycle, and even more so during pregnancy.

Sockets are normally made from a plaster cast of the stump. A positive plaster model of the stump is then made, and 'rectified' to increase loading in the pressure tolerant areas (such as the ischial tuberosity or patellar tendon) and to reduce loading in pressure intolerant areas (such as the adductor longus tendon or the head of the fibula). Various materials are used for sockets, such as polypropylene, fibreglass, leather and aluminium alloy. Plastic sockets are now most often employed, being vacuum formed over the rectified cast. Standard sockets are worn over a stump sock of cotton or wool, and the appropriate thickness of sock must be used to achieve the correct socket fit. No sock is used, however, with suction sockets or myoelectric upper limb prostheses. Some patients find that a very thin nylon sock next to the skin increases comfort by reducing friction; recent developments, such as silicone impregnated socks, and socks incorporating a layer of polyurethane gel, also reduce shear on the skin and sweating of the stump, which is a major source of discomfort for amputees.

The prosthesis requires suspension to hold it in place. This may be provided by a belt, cuff or sleeve. Some sockets are self-suspending, either by mechanical means (e.g. by moulding the socket over the femoral condyles) or by suction. The alignment of the various parts of the prosthesis also has a profound effect on comfort, as well as stability. Rotational alignment around the central axis of the limb, angular alignment in the coronal and sagittal planes, and shift (mediolateral and anteroposterior) must all be optimized.

Surgery and prostheses for specific amputation levels

The most common levels of amputation are the transtibial (below-knee) and transfemoral (above-knee), and these will be described in some detail. A briefer description of other levels follows. In each case the particular advantages and disadvantages will be mentioned, together with a description of the types of prosthesis which are used.

BELOW-KNEE AMPUTATION

The knee should be preserved if the blood supply permits, unless the joint is severely damaged. More than 30° of fixed flexion at the knee generally contraindicates below knee amputation, as does arthrodesis of the knee or a total range of movement at the knee of less than 45°. Ligamentous instability does not necessarily contraindicate a below knee amputation, because it may be possible to control this by using a prosthesis with thigh corset.

The main advantage of below-knee amputation is that it is functionally much superior to any higher level; 75% of elderly dysvascular amputees gain useful long term walking ability over short distances with a below knee prosthesis, walking with bilateral below-knee prostheses is often possible, and the mortality in this group is relatively low at under 10% (Sethia *et al.*, 1986). The patellar tendon bearing prosthesis is easy to don and doff, even for the elderly, and a good cosmetic result is usual. Younger patients can walk with a normal gait pattern, although their comfortable walking distance will be much less than a two-legged individual, can enjoy sports, and have good prospects of returning to work (Purry and Hannon, 1989).

The disadvantage of below-knee amputation is that healing can be a problem if vascular disease is present. Although recent work has shown that it should be possible to achieve a healed below-knee amputation in at least 60% of patients with peripheral vascular disease, and a higher proportion of diabetics (McWhinnie *et al.*, 1994), most published series show that this is rarely achieved (Fyfe, 1990). If there is a small area of skin necrosis in a generally sound stump, it is well worth locally excising and resuturing the affected area; sometimes a minor shortening of the tibia will be necessary to permit skin closure without tension. Because the stump does not tolerate end weight-bearing, the fit of a patellar tendon bearing below-knee socket is extremely critical, and particularly during the first year after amputation, frequent adjustments are likely to be required.

The ideal length of tibial stump for optimum function with a prosthesis (measured from the knee joint line) is 15–18 cm (6–7 inches), depending on the patient's height; stumps longer than this are prone to problems of alignment, impaired cosmesis and discomfort over the distal tibia, and there is no proportionate advantage from the longer lever. In vascular disease, however, the tibial length of choice is 12 cm (4.5 inches) as this will still allow good control of a prosthesis, but will be much more likely to heal. The minimum useful length of tibial stump is about 9 cm (3.5 inches), depending on the build of the patient (a stump this short in an obese patient is unlikely to be successful). A good test is to flex the knee to a right angle; if the residual tibia (not the soft tissues) extends at least three fingerbreadths beyond the insertion of the medial hamstring tendons, the patient can be fitted with a below-knee prosthesis.

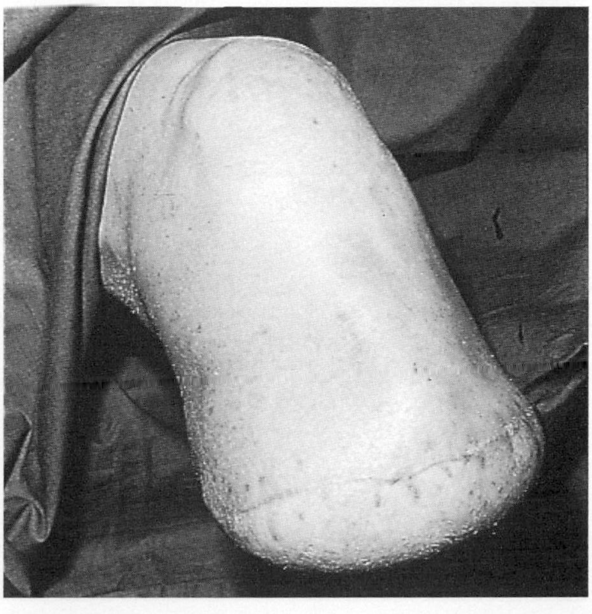

Figure 18.5 Anterior view of healed below-knee stump; long posterior flap method.

The two standard techniques of below-knee amputation, and the only ones which can be recommended in the presence of vascular disease, are the Burgess long posterior flap method (Burgess *et al.*, 1971) and the newer 'skew-flap' technique advocated by Robinson *et al.* (1982). The main advantage of the latter is that it intrinsically produces a tapered stump, and it is therefore easier to fit a definitive prosthesis at an early stage. The long posterior flap method tends to produce a stump which is bulbous at the medial end, unless special steps are taken to avoid this. A bulbous soft tissue end, particularly if there is redundant floppy tissue, will delay and complicate limb fitting; even when correct fitting is achieved, the limb will be more difficult for the patient to don and doff, and probably less comfortable.

For the long posterior flap method (Figure 18.5) the skin and anterior muscles are divided 1 cm proximally to the desired level of bone section for just over half the circumference of the leg to form the short anterior flap. The incision is extended down the long axis of the leg both medially and laterally for a distance 3–4 cm greater than the diameter of the calf at the level of tibial section to form the long posterior flap. The tibia is divided transversely and the entire circumference of the cut tibia is well rounded off with a file, particularly anteriorly, to avoid a prominent end of tibia which would give rise to problems with the overlying skin when using a prosthesis. The fibula is divided 1 cm proximally to the tibia. To avoid unwanted bulk in the posterior flap, and because it is prone to become the seat of deep venous thrombosis, the soleus should be excised beyond the level of tibial section; the gastrocnemius should be thinned, particularly medially, to avoid a bulbous stump end, and trimmed to the required length. A myoplasty is then fashioned by suturing the aponeurosis of the gastrocnemius to the tibial periosteum and fascia anteriorly under slight tension. A suction drain should be inserted deep to the muscle. The posterior skin flap is then trimmed and closed without tension.

In cases where the blood supply is good, and there is no infection, alternatives are to form a bone bridge between the lower ends of the tibia and fibula, using part of the distal fibula, and to employ a myodesis rather than a myoplasty. In this technique, the anterior cut end of the tibia is drilled, and the gastrocnemius is sutured to the tibia using these holes. These techniques provide a more stable distal stump, which may be of benefit to the more active prosthetic users.

The skew-flap method (Figure 18.6) also uses a gastrocnemius myoplasty, and indeed is similar to

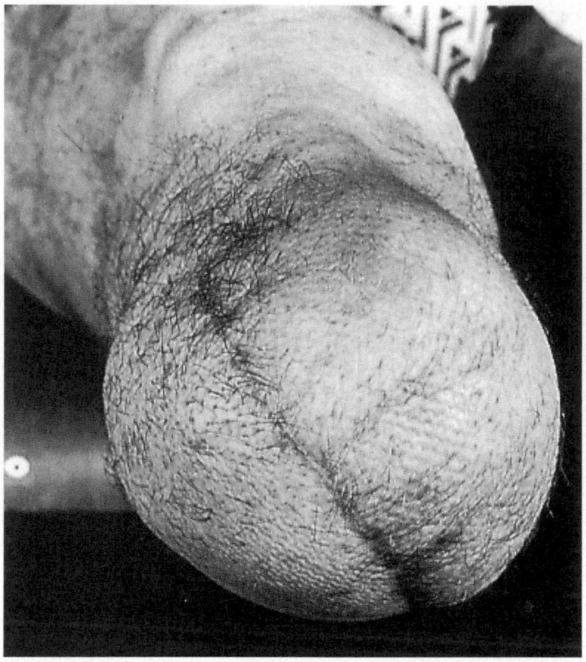

Figure 18.6 End view of right below-knee stump, to show the oblique scar of the skew-flap method.

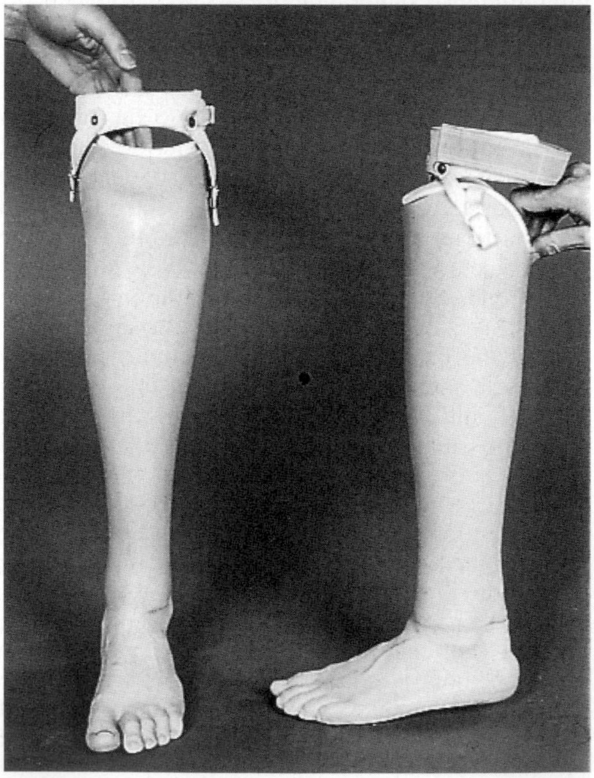

Figure 18.7 Patellar tendon-bearing prosthesis with cuff suspension.

the long posterior flap method except for the skin flaps, and the need to remove more of the medial and lateral portions of the gastrocnemius. The rationale for the use of skewed sagittal flaps is that the saphenous nerve artery and the sural nerve artery provide the main blood supply to the skin at this level, rather than the perforating arteries from the gastrocnemius as was previously thought (McCollum *et al.*, 1985), and skewing the (equal sized) flaps by 15° keeps the anterior scar lateral to the crest of the tibia, and thus it is less vulnerable in a prosthesis. Accurate measurement and marking of the skin flaps is important. The level of bone section is drawn round the circumference of the limb, and a mark made 2 cm lateral to the subcutaneous crest of the tibia, representing the position of the anterior incision. The position of the posterior incision is marked by halving the circumferential measurement. Semicircular flaps are then drawn between these points, their length being a quarter of the circumference.

Most below-knee amputees who are capable of using a prosthesis can and should be fitted with a patellar tendon-bearing (PTB) prosthesis, or one of its variants (Figure 18.7). With this type of limb, all the weight is borne below the knee, the patient controls the prosthesis with his own knee movement, and the prosthesis only places minor restrictions on the range of knee movement. As the name implies, the patellar tendon is the key weight-bearing area within the socket, but the posterior aspect of the stump up to the popliteal fossa represents an important counterpressure area, to ensure that the patellar tendon does not slip off the tendon bar of the socket. The medial and lateral paratibial areas and the medial condylar flare also carry significant load (Figure 18.8).

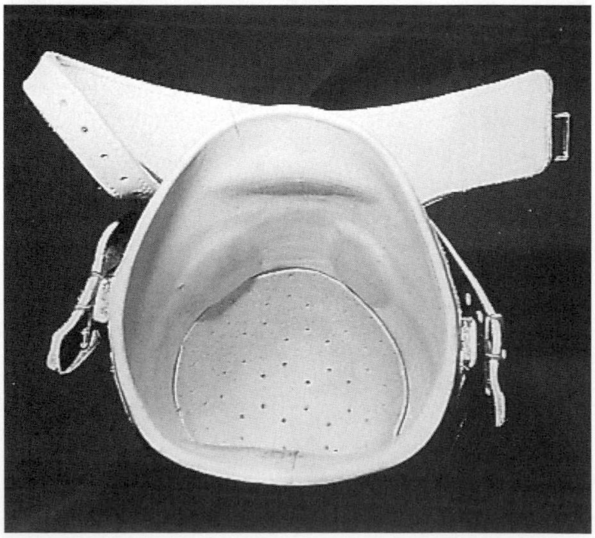

Figure 18.8 PTB socket, emphasizing the loading of the patellar tendon, popliteal and paratibial areas.

The pressure-intolerant areas of the stump are the head of the fibula, the tibial tubercle and anterior crest of the tibia, and the cut ends of both tibia and fibula; the socket must have precise relief areas in these places.

Usually a plaster cast of the stump is taken by hand, after marking key areas, and the cast is then rectified to ensure that the volume, areas of loading, and relief areas are correct. It has been shown that the technique of computer assisted design (CAD) can be used to design sockets which are comparable in terms of comfort with those using conventional methods of rectification (Topper and Fernie, 1990); CAD is usually combined with an automated socket manufacturing process (computer assisted manufacture or CAM), hence the term 'CAD-CAM socket', which must not be confused with the 'CAT-CAM socket' which is totally unrelated and will be discussed later! The main advantages of CAD-CAM so far apparent are that comfortable sockets can be duplicated very accurately, and that local modifications to an existing socket shape can be made without introducing other unwanted changes. In order to achieve correct loading of the patellar tendon, the socket is usually set in about 5° of knee flexion. The socket is made from thermoplastic or laminated plastic, and normally has a compliant liner of closed cell polyethylene foam such as Pelite™.

The traditional, and still very effective, type of suspension for a PTB prosthesis is a leather cuff strap above the femoral condyles (Figure 18.7), but ladies may prefer an elastic stocking for cosmetic reasons, while a neoprene sleeve may give greater security and comfort for active amputees. Many patients can be fitted with self-suspending sockets; until recently, most self-suspending below-knee sockets used mechanical means, by extending the proximal part of the socket above the femoral condyles medially and laterally ('supracondylar socket' – Figure 18.9) or additionally extending proximally above the patella ('suprapatellar socket'), these are worn with a stump sock. The supracondylar socket is specifically indicated for short stumps so that the stump loading can be spread over a wider area, and for stumps with sensory loss, because movement of the stump within the socket (and therefore skin friction) is minimized. True suction sockets can now be successfully made for below-knee amputees, by using a silicone socket liner worn next the skin (Fillauer *et al.*, 1989); such sockets are particularly useful for stumps with extensive scarring or skin grafting. A pressure casting method is sometimes used for this type of socket.

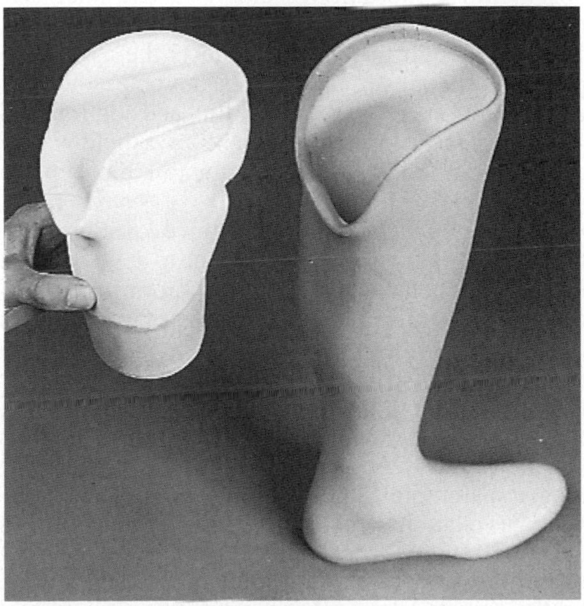

Figure 18.9 PTB prosthesis with self-suspending supracondylar socket (liner removed).

In a conventional patellar tendon-bearing socket, although the distal soft tissues should be supported to prevent oedema, little weight is borne on the distal end; the cast is taken with the patient seated. Some stumps, however, will tolerate a total contact fit, in which case the patellar tendon bears a lower proportion of body weight. Such sockets are made from a weight-bearing cast, taken while the patient stands with the stump in a casting frame.

In England, the majority of patellar tendon bearing sockets are mounted on endoskeletal limbs, but laminated plastic exoskeletal PTB limbs are also widely used. The type of foot selected will depend on the patient's activity level and pattern of use; the elderly require a lightweight foot, the solid ankle cushioned reel ('SACH') foot needs minimal maintenance, multiaxial ankles optimize gait and facilitate walking on rough ground, more active users may benefit from an 'energy-storing' foot, in which the ankle joint is replaced by a plastic 'spring' in the foot (Figure 18.10), while very specialized (and expensive) laminated plastic energy-storing shin and foot sections can be made for serious athletes.

A minority of below-knee amputees cannot tolerate full weight-bearing below the knee, for example because of extensive scarring, the presence of split skin grafts, loss of protective sensation, a severely damaged or arthritic knee, or because the physical demands of their work place excessively high loads on the skin below the knee. Such patients can be fitted with a prosthesis incorporating a leather thigh corset (Figure 18.11), which is joined to the lower part of the prosthesis by sidesteels incorporating joints at knee level, so that about 40% of the body

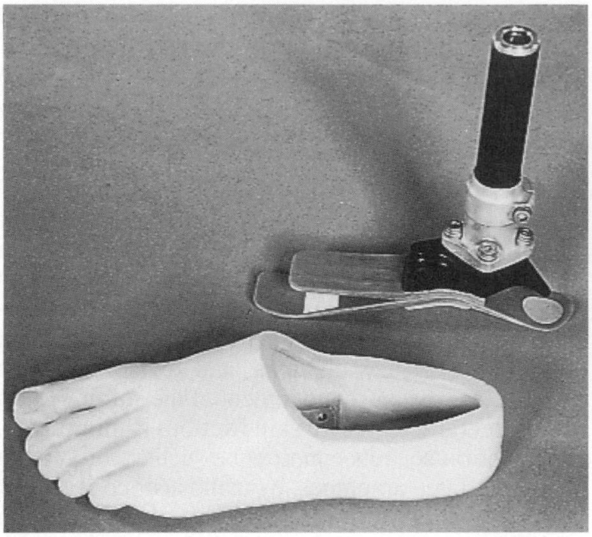

Figure 18.10 Prosthetic foot with internal plastic laminate spring and alignment device removed from outer flexible cosmetic cover.

weight is taken above the knee, but full knee movement and control are maintained. In extreme cases an ischial tuberosity bearing corset can be used to reduce weight-bearing below the knee still further.

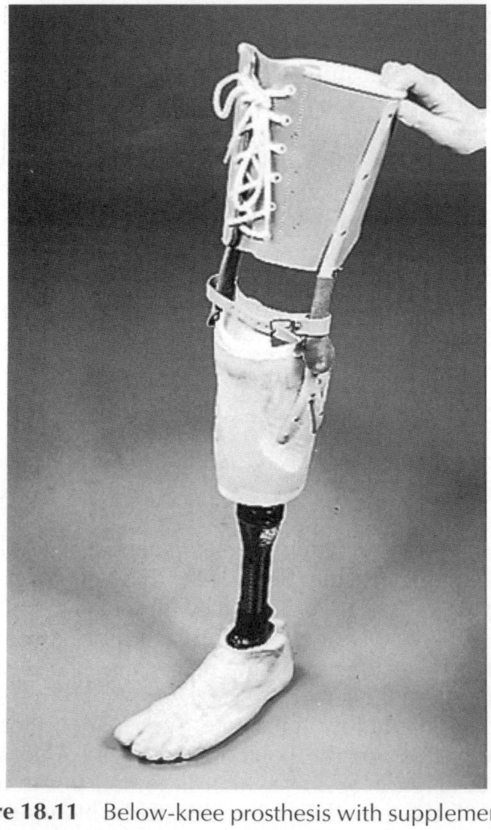

Figure 18.11 Below-knee prosthesis with supplementary thigh corset (cosmetic cover removed).

A thigh corset can be used either in conjunction with a normal PTB socket, or a leather below-knee socket can be used, as in the traditional metal below-knee prosthesis. A prosthesis with thigh corset may also be required if there is major ligamentous instability at the knee. This type of limb is inevitably heavier and more awkward to don than a PTB limb, and should be avoided if possible in the elderly.

ABOVE-KNEE AMPUTATION

Above-knee amputation should only be carried out if below-knee amputation is impossible. Whereas a unilateral below-knee amputee expends about 10% more energy when walking than a normal subject, a unilateral above-knee amputee expends about 50% extra, and a bilateral above-knee amputee expends at least four times as much (Huang *et al.*, 1979). In addition, the prosthesis is heavier, more restrictive and less comfortable, and much more difficult to walk in safely than a below-knee limb. Of particular concern to the elderly, the above-knee prosthesis is more difficult to don, and greatly complicates dressing and use of the lavatory. For these various reasons, only about one third of elderly dysvascular above-knee amputees will make effective use of a prosthesis, and the majority of these will use a wheelchair in addition (Sethia *et al.*, 1986). Very few elderly bilateral above-knee amputees benefit from the supply of functional prostheses, although some may be helped psychologically by purely cosmetic lightweight limbs for use when seated. The early postoperative mortality of elderly above-knee amputees is high, at around 25% percent (Sethia *et al.*, 1986), although this in part reflects the associated pathology. Younger above-knee amputees will of course fare better, but their mobility and comfort will still be greatly inferior to those of a below-knee amputee (although much superior to a through-hip disarticulation).

Unless infection is present, above-knee amputations usually heal well, but are prone to develop fixed flexion contractures at the hip. The shortest length of above-knee stump for effective use of a prosthesis is 8 cm (3 inches), measured from the origin of adductor longus on the pubis to the cut end of the femur. In general, the longer the above-knee stump, the better will be the patient's function, and the less will be the tendency to flexion deformity, but very long transfemoral amputations have certain disadvantages from the prosthetic point of view. If there is at least 10 cm (4 inches) of clearance, measured from the most distal point of the soft tissues of the stump, to the (contralateral) knee joint line, all normal prosthetic knee joint types, and adequate alignment facilities, can be accommodated. This is equivalent to a level of femoral section 13 cm (5 inches) above the knee, provided there is a snug myoplasty and no excess of distal soft tissue. If the stump is longer than this, the choice of knee joint mechanisms is restricted. If there is less than 5 cm (2 inches) of clearance above the knee, even the compact polycentric (e.g. 'four-bar') internal prosthetic knee mechanisms cannot be accommodated without causing excessive thigh length when seated; external knee hinges can be used but these have functional and cosmetic drawbacks.

Equal anterior and posterior skin flaps are normally chosen for above-knee amputation, the length of each flap being approximately one quarter of the circumference of the thigh at the level of femoral section (Figure 18.12). The muscles are divided into anterior, posterior, medial and lateral groups and trimmed as required to permit a myoplastic closure. The cut end of the femur must be well rounded with a file, particularly anteriorly, to avoid high pressure on the overlying skin. In dysvascular patients, a simple myoplasty is carried out, suturing the adductor muscles to the iliotibial tract over the bone end, and then the quadriceps is sutured to the hamstrings, maintaining physiological length. For elective procedures in younger patients, periosteal flaps should be reflected, and subsequently closed over the end of the femur, and the muscles should be located by sutures passed through drill holes in the cortex of the femur.

The ischial tuberosity is the key weight-bearing part of the above-knee stump, although sockets should be of total contact type to spread the load as widely as possible and to prevent distal oedema, unless the end of the femur is too prominent to permit this. Above-knee stumps are cast either by hand or by using a brim system to produce the shape of the proximal part of the socket. The brims are of various sizes, and each is adjustable in the anteroposterior dimension. The 'quadrilateral' brim shape is most widely used, and is designed to locate the ischial tuberosity positively on the posterior flat seating, while minimizing pressure on the inferior pubic ramus and adductor longus tendon (Figure 18.13). In order to stop the ischial tuberosity from slipping off the seating, the anterior wall of the socket must extend more proximally than the level of the ischial seating. The socket is usually made in rigid plastic, but an alternative, the so-called ISNY or Iceland Sweden New York socket (Jendrzejczyk, 1985) employs a flexible plastic liner supported in a rigid carbon fibre reinforced frame, which controls the shape of the socket brim and extends down the

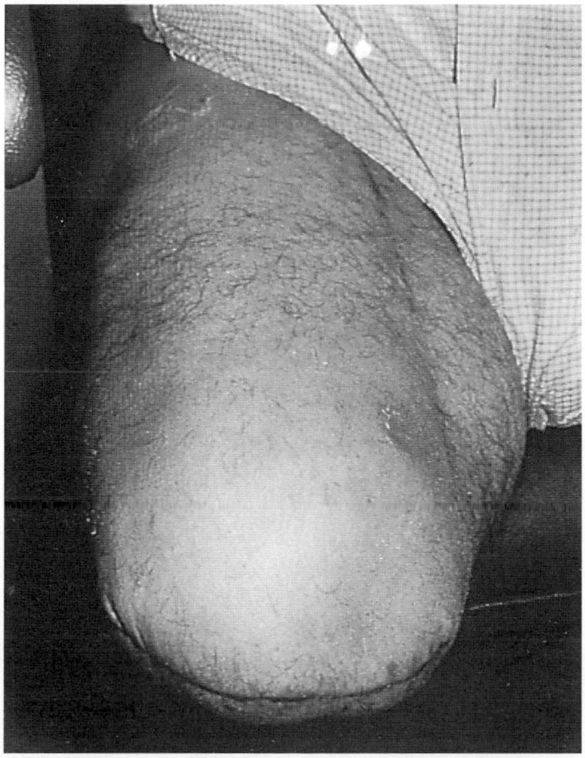

Figure 18.12 Above-knee stump (note scar of previous arterial bypass).

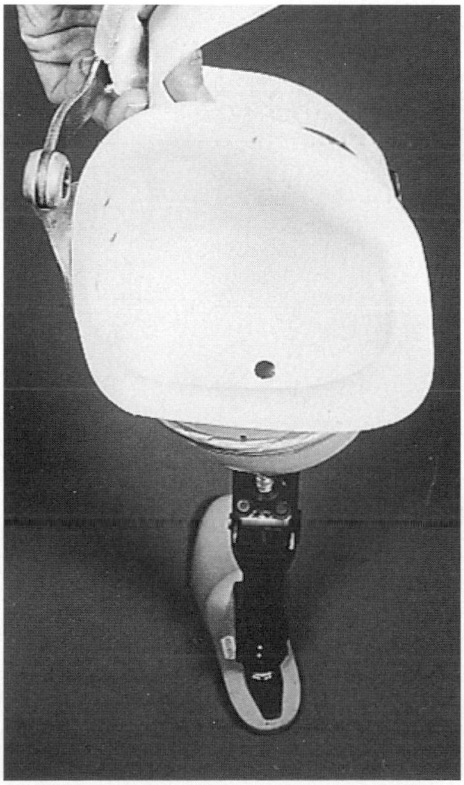

Figure 18.13 Looking down into left quadrilateral above-knee socket.

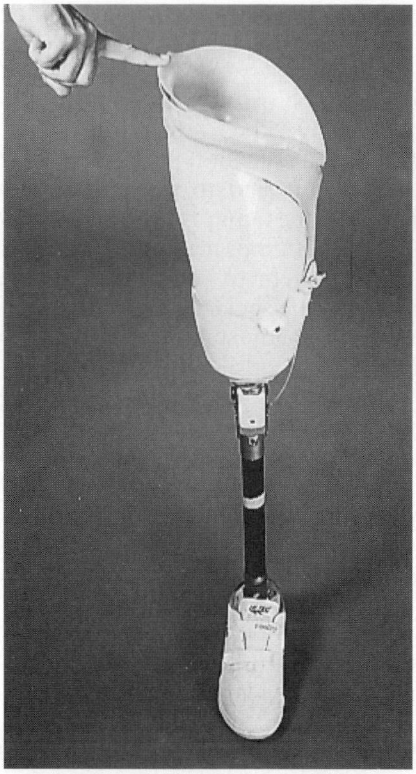

Figure 18.14 Right above-knee prosthesis with ISNY suction socket.

medial side of the socket only as a narrow strut to provide strength and attachment to the knee mechanism (Figure 18.14).

A recent development, which may have advantages for some active patients, is the ischial containment socket (Sabolich, 1985), which is also known as the 'CAT-CAM' or contoured adducted trochanteric-controlled alignment method socket (Figure 18.15). This socket relies less on the ischial tuberosity for weight-bearing, but stabilizes the stump in the coronal plane by providing a bony lock between the medial aspect of the ischial tuberosity and the greater trochanter, and is therefore relatively much narrower mediolaterally than the quadrilateral socket, and the lateral aspect of the shaft of the femur is specifically loaded, the femur being held in an adducted position.

Elderly mid-thigh amputees generally walk with a locked prosthetic knee, which flexes for sitting, but there is a considerable choice of knee mechanisms available for fitter subjects, who are physically capable of walking with a free knee gait. Stance phase stability is obtained by ensuring that the weight line passes anteriorly to the axis of the knee

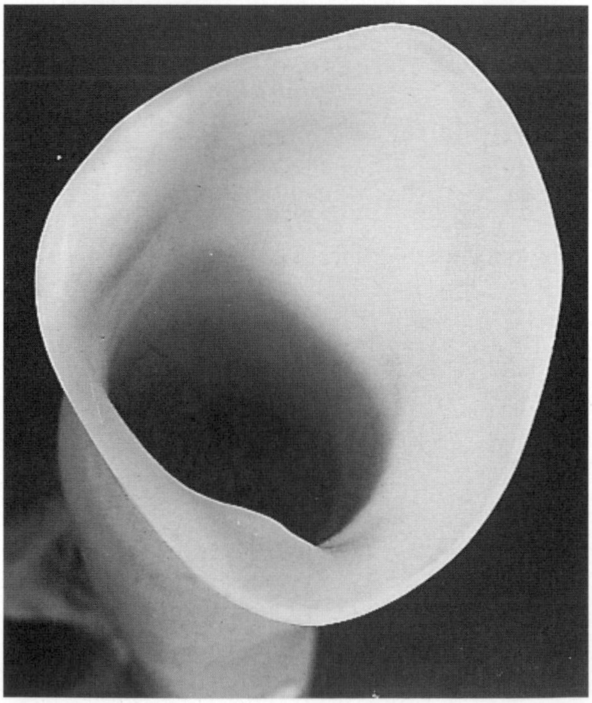

Figure 18.15 Posteromedial view, looking down into right ischial containment suction socket.

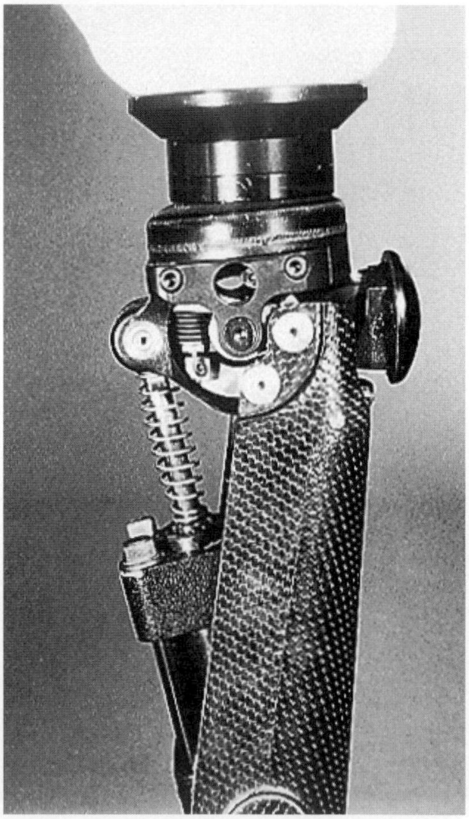

Figure 18.16 Stabilized prosthetic knee with pneumatic swing phase control (lateral view).

joint, but can be enhanced by using so-called 'safety' or 'stabilized' knee units (Figure 18.16). Swing phase control can be provided by simple friction systems, often combined with a spring to assist extension, or by a pneumatic unit (Figure 18.16). Hydraulic units can provide excellent control of stance and swing phase, but are heavier and more expensive (Figure 18.17). Most knee joints are of uniaxial geometry, but as mentioned above, polycentric 'four bar' knee units have particular advantages for long above-knee stumps, but are less versatile in terms of the control systems which can be used with them (see Figure 18.25).

For elderly patients or recent amputees, suspension is usually by means of a soft neoprene or leather waist belt (Figure 18.18), although a rigid pelvic band and/or a shoulder brace are occasionally required. Fit patients with sound stumps which are stable in volume, can use a self-retaining suction socket, which is worn next to the skin without the usual stump sock (see Figures 18.1 and 18.2). Active contraction of the thigh muscles (by increasing their girth) contributes to suspension when walking. Most above-knee prostheses in the United Kingdom are of carbon fibre endoskeletal construction, usually with a one-piece cosmetic cover, and as for below-knee

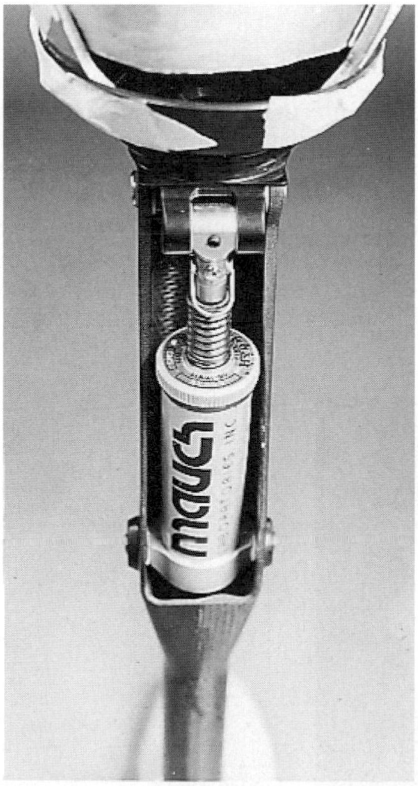

Figure 18.17 Uniaxial prosthetic knee with hydraulic stance and swing phase control (posterior view).

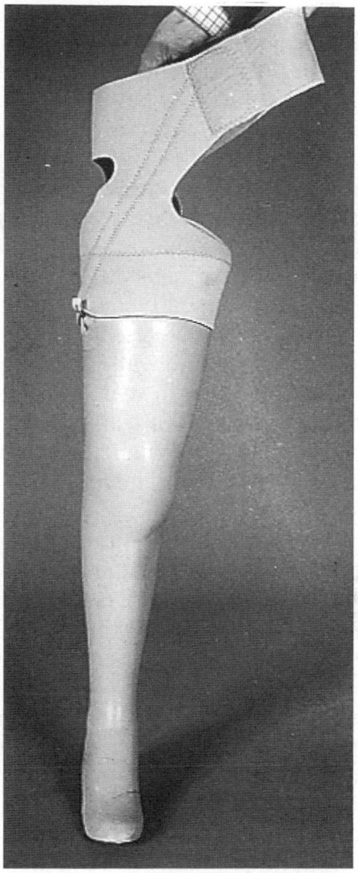

Figure 18.18 Completed above-knee endoskeletal prosthesis with neoprene belt suspension (Velcro fastening). Note knee-lock release lever.

prostheses, a wide range of ankle and foot units can be used.

PARTIAL FOOT AMPUTATIONS

Removal of part of the foot may be required as a result of trauma, gross deformity of the toes, or ischaemia, particularly when this is due to small vessel disease, as in diabetes mellitus. Partial foot amputations are less often successful in cases of arteriosclerotic vascular disease, because the likelihood of primary healing is low, but a transmetatarsal amputation combined with a distal arterial bypass (e.g. femoro-posterior tibial) may sometimes avoid the need for a transtibial amputation, and should be considered in a patient who has already lost the contralateral limb. It is important, however, to avoid the situation of 'creeping amputation', in which the patient has a partial foot amputation which fails to heal, followed by a below-knee which is also unsuccessful (perhaps due to infection of a synthetic arterial graft), and then requires revision to above-knee level. Nothing is surer to deplete the patient's physical and mental capacity to recover, and successful rehabilitation is unlikely. Beware too of removing a single gangrenous toe, unless this is essential due to sepsis; it is better to allow time for natural demarcation and separation to occur.

Amputation through the distal shafts of all the metatarsals is a good procedure, provided that the distal end of the stump can be covered with sole skin. Split skin grafts in this situation are almost certain to break down when the patient starts to walk. A simple shoe-filler appliance, usually made of soft leather with a foam (e.g. Plastazote™) toe section, will restore good balance and walking ability (Figure 18.19). Ray amputations, in which a single toe and its metatarsal are removed, are also worthwhile procedures, for example in the diabetic foot where poor blood supply combined with neuropathy have led to ulceration and osteomyelitis.

In general, hindfoot amputations such as Lisfranc (between the tarsals and metatarsals) and Chopart (in which only the talus and calcaneum are preserved) are best avoided (Figure 18.20). They usually develop an equinovarus deformity, which can result in pain and skin breakdown distally, and it is difficult to provide a sufficiently stable prosthesis without obliterating ankle movement (Figure 18.21). In most cases a Syme's amputation is preferable. It is well recognized that over half of patients receiving a partial foot operation for dysvascular conditions will require a higher revision at a later date.

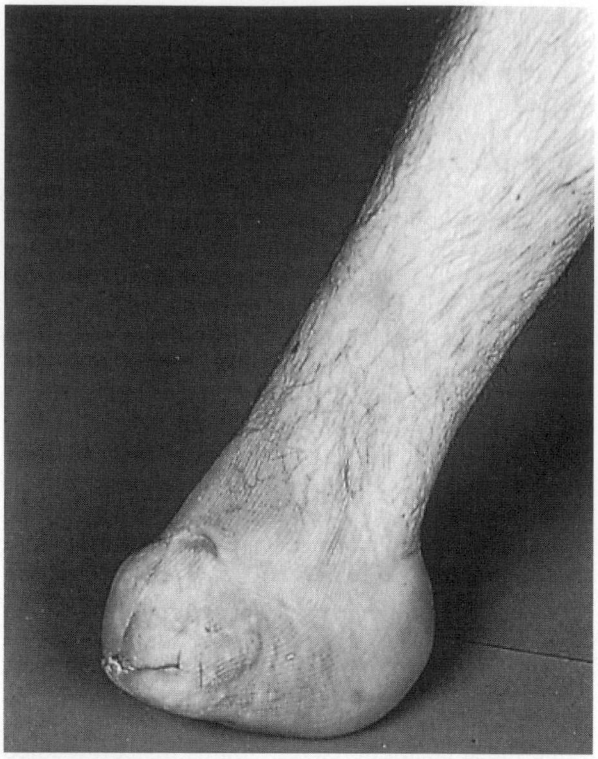

Figure 18.20 Chopart amputation stump.

SYME'S AMPUTATION

Unlike amputations through the diaphysis, amputations through a joint (correctly referred to as disarticulations), or immediately proximal to a joint where the cross sectional area of the bone is large, usually result in a stump which is tolerant of substantial, if not total, end weight-bearing. This simplifies prosthetic fitting, reduces the frequency of socket adjustments needed, and enhances the amputee's comfort. This is a major advantage of a well fashioned Syme's stump, compared with a mid-tibial amputation; indeed, many Syme's amputees can walk for short distances indoors without a prosthesis, and can take a bath or shower with much greater ease and safety. The prosthetic problems associated with bulbous soft tissue at the distal end of stumps have been mentioned in the section relating

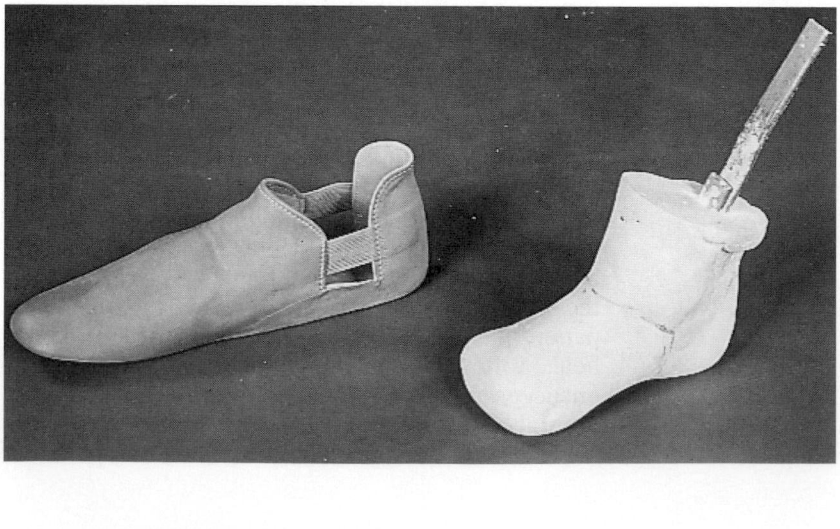

Figure 18.19 Cast of, and prosthesis for, transmetatarsal amputation.

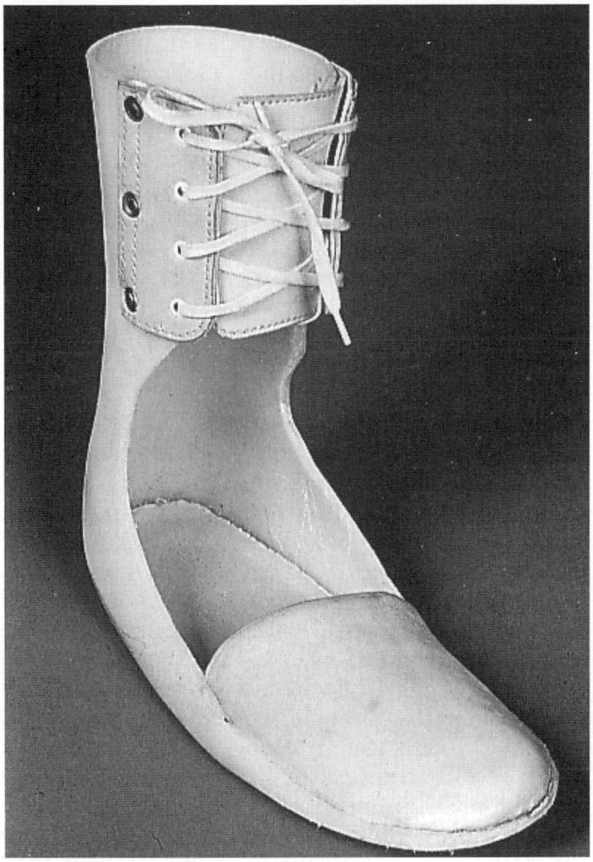

Figure 18.21 Polypropylene prosthesis for Chopart amputation.

to below-knee amputation; a bulbous bony end to a stump, by contrast, is a considerable advantage, since it allows the fabrication of a simple self-suspending socket, and helps to prevent rotation of the socket on the stump (Figure 18.22). An additional reason why disarticulations are always preferable to amputations through the diaphysis in children is that the problem of relative overgrowth of the residual bone compared to the skin, which characterizes below-knee and above-elbow amputations in children, and which usually necessitates several bony retrims during the growth period, is avoided. Another possible method of avoiding the problem of bony overgrowth in the stump is the stump-capping procedure, developed by Marquardt (Pfeil *et al.*, 1991). The activity level following Syme's amputation is potentially high, and when it is carried out for an isolated congenital deformity, the patient can enjoy a virtually normal life, including participation in contact sports (Fergusson *et al.*, 1987). Klippenstein and Lyttle (1992) have confirmed the very good everyday living activities in 18 children at 14 years average follow-up with no pain, although running was considered to be abnormal.

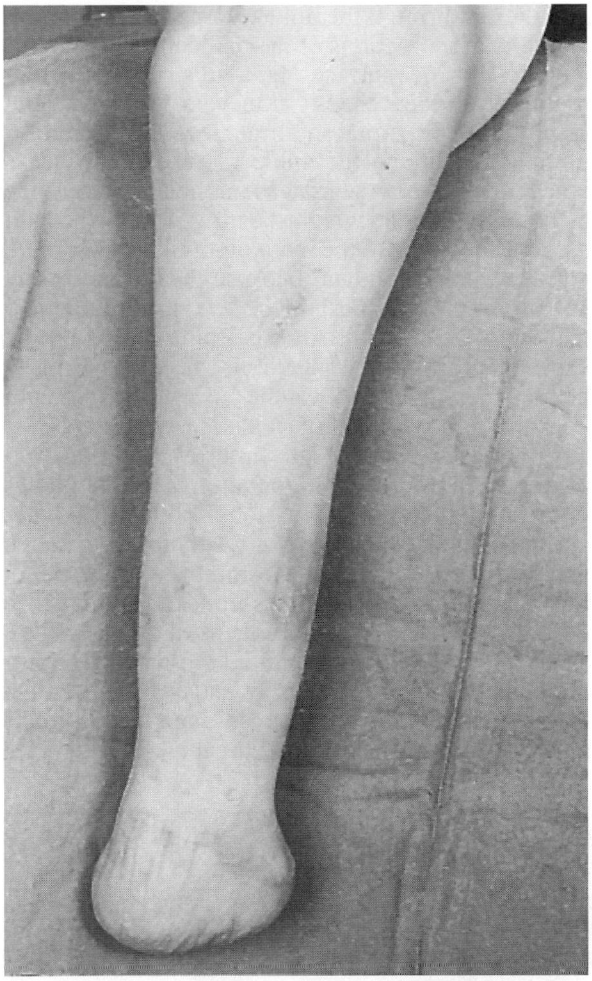

Figure 18.22 Anterior view of Syme's stump; note favourable bulbous bony end and position of heel pad.

Preservation of a healthy heel pad is essential to ensure healing and optimal function. The heel pad (which is raised as a posterior flap) is dependent on the posterior tibial artery for its viability, and it is imperative that this vessel is not damaged during the operation. Unfortunately, poor healing limits the usefulness of Syme's amputation in vascular disease. The heel pad must be properly located at the time of surgery, directly under the distal tibia; a percutaneous pin passed through the centre of the heel pad into the tibia helps to ensure this. A loose heel pad which can displace medially can cause major prosthetic problems. In children with congenital shortening of the tibia, however, the gradual posterior displacement of the heel pad which often occurs with growth (due to relative shortening of the Achilles tendon) is rarely a problem (Fergusson *et al.*, 1987).

In children, Syme's amputation is really a disarticulation through the ankle, with slight trimming of the distal projections of the malleoli, to produce a flat end-bearing surface. In adults, the tibia and fibula are divided exactly transversely (so that the bony end is horizontal in all planes when standing) immediately above the ankle mortice, to leave as large a cross-sectional area as possible to maximize the potential for end weight-bearing. The medial and lateral projections of the malleoli must be preserved, both for this reason, and because the bulbous bony end allows the prosthesis to be self-suspending, and helps to prevent the prosthesis from rotating on the stump. Unfortunately, in adults the Syme's prosthesis is inevitably bulky at the ankle compared with the sound limb; for this reason, some young women may prefer to accept the inferior function and comfort of a mid-tibial amputation, and this matter requires preoperative discussion. Another disadvantage is that, because there is very little clearance between the end of a Syme's stump and the ground, the choice of prosthetic feet is limited. For the same reason, although their subsequent function will be superior, paradoxically the initial prosthetic rehabilitation of Syme's amputees is usually slower than that of comparable below-knee amputees. Syme's amputees cannot use the pneumatic early walking aid (see below) and while the stump is still tender and swollen, it is impossible to fit a definitive prosthesis. The ugly but effective leather 'elephant boot' peg appliance may still have a place at this early stage; a more modern alternative, along the lines of a plastic ankle–foot orthosis, will allow partial weight-bearing. If tibial (or femoral) shortening is present, as it will be in most of the cases with congenital abnormalities, these problems do not arise.

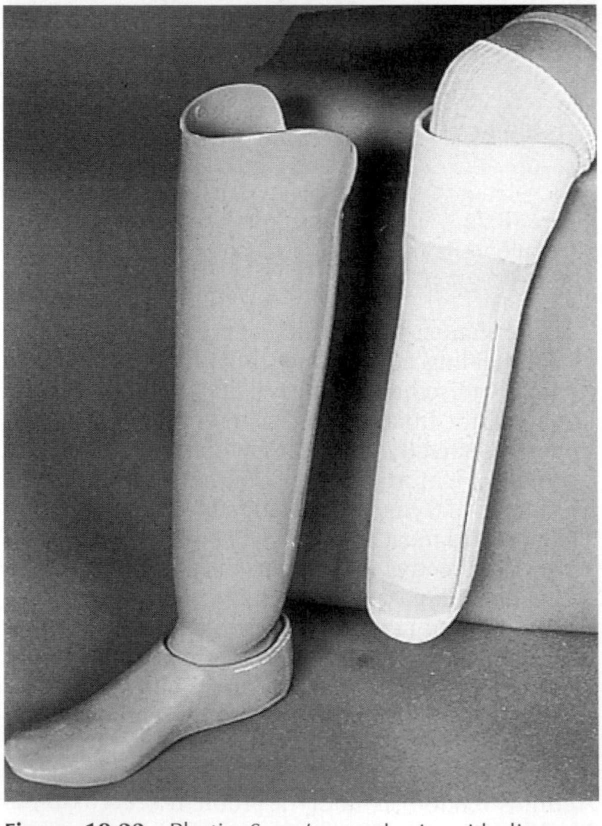

Figure 18.23 Plastic Syme's prosthesis with liner removed (note longitudinal slit).

The standard prosthesis for Syme's amputation consists of a closely fitting compliant liner, usually made of polyethylene foam, which is built up on the outside where the stump is narrower above the malleoli so that the liner is roughly cylindrical externally, and can therefore be slid in and out of the outer rigid plastic socket. The liner has a longitudinal slit cut along most of the medial wall so that the bulbous stump end can be introduced, and then the stump plus liner are pushed into the outer socket (Figure 18.23). Normally the socket is designed for end weight-bearing, but should extend proximally to the level of the patellar tendon to avoid excessive moments over the shaft of the tibia during walking. If necessary, some weight may also be taken by the patellar tendon. A variant of the SACH foot is usually employed. An alternative, which results in a less bulky limb, is to dispense with the built-up liner, and to cut a window in the medial wall of the rigid socket to allow donning and doffing. These prostheses, however, have their own cosmetic drawbacks, and most patients find them less comfortable.

THROUGH-KNEE DISARTICULATION

The through-knee disarticulation has many of the same advantages and disadvantages compared to an above-knee amputation, as the Syme's does relative to below-knee amputation. However, it must be stressed that although the through-knee has functional advantages compared to the above-knee, both are enormously inferior to below-knee (or Syme's), if ambulation is the goal. Most through-knee stumps tolerate partial end weight bearing, and the condyles and patella (which should not be removed or trimmed) aid suspension and control of the prosthesis (Figure 18.24). Although it needs to extend to groin level, to avoid long term skin problems such as epidermoid cysts, the proximal part of the socket is less restricting and more comfortable than that of an ischial-bearing limb. The long stump provides good leverage, and unless present before amputation (in which case a through-knee amputation should be avoided if prosthetic use is planned), the development of fixed flexion at the hip is unlikely.

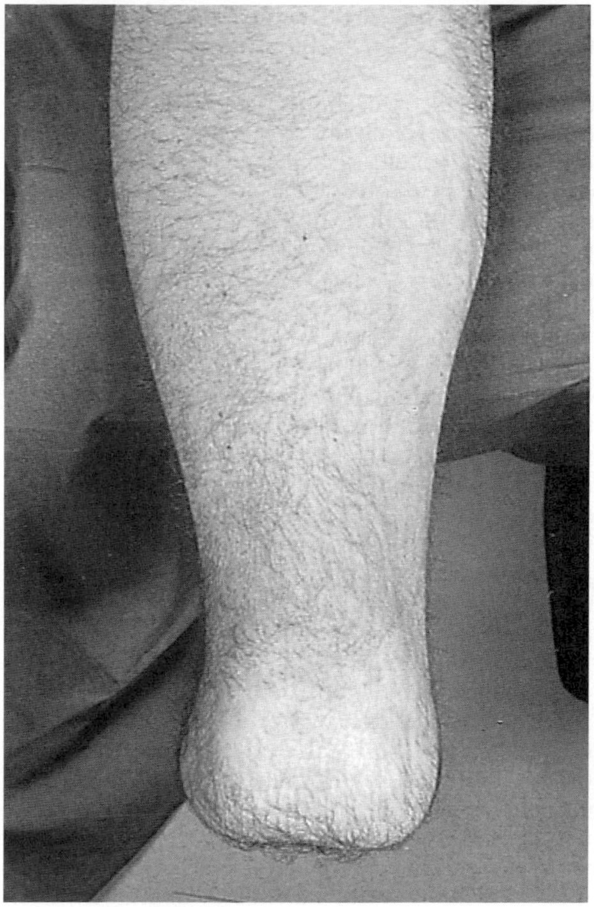

Figure 18.24 Through-knee stump; bulbous bony end will allow supracondylar suspension.

The main disadvantage of through-knee disarticulation is that the cosmetic result with any type of prosthesis is poor, and unless multiple injuries are present, it is best avoided in young women. With an endoskeletal prosthesis, the problem is that the prosthetic thigh length will be appreciably longer than the natural side when seated. This can be minimized, but not eliminated, by the use of a 'four bar' polycentric knee, with which most of the knee mechanism is contained within the shin section (Figure 18.25). The choice of sophisticated swing and stance phase knee controls available for this level of amputation is more restricted than for shorter stumps, but on the other hand, the need for these is less. The alternative is to use an exoskeletal prosthesis, with external simple hinge knee joints, which virtually eliminates this problem, but results in excess width at the knee, poorer knee control, increased wear on clothing, and the lack of a one-piece cosmetic cover (Figure 18.26).

The most usual type of socket is similar in principle to that for a Syme's amputation, with a

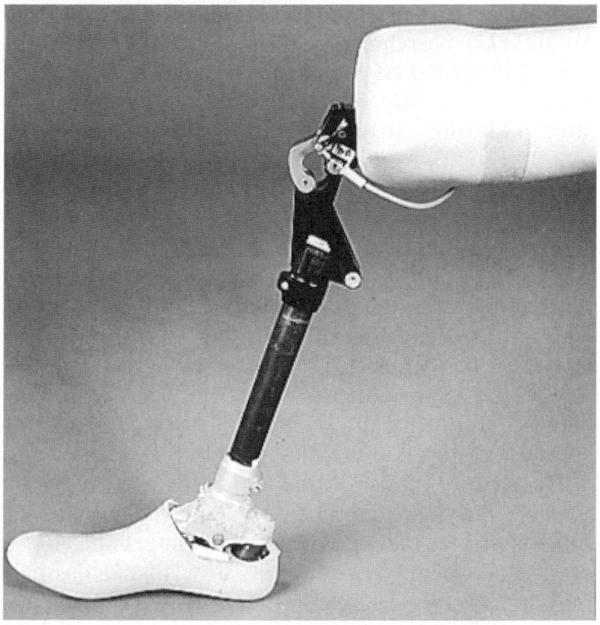

Figure 18.25 Endoskeletal prosthesis with four-bar knee for through-knee disarticulation, cosmetic cover removed. (prosthesis for Gritti–Stokes would look similar).

built-up compliant liner inside a rigid plastic outer socket. The part of the liner beneath, around, and immediately above the condyles must fit very accurately to minimize movement of the stump

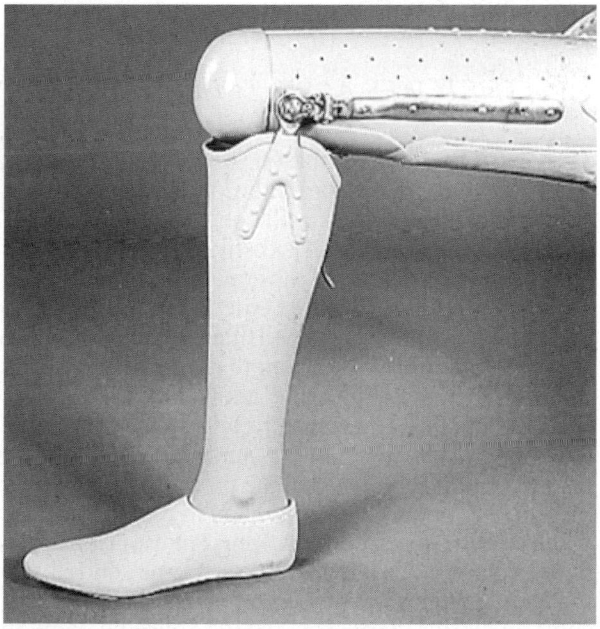

Figure 18.26 Exoskeletal prosthesis with external knee joints and metal socket for Gritti–Stokes amputation (prosthesis for through-knee would look similar, but would normally have a plastic socket).

within the socket, which would lead to pain and skin breakdown over the bony prominences. Alternatives include the use of a flexible plastic liner and the traditional lace-up leather socket. If the patient is slim, additional suspension may not be needed, but many patients require a soft (neoprene or leather) waist belt. A through-knee stump is not normally suitable for a true suction socket.

Equal sagittal flaps, extending 5–7 cm (2–3 inches) distally to the knee joint line are used. Anteriorly, the incision starts 2 cm (one inch) distally to the tibial tubercle, and finishes at the level of the knee joint posteriorly, so that the resultant scar lies in the intercondylar notch. The patellar tendon is sutured to the cruciate ligaments and hamstrings.

Because long skin flaps are needed to cover the bulky condyles, and because leakage of synovial fluid is sometimes a problem, healing tends to be poor, and there are relatively few instances, particularly in dysvascular patients, when a through-knee disarticulation is indicated, because a short below-knee amputation would usually be a possible, and preferable alternative. However, as previously mentioned, through-knee disarticulation is preferable to both mid-thigh and below-knee amputation for those elderly patients for whom prosthetic rehabilitation is not being considered, and may also be indicated for the extremely ill or frail patient for whom the quickest, least surgically traumatic (because there is no cutting of bone and little division of muscle) operation is required.

GRITTI–STOKES AMPUTATION

The Gritti–Stokes amputation, which is quite distinct from through-knee disarticulation although the resultant stumps are of similar length, remains controversial. It is generally disliked by prosthetists and has little place in orthopaedic practice, but does have indications in the elderly vascular patient, in whom it should be considered as a possible alternative to mid-thigh amputation. The femur is divided at the level of the adductor tubercle (the line of the cut should slope slightly upwards towards the back when the patient stands to increase the stability of the patella), and the patella, after removal of its articular surface, is stitched in place under the distal end of the femur. A long anterior skin flap, extending from just above the femoral condyles to the level of the tibial tubercle, is used, with a very short posterior flap. The patella must be kept in continuity with the anterior flap.

Unless skin ischaemia or cellulitis extends above the knee, the healing rates for Gritti–Stokes amputation are comparable to mid-thigh amputation (Sethia *et al.*, 1986), and are significantly better than for through-knee disarticulation (Campbell and Morris, 1987). The tendency to develop fixed flexion at the hip is less than for higher amputations, and the mortality in several published series is less than for mid-thigh amputation, and indeed at about 10% is comparable with that for below-knee amputation (Beacock *et al.*, 1983; Sethia *et al.*, 1986). However, it is probable that some of the difference is because the most severely ill patients tended to have the higher amputations.

Because the stump is of similar length, the prosthesis superficially resembles that for a through-knee disarticulation (Figures 18.25 and 18.26), and the cosmetic disadvantages are similar, but an ischial tuberosity-bearing socket (without liner) should be used, as for a mid-thigh amputation, because the condylar shape has been lost, although limited end weight-bearing is sometimes tolerated. Union of the patella to the distal femur is usually fibrous rather than bony, and sometimes the patella remains mobile and tender. This is not usually a major problem, and frank dislocation is rare.

The longer lever provided by the Gritti–Stokes stump, compared to a mid-thigh stump, does make control of a prosthesis easier, but the main advantage of the Gritti–Stokes amputation in these elderly vascular patients is for the two-thirds who will not use a prosthesis, and even more so, for the one-third who will have the contralateral leg amputated within the following 3 years. Balance in bed, in a wheelchair, or on the lavatory, and transfers between these, are much easier and safer with the longer Gritti–Stokes stump, the difference being even more marked in bilateral cases.

THROUGH-HIP AND HINDQUARTER AMPUTATIONS

Through-hip disarticulation (in which the pelvis is preserved) and hindquarter amputation, in which the hemipelvis is excised, will only be carried out in extreme situations, such as malignant disease or severe trauma. The surgical technique will vary, depending upon the pathology to be removed, but normally a long posterior buttock flap is used, with the anterior incision being 2 cm (1 inch) distal (through-hip) or 2 cm (1 inch) proximal (hindquarter) to the inguinal ligament. Current endoskeletal prostheses are relatively light (about 4 kg), and provide acceptable cosmesis (Figures 18.27 and 18.28). Frequent minor adjustments are usually needed to maintain comfort; through-hip patients take weight through the ischial tuberosity and buttock on the amputated side, but hindquarter amputees usually weight-bear on the remaining

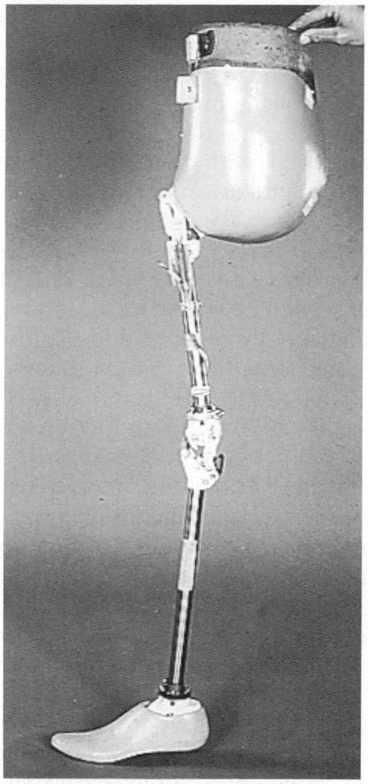

Figure 18.27 Through-hip prosthesis without cosmetic cover; note anterior position of hip joint and hyperextension of knee.

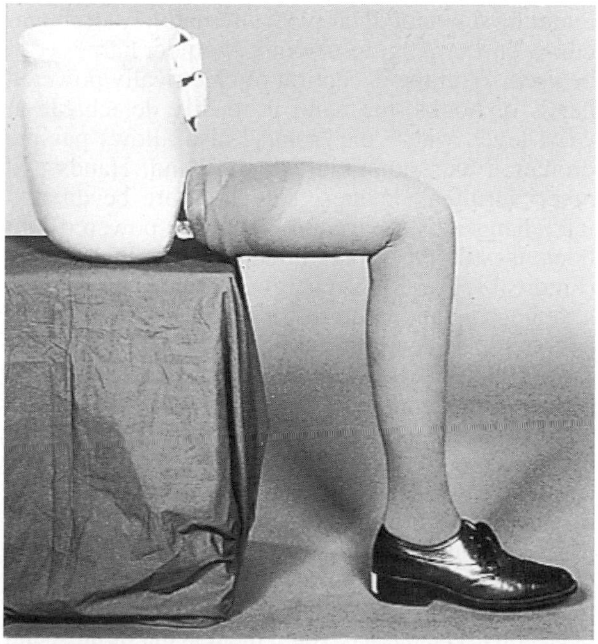

Figure 18.28 Completed through-hip prosthesis in seated position.

(contralateral) ischial tuberosity, although some weight may be taken through the soft tissues on the amputated side, the coccyx, and any bony remnants if the hemipelvectomy has been incomplete. The socket wraps around both iliac crests in through-hip patients, and is normally self-suspending, but hindquarter amputees usually require a shoulder brace. Fit patients can walk surprisingly well with a prosthesis, some managing to control both a free prosthetic hip and knee, while others require the stability of a hip limiter and/or a knee lock, but many find that they can move around faster by using crutches without a prosthesis.

Sherman and Duthie (1960) described a modified hemipelvectomy with preservation of the pubic bones and upper iliac leaf for malignant tumours of the upper femur, involving the hip joint. It allows excision to be within the compartment but produces less deformity and dysfunction as well as complications.

OUTCOME OF AMPUTATION

Amputation with prosthetic fitting is an important therapeutic procedure even in the elderly. De Luccia *et al.* (1992), from a follow-up study of 128 lower limb amputees over an 8-year period, described the importance of preserving the knee. Vascular disease was the main cause for amputation; over 60% of bilateral lower limb amputees used their prostheses successfully. When carried out for diabetes the mortality rate was six times greater. Pinzur *et al.* (1993), from a multicentre study, found that over a 3-year period 87% were still using their prostheses even though 29% were bilateral, when the life expectancy of this latter group was about 36%, most having died within two years.

THE HAND

Whereas the main functions of the lower limb are to support the body weight, and to provide locomotion, that is to position the individual in the environment, the main function of the hand is to interact with and influence that environment, by means of tactile sensation and the performance of manipulative tasks. The function of the rest of the upper limb is to place the hand optimally with respect to the individual. Upper limb prostheses can provide grip, but only very limited (proprioceptive) sensation, and their movements are crude compared with the delicate and complex movements of which the natural hand is capable. As little as possible of the hand should be removed; unless it is devoid of both movement and sensation, even a severely mutilated hand is worth preserving. Loss of a single finger is mainly a cosmetic problem, unless one is a musician, but loss of a thumb is very serious, since pinch grip is lost. A prosthetic opposition post can be very helpful, but as much natural skin as possible should be left exposed to minimize sensory impairment. Even if all the digits are lost the residual part of the hand should be preserved; if the wrist joint is functional, sensate pinch grip can be restored by means of an opposition plate attached immediately above the wrist. Cosmetic partial hand prostheses can help psychologically, but in general impair function.

Unlike the lower limb, trauma accounts for the majority of upper limb amputations, and congenital loss is the other major reason for requiring an upper extremity prosthesis. Industrial injuries are usually isolated, but upper limb injuries sustained in motor cycle accidents, which result in amputation, are frequently associated with head, spinal or brachial plexus injuries, and with fractures elsewhere, with corresponding effects on the patient's overall rehabilitation.

Because of the relatively recent development of microvascular replantation and revascularization techniques, fewer amputations – particularly in the upper limbs – are being carried out. Ipsen *et al.* (1990) have reviewed after 4.5 years, a small series of patients who had replantation of various components of the upper limb – e.g. half were above the elbow. There was an 85% survival rate with four patients requiring subsequent amputation. Over half of all patients had an excellent result with a much greater functional level of activity than when compared with four amputees with prostheses.

THROUGH-WRIST DISARTICULATION

Loss of a mobile wrist joint is a serious problem. Through-wrist disarticulation has the theoretical advantage over mid-forearm (below-elbow) amputation of preserving supination and pronation, but there is insufficient space to incorporate the newer types of functional hand and cosmesis tends to be poor. Good function, can, however be achieved with a split hook.

BELOW-ELBOW AMPUTATION

Just as it is vital to preserve the knee joint whenever possible, so it is justified to go to extreme lengths to save the elbow joint. Because the loads imposed on the stump are not as great in the upper limb and the blood supply is usually good, it is easier to find suitable skin cover, although anaesthetic skin will still be at risk of breakdown. Muscle transfers, free myocutaneous flaps and split skin grafts are all worth considering if at least 8 cm (3 inches) of ulna remain, measured from the tip of the olecranon. This is equivalent to about 4 cm (1.5 inches) of stump on the flexor aspect beyond the insertion of the biceps tendon, measured with the elbow flexed to 90°. No major problem arises if the radius cannot be preserved.

The optimum level of below-elbow amputation, which will provide a strong lever and at the same time leave sufficient space to incorporate the full range of both body-powered and electrically powered hands and other terminal appliances, is 9 cm (3.5 inches) above the wrist joint. This is roughly at the junction of the middle and distal thirds of the forearm. The choice of skin flaps may be determined by the site of injury, but ideally equal flaps, extending some 4 cm (1.5 inches) beyond the level of bone section, on the flexor and extensor aspects, with the forearm midway between supination and pronation, are used. It is best to divide the more mobile radius before the ulna, the cut bone ends must be well rounded with a file to eliminate any sharp edges, and the muscles are sutured over the bone ends so that they do not retract leaving the bone ends subcutaneously. Particularly in the proximal forearm, care should be taken to avoid excessive or loosely attached muscles, which could hinder prosthetic fitting.

The prosthesis and socket are usually of plastic laminate construction; a liner is not normally used, but the arm is worn over a cotton sock (Figure 18.29). In favourable cases the socket can be of self-retaining supracondylar type; alternatively an above-elbow cuff or a figure-of-eight shoulder harness can be used. With the exception of electrically powered hands or hooks, the hand is readily detachable at wrist level, where the 'rotary' also allows passive pronation and supination of the hand. Hands and other 'terminal devices' can therefore be quickly interchanged by the wearer. The body-powered split hook is still the most functional terminal device (Figure 18.30). It is very light, provides precise yet strong grip, and requires little physical effort to operate. The mobile half of the split hook is connected, via the operating cord which passes round the patient's back to a loop which lies in the contralateral axilla. Shoulder flexion tightens the operating cord and opens the hook ('voluntary opening'), which is passively closed by graduated elastic bands; extra bands are added for a stronger grip. 'Voluntary closing' grippers are favoured by some users. Many patients prefer to exchange the hook or gripper for a cosmetic hand for social occasions. The passive foam hand is the lightest and most natural in appearance but has no active movement, whereas the mechanical hand provides an

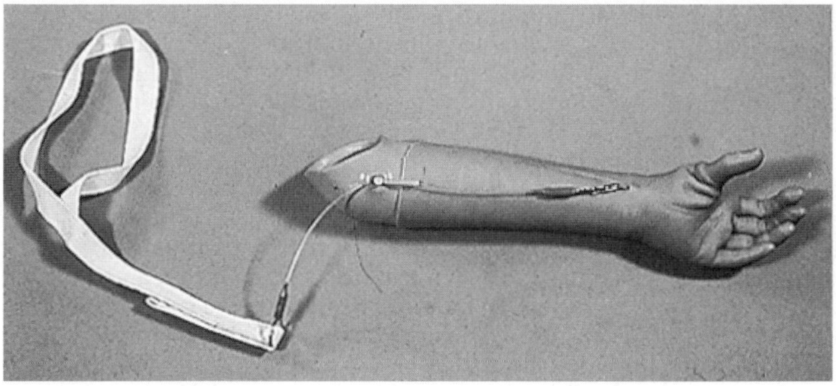

Figure 18.29 Below-elbow prosthesis with mechanical hand; note the operating cord with shoulder loop.

active three-point grip between the thumb and the index and middle fingers. The mechanical hand, however, requires considerably more effort to operate than the split hook, provides a less precise grip, and is heavier than the hook or the passive hand. A variety of terminal appliances is available to assist specific tasks, such as driving, gardening, typing, sports and workshop activities. Some patients only use their arm prosthesis for cosmetic purposes, in which case a very light one-piece arm with a more natural wrist shape (the standard prosthetic wrist is round to allow rotation) can be supplied.

The myoelectric hand has the advantage of not requiring the use of any physical effort or unphysiological movement to operate it, nor does it need an operating cord. Electrical signals are picked up by skin electrodes placed close to the common flexor and common extensor origins within the socket, which is worn without a stump sock. A self-suspending socket is normally used so the prosthesis requires no appendages, except in the case of small children who need to carry the battery remotely (Figure 18.31). The electric hand provides similar movements to the mechanical hand, that is a three point grip, although powered wrist rotation is also now possible, and electrically powered split hooks (or 'grippers') have recently become available. The disadvantages of electrically powered hands are that they are heavy, cannot be fitted to long forearm stumps, need more maintenance and are much more costly than simpler appliances, and lack the proprioceptive feedback of a body-powered hook or hand.

THROUGH-ELBOW DISARTICULATION

Through-elbow disarticulation is rarely undertaken. The function with or without a prosthesis is much poorer than for the below-elbow level, and the prosthesis is less satisfactory than that for an above-elbow amputation in that it is less attractive, being bulkier and having external elbow hinges with a less satisfactory locking arrangement. It also lacks the ability to rotate the elbow on the distal forearm, with which the above-elbow prosthesis compensates for shoulder rotation, which is restricted by the pros-

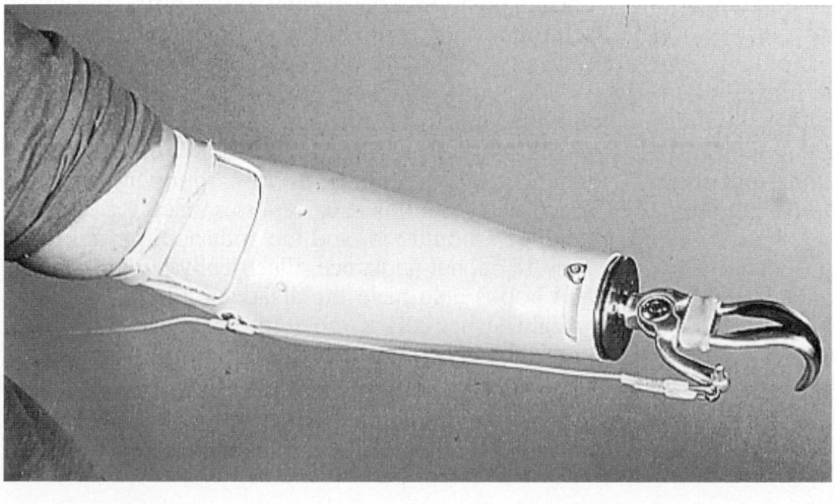

Figure 18.30 Below-elbow prosthesis with split hook and self-retaining socket.

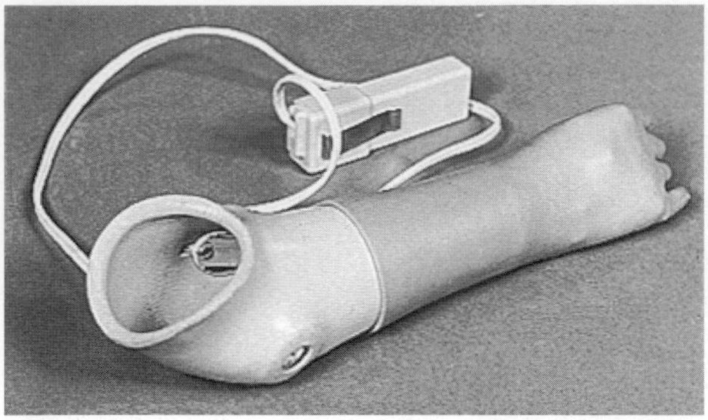

Figure 18.31 Child's myoelectric below-elbow prosthesis; note electrodes and remote battery.

thetic socket. However, the through-elbow stump does provide extra length and leverage, and in some cases it is possible to suspend the limb above the humeral condyles (usually by means of a leather socket) so that a simpler harness can be used. It should be considered, as an alternative to the above-elbow level, for those patients who want to return to heavy work and are prepared to accept inferior cosmesis.

ABOVE-ELBOW AMPUTATION

Above-elbow amputation is most frequently required because of trauma, in which case the aim is normally to retain as much length as possible, and to use whatever skin is available for closure. However, if there is less than 9 cm (3.5 inches) of clearance between the end of the stump and the tip of the olecranon (measured with the elbow flexed to a right angle), the optimal type of prosthetic elbow mechanism cannot be used without adversely affecting cosmesis. Ideally, equal anterior and posterior flaps should be used, their length beyond the level of bone section being approximately one-quarter of the circumference of the arm. In a similar way to other levels, the end of the humerus must be well rounded with a file, a myoplasty should be performed by suturing biceps to triceps, and a bulbous soft tissue end to the stump should be avoided. Postoperative shoulder exercises are important as stiffness is likely, and will impair long-term function. The minimum length of stump for functional use of an above-elbow prosthesis is one in which the distal end of the residual humerus extends three fingerbreadths beyond the anterior axillary fold, measured with the arm at the side. However, even the humeral head is worth preserving, as it maintains the normal shoulder contour so that clothes hang more naturally than after a through-shoulder disarticulation.

Not infrequently, an injury to the brachial plexus coexists with the need to carry out an above-elbow amputation. In this situation, function with a prosthesis is likely to be poor, due to the combination of little or no power, muscle wasting making the skin overlying the bony prominences vulnerable, and sensory loss. If good scapular movements are preserved, there is some advantage in arthrodesis of the glenohumeral joint. Brachial plexus injury on its own, however, is no longer considered an indication for amputation.

The prosthesis for above-elbow amputation is much heavier and bulkier than that for below-elbow loss, considerably more difficult to learn to use to the full, and the likely functional outcome is poorer and more variable (Figure 18.32). Thus the very well motivated individual who needs to maintain bimanual activities for work or hobbies can achieve surprisingly good function, but many above-elbow amputees only use a prosthesis for cosmetic purposes (Millstein *et al.*, 1986). Functional prostheses are normally of plastic exoskeletal construction, but if the arm is only required for cosmetic purposes endoskeletal limbs provide a better appearance and are slightly lighter. The socket, made of plastic or leather, normally has to extend over the top of the shoulder to provide sufficient comfort and stability, and this restricts shoulder movements. The limb is suspended by a figure-of-eight harness passing round the back to the contralateral axilla. The operating cord controls the hand or other terminal appliance in a similar manner to that for a below-elbow amputee, but in addition controls elbow flexion. Elbow extension is produced by gravity. In order to operate the terminal device without producing unwanted elbow flexion, the elbow needs to be locked. This is done by means of an additional control strap on the anterior aspect of the upper arm, which is tightened by a sharp extension movement of the shoulder, which alternately locks and then unlocks the elbow in the chosen position. This means of controlling the elbow requires considerable skill, and many patients prefer to use the sound hand to operate the lock.

The same range of hands and other terminal appliances can be fitted to the above-elbow prosthesis as to the below-elbow, but because of the weight and the effort needed to operate it, the mechanical hand is usually less satisfactory for this level of amputation, and the split hook remains the best functional appliance. Electrically powered hands and hooks also have the disadvantage of excessive weight, especially if the stump is short, but have a particular advantage in that the means of operating the hand and the elbow are separated. The activation of electric hands for above-elbow amputees is usually by a servo system, with a switch requiring a

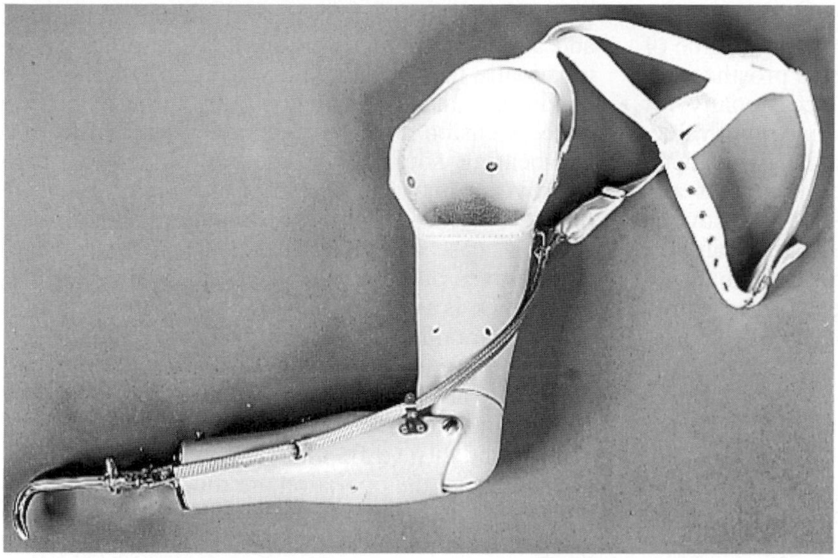

Figure 18.32 Above-elbow prosthesis with split hook; note operating cord and harness.

very small movement incorporated in the harness, rather than by the myoelectric method. Electric elbows are not widely used because the large mechanical disadvantage imposed on them by the geometry of the human elbow limits their effective power, and they are very expensive, but electrical actuation of the elbow lock may be a useful development.

THROUGH-SHOULDER DISARTICULATION

Disarticulation through the glenohumeral joint, retaining the scapula, is significantly less disfiguring than forequarter amputation, but functional use of a prosthesis is unlikely. A full cosmetic endoskeletal prosthesis can be fitted, but some patients find even the weight of this excessive in the context of minimal functional benefit, and prefer to use a lightweight foam cap, which re-establishes shoulder and upper arm contour only, but allows clothes to hang correctly.

FOREQUARTER AMPUTATION

This very mutilating procedure will normally only be carried out for malignant disease. A formal prosthesis is rarely tolerated, but a foam shoulder cap with upper arm extension, as mentioned above, can be helpful.

Prostheses for congenital limb deficiency

In general, children born with all or part of a limb or limbs missing manage very well with or without a prosthesis, and the psychological reaction (for the patient but not necessarily for the parents) is very different from that associated with surgical amputation in later life. Children with major bilateral upper limb deficiencies, for example, may derive better function by using their feet than by using prostheses. If only the hand is affected, a simple appliance to improve grip can be helpful; often this takes the form of an opposition plate against which the patient grips with a digit, or if no fingers are present, wrist movement is employed to provide grip against the palm.

Gillespie (1990) has emphasized three important factors when operating upon limb-deficient children. Surgical treatment is aimed at improving prosthetic function, but every consideration must be given to:

- growth
- stump overgrowth
- wound healing.

Therefore, growth epiphyses should be preserved for achieving the future growth potential of the stump, e.g. preserving the lower femoral epiphysis will contribute to 70% of total femoral length. Stump overgrowth of bone will produce abnormal pressure effects on overlying soft tissues, e.g. inflammation, tenderness and pain.

The most common congenital upper limb deficiency presenting for prosthetic management is the transverse below-elbow loss. Although some of these patients will choose not to use a prosthesis in adult life, or will only wear one occasionally for cosmetic purposes, a prosthesis is definitely of value, and such children should be seen in a prosthetic clinic when very young so that the prognosis and prosthetic possibilities can be discussed with the parents, and so that they may meet other families with similarly affected children. Prosthetic management starts at about 6 months of age, with the supply of a one-piece cosmetic arm. At around 18 months of age a functional arm, with interchangeable split hook and cosmetic hand is substituted (the 'CAPP' gripper with rounded jaws is an alternative to the split hook), and from about 4 years of age either a mechanical or myoelectric hand can be used if preferred (Figure 18.31). Scott (1990) has emphasized that, although modern designs for achieving velocity, force and appropriate joint angles and torques, are now available, an appropriate sensory feedback system is still required to be developed, as well as proprioceptive and other pressure sensors. These developments would lead to greater acceptability and use of the appliance.

Congenital deficiencies of the lower limb usually present for prosthetic management on account of progressive leg length discrepancy which is not suitable for leg lengthening surgery. The most common such abnormality encountered in limb-fitting clinics is the lateral longitudinal deficiency of the leg and foot, commonly referred to as 'fibular hemimelia'. In this the tibia is short and often bowed (convex anteriorly), the fibula is either absent or rudimentary, the ankle is unstable on the lateral side and adopts a valgus position, and the foot characteristically has only three rays (Figure 18.33). This condition can be managed by providing a below-knee extension prosthesis, using a plastic or leather end-bearing socket with the foot in equinus (to improve cosmesis) and the valgus deformity corrected. However, the better treatment in terms of comfort, ease of fitting, function and appearance, which gives predictably good results (Fergusson *et al.*, 1987), is to carry out a Syme's amputation at about 18 months of age, or shortly after the child is starting to try to walk and then to supply a standard plastic Syme's prosthesis. The amputation can be carried out at an even younger age, but parents always find this a difficult decision to make, and the advantages of the operation are much more obvious if the parents have actually seen their child struggling to walk on the short leg.

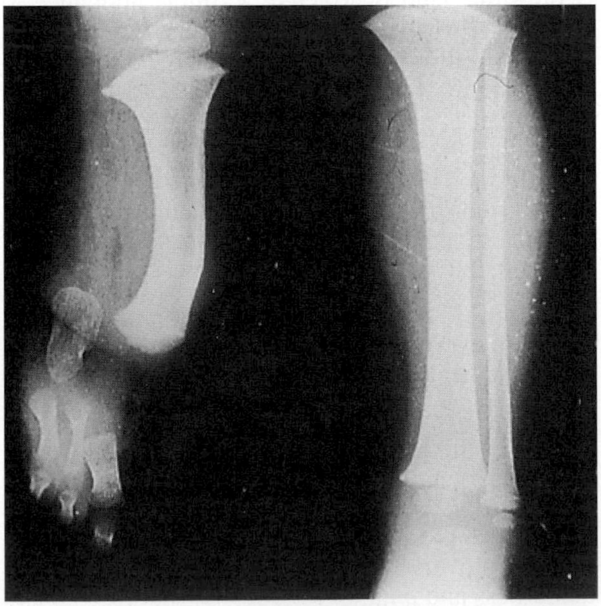

Figure 18.33 x-Ray showing right fibular hemimelia.

Proximal focal femoral deficiency (PFFD) is the other main condition which requires prosthetic treatment; the indications for reconstructive or ablative surgery are much less clear cut, but for the more severe forms which are not suitable for leg lengthening, surgery may be helpful to make the short limb more suitable for use with a prosthesis. It should be remembered that PFFD and fibular hemimelia may coexist. For Aitken type A cases (Aitken, 1969), in which the hip joint is well preserved with little fixed flexion, and in which the knee, although high, is at an acceptable level, a below-knee extension prosthesis, with leather or bivalved plastic socket to accommodate the foot in equinus, will give reasonable cosmesis and acceptable function. Syme's amputation may be indicated to improve cosmesis, simplify limb fitting, improve comfort and slightly enhance function, but cannot be advised as strongly as for fibular hemimelia.

The most severe cases of PFFD (Aitken type D), in which the hip is grossly deficient, with fixed flexion approaching 90°, and the knee lies very close to the hip, may require surgery to the hip. A partially ischial tuberosity bearing prosthesis is necessary, and socket design may call for considerable ingenuity. The knee should not be arthrodesed in this situation as its mobility is essential to compensate for the lack of hip extension. If the tibia is also short, the natural foot can be accommodated in the prosthetic thigh, but if the tibia is of normal length the foot may prevent the incorporation of a prosthetic knee joint at a reasonable level (Figure 18.34). The choice is then between a rigid full length prosthesis, which can nevertheless be given a very pleasing external shape, and a Syme's amputation which will allow space for a prosthetic knee joint and allow the use of a more standard type of socket, either in leather or in plastic with a compliant liner.

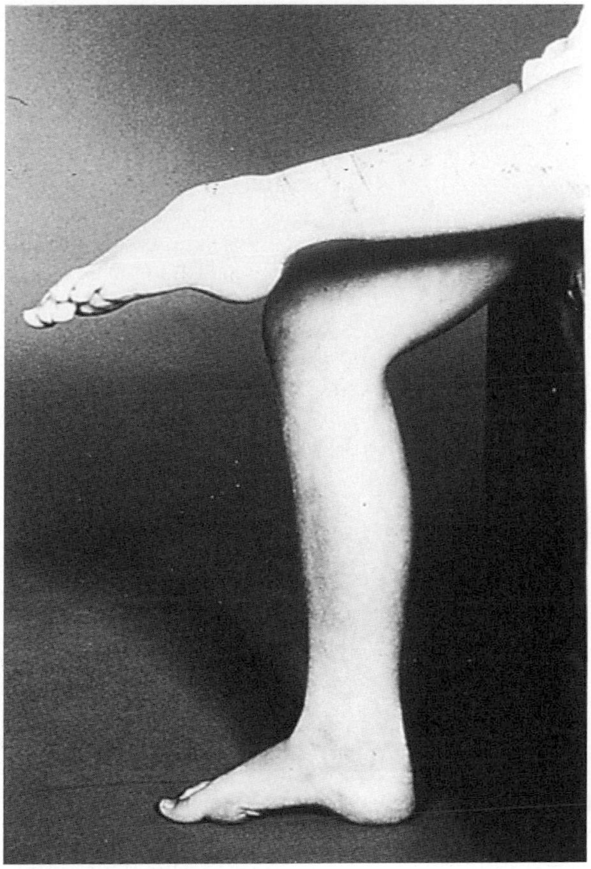

Figure 18.34 Aitken type D PFFD with normal tibia. Later treated by Syme's amputation.

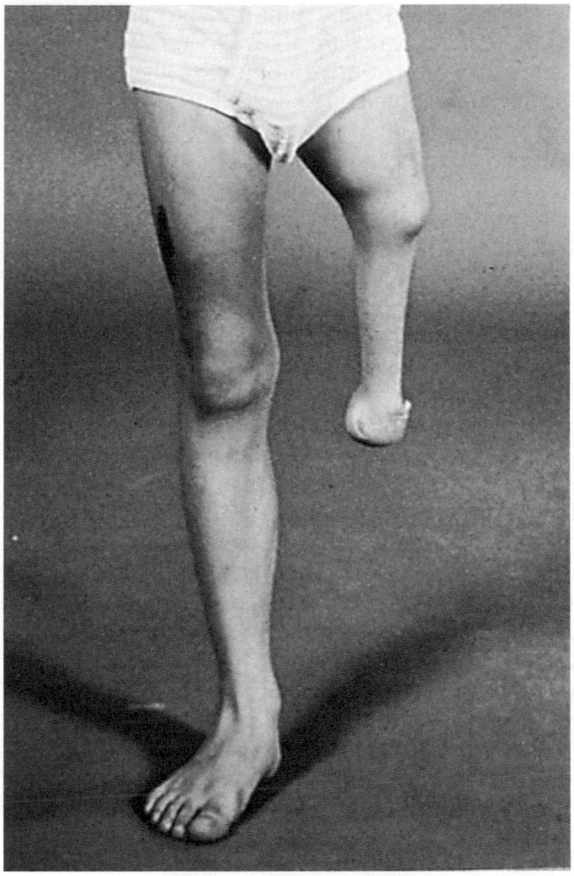

Figure 18.35 Aitken type B PFFD with fibular hemimelia, after treatment by arthrodesis of the knee and Syme's amputation.

Arthrodesis of the knee combined with Syme's amputation is sometimes helpful in those intermediate cases in which hip extension is good, the knee is at roughly mid-thigh level, and the tibia is also short, so that the ankle joint of the affected limb approximates to knee level on the normal side (Figure 18.35). This allows the use of a prosthesis similar to that for a through-knee amputee. Another possibility, if the ankle of the short limb is approximately at knee level is the Van Nes rotationplasty; this is a 180° rotational osteotomy through the tibia, designed so that the reversed ankle joint acts as a 'knee', and the patient can then wear a prosthesis similar to a below-knee prosthesis with thigh corset (Van Nes, 1950). The limb tends to derotate with growth and therefore the operation should not be carried out before 12 years of age. This somewhat bizarre procedure can also be used for some cases of tumour resection. Although an unusually demanding operation for the patients and parents as well as for the surgeon, it has been performed over the past 40 years with gratifying results. Krajbick and Carrol (1990) have reported on 21 children receiving this operation for malignant tumours, and concluded that the functional results were better than an above-knee amputation or hip disarticulation. A recent gait analysis of patients having received a Van Nes rotationplasty showed that they walked well, although abnormally.

There is no place for trans-tibial, transfemoral or through-knee amputation in the treatment of PFFD, and they are rarely indicated in other congenital conditions, although through-knee disarticulation may be required for tibial (never for fibular) aplasia.

Rehabilitation after amputation

Young and otherwise fit lower-limb amputees may be able to mobilize safely with crutches until they are ready for a prosthesis, but this is hazardous for elderly patients who are likely to fall. Even in the absence of other injuries, a blow to the stump will cause persistent pain and swelling or possibly stump breakdown, any of which will delay limb-fitting by several weeks. In the elderly, the initial aim should be to make the patient sufficiently independent with the aid of a wheelchair to return home at an early stage. Once this has been achieved, the patient should be assessed to see if a prosthesis will be beneficial, bearing in mind his cognitive function and the other medical and social difficulties which are likely to exist. A good idea of the below-knee amputee's ability to use a prosthesis safely can be obtained by studying his ability to use the pneumatic pylon (pneumatic post-amputation mobility aid or 'PPAMAID' – Figure 18.36) in the physiotherapy department (Redhead *et al.*, 1978). For above-knee amputees, a rapidly adjustable multi-use assessment prosthesis such as the Femurett™, which simulates a definitive prosthesis much more closely, should be used (Parry and Morrison, 1989). The adjustments available are shown in Figures 18.37 and 18.38. Both these appliances are also valuable walking training aids.

Upper-limb amputees need to be taught one-handed techniques for basic activities, such as dressing, and to be shown simple appliances, such as non-slip mats, which will assist everyday household tasks, at an early stage. For both upper- and lower-limb amputees, a home visit in the company of therapy and social work staff should be carried out prior to discharge from hospital, to determine what alterations, such as the installation of ramps, or appliances (bathing aids or a commode), are required, bearing in mind that most elderly amputees will be unable to negotiate stairs in the early stages.

Assuming that healing is not delayed and that the patient's general condition is favourable, 4 weeks after amputation is the optimum time to cast and measure the patient for his first definitive prosthesis. Before that time the stump is usually shrinking rapidly as the normal postoperative oedema resolves, so a socket made earlier can become a poor fit in a matter of days. If a modular limb is being used, it will be ready for fitting within a week, and can sometimes be finished on the day of fitting. The new amputee should only wear the first limb for short periods initially (e.g. half an hour, four times per day), to avoid soreness and skin problems, increasing gradually to full time wear after about a month. Although amputees should be encouraged to don their prosthesis themselves from the outset, lower-limb amputees should undertake their initial walking practice

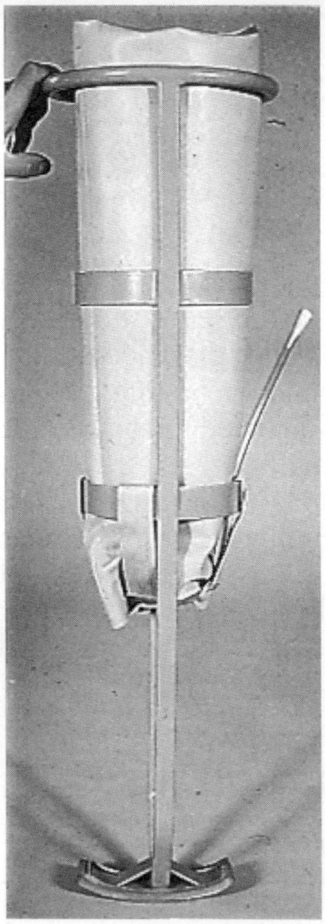

Figure 18.36 Pneumatic post-amputation mobility aid (PPAMAID).

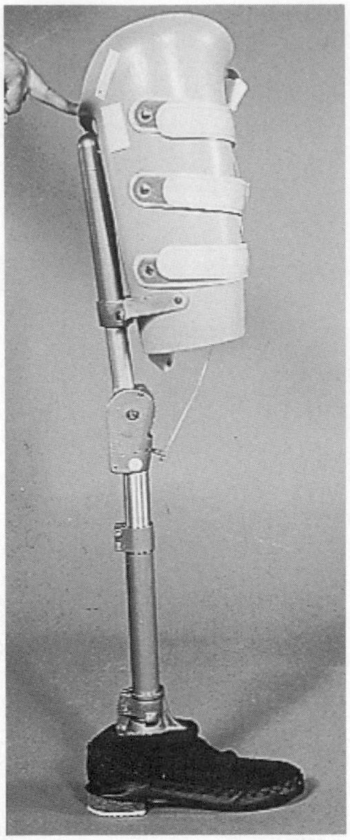

Figure 18.37 Above-knee assessment prosthesis, lateral view. Note adjustable (and interchangeable) socket.

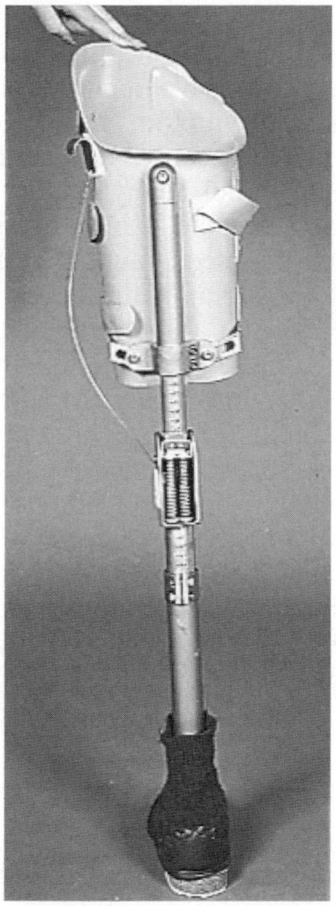

Figure 18.38 Above-knee assessment prosthesis; note the adjustment for length, rotation, and socket adduction and abduction.

under the supervision of a physiotherapist familiar with their particular problems and limitations.

Unless the patient has lost weight around the time of the amputation, the stump is likely to shrink progressively over the first few months, although the shrinkage is less marked if a total contact socket is used. The patient can compensate for this by wearing extra, and/or thicker stump socks, and greater changes can be allowed for by the prosthetist by adding pads or a leather lining to the socket. Usually a new socket will be needed after 2–3 months to ensure an optimal fit. Most lower-limb amputees should be taught to walk with sticks (canes) initially, although some elderly above-knee amputees need the stability of a walking frame; in general crutches should be avoided as they discourage correct weight-bearing through the prosthesis. Fitter patients will soon dispense with their sticks. Few amputees are ready to return to full time work earlier than 6 months after surgery. Swimming is an excellent sport and means of exercise for amputees as it places little demand on the stump skin. Most amputees swim without a prosthesis, but special waterproof limbs of controlled buoyancy can be made for swimming, and are particularly beneficial for below-knee amputees (most above-knee amputees find swimming easier without a prosthesis).

Common problems following amputation

Stump shrinkage is the most common cause of socket discomfort; the upper-limb amputee will feel that the socket has become loose, but paradoxically the inexperienced lower-limb amputee may complain that the socket feels too tight. This is because on weight-bearing the stump slips too far into the socket so the body weight is taken through pressure-intolerant areas. In this situation the above-knee amputee will usually complain of pain in the groin adjacent to the adductor longus tendon, whereas the below-knee amputee will experience pain or skin rubbing over the head of the fibula and under the distal tibia.

Other problems which can arise include epidermoid cysts, caused by a combination of pressure and friction where the skin crosses the socket brim, particularly in active amputees. They can become infected and tend to recur after surgical removal. Backache is likely to occur if the length of the prosthesis is incorrect. On the face of it, this should be easily avoided, but many amputees find walking easier if the prosthesis is shorter than the sound limb. The most practical way to assess prosthetic length is to compare the heights of the iliac crests or anterior superior iliac spines with the patient

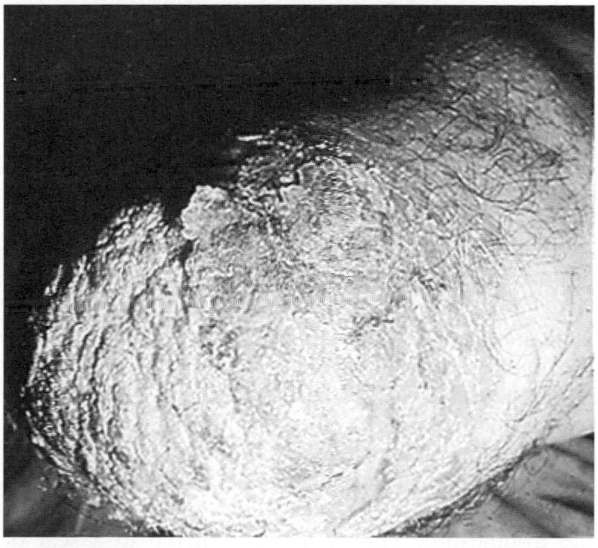

Figure 18.39 Below-knee stump with marked verrucose hyperplasia.

standing; these should be level for below-knee amputees, but 0.5 cm (0.25 inch) lower on the amputated side for above-knee amputees. Verrucose hyperplasia (Figure 18.39) is a dramatic form of chronic distal oedema of the stump, which develops a gross warty appearance, sometimes associated with exudation from the skin. It is caused by proximal constriction within the socket and inadequate distal tissue support; correction of these factors will allow gradual resolution of the problem. Allergy to the various components of the prosthesis can occur, and the enclosed damp environment within the socket can exacerbate other skin problems.

PHANTOM LIMB PAIN

As mentioned earlier, almost all amputees experience the phenomenon of phantom limb – a feeling that the amputated limb is still present, sometimes in contorted positions. New amputees may try to stand on the absent limb. In the early weeks or months, the phantom limb is usually painful, and this pain should be treated with standard analgesics. Usually the pain subsides, to be replaced by intermittent paraesthesia, and later merely an awareness of the absent limb with occasional painful episodes. A minority of amputees, however, experience persistent distressing phantom limb pain, which is sometimes accompanied by involuntary jerking movements of the stump, referred to as jactitation, and this type of pain can be very resistant to treatment. It is more likely to be a problem in those who had severe chronic pain or sepsis before amputation, and is usually worse when the patient is relaxing or at night when there is less other afferent nervous activity to inhibit the pain pathways. Limb-wearing usually reduces phantom limb pain; if the pain is worse on walking, this may be because the general socket fit is poor, or there may be pressure over a neuroma which can be eased by local socket adjustment.

Phantom limb pain, particularly if episodic, can often be controlled adequately by simple analgesics or by light massage of the stump. It is helpful to determine whether a 'trigger point' is present on the stump, that is to say a localized area, pressure over which brings on the pain. If there is, physical treatment such as daily local ultrasound for a week may relieve the pain on a long term basis. Alternatively, transcutaneous electrical nerve stimulation may provide symptomatic relief; small stimulators which can be carried in a pocket are available, but this treatment is rarely curative. Neuromas recur after excision, so their removal is only likely to provide long term benefit if the troublesome neuroma was tethered to a scar or subject to pressure against bone, and the revised cut end of the nerve can be positioned in a well protected situation to avoid this. If no trigger point is detectable, drugs such as the anti-epileptic carbamazepine or tricyclic antidepressants like amitriptyline, taken regularly, may make the symptoms more tolerable.

Davis (1993) has recently reviewed the phantom syndrome which is not solely due to psychological factors. He described the pain as arising from pain transmitting neurons, accepting the Melzach explanation of the mechanism behind this phenomenon. Originally before the amputation, there may have been irritation of the centrally conducting axons, bringing messages to the higher centres, via abnormal sensory reflexes within the internuncial pools of the spinal cord. These persist even though all the known afferent somatic and autonomic pathways from the stump have been severed.

Reamputation at a higher level rarely, if ever, gives lasting relief – nor does nerve section or block, spinal cord tract surgery – and all such procedures should be avoided.

WHEELCHAIRS

Wheelchairs may be classified as three main types: pushchairs, occupant-propelled chairs, and powered chairs.

Pushchairs

These may be required by elderly people, who can walk sufficiently to provide independent indoor mobility, but are unable to walk the longer distances necessary outside, and who have an able-bodied helper. Chairs for this purpose usually have a folding steel tubular frame to ease storage, folding push-handles (to facilitate transport by car), relatively small (e.g. 30 cm) diameter rear wheels with pneumatic tyres (to reduce weight and provide a comfortable ride), and front castor wheels to improve manoevrability, bearing in mind the relatively heavy occupant. Brakes are fitted to the rear wheels. A simple seating system with vinyl covered hammock-type seat and backrest and a foam cushion usually suffice. Hinged and/or removable footplates are normally provided.

Pushchairs may also be needed by very severely disabled children and younger adults who are totally unable to walk, and indeed may be dependent on others for all aspects of their care. The frame of such a chair may be similar to that described above, or in the case of children may resemble, or indeed be, a 'baby buggy' (usually with an aluminium frame) or the type of pushchair used by healthy young children. Often, however, these severely disabled people will require adaptations of the basic chair to fulfil their individual needs, either to provide additional postural support (e.g. for muscular dystrophy) or to accommodate fixed deformity (e.g. cerebral palsy) or both. Extra support may be provided by shaped foam pads, or one of the proprietary 'modular' seating systems, designed to support the patient in such a position that his or her limited sitting ability, strength and balance are utilized to the best advantage. A lap strap may be necessary for safety. Those with complex fixed deformities (e.g. the 'windswept' child with cerebral palsy) may require the total postural support provided by a custom moulded seat, which is usually made in fibreglass from a plaster cast, an alternative being a 'matrix' seat made up of many interlocking plastic components, each of approximately 2 cm diameter.

Occupant-propelled wheelchairs

These are often referred to as 'self-propelling' wheelchairs, meaning that the *user* propels the chair him- or herself. A chair of this type is required for full time use by people who are totally unable to walk (e.g. paraplegics), or for part time use (e.g. by the elderly amputee whose walking ability in, or tolerance of, his prosthesis is limited), and such people can be fully independent provided their upper-limb function is good. The majority of such chairs have a tubular frame, which folds from side to side, and are similar in construction to the adult-type pushchair, except that the rear wheels are of larger diameter (about 60 cm) and are equipped with propelling rims, operated by the hands, which serve both to propel and to steer the chair.

Because of the wide variety of people using such chairs, there are many sizes and differing designs. The environment in which the chair is to be used must also be considered when recommending a particular chair to an individual, particularly if space at home is limited, and sometimes compromises are necessary. Removable armrests are usually specified to make transfers to and from the chair easier, and special cushions may be needed, either to improve comfort in prolonged sitting or to prevent pressure sores; examples are gel cushions and air-flotation cushions. Accessories, such as elevating leg rests, supports for below-knee amputation stumps, or extended backrests may be needed. The axis of the rear wheels is usually just behind the position of the backrest. If extra stability against tipping backwards is required (e.g. for the bilateral transfemoral amputee), the rear wheels of the chair should be set further back (usually 7.5 cm), but this makes the chair bulkier and harder to propel.

By contrast, the very active user (e.g. the otherwise fit paraplegic) may prefer to have the rear wheels set further forward than usual to facilitate rear wheel balancing, which will allow the skilled wheelchair user to negotiate kerbs and other obstructions; the wheels are usually set with marked negative camber (i.e. the rims are closer at the top than the bottom) to give greater stability when cornering. Some such users prefer a rigid (non-folding) frame to give improved handling and lighter weight, usually with quickly detachable wheels and a low or folding backrest so that the chair is still compact enough to be loaded into a car without assistance. For the permanent wheelchair user, the style and appearance of the chair are of great psychological importance, in terms of body image.

Powered wheelchairs

Electrically powered wheelchairs are indicated for patients who are unable to walk *and* are unable to propel a non-powered chair (e.g. with progressive neurological conditions or very severe arthritis), provided they are alert and orientated. Such chairs are usually controlled by a joystick attached to the armrest of the chair, but in extreme cases (e.g. motor neuron disease) almost any remaining controllable voluntary movement can be harnessed. Examples include head movements and breathing (blow and suck). Electric wheelchairs are heavy and not usually readily transportable, and the user or assistant must be able to recharge the battery. Some powered wheelchairs can be used both indoors and outside, but many of the larger chairs, with the ability to negotiate kerbs and longer range per charge, are too bulky for use in the house, while the compact chairs most suitable for indoor use usually have limited ability outside.

References

Aitken, J.G. (1969) In: *Proximal Femoral Focal Deficiency; a Congenital Anomaly*, pp. 1–22. Symposium National

Academy of Sciences. National Research Council: Washington D.C.

Beacock, C.J.M., Doran, J., Hopkinson, B.R. and Makin, G.S. (1983) A modified Gritti–Stokes amputation: its place in the management of peripheral vascular disease. *Annals of the Royal College of Surgeons of England* **65**, 90–92

Burgess, E.M., Romano, R.L., Zettl, J.H. and Schrock, R.D. (1971) Amputations of the leg for peripheral vascular insufficiency. *Journal of Bone and Joint Surgery* **53A**, 874–890

Campbell, W.B. and Morris, P.J. (1987) A prospective randomized comparison of healing in Gritti–Stokes and through-knee amputations. *Annals of the Royal College of Surgeons of England* **69**, 1–4

Clyne, C.A.C. (1991) Selection of level for lower limb amputation in patients with severe peripheral vascular disease. *Annals of the Royal College of Surgeons of England* **73**, 148–151

Davis, R.W. (1993) Phantom sensation, phantom pain and stump pain. *Archives of Physical Medicine and Rehabilitation* **74**, 79–91

De Luccia, N., Pinto, M.A.G. and Guedes, J.P. (1992) Rehabilitation after amputation for vascular disease. A follow-up study. *Prosthetics and Orthotics International* **16**, 124–128

Fergusson, C.M., Morrison, J.D. and Kenwright, J. (1987) Leg-length inequality in children treated by Syme's amputation. *Journal of Bone and Joint Surgery* **69B**, 433–436

Fillauer, C.E., Pritham, C.H. and Fillauer, K.D. (1989) Evolution and development of the silicone suction socket (3S) for below-knee prostheses. *Journal of Prosthetics and Orthotics* **1**, 92–103

Fyfe, N.C.M. (1990) An audit of amputation levels in patients referred for prosthetic rehabilitation. *Prosthetics and Orthotics International* **14**, 67–70

Georgiadis, G.M., Behrens, A., Joyce, M. and Earle, A.S. (1992) End results after severe open tibial shaft fractures treated by limb salvage or early below-knee amputations. *Orthopedic Transactions* **16**, 676

Gillespie, R. (1990) Principles of amputation surgery in children with longitudinal deficiencies of the femur. *Clinical Orthopaedics and Related Research* **256**, 29–38

Gregory-Dean, A. (1991) Amputations: statistics and trends. *Annals of the Royal College of Surgeons of England* **73**, 137–142

Huang, C.T., Jackson, J.R., Moore, N.B. *et al.* (1979) Amputation: energy cost of ambulation. *Archives of Physical Medicine and Rehabilitation* **60**, 18–24

Ipsen, T., Lindquist, L., Barfred, T. and Ples, J. (1990) Principles of evaluation and results in microsurgical treatment of major limb replantations. *Scandinavian Journal of Plastic and Reconstructive Surgery and Hand Surgery* **24**, 75–80

Jendrzejczyk, D.J. (1985) Flexible socket systems. *Clinical Prosthetics and Orthotics* **9**(4), 27–31

Klippenstein, N. and Lyttle, D. (1992) Syme amputation in children. A good functional level? *Orthopedic Transactions* **16**, 107

Krajbick, J.I. and Carrol, N.C. (1990) Van Nes rotationplasty with segmental limb resection. *Clinical Orthopaedics and Related Research* **256**, 7–13

McCollum, P.T., Spence, V.A., Walker, W.F. and Murdoch, G. (1985) A rationale for skew flaps in below-knee amputation surgery. *Prosthetics and Orthotics International* **9**, 95–99

McWhinnie, D.L., Gordon, A.C., Collin, J., Gray, D.W.R. and Morrison, J.D. (1994) Rehabilitation outcome 5 years after 100 lower-limb amputations. *British Journal of Surgery* **81**, 1596–1599

Millstein, S.G., Heger, H. and Hunter, G.A. (1986) Prosthetic use in adult upper limbs amputees: a comparison of the body powered and electrically powered prostheses. *Prosthetics and Orthotics International* **10**, 27–34

Parry, M. and Morrison, J.D. (1989) Use of the Femurett adjustable prosthesis in the assessment and walking training of new above-knee amputees. *Prosthetics and Orthotics International* **13**, 36–38

Pfeil, J., Marquardt, E., Holtz, T., Neithard, F.U., Schneider, E. and Carstens C. (1991) The stump capping procedure to prevent or treat terminal osseous overgrowth. *Prosthetics and Orthotics International* **15**, 96–99

Pinzur, M.S., Gottsehalk, F., Smith, D. *et al.* (1993) Functional outcome of below-knee amputation in peripheral vascular insufficiency. A multicentre review. *Clinical Orthopaedics and Related Research* **286**, 247–249

Purry, N.A. and Hannon, M.A. (1989) How successful is below-knee amputation for injury? *Injury* **20**, 32–36

Redhead, R.G., Davis, B.C., Robinson, K.P. and Vitali, M. (1978) Post-amputation pneumatic walking aid. *British Journal of Surgery* **65**, 611–612

Robinson, K.P., Hoile, R. and Coddington, T. (1982) Skew flap myoplastic below-knee amputation: a preliminary report. *British Journal of Surgery* **69**, 554–557

Sabolich, J. (1985) Contoured adducted trochanteric-controlled alignment method (CAT-CAM). Introduction and basic principles. *Clinical Prosthetics and Orthotics* **9**(4), 15–26

Scott, R.N. (1990) Feedback in myoelective prostheses. *Clinical Orthopaedics and Related Research* **256**, 58–63

Sethia, K.K., Berry, A.R., Morrison, J.D., Collin, J., Murie, J.A. and Morris, P.J. (1986) Changing pattern of lower limb amputation for vascular disease. *British Journal of Surgery* **73**, 701–703

Sherman, C.D. and Duthie, R.B. (1960) A modified hemipelvectomy. *Cancer* **13**, 51–54

Topper, A.K. and Fernie, G.R. (1990) An evaluation of computer aided design of below-knee prosthetic sockets. *Prosthetics and Orthotics International* **14**, 136–142

Van Nes, C.P. (1950) *Journal of Bone and Joint Surgery* **32B**, 12–16

CHAPTER 19

Physical Therapy, Rehabilitation and Orthotics

DAVID C. REID

Introduction

The term rehabilitation has many different meanings, but from an orthopaedic perspective it has been defined as signifying the whole process of restoring a disabled person to a condition in which he or she is able, as early as possible, to resume a normal life, or at least achieve his/her physical potential (Tunbridge, 1972) In recent years there has been a worldwide increase in awareness of the value of rehabilitation but there is still a general lack of understanding of the detailed application of physical therapy, its prescription and practice. Frequently the conditions and disorders treated by physical methods are subject to natural remissions and exacerbations and not easily amenable to scientific evaluation. Many therapeutic protocols are unproven and empirical and there is still a great need for therapists to develop new techniques, to challenge traditional methods, and to widen their theoretical understanding of the modalities they use. With the growth of applied biomechanics of the musculoskeletal system as well as the understanding of functional disability, external appliances, or orthoses, are much more frequently being prescribed and used by patients.

Therapy of the musculoskeletal system has its advocates and its adversaries but the surgeon would do well to remember the words of Moynihan who stated: 'The operation is but one incident, no doubt the most dramatic, yet still only one in a long series of events which must stretch between illness and recovery.' Just as ill-advised and poorly directed therapy can lessen and reverse the outcomes of well performed surgery, a thorough, appropriate rehabilitation protocol can obtain functional results from many of the orthopaedic procedures commonly carried out today.

In its broader sense, the sphere of rehabilitation includes the physical therapist, occupational therapist, remedial gymnast, orthotist and prosthotist. These areas combine in very different ways to address the special needs of the orthopaedic patient, the neurologically injured person, those with chronic debilitating diseases, and those with primarily psychiatric disturbances. This chapter will focus on physical therapy as it relates to orthopaedics.

General principles of physiotherapy

Physiotherapy can be broadly divided into passive (i.e. directed towards the alleviation of symptoms) and active physical therapy (the restoration of function by activity). In addition, there is an expanding role of the therapist in the assessment of the patient's disability, functional progression and fitness to return to specific recreational and occupation tasks. In many centres the therapist is involved in the provision and training in the use of prosthetics as well as the prescription and fitting of orthotics.

Therapists are trained with a solid background in anatomy, biomechanics and pathology, and therefore are in a unique position to adapt to fill numerous different roles in varying health care environments. Thus the tasks demanded of therapists will depend very much on the institution and even the country in which they practise. Many therapists have subspecialized in the area of manipulative therapy, sports therapy, and the care of the neurologically or orthopaedically injured patient.

Passive physical therapy

Passive treatments are administered by the therapist to the patient and are directed at relief of pain, gaining range of motion, reducing oedema, and assisting in gaining muscle control. The methods utilized include the application of various modalities of heat or cold, electrical stimulation, techniques of counter-irritation, massage, mobilization and manipulation. Many of the therapeutic benefits are still poorly documented and it is exceedingly difficult to separate placebo effect from therapeutic changes induced by the modalities. Prolonged patient contact afforded during the application of these techniques serves to emphasize the importance of the clinical approach and the personality of the therapist. The placebo effect, where it exists, therefore should not be ridiculed but recognized for what it is and utilized. By the same token this fact should not be used as an excuse to refer patients without a sound diagnosis, therapeutic goal or treatment end point.

Many of the conditions traditionally treated with physical measures are degenerative, chronic, and episodic, subject to characteristic patterns of remissions and exacerbations. Conditions are unlikely to respond with universally good results to any single treatment. Naturally each condition will go through a phase during which physical therapy can be used to its greatest advantage, and timing of treatment is best determined by good communication between physician and therapist.

In most conditions passive physical treatments are used to enhance the effects achieved by active therapy. There are very few instances in which passive therapy alone will constitute an effective treatment. Exercise and its modification is the cornerstone of physiotherapy.

REMEDIAL GYMNASTICS

Very largely because of the needs and influence of orthopaedic rehabilitation units, a separate profession of remedial gymnasts was created. The dividing line between the two professions is often difficult to delineate as far as exercise therapy is concerned. Broadly speaking, physiotherapists may be more concerned with individual patients and remedial gymnasts are particularly expert at the use of exercise as a form of group therapy. Remedial gymnasts have a special role to play in rehabilitation centres and in those centres which cater for particular types of disabilities (e.g. paraplegia, fractures). In some units, the boundaries between the activities of the two professions are clearly marked, whereas in many others they are merging.

ACTIVE PHYSICAL TREATMENT

Active physical treatment is largely the application and modification of exercises. This may range from minimal movement of single muscles, encouraged during the stage of recovery from paralysis or severe injury, to intensive exercise routines akin to those practised by athletes. These exercises may be given as individual instruction or as group activities. The exercises may be tailored to influence specific muscles, muscle groups, or mass movement patterns. Where poor control exists because of pain inhibition or pathologically generated movement patterns, biofeedback techniques can be put into play in order to restore adequate motion, movement patterns or phase of firing of muscles (DeAndrade *et al.*, 1965). In addition, strong functional emphasis can be placed on the exercise activities, which requires a detailed knowledge of the patient's occupation and requirements for daily living. More recently, the full significance of proprioceptive deficit following ligament injury and joint dysfunction, and the ability to retrain these reflexes or at lease compensate for them, have altered the approach to many joint instabilities and the associated functional problems (Reid, 1992).

It is in the area of functional training and proprioceptive rehabilitation that the most dramatic strides have been made in the application to orthopaedics of the knowledge acquired by the basic scientist.

Physiotherapists are concerned with the maintenance of function during acute illness, not only by maintaining joint and range of muscle power, but also by ensuring effective early mobilization and short-term rehabilitation. Following all orthopaedic surgery they play a role in minimizing chest complications and deep vein thrombosis, mobilization and strengthening and overall patient education. During a chronic illness, physiotherapists are similarly concerned with the maintenance of maximal function of a locomotor system and the long-term rehabilitation of those with residual permanent disability.

More and more the emphasis is on the active participation of the patient. There is a move away from hospital-based therapy to much more cost-effective home programmes. This means that the therapist must assume the role of teacher and spend a great deal of time educating the patient to understand the needs, aims and the safe conduct of the required exercises. It is important that the therapist raise the motivational level of the patient and thus ensure compliance. With the more acute joint problems and post-surgical fracture care, it is more likely that therapy programmes will be set up with a few intense initial treatments followed by follow-up visits to ensure the patient is carrying out an effective home programme. It is here that the surgeon may be of significant value in supporting and enhancing the suggestions of the therapist as well as ensuring the patient is being compliant with the programme.

ASSESSMENT

Physiotherapists have an excellent training in neuromuscular anatomy and with experience, this expertise may be used in the area of assessment. Muscle testing following spine trauma is an obvious example. Scoliosis screening in the community and ongoing documentation of the neuromuscular control of cerebral palsy infants are other examples. Short- and longer-term follow up of the functional outcomes of joint surgery for unstable shoulders, fracture care, prosthetic replacement of the joints, and post-ligamentous surgery to the knee are excellent examples of situations in which the therapist's skills may be used maximally to serve, not only as quality control of treatment, but also to establish the effectiveness of different surgical techniques.

Orthotics and prosthetics are specialized areas in their own rights. However, there are many clinical situations in which the therapist, with additional training, may be involved in the provision of aids and appliances associated with locomotive function (splints, calipers, artificial limbs, spinal supports, corrective casts and wheelchairs). Furthermore, they are vitally involved in the training of patients in their use.

Physical modalities

HEAT

Heat is transmitted in three ways: by conduction, by convection, and by radiation. Conduction is the movement of heat within a substance, flowing from warmer to cooler parts. Convection is transmission of heat by the actual flow of the liquid or gas heated. Both of these forms of heat transmission are accomplished by the transfer of energy by molecular activity, whereas the radiation of heat depends on electromagnetic radiation.

Skin and fat are poor conductors of heat and any modality utilizing forms of conducted heat produces mainly superficial temperature change. Skin temperature rises rapidly when in contact with a heat source, but the underlying tissues show a temperature rise of lesser degree depending on:

1. The heat dissipated on the skin surface (sweat and convection).
2. The conductivity of the subcutaneous tissue (thickness of fat).
3. The amount of heat carried away by the circulating blood.

The local effect of heat (temperatures of up to 42°C) is vasodilation of the blood vessels with blood flow increasing by four to five times that of resting level. Subcutaneous blood flow follows the changes in cutaneous blood flow. Muscle and joint temperature are, however, usually unaltered by conductive and convective types of heating. They may show delayed rise in temperature if large body areas are heated for 20–30 minutes. This local rise in joint temperature is related to the general rise in body temperature and may be in the order of 1–2°C.

Surface heating is limited by the direct effect of heat on the tissues and the comparatively low temperatures which can be comfortably tolerated. Skin temperature of over 43°C is associated with pain and a temperature of over 45°C will rapidly produce discomfort and arteriolar flare and wheal (Reid, 1992).

Various therapeutic effects of heat have been claimed and in general include:

1. Metabolic rate is increased by an average of 13% for rise of 1°C. This may decrease local stasis and assist tissue nutrition. While useful in

subacute situations, there is, however, little direct evidence in the literature of the results of these changes in terms of long-term clinical effects.
2. It is possible to influence the extensibility of collagen. At normal tissue temperatures, collagen exhibits primarily elastic properties and only minimal viscous flow. However, when heated to 39–44°C the viscous flow becomes more dominant and therefore the tissue becomes more extensible. This fact is utilized in preparing tissue for mobilizing scar, adhesions and contractures by exercise techniques (Kottke *et al.*, 1966).
3. Relief of pain and spasm is an easily documented short-term effect. Apart from stimulating the sensation of hot and cold, heat produces a definite sedative effect. This in turn may promote decreased muscle spasm. Whether this effect is related to increased blood flow, or due to the so-called 'counter-irritant' effect of the two sensations simultaneously reaching the central nervous system, is not well documented (Downey, 1964).

Heating by radiation

Radiant heat lamps, using emitters similar to various electric light bulbs, are a convenient and a relatively cheap source of heat. Electric pads and infrared lamps provide heat from a mainly longer wavelength than the radiant heat lamps and these forms of heat emit little, if any, visible light. They have the disadvantage that they take longer to heat up and reach an even temperature and therefore are less efficient. Unless a very large area is being heated, radiant heat lamps must be considered a very superficial form of application.

Conductive and convective heating

Hot water is probably the most widely used agent for conductive heating, either in the form of hot packs, hot soaks, compresses, or hydrotherapy pools of various sizes. The commonly used hot packs are usually canvas containers filled with a silicone gel and heated in warm water baths to temperatures between 76 and 80°C. The main properties of the gel is its capability to absorb many times its own volume of water, when heated it gives off moist heat for approximately 30–40 minutes (Borrell *et al.*, 1980). The packs have the advantage that they can be moulded into the various contours of different parts of the body. Whirlpools and hot baths may be selected as the treatment of choice in situations where it is desirable to exercise the part while heat is being applied, or the area to be heated is extremely large.

Wax baths are a convenient form of heating for the extremities, particularly the hand. Paraffin wax is melted in an electrically heated bath and applied to the skin either by immersion of the part, or by application with a brush at approximately 48–49°C. Usually six or seven coats of wax are used and towels wrapped around the limb for further insulation for a period of 20–30 minutes. At the end of the treatment, the wax is easily peeled off and manipulation of the wax then may form part of the exercise therapy for mobilizing and strengthening of the hand. This modality is extremely effective in the treatment of the rheumatoid hand. Prolonged heating effect is mainly due to the latent heat of solidification and to the specific heat of the wax. Overall, there is no evidence that immersion in wax is any more beneficial than immersion in warm water (Magee, 1976).

Contraindications and precautions to heat therapy

There are some general contraindications to all modalities that produce heat. These include:

1. Impaired skin sensation.
2. The coexistent use of strong narcotic analgesics which may alter both sensation and judgement.
3. Circulatory dysfunction, which may inhibit the necessary vasodilation and dispersal of heat.
4. Poor quality and fragile skin.
5. Deep x-ray therapy during the preceding 3 months with atrophic skin and altered sensation.
6. Inability of the patient to comprehend adequately the dangers of these specific therapies.

In addition, there must be special consideration when treating open or contaminated wounds, particularly with wax bath. The presence of certain dermatological conditions may also present difficulties. Some liniments and creams may increase the risk of damages to the skin and the area must be appropriately prepared. Essentially most of these modalities are safe if the therapist takes sufficient care and the patient is adequately instructed.

While some modalities such as the conductive and convective heating (infrared lamps) have their physiological effect directly through their ability to heat the tissues, others such as shortwave diathermy and ultrasonics, may indeed affect the tissues in other ways. They are capable of producing effects by disturbance of electromagnetic fields or the mechanical agitation of extracellular particles, cell walls, and intracellular molecules.

HIGH-FREQUENCY CURRENTS

Shortwave diathermy

The heating effects of diathermy are produced by placing the patient within an electric field created by a high-frequency alternating current. The assigned frequency is 1.2 megacycles with a wavelength of 11 metres. Thus the patient forms part of the secondary circuit of a high-frequency generator. The rapidly alternating current agitates, vibrates and rotates various molecules and ions within the tissues, and a secondary heating effect is produced. It is unknown whether these secondary mechanical effects on the molecules of the tissues have any therapeutic effect of their own, such as the dispersal of tissue oedema, alteration of oxidation–reduction potentials or influencing ionic transfer across cell membranes.

In current clinical practice, it is impossible to measure the current input into the patient and therefore the only control of intensity depends on the patient's skin sensation of heat. Theoretically deep heating will occur in the field of a shortwave diathermy emitter if the medium is homogenous and there is no heat loss by conduction to untreated areas. In practice, it is impossible to achieve an even distribution of current in the body and heat is dissipated by blood and tissue both by physical conduction and by electrical conduction.

Therefore, the greatest current density and the maximum heating effect usually occurs at the surface of the skin under the electrodes. However, it is possible to minimize the superficial heating by special arrangements of the electrodes. Shortwave diathermy is potentially the most efficient way of heating large areas of subcutaneous tissue and muscle and is even capable of some significant deep heating.

Contraindications and precautions of shortwave diathermy include:

1. Over any part of the body in the presence of a cardiac pacemaker.
2. Over malignant tumours because of the potential and theoretical danger of metastasis.
3. In areas where circulation is not sufficient to disperse heat or accommodate increased metabolism.
4. Over wet dressings, adherent tape or through casts.
5. If there is metal in the tissue.
6. If there is impairment of thermal sensation.
7. Over a pregnant uterus or over the abdomen during menstruation.
8. In cases of severe cardiac conditions where the potential increased circulating demand would stress the limited cardiac output.
9. Over the chest of pulmonary tuberculosis.
10. In the patients who is unable to appreciate the dangers or concentrate sufficiently to sit still during the treatment.

Microwave diathermy

The microwave has two assigned frequencies, 2456 and 915 MHz, giving it a higher frequency and shorter wavelength than shortwave diathermy. The microwave antenna, or director, beams energy that is both absorbed and reflected. The limiting factor with heating may be the temperature rises to the superficial fat which then produces discomfort. Tissue heating is generated in much the same way as with shortwave diathermy and the same contraindications should be observed.

Pulse electromagnetic energy

It has never been conclusively demonstrated that the many mechanical and non-thermal effects that undoubtedly occur with shortwave diathermy and microwave therapy have any specific isolated therapeutic function. Nevertheless the rationale behind a non-thermal pulse electromagnetic equipment assumes that there may be useful clinical effects other than heating. Therefore, the shortwaves are pulsed in packages with sufficient rest intervals that the small amounts of heat generated are rapidly dissipated. This prevents a cumulative rise in tissue temperature. All apparatus in this category uses a base frequency of 27.12 MHz. There are a large number of instruments available, each with a number of output options in terms of pulse widths, pulse repetition rates, intensity settings, and shape of the electromagnetic field generated. These apparatus are all used for their potential effect on promoting tissue healing, decreasing inflammation, reducing muscle spasms and decreasing pain.

Although there is a certain amount of substantiation of the effect on inflammation and on subcellular and cellular events, the efficacy, cost-effectiveness and superiority of these apparatus, one over another, has yet to be conclusively demonstrated (Griffin and Karselis, 1982). Each has its special advocates and champions and it remains for more carefully generated research to elicit their true place in the physiotherapy protocols.

ULTRASONICS

Therapeutic ultrasound is a physical agent with its effect being due to heating and to mechanical phenomenon within the tissues. The upper limit of man's audibility is in the range of 15–20 kHz.

Frequencies above these upper limits are referred to as ultrasound although many animals can in fact hear in these ranges. Ultrasonic energy is produced via the piezoelectric effect of a voltage applied to a ceramic disc or crystal. This is contained within a treatment head which is applied to the patient's skin. Some form of liquid or gel coupling medium is used to exclude air and ensure good contact of the treatment head with the tissues, since high-frequency sound waves are not conducted well by air. The speed at which sound propagates is the characteristic of medium through which it is passing, and in human tissue this is about 457 metres (1500 feet) per second. The ultrasound frequency most commonly used is 1 MHz, although the range of therapeutic apparatus is from 750 kHz through to 3 MHz. In many ways, sound of this frequency behaves similarly to light in that the energy may be absorbed, transmitted or reflected. These properties influence the type and magnitude of response of the various tissues to ultrasound.

High-frequency sound is transmitted through the tissues as an alternating band of compression and rarefaction. Absorption is mainly a molecular phenomenon and the forces generated in the tissues have been shown to be of considerable magnitude. Pressure amplitudes are in the range of 1–4 atmospheres and in small cells and elementary particles may be subjected to rapidly accelerating and decelerating forces of up to 10^5 times that of gravity. Because of the potentially destructive effect on tissue, therapeutic machines have an output restricted to a maximum of 3 watts/cm^2. At this level of intensity, there is evidence that significant heating can be produced at a depth of 1–3 cm although even penetration of 5 cm is possible with the correct technique and application. Ultrasound therapy may be applied in a continuous or pulse mode, the latter allowing for heat dissipation and thus minimizing rising tissue temperature.

While temperature changes induced by ultrasound are well documented, it is only more recently that the mechanical phenomena have been carefully linked to potentially therapeutic effects within the tissues (Reid, 1992). Heating of the tissues induces compensatory circulatory adjustments in order to prevent excessive temperature rise. This may give an acceleration of local metabolism and a more efficient turnover of nutrients. It may be possible to interrupt the 'pain–spasm' cycle via the vasodilatory effect, and also by alteration of tissue excitability. A particularly useful physiological effect of heat is the ability to increase the extensibility of scar and connective tissues (Gernsten, 1955).

The mechanical effects of ultrasound consist of both cyclic and cyclic averaging phenomena. The cyclic effects involve vibration of cells and cellular particles. This mechanical agitation of cells may be capable of inducing release of potent cellular enzymes such as prostaglandins. The significance of this in producing clinical effects is at this time speculative. Other cyclic effects include an alteration in ionic gradients due to the agitation of the environment adjacent to the cell membranes as well as internal stressing of large molecules and cells. At present the only known cyclic averaging effect is acoustic streaming, which is the motion of particles free to move under the influence of radiation pressure.

There is sufficient evidence to demonstrate that the effect of ultrasound on tissues may vary widely within the range of intensities clinically available. However, it is not yet possible to know exact dosage delivered to a certain structure or its specific depth in the tissues. While the physiological effects of ultrasound have been well documented, proof of more major therapeutic effects are more tenuous. The lack of availability of good clinical studies is disappointing. Nevertheless, the current literature will probably support the use of ultrasound in facilitating haematoma resorption and assisting tissue regeneration. The area of scar softening and contracture mobilization depends mainly on the heating effects of ultrasound. There is very little experimental support for ultrasound as an agent for reducing and relieving inflammation. Paradoxically, this is the area of most frequent clinical use. Ultrasound has the drawback of requiring the individual attention of the therapist throughout the duration of the treatment, and thus it is expensive in manpower. For this reason its use should be restricted to the areas best supported by experimental evidence. Furthermore, if good therapeutic results are not obtained in a period of 2–3 weeks, it is unlikely that continued treatment over a further period will produce desirable results. Lastly, it must be remembered that the forces generated in the tissues are of considerable magnitude and therefore ultrasound is a potentially dangerous treatment and should be applied only by trained personnel (Reid and Cummings, 1973).

Contraindications and precautions

A series of standard precautions and contraindications associated with ultrasound application have been developed. The vulnerable tissues are neural, reproductive organs and fluid-filled cavities, the latter because of the danger of cavitation. There are conflicting reports that the effects of ultrasound on open epiphyses and prolonged exposures are probably inadvisable. Although metal in the tissues is not a direct contraindication, because of its excellent ability to dissipate heat, good protective sensation is required. The potential for ultrasound to loosen implants is an unanswered issue. Most of the harmful effects of ultrasound are reduced by the low output of the therapeutic range. Risks are further minimized by continuously moving the treatment head during therapy. This action smoothes out the extremes of energy intensity in the near and far fields and prevents formation of hot spots.

LASER THERAPY

Lasers (light amplification by stimulated emissions of radiation) are light amplifiers that emit energy in the invisible infrared regions of the electromagnetic spectrum. Laser light is generated by the stimulated emission of photons (light energy) from gases usually helium-neon (HeNe) or gallium arsenide (GaAs). The three main characteristics of laser light are monochromaticity, coherence, and divergence (Krikorian *et al.*, 1986). Monochromaticity means that the light is of a single well defined wavelength. The infrared GaAs laser has a specific wavelength at 904 nm which is beyond the visible spectrum of 400–770 nm. Frequently a filter is introduced to make a visible beam. Normal light is made up of numerous wavelengths superimposing their phases on one another. By contrast, lasers with a single specific wavelength travel with the phases in synchrony. The beam progresses unidirectionally and symmetrically, which produces the second characteristic of coherence. The third characteristic is the minimal divergence of the emitted light so that it maintains a concentrated beam.

Laser devices emit their energy in pulses that correspond to some degree to the natural resonating frequencies of the tissues. The specific physiological effects of laser light at a subcellular level are still a subject of considerable speculation. The resonance of human tissue is such that it absorbs laser emission well, although there is some reflection and dispersion. Generally the higher the water content of the tissue, the greater is the absorption of laser.

The HeNe laser may have a direct penetration of 0.8 mm and indirect penetration and absorption up to 10–15 mm. The GaAs laser with a longer wavelength has a direct penetration of 15 mm and an indirect penetration about 5 cm. Hence penetration is directly proportional to wavelength. The following tissue effects have been reported in the literature:

1. The possible alteration of the level of various tissue prostaglandins and hence modifying the inflammatory phase of trauma.
2. Reduction of oedema possibly secondary to the effects on membrane potentials and active transport across cell walls.
3. Increased mitochondrial activity and associated elevated production of the energy-rich phosphate, adenosine triphosphate (ATP), possibly related to enhancing electron transfer in the inner membrane of the mitochondria.
4. Increased levels of RNA in the endoplasmic reticulum of animals.
5. Stimulation of fibroblast proliferation and early increase in collagen production in wounds, the mechanism for which is unknown.
6. Increased vascularization of wounds.

When attempting to reduce oedema, stimulate tissue function and promote healing, a technique called gridding is used. Essentially the area to be treated is divided into approximately 1 cm squares or grids. The unit of therapy is then applied to each square, usually 10–15 seconds per unit area for the GaAs laser and 20–30 seconds for HeNe device. Other techniques are available and laser therapy is in a state of evolution, as far as clinical application is concerned, at the present time.

Although the traditional short periods are well accepted, there are proponents of treatments that last much longer. Realistically, the limited depth of penetration of the laser beam makes it an unsuitable modality for many soft tissue lesions. Although the indirect effects of the laser have been reported to significant depths, 99% of the beam is absorbed directed by about 1 cm of the epidermis.

Contraindications and precautions

Lasers probably should either not be used or precautions taken in the following situations:

1. Overstimulation: exposing tissue to laser energy densities of more than 8–9 joules/cm^2 during one treatment session.
2. The effect of laser application during the first trimester of pregnancy has not been established.
3. Photosensitizing medications may enhance or produce an unpredictable effect.
4. Laser should never be applied over the unclosed fontanelles of infants.
5. The results of laser applied over tumorous tissue are unknown and hence contraindicated.
6. Treatment should be suspended in situations where prolonged or repeated nausea or dizziness is experienced either during or immediately after treatment.
7. It is undesirable to stare into the laser beam for any significant period of time, as it may affect the retina.
8. It is unwise to apply the laser to tissue if underlying pathology has not been established.

In summary, laser, like some many of the physical therapy modalities, is a powerful energy source being harnessed in the hope of producing a desirable therapeutic effect. The ability to calculate optimal dosages and the delivery of this quantum of energy to the appropriate tissue, however, is a formidable task still in its infancy. It means that the empirical application of this modality requires experience, keen observation, and careful record keeping, if successful results are to be duplicated (Reid, 1992).

CRYOTHERAPY

Symptoms of musculoskeletal disorders may be considerably reduced by the application of ice in one its many forms. There is mounting physiological and clinical evidence that the therapeutic use of ice, whether by local application or by immersion of limbs in ice water, can decrease the spasm of spastic muscles and is also capable of producing vasodilatation in the deep tissues (Sloan *et al.*, 1988). Ice is widely used in three main situations:

1. As a first-aid measure to produce a vasoconstriction and promote clotting and haemostasis.
2. To reduce pain and oedema, whether associated with recent trauma, following surgery, or during an exacerbation of arthritis.
3. To reduce spasticity and thereby enable a physiotherapist to proceed with mobilizing activities (Kirk and Kersley, 1968).

The physiological responses to ice application are complex but show the following sequence:

1. *Initial vasoconstriction*. During the first 5–15 minutes of cold application, the treated area undergoes a reduction in blood flow due to vasoconstriction and increased blood viscosity. The vasoconstriction is mediated both locally and via reflexes in the central nervous system. Local oedema is reduced and haematoma formation controlled in the acute phase of injury involving the torn muscle (e.g. quadriceps contusion or strain), ligamentous injury or a haematoma after mild injury in haemophilia.
2. *Vasodilatation*. If the cold application is continued, a sudden deep vasodilatation lasting some 4–6 minutes will ensue. This circulatory adaption is viewed as a defence against thermal insult and is capable of raising local temperature by several degrees.
3. *Vasoconstriction* is then usually re-established followed by a further period of vasodilatation in 15–30-minute cycles. This so-called 'hunting' response is a combination of limb preserving and core-preserving reflexes and can be kept up for hours.
4. *Reduction in muscle spasm*. Muscle spasm can be reduced in both neurological disease (e.g. stroke or paraplegia) and acute traumatic situations (e.g. a hamstring tear). Indirectly, therefore, pain is also decreased and the muscle prepared for further rehabilitation. With cooling, it can be demonstrated that there is a reduction of action potential firing and diminishing of deep tendon reflexes.
5. *Limited anaesthesia*. This effect is achieved after 5–10 minutes of direct application of ice, usually through a technique referred to as ice massage. As the ice is rubbed on the patient's skin, there is an initial feeling of intense cold followed by a burning and aching before some mild thermal anaesthesia takes effect. This effect can be demonstrated to last to some degree for as long as 30 minutes. This is an adequate period of time for rehabilitation (Olson and Stravins, 1972).

Cold therapy can be applied in the form of ice massage, ice baths, ice towels or cold packs (Table 19.1). Each of these techniques can be used in a slightly different situation and makes cryotherapy a versatile form of treatment.

The exact physiological effects of therapeutic heat or cold are by no means clear. There is a certain amount of individual response, and for this reason it is difficult to postulate the relative values in the various forms of treatment. It is preferable instead to leave the selection to the physiotherapist, provided he or she has been trained to develop a critical and discerning approach, recognizing the empirical nature of the treatment and understanding the need to combine the alleviation of symptoms with the objective improvement.

The precautions and contraindications of the use of cryotherapy include Raynaud's phenomenon, peripheral vascular disease, cold allergy, severe cold-induced urticaria, cryoglobulinaemia, and paroxysmal cold haemoglobinuria. Awareness

Table 19.1 Approximate reduction in tissue temperature with cooling agents

	Intramuscular temperature decrease (°C), by time after application			
Modality	15 min	30 min	45 min	60 min
Ice*	3.4	6.9	9.2	11.3
Gel	1.8	4.4	6.5	3.4
Chemical	1.6	2.9	3.0	3.5
Freon	0.2	0.9	1.2	1.7

*Supporting studies show decrease of temperature in tissues of 3.0° to 12.5° at 2 cm after 10 minutes of ice massage.

of the potential for frostbite and observing precautions, such as limiting the time of direct application of cold, thus minimizes such risks. Prolonged periods of cryotherapy directly over superficial nerve trunks have on rare occasion been associated with paralysis. Usually these nerve lesions are transient and full recovery is the norm. Some individuals have severe sensitivity to cold and may respond to ice pack therapy with an elevation of blood pressure, systolic and diastolic, in the range of 15–20 mmHg. Freon sprays have the most potential for abuse. Used sensibly, cryotherapy is one of the safest modalities, although carelessness may produce some severe circulatory problems.

ELECTRICAL MUSCLE STIMULATION

Electricity is a form of energy that can be made to exhibit magnetic, chemical, mechanical, thermal and electrostatic effects. An enormous variety of waveforms, pulse widths and frequencies are available allowing a variety of physiological responses within the tissues. The original muscle stimulator produced a faradic current that was an uneven alternating current with a pulse duration of about 1 ms and a frequency of 50 Hz. From this beginning was derived the more versatile and comfortable muscle stimulating current with a variety of pulse shapes and widths that generates muscle contraction via the motor nerve.

Other currents have been adopted for their effect on sensory nerve and their ability to alter intensity of pain impulses. These include transcutaneous nerve stimulators, interferential currents and high-voltage pulsed galvanic stimulators.

Electrical muscle stimulation (EMS) is used:

1. To enhance contraction where there is reflex inhibition.
2. To supplement contraction in post-injury or post-surgical states where the limb is immobilized.
3. To reinforce contraction, particularly towards the end of a training session when voluntary effort may decline.
4. As an adjunct to strengthening programmes.
5. As a mean of promoting normal physiology in paralyzed muscle.

In addition, EMS may be used to maintain or gain range of motion and to break down or stretch adhesions. Indirectly it may influence pain, particularly when the pain is secondary to muscle spasm (Reid, 1992). There is some discrepancy as to classification. Low-frequency stimulation is usually in the range of 10–500 or 1000 Hz and the range 1000–10 000 Hz has been variously called medium or high frequency. Electrical stimulus by a combination of intradural and extradural electrode implantation on the anterior sacral outflow has proved to be most successful in the control of urinary incontinence after spinal injury. The pelvic floor and urethral sphincter muscles are reduced in tone with regular voiding (Wheeler *et al.*, 1993).

There are numerous protocols, some designed for strengthening and others designed for endurance. Muscle contraction induced by EMS is different from voluntary contraction in that the area stimulated is usually localized to the area of current flow. This area may be relatively small and superficial. Furthermore, there tends to be a synchronous nerve recruitment and hence an unphysiological mode of firing of motor units. This situation, with the constant nerve discharge frequency, may lead to fairly rapid fatigue and this has to be accommodated in treatment protocols.

There is great discussion about the ability to strengthen normal muscle more efficiently by electrical stimulation than simple resisted exercise. However, there is little good evidence that functional electrical stimulation, i.e. to restore the movements in paralysed lower and upper limbs, has any advantage over resisted voluntary exercise unless there is some mitigating factor such as reflex inhibition from pain or effusion, disuse atrophy from immobilization, oedema, intramuscular adhesions or some degree of denervation. Whenever possible, the electrical stimulation should be combined with voluntary muscle contraction. In the correct clinical circumstances, however, the effect of EMS may be dramatic. Granat (1993) has reviewed the use of functional electrical stimulation with hybrid orthosis systems, particularly for reciprocating gait in paraplegia and some upper limb neuroprostheses. Reduction in energy expenditure can be achieved at the patient's preferred walking speed.

For restoring some form of locomotion in the paraplegic or quadraplegic, functional electrical stimulation (FES) with dynamic activation of muscle is now possible. Kralj and Bajd (1991) have pointed out that FES can promote cardiovascular conditioning and general improvement in metabolism. They emphasize that a dynamic weight transfer phase must be incorporated to improve gait efficiency and velocity but because of lack of balance control FES assisted gait required balancing aids, e.g. crutches or orthosis such as the hip guidance orthosis of Oswestry or reciprocating gait orthosis of Orleans.

The hybrid system is defined as applying mechanical forces to give stability and using FE stimulated muscles to provide the propulsive forces. However, safety, comfort, cosmesis, its use in a home or work setting, its durability and backup equipment, and finally the fast fatiguing of electrically stimulated muscle, all are important in its design, development and use outside the laboratory.

TRANSCUTANEOUS ELECTRICAL NEURAL STIMULATION (TENS, TNS, TCNS)

Transcutaneous electrical neural stimulation (TENS) is also referred to as transcutaneous neural stimulation (TNS). Initially during the 1960s, TENS were used as a screening test to identify patients who might benefit from implanted dorsal column stimulators for the treatment of chronic pain. Many patients, however, experienced considered relief after TENS application itself, thus raising the interest in this as a pain-relieving modality.

The contemporary era of electrical stimulation began with the publication of a theory on pain by Melzac and Wall (1965) (Figure 19.1). This 'gate' theory proposed that both large and small diameter fibres synapse on common cells in the dorsolateral horns of the spinal cord. Input travelling along small fibres is thought to facilitate transmission of pain sensation to the central pathways. However, input along the large diameter fibres, which are more commonly associated with mechanical reception, can inhibit the small fibre input by interaction at the dorsolateral horn level. More recent experiments have shown that a variety of other influences are at work both at the spinal level and even within the brain stem and brain itself. Indeed, several gates may affect the perception of pain and other sensory input. It has been shown that stimulation of the spinal cord can inhibit the passage of sensory inflow to the cortex, as demonstrated by decrease in sensory somatocortical potentials. While the exact mechanism of pain transmission is still poorly understood, most neurophysiologists would now accept the phenomenon of pain inhibition by electrical stimulation of peripheral and central neural structures. For this reason neurostimulators have been developed and are now being widely used for low back pain syndromes, neck pain, etc.

There is also some possibility that electrical stimulation may produce pain relief via endorphin production. Indeed, if the suggestion that endorphin and enkephalin production can be stimulated by TENS is true, then the chemical effect could outlast the period of stimulation, thus explaining some of the longer-term relief.

There are two basic forms of TENS, low- and high-intensity. Low-intensity TENS, applied to high pulse rate (up to 100 pulses per second), does not cause muscle contraction. It is usually comfortable and barely perceivable. High-intensity TENS is applied at a tolerable level of approximately 10 pulses per second and is likely to be less comfortable and usually is modulated to achieve the desired pain-relieving effect.

Pain relief

High-frequency TENS mainly between 100 and 500 Hz is set at a frequency that produces a distinct tingling sensation. This frequency gives the fastest pain relief of all techniques of TENS application although it may be of short duration. In this regard it is often used as a pretreatment for other exercise modalities. In the acute situation it may supplement the standard ice, rest, and elevation protocol and in chronic pain situations, it is applied for 30 minutes up to 24 hours.

By contrast, low-frequency high-intensity stimulation, often referred as acupuncture-like low-frequency TENS, may bring about an associated muscle contraction. It is felt that it is this pattern

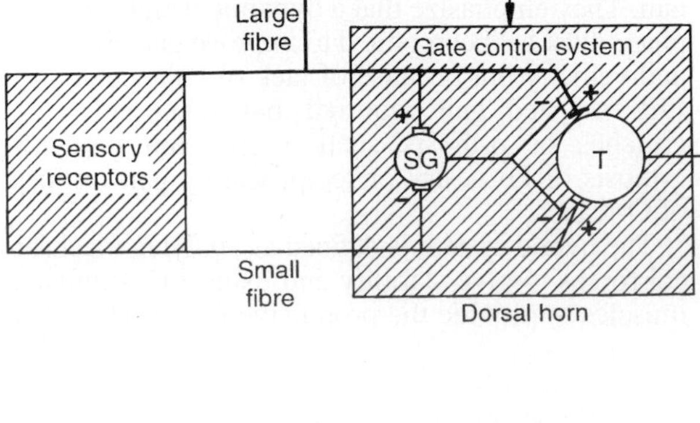

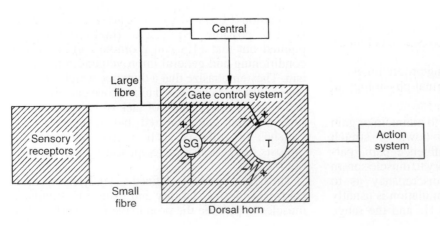

Figure 19.1 Cells of the substantia gelatinosa (SG) serve as a modifying or grading system for sensory input. Large fibre activity closes the gate, and an increase in small fibre activity opens the gate to the transmission of nociceptive information by the transmission cells (T) and brain. (After Melzack and Wall, 1965)

of TENS that has some systemic effect via the endorphins.

The individual response to transcutaneous nerve stimulators is very variable, but many people suffering from chronic pain syndromes have reported benefit from the intermittent use of this type of apparatus. While the exact indications for the use of TENS are still to be defined, this mode of therapy has the advantage in that the apparatus is compact, can be applied by the patients themselves at any convenient time, does not appear to be associated with any serious side-effects in the central nervous system, and perhaps presents a welcome alternative to the chronic use of pain-relieving medication. The disadvantage is, of course, the cost of supplying each patient with such an apparatus and the efficacy of this treatment will have to be more clearly delineated before it is cost-effective (Ray, 1977).

IONIZATION

The process of driving ions into the tissues by an electric current is referred to as ionization or iontophoresis. This is not a frequently practised therapy at the present time but in the past histamine has been used as a counter-irritant. Experiments using radioactive isotope clearance techniques show that both the application of a direct current and the production of a histamine iontophoresis bring about an increase in the skin circulation, the increase due to histamine iontophoresis being about 100% greater than that due to direct current alone. However, the changes in the underlying blood flow are of an insignificant quantity. An increase in circulation in the deeper tissues occurs as part of a generalized histamine reaction. Thus the main effect of both direct current and histamine iontophoresis is superficial. Neither technique produces a circulatory effect deep to the skin. Both techniques are capable of giving counter-irritation but, since this can also be achieved quite efficiently by the application of histamine ointment, it is questionable whether ionization techniques are justified.

Currently there is interest in using cortisol and some non steroidal anti-inflammatories as topical agents and using iontophoresis to increase efficacy (Griffin and Karselis, 1982). There are few data available to evaluate this form of therapy.

Depending on the desired effect, electrodes may be placed directly over the painful area, over nerve plexus and trunks or over motor, trigger or acupuncture points. The latter technique is referred to as electroacupuncture.

Therapeutic exercise

Wasting and weakness of muscles occurs rapidly when adjacent joints are involved in a disease process, are injured, or are immobilized. Tone, power and muscle bulk diminish early in muscles such as the quadriceps and the interossei, and can be detected clinically, but similar changes are associated to a greater or lesser degree with all acute and chronic joint disease. In particular, this wasting is very dramatic wherever there is significant pain or effusion present in the joint, and this is particularly true following surgery. This wasting is not simply a disuse atrophy but is compounded to some degree by reflex neural mechanisms as some systemic hormonal responses which seem to aggravate the process of muscle wasting (Haggmark *et al.*, 1978). This wasting and atrophy can be minimized by prompt reduction of pain and a programme of static (muscle-setting) exercises in the most comfortable range practised regularly several times a day. However, once muscle weakness or wasting is established, a more elaborate programme of exercises becomes necessary.

There are two recent areas of research and interest which have greatly affected the approach to rehabilitation of the unstable joint as well as following ligament surgery. The first is the appreciation of potential proprioceptive deficits compounding mechanical instability of joints, exaggerating and producing increasing functional instability. The second is the increasing knowledge of the fine control of muscles around a joint, the so-called intrinsic muscle balance, that is altered by pain and trauma and may manifest itself by persistent dysfunction and pain. This in turn can contribute to functional instability, even further pain, and thus establishment of a vicious cycle of more inhibition of muscle control. These two new areas, particularly in the field of sports medicine, have generated interest in developing numerous protocols involving either balance and proprioceptive training or, alternatively, the use of biofeedback techniques for intrinsic muscle control adopted to functional movement patterns. Specific examples will be given later in the chapter.

PASSIVE MOVEMENTS

The movement of joints and muscles by a therapist, unaided by voluntary contraction of the muscle by the patient, is known as 'passive movement'. Passive movement maintains joint mobility and proprioceptive sense, when muscles are excessively weak or paralysed. This technique may also be used to re-establish mobility in joints which have stiffened up. Such movements are particularly useful in the early phases of management after paralysis. The need for a full range of motion at a paralysed joint, however, must be carefully assessed. For instance, in spinal cord injuries it may indeed be desirable in some cases to allow a certain amount of stiffness to occur within the wrist and fingers so that good tenodesis action may be used to supplement a weak grip. By contrast, a stiff, painful, fixed shoulder will occur rapidly after a stroke if passive mobilization is not introduced very early and maintained for several weeks. In this later situation, the stiffness produces a significant handicap. Similarly, stiff fingers are common after brachial plexus lesions, if the hand and arm are not passively mobilized early and if oedema is allowed to become established and organized. In general, passive movements have little part to play in the management of arthritis, although gentle passive mobilization – particularly as part of a hydrotherapy programme – may often help to increase the range of motion in the shoulder, hips and knees. By contrast, the elbow and the finger joints usually react badly to passive movement in arthritic conditions. Indeed, passive stretching of the elbow is rarely appropriate unless it is of the prolonged stretching technique variety as practised with the haemophilic joint using a balanced suspension and continued traction (Duthie *et al.*, 1994).

ASSISTED MOVEMENTS

During assisted movements, the patient actively collaborates with the therapist by contracting the muscles while the therapist assists the movement. This type of exercise is particularly useful during early recovery after paralysis and in the early mobilization of joints after injury or operation when the movements are inhibited by pain as well as weakness.

FREE MOVEMENTS

As the patient progresses, movement may be achieved without assistance from the therapist and the patient. Free movements may be undertaken with the assistance of springs or water to eliminate the effects of gravity, and, as joint range and muscle power increase, the exercises can often be carried out against gravity.

Often in the early stages of rehabilitation, the patient can achieve a greater range of movement when gravity has been eliminated. Judgement is needed on the part of the therapist to decide the point at which resisted exercises are to be introduced, since in some circumstances premature introduction of resisted work may prevent restoration of adequate joint range.

RESISTED EXERCISES (STRENGTHENING TECHNIQUES)

Resisted exercises may be classified as:

1. Isometric – increasing muscle tension without altering the muscle length.
2. Isotonic – exercises performed against resistance with joint movement occurring.

Isotonic exercise has several broad patterns: concentric, eccentric and isokinetic. With concentric exercise, as the muscle contracts the two bones involved in the joint move closer together. With eccentric exercise the muscle ‘pays out’ against resistance and the muscle lengthens. The best example is the hamstring muscle slowing the swinging leg in walking and running.

Isometric exercises

These exercises are performed when movement is not desirable or possible. The are particularly applicable to limbs immobilized in plaster casts, whether because of fractures, orthopaedic procedures or joint inflammation (Partridge and Duthie, 1963). There is good evidence that even in acute arthritis from whatever cause (e.g. rheumatoid arthritis or haemophilic haemarthrosis), muscle bulk can be maintained and wasted muscle encouraged to increase in bulk by isometric exercises provided the joint is adequately splinted and pain relieved. The advantage of this type of resisted exercise is that maximum resistance may be applied in the most comfortable part of the range. For example, with retropatellar chondromalacia, maximal resisted work usually may be given in full extension without retropatellar discomfort.

Isotonic exercises

This type of resisted exercise can be used for developing either muscle power or muscle endurance, or a combination of both. There are many different techniques, some using increasing loads, some using decreasing loads and some keeping the resistance constant for each set. In addition, it is usually recognized that low repetitions up to a maximum of 12 can be used for maximum gains in strength while repetitions in the region of 15–30 or more can be used for building endurance. There has been much new literature concerning the physiology of muscle wasting and re-education as influenced by isotonic exercise. Human muscle consists of several different fibre types, of which type I (also referred to as red or slow-twitch fibre) seems to waste disproportionately with disuse or joint pain (Haggmark *et al.*, 1978). It is the type I muscle fibre that is mainly involved in postural activity and high repetition work, and is very resistant to fatigue, provided adequate oxygen is supplied, since the basic energy source is aerobic for this type of muscle fibre. Conversely, the other major muscle type in human muscle, type IIa (also called white or fast-twitch fibre), is mainly involved in the production of maximal power but has the characteristics of easy fatigue and depends on glycolytic anaerobic energy sources. It has become apparent that different types of exercises influence these different fibre types, and therefore in a complete rehabilitation programme it is often necessary to have a mixture of high resistance, low repetition work leading to eventually high repetition endurance muscle exercise towards the end of the rehabilitation programme (Eriksson, 1980). It must be remembered that uncontrolled weight-resisted exercises may well give rise to complications of a joint in the form of effusion, exacerbation of pain, and even ligamentous laxity.

Concentric and eccentric muscle work influence the muscle slightly differently. Delayed muscle soreness is usually greater with eccentric work; however, it is important in that many functional movement patterns use this type of contraction. Furthermore, in conditions with an element of joint pain, one or the other type of contraction may be more comfortable for the patient and this would dictate the choice of technique.

When the resistance is applied to a long lever arm the joint forces may be exceedingly high. For example, retropatellar forces may be several times body weight with traditional leg extensions with resistance added. Furthermore, these techniques may produce undesirable shear on ligaments. For instance, in the last 30° of knee extension there is a large shearing force on the anterior cruciate ligament. This may be undesirable following cruciate surgery and thus these techniques of 'open kinematic chain' are not always appropriate. By applying the resistance to the sole of the foot (weight-bearing or leg-press apparatus), the kinematic chain is closed and the anterior tibial shear is reduced.

Each ligament (static joint support) has a dynamic muscle counterpart. The quadriceps, for instance, are posterior cruciate analogues and the hamstrings are anterior cruciate analogues at the knee. Thus the therapist appropriately elects to emphasize one group over another in specific ligament-deficient situations at each joint.

In other situations co-contraction of agonist and antagonist muscles enhances early strength following surgery to a joint while reducing undesirable shear in one or other direction. This is another principle used in rehabilitation following anterior cruciate surgery.

At present there are many new forms of resisted exercise equipment available, each with its special advantage. For instance, some forms of equipment, referred to as isokinetic, are specially designed to alter their resistance to match the speed and power of the movement in different parts of the range and thus accommodate to painful arcs of movement. The best known of this type of equipment is the Cybex isometric apparatus. Nevertheless, while these sophisticated types of equipment offer certain advantages over the normal resisted exercise against gravity, it still requires care and imagination in the selection of the correct exercise routine and particularly in the progression of these routines as the muscle gains in power and endurance. The most important component of this type of accommodating resistance apparatus is that computerization has allowed quantification and visualization of the patient's effort. This information may be used to record progress, develop biofeedback or as outcome measures and standards for both research and clinical situations.

Isokinetic exercises and testing

Isokinetic exercise is said to occur when the speed of contraction is set and the resistance is adjusted through out the range to balance the muscle effort. This is usually achieved either hydraulically or in some cases electrically. The concept of isokinetic exercise was popularized initially by Hislop and Thistle in 1967 (Hislop and Perrine, 1967; Thistle *et al.*, 1967). It was followed by the appreciation that torque values could be graphed, accurately measured, reproduced and computerized, giving a more objective assessment method than the time honoured manual muscle test and free-weight systems. Many of these apparatus measure strength (slow torque), power (maximum torque developed at faster velocities) and endurance (Figure 19.2). Despite spectacular advances in technology, the implications of these measurements are not universally accepted, and the information obtained on one machine is not transferable to a different system.

A large variety of omnikinetic and isokinetic instruments have been developed that allow reciprocal varying speed muscle action and there are also devices that allow omnikinetic, eccentric, and concentric muscle action. Each company has developed an accompanying computer package, and in reality it would be fair to say that the ability to generate

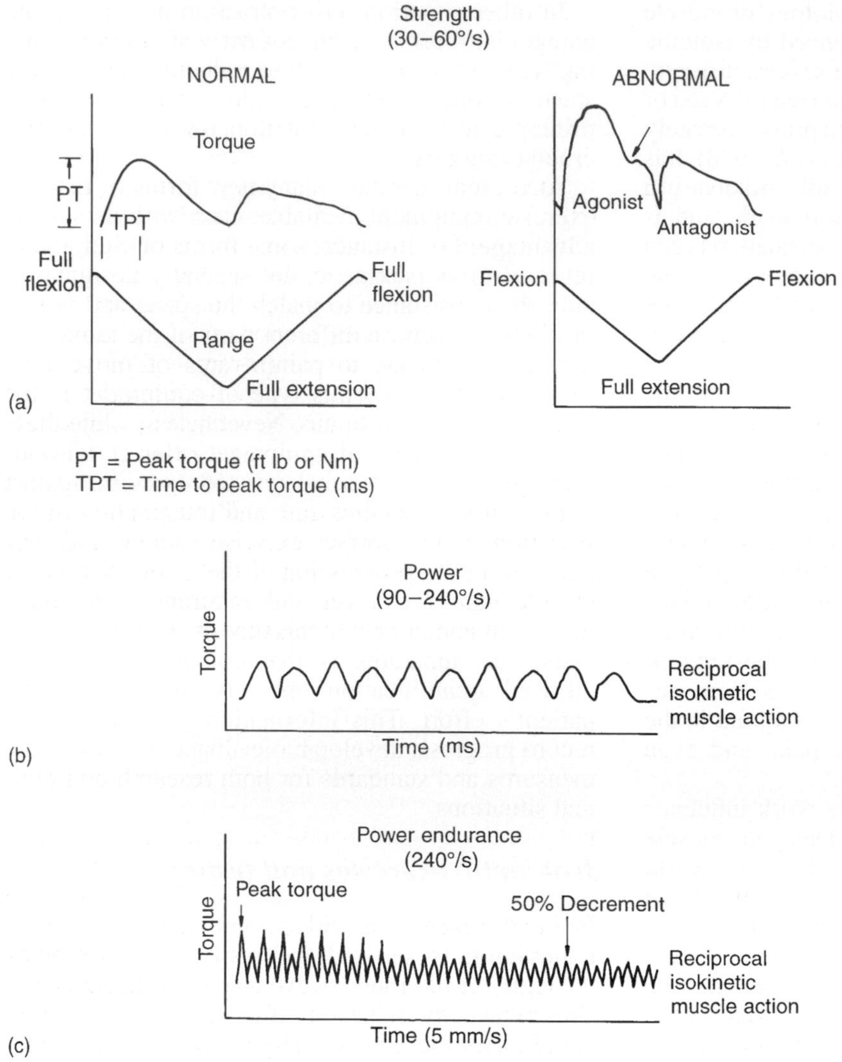

Figure 19.2 Isokinetic tracings. (a) At 30–60° per second, peak torque and time to peak torque are indications of strength. (b) Reciprocal contraction at higher speeds measure power. (c) Measurements of the decrement by 50% gives an indication of endurance. (Afer Reid, 1992)

numbers has fast surpassed our grasp for what they mean in terms of function, performance and safe return to employment and activity.

Normal values have been established for specific populations, specific muscle actions and specific speeds of limb segment movement. These normals are specific for each machine and are not directly transferable. To some degree these problems are circumvented by considering ratios of strength and endurance between the muscle groups within a limb rather than between apparatus. Nevertheless, in view of the ability of these machines to provide a visual feedback and permanent record that can be used to assess patient progress and to supplement biofeedback training as well as the ability to measure safely muscle action throughout a range of motion, they have become very important clinical and research tools in the rehabilitation world.

PROPRIOCEPTIVE TRAINING

One of the most exciting recent advances in therapeutic exercises is the emphasis on retraining proprioceptive reflexes. Definite position sense and balance deficiencies may be demonstrated in the unstable shoulder, the cruciate-deficient knee and the functional unstable ankle. While improving strength is still a key goal in the rehabilitation of these joints, improved proprioceptive reflexes sometimes has a greater impact on functional stability and hence becomes a major thrust in rehabilitation protocols (Reid, 1992).

MOBILIZING EXERCISES

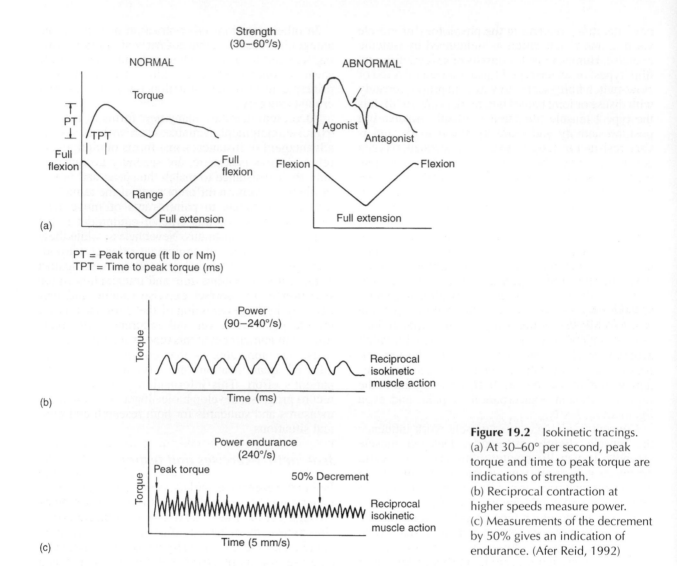

These are aimed at increasing joint movement and

are best delayed until active joint reactions have settled. Progressed at optimal speed there should be no recurrence of joint symptoms or evidence of any flare up of joint pain, effusion or indeed loss of range. Mobilizing exercises are often preceded by the application of heat or ice packs, or they may be performed in water (hydrotherapy) or in suspension apparatus, or using various apparatus such as wall bars or parallel bars. The technique of the exercise is adapted to the particular clinical situation. The physiotherapist responsible for the treatment needs careful guidance as to the restrictions necessary and the expected response to activity. An important part of the physiotherapist's treatment is the on-going assessment of the functional capability with regard to joint range achieved and the resistance overcome. In this way, therapist, clinician and patient have an objective record of progress.

As recovery proceeds, the specific exercise usually should give way to more purposeful activities. Acts of walking, getting in and out of bed, on and off the lavatory, dressing and gradually increasing activities up to the level of normal living and work provide an area for collaboration between physiotherapist and occupational therapist.

FUNCTIONAL ACTIVITIES

Functional or purposive activities may persuade a patient to greater effort than repetitive exercises in the gymnasium, and enable all concerned to obtain a realistic assessment of the patient's functional capabilities. These exercises may be occupation specific (work hardening) or sport specific. It requires a detailed knowledge of the activity in order to evolve functional training programmes that progress safely towards achieving a functional goal without jeopardizing the healing structure. These activities emphasize skills along with strength and endurance in specific ranges.

It is a basic skill of the therapists, reinforced by experience, that allows maximum progression of ability towards functional independence without flaring up the underlying pathology or damaging healing tissue.

The intensity and duration of exercise and activity routines varies considerably with the clinical problem.

Manipulation and mobilization

Many of the joints of the body have small gliding motions that occur in conjunction with the better recognized primary motion of the joint. These small gliding motions are necessary for normal joint patterns and are referred to as joint play. These movements can be quite subtle, as in the intercarpal motion at the wrist, the intertarsal motion in the foot or the facet joint motion in the spine. Indeed, some of this joint play may be lost following trauma, surgery or inflammation. To restore normal motion to the joint it may be necessary to restore joint play. While this can often be achieved by normal active motion, joint play can be restored by small repetitive low amplitude and pressure motions referred to mobilizations (as for spinal arthritis) or by larger amplitude more forceful movements called manipulation. Skill is necessary to achieve the necessary relaxation required for these motions, and a good knowledge of functional anatomy and of the underlying pathology in order to localize the forces (Maitland, 1973) and prevent further damage. While the exact indications and contraindications for many of these techniques are yet to be standardized, there is undoubtedly a role for this modality in orthopaedic treatments.

Occupational therapy

In the past, occupational therapy has been concerned particularly with diversional activities; however, the emphasis is now being increasingly laid on the functional assessment of the patient's capabilities, exploitation of residual skills, and the institution of planning retraining to compensate for permanent disability. In addition, the involvement of the occupational therapist with many aspects of assessment and treatment of the mentally ill patients now forms a significant role in some hospitals. With a background training in the relationship of crafts, skills and daily activities to normal and pathological anatomy, the occupational therapist can undertake the integrated functional assessment of the physically handicapped. Practical functional assessment should precede the planning of the final stages of rehabilitation and resettlement, and repeated assessments provide an objective record of the patient's progress. Some of this assessment is carried out in the patient's home environment or work situation (Haworth *et al.*, 1981).

Occupational therapy aims at achieving improvement in muscle power, joint range and functional achievement through purposeful movement and activities. This may involve the use of splints or appliances. For example, the patient with rheumatoid arthritis may not be able to hold conventional cutlery, but may be able to feed herself either by using adapted cutlery or with the conventional appliances when wrist, thumb and finger are stabilized in a lightweight plastic splint.

Careful evaluation of the patient's functional capabilities and activities of daily living, leisure activities and at work, or in a work simulating situation, provide essential background information for the overall management of the patient. Repeated evaluation of functional capabilities provides an objective measure of improvement or deterioration often not clearly interpreted from muscle power charts or joint range measurements.

Although by its very nature, occupational therapy tends to be more concerned with upper-limb function, it has a considerable contribution to make to lower-limb function and to general activities. Many of the conventional craft techniques can be exploited to provide graduated exercises for the lower limbs and many activities of daily living (dressing and toilet activities) require a co-ordinated action of upper limbs, lower limbs and trunk.

The majority of older patients undergoing orthopaedic care will have some impairment of function, and, although often not essential, the careful assessment of their activities of daily living by an occupational therapist may enable the patient to achieve many important goals leading to independence (Table 19.2). Getting in and out of bed, getting on and off the toilet, dressing, housework and leisure activities may all involve complex manoeuvres for the elderly, the arthritic or modifications of habit pattern can make life easier, and complement the orthopaedic management of the disability (Haworth *et al.*, 1981).

In the care of the more severely and chronically disabled, diversional activities, craft work, hobbies and general activities each have a specific value, but more important is the functional assessment and improvement of functional activities. Most patients in the orthopaedic wards will require some help in regaining maximal functional recovery. Depending on the personnel available, some occupational therapists develop special expertise in the production and fitting of various orthotic appliances, particularly functional splints for the upper limb. Naturally there is an overlap of function in several areas of occupational therapy with the orthotists, physiotherapist and social worker. In fact, collaboration within the rehabilitation team is absolutely vital, and must include the speech therapist and the occupational psychologist.

Table 19.2 Comparison of satisfaction/disappointment of 145 patients who received total hip replacement (Haworth *et al.*, 1981)

Area of daily living	Satisfied with improvement (%)	Disappointed because expectations not fulfilled (%)
Relief of pain	97	10
Mobility	92	15
Personal care	86	3
Leisure/social activities	73	3
Transport	64	6
Domestic activities	64	2
Work	31	1

Special rehabilitation problems

Patients who require special rehabilitation facilities include those who need a high degree of physical fitness for their work; for their sporting activities; those with multiple injuries, those with complex lesions (such as crush injuries of the hand, spinal injuries and head injuries); and those with lesions or diseases which give rise to severe residual disability. All such patients benefit from the intensive full time regimen of special rehabilitation centres and from the integration of a retraining programme for work at the final stages of their rehabilitation.

The number of patients in these categories with lesions of traumatic origin is small compared with the total number of patients with medical locomotor disorders in the population as a whole. Whether or not such patients need rehabilitation in a special unit is dictated by the severity of the causative disease.

REHABILITATION TECHNIQUES AND PERSONNEL

There are five main groups of physically disabled patients, each having its own particular rehabilitation problems:

1. Those patients for whom full recovery is to be expected.
2. Those with permanent but stable disabilities, such as amputation.
3. Those with unstable disabilities, such as rheumatoid arthritis.
4. Those with chronic and degenerative disorders, such as osteoarthritis and disseminated sclerosis.
5. Those with sports injuries and requiring to return to full fitness.

The key to full development of rehabilitation in the hospital service is the attitude of the hospital medical staff. Comparatively few patients need special measures of rehabilitation. All of them, however, benefit to the fullest extent from hospital treatment only when that treatment is conceived and planned from the outset with the effect on the patient's working capacity and his home life in mind. The clinician's responsibility is not restricted simply to the diagnosis and care of the patient. There is the further responsibility of assessing the patient's capacity and recommending the appropriate rehabilitation and training for any patient likely to be left with some residual disability. These patients will need assessment of:

1. What work can be done.
2. Whether new employment is necessary and, if so, whether retraining is indicated.
3. What assistance is needed in the home.
4. What sporting activity is to be achieved.

The team approach to such problems is mandatory and may involve the surgeon, the physician, the medical social workers, the disablement resettlement officers, physiotherapists, occupational therapists, speech therapists, psychologists and the nursing staff. It is obvious that total rehabilitation in its fullest sense is a multifaceted problem and requires thorough record keeping and good co-ordination.

MOTIVATION IN REHABILITATION

Illness and injury always induce some anxiety in the patient and relatives, and the response to incapacity depends on the patient's personality, education, and social and economic situation. Motivation may be described as the expression of the patient's personality when striving to overcome adversity, and thus it is also an expression of his response to rehabilitation. Evaluation of the premorbid personality and adequate assessment of the social, educational and economic circumstances are as important in rehabilitation as a realistic delineation of the prognosis and likely functional handicap. It is within this area that the art of medicine is as important as the science, for the methodology available for the quantitative assessment of personality and motivation of the physically disabled is not readily achieved and no generally acceptable and simply applied techniques have been devised.

Indeed, there is little available literature on this important subject, although there is a great deal of psychological literature, dealing with motivation in a more general manner. There is no evidence that there are particular personalities associated with specific disabilities, but many physical disorders are associated with organic changes in the brain, thus inducing intellectual and personality changes.

Painful conditions and physical disabilities undoubtedly bring about reactive depression. Severe disability limiting social activities and contacts will clearly be accompanied by personality changes. The psychological trauma of amputation is obvious and the appropriate preparation of patients for ablative surgery is being increasingly introduced.

Lastly, the reactions of patients to minor injury, their reaction to minor handicap, and the factors which determine a patient's return to work are subjects of considerable clinical, psychological and economic interest, and as yet there is little advice and information available.

Orthotics and prosthetics

Orthotics is the application of an orthosis to the body after assessment, prescription, manufacture and fitting.

The traditional splint, surgical appliance or orthopaedic brace are now covered by the term 'orthosis' (plural, 'orthoses') but this is difficult to define in a comprehensive and meaningful way. For example, the British Orthopaedic Association Committee define it as 'a device or external appliance which promotes limb function, excluding prosthesis', and Rose has defined it as 'an external appliance designed to apply forces to the body in a controlled manner, to perform one or both of two basic functions – the control of body motion and alteration of body tissue shape'. The second definition requires understanding of basic concepts of mechanics such as force, equilibrium, pressure, movement and torque which must apply to the manufacture and fitting of all orthoses. Basically, orthotic devices are used to assist joints which are unstable, lack power or are painful. They should provide freedom to move in all the axes of the natural joint concerned.

Prosthesis is the term used to define a replacement of a body part by a mechanical substitute. Depending on the circumstance these prostheses may be directly controlled and driven by muscle action or via electrical potential from selected muscle groups. These electrical sequels are amplified and used to trigger electric motors (myoelectric limbs). Newer computer technology has encouraged the evolution of new electric limbs and braces with implanted neural electrodes. In addition, computerized patterned activities in braces are being evolved to assist motion of paralysed extremities. The material of limb orthoses varies considerably from country to country but there are two basic types available:

1. Conventional metal and leather.

2. Moulded plastics, with or without reinforcement by carbon fibres, graphite, etc.

Plastics and polypropylene have begun to attain popularity in the fabrication of many types of lower limb orthoses – especially in the correction of ankle and foot problems – for their lightness and for being more hygienic and cosmetically acceptable. Today there are over a hundred different suitable materials available for strong lightweight construction.

BIOMECHANICS

No orthosis can exert an influence on body position or motion except by applying stress to the body, which must be either pressure (i.e. stress applied at right angles to the surface) or shear, which is stress applied parallel to the surface of the orthosis against the skin, subcutaneous tissue and deeper tissues.

Shear can be very destructive, particularly in a scarred area. Obviously, to reduce pressure – especially in a dynamic situation – it must be spread over a large area (e.g. weight-bearing over superficial bony points). Failure to distinguish pressure from shear causes many problems in orthotic mechanics as well as for the patient's skin surface, resulting in pressure sores, pain, etc. Therefore shear should be prevented by applying a sliding membrane between the skin and the contact area (e.g. a nylon stocking beneath a woollen one).

CLASSIFICATION OF ORTHOSES

Appliances can be classified as:

1. Devices which rest a joint or fracture in an acceptable and functional position. For example, a Thomas splint or cast bracing (e.g. patellar-bearing, hip hinge thigh brace); such a device made up of a plastic quadrilateral thigh cast with a rigid pelvic band through a stable uniplanar hip hinge, has been shown to be efficacious and economical for fractures involving the proximal half of the femur as well as for fractures below a total hip replacement (Meggitt and Vaughan-Lane, 1980).
2. Devices which totally or partially relieve weight from a joint (e.g. caliper, spinal braces in muscular dystrophy).
3. Stabilizing a joint/joints (e.g. long leg caliper).
4. Correcting or preventing deformity – i.e. those which change the shape of body tissues. This group is difficult to use, as high forces can be generated on the skin (e.g. modified Milwaukee brace).
5. Exercising muscles (e.g. a lively splint for a paralysed hand or a quadriceps enhancing splint for the knee.
6. Controlling joint range and/or direction (e.g. articulated knee caliper with stops to provide range control – active or passive.
7. Re-educating phasic muscle activity (e.g. in cerebral palsy).
8. Transmitting forces (e.g. in scoliosis).
9. Providing cosmetic or protective coverage (e.g. a glove).

An orthotics terminology, developed in the USA by a committee of the National Academy of Sciences (Harris, 1973), is now widely used in North America and is gaining acceptance elsewhere. The basis of the terminology is that orthoses are described by the joints they encompass – in the lower limb, hip, knee, ankle and foot. Thus, for example, an orthosis spanning the knee, ankle or foot is a knee–ankle–foot orthosis (KAFO). The orthosis is further described by the control which it imposes on motion at each point:

- F Free – free motion permitted in any direction.
- A Assist – application of external force for the purpose of increasing the range, velocity of force of a motion (e.g. spring, use of gravity).
- R Resist – application of an external force to decrease the force of velocity of a desired motion.
- S Stop – prevention of an undesired motion in one direction.
- H Hold – elimination of all movement in a prescribed plane.
- L Lock – device includes an optional lock.
- V Variable – a unit which can be adjusted without making any structural change.

Such a schedule helps not only to define the orthotic vocabulary but also to build up an understanding between the doctors prescribing and the orthotist.

ASSESSMENT OF THE PATIENT

Accurate assessment of the patient is required in order to prescribe the orthosis best suited to a particular patient's needs. It is vital that the surgeon understands the details of normal gait or upper limb function or spinal factors and communicates this to the orthotist. His main task is the clinical assessment of the patient's abnormal gait or altered function. Because each orthosis presents its own anatomic restraints, these must be balanced against the benefit it offers.

Lower limb

A wide range of disorders interfere with walking –

cerebral palsy, stroke, myelomeningocele, brain injury, muscular dystrophy, arthritis, trauma and congenital abnormality. It is no longer sufficient to memorize a list of typical limps. Rather, the actions of each body segment must be identified and their deviation from normal noted.

The clinical analysis of abnormal gait is difficult because of problems of visualizing changes occurring simultaneously at a number of joints. Perry (1975, personal communication) regarded walking as a changing sequence of standing postures, the two basic requirements of which are stance stability and stride length. The patient's potential for walking may be determined more easily by assessing stability at three levels: standing, single limb standing and walking.

The interdependence of the hip, knee and ankle require the examiner to consider all three joints even when his attention is directed chiefly to one. Distinction must be made between primary and secondary abnormalities – if an orthosis is prescribed to control a secondary abnormality, while ignoring the primary one, gait deteriorates. For example, equinus deformity at the ankle may be accompanied by hyperextension at the knee, allowing the trunk to be aligned over the feet, and maintaining a stable position. If hyperextension of the knee is prevented by an inappropriate orthosis, the entire limb is directed posteriorly, aligning the trunk behind the heels. In order to retain stability, the patient must flex at the hips, and even with strong hip extensors or crutch support this is an insecure position.

Major *et al.* (1981) have described the complex dynamics of walking for spinal paraplegics, in which, by stabilizing the knees and using the hip guidance orthosis, bilateral crutches provide control for forward movements. In addition, small propulsive forces are produced which reduce somewhat the high energy consumption of this severe disability. The swing-through gait with the bracing of back, hips and knees in heavy long length calipers attached to the body brace produces enormous energy consumption.

Upper limb

In the upper extremity, the main purpose of supporting the weight of the arm and of stabilizing the joints is to assist some of the functions of the hand – grip or pinch, to position the hand through the shoulder, elbow and wrist joints for some function in relationship to the surfaces of the body (e.g. for eating and drinking, for toilet purposes) or to position the hand for working on flat surfaces in front of the body or to provide stability and/or power for movement of the body. Various components of this total upper limb function can be provided by single (e.g. wrist support) or more complex total orthotic devices (e.g. the pivotal mobile arm support on a wheelchair or working surface or a free-standing upper extremity pneumatic mobile arm support (Radulovic *et al.*, 1980). Myoelectric control and power with sensory feedback mechanisms are being developed to assist upper-limb orthotics in their complex role. Electrical stimulation and substitution by electrically programmed orthosis in the severely paralysed patient (e.g. with quadriplegia or following a stroke) are being developed.

Spine

Greater understanding of the biomechanics of the spine – not only for posture but also for loading and for movement – has permitted improvement in spinal support (e.g. modification of the original Milwaukee brace, corsets, traction devices such as the halo–thoracic–pelvic). For extensive description and illustration of all orthotics, the *Atlas of Orthotics* by the American Academy of Orthopaedic Surgeons (1985) is recommended.

PRESCRIPTION

McCullough (1985) has described a systematic approach to orthotic prescription, which has been adopted by the Committee on Orthotics and Prosthetics of the American Academy of Orthopaedic Surgeons. The essential steps are:

1. Biomechanical analysis of the patient.
2. Summary of function disability.
3. Identity of objectives of treatment.
4. Specify orthotic controls at each level.
5. Select appropriate orthotic components.
6. Combine components into orthosis.

Although this analysis cannot be applied to all patients, McCullough believes that the concept of a biomechanical approach of this nature is essential to writing an orthotic prescription.

Foot orthoses should provide to correct mobile deformity, accommodate fixed deformity, and where necessary limit movement.

Ankle–foot orthoses should limit movement, provide stability, relieve stress or give some dorsiflexion assistance.

Knee orthoses should stabilize the knee, especially in the sagittal and coronal planes, provide relief from the longitudinal stress of weight-bearing or torsional force but usually limit movement. Knee orthoses have been further divided as to their function, namely prophylactic, postoperative and functional. The role of prophylactic knee orthosis is questionable and while protecting some ligaments from outside forces in sport, others may be placed at risk. The more complex, expensive braces may give some measure of protection for sport related stresses. Postoperative braces are usually designed in such a way that range of motion is controlled according to the surgeon's protocol. Functional braces are designed to compensate for instability. These may produce their effect via psychological (confidence) and physiological (enhancing proprioception) means as well as biomechanically enhancing stability. In many situations the latter is the least important.

Hip orthoses should provide stabilization of the hip in ambulation, but this is a complex problem and orthotic substitution for hip musculature is difficult. Adult patients who lack trunk stability and pelvic and trunk control do not usually become outdoor walkers. A particular problem is that pelvic and trunk control orthoses may block substitution mechanisms (e.g. Trendelenburg) which the patient uses to maintain stability during gait. They should provide weight relief through an ischial ring or quadrilateral socket or pattern-ended calipers, provide position, and guide hips in ambulation, or correct deformity.

Myoelectric prostheses

Silcox *et al.* (1993) have reviewed their large series of 44 patients over a 17-year experience and a 5-year follow-up. Initially their indications in prescribing a myoelectric prosthesis were for patients who used a conventional prosthesis very well, who had a keen interest and a stump with excellent sensation and good skin. Later these were extended to all patients who had had an acute amputation. The average age of fitting was 38 years. Ninety-one per cent of patients had received a traumatic amputation (work related accident, 28; military service, 7; motor vehicle injury, 5), the remaining patients had vascular insufficiency, tumour and congenital abnormalities.

Fifty per cent rejected the myoelectric prosthesis completely against 32% who had rejected the conventional prosthesis; and 55% wearing cosmetic prostheses also rejected them. Factors associated with rejection were subjects receiving or seeking workers' compensation, those employed in manual occupations, e.g. repetitive manual labour, lifting more than 10 lbs.

Age, sex, dominant limb, length of time before fitting prosthesis, were not found to be significant. In this study 50% of the patients who owned two prostheses preferred the conventional and only 33% preferred the myoelectric type. These authors also commented that they did not find any association between the belief that the sensory feedback was better with the myoelectric prosthesis and its better usage.

References

American Academy of Orthopedic Surgeons (1985) *Atlas of Orthotics*. C.V. Mosby: St Louis

Borrell, R.M., Parker, R., Henley, E.J., Masley, D. and Repinecz, M. (1980) Comparison of *in vivo* temperatures produced by hydrotherapy, paraffin wax treatment and fluidotherapy. *Physical Therapy* **60**, 1273–1276

DeAndrade, J.R., Grant, C. and Dixon, A. StJ. (1965) Joint distension and reflex muscle inhibition in the knee. *Journal of Bone and Joint Surgery* **47A**, 313–316

Downey, J.A. (1964). Physiological effects of heat and cold. *Journal of the American Physical Therapy Association* **44**, 713–717

Duthie, R.B., Rizza, C., Giangrande, P. and Dodd, C. (1994). *The Management of Haemophiliac Disorders of the Musculo-skeletal System.* Oxford University Press: Oxford

Eriksson, E. (1980). Muscle physiology. Adaptation of the musculoskeletal system to exercise. *Contemporary Orthopaedics* **2**, 228–232

Gernsten, J.W. (1955). Effect of ultrasound on tendon extensibility. *American Journal of Physical Medicine* **34**, 362–369

Granat, M.H. (1993) Functional electrical stimulation and hybrid arthrosis systems. *Current Science. Current Opinion in Orthopaedics* **4**, 105–109

Griffin, J.E. and Karselis, T.C. (1982). The diathermies. *Physical Agents for Physical Therapists*, 2nd edn, pp. 177–216. Charles C. Thomas: Springfield, IL

Haggmark, T., Jansson, E. and Svane, B. (1978). Cross-sectional area of the thigh muscle in man measured by computed tomography. *American Journal of Clinical Laboratory Investigation* **38**, 355–360

Harris, E. (1973) A new orthotics terminology. *Orthotics and Prosthetics* **27**, 6

Haworth, R.J., Hopkins, J., Ells, P., Ackroyd, C.E. and Mowat, A.G. (1981) Expectations and out-come of total hip replacement. *Rheumatology and Rehabilitation* **20**, 65–70

Hislop, H. and Perrine, J.J. (1967) The isokinetic concept of exercise. *Physical Therapy* **47**, 114–8

Kirk, J.A. and Kersley, G.D. (1968) Heat and cold in the physical treatment of rheumatoid arthritis of the knee. *Annals of Physical Medicine* **9**, 270–273

Kottke, F.J., Pauley, D.L. and Ptak, R.A. (1966) The rationale for prolonged stretching for correction of shortening of connective tissue. *Archives of Physical Medicine and Rehabilitation* **47**, 345–348

Kralj, A.R. and Bajd, T. (1991) Functional electrical stimulation. *Clinical Science. Current Opinion in Orthopaedics* **2**, 830–837

Krikorian, D.J., Hartshorne, M.F. and Stratton, S.A. (1986) Use of He-Ne laser for treatment of soft tissue trauma: evaluation by gallium-67 citrate scanning. *Journal of Orthopaedic Sports Physical Therapy* **8**, 93–101

McCullough, N. (1985) *Atlas of Orthotics*, p. 169, edited by the American Academy of Orthopedic Surgeons. C.V. Mosby: St Louis

Magee, D.J. (1976) Therapeutic modalities. *Canadian Journal of Applied Sport Sciences* **1**, 219–222

Maitland, G.D. (1973) *Vertebral Manipulation*, 3rd edn. Butterworths: London

Major, R.E., Stallard, J. and Rose, G.K. (1981) The dynamics of walking using the hip guidance orthosis (hgo) with crutches. *Prosthetics and Orthotics International* **5**, 19

Meggitt, B.F., Vaughan-Lane, T. (1980) Hip hinge thigh brace for early mobilization of proximal femoral shaft fractures. *Prosthetics and Orthotics International* **4**, 150–155

Melzac, R. and Wall, P.D. (1965) Pain mechanisms: a new theory. *Science* **150**, 971–979

Olson, J.E. and Stravins, R.A. (1972) A review of cryotherapy. *Physical Therapy* **52**, 840–844

Partridge, R.E.H. and Duthie, J.J.R. (1963) Controlled trial of the effect of complete immobilization of joints in rheumatoid arthritis. *Annals of the Rheumatic Diseases* **22**, 91–94

Radulovic, R., Piera, J.B., Cassagne, B., Grossiord, A. and Boruchowitsch, G. (1980) The mobile arm support. *Prosthetics and Orthotics International* **4**, 101–105

Ray, C.D. (1977) New electrical stimulation methods for therapy and rehabilitation. *Orthopaedic Review* **6**, 29–34

Reid, D.C. (1992) Physical modalities. *Sports Injury, Assessment and Rehabilitation*, pp. 31–65. Churchill Livingstone: New York

Reid, D.C. and Cummings, G.E. (1973) Factors in selecting dosage of ultrasound. *Physiotherapy Canada* **25**, 5–8

Silcox, D.H., Rooks, M.D., Vogel, R.R. and Fleming, L.L. (1993) Myoelectric prostheses. *Journal of Bone and Joint Surgery* **75A**, 1781–1789

Sloan, J.P., Giddings, P. and Hain, R. (1988) Effects of cold and compression on edema. *Physician and Sportsmedicine* **16**, 116–120

Thistle, H.G., Hislop, H.J., Moffroid, N. *et al.* (1967) Isokinetic contraction: a new concept of exercise. *Archives of Physical Medicine* **48**, 279–283

Tunbridge, R. (1972) *Rehabilitation*. HMSO: London

Wadsworth, H. and Chanmugam, A. (1980) *Electrophysical Agents in Physiotherapy*, p. 28. Science Press: Marrickville, Australia

Wheeler, J.S., Walter, J.S. and Cai, W. (1993) Electrical stimulation for urinary incontinence. *Critical Review of Physical and Rehabilitation Medicine* **5**, 31–55

Index

vs denotes differential diagnoses or comparisons